Manual Therapy for Musculoskeletal Pain Syndromes

an evidence- and clinical-informed approach

For Elsevier
Content Strategist: Rita Demetriou-Swanwick
Content Development Specialist: Nicola Lally
Project Manager: Shereen Jameel
Designer/Design Direction: Miles Hitchen
Copy Editor: Chris Wyard
Illustration Manager: Emily Constantino
Illustrators: Graeme Chambers and Wendy Beth Jackelow

Manual Therapy for Musculoskeletal Pain Syndromes

an evidence- and clinical-informed approach

Edited by

César Fernández-de-las-Peñas PT, MSc, PhD
Head, Physical Therapy, Occupational Therapy, Rehabilitation and Physical Medicine,
Universidad Rey Juan Carlos, Alcorcon, Madrid, Spain
Researcher, Center for Sensory-Motor Interaction (SMI), Aalborg University, Aalborg, Denmark

Joshua A. Cleland PT, PhD
Professor, Physical Therapy, Franklin Pierce University, Manchester, NH, USA

Jan Dommerholt PT, DPT
Physical Therapist, Bethesda Physiocare/Myopain Seminars, Bethesda, MD, USA

Forewords by

Ola Grimsby PT, DMT, FAAOMPT
The Ola Grimsby Institute Consortium Inc.

Rob A.B. Oostendorp PhD, PT, MPT
Emeritus professor of Manual Therapy, Faculty of Medicine and Pharmacy, Vrije Universiteit Brussel, Brussels, Belgium
Emeritus professor of Allied Health Sciences, Faculty of Medical Sciences, Radboud University Nijmegen, Nijmegen, The Netherlands

Prof. Dr. Andry Vleeming PT, PhD
Department of Anatomy, Medical College of the University of New England, Maine, USA
Department of Rehabilitation Sciences and Physiotherapy, Faculty of Medicine and Health Sciences, Ghent University, Belgium

ELSEVIER

ELSEVIER

First edition 2016

ISBN 978-0-7020-5576-8

Notices
Knowledge and best practice in this field are constantly changing. As new research and experience broaden our understanding, changes in research methods, professional practices, or medical treatment may become necessary.

Practitioners and researchers must always rely on their own experience and knowledge in evaluating and using any information, methods, compounds, or experiments described herein. In using such information or methods they should be mindful of their own safety and the safety of others, including parties for whom they have a professional responsibility.

With respect to any drug or pharmaceutical products identified, readers are advised to check the most current information provided (i) on procedures featured or (ii) by the manufacturer of each product to be administered, to verify the recommended dose or formula, the method and duration of administration, and contraindications. It is the responsibility of practitioners, relying on their own experience and knowledge of their patients, to make diagnoses, to determine dosages and the best treatment for each individual patient, and to take all appropriate safety precautions.

To the fullest extent of the law, neither the Publisher nor the authors, contributors, or editors, assume any liability for any injury and / or damage to persons or property as a matter of products liability, negligence or otherwise, or from any use or operation of any methods, products, instructions, or ideas contained in the material herein.

Printed in United Kingdom

Contents

Dedication viii
Acknowledgements ix
Contributors x
Forewords xiv
Preface xvii

Part 1 General introduction

1. **Epidemiology of upper extremity pain syndromes** 3
Louise Thwaites and Karen Walker-Bone
2. **Epidemiology of lower extremity pain disorder** 13
Adam P. Goode and Sean D. Rundell
3. **History taking** 22
Peter A. Huijbregts
4. **History taking for patients with lower extremity syndromes** 36
Megan Burrowbridge Donaldson and Kristina Averell
5. **Physical examination** 47
Shane Koppenhaver, Timothy Flynn and Jennifer Crane
6. **Treating the brain in chronic pain** 66
Adriaan Louw
7. **Mechanical diagnosis and therapy for the spine: McKenzie method** 76
Stephen May and Richard Rosedale
8. **Mechanical diagnosis and therapy for extremity problems: McKenzie method** 85
Stephen May and Grant Richard Burges Watson

Part 2 Cervicothoracic spine in upper extremity pain syndromes

9. **Mechanical neck pain** 95
Bryan S. Dennison and Michael H. Leal
10. **Whiplash-associated disorders** 110
Michele Sterling
11. **Differential diagnosis and treatment of cervical myelopathy, cervical radiculopathy and cervical myeloradiculopathy** 118
Chad Cook and Amy Cook
12. **Thoracic outlet syndrome** 132
Susan W. Stralka
13. **Thoracic spine manipulation** 142
William Egan, Paul E. Glynn and Joshua A. Cleland
14. **Joint mobilization and manipulation of the cervical spine** 158
John R. Krauss, Douglas S. Creighton, Joshua A. Cleland and César Fernández-de-las-Peñas
15. **Therapeutic exercise for mechanical neck pain** 174
Carol Kennedy

Part 3 Lumbar spine pain syndromes

16. **Mechanical low back pain** 191
Scott Burns, Edward Foresman, Stephenie Kraycsir and Joshua A. Cleland
17. **Lumbar radiculopathy** 199
Chad Cook and Mark Wilhelm
18. **Lumbar spine instability** 210
Bryan S. Dennison and Michael H. Leal
19. **Lumbar spine in lower extremity pain syndromes** 221
Scott Burns, Paul E. Glynn, Edgar Savidge and Joshua A. Cleland
20. **The contribution of the pelvic floor muscles to pelvic pain** 226
Ruth Jones
21. **Chronic low back pain** 236
Mark D. Bishop, Joel E. Bialosky and Charles W. Gay
22. **Joint mobilization and manipulation of the lumbar spine** 245
Emilio J. Puentedura
23. **Therapeutic exercise for mechanical low back pain** 255
Carol Kennedy and Lenerdene Levesque
24. **Sacroiliac joint as a source of pain: diagnosis and management** 274
Kenneth E. Learman

Part 4 The shoulder region in upper extremity pain syndromes

25. **Acromioclavicular joint** 293
Janette W. Powell, Ian Shrier and Peter A. Huijbregts
26. **Sternoclavicular joint** 302
Erland Pettman
27. **Rotator cuff lesions: shoulder impingement** 309
Peter A. Huijbregts and Carel Bron
28. **Glenohumeral instability** 321
Steven C. Allen, Russell S. VanderWilde and Peter A. Huijbregts
29. **Superior labrum anterior-to-posterior (SLAP) lesions** 333
Janette W. Powell and Peter A. Huijbregts
30. **Frozen shoulder** 344
Carel Bron, Arthur de Gast and Jo L.M. Franssen

31. Joint mobilization of the shoulder 350
Wayne Hing, Jack Miller and César Fernández-de-las-Peñas

32. Motor control of the shoulder region 358
Mary E. Magarey, Mark A. Jones and Samuel R. Baida

33. Therapeutic exercises for the shoulder region 373
Johnson McEvoy, Kieran O'Sullivan and Carel Bron

Part 5 The hip region in lower extremity pain syndromes

34. Hip osteoarthritis 389
Alexis A. Wright

35. Other hip disorders: muscle, labrum and bursa 397
John Dewitt and David Kohlrieser

36. Postoperative management of hip disorders 413
Robert C. Manske and Erik Meira

37. Joint mobilization and manipulation of the hip 421
Jack Miller and Wayne Hing

38. Therapeutic exercises for the lower quadrant 426
Carol Kennedy and Lenerdene Levesque

Part 6 The elbow region in upper extremity pain syndromes

39. Elbow tendinopathy: lateral epicondylalgia 445
Bill Vicenzino

40. Other elbow disorders: elbow instability, arthritic conditions 451
Chris A. Sebelski

41. Joint mobilization and manipulation of the elbow 458
Helen Slater and César Fernández-de-las-Peñas

Part 7 The knee region in lower extremity pain syndromes

42. Ligamentous and meniscal injuries of the knee 467
Carol A. Courtney and Craig P. Hensley

43. Knee osteoarthritis 482
Lars Arendt-Nielsen and César Fernández-de-las-Peñas

44. Patellofemoral pain syndrome 493
Johnson McEvoy and Caroline MacManus

45. Postoperative management of the knee: ligamentous, meniscal and total joint replacement 514
Jodi Young and Ellen Pong

46. Joint mobilization and manipulation of the knee 525
Cody Weisbach, William Egan, Paul E. Glynn and Joshua A. Cleland

47. Tendinopathy of the knee 531
Ellen Pong

Part 8 The wrist and hand regions in upper extremity pain syndromes

48. Tendinopathies of the wrist and hand 545
C. Joseph Yelvington and Ellen Pong

49. Carpal instability 558
Ellen Pong

50. Carpal tunnel syndrome 566
Luca Padua, Daniele Coraci and César Fernández-de-las-Peñas

51. Other entrapment neuropathies 575
Joy C. MacDermid and David M. Walton

52. Joint mobilization and manipulation 584
Peter A. Huijbregts, Freddy M. Kaltenborn and Traudi Baldauf Kaltenborn

53. Finger and thumb pathology 594
Joy C. MacDermid, Ruby Grewal and B. Jane Freure

Part 9 The foot and ankle in lower extremity pain syndromes

54. Ankle sprains 605
Thomas Denninger and Gary Austin

55. Plantar heel pain 616
Matthew P. Cotchett

56. Postoperative management of foot and ankle disorders 623
Stephanie Albin, Mark W. Cornwall and Thomas G. McPoil

57. Manipulation of the foot and ankle 637
William Egan, Wayne Hing, Jack Miller and Joshua A. Cleland

58. Tendinopathy of the foot and ankle 646
Ellen Pong

Part 10 Soft tissues in the upper and lower quadrants

59. Referred pain from myofascial trigger points 659
César Fernández-de-las-Peñas, Hong-You Ge, Lars Arendt-Nielsen and Jan Dommerholt

60. Manual treatment of myofascial trigger points 678
César Fernández-de-las-Peñas, Jaime Salom-Moreno, Hong-You Ge and Jan Dommerholt

61. Dry needling of trigger points 690
Jan Dommerholt and Erik H. Wijtmans

62. Muscle energy approaches 710
Gary Fryer

63. Myofascial induction approaches 729
Andrzej Pilat

Part 11 Neurodynamics in the upper and lower quadrants

64. Peripheral nerve mechanisms of chronic upper limb pain: dynamics, inflammation and neurophysiology 765
Jane Greening and Andrew Dilley

65. Clinical neurodynamics in the upper and lower quadrants 781
Emilio J. Puentedura, Paul E. Mintken and Adriaan Louw

Index 799

Dedication

César Fernández-de-las-Peñas would like to dedicate this book to:

Cristina for her love and support during her life

Marta for not permitting me to write during the day

Miguel Angel for his love from heaven

Sofia for her love and smiles during the day and waking me up too early

My fourth child, Estella, who has born during this process

My parents for their love dedicated to the family

My colleagues and friends of the Department of Physical Therapy, Occupational Therapy, Rehabilitation and Physical Medicine for their support during my professional life

My patients for permitting my personal and professional growth

Joshua Cleland would like to dedicate this book to:

Kelley-Jaye for all her love and support

My patients who have provided a world of insight

My friends and colleagues for the intellectual conversations that have kept my passion burning

Jan Dommerholt would like to dedicate this book to:

Mona, Taliah and Aram for their love, support and understanding

My patients for giving me the inspiration to continue to improve my understanding of pain and pain mechanisms, and therapeutic interventions

Acknowledgements

While enjoying a beer during a 2011 conference in Madrid, we agreed that the time had come to put together a book about the lower quadrant. At that time, we did not really grasp how many people would eventually become involved with this project. In fact, our first aim was to write just a lower quadrant textbook, complementary to our previous text entitled *Neck and Arm Pain Syndromes: Evidence-Informed Screening, Diagnosis, and Management in Manual Therapy*. In communication with Elsevier, the publisher, we agreed that it was time to update the first text and include new materials about lower quadrant pain syndromes. The result is the current publication, made possible through the efforts of many individuals.

First, we would like to thank all the co-authors, who prepared numerous chapters and graciously considered the editorial comments after submitting the draft versions of their chapters. The authors come from all corners of the world, making this a truly international collaboration. Secondly, we would also like to acknowledge our patients who have taught us so much about what it is like to live with acute and persistent pain. Thirdly, we cannot forget to acknowledge Elsevier, the publisher, for trusting us to prepare this textbook. As always, we are very impressed with the professionalism and enthusiasm of the folks at Elsevier. We very much appreciate their guidance and attention to detail.

Lastly, we recognize our families and friends. We realize that our professional activities, such as writing book chapters and teaching courses, do take us away from our families and friends. We appreciate the understanding and positive support of our endeavours.

Contributors

Stephanie Albin
PT, DPT, OCS, FAAOMPT
Physical Therapist, Intermountain Healthcare, PhD Student, Rehabilitative Science, University of Utah, Salt Lake City, UT, USA

Steven C. Allen
PT, MSc, OCS, FAAOMPT
Clinic Director, Liberty Lake Physical Therapy, Therapeutic Associates, Inc., Liberty Lake, WA, USA

Lars Arendt-Nielsen
Dr.Med.Sci., Ph
Director, Professor, Center for Sensory-Motor Interaction (SMI), Aalborg University, Aalborg, Denmark

Gary P. Austin
PT, PhD, OCS, FAFS, FAAOMPT
Associate Professor, Physical Therapy, Lynchburg College, Lynchburg, VA, USA

Kristina Averell
SPT, ATC
Graduate Student, Doctor of Physical Therapy, Walsh University, North Canton, OH, USA

Samuel R. Baida
BAppSc (Human Movement), BScPT, MPT (MSK & Sports)
Olympic Sports Clinic, Adelaide Sports Physiotherapy, Adelaide, South Australia

Joel E. Bialosky
PhD, PT
Clinical Assistant Professor, Department of Physical Therapy, University of Florida, Gainesville, FL, USA

Mark D. Bishop
PT, PhD
Associate Professor, Department of Physical Therapy, University of Florida, Gainesville, FL, USA

Carel Bron
PT, PhD
Private Practice for Physical Therapy for Neck, Shoulder and Arm Disorders, Groningen, The Netherlands

Scott Burns
PT, DPT, OCS, FAAOMPT
Assistant Professor, Physical Therapy, Temple University, Philadelphia, PA, USA

Joshua A. Cleland
PT, PhD
Professor, Physical Therapy, Franklin Pierce University, Manchester, NH, USA

Amy Cook
PT, MS
Physical Therapist HCR Manor Care Rehabilitation, Canton, OH, USA

Chad Cook
PhD
Professor, Department of Orthopedics, Duke University, USA

Daniele Coraci
MD
Board of Physical Medicine and Rehabilitation, Department of Orthopedic Science, Sapienza University, Rome, Italy
Neurorehabilitation, Don Carlo Gnocchi Onlus Foundation, Milan, Italy

Mark W. Cornwall
PT, PhD
Professor, Physical Therapy and Athletic Training, Northern Arizona University, Flagstaff, AZ, USA

Matthew P. Cotchett
BSc BPod (Hons)
Lecturer, Allied Health, La Trobe University, Bendigo, Victoria, Australia

Carol A. Courtney
PT, PhD, ATC, FAAOMPT
Clinical Associate Professor, Department of Physical Therapy, University of Illinois at Chicago, Chicago, IL, USA

Jennifer Crane
PT, DPT, ATC
Research Physical Therapist, Adjunct Faculty, US Army
Baylor University Doctoral Program in Physical Therapy, San Antonio, TX, USA

Douglas S. Creighton
MS, PT, DPT OCS FAAOMPT
Associate Professor, Oakland University, Rochester Michigan, USA

Arthur de Gast
MD, PhD
Head, Clinical Orthopedic Research Center Midden-Nederland
Department of Orthopedics, Diakonessenhuis, Utrecht/Zeist Doorn, The Netherlands

Thomas Denninger
DPT, OCS, FAAOMPT
Clinic Director, Proaxis Therapy, Greenville, SC, USA

Bryan S. Dennison
PT, DPT, OCS, CSCS, FAAOMPT
Owner, Summit Physical Therapy, Mammoth Lakes, CA, USA

John Dewitt
PT, DPT, SCS, ATC
Assistant Clinical Professor, OSU Division of Physical Therapy, Ohio State University, Columbus, OH, USA
Rehab Manager, OSU Sports Medicine, Ohio State University's Wexner Medical Center, Columbus, OH, USA

Andrew Dilley
BSc, PhD
Lecturer in Anatomy, Brighton and Sussex Medical School, University of Sussex, Brighton, UK

Jan Dommerholt
PT, DPT, DAAPM
Physical Therapist, Bethesda Physiocare/Myopain Seminars, Bethesda, MD, USA
Lecturer, University of Maryland, Baltimore, MD, USA
Lecturer, Universidad CEU Cardenal Herrera, Valencia, Spain

Megan Burrowbridge Donaldson
PT, PhD, FAAOMPT
Associate Professor, Assistant Program Director of Physical Therapy, Walsh University, North Canton, OH, USA

William Egan
PT, DPT, OCS, FAAOMPT
Clinical Associate Professor, Physical Therapy, Temple University, Philadelphia, PA, USA

César Fernández-de-las-Peñas
PT, MSc, PhD, DMSc
Head Division, Physical Therapy, Occupational Therapy, Rehabilitation and Physical Medicine, Universidad Rey Juan Carlos, Alcorcon, Madrid, Spain
Clinical Researcher, Center for Sensory-Motor Interaction (SMI), Aalborg University, Aalborg, Denmark

Timothy Flynn
PT, PhD, OCS, FAAOMPT
Distinguished Professor, Physical Therapy, Rocky Mountain University of Health Professions, Provo, UT, USA
Owner, Colorado Physical Therapy Specialists, Fort Collins, CO, USA
Principal, Evidence in Motion, Louisville, KY, USA

Edward Foresman
PT, DPT, OCS
Staff Physical Therapist, Cherry Creek Wellness Center, Denver, CO, USA

Jo L.M. Franssen
PT
Private Practice for Physical Therapy for Neck, Shoulder and Arm Disorders, Groningen, The Netherlands

B. Jane Freure
BSc (PT), MManipTher (AU), FCAMT, Dip. Sport PT Physiotherapist, D3 Physiotherapy, St. Joseph's Health Care London, London, Ontario, Canada

Gary Fryer
PhD, BSc (Osteopathy)
Associate Professor, College of Health & Biomedicine, Victoria University, Melbourne, Victoria, Australia
Research Associate Professor, A.T. Still Research Institute, A.T. Still University, Kirksville, MO, USA

Charles W. Gay
DC, PhD
Postdoctoral Research Fellow, Rehabilitation Science PhD Program, University of Florida, Gainesville, FL, USA

Hong-You Ge
MD, PhD
Center for Sensory-Motor Interaction (SMI), Aalborg University, Aalborg, Denmark

Paul E. Glynn
PT, DPT, OCS, FAAOMPT
Director of Rehabilitation and Orthopedic Surgical Services, Newton-Wellesley Hospital, Newton, MA, USA

Adam P. Goode
PT, DPT, PhD
Assistant Professor, Department of Orthopedic Surgery, Duke University School of Medicine, Durham, NC 27705, USA

Jane Greening
MCSP, MSc, PhD, FMACP
Visiting Research Fellow, Brighton and Sussex Medical School, University of Sussex, Brighton, UK

Ruby Grewal
MD, MSc, FRCSC
Assistant Professor, Department of Surgery, University of Western Ontario, London, Canada
Hand and Upper Limb Center, St. Joseph's Health Care London, London, Ontario, Canada

Craig P. Hensley
PT, DPT, OCS, FAAOMPT
Physical Therapist, Clinical Faculty, Therapy Services, University of Chicago Medicine, Chicago, IL, USA

Wayne Hing
PhD, MSc, ADP (OMT), DipMT, DipPhys, FNZCP
Professor, Physiotherapy, Bond University, Gold Coast, Queensland, Australia

Peter A. Huijbregts – deceased

Mark A. Jones
BS (Psychology), Certificate Physical Therapy, Graduate Diploma in Advanced Manipulative Therapy, Master of Applied Science (Manipulative Therapy), Program Director Postgraduate Physiotherapy, Senior Lecturer, School of Health Sciences, University of South Australia, Adelaide, Australia

Ruth Jones
PhD, MCSP
External Lecturer, University of Southampton; European University, Madrid
Specialist Physiotherapist, The Place for Movement & Health, UK

Freddy M. Kaltenborn
PT, OMT, ATC, PhD (Hon)
Orthopaedic Manipulative Therapist, Chiropractor, Osteopath, Scheidegg, Germany

Traudi Baldauf Kaltenborn
PT, OMT
Orthopaedic Manipulative Therapist, Scheidegg, Germany

Carol Kennedy
BScPT, MClSc (manipulation), FCAMPT
Clinical Specialist – Musculoskeletal Physiotherapy
Chief Examiner, Orthopaedic Division, Canadian Physiotherapy Association
Clinical Physiotherapist / Partner, Treloar Physiotherapy Clinic, Vancouver, BC, Canada

David Kohlrieser
DPT, OCS, SCS
Staff Physical Therapist, Ohio State University, Columbus, OH, USA

Shane Koppenhaver
PT, PhD, OCS, FAAOMPT
Associate Professor, U.S. Army/Baylor Doctoral Physical Therapy Program Fort Sam Houston, Texas

John R. Krauss
PhD, PT, OCS, FAAOMPT
Associate Professor, School of Health Sciences, Oakland University, Rochester, MI, USA

Stephenie J. Kraycsir
PT, DPT, OCS
Director, Saddle Horn Physical Therapy, Gillette, WY, USA

Michael H. Leal
PT, DPT, OCS, FAAOMPT
Assistant Professor, Department of Physical Therapy, West Coast University, Los Angeles, CA, USA
Clinical Specialist II, Department of Physical Medicine, Kaiser Permanente, Fontana, CA, USA

Kenneth E. Learman
PhD, PT, OCS, COMT, FAAOMPT
Professor, Physical Therapy, Youngstown State University, Youngstown, OH, USA

Lenerdene Levesque
BScPT, MClSc (manipulative field), FCAMPT
Adjunct Professor, School of Physical Therapy, Western University, London, ON, Canada
Chief Examiner, Orthopaedic Division, Canadian Physiotherapy Association, Ottawa, ON, Canada
Clinical Physiotherapist, Physiofirst Orthopaedic and Sports Centre, Ottawa

Adriaan Louw
PhD, PT
International Spine and Pain Institute, Story City, IA, USA

Joy C. MacDermid
BSc, BScPT, MSc, PhD
Associate Professor, School of Rehabilitation Science, McMaster University Hamilton, Ontario, Canada
Co-director of Clinical Research Hand and Upper Limb Centre, London, Ontario, Canada

Caroline MacManus
BSc (Sport), MHSc (ExSpSci), BSc (PT)
Head of Performance Science, Irish Institute of Sport, Dublin, Ireland
Chartered Physiotherapist, United Physiotherapy Clinic, Limerick, Ireland

Mary E. Magarey
Dip Tech Physio, Grad Dip Advanced Manip Therapy, PhD, FACP, FASMF
Adjunct Senior Lecturer, School of Health Sciences, University of South Australia, Adelaide, Australia
Specialist Musculoskeletal & Sports Physiotherapist, Flex Rehabilitation Clinic, Adelaide, Australia

Robert C. Manske
DPT, MEd
Professor and Chair, Wichita State University Department of Physical Therapy
Via Christi Sports and Orthopedic Physical Therapy, Wichita, KS, USA

Stephen May
MA, FCSP, Dip MDT, MSc, PhD
Faculty of Health and Wellbeing, Sheffield Hallam University, Sheffield, UK

Johnson McEvoy
BSc, MSc, DPT, MISCP, PT
External Lecturer, Sports Science, University of Limerick, Ireland
Lead Physiotherapist, High Performance Boxing Unit, Irish Amateur Boxing, Dublin, Ireland
Chartered Physiotherapist, United Physiotherapy Clinic, Limerick, Ireland

Thomas G. McPoil
PT, PhD
Professor, Physical Therapy, Regis University, Denver, CO, USA

Erik Meira
PT, DPT, SCS, CSCS
Clinic Director, Black Diamond Physical Therapy, Portland, OR, USA

Jack Miller
BSc (PT), DipMT (NZ), MClSc, DPT, FCAMPT
Clinical Associate Professor, Rehabilitation Science, McMaster University, Hamilton, ON, Canada
Adjunct Clinical Professor, Health Science, Western University, London, ON, Canada
Lecturer, Rehabilitation Medicine, University of Toronto, Toronto, ON, Canada

Paul E. Mintken
PT, DPT, OCS, FAAOMPT
Associate Professor, School of Medicine, University of Colorado, Aurora, CO, USA
Lead Clinician, Sports Medicine, Wardenburg Health Center, Boulder, CO, USA

Kieran O'Sullivan
BScPT (Hons), MManipTher
Lecturer in Physiotherapy, University of Limerick, Limerick, Ireland

Luca Padua
MD, PhD
Neurosciences, Università Cattolica del Sacro Cuore, Rome, Italy
Neurorehabilitation, Don Carlo Gnocchi Onlus Foundation, Milan, Italy

Erland Pettman
PT, OMT, FCAMT
Associate Professor, Post-professional Program, Department of Physical Therapy, Andrews University, Berrien Springs, MI, USA

Andrzej Pilat
PT
Director, Myofascial Therapy School 'Tupimek', Madrid, Spain
Masters Degree Program, Physiotherapy School ONCE, Universiad Autónoma, Madrid, Spain

Ellen Pong
DPT, MOT, BA
Adjunct Instructor and Coursewriter, University of St. Augustine for Health Sciences, St Augustine, FL, USA
Contract Therapist for Clinical Research Group, Child Neurology Center of Northwest Florida, Gulf Breeze, FL, USA
Occupational and Physical Therapist, Private Contract, Pensacola, FL, USA

Janette W. Powell
PT, MHSc, OCS, STC
Supervisor of Performance Medicine Cirque du Soleil 'O', Las Vegas, NV, USA

Emilio J. Puentedura
PhD, DPT, BAppSc (Phty), Grad Dip Manip Physio, OCS, FAAOMPT
Associate Professor, Physical Therapy, University of Nevada Las Vegas, Las Vegas, NV, USA

Richard Rosedale
PT, BSc, Dip MDT
Senior Instructor, Canadian Branch, McKenzie Institute International, Raumati Beach, New Zealand
Physiotherapist, Occupational Health and Safety Services, London Health Sciences Centre, London, Ontario, Canada

Sean D. Rundell
PT, DPT, PhD
Acting Assistant Professor, Department of Rehabilitation Medicine, University of Washington, Seattle, WA, USA

Jaime Salom-Moreno
PT, MSc, PhD
Professor, Physical Therapy, Occupational Therapy, Rehabilitation and Physical Medicine, Universidad Rey Juan Carlos, Alcorcon, Madrid, Spain

Edgar Savidge
PT, DPT, OCS
Outpatient Rehabilitation Manager, Rehabilitation Services, Newton-Wellesley Hospital, Newton, Massachusetts, USA

Chris A. Sebelski
PT, DPT, OCS
Assistant Professor, Department of Physical Therapy and Athletic Training, Saint Louis University, St Louis, MO, USA

Ian Shrier
MD, PhD, Dip Sport Med, FACSM
Associate Professor, Centre for Clinical Epidemiology and Community Studies, Lady Davis Institute for Medical Research Jewish General Hospital, McGill University, Montreal, Canada

Helen Slater
BAppSc (Phty), MAppSc (Phty), PhD, FACP
Associate Professor, School of Physiotherapy and Exercise Science, Curtin University, Perth, Western Australia, Australia

Michele Sterling
PhD, MPhty, BPhty, Grad Dip Manip Physio, FACP
Professor and Associate Director of the Centre of National Research on Disability and Rehabilitation Medicine (CONROD), Queensland, Australia
School of Allied Health, Griffith University, Queensland, Australia

Susan W. Stralka
PT, DPT, MS, ACHE
CEO/Administrator, Baptist Rehabilitation Hospital, Germantown, Tennessee
Clinical Instructor, University of Tennessee Health Sciences Center College of Allied Health, Department of Physical Therapy, Memphis, TN, USA

Louise Thwaites
BSc, MBBS, MD
Clinical Research Fellow, Oxford University Clinical Research Unit, Hospital For Tropical Diseases, Ho Chi Minh City, Vietnam

Russell S. VanderWilde
MD
Orthopedic Surgeon, Northwest Orthopedic Specialists, Spokane, WA, USA

Bill Vicenzino
PhD, MSc, BPhty, GradDipSportsPhty
Chair of Sports Physiotherapy, Chair of the Medical Research Ethics Committee, and Head of the Sports Injury Rehabilitation and Prevention for Health Research Unit in the School of Health and Rehabilitation Sciences, University of Queensland, Australia

Karen Walker-Bone
BM, FRCP, PhD, Hon FFOM
Reader and Honorary Consultant in Occupational Rheumatology, MRC Lifecourse Epidemiology Unit, University of Southampton Medical School, Southampton, UK

David M. Walton
PT, PhD
Assistant Professor, School of Physical Therapy, The University of Western Ontario, London, Ontario, Canada

Grant Richard Burges Watson
Dip Phys, ADP (OMT), Dip MDT
Clinical Physiotherapy Specialist, Connect Physical Health, Newcastle upon Tyne, Tyne and Wear, UK

Cody Weisbach
PT, DPT, OCS, FAAOMPT
Senior Physical Therapist, Physical Therapy Associates of Concord, Concord, MA, USA

Erik H. Wijtmans
PT, MTC, CGIMS, CMTPT
Physical therapist, Manual Therapist, Partner, The Therapy Network, Virginia Beach, VA, USA
Adjunct Clinical Professor, College of Health Sciences, School of Physical Therapy, Old Dominion University, Norfolk, VA, USA
Lecturer, Myopain Seminars, Bethesda, MD, USA

Mark Wilhelm
PT, DPT
PhD Student, Rehabilitation Sciences, Texas Tech University Health Sciences Center, Lubbock, TX, USA

Alexis A. Wright
PT, PhD, DPT, FAAOMPT
Assistant Professor, Department of Physical Therapy, High Point University, High Point, NC, USA

C. Joseph Yelvington
PT, BA
Physical Therapist, Sacred Heart Rehabilitation at Pace, Pace, FL, USA

Jodi Young
PT, DPT, OCS, FAAOMPT
Assistant Professor, Physical Therapy, Franklin Pierce University, Goodyear, AZ, USA

Forewords

Foreword by Ola Grimsby

Manual therapy has developed from a selection of techniques from Hippocrates through various schools of thought for many generations. It has documented its validity simply by surviving the scrutiny of time. From the skill of its practitioners, new generations have refined and modified the performance and over time it has emerged as a scientific, multidisciplinary, evidence-guided approach to rehabilitation medicine.

The evaluation and treatment of functional range of motion followed the principles of joint biomechanics up to the 1970s. In the 1980s we then learned to understand and assess pain concepts and how manual therapy influences inhibition and facilitation through neurophysiology. From histology and the cellular repair curriculum, we added the optimal stimuli for tissue rehabilitation and thus widened the concept of manual therapy interventions in the 1990s. As our understanding grew of the biomechanical and nutritional energy essential for cellular repair, supplements such as vitamins, herbs and minerals became an important addition to the patient's healthcare. In the last 15 years, medical technology from imagery and electroneuromyography, as well as clinical competencies from psychology, diagnostic methodology and pharmacology, have shed light on our patient care and our outcome studies. A growing volume of multidisciplinary research is assisting the evolution of the scientific basis for modern manual therapy assessment and interventions.

Within this community of rehabilitation schools of thought, we have today a number of 'families'. Manual therapy has become an umbrella of integrated rehabilitation services, and it is of great importance to understand how the contributors of this textbook exhibit sufficient commonality to be united under this one headline. It is even more important to appreciate how these schools of thought differ from each other while still contributing to the complete, complex picture of the community of manual therapy.

The three editors of *Manual Therapy for Musculoskeletal Pain Syndromes: an evidence- and clinical-informed approach* have authored and also coordinated the efforts of some of the most prominent authors, scientists and clinicians in the international world of manual therapy. The chapters are clinically relevant, well referenced and cover a wide variety of essential topics. Each chapter speaks of personal experience and grounded theory with passion and purpose.

It is with admiration and respect that I recognize the efforts behind this monumental task. The book is an asset to the manual therapy community, a reference of current achievements and a triumph in the process of interacting and coordinating the different components of musculoskeletal assessment and rehabilitation. It is a document that should be found on the shelves of every clinician, educator, scientist and library and it should serve as a compass for clinical competencies, research as well as future developments.

My warmest congratulations go to the authors and editors.

Ola Grimsby, PT, DMT, FAAOMPT
The Ola Grimsby Institute Consortium, Inc.

Foreword by Rob A.B. Oostendorp: Learning from the past as a bridge to the future of manual therapy

With a request to write a foreword, before me lies the substantial manuscript of *Manual Therapy for Musculoskeletal Pain Syndromes: an evidence- and clinical-informed approach.*

The history of this book has a particular and very special meaning for me. Peter Huijbregts, a fellow countryman, one of my closest friends and one of my best students during my time at the Free University of Brussels, Belgium, made a special contribution to the creation of this book. Although Peter sadly passed away at far too young an age on 6 November 2010, something of his spirit permeates this book and embodies his knowledge of the field of manual therapy and his enthusiasm in sharing this knowledge with others. The editors, along with a large number of prominent authors, do him a great honour by dedicating this book to him. A wonderful gesture!

Manual therapy has undergone rapid development over recent decades and this fascinating journey is reported in the book before you. However, and despite the significant accrual of knowledge, manual therapy still struggles with significant uncertainties concerning the manual assessment of patients with musculoskeletal disorders. While this book describes the state of the art for manual therapy as of 2014, the current status of the field serves to underline the urgent need for valid diagnostic and classification criteria, together with the need for international harmonization in order to increase the comparability of clinical trial data. Further uncertainties relate to treatment regimens per se. It is striking that randomized clinical trial (RCT) reports devote substantial attention to the design and methodology of the study, but relatively little attention to the manual diagnostic and therapeutic interventions. Whereas the description of the study design and methods generally form a substantial part of a manuscript, manual therapy interventions are often described in only a few sentences. Many current RCTs even lack crucial details on the manual therapy intervention examined. In order to interpret results from individual studies to clinical practice it is important to have more detailed information about the 'who, what, when and where' of the intervention, especially given that interventions are generally tailored to meet the needs of the individual patient. Although it is widely accepted that manipulation and mobilization are the mainstay of treatment, there is still a notable lack of proven information on treatment. The goal of the CIRCLe SMT (Consensus on Interventions Reporting Criteria List Spinal Manipulative Therapy) study is therefore to develop a minimum set of criteria for the description of spinal manipulative therapy in RCT reports.

Important aspects of the transition from the past as a bridge to the future of manual therapy are: (1) the transition from authority-based practice to evidence-based practice, (2) the transition from the International Classification of Diseases (ICD) to the International Classification of Functioning, Disability and Health (ICF), and (3) the transition from manual therapy as a unimodal treatment to an integration of manual therapy into the current understanding of the neurophysiology and psychology in relation to pain (multimodal manual therapy).

The transition from authority-based practice to evidence-based practice

Whereas in the past the practice of manual therapy was almost exclusively authority based, today the practice is based on the best-available evidence. Within the definition of evidence-based medicine (EBM), three dimensions define evidence from clinical practice: external scientific evidence, clinical expertise of the practitioner and the wishes, values and expectations of the patient. The relative allocation of attention to these three dimensions in education, clinical practice and research ultimately determines the quality of manual therapy. Within this comprehensive book, the various chapters aim to reflect this proportional distribution and in most chapters particular attention is paid to the transparency of clinical reasoning based on clinical expertise. This book will certainly contribute to an increase in the transparency of manual therapy.

The transition from the International Classification of Diseases (ICD) to the International Classification of Functioning, Disability and Health (ICF)

In the past, manual therapy was chiefly organized around the ICD (this traditional classification is also followed by the chapters of this book), whereas today the components of the ICF (in addition to the ICD) increasingly form the basis for patient health profiles. In addition to a focus on body function and structure, there is an increasing focus on participation in society and on personal and environmental factors in the onset and persistence of health problems. Over the past decades, clinical and scientific understanding of (chronic) musculoskeletal pain has increased substantially and it is now well established that a model restricted to body function and structure falls far short in diagnosing and treating patients with musculoskeletal pain. However, the majority of manual therapists were educated in this biomedical model, and manual therapy has a very long history of biomechanical diagnostics and treatment. Many of the authors of this book now advocate a transition to a biopsychosocial model in patients with musculoskeletal disorders. This model does not imply ignoring body function and structure. Rather, these biological issues are integrated into a wider and more comprehensive biopsychosocial model.

The transition from unimodal manual therapy to an integration of manual therapy into the current understanding of the neurophysiology and psychology of pain

Consideration of the conflicting scientific assessments found in publications that have evaluated the effectiveness of manual therapy shows that those carrying out the evaluation focus mainly on the methodological quality of the studies (including study design, randomization, blinding and outcome measures) and hardly touch upon possible theoretical explanations for the limited effectiveness of manual therapy. Valuable insights could be gained from a deeper inquiry into the theoretical background to the question of why the effectiveness of manual therapy in patients with chronic pain appears to be limited.

Patients with chronic pain who request help from a manual therapist often experience a reduction in pain during the initial treatment period but notice that the effect of treatment declines and that the period between treatments becomes shorter. It is therefore advisable to document accurately a history of previous treatment when taking a patient's history because previous treatment may have either a positive or a negative effect on the outcome.

The logical response of most patients during a (sub)acute stage of pain, a new episode of pain or an increase in pain is to avoid movements and activities in the expectation that increased pain can thereby be prevented. These behaviours often appear to be effective and pain usually decreases after a few hours or days. However, in a limited number of patients a fear of certain movements and activities gradually develops, owing to an attributing cognition that pain translates to an increase in tissue damage and damage to muscles and joints. This increasing fear leads to less and less time being dedicated to activities, and results in a vicious circle of fear, passivity, disuse and depression. A patient's experience of pain can result in loneliness, fears of never being pain free, and a sense of feeling trapped within a painful body. These patients often experience severe effects, manifesting as signs of sensitization of the central nervous system. Under the condition of central sensitization, the central nervous system is insufficient or no longer able to orchestrate peripheral and central nociceptive pain mechanisms, including a sustained inhibition of motor function, physical activities and general activities. The development, implementation and evaluation of clinical guidelines for therapeutic education based on actual pain–neurophysiological and psychological insights, before and during the active rehabilitation process, stand in the spotlight in multimodal manual therapy. The editors and the authors of this book have clearly understood that the transition of manual therapy to a multimodal approach is a necessary prerequisite for a bright future for manual therapy.

Manual physical therapists should be familiar not only with the biopsychosocial context of pain, but also with modern insights derived from pain neuroscience and psychology concerning reconceptualization of pain. In fact, a sustained biomedical approach can even lead to an iatrogenic effect, which results in an increase in pain. Although increasing evidence supports a role for psychological and social factors in the emergence and persistence of chronic musculoskeletal pain, the majority of clinicians have received an education with a solely biomedical focus – a focus that is also evident in the profession of manual physical therapy. This focus is reflected in a long tradition of treatment options for patients with musculoskeletal disorders based on biomechanical principles. This emphasis on biomedical aspects appears to shape a therapist's knowledge, attitudes, beliefs and behaviour towards (chronic) musculoskeletal pain. An additional barrier to the acceptance of the emerging biopsychosocial model is that the emergence of new or revised theory and subsequent changes in practice are often characterized by a significant time-lag. This book makes an important contribution to the transition from manual therapy in a narrow sense to manual therapy in a broader sense, including the application of modern neurophysiological and psychological insights. This book therefore forms a bridge from the past to the future, and will benefit not only patients but also manual physical therapists worldwide.

The book now in front of you also documents how the theory and practice of manual therapy have changed over time. Current knowledge often has a half-life of only a few years and what is now standard practice in manual therapy may quickly become outdated. Experimental and clinical questions that are now unanswered can be expected to be answered in the near or not-too-distant future. This ongoing progress bodes well for future editions of this excellent book.

The authors who contributed to the present volume have each brought deep knowledge of manual therapy to their individual chapters, just as the editors, César Fernández-de-las-Peñas, Joshua Cleland and Jan Dommerholt, have used their skill and understanding to maintain consistency between chapters. I would therefore like to congratulate both the authors and the editors on the appearance of this standard work in the field of manual therapy.

Rob A.B. Oostendorp, PhD, PT, MPT, Emeritus professor of Manual Therapy,
Faculty of Medicine and Pharmacy, Vrije Universiteit Brussel, Brussels, Belgium
Emeritus professor of Allied Health Sciences, Faculty of Medical Sciences,
Radboud University Nijmegen, Nijmegen, The Netherlands

Foreword by Prof. Dr Andry Vleeming

This textbook was conceived by a resourceful editorial team with a straightforward ambition: to create a manual treatment book of musculoskeletal pain syndromes. A diversified international group of colleagues with clinical and scientific experience have contributed to specified chapters on the basis of both evidence- and clinical-informed knowledge and experience.

The ambitions for the textbook are well defined to conceive an integrated approach of effective manual treatment and to bridge apparent differences in therapeutic opinions. In particular, the text emphasizes that manual techniques need to be intrinsically related to neuroscience concepts, which requires an integrated clinical approach. It encourages the substitution of manual techniques from 'hands on' to 'hands with the involvement of the patient'. This commences a joint partnership between the clinician and the patient, enabling them to fathom their pain and problems. The patient is challenged and engaged in their rehabilitation, with sufficient understanding of how integrated treatment and training adherence is the core of a successful treatment approach.

Clinicians working with any kind of manual treatment modality should study this textbook, particularly to deepen their knowledge and to realize that during manual treatment the nervous system is surely involved. Therefore manual techniques should be combined with a cognitive approach such as therapeutic neuroscience education.

This informational textbook is a profound and accessible composition of many knowledgeable clinicians, recommending an integrated treatment approach to rehabilitate patients effectively. Likewise, it is an innovative approach to manual treatment techniques and clearly reflects how patients can benefit from it.

This book is a fascinating and highly readable account of manual treatment practices that should be endorsed to many clinicians. Pass this textbook on to your colleagues!

Prof. Dr Andry Vleeming, PT, PhD, Department of Anatomy, Medical College of the University of New England, Maine, USA
Department of Rehabilitation Sciences and Physiotherapy, Faculty of Medicine and Health Sciences, Ghent University, Belgium

Preface

What inspired us to invite a wide variety of contributors from all over the world to this book is the realization that manual therapy can no longer be separated from the emerging concepts and knowledge coming from pain neurosciences. In fact, manual therapy is probably the most-used treatment approach by many healthcare professionals, including physical therapists, osteopaths, chiropractors, massage therapists, medical doctors, etc. Whereas, traditionally, some manual physiotherapists would advocate that they would not be treating pain conditions, but instead focus only on dysfunctional movement patterns, in fact manual therapy can be understood only when we consider both the mechanical and the neurophysiological underlying mechanisms (Bialosky et al 2009). Not only can manual therapy interventions trigger peripheral and central nervous system responses in acute and especially chronic pain conditions, but the central nervous system itself plays a critical role in the personal experience and presentation of pain.

Before we discuss the details of this textbook, we would like to take a moment to acknowledge the contributions to this book by our dear friend and colleague Peter Huijbregts, who not only contributed as an author or co-author of several chapters, but also conceived the need to put together a book of this magnitude and focus. Unfortunately, Peter passed away unexpectedly long before this book came to fruition, but, throughout the preparatory work, his spirit and inspiration permeated our efforts. We are saddened that countless people will never have a chance to be personally influenced by him. Peter was one of those persons you could not forget if you were fortunate enough to have him cross your path. He was always up for discussing the historical origins of manual therapy or the current evidence supporting the effectiveness of interventions. We will never forget his sense of humour – many times Peter entertained the room with his wit and comedy. He has had a remarkable influence on many professionals who have been fortunate enough to encounter him. His passing has left a huge void in the manual therapy community around the world. We are proud to dedicate this book to the memory of Peter Huijbregts and we hope we have succeeded in making his dream a reality.

The paradigm we have chosen for this book is the evidence- and clinical-informed paradigm. It has been more than 30 years since a group of clinical epidemiologists at McMaster University introduced the evidence-based practice paradigm to replace the traditional paradigm (Guyatt 2008). According to the traditional paradigm, diagnosis and management were guided mainly by a pathophysiological rationale and by knowledge provided by respected authorities in the field. The main feature of the evidence-based paradigm is that the diagnosis and management should be guided mainly by the best-available scientific evidence; however, the evidence-based practice paradigm has been met with and continues to meet considerable resistance from the clinical field. Its early definition as the 'conscientious, explicit, and judicious use of current best evidence in making decisions about the care of individual patients' (Sackett et al 1996, p 71) seemed to mirror the often-heard criticisms of over-reliance on research evidence at the expense of clinical experience and disregard of social context. Although evidence-based practice has now evolved to where it adopts a more inclusive view of scientific evidence, recognizing not only the value of different research designs, but also of clinical expertise, patient values and preferences and even contextual factors in the clinical decision-making process (Rycroft-Malone 2008), the evidence-informed paradigm is a more appropriate paradigm in which the clinician takes the available evidence from research into account when making a clinical decision with regard to individual patient management but where evidence does not completely dictate this decision (Pencheon 2005).

Throughout this textbook, the chapter authors have integrated clinical experience and expertise and reasoning based on a neurophysiological rationale with the most updated evidence, thereby in effect combining the best of the traditional and evidence-based paradigms in a new paradigm that is truly representative of what clinicians do in everyday clinical practice. We believe that this approach has created a book that provides practising clinicians with what they need to know for real-life screening, diagnosis and management of patients with musculoskeletal pain.

The textbook is divided into 11 parts. In the general introduction, several authors review the epidemiology of upper and lower extremity pain syndromes and the process of taking a comprehensive history in patients affected by pain. In Chapter 5, the basic principles of the physical examination are covered, while Chapter 6 places the field of manual therapy within the context of contemporary pain neurosciences and therapeutic neuroscience education. For the remaining sections, the textbook alternates between the upper and lower quadrants. Parts 2 and 3 provide state-of-the-art updates on mechanical neck pain, whiplash, myelopathy, radiculopathy, thoracic outlet syndrome, peripartum pelvic pain, joint mobilizations and manipulations and therapeutic exercises, among others. Parts 4 to 9 review pertinent and updated aspects of the shoulder, hip, elbow, knee, the wrist and hand, and finally the ankle and foot. The last two parts of the book are devoted to muscle-referred pain and neurodynamics, which are two often-undervalued areas pertinent to manual physiotherapy.

We anticipate that this textbook will become the standard in manual therapies and we hope that it will bridge apparent differences in opinions. We aim to unite different healthcare disciplines using manual therapy as their therapeutic approach. In the end, the welfare of our patients needs to be the guiding principle. We hope that the current textbook will ultimately benefit many patients worldwide.

César Fernández-de-las-Peñas
Madrid, Spain
Joshua A. Cleland
Concord, NH, USA
Jan Dommerholt
Bethesda, MD, USA

References

Bialosky JE, Bishop MD, Price DD, et al. 2009. The mechanisms of manual therapy in the treatment of musculoskeletal pain: a comprehensive model. Man Ther 14: 531–538.

Guyatt G. 2008. Preface. In: Guyatt G, Rennie D (eds) User's guide to the medical literature: a manual for evidence-based clinical practice, 2nd edn. Chicago: AMA Press, p xxi.

Pencheon D. 2005. What's next for evidence-based medicine? Evid Based Health Care Public Health 9: 319–321.

Rycroft-Malone J. 2008. Evidence-informed practice: from individual to context. J Nurs Manag 16: 404–408.

Sackett D, Rosenberg WMC, Gray JAM, et al. 1996. Evidence based medicine: what it is and what it isn't. BMJ 312: 71–72.

In Memoriam

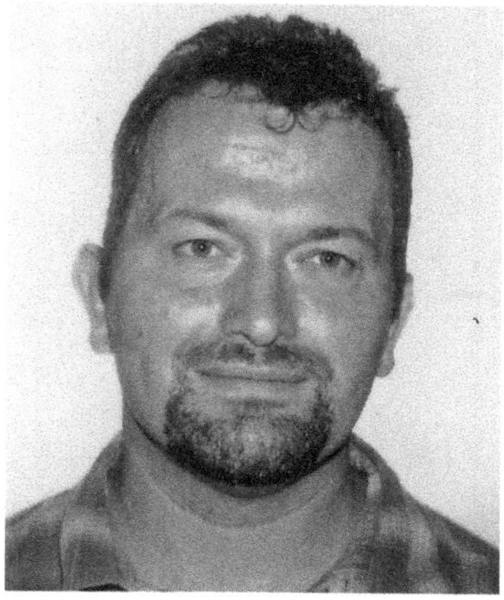

Peter Huijbregts

PART 1

General Introduction

1 Epidemiology of Upper Extremity Pain Syndromes 3
Louise Thwaites and Karen Walker-Bone

2 Epidemiology of Lower Extremity Pain Disorder 13
Adam P. Goode and Sean D. Rundell

3 History Taking 22
Peter A. Huijbregts

4 History Taking for Patients with Lower Extremity Syndromes 36
Megan Burrowbridge Donaldson and Kristina Averell

5 Physical Examination 47
Shane Koppenhaver, Timothy Flynn and Jennifer Crane

6 Treating the Brain in Chronic Pain 66
Adriaan Louw

7 Mechanical Diagnosis and Therapy for the Spine: McKenzie Method 76
Stephen May and Richard Rosedale

8 Mechanical Diagnosis and Therapy for Extremity Problems: McKenzie Method 85
Stephen May and Grant Richard Burges Watson

Chapter 1

Epidemiology of Upper Extremity Pain Syndromes

Louise Thwaites, Karen Walker-Bone

CHAPTER CONTENTS

Introduction	3
Epidemiological issues	3
Terminology	3
Non-specific pain	4
Classification criteria	4
Study design	5
Population	5
Measurement of exposure	5
Occurrence of upper extremity disorders	6
Prevalence of upper extremity pain	6
Prevalence of specific upper extremity disorders	6
Health care utilization and impact	9
Risk factors for upper extremity disorders	9
Gender	9
Age	10
Anthropometry	10
Hand dominance	10
Hormonal factors	10
Occupational risk factors: physical/mechanical factors	10
Occupational risk factors: psychosocial	10
Conclusion	11

Introduction

In the 21st century, upper extremity pain syndromes are common and cause substantial disability. Their greatest impact is often felt in the workplace because these conditions commonly affect working-age adults, in whom they may cause absence through sickness as well as restricted workplace performance. Upper extremity pain may result from a very wide range of clinical conditions; however, this text focuses on pain arising from non-traumatic non-articular soft tissues – that is, excluding pain resulting from acute trauma, malignancy and chronic inflammatory rheumatic diseases such as rheumatoid arthritis (Box 1.1). Non-articular soft tissue disorders include some relatively well-defined 'specific' pathoanatomical conditions such as lateral epicondylalgia, de Quervain's tenosynovitis and carpal tunnel syndrome (CTS). However, upper extremity pain may also be referred from pathology occurring in the cervical spine (cervicobrachial disorders). Moreover, upper extremity pain can also commonly occur in the absence of distinct pathoanatomical physical signs, when it is most usefully described as 'non-specific' regional pain so as to avoid implied causation.

The results of epidemiological studies in general population samples suggest that, at any given point in time, 20–53% of the adult population in Western countries experience upper extremity pain symptoms. Over a lifetime, the estimated prevalence is >70% (Walker-Bone et al 2003a; Huisstede et al 2006). These disorders occur commonly in the working population, causing considerable morbidity and sickness absence, and thereby a significant economic impact (Silverstein et al 1998). In the developed world, musculoskeletal disorders cause the majority of occupational ill-health, and upper extremity pain is second only to back pain as a cause of work-related illness (Palmer 2006). According to a recent UK estimate, upper extremity disorders were responsible for an estimated annual loss of 3.64 million working days in 2009 / 10 (Health and Safety Executive 2012) and this appears to have been relatively constant over at least the past decade (Jones & Clegg 1998). This compares with an estimated 52 million working days lost because of low back pain (Macfarlane et al 2009). Using published criteria for examining work-relatedness of upper extremity disorders, approximately 70–95% of upper extremity musculoskeletal pain in working populations could be classified as 'work related' (Roquelaure et al 2006), but this may not imply a causal relationship.

Given these rates of occurrence and the associated levels of disability, it could be reasonably expected that the epidemiology of these conditions would be thoroughly investigated and understood. Unfortunately, for many reasons, this is not currently the case. In fact, high-quality epidemiological research in this field has been hampered in several different ways resulting in the confusion and controversy that beset this field. In order to understand the available epidemiological data that make up the majority of this chapter, we will briefly explain the epidemiological issues in the next section.

Epidemiological Issues

Terminology

As with other branches of medicine, the origins of much of the terminology for specific upper extremity disorders are to

Box 1.1 Causes of upper extremity pain

Outside the scope of this text

Rheumatological conditions
Inflammatory arthritis, e.g. rheumatoid arthritis, ankylosing spondylitis
Osteoarthritis
Systemic lupus erythematosus (SLE)
Fibromyalgia syndrome
Polymyalgia rheumatica/temporal arteritis

Systemic conditions
Malignancy (primary or secondary)
Stroke
Myocardial infarction and coronary artery syndromes
Multiple sclerosis
Diabetes mellitus
Diaphragmatic irritation (liver disease, splenic disease)

Acute trauma
Fracture/dislocation

Within the scope of this text

Specific non-articular conditions
Adhesive capsulitis
Rotator cuff syndrome
Subacromial bursitis
Acromioclavicular joint dysfunction
Lateral epicondylitis
Medial epicondylitis
Tenosynovitis
De Quervain's disease
Carpal tunnel syndrome

Non-specific pain syndromes
Occupational cervicobrachial disorder
Cumulative trauma disorder (CTD)
Repetitive strain injury (RSI)
Work-related upper limb disorder (WRULD)
Work-related upper extremity musculoskeletal disorder (WRUEMSD)
Non-specific forearm pain

be found in medical history, dating back from the original publications of the findings associated with an individual clinical syndrome (e.g. 'lawn tennis arm' (Morris 1882)). Some conditions have eponyms (de Quervain's tenosynovitis) and others have names based on the presumed pathoanatomical basis of the condition (tendonitis, epicondylitis, tenosynovitis). Controversy has ensued because of the multiplicity of disease labels and diagnostic criteria adopted both in clinical practice and in research, frequent ambiguity in the coverage and boundaries of case definition, and a lack of reference standards (Palmer et al 2012). Recently there have been attempts to standardize some of these terms aiming to suit more closely our modern view of the underlying pathophysiology (Hutson 2006). For example, in non-rheumatological conditions that affect tendons (tendonitis) and present with pain, there is growing evidence that true inflammation is rarely present. Rather, histopathological studies suggest that repetitive mechanical overload produces degenerative changes within the tendon substance leading to eventual collagen fibril micro-failure. A similar pathological picture is seen in tendons as they pass through the synovial-lined fibro-osseous tunnels at the wrist. Thus technically 'tendinosis' would be a much more accurate clinical term then tendonitis – reserving the latter term and 'tenosynovitis' for use only in the presence of true synovial inflammation (e.g. in rheumatoid arthritis). However, it should be borne in mind that histology is rarely available in the diagnosis or management of these conditions in practice and the clinician may be faced with patients presenting with a secondary inflammatory reaction visible in the paratenons overlying degenerate tendons. It is unsurprising, therefore, that terms that may be technically inaccurate pathologically nevertheless continue to prevail in clinical practice.

Non-specific pain

Upper extremity pain frequently occurs in the absence of clinical signs that fit into the conventional anatomical–pathological model ('non-specific' pain). As long ago as 1713, Ramazzini described an upper extremity disorder related to 'constant sitting, perpetual motion of the hand in the same manner and the attention and application of the mind' (Ramazzini 1940). Since then, upper extremity pain has been described occurring among different groups of workers many times (e.g. writer's cramp (British Civil Service 1830s) and telegraphist's cramp (UK 1908)). In the last half of the 20th century, occupational cervicobrachial disorders (Japan), cumulative trauma disorders (CTDs) (USA), repetitive strain injury (RSI) (Australia) and work-related upper limb disorders (WRULD) (UK) were terms used in different countries for syndromes similar to each other occurring in various groups of workers. These terms have similarly been used to describe pain at different sites in the neck and upper limb with no confirmed pathoanatomical abnormality, but they were overlapping and their usage varied (Robinson & Walker-Bone 2009). It is now widely believed that terms such as these with implied causation have impacted negatively on research in this field (Helliwell 1995; Palmer et al 2012). For one thing, such tautological terms imply blame or even negligence by an employer and so this is now a field where much of the investigation has moved into the law courts rather than the research laboratories. Secondly, if a pain has, because of its nomenclature, been attributed to a type of occupation, it is very difficult to investigate any other possible aetiological factors systematically as the affected individual already has fixed preconceptions.

Classification criteria

In clinical practice, diagnostic criteria are used to separate types of disease with different causation, treatment or prognosis. It is an absolute requirement of epidemiological research that the problem under study is clearly defined. We have already seen that non-specific pains are widely classified using different systems in different countries. However, even amongst the specific upper extremity conditions, classification criteria may differ widely and few have a 'gold standard' diagnostic test. Therefore, case definitions used in epidemiological studies have historically used textbook definitions or authors' personal opinions. A review by Van Eerd et al (2003) identified 27 classificatory schemes for upper limb disorders that were proposed following multidisciplinary workshops and consultations with experts, none of which were identical. In a systematic review of studies investigating incidence and prevalence of upper extremity disorders, Huisstede et al (2008) found variation in point prevalence from 1% to 53%, largely due to disparity of case definitions. Without consistent and clear classification, reliable data regarding disease burden and its health and socioeconomic impact are impossible to obtain. This in turn impacts upon treatment and prevention strategies and future research.

Buchbinder et al (1996) examined existing classification schemes for soft tissue disorders of the neck and upper limb. They found major inadequacies such as failure to be comprehensive and overlap of categories, and consequently suggested criteria by which future classification systems might be better assessed. In an attempt to improve consensus over classification, several multidisciplinary groups convened and produced their own classifications systems (Harrington et al 1998; Sluiter et al 2001). However, these too have been criticized for reflecting the opinions of workshop participants without clear definitions of extent or duration of symptoms and without any formal testing. A systematic review of 117 articles showed very few attempts to establish the validity of classification systems, with only one showing rigorous testing of validity and reliability (Walker-Bone et al 2003b).

The Southampton examination schedule was developed from the multidisciplinary UK workshop consensus statement on classification of musculoskeletal disorders of the upper limb and was tested in both hospital and general populations (Fig. 1.1) (Palmer et al 2000; Walker-Bone et al 2002). Overall findings showed a valid reproducible system for the examination of upper limb disorders that was suitable for use in large-scale epidemiological research, although it performed better in hospital patients (Palmer et al 2000) with the most clear-cut clinical presentations compared with community patients (Walker-Bone et al 2002).

More recently a 'complaints of the arm, neck and/or shoulder' (CANS) classification was proposed by a group comprising 11 medical and paramedical disciplines, which aimed to obtain consensus and establish a category of specific and non-specific conditions defined as musculoskeletal complaints of the arm, neck and shoulder not caused by acute trauma or any systemic disease (Huisstede et al 2007). A final group of 23 conditions, categorized as specific disorders, was produced; all other conditions were classified as non-specific disorders.

Study design

Neck and upper limb disorders are frequently episodic and recurrent; therefore most studies examine prevalence, rather than incidence, using a cross-sectional design. Investigators often choose different period prevalence case definitions; for example, 'neck pain lasting >1 day in the past 7 days' (1-week prevalence) is one possible case definition, which will yield a different prevalence estimate from 'neck pain lasting >6 months in the past year' (1-year prevalence of chronic neck pain) and also from 'neck pain ever' (lifetime prevalence of neck pain). Many of the studies have eschewed the difficulties of classification and chosen instead to measure the prevalence of self-reported pain at different sites of the neck and/or upper limb, using this as the outcome (Walker-Bone et al 2003b).

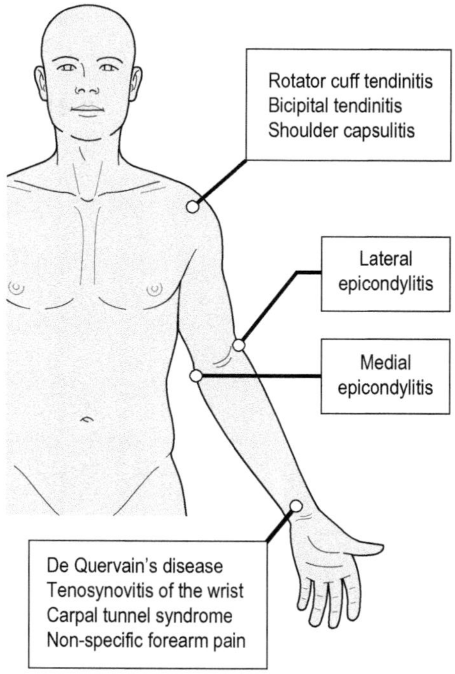

Figure 1.1 Upper extremity disorders for which consensus criteria were developed by the HSE Delphi workshop.

Population

Much of the available epidemiological research has been carried out in workplace or occupational groups, rather than in general population samples. This choice of setting, however, incurs the risk of results biased by the 'healthy worker' effect, in which those most severely affected are off sick or medically retired and therefore are not present in the workplace. Moreover, many studies have reported on upper extremity syndromes by referring to workers' compensation claims, which again may underestimate the true occurrence of disorders and bias results towards the most severe types of conditions causing the worst levels of disability (Roquelaure et al 2006).

Measurement of exposure

One of the greatest challenges to occupational research lies in measuring the exposure to different types of occupational factors. It is relatively uncommon in any particular occupation for there to be exposure to only a single type of physical risk factor; manual occupations frequently involve combinations of exposure (e.g. force and vibration, or pulling and pushing) thus making the exposure difficult to define and measure objectively. Direct observation and video surveillance are preferred methods for quantifying these but they are time consuming and expensive, so are not practicable for large studies. Surrogate markers such as job title or occupation classification have been regularly employed in studies, but are generally less sensitive. Thus subjective, retrospective reporting of exposure is frequently used; however, this relies on individuals' recall and estimation of times, forces and other physical factors and may also be influenced by their personal beliefs about the causation of their symptoms. Some investigators have attempted to overcome these by using a combination of subjective reporting and direct observation validation (Andersen et al 2007).

To summarize, there is little doubt that upper extremity pain is common, recurrent and disabling. There are several weaknesses inherent in our knowledge and understanding of the occurrence, risk factors and impact of these conditions, which have arisen for methodological reasons. This has produced a field that is both confusing and contentious, and controversy remains over even basic aspects. The reader must therefore put the following section into this context.

Occurrence of Upper Extremity Disorders

Prevalence of upper extremity pain

The results of epidemiological surveys suggest that neck pain may affect 10–17% of adults at any point in time, and as many as 71% during a lifetime, and that pain in the upper limb has a point prevalence of 7–26% (Walker-Bone et al 2004a). Many of the studies are poorly comparable owing to wide variation in the case definition and population characteristics. Shoulder pain lasting >1 day in the previous month, for example, was estimated to affect 13% of men and 15% of women aged 53 years in one study (Bergenudd et al 1988), whereas in another 26% of men and 19% of women aged 31–74 years reported current shoulder pain and restricted movement (Allander 1974). Point prevalence and period prevalence estimates for the occurrence of upper extremity pain, together with their case definitions, are summarized in Table 1.1. Although few specific conclusions can be drawn, the available data suggest that all upper extremity pain syndromes are common, are generally reported more often by women than by men and tend overall to occur more frequently in proximal (neck / shoulder) than in distal areas – although hand / wrist pain is more frequent than elbow pain. Broadly, these demographic findings from general population studies have been replicated in working populations. French workforce data showed a 12-month prevalence of upper extremity musculoskeletal symptoms of 35% in women compared with 27% in men (Roquelaure et al 2006) and similar Danish data estimated the prevalence rates of chronic upper extremity symptoms as 11.3% among women compared with 7.7% among men (Huisstede et al 2008).

In general, where studies have compared different types of workers, prevalence rates are higher in current workers than the non-working general population (8.1 vs 6.1% in The Netherlands). Rates also vary according to the specific occupational group. In one study in the USA, 50% of college students reported upper extremity musculoskeletal symptoms (Menendez et al 2008). Similarly high prevalence rates have been reported in computer workers (Tornqvist et al 2009) and textile workers (Huisstede et al 2006). In Denmark, 37% of working adults reported moderately severe neck and shoulder pain, compared with 49% of kitchen and cleaning workers and 22% of skilled workers (Andersen et al 2007). In French workers undergoing routine medical examinations, upper extremity pain disorders were most common in those working in the manufacturing industries and public administration; the highest rates of occurrence were in unskilled industrial and agricultural workers, drivers and male public service employees and female personal care workers (Roquelaure et al 2006). The highest risk seen amongst these occupational groups in France was consistent with those occupations at highest risk for compensation claims in the USA (Silverstein et al 1998).

Although most data on upper extremity symptoms comes from the Developed World, it is interesting that one study amongst office workers in Sudan using the CANS classification system has shown similar prevalence rates to those seen in Western populations (Eltayeb et al 2008).

Prevalence of specific upper extremity disorders

There are relatively few population-based surveys aimed at determining anatomical locations or specific causes of upper extremity pain. Differences in diagnostic and classification procedures, as discussed earlier, add to the difficulty in interpretation. Table 1.2 summarizes the results of the available population-based prevalence studies for specific conditions, together with the case definitions utilized. Shoulder conditions appear to occur most frequently, in line with the relative frequency of shoulder pain; CTS and epicondylitis are the next most commonly observed. There is a preponderance of data available on the occurrence of CTS, probably because of its relative frequency and the availability of nerve conduction studies as a test that is to some extent standardized. The incidence of CTS has been estimated at approximately 1 per 1000 of the general population, with higher rates among women than among men (1.5 per 1000) (Walker-Bone et al 2004a). Rates of prevalence range from 0.9% to 5% depending upon the case definition utilized.

There is a much greater body of literature on specific conditions studied in different occupational settings – which generally compares the prevalence of one or more specific upper extremity diagnoses in groups of workers with different types of occupational exposure (e.g. rates of prevalence of epicondylitis were compared between meat packers and cutters and those working in administration in meat factories in the study by Viikari-Juntura (1983)). These studies were extensively and critically reviewed in 1993 by the US NIOSH organization (Bernard 1997); this report highlighted the ubiquitous nature of the methodological shortcomings in the available studies, drawing attention to the same issues as in the occupation-based studies described above.

Despite these inherent weaknesses, it is notable that a French study, in which data were collected by a regional network of occupational physicians, showed that >50% of a sample of 2685 working adults experienced non-specific upper extremity musculoskeletal symptoms in the preceding

Table 1.1 **Population-based prevalence estimates for the occurrence of upper extremity regional pain**

	Case definition	Size of population sampled	Age (years)	Prevalence estimate men (%)	Prevalence estimate women (%)	Prevalence estimate all (%)
Neck pain						
Period prevalence	Pain lasting >1 week in past month	5752	>16	11	17	14
	Neck pain, tenderness or stiffness in past year	537	18–65	–	–	12
	Troublesome neck pain in the past year	7648	18–67	29	40	34
	Pain lasting >1 day in past year	800	>30	15	17	–
	Pain lasting >1 day in past week (Walker-Bone et al 2004a)	9698	25–64	21	26	24
Point prevalence	Currently suffering from neck pain	10532	20–65	10	18	–
	Pain lasting >1 month	1806	25–74	15	19	17
Shoulder pain						
Period prevalence	Pain lasting >1 week in past month	5752	>16	14	17	16
	Pain lasting >1 day in past month	574	53	13	15	14
	Pain lasting >1 day in past week (Walker-Bone et al 2004a)	9698	25–64	21	26	24
Point prevalence	Current pain lasting >3 months	1806	25–74	–	–	7
	Current pain and restricted movement	15268	31–74	26	19	20
	Current shoulder pain	644	>70	–	–	26
Elbow pain						
Period prevalence	Pain lasting >1 week in past month	5752	>16	6	6	6
	Pain lasting >1 day in past week (Walker-Bone et al 2004a)	9698	25–64	12	10	11
Point prevalence	Pain lasting >3 months in elbow/forearm	1806	25–74	8	12	11
Wrist/hand pain						
Period prevalence	Pain in the hand lasting >1 week in the past month	5752	>16	12	20	–
	Pain lasting >1 day in past week (Walker-Bone et al 2004a)	9698	25–64	19	23	21
Point prevalence	Current pain in hand/wrist lasting >3 months	1806	25–74	9	17	13

(Updated from Walker-Bone et al (2003a).)

year, with approximately 30% affected in the preceding week (Roquelaure et al 2006). Overall, the 12-month prevalence of 'specific' upper limb musculoskeletal disorders (rotator cuff syndrome, lateral epicondylitis, ulnar tunnel syndrome, CTS, de Quervain's disease, and flexor–extensor peritendinitis or tenosynovitis of the forearm–wrist defined according to specific criteria) was found to be 13%.

Another important emerging finding is that concurrent pain at different anatomical locations in the upper limbs is common (Walker-Bone et al 2004b). In a recent Dutch study, 33% of adults reported pain at two different anatomical sites in the upper extremity, with a further 8.5% experiencing pain at three separate sites (Huisstede et al 2008). In addition, 'specific' and 'non-specific' causes of pain commonly occur together; for example, features of hypersensitivity and allodynia have been shown to occur with lateral epicondylitis and trigger points are widespread in other arm pain syndromes (Huisstede et al 2008; De-la-Llave-Rincón et al 2009). It appears that musculoskeletal pain syndromes cluster within an individual, but it is currently unclear whether this is an effect of enhanced predisposition to the risk factors, or psychosocial factors such as somatization, or whether it occurs as a consequence of changed use of the musculoskeletal system precipitated by the onset of pain at one site.

Table 1.2 **Population-based occurrence of specific upper extremity musculoskeletal disorders**

	Case definition (reference for original data in parentheses)	Size of population sampled	Age (years)	Prevalence estimate men (%)	Prevalence estimate women (%)	Prevalence estimate all (%)
Shoulder						
Rotator cuff disorder	Pain in the shoulder region accompanied by pain on resisted abduction, external rotation or internal rotation (Chard et al 1991)	644	>70	–	–	15
Rotator cuff tendinitis	Pain in the deltoid region and pain on resisted active movement (Walker-Bone et al 2004b)	9698	25–64	4.5	6.1	–
Adhesive capsulitis	Pain in the deltoid area and equal restriction of active and passive glenohumeral movement with a capsular pattern (Walker-Bone et al 2004b)	9698	25–64	8.2	10.1	–
Acromioclavicular joint dysfunction	Pain over the acromioclavicular joint and tenderness over the joint and a positive acromioclavicular stress test (Walker-Bone et al 2004b)	9698	25–64	1.0	1.0	–
Elbow						
Lateral epicondylitis	History of pain in the elbow region for >1 month, tenderness over lateral epicondyle and pain increased when hand pronated against resistance and increased pain on carrying (Allander 1974)	15268	31–74	–	–	2.5
Lateral epicondylitis	Lateral epicondylar pain and tenderness and pain on resisted extension of the wrist (Walker-Bone et al 2004b)	9698	25–64	1.3	1.1	–
Lateral epicondylitis	Not stated (Verhaar 1994)	708	20–80	–	–	4.4
Medial epicondylitis	Medial epicondylar pain and tenderness and pain on resisted flexion of the wrist (Walker-Bone et al 2004b)	9698	25–64	0.6	1.1	
Wrist/hand						
De Quervain's disease	Pain over the radial styloid and tender swelling of the first extensor compartment and either pain reproduced by resisted thumb extension or positive Finkelstein's test (Walker-Bone et al 2004b)	9698	25–64	0.5	1.3	–
Tenosynovitis	Pain on movement localized to the tendon sheaths in the wrist and reproduction of the pain on resisted active movement (Walker-Bone et al 2004b)	9698	25–64	1.1	2.2	–
Carpal tunnel syndrome	Pain or paraesthesia or sensory loss in the median nerve distribution and one of: Phalen's test positive, Tinel's test positive, nocturnal exacerbation of symptoms, motor loss with wasting of abductor pollicis brevis (Walker-Bone et al 2004b)	9698	25–64	1.2	0.9	–

Continued

Table 1.2 Population-based occurrence of specific upper extremity musculoskeletal disorders—cont'd

	Case definition (reference for original data in parentheses)	Size of population sampled	Age (years)	Prevalence estimate men (%)	Prevalence estimate women (%)	Prevalence estimate all (%)
Carpal tunnel syndrome	Clinical diagnosis of CTS (Atroshi et al 1999)	2466	25–74	3	5	4
Carpal tunnel syndrome	Electrophysiological diagnosis of CTS (Atroshi et al 1999)	2466	25–74	4	5	5
Carpal tunnel syndrome	Clinical and electrophysiological diagnosis of CTS (Atroshi et al 1999)	2466	25–74	2	3	3
Carpal tunnel syndrome	Electrophysiological diagnosis of CTS (de Krom et al 1992)	715	25–74	1	6	5
Carpal tunnel syndrome	Electrophysiological motor latency >4.5 ms (Ferry et al 1998)	820	18–75	8	6	7

Healthcare Utilization and Impact

As stated above, upper extremity disorders can cause considerable disability; therefore they frequently lead to healthcare use and presentation in primary care or rheumatology clinics (Turk & Rudy 1990). Chronic symptoms (lasting usually at least 3 months) are associated with greater healthcare use and higher levels of disability. Dutch population data show that, in individuals meeting the CANS criteria for chronic symptoms (pain lasting more than 3 months in the last 12 months), 58% reported use of healthcare in the last 12 months – 81% of these patients consulted their general practitioner, 59% a medical specialist and 54% a physiotherapist (Huisstede et al 2008). Comparable data were seen for respondents to a British population-based study, such that 39% of those with pain had seen a doctor in the preceding 12 months, 11% a physiotherapist and 10% a chiropractor, while 24% had been prescribed medication for their complaint (Walker-Bone 2002). In the Dutch study, healthcare users reported more sickness absence than non-healthcare users; 37.2% reported sickness absence due to upper extremity symptoms, compared with 9.3% non-healthcare users, and 12.4% reported sickness absence for more than 4 weeks. Healthcare users also reported more recurrent and constant pain and more limitation in daily life due to their symptoms (48.9% compared with 8.5%).

In a comparision of specific and non-specific upper extremity disorders in the UK, specific diagnoses were also associated with more healthcare use – although use of self-prescribed medication in people with specific diagnoses was similar to that in those with non-specific pain. In total, 69% of subjects with upper extremity pain reported difficulty with their work, hobbies or housework (Table 1.3) and 59% reported difficulty sleeping due to their pain. Specific upper limb conditions were reported by those affected to be more disabling than non-specific pain (Walker-Bone et al 2004a). As an example, 11.5% of people with specific shoulder diagnoses reported difficulty in carrying a shopping bag, compared with just 6.1% of people with non-specific shoulder pain (Walker-Bone 2002).

Table 1.3 Disability associated with upper extremity pain

	No difficulty (%)	Some difficulty (%)	Impossible to do (%)
Impact of regional pain at different sites on ability to perform normal daily activities (e.g. work, hobbies, housework)			
Neck pain	30	59	11
Shoulder pain	28	48	11
Elbow pain	29	58	12
Wrist/hand pain	28	58	13
Pain at any site	31	56	13
Impact of pain at any site on sleeping	41	55	4
Impact of pain at any site on driving	34	46	5
Impact of pain at any site on dressing	30	58	8
Impact of pain at any site on carrying bags	67	34	3

NB Not all rows add up to 100% as not all respondents completed every question.
(Adapted from Walker-Bone 2002.)

Risk Factors for Upper Extremity Disorders

Gender

As with other sites of musculoskeletal pain, there is a higher prevalence of women reporting upper extremity pain compared with men. However, in primary care women also tend to consult more frequently than men with a range of other symptoms, hence these differences may reflect a gender difference in the threshold for seeking help. Alternatively, women may be more vulnerable to factors causing musculoskeletal pain, because of either their physical size and strength or constitutional differences such as hormonal factors (Walker-Bone et al 2003a). Fewer data are available comparing prevalence rates between men and women for specific conditions, but there is some evidence that women are more commonly affected by tenosynovitis, de Quervain's disease, shoulder capsulitis and CTS. However, epicondylitis has generally been found to be more common among men than women.

Age

Musculoskeletal pain is reported more frequently with age in both genders, with a peak in the middle years (50–60 years) and a modest reduction in prevalence in subsequent decades of life. The pattern in specific conditions is less well studied, but there is evidence of a similar age curve for lateral epicondylitis, CTS among women and possibly de Quervain's disease and tenosynovitis.

Anthropometry

Obesity is associated with an increased frequency of reporting neck and upper extremity pain. Moreover, the disability caused by painful conditions also increases with body mass index (BMI). It is a consistent finding that the risk of CTS increases with BMI such that, in one US survey, the risk of CTS increased by 8% for every 1 unit of increase in BMI.

Hand dominance

Often used as a surrogate for occupational stressors, hand dominance has been included in some of the more recent workplace studies (Shiri et al 2007). In particular, epicondylitis has been demonstrated to occur more frequently in the dominant arm than in the non-dominant arm.

Hormonal factors

CTS occurs more frequently in women during pregnancy and lactation and soon after the menopause than at other times (Walker-Bone et al 2003a). Hysterectomy without oophorectomy has been found to lead to a doubling of the risk of CTS, compared with hysterectomy and oophorectomy. Both the oral contraceptive pill and hormone replacement therapy (HRT) have also been associated with an increased risk of CTS. Case reports also suggest that de Quervain's disease is more common during pregnancy or early post-partum. These relationships imply a hormonal effect, perhaps related to oedema of the non-articular tissues, but the underlying mechanism remains to be elucidated.

Occupational risk factors: physical / mechanical factors

Occupational and physical workplace exposures have been shown to be risk factors for upper extremity pain disorders, although the difficulties in accurately estimating these have already been discussed. Many epidemiological studies have investigated these factors and this literature has been the subject of several comprehensive reviews, all of which comment on the heterogeneity of design, and variation in assessment of outcomes and exposures, mode of analysis and presentation. Few stand up to rigorous methodological examination (Buchbinder et al 1996).

As with low back pain, mechanical load, repetitive work and abnormal working postures are all associated with the development of upper extremity symptoms (Macfarlane et al 2000). Lifting heavy loads, standing for long periods and pushing / pulling are more likely to be associated with low back pain than upper extremity symptoms (Andersen et al 2007). Nevertheless, standing for long periods has been shown to be associated with an increased risk of regional musculoskeletal pain at any anatomical site (hazard ratio (HR) 1.6, 95% confidence interval (CI) 1.2–2.3) (Andersen et al 2007).

The findings of several systematic reviews conclude that there is strong evidence that neck pain is associated with working in sustained and abnormal postures, such as prolonged sitting with the neck or trunk held in flexion or rotation, or a combination of both (Bernard 1997). There is also evidence suggesting that neck and neck / shoulder symptoms are increased when work involves forceful and / or repetitive tasks; however, to date there is no convincing evidence that vibration increases the risk of neck or neck / shoulder problems. Shoulder pain is also associated with heavy physical work – intensive and repetitive shoulder work, especially overhead, both increase the risk. Furthermore, the level of risk appears to be maximal in occupations that involve combinations of exposures, such as working overhead using a heavy tool. Elbow conditions have also been associated with exposure to intensive forces in the workplace, particularly when workers are regularly exposed to combinations of repetition, force and abnormal postures. Repetitious movements may increase the risk of CTS, as may forceful work and exposure to vibration (Bernard 1997). Once again, however, the evidence is strongest that occupations involving combinations of force, vibration and repetition are most likely to increase the risk of CTS syndrome (Abbas et al 1998). When a job involves exposure to awkward forearm, wrist and finger postures, this too may play a role. However, prolonged use of a keyboard at work has not been convincingly demonstrated to be a risk factor for CTS.

Hand / wrist tendonitis or tenosynovitis has been observed in a wide range of different occupational groups ranging from tobacco packers to factory workers during World War II, automobile assembly workers, scissor manufacturers and textile workers (Walker-Bone et al 2003a). It appears that exposure to high levels of force, repetitious tasks and sustained abnormal finger / wrist postures are the most risky. The underlying mechanism is poorly researched, but it may well represent a physiological / mechanical response of the tendon to chronic mechanical stressors.

Occupational risk factors: psychosocial

Psychosocial factors such as perceived workload, psychological stress and support have been consistently shown to be important risk factors for upper extremity pain disorders. However, exposure to psychosocial risk factors is also difficult to measure accurately and lacks any standard measurement system, and it is therefore usually estimated from subjective reports. The European League against Rheumatism (EULAR) reviewed the literature on these factors with the aim of establishing whether reviews of risk factors for work-related musculoskeletal disorders reached consistent conclusions (Macfarlane et al 2009). The resulting paper looked at four regional pain syndromes, two of which were of the upper extremity, and reported that the most consistent conclusions related to psychosocial exposures: high work demands and low job demands (monotonous or insufficient use of skills), and low work control (Bongers et al 2006). In a prospective UK study of risk factors for non-specific forearm pain, Macfarlane et al (2000) found that psychosocial factors were important predictors of the development of upper extremity symptoms, including psychological distress (odds ratio (OR) 1.8, 95% CI 0.8–4.0) and aspects of illness behaviour (OR 6.6, 95% CI 1.5–29) as well as exposure to repetitive physical tasks (OR 2.9, 95% CI 1.2–7.3). Another British study similarly found that minimal job control and little supervisor support were important risk factors (OR 1.6, 95% CI 1.3–1.8 and OR 1.3, 95% CI 1.1–1.5, respectively) (Sim et al 2006).

Conclusion

Upper extremity pain syndromes are common in both the general population and the workplace and are associated with high levels of morbidity and disability. Until recently, epidemiological research has been hampered by lack of clear case definitions; however, increasing use of standardized classification schemes allows for more meaningful analysis and comparisons between settings and over time. Much of the upper extremity pain that occurs is best classified as 'non-specific' as there are no clear-cut pathoanatomical features; however, there is an expanding literature exploring aetiological factors in non-specific pain. It is clear that many upper extremity pain conditions can be classified as 'work related' and that there is a number of potentially modifiable workplace risk factors. Although physical workplace factors (such as force, abnormal posture and repetition, particularly in combination) are implicated in the exacerbation or even causation of these conditions, there is growing evidence that psychosocial factors also play a significant role. This suggests that interventions in the workplace based solely upon mechanical exposures (e.g. ergonomic keyboards and workstations) may not be 100% successful unless attention is also paid to psychosocial risk factors such as control over work, demands of the job and support in the workplace.

References

Abbas MA, Afifi AA, Zhang ZW, et al. 1998. Meta-analysis of published studies of work-related carpal tunnel syndrome. Int J Occup Environ Health 4: 160–167.

Allander E 1974. Prevalence, incidence and remission rates of some rheumatic diseases and syndromes. Scand J Rheumatol 3: 145–153.

Andersen JH, Haahr JP, Frost P. 2007. Risk factors for more severe regional musculoskeletal symptoms: a two-year prospective study of a general working population. Arthritis Rheum 56: 1355–1364.

Atroshi I, Gummesson C, Johnsson R, et al. 1999. Prevalence of carpal tunnel syndrome in the general population. JAMA 282: 153–158.

Bergenudd H, Lindgarde F, Nilsson B, et al. 1988. Shoulder pain in middle age. Clin Orthop 231: 234–238.

Bernard BP (ed). 1997. Musculoskeletal disorders (MSDs) and workplace factors. Cincinnati, OH: US Department of Health and Human Services.

Bongers PM, Ijmker S, van den Heuvel S, et al. 2006. Epidemiology of work related neck and upper limb problems: psychosocial and personal risk factors (part I) and effective interventions from a bio behavioural perspective (part II). J Occup Rehabil 16: 279–302.

Buchbinder R, Goel V, Bombardier C, et al. 1996. Classification systems of soft tissue disorders of the neck and upper limb: do they satisfy methodological guidelines? J Clin Epidemiol 49: 141–149.

Chard MD, Hazelman R, Hazelman BL, et al. 1991. Shoulder disorders in the elderly: a community survey. Arthritis Rheum 34:766–769.

De-la-Llave-Rincón AI, Fernández-de-las-Peñas C, Fernández-Carnero J, et al. 2009. Bilateral hand / wrist heat and cold hyperalgesia, but not hypoesthesia in unilateral carpal tunnel syndrome. Exp Brain Res 198: 455–463.

De Krom M, Knipschild PG, Kester ADM, et al. 1992. Carpal tunnel syndrome: prevalence in the general population. J Clin Epidemiol 45: 373–376.

Eltayeb SM, Staal JB, Hassan AA, et al. 2008. Complaints of the arm, neck and shoulder among computer office workers in Sudan: a prevalence study with validation of an Arabic risk factors questionnaire. Environ Health 7: 33

Ferry S, Silman A, Pritchard T, et al. 1998. The association between different patterns of hand symptoms and objective evidence of median nerve compression. Arthritis Rheum 41: 720–724.

Harrington JM, Carter JT, Birrell L, et al. 1998. Surveillance case definitions for work related upper limb pain syndromes. Occup Environ Med 55: 264–271.

Health and Safety Executive. 2012. Self-reported work-related illness (SWI) and workplace injuries: results from the Labour Force Survey (LFS). All illnesses – last updated 10 / 12. Online. Available: http://www.hse.gov.uk/statistics/lfs/index.htm#neck.

Helliwell P. 1995. Diagnostic criteria for work-related upper limb disorders. Br J Rheumatol 35: 1195–1196.

Huisstede BM, Bierma-Zeinstra SM, Koes BW, et al. 2006. Incidence and prevalence of upper-extremity musculoskeletal disorders. A systematic appraisal of the literature. BMC Musculoskelet Disord 7: 7.

Huisstede BM, Miedema HS, Verhagen AP, et al. 2007. Multidisciplinary consensus on the terminology and classification of complaints of the arm, neck and / or shoulder. Occup Environ Med 64: 313–319.

Huisstede BM, Wijnhoven HA, Bierma-Zeinstra SM, et al. 2008. Prevalence and characteristics of complaints of the arm, neck, and / or shoulder (CANS) in the open population. Clin J Pain 24: 253–259.

Hutson M. 2006. Upper limb disorders. In: Hutson E, Ellis R (eds) Textbook of musculoskeletal medicine. New York: Oxford University Press, pp 249–268.

Jones JRHJT, Clegg TA. 1998. Self-reported work-related illness in 1995. London: HMSO.

Macfarlane GJ, Hunt IM, Silman AJ. 2000. Role of mechanical and psychosocial factors in the onset of forearm pain: prospective population based study. BMJ 321: 676–679.

Macfarlane GJ, Pallewatte N, Paudyal P, et al. 2009. Evaluation of work-related psychosocial factors and regional musculoskeletal pain: results from a EULAR Task Force. Ann Rheum Dis 68: 885–891.

Menendez CC, Amick BC 3rd, Chang CH, et al. 2008. Computer use patterns associated with upper extremity musculoskeletal symptoms. J Occup Rehabil 18: 166–174.

Morris H. 1882. Riders sprain. Lancet 2: 557.

Palmer KC. 2006. Work related disorders of the upper limb. Topical Reviews 10: 1–7.

Palmer K, Walker-Bone K, Linaker C, et al. 2000. The Southampton examination schedule for the diagnosis of musculoskeletal disorders of the upper limb. Ann Rheum Dis 59: 5–11.

Palmer KT, Harris EC, Linaker C, et al. 2012. Optimal case definitions of upper extremity disorder for use in the clinical treatment and referral of patients. Arthritis Care Res 64: 573–580.

Ramazzini B. 1940 (first published 1713). De morbis artificum. Chicago IL: University of Chicago.

Robinson H, Walker-Bone K. 2009. Occupation and disorders of the neck and upper limb. Rheumatol Practice 7: 7–10.

Roquelaure Y, Ha C, Leclerc A, et al. 2006. Epidemiologic surveillance of upper-extremity musculoskeletal disorders in the working population. Arthritis Rheum 55: 765–778.

Shiri R, Varonen H, Heliövaara M, et al. 2007. Hand dominance in upper extremity musculoskeletal disorders. J Rheumatol 34: 1076–1082.

Silverstein B, Welp E, Nelson N, et al. 1998. Claims incidence of work-related disorders of the upper extremities: Washington State, 1987 through 1995. Am J Pub Health 88: 1827–1833.
Sim J, Lacey RJ, Lewis M. 2006. The impact of workplace risk factors on the occurrence of neck and upper limb pain: a general population study. BMC Public Health 6: 234
Sluiter JK, Rest KM, Frings-Dresen MH. 2001. Criteria document for evaluating the work-relatedness of upper-extremity musculoskeletal disorders. Scand J Work Environ Health 27: 1–102.
Tornqvist EW, Hagberg M, Hagman M, et al. 2009. The influence of working conditions and individual factors on the incidence of neck and upper limb symptoms among professional computer users. Int Arch Occup Environ Health 82: 689–702.
Turk DC, Rudy TE. 1990. Neglected factors in chronic pain treatment outcome studies – referral patterns, failure to enter treatment, and attrition. Pain 1: 7–25.
Van Eerd D, Beaton D, Cole D, et al. 2003. Classification systems for upper-limb musculoskeletal disorders in workers: a review of the literature. J Clin Epidemiol 56: 925–936.
Verhaar JAN. 1994 Tennis elbow. Int Orthop 18: 263–267.
Viikari-Juntura E. 1983. Neck and upper limb disorders among slaughterhouse workers. Scand J Work Environ Health 9: 283–290.
Walker-Bone K. 2002. Prevalence of and risk factors for musculoskeletal disorders of the neck and upper limb. Southampton, UK: University of Southampton. [PhD thesis.]
Walker-Bone K, Byng P, Linaker C, et al. 2002. Reliability of the Southampton examination schedule for the diagnosis of upper limb disorders in the general population. Ann Rheum Dis 61: 1103–1106.
Walker-Bone KE, Palmer KT, Reading I, et al. 2003a. Soft-tissue rheumatic disorders of the neck and upper limb: prevalence and risk factors. Semin Arthritis Rheum 33: 185–203.
Walker-Bone KE, Palmer KT, Reading I, et al. 2003b. Criteria for assessing pain and nonarticular soft-tissue rheumatic disorders of the neck and upper limb. Semin Arthritis Rheum 33, 168–184.
Walker-Bone K, Palmer K, Reading I, et al. 2004a. Prevalence and impact of musculoskeletal disorders of the upper limb in the general population. Arthritis Rheum 51: 642–651.
Walker-Bone K, Reading I, Coggon D, et al. 2004b. The anatomical pattern and determinants of pain in the neck and upper limbs: an epidemiologic study. Pain 109: 45–51.

Chapter 2

Epidemiology of Lower Extremity Pain Disorder

Adam P. Goode, Sean D. Rundell

CHAPTER CONTENTS

Introduction	13
Prevalence and incidence of specific lower extremity disorders	13
Lumbar conditions	13
Hip conditions	16
Labral tears	17
Greater trochanteric pain syndrome	17
Knee conditions	17
Foot and ankle conditions	18
Healthcare utilization and impact	19
Conclusion	20

Introduction

Musculoskeletal diseases are a major public health problem and are the leading cause of physical disability (Weinstein 2000). The Bone and Joint Initiative has reported a rapid increase in musculoskeletal chronic conditions, many of which may result in chronic pain (Jacobs 2011). As with many chronic conditions, musculoskeletal pain and disease can have long-term impacts on people's quality of life, place a large burden on healthcare systems and affect society as a whole.

Musculoskeletal conditions affect many people. The estimated prevalence of musculoskeletal disease varies substantially between 2% and 65% depending on the condition (Picavet & Hazes 2003). Gender differences also exist, with chronic musculoskeletal conditions affecting approximately 53 in every 100 females and 45 in every 100 males (Jacobs 2011).

This chapter describes some of the most common musculoskeletal conditions in the lower extremity (Fig. 2.1). Many of these conditions can lead to chronic symptoms greatly impacting daily function and leading to disability. Pain in the lower extremity makes up a substantial amount of the musculoskeletal diseases and is one of the most common reasons for seeking care from a medical provider. In 2008, three of the four most common medical conditions reported were musculoskeletal conditions impacting the lower extremity (i.e. low back pain (LBP), chronic joint pain and arthritis) (Pleis et al 2009). Back pain, the most prevalent condition impacting the lower extremity, accounted for over 45 million healthcare visits annually, and of those reporting chronic joint pain the most common joint affected was the knee (Pleis et al 2009). Within the lower extremity, pain syndromes may take on many forms and present in many different joints, muscles or tendons. The focus of this chapter is on those lower extremity pain disorders (i.e. chronic pain, osteoarthritis (OA), sprains and strains) that are commonly treated by techniques such as manual therapy and exercise. Conditions such rheumatic diseases, work-related musculoskeletal disorders and malignancy or systemic issues will not be covered.

An estimated 7.4% of the United States gross domestic product is spent on annual direct and indirect costs for bone and joint health. Despite the impact on healthcare costs and personal financial burden, an estimated 2% of the National Institutes of Health budget is spent on musculoskeletal conditions (Jacobs 2011). The majority of research in the area of lower extremity pain disorders has been towards understanding their prevalence. Many studies are conducted using retrospective chart reviews, secondary data analysis and samples of convenience; however, these factors limit the ability to understand the true burden of disease. Many epidemiological studies have inconsistent case definitions or methodological differences in study design that result in variable estimates. Another limited area of research is that of incidence, or new cases of disease in a given period. Due to the limited number of these studies, in this chapter we focus on the burden (prevalence) of disease from population-based studies or report limitations in sampling from non-population-based studies; we report incidence estimates when they are available.

Prevalence and Incidence of Specific Lower Extremity Disorders

Lumbar conditions

Prevalence

Table 2.1 summarizes selected studies, their outcome measures, overall prevalence estimates and stratified prevalence estimates by gender for LBP, sciatica and lumbar spinal stenosis. Back pain has a large impact on society and individuals. The Global Burden of Diseases, Injuries, and Risk Factors Study in 2010 found that back pain continues to be the number one health condition in terms of years lived with disability,

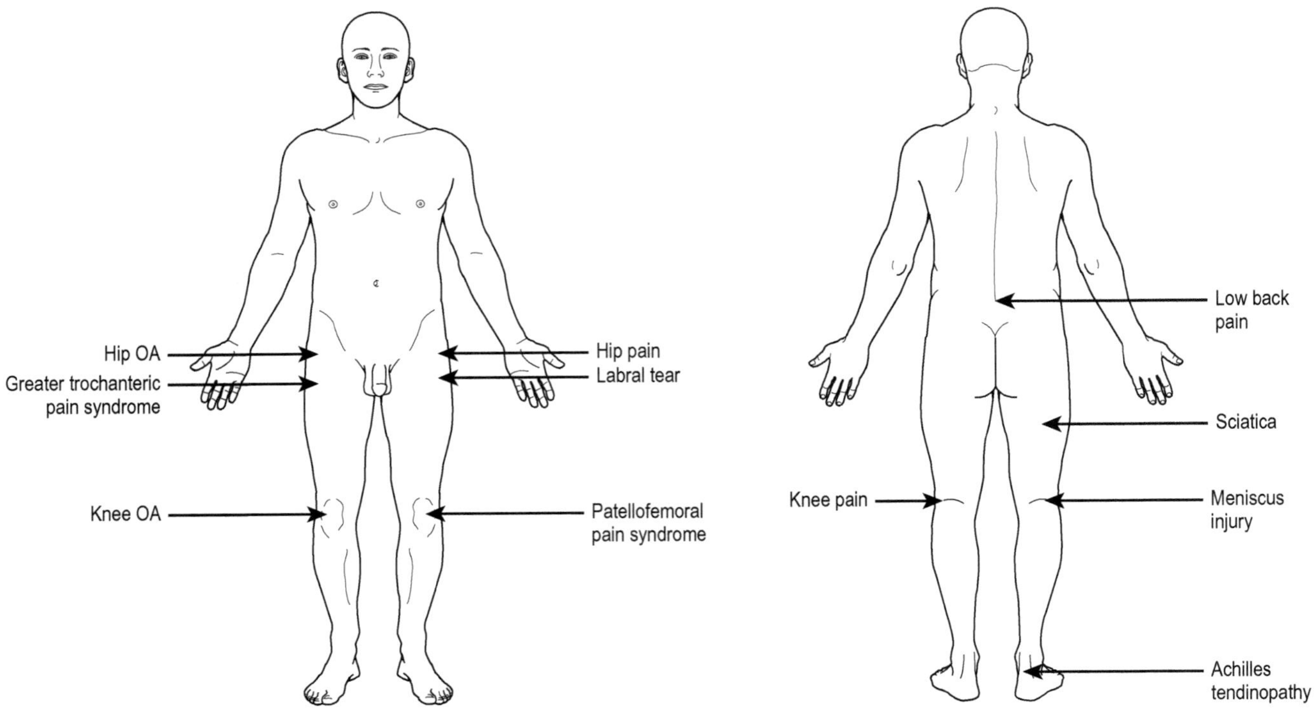

Figure 2.1 Musculoskeletal conditions in the lower extremity covered in this chapter. OA, osteoarthritis.

Table 2.1 Prevalence of lumbar-related conditions

Author year	Definition	Sample size	Prevalence estimate (men) (%)	Prevalence estimate (women) (%)	Overall prevalence (%)
Low back pain					
Hoy et al 2012	Mean prevalence for any definition	Systematic review of 165 studies	29.4	35.3	31.0
Deyo et al 2006	Prevalence of LBP within past 3 months	31 044	24.3	28.3	26.4
Cassidy et al 1998	Point prevalence Lifetime prevalence	1131	N/R	N/R	28.7 84.0
Sciatica					
Heliövaara et al 1987a	Point prevalence of lumbar-disc-related leg pain	7217	5.1	3.7	4.8
Hillman et al 1996	Any leg pain or related paraesthesiae within the previous year	3184	N/R	N/R	17.8
Spinal stenosis					
Kalichman et al 2009	Lumbar spinal stenosis seen on CT scan	191	N/R	N/R	23.6

N/R=not reported.

both worldwide and in the United States (Murray et al 2013; Vos et al 2013). Prevalence is an important component for determining the burden of disease. However, the prevalence of LBP is often described variously in the literature – various methods, definitions and time-periods of prevalent LBP have been used. Consequently, this produces a wide variation in the estimated prevalence of LBP. Hoy et al (2012) conducted a systematic review on the prevalence of LBP, and found estimates ranging from 1.2% to 85.5%. From these studies, the estimated overall mean prevalence of back pain was 31.0%. The mean point prevalence was 18.7%, and the mean 1-year prevalence was 38.0%. Prevalence estimates differ depending on study quality, definition of back pain and time-period. The above authors recommend caution when interpreting a single summary measure of prevalence due to this heterogeneity (Hoy et al 2012).

The same systematic review also found that the prevalence of LBP was greater in females than in males. The mean overall prevalence of LBP for females was 35.3%, whereas males had a mean overall prevalence of 29.4%. The prevalence of LBP also varied over the lifespan. The overall prevalence of LBP was highest for 40–69-year olds compared with those who were 20–29 or 80–89 years old. Adolescents had a higher prevalence of LBP compared with 20–29-year olds, although this difference was not significant (Hoy et al 2012). These findings are consistent with a systematic review by Jeffries et al (2007) on adolescent spinal pain, which suggests that 7–51% of adolescents report LBP within the previous year, and 7–72% report ever having had LBP during their lifetime.

Recent evidence since the systematic review by Hoy et al (2012) indicates that the difference in prevalent LBP between older and younger adults is still unclear. Macfarlane et al (2012) conducted a population-based study in the United Kingdom and found that the prevalence of back pain within the previous month peaked for adults aged 41–50 years (29.8%) and decreased to 25.5% for adults >80 years of age. These findings mirror the curvilinear pattern of prevalent LBP with increasing age observed by Hoy et al (2012). However, Macfarlane et al (2012) also reported that the prevalence of high-grade back pain, measured using the Chronic Pain Grade (CPG) scale, progressively increased with older age – the highest prevalence of high-grade pain being 10.0% among people aged >80 years.

In the United States, Deyo et al (2006) estimated that the prevalence of LBP during the previous 3 months was fairly similar to the studies discussed above. The age-adjusted prevalence was 26.4%. The prevalence of LBP was highest among those 45–64 years old (29.8%), and it dropped slightly for those aged 65 and older – it was 28.8% for those aged 65–74 years and 28.7% for those aged >74 years.

Overall, the variety of LBP definitions and research methods used for prevalence studies makes comparisons between studies and between age groups challenging. However, the evidence clearly demonstrates that LBP is a common health condition and has a large burden worldwide.

Similar to back pain, sciatica is a symptom. Although there is no standard definition, it typically involves low-back-related leg pain. Sciatica is commonly associated with spinal nerve root involvement, but this is not always necessary according to some definitions (Alexopoulos et al 2008). Consistent with the lack of a common definition, there are variable estimates for the prevalence of sciatica. A review by Konstantinou and Dunn (2008) found prevalence estimates for sciatica ranging from 1.2% to 43%. A Finnish population-based study estimated the point prevalence of lumbar-disc-related leg pain, diagnosed using symptoms and a physical exam, to be 4.8% (95% confidence interval (CI) 4.3–5.2%) (Heliövaara et al 1987a). Males had a higher prevalence of lumbar-disc-related leg pain than females: 5.1% and 3.7% respectively. These authors also found the prevalence was highest among those aged 45–64 years (Heliövaara et al 1987a). The prevalence of any leg pain or related paraesthesiae within the previous year was estimated to be 17.8% in the British population, and 45.6% of those reporting back pain within the previous year also reported leg pain (Hillman et al 1996).

Lumbar spinal stenosis is one of the few radiographic features associated with back pain (Jarvik & Deyo 2002; Suri et al 2010). There is no commonly accepted definition of lumbar spinal stenosis (Mamisch et al 2012), but the North American Spine Society defines it as 'buttock or lower extremity pain, which may occur with or without LBP, associated with diminished space available for the neural and vascular elements in the lumbar spine' (North American Spine Society (NASS) 2007). Kalichman et al (2009) studied lumbar spinal stenosis in a small subsample of the Framingham Study who received computed tomography (CT) scans. They found up to 23.6% of adults may have anatomical lumbar spinal stenosis, and the prevalence increased to 38.8% in those over 60 years of age (Kalichman et al 2009). There was no difference in prevalence between females and males. Older age and higher body mass index (BMI) were factors associated with having lumbar spinal stenosis ≤12 mm, and LBP was associated with having lumbar spinal stenosis ≤10 mm (Kalichman et al 2009). A Japanese study measured symptomatic lumbar spinal stenosis using a questionnaire / diagnostic support tool (Yabuki et al 2013). The prevalence of symptomatic lumbar spinal stenosis was 5.7% and increased with older age; of those aged 70–79 years, 10.8% had symptomatic lumbar spinal stenosis. As with other studies, differences in definitions and measurement of lumbar spinal stenosis make comparing prevalence estimates a challenge. However, the prevalence of lumbar spinal stenosis does appear to increase with advancing age.

Incidence

Studies on the incidence of LBP are less common. 'Incident LBP' is typically measured as the first-ever episode of LBP or any episode of LBP (whether new or recurrent). The cumulative incidence for first-ever episodes of LBP may range from 6.3% to 15.4% (Hoy et al 2010). Croft et al (1999) conducted a 1-year cohort study of 2715 back-pain-free adults aged 18–75 years in the United Kingdom and found that the cumulative incidence of a first-ever LBP episode was 15.4%.

The 1-year incidence of any back pain episode may range from 1.5% to 36.5% of a population (Hoy et al 2010). A population-based survey of adults 20–69 years old from Saskatchewan, Canada, found the cumulative incidence for a back pain episode to be 18.6% (95% CI 14.2–23.0%), an incidence that did not differ according to age or gender (Cassidy et al 2005). The above estimates suggest that new episodes of back pain are also fairly common at a population level.

Specific to older adults, a cohort study of community-dwelling adults 70 years of age or more found the cumulative incidence of restricting LBP over 10 years to be 77% in males and 82% in females. The incidence rate was 32.9 per 1000 person-months, and the vast majority of episodes (80%) were less than 1 month (Makris et al 2011).

There are few population-based studies on the incidence of sciatica. Heliövaara et al (1987b) estimated the incidence of sciatica from a herniated disc that resulted in a hospitalization within the Finnish population; they found an incidence of only 2.75 per 1000 person-years, and a cumulative incidence of 0.65%. A more recent Finnish study of city employees found a cumulative incidence of back pain radiating into the calf and foot of 35% among females and 37% among males over a 5–7-year span (Kaila-Kangas et al 2009). Sciatic symptoms were ascertained using a questionnaire, so recall bias is likely. Additionally, this study was limited to participants aged 40 years or older. Incident sciatica appears much less common than incident back pain, but the limited quantity of studies makes it difficult to draw firm conclusions or comparisons.

Hip conditions

Hip symptoms and osteoarthritis

Table 2.2 describes the studies, measures, overall and stratified prevalence estimates by gender for the hip joint. Hip pain and osteoarthritis (OA) have received little attention in population-based studies despite their importance and impact on general physical function. Both the National Health and Nutrition Survey (NHANES) and the Johnston County Osteoarthritis (JoCo OA) Project have been determining the prevalence and incidence of hip pain and OA since the 1990s (Tepper & Hochberg 1993; Jordan et al 2009). In the JoCo OA Project (Jordan et al 2009), the overall prevalence of hip OA was 28.0%, with a higher prevalence among Caucasian women (29.1%) and African-American men (33.2%). In contrast, in the NHANES-I study (Tepper & Hochberg 1993), the estimated prevalence of hip OA was 3.1%, with similar estimates for men and women.

There are also wide variations in the estimated prevalence of hip symptoms between the JoCo OA Project and the NHANES study. In the JoCo OA Project (Jordan et al 2009), the estimated prevalence of hip pain was 36.0%, with a higher prevalence among women but similar estimates in Caucasians and African-Americans. In contrast, the prevalence of hip pain in the NHANES-III study was 14.3%, but similar to the JoCo OA Project there was a higher prevalence in women (Lawrence et al 2008). Differences in the questions used to ascertain hip symptoms are a likely reason for the variations. The JoCo OA Project applied a broader case definition; it included aching and stiffness as well as pain in the case question. There are also large differences in the prevalence of hip OA between the JoCo OA Project and NHANES. Possible reasons for these discrepancies include variability in radiograph readings by the radiologists (the NHANES-I radiographs may not reflect the true prevalence of hip OA owing to under-reading of films), a higher prevalence of radiographic hip OA among rural men in the JoCo OA Project, and geographic variations in risk factors (Jordan et al 2009). Nevitt et al (1995) estimated the prevalence of hip pain and OA in a population of postmenopausal women (and therefore the findings from this study are generalizable only to women). They found a prevalence of hip pain (35.0%) consistent with the JoCo OA Project. However, their hip OA estimates were closer to NHANES. The emphasis of this study was on osteoporosis and therefore their study sample was markedly different from the general community-based samples in the JoCo OA Project and NHANES. Despite the differences in study samples and questions to define hip symptoms and OA, these conditions are also common in the general population and have substantial impact on general physical function.

Table 2.2 **Prevalence of hip-related pain conditions**

Author year	Definition	Sample size	Prevalence estimate (men) (%)	Prevalence estimate (women) (%)	Overall prevalence (%)
Hip OA					
Jordan et al 2009	K-L score 2–4	3068	Caucasian 23.8 African-American 33.2	Caucasian 29.1 African-American 31.2	28.0
Nevitt et al 1995	Score of 2–4	4855	N/A	11.9	N/A
NHANES-I (Tepper & Hochberg 1993)	K-L score 2–4	2358	3.2	3.0	3.1
Hip pain					
Jordan et al 2009	'On most days, do you have pain, aching, or stiffness in your (right, left) hip?'	3068	Caucasian 31.7 African-American 32.0	Caucasian 39.4 African-American 40.3	36.0
Nevitt et al 1995	'Hip pain on most days for 1 month'	4855	N/A	35.0	N/A
NHANES-III (Lawrence et al 2008)	'Significant pain on most days over the preceding 6 weeks'	6596	11.9	16.2	14.3
Labral tear					
Narvani et al 2003	MRI	18	N/R	N/R	22
McCarthy et al 2001	Arthroscopy	436	54.4	45.6	55.0
Greater trochanteric pain syndrome					
Segal et al 2007	Tenderness to palpation	3206	1.9	6.6	Unilateral 15.0 Bilateral 8.5
Tortolani et al 2002	Clinical examination	252	N/R	N/R	20.2

K-L=Kellgren and Lawrence; N/A=not available; N/R=not reported.

Incidence

The incidence of hip OA has only recently been estimated, and differences have been found between African-Americans and Caucasians. The age- and sex-standardized incidence of hip OA is estimated to be 88 per 100 000 person-years (Oliveria et al 1995). The adjusted incidence of hip OA in African-Americans is significantly lower (hazard ratio (HR) 0.44, 95% CI 0.27–0.71) than in Caucasians (Kopec et al 2013).

Labral tears

Acetabular labral tears have received increasing attention in recent years, and particularly the role that labral tears may play in chondral damage and development of hip OA. In one study the prevalence of hip labral tears was estimated at 22–55% (McCarthy et al 2001), but as this study was conducted in a sample of patients with existing groin or hip pain a population-based estimate of hip labral tears is still unavailable. Similarly, there are as yet no population-based studies on the incidence of hip labral tears.

Greater trochanteric pain syndrome

Greater trochanteric pain syndrome (GTPS) can be a challenging condition to diagnose and treat. Few studies have been conducted within a well-defined population. Tortolani et al (2002) estimated the prevalence of GTPS, using a medical chart review, to be approximately 20% among patients seeking care for LBP. Segal et al (2007) conducted the only population-based study of GTPS in 2954 subjects within the Multicenter Osteoarthritis Study. They used a clinical examination with a standardized dolorimeter to calibrate finger pressure prior to examination, and found the prevalence of unilateral GTPS to be 11.7%, with a higher prevalence in women (15.0%) than in men (6.6%) (Segal et al 2007). The higher prevalence estimate of 20% in the Tortolani et al (2002) study is most likely to be due to the differences in selection of subjects and the broad definition of GTPS, as the study participants were identified through a retrospective medical chart review and were therefore seeking care. No population-based studies have been conducted on the incidence of greater trochanteric pain syndrome.

Knee conditions

Knee symptoms and osteoarthritis

Table 2.3 describes the studies, measures, overall prevalence and stratified prevalence estimates by gender for pain related to the knee joint. Similar to the prevalence estimates for the hip, substantial variability exists in those for knee symptoms. In the JoCo OA Project the overall prevalence of knee symptoms was 43.3%, with a higher prevalence in women (47.6%)

Table 2.3 **Prevalence of knee-related pain conditions**

Author year	Definition	Sample size (*n*)	Prevalence in men (95% CI) (%)	Prevalence in women (95% CI) (%)	Overall prevalence (95% CI) (%)
Knee pain					
Jordan et al 2007	'On most days, do you have pain, aching, or stiffness in your (right, left) knee?'	3018	37.4 (35.4–39.4)	47.6 (45.7–49.6)	43.3 (41.7–44.9)
NHANES-III (Andersen et al 1999)	'Significant knee pain on most days over the preceding 6 weeks'	6596	18.1	23.5	N/A
Framingham Osteoarthritis Study (Felson et al 1987)	'Ever had pain in or around a knee of most days for at least a month'	1805 symptoms 1424 radiographs	6.8 (symptomatic OA)	11.4 (symptomatic OA)	16.1
Knee OA					
Jordan et al 2007	K-L score 2–4	3018	23.7 (26.5–29.2)	31.0 (29.2–32.8)	27.8 (26.5–29.2)
NHANES-III (Andersen et al 1999)	K-L score 2–4	2415	31.2 (26.4–35.9)	42.1 (38.2–46.0)	37.4 (35.0–39.8)
Framingham Osteoarthritis Study (Felson et al 1987)	K-L score 2–4	1420	30.9	34.4	33.0
Meniscus tear					
Englund 2008	MRI	991	33 (28.0–37.0)	19 (15.0–24)	35 (32.0–38.0)
Patellofemoral pain syndrome					
Boling et al 2010	Medical record review	1525	15.3 (13.7–16.9)	12.3 (11.1–13.4)	13.5 (11.7–15.3)

N/A=not available; K-L=Kellgren and Lawrence.

(Jordan et al 2009). In the NHANES-III study there was also a higher prevalence of knee symptoms in women (23.5%) (Lawrence et al 2008); however, the estimates across the genders were substantially lower than those found in the JoCo OA Project. Variability in knee symptom questions is the reason for this inconsistency.

The prevalence estimates for knee OA are more similar across studies. In the JoCo OA Project the overall prevalence of knee OA was 27.8%, with a higher prevalence found in women (31.0%) (Jordan et al 2009). Similarly, in the NHANES-III study the overall prevalence was 37.4% (Lawrence et al 2008) and in the Framingham OA Study it was 33.0% (Felson et al 1987). Both the NHANES-III and the Framingham OA Study reported a higher prevalence in women. The differences between knee OA found in the JoCo OA Project compared with the NHANES-III study are thought to be primarily due to the use of non-weight-bearing radiographs in the NHANES study. Symptomatic knee OA was very prevalent in the JoCo OA Project (men 13.5% and women 18.7%) (Jordan et al 2007). Similarly, findings from the Framingham OA Study indicate a higher prevalence of symptomatic OA in women (11.4%); however, these estimates are much greater than those in the JoCo OA Project. The increasing rate of obesity over the time periods when these studies were conducted is a possible reason for this discrepancy (Jordan et al 2007).

Incidence of knee osteoarthritis

Age- and sex-standardized incidence rate of symptomatic knee OA is 240 per 100 000 person-years (Oliveria et al 1995). These rates increase with age and level off around the age of 80 years (Buckwalter et al 2004). The lifetime risk of developing symptomatic knee OA is estimated to be approximately 40% in men and 47% in females.

Meniscus injury

Meniscal injuries are extremely prevalent, but population-based studies are rare. The majority of meniscal injuries occur in the athletic population from contact and non-contact injury, but degenerative meniscal injury is also possible. The variety of potential injury exposures occurring across sports leads to substantial variability in meniscal injury prevalence estimates across studies. One previous study conducted within the Framingham census tract estimated the prevalence (35%) of right knee lateral or medial meniscus damage among a sample of middle-aged and elderly adults (Englund et al 2009b). This study found that men had a substantially greater prevalence (33%) of meniscal tear compared with women (19%). Since these results were derived from a population-based sample, these authors were able to identify that 23% of subjects had a meniscal tear without reporting knee symptoms. A common question is whether meniscal damage may lead to knee OA. In this study a large proportion (63%) of subjects with symptomatic OA had evidence of a meniscus tear. Other studies have also noted the presence of meniscus injury to be a potent risk factor for the development of knee OA (Englund 2008; Englund et al 2009a).

Patellofemoral pain syndrome

Anterior knee pain, caused from patellofemoral pain syndrome (PFPS), is one of the most common knee complaints (Davis & Powers 2010). PFPS is a common diagnosis within the athletic population, and runners in particular (Devereaux & Lachmann 1984). There are few population-based studies. Boling et al (2010) conducted an epidemiological study to determine the prevalence and incidence of PFPS among 1525 military cadets at the United States Naval Academy. Given previous reports of a gender difference, with females having a higher prevalence, these authors examined gender differences with a sample that was approximately one-half female. Participants underwent a clinical examination at baseline and were followed prospectively. The prevalence of PFPS was 13.5% (95% CI 11.7–15.3%) in the sample, with a higher prevalence in women (15.3%, 95% CI 13.7–16.9%) than in men (12.3%, 95% CI 11.1–13.4%). In adjusted longitudinal analyses, women were 2.23 (95% CI 1.16–4.10) times more likely to develop PFPS (Boling et al 2010).

Foot and ankle conditions

Ankle sprains

Table 2.4 presents selected studies, their measures, overall and stratified prevalence estimates by gender for common musculoskeletal conditions at the ankle and foot. Ligament sprains are a common injury at the ankle. Doherty et al (2014) performed a large meta-analysis of ankle sprain injuries. They found the pooled prevalence of ankle sprains was 11.88% (95% CI 10.56–13.19%) when using estimates from high-quality studies only. The pooled prevalence estimates were similar between males and females. The prevalence of ankle sprains was greatest in children (12.62%, 95% CI 11.81–13.43%), whereas the prevalence estimates in adolescents (10.55%, 95% CI 9.92–11.17%) and adults (11.41%, 95% CI 11.28–11.54%) were slightly lower (Doherty et al 2014).

The meta-analysis by Doherty et al (2014) also created pooled estimates for the incidence of ankle sprains. The overall incidence was 11.55 per 1000 exposures (95% CI 11.54–11.55) among their high-quality studies. Females had more than double the estimated incidence of ankle sprains: 13.6 per 1000 exposures (95% CI 13.25–13.94) versus 6.94 per 1000 exposures (95% CI 6.–7.09) for males. Furthermore, adolescents and children have more incident ankle sprains than adults: 1.94 (95% CI 1.73–2.14) and 2.85 (95% CI 2.51–3.19) ankle sprains per 1000 exposures respectively, whereas adults had 0.72 ankle sprains per 1000 exposures (95% CI 0.67–0.77) (Doherty et al 2014).

The incidence of ankle sprains requiring an emergency department visit in the United States population is 2.15 per 1000 person-years (Waterman et al 2010). Teenagers (15–19 years old) had the highest incidence of any age group, at 7.2 per 1000 person-years. Overall, there was no difference in incident ankle sprain between males and females (Waterman et al 2010). These estimates probably underestimate the true incidence of ankle sprains in the United States, however, since many people experiencing an ankle sprain may not seek care in an emergency department.

Lateral ankle sprain is the most common site for incident sprains; there were 0.93 lateral ankles sprains per 1000 athletic exposures. Syndesmotic sprains were the next most common, with 0.38 per 1000 athletic exposures, and medial ankle sprains were least common, with 0.06 per 1000 athletic exposures (Doherty et al 2014).

Table 2.4 **Prevalence of foot/ankle pain conditions**

Author year	Definition	Sample size (*n*)	Prevalence in men (95% CI) (%)	Prevalence in women (95% CI) (%)	Overall prevalence (95% CI) (%)
Ankle sprains					
Doherty et al 2014	Pooled prevalence of ankle sprains	Meta-analysis of 181 studies	11.0 (10.8–11.2)	10.6 (10.8–11.2)	11.9 (10.56–13.19)
Achilles tendinopathy					
de Jonge et al 2011	Achilles pain above the insertion	57 725	N/R	N/R	0.2
McKean et al 2006	Self-reported Achilles injuries	981 runners over 40	N/R	N/R	6.2
Plantar fasciitis					
McKean et al 2006	Self-reported plantar fasciitis	2886 runners	N/R	N/R	8.4

N/R=non-reported.

Achilles tendinopathy

There are few population-based estimates for the prevalence of Achilles tendinopathy. In the Dutch population, de Jonge et al (2011) reported that 0.2% of registered general practice patients have Achilles tendinopathy. However, its prevalence may be higher in distance runners. One study found that 6.2% of runners aged over 40 years at a relay race had self-reported Achilles tendinopathy over the previous 12 months (McKean et al 2006). Also, runners aged over 40 years had a greater prevalence than those aged less than 40 years (McKean et al 2006). Jacobs & Berson (1986) found the prevalence in runners was 2.9% over a 2-year span.

Population-based estimates for the incidence of Achilles tendinopathy are also rare. The study by de Jonge et al (2011) looked at incident general practitioner visits for mid-portion Achilles tendinopathy in their Dutch population sample. These authors found an incidence rate of 1.85 per 1000 registered general practice patients. The incidence was similar between males and females. Patients aged 41–65 years had the highest incidence, at 2.4 per 1000 (de Jonge et al 2011). Although very generalizable to the Dutch population, this study may underestimate the real incidence of Achilles tendinopathy since not all individuals may seek care for their injury.

Incident Achilles tendinopathy has been estimated to occur in 10.9% of runners (Lysholm & Wiklander 1987). In fact, Knobloch et al (2008) found incident Achilles tendinopathy to be the most common injury in a cohort of runners. The incidence rate was 0.16 per 1000 kilometres run (Knobloch et al 2008). A study looking at elite track and field athletes during a 2009 world championship meet found the cumulative incidence of Achilles tendinopathy to be 6.1 per 1000 athletes during the meet (Alonso et al 2010; Sobhani et al 2013).

Plantar fasciitis

Plantar fasciitis is a frequent reason for physician visits and one of the most common reasons for heel pain. During the years 1995 to 2000, the average number of physician visits for plantar fasciitis was 1 005 000 per year in the USA (Riddle & Schappert 2004). Despite being a fairly common reason for seeking healthcare, population estimates for the prevalence of plantar fasciitis are scarce. However, within sporting populations some studies have estimated the proportion of people with plantar fasciitis. The 1-year prevalence in triathletes is estimated to be 3.9% (Collins et al 1989). In distance runners it is estimated to be 8.4%, and there is no difference in prevalence for runners aged 40 years or older compared with those less than 40 years of age (McKean et al 2006). In another study, the prevalence in runners was reported to be 2.4% over 2 years (Jacobs & Berson 1986).

There are a few estimates of incident plantar fasciitis in active or athletic populations. In the study by Kochen et al (2009), the incidence of plantar fasciitis for an active-duty military population in the United States was 10.5 per 1000 person-years. Females had almost twice the incidence rate of plantar fasciitis compared with males: 18.0 per 1000 person-years and 9.2 per 1000 person-years respectively. Service members who were 40 years old or more had the highest rate of plantar fasciitis, at 16.6 per 1000 person-years; this was more than three times as high as for 20–24-year-olds. In other studies, the incidence rate of plantar fasciitis among runners was 0.004 per 1000 kilometres run (Knobloch et al 2008). In elite track athletes, incident plantar fasciitis was less common than Achilles tendinopathy, at 0.7 per 1000 participating athletes (Alonso et al 2010; Sobhani et al 2013).

Healthcare Utilization and Impact

The population is ageing and therefore chronic conditions are becoming more prevalent, leading to increased morbidity. With increasing longevity, the healthcare system is sustaining severe financial pressure to maintain care. An estimated $950 billion dollars in direct and indirect dollars costs are spent on musculoskeletal disease. Individuals with musculoskeletal diseases have a large impact on the healthcare system, with costs increasing from $5151 per person in 1996–98 to $6429 in 2004–06, representing a 25% increase in expenditure (Jacobs 2011).

The economic burden of LBP is extensive. For the entire United States population, the annual medical costs for LBP were $86 billion in 2005 and estimated to be over $100 billion in 2010 (Martin et al 2008). LBP-associated costs and healthcare utilization among Medicare beneficiaries have increased disproportionately, compared with Medicare enrollment (Weiner et al 2006). As the population ages and Medicare coverage grows, the US healthcare system will have an increased burden.

LBP is the second most common reason for physician visits in the United States (Hart et al 1995). Mafi et al (2013) have recently examined trends from 1999–2000 to 2009–10 in the United States for specific types of back-related healthcare use. Physical therapy utilization has remained relatively stable over the 10-year period; approximately 15–20% of patients with back pain utilized physical therapy services during this time-period. The proportion of patients receiving radiographs has also remained fairly stable (approximately 13–17%), but the use of advanced imaging for individuals with LBP had increased from 7% to about 11% by 2010. Use of non-steroidal anti-inflammatory medication for back pain has actually decreased, whereas the use of opioids has increased from 19.3% to 29.1% of patients. Other studies show that the use of lumbosacral injections for back pain (Friedly et al 2007) and complex spinal fusion surgeries for spinal stenosis (Deyo et al 2010) also have trends of increasing usage.

Osteoarthritis is one of the most common musculoskeletal conditions leading to functional impairment and disability. OA, in general, accounts for substantial morbidity, healthcare utilization, and high annual direct and indirect costs. Patients with OA are subject to roughly double the healthcare costs of those without OA. Yelin et al (2007) reported no changes in total healthcare costs among patients with OA from 1997 to 2003. However, a previous study (MacLean et al 1998) from 1991 to 1993 reported that medication costs had more than doubled and outpatient charges increased substantially over that period.

The most common site for lower extremity OA is the knee and hip. A common treatment for end-stage OA in the knee and hip is total joint arthroplasty. Kurtz et al (2007) anticipated that such surgeries would increase at a rapid rate between 2005 and 2030 – by 174% for total hip joint arthroplasty and 673% for knee arthroplasty. In 2007, the estimated annual cost of knee and hip arthroplasty was $15.6 billion dollars (Ong et al 2006). Despite the high volume and cost associated with hip and knee arthroplasty, the improvements in pain and function appear to be justified, however.

Ankle sprain is a common musculoskeletal condition that often becomes chronic or recurrent (Verhagen et al 2000), and the associated healthcare costs and utilization create a large burden on the healthcare system. It is the most common lower extremity injury responsible for emergency visits in the United States, at 206 per 100 000 visits (Lambers et al 2012). Although no recent data on healthcare costs associated with ankle sprains in the United States are available, in the Netherlands it was estimated that sports-related ankle sprains may cost 187.2 million Euros (Hupperets et al 2010). Clearly, more work is needed to understand better the healthcare utilization and associated costs for ankle sprains.

Conclusion

Understanding the epidemiology of lower extremity pain syndromes is clearly important for practitioners as the prevalence of disease has implications for accurate diagnosis. Prevalence is often the basis for pre-test probabilities of diagnostic tests. The prevalence of lower extremity pain syndromes varies substantially with respect to location and diagnosis. In some cases, the prevalence and incidence estimates from population-based studies contradict one another, and this is in large part due to the questions used to ascertain case definitions. Although musculoskeletal lower extremity pain syndromes are increasing, population-based research on the incidence, prevalence and risk factors is insufficiently studied and rare. Not only does more work need to be done in this area to understand the disease burden better, but uniformity in question design and diagnosis are critical to achieve better consistency between estimates. The impact of disease incidence and prevalence on healthcare utilization and costs makes it imperative to understand further the epidemiology of lower extremity pain syndromes.

References

Alexopoulos EC, Konstantinou EC, Bakoyannis G, et al. 2008. Risk factors for sickness absence due to low back pain and prognostic factors for return to work in a cohort of shipyard workers. Eur Spine J 17: 1185–1192.

Alonso JM, Tscholl PM, Engebretsen L, et al. 2010. Occurrence of injuries and illnesses during the 2009 IAAF World Athletics Championships. Br J Sports Med 44: 1100–1105.

Andersen RE, Crespo CJ, Ling SM, et al. 1999. Prevalence of significant knee pain among older Americans: results from the Third National Health and Nutrition Examination Survey. J Am Geriatrics Society 47: 1435–1438.

Boling M, Padua D, Marshall S, et al. 2010. Gender differences in the incidence and prevalence of patellofemoral pain syndrome. Scand J Med Sci Sports 20: 725–730.

Buckwalter JA, Saltzman C, Brown T. 2004. The impact of osteoarthritis: implications for research. Clin Orthop Relat Res 427 (Suppl): S6–S15.

Cassidy JD, Carroll LJ, Cote P. 1998. The Saskatchewan health and back pain survey. The prevalence of low back pain and related disability in Saskatchewan adults. Spine 23: 1860–1866.

Cassidy JD, Cote P, Carroll LJ, et al. 2005. Incidence and course of low back pain episodes in the general population. Spine 30: 2817–2823.

Collins K, Wagner M, Peterson K, et al. 1989. Overuse injuries in triathletes: a study of the 1986 Seafair Triathlon. Am J Sports Med 17: 675–680.

Croft PR, Papageorgiou AC, Thomas E, et al. 1999. Short-term physical risk factors for new episodes of low back pain: prospective evidence from the South Manchester Back Pain Study. Spine 24: 1556–1561.

Davis IS, Powers CM. 2010. Patellofemoral pain syndrome: proximal, distal, and local factors, an international retreat, April 30–May 2, 2009, Fells Point, Baltimore, MD. J Orthop Sports Phys Ther 40: A1–16.

de Jonge S, van den Berg C, de Vos RJ, et al. 2011. Incidence of midportion Achilles tendinopathy in the general population. Br J Sports Med 45: 1026–1028.

Devereaux MD, Lachmann SM. 1984. Patello-femoral arthralgia in athletes attending a Sports Injury Clinic. Br J Sports Med 18: 18–21.

Deyo RA, Mirza SK, Martin BI. 2006. Back pain prevalence and visit rates, estimates from US national surveys, 2002. Spine 31: 2724–2727.

Deyo RA, Mirza SK, Martin BI, et al. 2010. Trends, major medical complications, and charges associated with surgery for lumbar spinal stenosis in older adults. JAMA 303: 1259–1265.

Doherty C, Delahunt E, Caulfield B, et al. 2014. The incidence and prevalence of ankle sprain injury: a systematic review and meta-analysis of prospective epidemiological studies. Sports Med 44: 123–140

Englund M. 2008. The role of the meniscus in osteoarthritis genesis. Rheumatic Dis Clinics North Am 34: 573–579.

Englund M, Guermazi A, Lohmander SL. 2009a. The role of the meniscus in knee osteoarthritis: a cause or consequence? Radiologic Clinics North Am 47: 703–712.

Englund M, Guermazi A, Roemer FW, et al. 2009b. Meniscal tear in knees without surgery and the development of radiographic osteoarthritis among middle-aged and elderly persons: the Multicenter Osteoarthritis Study. Arthritis Rheum 60: 831–839.

Felson DT, Naimark A, Anderson J, et al. 1987. The prevalence of knee osteoarthritis in the elderly: the Framingham Osteoarthritis Study. Arthritis Rheum 30: 914–918.
Friedly J, Chan L, Deyo R. 2007. Increases in lumbosacral injections in the Medicare population: 1994 to 2001. Spine 32: 1754–1760.
Hart LG, Deyo RA, Cherkin DC. 1995. Physician office visits for low back pain. Frequency, clinical evaluation, and treatment patterns from a U.S. national survey. Spine 20: 11–19.
Heliövaara M, Impivaara O, Sievers K, et al. 1987a. Lumbar disc syndrome in Finland. J Epidemiol Community Health 41: 251–258.
Heliövaara M, Knekt P, Aromaa A. 1987b. Incidence and risk factors of herniated lumbar intervertebral disc or sciatica leading to hospitalization. J Chronic Dis 40: 251–258.
Hillman M, Wright A, Rajaratnam G, et al. 1996. Prevalence of low back pain in the community: implications for service provision in Bradford, UK. J Epidemiol Community Health 50: 347–352.
Hoy D, Brooks P, Blyth F, et al. 2010. The epidemiology of low back pain. Best Pract Res Clin Rheumatol 24: 769–781.
Hoy D, Bain C, Williams G, et al. 2012. A systematic review of the global prevalence of low back pain. Arthritis Rheum 64: 2028–2037.
Hupperets MD, Verhagen EA, Heymans MW, et al. 2010. Potential savings of a program to prevent ankle sprain recurrence: economic evaluation of a randomized controlled trial. Am J Sports Med 38: 2194–2200.
Jacobs J. 2011. United States Bone and Joint Initiative. The burden of musculoskeletal diseases in the United States. Rosemont, IL: American Academy of Orthopedic Surgeons.
Jacobs SJ, Berson BL. 1986. Injuries to runners: a study of entrants to a 10,000 meter race. Am J Sports Med 14: 151–155.
Jarvik JG, Deyo RA. 2002. Diagnostic evaluation of low back pain with emphasis on imaging. Ann Intern Med 137: 586–597.
Jeffries LJ, Milanese SF, Grimmer-Somers KA. 2007. Epidemiology of adolescent spinal pain: a systematic overview of the research literature. Spine 32: 2630–2637.
Jordan JM, Helmick CG, Renner JB, et al. 2007. Prevalence of knee symptoms and radiographic and symptomatic knee osteoarthritis in African Americans and Caucasians: the Johnston County Osteoarthritis Project. J Rheumatol 34: 172–180.
Jordan JM, Helmick CG, Renner JB, et al. 2009. Prevalence of hip symptoms and radiographic and symptomatic hip osteoarthritis in African Americans and Caucasians: the Johnston County Osteoarthritis Project. J Rheumatol 36: 809–815.
Kaila-Kangas L, Leino-Arjas P, Karppinen J, et al. 2009. History of physical work exposures and clinically diagnosed sciatica among working and nonworking Finns aged 30 to 64. Spine 34: 964–969.
Kalichman L, Cole R, Kim DH, et al. 2009. Spinal stenosis prevalence and association with symptoms: the Framingham Study. Spine J 9: 545–550.
Knobloch K, Yoon U, Vogt PM. 2008. Acute and overuse injuries correlated to hours of training in master running athletes. Foot Ankle Int 29: 671–676.
Kochen MM, Blozik E, Scherer M, et al. 2009. Imaging for low-back pain. Lancet 373: 436–437.
Konstantinou K, Dunn KM. 2008. Sciatica: review of epidemiological studies and prevalence estimates. Spine 33: 2464–2472.
Kopec JA, Sayre EC, Schwartz TA, et al. 2013 Occurrence of radiographic osteoarthritis of the knee and hip among African Americans and whites: a population-based prospective cohort study. Arthritis Care Res 65: 928–935.
Kurtz S, Ong K, Lau E, et al. 2007. Projections of primary and revision hip and knee arthroplasty in the United States from 2005 to 2030. J Bone Joint Surgery Am 89: 780–785.
Lambers K, Ootes D, Ring D. 2012. Incidence of patients with lower extremity injuries presenting to US emergency departments by anatomic region, disease category, and age. Clin Orthop Relat Res 470: 284–290.
Lawrence RC, Felson DT, Helmicj CG, et al. 2008. Estimates of the prevalence of arthritis and other rheumatic conditions in the United States. Part II. Arthritis Rheum 58: 26–35.
Lysholm J, Wiklander J. 1987. Injuries in runners. Am J Sports Med 15: 168–171.
Macfarlane GJ, Beasley M, Jones EA, et al. 2012. The prevalence and management of low back pain across adulthood: results from a population-based cross-sectional study (the MUSICIAN study). Pain 153: 27–32.
MacLean CH, Knight K, Paulus H, et al. 1998. Costs attributable to osteoarthritis. J Rheumatol 25: 2213–2218.
Mafi JN, McCarthy EP, Davis RB, et al. 2013. Worsening trends in the management and treatment of back pain. JAMA Intern Med 173: 1573–1581.
Makris UE, Fraenkel L, Han L, et al. 2011. Epidemiology of restricting back pain in community-living older persons. J Am Geriatr Soc 59: 610–614.
Mamisch N, Brumann M, Hodler J, et al; Zurich LSSOSWG. 2012. Radiologic criteria for the diagnosis of spinal stenosis: results of a Delphi survey. Radiology 264: 174–179.
Martin BI, Deyo RA, Mirza SK, et al. 2008. Expenditures and health status among adults with back and neck problems.JAMA 299: 656–664.
McCarthy JC, Noble PC, Schuck MR, et al. 2001. The Otto E. Aufranc Award: The role of labral lesions to development of early degenerative hip disease. Clin Orthop Related Res 393: 25–37.
McKean KA, Manson NA, Stanish WD. 2006. Musculoskeletal injury in the masters runners. Clin J Sport Med 16: 149–154.
Murray CJ, Abraham J, Ali MK, et al. 2013. The state of US health, 1990–2010: burden of diseases, injuries, and risk factors. JAMA 310: 591–608.
Narvani AA, Tsiridis E, Tai CC, et al. 2003. Acetabular labrum and its tears. Br J Sports Med 37: 207–211.
Nevitt MC, Lane NE, Scott JC, et al. 1995. Radiographic osteoarthritis of the hip and bone mineral density. The Study of Osteoporotic Fractures Research Group. Arthritis Rheum 38: 907–916.
North American Spine Society (NASS). 2007. Evidence based clinical guidelines for multidisciplinary spine care: diagnosis and treatment of degenerative lumbar spinal stenosis. Burr Ridge, IL: North American Spine Society.
Oliveria SA, Felson DT, Reed JI, et al. 1995. Incidence of symptomatic hand, hip, and knee osteoarthritis among patients in a health maintenance organization. Arthritis Rheum 38: 1134–1141.
Ong KL, Mowat FS, Chan N, et al. 2006. Economic burden of revision hip and knee arthroplasty in Medicare enrollees. Clin Orthop Related Res 446: 22–28.
Picavet HS, Hazes JM. 2003. Prevalence of self reported musculoskeletal diseases is high. Ann Rheum Dis 62: 644–650.
Pleis JR, Lucas JW, Ward BW. 2009. Summary health statistics for U.S. adults: National Health Interview Survey, 2008. Vital Health Stat 10: 1–157.
Riddle DL, Schappert SM. 2004. Volume of ambulatory care visits and patterns of care for patients diagnosed with plantar fasciitis: a national study of medical doctors. Foot Ankle Int 25: 303–310.
Segal NA, Felson DT, Torner JC, et al. 2007. Greater trochanteric pain syndrome: epidemiology and associated factors. Arch Phys Med Rehabil 88: 988–992.
Sobhani S, Dekker R, Postema K, et al. 2013. Epidemiology of ankle and foot overuse injuries in sports: a systematic review. Scand J Med Sci Sports 23: 669–686.
Suri P, Morgenroth DC, Kwoh CK, et al. 2010. Low back pain and other musculoskeletal pain comorbidities in individuals with symptomatic osteoarthritis of the knee: data from the osteoarthritis initiative. Arthritis Care Res 62: 1715–1723.
Tepper S, Hochberg MC. 1993. Factors associated with hip osteoarthritis: data from the First National Health and Nutrition Examination Survey (NHANES-I). Am J Epidemiol 137: 1081–1088.
Tortolani PJ, Carbone JJ, Quartararo LG. 2002. Greater trochanteric pain syndrome in patients referred to orthopedic spine specialists. Spine J 2: 251–254.
Verhagen EA, van Mechelen W, de Vente W. 2000. The effect of preventive measures on the incidence of ankle sprains. Clin J Sport Med 10: 291–296.
Vos T, Flaxman AD, Naghavi M, et al. 2013. Years lived with disability (YLDs) for 1160 sequelae of 289 diseases and injuries 1990–2010: a systematic analysis for the Global Burden of Disease Study 2010. Lancet 380: 2163–2196.
Waterman BR, Owens BD, Davey S, et al. 2010. The epidemiology of ankle sprains in the United States. J Bone Joint Surg Am 92: 2279–2284.
Weiner DK, Kim YS, Bonino P, et al. 2006. Low back pain in older adults: are we utilizing healthcare resources wisely? Pain Med 7: 143–150.
Weinstein SL. 2000. 2000–2010: the bone and joint decade. J Bone Joint Surg Am 82: 1–3.
Yabuki S, Fukumori N, Takegami M, et al. 2013. Prevalence of lumbar spinal stenosis, using the diagnostic support tool, and correlated factors in Japan: a population-based study. J Orthop Sci 18: 893–900.
Yelin E, Murphy L, Cisternas MG, et al. 2007. Medical care expenditures and earnings losses among persons with arthritis and other rheumatic conditions in 2003, and comparisons with 1997. Arthritis Rheum 56: 1397–1407.

3 Chapter

History Taking

Peter A. Huijbregts

CHAPTER CONTENTS

Introduction 22
Patient profile 23
Location and description of symptoms 24
Symptom behaviour 26
Symptom history 27
Medical history 28
Systems review 29
Conclusion 34

Introduction

In all healthcare professions including physical therapy there are five elements to patient management. An examination is usually followed by evaluation of the examination findings, establishing a diagnosis, producing a prognosis and a plan of care and, finally, performing the interventions (American Physical Therapy Association (APTA) 2001). In physical therapy the examination usually consists of history taking, systems review, and tests and measures and it serves to provide data used in the clinical-reasoning process. During this process the clinician develops, in an ongoing manner, multiple competing diagnostic hypotheses. Data acquired during the examination are then used to support or refute these various hypotheses. This hypothesis-testing process guides the format and content of the ongoing examination process until the clinician decides that sufficient information is obtained to make a diagnostic or management decision (Jones 1995).

Within the profession of physical therapy there are many distinct approaches to patient management. The specific information that a clinician looks for, the order in which it is obtained and the emphasis that is given to the data collected will all vary depending on the philosophy to which the individual clinician subscribes. However, all approaches end up testing hypotheses related to (Jones 1995):

1. Source of the symptoms
2. Contributing factors including environmental, behavioural, emotional, psychosocial, systemic / pathological and musculoskeletal factors
3. Precautions or contraindications to examination and management
4. Management
5. Prognosis.

Irrespective of management philosophy, the need to test the above-mentioned types of hypotheses leads to a consistent content of the history component of examination, with history items related to six categories (Boissonnault & Janos 1995) (Box 3.1):

1. Patient profile
2. Location and description of symptoms
3. Symptom behaviour
4. Symptom history
5. Medical history
6. Review of systems.

In the examination, history taking and physical examination are inextricably linked. History taking allows the clinician to gather information that is used in the subsequent physical examination to establish the patient's concordant or comparable signs. A concordant sign consists of pain or other symptoms reproduced upon physical examinations that are indicated by the patient as his or her chief complaint – that is, the reason for seeking out therapy (Laslett et al 2003). Without this information derived from history taking, the clinician would be unable during the examination to distinguish between concordant and discordant signs. Discordant signs are findings on physical examination seemingly implicating a source of symptoms that are, however, in no way related to the chief complaint (Cook 2007).

During history taking the clinician also should seek to get an impression of patients' communication ability, affect, cognition, language, and learning style (APTA 2001). In addition, the history allows the clinician to gain insight into patients' understanding of their own health problem, underlying pathology or dysfunction, mechanism of injury or aetiology, and contributing factors. It provides information on patient goals (that may or may not be realistic or attainable with interventions within the physical therapy scope of practice) and patient motivation and willingness to change (Brouwer et al 1999).

Data collection in the history also establishes a baseline against which to compare the results of the treatment (Cook 2007). Baseline data can, of course, consist of answers to questions asked during the history and findings on physical examination tests; however, the often-dichotomous (and even most continuous) variables of this nature usually lack the sufficient

Box 3.1 History-taking content

Patient profile

- Age
- Sex
- Ethnic origin
- Marital status
- Social situation
- Occupation
- Leisure activities

Location and description of symptoms

- Chief complaint
- Presence and location of pain, sensory abnormalities, strength deficits, range of motion deficits, inflammatory symptoms
- Character of symptoms

Symptom behaviour

- Constant, episodic, or intermittent
- Aggravating factors
- Easing factors
- Diurnal variation

Symptom history

- Nature/mechanism of onset
- Symptom change since onset
- Treatment received

Medical history

- Current and past illnesses
- Hospitalizations
- Family medical history
- Medication use
- Substance abuse
- Nutritional status
- Medical tests and results (imaging, blood work, urinalysis, electrodiagnosis, cerebrospinal fluid analysis, biopsies, etc.)

Review of systems

- Gastrointestinal system
- Urogenital system
- Cardiovascular system
- Pulmonary system
- Musculoskeletal system
- Neurological system
- Integumentary system
- Psychosocial factors

responsiveness required of an outcome measure. Therefore, outcomes are preferably collected using reliable, valid and responsive questionnaire-type outcomes. These outcome measures can be generic – that is, collect data on general health status, such as the Short Form (SF)-36 (Ware et al 1993) – or they can be more specific to a condition. Examples of condition-specific outcome measures relevant to patients with neck and arm pain include the Neck Disability Index (Vernon & Mior 1991) and the DASH (Disabilities of the Arm, Shoulder, and Hand) tools (Hudak et al 1996). Subsequent chapters will discuss various relevant condition-specific outcome measures. Some validated measures collected as part of history taking serve a prognostic purpose; the Tampa Scale of Kinesiophobia (TSK) is a good example of such a prognostic tool relevant to patients with neck pain (Vlaeyen et al 1995).

In addition to data collection, the history (and subsequent physical examination) also serves another important purpose. A skilfully applied funnel sequence where open-ended questions are followed by specific closed-ended follow-up questions, paraphrasing by the therapist of information provided by the patient to establish effective and accurate communication, appropriate intonation, and attentive non-verbal communication, including appropriate therapist body posture and facial expression, all allow the clinician to establish a professional relationship based on mutual cooperation, respect, and trust (Goodman & Snyder 1995; Brouwer et al 1999).

Patient Profile

During this portion of the history the clinician collects and records demographic data on patient age, sex, ethnic origin, marital status, social situation, occupation and leisure activities. Various pathologies are more common based on age and sex (Table 3.1). There is strong evidence for older age as a poor prognostic indicator with regard to mechanical neck pain (McLean et al 2007; Carroll et al 2008b). Sex also seems to affect prognosis for some neck and arm pain syndromes. Women are at a greater risk than men for developing persistent problems after cervical whiplash injury (odds ratio (OR) 1.54, 95% confidence interval (CI) 1.16–2.06) (Walton et al 2009), whereas men are at higher risk of developing persistent arm and especially elbow pain (OR 1.9, 95% CI 1.2–3.2) (Ryall et al 2007).

Ethnicity may also predispose patients to certain diseases with, for example, sickle cell disease (and its musculoskeletal presentation) more prominent in the Black population and skin cancer more prominent in the White population (Boissonnault & Janos 1995). White, Asian or Hispanic ethnic origin predisposes women to osteoporosis, whereas Black women are less likely to be osteopenic (Huijbregts 2001; Siris et al 2001; South-Paul 2001).

Information on marital status and social situation (including questions on the available support network, adaptations in home and work situation, durable medical equipment availability and disposable income) helps the therapist establish realistic goals, but may also indicate areas relevant to intervention. Questions on leisure activities and occupation can identify causative or contributing factors, but also establish loading requirements and thus appropriate rehabilitation goals. Occupational exposure to industrial toxins (e.g. asbestos, lead, agricultural pesticides or arsenic), extreme temperatures, repetitive or sustained postures and movements, or excessive emotional or mental pressure may predispose patients to pathology. For example, exposure to silica, coal dust, flour dust, or asbestos can lead to pulmonary pathology (Boissonnault & Janos 1995; Goodman & Snyder 1995). Occupational variables can also affect prognosis. Prognosis with regard to neck pain is better for white-collar than for blue-collar workers and worse if patients have little influence on their work situation (Carroll et al 2008a).

Table 3.1 Some age- and sex-related medical conditions

Diagnosis	Age (years)	Sex
Musculoskeletal		
Rotator cuff degeneration	30+	
Spinal stenosis	60+	Men>women
Costochondritis	40+	Women>men
Neurological		
Guillain–Barré syndrome	Any age (history of infection)	
Multiple sclerosis	15–50	
Neurogenic claudication	40–60+	
Systemic		
AIDS/HIV	20–49	Men>women
Coronary artery disease	40+	Men>women
Mitral valve prolapse	Young	Women>men
Bürger disease	20–40 (smokers)	Men>women
Aortic aneurysm	40–70	Men>women
Breast cancer	45–70	Women>men
Hodgkin lymphoma	20–40; 50–60	Men>women
Osteoid osteoma	10–20	Men>women
Pancreatic cancer	50–70	Men>women
Skin cancer	Rarely before puberty	Men=women
Gallbladder disease	40+	Women>men
Gout	40–59	Men>women
Gynaecological conditions	20–45	Women
Prostatitis	40+	Men
Primary biliary cirrhosis	40–60	Women>men
Reiter syndrome	20–40	Men>women
Rheumatic fever	4–8; 18–30	Women>men
Shingles	60+	
Spontaneous pneumothorax	20–40	Men>women
Thyroiditis	30–50	Women>men
Vascular claudication	40–60+	
Osteoporosis	50+	Women>men

Sources: Boissonnault & Bass 1990a, 1990b; Goodman & Snyder 1995; Huijbregts 2001; South-Paul 2001.

Location and Description of Symptoms

Although a patient's chief complaint often revolves around pain and pain-related functional limitations, symptoms that need to be investigated with regard to location and description also include sensory abnormalities, strength deficits, range of motion deficits and inflammatory symptoms. The subsequent chapters will address location and description of symptoms relevant to the respective neuro-musculoskeletal dysfunctions in more detail.

Inherent in testing competing hypotheses with regard to the source of symptoms is ruling out various conditions that can result in a similar presentation. These conditions are not limited to the mechanical neuro-musculoskeletal dysfunctions with an indication for physical therapy management, but also include visceral or other systemic pathology that may indicate a need for referral or at the very least affect physical therapy management and prognosis. Note that the role of the physical therapist is not to establish a specific disease-level medical diagnosis but rather to screen for disease using a systems approach (Boissonnault & Janos 1995).

Although in physical therapy clinical practice we certainly encounter patients with cutaneous pain related to the skin and other superficial structures, deep somatic, true visceral and neuropathic pain are more relevant to physical therapy differential diagnosis. Neuropathic pain results from a primary lesion or dysfunction in the peripheral or central nervous system. Painful neuropathies are characterized by spontaneous and / or abnormal stimulus-evoked pain related to the presence of allodynia, whereby pain is caused by normally innocuous stimuli, and / or hyperalgesia, in which case pain intensity evoked by normally painful stimuli is increased (Merskey & Bogduk 1994). Deep somatic pain can originate in the bone, muscle, tendon, capsule and ligament, periosteum, artery and nerve connective tissue structures (Boissonnault & Janos 1995). It can also be the result of visceral pathology with irritation of the parietal peritoneum. True visceral pain is a deep pain felt at the site of nociceptive stimulation of the affected internal organ (McCowin et al 1991; Goodman & Snyder 1995). The predominant clinical presentation of both deep somatic and visceral pain is the associated referred pain pattern. Related to convergence of a greater number of primary afferent neurons on a lesser number of secondary afferent neurons and subsequent cortical misinterpretation of the true location of nociceptive afferent input, the patient will report referred pain more superficially in tissues that are segmentally related to the dysfunctional tissue or organ (Van der El 2010).

Referred pain patterns have been established for muscles and will be discussed in detail in Chapter 59, as will neuropathic (including radicular) pain. Chapter 9 (Mechanical neck pain) discusses referral patterns established for cervical zygapophyseal joints, dorsal rami, and discs (Fukui et al 1996; Grubb et al 2000; Cooper et al 2007). Most relevant for suggesting possible visceral pathology in patients presenting with neck, thoracic and arm pain are the referral patterns related to the cardiovascular, pulmonary and gastrointestinal systems, although a thorough examination even of patients with predominant neck and arm symptoms cannot a priori exclude pathology in other systems. Figure 3.1, therefore, provides visceral referral patterns to the neck, arm and trunk from all systems (Boissonnault & Janos 1995).

Although serious gastrointestinal disease rarely causes pain without concomitant digestive symptoms, it is important to know that both a peptic ulcer and oesophagitis can cause pain in the upper and mid-abdomen, mid-thoracic region, anterior chest, neck and bilateral shoulders. The mechanism for referral from the stomach and oesophagus to

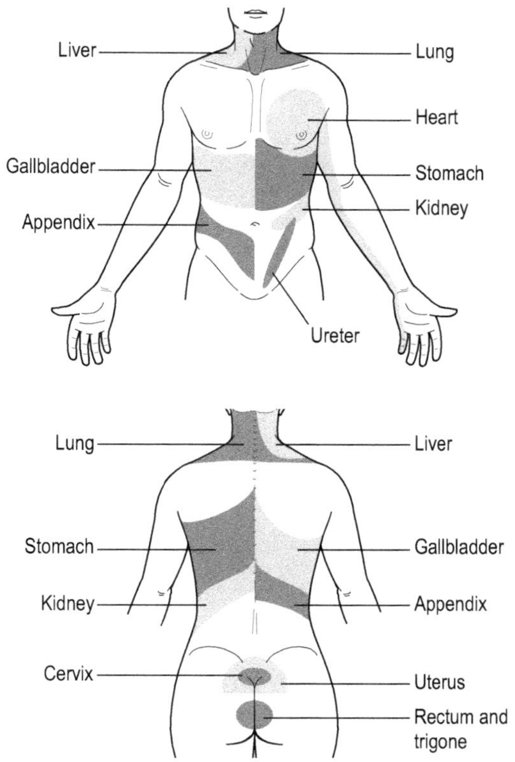

Figure 3.1 Visceral referral patterns.

Table 3.2 Diagnostic accuracy data pain location and description in the diagnosis of acute myocardial infarction

Pain descriptor	Positive likelihood ratio (95% CI)
Increased likelihood of myocardial infarction	
Radiation to right arm or shoulder	4.7 (1.9–12)
Radiation to both arms or shoulders	4.1 (2.5–6.5)
Radiation to left arm	2.7 (1.7–3.1)
Worse than previous angina or similar	1.8 (1.6–2.0)
Described as pressure	1.3 (1.2–1.5)
Decreased likelihood of myocardial infarction	
Described as pleuritic	0.2 (0.1–0.3)
Described as sharp	0.3 (0.2–0.5)
Inframammary location	0.8 (0.7–0.9)

(Adapted from Swap & Nagurney 2005.)

the neck and shoulders is related to irritation of the adjacent diaphragm with its segmental innervation derived from C3 to C5 through to the phrenic nerve. The liver and pancreas normally refer to the right upper and mid-thoracic spine or to the thoracolumbar and upper abdominal region respectively, but again through irritation of the diaphragm can also cause neck and shoulder pain, with the liver referring the right side of the anterior, lateral and posterior neck (Boissonnault & Bass 1990a). The gallbladder generally refers to the right costal margin or epigastrium, but in some patients also refers pain to the bilateral or unilateral infrascapular region (Vestergaard-Middelfart et al 1998). Grieve (1994) noted that a hiatal hernia can present with widespread chest and bilateral shoulder pain.

Cardiovascular pathology can also be the cause of pain in patients with neck and arm symptoms. Pain originating in the heart can refer to the face, jaw, neck, the precordial region, epigastrium and less commonly the posterior thorax. Upper extremity referral can be bilateral or unilateral, but is most commonly in a left C8 distribution (Boissonnault & Bass 1990b; Grieve 1994). Swap & Nagurney (2005) provided diagnostic accuracy data for history items related to pain description and location in the clinical diagnosis of acute myocardial infarction (Table 3.2). Diffuse throbbing or aching pain in the mid-back, abdomen, chest and left shoulder may indicate a symptomatic aortic aneurysm (Boissonnault & Bass 1990b). A sudden tearing chest pain radiating into the neck, dorsal trunk, abdomen and legs may indicate a dissection of the ascending aorta or aortic arch (Grieve 1994). Pain from internal carotid artery dissection is felt in the ipsilateral frontotemporal and periorbital region, whereas pain from vertebral artery dissection is reported in the ipsilateral occipital region (Triano & Kawchuk 2006). Figures 3.2 and 3.3 show pain referral patterns for major vascular structures.

The pulmonary system produces local thoracic and chest pain, but can also cause referred pain to the neck and shoulders. As with serious gastrointestinal pathology, noted pulmonary pathology in addition to pain will generally present with other symptoms including stridor, coughing, wheezing, dyspnoea, hoarseness, fever or a sore throat. Pleurisy originating in the parietal pleura refers to the scapular, axillary and nipple regions (Boissonnault & Bass 1990b; Grieve 1994). A Pancoast tumour of the apex of the lung may cause neck, shoulder and upper extremity pain in a C8–T1 distribution mimicking thoracic outlet syndrome or low cervical radiculopathy (Boissonnault & Bass 1990b, 1990c).

With both visceral and deep somatic structures causing the same poorly localized, vague and deep-aching somatic pain, the description or character of pain is less relevant in the differential diagnosis between mechanical neuro-musculoskeletal dysfunction and visceral pathology (Boissonnault & Bass 1990a; Goodman & Snyder 1995). However, some pain descriptors have been suggested or shown to have diagnostic value. Pressure-like pain is indicative of acute myocardial infarction, whereas pain described as sharp or pleuritic decreases the likelihood of this condition (Swap & Nagurney 2005). Goodman & Snyder (1995) suggested pain characterized as knife-like, boring, colicky, coming in waves, or deep aching as possibly indicative of visceral problems. Cramping or colicky pain may be related to the rhythmic contraction and relaxation of the smooth muscle wall of a hollow viscus that may last up to a few minutes per cycle. Throbbing, cramping or aching pain may also be suggestive of cardiovascular involvement, as is pain described as pressure, tightness or heaviness (Boissonnault & Janos 1995). Tearing pain has been associated with aortic dissection (Grieve 1994). A stabbing, pulsating, aching, thunderclap-like headache may indicate cervical (vertebral and internal carotid) artery dissection

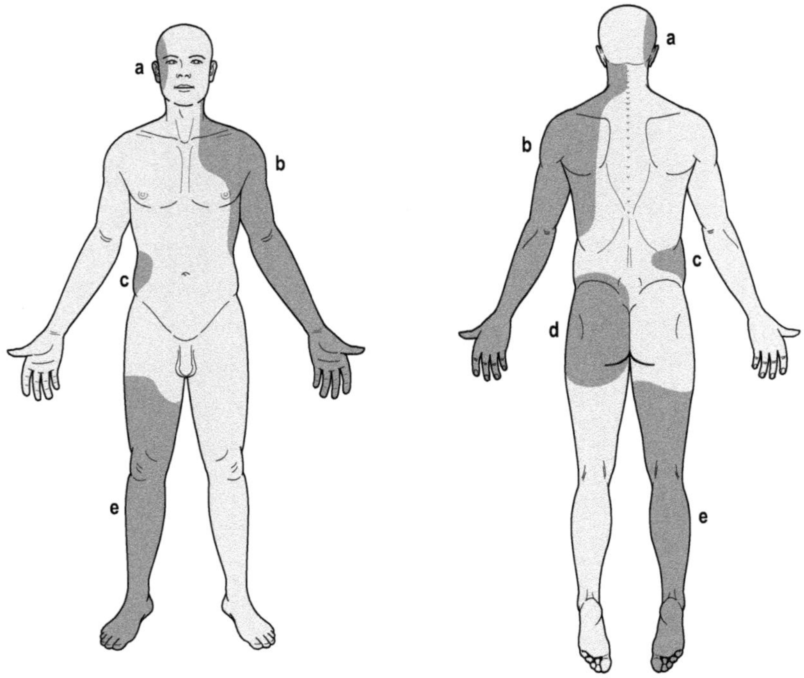

Figure 3.2 Vascular referral patterns: a, common carotid artery; **b,** subclavian artery; **c,** descending aorta; **d,** internal iliac artery, **e,** external iliac artery.

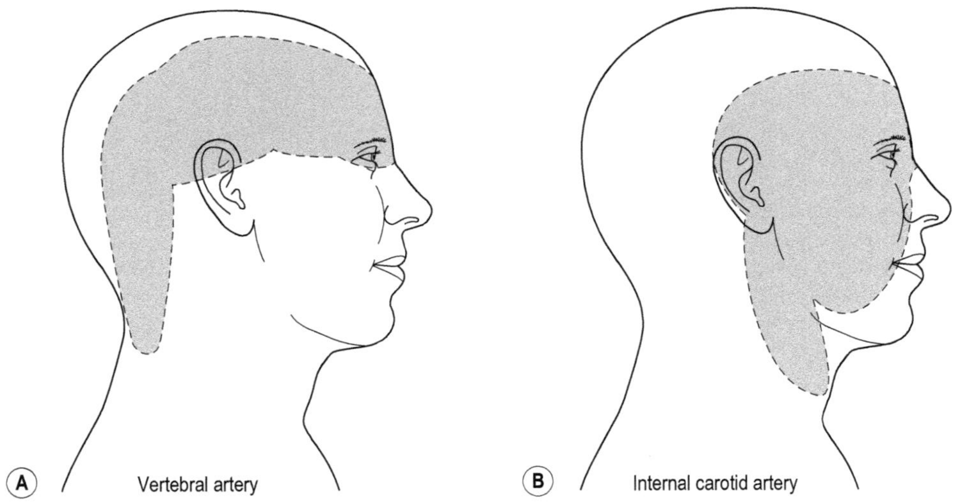

Figure 3.3 Vascular referral patterns: (**A**) vertebral artery, (**B**) internal carotid artery.

(Triano & Kawchuk 2006). Clinicians should note, however, the overlap of at least a number of these pain descriptors with pain of myofascial or other somatic aetiology.

Symptom Behaviour

Symptom behaviour can be defined as a change in location, intensity and / or quality of symptoms related to aggravating and easing factors (Boissonnault & Janos 1995). When investigating symptom behaviour, the clinician seeks to find out whether symptoms are intermittent, episodic or constant, if there is a 24-hour or diurnal pattern to the symptoms, and to get information about aggravating or easing factors.

Physical therapists should expect that pain associated with mechanical neuro-musculoskeletal dysfunction is aggravated and eased by postures and activities. This is not to say that the pain and symptoms from mechanical dysfunction are always intermittent, as especially in the acute stage where inflammation is predominant the symptoms can be constant, although intensity will still be affected by postures or activities (Boissonnault & Janos 1995). Episodic symptoms are suggestive of systemic disease, especially a progressive pattern with cyclical periods where the patient feels better and then again worse, should raise the clinician's index of suspicion with regard to systemic aetiology (Goodman & Snyder 1995).

A diurnal pattern when not related to consistent mechanical aggravation (as may sometimes occur with occupational demands) also suggests systemic pathology. Examples are the pain related to a duodenal ulcer that will consistently start some 2 hours after eating (Boissonnault & Bass 1990a). Particularly ominous in this regard is night pain. In this context, we do not think of the pain that wakes up the patient but is easily relieved by changing positions. Various studies have reported an association of this type of night pain with osteoarthritis especially of the lumbar, hip and knee joints (Acheson et al 1969; Siegmeth & Noyelle 1988; Foldes et al 1992; Jonsson & Stromqvist 1993). Night pain becomes relevant as a red flag indicating the need for medical referral if the patient reports that this pain is the worst pain over a 24-hour period and / or if this night pain results in their being unable, or requiring considerable effort, to get back to sleep (Boissonnault & Janos 1995; Goodman & Snyder 1995).

Symptoms of visceral pathology can often be elicited and relieved by factors that are clearly not mechanical in nature. We discussed above the pain from a duodenal ulcer occurring some 2 hours after eating. Duodenal pain can often be relieved by eating again or by taking antacid medication. Gastrointestinal pathology should be suspected if the patient reports that ingestion of certain foods, or food in general, precipitates or alleviates symptoms. Pain in the right costal margin or epigastrium and the infrascapular region(s) after eating high-fat food may implicate the gallbladder as the source of pain symptoms (Boissonnault & Bass 1990a). Pain decreased with fasting, after a bowel movement, or after vomiting also implicates the gastrointestinal system. Ingestion of caffeine, especially when combined with smoking, raises the blood pressure for some 2 hours, which may lead to cardiovascular symptomatology in hypertensive patients. Alcohol consumption and fever increase the systolic thrust and may elicit pain originating in arteries. Increased metabolic demand not related to physical activity, as occurs with emotion or exposure to extreme temperatures, may elicit cardiovascular symptoms (Goodman & Snyder 1995).

Associating symptoms aggravated with postures and activities solely with benign mechanical dysfunction is, however, a dangerous oversimplification of the clinical picture (Grieve 1994). Activity-related cardiovascular symptoms including vascular claudication and pain due to coronary ischaemia in patients with coronary artery disease or pulmonary system pain from the pleura and trachea with respiratory movement require no further explanation. Perhaps less obvious is pain due to distension of a hollow organ aggravated by increased intra-abdominal pressure and relieved by positions that reduce pressure or support the painful organ. For example, the pain from acute gallbladder distension decreases with slight trunk flexion, whereas flexion and ipsilateral side-bending may relieve kidney pain. Seated flexion or bringing the knees to the chest in supine may decrease pancreatic pain. Bending over increases the systolic thrust and may aggravate pain arising from arteries (Goodman & Snyder 1995). The pain from pericarditis is aggravated by coughing or changing position and relieved by leaning forward.

Pain with swallowing or breathing may be related to the mechanical compression of the oesophagus or bronchi caused by an aortic aneurysm. Although dyspnoea would lead a clinician to suspect cardiovascular or pulmonary pathology, a patient report of nocturnal shortness of breath relieved by sitting up or sleeping with multiple pillows (orthopnoea) should raise even greater suspicion. Swap & Nagurney (2005) provided diagnostic accuracy data for history items related to (non)-mechanical symptom behaviour in the clinical diagnosis of acute myocardial infarction (Table 3.3). One system often overlooked when screening for pathology using a systems approach is the musculoskeletal system; systemic inflammatory conditions, infection and fractures are all likely to be aggravated and eased mechanically and may thereby be mistaken for benign mechanical dysfunctions (Boissonnault & Bass 1990c).

Table 3.3 **Diagnostic accuracy data symptom behaviour (and associated symptoms) in the diagnosis of acute myocardial infarction**

Symptom behaviour	Positive likelihood ratio (95% CI)
Increased likelihood of myocardial infarction	
Associated with exertion	2.4 (1.5–3.8)
Associated with diaphoresis	2.0 (1.9–2.2)
Associated with nausea or vomiting	1.9 (1.7–2.3)
Decreased likelihood of myocardial infarction	
Described as positional	0.3 (0.2–0.5)
Reproducible with palpation	0.3 (0.2–0.4)
Not associated with exertion	0.8 (0.6–0.9)

(Adapted from Swap & Nagurney 2005.)

An inventory of pain symptom behaviour also serves the purpose of identifying limitations in activities and restrictions in participation resulting from dysfunction or pathology. This way the clinician gets an impression of severity, which is the subjective identification of how significantly the patient has been affected by this current health problem. In addition, questioning the patient with regard to symptom behaviour also provides the clinician with information on irritability. Irritability or reactivity is a concept that tries to quantify how stable a condition is – in other words, how quickly does a stable presentation degenerate in the presence of aggravating factors? Irritability is a three-dimensional concept. The clinician collects information not only (1) on aggravating factors but also (2) on duration and severity of a condition once aggravated and (3) on what the patient needs to do to again relieve or decrease symptoms (Cook 2007).

Symptom History

In the symptom history portion the therapist constructs a chronological description of the current health problem including information on onset, changes in symptoms since onset, and treatment received for the current problem (Boissonnault & Janos 1995). This allows determination of the stage of the health problem, which reflects the patient's interpretation of current complaints and impairments as compared with a given point in the past. Health problems can be worse, better or the same with regard to symptoms and impact on function, leading the clinician to characterize a condition as stabilized, stagnated or progressed (for better or worse). Together with information on severity and irritability gained from the symptom behaviour portion, knowledge with regard to the stage of a condition determines precautions with regard to subsequent examination and guides management (Cook 2007). If the stage, severity and irritability of a condition do not match the expected normal course of a mechanical dysfunction of traumatic aetiology, where an acute inflammatory stage with moderate to high severity and high irritability is followed by a progressively less irritable and severe subacute and / or chronic stabilized, stagnated or improved presentation, systemic pathology may be suspected. Likewise, a cyclical or episodic presentation should raise suspicion with regard to non-mechanical problems.

Although clinicians might associate an insidious, slow, progressive onset more with systemic pathology and a clear traumatic mechanism of acute injury with mechanical dysfunction, the clinician needs to consider systemic pathology even when complaints seem to have been brought on acutely by trauma. For example, pathological fractures in bones weakened by osteoporosis, osteomalacia, infection and tumours may result from similar traumatic mechanisms that can also cause mechanical neuro-musculoskeletal dysfunctions (Boissonnault & Janos 1995). Acute-onset monoarthritis has to be considered infective until proven otherwise (Woolf & Åkesson 2008). In contrast, mechanical dysfunctions related to overuse or chronic pain syndromes associated with peripheral and central sensitization are characterized by an insidious onset and a slow, progressive presentation.

Collecting information on the nature and the results of previous treatments provides guidance with regard to management. After all, replicating previously unsuccessful treatment makes little sense. However, when the patient reports no improvement despite seemingly appropriate previous treatments then once again the index of suspicion for systemic pathology is raised (Goodman & Snyder 1995).

Medical History

In the medical history portion the physical therapist collects information on the patient's current and past illnesses, hospitalizations, family medical history, medication use, substance abuse, nutritional status and medical tests and results.

Current illnesses may affect physical therapy diagnosis, prognosis and management (Boissonnault & Janos 1995). Cardiovascular and pulmonary pathology of course often affect exercise tolerance. Although less acutely, gastrointestinal pathology, especially if it results in malabsorption, also limits how much exercise a patient can perform. Knowledge of past and concurrent illnesses affects diagnosis. A medical history of previous cancer with a presentation not indicative of mechanical dysfunction should raise the clinician's index of suspicion. Metastases from primary tumours in the prostate, lung, breast, kidney and colon preferentially occur in the spine (Boissonnault & Bass 1990c). In fact, patients with breast cancer have an 85% lifetime incidence of bony metastases, especially in the thoracic spine (Greenhalgh & Selfe 2004). A history of, for example, rheumatic fever increases the risk of valvular heart disease (Boissonnault & Bass 1990b). Previous surgery, even in the absence of constitutional symptoms, carries an increased risk of iatrogenic infection up to several months after the surgery. Cancer, certain cardiovascular conditions, diabetes, osteoporosis and kidney disease all have a familial tendency (Boissonnault & Bass 1990a). A thorough questioning with regard to medication often uncovers additional concurrent pathology but, conversely, the therapist also needs to be aware of adverse effects of medication that may mimic mechanical dysfunction or predispose the patient to pathology. The depth and breadth of knowledge required for the therapist to elicit and be able to interpret a comprehensive medical history is well illustrated when, for example, reviewing the various causes described for secondary osteoporosis as one of the relevant pathologies to be considered in patients complaining of neck, trunk and arm pain (Box 3.2).

The medical history may also provide less ominous prognostic indicators. Concurrent chronic pain at sites other than the arm increases the risk of arm pain continuing up to 12 months after initial onset (OR 1.6–2.4 based on the site of pain) (Ryall et al 2007). Shoulder pain concomitant with neck pain indicates a poorer prognosis for resolution of the neck pain (McLean et al 2007). Concomitant neck pain is a predictor of shoulder pain at 6 weeks, whereas concomitant low back pain is a predictor for continued shoulder pain at 6 months (Kuijpers et al 2006). Concomitant low back pain also serves as a poor prognostic indicator in patients with neck pain (Hill et al 2004; Hoving et al 2004). Previous neck pain indicates a poorer prognosis for occupational neck pain (Carroll et al 2008b) and a higher risk of chronic pain post-whiplash injury (OR 1.7, 95% CI 1.17–2.48) (Walton et al 2009).

Although patients are less likely to freely discuss this, the therapist needs to also be attentive of indications of substance abuse. Excessive alcohol use increases not only the risk of osteoporosis but also that of cirrhosis and neurodegenerative conditions. It can also cause osteonecrosis and subsequent pathological fractures. The therapist also needs to be aware of an alcohol-related altered perception of pain and fatigue and of the interaction of alcohol with numerous medications (Goodman & Snyder 1995; Huijbregts 2000; Huijbregts & Vidal 2004). As an example of the effects of illicit drugs, cocaine and amphetamines increase the production of adrenaline (epinephrine) causing systemic vasoconstriction, resulting in increased blood pressure and possibly seizures, dysrhythmia and tachycardia. Cocaine use has also been associated with an increased risk of stroke, aortic rupture, pulmonary oedema and clotting disorders (Goodman & Snyder 1995). Intravenous drug use increases the chances of blood-borne infections (Boissonnault & Bass 1990c). Cardiovascular health risks of smoking need no further discussion, but smoking also increases the risk of gastrointestinal pathology and osteoporosis (Boissonnault & Bass 1990a; Huijbregts 2001; South-Paul 2001). Smoking also generally retards musculoskeletal healing. For example, a current smoking habit is a poor prognostic indicator for continued arm pain at 12 months (OR 3.3, 95% CI 1.6–6.6) (Ryall et al 2007).

Nutritional status affects diagnosis and prognosis and the therapist needs to have at least a basic knowledge base in this area. General malnutrition in the sense of insufficient dietary

Box 3.2 Secondary causes of osteoporosis

Nutritional deficiencies

- Excessive consumption of phosphates, oxalates, alkalis, fatty acids, dietary fibre, proteins, refined sugar, caffeine, alcohol and sodium
- Insufficient intake of calcium and/or vitamin D

Endocrine diseases

- Acromegaly
- Anorexia nervosa
- Athletic amenorrhoea
- Cystic fibrosis
- Delayed puberty
- Diabetes mellitus (untreated)
- Female hypogonadism
- Growth hormone deficiencies
- Haemochromatosis
- Hypercortisolism (Cushing disease)
- Hyperparathyroidism
- Hyperprolactinaemia
- Hyperthyroidism
- Hypothalamic amenorrhoea
- Idiopathic hypogonadotrophic hypogonadism
- Klinefelter syndrome
- Male hypogonadism
- Oophorectomy
- Premature and primary ovarian failure
- Primary gonadal failure

Gastrointestinal diseases

- Alactasia
- Chronic obstructive jaundice
- Malabsorption syndromes
- Primary biliary cirrhosis and other cirrhoses
- Subtotal gastrectomy

Bone marrow disorders

- Disseminated carcinoma
- Haemolytic anaemias
- Leukaemia
- Lymphoma
- Multiple myeloma
- Systemic mastocytosis

Connective tissue diseases

- Ehlers–Danlos syndrome
- Glycogen storage diseases
- Homocystinuria
- Hypophosphatasia
- Marfan syndrome
- Osteogenesis imperfecta

Medication

- Anticonvulsants
- Chemotherapy
- Ciclosporin
- Glucocorticoids
- Gonadotrophin-releasing hormone (GnRH) agonists
- Heparin
- Methotrexate
- Phenobarbital
- Phenothiazines
- Thyroxine

Miscellaneous

- Immobilization
- Rheumatoid arthritis
- Smoking

(Sources: Huijbregts 2001; South-Paul 2001.)

glucose and protein intake retards musculoskeletal healing, but high-protein diets used to combat malnutrition especially in the elderly can cause dehydration, which also impairs healing (Posthauer 2006). Amino acid deficiencies (e.g. arginine, methionine and glutamine) negatively affect the course of the normal inflammatory process. Deficiencies in the trace minerals manganese, copper, calcium, magnesium and iron decrease collagen synthesis. Deficiencies in zinc and vitamins A, B, C and E impair the immune response relevant to musculoskeletal healing (Arnold & Barbul 2006; Broughton et al 2006; Campos et al 2008). If nutritional deficiencies are suggested in the history then a nutritional wellness assessment by the therapist and, if indicated, referral to a dietitian are indicated (Fair 2010).

Finally, the therapist should ask the patient about medical diagnostic procedures that may have been done (e.g. imaging, blood work, urinalysis, electrodiagnosis, cerebrospinal fluid analysis and biopsies). Knowing which tests have already been done with knowledge of their findings is obviously helpful in diagnosis and management.

Systems Review

Screening for systemic pathology occurs as part of the history and physical examination but also throughout the management process, where we continuously monitor the patient's condition and also response to seemingly appropriate treatment (Cook 2007). We have discussed how therapists screen for medical disease at the systems level, unlike medical physicians, who seek to diagnose patients at the disease level (Boissonnault & Janos 1995). Despite this distinction, the therapist needs to have considerable acumen with regard to knowledge of pathology so as to screen optimally even at the systems level.

The medical-screening or systems review portion of the history (and physical examination) serves a number of purposes. First and foremost, by way of ruling out systemic pathology it allows for sufficient confidence that a patient presentation is in fact based on a mechanical neuromusculoskeletal dysfunction and, therefore, may pose an

Box 3.3 Checklist for review of general health status

- Fever/chills
- Unexplained perspiration
- Night sweats
- Recent infection
- Unexplained weight change
- Malaise
- Nausea/vomiting
- Bowel dysfunction
- Numbness
- Weakness
- Pallor
- Dizziness/lightheadedness
- Syncope
- Night pain
- Difficulty in breathing
- Difficulty urinating
- Urinary frequency changes
- Sexual dysfunction

(Sources: Boissonnault & Janos 1995; Goodman & Snyder 1995.)

indication for physical therapy management. Secondly, the systems review may raise the index of suspicion with regard to a systemic aetiology of the patient presentation and indicate the need for referral for medical–surgical evaluation. Starting a systems review with a list of general health status indicators, either as part of the patient–therapist face-to-face encounter or in the form of an intake questionnaire reviewed prior to the examination by the clinician, can indicate the need for a more in-depth systems review (Box 3.3). A number of these general health status indicators have been discussed above and some return in more specific systems-based questions. Fever and night sweats are characteristic symptoms of systemic disease. Weight loss of 10% over a 4-week period not related to lifestyle changes (diet, exercise) may indicate diabetes, hyperthyroidism, depression, anorexia nervosa or neoplastic disease. However, an unexplained weight gain may also be relevant in that it can be the result of congestive heart failure and again neoplastic disease or hyperthyroidism (Goodman & Snyder 1995). The need for a more in-depth systems review becomes greater if, as the history taking progresses, other portions of the history as discussed above also yield indicators of systemic aetiology or contribution to patient presentation. Although no such list can ever be comprehensive, Table 3.4 provides suggestions for more specific systems-based questions. Positive findings on any of the questions in the systems-based review should again prompt further investigation. Table 3.5 provides an example for further investigation of indicators for the need for urgent medical referral (red flags) in the case of a patient reporting headache (Huijbregts 2009).

The third and final purpose of medical screening is to also provide the clinician with information on systemic pathology that can affect prognosis / rehabilitation potential or that dictates choice and progression of physical therapy interventions (Boissonnault & Janos 1995).

Box 3.4 Diagnosis of panic disorder

Signs and symptoms (diagnosis requires four)

- Sweating
- Rapid heart rate, palpitations, pounding heart
- Tremor
- Shortness of breath
- Feeling of choking
- Chest pain
- Nausea/abdominal distress
- Dizziness
- Lightheadedness
- Feeling of unreality
- Fear of losing control
- Fear of dying
- Paraesthesiae
- Hot flashes

Associated signs and symptoms

- Insomnia
- Anxiety
- Depression
- Chronic fatigue
- Gastro-oesophageal reflux

(Adapted from Huijbregts & Vidal 2004.)

Relevant to the differential diagnosis of a multitude of symptoms suggestive of visceral pathology and within the context of screening for psychosocial factors in patients with neck and arm pain is the diagnosis of panic disorder (Box 3.4) (Huijbregts & Vidal 2004). Psychosocial factors often serve as prognostic indicators. Depression is an independent risk factor for developing subsequent low back or neck pain (Carroll et al 2004) but also predicts poorer outcome after cervical whiplash injury (Carroll et al 2008c). Passive coping and fear of movement also serve as poor prognostic indicators after whiplash injury (Carroll et al 2008c) and fear of movement is also a consistent impediment to recovery from subacute neck pain at both the 12- and 52-week marks (Pool et al 2010). Fear of movement can be quantified using the Tampa Scale of Kinesiophobia tool (Vlaeyen et al 1995). It will also serve the clinician well to be familiar with the presentation of depression (Box 3.5). Arroll et al (2003) reported a sensitivity of 97% and a specificity of 67% in the clinical diagnosis of depression in primary care for the following two questions:

1. During the last month have you often been bothered by feeling down, depressed, or hopeless?
2. During the last month have you often been bothered by little interest or pleasure in doing things?

Although as therapists we tend to concentrate on mechanical dysfunction of the musculoskeletal system, in our systems review we should not overlook the possibility of musculoskeletal pathology including fractures and infectious, inflammatory and neoplastic disease. Indicators for neoplastic disease have been discussed above. Chapter 11 discusses cervical myelopathy as a differential diagnostic possibility in patients with neck and arm pain. In this era of direct access to physical

Table 3.4 **Suggested questions for systems review**

System	Questions
Cardiovascular	Do you ever experience chest pain (angina)? Do you experience excessive unexplained fatigue? Do you have shortness of breath? Do you ever note chest palpitations? Have you noted lightheadedness? Have you ever fainted? Do you experience widespread leg pains? Have you noted swelling in the feet, ankles or perhaps the hands?
Pulmonary	Do you ever experience chest pain? Do you have shortness of breath? Have you been coughing more lately? Have you noticed a change in your breathing? Do you have difficulty catching your breath when lying flat; do you have to sleep propped up on multiple pillows?
Gastrointestinal	Have you had difficulty swallowing? Have you noticed intolerance to specific foods? Have you had abdominal pain? Has your stool been black in colour? Have you had rectal bleeding? Has your stool been different in consistency (diarrhoea, tarry stool)? Have you been constipated?
Genitourinary	Any difficulty urinating? Have you noted blood in your urine? Have you noted an increased frequency with regard to urination? Have you noted an increased urgency with regard to urination? Have you noted an increased difficulty with initiating urination? Have you noted decreased force with urination? Have there been episodes of impotence? Have there been any changes with regard to menstruation? Have you experienced pain with intercourse? Have you noted incontinence for urine and/or stool?
Integumentary	Have you recently experienced any rashes? Have you noticed any enlargement or bleeding of moles? Have you noted any itching or burning of the skin? Have you noticed any areas of blistering?
Neurological	Have you been experiencing headaches or vision changes? Have you noted dizziness or vertigo? Have you been experiencing seizures or unconsciousness? Do you ever experience weakness or paraesthesiae?

(Sources: Boissonnault & Bass 1990a; Goodman & Snyder 1995; Flynn et al 2008.)

Box 3.5 Symptoms associated with depression

- Persistent sadness or feelings of emptiness
- Sense of hopelessness
- Frequent or unexplained crying spells
- Problems with sleeping
- Feelings of guilt
- Loss of interest or pleasure in normal activities
- Fatigue or decreased energy
- Difficulty in concentrating, remembering and decision making
- Appetite loss (or overeating)

(Adapted from Goodman & Snyder 1995.)

therapy services, therapists need to be able to screen for the presence of fractures. With regard to cervical spine injuries, both the NEXUS (National Emergency X-radiography Utilization Study) and the Canadian cervical (C)-spine rule need to be considered (Eyre 2006). The NEXUS rule recommends cervical plain-film radiography unless all five criteria below are met:

1. Absence of posterior midline cervical spine tenderness
2. No evidence of intoxication
3. Normal level of alertness / consciousness
4. Absence of focal neurological deficit
5. Absence of distracting injuries.

Although the NEXUS rule has shown a sensitivity of 99.6% and a specificity of 12.9% and also 100% sensitivity in separate

Table 3.5 **Red flag indicators in the history taking of patients with headaches indicating the need for urgent referral**

Factor	'Red flag' indicators
Demographics	New onset of headache or change in existing headache pattern in patients over 50
Location of pain	Persistent unilateral location of headaches
Onset and course of headache	New-onset headache Onset of a new headache type Unexplained change for the worse in pattern of existing headache Progressively worsening headache Abrupt, split-second onset of headache: thunderclap headache
Character and intensity of headache	New pain level, especially when described as worst-ever Cluster-type headache
Aggravating and easing factors	Headache aggravated or brought on by physical exertion, coughing, sneezing, straining or sexual activity Noted effect of position changes on pain No response to seemingly appropriate treatment
Neurological symptoms	Seizures, confusion, changes in alertness, apathy, clumsiness, unexplained inappropriate behaviour, brainstem symptoms, bowel and bladder symptoms, neck flexion stiffness, aura preceding the headache (especially one with quick diffusion), or weakness (not consistent with an existing diagnosis of migraine headaches or other pathology explaining these symptoms) Pre-syncope or syncope starting off headache
Otolaryngological symptoms	Associated eye pain and simultaneous vision changes
Systemic symptoms	Fever, weight loss, temporal artery tenderness, profuse vomiting (especially when not associated with nausea), photophobia, phonophobia, or developing rash (not consistent with an existing diagnosis of migraine headaches) Headache that awakens a patient from night sleep (especially in children)
Medical history	Medical history of cancer and human immunodeficiency virus (HIV) infection Head or neck injury Uncontrolled hypertension
Medication history	Use of anticoagulant medication in combination with even minor trauma
Family history	Absence of a family history of migraine in children with migraine-like symptoms

(Adapted from Huijbregts 2009.)

studies in a geriatric and a paediatric population, with distracting injuries defined as long-bone fractures, degloving injuries, and extensive burns and lacerations, it was obviously developed and validated in an emergency room and not in a primary care physical therapy setting (Eyre 2006). The Canadian C-spine rule, although suffering from the same spectrum bias and thereby expected to overestimate sensitivity and underestimate specificity when applied in a physical therapy primary care setting (Cook et al 2007), still seems more relevant to therapists (Fig. 3.4). When compared in nine Canadian emergency departments the Canadian C-spine rule showed 99.4% sensitivity and 45.1% specificity, versus 90.7% sensitivity and 36.8% specificity for the NEXUS rule (Eyre 2006).

We discussed osteoporosis in the medical history portion above (see Box 3.2). Cadarette et al (2000) developed the Osteoporosis Risk Assessment Instrument (ORAI) (Table 3.6). Screening women with a score ≥9 yielded a sensitivity of 93.3% (95% CI 86.3–97.0%) and a specificity of 46.4% (95% CI 41.0–51.8%) for osteopenia. The sensitivity for a diagnosis of osteoporosis was 94.4% (95% CI 83.7–98.6%). A score <9 on this instrument would thus seem to reduce the likelihood of a suspected osteoporotic fracture in female patients.

We discussed surgery as a risk factor for subsequent blood-borne or haematogenous infection. Recent infection was an

Table 3.6 **ORAI scoring system**

Variable	Score
Age (years)	
≥75	15
65–74	9
55–64	5
45–54	0
Weight (kg)	
<60	9
60–69	3
≥70	0
Current oestrogen use	
Yes	0
No	2

(Adapted from Cadarette et al 2000.)

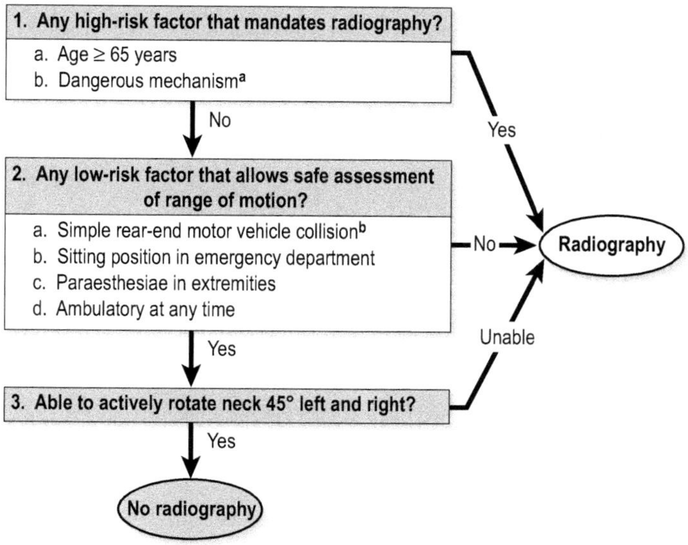

[a] A dangerous mechanism is considered to be a fall from an elevation ≥3 ft or 5 stairs, an axial load to the head (e.g. diving), a motor vehicle collision at high speed (>100 km/h), or with rollover or ejection

[b] A simple rear-end motor vehicle collision excludes being pushed into oncoming traffic, being hit by a bus or a large truck, a rollover, and being hit by a high-speed vehicle

Figure 3.4 Canadian cervical-spine rule.

item included in our general health status checklist (see Box 3.3). Risk factors for, for example, discitis also include intravenous drug use and immunosuppression (as occurs for example in patients with AIDS and HIV). Infection can also lead to vertebral osteomyelitis. Risk factors for pyogenic (bacterial) osteomyelitis include (Vincent & Benson 1991; Heggeness et al 1993):

- intravenous drug use
- diabetes
- urinary tract infection
- stab wounds
- gunshot wounds
- sickle cell disease
- immunodeficiency
- pre-existing paraplegia
- non-operatively treated thoracolumbar fractures
- metal implants
- polymethylmethacrylate
- urology or dental procedures in patients with metal implants without antibiotic prophylaxis.

The most common systemic inflammatory diseases relevant to patients with neck and arm pain include rheumatoid arthritis and seronegative spondyloarthropathies. Pathological changes in spondyloarthropathies involve joints but also entheses or insertions of ligaments, tendons and capsule to the bone. Especially these enthesopathies and initially the spinal articular manifestations may be mistaken for mechanical dysfunctions in patients with neck and arm pain. Table 3.7

Table 3.7 **Clinical findings in seronegative spondyloarthropathies**

Disease	Clinical presentation
Ankylosing spondylitis	Affects sacroiliac, zygapophyseal and costovertebral joints Pain in heels, ischial tuberosities, iliac crests, humeral epicondyles, and shoulders Nocturnal pain Morning pain and stiffness Asymmetric peripheral arthritis yet often symmetric arthritis in both hips Uveitis with pain and photophobia
Psoriatic arthritis	Asymmetric oligoarthritis, symmetric polyarthritis Back or peripheral joint initial symptom Unilateral sacroiliac involvement More frequent in patients with psoriatic skin involvement
Enteropathic arthritis	Occurs in patients with Crohn disease or ulcerative colitis Morning pain and stiffness Affects sacroiliac, zygapophyseal and costovertebral joints May include periostitis, osteonecrosis, septic hip arthritis, granulomatous inflammation of the bone, synovium and muscle May include ulceration of the perineum, oropharynx and rectum Erythema nodosum and pyoderma gangrenosum
Reiter syndrome	Can develop after or during infection elsewhere in body Lumbopelvic and lower limb arthritis Genitourinary symptoms: mucopurulent discharge, dysuria, vaginitis, cervicitis Ocular disease: conjunctivitis or iritis Systemic symptoms: fever, anorexia, weight loss, fatigue Heel pain, Achilles tendonitis, dactylitis Mucocutaneous lesions of oropharynx, soles, palms and nails

(Sources: Katz & Liang 1991; McCowin et al 1991.)

provides information on clinical findings in patients with inflammatory joint disease (Katz & Liang 1991; McCowin et al 1991).

Conclusion

History taking is inextricably linked to physical examination in the examination phase of patient management. Although various approaches to patient management within physical therapy differ with regard to the specific information they seek to collect during history taking, the order in which they collect these data and the importance they place on them, clinicians can still identify six consistent and distinct categories in all history taking. Within this chapter we have addressed this general content of history taking with specific attention to the systems review component and to screening for systemic pathology in patients with neck and arm pain during their history. Subsequent chapters will address in more detail the history findings specific to the dysfunctions discussed. With a paucity of data on diagnostic accuracy relevant to history items, history taking still heavily relies on extrapolation of basic science knowledge, experience and authority-based knowledge. Rather than devaluing the role of the history within the evidence-informed paradigm as a result of this absence of diagnostic accuracy research, this chapter has sought to indicate the depth and breadth of knowledge required from the clinician when the goal is to elicit from the patient a comprehensive and clinically useful history.

References

Acheson RM, Chan YK, Payne M. 1969. New Haven survey of joint diseases: the interrelationships between morning stiffness, nocturnal pain and swelling of the joints. J Chronic Dis 21: 533–542.

American Physical Therapy Association (APTA). 2001. Guide to physical therapist practice, 2nd edn. Phys Ther 81: 9–746.

Arnold M, Barbul A. 2006. Nutrition and wound healing. Plast Reconstr Surg 117: 42S–58S.

Arroll B, Khin N, Kerse N. 2003. Screening for depression in primary care with two verbally asked questions: cross-sectional study. BMJ 327: 144–146.

Boissonnault WG, Bass C. 1990a. Pathological origins of trunk and neck pain: Part I. Pelvic and abdominal visceral disorders. J Orthop Sports Phys Ther 12: 192–207.

Boissonnault WG, Bass C. 1990b. Pathological origins of trunk and neck pain: Part II. Disorders of the cardiovascular and pulmonary systems. J Orthop Sports Phys Ther 12: 208–215.

Boissonnault WG, Bass C. 1990c. Pathological origins of trunk and neck pain: Part III. Diseases of the musculoskeletal system. J Orthop Sports Phys Ther 12: 216–221.

Boissonnault WG, Janos SC. 1995. Screening for medical disease: physical therapy assessment and treatment principles. In: Boissonnault WG (ed) Examination in physical therapy practice, 2nd edn. New York: Churchill Livingstone, pp 1–30.

Broughton G, Janis JE, Attinger CE. 2006. Wound healing: an overview. Plast Reconstr Surg 117: 1eS–32eS.

Brouwer T, Boiten JC, Uilenreef-Tobi FC, et al. 1999. Diagnostiek in de fysiotherapie: proces en werkwijze, 2nd edn. Maarssen: Elsevier / Bunge.

Cadarette SM, Jaglal SB, Kreiger N, et al. 2000. Development and validation of the osteoporosis risk assessment instrument to facilitate selection of women for bone densitometry. Can Med Assoc J 162: 1289–1294.

Campos ACL, Groth AK, Branco AB. 2008. Assessment and nutritional aspects of wound healing. Curr Opin Clin Nutr Metab Care 11: 281–288.

Carroll LJ, Cassidy JD, Côté P. 2004. Depression as a risk factor for the onset of an episode of troublesome neck and low back pain. Spine 107: 134–139.

Carroll LJ, Hogg-Johnson S, Côté P, et al. 2008a. Course and prognostic factors for neck pain in workers. Spine 33 (4S): S93–S100.

Carroll LJ, Hogg-Johnson S, Van der Velde G, et al. 2008b. Course and prognostic factors for neck pain in the general population. Spine 33 (4S): S75–S82.

Carroll LJ, Holm LW, Hogg-Johnson S, et al. 2008c. Course and prognostic factors for neck pain in whiplash-associated disorders (WAD). Spine 33 (4S): S83–S92.

Cook CE. 2007. Orthopaedic manual therapy: an evidence-based approach. Upper Saddle River, NJ: Pearson Prentice Hall.

Cook C, Cleland J, Huijbregts PA. 2007. Creation and critique of studies of diagnostic accuracy: use of the STARD and QUADAS methodological quality assessment tools. J Man Manip Ther 15: 93–102.

Cooper G, Bailey B, Bogduk N. 2007. Cervical zygapophysial joint pain maps. Pain Med 8: 344–353.

Eyre A. 2006. Overview and comparison of the NEXUS and Canadian C-spine rules. Am J Med 8: 12–15.

Fair SE. 2010. Wellness and physical therapy. Sudbury: Jones & Bartlett.

Flynn TW, Cleland JA, Whitman JM. 2008. User's guide to the musculoskeletal examination: fundamentals for the evidence-based clinician. Buckner: Evidence in Motion.

Foldes K, Balint P, Gaal M, et al. 1992. Nocturnal pain correlates with effusions in diseased hip. J Rheumatol 19: 1756–1758.

Fukui S, Osheto K, Shiotani M, et al. 1996. Referred pain distribution of the cervical zygapophyseal joints and cervical dorsal rami. Pain 68: 79–83.

Goodman CC, Snyder TEK. 1995. Differential diagnosis in physical therapy, 2nd edn. Philadelphia: WB Saunders.

Greenhalgh S, Selfe J. 2004. Margaret: a tragic case of spinal red flags and red herrings. Physiotherapy 90: 73–76.

Grieve GP. 1994. The masqueraders. In: Boyling JD, Palastanga N (eds) Grieve's modern manual therapy, 2nd edn. Edinburgh: Churchill Livingstone, pp 841–856.

Grubb SA, Kelly CK, Bogduk N. 2000. Cervical discography: clinical implications from 12 years of experience. Spine 25(11): 1382–1389.

Heggeness MH, Esses SI, Errico T, et al. 1993. Late infection of spinal instrumentation by hematogenous seeding. Spine 18: 492–496.

Hill J, Lewis M, Papageorgiou AC, et al. 2004. Predicting persistent neck pain: a 1-year follow-up of a population cohort. Spine 29: 1648–1654.

Hoving JL, De Vet HCW, Twisk JWR, et al. 2004. Prognostic factors for neck pain in general practice. Pain 110: 639–645.

Hudak PL, Amadio PC, Bombardier C. 1996. The Upper Extremity Collaborative Group (UECG): development of an upper extremity outcome measure: the DASH (Disabilities of the Arm, Shoulder, and Hand). Am J Ind Med 29: 602–608.

Huijbregts PA. 2000. Osteonecrosis of the humeral head: a literature review and two case studies. J Man Manip Ther 8: 175–182.

Huijbregts PA. 2001. Osteoporosis: diagnosis and conservative management. J Man Manip Ther 9: 143–153.

Huijbregts PA. 2009. Clinical reasoning in the diagnosis: history taking in patients with headache. In: Fernández-de-las-Peñas C, Arendt-Nielsen L, Gerwin R (eds) Diagnosis and management of tension-type and cervicogenic headache. Sudbury: Jones & Bartlett, pp 133–152.

Huijbregts P, Vidal P. 2004. Dizziness in orthopaedic physical therapy: classification and pathophysiology. J Man Manip Ther 12: 199–214.

Jones MA. 1995. Clinical reasoning process in manipulative therapy. In: Boyling JD, Palastanga N (eds) Grieve's modern manual therapy, 2nd edn. Edinburgh: Churchill Livingstone, pp 471–490.

Jonsson B, Stromqvist B. 1993. Symptoms and signs in degeneration of the lumbar spine: a prospective, consecutive study of 300 operated patients. J Bone Joint Surg 75B: 381–385.

Katz JN, Liang MH. 1991. Differential diagnosis and conservative treatment of rheumatic disorders. In: Frymoyer JW (ed) The adult spine: principles and practice. New York: Raven Press, pp 699–718.

Kuijpers T, Van der Windt DAWM, Boeke AJP, et al. 2006. Clinical prediction rules for the prognosis of shoulder pain in general practice. Pain 120: 276–285.

Laslett M, Young SB, Aprill CN, et al. 2003. Diagnosing painful sacroiliac joints: a validity study of a McKenzie evaluation and sacroiliac provocation tests. Aust J Physiother 49: 89–97.

McCowin PR, Borenstein D, Wiesel SW. 1991. The current approach to the medical diagnosis of low back pain. Orthop Clin North Am 22: 315–325.

McLean SW, May SW, Klaber-Moffett J, et al. 2007. Prognostic factors for progressive non-specific neck pain: a systematic review. Phys Ther Rev 12: 207–220.

Merskey H, Bogduk H. 1994. Classification of chronic pain: descriptions of chronic pain syndromes and definitions of pain terms. Seattle, WA: IASP Press, pp 209–213.
Pool JJ, Ostelo RW, Knol D, et al. 2010. Are psychological factors prognostic indicators of outcome in patients with sub-acute neck pain? Man Ther 15: 111–116.
Posthauer ME 2006. Hydration: does it play a role in wound healing? Adv Skin Wound Care 19: 74–76.
Ryall C, Coggon D, Peveler R, et al. 2007. A prospective cohort study of arm pain in primary care and physiotherapy: prognostic determinants. Rheumatology 46: 508–515.
Siegmeth B, Noyelle RM. 1988. Night pain and morning stiffness in osteoarthritis: a crossover study of flurbiprofen and diclofenac sodium. J Int Med Res 16: 182–188.
Siris ES, Miller PD, Barrett-Connor E, et al. 2001. Identification and fracture outcomes of undiagnosed low bone mineral density in postmenopausal women. JAMA 286 (22): 2815–2822.
South-Paul JE. 2001. Osteoporosis: part I. Evaluation and assessment. Am Fam Physician 63: (5), 897–904.
Swap CJ, Nagurney CJ. 2005. Value and limitations of chest pain history in the evaluation of patients with suspected acute coronary syndromes. JAMA 294: 2623–2629.
Triano JJ, Kawchuk G (eds). 2006. Current concepts: spinal manipulation and cervical arterial incidents. West Des Moines, IA: NCIMC Chiropractic Solutions.
Van der El A. 2010. Orthopaedic manual therapy diagnosis: spine and temporomandibular joints. Sudbury: Jones & Bartlett.
Vernon H, Mior S. 1991. The Neck Disability Index: a study of reliability and validity. J Manipulative Physiol Ther 14: 409–415.
Vestergaard-Middelfart H, Jensen P, Højgaard L, et al. 1998. Pain patterns after distension of the gallbladder in patients with acute cholecystitis. Scand J Gastroenterol 33: 982–987.
Vincent KA, Benson DR. 1991. Differential diagnosis and conservative management of infectious diseases. In: Frymoyer JW (ed) The adult spine: principles and practice. New York: Raven Press, pp 763–785.
Vlaeyen J, Kole-Snijders A, Boeren R, et al. 1995. Fear of movement / (re) injury in chronic low back pain and its relation to behavioral performance. Pain 62: 363–372.
Walton DM, Pretty J, MacDermid JC, et al. 2009. Risk factors for persistent problems following whiplash injury: results of a systematic review and meta-analysis. J Orthop Sports Phys Ther 39: 334–350.
Ware JE, Snow KK, Kosinki M, et al. 1993. The MOS 36-item Short-Form Health Survey (SF-36): manual and interpretation guide. Boston: The Health Institute, New England Medical Center.
Woolf AD, Åkesson K. 2008. Primer: History and examination in the assessment of musculoskeletal problems. Nat Clin Pract Rheumatol 4: 26–33.

4 Chapter

History Taking for Patients with Lower Extremity Syndromes

Megan Burrowbridge Donaldson, Kristina Averell

CHAPTER CONTENTS

Purpose of the interview 36
Communication style and approach 37
Medical interview content 37
Systems review and differential diagnosis inquiry 37
Neurological screen 38
Cardiovascular screen 38
Gastrointestinal screen 39
Non-mechanical pathologies: differential diagnosis 39
Psychosocial factors 40
Red flags 40
Symptom investigation 40
Nature and behaviour of the problem 41
History-taking questions specific to lower extremity pain syndromes 42
Central and peripheral nerve sensitization 42
Specific low-back-associated musculoskeletal pain syndromes 42
Lumbar spinal stenosis 42
Nerve root compression/radiculopathy 43
Lumbar disc herniation 43
Clinical lumbar instability 43
Specific lower-extremity-associated musculoskeletal pain syndromes 43
Hip osteoarthritis 43
Other hip pathology 43
Knee osteoarthritis 43
Patellofemoral pain syndrome 43
Knee meniscal injury 44
Knee ligamentous injury 44
Achilles tendinopathy 44
Heel pain/plantar fasciitis 44
Conclusion 44

Purpose of the Interview

Within the United States, most states allow physical therapists to evaluate patients without a referral from another healthcare professional. The majority of those states further improve accessibility by allowing physical therapists to evaluate and treat, under certain conditions, patients without a referral. Patients with lower extremity syndromes may present with a myriad of clinical presentations for physical therapy to differentiate; some may be well defined and some range to very complex. In many instances, physical therapists are involved in primary care settings that require advanced skill sets of differential diagnosis and decision making to treat this population appropriately.

The examination process has three components that are closely related, in that they often occur concurrently: (1) patient history, (2) systems review and (3) tests and measures (Jarvik & Deyo 2002). A thorough examination beginning with a well-constructed interview that helps to develop a plan for the physical examination can provide diagnostic value for both the clinician and the patient (Edwards et al 2004). The medical interview is a critical component of an examination for decision making, screening and differential diagnosis. A well-structured history-taking practice involving a screening process and / or differential diagnosis provides critical information regarding the general health status, lifestyle and well-being of the patient. Although the medical interview occurs in most medical interactions, it remains widely understudied with respect to the best type of approach and the most accurate questions for yielding a diagnosis.

There are a variety of medical interview approaches described within the literature. However, a patient-centred approach or collaborative interview is a style of interviewing that has led to better interventions and improved patient outcomes (Dwamena et al 2012).

Centring the care around the patient encourages: (a) shared control of the consultation, decisions about interventions or management of the health problems with the patient, and / or (b) a focus in the consultation on the patient as a whole person who has individual preferences situated within social contexts (Dwamena et al 2012). This can be a challenge for every clinician, and although it is learned during entry-level education, it is not enough simply to learn these skills without significant practice (Beck et al 2002). Current literature provides evidence that clearly illustrates the fundamental relationships existing between effective communication and the quality of working relationships, the degree of patient safety, and the satisfaction levels both of the patient and of the healthcare providers (Walter et al 2005; Asnani 2009; Dwamena et al 2012).

Communication Style and Approach

Although there are many purposes to taking an effective history, the style and approach in which the medical interview or history taking is conducted appears to impact on the patient's clinical outcome based on systematic review and meta-analysis (Henry et al 2012). The interview is a process of the clinician seeking information, reflective listening and exploration of a variety of related medical conditions based on the patient's clinical presentation / symptoms (Taylor 2009). The Calgary–Cambridge guides provide suggestive models for conducting the medical interview and are used widely throughout Europe and North America for teaching and assessment (Kurtz et al 2003; Silverman et al 2011). These guides have been presented and substantiated within the literature and should be considered for educational training of clinicians and for use in clinical practice. These interview guides simultaneously provide structure and emphasize relationship building with the patient (Kurtz & Silverman 1996; Kurtz et al 1998). The basic process includes: (1) initiating the session, (2) gathering information, (3) performing the physical examination, (4) explanation and planning, and (5) closing the session. Continuous attention to providing structure to the interview and building a relationship must be maintained through this framework.

This communication guide identifies the role that patients' perceptions may have regarding their medical condition. Open conversation regarding the patient's fears and motivation, and commitment level to participating in care, allows the clinician to explore barriers to care with the patient (Britt et al 2004). This type of medical interviewing is also known as motivational interviewing (MI) – a collaborative conversation style that is a patient-centred approach acknowledging the patient's expertise in his / her own problems and empowering the patient (Rollnick et al 2008). Beginning with the medical interview and subsequent interactions, it is important to encourage patients to be able to solve problems, make decisions and overcome barriers and setbacks within a supportive relationship from the medical care provider. A meta-analysis and systematic review on MI found that it appeared to be useful in clinical settings, and that only one session could be effective in enhancing readiness to change and action that is directed toward reaching health behaviour-change goals (VanBuskirk & Wetherell 2014). Additionally, a large body of literature supports the notion that involving patients in the interview may improve adherence with prescription and treatment (Street et al 2009; Street & Haidet 2011; VanBuskirk & Wetherell 2014).

Medical Interview Content

The value of the medical interview has been significant in primary care, with physicians reporting that the history alone was sufficient to make a diagnosis in around 75% of patients, physical examination in around 10% and lab or imaging investigation in a further 10% (Hampton et al 1975; Peterson et al 1992; Goodman & Snyder 2009). The diagnostic value of the clinical subjective report is widely understudied throughout the literature within study design types for diagnostic accuracy. However, based on the best evidence that exists to date, there are some questions or content items contained within the medical interview that should help the clinician differentiate lower extremity pain syndromes from other conditions. Regardless of the content-specific questions, the interview should be planned carefully and should utilize a good intake form / strategy that includes many key questions about the patient's condition.

In many of lower extremity pain syndromes, there are a variety of clinical presentations; therefore it is suggested to take a systems approach to the content of items in the medical interview. The systems approach should be screened as an initial process to aid in a differential diagnosis and rule out other systems as potential pain generators. Typically there are three goals at the end of the interview: (1) understanding the patient's problem and potential causes, (2) identifying the effect of the problem on the patient's lifestyle, and (3) planning the objective examination (Woolf 2003).

The use of intake forms to gain information regarding demographics and medical history for the patient may save significant time when completed outside of the medical interview. Integrating the findings from the patient intake form, self-reported outcome forms, initial referral (if one exists) and observations of the patient in the waiting room can evoke a wide range of clinical hypotheses for consideration (Goodman & Snyder 2009). These forms should help initiate the conversation and allow the therapist to generate additional questions to assist in the decision-making process. Clearly, the initial hypotheses are derived from clinicians' knowledge base and clinical experience, and differences exist between novice and expert clinicians (Higgs 1992).

Many of these conditions, including major healthcare burdens such as low back pain (LBP) and osteoarthritis (OA) of the hip, knee and ankle, are often recurrent, progressive and lead to a significant decrease in quality of life. The practitioner should consider the physical diagnostic possibilities contributing to the problem, but must also explore the full range of factors that may contribute to the patient's health and impact of the condition on the patient's life. Self-reported outcome measures capture information contained within the domains of pain, disability, function, quality of life, job satisfaction, fear and / or psychosocial concerns, which are important for the complexity of lower extremity syndromes (Harris-Hayes et al 2013). Capturing information from more than one domain may be helpful in understanding and managing the patient with lower extremity pain syndromes (Table 4.1).

Systems Review and Differential Diagnosis Inquiry

The goal of the screening process is recognition of the need for a physician referral, speeding up the diagnosis of systemic and other pathological processes (Boissonnault 2011). A primary purpose of the screen is to identify symptoms unusual for neuro-musculoskeletal conditions that may have been overlooked during the investigation of the patient's chief presenting symptoms. There is considerable overlap of symptoms between disease and neuro-musculoskeletal conditions (Koes et al 2006); therefore the history should aim to

Table 4.1 Self-reported outcome measures for patients with lower extremity pain syndromes

Name of outcome measure	Description
Short Form 36 (MOS SF-36)	A self-report questionnaire consisting of 36 questions, an eight-scale profile of physical, mental health and well-being; highly used throughout physical therapy research; most well-known to evaluate health-related quality of life (HRQOL) (Ware et al 1993).
Patient-specific Functional Scale (PSFS)	Investigates functional status by asking patient to nominate activities that are difficult to perform based on their condition and rate the level of limitation with each activity. This measure is valid and responsive to change in patients with knee pain, LBP, neck pain and cervical radiculopathy (Stratford et al 1995).
Oswestry Low Back Disability Questionnaire (OLBDQ)	This tool quantifies a patient's functional status by assessing pain-related disability in person's with LBP. This measure has been studied and is a reliable and valid tool (Fairbank et al 1980).
The Functional Rating Index (FRI)	This measure is specifically designed to measure quantitatively the subjective perception of function and pain of the spinal musculoskeletal system in a clinical environment. The measure appears to have good reliability and validity (Feise & Menke 2001).
Roland–Morris Disability Questionnaire	This is a health status measure, designed to assess physical disability due to LBP. Correlates well with OLBDQ and SF-36 (Roland & Morris 1986; Roland & Fairbank 2000).
Fear-avoidance Belief Questionnaire (FABQ)	The FABQ assesses patient beliefs with regard to the effect of physical activity and work on their LBP. It consists of 16 items and patients rate their agreement with each statement on a 7-point Likert scale. A higher score indicates more strongly held fear-avoidance beliefs. Two subscales are contained: 7-item work subscale and 4-item physical activity scale. Previous studies have found FABQ work subscale to be associated with current and future disability and work loss in patients with chronic and acute LBP (Waddell et al 1993; Williamson 2006).
WOMAC (Western Ontario and McMaster University Osteoarthritis Index)	This tool measures symptoms and physical disability, originally developed for people with OA of the hip and knee. It has been studied with reliability and validity for OA (Bellamy et al 1988).
Knee Outcome Survey	There is an indication to use this tool with patients with a non-specific knee injury. It has reliability and validity. It is responsive for functional limits for a variety of impairments (Irrgang et al 1998).
Lower Extremity Functional Scale (LEFS)	Indications: all lower extremity conditions; reliability and validity: strong for hip and knee total arthroplasty; useful with patients following arthroplasty. In a 1999 study, this scale was administered with the SF-36, the acute version. In the conclusion of the study, retest reliability of the LEFS scores was found to be excellent. The minimal detectable clinical change within the score was at least 9 scale points and this scale was recommended over the SF-36 (Binkley et al 1999; Stratford et al 1999).

differentiate between these potential causes. Often a planned list of general health status indicators to be used at the initial physical therapy visit during intake may lead to an indication of a more in-depth systems review during the subsequent history taking or physical examination (Table 4.2).

General reports of fatigue, fever, chills, sweats and weight loss are common concerns if reported on intake or in subjective complaints, as these are commonly associated with serious illnesses, infections, cancer, and endocrine and connective tissue disorders. Infective spondylitis (a non-mechanical condition) is commonly associated with fever and has a sensitivity of 98% and a specificity of 50% (Lurie 2005). Unexplained weight changes can be related to diabetes, hyperthyroidism, depression, anorexia nervosa or neoplastic disease and should prompt further inquiry. Excessive weight gain is often associated with fluid retention (oedema, ascites), which can be a manifestation of conditions such as congestive heart failure, liver or renal disease and preeclampsia (Hall 2003).

Neurological screen

Neurological symptoms such as progressive leg paraesthesiae, numbness and / or weakness may be caused by a peripheral nerve entrapment or spinal nerve root lesion and require further inquiry. Any unusual descriptions of altered sensation, bilateral extremity deficit, difficulty in urinating, or change in its frequency, also require further neurological investigation, as concerns about bilateral symptoms and / or urination relate to the medical diagnosis of cauda equina. Questions regarding the symptom of urinary retention have a sensitivity of 90% and specificity of 95% (Deyo et al 1992). Cauda equina also presents with unilateral or bilateral leg pain, numbness and / or weakness in over 80% of cases (Deyo et al 1992).

Cardiovascular screen

The cardiovascular system can also refer pain and or symptoms (including oedema) into the lower extremity, so requires differential diagnosis. In peripheral oedema the clinician will need to rule out venous insufficiency, congestive heart failure and pulmonary hypertension as causes, as well as deep-vein thrombosis, which is more associated with unilateral oedema (Boissonnault 2011). Occlusive arterial disease is a common problem in the elderly and in smokers, and may present as claudication (Siracuse et al 2012). The presentation may be similar to other lower extremity syndromes with pain,

Table 4.2 **General systems review questions**

Cardio/peripheral vascular and pulmonary system questions regarding the following	Gastrointestinal system questions regarding the following
Dyspnoea Cough Palpitations Syncope Sweats Cold distal extremities Skin discoloration Open wounds/ulcers Clubbing of the nails Wheezing, stridor	Swallowing difficulties Indigestion, heartburn Food intolerance Bowel dysfunction Colour of stool Shape, calibre of stool Constipation Diarrhoea Difficulty in initiating eating Incontinence
Genitourinary system questions regarding the following	**Reproductive system questions regarding the following**
Urinary changes Colour Flow Reduced calibre or force of urine stream Incontinence	Male gender Urethral discharge Sexual dysfunction Pain during intercourse Female gender Vaginal discharge Pain with intercourse Menstruation changes Menopause

(Adapted from Boissonnault 2011.)

oedema and/or cramping sensations in the buttocks, thighs or calves. However, claudication pain is typically associated with increased physical activity and is relieved by rest (Siracuse et al 2012). Aortic aneurysms are potentially dangerous conditions and may present as deep, diffuse, throbbing, or aching mid-back, chest, left shoulder or abdominal pain (de Virgilio & Chan 2010). If related to a recent surgical event or a reduced level of activity, the clinician will need to ask questions related to deep-vein thrombosis (Wells et al 1997). The Wells clinical prediction rule has been shown to be a reliable and valid tool for clinical assessment for predicting the risk of deep-vein thrombosis in the lower extremity (Table 4.3).

Table 4.3 **Wells' clinical decision rule for deep-vein thrombosis**

Clinical presentation (questions and observation)	Score
Do you have active cancer (within 6 months of diagnosis or receiving palliative care)?	1
Do you have paralysis, paresis or recent immobilization of the lower extremity?	1
Have you been bedridden for more than 3 days or had major surgery in the last 4 weeks?	1
Do you have localized tenderness in the centre of the posterior calf, the popliteal space, or along the femoral vein in the anterior thigh/groin?	1
Have you noticed entire lower extremity swelling?	1
Observation: unilateral calf swelling (>3 mm compared with contralateral side)	1
Observation: collateral superficial veins	1
An alternative diagnosis is more likely (cellulitis, calf strain, postoperative swelling)	−2

(Source: Wells et al 1997.)

Gastrointestinal screen

The gastrointestinal system can also refer pain and/or symptoms into the lower extremity and needs to be ruled out as a source of pain in patients presenting with lower extremity pain syndromes. Questions on intake regarding changes in bowel habits should act as an initial screen. If such changes are reported then the clinician should ask additional questions about the presence of blood in stools, or black stools, to screen for colon cancer (Goodman & Synder 2009). Also, visceral organ symptoms vary depending on the function of the particular organ. Reports of fluctuating symptoms may be related either to eating habits or to bowel or bladder function. Certain foods may precipitate the onset of symptoms or may affect their intensity. Some disorders may be associated with bladder fullness or constipation, urination or defecation. It is therefore important to ask about the total area in which the pain and related symptoms occur to pinpoint the contributing causes when patients report gastrointestinal changes (Goodman & Synder 2009).

Non-mechanical pathologies: differential diagnosis

There are other non-mechanical pathologies that need to be considered in differential diagnosis and screening of the lower extremity (Koes et al 2006). Many of these conditions can worsen at night, although presenting as common lower extremity pain syndromes and behaving similarly to mechanical pain presentations. For example, seronegative spondyloarthropathies need to be considered when progressive back pain is present in a young patient with fluctuating inflammatory symptoms manifesting as morning stiffness or improvement with exercise. Conditions including ankylosing spondylitis (AS), Reiter's syndrome, psoriatic arthritis and the arthritis of inflammatory bowel disease all require additional medical testing to establish a diagnosis (Atlas & Deyo 2001). However, AS may be elicited from questions that establish a slow onset, age <40, long-term discomfort (>3 months) and a fluctuating inflammatory pattern (i.e. morning stiffness and improvement of discomfort with exercise). These questions helping to rule in AS have a sensitivity of 23% and a specificity of 82% (Deyo 1991).

Psychosocial factors

Psychosocial factors also may manifest in the presentation of musculoskeletal pain, both regional and general. A systematic review (Chou & Shekelle 2010) identified the baseline predictors of persistent disabling LBP to be maladaptive pain-coping behaviour, non-organic signs, functional impairment, low general health status, and the presence of psychiatric comorbidities; conversely, low levels of fear avoidance and functional impairment predicted recovery at 1 year. Consistent evidence has been found to support the role of various psychological factors in prognosis, although the literature is less consistent regarding which of these factors are most prognostic (Nicholas et al 2011; Grovle et al 2013).

Red Flags

The presence of any of the 'red flags' should be noted at the initial assessment. This step is critical in determining who is and who is not a candidate for physical therapy, and requires both recognizing and ruling out the presence of red flags (Koes et al 2006). Such flags are, by definition, signs and symptoms that may relate a disorder to a serious pathology but may also reflect a musculoskeletal condition (Sizer et al 2007). Typically, they are features from a patient's clinical history and physical examination that are thought to be associated with a higher risk of serious pathology or malignancy (Boissonnault 2011). There are several regional screening tools to help recognize potential serious disorders (red or yellow flags) that aid in differential diagnosis of musculoskeletal conditions commonly encountered by physical therapists and that require questions from the medical interview (Fritz & Flynn 2005).

Low back pain, buttock pain and / or pain in the lower extremity may be related to spinal malignancy, which is the most common site for bony metastases, affecting up to 30–70% of patients (Cook et al 2011a). However, lumbar movement restrictions may reproduce mechanical pain in patients with or without cancer (Cook et al 2011b). Recently, a well-conducted systematic review found that a previous history of cancer meaningfully increased the likelihood of malignancy, with a high positive likelihood ratio (Henschke et al 2013). Additionally, the same Cochrane systematic review found that other red flags have high false-positive rates leading to unnecessary and potentially harmful investigations, such as radiation. It concluded that, at this time, there is a lack of evidence and studies with sufficient statistical power to produce precise estimates of sensitivity and specificity of red flags (Henschke et al 2013); despite their inclusion in the guidelines, the usefulness of screening for 'red flags' for malignancy in patients with LBP continues to be debated and there remains very little information on their diagnostic accuracy and how best to use them in clinical practice (Underwood 2009). It is therefore recommended that clinicians utilize more than one of the single red flag questions that are presented in Table 4.4 (Downie et al 2013; Henschke et al 2013).

Table 4.4 **Red flags to screen for malignancy in patients with low back pain**

Clinical history questions	Post-test probability (%)
Do you have a previous history of cancer?	4.6
Have you experienced any unexplained weight loss?	1.2
Have your symptoms improved after 1 month (if the result is negative)?	0.9
Age >50 years?	0.8
Have you had symptoms (this episode) >1 month?	0.8
Do you have severe pain?	0.5
Have you tried bedrest with no relief?	0.6

(Source: Henschke et al 2013.)

Fractures are also a common red flag and are often a cause for LBP and related leg symptoms. Vertebral compression fractures are the most common osteoporosis-related spinal fractures, presenting with clinical symptoms of back pain, posture changes, loss of height, functional impairment, disability and diminished quality of life. A recent systematic review (Downie et al 2013) identified three red flags with potentially useful positive likelihood ratios that would be useful to capture in primary care settings; these are significant trauma, older age and corticosteroid use. Additionally, metatarsal insufficiency fractures in both men and women have been identified as early sign of osteoporosis (Tomaczak & VanCourt 2000). It has been reported, however, that many red flags in current guidelines either provide virtually no change in probability of fracture or have untested diagnostic accuracy (Downie et al 2013).

Symptom Investigation

During intake and / or during the medical interview, it is imperative to identify specific movement patterns that alter the patient's symptoms for better and / or worse. Conditions associated with inflammation may worsen either when at rest or during aggressive movements (Maitland 2001). To streamline the medical interview, some of the initial symptom investigation can be completed on the medical history intake form (Table 4.5). On this, the patient needs to characterize the

Table 4.5 **Intake information for patients with lower extremity pain syndromes**

Intake questions related to	Purpose of the content
Patient profile and demographics	Relates to the epidemiology with prevalence and incidence of related conditions based on age, gender and ethnicity
Description of the problem	Characterize the problem and determine cause (if one exists), determine chief complaint, and other related concerns Concordant/familiar/comparable sign – movement associated with the pain in which the patient is seeking care Patient's perspective of the condition (concerns, expectations, feelings, beliefs)
Nature and behaviour of the condition	Severity: intensity of the patients symptoms as they relate to a functional activity or time of day Irritability: how quickly a stable condition degenerates in the presence of pain-causing inputs Nature: represents the structures at fault, or involved in the syndrome; may also inquire as to the aggravating factors or relieving factors; may also inquire as to presentation: constant, intermittent, and/or episodic Stage of pathology: assessment of the stage of healing in which the condition is presenting Stability: symptom progression over time (better, worse, staying the same)
Pertinent medical history	Use intake forms to minimize questions for screening Review of systems for differential diagnosis of viscerogenic, vasculogenic, spondylogenic, neurogenic and/or psychogenic pain generators Determine whether potential related medical components may be related to clinical presentation Baseline for current medication use, general wellness, activity level, current medical conditions and/or medical test for present condition
Patient goals and barriers to care	Commonly used to identify motivation to improving current health status Related to adherence to plan of care and self-efficacy, which are prognostic variables to successful outcomes Treatment alternatives in accordance to patient-centred care

problem and determine the cause (if one exists), the chief complaint, and other related concerns. Symptoms that vary over the course of the day have been associated with neuromusculoskeletal impairments or movement disorders. Such conditions typically fluctuate as the mechanical loads on the body increase or decrease with time of day, onset or cessation of specific activities, and adoption or avoidance of certain postures. Some spinal and / or extremity pain syndromes can also present with alteration in pain presentation (including peripheralization or centralization) in various postures or positions with repetition of movement (Maitland 2001).

History questions that identify alleviating and aggravating positions can help the clinician to pinpoint mechanical conditions associated with musculoskeletal conditions. For instance, non-inflammatory conditions may worsen during very aggressive unguarded movements. However, if, upon a complete examination, the patient does not report or present with a symptom pattern consistent with a musculoskeletal condition, further screening for conditions related to specific body systems should then be conducted. A pain pattern associated with systemic disease is often a progressive pattern with a cyclical onset (Goodman & Snyder 2009). Additionally, an insidious onset of symptoms and / or reports of atypical symptoms or symptom behaviour may raise suspicions of a serious underlying condition.

During the interview, it is important to help the patient identify the primary reason for seeking care. In the physical examination this is termed the concordant sign, which is distinguished from other symptoms produced during the physical assessment. The concordant sign needs to be identified during the interview to allow both the patient and the clinician to ascertain the key complaint (Maitland 2001; Laslett et al 2003). A patient with a lower extremity syndrome may also present with one or more discordant signs; this may be described as painful or abnormal, but not related to concordant sign. The discordant sign is unlike the pain for which the patient has sought treatment (Maitland 2001).

Nature and Behaviour of the Problem

It is important to construct the symptom history during the history-taking session. This involves determining the stage of the health problem. The primary purpose is for the clinician to determine the cause of injury and to elicit a careful explanation of the symptoms. Discussion of the concordant sign and nature of the problem is further investigated, while the timing of the event is closely associated with the stage of the disorder (Maitland 2001).

The nature and behaviour of the condition require the clinician to ask questions regarding the severity, nature, irritability, stage of pathology and stability of the symptoms. Again, as with many other history-taking components, many of these concepts have not been well described or studied within the literature. The severity describes the intensity of the patient's symptoms in relation to a functional activity or time of day; this typically involves the patient rating the pain severity on a rating scale (e.g. the numeric pain rating scale) to provide a baseline for comparison with that elicited by various movements during the physical examination (Farrar et al 2001). The nature of the patient's symptoms refers to the pain presentation as being constant, intermittent, and / or episodic in behaviour; the clinician should also ask the patient about factors that aggravate or relieve the pain.

Irritability is another pain behaviour concept that relates to how quickly a stable condition degenerates in the presence of pain-causing inputs. This concept can be operationally defined by three criteria: (1) what does the patient have to do to set this condition off, (2) how long do the symptoms last and how severe are the symptoms, and (3) what does the patient have to do to calm the symptoms down. Patients with high levels of irritability may often be cautious of aggressive treatment because they will typically worsen with selected activities (Zusman 1998; Maitland 2001).

The stage of the pathology or condition relates specifically to the stage of healing for the injury or symptom presentation, whereas the stability of the symptom presentation refers to the symptom progression over time as improving, worsening, or staying the same.

History-taking Questions Specific to Lower Extremity Pain Syndromes

Leg pain is a frequent accompaniment to LBP, but can also often present in the absence of LBP and can be quite debilitating. The structures often involved with leg pain (with or without LBP) will be presented and classified in this chapter as (1) central sensitization, (2) peripheral nerve sensitization (with or without denervation), and (3) musculoskeletal pain from non-neural structures (Schafer et al 2009). Each of the various structures involved can present with a distinct pattern of signs and symptoms that the patient may describe during the interview or on the intake form, although further research in pain science is indicating that there is significant crossover between the patterns (Schafer et al 2009).

The sections below deal with specific questions that clinicians may ask during history taking to assist their hypothesis generation and decision making. Where possible, along with the characterization statements, subjective history questions and / or self-report questionnaire items affiliated with a specific condition, the diagnostic odds ratios (DOR), sensitivity (SN, the ability of the test to identify positively an individual who has the problem according to the reference test), specificity (the ability of the test to positively exclude an individual who does not have the problem according to the reference test) and likelihood ratios (+LR or –LR) are included (Cook et al 2007; see also Ch 5). However, in many instances such statistical information is not available, and in such cases the text reports the best available evidence regarding history taking related to specific lower extremity pain syndromes.

Central and peripheral nerve sensitization

The research literature indicates there are certain history-taking questions that can be used to examine lower extremity syndromes including conditions associated with central sensitization, peripheral nerve sensitization and musculoskeletal pain. (For purposes of this chapter, central sensitization is operationally defined as an amplification of neural signalling within the central nervous system (CNS) that elicits pain hypersensitivity (Woolf 2011); peripheral sensitization is operationally defined as increased responsiveness and reduced threshold of nociceptors to stimulation of their receptive fields. This includes nociceptive pain, which refers to pain conditions assumed to be predominantly driven by the activation of peripheral nociceptive sensory fibres.) Two studies have examined low back with leg pain that could not be traced back to an anatomical abnormality, including central sensitization and nociceptive LBP with or without leg pain. Patients experiencing pain disproportionate to injury, disproportionate aggravating / easing factors and other psychosocial symptoms were very likely to be diagnosed with central sensitization (DOR 15.19, 30.69 and 7.65 respectively) (Smart et al 2012a, 2012b). Individuals complaining of localized or intermittent pain were more likely to be diagnosed with nociceptive LBP (DOR 69.79 and 4.25 respectively) (Smart et al 2012a, 2012b).

Specific Low-back-associated Musculoskeletal Pain Syndromes

There are a variety of low back or spinal conditions that should be considered when addressing patients with lower extremity pain syndromes. In the many studies on these syndromes, a variety of questions have been used by the researchers / authors to identify a specified lower quarter condition. Specifically for the lumbar spine, several studies have examined the diagnostic accuracy of history-taking items for lumbar spinal stenosis (LSS), lumbar sacral nerve root compression / radiculopathy, lumbar disc herniation, and clinical lumbar instability.

Lumbar spinal stenosis

A variety of subjective history questions / self-report items have been studied for their usefulness in the diagnosis of LSS; all of the following met criteria for at least a small increase in the probability of an LSS diagnosis. In the study by Cook et al (2011a), the most strongly diagnostic combination of self-report items comprised: (1) bilateral symptoms, (2) leg pain more than back pain, (3) pain during walking / standing, (4) pain relief upon sitting, and (5) age >48 years. Failure to meet the condition of any one of these five positive examination findings demonstrated a high sensitivity (0.96) and a low LR– (0.19); meeting the condition of four of the five yielded a LR+ of 4.6 and a post-test probability of 76%. Other studies have identified that increasing patient age (older than 48 years) increased the LR+ of having the condition (Katz et al 1995; Konno et al 2007; Sugioka et al 2008). Katz et al (1995) also found the following questions helpful: does the patient have the following: severe leg pain (LR+ 2.00), no pain when seated (LR+ 6.60), symptoms that improve when seated (LR+ 3.10), or leg numbness (LR+ 2.62)? Konno et al (2007) identified additional questions including: pain that is worse when walking but relieved by taking a rest (DOR 70.77), pain that is worse on standing (DOR 11.38), and numbness around the buttocks (DOR 77.0). Additionally, Sugioka et al (2008) inquired whether the pain was reported as lasting for more than 6 months (DOR 2.17), the patient was walking more slowly than usually (DOR 2.28), was sitting down because of lower extremity pain (DOR 2.01), or needed to wake up to urinate at night (DOR 2.34); positive responses related to a slightly to moderately increased probability of having LSS.

Nerve root compression / radiculopathy

The most significant history component for nerve root compression is the location of pain, whether the symptoms present within a dermatome distribution, and / or whether symptom radiation was the most significant history complaint (DOR 24.29) (Smart et al 2012a, 2012b). Furthermore, questions about whether the patient experienced more pain with coughing, sneezing or straining (DOR 3.20), as well as self-reports of muscle weakness (DOR 2.20), sensory loss (DOR 2.10) or of disturbed urinary passage (DOR 2.3), have been associated with the diagnosis of lumbar sacral nerve root compression / radiculopathy (Coster et al 2010). Additionally, there appears to be an age relationship as older-aged patients (51–81 years) have an increased probability of being diagnosed with this condition (DOR 2.2) (Vroomen et al 2002).

Lumbar disc herniation

In the diagnosis of lumbar disc herniation, only a few studies have compared findings with a reference standard, and some studies have significant risk of bias. At this point, some of the key history items that yield some benefit in screening for possible lumbar disc herniation include previous non-spinal surgery (DOR 3.52), education level (DOR 3.22), and progressive sciatic pain (DOR 2.77) (Vucetic et al 1997).

Clinical lumbar instability

Although within the literature there are some studies testing the accuracy of clinical tests for lumbar stability / instability, no studies have uniquely analysed history taking. A systemic review by Alqarni et al (2011) found that physical therapists typically utilize tests such as the posterior shear test, the prone instability test, the Beighton hypermobility scale, the prone leg extension test, and tests for the instability catch sign, the painful catch sign and the apprehension sign (presented later in this book). Other possibly useful questions that need to be studied for their diagnostic accuracy are based on a Delphi study (by a panel of clinical experts): clinicians typically inquire about episodes of giving way or the back giving out, pain through the range of motion, painful locking or catching during twisting or bending of the spine during transitional activities, pain during sudden activities, and pain with lifting, sneezing and / or returning from a flexed-forward position (Cook et al 2006).

Specific Lower-extremity-associated Musculoskeletal Pain Syndromes

Hip osteoarthritis

For the diagnosis of hip osteoarthritis (OA), some of the key history items that should be included are as follows (Sutlive et al 2008; Morvan et al 2009). Does the patient have buttock pain / hip / groin pain (which yields a LR+ range from 1.74 to 6.4 and LR– of 0.52)? Does the patient complain of pain when climbing stairs or walking down slopes (yields an LR+ of 2.10)? Does the patient self-report squatting as an aggravating factor (yields an LR+ of 1.8 and LR– of 0.42)? Does the patient have posterior hip pain (yields an LR+ of 6.1 and LR– of 0.79)? Lastly, does the patient self-identify limited motion of the hip (yielded a small LR+ of 2.86)?

Other hip pathology

A systematic review by Burgess et al (2011) examined the diagnostic accuracy of patients' subjective statements associated with labral pathology. They identified two studies that found patients with labral pathology presented with anterior groin pain (sensitivity of 100% and a specificity of 40%), or reported clicking (with sensitivity ranging from 57% to 100%). Tijssen et al (2012) conducted a second systematic review; these authors grouped patients exhibiting the mechanical symptoms of clicking, locking, popping or giving way together from a combination of three of their included studies (Farjo et al 1999; O'Leary et al 2001; Burnett et al 2006) and found that reports of mechanical symptoms yielded a range of sensitivity of 53% to 100%. Little is known about the diagnostic accuracy of not only the history taking but also the physical examination in screening for femoro-acetabular impingement (FAI), although this condition is now increasingly recognized as a causative factor of many intra-articular hip lesions and labral pathology. Some studies have described the clinical characteristics and symptoms; however, no studies have examined the diagnostic accuracy of history questions related to these for FAI.

Knee osteoarthritis

The knee is a significant target of osteoarthritis (OA). Morvan et al (2009) found three questions during the interview to be useful, as they were related to a small increase in the probability of having knee OA. These questions included having had pain for at least 4 weeks (which yielded a sensitivity of 0.95, specificity of 0.46, LR+ of 1.77, and LR– of 0.10), having pain while climbing stairs or walking down slopes (a sensitivity of 0.81, specificity of 0.63, LR+ of 2.19 and LR– of 0.30), and having swelling in one or both knees (a sensitivity of 0.47, specificity of 0.84, LR+ of 3.10 and LR– of 0.62) (Morvan et al 2009).

Patellofemoral pain syndrome

Cook et al (2012) conducted a systematic review that identified some questions that may be helpful in identifying patients with patellofemoral pain syndrome (PFPS). Within their included studies they identified that self-reported pain during squatting presents with a range of low LR+ (from 1.3 to 1.8) and LR– (between 0.9 and 0.1) from three studies reported in a systematic review. Further, self-reports of pain during kneeling also have a low LR+ (1.7) and LR– (0.3). Self-reported pain during prolonged sitting or flexion of the knee was captured in three studies and ranged from low to moderate shifts in probabilities from LR+ (1.7 to 7.4) and LR– (0.3 to 0.5). Pain reports during stair climbing had a wider range of LR+ (from 1.3 to 11.6) and LR– (from 0.6 to 0.1) from three studies that captured this item. The wide ranges of differential diagnosis identified by the authors of the systematic review may be due to the high variability in reference standards for diagnosis as well as in the definitions of PFPS amongst the studies included (Cook et al 2012).

Knee meniscal injury

There are two history-taking items that have been identified for diagnosing knee meniscal injuries. One study found that the self-reported sensations of giving way and locking during history taking had a diagnostic accuracy of 49.2% and 60.9% respectively, compared with MRI findings, with specificities of 0.84 and 0.96 respectively (Yan et al 2011). Wagemakers et al (2008), in another diagnostic accuracy study, identified that a question cluster of being older ('age over 40 years'), 'continuation of activity impossible', and reports of 'weight-bearing during trauma' was associated with a slightly increased probability (LR+ 2.0) of meniscal injury.

Knee ligamentous injury

More diagnostic accuracy studies have examined anterior cruciate ligament (ACL) injury than many of the other types of ligamentous injuries (Benjaminse et al 2006). One study separated history components within the examination from the physical examination, to identify the diagnostic value (Wagemakers et al 2012). This study further examined history-taking clusters for both partial and complete ACL lesions. The history-taking items of reported swelling / effusion yielded an LR+ of 1.6, LR– of 0.8 for identifying partial tears and LR+ of 2.0, LR– of 0.6 for identifying complete tears. Reports of a 'popping sensation' yielded an LR+ of 2.3, LR– of 0.5 for partial tears, and LR+ of 2.1, LR– of 0.5 for complete tears. The self-reported sensation of 'giving way' yielded a small shift in probability (with an LR+ of 1.6, LR– of 0.6 for partial tears, and LR+ of 1.7, LR– of 0.6 for complete tears). When combined in a cluster, the history findings yielded a specificity of 0.99, a sensitivity of 0.18 and LR+ of 17.7 for partial tears compared with MRI. Complete ACL tears yielded a large, albeit slightly smaller shift compared with partial tears, with an LR+ of 9.8, an LR– of 0.8 and similar specificity (0.98) and sensitivity (0.18). Many other items were evaluated, including swelling, crepitation, pain score, type of injury and others; however, none of these were included within the final diagnostic model for assessing ACL lesions (Wagemakers et al 2012).

Achilles tendinopathy

Differential diagnosis of Achilles pathology can be very challenging within the research literature and clinical practice. The reference standard for this diagnosis is ultrasound and there was one study that presented data on the diagnostic accuracy of self-reported items or questions for this condition (Hutchison et al 2013). Self-reported pain with palpation of the tendon presented with a sensitivity of 0.84 and specificity of 0.73. Additionally, the subjective report of pain at 2–6 cm above the insertion into the calcaneus showed a sensitivity of 0.78 and specificity of 0.77. Although not well examined within the literature, these two key history-taking items may prove to be useful in screening for this condition.

Heel pain / plantar fasciitis

There are several common history items that clinicians have used for years to help with the differential diagnosis of this condition. Clinically, patients often report pain during their first steps in the morning or after prolonged sitting, and may also report sharp pain when the medial plantar calcaneal region is touched / palpated. However, there are many other conditions that can also cause heel pain, including (but not limited to) nerve entrapment, lumbar spine conditions and neuropathies (Cole et al 2005). No diagnostic accuracy studies have been found to date that examine the patient history for plantar fasciitis. Interestingly though, the history taking is nevertheless significantly valued in the classification and / or diagnosis of heel pain / plantar fasciitis within clinical practice guidelines for physical therapy (McPoil et al 2008).

Conclusion

As evidence-based clinicians, physical therapists need to utilize the best evidence with regards to developing the subjective interview. The history-taking approach / style and content of questions are both understudied within the current literature in physical therapy. However, in this chapter several questions that should aid in decision making have been presented based on body structures often involved with leg pain (with or without low back pain), including questions to differentiate and screen for red flags and pain referral to other systems. Pain / symptoms that are not generated from other systems or due to red flag / pathological conditions have also been presented as questions to identify central sensitization, peripheral nerve sensitization (with or without denervation) and musculoskeletal pain. Although in clinical practice the history and clinical examination are not isolated, the form of history questions within the medical interview and their contributing value for decision making remain understudied within the literature compared with studies of the physical examination testing. We may not know the real value of the history with regards to diagnostic accuracy. However, literature does support its value within a tailored, patient-centred approach to improving patient satisfaction with care and patient outcomes in many musculoskeletal conditions.

References

Alqarni AM, Schneiders AG, Hendrick PA. 2011. Clinical tests to diagnose lumbar segmental instability: a systematic review. J Orthop Sports Phys Ther 41: 130–140.

Asnani MR. 2009. Patient–physician communication. West Indian Med J 58: 357–361.

Atlas SJ, Deyo RA. 2001. Evaluating and managing acute low back pain in the primary care setting. J Gen Int Med 16: 120–131.

Beck RS, Daughtridge R. Sloane PD. 2002 Physician–patient communication in the primary care office: a systematic review. J Am Board Fam Pract 15: 25–38.

Bellamy N, Buchanan WW, Goldsmith CH, et al. 1988. Validation study of WOMAC: a health status instrument for measuring clinically important patient-relevant outcomes following total hip or knee arthroplasty in osteoarthritis. J Orthop Rheumatol 1: 95–108.

Benjaminse A, Gokeler A, van der Schans CP. 2006. Clinical diagnosis of an anterior cruciate ligament rupture: a meta-analysis. J Orthop Sports Phys Ther 36: 267–288.

Binkley JM, Stratford PW, Lott SA, et al. 1999. The Lower Extremity Functional Scale (LEFS): scale development, measurement properties, and clinical

application: North American Orthopaedic Rehabilitation Research Network. Phys Ther 79: 371–383.
Boissonnault WG. 2011. Primary care for the physical therapist: examination and triage, 2nd edn. St Louis: Elsevier Saunders.
Britt E, Hudson SM, Blampied NM. 2004. Motivational interviewing in health settings: a review. Patient Educ Couns 53: 147–155.
Burgess RM, Rushton A, Wright C, et al. 2011. The validity and accuracy of clinical diagnostic tests used to detect labral pathology of the hip: a systematic review. Man Ther 16: 318–326.
Burnett R, Della Rocca G, Prather H, et al. 2006. Clinical presentation of patients with tears of the acetabular labrum. J Bone Joint Surgery 88: 1448–1457
Chou R, Shekelle P. 2010. Will this patient develop persistent disabling low back pain? JAMA 303: 1295–1302.
Cole C, Seto C, Gazewood J. 2005. Plantar fasciitis: evidence-based review of diagnosis and therapy. Am Fam Physician 72: 2237–2242.
Cook CE, Brismee JM, Sizer PS. 2006. Subjective and objective descriptors of clinical lumbar spine instability: a Delphi study. Man Ther 11: 11–21.
Cook C, Cleland J, Huijbregts P. 2007. Creation and critique of studies of diagnostic accuracy: use of the STARD and QUADAS methodological quality assessment tools. J Man Manip Ther 14: 93–100.
Cook C, Brown C, Michael K, et al. 2011a. The clinical value of a cluster of patient history and observational findings as a diagnostic support tool for lumbar spine stenosis. Physiother Res Int 16: 170–178.
Cook C, Ross MD, Isaacs R. et al. 2011b. Investigation of non-mechanical findings during spinal movement screening for identifying and / or ruling out metastatic cancer. Pain Pract 12: 426–433.
Cook C, Mabry L, Reiman MP, et al. 2012. Best test / clinical findings for screening and diagnosis of patellofemoral pain syndrome: a systematic review. Physiotherapy 98: 93–100.
Coster S, de Bruijn SF, Tavy DL. 2010. Diagnostic value of history, physical examination and needle electromyography in diagnosing lumbosacral radiculopathy. J Neurol 257: 332–337.
de Virgilio C, Chan T. 2010. Assessment of vascular patients and indications for therapy. In: Fogarty TJ, White RA (eds) Peripheral endovascular interventions. New York: Springer-Verlag, pp 37–44.
Deyo RA. 1991. Nonsurgical care of low back pain. Neurosurg Clinics North Am 2: 851–862.
Deyo RA, Rainville J, Kent DL. 1992. What can the history and physical examination tell us about low back pain? JAMA 268: 760–765.
Downie A, Williams CM, Henschke N, et al. 2013. Red flags to screen for malignancy and fracture in patients with low back pain: systematic review. BMJ 347: f7095.
Dwamena F, Holmes-Rovner M, Gaulden CM, et al. 2012. Interventions for providers to promote a patient-centered approach in clinical consultations. Cochrane Database Syst Rev 12: CD003267.
Edwards I, Jones M, Carr J, et al. 2004. Clinical reasoning strategies in physical therapy. Phys Ther 84: 312–330.
Fairbank J, Couper J, Davies J, et al. 1980. The Oswestry Low Back Pain Questionnaire. Physiotherapy 66: 271–273.
Farjo L, Glick J, Sampson T. 1999. Hip arthroscopy for acetabular labral tears. Arthroscopy 15:132–137.
Farrar JT, Young JP, LaMoreaux L, et al. 2001. Clinical importance of changes in chronic pain intensity measured on an 11-point numerical pain rating scale. Pain 94: 149–158.
Feise RJ, Menke J. 2001. Functional Rating Index: a new valid and reliable instrument to measure the magnitude of clinical change in spinal conditions. Spine 26: 78–86.
Fritz J, Flynn TW. 2005. Autonomy in physical therapy: less is more. J Orthop Sports Phys Ther 35: 696–968.
Goodman CC, Snyder TE. 2009. Differential diagnosis in physical therapy, 3rd edn. Philadelphia: WB Saunders.
Grovle L, Haugen AJ, Keller A, et al. 2013. Prognostic factors for return to work in patients with sciatica. Spine 13: 1849–1857.
Hall JE. 2003. The kidney, hypertension, and obesity. Hypertension 41: 625–633.
Hampton JR, Harrison MJ, Mitchell JR, et al. 1975. Relative contributions of history-taking, physical examination and laboratory investigations to diagnosis and management of medical out-patients. BMJ 2: 486–489.
Harris-Hayes M, McDonough CM, Leunig M. 2013. Clinical outcomes assessment in clinical trials to assess treatment of femoroacetabular impingement: use of patient-reported outcome measures. J Am Acad Orthop Surg 21: S39–S46.
Henry SG, Fuhrel-Forbis A, Rogers M, et al. 2012. Association between nonverbal communication during clinical interactions and outcomes: a systematic review and meta-analysis. Patient Educ Couns 86: 297–315.
Henschke N, Maher CG, Ostelo RW, et al. 2013. Red flags to screen for malignancy in patients with low-back pain. Cochrane Database Syst Rev 2: CD008686.
Higgs J. 1992. Developing knowledge: a process of construction, mapping and review. N Z J Physiother 20: 23–30.
Hutchison AM, Evans R, Bodger O, et al. 2013. What is the best clinical test for Achilles tendinopathy? Foot Ankle Surg 19: 112–117.
Irrgang JJ, Snyder-Mackler L, Wainner RS, et al. 1998. Development of a patient-reported measure of function of the knee. J Bone Joint Surg 80: 1132–1145.
Jarvik JG, Deyo RA. 2002. Diagnostic evaluation of low back pain with emphasis on imaging. Ann Intern Med 137: 586–597.
Katz JN, Dalgas M, Stucki G, et al. 1995. Degenerative lumbar spinal stenosis: diagnostic value of the history and physical examination. Arthritis Rheum 38:1236–1241.
Koes BW, van Tulder MW, Thomas S. 2006. Diagnosis and treatment of low back pain. BMJ 332: 1430–1434.
Konno SI, Kikuchi SI, Tanaka Y, et al. 2007 A diagnostic support tool for lumbar spinal stenosis: a self-administered, self-reported history questionnaire. BMC Musculoskeletal Dis 8: 102.
Kurtz SM, Silverman JD. 1996. The Calgary–Cambridge observation guides: an aid to defining the curriculum and organizing the teaching in communication training programmes. Med Educ 30: 83–89.
Kurtz SM, Silverman JD, Draper J. 1998. Teaching and learning communication skills with patients. Oxford, UK; Radcliffe Medical Press.
Kurtz SM, Silverman JD, Benson J, et al. 2003. Marrying content and process in clinical method teaching: enhancing the Calgary–Cambridge Guides. Acad Med 78: 802–809.
Laslett M, Young S, April C, et al. 2003. Diagnosing painful sacroiliac joints: a validity study of a McKenzie evaluation and sacroiliac provocation tests. Aust J Physiother 49: 89–97.
Lurie JD. 2005. What diagnostic tests are useful for low back pain? Best Pract Res Clin Rheumatol 19: 557–575.
Maitland GD. 2001. Maitland's vertebral manipulation, 6th edn. London: Butterworth-Heinemann.
McPoil TG, Martin RL, Cornwall MW, et al. 2008. Heel pain–plantar fasciitis: clinical practice guidelines linked to the international classification of function, disability, and health from the orthopaedic section of the American Physical Therapy Association. J Orthop Sports Phys Ther 38: A1–A18.
Morvan J, Roux CH, Fautrel B, et al. 2009. A case-control study to assess sensitivity and specificity of a questionnaire for the detection of hip and knee osteoarthritis. Arthritis Rheum 61:92–99.
Nicholas MK, Linton SJ, Watson PJ, et al; 'Decade of the Flags' Working Group. 2011. Early identification and management of psychological risk factors ('yellow flags') in patients with low back pain: a reappraisal. Phys Ther 91: 737–753.
O'Leary J, Berend M, Parker T. 2001. The relationship between diagnosis and outcome in arthroscopy of the hip. Arthroscopy 17(2): 181–188.
Peterson MC, Holbrook JH, Von Hales D, et al. 1992. Contributions of the history, physical examination and laboratory investigation in making medical diagnoses. West J Med 156: 163–165.
Roland M, Fairbank J. 2000. The Roland–Morris Disability Questionnaire and the Oswestry Disability Questionnaire. Spine 25: 3115–3122.
Roland M, Morris R. 1986. A study of the natural history of back pain, part I: the development of a reliable and sensitive measure of disability of low back pain. Spine 8: 141–144.
Rollnick S, Miller WR, Butler CC. 2008. Motivational interviewing in health care. New York: Guilford Press.
Schafer A, Hall T, Briffa K. 2009. Classification of low back-related leg pain: a proposed patho-mechanism-based approach. Man Ther 14: 222–230.
Silverman J, Archer J, Gillard S. 2011. Initial evaluation of epscale, a rating scale that assesses the process of explanation and planning in the medical interview. Patient Educ Couns 82: 89–93.
Siracuse JJ, Giles KA, Pomposelli FB. 2012. Results for primary bypass versus primary angioplasty / stent for intermittent claudication due to superficial femoral artery occlusive disease. J Vascular Surg 55: 1001–1007.
Sizer P, Brismee JM, Cook C. 2007. Medical screening for red flags in the diagnosis and management of musculoskeletal spine pain. Pain Pract 7: 53–71.
Smart KM, Blake C, Staines A, et al. 2012a. Mechanisms-based classifications of musculoskeletal pain: part 1 of 3: symptoms and signs of central sensitization in patients with low back (±leg) pain. Man Ther 17: 336–344.
Smart KM, Blake C, Staines A, et al. 2012b. Mechanisms-based classifications of musculoskeletal pain: part 3 of 3: symptoms and signs of nociceptive pain in patients with low back (±leg) pain. Man Ther 17: 352–357.

Stratford P, Gill C, Westway M, et al. 1995. Assessing disability and change on individual patients: A report of a patient specific measure. Physiother Can 47: 258–263.

Stratford P, Binkley J, Lott S, et al. 1999. The Lower Extremity Functional Scale (LEFS): scale development, measurement properties, and clinical application. J Am Phys Ther Assoc 79: 371–383.

Street RL, Haidet P. 2011. How well do doctors know their patients? Factors affecting physician understanding of patients' health beliefs. J Gen Intern Med 26: 21–27.

Street RL, Richardson MN, Cox V, et al. 2009. (Mis)understanding in patient-health care provider communication about total knee replacement. Arthritis Rheum 61: 100–107.

Sugioka T, Hayashino Y, Konno S, et al. 2008. Predictive value of self-reported patient information for the identification of lumbar spinal stenosis. Fam Pract 25: 237–244.

Sutlive TG, Lopez HP, Schnitker DE, et al. 2008. Development of a clinical prediction rule for diagnosing hip osteoarthritis in individuals with unilateral hip pain. J Orthop Sports Phys Ther 38: 542–550.

Taylor K. 2009. Paternalism, participation, and partnership: the evolution of patient centeredness in the consultation. Patient Educ Couns 74: 150–155.

Tijssen M, van Cingel R, Willemsen L, et al. 2012. Diagnostics of femoroacetabular impingement and labral pathology of the hip: a systematic review of the accuracy and validity of physical tests. Arthroscopy 28(6): 860–871.

Tomaczak RL, VanCourt R. 2000. Metatarsal insufficiency fractures in previously undiagnosed osteoporosis patients. J Foot Ankle Surg 39: 174–183.

Underwood M 2009. Diagnosing acute nonspecific low back pain: time to lower the red flags? Arthritis Rheum 60: 2855–2857.

VanBuskirk KA, Wetherell JL. 2014 Motivational interviewing with primary care populations: a systematic review and meta-analysis. J Behav Med 37(4):768–780. doi: 10.1007/s10865-013-9527-4.

Vroomen PC, de Krom MC, Wilmink JT, et al. 2002. Diagnostic value of history and physical examination in patients suspected of lumbosacral nerve root compression. J Neurol Neurosurg Psychiatry 72: 630–634.

Vucetic N, Bri ED, Svensson O. 1997. Clinical history in lumbar disc herniation: a prospective study in 160 patients. Acta Orthop Scand 68: 116–120.

Waddell G, Newton M, Henderson I. 1993. A Fear Avoidance Beliefs Questionnaire (FABQ) and the role of fear-avoidance beliefs in chronic low back pain and disability. Pain 52: 157–168.

Wagemakers HP, Heintjes EM, Boks SS, et al. 2008. Diagnostic value of history-taking and physical examination for assessing meniscal tears of the knee in general practice. Clin J Sport Med 18: 24–30.

Wagemakers HP, Luijsterburg PA, Boks SS, et al. 2012 Diagnostic accuracy of history taking and physical examination for assessing anterior cruciate ligament lesions of the knee in primary care. Arch Phys Med Rehabil 91: 1452–1459.

Walter A, Bundy C, Dornan T. 2005. How should trainees be taught to open a clinical interview? Med Educ 39: 492–496.

Ware JE, Snow KK, Kolinsky M, et al. 1993. SF-36 health survey: manual and interpretation guide. Boston: The Health Institute.

Wells PS, Anderson DR, Bormanis J, et al. 1997. Value of assessment of pretest probability of deep-vein thrombosis in clinical management. Lancet 350: 1795–1798.

Williamson E. 2006. Fear Avoidance Beliefs Questionnaire (FABQ). Austr J Physiother 52: 149.

Woolf AD. 2003. How to assess musculoskeletal conditions: history and physical examination. Best Pract Res Clin Rheumatol 17: 381–402.

Woolf CJ. 2011. Central sensitization: implications for the diagnosis and treatment of pain. Pain 152: S2–S15.

Yan R, Wang H, Yang Z, et al. 2011. Predicted probability of meniscus tears: comparing history and physical examination with MRI. Swiss Med Wkly 141: w13314.

Zusman M. 1998. Irritability. Man Ther 3(4): 195–202.

Chapter 5

Physical Examination

Shane Koppenhaver, Timothy Flynn, Jennifer Crane

CHAPTER CONTENTS

Introduction	47
Observation and screening for medical conditions	48
Screening for severe injuries to the spine	50
Screening for neurological deficits	51
Nerve root examination	51
Upper motor neuron examination	59
Cranial nerve examination	60
Clearing the spine	60
Region-specific examination	63

Introduction

The physical examination is a continuation of a comprehensive patient history and interview. No matter how thorough the physical examination is, it cannot substitute for an incomplete patient history. After completing the history and patient interview, the examiner should have an appreciation of the severity of symptoms, the potential irritability of the condition (once provoked, how long do symptoms take to ease?) and the stage of the process (acute, subacute, or chronic). The clinician should also have formed a reasonable hypothesis, or several competing hypotheses, about the likely pathology or treatment classification, as well as an initial prognostic assessment. Furthermore, the clinician should have an initial understanding of the social, environmental and behavioural factors influencing the patient's status. The physical examination then focuses on testing these initial hypotheses formed during the history taking and on gaining any additional information necessary to establish an appropriate treatment plan and patient prognosis. It should be systematic, yet adaptable to the individual patient findings that support or refute the examiner's primary and alternative hypotheses. Finally, the real power of a comprehensive physical examination to aid in healing cannot be underestimated. An examination is a therapy in that, if performed in a competent and compassionate fashion, facilitates a positive clinician–patient relationship.

A comprehensive physical examination consists first of using various tests and measures to screen the neuromotor and vascular systems and subsequently focusing on region-specific procedures. However, before discussing the tests involved in the physical clinical exam, this chapter discusses the psychometric properties of the various tests and measures the clinician must understand in order to select the most useful tests, accurately interpret their results, and move forward with appropriate treatment (see also Ch 4).

The assessment of diagnostic tests involves examining several different properties, including reliability and diagnostic accuracy. **Reliability** describes the degree of consistency with which an instrument or rater measures a particular attribute (Portney & Watkins 2009). The reliability of a test tells the clinician the proportion of the measure that is a true representation, and the proportion that is a result of measurement error. Intra-rater reliability is the consistency between different measurements taken by one person, whereas inter-rater reliability is the consistency between measurements taken by two or more people. Reliability is most often quantified by the use of reliability coefficients that range between 0 (no agreement) to 1 (perfect agreement). Intra-class correlation coefficients (ICCs) are the most common reliability coefficients used to estimate reliability of data that is measured on a continuous scale (e.g. degrees of range of motion). Kappa (κ) coefficients are the preferred reliability coefficients used with categorical data (e.g. positive vs negative) as they statistically correct for change associations. Interpretations of reliability coefficients vary, but generally are as follows: < 0.50 represents poor reliability, 0.50–0.74 represents moderate reliability, and greater than 0.75 represents good reliability (Portney & Watkins 2009).

The **diagnostic accuracy** of a test is most often quantified by the measure of agreement between the test and a reference standard, which is the criterion that is considered the closest representation of whether or not a disorder is present. The results of the reference standard are compared with the results of the clinical test being studied, to determine the percentage of people who were correctly diagnosed with the test under investigation. When interpreting the reported diagnostic utility of a test, it is vital for clinicians to keep in mind both the reference standard used and the population that was studied; this will help them to decide whether the results are applicable to their own patient population. Diagnostic accuracy is typically expressed in terms of sensitivity and specificity, and positive–negative likelihood ratios. **Sensitivity** (true positive rate) is defined as the ability of a test to identify correctly patients who have a particular disorder (Portney & Watkins 2009; Straus 2011). A highly sensitive test is most valuable when it is negative, as this can help to rule out a specific diagnosis. However, highly sensitive tests will often be positive in a number of individuals that do not have the disorder being studied. Therefore a positive result of a highly sensitive test is of less value than a negative result. **Specificity** (true negative rate), in contrast, is the ability of a test to identify correctly patients who do not have a particular disorder. Highly specific tests are good at ruling in a condition and, as such, a positive finding would probably be a true positive. A perfect predictor would be described as 100% sensitive (i.e. predicting all people from the sick group as sick) and 100% specific (i.e. not predicting anyone from the healthy group as sick).

Likelihood ratios (LRs) are often more clinically useful than sensitivity and specificity as they determine shifts in the probability of the patient having a specific disorder (Hayden & Brown 1999). LRs are calculated by incorporating both the sensitivity and specificity of a test and can be used to estimate directly the likelihood that the disorder is present. If the test under investigation is positive, then the positive likelihood ratio (+LR) is used to determine the increased likelihood that the patient has the disorder. If the test is negative, the negative likelihood ratio (−LR) is used to determine the decreased probability of the patient having the disorder. The following scale is used to determine the significance of +LRs: 10 or greater generates a large and often conclusive shift in probability, 5–10 generates moderate shifts in probability, 2–5 indicates small but occasionally important shifts, and less than 2 indicates a rarely important shift in probability (Portney & Watkins 2009). With −LRs, less than 0.1 indicates a large shift in probability, 0.1–0.2 demonstrates a moderate shift, 0.2–0.5 indicates a small shift, and 0.5–1 shows a rarely important shift (Portney & Watkins 2009).

Clinicians should select tests and measures that are reliable and have high diagnostic utility. For example, screening tests refer to a group of tests that can be used to decrease the likelihood of a particular condition being present. Therefore a screening test should be highly sensitive and have a small −LR. The real value in a screening test is that a negative result, when using a highly sensitive test with a very small −LR, dramatically lowers the probability that the patient has the condition (i.e. the clinician can confidently 'rule it out'). Typically, screening tests will have an increased number of false positives (since they are highly sensitive) and thus a positive screening test should alert the clinician to perform a more thorough investigation to rule in or rule out the condition. On the other hand, region-specific procedures are generally deductive in nature, and should be highly specific and have large +LRs. It is imperative therefore that clinicians understand the diagnostic properties of the clinical examination tests they perform. For example, frequently clinicians will get a positive test result when utilizing a highly sensitive test (−LR is small) and immediately label the patient with that disorder without considering the possibility of a false-positive test result. This is often why novice clinicians become more confused the more testing they do, as more testing will increase the number of false positives.

The screening portion of the physical examination is a continuation of the review of systems that occurs during the patient history. Whereas some elements should be routinely performed on all patients, the inclusion of other components will be driven by findings from the history and other physical examination. Most inclusively, a comprehensive screening examination will consist of:

- observation
- screening for known and unknown medical diseases or conditions
- screening for severe injuries to the spine
- screening for neurological deficits
- 'clearing' the spine (in other words, removing the cervical or lumbar spine structures as prime contributors to the patient's complaints).

The region-specific portion of the physical examination should also be tailored by the history and other findings during the physical examination. A comprehensive region-specific examination, however, will always consist of:

- active movements
- passive movements (with and without overpressure)
- palpation
- clinical special tests.

Because the screening portion of the physical examination is basically the same regardless of the specific location of primary symptoms, it will be the focus of this general physical examination chapter. Although the region-specific part of any examination should include the same general components, the specific evaluative procedures will depend on the location of primary symptoms and the potential joints and soft tissues involved. However, emerging evidence demonstrates that many spine and extremity pain syndromes are appropriately managed with manual techniques targeted at the spine (Hurwitz et al 2002; Childs et al 2004; Cleland et al 2007; Iverson et al 2008; Boyles et al 2009) and thus those regions that will be treated require screening prior to performing manual interventions. Subsequent chapters will focus on the relevant pathology-specific examination procedures for specific disorders.

Observation and Screening for Medical Conditions

The initial questions that should be at the forefront of a musculoskeletal practitioner's mind during the physical examination is whether or not the patient's symptoms are consistent with neuro-musculoskeletal pathology and whether the patient may require immediate referral to another specialist. As discussed in Chapters 3 and 4, many visceral pathologies can cause symptoms that may be confused with neuro-musculoskeletal conditions, screening for which is primarily done by conducting a comprehensive and detailed patient history and interview. However, symptoms from neuro-musculoskeletal pathology should also be able to be reproduced and / or exacerbated during a comprehensive neuro-musculoskeletal physical exam. When patients report symptoms of moderate to severe intensity that the examiner is unable to reproduce and / or exacerbate during the physical exam, he or she should be highly suspicious of underlying medical pathology.

Signs of non-neuro-musculoskeletal pathology can often be noted during the initial observation portion of the physical examination. For this reason, the clothing over any region of symptoms should be removed and the area should be closely inspected for any abnormalities. Primary skin lesions (e.g. a macule, papule, patch, wheal, or cyst) may be immediately discoverable during observation. Although most primary skin lesions are not emergent, a musculoskeletal practitioner may be the first provider to discover the lesion, and at a minimum the patient should be told to discuss the lesion with their primary care provider. However, primary skin lesions that are associated with fever, difficulty in breathing or swallowing, or tenderness with mucosal involvement may be life threatening and require immediate emergent referral (Cole & Gray-Miceli 2002).

During observation, providers may additionally discover signs of fever, an abdominal mass or atraumatic swelling. The presence of a pulsatile abdominal mass may represent an abdominal aortic aneurysm and this requires immediate emergent referral. Atraumatic swelling, especially joint effusion, may signify an infectious or malignant process and should prompt further examination and / or immediate referral to another specialist.

Vascular disorders of the cervical arterial system (i.e. vertebrobasilar and carotid arteries) can present as head and neck pain. Occlusion of these arteries may lead to ischaemia with symptoms ranging from dizziness, diplopia, dysarthria, dysphagia, drop attacks, nausea, nystagmus, facial numbness, ataxia, vomiting, hoarseness, loss of short-term memory, vagueness, hypotonia / limb weakness, anhidrosis (lack of facial sweating), hearing disturbances, malaise, perioral dysaesthesia, photophobia, papillary changes, clumsiness and agitation to permanent neurological damage and death (Kerry & Taylor 2009). Damage to the arterial system, particularly the vertebrobasilar artery, has been linked to cervical manipulation (Ernst 2007). Several screening procedures have been advocated to identify patients at risk for vertebrobasilar insufficiency. The tests usually involve cervical postures that put stress on the vertebrobasilar system and monitor for signs and symptoms suggestive of such compromise (e.g. dizziness, diplopia, dysarthria, nystagmus, etc.) (Childs et al 2005). Unfortunately no studies have demonstrated the ability of such tests to identify effectively either those patients with vertebrobasilar insufficiency or those at risk of having a cerebrovascular accident. Table 5.1 provides a summary of physical examination procedures designed to differentiate vascular head and neck pain. Kerry and Taylor (2009) have provided prudent advice to clinicians by encouraging them to develop a high index of suspicion for cervical vascular pathology, particularly in cases of cervical trauma. More recently, an international framework for examining the cervical region prior to manual interventions has been developed (Rushton et al 2014). However, the clinician must balance this 'alertness' with the knowledge that the chronic-pain mentality and psychological factors are major issues in this patient group and should, therefore, be sensitive to the possible impact of reinforcing biomedical beliefs about a chronic-pain episode.

At a minimum, screening for cervical artery dysfunctions should include a detailed historical exam (when the patient reports of trauma and / or signs or symptoms consistent with compromise to the vascular system), and the physical exam portion of screening should include routine physical

Table 5.1 **Important physical examination procedures for differentiating vasculogenic head and neck pain**

Test	Purpose	Evidence status	Limitation and advantages
Functional positional test, cervical rotation	Affects flow in contralateral vertebral artery. Limited effect on internal carotid artery.	Poor sensitivity, variable specificity. Blood-flow studies support effect on vertebral artery flow.	Only assesses posterior circulation. Results should be interpreted with caution. Recommended by existing protocols. Cannot predict propensity for injury.
Functional positional test, cervical extension	Affects flow in internal carotid arteries. Limited effect on vertebral arteries.	No specific diagnostic utility evidence available. Blood-flow studies support effect on internal carotid artery flow.	Primarily assesses anterior circulation.
Blood pressure examination	Measure of cardiovascular health.	Correlates to cervical arterial atherosclerotic pathology.	Reliability dependent on equipment, environment and experience. Continuous, not categorical, measure.
Cranial nerve examination	Identifies specific cranial nerve dysfunction resulting from ischaemia or vessel compression.	No specific diagnostic utility evidence available.	Reliability dependent on experience.
Eye examination	Assists in diagnosis of possible neural deficit related to internal carotid artery dysfunction.	No specific diagnostic utility evidence available.	Eye symptoms may be early warning of serious underlying pathology.
Handheld Doppler ultrasound	Direct assessment of blood-flow velocity.	Limited manual therapy specific evidence. Existing studies suggest good to require further study.	Reliability dependent on equipment, environment and experience.

(Modified and adapted from Kerry R, Taylor AJ. 2006. Cervical arterial dysfunction assessment and manual therapy. Man Ther 11: 243–253.)

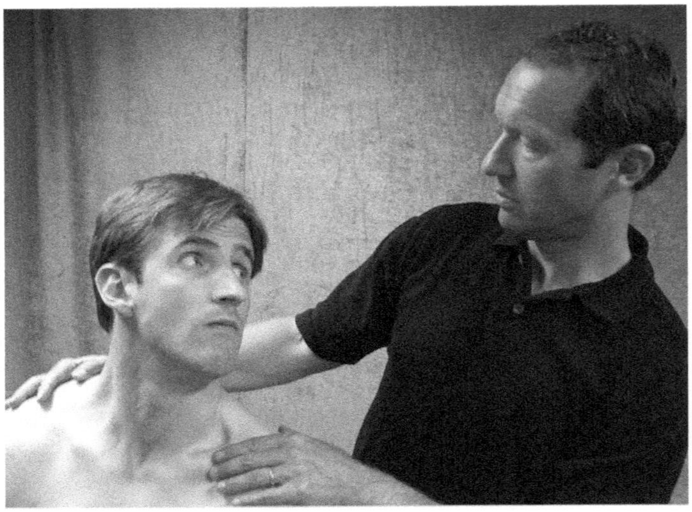

Figure 5.1 Observing eyes during combined extension, rotation and side-bending motion. (From Flynn et al 2008, with permission.)

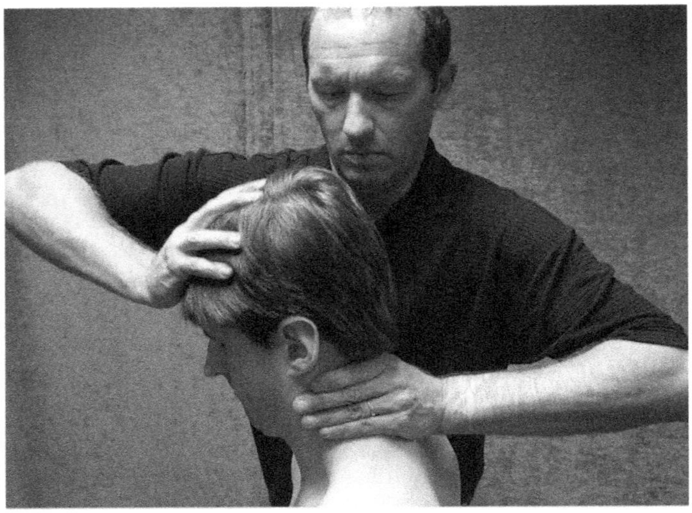

Figure 5.2 Sharp–Purser test. (From Flynn et al 2008, with permission.)

assessment using incrementally greater movements and loads of the cervical spine (Rushton et al 2014). When 'clearing' the cervical spine (see later section), the examiner should constantly observe the patient's response during cervical range of motion, especially during rotation and combined extension, rotation and side-bending motions (Fig. 5.1). In addition to assessing for nystagmus, the examiner should also note the presence of dizziness, lightheadedness, impaired sensation to the face, blurred vision, or other signs or symptoms consistent with compromise to the vertebrobasilar complex.

A thorough history is vital when screening the lumbar spine for medical conditions such as spinal tumour or infection. Most red flags for both malignancy and infection are discovered during the patient interview, and are more diagnostically valuable when combined with the findings of the physical examination, as opposed to in isolation (Henschke et al 2007, 2009). As always, the clinician should learn to be suspicious whenever the patient demonstrates symptoms or exam findings inconsistent with neuro-musculoskeletal pathology.

Screening for Severe Injuries to the Spine

Undiagnosed vertebral fracture should be a concern to the clinician when differentiating the origin of symptoms in the spine, especially after any sort of trauma. The Canadian C-spine rule and the NEXUS low-risk criteria are clinical decision rules that indicate when to order cervical spine radiographs to rule out cervical fractures (Stiell et al 2003) and these have been detailed in Chapter 3. Both criteria are excellent at ruling out clinically important cervical spine fractures (Stiell et al 2003) and the Canadian C-spine rule has been shown to be superior to clinician judgement in ordering radiography (Bandiera et al 2003).

In screening for fracture in the lumbar spine, most red flags should be discovered whilst taking the patient history. A systematic review (Henschke et al 2008) discussed five red flags that are essential to the history when screening for lumbar vertebral fracture: acute trauma, acute pain and tenderness, age > 50 years, female gender and distracting painful injury. A further study (Henschke et al 2009) derived a clinical prediction rule identifying four features that were reported to predict lumbar spinal fracture: age > 70 years, female gender, significant trauma and prolonged use of corticosteroids. The researchers found that the presence of three or more of these factors increased the post-test probability of vertebral fracture from 0.5% to 52%; however, this finding has not been validated at this time. These studies accentuate the importance of taking a thorough history in patients with low back pain.

In addition, upper cervical spine instability should be screened for in the presence of any predisposing factors, especially before administering any mechanical treatment such as mobilization, manipulation, or traction of the upper cervical spine. Upper cervical spine instability has been associated with trauma and infection, and is also commonly reported in patients with rheumatoid arthritis because of the chronic inflammation and subsequent tissue degeneration in this condition (Sizer et al 2007). Additionally, people with congenital disorders such as Down syndrome (Salman Riaz 2007), Marfan syndrome (Demetracopoulos & Sponseller, 2007) and other skeletal dysplasias (Song & Maher 2007) are at increased risk of experiencing upper cervical spine instability.

Several clinical tests have been purported to screen for upper cervical spine instability by testing for laxity of the transverse ligament of the atlas (TLA), of which the TLA test and the Sharp–Purser test are perhaps the most widely known. To perform the TLA test, the examiner grasps the cranium of a sitting patient with one hand whilst stabilizing C2 against C3 in a ventral–caudal direction. The examiner then translates the cranium and C1 in a ventral direction. The test is repeated in each lateral direction and considered to be positive when symptoms are reproduced during the test (Sizer et al 2007). The Sharp–Purser test is performed on a patient who is sitting with the neck in a semiflexed position. With one hand on the patient's forehead and the index finger of the other hand on the spinous process of axis, the examiner applies posterior pressure through the patient's forehead (Fig. 5.2). A sliding motion of the head posteriorly in relation to the axis indicates a positive test for atlanto-axial instability. Although the diagnostic utility of the TLA test is unknown, the single study to investigate the Sharp–Purser test found it to be highly specific in identifying upper cervical spine instability as defined by radiographic evidence of an atlantodens interval of greater than 3 mm (Uitvlugt & Indenbaum 1988). The resulting +LR of 17.3 and −LR of 0.32 suggest that the Sharp–Purser test may be very helpful in both ruling in and ruling out upper cervical spine instability. However, this was studied only in subjects with rheumatoid arthritis, so it is not known how this test would perform in a different population.

Furthermore, as with most screening tests, the paucity of studies investigating tests for upper cervical spine instability should not prevent clinicians from performing them or, perhaps more importantly, using robust clinical reasoning during screening for such disorders. The importance of clinical reasoning and upper cervical ligament testing has been well documented in case studies (Elliott & Cherry 2008; Mintken et al 2008) that illustrate the potential effects of upper cervical spine instability as well as how positive outcomes can be obtained if properly diagnosed.

Screening for Neurological Deficits

In addition to screening for more serious neurological diseases, musculoskeletal providers should attempt to screen for radiculopathies and myelopathies. Radiculopathies are disorders of the spinal nerve roots as they exit the spinal column. They are most commonly caused by disc herniation or other space-occupying lesions and result in inflammation and / or impingement of the nerve root (Wainner et al 2003). Patients with cervical radiculopathy may or may not experience pain, which if present commonly occurs in the neck, upper extremity and thoracic regions (Slipman et al 1998). Pain associated with lumbar radiculopathy is often described as 'aching', 'burning' or 'sharp' pain that typically presents in the low back, buttocks, and one or both legs (Tomić et al 2009). Additionally, both cervical and lumbar radiculopathy commonly cause unilateral extremity strength, sensation and reflex deficits that are confined to the distribution of the affected nerve root(s) (Murphy et al 2009; Tomić et al 2009). With lumbar radiculopathy (with the exception of S1), the symptoms are less likely to follow specific dermatomal patterns than with cervical radiculopathy (Murphy et al 2009).

Myelopathies, as opposed to radiculopathies, are disorders of the spinal cord and are discussed in detail in Chapter 11. Theoretically, they can occur at any vertebral level from C1 to where the spinal cord terminates at approximately L1 (Macdonald et al 1999); however, they are most common in the cervical spine. Initial symptoms of cervical myelopathy tend to be described as generalized neck pain or stiffness. Myelopathies of the mid-cervical spine (C3–C5) often progress to cause more distal pain and symptoms of numb and / or 'clumsy' hands. In the lower cervical spine (C6–T1), symptoms typically also include weakness and proprioceptive losses in the legs that can result in gait disturbances.

Myelopathies and radiculopathies can often be difficult to distinguish from one another. Moreover, they are not mutually exclusive as many patients have disorders that affect both the nerve roots and the spinal cord. That said, the two most obvious discriminators between the conditions are the presence of bilateral or unilateral symptoms and of upper motor neuron or lower motor neuron symptoms. Patients with simple (single unilateral level) radiculopathies classically present with unilateral lower motor symptoms only, whereas patients with myelopathies typically present with bilateral symptoms that include upper motor neuron signs. Moreover, a radiculopathy affecting a single nerve root can theoretically be identified by the pattern and location of dermatomal and myotomal symptoms. (Readers are referred to Chs 11 and 17 for further discussion on these conditions.)

Cauda equina syndrome is a related neurological condition in which compression to the cauda equina causes acute damage to the lumbar plexus (nerve roots) of the spinal canal below the termination of the spinal cord at L1 (Macdonald et al 1999). Like many other red flags in patient care, this syndrome should be discovered during a thorough patient history taking and is considered a medical emergency. The lower motor nerves comprising the cauda equina supply the majority of the sensory and motor innervation to most of the lower extremities and pelvic region and, as such, the symptoms include multisegment sensory and motor changes. The most common symptoms that the clinician should inquire about include bilateral leg pain, saddle region anaesthesia, loss or change in bowel and bladder control, and severe back pain (Fraser et al 2009; Shi et al 2010). The clinician should make it a priority to screen for this condition, as it is a medical emergency frequently requiring immediate surgical intervention.

Nerve root examination

Traditional neurological screening consists of sensation, muscle stretch reflex and manual muscle testing. Although for decades it has been considered a key component of any standard neuro-musculoskeletal examination, very little evidence exists regarding the diagnostic utility of traditional neurological screening. The one study (Wainner et al 2003) to investigate the diagnostic utility of neurological testing in the upper quarter did so by comparing findings with a diagnosis of cervical radiculopathy via needle electromyography and nerve conduction studies. The findings from this study suggested that neurological testing in the upper quarter is of only moderate benefit, and is most robust when combining multiple positive findings, as opposed to taking the results in isolation.

Studies investigating the diagnostic utility of neurological testing of the lower quarter report similar findings. In a Cochrane review (van der Windt et al 2010), authors appraised the available evidence of neurological testing to identify radiculopathy due to lumbar disc herniation. Sensation, muscle strength and reflexes were of little help when used in isolation, but were of moderate utility if used in combination in screening for lumbar radiculopathy. These results, however, were obtained in populations with a very high prevalence of disc herniation (> 75% in nearly all studies); therefore they cannot necessarily be generalized to populations with a lower prevalence of that condition.

Although findings from these studies suggest that neurological exam testing may be marginally helpful in identifying radiculopathy, it is important to note the challenges of performing such research. First of all, there is no universally agreed-upon definition of radiculopathy; some sources define it solely by the clinical exam (Magee 2008), whereas others use imaging or electrophysiological findings as the criterion standard (Rubinstein et al 2007; van der Windt et al 2010). Additionally, there is wide individual anatomical variation in nerve root innervations (Magee 2008), which means that operational definitions of what constitutes positive findings for each nerve root may greatly affect the reported diagnostic utilities of the tests. Lastly, the symptoms associated with radiculopathies have been reported to be highly variable and somewhat unpredictable (Slipman et al 1998; Cook 2007; Murphy et al 2009; Tomić et al 2009); this naturally decreases the ability of even a highly reliable test to identify underlying pathologies.

Therefore, we advocate that sensation, muscle stretch reflex and manual muscle test screening be routinely performed as a part of every musculoskeletal examination. In addition to being prudent from a neurological perspective, sensation, muscle stretch reflex and manual muscle testing is largely considered the standard of care and therefore should also be performed from a legal / ethical perspective. Finally, the results of the neurological screening can be used as interim outcome measures to judge a patient's response to treatment.

Sensation

Although light touch and pin-prick are the most common testing procedures, sensation can also be tested by various other methods including two-point discrimination, vibration and temperature testing. In general, dermatomal patterns of sensory changes are thought to be associated with radiculopathies, whereas multiple-level and / or bilateral patterns of dermatomal changes are associated with myelopathies (Sizer et al 2007). Although there is some individual anatomical variation in dermatomal nerve root innervations (Magee 2008), Figure 5.3 illustrates a typical dermatomal map. Wainner et al (2003) tested pin-prick sensation graded as normal or abnormal, and found poor diagnostic utility for identifying cervical radiculopathy at all dermatomal levels. With the exception of the C5 dermatome, decreased sensation demonstrated +LR point estimates of < 1 and −LR estimates of > 1. However, the fact that both +LR and −LR confidence intervals included '1' for all dermatomal levels indicates that the presence of decreased sensation in isolation is not a robust measure of the probability of having cervical radiculopathy.

In the lumbar spine, sensory exam findings are similar. Many studies have assessed the diagnostic utility of sensory testing, with unremarkable results. One study (Lauder et al 2000a) assessed sensation via pin-prick and vibration, and reported the finding as abnormal when either sensation was reduced on the side of the lesion. They reported a sensitivity of 0.50, specificity of 0.62, +LR of 1.32 and −LR of 0.81. In isolation, this gives the clinician very little confidence when using sensory testing to assess nerve root involvement. Similarly, a Cochrane review (van der Windt et al 2010) reported a range of sensitivities for sensory testing from 0.39 to 0.68, and

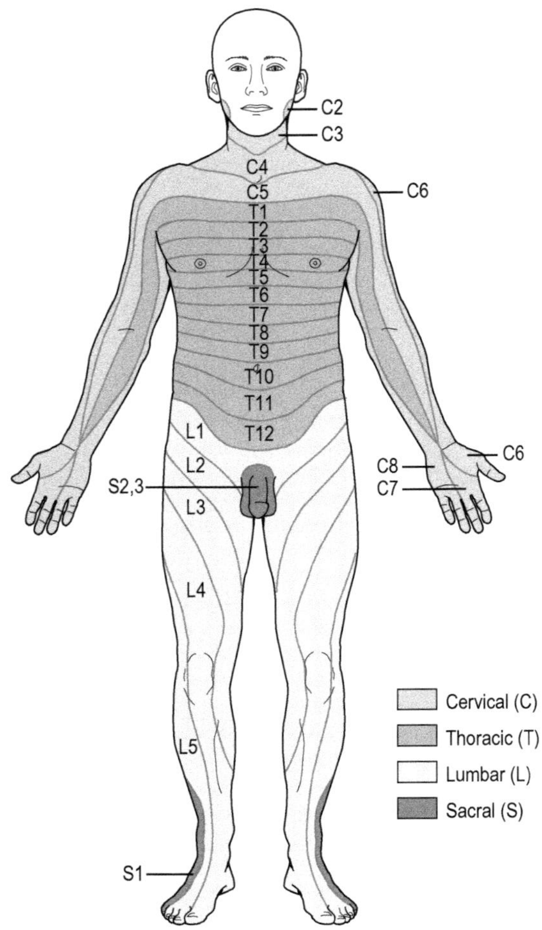

Figure 5.3 Typical dermatomes.

specificities ranging from 0.62 to 0.89. As discussed earlier in this chapter, screening tests should ideally be more sensitive than specific, so that clinicians can confidently rule out the disorder in the presence of a negative test. The fact that most studies have found higher specificity than sensitivity in sensory testing suggests that, when conducting a lumbar sensory exam, the clinician should be sceptical of a negative result as it may, in fact, be a false negative.

Nevertheless, a sensory screen provides a baseline level of patient presentation and should drive the examiner's subsequent testing, particularly if there is multisegmental or bilateral loss of sensation.

Myotomes

Like sensation, manual muscle testing has also been reported using various methods. Mostly commonly, isometric strength is tested by providing manual resistance to the muscle in the midrange of a joint's range of motion. The patient is instructed to 'not let me move you' as the examiner exerts enough force to surpass (break) the patient's maximal isometric resistance. The patient's maximum resistance is generally graded on a scale from 0 to 5, with some clinicians adding + or − to delineate the scale further:

- **5 (normal):** complete range of motion against gravity with full resistance

Table 5.2 **Manual muscle testing for the cervical nerve roots**

Nerve root	Primary muscles innervated	Test procedure
C1 and C2	Muscles that flex the neck	The examiner stabilizes the trunk with one hand and applies a posteriorly directed force through the patient's forehead while matching the resistance.
C3	Muscles that side-bend the neck	The examiner stabilizes the shoulder with one hand and applies a force away from the side to be tested while the patient is instructed to match the resistance.
C4	Muscles that elevate the shoulders	The patient is instructed to elevate the shoulders. The examiner applies an inferiorly directed force through the shoulders while the patient is instructed to match the resistance.
C5	Deltoids	The patient is instructed to abduct their shoulders to 90°. The examiner applies a force into adduction while the patient resists.
C6	Biceps braquii and extensor carpi radialis brevis and longus	The patient's elbow is flexed to 90° and the forearm supinated. The examiner applies a force into extension while the patient resists. The patient's elbow is flexed to 90°, forearm pronated, and wrist extended and radially deviated. The examiner applies a force into flexion and ulnar deviation while the patient resists.
C7	Triceps braquii and flexor carpi radialis	The patient's elbow is flexed to 90° and the examiner applies a force into elbow flexion while the patient resists. The patient's elbow is flexed to 90° with the wrist flexed and radially deviated with forearm supinated. The examiner applies a force into wrist extension and ulnar deviation while the patient resists.
C8	Abductor pollicis brevis	The examiner places the thumb in abduction. The examiner applies a resistance through the proximal phalanx in the direction of abduction while the patient resists.
T1	First dorsal interossei	The examiner separates the index and middle finger and applies a force against the lateral aspect of proximal phalanx of the index finger into adduction.

- **4 (good):** complete range of motion against gravity with some resistance
- **3 (fair):** complete range of motion against gravity
- **2 (poor):** complete range of motion gravity eliminated
- **1 (trace):** evidence of slight muscle contraction
- **0 (zero):** no evidence of muscle contraction.

Although all muscles are innervated by multiple nerve roots, those muscles that are primarily innervated by each level are selected to screen the cervical and lumbar nerve roots and these are listed in Tables 5.2 and 5.3; the testing of each muscle is illustrated in Figures 5.4–5.18.

Wainner et al (2003) tested manual muscle testing dichotomized as either normal or abnormal, and generally found poor diagnostic utility for identifying cervical radiculopathy. Although the +LR point estimates for the deltoids and biceps were 2.1 and 3.7 respectively, LR confidence intervals for every muscle included '1', indicating that the presence of isolated weakness may not alter the probability of having cervical radiculopathy.

A Cochrane review assessed seven studies that looked at strength of muscles innervated by lumbar nerve roots. They found similar results, with sensitivities ranging from 0.29 to 0.62, and specificities ranging from 0.50 to 0.89 (van der Windt et al 2010). In both the cervical and lumbar spine, weakness in one myotome alone does not provide adequate information. However, findings of gross weakness or multi-segmental weakness have not been studied, and these are more likely to be suggestive of myelopathy, peripheral nerve injury or neuromuscular disease.

Reflexes

Attenuated muscle stretch reflexes (MSRs) suggest lower motor neuron problems, mostly commonly of the spinal nerve roots (i.e. radiculopathy). Hyperactive muscle stretch reflexes can present an increased single response and / or repetitive response (clonus). Generally, the cervical nerve roots are screened by testing the biceps, brachioradialis and triceps MSRs and the lumbar nerve roots are assessed by testing the patellar and Achilles MSRs. These are illustrated in Figures 5.19–5.23. As with myotomes and sensation, MSR testing has been reported to be poorly sensitive for identifying (i.e. ruling out) cervical and lumbar radiculopathy (Lauder et al 2000b; Wainner et al 2003; van der Windt et al 2010), perhaps because many abnormalities of both efferent and afferent pathways via electromyography have been found to be subthreshold during MSR testing (Miller et al 1999). However, two studies (Lauder et al 2000b; Wainner et al 2003) found that the presence of a decreased biceps reflex substantially increased the probability of patients having (i.e. ruling in) a cervical radiculopathy (+LR 4.9–10). The findings of the studies conflicted, however, regarding the utility of a decreased brachioradialis or triceps reflex. Lauder et al (2000b) found +LRs of 2.0 for a decreased triceps reflex and 8.0 for a decreased brachioradialis reflex, whereas Wainner et al (2003) found +LRs that did not alter the probability of having cervical radiculopathy.

In assessing the lumbar nerve roots, Lauder et al (2000a) found the patellar reflex to have high specificity at 0.93, with a +LR of 7.14. However, a Cochrane review (van der Windt et al 2010) found a wide range for both Achilles and patellar

Table 5.3 Manual muscle testing for the lumbar nerve roots

Nerve root	Primary muscles innervated	Test procedure
L2–L3	Hip flexors	The patient flexes the hip to near end range and the examiner applies a force to the anterior thigh into hip extension while the patient resists.
L3–L4	Knee extensors	The patient extends the knee to a position slightly less than full extension. The examiner stabilizes the patient's thigh with one hand and applies pressure on the anterior distal tibia into knee flexion with the other while the patient resists. Step-up: the patient is instructed to step up onto a step stool. If the patient exhibits difficulty this could suggest involvement of the L3–L4 nerve root.
L4	Ankle dorsiflexors	The patient dorsiflexes the ankle with slight inversion. The examiner stabilizes the distal tibia with one hand and the other hand applies pressure on the dorsum of the foot into plantarflexion with some eversion while the patient resists.
L5	Hallux extension	The great toe is placed into extension. The examiner stabilizes the foot with one hand and applies pressure on the dorsum of the distal phalanx of the big toe into flexion while the patient resists.
L5–S1	Ankle plantar-flexors	The patient is asked to rise up on the toes. Inability or difficulty to do so in relation to the opposite side may be indicative of involvement of the L5–S1 nerve root.
S1–S2	Ankle evertors	The ankle is placed in full eversion and dorsiflexion. The examiner stabilizes the distal tibia with one hand and with the other hand applies pressure on the lateral aspect of the foot into plantarflexion and inversion while the patient resists.

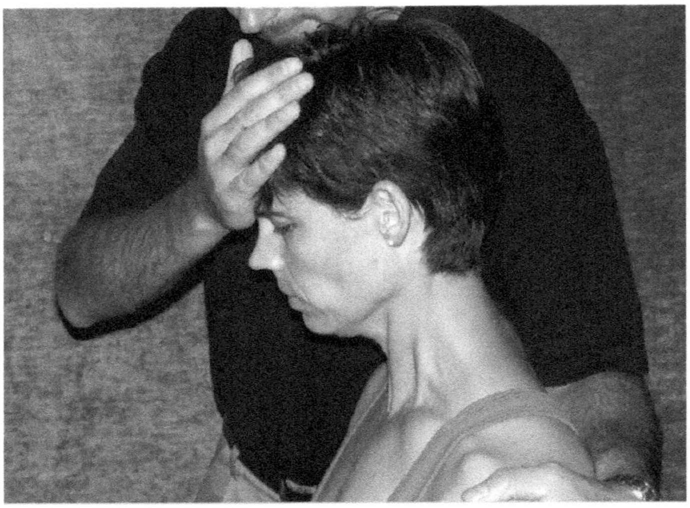

Figure 5.4 Cervical flexion (C1–C2). (From Flynn et al 2008, with permission.)

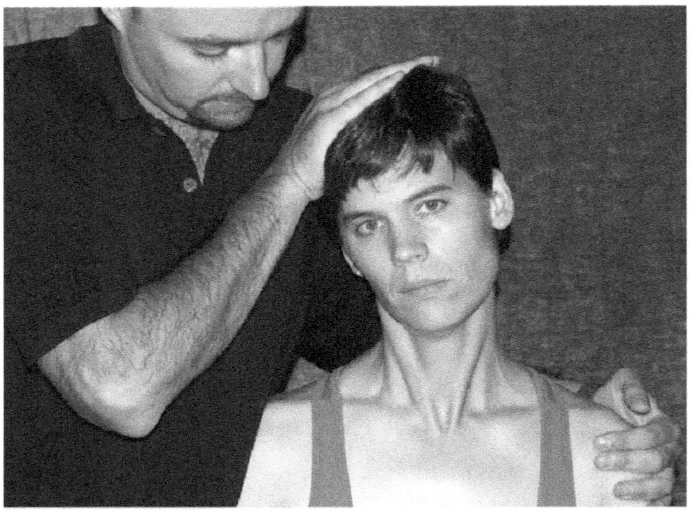

Figure 5.5 Cervical side-bending (C3). (From Flynn et al 2008, with permission.)

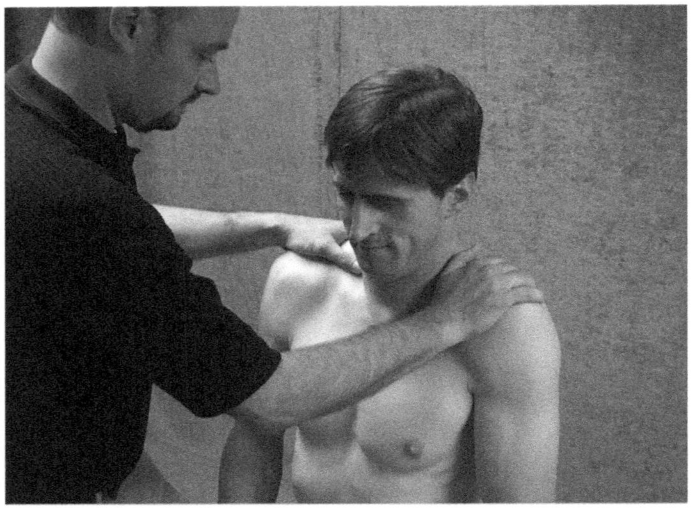

Figure 5.6 Shoulder elevation (C4). (From Flynn et al 2008, with permission.)

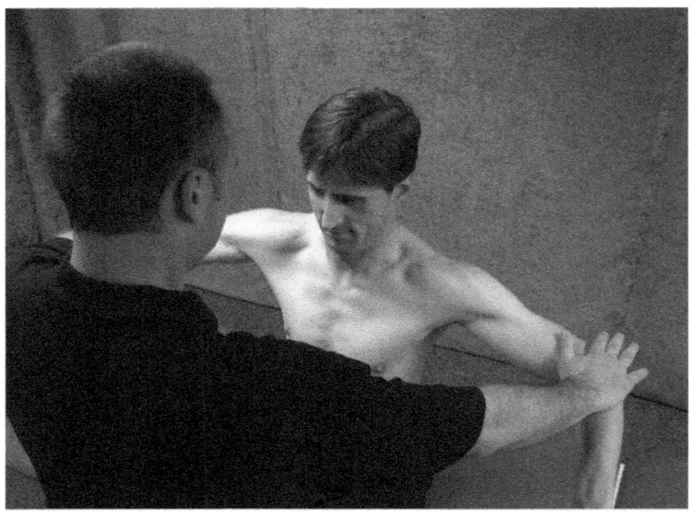

Figure 5.7 Shoulder abduction (C5). (From Flynn et al 2008, with permission.)

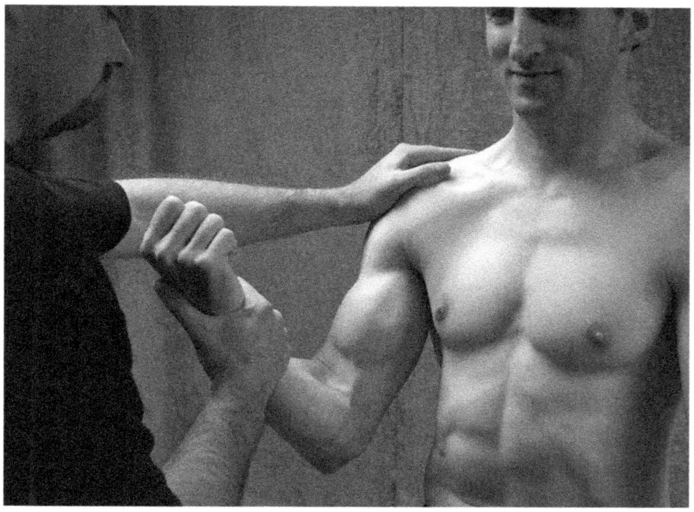

Figure 5.8 Elbow flexion (C6). (From Flynn et al 2008, with permission.)

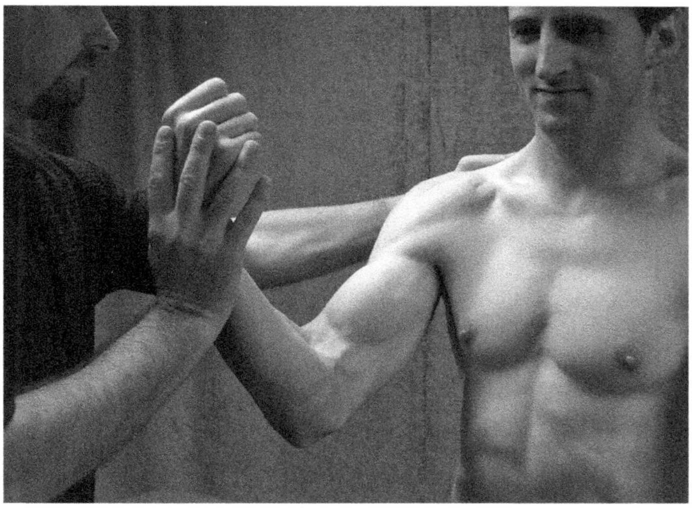

Figure 5.9 Elbow extension (C7). (From Flynn et al 2008, with permission.)

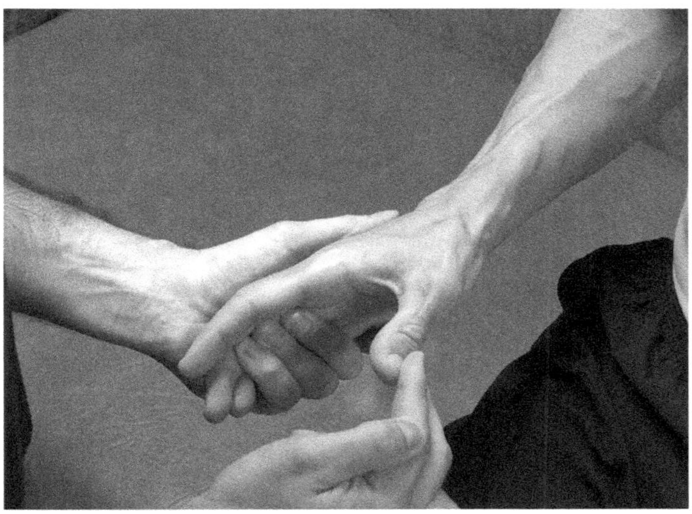

Figure 5.10 Thumb abduction (C8). (From Flynn et al 2008, with permission.)

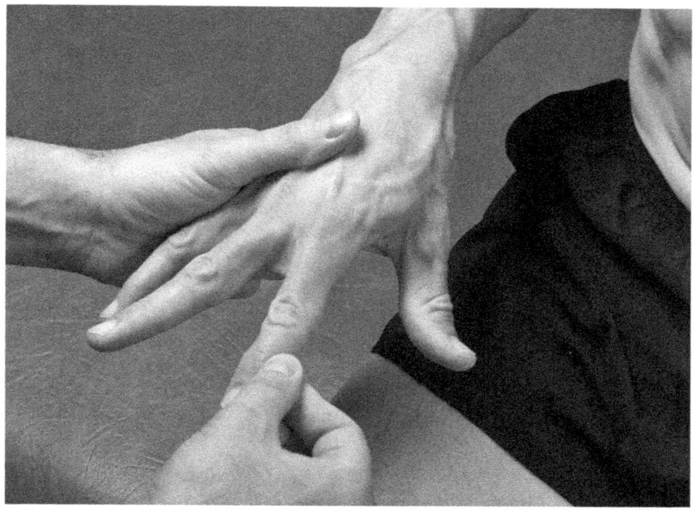

Figure 5.11 Finger abduction (T1). (From Flynn et al 2008, with permission.)

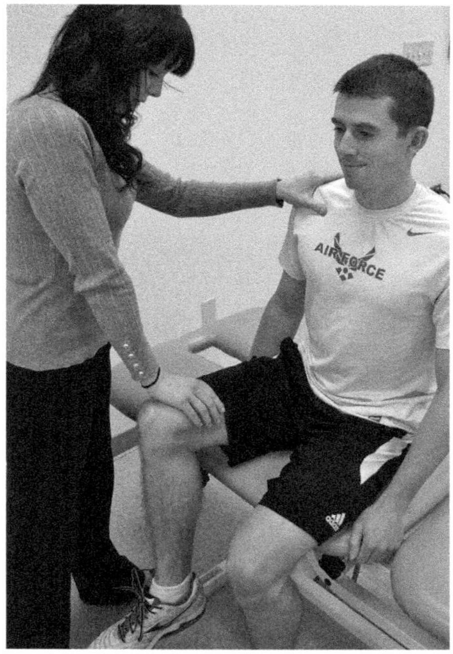

Figure 5.12 Hip flexion (L2–L3).

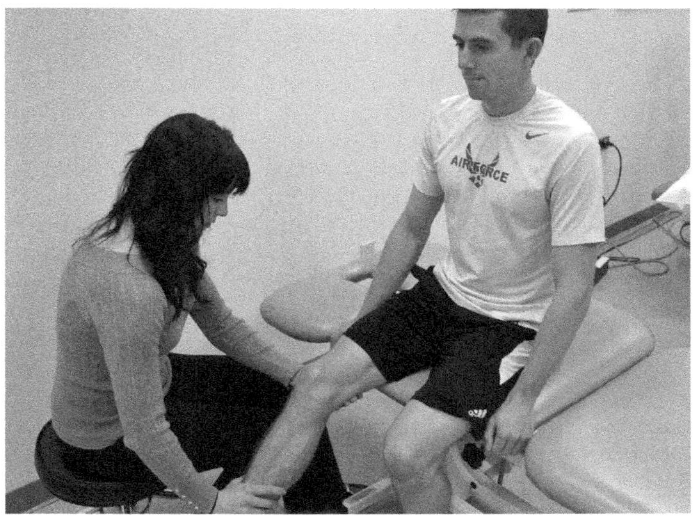

Figure 5.13 Knee extension (L3–L4).

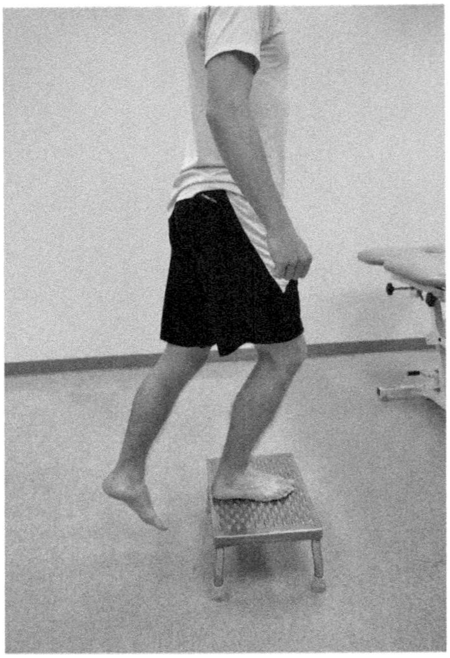

Figure 5.14 **Step up (L3–L4).**

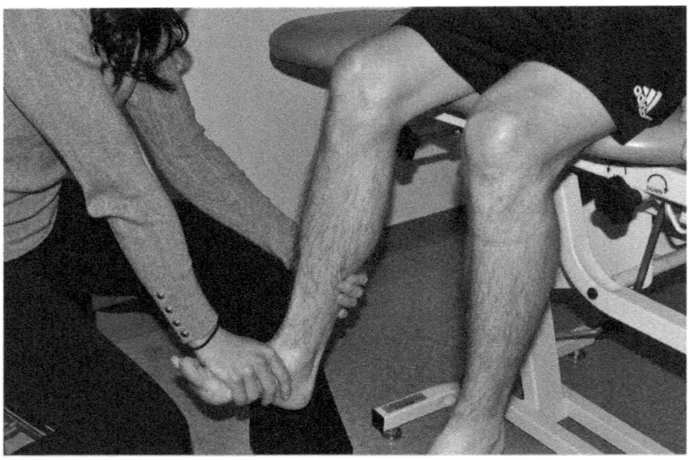

Figure 5.15 **Ankle dorsiflexion (L4).**

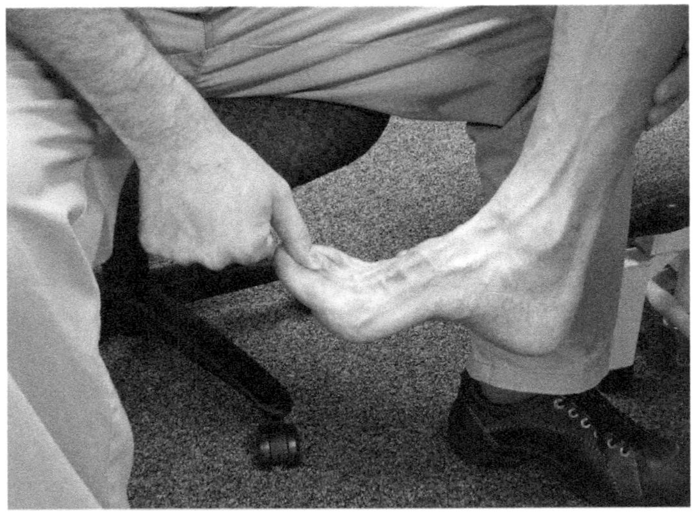

Figure 5.16 **Hallux extension (L5).** (From Flynn et al 2008, with permission.)

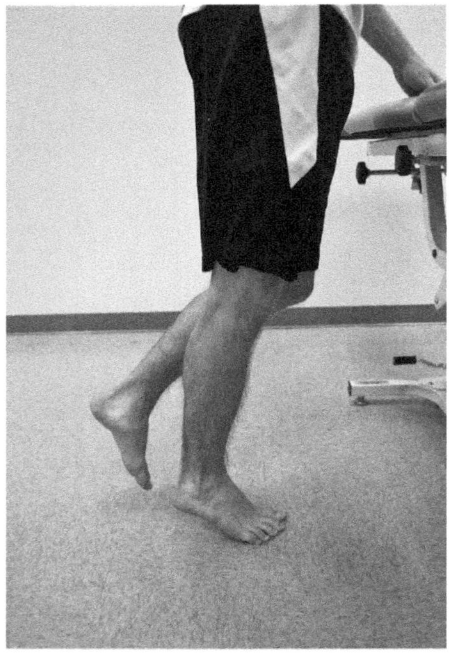

Figure 5.17 **Plantarflexion (L5–S1).**

reflexes. Achilles MSR, as assessed in seven different studies, demonstrated sensitivities ranging from 0.31 to 0.62, and specificities ranging from 0.60 to 0.89. Patellar MSR values also varied greatly in the studies assessed, making conclusions difficult to draw. Given the challenges of performing such studies and the lack of a superior evidence-based alternative, however, it is recommended that sensation testing, manual muscle testing and reflex testing are performed for all patients with spinal or extremity disorders.

Neurodynamic assessment

In addition to assessing sensation, manual muscle testing and MSRs, there are several tests that have been supported in literature to help rule out radiculopathy in both the cervical and lumbar spine. In the cervical neurological exam, two additional tests have been identified that, when performed in conjunction with cervical range of motion with overpressure, substantially alter the probability of a patient's symptoms originating from the cervical spine, or more specifically the presence of cervical radiculopathy. Wainner et al (2003) reported that when patients were found to have a positive upper limb tension test A, distraction test, Spurling's test, and cervical rotation less than 60° to the ipsilateral side, their probability of having a cervical radiculopathy was increased from 23% to 90% (+LR 30.3). If three of these four tests were positive, the probability of having cervical radiculopathy changed from 23% to 65% (+LR 6.1). Spurling's test is cervical side-bending with a downward and medially directed overpressure, and is therefore included in the general cervical screening

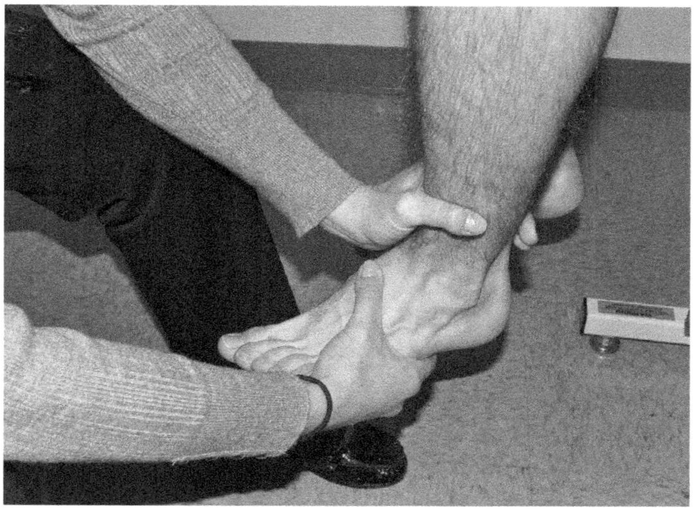

Figure 5.18 Ankle eversion (S1–S2).

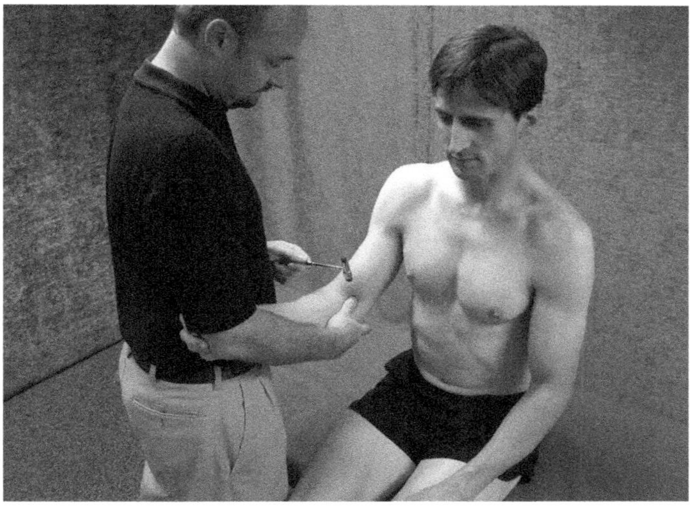

Figure 5.19 Testing biceps muscle stretch reflex. (From Flynn et al 2008, with permission.)

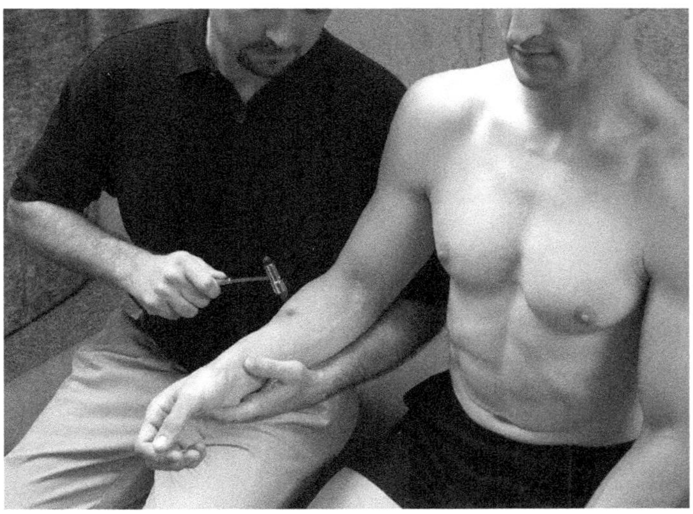

Figure 5.20 Testing brachioradialis muscle stretch reflex. (From Flynn et al 2008, with permission.)

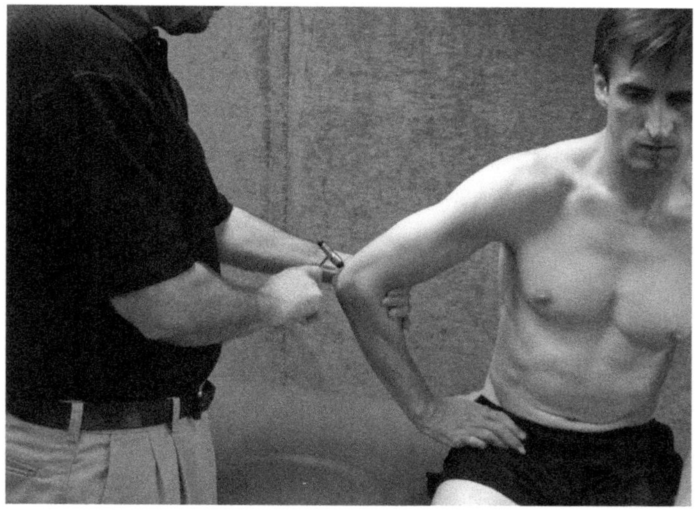

Figure 5.21 Testing triceps muscle stretch reflex. (From Flynn et al 2008, with permission.)

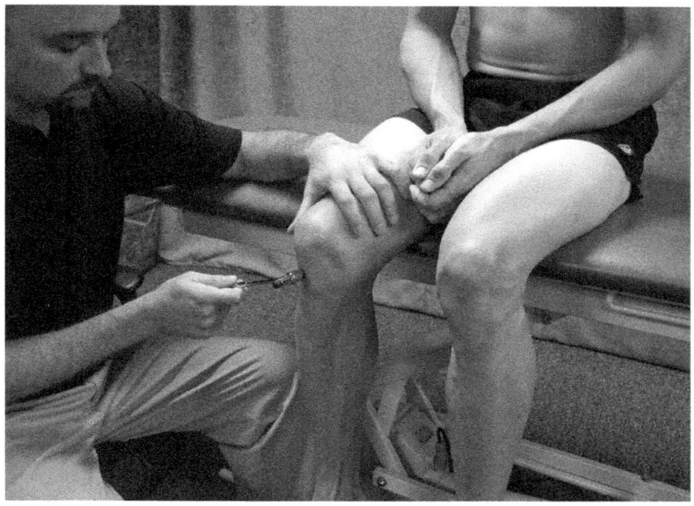

Figure 5.22 Testing patellar muscle stretch reflex. (From Flynn et al 2008, with permission.)

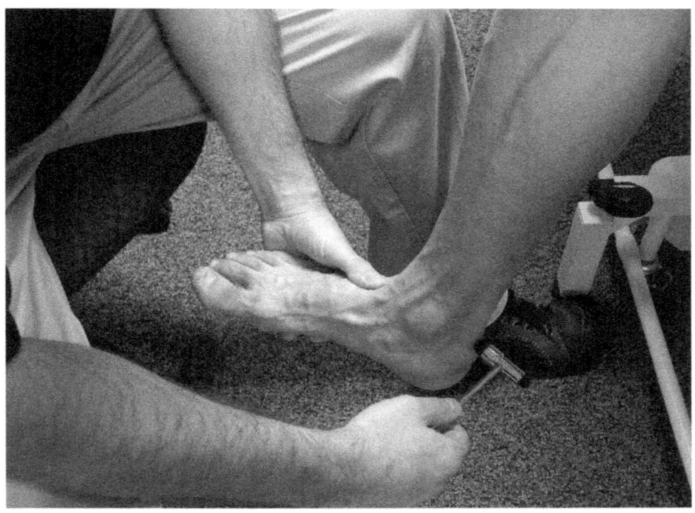

Figure 5.23 Testing Achilles muscle stretch reflex. (From Flynn et al 2008, with permission.)

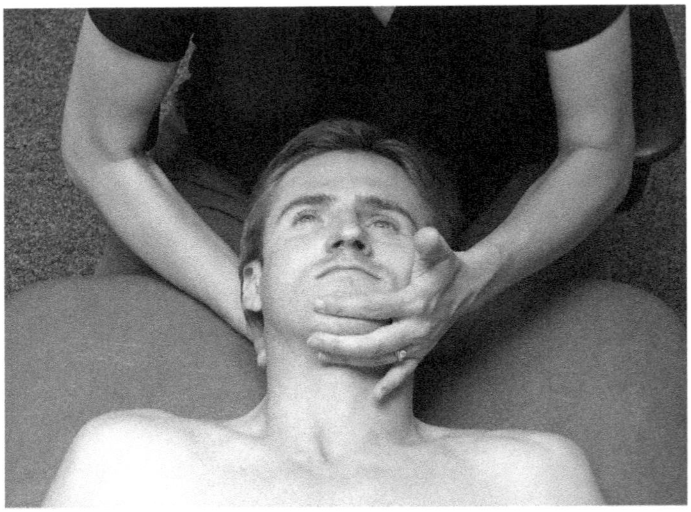

Figure 5.24 Cervical distraction. (From Flynn et al 2008, with permission.)

examination (see Ch 11). To perform cervical distraction, the examiner grasps a supine patient under the chin and occiput while slightly flexing the patient's neck and applies a distraction force of approximately 14 pounds (6 kg) (Fig. 5.24). The test is considered positive if the patient's symptoms are reduced during the manoeuvre. The upper limb tension test A is also performed with the patient supine. The examiner then performs the following movements in order (Fig. 5.25):

1. Scapular depression
2. Shoulder abduction
3. Forearm supination
4. Wrist and finger extension
5. Shoulder lateral rotation
6. Elbow extension
7. Contralateral / ipsilateral cervical side-bending.

A positive response is defined by any of the following:

1. Patient symptoms reproduced
2. Side-to-side differences in elbow extension > 10°
3. Contralateral cervical side-bending increases symptoms or ipsilateral side-bending decreases symptoms.

The upper limb tension test A (median nerve bias) used in isolation is helpful for ruling out cervical radiculopathy. The diagnostic accuracy has been demonstrated to be substantial (sensitivity 0.97, –LR 0.12) and thus a negative test significantly reduces the likelihood that a cervical radiculopathy is present. (Readers are referred to Ch 65 for further discussion of neurodynamic testing.)

In the lumbar spine, the straight leg raise (SLR) has been shown to be a good screening tool for ruling out lumbar radiculopathy (Devillé et al 2000). Pooled estimates from a meta-analysis of 11 patients (Devillé et al 2000) yielded a sensitivity of 0.91, specificity of 0.26, +LR of 1.23 and –LR of 0.35, indicating that a negative result is likely to be a true negative. The SLR is typically performed with the patient supine and knees fully extended, with their ankles in neutral dorsiflexion. The examiner passively flexes the hip while maintaining the knee in extension. The amount of hip flexion is recorded at the point of pain or paraesthesia in the back or leg (Fig. 5.26). A positive result is described as reproduction of symptoms at

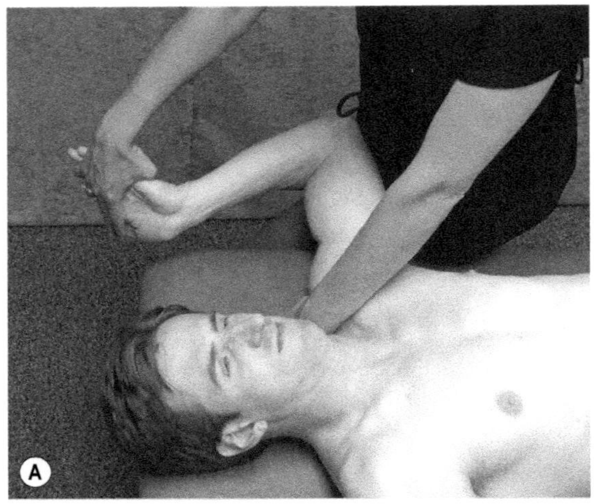

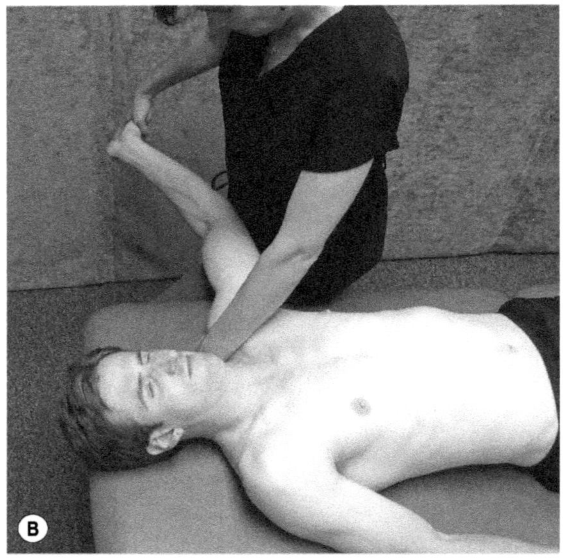

Figure 5.25 Upper limb tension test: (**A**) starting position, (**B**) ending position. (From Flynn et al 2008, with permission.)

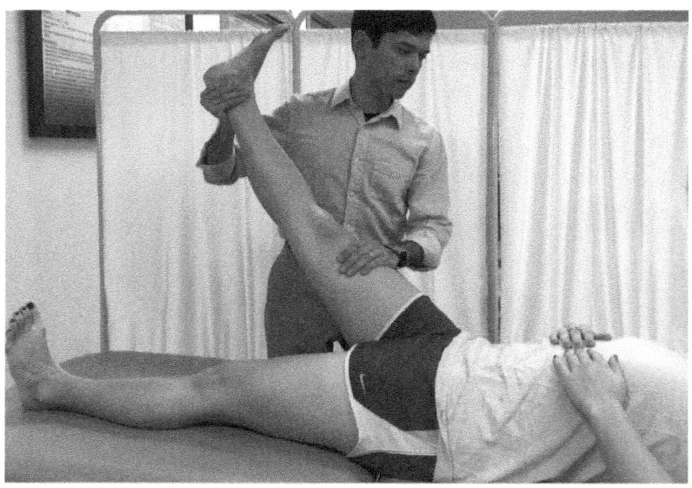

Figure 5.26 Straight leg raise. (From Flynn et al 2008, with permission.)

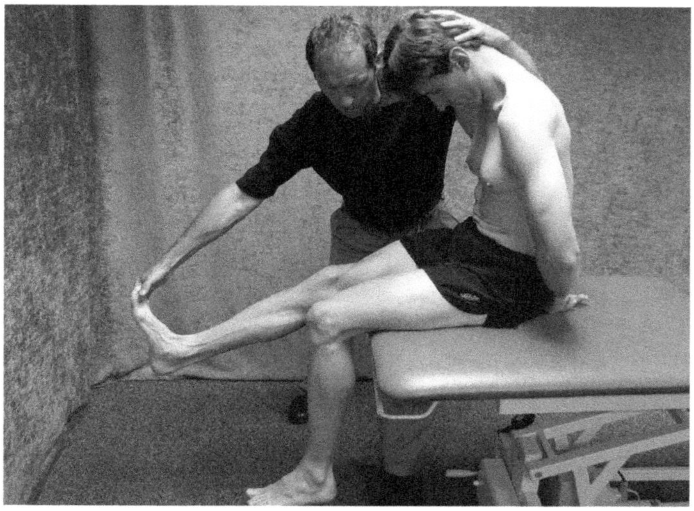

Figure 5.27 Slump test. (From Flynn et al 2008, with permission.)

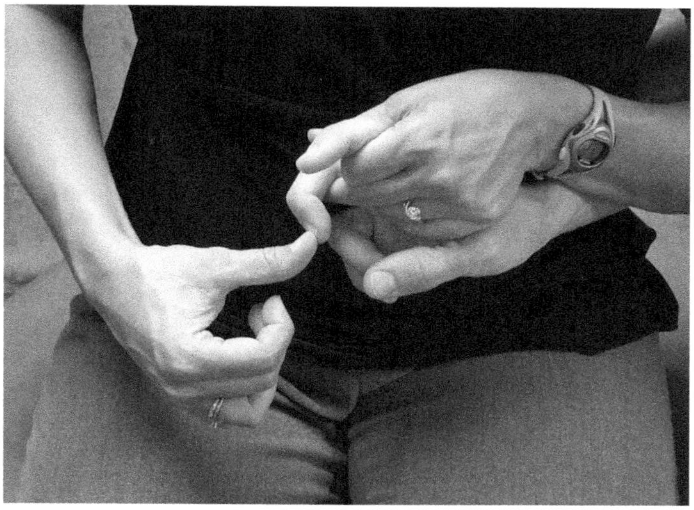

Figure 5.28 Hoffman's reflex. (From Flynn et al 2008, with permission.)

40° or less. The slump test is another useful screening tool to help the clinician rule out lumbar radiculopathy, with an estimated sensitivity of 0.84 and a +LR of 4.94 (Majlesi et al 2008). It is performed with the patient sitting with the back straight. From here, the patient is instructed to slump into lumbar and thoracic flexion while looking straight ahead, then to flex the neck fully and extend one knee, and finally to dorsiflex the ipsilateral foot (Fig. 5.27). The test is considered positive if it reproduces the patient's familiar pain. (Ch 65 of this textbook describes the slump test in more detail.)

Upper motor neuron examination

Although probably not required for all patients, further neurological examination should be performed when indicated by the history, observation or a traditional neurological screen. For example, if a patient reports subjective complaints of bilateral neurological involvement, a history of neck trauma and / or problems with balance or walking, the examiner should include an upper motor neuron examination as a part of the neurological screen. Moreover, if the examiner witnesses problems with coordination or gait disturbances during visual observation or clonus during muscle stretch reflex testing, he / she may suspect disturbances of the corticospinal and spinocerebellar tracts within the spinal cord and further testing is also indicated. Whereas disruptions of the spinal nerve roots generally cause attenuation of motor reflexes, disorders of the central nervous system usually result in disruption of the upper motor neuron's regulatory control over the motor reflexes and they become hyper-reflexive. Although no studies, to our knowledge, have investigated the diagnostic utility of tests of the upper motor neuron system, the following are a prudent set of procedures that have been advocated to identify upper motor neuron problems.

Hoffman's reflex (Fig. 5.28) is tested with the patient seated and with the head in a neutral position. The examiner flicks the distal phalanx of the middle finger and the test is considered positive if there is flexion of the interphalangeal joint of the thumb, with or without flexion of the index finger's proximal or distal interphalangeal joints.

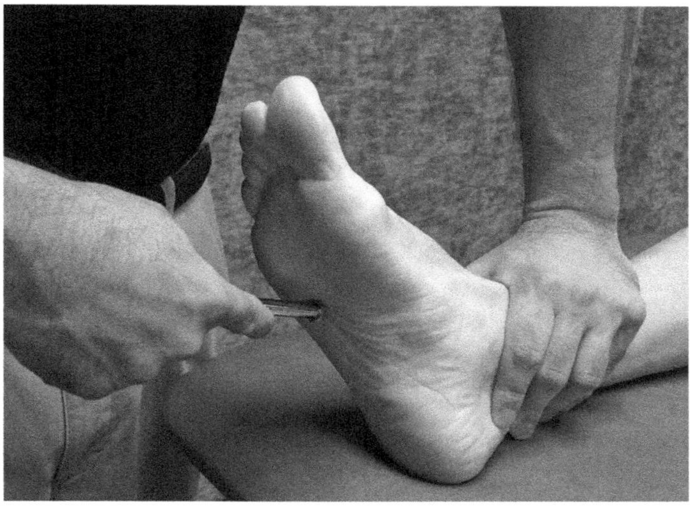

Figure 5.29 Babinski sign. (From Flynn et al 2008, with permission.)

Babinski sign (Fig. 5.29) is tested with the patient supine. The examiner strokes the plantar surface of the foot with a fingernail or instrument from the posterior lateral surface towards the ball of the foot. The test is considered positive if the great toe extends and the other toes fan out.

Clonus (Fig. 5.30) is generally assessed in the gastrocnemius and soleus muscles and can be assessed with the patient either seated or supine. The examiner rapidly dorsiflexes the ankle and the test is considered positive if the quick stretch results in reflexive twitching of the plantar-flexors.

Romberg test (Fig. 5.31) is performed with the patient standing with feet close together. The patient is then instructed to close the eyes and the test is considered positive if the amount of sway is increased when the eyes are closed, or if the patient loses balance.

The scapulohumeral reflex is evaluated from upper motor neuron signs from the upper cervical spine (C1–C4). The examiner strikes the superior tip of the patient's lateral acromion process and / or the superior midpoint of the scapular spine with a reflex hammer. A test is considered positive when the patient involuntarily shrugs and / or abducts the shoulder (Shimizu et al 1993; Sizer et al 2007).

Lhermitte's sign is elicited when cervical flexion causes tingling and / or an 'electrical shock' in the midline of the thoracic spine; it is thought to signify the possible presence of spinal cord conditions including multiple sclerosis, tumours or other space-occupying lesions (Sizer et al 2007; Gemici 2010).

Cranial nerve examination

The 12 cranial nerves are peripheral nerves carrying motor and sensory information to the head, face and neck. Like the upper motor neuron screen, a cranial nerve examination is recommended when indicated by the history, observation or traditional neurological screen. Some examples of indications are if patients report significant trauma to the head or neck, symptoms such as pain, weakness or numbness in the head, face or neck, visual or other sensory disturbances, or trouble with eating, drinking or swallowing. Table 5.4 lists the 12 cranial nerves and a typical examination of each.

Clearing the Spine

Even in the absence of neurological deficit, it is not uncommon for symptoms anywhere in the upper or lower

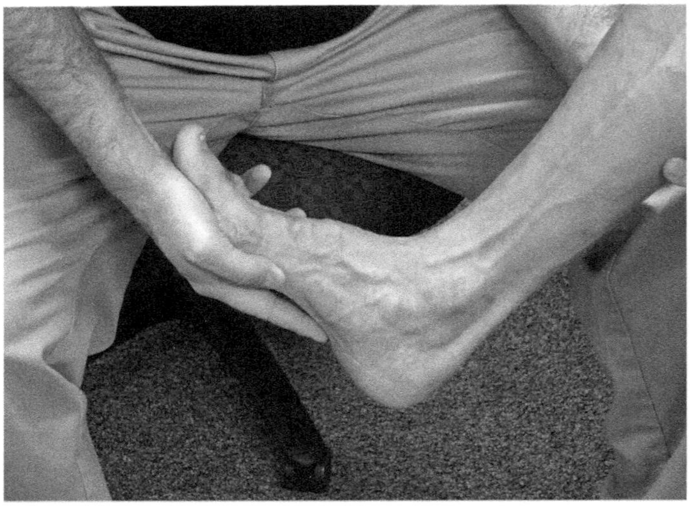

Figure 5.30 Testing for clonus. (From Flynn et al 2008, with permission.)

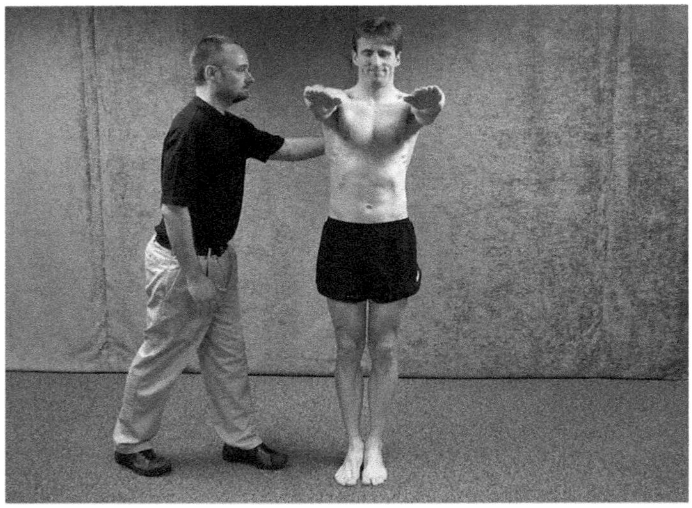

Figure 5.31 Romberg test. (From Flynn et al 2008, with permission.)

Table 5.4 **Cranial nerves and cranial nerve examination**

Cranial nerve number	Function	Test
I: Olfactory	Sensory from olfactory epithelium	Assess the ability to smell common scents.
II: Optic	Sensory from retina of eyes	Assess peripheral vision by having person read an eye chart.
III: Oculomotor	Motor to muscles controlling upward, downward, and medial eye movements, as well as pupil constriction	Assess pupil constriction as a reaction to light.
IV: Trochlear	Motor to muscles controlling downward and inward eye movements	Assess the ability to move eye downward and inward by asking patient to follow your finger.
V: Trigeminal	Sensory from face and motor to muscles of mastication	Test sensation of face and cheeks as well as corneal reflex. Assess the patient's ability to clench the teeth.
VI: Abducens	Motor to muscles that move eye laterally	Assess patient's ability to move eyes away from midline by asking him to follow your finger with his eyes.
VII: Facial	Motor to muscles of facial expression and sensory to anterior tongue	Assess symmetry and smoothness of facial expressions. Test taste on anterior two-thirds of tongue.
VIII: Vestibulocochlear	Hearing and balance	Assess by rubbing fingers by each ear. Patient should hear both equally. Can also ask patient to perform balance test.

Continued

Table 5.4 **Cranial nerves and cranial nerve examination—cont'd**

Cranial nerve number	Function	Test
IX: Glossopharyngeal	Controls gag reflex and sensory to posterior tongue	Assess gag reflex and taste on the posterior tongue.
X: Vagus	Controls muscles of pharynx, which facilitate swallowing Provides sensory to thoracic and abdominal visceral region	Ask patient to say 'ah' and watch for elevation of soft palate.
XI: Accessory	Motor to trapezius and sternocleidomastoid muscles	Muscle testing of trapezius.
XII: Hypoglossal	Motor to muscles of the tongue	Ask patient to stick tongue straight out. Tongue will deviate towards injured side.

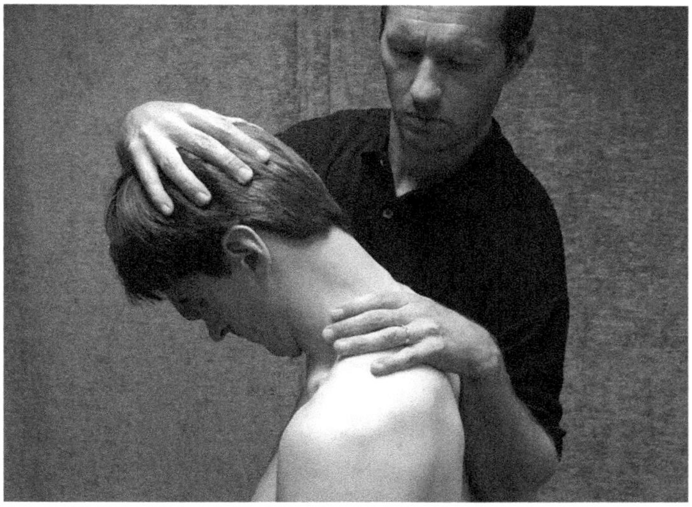

Figure 5.32 Cervical flexion with overpressure. (From Flynn et al 2008, with permission.)

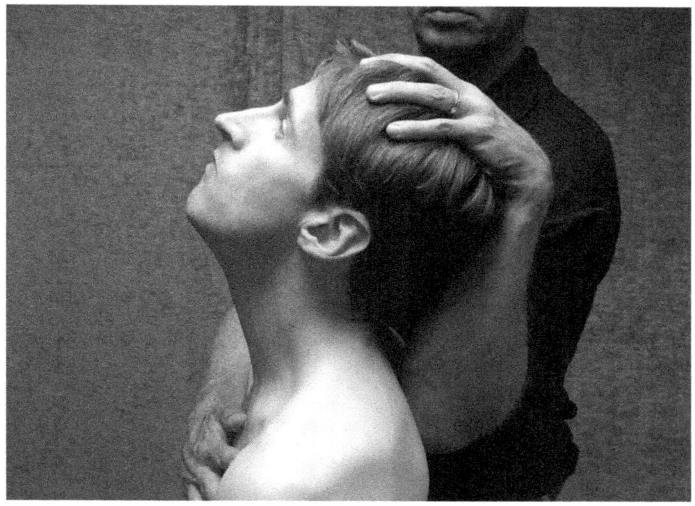

Figure 5.33 Cervical extension with overpressure. (From Flynn et al 2008, with permission.)

extremities to originate more proximally, especially from the spine. Therefore, it is recommended that examiners perform a screening examination of the region proximal to the primary area of symptoms and, at a minimum, ensure that distal symptoms are not primarily altered with movements of the spine. The cervical- and lumbar-screening examination should consist of active range of motion of flexion, extension, bilateral side-bending, bilateral rotation, and combined extension, side-bending and rotation (quadrant). If no symptoms are produced with a full active range of motion, the examiner should then add slow overpressure to each motion (Figs 5.32–5.39).

The next component of 'clearing' the cervical or lumbar spine as the prime contributor to the patient's symptoms is a central posterior-to-anterior accessory glide of each vertebra. This is commonly referred to as 'spring testing', which tests for segmental movement and pain response. In both the cervical and lumbar spine, this is tested with the patient in prone position. When testing the cervical spine, the examiner contacts the spinous process with the thumbs. The lateral neck musculature is gently pulled posteriorly with the fingers. At this point, a posterior-to-anterior force is imparted in a progressive and oscillatory fashion over the spinous process (Fig. 5.40). The test is positive if the patient reports reproduction

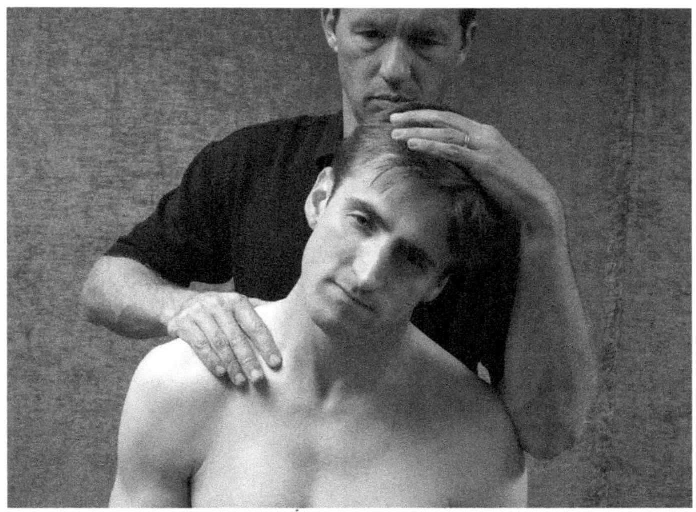

Figure 5.34 Cervical side-bending with overpressure. (From Flynn et al 2008, with permission.)

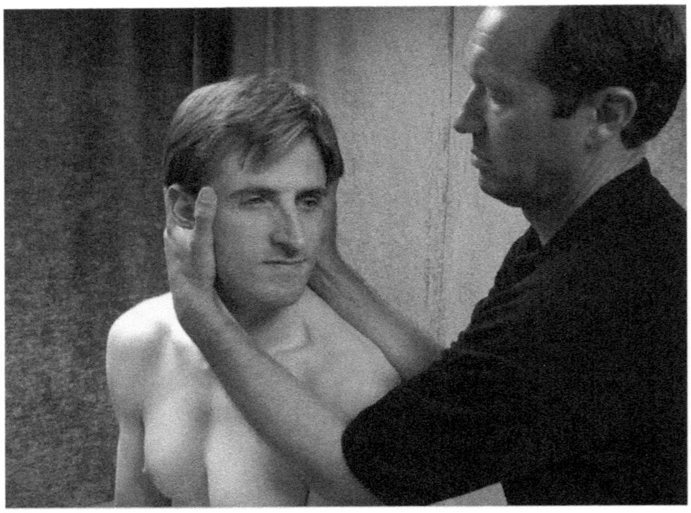

Figure 5.35 Cervical rotation with overpressure. (From Flynn et al 2008, with permission.)

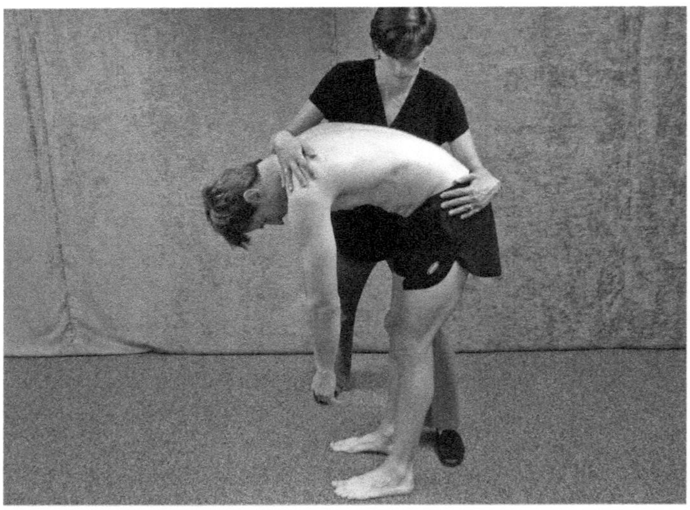

Figure 5.36 Lumbar flexion with overpressure. (From Flynn et al 2008, with permission.)

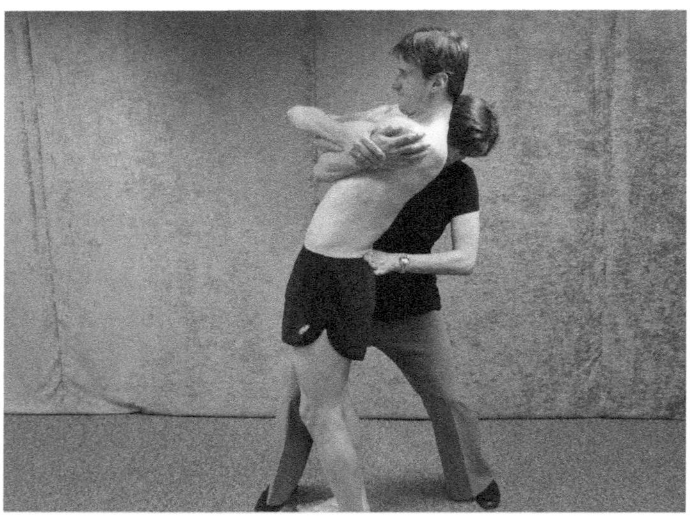

Figure 5.37 Lumbar extension with overpressure. (From Flynn et al 2008, with permission.)

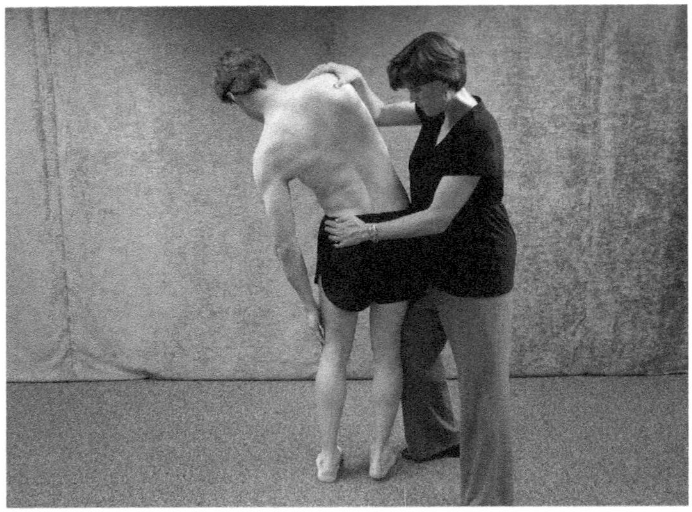

Figure 5.38 Lumbar side-bending with overpressure. (From Flynn et al 2008, with permission.)

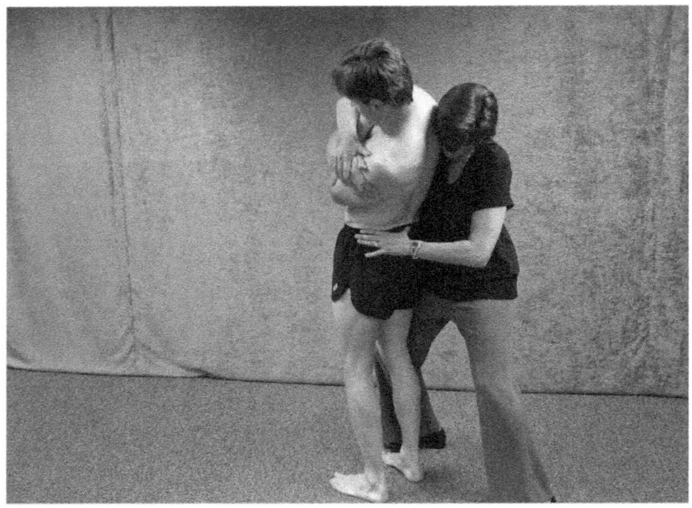

Figure 5.39 Combined lumbar extension, rotation and side-bending with overpressure. (From Flynn et al 2008, with permission.)

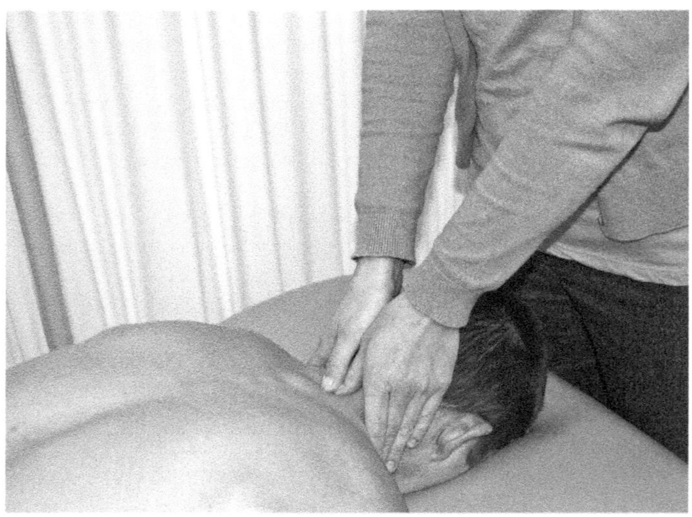

Figure 5.40 Posterior–anterior mobility of cervical spine. (From Flynn et al 2008, with permission.)

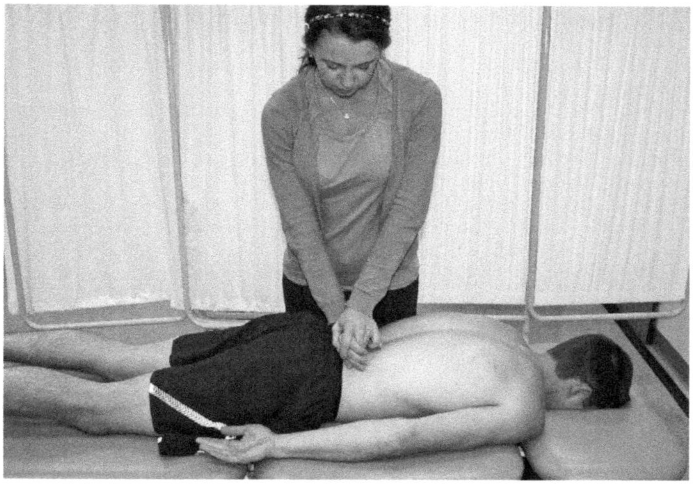

Figure 5.41 Posterior–anterior mobility of lumbar spine. (From Flynn et al 2008, with permission.)

of their pain or symptoms. The clinician then additionally judges the segment to be hypomobile, normal or hypermobile. This test has been shown to be a good screening tool in patients with neck pain, with a sensitivity of 0.82 and a −LR of 0.23 (Sandmark & Nisell 1995).

To assess posterior–anterior mobility of the lumbar spine, the patient is positioned in prone. The examiner contacts the spinous process with the hypothenar eminence just distal to the pisiform. The examiner should be directly over the contact area and, keeping the elbows extended, use their upper body to impart a posterior-to-anterior force in a progressive and oscillatory fashion (Fig. 5.41). This is repeated with all lumbar segments. The clinician judges each segment as being hypomobile, normal or hypermobile, and reports whether or not it reproduced the patient's familiar pain. One study (Fritz et al 2005) has shown this test to be specific (specificity 0.95, +LR 8.86) in patients with radiographic evidence of lumbar instability. The clinician should bear in mind, however, that in the event of a negative result it may be a false negative. It is noteworthy that this study was not looking at patient with traumatic instability requiring medical or surgical attention; instead it was used in directing treatment later, after a complete regional exam.

The final component of 'clearing' the cervical or lumbar spine as the prime contributor to the patient's symptoms includes palpatory examination of the joint and muscle structures. Specifically, palpating for trigger points within the spine and trunk musculature that may refer pain distally is appropriate. (Ch 59 of this textbook includes further information on referred pain from trigger points.)

Region-specific Examination

Like the screening portion, the clinician should focus the region-specific portion of the physical examination on testing hypotheses formed during the patient history. Unlike the screening portion, however, the region-specific portion of the physical examination generally consists of deductive procedures aimed at (1) narrowing in on a patient's concordant sign and (2) gathering knowledge of how specific movements affect the patient's symptoms. As described in Chapters 3 and 4, a patient's concordant sign consists of the familiar symptoms that caused them to seek medical care (Laslett et al 2003). During the region-specific examination, concordant signs are distinguished from discordant signs, which are symptoms that are unlike the pain or other symptoms that caused the patient to seek treatment (Laslett et al 2003). Clearly establishing a patient's concordant sign and knowing specifically what movements or procedures primarily reproduce such symptoms is a pragmatic method for establishing a pathoanatomical diagnosis. However, even when establishment of a specific pathoanatomical diagnosis is not possible, knowledge of a patient's concordant sign and the movements or procedures that specifically reproduce that sign can be used to guide patient management and evaluate treatment effectiveness. As will be detailed in later chapters, reassessing a patient's concordant sign immediately after each treatment procedure is an objective method of evaluating the effectiveness of the procedure and guiding the choice of which treatment procedure to perform next. Therapeutic benefits obtained using this method within a single treatment session have been shown to be predictive of longer-term clinical benefits (Hahne et al 2004).

The region-specific portion of the physical examination should generally consist mostly of:

- active movements
- passive movements
- palpation
- clinical special tests.

Active movements are physiological movements performed exclusively by the patient in each motion plane for a selected joint. The goals of active movements are both to identify concordant versus discordant signs and to determine the effect of the specific active movements on those signs. Since all active movements are within the patient's complete control, starting an examination with active movements begins the deductive examination process in a safe and gradually more aggressive manner. Consistent with this concept of incrementally increasing loads, the examiner will follow active movements that do not cause symptoms with overpressure, which is manual pressure in each direction at the end range of motion. The overpressure should start gently and the pressure will be gradually progressed while carefully monitoring the patient's response.

Passive movements include both passive physiological movements and passive accessory movements performed exclusively by the examiner. Physiological movements are joint movements that can be performed actively by the patient, such as flexion, extension, side-bending and rotation. Accessory movements are joint movements that cannot be performed by the patient and generally occur across joint planes, such as anterior or posterior glides. Comparing symptom response during passive physiological movements with that of active physiological movements gives the examiner information about the nature of the affected tissue and whether it is likely to be contractile (e.g. muscle, tendon) or not (e.g. ligament, bone, cartilage, nerve). Additionally, assessing passive physiological motion allows the examiner to assess the true full range of motion without the limitations of muscle function and patient motivation, and also permits the examiner to assess the type of resistance encountered at the end of joint motion ('end feel'). Assessment of passive accessory motion is helpful to localize more precisely the tissues and area responsible for the concordant sign. In the spine, for example, passive accessory intervertebral motions help the examiner isolate the side and specific spinal level(s) of primary symptoms. Additionally, many manual practitioners use assessments of both the amount and quality of accessory motions to make treatment decisions about how and where to deliver joint mobilization and / or manipulation. Although assessments of joint mobility have consistently been shown to be unreliable (Mootz et al 1989; Binkley et al 1995; Maher et al 1998; Smedmark et al 2000; Hicks et al 2003; Fritz et al 2005; Arab et al 2009), there is some evidence that such assessments are helpful in treatment selection and patient management (Flynn et al 2002; Fritz et al 2005; Hicks et al 2005; Brennan et al 2006).

Palpation is a standard procedure for almost any sort of medical examination. Like passive accessory motion testing, it can help further localize the tissues and areas responsible for the concordant sign. Also, like passive accessory motion testing, palpation can help differentiate whether an area of symptoms represents the primary source of symptoms or is more likely to comprise referred symptoms that actually originate in another location. For example, pain in the proximal lateral forearm may be caused by local tissues underlying the area (tendonopathy or epicondylalgia) or may be referred from the cervical spine or shoulder.

Clinical special tests are procedures used to identify specific diagnoses further. They include combinations of active and passive movements, resistive tests and functional tests, and are generally both region and diagnosis specific. Hundreds (perhaps thousands) of special tests have been advocated based on clinician experience and biological plausibility. A growing number of special tests have been scrutinized in diagnostic research by comparing their outcomes with those of reference standard tests. Whenever possible, it is recommended that clinicians select special tests and procedures with known diagnostic utility that have demonstrated high specificity and large +LRs.

References

Arab AM, Abdollahi I, Joghataei MT, et al. 2009. Inter- and intra-examiner reliability of single and composites of selected motion palpation and pain provocation tests for sacroiliac joint. Man Ther 14: 213–221.

Bandiera G, Stiell IG, Wells GA, et al. 2003. The Canadian C-spine rule performs better than unstructured physician judgment. Ann Emerg Med 42: 395–402.

Binkley J, Stratford PW, Gill C. 1995. Interrater reliability of lumbar accessory motion mobility testing. Phys Ther 75: 786–792.

Boyles RE, Ritland BM, Miracle BM, et al. 2009. The short-term effects of thoracic spine thrust manipulation on patients with shoulder impingement syndrome. Man Ther 14: 375–380.

Brennan GP, Fritz JM, Hunter SJ, et al. 2006. Identifying subgroups of patients with acute / subacute 'nonspecific' low back pain: results of a randomized clinical trial. Spine 31: 623–631.

Childs JD, Fritz JM, Flynn TW, et al. 2004. A clinical prediction rule to identify patients with low back pain most likely to benefit from spinal manipulation: a validation study. Ann Intern Med 141: 920–928.

Childs JD, Flynn TW, Fritz JM, et al 2005. Screening for vertebrobasilar insufficiency in patients with neck pain: manual therapy decision-making in the presence of uncertainty. J Orthop Sports Phys Ther 35: 300–306.

Cleland JA, Childs JD, Fritz JM, et al. 2007. Development of a clinical prediction rule for guiding treatment of a subgroup of patients with neck pain: use of thoracic spine manipulation, exercise, and patient education. Phys Ther 87: 9–23.

Cole JM, Gray-Miceli D. 2002. The necessary elements of a dermatologic history and physical evaluation. Dermatol Nurs 14: 377–383.

Cook C. 2007. Orthopedic manual therapy: an evidence based approach. Upper Saddle River, NJ: Pearson / Prentice Hall.

Demetracopoulos CA, Sponseller PD. 2007. Spinal deformities in Marfan syndrome. Orthop Clin North Am 38: 563–572.

Devillé WL, van der Windt DA, Dzaferagić A, et al. 2000. The test of Lasègue: systematic review of the accuracy in diagnosing herniated discs. Spine 25: 1140–1147.

Elliott JM, Cherry J. 2008. Upper cervical ligamentous disruption in a patient with persistent whiplash associated disorders. J Orthop Sports Phys Ther 38: 377.

Ernst E. 2007. Adverse effects of spinal manipulation: a systematic review. J R Soc Med 100: 330–338.

Flynn T, Fritz J, Whitman J, et al. 2002. A clinical prediction rule for classifying patients with low back pain who demonstrate short-term improvement with spinal manipulation. Spine 27: 2835–2843.

Flynn T, Cleland JA, Whitman J. 2008 Users' guide to the musculoskeletal examination: fundamentals for the evidence-based clinician. Louisville: Evidence in Motion.

Fraser S, Roberts L, Murphy E, 2009. Cauda equina syndrome: a literature review of its definition and clinical presentation. Arch Phys Med Rehabil 90: 1964–1968.

Fritz JM, Piva SR, Childs JD. 2005. Accuracy of the clinical examination to predict radiographic instability of the lumbar spine. Eur Spine J 14: 743–750.

Gemici C. 2010. Lhermitte's sign: review with special emphasis in oncology practice. Crit Rev Oncol Hematol 74: 79–86.

Hahne AJ, Keating JL, Wilson SC. 2004. Do within-session changes in pain intensity and range of motion predict between-session changes in patients with low back pain? Aust J Physiother 50: 17–23.

Hayden SR, Brown MD. 1999. Likelihood ratio: a powerful tool for incorporating the results of a diagnostic test into clinical decision making. Ann Emerg Med 33: 575–580.

Henschke N, Maher CG, Refshauge KM. 2007. Screening for malignancy in low back pain patients: a systematic review. Eur Spine J 16: 1673–1679.

Henschke N, Maher CG, Refshauge KM. 2008. A systematic review identifies five 'red flags' to screen for vertebral fracture in patients with low back pain. J Clin Epidemiol 61: 110–118.

Henschke N, Maher CG, Refshauge KM, et al. 2009. Prevalence of and screening for serious spinal pathology in patients presenting to primary care settings with acute low back pain. Arthritis Rheum 60: 3072–3080.

Hicks GE, Fritz JM, Delitto A, et al. 2003. Interrater reliability of clinical examination measures for identification of lumbar segmental instability. Arch Phys Med Rehabil 84: 1858–1864.

Hicks GE, Fritz JM, Delitto A, et al. 2005. Preliminary development of a clinical prediction rule for determining which patients with low back pain will respond to a stabilization exercise program. Arch Phys Med Rehabil 86: 1753–1762.

Hurwitz EL, Morgenstern H, Harber P, et al. 2002. A randomized trial of chiropractic manipulation and mobilization for patients with neck pain: clinical outcomes from the UCLA neck-pain study. Am J Public Health 92: 1634–1641.

Iverson CA, Sutlive TG, Crowell MS, et al. 2008. Lumbopelvic manipulation for the treatment of patients with patellofemoral pain syndrome: development of a clinical prediction rule. J Orthop Sports Phys Ther 38: 297–309.

Kerry R, Taylor AJ. 2006. Cervical arterial dysfunction assessment and manual therapy. Man Ther 11: 243–253.

Kerry R, Taylor AJ. 2009. Cervical arterial dysfunction: knowledge and reasoning for manual physical therapists. J Orthop Sports Phys Ther 39: 378–387.

Laslett M, Young SB, Aprill CN, et al. 2003. Diagnosing painful sacroiliac joints: a validity study of a McKenzie evaluation and sacroiliac provocation tests. Aust J Physiother 49: 89–97.

Lauder TD, Dillingham TR, Andary M, et al. 2000a. Effect of history and exam in predicting electrodiagnostic outcome among patients with suspected lumbosacral radiculopathy. Am J Phys Med Rehabil 79: 60–68

Lauder TD, Dillingham TR, Andary M, et al. 2000b. Predicting electrodiagnostic outcome in patients with upper limb symptoms: are the history and physical examination helpful? Arch Phys Med Rehabil 81: 436–441.

Macdonald A, Chatrath P, Spector T, et al. 1999. Level of termination of the spinal cord and the dural sac: a magnetic resonance study. Clin Anat 12: 149–152.

Magee DJ. 2008. Orthopedic physical assessment. St Louis, MO: Saunders Elsevier.
Maher CG, Latimer J, Adams R. 1998. An investigation of the reliability and validity of posteroanterior spinal stiffness judgments made using a reference-based protocol. Phys Ther 78: 829–837.
Majlesi J, Togay H, Unalan HT et al. 2008. The sensitivity and specificity of the Slump and the Straight Leg Raising tests in patients with lumbar disc herniation. J Clin Rheumatol 14: 87–91.
Miller TA, Pardo R, Yaworski R. 1999. Clinical utility of reflex studies in assessing cervical radiculopathy. Muscle Nerve 22: 1075–1079.
Mintken PE, Metrick L, Flynn TW. 2008. Upper cervical ligament testing in a patient with os odontoideum presenting with headaches. J Orthop Sports Phys Ther 38: 465–475.
Mootz RD, Keating JC, Kontz HP, et al. 1989. Intra- and interobserver reliability of passive motion palpation of the lumbar spine. J Manipulative Physiol Ther 12: 440–445.
Murphy DR, Hurwitz EL, Gerrard JK, et al. 2009. Pain patterns and descriptions in patients with radicular pain: does the pain necessarily follow a specific dermatome? Chiropr Osteopat 17: 9.
Portney LG, Watkins MP. 2009. Foundations of clinical research: applications to practice. Upper Saddle River, NJ: Pearson / Prentice Hall.
Rubinstein SM, Pool JJM, van Tulder MW, et al. 2007. A systematic review of the diagnostic accuracy of provocative tests of the neck for diagnosing cervical radiculopathy. Eur Spine J 16: 307–319.
Rushton A, Rivett D, Carlesso L, et al. 2014. International framework for examination of the cervical region for potential of cervical arterial dysfunction prior to Orthopaedic Manual Therapy intervention. Man Ther 19(3): 222–228. doi: 10.1016/j.math.2013.11.005.
Salman Riaz JMD. 2007. Images in spine surgery: atlantoaxial instability in Down syndrome. J Pak Med Assoc 57: 213–215.
Sandmark H, Nisell R. 1995. Validity of five common manual neck pain provoking tests. Scand J Rehabil Med 27: 131–136.
Shi J, Jia L, Yuan W, et al. 2010. Clinical classification of cauda equina syndrome for proper treatment. Acta Orthop 81: 391–395.
Shimizu T, Shimada H, Shirakura K. 1993. Scapulohumeral reflex (Shimizu): its clinical significance and testing maneuver. Spine 18: 2182–2190.
Sizer PS, Brismée JM, Cook C. 2007. Medical screening for red flags in the diagnosis and management of musculoskeletal spine pain. Pain Pract 7: 53–71.
Slipman CW, Plastaras CT, Palmitier RA, et al. 1998. Symptom provocation of fluoroscopically guided cervical nerve root stimulation. Are dynatomal maps identical to dermatomal maps? Spine 23: 2235–2242.
Smedmark V, Wallin M, Arvidsson I. 2000. Inter-examiner reliability in assessing passive intervertebral motion of the cervical spine. Man Ther 5: 97–101.
Song D, Maher CO. 2007. Spinal disorders associated with skeletal dysplasias and syndromes. Neurosurg Clin North Am 18: 499–514.
Stiell IG, Clement CM, McKnight RD, et al. 2003. The Canadian C-spine rule versus the NEXUS low-risk criteria in patients with trauma. N Engl J Med 349: 2510–2518.
Straus SE. 2011. Evidence-based medicine: how to practice and teach it. Edinburgh: Elsevier Churchill Livingstone.
Tomić S, Soldo-Butković S, Kovac B, et al. 2009. Lumbosacral radiculopathy: factors effects on it's severity. Coll Antropol 33: 175–178.
Uitvlugt G, Indenbaum S. 1988. Clinical assessment of atlantoaxial instability using the Sharp–Purser test. Arthritis Rheum 31: 918–922.
van der Windt DA, Simons E, Riphagen II, et al 2010. Physical examination for lumbar radiculopathy due to disc herniation in patients with low-back pain. Cochrane Database Syst Rev 2: CD007431.
Wainner RS, Fritz JM, Irrgang JJ, et al. 2003. Reliability and diagnostic accuracy of the clinical examination and patient self-report measures for cervical radiculopathy. Spine 28: 52–62.

6 Chapter

Treating the Brain in Chronic Pain

Adriaan Louw

CHAPTER CONTENTS

Changes in the nervous system and brain in people with chronic pain	66
Neuromatrix	66
Structural changes in the brain	68
Functional changes in the brain	69
Descending pathways	69
Treatment	70
Therapeutic neuroscience education – restricting meaning	71
Graded motor imagery – restructuring brain/body maps	73
Conclusion	73

Changes in the Nervous System and Brain in People with Chronic Pain

People's pain experience is complex, individualized and 100% produced by their brain (Moseley 2003a, 2007). Pain is a decision taken by the brain, based on the perception of threat (Moseley 2007; Louw & Puentedura 2013). In contrast to pain, of which the individual will always be aware, nociception can be present without any awareness. This dichotomy is the basis of the Cartesian model of pain (1654), which assumes that tissue injury or disease states are synonymous with pain (Haldeman 1990; Goldberg 2008; Louw & Puentedura 2013). Not only is this false, but it still seems to be the prevailing model for treating pain (Goldberg 2008). Furthermore, this model of seeking 'what tissues to blame' may in fact be a significant source for the increased epidemic of chronic pain worldwide (Haldeman 1990; Goldberg 2008; Louw & Puentedura 2013). For any clinician interested in treating people in pain, especially chronic pain, the brain should be the primary target for directing treatment (Melzack 2001). It is now well established that the central nervous system (CNS) and brain undergo several significant changes in individuals experiencing chronic pain and may contribute to the development and maintenance of chronic pain states (Flor et al 1997; Flor 2000; Schmidt-Wilcke et al 2006; Apkarian et al 2009; Tracey & Bushnell 2009). It is thus proposed that treatment should aim to restore these changes in the brain and CNS as a means to ease the pain and suffering of the patient with chronic pain. Four key changes are discussed in this chapter: the pain neuromatrix, structural changes in the brain, functional changes in the brain, and alteration of descending antinociceptive pathways.

Neuromatrix

It is now well established that, during a pain experience, multiple areas of the brain are activated (Fig. 6.1) (Flor 2000, 2003; Melzack 2001; Moseley 2003a). This finding is contrary to a flawed historical view of a single pain area in the brain (Melzack 2001). This widespread brain activation during a pain experience has become known as the 'pain neuromatrix', a term introduced by Ron Melzack in 1996. The pain neuromatrix is defined as a pattern of nerve impulses generated by a distributed neural network in the brain (Melzack 2001). Pain then, is produced by the output of this widely distributed neural network in the brain rather than directly by sensory input evoked by injury, inflammation or other pathology (Melzack 2001; Moseley 2003b). Although care should be taken in generalization, it is now well established that common areas are activated during various pain experiences and these areas have become synonymous with the pain neuromatrix (Melzack 2001; Flor 2003; Moseley 2003b; Puentedura & Louw 2012). The most common areas associated with the pain neuromatrix are the anterior cingulate, primary sensory cortex, thalamus, anterior insula, and the prefrontal and posterior parietal cortices (Flor 2000, 2003; Moseley 2003b). During a painful task, it is believed that these increasingly active brain areas communicate with each other, developing in essence a pain map (Fig. 6.2) (Louw & Puentedura 2013).

The pain neuromatrix provides two immediate clinically important features. First, there are no specific pain areas in the brain and secondly, during a pain experience, pain activates several areas of the brian. In chronic pain these areas are likely to be 'enslaved' by pain (Puentedura & Louw 2012; Louw & Puentedura 2013). For example, a patient engaging in motor control exercises such as a co-contraction of the transversus abdominis and multifidus (specific spinal stabilization exercises) (Richardson et al 2004) may have a hard time executing the precise motor control activities prescribed by this approach, since the motor cortex is being utilized as part of the pain neuromatrix (Moseley & Hodges 2002). From a clinical point of view, this statement is profound. For too long have patients who are unable to perform these precise and intricate exercises been accused of malingering, or being lazy

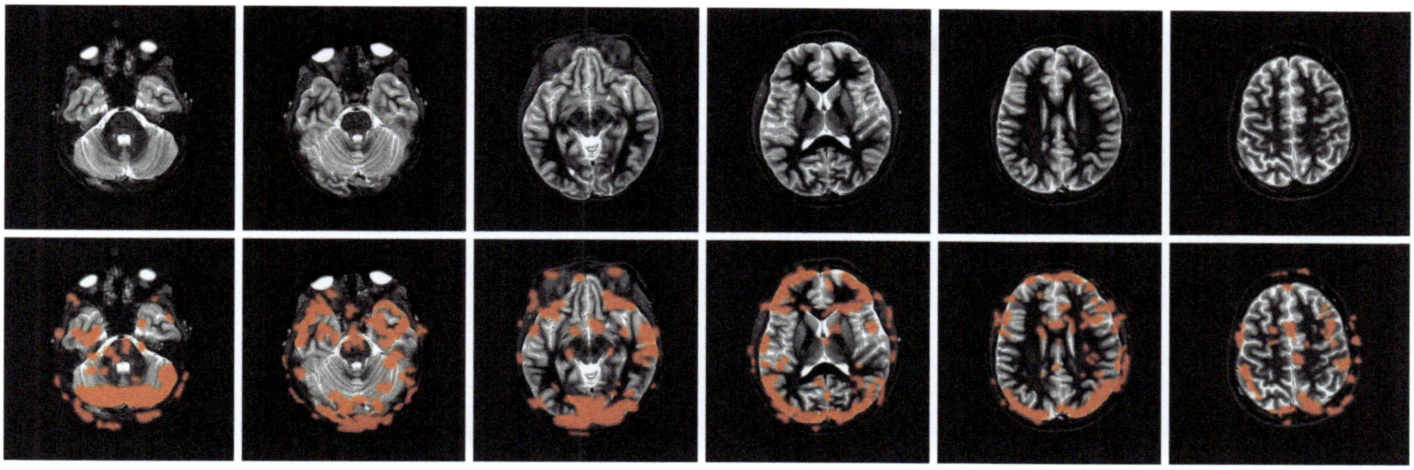

Figure 6.1 A single case functional magnetic resonance imaging (fMRI) study of a patient with low back pain. The first row indicates the brain activity while the subject is in a rested state and the second row indicates the same subject's scan while performing a painful task (anterior pelvic tilt). Note the widespread activity in the brain during a painful task.

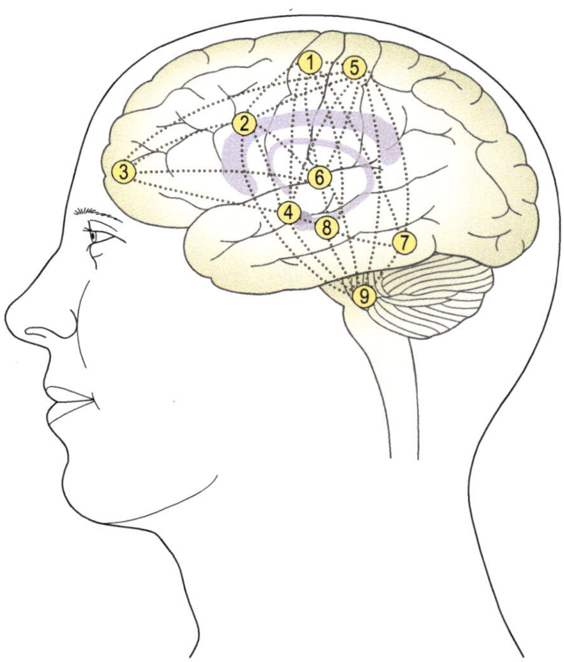

Area	Primary function
① Premotor cortex	Organize and prepare movements
② Cingulate cortex	Concentration and focus
③ Prefrontal cortex	Problem solving and memory
④ Amygdala	Fear, conditioning and addictions
⑤ Sensory cortex	Sensory discrimination
⑥ Hypothalamus/ thalamus	Stress responses, automonic regulation and motivation
⑦ Cerebellum	Movement and cognitions
⑧ Hippocampus	Memory, spatial recognition and fear conditioning
⑨ Spinal cord	Gating from the periphery

Figure 6.2 An illustration of the pain neuromatrix theory. (Image adapted from Louw A, Puentedura EJ. 2013. Therapeutic neuroscience education, Vol 1. Minneapolis, MN: OPTP. p 76. Copyright Adrian Louw.)

or not motivated, yet from a neuroscience perspective there is a justified reason for their difficulty with these exercises. Similarly, the pain neuromatrix theory of pain using other areas explains many issues commonly seen in patients with chronic pain – such as problems with focus, concentration and regulating body temperature, sleep disturbances, or short-term memory issues (Sapolsky 1994; Luerding et al 2008). More importantly, understanding these issues and being able to explain this to patients with chronic pain is the cornerstone of therapeutic neuroscience education (TNE) (Louw et al 2011a).

The second key issue of the pain neuromatrix is the individual's experience of pain (Moseley 2003a). Given the enormous complexity of neuronal activation, synaptic activity, neurotransmitters and modulators, the primary pain map can also be influenced by neighbouring neural circuits, which will probably influence the individual pain experience (Fig. 6.3) (Puentedura & Louw 2012).

The fact that an individual's pain map can be tuned up or down by the adjacent maps with regards their knowledge, experiences, beliefs, etc. makes each person's pain experience even more individualized and complicated. A skilled clinician should realize that a pain experience is associated with various such issues, which may need to be addressed in treatment as well. The pain neuromatrix allows, in essence, a neuroscience view of the interaction of a pain circuit with various bio-psychosocial factors (yellow flags) that have been associated with poor outcomes (Kendall et al 1997; Kendall &

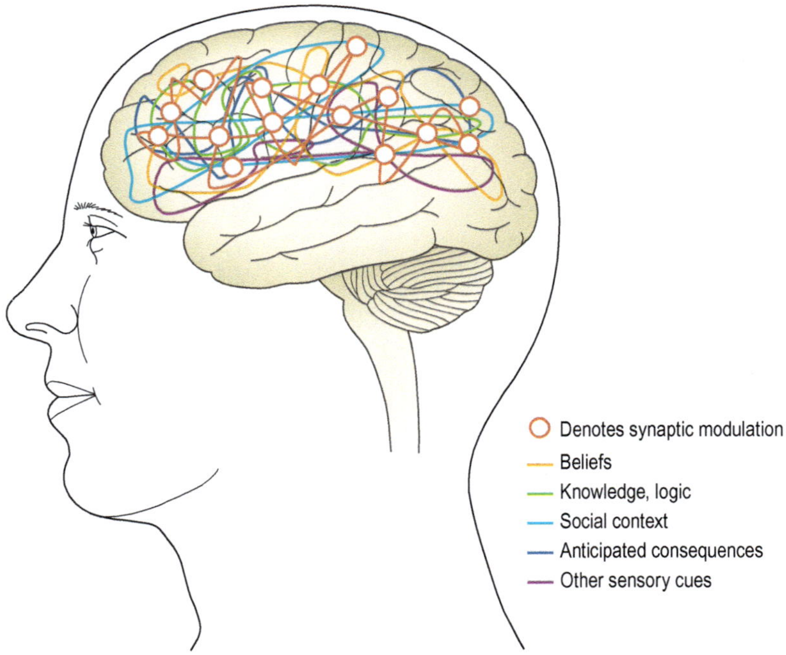

Figure 6.3 The primary pain map can also be influenced by neighbouring neural circuits. (Image adapted from Louw A, Puentedura EJ. 2013. Therapeutic neuroscience education, Vol 1. Minneapolis, MN: OPTP. p 77. Copyright Adrian Louw.)

Watson 2000). Adding further to the complexity of the neuromatrix and adjacent maps is the Hebbian theory, which proposes that 'neurons that fire together wire together' (Amit et al 1994). This is a scientific theory in neuroscience that explains the adaptation of neurons in the brain during the learning process. It describes a basic mechanism for synaptic plasticity wherein an increase in synaptic efficacy arises from the presynaptic cell's repeated and persistent stimulation of the postsynaptic cell. The theory further suggests that when an axon of cell A is near enough to excite a cell B and repeatedly or persistently takes part in firing it, some growth process or metabolic change takes place in one or both cells such that A's efficiency, as one of the cells firing B, is increased (Doidge 2007). It is believed that the neurotransmitter dopamine, which plays a major role in reward-driven learning, may also play a significant role in wiring pathways together. Every type of reward that has been studied increases the level of dopamine transmission in the brain, and a variety of highly addictive drugs, including stimulants such as cocaine and methamphetamine, act directly on the dopamine system. A chronic pain patient's brain may thus, in effect, become more proficient in running its pain map. In clinical terms, less stimulation may be needed to activate the pain map, which is the hallmark of central sensitization (Woolf 2007; Nijs et al 2010).

Structural changes in the brain

Several studies have compared the brain structure (volume of grey and white matter) of healthy individuals with those suffering from chronic pain (Apkarian et al 2004; Schmidt-Wilcke 2008; Schmidt-Wilcke et al 2008). It is now well established that, in people with chronic pain, various areas of the brain undergo volume changes including the dorsolateral prefrontal cortex, right anterior thalamus, brainstem, somatosensory cortex and the posterior parietal cortex (Apkarian et al 2004; Schmidt-Wilcke et al 2008). Several key issues are raised that impact on the treatment of patients with chronic pain. First, it is interesting to note that there is a relationship between the extent of brain density changes and pain intensity (Schmidt-Wilcke et al 2006). This finding correlates with a growing body of research indicating that acute pain, especially pain intensity, may indeed by a big predictor in the development of chronic pain (Woolf & Salter 2005; Jull et al 2007; Woolf 2007). It is now well established that persistent and high-intensity nociceptive bombardment of the CNS leads to significant, long-lasting neuroplastic changes that may be irreversible (Woolf & Mannion 1999; Woolf & Salter 2005; Woolf 2007; Latremoliere & Woolf 2009). The more interesting phenomenon of structural changes in the brain is the ability to restore grey matter; hence changes in grey matter found in chronic pain patients may not reflect true brain damage but rather a reversible consequence of the pain experience (Rodríguez-Raecke et al 2009). Treatments aimed at altering information to the brain (affecting nociception, education, etc.) have demonstrated an ability to restore grey matter to the brain in chronic pain states (de Lange et al 2008; Rodríguez-Raecke et al 2009; Gwilym et al 2010; Seminowicz et al 2011, 2013); it is also interesting to note that, apart from the increase in grey matter in the brain, a positive effect on pain, pain catastrophization and disability was also achieved in these treatments. Although care should be taken to interpret the correlations found in these results, the above studies along with a growing body of evidence suggest that strategies aimed at structural reorganization of the brain might be utilized as a means of treating chronic pain (Apkarian et al 2004; de Lange et al 2008; Schmidt-Wilcke 2008; Schmidt-Wilcke et al 2008; Rodríguez-Raecke et al 2009; Gwilym et al 2010; Seminowicz et al 2011; Wand et al 2011; Seminowicz et al 2013).

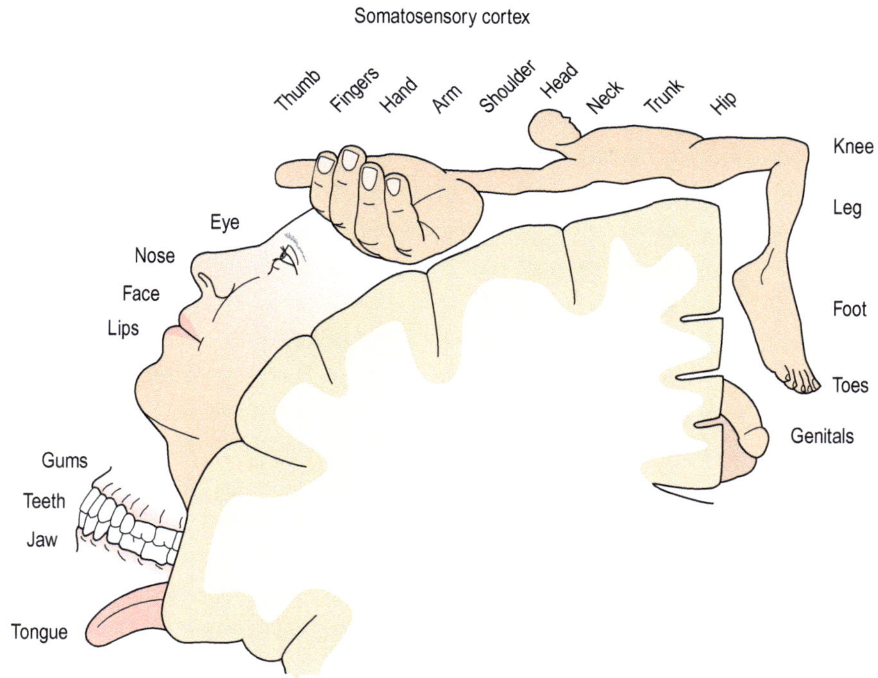

Figure 6.4 Somatosensory homunculus. (Image adapted from Louw A, Puentedura EJ. 2013. Therapeutic neuroscience education, Vol 1. Minneapolis, MN: OPTP. p 70. Copyright Adrian Louw.)

Functional changes in the brain

It is well established that the physical body of a person is represented in the brain by a network of neurons, which is often referred to as a representation of that particular body part in the brain (Penfield & Boldrey 1937; Flor 2000; Wand et al 2011). This representation refers to the pattern of activity that is evoked when a particular body part is stimulated. The most famous area of the brain associated with representation is the primary somatosensory cortex (S1) (Fig. 6.4) (Penfield & Boldrey 1937; Flor 2000; Stavrinou et al 2007; Wand et al 2011).

These neuronal representations of body parts are dynamically maintained (Flor et al 1997, 1998; Maihofner et al 2003; Moseley 2005a, 2008a; Lotze & Moseley 2007). It has been shown that patients with chronic pain display different S1 representations to those in people with no pain (Flor et al 1997, 1998; Maihofner et al 2003; Moseley 2005b, 2008a; Lotze & Moseley 2007). The interesting phenomenon associated with cortical restructuring is the fact that the body maps expand or contract, in essence increasing or decreasing the body map representation in the brain. Furthermore, these changes in shape and size of body maps seem to correlate to increased pain and disability (Flor et al 1997; Lloyd et al 2008). Although various factors have been linked to the development of this altered cortical representation of body maps in S1, such as neglect and decreased use of the painful body part (Marinus et al 2011), it is believed that altered immune activity may be a significant source of the 'smudging' of body maps (Flor et al 1997; Beggs et al 2010). An astounding fact of this reorganization of body maps is the fact that it occurs fast. It has been shown that, when four fingers are webbed together for just 30 minutes, cortical maps change in association with the fingers (Stavrinou et al 2007). This finding has significant clinical importance as it underscores the importance of strategies such as movement, tactile and visual stimulation of the CNS and brain early in a pain experience to help maintain S1 representation. Furthermore, it has now also been shown that patients with chronic pain struggle when identifying left and right body parts (left–right discrimination) (Moseley 2004a; Moseley et al 2005). Although most recent pain research has focused on the S1 reorganization, it is also important from a rehabilitation perspective to realize that changes also occur in the primary motor cortex (M1) (Tsao & Hodges 2007; Tsao et al 2008), which is organized according to movements, not muscles (Wolpert et al 2001). For example, in spinal stabilization exercises, it was found that the M1 representation of contraction of the transversus abdominis muscle was shifted and enlarged in patients with recurrent low back pain, and that both the location and size of the map volume were associated with slower onset of transversus abdominis muscle activity as part of the postural adjustment associated with rapid arm movement (Tsao et al 2008). People with chronic low back pain also exhibit an expanded area of cortical activity in preparation for arm movement and a decrease in specific cortical responses in relation to observed delayed onset of deep abdominal muscle activity (Jacobs et al 2010).

Descending pathways

A person's pain experience is complex and multifactorial, one factor of which is the CNS and brain's descending antinociceptive system (Fields et al 2005; Giesecke et al 2006). It is well established that various neurophysiological mechanisms in the CNS and brain, especially the midbrain, control the amount of information that the brain may receive from the

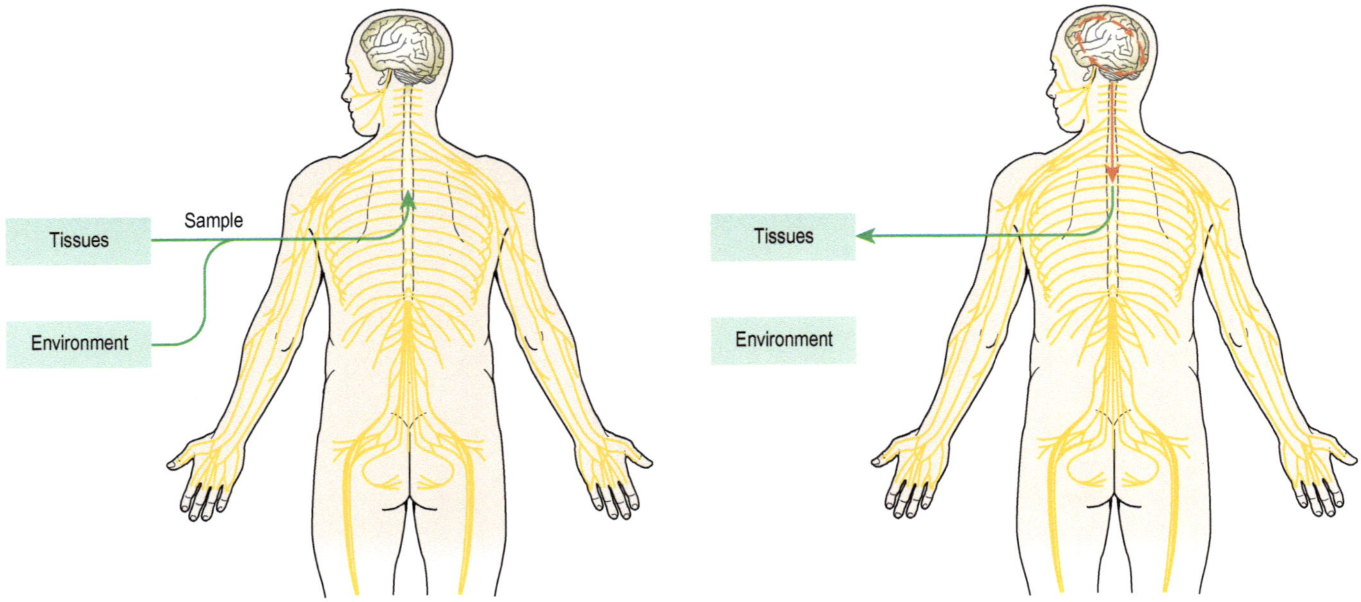

Figure 6.5 The bidirectional top-down and bottom-up approach to treating pain. (Modified and adapted from Gifford LS. 1998. Pain, the tissues and the nervous system. Physiotherapy 84: 27–33.)

tissues. This bidirectional system may allow information to be enhanced (facilitation) or down-regulated (inhibition); for example, during sporting events or war, severe injuries are often reported as almost painless (Melzack et al 1982). One area that has gained much interest is the midbrain periaqueductal grey (PAG). The PAG integrates inputs from the limbic forebrain and diencephalon with the nociceptive input received by the dorsal horn (Bandler & Keay 1996). Furthermore, functional neuroimaging studies in humans indicate that PAG activation by nociceptive inputs is modulated by attention, emotion, expectation of pain, and expectation-related placebo analgesia (Tracey et al 2002; Parry et al 2008; Wiech & Tracey 2009). Considering that patients with chronic pain display a decreased ability to engage the endogenous mechanisms of the brain, it is commonly believed that the PAG is negatively affected in patients with chronic pain (Peyron et al 2000; Sterling et al 2001; Nijs et al 2012). For example, it has been shown that in patients with chronic low back pain there are lesser increases in blood flow in the PAG compared with controls when exposed to equally painful stimuli (Giesecke et al 2006). The decreased ability of the PAG to alter sensory information, such as touch, is likely to be a part of the clinical manifestation of central sensitization (Woolf 2007; Nijs et al 2011).

Treatment

Many changes occur to the CNS and brain in people with chronic pain, and this chapter focuses on four key changes. Addressing and correcting these changes may be key in helping people with chronic pain – a statement that is validated by the emerging and growing evidence for the use of treatments aimed at restoring these changes in the CNS and brain, such as graded motor imagery (GMI) (Moseley 2004b, 2006; Daly & Bialocerkowski 2009; Bowering et al 2013), sensory discrimination (Moseley & Wiech 2009) and TNE (Moseley 2002; Moseley et al 2004; Louw et al 2011b). Understanding that pain is an output produced by the brain, based on perception of threat, is key when it comes to selecting appropriate treatments The brain, CNS and peripheral nervous system along with the immune and endocrine systems should be seen as a living organism seeking information at all times and adapting as needed. Feeding the brain information (sensory, visual, auditory, tactile, etc.) is important for how the brain may perceive threat: it creates an opportunity to lessen that threat and ultimately the pain experience. This brain-feeding process can be performed through various avenues, which can be categorized into a top-down and bottom-up approach to influencing the pain experience (Fig. 6.5).

Traditionally, clinicians have either followed a top-down (cognitive) or a bottom-up approach (such as manual therapy) to treat pain. It is strongly suggested, however, that the two approaches are not mutually exclusive and clinicians are therefore urged to consider a combination of the two. Viewing this as either a tissue or a cognitive issue would be contrary to the modern neuroscience view of pain and propagates the Cartesian model of pain, which seeks to determine whether pain is either physical or psychological in nature. Pain involves both processes and so requires treatment that addresses both. For example, studies on TNE have shown compelling evidence of benefit in treating people with chronic pain (Louw et al 2011a), but also that TNE works best if combined with movement-based therapies such as manual therapy and exercise, thus feeding the brain information 'from both ends' (Ryan et al 2010; Louw et al 2011b). Likewise, cervical spine manipulation has been shown to be efficacious in treating acute neck pain, but a paramount predictor of success is patients' beliefs that spinal manipulation will help their pain (Puentedura et al 2012). A skilled clinician will therefore aim to address both approaches in people with chronic pain.

This neuroscience view of altering the information that the CNS and brain receive opens the doorway to many therapies, and it is further proposed that any treatment aimed at altering the information the brain gets may indeed be of therapeutic value. For instance, it has long been established that treatments such as transcutaneous electrical neuromuscular stimulation (TENS) and electrical stimulation, via the pain gate, can have an effect on the information received by the dorsal horn of the spinal cord and ultimately the brain, pain neuromatrix and the person's pain experience (Wall 1996; Melzack 1999). Likewise, a number of studies have found that various manual treatments such as spinal mobilization and spinal manipulation, exercise, needling techniques and so forth can elicit an endogenous process and thus positively affect a person's pain state (Vicenzino et al 1996; Sterling et al 2001; George et al 2006; Fernández-Carnero et al 2008). This is especially true in more acute, subacute and peripherally evoked pain states. Nevertheless, a well-meaning clinician utilizing sound clinical reasoning and an updated knowledge of pain science and pain mechanisms should view any and all treatments from a perspective of altering danger information being relayed to the CNS and brain so as to lessen perceived threat and therefore ultimately the patient's pain experience. The treatments described below will focus on two of the emerging therapies associated with restructuring the CNS and brain in patients with chronic pain.

Therapeutic neuroscience education – restricting meaning

Recent research into educational strategies for patients with chronic pain shows an increased usage of TNE (Moseley 2003a, 2004c, 2005a; Moseley et al 2004). TNE aims to reduce pain and disability by helping patients gain an increased understanding of the biological and physiological processes involved in their pain experience (Ryan et al 2010; Louw et al 2011b). TNE differs from traditional education strategies by focusing not on anatomical or biomechanical explanations for pain, but rather on the neurophysiological and neurobiological processing and representation, and meaning of pain (Moseley 2005a; Meeus et al 2010; Ryan et al 2010). It has further been demonstrated that patients are capable of understanding the neurophysiology of their pain, whereas professionals tend to underestimate their patient's ability to understand the complex issues related to it (Moseley 2003c). A recent systematic review provides strong suggestive evidence with respect to the efficacy of TNE in addressing pain, disability and physical performance in musculoskeletal pain, particularly spinal disorders (Louw et al 2011a). Studies of treatment utilizing TNE have, furthermore, shown it to decrease fear and to change patients' perception of their pain (Moseley 2003c), to have an immediate effect in improving patients' attitudes about pain (Moseley 2003b), and show improvements in pain, cognition and physical performance (Moseley 2004c), increase pain thresholds during physical tasks (Moseley et al 2004), improve outcomes of therapeutic exercises (Moseley 2002), and significantly reduce widespread brain activity characteristic of a pain experience (Moseley 2005a).

A very important clinical issue regarding TNE needs discussion, however. As pointed out earlier, in line with the Cartesian model of pain (1654), many clinicians still seem to decide that a patient's pain is either physical or psychological, and if more psychological then TNE is the approach that is more suited. TNE has therefore become synonymous with lengthy one-on-one psychoeducational sessions between a patient and therapists around a table, the latter trying to get the patient to 'believe'. TNE should, rather, be used in conjunction with movement-based treatments and seen as a dual process that constantly feeds the brain and CNS with information. Furthermore movement, when applied and utilized within a TNE model, is better understood, less feared and has a different meaning, as pain experienced during a movement is understood as arising not so much from the injury itself as from an oversensitized nervous system (Louw et al 2013).

The original question now arises: if in patients with chronic pain there are CNS and brain changes such as increased brain activity (pain neuromatrix), structural and functional changes within the brain and altered antinociceptive activity of the PAG, does TNE have the ability to impact these changes positively? To date, two single-case fMRI (functional magnetic resonance imaging) studies have investigated the specific effect of TNE on brain activity (Moseley 2005a; Louw et al submitted for publication). Although care should be taken in extrapolating the findings of these two single-case studies, both found a similar reduction in widespread brain activity associated with performing a painful task after a TNE session, compared with performing the same task prior to TNE (Fig. 6.6). These preliminary findings may indeed indicate that TNE lessens threat, leading to a deactivation of the pain neuromatrix (Moseley 2005b). The findings from these fMRI studies, along with the authors' interpretation of its effect on the pain neuromatrix, are underscored by studies finding that TNE has a positive effect on pain, pain catastrophization and disability (Moseley 2002, 2003a; Moseley et al 2004; Louw et al 2011b).

With regards to structural changes, no studies specific to TNE have been conducted; however, recent cognitive behavioral therapy (CBT) studies have found grey matter increases in the brain following CBT (de Lange et al 2008; Seminowicz et al 2013). How does this apply to TNE? TNE is cognitive therapy and its ability to restructure the meaning of pain probably represents the 'C' of CBT. TNE aims to restructure threat and the meaning of pain, which is a cornerstone of CBT (Bennett & Nelson 2006; Ang et al 2010). Future studies should investigate whether the increases in grey matter do correlate with cognitive restructuring and so are more directly specific to TNE. To date, however, no studies have been conducted to determine whether TNE is associated with functional changes in body maps in the brain. It may, however, have an effect on the PAG and the antinociceptive system. TNE is indirectly associated with decreased levels of pain experience, and increases in pressure pain thresholds and the ability to exercise and move more despite pain (Louw et al 2011b). These findings may give an insight into the effect of TNE on the antinociceptive system of the PAG. In a recent fMRI case study using TNE preoperatively for lumbar radiculopathy, pre- and post-TNE changes to the PAG were observed (Louw et al submitted for publication). During a painful task, the patient with low back pain displayed widespread brain activity (see Fig. 6.6). Closer analysis revealed significant activation of the PAG (Fig. 6.7A). Although care should be taken to extrapolate from one case study as well as with respect to the various unknowns regarding fMRI (Moseley 2008a), it is

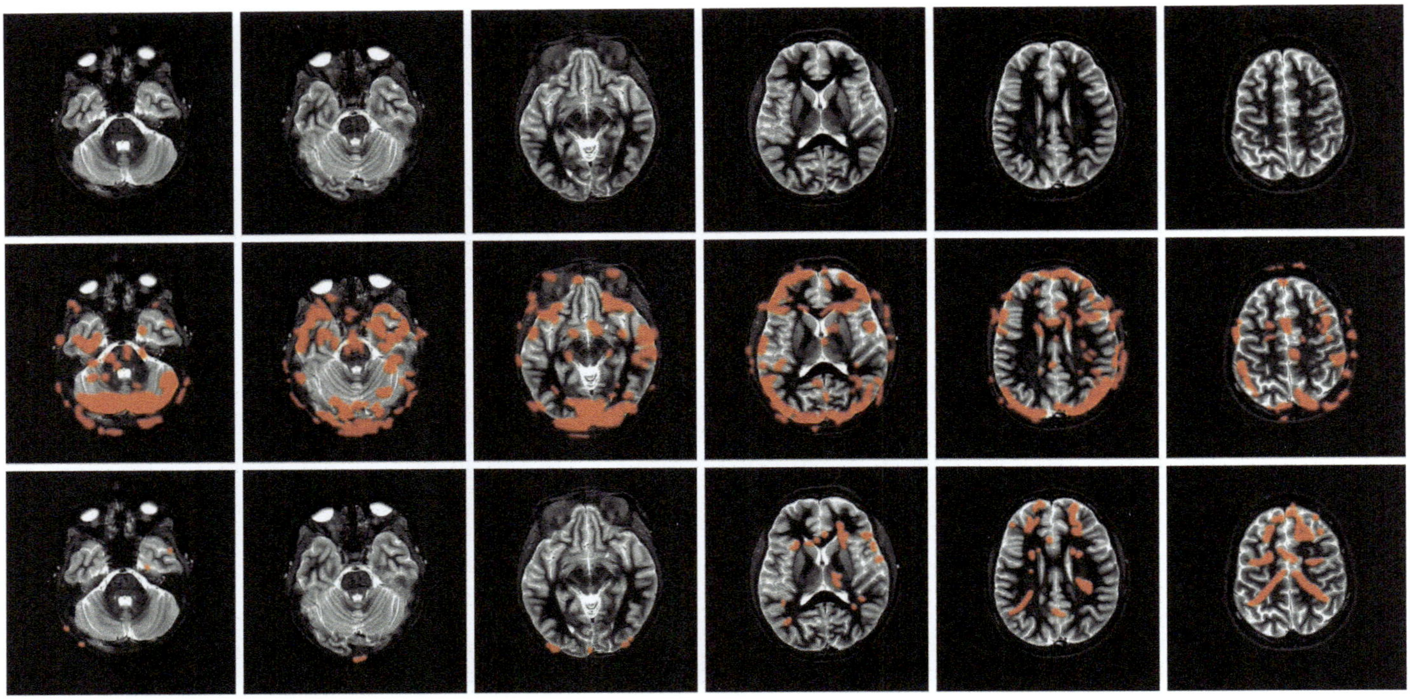

Figure 6.6 **A single-case functional magnetic resonance imaging (fMRI) study of a patient with low back pain.** The first row indicates the brain activity while the subject is in a rested state and the second row indicates the same subject's scan while performing a painful task (anterior pelvic tilt). The third row indicates the same painful task performed after a 30-minute TNE session.

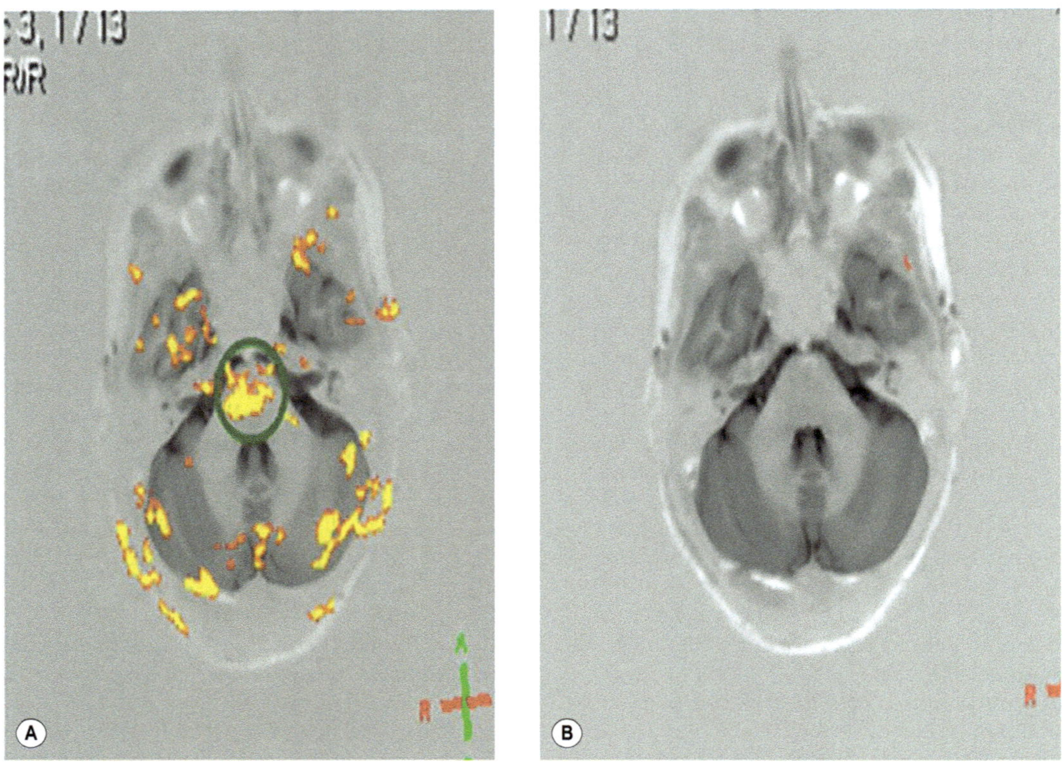

Figure 6.7 **(A) Brain activity during a painful task. Scan showing activation of the PAG (green circle). (B) The brain scan of the same patient, performing the same task following a TNE session, showing a deactivated PAG.**

plausible that the PAG was activated in response to a 'threatening' movement that this patient associated with a painful task. Following TNE, however, the same painful task did not result in a similar activation of the PAG (Fig. 6.7B). In line with current beliefs that TNE reconceptualizes pain and decreases fear associated with movement, one could interpret this single case as showing that the PAG no longer needed activation, as the incoming nociception was understood after the TNE session. However, future larger studies are needed to investigate the specific effect of TNE on the antinociceptive systems, such as the PAG.

Graded motor imagery – restructuring brain/body maps

Therapeutic treatments directly aiming at correcting functional changes in the brain have gained increased attention, especially in advanced pain states such as complex regional pain syndrome (CRPS) (Daly & Bialocerkowski 2009; Wand et al 2011). Graded motor imagery (GMI), a structured, sequential series of cortical exercises, aims to re-establish the cortical deficits described previously (Moseley 2004b, 2006; Daly & Bialocerkowski 2009; Bowering et al 2013). GMI contains strategies such as normalizing a person's ability to recognize left or right body parts or movements (laterality), motor imagery or visualization of static and dynamic use of a body part and mirror therapy. Apart from the increased interest, GMI has shown increasing evidence of efficacy as a means to influence positively such pain states such as CRPS (McCabe et al 2003; Moseley 2004b, 2006; Daly & Bialocerkowski 2009; Bowering et al 2013). Additional strategies aimed at restructuring cortical maps, such as sensory discrimination, graphesthesia and two-point discrimination, have been proposed and utilized alongside GMI to help facilitate these cortical changes (Moseley 2008b; Moseley et al 2008; Moseley & Wiech 2009; Luomajoki & Moseley 2011). Despite these early results and growing evidence, readers are cautioned that many unknowns still remain in this early thought process of cortical restructuring, although early findings do show promise. Traditional treatments such as manual therapy and being precise, specific and even vocalizing the intent and findings, such as a central posterior–anterior mobilization on the C4 spinal level, could also be seen as a form of cortical restructuring. As we gain more and more insight into the exact cortical changes that occur (i.e. two-point discrimination), treatments can become more deliberate and targeted towards creating a bottom-up feeding of the brain – in which the senses (touch, sight, sound, etc.) are used to help the brain understand more, lessening perceived threat and restoring body parts.

Conclusion

The decade of the brain has come and gone, yet we have barely scratched the surface. The new neuroscience view of pain, especially musculoskeletal pain, has created significant advances for patients and clinicians. For patients, neuroplasticity gives hope and people with advanced pain states such as CRPS can receive much-needed non-surgical and non-pharmacological help. For the clinician there is also hope. For too long has chronic pain been seen as a black hole from which there is no return. The advances described in this chapter allow clinicians to cease fearing chronic pain patients, but instead to create both new paradigms and new treatments. No human structure can have an impact on pain as much as the brain: 'no brain, no pain'.

References

Amit DJ, Brunel N, Tsodyks MV. 1994. Correlations of cortical Hebbian reverberations: theory versus experiment. J Neurosci 14: 6435–6445.

Ang DC, Chakr R, Mazzuca S, et al. 2010. Cognitive–behavioral therapy attenuates nociceptive responding in patients with fibromyalgia: a pilot study. Arthritis Care Res 62: 618–623.

Apkarian AV, Sosa Y, Sonty S, et al. 2004. Chronic back pain is associated with decreased prefrontal and thalamic gray matter density. J Neurosc 24: 10410–10415.

Apkarian AV, Baliki MN, Geha PY. 2009. Towards a theory of chronic pain. Progress Neurobiol 87: 81–97.

Bandler R, Keay KA. 1996. Columnar organization in the midbrain periaqueductal gray and the integration of emotional expression. Progress Brain Res 107: 285–300.

Beggs S, Liu XJ, Kwan C, et al. 2010. Peripheral nerve injury and TRPV1-expressing primary afferent C-fibers cause opening of the blood–brain barrier. Mol Pain 6: 74.

Bennett R, Nelson D. 2006. Cognitive behavioral therapy for fibromyalgia. Nat Clin Pract Rheumatol 2: 416–424.

Bowering KJ, O'Connell NE, Tabor A, et al. 2013. The effects of graded motor imagery and its components on chronic pain: a systematic review and meta-analysis. J Pain 14: 3–13.

Daly AE, Bialocerkowski AE. 2009. Does evidence support physiotherapy management of adult complex regional pain syndrome type one? A systematic review. Eur J Pain 13: 339–353.

de Lange FP, Koers A, Kalkman JS, et al. 2008. Increase in prefrontal cortical volume following cognitive behavioural therapy in patients with chronic fatigue syndrome. Brain 131: 2172–2180.

Doidge N. 2007. The brain that changes itself. New York: Penguin Books.

Fernández-Carnero J, Fernandez-de-las-Peñas C, Cleland JA. 2008. Immediate hypoalgesic and motor effects after a single cervical spine manipulation in subjects with lateral epicondylalgia. J Manipulative Physiol Ther 31: 675–681.

Fields HL, Basbaum AI, Heinricher MR. 2005. Central nervous system mechanisms of pain modulation. In: McMahon S, Koltzenburg M (eds) Wall and Melzack's textbook of pain. Edinburgh: Elsevier, pp 125–142.

Flor H. 2000. The functional organization of the brain in chronic pain. Prog Brain Res 129: 313–322.

Flor H. 2003. The image of pain. Annual scientific meeting of The Pain Society (Britain). Glasgow, Scotland. [Verbal presentation.]

Flor H, Braun C, Elbert T, et al. 1997. Extensive reorganization of primary somatosensory cortex in chronic back pain patients. Neurosci Lett 224: 5–8.

Flor H, Elbert T, Muhnickel W, et al. 1998. Cortical reorganisation and phantom phenomena in congenital and traumatic upper-extremity amputees. Exp Brain Res 119: 205–212.

George SZ, Bishop MD, Bialosky JE, et al. 2006. Immediate effects of spinal manipulation on thermal pain sensitivity: an experimental study. BMC Musculoskelet Disord 7: 68.

Giesecke T, Gracely RH, Clauw DJ, et al. 2006. Central pain processing in chronic low back pain. Evidence for reduced pain inhibition. Schmerz 20: 411–414.

Gifford LS. 1998. Pain, the tissues and the nervous system. Physiotherapy 84: 27–33.

Goldberg JS. 2008. Revisiting the cartesian model of pain. Med Hypotheses 70: 1029–1033.

Gwilym SE, Filippini N, Douaud G, et al. 2010. Thalamic atrophy associated with painful osteoarthritis of the hip is reversible after arthroplasty: a longitudinal voxel-based morphometric study. Arthr Rheum 62: 2930–2940.

Haldeman S. 1990. Presidential address, North American Spine Society: failure of the pathology model to predict back pain. Spine 15: 718–724.

Jacobs JV, Henry SM, Nagle KJ. 2010. Low back pain associates with altered activity of the cerebral cortex prior to arm movements that require postural adjustment. Clin Neurophysiol 121: 431–440.

Jull G, Sterling M, Kenardy J, et al. 2007. Does the presence of sensory hypersensitivity influence outcomes of physical rehabilitation for chronic whiplash? A preliminary RCT. Pain 129: 28–34.

Kendall N, Watson P. 2000. Identifying psychosocial yellow flags and modifying management. In: Gifford LS (ed) Topical issues in pain 2. Falmouth: CNS Press, pp 131–139.
Kendall NAS, Linton SJ, Main CJ. 1997. Guide to assessing psychosocial yellow flags in acute low back pain: risk factors for long term disability and work loss. Wellington: Accident Rehabilitation and Compensation Insurance Corporation of New Zealand and the National Health Committee.
Latremoliere A, Woolf CJ. 2009. Central sensitization: a generator of pain hypersensitivity by central neural plasticity. J Pain 10: 895–926.
Lloyd D, Findlay G, Roberts N, et al. 2008. Differences in low back pain behavior are reflected in the cerebral response to tactile stimulation of the lower back. Spine 33: 1372–1377.
Lotze M, Moseley GL. 2007. Role of distorted body image in pain. Curr Rheumatol Rep 9: 488–496.
Louw A, Puentedura EJ. 2013. Therapeutic neuroscience education. Minneapolis, MN: OPTP.
Louw A, Diener I, Butler DS, et al. 2011a. The effect of neuroscience education on pain, disability, anxiety, and stress in chronic musculoskeletal pain. Arch Phys Med Rehabil 92: 2041–2056.
Louw A, Puentedura EL, Mintken P. 2011b. Use of an abbreviated neuroscience education approach in the treatment of chronic low back pain: a case report. Physiother Theory Pract 28: 50–62
Louw A, Butler DS, Diener I, et al. 2013. Development of a preoperative neuroscience educational program for patients with lumbar radiculopathy. Am J Phys Med Rehabil 92: 446–452.
Luerding R, Weigand T, Bogdahn U, et al. 2008. Working memory performance is correlated with local brain morphology in the medial frontal and anterior cingulate cortex in fibromyalgia patients: structural correlates of pain-cognition interaction. Brain 131: 3222–3231.
Luomajoki H, Moseley GL. 2011. Tactile acuity and lumbopelvic motor control in patients with back pain and healthy controls. Br J Sports Med 45: 437–440.
Maihofner C, Handwerker HO, Neundorfer B, et al. 2003. Patterns of cortical reorganization in complex regional pain syndrome. Neurology 61: 1707–1715.
Marinus J, Moseley GL, Birklein F, et al. 2011. Clinical features and pathophysiology of complex regional pain syndrome. Lancet Neurol 10: 637–648.
McCabe CS, Haigh RC, Ring EFR, et al. 2003. A controlled pilot study of the utility of mirror visual feedback in the treatment of complex regional pain syndrome (type 1). Rheumatology 42: 97–101.
Meeus M, Nijs J, Van Oosterwijck J, et al. 2010. Pain physiology education improves pain beliefs in patients with chronic fatigue syndrome compared with pacing and self-management education: a double-blind randomized controlled trial. Arch Phys Med Rehabil 91: 1153–1159.
Melzack R. 1999. From the gate to the neuromatrix. Pain Suppl 6: S121–S126.
Melzack R. 2001. Pain and the neuromatrix in the brain. J Dent Educ 65: 1378–1382.
Melzack R, Wall PD, Ty TC. 1982. Acute pain in an emergency clinic: latency of onset and descriptor patterns related to different injuries. Pain 14: 33–43.
Moseley L. 2002. Combined physiotherapy and education is efficacious for chronic low back pain. Aust J Physiother 48: 297–302.
Moseley GL. 2003a. A pain neuromatrix approach to patients with chronic pain. Man Ther 8: 130–140.
Moseley GL. 2003b. Unraveling the barriers to reconceptualization of the problem in chronic pain: the actual and perceived ability of patients and health professionals to understand the neurophysiology. J Pain 4: 184–189.
Moseley GL. 2003c. Joining forces – combining cognition-targeted motor control training with group or individual pain physiology education: a successful treatment for chronic low back pain. J Manual Manipulative Ther 11: 88–94.
Moseley GL. 2004a. Why do people with complex regional pain syndrome take longer to recognize their affected hand? Neurology 62: 2182–2186.
Moseley GL. 2004b. Graded motor imagery is effective for long standing complex regional pain syndrome. Pain 108: 192–198.
Moseley GL. 2004c. Evidence for a direct relationship between cognitive and physical change during an education intervention in people with chronic low back pain. Eur J Pain 8: 39–45.
Moseley GL. 2005a. Widespread brain activity during an abdominal task markedly reduced after pain physiology education: fMRI evaluation of a single patient with chronic low back pain. Aust J Physiother 51: 49–52.
Moseley GL. 2005b. Distorted body image in complex regional pain syndrome. Neurology 65: 773.
Moseley GL. 2006. Graded motor imagery for pathologic pain: a randomized controlled trial. Neurology 67: 2129–2134.
Moseley GL. 2007. Reconceptualising pain acording to modern pain sciences. Phys Ther Rev 12: 169–178.
Moseley GL. 2008a. I can't find it! Distorted body image and tactile dysfunction in patients with chronic back pain. Pain 140: 239–243.
Moseley GL. 2008b. Pain, brain imaging and physiotherapy: opportunity is knocking. Man Ther 13: 475–477.
Moseley GL, Hodges PW. 2002. Chronic pain and motor control. In: Jull G, Boyling J (eds) Grieve's modern manual therapy of the vertebral column. Edinburgh: Churchill-Livingstone, pp 215–231.
Moseley GL, Wiech K. 2009. The effect of tactile discrimination training is enhanced when patients watch the reflected image of their unaffected limb during training. Pain 144: 314–319.
Moseley GL, Nicholas MK, Hodges PW. 2004. A randomized controlled trial of intensive neurophysiology education in chronic low back pain. Clin J Pain 20: 324–330.
Moseley GL, Sim DF, Henry ML, et al. 2005. Experimental hand pain delays recognition of the contralateral hand – evidence that acute and chronic pain have opposite effects on information processing? Brain Res Cogn Brain Res 25: 188–194.
Moseley GL, Zalucki NM, Wiech K. 2008. Tactile discrimination, but not tactile stimulation alone, reduces chronic limb pain. Pain 137: 600–608.
Nijs J, Van Houdenhove B, Oostendorp RA. 2010. Recognition of central sensitization in patients with musculoskeletal pain: application of pain neurophysiology in manual therapy practice. Man Ther 15: 135–141.
Nijs J, Meeus M, Van Oosterwijck J, et al. 2011. Treatment of central sensitization in patients with 'unexplained' chronic pain: what options do we have? Expert Opin Pharmacother 12: 1087–1098.
Nijs J, Kosek E, Van Oosterwijck J, et al. 2012. Dysfunctional endogenous analgesia during exercise in patients with chronic pain: to exercise or not to exercise? Pain Phys 15: ES205–ES213.
Parry DM, Macmillan FM, Koutsikou S, et al. 2008. Separation of A- versus C-nociceptive inputs into spinal–brainstem circuits. Neuroscience 152: 1076–1085.
Penfield W, Boldrey E. 1937. Somatic, motor and sensory representation in the cerebral cortex of man as studied by electrical stimulation. Brain 60: 389–448.
Peyron R, Laurent B, Garcia-Larrea L. 2000. Functional imaging of brain responses to pain. A review and meta-analysis (2000). Neurophysiol Clin 30: 263–288.
Puentedura EJ, Louw A. 2012. A neuroscience approach to managing athletes with low back pain. Phys Ther Sport 13: 123–133.
Puentedura EJ, Cleland JA, Landers MR, et al. 2012. Development of a clinical prediction rule to identify patients with neck pain likely to benefit from thrust joint manipulation to the cervical spine. J Orthop Sports Phys Ther 42: 577–592.
Richardson C, Hodges P, Hides J. 2004. Therapeutic exercise for lumbopelvic stabilization. London: Churchill Livingstone.
Rodríguez-Raecke R, Niemeier A, Ihle K, et al. 2009. Brain gray matter decrease in chronic pain is the consequence and not the cause of pain. J Neurosci 29: 13746–13750.
Ryan CG, Gray HG, Newton M, et al. 2010. Pain biology education and exercise classes compared to pain biology education alone for individuals with chronic low back pain: a pilot randomised controlled trial. Man Ther 15: 382–387.
Sapolsky RM. 1994. Why zebras don't get ulcers. New York: Freeman.
Schmidt-Wilcke T. 2008.Variations in brain volume and regional morphology associated with chronic pain. Curr Rheumatol Rep 10: 467–474.
Schmidt-Wilcke T, Leinisch E, Ganssbauer S, et al. 2006. Affective components and intensity of pain correlate with structural differences in gray matter in chronic back pain patients. Pain 125: 89–97.
Schmidt-Wilcke T, Ganssbauer S, Neuner T, et al. 2008. Subtle grey matter changes between migraine patients and healthy controls. Cephalalgia 28: 1–4.
Seminowicz DA, Wideman TH, Naso L, et al. 2011. Effective treatment of chronic low back pain in humans reverses abnormal brain anatomy and function. J Neurosci 31: 7540–7550.
Seminowicz DA, Shpaner M, Keaser ML, et al. 2013. Cognitive–behavioral therapy increases prefrontal cortex gray matter in patients with chronic pain. J Pain 14: 1573–1584.
Stavrinou ML, Della Penna S, Pizzella V, et al. 2007. Temporal dynamics of plastic changes in human primary somatosensory cortex after finger webbing. Cereb Cortex 17: 2134–2142.
Sterling M, Jull G, Wright A. 2001. Cervical mobilisation: concurrent effects on pain, sympathetic nervous system activity and motor activity. Man Ther 6: 72–81.

Tracey I, Bushnell MC. 2009. How neuroimaging studies have challenged us to rethink: is chronic pain a disease? J Pain 10: 1113–1120.
Tracey I, Ploghaus A, Gati JS, et al. 2002. Imaging attentional modulation of pain in the periaqueductal gray in humans. J Neurosci 22: 2748–2752.
Tsao H, Hodges PW. 2007. Immediate changes in feedforward postural adjustments following voluntary motor training. Exp Brain Res 181: 537–546.
Tsao H, Galea MP, Hodges PW. 2008. Reorganization of the motor cortex is associated with postural control deficits in recurrent low back pain. Brain 131: 2161–2171.
Vicenzino B, Collins D, Wright A. 1996. The initial effects of a cervical spine manipulative physiotherapy treatment on the pain and dysfunction of lateral epicondylalgia. Pain 68: 69–74.
Wall PD. 1996. Comments after 30 years of the gate control theory. Pain Forum 5: 12–22.
Wand BM, Parkitny L, O'Connell NE, et al. 2011. Cortical changes in chronic low back pain: current state of the art and implications for clinical practice. Man Ther 16: 15–20.
Wiech K, Tracey I. 2009. The influence of negative emotions on pain: behavioral effects and neural mechanisms. Neuroimage 47: 987–994.
Wolpert DM, Ghahramani Z, Flanagan JR. 2001. Perspectives and problems in motor learning. Trends Cognitive Sci 5: 487–494.
Woolf CJ. 2007. Central sensitization: uncovering the relation between pain and plasticity. Anesthesiology 106: 864–867.
Woolf CJ, Mannion RJ. 1999. Neuropathic pain: aetiology, symptoms, mechanisms, and management. Lancet 353: 1959–1964.
Woolf CJ, Salter MW. 2005. Plasticity and pain: the role of the dorsal horn. In: McMahon S, Koltzenburg M (eds) Wall and Melzack's textbook of pain. Edinburgh: Elsevier, pp 91–105.

7 Chapter

Mechanical Diagnosis and Therapy for the Spine: McKenzie Method

Stephen May, Richard Rosedale

CHAPTER CONTENTS

Introduction	76
The literature base for MDT	77
Epidemiological perspective	77
Review of anatomy and biomechanics in MDT	78
Review of proposed pathology and anatomy in MDT	79
Evidence regarding diagnosis in MDT	80
Evidence regarding prognosis in MDT	80
Evidence regarding conservative treatment with MDT	80
Conclusion	82

Introduction

The method of Mechanical Diagnosis and Therapy (MDT) was devised by Robin McKenzie, a New Zealand physiotherapist, during the 1950s and 1960s following a chance clinical encounter. A patient had lain on a treatment couch with the head end raised in a prone position following several episodes of unsuccessful treatment for his back and leg pain. When Robin McKenzie entered the room several minutes later he was shocked to see the patient lying in this position, as in those days extension was considered a very unsuitable position for patients with leg pain. However, before McKenzie could say anything the patient volunteered the information that his leg pain 'had not felt so good in weeks and most of it had gone, although the back felt a bit worse'. It was McKenzie's first encounter with what he came to term **centralization**.

Over the ensuing years Robin McKenzie continued to experiment with sustained positions and then more commonly with repeated movements. He used repeated movements so that patients were able to continue the exercises independently at home by repeating them every few hours. Self-management was to become a central tenet of the method. Robin McKenzie found that extension did not help all patients; in fact, it made some worse, so he experimented with flexion and frontal plane movements. He found that some patients were effectively treated with these other directions of movement and so his assessment developed to explore the potential for different directions of movement to produce a positive effect on symptoms.

In attempting to adapt his findings from the lumbar spine to the cervical spine, McKenzie found that his initial success was somewhat more limited. However, his efforts were assisted when he was made aware of the work of Dr Laurens Penning, a neuroradiologist from Amsterdam. This led Robin McKenzie to begin also to explore the effects of retraction and protrusion as well as flexion and extension motions, culminating in his finding much greater success when using retraction prior to moving the neck into extension (Ordway et al 1999).

Positive effects in the lumbar and cervical spine included centralization or a lasting decrease in symptoms and an increase in the reduced range of movement in response to repeated movements or sustained positions. The movements or postures that produced these responses became known as the **directional preference**. The key to directional preference was that these positive therapeutic effects were apparently the result of therapeutic interventions, and not simply the effect of a natural history. Centralization and directional preference in response to repeat movements are now central tenets of the method, and are characteristic of what Robin McKenzie termed **derangement syndrome**. These phenomena have subsequently become the focus of some research over the years as the implications of this response to simple end-range exercises and loading strategies are wide ranging and sometimes clinically significant.

Thus grew an assessment and management process that was based on a hands-off, patient-centred exercise-based approach, without emphasis on therapist-centred palpation or mobilization procedures. If, however, the patient either did not demonstrate a positive directional preference or came to a plateau after initial improvement then therapist-generated forces could be added into the patient-generated forces. This principle of the method was termed **force progression**. The use of different starting positions or different directions of movement, such as standing or lying, or frontal plane movements as opposed to sagittal plane movements, were termed **force alternatives**.

McKenzie also recognized that not everybody showed a rapid pain-change response. A subgroup of patients responded well to repeated painful end-range movements, but only gradually improved and restored a reduced range of movement over time. This subgroup of mechanical classification was known as **dysfunction syndrome**. An even smaller group, often young patients with very poor posture, had a normal physical examination with only sustained postures provoking the symptoms. These patients responded to postural correction, and therefore this subgroup was named **postural syndrome**. McKenzie hypothesized that this group might represent the mild end of the back and neck pain continuum before progression to more disabling conditions such as derangement. The key was that McKenzie recognized that spinal pain conditions presented in different, but very distinct, ways. Another core aspect of the method was set in motion – that of subclassification. Robin McKenzie also recognized that not everybody could be classified within one of the above three syndromes; those outside these subgroups were termed **non-mechanical syndromes** and now represent the MDT 'other' classifications. However, it is important to note that not all patients with spinal pain conditions can be properly included in any of these subgroups.

The Literature Base for MDT

After many years developing and then teaching the method, McKenzie started to describe it; first in a series of *Treat Your Own Back / Neck* booklets aimed at patients (McKenzie 1980, 1983), and then in two textbooks for clinicians describing the management strategy for the lumbar and then the cervical and thoracic spines (McKenzie 1981, 1990). At these points in time there was limited scientific evidence to support the concepts outlined above and their relevance to clinical practice. However, since 1990 there has been a growing body of evidence that has endorsed certain aspects of the method, especially in the lumbar spine. Evidence is still limited with respect to the cervical spine and the extremities, but is becoming more substantial. During the early to mid 2000s the original textbooks were carefully revised, including the contextual background for back and neck pain, describing the technical aspects of using the approach, and giving the evidence relevant to the method (McKenzie & May 2003, 2006).

McKenzie had always recommended that the concepts he described were equally applicable to extremity problems and the first of the last series of books was about the application of this approach to musculoskeletal problems in the upper and lower extremities (McKenzie & May 2000). This development also included distinguishing between articular and contractile dysfunctions; articular dysfunctions present with painful end-range restrictions of movement at joints, whereas contractile dysfunctions present with pain on loading contractile tissues, notably tendons, with resisted or active movements. Instruction in the use of the methods as applied to extremity problems is now included in the training courses. (The use of MDT in the extremities is dealt with in more detail in Ch 8.)

When McKenzie began to describe the method of MMDT he was initially met with considerable scepticism, especially by medical colleagues. In order to confront or challenge these criticisms, a series of models to describe the subclassification syndromes were developed. However, these were very much theoretical models rather than clear-cut pathological scenarios. It must be recognized that the operational definitions for all mechanical syndromes and for the other syndromes are based entirely on clinical presentations and responses (Table 7.1). The method is not reliant on diagnostic modelling, although pathological criteria can be suggested in certain instances, especially amongst the other categories. The following sections will focus on the application of the McKenzie method in the lumbar and the cervical spine.

Epidemiological Perspective

The epidemiological nature of low back pain and other musculoskeletal problems is well known. Despite early claims that the majority of low back pain is acute and only a small proportion is chronic, more recent evidence contradicts this perspective. Low back pain is frequently protracted and chronic, and shows limited improvement between 3 months and 1 year (Abbott & Mercer 2002; Pengel et al 2003; Hayden et al 2010). This persistence is seen in over 50% of those with acute low back pain (Pengel et al 2003; Hayden et al 2010). Furthermore, even in those who recover quickly, recurrence in the subsequent year is extremely common – happening in about 70% of those with an initial episode (Abbott & Mercer 2002; Pengel et al 2003). One survey of nearly 600 patients with low back pain found that 73% reported previous episodes, and over 60% reported a worsening of symptoms over time with subsequent episodes (Donelson et al 2012).

Although there are fewer studies related to the cervical spine, the pattern appears to be mirrored there. A systematic review of the prognosis of acute neck pain reported that the outcome is relatively poor and resolution commonly incomplete with regards to both pain and disability (Hush et al 2011). In fact, improvement in both pain and disability appeared to cease after 6.5 weeks with no further improvements up to 1 year. The remaining symptoms were severe enough to interfere with daily life activities and adversely affect quality of life (Hush et al 2011) and even compared unfavourably with the outcomes reported for low back pain (Pengel et al 2003).

Hence, despite the fact that spinal pain is more commonly cared for conservatively, because of the extremely large population numbers the impact on healthcare is enormous. It is difficult to estimate the cost for such a common condition, for which patients might seek a myriad of healthcare providers; however, one review (Dagenais et al 2008) found that physical therapy absorbed the largest proportion of direct medical costs (17%), but indirect, societal costs represented the majority of overall costs associated with back pain. It was estimated that in 2005 the mean medical expenditure in the USA for those with spine problems was over $6000 – nearly double that of those without spine problems (Martin et al 2008); this represented a 65% increase from 1997, despite which limitations in physical function had increased.

Clinicians should explore all possible avenues for patients with spinal pain to treat their symptoms effectively and to involve them in their own treatment. The physical therapist's primary role should be to assess, diagnose and guide the patient in the therapeutic process. As much as is possible, patients should actually be involved in their own therapeutic process. In that way, they should be able to manage the current and future episodes. For instance, if the main problem

Table 7.1 Operational definitions for mechanical syndromes and 'other'

Mechanical syndromes	
Derangement	Centralization or progressive abolition of distal pain in response to therapeutic loading Each progressive abolition retained over time until all symptoms are abolished Back pain is also abolished Changes in pain remain better Accompanied by changes in mechanical presentation, such as increase in range of movement
Articular dysfunction	Local pain only Intermittent pain only At least one movement is restricted and restricted movement consistently produces concordant pain at end range No rapid reduction or abolition of symptoms No lasting production or peripheralization of symptoms
Contractile dysfunction	Intermittent pain only Concordant pain reproduced with resisted movement Active movements may also be painful
Postural syndrome	Local pain only Intermittent pain only Concordant pain with static loading Abolition of pain with postural correction No pain with repeated movements No loss of range of movement No pain during movement
'Other'	
Spinal stenosis	Leg symptoms when walking, eased in flexion Minimal extension Sustained extension provokes leg symptoms
Isthmic spondylolisthesis	Sports-related injury in adolescence Worse with static loading
Hip	Pain on walking, eased with sitting Specific pain pattern Positive hip tests
Sacroiliac joint (SIJ)	Three or more positive SIJ pain provocation tests
Mechanically inconclusive	Inconsistent response to loading strategies No obstruction to movement
Chronic pain	Persistent widespread pain Aggravation with all activity Exaggerated pain behaviour Inappropriate beliefs and attitudes about pain

conforms to the typical natural history, then during reoccurrences the patient should be able to apply the same principles and exercise programmes they found successful with their previous episode to treat and manage the current one. Other approaches that encourage therapist dependency and leave the patient as only a passive recipient of care should be complemented with more active approaches including the McKenzie method and exercise programmes. Therapists need to consider the broader implications of the available management strategies and ask themselves whether they have fully explored the potential therapeutic options for teaching patients to participate in their own management.

Review of Anatomy and Biomechanics in MDT

Mechanical Diagnosis and Therapy uses the physiological movements that are available at the joints concerned. For instance, in the examination of spinal problems, sagittal plane movements, flexion and extension motions are always examined first as most spinal problems respond in this plane of movement. Extension is the movement that is the most common direction of preference. This was confirmed in a study of New Zealand patients from 34 physical therapists (Hefford 2008); this study of 340 patients looked at the profile of syndromes and the directional preference prevalence. Of the 187 lumbar spine patients in the derangement category 70%, 6% and 24% were given extension, flexion and lateral movements respectively to centralize or to have a lasting positive symptomatic effect. For the 111 cervical spine patients, treatment directions for the derangements were similar: 72%, 9% and 19% for extension, flexion and lateral movements respectively (Hefford 2008). The one exception to starting always with sagittal plane movements is those few patients who present with a lateral shift or acute wry neck, in which case management is initiated in the frontal plane.

The frontal plane movement that is utilized in McKenzie assessment of the lumbar spine is the side-glide in standing. This movement tends to focus movement on the lower lumbar spine where most of the issues occur, whereas with side-flexion the upper lumbar spine is more engaged (Mulvein & Jull 1995). When a patient presents with a lateral shift it is the side-glide in standing movement that is the one most obstructed, so in assessing this movement the therapist is able to reveal whether there is any loss and tendency towards this particular lumbar deformity.

In the cervical spine it is important to remember that protrusion and retraction are part of sagittal plane movements. Retraction fully flexes the upper cervical spine and extends the lower cervical spine; conversely, protrusion fully extends the upper cervical spine and flexes the lower (Penning 1998). One of the clinical implications is that fully restoring retraction is a prerequisite to recovering full extension. If retraction has not been restored, extension may not have the desirable symptomatic effect. Frontal plane movements are tested only when the sagittal plane has been fully exhausted and they are required in a smaller subgroup of patients. Rotation or lateral flexion is tested during the assessment in this circumstance, and in a minority of patients either one of these may provide a directional preference for the lateral principle.

Review of Proposed Pathology and Anatomy in MDT

The system of MDT is essentially based on non-pathology-specific mechanical syndromes whose operational definitions are derived from the symptomatic and mechanical responses (see Table 7.1). However, some conceptual models that might explain these symptomatic responses have been suggested (McKenzie & May 2000, 2003, 2006; May 2006).

The conceptual model offered to explain derangement syndrome in the spine relates to the dynamic disc model (Wetzel & Donelson 2003; Kolber & Hanney 2009). Within this model it is suggested that internal intervertebral disc disruption and displacement of disc material can result in pain and impaired movement. The end of the pathological continuum would be extrusion or sequestration of disc material through the outer restraining annulus fibrosus. This frank herniation causes sciatica or cervical radiculopathy. However, at the mild end of the continuum, there would be easily reversible internal disc displacement resulting in back or neck pain, with or without some referred symptoms. With increasing disc displacement there would be more signs and symptoms. The direction of the displacement would indicate the therapeutic loading necessary; most commonly posterior and posterior–lateral displacements would require extension forces, anterior displacement would require flexion forces, and lateral displacement would require frontal plane procedures.

The conceptual model in no way implies that the McKenzie method can be used only to treat discogenic pain, as has been misinterpreted by some clinicians and researchers. Although it is only a conceptual model, there are a number of studies that validate it. The disc is a common source of back and leg pain (Ohnmeiss et al 1997; Milette et al 1999), centralization has been associated with discogenic pain (Donelson et al 1997; Werneke et al 1999), and in vivo studies have shown the disc to be mobile with loading strategies (Brault et al 1997; Edmondston et al 2000). Numerous other studies supporting the dynamic disc model as a source of symptoms have been described (Wetzel & Donelson 2003). A systematic review supported the dynamic disc model in the lumbar spine, although noted some inconsistencies in its application to the presence of disc degeneration (Kolber & Hanney 2009).

There has been some controversy over the application of this conceptual disc model in the cervical spine (Mercer & Jull 1996). This was provoked with the recognition that the cervical disc is morphologically and biochemically distinct from the lumbar disc (Mercer & Bogduk 1999). Despite these differences, a more recent stress profilometry study showed that cervical discs usually have a hydrostatic nucleus. The discs exhibit a high concentration of compressive force anteriorly with flexion and high compressive stress posteriorly in extension (Skrzpiec et al 2007). These findings of similarities in properties between the cervical and lumbar discs may go some way to explain similarities in the clinical response observed between the two regions. It is clear that we cannot so readily dismiss the disc model despite other documented differences. Similarities and differences aside, in the cervical as in the lumbar spine, it is the symptomatic and mechanical responses that determine classification and the appropriate therapeutic choice. The diagnosis of derangement remains non-pathoanatomical.

The conceptual model underlying the dysfunction syndrome is the mechanical deformation of structurally impaired soft tissue. This is caused by trauma, previous derangement or degenerative changes. After this initial event, full rehabilitation or remodelling does not happen sufficiently or appropriately (Hunter 1994); there follows a lengthy history of several months in which the patient may be left with a painful impairment associated with restricted movement in a single direction, or less commonly in multiple directions. Dysfunctions may affect articular or peri-articular structures, such as occurs in early osteoarthritis (McCarthy et al 1994). They also may affect contractile tissue, most commonly tendons, such as the common extensor origin at the elbow, the tendons at the shoulder or the Achilles tendon, leading to tendinopathy (Littlewood 2012). Dysfunction also, rarely, affects neural structures; this would be classified as an adherent nerve root and might occur after the partial resolution of an episode of sciatica (Melbye 2010). Adherent nerve root presents with very limited range of flexion in standing, which produces leg symptoms at end range. In the direction of the dysfunction the pain is produced consistently each time, regardless of how many repetitions are done, but ceases when the movement is ended. (Readers are referred to Ch 65 for further discussion on neurodynamics.) Articular dysfunctions typically present with restricted and painful end-range movements in certain patterns – for instance at the knee with loss of flexion and / or extension, or at the hip with loss of medial rotation and flexion. Contractile dysfunction presents usually with full, but possibly painful, active movement; the patient's familiar pain is produced when the relevant movement is resisted, such as resisted wrist extension or resisted shoulder abduction.

The conceptual model for the postural syndrome relates to pain that is induced because soft tissues are overstretched, blood flow is restricted and the tissue is starved of oxygen. This occurs with sustained loading over the tissue for a period of time. It is not frequently seen in the clinic as the symptoms are relatively mild, but is commonly found in student-age populations (Womesley & May 2006; May et al 2011). It is associated with poor posture and is hypothesized to lead to the more disabling syndromes associated with later life. (Readers can find further information on soft tissue disorders in Part 10.)

Again, it is important to emphasize the fact that these mechanical syndromes are classified by their symptomatic and mechanical responses (see Table 7.1); therefore, these mechanical syndromes are defined by their response to repeated movements. The conceptual models suggested above are no more than that: conceptual models.

Evidence Regarding Diagnosis in MDT

Diagnostic accuracy depends on two psychometric properties: validity and reliability. In order to establish the validity, both the sensitivity and the specificity (see Ch 5) are evaluated so as to gauge how accurate specific criteria or clinical tests are in making a pathology-specific orthopaedic diagnosis. In the McKenzie system a specific pathological diagnosis is not being sought; therefore, the main requirement is to know whether the assessment process is reliable between clinicians. In a systematic review of 48 reliability studies on physical examination procedures for patients with non-specific low back pain (May et al 2006) most procedures showed limited reliability. With an upper threshold of kappa / intra-class correlation coefficient of 0.85, most procedures demonstrated either conflicting evidence or moderate to strong evidence of low reliability. When a lower threshold was used – a kappa (κ) / intra-class correlation coefficient of 0.70 – the procedure of pain response to several repeated movements demonstrated moderate evidence for high reliability.

In fact, several exploratory procedures including manual palpation, visual observation and mobility assessments have also shown weak reliability. An inaccurate diagnosis is the likely sequel and management strategies should be based on reliable assessment outcomes. In such a scenario – that is, pain responses to repeated movements – as testing used for directional preference and centralization has demonstrated reasonably good levels of reliability it therefore can constitute a proper method of establishing a classification and determining management strategies. Five studies have examined the reliability of the McKenzie classification system itself; of these, three reported kappa values of 0.7 or greater, one reported moderate agreement on cervical classification (Dionne et al 2006) and one reported poor kappa values but the therapists involved had limited knowledge of the classification system (May et al 2006).

Evidence Regarding Prognosis in MDT

Within physical therapy examination procedures, centralization has been demonstrated to be a good prognostic factor. Centralization is defined as the abolition of distal pain *in response to therapeutic loading*. Distal or leg pain can come or go during the natural history of back pain; this is not the same as centralization or directional preference, which by definition must be demonstrated during repeated movements or other therapeutic interventions. This distinction is important as most of the evidence about these clinical phenomena derives from their clinically driven nature.

One systematic review of 22 articles investigating prognostic value (Chorti et al 2009) revealed that directional preference (i.e. changes in pain location and / or intensity induced by repeated spinal movements) showed evidence supporting the use of these responses to inform management. A more recent systematic review located 54 articles for centralization and eight for directional preference (May & Aina 2012). Centralization showed a prevalence rate of 44% in a total of 4745 patients, with a higher rate in acute (74%) than in subacute or chronic patients (42%). The prevalence rate of directional preference was 70% in 2368 patients. It is clear that these clinical phenomena are commonly encountered in spinal patients. Out of 23 studies investigating the prognostic validity of centralization, 21 demonstrated a positive effect in those patients who demonstrated centralization, compared with those who did not. For both centralization and directional preference, in seven out of eight studies there is evidence that they are useful treatment-effect modifiers. The implications of these findings are that these clinical responses, based on this mechanical assessment, are evidence-based ways of establishing appropriate management strategies for subgroups of patients with spinal problems.

Evidence Regarding Conservative Treatment with MDT

When evaluating treatment efficacy the ideal study design is the randomized controlled trial (RCT). Systematic reviews are used to summarize this evidence analytically and guidelines then use these systematic reviews to make their prescriptive management suggestions. A number of systematic reviews related to he McKenzie method have been published (Table 7.2), all of which provide some support for the efficacy of MDT or classification-based management of lumbar spine problems.

A few of the randomized controlled trials on the use of the McKenzie system in the lumbar spine are worth highlighting. A multicentre trial of individuals with acute and chronic low back pain challenged the guideline advice that no one specific exercise or repeated movement is better than any other (Long et al 2004). This was the first clinical trial to subgroup patients prior to randomization using the derangement

Table 7.2 **Conclusions from systematic reviews regarding evidence for the McKenzie method and classification systems**

Reference	Number of RCTs	Remit	Conclusions
Clare et al 2004	6	Use of McKenzie principles Meta-analysis of data	Short-term 8.6% greater reduction in pain, 5.4% greater reduction in disability than controls
Cook et al 2005	5 – high quality (PEDro)	Therapeutic exercises with patients classified using symptom responses	4 / 5 significantly better than control group
Machado et al 2006	11 – mostly high quality	McKenzie method Meta-analysis of data	Short-term 4.2% greater reduction in pain, 5.2% greater reduction in disability than controls
Slade & Keating 2007	6 – high quality	Unloaded exercises; 4 / 6 McKenzie exercises	Short-term mean difference favoured McKenzie for pain 0.36–0.63 and for function 0.45–0.47
Fersum et al 2009	5	Subclassification systems and matched interventions for manual therapy and exercise	Subclassification systems significantly better reduction in pain and disability short term, long term for pain
Kent et al 2010	4 – high quality	Targeted manual therapy or exercise therapy	One study showed McKenzie method had significantly better effects short term
Slater et al 2012	7 – quality of evidence low	Subclassification systems and matched intervention for manual therapy	Significant treatment effects favoured the classification-based treatment compared with controls in pain and disability short and medium term
Surkitt et al 2012	6 – 5 high quality	Management using directional preference (DP)	Moderate evidence that DP is significantly more effective than controls in short and long term

classification. Two hundred and thirty patients classified with derangement syndrome were randomized into three groups: one in which they performed the matched exercise to their directional preference, one in which they exercised in the opposite direction to their directional preference and one in which they were given 'evidenced-based' general exercises. The matched group improved to a significantly greater degree for all outcomes, which included leg pain, back pain, disability, medication use, depression and interference with activity. Over 90% of the matched group rated themselves as better or resolved at 2 weeks, compared with just over 20% of the opposite group and just over 40% of the evidenced-based group. The magnitude of differences between the groups demonstrates clearly that, in this sample of patients with low back pain, the direction of exercises they were given did matter. All of the patients included in the study had a favourable prognosis, so the dramatic differences in outcomes were highly dependent on the matching of the exercises to the specific patient direction. A follow-up study showed the results of the introduction of directional preference exercises to those patients who were worse or unchanged during the initial 2-week trial period (Long et al 2008). Substantial improvements in pain and functional outcomes were the result, mirroring the effect on the original directional preference group in the trial.

Another high-quality randomized controlled clinical trial compared the McKenzie method with chiropractic manipulation in 350 patients who demonstrated either centralization or peripheralization (Petersen et al 2011). Both groups improved, but the number of patients within the McKenzie group reporting success was greater. The McKenzie group had significantly greater improvement than the manipulation group in regards to function and global perceived effect at both 2 months and 12 months. A greater number of withdrawals in the manipulation group reinforced the conclusion that McKenzie therapy is a suitable method for individuals showing either centralization or peripheralization. A possible implication of this study is related to the fact that, in patients exhibiting centralization or peripheralization, an active intervention such as McKenzie therapy (where the forces are applied by the patients themselves) can be more effective than a passive intervention such as manipulative therapy (where it is the clinician who applies the forces).

The last high-quality trial was conducted on individuals reporting severe sciatica (Albert & Manniche 2012), in which 181 patients were randomized into two treatment groups: a 'symptom-guided' exercise group that utilized the McKenzie system and were given stabilization exercises, and a sham exercise group in which patients were given low-dose exercises. Despite patients' expectations of having greater improvement with the low-dose exercises, significantly more patients in the group given McKenzie stabilization exercises experienced improvement and there was a trend towards significance in leg pain reduction compared with the sham group. Perhaps the most dramatic differences were exhibited in the neurological signs at the end of treatment and at 1 year. There was a significant 40% and 43% reduction in the number of individuals with motor deficit and sensory disturbance respectively by the end of McKenzie treatment, versus a 13% and 30% reduction respectively in the sham group. These differences remained significant at 1 year. Nevertheless, there is certainly the need for further high-quality trials in the lumbar

Table 7.3 **Guideline recommendations for the McKenzie system**

Guideline	Aspect of McKenzie system recommended	Degree of recommendation
Danish Institute for Health Technology Assessment (1999)	Assessment, treatment and prognosis	As a diagnostic and prognostic method for both acute and chronic low back pain (LBP) Treatment recommended for certain conditions
American College of Occupational and Environmental Medicine (2005)	McKenzie approach	Supported as a classification system for acute and subacute LBP
Quebec CLIP guidelines (Rossignol et al 2007)	McKenzie approach	Low recommendation for acute LBP Moderate recommendation for subacute LBP Low recommendation for chronic LBP
Work Loss Data Institute (2008)	Assessment, subgrouping using centralization, treatment effects	Recognized reliability of assessment, the value of subgrouping using centralization Treatment recommended for acute and chronic for pain and disability in the short term
Michigan Quality Improvement Consortium Guideline (Goertz et al 2012)	McKenzie exercises	Level A evidence for pain radiating below knee
Journal of Family Practice Guideline (Bach & Holten 2009)	McKenzie exercises	Grade A recommendation for pain radiating below knee
APTA Guideline (Delitto et al 2012)	Centralization and directional preference exercises	Supported by strong, level-A evidence

spine but, as can be seen from the examples above and the systematic reviews (see Table 7.2), significant progress has been made. In fact, this progress is reflected by some of the recommendations in low back pain guidelines published by various institutions (Table 7.3).

The evidence base for the efficacy of the McKenzie system in the cervical spine is more limited at this point in time, but three trials are worthy of mention. A Swedish randomized controlled trial compared general exercise, McKenzie therapy and a control group in patients with neck pain (Kjellman & Oberg 2002). The only significant resultant differences in this three-group comparison were in general health and a psychosomatic and depressive scale, where only the McKenzie group showed significant improvements. In a further two-group analysis, the McKenzie group showed significantly greater improvements than the control group for pain intensity at 3 and 6 months and for disability post treatment. Additional healthcare use was much less in the McKenzie group. In a Polish clinical trial including 61 individuals with chronic cervical derangement, McKenzie therapy was compared with 'traditional therapy' and found to be significantly more effective in terms of reductions in head, upper extremity and overall pain as well as in the number of pain-free days (Guzy et al 2011). The other trial of significance in the cervical spine was conducted on 97 patients suffering from whiplash-associated disorders (Rosenfeld et al 2000). In this high-quality trial, patients were randomized into an active intervention group based on McKenzie principles and a 'standard' intervention group. At the 6-month follow-up, the pain was significantly less in the McKenzie active group. The patients were then followed up for 3 years and the McKenzie active group still had significantly less pain, less need for sick leave and a better chance of regaining the former range of cervical motion (Rosenfeld et al 2003). An economic analysis of the study demonstrated lower costs for the McKenzie active group both for healthcare and for lost productivity (Rosenfeld et al 2006).

With the finding regarding the high prevalence of derangements in the cervical and thoracic spine (Hefford 2008), and thus the potential for a significant population that may experience a rapid response to simple end-range exercises, the need for clinical trials exploring the McKenzie system with the cervical spine is compelling.

Conclusion

The system of MDT has scientific evidence supporting its use, especially in regards to its reliability, its prognostic validity and its effectiveness for treating patients with low back pain. It is an assessment and management system that can be used as a screening tool for several patients with musculoskeletal problems, and is able to broadly distinguish responders from slow responders and from non-responders to a specific therapy. The three mechanical syndromes respond in a predictable way, the biggest proportion of which will be derangement, which will respond rapidly to repeated movements with centralization or a lasting decrease in symptoms. These responses of centralization and directional preference are supported in the literature with respect to their prognostic value. A few patients will present with dysfunction, which will respond more slowly to repeated movements, and a very few will present with postural syndrome. Patients not classifiable in one of the mechanical syndromes might be classified as one of the 'other' classifications. The response of the 'others' to intervention is less predictable: some may respond well, some partially and some may need a referral for other interventions. Classification is based on the operational definitions presented. The evidence base is substantial regarding the lumbar spine, but less, though accumulating, regarding the cervical spine and the use of MDT in the extremities.

Given the confines of the chapter, only a limited reference base has been cited. (For full access to reference citations see Core reference list at www.mckenziemdt.org.)

Acknowledgements

In memory of Robin McKenzie 1931–2013.

References

Abbott JH, Mercer SR. 2002. The natural history of acute low back pain. N Z J Physiother 30: 8–16.

Albert HB, Manniche C. 2012. The efficacy of systematic active conservative treatment for patients with severe sciatica: a single-blind, randomized, clinical, controlled trial. Spine 37: 531–542.

American College of Occupational and Environmental Medicine. 2005. Exercise and manipulative therapies for treatment of acute and sub-acute low back pain. Elk Grove Village, IL: ACOEM.

Bach SM, Holten KB. 2009. Guideline update: what's the best approach to acute low back pain? J Fam Pract 58: 12.

Brault JS, Driscoll DM, Laakso LL. 1997. Quantification of lumbar intradiscal deformation during flexion and extension, by mathematical analysis of MRI pixel intensity profiles. Spine 22: 2066–2072.

Chorti AG, Chortis AG, Strimpakos N, et al. 2009. The prognostic value of symptom responses in the conservative management of spinal pain: a systematic review. Spine 34: 2686–2699.

Clare HA, Adams R, Maher CG. 2004. A systematic review of efficacy of McKenzie therapy for spinal pain. Aust J Physiother 50: 209–216.

Cook C, Hegedus EJ, Ramey K. 2005. Physical therapy exercise intervention based on classification using the patient response method: a systematic review of the literature. J Manual Manip Ther 13: 152–162.

Dagenais S, Caro J, Haldeman S. 2008. A systematic review of low back pain cost of illness studies in the United States and internationally. Spine J 8:8–20.

Danish Institute for Health Technology Assessment. 1999. Low back pain. Frequency, management and prevention from an HTA perspective. [In Danish.] Copenhagen: National Board of Health.

Delitto A, George SZ, Van Dillen L, et al. 2012. Low back pain: clinical practice guidelines linked to the international classification of functioning, disability, and health from the orthopaedic section of the American Physical Therapy Association. J Orthop Sports Phys Ther 42: A1–A57.

Dionne C, Bybee R, Tomaka J. 2006. Inter-rater reliability of McKenzie assessment in patients with neck pain. Physiotherapy 92: 75–82.

Donelson R, Aprill C, Medcalf R, et al. 1997. A prospective study of centralization of lumbar and referred pain: a predictor of symptomatic discs and annular competence. Spine 22: 1115–1122.

Donelson R, McIntosh G, Hall H. 2012. Is it time to rethink the typical course of low back pain? Phys Med Rehab 4: 394–401.

Edmondston SJ, Song S, Bricknell RV. 2000. MRI evaluation of lumbar spine flexion and extension in asymptomatic individuals. Man Ther 5: 158–164.

Fersum KV, Dankaets W, O'Sullivan PB, et al. 2009. Integration of subclassification strategies in randomised controlled clinical trials evaluating manual therapy treatment and exercise therapy for non-specific chronic low back pain: a systematic review. Br J Sports Med 44: 1054–1062.

Goertz M, Thorson D, Bonsell J, et al. 2012. Adult acute and sub-acute low back pain. Bloomington, MN: Institute for Clinical Systems Improvement (ICSI).

Guzy G, Franczuk B, Krakowska A. 2011. A clinical trial comparing the McKenzie method and a complex rehabilitation program in patients with cervical derangement syndrome. J Orthop Trauma Surg Rel Res 2: 32–38.

Hayden JA, Dunn KM, van der Windt DA, et al. 2010. What is the prognosis of back pain? Best Pract Res Clin Rheum 24: 167–169.

Hefford C. 2008. McKenzie classification of mechanical spinal pain: profile of syndromes and directions of preference. Man Ther 13: 75–81.

Hunter G 1994. Specific soft tissue mobilisation in the treatment of soft tissue lesions. Physiotherapy 80: 15–21.

Hush J, Lin C, Michaleff Z, et al. 2011. Prognosis of acute idiopathic neck pain is poor: a systematic review and meta-analysis. Arch Phys Med Rehabil 92: 824–829.

Kent P, Mjosund HL, Petersen DHD. 2010. Does targeting manual therapy and / or exercise improve patient outcomes in nonspecific low back pain? A systematic review. BMC Med 8: 22.

Kjellman G, Oberg B. 2002. A randomized clinical trial comparing general exercise, McKenzie treatment and a control group in patients with neck pain. J Rehabil Med 34:183–190.

Kolber MJ, Hanney WJ. 2009. The dynamic disc model: a systematic review of the literature. Phys Ther Rev 14: 181–295.

Littlewood C. 2012. Contractile dysfunction of the shoulder (rotator cuff tendinopathy): an overview. J Man Manip Ther 20: 209–213.

Long A, Donelson R, Fung T. 2004. Does it matter which exercise? A randomized control trial of exercises for low back pain. Spine 29: 2593–2602.

Long A, May S, Fung T. 2008. Specific directional exercises for patients with low back pain: a case series. Physiother Can 60: 307–317.

Machado LAC, de Souza MvS, Ferreira PH, et al. 2006. The McKenzie method for low back pain: a systematic review of the literature with a meta-analysis approach. Spine 31: E254–E262.

Martin BI, Deyo RA, Mirza SK, et al. 2008. Expenditure and health status among adults with back and neck problems. JAMA 299: 656–664.

May S. 2006. Classification by McKenzie mechanical syndromes: a survey of McKenzie-trained faculty. J Manip Physiol Ther 29: 637–642.

May S, Aina A. 2012. Centralization and directional preference: a systematic review. Man Ther 17: 497–506.

May S, Littlewood C, Bishop A. 2006. Reliability of procedures used in the physical examination of non-specific low back pain: a systematic review. Aust J Physiother 52: 91–102.

May S, Nanche G, Pingle S. 2011. High frequency of McKenzie's postural syndrome in young population of non-care seeking individuals. J Man Manip Ther 19: 48–54.

McCarthy C, Cushnaghan J, Dieppe P. 1994. Osteoarthritis. In: Wall PD, Melzack R (eds) Textbook of pain, 3rd edn. Edinburgh: Churchill Livingstone, Edinburgh, pp 387–396.

McKenzie RA. 1980. Treat your own back pain. Waikanae, New Zealand: Spinal Publications.

McKenzie RA. 1981. The lumbar spine Mechanical Diagnosis and Therapy. Waikanae, New Zealand: Spinal Publications.

McKenzie RA. 1983. Treat your own neck pain. Waikanae, New Zealand: Spinal Publications.

McKenzie RA. 1990. The cervical and thoracic spine Mechanical Diagnosis and Therapy. Waikanae, New Zealand: Spinal Publications.

McKenzie RA, May S. 2000. The human extremities Mechanical Diagnosis and Therapy. Waikanae, New Zealand: Spinal Publications.

McKenzie RA, May S. 2003. The lumbar spine Mechanical Diagnosis and Therapy. Waikanae, New Zealand: Spinal Publications.

McKenzie RA, May S. 2006. The cervical and thoracic spine Mechanical Diagnosis and Therapy. Waikanae, New Zealand: Spinal Publications.

Melbye M. 2010. An adherent nerve root: classification and exercise therapy in a patient diagnosed with lumbar disc prolapse. Man Ther 15: 126–129.

Mercer S, Bogduk N. 1999. The ligaments and annulus fibrosus of human adult cervical intervertebral discs. Spine 24: 619–628.

Mercer S, Jull G. 1996. Morphology of the cervical inter-vertebral disc: implications for McKenzie's model of the disc derangement syndrome. Man Ther 2: 76–81.

Milette PC, Fontaine S, Lepanto L, et al. 1999. Differentiating lumbar disc protrusions, disc bulges, and discs with normal contour but abnormal signal intensity: MRI with discographic correlations. Spine 24: 44–53.

Mulvein K , Jull G. 1995. Kinematic analysis of the lumbar lateral flexion and lumbar lateral shift movement techniques. J Manual Manip Ther 3: 104–109.

Ohnmeiss DD, Vanharanta H, Ekholm J. 1997. Degree of disc disruption and lower extremity pain. Spine 22: 1600–1605.

Ordway NR, Seymour RJ, Donelson RG, et al. 1999. Cervical flexion, extension, protrusion, and retraction: a radiographic segmental analysis. Spine 24: 240–247.

Pengel LHM, Herbert RD, Maher CG, et al. 2003. Acute low back pain: systematic review of its prognosis. BMJ 327: 323–325.

Penning L 1998. Normal kinematics of the cervical spine. In: Giles LGF, Singer KP (eds) Clinical anatomy and management of cervical spine pain. Oxford: Butterworth Heinemann, pp 53–70.

Petersen T, Larsen K, Nordsteen J, et al. 2011. The McKenzie method compared with manipulation when used adjunctive to information and advice in low back pain patients presenting with centralisation or peripheralization: a randomised controlled trial. Spine 36: 1999–2010.

Rosenfeld M, Gunnarsson R, Borenstein P. 2000. Early intervention in whiplash-associated disorders. A comparison of two treatment protocols. Spine 25: 1782–1787.

Rosenfeld M, Seferiadis A, Carlsson J, et al. 2003. Active intervention in patients with whiplash-associated disorders improves long-term prognosis. Spine 28: 2491–2498.

Rosenfeld M, Seferiadis A, Gunnarsson R. 2006. Active involvement and intervention in patients exposed to whiplash trauma in automobile crashes reduces costs: a randomized, controlled clinical trial and health economic evaluation. Spine 31: 1799–1804.

Rossignol M, Arsenault B, Dionne C, et al. 2007. Clinic on low back pain in interdisciplinary practice (CLIP) guidelines. Montréal, Canada: Agence de la Santé et des Services Sociaux.

Skrzpiec D, Pollintine P, Przybla A, et al. 2007. The internal mechanical properties of cervical intervertebral discs as revealed by stress profilometry. Eur Spine J 16: 1701–1709.

Slade SC, Keating J. 2007. Unloaded movement facilitation exercise compared to no exercise or alternative therapy on outcomes for people with nonspecific chronic low back pain: a systematic review. J Manip Physiol Ther 30: 301–311.

Slater SL, Ford JJ, Richards MC, et al. 2012. The effectiveness of sub-group specific manual therapy for low back pain: a systematic review. Man Ther 17: 201–212.

Surkitt LD, Ford JJ, Hahne AJ, et al. 2012. Efficacy of directional preference management for low back pain: a systematic review. Phys Ther 92: 652–665.

Werneke M, Hart DL, Cook D. 1999. A descriptive study of the centralisation phenomenon: a prospective analysis. Spine 24: 676–683.

Wetzel FT, Donelson R. 2003. The role of repeated end-range / pain response assessment in the management of symptomatic lumbar discs. Spine J 3: 146–154.

Womersley L, May S. 2006. Sitting posture of subjects with postural backache. J Manip Physiol Ther 29: 213–218.

Work Loss Data Institute. 2008. Low back – lumbar and thoracic (acute and chronic). Corpus Christi, TX: Work Loss Data Institute, p 481.

Chapter 8

Mechanical Diagnosis and Therapy for Extremity Problems: McKenzie Method

Stephen May, Grant Richard Burges Watson

CHAPTER CONTENTS

Introduction	85
Brief epidemiology of extremity musculoskeletal pain conditions	85
Medical diagnosis for extremity conditions	86
Anatomy and biomechanics in MDT	86
Proposed pathological model in MDT	87
Evidence regarding diagnosis in MDT	88
Evidence regarding prognosis in MDT	88
Evidence regarding treatment of extremity conditions with MDT	88
Conclusion	89

Introduction

In the introduction to his first textbook, Robin McKenzie (1981, p xix) wrote: 'the procedures for the lumbar spine to arrive at appropriate conclusions regarding diagnosis and treatment may also be applied successfully to the thoracic and cervical spine, and indeed to all peripheral joints and their surrounding soft tissues. Irrespective of the presenting pathology, the principles of diagnosis and treatment remain the same.' However, the system of mechanical diagnosis and therapy (MDT) was generally not applied to peripheral or extremity musculoskeletal problems in the early years after this publication. This changed after 2000, when a text describing and illustrating the use of MDT principles for extremity problems was finally published (McKenzie & May 2000). Over the following decade, literature has been published that is gradually giving some scientific support to the McKenzie method in the extremities (McKenzie et al 2009, 2012). This chapter will introduce the use of MDT in the extremities and describe the existing literature.

In terms of the issues being discussed in this chapter, the general comments refer to all extremity conditions, but shoulder and knee problems are frequently identified as the most common extremity problems seen in clinical practice. For instance, in an audit of 1713 patients discharged from an outpatient department in primary care in the UK, about half the patients had spinal pain and about half had extremity pain. Patients with shoulder and knee problems represented 11% and 13% of the total respectively, with other extremity joints comprising about 4% each (May 2003). There are a number of epidemiological aspects to extremity musculoskeletal problems that require elaboration, as some of the traditional perceptions of extremity problems have not stood up to the actual evidence that exists. For instance, it used to be considered that most extremity problems were short lived, easily cured and could be easily diagnosed with valid and reliable physical examination procedures, but increasingly the evidence suggests this is not the case. (Chs 1 and 2 discussed epidemiological issues for the upper and lower extremity respectively.)

Brief Epidemiology of Extremity Musculoskeletal Pain Conditions

Musculoskeletal problems in general are a massive burden in the general population. In a survey of nearly 6000 participants conducted across eight European countries, over 60% of female participants and over 40% of those over 60 years of age reported musculoskeletal symptoms of some kind (Woolf et al 2004). Although substantial differences in the prevalence rates of upper extremity disorders were reported in one systematic review across 13 studies, one study reported a lifetime prevalence rate of 29% (Huisstede et al 2006). In 2005 in Japan, in those over 30 years of age the prevalence rate of back, hip and knee pain was reported as 24%, 4% and 10% respectively (Suka & Yoshida 2009). In a survey of over 800 people aged 58 years in Scotland, 31% reported knee pain, 21% shoulder pain, 16% hip pain, 13% hand pain, 23% pain in the ankles or the toes and less than 10% pain in the elbow or the wrist (Adamson et al 2006).

Despite the fact that not everybody with musculoskeletal problems seeks care for treatment, they constitute a major healthcare expenditure, as they account for 15% of all consultations in general practice in the UK (McCormick et al 1995). In fact, typically in a primary care physical therapy department, half the patients attend with an extremity problem (May 2003). It has generally been thought that the natural history of extremity musculoskeletal problems is good, but current evidence suggests that extremity problems have a similar history of protracted episodes, recurrence and failed treatments as lumbar spine problems. For instance, of 251 patients who presented with a new episode of knee pain, only 25% and 44% reported full recovery at 3 and 12 months respectively (van der Waal et al 2005). Forty per cent of individuals with shoulder problems still report problems 1 year after seeking care, despite treatment including physiotherapy, corticosteroid injections and non-steroidal anti-inflammatory drugs (Croft et al 1996). Similarly, from 181 patients with elbow pain followed up in primary care, 13% reported recovery at 3 months and only 34% at 12 months (Bot et al 2005). Furthermore, Vincenzino and Wright (1996) found that elbow pain had a recurrence rate of 25–50%.

Medical Diagnosis for Extremity Conditions

The other myth that has persisted in extremity problems is that a structural diagnosis is easy to make using standard orthopaedic tests. Unfortunately this is not as simple as suspected. For shoulder pathology, the literature related to medical diagnosis is extensive and includes multiple systematic reviews; consequently only a few are referenced here. In a meta-analysis of 45 studies (Hegedus et al 2008), only half of them demonstrated high quality and only two had adequate sample size; in addition, all tests exhibited either reasonable or poor sensitivity but poor specificity, or vice versa. The authors of this review concluded that currently there is a lack of clarity with regard to whether common orthopaedic special tests used routinely in clinical examination are clearly useful in differential diagnosis at problems of the shoulder. Reviews about tests for specific pathologies are very similar. For instance, for superior labral anterior–posterior tears, it was concluded that none of the tests exhibited strong validity (Dessaur & Margarey 2008; Walton & Sadi 2008; Munro & Healy 2009). Similarly, most tests attempting to identify rotator cuff pathology are not useful and cannot be recommended for clinical practice (Hughes et al 2008). (Readers are referred to other chapters in this book for further information on clinical diagnosis of upper extremity conditions.)

The situation is similar for knee problems. Systematic reviews concluded that no single test appears to diagnose a torn meniscus accurately since pooled sensitivity and pooled specificity for McMurray's, Apley's and joint line tenderness were respectively 70% and 71%, 60% and 70%, and 63% and 77% (Hegedus et al 2007). The review conducted by Hing et al (2009) concluded that the McMurray's test is of limited clinical value owing to low sensitivity. Another review summarized the diagnostic odds ratios (ORs) and found joint line tenderness to be the most accurate (OR 10.98), but McMurray's test (OR 3.99) and Apley's test (OR 2.2) were weak (Meserve et al 2008).

A systematic review investigating reliability studies of individuals with shoulder problems found that the majority of high-quality studies reported poor reliability for the procedures investigated (May et al 2010). For instance, kappa values for the Hawkins–Kennedy test ranged from 0.18 to 0.91, for Neer's sign they ranged from 0.10 to 1.00, for the empty can test from 0.44 to 0.49, and for Gerber's lift-off test from 0.18 to 0.45. In an assessment of the physical examination of the knee, inter-tester reliability for dichotomous and ordinal examination items was found to be generally poor, ranging from −0.08 to 0.43 (Wood et al 2006). In the assessment of four tests for patellofemoral alignment, kappa values were 0.10–0.36 (Fitzgerald & McClure 1995).

Obviously any history taking and examination focusing on making a diagnostic conclusion will involve multiple items from all aspects of the assessment process, but the evidence suggests that standard orthopaedic tests have shortcomings in terms of both validity and reliability. One review that looked at the value of diagnostic labelling at the shoulder in terms of consistency and treatment outcomes (Schellingerhout et al 2008) concluded that a group classification based on prognostic and reliable treatment indicators should be used instead. In such a scenario, MDT can help to address some of these criteria.

Anatomy and Biomechanics in MDT

As already stated the MDT method uses non-specific classifications, which are defined by clinical operational definitions (Table 8.1) and not by structurally specific anatomical diagnoses. One survey of experienced therapists' classification of 388 patients found that although the derangement category

Table 8.1 Operational definitions for MDT classifications and other

Derangement	Lasting abolition or decrease of symptoms, and/or an increase in restricted range of movement in response to repeated movements
Articular dysfunction	Intermittent pain consistently produced at a restricted end range with no rapid change of symptoms or range
Contractile dysfunction	Intermittent pain, consistently produced by loading the musculotendinous unit, for instance with an isometric contraction against resistance
Postural syndrome	Only produced by sustained loading, which, once avoided, the rest of the physical examination would be normal
Other categories*	Failure to classify as one of the above mechanical syndromes and considered to be non-mechanical according to operational definitions (see below), such as recent trauma, post surgery or chronic pain state

*Before any of these other categories are considered a full mechanical evaluation must be conducted, which may occur over several days. The mechanical syndromes (derangement, articular dysfunction, contractile dysfunction and postural syndrome) must be absolutely rejected before any of these categories are considered. To meet other categories, patients must fail to meet operational definitions for mechanical syndromes *and* meet operational definitions for other categories as described.

was most common (37%), as in the spine, dysfunctions were also not uncommon (May & Rosedale 2012) (Fig. 8.1). In the spine, directional preference for derangement syndrome is predominantly in the sagittal plane (Ch 7). Within the extremities, although extension and flexion still featured strongly loading, strategies were more varied for both derangement and dysfunctions (May & Rosedale 2012). In the large group classified as 'other', 20% of the 36% occurred after either surgery or trauma. Figure 8.2 provides examples from the shoulder and knee problems, which were the two most common extremity problems. It is hypothesized that the greater number of loading strategies used in the extremities is a product of the number of degrees of freedom available at some of the extremity joints, especially at the shoulder and the hip. Figure 8.2 shows much more varied loading strategies at the shoulder compared with the knee, where only extension and flexion were used. Other common patterns emerged in contractile dysfunctions, such as abduction at the shoulder (9 / 14), wrist extension at the elbow (9 / 14), and extension at the knee (7 / 9).

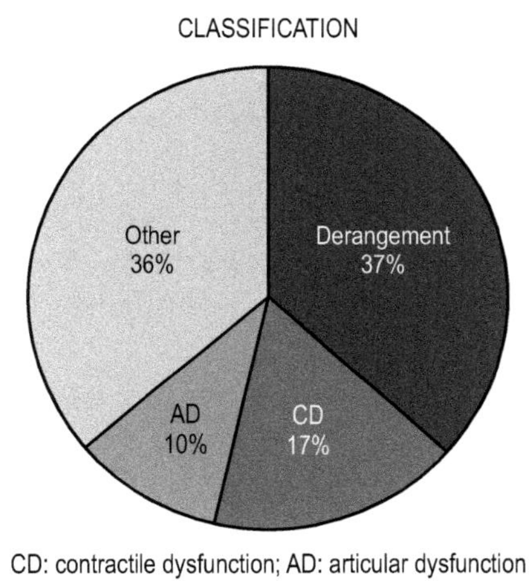

Figure 8.1 Final classification recorded by 30 therapists on 388 extremity patients. (Source: May & Rosedale 2012.)

Proposed Pathological Model in MDT

The proposed system of MDT is mainly based on non-specific mechanical syndromes whose operational definitions are derived from symptomatic and mechanical responses (see Table 8.1). However, conceptual models explaining these symptomatic responses have been proposed (McKenzie & May 2000, 2003, 2006).

In spinal problems the McKenzie method of MDT has been associated with intervertebral disc pathology, even though this has been used as a conceptual model only for derangements. Clearly the dynamic disc model does not fit in with patients with extremity problems, in which inter-joint discs are few, though they do exist – such as at the temporomandibular joint (Krog & May 2012). However, *intra-articular inclusions are characteristic of complex synovial joints*, such as the fat pads and fibroadipose meniscoids found in cadaver elbow joints (Mercer & Bogduk 2007). It is conceivable that such structures may cause problems: '*internal displacement of articular tissue of whatever origin will cause pain … and obstruct movement*' (McKenzie & May 2000, p 84). Again, it should be emphasized that this is a theoretical and conceptual model suggested for giving biological plausibility and that the operational definition is not at all dependent on this, but rather on symptomatic and mechanical responses.

The conceptual model underlying the dysfunction syndrome is that there has been some trauma, previous derangement or degenerative changes in the affected tissue. There is always a lengthy history of months, but after the initial event no effective remodelling has occurred (Hunter 1994; Scott et al 2004). Because of this the patient is left with a painful impairment, which may be associated with restricted movement depending on the type of dysfunction. Dysfunctions may affect articular or periarticular structures, such as occurs in early osteoarthritis (McCarthy et al 1994). Articular dysfunctions typically present with restricted and painful end-range movements in certain patterns – for instance, at the knee with loss of flexion and / or extension, or at the hip with loss of medial rotation and flexion. This is similar to the concept of capsular patterns outlined by Cyriax (1982), in which irritation of the joint causes painful and restricted range of movement, typically but not always in certain patterns at different joints.

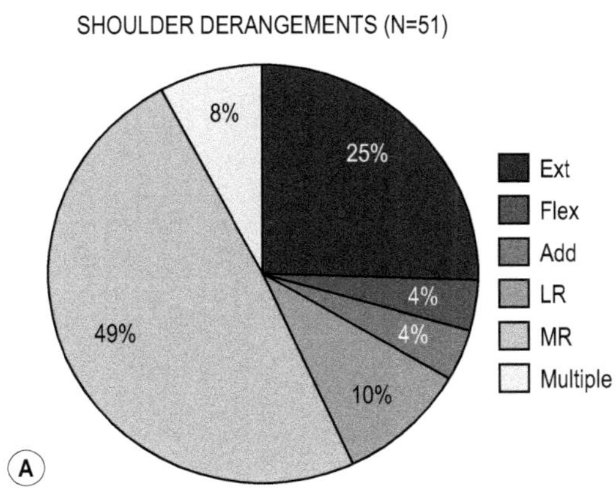

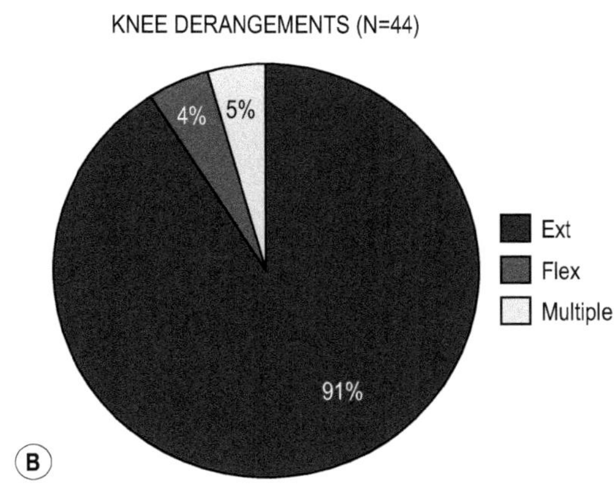

Figure 8.2 Direction of loading strategies in derangements: (A) at the shoulder and **(B)** at the knee. (Source: May & Rosedale 2012.)

Both active and passive movements will produce pain at a restricted range of movement in one or more directions, which will be consistently reproduced every time the joint is moved.

Dysfunction may also affect contractile tissue, most commonly tendons, such as in lateral epicondylalgia, shoulder tendinopathy or Achilles tendinopathy (Littlewood 2012). Muscle can be also affected (see Part 10). Contractile dysfunction presents usually with full but possibly painful active movement and the patient's pain is reproduced when the relevant movement is resisted (e.g. resisted wrist extension in lateral epicondylalgia, or a resisted shoulder abduction in tendinopathy at the shoulder).

With all dysfunctions, pain is elicited by active, passive or resisted movements; the pain comes on each time, however many times it is repeated, and ceases when the movement is ended. Again it should be emphasized that the operational definitions are based on the symptomatic and mechanical responses outlined above, but clinical definitions are not dependent on the conceptual models suggested above. Postural syndrome (described in Ch 7) is rarely used in the classification of patients with extremity problems. Nevertheless, the conceptual models above are indeed no more than conceptual models; they may or may not be entirely accurate, but ultimately are not relevant to the effectiveness of the method.

Evidence Regarding Diagnosis in MDT

The MDT system is not seeking to make specific pathoanatomical diagnoses in terms of the MDT non-specific mechanical syndromes; these are established using the operational definitions laid out in Table 8.1. Some reliability studies have explored the ability of clinicians to agree on MDT classifications. Kelly et al (2008), in a pilot study, evaluated the agreement on extremity McKenzie assessment and found reasonable agreement (82% agreement, kappa 0.70). In a follow-up study with 97 experienced McKenzie clinicians evaluating 25 patient vignettes, the overall agreement was 92%, with kappa scores of 0.83 (May & Ross 2009). These studies would suggest that clinicians experienced in the method are sufficiently able to agree on the classification.

Two studies showed that, from 1000 patients with extremity problems, between 64% and 72% were classified with a mechanical syndrome, attesting to the clinical utility of the system (May 2006; May & Rosedale 2012). If patients do not meet the operational definition of one of the mechanical syndromes after several assessment sessions, then one of the 'other' classifications can be considered (see Table 8.1).

Evidence Regarding Prognosis in MDT

Since the use of the MDT system in the extremities is relatively recent, practitioners were initially unfamiliar with these classifications applied to the extremities. From surveys including multiple practitioners utilizing the MDT method in the extremities and including data from 753 patients (May 2006), the prevalence of MDT classifications in the extremities was as follows: derangement 19%, articular dysfunction 26%, contractile dysfunction 27% and other 28%. In this study, 72% were classified with a mechanical syndrome (May 2006). In a more recent survey involving 30 therapists worldwide and data on 388 consecutive patients (May & Rosedale 2012), a similar proportion (64%) was classified with MDT syndromes, but the proportions within this category were dramatically different: derangement 37%, articular dysfunction 10%, contractile dysfunction 17% and other 36%. The rise in those classified with derangement may indicate a learning process in recognition of this syndrome, and the importance of experience in and continued application of the system to maximize its potential.

The reason why a doubling of recognition of derangement and a subsequent decrease in the 'other' mechanical classifications was found can be related to the fact that, by definition, derangement is associated with a rapid response to repeated movements, and in the spine this classification has been associated with a good prognosis (Ch 7). The data provided in the next section attests to early evidence that the classification of derangement in the extremities is also associated with rapid positive changes in symptoms, such as in case studies at the shoulder joint (Aina & May 2005), or temporomandibular joint (Krog & May 2012), and in a randomized controlled trial with patients with osteoarthritis of the knee (Rosedale et al 2014).

The prognosis of patients with articular and contractile dysfunctions is, by the very nature of their problems, slower – but generally equally good. Rapid changes are not expected in these groups, but change is generally forthcoming over a longer time period, possibly a few months, as the tissues are remodelled with the appropriate loading strategy. So management in these cases must emphasize the importance of maintaining the appropriate rehabilitation routine to determine a long-term return to full and pain-free function.

Evidence Regarding Treatment of Extremity Conditions with MDT

Conservative treatment based on the McKenzie method is founded on the classification as per the operational definitions in Table 8.1. A patient with derangement performs repeated movements that decrease and can abolish symptoms and restore a full range of movement, which is the directional preference. Sometimes opposite movements aggravate symptoms; therefore temporary avoidance of certain movements might also be indicated. A patient with articular dysfunction repeats movements into the restricted painful motion, and in one patient with a contractile dysfunction the repeated resisted movements reproduce the symptoms. These movements may be isometric exercises, active movements or eccentric exercises; the degree of loading is determined by the level of pain response. Some pain or discomfort may be produced, but any aggravation should disappear quickly when the loading is removed.

The emphasis for all syndromes should include self-management, with a patient-centred approach to management and with an emphasis on education to ensure that patients know what exercise they need to perform, the number of repetitions and the rationale. Generally a few exercises at a time are given, and patients demonstrate that they know what they are doing before leaving the session, which tends to increase compliance. The actual direction of loading will depend on the therapist's clinical-reasoning process. In fact, there are certain patterns that are more common, but the MDT system allows variability in the prescription of specific exercises.

As discussed in the introduction, scientific evidence base for the use of MDT in the extremities is relatively new. After the textbook by McKenzie and May (2000), a number of case studies began to emerge in the scientific literature. These case studies included individuals classified with derangement at the shoulder (Aina & May 2005), the radiocarpal joint (Kaneko et al 2009), the temporomandibular joint (Krog & May 2012), and the knee joint (Lynch & May 2013). There are a number of features that stand out from these studies, particularly the possible length of the previous history and past unsuccessful treatments, but a rapid and lasting response to MDT. The patient with a temporomandibular derangement exhibited symptoms for many years, but remained resolved at long-term follow-up at 1 year (Krog & May 2012). Several of the other case studies also had 1-year follow-ups where patients remained fully asymptomatic (Kaneko et al 2009; Lynch & May 2013), or where minor symptoms had returned but which had been swiftly resolved by self-management using MDT repeated movements (Kaneko et al 2009). However, cause-and-effect relationships cannot be inferred from case reports. In all these case studies, resolution of the derangement meant reduction, and sometimes abolition, of pain and return to function, including in 1 subject return to an intense swimming training programme (Lynch & May 2013). Treatment of these individuals was accomplished by clinical reasoning on the part of the therapist to determine the appropriate directional preference that reduced or abolished the pain. In the various studies this involved: hand behind the back with overpressure at the shoulder (Aina & May 2005), distraction with lateral movement at the wrist (Kaneko et al 2009), lateral overpressure to the jaw (Krog & May 2012) and extension with overpressure at the knee (Lynch & May 2013). It was also found that repeated movements opposite to the directional preference could cause the symptoms to return temporarily (Aina & May 2005).

One case study also described how a patient with pain at the tip of his shoulder, involved in lifting heavy loads during his work, and with a positive magnetic resonance imaging showing a complete tear of subscapularis muscle and a type 2 SLAP lesion, improved his symptoms with repeated movements of retraction and extension of the neck (Menon & May 2013). At 1-year telephone follow-up, the patient reported that he had generally remained asymptomatic.

Another case study described a contractile dysfunction of the shoulder in a 57-year old man with a 1-year history of symptoms (Littlewood & May 2007). There was no pain at rest; he had complete active and passive range of movement, a painful arc on abduction, and pain on resisted abduction and lateral rotation. The patient was instructed to perform active abduction exercises where pain was felt. One month later, he reported a reduction in symptoms, and at 10 weeks from initial consultation he reported no pain or functional disability. (Note here the longer time-frame to resolution, as would be expected with this type of classification.)

One trial involved patients with contractile dysfunction at the shoulder, but at present this trial is ongoing and the only published material for this involves the trial protocol (Littlewood et al 2012), the development of the exercise programme (Littlewood et al 2013a) and the pilot study (Littlewood et al 2013b). The self-managed component of this trial comprised an initial assessment to consider baseline functional problems, exercise loading, barriers to implementation and possible solutions, and possible follow-up appointments or telephone follow-ups if thought necessary. The standard physiotherapy consisted of multiple interventions and multiple treatment sessions. The self-managed group received an average of 3.9 sessions, whereas the standard physiotherapy group received 7.6 sessions. The pilot study found no significant differences between the groups, in terms of shoulder disability and general heath measures. The mechanical syndrome of contractile dysfunction could also be referred to in specific terms as a rotator cuff tendinopathy (Littlewood 2012); this paper explores current understanding in relation to pathology, diagnosis, treatment and prognosis related to contractile dysfunction and rotator cuff tendinopathy. It also explores the strengths of this subclassification as well as issues where further progress needs to be made. The review highlights the importance of loaded exercises for this condition.

The use of loaded exercises for contractile dysfunction, especially but not only eccentric exercises, is well established in this group. Other studies on this dysfunction in the extremities involved the shoulder (Holmgren et al 2012), groin (Holmich et al 2011), elbow (Raman et al 2012), patella tendon (Bolgla & Boling 2011) and Achilles tendon (Scott et al 2011) – all common sites of tendon problems. (Readers are referred to Parts 4–9 for appropriate exercise programmes targeted at these different regions and conditions.)

The strongest evidence for the use of MDT in the extremities for derangement classification comes from a single randomized controlled trial (Rosedale et al 2014). Patients with established knee osteoarthritis ($n=180$) were recruited from a tertiary centre where they had been referred for possible knee replacement, and randomized to an intervention or a control group. The intervention group received an MDT assessment, and those classified as derangement were given directional preference exercises, whereas those classified as MDT non-responders were given evidence-based exercises. The control group remained on the waiting list. Pain and function were assessed at 2 weeks and 3 months using established outcome measures. At 2 weeks and 3 months, the MDT group had significantly lower pain and better function than both the control group and the MDT non-responders. Despite being a group of patients with established osteoarthritis in their 60s and referred for total knee replacement, 40% of those individuals who received MDT assessment were classified as derangement. This is a very similar proportion to the 43% of patients with knee problems classified as derangement in the previously quoted survey (May & Rosedale 2012), which was in mostly private, standard outpatient clinics. It is remarkable that, despite very different population groups, the prevalence of derangement was so similar, which indicates the importance of this population group in musculoskeletal problems in general.

Conclusion

Mechanical Diagnosis and Therapy uses a non-specific classification for extremity pain conditions including derangement, articular and contractile dysfunction, postural and other, which indicates how the problem can be managed: for derangement establish the directional preference, for articular dysfunction apply end-range loading, and for contractile dysfunction apply resisted or active loading. Derangements generally respond quickly to self-applied exercise programmes. The operational definitions of these syndromes are all based on clinical symptomatic and mechanical presentations.

The McKenzie approach has been well established for spinal problems for many decades, whereas its use in extremity problems is more recent. Some differences apply, most notably in the prevalence rates of the different syndromes, with derangement being the most prominent subclassification in spinal problems, whereas dysfunctions seem to be more common in extremity problems. Despite these differences, the same management strategies apply to both extremity and spinal problems. The evidence base for the use of MDT in extremity problems is clearly limited at this moment. There exist numerous case studies, and some reliability and survey studies, and trials into its effectiveness begin to be published.

Acknowledgement

In memory of Robin McKenzie 1931–2013.

References

Adamson J, Ebrahim S, Dieppe P, et al. 2006. Prevalence and risk factors for joint pain among men and women in the West of Scotland Twenty-07 study. Ann Rheum Dis 65: 520–524.

Aina A, May S. 2005. Case report: a shoulder derangement. Man Ther 10: 159–163.

Bolgla LA, Boling MC. 2011. An update for the conservative management of patellofemoral pain syndrome: a systematic review of the literature from 2000 to 2010. Int J Sports Phys Ther 6: 112–125.

Bot SDM, van der Waal JM, Terwee CB, et al. 2005. Course and prognosis of elbow complaints: a cohort study in general practice. Ann Rheum Dis 64: 1331–1336.

Croft P, Pope D, Silman A. 1996. The clinical course of shoulder pain: prospective cohort study in primary care. BMJ 313: 601–602.

Cyriax J. 1982. Textbook of orthopaedic medicine. Vol 1: Diagnosis of soft tissue lesions, 8th edn. London: Baillière Tindall.

Dessaur WA, Margarey ME. 2008. Diagnostic accuracy of clinical tests for superior labral anterior posterior lesions: a systematic review. J Orthop Sports Phys Ther 38: 341–352.

Fitzgerald GK, McClure PW. 1995. Reliability of measurements obtained with four tests for patellofemoral alignment. Phys Ther 75: 84–92.

Hegedus EJ, Cook C, Hasselblad V, et al. 2007. Physical examination tests for assessing a torn meniscus in the knee: a systematic review with meta-analysis. J Orthop Sports Phys Ther 39: 541–550.

Hegedus EJ, Goode A, Campbell S, et al. 2008. Physical examination tests of the shoulder: a systematic review with meta-analysis of individual tests. Br J Sports Med 42: 80–92.

Hing W, White S, Reid D, et al. 2009. Validity of the McMurray's test and modified versions of the test: a systematic literature review. J Man Manip Ther 17: 22–35.

Holmgren T, Hallgren HB, Oberg B, et al. 2012. Effect of specific exercise strategy on need for surgery in patients with subacromial impingement syndrome: randomised controlled study. BMJ 344: e787.

Holmich P, Nyvold P, Larsen K. 2011. Continued significant effect of physical training as treatment for overuse injury. 8-to-12-year outcome of a randomized clinical trial. Am J Sports Med 39: 2447–2451.

Hughes PC, Taylor NF, Green RA. 2008. Most clinical tests cannot accurately diagnose rotator cuff pathology: a systematic review. Aust J Physiother 54: 159–170.

Huisstede BMA, Bierma-Zeinstra SMA, Koes BW, et al. 2006. Incidence and prevalence of upper-extremity musculoskeletal disorders: a systematic appraisal of the literature. BMC Musculoskel Dis 7: 7.

Hunter G. 1994. Specific soft tissue mobilisations in the treatment of soft tissue lesions. Physiotherapy 80: 15–21.

Kaneko S, Takasaki H, May S. 2009. Application of mechanical diagnosis and therapy to a patient diagnosed with de Quervain's disease: a case study. J Hand Ther 22: 278–284.

Kelly E, May S, Ross J. 2008. The reliability of the McKenzie classification system using extremity McKenzie assessment forms. Int J Mech Diagnosis Ther 3: 3–6.

Krog C, May S. 2012. Derangement of the temporomandibular joint: a case study using mechanical diagnosis and therapy. Man Ther 17: 1–4.

Littlewood C. 2012. Contractile dysfunction of the shoulder (rotator cuff tendinopathy): an overview. J Man Manipul Ther 20: 209–213.

Littlewood C, May S. 2007. A contractile dysfunction of the shoulder. Man Ther 12: 80–83.

Littlewood C, Ashton J, Mawson S, et al. 2012. A mixed methods study to evaluate the clinical and cost-effectiveness of a self-managed exercise programme versus usual physiotherapy for chronic rotator cuff disorders: protocol for SELF study. BMC Musculoskel Dis 13: 62.

Littlewood C, Malliaris P, Mawson S, et al. 2013a. Development of a self-managed loaded exercise programme for rotator cuff tendinopathy. Physiotherapy 99: 358–362.

Littlewood C, Malliaras P, Mawson S, et al. 2013b. Self-managed loaded exercise versus usual physiotherapy treatment for rotator cuff tendinopathy: a pilot randomised controlled trial. Physiotherapy 100(1): 54–60. doi:10.1016/j.physio.2013.06.001.

Lynch G, May S. 2013. Directional preference at the knee: a case report using mechanical diagnosis and therapy. J Man Manip Ther 60–66.

May S. 2003. An outcome audit for musculoskeletal patients in primary care. Physiother Theory Pract 19: 189–198.

May S. 2006. Classification by McKenzie's mechanical syndromes: report on directional preference and extremity patients. Int J Mech Diagnosis Ther 3: 7–11.

May SJ, Rosedale R. 2012. A survey of the McKenzie classification system in the extremities: prevalence of the mechanical syndromes and preferred loading strategy. Phys Ther 92: 1175–1186.

May S, Ross J. 2009. The McKenzie classification system in the extremities: a reliability study using McKenzie assessment forms and experienced clinicians. J Manip Physiol Ther 32: 556–563.

May S, Chance-Larsen K, Littlewood C, et al. 2010. Reliability of physical examination tests used in the assessment of patients with shoulder problems: a systematic review. Physiotherapy 96: 179–190.

McCarthy C, Cushnaghan J, Dieppe P. 1994. Osteoarthritis. In: Wall PD, Melzack R (eds) Textbook of pain, 3rd edn. Edinburgh: Churchill Livingstone, pp 387–396.

McCormick A, Charlton J, Fleming D. 1995. Assessing health needs in primary care. Morbidity study from general practice provides another source of information. BMJ 310: 1534.

McKenzie RA. 1981. The lumbar spine Mechanical Diagnosis and Therapy. Waikanae, New Zealand: Spinal Publications.

McKenzie RA, May S. 2000. The human extremities Mechanical Diagnosis and Therapy. Waikanae, New Zealand: Spinal Publications.

McKenzie RA, May S. 2003. The lumbar spine Mechanical Diagnosis and Therapy. Waikanae, New Zealand: Spinal Publications.

McKenzie RA, May S. 2006. The cervical and thoracic spines Mechanical Diagnosis and Therapy. Waikanae, New Zealand: Spinal Publications.

McKenzie R, Watson G, Lindsay R. 2009. Treat your own shoulder. Waikanae, New Zealand: Spinal Publications.

McKenzie R, Watson G, Lindsay R. 2012. Treat your own knee. Waikanae, New Zealand: Spinal Publications.

Menon A, May S. 2013. Shoulder pain: differential diagnosis with mechanical diagnosis and therapy extremity assessment: a case report. Man Ther 18: 354–357.

Mercer SR, Bogduk N. 2007. Intra-articular inclusions of the elbow joint complex. Clin Anat 20: 668–676.

Meserve BB, Cleland JA, Boucher TR. 2008. A meta-analysis examining clinical test utilities for assessing meniscal injury. Clin Rehab 22: 143–161.

Munro W, Healy R. 2009. The validity and accuracy of clinical tests used to detect lateral pathology of the shoulder. Man Ther 14: 119–130.

Raman J, MacDermid JC, Grewal R. 2012. Effectiveness of different methods of resistance exercises in lateral epicondylosis: a systematic review. J Hand Ther 25: 5–26.

Rosedale R, Rastogi R, May S, et al. 2014. Efficacy of exercise interventions as determined by the McKenzie system of Mechanical Diagnosis and Therapy for knee osteoarthritis: a randomized controlled trial. J Orthop Sports Phys Ther 44(3): 173–181, A1–A6. doi:10.2519/jospt.2014.4791.

Schellingerhout JM, Verhagen AP, Thomas S, et al. 2008. Lack of uniformity in diagnostic labeling of shoulder pain: time for a different approach. Man Ther 13: 478–483.
Scott A, Khan KM, Roberts CR, et al. 2004. What do we mean by the term 'inflammation'? A contemporary basic science update for sports medicine. Br J Sports Med 38: 372–380.
Scott A, Huisman E, Khan K. 2011. Conservative treatment of chronic Achilles tendinopathy. Can Med Assoc J 183: 1159–1165.
Suka M, Yoshida K. 2009. The national burden of musculoskeletal pain in Japan. Clin J Pain 25: 313–319.
Van der Waal JM, Bot SDM, Terwee CB, et al. 2005. Course and prognosis of knee complaints in general practice. Arthritis Rheum 53: 920–930.
Vincenzino B, Wright A. 1996. Lateral epicondylalgia: epidemiology, pathophysiology, aetiology and natural history. Phys Ther Rev 1: 23–34.
Walton DM, Sadi J. 2008. Identifying SLAP lesions: a meta-analysis of clinical tests and exercise in clinical reasoning. Phys Ther Sport 9: 167–176.
Wood L, Peat G, Wilkie R, et al. 2006. A study of the noninstrumented physical examination of the knee found high observer variability. J Clin Epidemiol 59: 512–552.
Woolf AD, Zeidler H, Haglund U, et al. 2004. Musculoskeletal pain in Europe: its impact and a comparison of population and medical perceptions of treatment in eight European countries. Ann Rheum Dis 63: 342–347.

PART 2

Cervicothoracic Spine in Upper Extremity Pain Syndromes

9 Mechanical Neck Pain 95
Bryan S. Dennison and Michael H. Leal

10 Whiplash-associated Disorders 110
Michele Sterling

11 Differential Diagnosis and Treatment of Cervical Myelopathy, Cervical Radiculopathy and Cervical Myeloradiculopathy 118
Chad Cook and Amy Cook

12 Thoracic Outlet Syndrome 132
Susan W. Stralka

13 Thoracic Spine Manipulation 142
William Egan, Paul E. Glynn and Joshua A. Cleland

14 Joint Mobilization and Manipulation of the Cervical Spine 158
John R. Krauss, Douglas S. Creighton, Joshua A. Cleland and César Fernández-de-las-Peñas

15 Therapeutic Exercise for Mechanical Neck Pain 174
Carol Kennedy

Chapter 9

Mechanical Neck Pain

Bryan S. Dennison, Michael H. Leal

CHAPTER CONTENTS

Mechanical neck pain definition	95
Prevalence of mechanical neck pain	96
Financial impact of mechanical neck pain	97
Risk factors and prognosis in mechanical neck pain	97
Review of anatomy specific to mechanical neck pain	99
Causes of mechanical neck pain	99
Clinical presentation of neck pain	100
Proposed management of mechanical neck pain	100
First level of classification	101
Red flag screening	101
Yellow flag screening	103
Second level of classification	103
Cervical spine self-report measures of pain and function	105
Numerical Pain Rating Scale	106
Neck Disability Index	106
Patient Specific Functional Scale	106
Fear-avoidance Belief Questionnaire	107
Global Rating of Change scale	107
Conclusion	107

Mechanical Neck Pain Definition

Neck pain is a common problem, increasingly affecting individuals worldwide (Hogg-Johnson et al 2009). Prevalence data suggest that neck pain can span the ages, affecting children and the elderly alike, without gender discrimination. Similar to low back pain, neck pain is episodic in nature (Hogg-Johnson et al 2009). Recent analysis suggests that neck pain follows a 'chronic–episodic course' (Hoy et al 2010). Absolute resolution of symptoms evades the majority of neck pain sufferers (Carroll et al 2009) resulting in both quality-of-life and economic impacts (Borghouts et al 1999; Wright et al 1999).

Despite its common presence, there is wide variability in defining neck pain (Fejer et al 2006). This is due, in part, to the presence of both physical and psychosocial contributors to cervical spine pain. As a result of the multifactorial presentation of neck pain and the inability to identify the exact source of presenting cervical spine symptoms (Borghouts et al 1998), the label 'non-specific neck pain' has been assigned to any undiagnosable symptomatic disorder of the cervical spine. The vagueness of this descriptive term has resulted in further variance of what comprises non-specific neck pain. As such, descriptive terms such as occupational cervicobrachial disorder, tension neck syndrome, cervical spondylosis, thoracic outlet syndrome, cervical osteoarthritis and mechanical neck pain have been synonymously applied to non-specific neck pain (Koes & Hoving 2002). Contributing to this terminology confusion is the reality that specific, valid and reproducible diagnostic criteria are absent (Buchbinder et al 1996a, 1996b).

In an effort to standardize a working definition of neck pain, steps have been taken to identify the symptomatic boundaries that comprise the neck pain experience. The following definition for neck pain or cervical spinal pain was proposed (Fig. 9.1):

> *Pain perceived as arising from anywhere within the region bounded superiorly by the superior nuchal line, inferiorly by an imaginary transverse line through the tip of the first thoracic spinous process, and laterally by the sagittal planes tangential to the lateral borders of the neck.*
>
> (Merskey & Bogduk 1994, p 11)

In 2009, The Neck Pain Task Force put forth its working definition for neck symptoms covering non-descript terms such as non-specific, soft tissue and mechanical neck pain. The Task Force excluded neck pain associated with systemic or pathological disease, or neck pain as a result of 'skin lesions, throat disorders, tumour, infections, fractures and dislocations' (Guzman et al 2009). They defined neck pain as symptoms 'located in the anatomical region of the neck as outlined (Fig. 9.2), with or without radiation to the head, trunk and upper limbs' (Guzman et al 2009).

The definitions above are intended to provide a uniform definition for neck pain. However, the following operational definitions have been used in research to define mechanical neck pain. Cleland et al (2005) defined mechanical neck pain as 'non-specific pain in the area of the cervico-thoracic junction that is exacerbated by neck movements'. Others (Martínez-Segura et al 2006; Fernández-de-las-Peñas et al 2007b; González-Iglesias et al 2009a, 2009b; Mansilla-Ferragut et al 2009) have used the following definition of mechanical neck pain by Fernández-de-las-Peñas et al (2007a), or a slight variation thereof: 'generalized neck and / or shoulder pain with mechanical characteristics including: symptoms

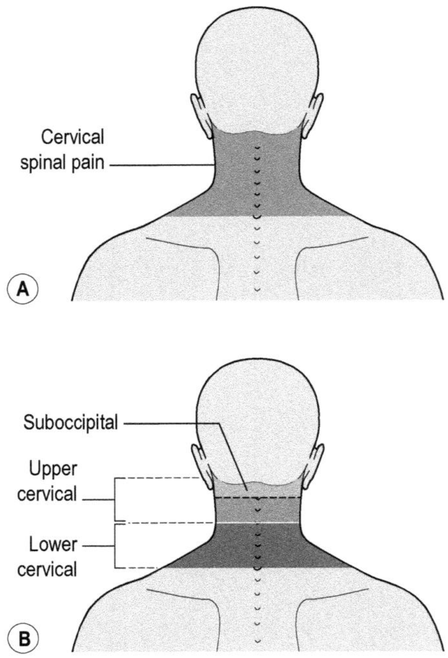

Figure 9.1 Topographical definition of mechanical neck pain.

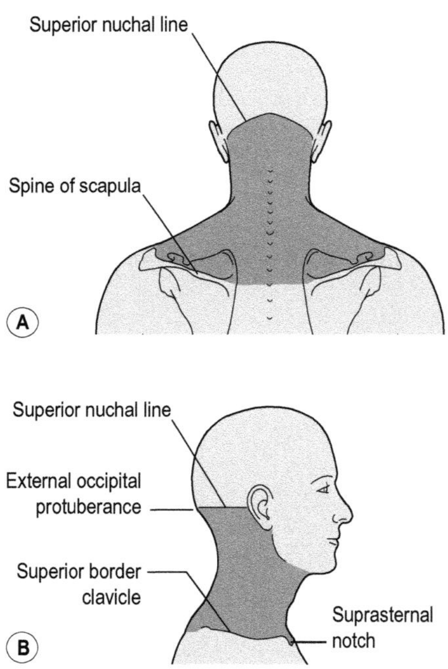

Figure 9.2 A new conceptual model of mechanical neck pain. (Based on Guzman et al 2009, with permission.)

provoked by maintained neck postures or by movement, or by palpation of the cervical muscles'. Still others have grouped symptoms like headache of cervical origin, mechanical neck disorder with radicular signs and symptoms, neck disorder associated with whiplash and neck disorder associated with degenerative changes as subsets of mechanical neck disorders (Gross et al 2002). Kanlayanaphotporn et al (2009) used the following definition of neck pain: 'pain primarily confined in the area on the posterior aspect of the neck that can be exacerbated by neck movements or by sustained postures'. In 2010, the Global Burden of Disease (GBD) study used the anatomical definition from the Neck Pain Task Force (as described Guzman et al 2009) along with the following case definition: 'neck pain (+ / – pain referred into the upper limb(s) that lasts for at least 1 day' (Hoy et al 2014).

These operational definitions of neck pain denote the location of and potential provocative manoeuvres for the patient's symptoms, but do not infer causation of the patient's perceived symptoms. This dilemma has led to efforts being made in current research to explain the neck pain experience and guide effective interventions.

Prevalence of Mechanical Neck Pain

Neck pain presents a global healthcare challenge to the medical profession with personal and economic impact. Prevalence estimates are of interest to researchers in order to help assess the population impact of neck pain and direct future investigations into the aetiology and management of this phenomenon. This ability to accurately analyse the worldwide impact of neck pain is challenged by the immense variation in the results and quality of the research to date.

In an effort to address the methodological issues noted in previous prevalence research, Hoy et al (2014) took on a 6-year challenge of estimating the global burden of neck pain. This study represented the first time global data for neck pain had been estimated. The intent of the 2010 GBD study was to report the global burden of neck pain while considering the risk of bias in the studies used to determine the burden estimates (Hoy et al 2014). The results of the study revealed a high prevalence and burden for neck pain globally. The study evaluated 291 global diseases and injuries. Neck pain ranked 'the 4th greatest contributor to global disability and 21st in terms of overall burden' (Hoy et al 2014). The global estimated point prevalence of neck pain was 4.9% for 0 years to 100 years of age. The prevalence was higher in women than in men, with a peak prevalence at about 45 years of age (Hoy et al 2014).

Other studies have looked at prevalence rates for neck pain, but efforts were not made, as in the GBD study, to control for the risk of bias. Methodological issues need to be recognized as they can overinflate analyses (i.e. mean prevalence rate) (Hoy et al 2012). Hence in the following studies the prevalence estimates need to be interpreted cautiously owing to the potential presence of methodological bias.

A systematic review by Fejer et al (2006) investigated the worldwide prevalence of neck pain as reported in the literature from 1980 to 2002. Their search resulted in 56 papers meeting their inclusion criteria from Scandinavia (46%), the rest of Europe (23%), Asia (16%) and North America (11%). Australia (two papers) and Israel (one paper) also made contributions investigating the prevalence of neck pain in their respective countries. Variation in the investigated studies was obvious. Various sample sizes were seen ranging from 300 to 51 050 subjects. Variation as to what constituted neck pain, in terms of both anatomical location and an operational definition, was present as well. However, in 79% of the studies investigated, unbiased and randomized population samples were used. Over half of the studies critiqued had sample sizes of over 1000 subjects. The most common categories of prevalence periods investigated and their collective results are shared below.

The point prevalence of neck pain was investigated in eight studies (13%) and ranged from 5.9% to 38.7%. These data were further broken down by age categories, resulting in prevalence ranges of 5.9–22.2% for individuals aged 15–74 years and 38.7% for individuals specifically over the age of 65.

One-week prevalence data were investigated in six studies (10%) with a range of 1.4–36%. However, one study used a unique definition of neck pain not used in others. Excluding this study resulted in five remaining studies with a range of 1.4–19.5% of individuals aged 15–90 years of age reporting a 1-week prevalence of neck pain.

One-month prevalence statistics were investigated in six studies (10%) resulting in a range of 15.4–41.1% for individuals between 16 and 79 years of age. One study by Wedderkopp et al (2001) investigated children (aged 8–10 years) and adolescents (aged 14–16 years) and reported a 1-month prevalence rate of neck pain of 6.9%.

Seven studies (11%) reported 6-month prevalence data for adults aged 18–80 years ranging from 6.9% to 54.2%. Three of these studies reported ranges from 6% to 45% for males of 12-year-old and females of 18-year-old females respectively.

The largest reported prevalence rate was in the 1-year category. Twenty-two studies (39%) reported ranges from 16.7% to 75.1% for individuals aged 17–70 years. Two studies reported ranges for adolescents. Niemi et al (1997) reported a 1-year prevalence rate of 15.8% for 714 high school students (408 girls, 306 boys – age ranges not specified). A second study by Holmen et al (2000) reported 1-year prevalence data for 4279 junior high and high school students aged 13–18 years. In this population, adolescents reported a 22.1% 1-year prevalence of neck and shoulder pain. In addition, the systematic critical review by Fejer et al (2006) went on to delineate a range of 8.8–11.6% 1-year prevalence as reported by three studies (Woo et al 1994; Isacsson et al 1995; Brochet et al 1998) in elderly populations (age >65, 68 years of age, and age >70 respectively).

Lifetime prevalence rates were reported in eight studies (13%), two of which were gathered from the Tokelau Islands in the South Pacific Ocean. There, lifetime prevalence rates ranged from 0.2% to 2.1%. The remaining six studies reported prevalence rates of 14.2–71% for individuals aged 18–84 years. One study (Aoyagi et al 1999) focused on 860 women of ages 60–79 years living in Japan or Hawaii. The results of this study reported a 14.8% lifetime prevalence (i.e. asking 'which of your joints have ever been painful?') of neck joint pain in the combined populations. However, in the systematic critical review by Fejer et al (2006), one of the inclusion criteria was to look at populations that were representative of the general population. In light of this, the Hawaiian–Japanese cohort was not considered representative of the Hawaiian population. Therefore, only the Japanese data were included, resulting in a lifetime prevalence for this group (n=222) of 17.1%.

In summary, the literature has revealed varying descriptors of neck pain, which can affect the quality of the studies. Interestingly, Fejer et al (2006) did not find a correlation between the variation in the studies they reviewed and prevalence estimates. This suggests that the quality of the studies (presence of heterogeneity) reviewed may not be a factor in neck pain prevalence estimates. In addition, the longer the duration of the prevalence period the higher are the reported prevalence estimates (i.e. 1-year prevalence estimates were higher than 1-month prevalence estimates). Gender differences were also seen: women consistently reported neck pain 83% more often than did men (25 out of 30 studies; Table 9.1).

Table 9.1 **Prevalence of mechanical neck pain**

Neck pain	Age (years)	World population (%)
Point prevalence	15–74 65+	5.9–22.2 38.7
One-week prevalence	15–90	1.4–19.5
One-month prevalence	16–79 8–10 and 14–16	15.4–41.1 6.9
Six-month prevalence	18–80 18 (female population) 12 (male population)	6.9–54.2 45 6
One-year prevalence	17–70 Secondary school and 13–18 65+	16.7–75.1 15.8–22.1 8.8–11.6
Lifetime prevalence	18–84 60–79	14.2–71 17.1
Global point prevalence	0–100	4.9

Financial impact of mechanical neck pain

In addition to disability, neck pain carries significant economic impact. In the Netherlands, total costs of neck pain were estimated to be $686.2 million, which comprised about 1% of the 1996 total healthcare expenditure in the Netherlands. Health service costs for patients with neck pain, denoted as 'direct (medical) costs', comprised $159.6 million of the $686.2 million total cost. The remaining $526.5 million represented 'wealth lost to society' or 'indirect (non-medical) costs' (Koopmanschap & Rutten 1996) as a result of neck pain (Borghouts et al 1999). In the US, cervical spine disorders present challenges to the healthcare system, accounting for billions of dollars spent on indemnity and medical costs in the workers' compensation system, which are second only to workers' compensation costs associated with lumbar spine disorders (Wright et al 1999).

Risk factors and prognosis in mechanical neck pain

In light of current evidence, neck pain cannot be looked at in isolation. Rather, this phenomenon is generally non-traumatic and multifactorial with evidence supporting the dual interaction of the physical and psychosocial arenas (Ariens et al 2001; Croft et al 2001; Côté et al 2009; Guzman et al 2009; Jull & Sterling 2009; Sterling 2009) as contributors to the pain experience. There seems to be a greater appreciation for the psychological contributors to neck pain, but a clinical tendency to continue to focus narrowly on the physical factors potentially involved in neck pain. The results of a recent international, multidisciplinary survey (Walton et al 2013a) suggested that clinician appreciation of psychological / behavioural factors had a large impact on patient prognosis. Despite this, the survey also reported physical findings as the most frequently analysed factors for patients with neck pain. These findings continue to highlight the discrepancy between current best evidence and clinical practice (Walton et al 2013a).

Identifying risk factors for, or predictors of, neck pain is useful in helping to direct both measures to prevent initial neck injury (primary prevention) and interventions for addressing factors that contribute to persistent symptoms and / or recurrent neck pain (secondary prevention) (Hill et al 2004). Historically, risk factors for neck pain have been broken down into categories: work-related or non-work-related risk factors. The categories can be broken down further into three basic subgroups: (1) physical risk factors, (2) psychosocial risk factors and (3) individual risk factors (i.e. coping behaviours) (Ariens et al 2000, 2001).

Early research (1966–1997) into risk factors (Ariens et al 2000, 2001), both physical and psychological, consisted primarily of methodology using cross-sectional study designs. However, this style of research inquiry limits the ability to establish cause-and-effect relationships (Croft et al 2001; Carroll et al 2009). Research has evolved over the last 10 years, improving upon this methodological dilemma by contributing larger numbers of prospective studies (Côté et al 2009). Prospective study designs allow a more confident establishment of relationships and thus contribute more significantly to the systematic review process.

Prevalence of neck pain in working individuals

A recent systematic review (Côté et al 2009) sought to investigate the prevalence of neck pain risk factors in working individuals. The researchers found that frequent or persistent neck disorders can develop in at least 5% of the workforce, with 10% of those that develop neck pain succumbing to activity limitation (due to neck pain) on at least one occasion. Over half of those workers (50%) who develop neck pain will go on to report it 1 year later (Carroll et al 2009). Identification of the factors contributing to neck pain has pointed researchers away from single risk factors and towards complex relationships involving interactions between individual, cultural and work-related variables. For instance, age, previous musculoskeletal pain, quantitative job demands, social support at work, job insecurity, low physical capacity, poor computer workstation design and work posture, sedentary work position, repetitive work and precision work are all factors contributing to an episode of neck pain. Other factors contributing to its development include gender, a history of headache, emotional problems, smoking, awkward work postures, physical work environment and ethnicity (Box 9.1).

Box 9.1 Risk factors for mechanical neck pain in working population

Risk factors: an episode of neck pain

- Age
- Previous musculoskeletal pain
- Quantitative job demands
- Social support at work
- Job insecurity
- Low physical capacity
- Poor computer workstation design and work posture
- Sedentary work position
- Repetitive work
- Precision work suggests an episode of neck pain

Risk factors: developing neck pain

- Gender
- History of headache
- Emotional problems
- Smoking
- Awkward work postures
- Physical work environment and ethnicity

Prognostic factors of neck pain in working individuals

Prognostic factors for workers with neck pain have also been investigated (Carroll et al 2009), revealing that 60% of workers still note persistent or recurrent neck pain 1 year after the onset of symptoms. Gender also plays a role in neck pain, with women more likely than men to report persistent or recurrent pain. Outcomes such as prior musculoskeletal pain, prior sick leave and occupational type (blue-collar versus white-collar work) were associated with poorer neck pain prognosis. The only psychosocial variable that demonstrated a prognostic role was a report of having little self-perceived control over one's work situation. This was associated with a further report of neck pain 4 years later. A challenge following the identification of these indicators of poor prognosis is the realization of the person's limited ability to modify these variables. However, improved outcomes have been noted after changing jobs (for sewing machine operators) and taking up exercise (Box 9.2).

Box 9.2 Prognostic variables for mechanical neck pain in working population

Poor prognostic variables

- Prior neck pain
- Musculoskeletal pain
- Prior sick leave and occupational type (blue-collar vs white-collar, etc.)
- Having little self-perceived influence over one's own work situation

Favourable prognostic variables

- Changing jobs (for sewing machine operators)
- Exercise

Prevalence of neck pain in the general population

Hogg-Johnson et al (2009) reviewed the literature on risk factors in the general population. Their review revealed

Box 9.3 Risk factors for mechanical neck pain in general population

Unfavourable risk factors

- Middle age
- Additional health complaints
- Psychological factors

Favourable risk factors

- Younger age

equivocal findings regarding age as a risk factor. The incidence of neck pain occurs across all ages, increasing in its prevalence as the years pass. There does, however, appear to be a peak in the prevalence of neck pain in the middle years of life, with lower prevalence in the most elderly.

Evidence has suggested a multifactorial presentation of neck pain. This includes additional health complaints (i.e. headache, low back pain, poorer self-rated health) that accompany the complaints of neck pain. Contrary to popular assumptions in medicine, cervical spine disc degeneration is not found to be a risk factor for neck pain. In addition to physical risk factors, psychological factors are predicted and presented with neck pain complaints (Box 9.3).

Prognostic factors for neck pain in the general population

Carroll et al (2008) investigated prognostic factors in the general population. Neck pain affects each sex, but with higher reports among women than men. However, gender only weakly predicts neck pain recovery. Younger age is associated with a more favourable prognosis. In contrast, old age is a predictor of poorer prognosis and a weak predictor of recovery. However, middle-aged individuals (45–59 years of age) were at the highest risk and carried the poorest prognosis for neck pain. Recovery is now being viewed as a multifactorial entity – much like the current thinking behind the causes of neck pain (i.e. that they are multifactorial in nature). Recovery likewise is dependent on symptom severity and quality, impairment, activity and participation-level interference, autonomy, spontaneity and satisfaction with the sense of self (Walton et al 2013b).

In studies of neck pain, physical activity and exercise are assessed by self-reported questionnaires. This poses challenges with regards the conclusions one is able to draw from this data. Regular physical activity is favourable for a number of musculoskeletal issues from a prophylactic perspective, including being a component of neck pain management. However, prognostic studies evaluating its effect have provided no relationship between the persistence or recurrence of neck pain when compared at the start and at the end of the studies.

Psychosocial health plays a factor in the prognosis of neck pain. For individuals who utilize a passive coping mechanism, the outcomes were worse compared those with greater social support and better psychological health. In contrast, neck pain is associated with poorer psychological health, which is also a risk factor for a new episode of neck pain (Box 9.4).

Box 9.4 Prognostic variables for mechanical neck pain in general population

Poor prognostic variables

- Middle age
- Passive coping mechanism

Favourable prognostic variables

- Younger age
- Greater social support
- Better psychological health

Review of Anatomy Specific to Mechanical Neck Pain

Any innervated structure in the cervical spine can contribute to a pain state – for example, the posterior musculature, cervical zygapophyseal joints, lateral atlanto-occipital joint, atlanto-occipital joint, median atlanto-axial joint, dura mater of the spinal cord, prevertebral and lateral muscles of the neck, intervertebral discs, vertebral artery, synovial joints, anterior and posterior longitudinal ligaments, atlanto-axial ligaments, and internal carotid artery (Bogduk 2003). The reader is referred elsewhere for more detailed discussions of the cervical spine anatomy and its associated innervations (Bogduk 2002, 2003; Bogduk & McGuirk 2006). However, it is important to note that, though these innervated structures can certainly be credited with the pain experience, the presence of innervation alone does not confirm the structure as the source of symptoms (Bogduk 2003).

Causes of Mechanical Neck Pain

Similar to low back pain, identifying the exact sources of neck pain is a challenging, if not impossible, task. The ability of any innervated structure in the cervical spine to contribute to a pain state makes identification of the source of neck pain a challenge (Bogduk 2002). Furthermore, pathological conditions (e.g. malignancy, cervical myelopathy, fracture, systemic disease and arterial dysfunction) can also contribute to neck pain.

Current spinal research, in both the low back and the cervical spine regions, is encouraging a shift in clinical decision making away from previously emphasized tissue-based models of pain towards multifactorial models of pain (Ariens et al 2000; Guzman et al 2009). The biomedical model is repeatedly found to account for only part of the pain experience in certain spinal conditions. The International Association for the Study of Pain (IASP) has therefore encouraged a broader clinical-reasoning framework when working with patients in pain. Specifically, it has encouraged clinicians to consider possible hypotheses beyond tissue-based sources. Assisting clinicians to move beyond simple tissue-based sources, the IASP has provided the following definition of pain: 'an unpleasant sensory and emotional experience associated with actual or potential tissue damage, or described in terms of such damage' (Merskey & Bogduk 1994, p 210).

Based on current evidence suggesting the failure of tissue-based models to explain accurately all the types of neck pain, today's clinician must be aware of both 'actual' and 'potential' sources of neck pain. Thus, a bio-psychosocial model is now being looked to as a more comprehensive model of spine pain. This model allows for a combination of biomedical, psychological and social contributors to neck pain. It has been introduced in an attempt to account more accurately for the multidimensional aspect of neck pain (Jull & Sterling 2009; Sterling 2009).

Neck pain and cervical radicular pain are two categories that have been identified in spine-related pain of the cervical region. Cervical radicular pain – pain that is perceived in the upper limb (Slipman et al 1998; Bogduk 2003) – emanates from the cervical spine. Due to the ability of the cervical spine to create pain locally in the neck as well as distally in the upper extremity, the terms 'cervical radicular pain' and 'neck pain' are used interchangeably. This association, however, is incorrect. Despite the commonality of the cervical anatomical region responsible for creating symptoms, neck pain and cervical radicular pain are not interchangeable terms. Adding to this confusion is the use of the term 'cervical radiculopathy' as a synonym for cervical radicular pain. Briefly, cervical radiculopathy is a 'neurologic condition, characterized by objective signs of loss of neurological function, that is, some combination of sensory loss, motor loss, or impaired reflexes in a segmental distribution' (Bogduk 2003, p 456). This is a result of pathology involving compression or compromise of the spinal nerve roots or the spinal nerve itself. It is objectively assessed as a loss of function and not pain. If pain is involved in a compressive condition in the cervical spine, it is due to compression of the dorsal root ganglion (see Ch 10). Compression of nerve roots does not cause illicit nociceptive activity (Howe et al 1977). Compression of the dorsal root ganglion evokes activity in the Aβ and C fibres (Howe et al 1977). This neural behaviour is more than nociceptive activity (which is predominantly Aδ- and C-fibre transmission). Because of the involvement of the Aβ fibres with dorsal root ganglion compression, this establishes a distinction between radiculopathy (a reflection of a loss of nerve function and not necessarily pain) and radicular pain (a reflection of dorsal root ganglion involvement beyond simple nociceptive function). Paraesthesia is associated with radicular pain, which reflects involvement of Aβ fibres (Bogduk 2003). From this perspective, the seemingly intuitive thought that pain results from 'pinched' or 'compressed' nerves does not hold true unless the dorsal root ganglion is involved in that compression.

Clinical Presentation of Neck Pain

Within a sound clinical reasoning framework, it is still important for physical therapists to have an appreciation for potential tissue-based contributors to neck pain. Epidemiological studies have provided support for prevalence rates of neck pain from around the world. This information is useful for helping clinicians to direct research and make predictions about this subgroup of patients. Although these studies are not useful for providing insight into the sources of neck pain, an appreciation of the possible contributors to neck pain can assist clinicians in identifying pre-test probabilities for neck

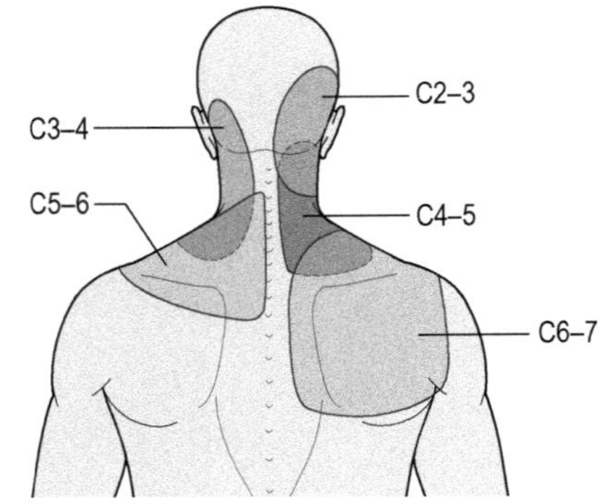

Figure 9.3 Referral patterns from spine zygapophyseal joints and intervertebral discs. (From Bogduk 2002, with permission.)

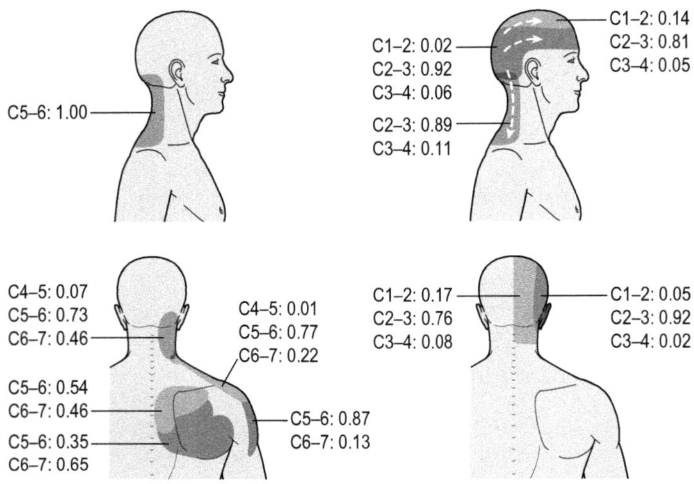

Figure 9.4 Referral patterns from spine zygapophyseal joints and intervertebral discs. (Data taken from Cooper & Bogduk 2005.)

conditions, which then allows them to prioritize their evaluation and match the patient to those interventions that are associated with a higher level of success (Yin & Bogduk 2008).

The patient with neck pain creates a clinical reasoning challenge owing to the vast number of possible causes behind the patient's chief complaint. Clinicians commonly evaluate their patients by looking for a familiar pattern of symptoms that will then lead them to hypothesize a particular tissue-based source of the patient's chief complaint. In this respect, research comparing normal and symptomatic patients has provided identifiable referral patterns for the cervical spine zygapophyseal joints and intervertebral discs (Figs 9.3–9.4), spinal nerves (Fig. 9.5) and soft tissue (Fig. 9.6). Nociceptive stimulation of the cervical spine, without involvement of cervical nerves or nerve roots, can refer symptoms to the upper limb, anterior chest wall, interscapular region and head (Grubb & Kelly 2000; Bogduk 2002, 2003; Bogduk & McGuick 2006) (Fig. 9.7).

Proposed Management of Mechanical Neck Pain

Current best evidence has advocated a treatment-based classification approach for the management of patients with neck pain. Emphasis has been placed on matching the patient to

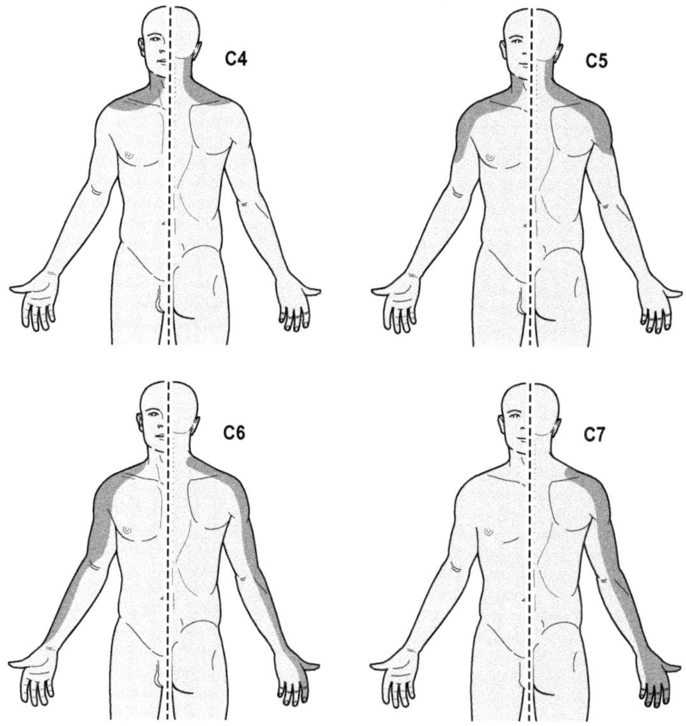

Figure 9.5 Referral patterns from C4, C5, C6 and C7 spinal nerves. (From Bogduk 2002, with permission.)

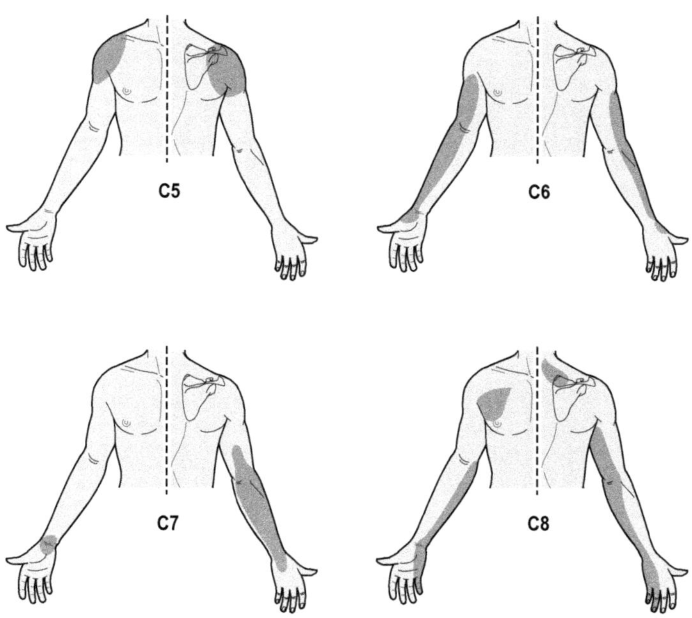

Figure 9.6 Referral patterns from interspinous muscles. (From Bogduk & McGuirk 2006, with permission.)

optimal interventions based on the identification of signs and symptoms collected during the patient interview and physical examination (Childs et al 2004, 2008; Cleland et al 2006; Fritz & Brennan 2007). The clinical decision-making process involved in applying this treatment-based classification strategy consists of two distinct levels (Cleland et al 2006). The first level requires that the therapist determine whether the patient will benefit from physical therapy services through a comprehensive medical screen including red and yellow flag assessments. The second level of the classification schema involves directing the patient to their matched intervention(s) or subgroup based on presenting signs and symptoms, as well as the respective physical examination findings (Cleland et al 2006; Fritz & Brennan 2007).

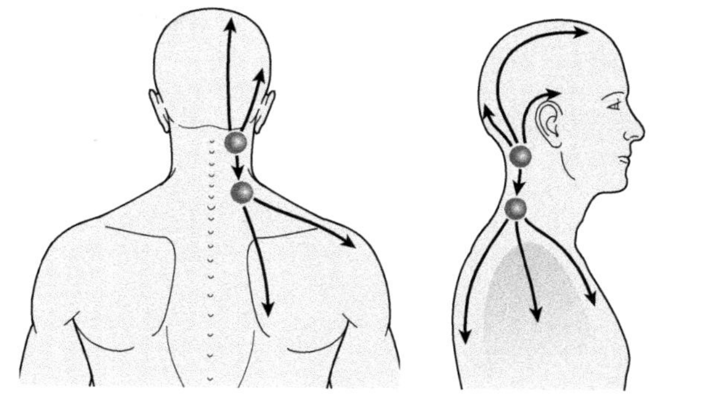

Figure 9.7 Referral patterns from nociceptive stimulation of the cervical spine.

First level of classification

Step one of this classification approach begins with a comprehensive review of the patient's medical history and a medical screen encompassing a review of both the general health and specific systems (Boissonnault 2005). General health questions should be asked of all patients by inquiring about the following: (1) fatigue, (2) malaise, (3) weakness, (4) unexplained weight loss / gain, (5) nausea, (6) paraesthesia or numbness, (7) dizziness or lightheadedness, (8) change in mentation or cognition and (9) chills, sweats, or fever.

Patient self-administered questionnaires can assist with this data collection. These have been shown to be accurate for reporting important health history information and for assisting the clinician to decide whether or not to proceed further to the second level of classification (Pecoraro et al 1979; Boissonnault 2005).

A specific system screen (cardiovascular, pulmonary, gastrointestinal, urogenital, endocrine, nervous system, integumentary) follows based on the initial information gathered from the general health questions review, including the body chart and self-administered questionnaires. The patient interview is a key component in attempting to recognize serious spinal pathology that may warrant additional concern, including appropriate medical follow-up with a primary care practitioner (Greene 2001; Greenhalgh & Selfe 2009).

Red flag screening

A screen for possible red flags (signs or symptoms that may suggest a more serious underlying pathology) is the first step in the classification process for determining whether physical therapy services are appropriate for the patient (Nordin et al 2009). It has been suggested that the clinician needs to determine one of three potential courses of action after the initial medical screening is complete: to treat the individual and proceed to the second level of classification, to treat the patient and proceed to the second level of classification with notification to the individual's physician regarding signs or symptoms that may warrant concern, or to refer the patient to a physician, without any form of treatment during the initial visit, for further diagnostic work-up due to the patient interview / examination findings (Boissonnault 2005). There is a small prevalence of more serious related sources such as spinal fractures, spinal or central cord compression, neoplastic conditions, vascular compromise, system or inflammatory disease, as well as upper cervical spine ligamentous instability, of which the practising clinician should be aware. The medical screening process, combined with a thorough red flag screen, alerts the clinician to the possibility of a more serious underlying condition (Cleland et al 2006).

Spinal fractures

Spinal fractures usually occur with some type of mechanical trauma or injury. Typically fractures occur from a fall, blunt trauma, the application of compressive or axial load force, or as the result of a motor vehicle collision. It has been shown that risk factors such as a patient's age, as well as the height of the fall (>3 m), are risk factors that increase the risk of cervical spine fractures. Incidents involving axial loads, diving incidents and collisions all raise the risk of potential cervical spine fracture. The highest occurrences take place with motor vehicle collisions at speeds >100 km / h (Thompson et al 2009). The Canadian cervical (C)-spine rule (see Ch 3) is a clinical prediction rule that is used to determine whether cervical spine radiography is needed for an alert and stable individual who has suffered a cervical spine injury (Stiell et al 2001, 2003). The rule is based on various high- and low-risk criteria as well as the ability of a patient to rotate the neck. If the rule is positive and the patient has not had any radiographs performed, the therapist should ensure that the appropriate radiographic evaluation is undertaken prior to the initiation of formal physical therapy services.

Cervical myelopathy

Cervical myelopathy is a disorder that involves compression of the spinal cord canal resulting in neurological compromise. Canal obstruction can be caused by a variety of factors, including degenerative changes of the intervertebral discs, hypertrophy of the ligamentum flavum, or osteophyte formation due to the degenerative processes occurring at the intervertebral disc level. Cervical myelopathy is reported as the most common form of spinal cord dysfunction in individuals over the age of 55, affecting 90% of individuals as they approach their seventies (Cook et al 2009). Common symptoms include sensory disturbances of the hands, gait disturbances or balance unsteadiness, decreased motor strength with associated muscle wasting in the upper extremities, as well as bowel and bladder disturbances. Current research has reported only moderate to substantial reliability for the clinical tests for cervical spine myelopathy. Furthermore, performing a cluster of commonly used tests for this disorder does not improve the diagnostic accuracy above that of the Babinski test alone (Cook et al 2009). (Readers are referred to Ch 11 for further information on cervical myelopathy.)

Primary neoplastic conditions

Primary neoplastic conditions are rare in the cervical spine, representing only 0.4% of all tumours and accounting for less than 5% of tumours that occur above the sacrum (Abdu & Provencher 1998). A more common clinical presentation may be from a Pancoast tumour, which is a malignant tumour of the upper apices of the lungs or within the superior pulmonary sulcus of the lung. It has been estimated that Pancoast tumours account for 2–5% of all cancers of the lung (Kovach & Huslig 1984). A common clinical presentation will include shoulder pain that radiates into the arm and / or hand with or without the presence of neck pain. These individuals may or may not have pulmonary signs or symptoms. Often a patient may exhibit a clinical presentation similar to Horner's syndrome or an ulnar nerve dermatomal pattern due to the close proximity of the tumour to the lower trunk of the brachial plexus (C8–T1). Pancoast tumours affect men more than women and typically show an increased incidence rate over the age of 50, especially in those with a history of tobacco usage. In the low back literature a systematic review that looked at screening for malignancy found that if four variables were absent in the patient evaluation process diagnostic sensitivity was 100%. The four variables were: age >50, a previous history of cancer, unexplained weight loss (more than 5-10% of the body weight within a month) and failure to improve after 1 month. (Henschke et al 2007). Given the fact that lung cancer is the leading cause of death among active cancers and is the second most common cancer in men and women in the United States (Centers for Disease Control 2014), it is important that clinicians screen for the disease appropriately.

Cervical arterial dysfunction

Cervical arterial dysfunction (CAD) is a recent term that describes the arterial events that can occur in both the anterior and posterior arterial systems of the cervical spine. The anterior system is composed of the internal carotid arteries and provides blood flow to the eyes as well as the cerebral hemispheres. The posterior system is composed of the vertebrobasilar arteries and provides blood flow to the hindbrain (Kerry & Taylor 2009). These pathologies can mimic cervicocranial pain. The clinician must be able to diagnose differentially between a likely arterial presentation and symptoms due to a musculoskeletal source based on physical examination findings encountered during a comprehensive screen and subsequent physical examination. The exact prevalence rate of spontaneous vertebral dissections and vertebrobasilar insufficiency is unknown. Therefore the clinician should have a high suspicion of CAD, especially in cases involving cervical spine trauma. Although the prevalence rate for these conditions is quite low, the clinician should be aware of the limitations surrounding the current objective examination for CAD. This awareness should lead to decreased clinical-reasoning errors, which occur when these tests are used in isolation during the differential diagnosis process.

This paradigm shift encourages the patient interview to include a thorough review of vascular risk factors such as hypertension, hypercholesterolaemia, diabetes mellitus, a history of smoking, infection, coagulation abnormalities and direct vessel trauma. During the objective component of the evaluation, additional tests such as a cranial nerve and eye examination can be used to assist the clinician to a comprehensive perspective on the patient's current haemodynamic status (Kerry & Taylor 2009). This comprehensive evaluation is extremely important as current literature supports the hypothesis that neck movements are not valid screening tools for determining who is at risk of a vertebrobasilar artery dissection (Haldeman et al 1999). The concept of premanipulative testing has also been discouraged when there is a strong suspicion of a vertebrobasilar artery dissection. It has also been suggested that premanipulative testing adds little to the clinical information needed for decision making. In light of this, clinicians should question whether or not provocation tests add any benefit to the patient-screening process and realize that a comprehensive approach to screening for cervical arterial dysfunction is the key to early identification (Thiel & Rix 2005). In 2012, the International Federation of Orthopaedic Manipulative (IFOMPT) came to a consensus regarding a framework for the clinical approach towards CAD. This international group established guidelines that clinicians could follow before applying manual therapy and giving exercises in patients with suspected CAD. The team, representing 22 countries, came to an agreement regarding the following: (1) although CAD and its side effects are rare it is a condition that clinicians should be aware of in their musculoskeletal assessment, (2) the presence or risk of CAD cannot be concluded from the result of one clinical test, and (3) a strong clinical-reasoning framework must be present in order both to understand all components of the patient's presentation, from the risk–benefit appreciation to the implications of informed consent and jurisdictionally specific requirements, and to enable the safe practice of manual therapy overall in the cervical spine region (Rushton et al 2014).

Clinical cervical spine instability

Clinical cervical spine instability (CCSI) can occur from a variety of traumatic and non-traumatic events. It has been difficult to diagnose owing to the subtle clinical features that are associated with this condition (Cook et al 2005), the relative low prevalence rate, and the lack of clinical tests that have shown reliability and validity in assisting clinicians in their clinical decision-making process (Mintken et al 2008). The clinician should undertake a screening process focused on ruling out ligamentous instability after injury to the cervical spine, especially after a fall, blunt trauma or a motor vehicle accident. There are also a variety of non-traumatic diagnoses of which clinicians should be aware that carry the potential for ligamentous instability – such as rheumatoid arthritis, Down syndrome, ankylosing spondylitis, as well as prolonged oral contraceptive or corticosteroid use (Boissonnault 2005). A combination of the application of the Canadian C-spine rule and a thorough history and physical examination aimed at identifying ligamentous structures is a key component of the clinician's examination process when attempting to rule out ligamentous instability. Despite the absence of strong empirical data for testing the integrity of the alar and transverse ligaments, these are considered essential components of the evaluation process, and are often performed because of potential medicolegal ramifications (Cleland et al 2006). From a clinical-reasoning perspective, however, it is helpful to understand that, because of the weak empirical evidence behind these tests, one must exercise caution in terms of ruling out the diagnosis when a negative result is obtained on either of these tests.

In addition to the physical examination findings, the patient interview may make revealing statements that increase the probability of CCSI. A large Delphi study (Cook et al 2005) reported common subjective identifiers as noted by expert physical therapists (Board Certified Orthopaedic Clinical Specialists (OCS) and Fellows of the American Academy of Orthopaedic Manual Physical Therapists (FAAOMPT)); a consensus of common patient complaints were noted as follows: 'intolerance to prolonged static postures', 'fatigue and inability to hold head up', 'better with external support, including hands or collar', 'frequent need for self-manipulation', 'feeling of instability, shaking, or lack of control', 'frequent episodes of acute attacks', and 'sharp pain, possibly with sudden movements'. These patient reports may assist the clinician in identifying patients with CCSI.

Yellow flag screening

After clinicians have completed the first level of classification and concluded that there are no red flags or systemic issues present, the next step in the evaluation process is to perform a yellow flag assessment. Yellow flags are defined as patient indicators that require further investigation by the clinician regarding the cognitive and behavioural aspects of the patient presentation (Pincus et al 2002). These psychosocial variables have been reportedly linked to neck pain in both the acute and the subacute tissue healing phases (Linton 2000; Bot et al 2005; Carroll et al 2008). Epidemiological studies have demonstrated that 47% of all individuals who experienced a neck pain episode had either continued persistent pain or a worsening of symptoms at an annual follow-up (Côté et al 2004).

Fear of movement has been identified in the research literature as a psychosocial indicator that can assist in predicting disability in the neck pain population. It may be a key variable in explaining why individuals continue to have pain up to a year after their initial episode. The Fear-avoidance Beliefs Questionnaire (FABQ) is a tool that the clinician can use to objectify the patient's fear of movement. Although primarily studied in the low back pain population, there is evidence to suggest there are similar prognostic capabilities, although with weaker statistical associations, for functional outcomes using this tool in the cervical spine population (George et al 2001). Once the clinician determines the presence of any yellow flags, the treatment plan can be adjusted accordingly (fear-avoidance-based model), which may include informing the patient's primary care physician or referring the individual regarding the clinical findings that may affect the patient's future prognosis.

Second level of classification

Once the patient has been evaluated for any potential red and yellow flags and the decision is made that the individual is appropriate for physical therapy services, the clinician can then move to the second level of classification (Fig. 9.8). Here the clinician can start to classify the patient in terms of key impairments, appropriately matching him or her to selected interventions. This current treatment-based classification system is based on presenting signs and symptoms obtained from the history and physical examination, with subsequent decision making using a clinical algorithm (Fritz & Brennan 2007). Individuals are then matched according to the most

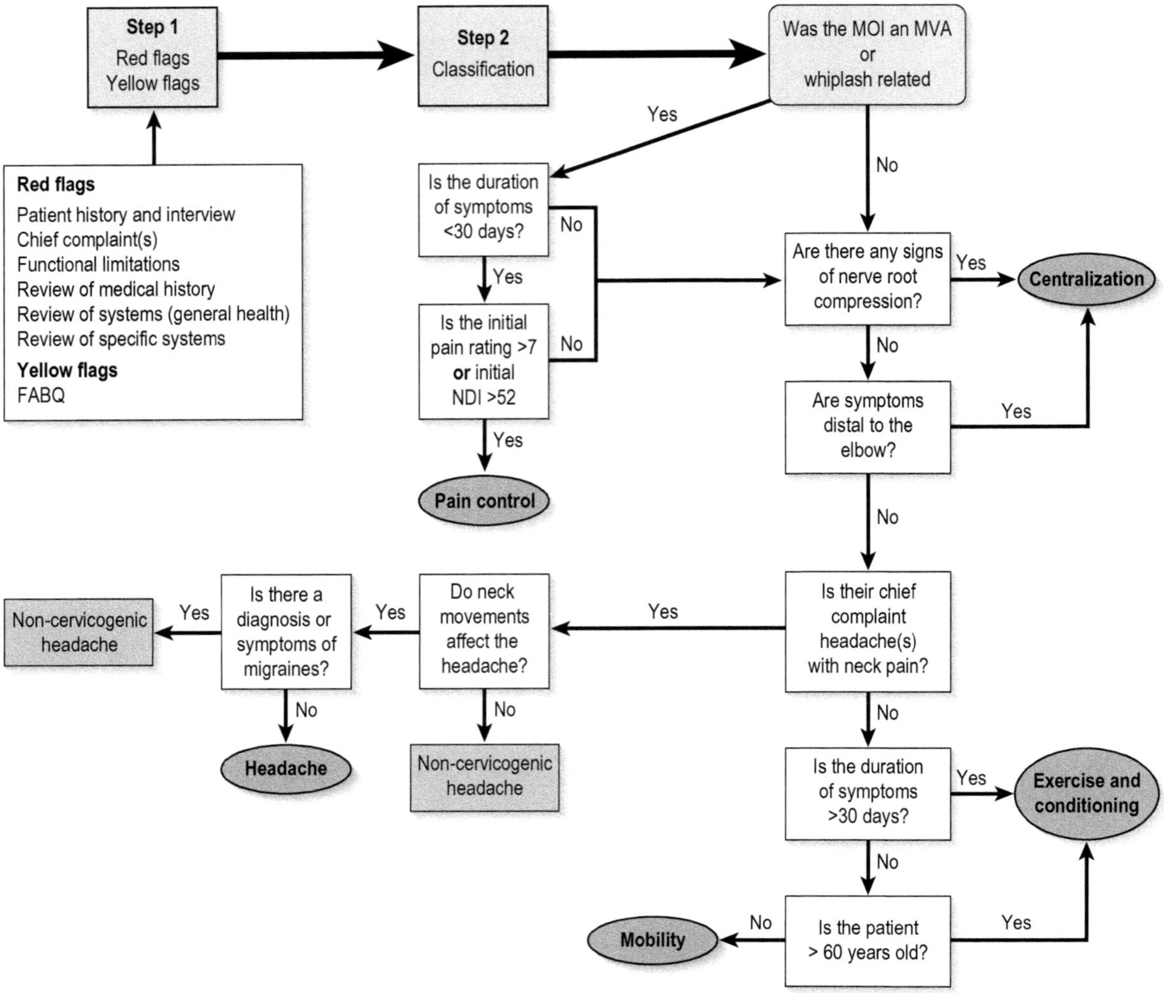

Figure 9.8 Treatment-based classification algorithm. FABQ=Fear-avoidance Beliefs Questionnaire; MOI=mechanism of injury; MVA=motor vehicle accident; NDI=Neck Disability Index. (Based on Fritz & Brennan 2007, with permission.)

appropriate interventions most likely to benefit their current clinical presentation (Childs et al 2004; Fritz & Brennan 2007). Preliminary studies of this treatment-based classification have shown that individuals receiving matched interventions were found to have strong associations with greater improvements in Neck Disability Index (NDI) scores, as well as pain ratings, than individuals receiving non-matched interventions (Fritz & Brennan 2007).

Mechanical neck pain classification

Mechanical neck pain is often managed with a conservative, non-surgical approach, which has traditionally been the mainstay of treatment interventions for this population. Physical therapists have historically used a variety of different interventions including modalities, joint mobilization and / or manipulation, therapeutic exercise and mechanical traction on the cervical spine (Cleland et al 2007). These interventions have largely been accepted as the standard practice of care, although high-quality evidence describing their usage is often absent or inconclusive (Childs et al 2004; Fritz & Brennan 2007). This individualized and personalized clinical decision-making approach to patient care has been described as professional uncertainty or Wennberg's hypothesis. Wennberg's hypothesis states that, when a clinician is faced with diagnostic uncertainty, treatment options are based on idiosyncratic factors. This outcome can lead to differences amongst providers in terms of the evaluative methods of their patients as well as subsequent treatment options (Wennberg et al 1982; Jette & Jette 1997). A previous critical appraisal revealed a scarcity of evidence for the treatment of individuals with neck pain. The researchers concluded that more decisive research was needed to support conclusions regarding the efficacy of physical therapy interventions for patients with neck pain (Hoving et al 2001).

A series of reviews from the Cochrane Library reported that exercise, mobilization, manipulation and electrotherapy had limited evidence of efficacy, and it was unclear whether there were any potential benefits of their use. Suggestions for improving the validity and statistical strength of future trials included obtaining larger patient sample sizes as well as establishing a model for the standardization of treatment in this population (Gross et al 2004; Kroeling et al 2005). Variability in practice and the absence of uniform professional decision making have been reported as key potential causes for the lack of high-quality studies within the neck pain population. Smaller effect sizes leading to a fair to moderate quality of evidence rating, combined with reported subsequent data with only moderate success in patient outcomes, could potentially be a result of this lack of standardization of care (Fritz & Brennan 2007).

Treatment-based classification

Due to the lack of high-quality evidence for the management of this population, a treatment-based classification (TBC) system was proposed that could assist practitioners in their clinical decision-making process (Wang et al 2003; Childs et al 2004; Fritz & Brennan 2007). This is different from a pathoanatomical approach to patient care, which is influenced by the search for the correct 'diagnosis' or tissue source. The pathoanatomical approach has been shown to largely be a failure based on the inadequacies of the medical model for low back pain (Fritz & Brennan 2007). Previous studies have shown that diagnostic uncertainty at the primary care level is as high as 85% in the low back population. One can therefore infer that this would be a similar statistic for the cervical spine population (Jarvik 2003). When a TBC system is not employed, clinicians apply physical therapy interventions with the perception that the patient has an equal chance of failure or success, largely based on a pathoanatomical model. The classification approach uses a clinical-reasoning process that focuses on classifying clinical data into certain categories for the purpose of making clinical decisions regarding therapeutic management. This current TBC model therefore assists the clinician in subgrouping larger groups of patients into smaller, similar homogeneous entities. The focus is less on the identification of a pathoanatomical source and more on recognizing key impairments gained from the patient history, self-report measures and the results of the physical examination to guide the treatment approach (Childs et al 2004; Fritz & Brennan 2007).

Classification categories

Although high-quality evidence is absent, there have been a series of studies that help guide intervention strategies once the patient has been classified into a subgroup. These interventions are the product of current best-available evidence. They are supplemented with expert opinion and common practice when necessary. The current treatment-based classification system for patients with neck pain comprises five classification categories (Fritz & Brennan 2007): mobility, centralization, exercise and conditioning, pain control, and headache. An algorithm is used to aid the clinician in determining which appropriate classification their patient should be assigned to (see Fig. 9.1). Interventions are applied according to best current evidence and standard practice of care.

Patients in the mobility classification will often present with a recent onset of symptoms, rarely have upper quarter symptoms (active range of motion does not peripheralize symptoms and no signs of nerve root compression) and usually demonstrate active range-of-motion discrepancies. In the mobility classification, matched interventions will include mobilization / manipulation directed at the cervical or thoracic spine. Neuromuscular re-education and strengthening of the deep neck flexors are also included as interventions within this subgroup (Cleland et al 2005, 2007, 2010; Masaracchio et al 2013).

The centralization classification typically consists of patients presenting with a referral pattern of pain into the upper extremity and / or hands, with or without concomitant neck pain. There may be pain radiating into one or both of the upper extremities, as well as peripheralization of symptoms with active range of motion. A test item cluster has been developed to assist the practitioner in determining whether the patient's presentation represents cervical radiculopathy. The four items of this cluster are: ipsilateral cervical spine rotation <60°, a positive upper limb median nerve neurodynamic test, relief of their current symptoms with manual distraction, and a positive Spurling's test (Wainner et al 2003). Typical interventions may include manual mechanical cervical traction (Raney et al 2009) and cervical retraction exercises based on the centralization phenomenon. Current research has also proposed a manual therapy approach including mobilization and manipulation techniques directed at the cervical and thoracic spine (Cleland et al 2007; Young et al 2009). Symptom response is then recorded for possible centralization or peripheralization of symptoms. This has been shown to assist in the clinician's prognostic reasoning (Werneke & Hart 2003; Werneke et al 2008). (See Ch 7 for details on the centralization phenomenon.)

Within the exercise and conditioning classification, patients will have lower pain and disability scores, a longer duration of symptoms (>30 days), no signs of nerve root compression, and no signs of peripheralization or centralization. Common interventions will include both general strengthening for the upper quarter as well as motor control exercises focused on the deep neck flexor muscle area (Bronfort et al 2001). Individuals often begin in one specific classification and then move into this category as they start to improve.

The pain control classification includes individuals who have higher initial pain and disability scores, a recent onset of symptoms, which is usually due to trauma, concomitant cervicogenic headaches and referred pain into the upper quarter, as well as poor tolerance to participation in the physical examination. Interventions include pain-relieving modalities and cervical spine range-of-motion exercises.

Finally, the headache classification includes patients who present with a one-sided or unilateral headache pattern with certain cervical spine motions exacerbating the symptoms. The following interventions have been recommended for this population: cervical spine manipulation or mobilization, motor control exercises for the deep neck flexor muscles, and strengthening of the upper quarter musculature (Jull et al 2002).

Cervical Spine Self-report Measures of Pain and Function

The administration and collection of self-report measures are gaining increased awareness in physical therapy clinical practice and published research. These health status questionnaires look at a variety of variables such as general health, functional limitations and current levels of the individual's self-perceived disability. It has been advocated that the use of these measures can assist the practitioner in their clinical performance as well as their overall professional accountability to the patient in providing the best care possible (Delitto 2006). Despite the critical importance of the integration of outcome tools into clinical practice, a recent international multidisciplinary survey showed that there continues to be a substantial need to implement more consistent outcome measurements in clinical practice (MacDermid et al 2013).

Common measures in the cervical spine population include the Numeric Pain Rating Scale (NPRS), Neck Disability Index (NDI), Patient Specific Functional Scale (PSFS), Fear-avoidance Belief Questionnaire (FABQ), and the Global Rating of Change scale (GRC). When applying these measures to a specific patient population it is helpful to know the tool's psychometric properties, especially the minimum detectable change (MDC) and the minimum clinically important difference (MCID). It is helpful to define MDC and MCID as their value is related to the clinical relevance of the measure used as well as determining whether a clinical meaningful change had occurred based upon a certain treatment approach. The MDC is defined as the least amount of change that falls outside of the normal measurement error (Kovacs et al 2008). MCID is the smallest amount of change, or difference that the patient perceives as being beneficial (Jaeschke et al 1989).

Currently there is a lack of published evidence suggesting an optimal time-frame for an appropriate follow-up when using self-report measures. The authors therefore recommend that a numeric pain rating (NPRS) and change between sessions (GRC) be measured at each visit. Tools that look at perceived functional limitations (PSFS) should be measured weekly. Fear-avoidance behaviour (FABQ) and self-reported disability (NDI) should be evaluated at the initial evaluation and at time of discharge (Table 9.2). One may administer these tools more often based on the patient's specific case presentation. These are general guidelines to assist the clinician in their preliminary usage of these tools in the clinical setting.

Numerical Pain Rating Scale

The Numerical Pain Rating Scale (NPRS) is a subjective measure in which individuals rate their pain on an 11-point numerical scale. The scale ranges from 0 (no pain at all) to 10 (worst imaginable pain). It has been shown that a composite scoring system including best, worse and current level of pain over the last 24 hours is sufficient to pick up changes in pain intensity with maximal reliability (Jensen et al 1999). The MCID has been found to be a change in score of 1.3 points or higher in the mechanical neck pain population (Cleland et al 2008). MacDermid et al (2013) reported that a single-item pain assessment (numeric or visual analogue scale) was performed in almost 75% of patient cases with neck pain across 24 countries in an international survey. It was by far the most common form of outcome measurement recorded on a patient-by-patient basis.

Neck Disability Index

The Neck Disability Index (NDI) is the most common region-specific tool in use for measuring neck-related disability. It has been shown to be both a reliable and a valid tool. In one study, there was no difference in NDI scores in patients with or without unilateral arm pain suggesting that the NDI adequately accounts for upper extremity symptoms in conjunction with neck pain (Young et al 2009). There are 10 questions, each scored with a possible 0–5 value, with the larger number indicating a higher self-reported disability status. The score on this questionnaire can therefore range from 0 to 50. In order to calculate a percentage, one simply multiplies the final value by 2. In this study the MCID was found to be 7.5 points and the MDC 10 points. It is recommended that the MDC be used as this exceeds the standard error of measurement that one would find with this tool if accepting the current MCID value (7.5 points) (Young et al 2009). It also has been reported that the natural course of neck pain under physical therapy management shows a linear progression in both pain and disability. Walton et al (2014) found that neck pain via numeric rating scale (NRS) improved by 0.5 points per week and the NDI improved at a rate of 1.5 points per week for the first 4 weeks of care. They also found two different mean trajectories within the NRS (stable and improving pain) and three within the NDI (worsening, rapid improvement and slow improvement in disability), again bringing importance to the fact that neck pain is a heterogeneous condition.

Patient Specific Functional Scale

The Patient Specific Functional Scale (PSFS) is an outcome measure that asks the patient to identify and rate limited functional activities. It is based on a 0–10 scale, with score of 10 establishing the patient's ability to perform the activity prior to injury and 0 representing a current inability to perform the activity at all. The PSFS has been shown to be highly reliable in the neck pain population (Westaway et al 1998). Currently there is a lack of evidence that supports an actual MCID for this tool in the mechanical neck pain population, but a study looking at individuals with suspected cervical spine

Table 9.2 **Self-reported measures for the cervical spine population**

Measure	Score	MCID / MDC	Frequency
Numeric Pain Rating Scale (NPRS)	0–10	1.3	Every session
Patient Specific Functional Scale (PSFS)	0–10	2	Weekly
Neck Disability Index (NDI)	0–50	7.5 / 10.2	Initial and discharge
Global Rate of Change (GROC)	(–5)–(+5)	+2	Every session
Fear-avoidance Beliefs Questionnaire (FABQ)	0–24 (PA)*	>19 (PA)*	Initial and discharge

*PA=physical activity subscale.

radiculopathy established an MCID of 2 points (Cleland et al 2006).

Fear-avoidance Beliefs Questionnaire

The Fear-avoidance Beliefs Questionnaire was originally developed in 1993. It was used to measure subjects' beliefs and fears about how their physical activity or work activity may contribute to their current pain state (Waddell et al 1993). The FABQ consists of a total of 16 questions, which can be scored from 0 to 6. Outlier questions are present, resulting in the work subscale (FABQW) containing a total of 42 points (questions 6, 7, 9, 10, 11, 12, 15) while the physical activity subscale (FABQPA) has a total of 24 points (questions 2, 3, 4, 5). One 2007 study used this tool in the development of a clinical prediction rule for those individuals with neck pain who may benefit from thoracic spine manipulation, exercise and patient education. The study found that a score of <12 on the FABQPA was one of the predictors of a successful outcome (Cleland et al 2007). An additional study in 2007 showed that a chronic neck pain subsample total score of 41/66 for the FABQ (T), 19/24 for the FABQPA and 19/42 for the FABQW could identify prolonged disability 6 months later (Landers et al 2008). Cleland et al (2008) looked at the psychometric properties of the FABQ for mechanical neck pain and found a fair but statistically significant correlation between concurrent measures of pain and disability. Overall there was a weaker relationship between measures of fear and avoidance with pain and disability in the mechanical neck pain population compared with studies regarding the low back population. However, the FABQW does appear to be an important factor to measure in mechanical neck pain patients. This is especially important with regards to looking at prognostic factors that may contribute to return to work ability and the risk of ongoing chronicity.

Global Rating of Change scale

The Global Rating of Change scale (GRC) is used to look at patients' self-perceived progress during the course of their treatment. This tool adds objectivity to the frequently asked clinical question, 'How are you feeling today – better, worse, or the same compared with when you first started physical therapy?' The GRC asks patients to rate their progress from a previous point in their care (often the initial evaluation) to their current state. The most common version of this scale used in the physical therapy literature is a 15-point scale that has data points ranging from −7 (a great deal worse) to +7 (a great deal better). The original literature that had described this tool was based on a patient population that was diagnosed with chronic lung or heart disease (Jaeschke et al 1989). The authors used the 15-point scale to define treatment success using an arbitrary cut-off system. A recent review of the GRC found that use of an 11-point scale ranging from −5 (very much worse) to +5 (completely recovered), as opposed to a 15-point scale as previously mentioned, yielded the same results in terms of responsiveness. Given the lack of empirical evidence for the arbitrary cut-off points used in the 15-point scale, it is the authors' opinion that the 11-point scale should be used with a corresponding MCID of 2 points (Kamper et al 2009).

Conclusion

Neck pain is a common occurrence that affects individuals around the world. Similar to low back pain, it is difficult to identify exact contributors to neck pain, strengthening the likelihood of a multifactorial presentation for this pain state. Epidemiological studies provide data to guide future research with the goal of optimizing management strategies. Physical therapists must be aware of current best-practice standards regarding neck pain. This includes screening patients for the appropriateness of physical therapy services prior to initiating treatment. Once the decision is made to proceed with physical therapy care, a treatment-based classification system is proposed as an ideal starting point for managing this population. Outcome measures provide objective data to support the clinical decision-making process for individuals with cervical spine pain. Future research is needed to provide further insight into the management of patients with neck pain.

References

Abdu WA, Provencher M. 1998. Primary bone and metastatic tumors of the cervical spine. Spine 23: 2767–2777.

Aoyagi K, Ross PD, Huang C, et al. 1999. Prevalence of joint pain is higher among women in rural Japan than urban Japanese–American women in Hawaii. Ann Rheum Dis 58: 315–319.

Ariens GA, van Mechelen W, Bongers PM, et al. 2000. Physical risk factors for neck pain. Scand J Work Environ Health 26: 7–19.

Ariens GA, van Mechelen W, Bongers PM, et al. 2001. Psychosocial risk factors for neck pain: a systematic review. Am J Ind Med 39: 180–193.

Bogduk N. 2002. Innervation and pain patterns of the cervical spine. In: Grant R (ed) Physical therapy of the cervical and thoracic spine, 3rd edn. Edinburgh: Churchill Livingstone, pp 399–412.

Bogduk N. 2003. The anatomy and pathophysiology of neck pain. Phys Med Rehabil Clin N Am 14: 455–472.

Bogduk N, McGuirk B. 2006. Management of acute and chronic neck pain: an evidence-based approach. Edinburgh: Elsevier.

Boissonnault WG. 2005. Primary care for the physical therapist examination and triage. St Louis: Elsevier Saunders, pp 53–104.

Borghouts JA, Koes BW, Bouter LM. 1998. The clinical course and prognostic factors of non-specific neck pain: a systematic review. Pain 77: 1–13.

Borghouts JA, Koes BW, Vondeling H, et al. 1999. Cost-of-illness of neck pain in The Netherlands in 1996. Pain 80: 629–636.

Bot SDM, van der Waal JM, Terwee CB, et al. 2005. Predictors of outcome in neck and shoulder symptoms: a cohort study in general practice. Spine 30: E459–E470.

Brochet B, Michel P, Barberger-Gateau P, et al. 1998. Population-based study of pain in elderly people: a descriptive survey. Age Ageing 27: 279–284.

Bronfort G, Evans R, Nelson B. 2001. A randomized clinical trial of exercise and spinal manipulation for patients with chronic neck pain. Spine 26: 788–797.

Buchbinder R, Goel V, Bombardier C. 1996a. Lack of concordance between the ICD-9 classification of soft tissue disorders of the neck and upper limb and chart review diagnosis: one steel mill's experience. Am J Ind Med 29: 171–182.

Buchbinder R, Goel V, Bombardier C, et al. 1996b. Classification systems of soft tissue disorders of the neck and upper limb: do they satisfy methodological guidelines? J Clin Epidemiol 49: 141–149.

Carroll LJ, Hogg-Johnson S, van der Velde G, et al. 2008. Course and prognostic factors for neck pain in the general population: results of the Bone and Joint Decade 2000–2010 Task Force on Neck Pain and Its Associated Disorders. Spine 33 (Suppl 4): S75–S82.

Carroll LJ, Hogg-Johnson S, Côté P, et al. 2009. Course and prognostic factors for neck pain in workers: results of the Bone and Joint Decade 2000–2010 Task Force on Neck Pain and Its Associated Disorders. J Manipulative Physiol Ther 32 (Suppl 2): S108–S116.

Centers for Disease Control. Lung cancer statistics. Online. Available: http://www.cdc.gov/cancer/lung/statistics/index.htm; accessed 2014.

Childs JD, Fritz JM, Piva SR, et al. 2004. Proposal of a classification system for patients with neck pain. J Orthop Sports Phys Ther 34: 686–700.
Childs JD, Cleland JA, Elliott JM, et al. 2008. Neck pain: clinical practice guidelines linked to the international classification of functioning, disability, and health from the orthopedic section of the American Physical Therapy Association. J Orthop Sports Phys Ther 38: A1–A34.
Cleland JA, Childs JD, McRae M, et al. 2005. Immediate effects of thoracic manipulation in patients with neck pain: a randomized clinical trial. Man Ther 10: 127–135.
Cleland JA, Fritz JM, Whitman JM, et al. 2006. The reliability and construct validity of the Neck Disability Index and patient specific functional scale in patients with cervical radiculopathy. Spine 31: 598–602.
Cleland JA, Childs JD, Fritz JM, et al. 2007. Development of a clinical prediction rule for guiding treatment of a subgroup of patients with neck pain: use of thoracic spine manipulation, exercise, and patient education. Phys Ther 87: 9–23.
Cleland JA, Childs JD, Whitman JM. 2008. Psychometric properties of the Neck Disability Index and Numeric Pain Rating Scale in patients with mechanical neck pain. Arch Phys Med Rehabil 89: 69–74.
Cleland JA, Mintken PE, Carpenter K, et al. 2010. Examination of a clinical prediction rule to identify patients with neck pain likely to benefit from thoracic spine thrust manipulation and a general cervical range of motion exercise: multi-center randomized clinical trial. Phys Ther 90: 1239–1250.
Cook C, Brismée J, Fleming R, et al. 2005. Identifiers suggestive of clinical cervical spine instability: a Delphi study of physical therapists. Phys Ther 85: 895–906.
Cook C, Roman M, Stewart KM, et al. 2009. Reliability and diagnostic accuracy of clinical special tests for myelopathy in patients seen for cervical dysfunction. J Orthop Sports Phys Ther 39: 172–178.
Cooper G, Bogduk N. 2005. Cervical zygapophyseal joint pain maps (Poster 97). Arch Phys Med Rehabil 86(9): e22–e23.
Côté P, Cassidy JD, Carroll LJ, et al. 2004. The annual incidence and course of neck pain in the general population: a population-based cohort study. Pain 112: 267–273.
Côté P, van der Velde G, Cassidy JD, et al. 2009. The burden and determinants of neck pain in workers: results of the Bone and Joint Decade 2000–2010 Task Force on Neck Pain and Its Associated Disorders. J Manipulative Physiol Ther 32 (Suppl 2): S70–S86.
Croft PR, Lewis M, Papageorgiou AC, et al. 2001. Risk factors for neck pain: a longitudinal study in the general population. Pain 93: 317–325.
Delitto A. 2006. Patient outcomes and clinical performance: parallel paths or inextricable links? J Orthop Sports Phys Ther 36: 548–549.
Fejer R, Kyvik KO, Hartvigsen J. 2006. The prevalence of neck pain in the world population: a systematic critical review of the literature. Eur Spine J 15: 834–848.
Fernández-de-Las-Peñas C, Alonso-Blanco C, Miangolarra JC. 2007a. Myofascial trigger points in subjects presenting with mechanical neck pain: a blinded, controlled study. Man Ther 12: 29–33.
Fernández-de-las-Peñas C, Palomeque-del-Cerro L, Rodríguez-Blanco C. 2007b. Changes in neck pain and active range of motion after a single thoracic spine manipulation in subjects presenting with mechanical neck pain: a case series. J Manipulative Physiol Ther 30: 312–320.
Fritz JM, Brennan GP. 2007. Preliminary examination of a proposed treatment-based classification system for patients receiving physical therapy interventions for neck pain. Phys Ther 87: 513–524.
George SZ, Fritz JM, Erhard RE. 2001. A comparison of fear-avoidance beliefs in patients with lumbar spine pain and cervical spine pain. Spine 26: 2139–2145.
González-Iglesias J, Fernández-de-las-Peñas C, Cleland JA, et al. 2009a. Inclusion of thoracic spine thrust manipulation into an electro-therapy / thermal program for the management of patients with acute mechanical neck pain: a randomized clinical trial. Man Ther 14: 306–313.
González-Iglesias J, Fernández-de-las-Peñas C, Cleland JA, et al. 2009b. Thoracic spine manipulation for the management of patients with neck pain: a randomized clinical trial. J Orthop Sports Phys Ther 39: 20–27.
Greene G. 2001.'Red Flags': essential factors in recognizing serious spinal pathology. Man Ther 6: 253–255.
Greenhalgh S, Selfe J. 2009. A qualitative investigation of red flags for serious spinal pathology. Physiotherapy 95: 224–227.
Gross AR, Kay T, Hondras M, et al. 2002. Manual therapy for mechanical neck disorders: a systematic review. Man Ther 7: 131–149.
Gross AR, Hoving JL, Haines TA, et al. 2004. A Cochrane review of manipulation and mobilization for mechanical neck disorders. Spine 29: 1541–1548.
Grubb SA, Kelly CK. 2000. Cervical discography: clinical implications from 12 years of experience. Spine 25: 1382–1389.
Guzman J, Hurwitz EL, Carroll LJ, et al. 2009. A new conceptual model of neck pain: linking onset, course, and care: the Bone and Joint Decade 2000–2010 Task Force on Neck Pain and Its Associated Disorders. J Manipulative Physiol Ther 32 (Suppl 2): S17–S28.
Haldeman S, Kohlbeck FJ, McGregor M. 1999. Risk factors and precipitating neck movements causing vertebrobasilar artery dissection after cervical trauma and spinal manipulation. Spine 24: 785–794.
Henschke N, Maher CG, Refshauge KM. 2007. Screening for malignancy in low back pain patients: a systematic review. Eur Spine J 16: 1673–1679.
Hill J, Lewis M, Papageorgiou AC, et al. 2004. Predicting persistent neck pain: a 1-year follow-up of a population cohort. Spine 29: 1648–1654.
Hogg-Johnson S, van der Velde G, Carroll LJ, et al. 2009. The burden and determinants of neck pain in the general population: results of the Bone and Joint Decade 2000–2010 Task Force on Neck Pain and Its Associated Disorders. J Manipulative Physiol Ther 32 (Suppl 2): S46–S60.
Holmen TL, Barrett-Connor E, Holmen J, et al. 2000. Health problems in teenage daily smokers versus nonsmokers, Norway, 1995–1997: the Nord-Trøndelag Health Study. Am J Epidemiol 151: 148–155.
Hoving JL, Gross AR, Gasner AR, et al. 2001. A critical appraisal of review articles on the effectiveness of conservative treatment for neck pain. Spine 26: 196–205.
Howe JF, Loeser JD, Calvin WH. 1977. Mechanosensitivity of dorsal root ganglia and chronically injured axons: a physiological basis for the radicular pain of nerve root compression. Pain 3: 25–41.
Hoy DG, Protani M, De R, et al. 2010. The epidemiology of neck pain. Best Pract Res Clin Rheumatol 24: 783–792.
Hoy DG, Bain C, Williams G, et al. 2012. A systematic review of the global prevalence of low back pain. Arthritis Rheum 64: 2028–2037.
Hoy DG, March L, Woolf A, et al. 2014. The global burden of neck pain: estimates from the Global Burden of Disease 2010 study. Ann Rheum Dis 73(7): 1309–1315. doi: 10.1136/annrheumdis-2013-204431.
Isacsson A, Hanson BS, Ranstam J. 1995. Social network, social support and the prevalence of neck and low back pain after retirement. A population study of men born in 1914 in Malmö, Sweden. Scand J Soc Med 23: 17–22.
Jaeschke R, Singer J, Guyatt GH. 1989. Measurement of health status. Ascertaining the minimal clinically important difference. Control Clin Trials 10: 407–415.
Jarvik JG. 2003. Imaging of adults with low back pain in the primary care setting. Neuroimaging Clin North Am 13: 293–305.
Jensen MP, Turner JA, Romano JM, et al. 1999. Comparative reliability and validity of chronic pain intensity measures. Pain 83: 157–162.
Jette DU, Jette AM. 1997. Professional uncertainty and treatment choices by physical therapists. Arch Phys Med Rehabil 78: 1346–1351.
Jull G, Sterling M. 2009. Bring back the biopsychosocial model for neck pain disorders. Man Ther 14: 117–118.
Jull G, Trott P, Potter H, et al. 2002. A randomized controlled trial of exercise and manipulative therapy for cervicogenic headache. Spine 27: 1835–1843, discussion 1843.
Kamper SJ, Maher CG, Mackay C. 2009. Global Rating of Change scales: a review of strengths and weaknesses and considerations for design. J Man Manip Ther 17: 163–170.
Kanlayanaphotporn R, Chiradejnant A, Vachalathiti R. 2009. The immediate effects of mobilization technique on pain and range of motion in patients presenting with unilateral neck pain: a randomized controlled trial. Arch Phys Med Rehabil 90: 187–192.
Kerry R, Taylor AJ. 2009. Cervical arterial dysfunction: knowledge and reasoning for manual physical therapists. J Orthop Sports Phys Ther 39: 378–387.
Koes BW, Hoving JL. 2002. Efficacy of manual therapy in the treatment of neck pain. In: Grant R (ed) Physical therapy of the cervical and thoracic spine, 3rd edn. Edinburgh: Churchill Livingstone, pp 399–412.
Koopmanschap MA, Rutten FF. 1996. A practical guide for calculating indirect costs of disease. Pharmacoeconomics 10: 460–466.
Kovach SG, Huslig EL. 1984. Shoulder pain and Pancoast tumor: a diagnostic dilemma. J Manipulative Physiol Ther 7: 25–31.
Kovacs FM, Abraira V, Royuela A, et al. 2008. Minimum detectable and minimal clinically important changes for pain in patients with nonspecific neck pain. BMC Musculoskelet Disord 9 43.
Kroeling P, Gross AR, Goldsmith CH. 2005. A Cochrane review of electrotherapy for mechanical neck disorders. Spine 30: E641–E648.
Landers MR, Creger RV, Baker CV, et al. 2008. The use of fear-avoidance beliefs and nonorganic signs in predicting prolonged disability in patients with neck pain. Man Ther 13: 239–248.
Linton SJ. 2000. A review of psychological risk factors in back and neck pain. Spine 25: 1148–1156.

MacDermid JC, Walton DM, Côté P, et al. 2013. Use of outcome measures in measuring neck pain: an international multidisciplinary study. Open Orthop J 7: 506–520.

Mansilla-Ferragut P, Fernández-de-Las Peñas C, Alburquerque-Sendín F, et al. 2009. Immediate effects of atlanto-occipital joint manipulation on active mouth opening and pressure pain sensitivity in women with mechanical neck pain. J Manipulative Physiol Ther 32: 101–106.

Martínez-Segura R, Fernández-de-las-Peñas C, Ruiz-Sáez M, et al. 2006. Immediate effects on neck pain and active range of motion after a single cervical high-velocity low-amplitude manipulation in subjects presenting with mechanical neck pain: a randomized controlled trial. J Manipulative Physiol Ther 29: 511–517.

Masaracchio M, Cleland JA, Hellman M, et al. 2013. Short-term combined effects of thoracic spine thrust manipulation and cervical spine nonthrust manipulation in individuals with mechanical neck pain: a randomized clinical trial. J Orthop Sports Phys Ther 43: 118–127.

Merskey H, Bogduk N. 1994. Classification of chronic pain. Description of chronic pain syndromes and definitions of pain terms, 2nd edn. Seattle: IASP Press, pp 11, 210.

Mintken PE, Metrick L, Flynn TW. 2008. Upper cervical ligament testing in a patient with os odontoideum presenting with headaches. J Orthop Sports Phys Ther 38: 465–475.

Niemi SM, Levoska S, Rekola KE, et al. 1997. Neck and shoulder symptoms of high school students and associated psychosocial factors. J Adolesc Health 20: 238–242.

Nordin M, Carragee EJ, Hogg-Johnson S, et al. 2009. Assessment of neck pain and its associated disorders: results of the Bone and Joint Decade 2000–2010 Task Force on Neck Pain and Its Associated Disorders. J Manipulative Physiol Ther 32 (Suppl 2): S117–S140.

Pecoraro RE, Inui TS, Chen MS, et al. 1979. Validity and reliability of a self-administered health history questionnaire. Public Health Rep 94: 231–238.

Pincus T, Vlaeyen JWS, Kendall NAS, et al. 2002. Cognitive–behavioral therapy and psychosocial factors in low back pain: directions for the future. Spine 27 E133–E138.

Raney NH, Petersen EJ, Smith TA, et al. 2009. Development of a clinical prediction rule to identify patients with neck pain likely to benefit from cervical traction and exercise. Eur Spine J 18: 382–391.

Rushton A, Rivett D, Carlesso L, et al. 2014. International framework for examination of the cervical region for potential of cervical arterial dysfunction prior to orthopaedic manual therapy intervention. Man Ther 19(3): 222–228. doi: 10.1016/j.math.2013.11.005.

Slipman CW, Plastaras CT, Palmitier RA, et al. 1998. Symptom provocation of fluoroscopically guided cervical nerve root stimulation. Are dynatomal maps identical to dermatomal maps? Spine 23 2235–2242.

Sterling M. 2009. Neck pain: much more than a psychosocial condition. J Orthop Sports Phys Ther 39: 309–311.

Stiell IG, Wells GA, Vandemheen KL, et al. 2001. The Canadian C-spine rule for radiography in alert and stable trauma patients. JAMA 286: 1841–1848.

Stiell IG, Clement CM, McKnight RD, et al. 2003. The Canadian C-spine rule versus the NEXUS low-risk criteria in patients with trauma. N Engl J Med 349: 2510–2518.

Thiel H, Rix C. 2005. Is it time to stop functional pre-manipulation testing of the cervical spine? Man Ther 10: 154–158.

Thompson WL, Stiell IG, Clement CM, et al. 2009. Association of injury mechanism with the risk of cervical spine fractures. CJEM 11: 14–22.

Waddell G, Newton M, Henderson I, et al. 1993. A Fear-Avoidance Beliefs Questionnaire (FABQ) and the role of fear-avoidance beliefs in chronic low back pain and disability. Pain 52: 157–168.

Wainner RS, Fritz JM, Irrgang JJ, et al. 2003. Reliability and diagnostic accuracy of the clinical examination and patient self-report measures for cervical radiculopathy. Spine 28: 52–62.

Walton DM, Macdermid JC, Santaguida PL, et al. 2013a. Results of an international survey of practice patterns for establishing prognosis in neck pain: the ICON Project. Open Orthop J 7: 387–395.

Walton DM, Macdermid JC, Taylor T, 2013b. What does 'recovery' mean to people with neck pain? Results of a descriptive thematic analysis. Open Orthop J 7: 420–427.

Walton DM, Eilon-Avigdor Y, Wonderham M. 2014. Exploring the clinical course of neck pain in physical therapy: a longitudinal study. Arch Phys Med Rehabil 95: 305–308.

Wang WTJ, Olson SL, Campbell AH, et al. 2003. Effectiveness of physical therapy for patients with neck pain: an individualized approach using a clinical decision-making algorithm. Am J Phys Med Rehabil 82: 203–218.

Wedderkopp N, Leboeuf-Yde C, Andersen LB, et al. 2001. Back pain reporting pattern in a Danish population-based sample of children and adolescents. Spine 26: 1879–1883.

Wennberg JE, Barnes BA, Zubkoff M. 1982. Professional uncertainty and the problem of supplier-induced demand. Soc Sci Med 16: 811–824.

Werneke M, Hart DL. 2003. Discriminant validity and relative precision for classifying patients with nonspecific neck and back pain by anatomic pain patterns. Spine 28: 161–166.

Werneke MW, Hart DL, Resnik L, et al. 2008. Centralization: prevalence and effect on treatment outcomes using a standardized operational definition and measurement method. J Orthop Sports Phys Ther 38: 116–125.

Westaway MD, Stratford PW, Binkley JM. 1998. The patient-specific functional scale: validation of its use in persons with neck dysfunction. J Orthop Sports Phys Ther 27: 331–338.

Woo J, Ho SC, Lau J, et al. 1994. Musculoskeletal complaints and associated consequences in elderly Chinese aged 70 years and over. J Rheumatol 21: 1927–1931.

Wright A, Mayer TG, Gatchel RJ. 1999. Outcomes of disabling cervical spine disorders in compensation injuries. A prospective comparison to tertiary rehabilitation response for chronic lumbar spinal disorders. Spine 24: 178–183.

Yin W, Bogduk N. 2008. The nature of neck pain in a private pain clinic in the United States. Pain Med 9: 196–203.

Young IA, Michener LA, Cleland JA, et al. 2009. Manual therapy, exercise, and traction for patients with cervical radiculopathy: a randomized clinical trial. Phys Ther 89: 632–642.

10 Chapter

Whiplash-associated Disorders

Michele Sterling

CHAPTER CONTENTS

Introduction 110
The whiplash condition 111
Classification of whiplash injury 111
Physical and psychological characteristics of the whiplash condition 111
Motor and sensorimotor control dysfunction 111
Augmented pain processing mechanisms in whiplash 112
Psychological factors in whiplash-associated disorders 113
The prediction of outcome following whiplash injury 113
Implications for assessment of whiplash 114
Implications for management of whiplash-associated disorders 114
Conclusion 115

Introduction

Whiplash-associated disorders (WAD) are common, disabling and costly conditions that usually occur as a consequence of a motor vehicle crash (MVC). Recent data indicate that rapid improvement in levels of pain and disability occur in the first 3 months post injury with little if any change after this period and that up to 50% of injured people will not fully recover (Carroll et al 2008; Kamper et al 2008; Sterling et al 2010). The associated cost secondary to whiplash injury, including medical care, disability, lost work productivity, as well as personal costs, is substantial (Crouch et al 2006; MAIC 2012).

Based on current data, whiplash in both the acute and the chronic stages is resistant to treatment. A review by Teasell et al (2010) of interventions for the management of acute whiplash identified only 16 randomized controlled trials of varying methodological quality and five non-randomized trials in the English literature over the past 30 years. The included trials involved eclectic approaches in various configurations, including advice to remain active or prescription of exercise in various forms (with or without manipulative therapy), immobilization in a collar, educational interventions, acupuncture and pulsed electromagnetic field therapy. The authors concluded on the available evidence that activity-based therapies seemed to be more effective. Nevertheless, inspection of these trials reveals that outcomes pertaining to recovery and non-recovery rates remain relatively consistent, in accord with the findings of the natural course of whiplash (Carroll et al 2008; Sterling et al 2010).

Since this review, two further randomized controlled trials for acute whiplash-associated disorders have been conducted. One trial in Australia investigated multidisciplinary (physiotherapy, medication and psychology) management compared with usual care. Again outcomes were equivocal with no additional benefit of early multidisciplinary care and still a chronicity rate of 50% for both groups – a proportion that is no different from the usual clinical pathway (Jull et al 2013). The second trial was conducted in accident and emergency departments in the UK. The results showed that a six-session physiotherapy programme of exercise and manual therapy provided only modest short-term benefit when compared with a single physiotherapy session comprising mainly advice on activity and exercise, and that this benefit was not cost effective (Lamb et al 2013). Moreover only 45–50% of the participants reported their condition as being 'much better' or 'better' – again a low recovery rate that is little different to the usual natural pattern of recovery following the injury.

Furthermore, trials of treatment for the chronic stage of the condition including various forms of exercise have offered only modest effects, with only 10–20% of individuals having a completely successful outcome – that is, minimal or no disability at the 12-month follow-up (Jull et al 2007; Stewart et al 2007). A recent large trial of a comprehensive exercise approach (specific neck, shoulder girdle and sensorimotor control exercises together with functional and general exercise) provided no additional benefit compared with a single physiotherapy advice session supplemented with telephone support (Michaleff et al 2014).

The disappointing results of recent randomized controlled trials for acute and chronic WAD demand a rethink of the condition and its management. There is a wealth of evidence available demonstrating the presence of complex physiological and psychological factors. Do these factors need to be taken into consideration in the development of new interventions for WAD, more than has so far been the case?

This chapter will review the whiplash condition, its classification and the prediction of outcomes following the injury before outlining current evidence for the physiological and psychological features of the condition. Finally, the implications of this research on the assessment and management of the condition will be discussed.

The Whiplash Condition

An MVC can lead to bony or soft tissue damage, which in turn may result in a variety of clinical manifestations called whiplash-associated disorders. The primary symptom is neck pain, although headache, arm pain, paraesthesia, dizziness and cognitive difficulties are also frequently reported (Spitzer et al 1995).

It is conceivable that virtually any cervical spine structure may sustain injury following whiplash. Bioengineering studies where cadavers were subjected to simulated rear-end crashes have demonstrated perturbations in segmental movement including intersegmental hyperextension, S-curve formation and differential acceleration of the upper cervical spine (Cusick et al 2001). This, together with evidence from autopsy and animal studies (Winkelstein et al 2000), indicates that lesions may occur to cervical structures including bony elements, intervertebral discs and zygapophyseal joints, ligaments, muscles and nerve tissues. Unfortunately, in vivo identification of structural pathology has proved to be difficult, which is probably due to the insensitivity of current radiological diagnostic imaging (Curatolo et al 2011). The best available evidence relates to the zygapophyseal joints and was demonstrated by placebo-controlled nerve blocks (Lord et al 1996; Curatolo et al 2011).

Whilst it could be argued to be beneficial if specific structural lesion(s) could be identified in whiplash-injured persons, at the current time this is usually not possible. Therefore, it is important to consider processes that may underlie the initiation of whiplash pain and also the maintenance of symptoms in those who do not recover (Sterling et al 2011c). This may allow for the development and testing of interventions to target these processes and improve outcomes. These processes may vary depending on the stage of the injury and so this will also need to be considered.

Classification of Whiplash Injury

Classification systems have been proposed in order to assist in the early assessment, prognosis and management of whiplash. The most commonly used classification system is the Quebec Task Force (QTF) system (Spitzer et al 1995). This broadly defines the condition into four groups: WAD I (neck complaint without musculoskeletal signs), WAD II (with musculoskeletal signs), WAD III (with neurological deficits) and WAD IV (with a fracture or dislocation). Although this system provides some necessary information related to condition classification, a major systematic flaw exists as the majority of whiplash-injured people are grouped within one classification (WAD II), which falsely assumes homogeneity of the most common complaints within this patient group (Sterling 2004). Nevertheless, the system at least provides a common language for effective communication between healthcare and non-healthcare providers involved in the management of people with WAD.

To date, neither the QTF classification system for WAD nor trials investigating various management approaches for this condition have fully considered both the physiological and psychological factors that are emerging as playing a role in the pain and disability of whiplash. It is apparent that whiplash is a more complex condition than had previously been assumed. Furthermore, it is also emerging that whiplash is in some ways different from neck pain conditions of a non-traumatic nature (mechanical idiopathic neck pain). In particular, chronic whiplash shows marked sensory features indicative of central nervous system hyperexcitability that have now consistently been shown not to be a feature of chronic non-traumatic neck pain (Scott et al 2005; Elliott et al 2009a; Chien et al 2010).

Physical and Psychological Characteristics of the Whiplash Condition

Historically much past research and certainly the clinical assessment of spinal pain conditions, including whiplash, has aimed to identify the pathoanatomical source(s) of the patient's reported symptoms. This approach has had limited success as a pathoanatomical diagnosis is not possible in the vast majority of patients with common musculoskeletal pain conditions, nor does such a diagnosis necessarily shed light on the most optimal intervention for a specific condition or patient. As a consequence, the focus has shifted in recent years more towards attempting to identify the underlying mechanisms or processes of the patient's pain syndrome. The purpose of this more specific diagnosis and classification of musculoskeletal pain syndromes is to help tailor interventions toward identifiable underlying processes so as to try to improve treatment success, particularly in some of the more recalcitrant conditions. Of all neck and upper quadrant conditions, there is arguably the most data available for motor, sensory and psychological characteristics of whiplash. One reason for this may be the easily defined onset of injury (MVC) compared with the more insidious onset often occurring in other conditions.

Motor and sensorimotor control dysfunction

One of the most common clinical characteristics of patients with WAD is that of either movement loss or decreased cervical range of movement (Dall'Alba et al 2001). Most prospective studies have shown that all whiplash-injured subjects have a loss of cervical active range of movement from soon after injury (Kasch et al 2001; Sterling et al 2003b) that persists in those who do recover (Sterling et al 2003b). Altered patterns of muscle recruitment in both the cervical spine and the shoulder girdle regions have been clearly shown to be features of chronic WAD (Nederhand et al 2002; Jull et al 2004). Longitudinal data demonstrate that these changes are apparent from very soon after injury (Sterling et al 2003b). Sterling et al (2003b, 2006) observed that the disturbed motor patterns persisted, not only in those with ongoing chronic symptoms but also in those with milder pain and disability and in those who reported full recovery, with these phenomena occurring at significant time-periods post injury – up to 2 years. These persisting deficits in muscle control may leave recovered individuals more vulnerable to future episodes of neck pain, but this proposal needs to be substantiated with further investigation. Altered patterns of muscle recruitment are not unique to whiplash and identical changes have also been observed in neck pain of insidious onset (idiopathic neck pain) (Nederhand et al 2002; Jull et al 2004; Woodhouse & Vasseljen 2008). These findings suggest that the driver of such motor changes may be more the nociceptive input than the injury mechanism itself.

Morphological changes to cervical spine muscles have also been demonstrated in people with chronic whiplash. Using magnetic resonance imaging (MRI), Elliott et al (2006, 2009b, 2010) demonstrated the presence of fatty infiltrate in both deep and superficial cervical extensor and flexor muscles in WAD patients compared with an asymptomatic control group. Although the fatty infiltrate was generally higher in all muscles investigated for the patient group, it was highest in the deeper muscles, the rectus capitis posterior minor and major and multifidi (Elliott et al 2006). In contrast to muscle recruitment changes, available data indicate that similar morphological changes are not apparent in individuals with chronic idiopathic neck pain (Elliott et al 2014). The relevance of these findings in terms of pain, disability or functional recovery and the cause of the muscle changes are not yet known.

Dysfunction of sensorimotor control is also a feature of both acute and chronic WAD. Greater joint-repositioning errors have been found in patients with chronic WAD and also in those within weeks of their injury (Sterling et al 2003b; Treleaven et al 2003). Loss of balance and disturbed neck-influenced eye movement control are present in patients with chronic WAD (Treleaven et al 2005a, 2005b). It is important to note also that sensorimotor disturbances seem to be greater in individuals who also report dizziness in association with their neck pain (Treleaven et al 2003).

Most of the documented motor deficits (movement loss, altered muscle recruitment patterns) seem to be present in whiplash-injured individuals irrespective both of reported pain and disability levels and of the rate or level of recovery (Sterling et al 2003b). Additionally, apart from cervical movement loss, motor deficits do not have predictive capacity (Daenen et al 2013). Furthermore, treatment directed at rehabilitating motor dysfunction and improving general movement shows only modest effects on reported pain and disability levels (Jull et al 2007; Stewart et al 2007; Michaleff et al 2014). Together these findings suggest that motor deficits, although present, may not play a key role in the development and maintenance of chronic or persistent symptoms following whiplash injury. This is not to say that management approaches directed at improving movement motor dysfunction should not be provided to patients with whiplash as these will be important to overall general health. Rather the identification of motor deficits alone may not equip the clinician with useful information to gauge either prognosis or potential responsiveness to physical interventions.

Augmented pain-processing mechanisms in whiplash

There is now considerable and consistent evidence of sensory disturbances in WAD that indicate the presence of augmented central nociceptive pain-processing mechanisms. Changes include sensory hypersensitivity (or decreased pain thresholds) to numerous stimuli such as pressure, thermal or electrical stimulation and light touch in both acute and chronic WAD (Sterling et al 2003a; Stone et al 2012; Van Oosterwijck et al 2013). Sensory hypersensitivity is found not only over the cervical spine (area of injury) but also at remote uninjured areas such as the upper and lower limbs (Koelbaek-Johansen et al 1999; Sterling et al 2003a). The absence of tissue damage at the site of testing suggests that central sensitization of nociceptive pathways is the cause of the pain sensitivity. Widespread hypoaesthesia (elevated detection thresholds) occurring concurrently with hypersensitivity, as well as less-efficacious conditioned pain modulation, has also been found in patients with WAD – indicating disturbances in central inhibitory processes as well (Chien et al 2009; Ng et al 2014).

Hypersensitivity has been shown to be present not only in testing involving a cognitive response from the participant; also, facilitated flexor withdrawal reflexes in the lower limbs of participants with chronic WAD have been demonstrated following electrical stimulation of the sural nerve (Lim et al 2011). In the latter test, reflex activity of the biceps femoris was measured and evidence of spinal cord hyperexcitability (central sensitization) was provided without relying on the subject's self-reported response to the stimuli, as is required with pain threshold testing. It has also been shown that the heightened reflex responses are not associated with psychological factors such as catastrophization and distress (Sterling et al 2008).

In contrast to the apparently uniform presence of motor dysfunction, sensory disturbances seem to differentiate whiplash from less severe neck pain conditions and whiplash subgroupings with higher or lower levels of self-reported pain and disability. Individuals with chronic WAD manifest a more complex presentation, involving lowered pain thresholds to pressure, heat and cold stimuli in areas remote to the cervical spine, which are not present in those with idiopathic (non-traumatic) neck pain (Scott et al 2005; Elliott et al 2009b; Chien et al 2010). Similarly, widespread hypoaesthesia to vibration, thermal and electrical stimulation, although present in WAD, is not a feature of idiopathic neck pain (Chien et al 2010). However, the presence of central hyperexcitability is not unique to whiplash; other painful musculoskeletal conditions such as fibromyalgia, tension-type headache and migraine also manifest such signs (Yunus 2007). With respect to the cervical spine and upper quadrant, widespread sensory hypersensitivity is a feature of cervical radiculopathy, as both patients with this condition and those with whiplash report similar pain and disability levels (Chien et al 2008). This finding suggests that chronic whiplash and chronic cervical radiculopathy share similar underlying mechanisms but differ from idiopathic neck pain – thus illustrating the diversity of processes involved in various neck pain conditions.

The reason why some whiplash-injured people develop a hypersensitive state is not clear. Numerous cervical spine structures are implicated as potential sources of nociception following whiplash injury (Curatolo et al 2011). It is possible that injuries to deep cervical structures do not rapidly heal and thus become a nociceptive 'driver' of central nervous system hyperexcitability; recent evidence supports this hypothesis (Smith et al 2014). Additionally, the sensory hypersensitivity seen in patients with whiplash is also associated with other disturbances such as impaired sympathetic vasoconstriction (Sterling 2006), stress-related factors (Sterling et al 2011b) and pain catastrophization (Rivest et al 2010). There is also emerging evidence that certain individuals may have a genetic vulnerability to higher levels of pain and the development of augmented central nociceptive processing (McLean et al 2011). The co-occurrence of these factors suggests that a complex interplay between various mechanisms may lead to this almost-systemic response in some individuals following whiplash injury. Research is now focusing on investigating such complex models that may in the future shed light on this intriguing issue (McLean et al 2005; Passatore & Roatta 2006; Sterling & Kenardy 2006).

Psychological factors in whiplash-associated disorders

There is no doubt that chronic whiplash is associated with psychological distress, including affective disturbances, anxiety, depression and behavioural abnormalities such as fear of movement (Williamson et al 2008). Psychological distress is also present in the acute post-injury stage, with most people showing some distress regardless of pain and disability levels (Sterling et al 2003c). Data from some studies indicate that the ongoing psychological distress is associated with non-resolving pain and disability. A large cross-sectional study showed an association between anxiety, depression and pain and disability in people whose accidents had occurred over 2 years previously, but not in those with acute injury, which suggests that symptom persistence is the trigger for psychological distress (Wenzel et al 2002). Longitudinal data indicate that initially elevated levels of distress decrease in those who recover, in a manner closely paralleling the decreasing levels of pain and disability (Sterling et al 2003c).

Unique psychological factors may be involved in the aetiology and development of chronic whiplash (Sterling et al 2003c) compared with other painful musculoskeletal conditions. For example, the role of fear-of-movement beliefs seems to be a less important factor in whiplash (Sterling et al 2005) than in low back pain (Vlaeyen et al 1995). The role of coping styles or strategies in whiplash is unclear, however. Some data indicate that a palliative reaction (e.g. seeking palliative relief of symptoms such as distraction, smoking or drinking) was associated with longer symptom duration (Buitenhuis et al 2003; Carroll et al 2006); in contrast, Kivioja et al (2005) found no evidence that different coping styles in the early stage of injury influenced the outcome at 1 year post accident. The different cohort inception times of these studies may account for the differences in findings, indicating that coping strategies may vary depending on the stage of the condition.

One factor that is likely to be unique to WAD (compared with other common musculoskeletal conditions), due to the mode of onset being a traumatic event, is that of post-traumatic stress. Symptoms of post-traumatic stress have been shown to be present in a proportion of people following a whiplash injury due to an MVC (Kongsted et al 2008; Sterling et al 2010) and these symptoms have shown prognostic capacity for poor functional recovery at 12 months and 2 years post MVC (Buitenhuis et al 2006; Sterling et al 2011b, 2012). These studies mostly utilized the Impact of Events Scale (IES) (Horowitz et al 1979), an instrument that measures distress associated with a specific event (in the case of whiplash an MVC), although it should be noted that a diagnosis of post-traumatic stress disorder cannot be made from IES scores. However, recent data utilizing a more robust tool, the Post-traumatic Diagnostic Scale (PDS) (Foa et al 1997), demonstrated that 22% of a prospective sample of 155 whiplash-injured people had a probable diagnosis of post-traumatic stress disorders at 3 months post MVC, with this figure dropping slightly to 17% by 12 months post injury (Sterling et al 2010). These findings indicate the need for further psychological evaluation of these patients, and clinicians should consider this factor in their assessment of whiplash-injured people.

The Prediction of Outcome Following Whiplash Injury

The capacity to predict those at risk of poor recovery following whiplash injury is important because it may allow the institution of appropriate early interventions targeted at modifiable risk factors. This could potentially reduce the transition to chronicity in those individuals deemed to be at risk. Numerous factors have been investigated for their prognostic capability, including sociodemographic status, crash-related variables, compensation and / or litigation, and psychosocial and physical factors. However, systematic reviews of prospective cohort studies on whiplash found that greater initial pain intensity and greater initial disability were the most consistent predictors of delayed functional recovery (Carroll et al 2008; Kamper et al 2008; Walton et al 2009, 2013b). A meta-analysis indicated that initial pain scores of greater than 5.5 on a visual analogue scale from 0 to 10 and scores of greater than 29% on the Neck Disability Index are useful cut-off scores for clinical use (Walton et al 2009).

Other factors reported by individual systematic reviews include post-injury psychological factors such as coping strategies (Carroll et al 2008), educational level no higher than secondary, female gender, a history of previous neck pain (Walton et al 2009), and symptoms of post-traumatic stress and poor self-efficacy (Williamson et al 2008). Whereas some of these factors such as pain intensity and psychological distress may be modifiable, many of the others (e.g. age, education) are not. Furthermore, when potentially modifiable factors of initial pain and disability levels are considered alone, although having high specificity they had relatively low sensitivity to predict those with ongoing moderate to severe symptoms at 6 months post-accident (Sterling et al 2005).

Cold hyperalgesia has been shown to predict disability and mental health outcomes at 12 months post injury (Sterling et al 2006, 2011b), and decreased cold pain tolerance measured with the cold pressor test predicted ongoing disability (Kasch et al 2005). A recent systematic review concluded that there is moderate evidence available to support cold hyperalgesia as an adverse prognostic indicator (Goldsmith et al 2012). Other sensory measures such as lowered pressure-pain thresholds (mechanical hyperalgesia) show inconsistent prognostic capacity, however. Walton et al (2011) reported that decreased pressure-pain thresholds over a distal site in the leg predicted neck-pain-related disability at 3 months post injury, but others have shown that this factor is not an independent predictor of later disability (Sterling et al 2006). The exact mechanisms underlying the hyperalgesic responses are not clearly understood, but are generally acknowledged to reflect augmented nociceptive processing in the central nervous system or central hyperexcitability (Curatolo et al 2004; Stone et al 2012).

The psychological factor of post-traumatic stress symptoms is emerging as a dominant one in poor outcome following whiplash injury (Buitenhuis et al 2006; Sterling et al 2012). Additional psychological factors such as high levels of pain catastrophizing, depressed mood and low expectations of recovery have also been identified, in some studies, as being predictive of poor functional recovery (Sterling et al 2011a).

The role of the controversial issue of compensation-related factors is inconclusive, with some studies finding that these have predictive capacity (Carroll et al 2008) and others reporting that they do not (Sterling et al 2005). A recent systematic meta-review outlined the limitations of research examining the influence of injury compensation on health outcomes, including the low quality of primary research papers in this area, the heterogeneous nature of compensation schemes studied and the lack of use of validated health outcome measures (Spearing et al 2012). These authors could find only one systematic review that could be considered both internally and externally valid and, based on this, their conclusion was that there is evidence of 'no association between litigation and poor health outcomes among people with whiplash' (Spearing & Connelly 2011, p 23).

Implications for Assessment of Whiplash

It is clear from current data that the whiplash condition involves complex interactions between physiological and psychological factors. Although the presence of high initial levels of pain and / or disability is a consistent predictor of poor outcome (Walton et al 2009, 2013b), the additional presence of sensory hypersensitivity (particularly cold hyperalgesia) and also post-traumatic stress symptoms has been shown to improve predictive capacity substantially (Sterling et al 2005). The long-term functional status following whiplash may be established within a few months of injury, with little further improvement after this time (Kamper et al 2008; Sterling et al 2010). This reiterates the important role that clinicians play in the early post-injury stage and even towards the prevention of chronicity.

The patient assessment will need to include an adequate history, such as previous history of neck pain and headache, as well as the possible mechanism of injury. The patient should be screened for the presence of any 'red flag' condition (WAD IV – fracture or dislocation). Although accident-related features have not been found to be consistent prognostic indicators of outcome (Walton et al 2009), they have shown some predictive capacity in certain studies (Sturzenegger et al 1995). Since pain and disability levels have been repeatedly demonstrated to be a consistent indicator of prolonged recovery (Walton et al 2013a, 2013b), it is essential that a validated measure, such as the Neck Disability Index (NDI) or Numeric Pain Rating scale, is used in the initial assessment. Certain physical factors, such as cold hyperalgesia and loss of neck movement, are predictive of poor recovery and so their presence must also be carefully assessed. With respect to whiplash injury, the psychological factor of post-traumatic stress appears to be involved in the transition from the acute to the chronic stage of the condition and so clinicians should include a measure of post-traumatic stress symptoms (e.g. using the IES) in their assessment of whiplash-injured patients.

At present, sensory examination such as that required to detect the variety of sensory disturbances outlined above is rarely performed, and if it is performed it is usually limited to rudimentary assessment of muscle power, deep tendon reflexes and light-touch sensation. More detailed assessment of sensory changes in patients with WAD may be helpful. The first stage of this assessment would be thorough recording of the patient's symptoms including the nature of pain. Although the usefulness of symptom classification as a way of clarifying pain mechanisms is debatable, it is a necessary part of the patient assessment (Jensen & Baron 2003). In recent times, questionnaires have been developed that aim to identify neuropathic-like pain specifically (Bennett et al 2007). Using the S-LANSS questionnaire (Bennett et al 2005), it has been shown that 20% of an acute whiplash cohort is likely have a predominantly neuropathic pain condition, certain questionnaire items being particularly associated with higher levels of pain and disability (Sterling & Pedler 2009).

Quantitative sensory testing can also be used. This could include the measurement of mechanical pain thresholds with pressure algometry and determination of the presence of allodynia with light tactile stimulation. There is moderate evidence for cold hyperalgesia as a predictor of poor recovery (Goldsmith et al 2012) and that it may be associated with lack of treatment responsiveness (Jull et al 2007), although a later more highly powered randomized controlled trial did not support this finding (Michaleff et al 2014). It is more difficult to measure clinically but a recent study comparing the use of ice application to the neck with cold pain thresholds obtained via the Somedic Thermotest® system indicated that pain >5 / 10 with ice was a good indication of cold hyperalgesia (Maxwell & Sterling, 2012), although further studies are required to further validate this measure.

However, it should be noted that, though such sensory assessments can provide useful information, at present there is no consensus over the most appropriate method to use and the reference standard with which to compare findings. The development of the most appropriate sensory examination of whiplash-injured patients is at an early stage and movement towards further development into clinically valid and useful measures is of vital importance.

Physiotherapists routinely assess the cervical range of movement and this will remain a mainstay of assessment of whiplash owing to the prognostic capacity of this measure. However, assessment will also need to include muscle recruitment patterns of the cervical and shoulder girdle regions. Furthermore, the assessment of sensorimotor control is relatively simple to undertake in the clinical situation and will be particularly important in whiplash-injured patients who report dizziness associated with their neck pain. Readers are referred to Jull et al (2008) for a detailed account of how to undertake these assessments.

Implications for Management of Whiplash-associated Disorders

An important aim for the treatment of acute WAD is the identification of people at risk of poor recovery, and then prevention of the development of chronic pain and disability. Currently, though, there is a paucity of evidence available to guide the clinician on how best to achieve this goal, which is frustrating for clinicians and researchers alike. Whereas there is now much better understanding of the characteristics of the condition and factors predictive of poor recovery, much less progress has been made in the development of improved and effective interventions. The next logical step in the research process is to determine the effectiveness of targeting these factors, many of which are potentially modifiable, with more specific interventions.

Education and advice to return to activity and exercise will remain the cornerstones of early treatment for WAD, but they require further investigation to determine the most effective form of exercise, its dosage and ways to deliver the approaches. Activity and exercise may be sufficient for patients at low risk of developing chronic pain (Ritchie et al 2013), although this proposition is yet to be formally tested. Those patients at higher risk of poor recovery will probably need additional treatments alongside the basic advice / activity / exercise approach. This may include medication to target pain and nociceptive process as well as methods of addressing early psychological responses to injury. However, a recent trial of multidisciplinary interventions for acute WAD demonstrated that this may not be so easy to achieve (Jull et al 2013); the participants in this trial not only found the side effects of medication unacceptable but were also less compliant with attendance to a clinical psychologist (46% of participants attended fewer than 4 of 10 sessions) compared with attendance with the physiotherapist (12% attended fewer than 4 sessions over 10 weeks). It is possible that people with acute whiplash injury see themselves as having a 'physical' injury and thus are more accepting of physiotherapy. The burden of requiring visits with several practitioners may also lead to poor compliance. Physiotherapists may therefore be the best-placed healthcare providers to deliver psychological interventions for acute WAD. This approach has been investigated in mainly chronic conditions such as arthritis (Hunt et al 2013) and in the management of acute low back pain (Hill et al 2011) with results showing some early promise. However, this is not to say that patients with a diagnosed psychopathology such as depression or post-traumatic stress disorder should be managed by physiotherapists; of course, such patients will require referral to an appropriately trained professional.

Physiotherapists may also need to take a greater role in the overall care plan of the patient with acute WAD. This would mean having expertise in the assessment of risk factors and an understanding of when additional treatments such as medication and psychological interventions may be required. Although in most jurisdictions this is still the role of general medical practitioners, physiotherapists may be better equipped in terms of time available for effective assessment, treatment planning and monitoring recovery and progress.

In the case of chronic WAD, more effective interventions need development and testing. It is becoming clear that management approaches focusing predominantly on physical rehabilitation are achieving only small effect sizes. However, it is important for the long-term general health of patients that they undertake regular activity and exercise and it is a concern if chronic pain prevents them from doing this. Randomized controlled trials are needed that combine activity / exercise approaches with other interventions such as psychological approaches, educational approaches and medication. The optimal combination and dosage of such approaches will need to be determined.

WAD, whether or acute or chronic, is a challenging and complex condition. With clear evidence emerging of a myriad of physical and psychological factors operating to varying degrees in individual patients, it is also clear that practitioners involved in the management of WAD will need specific skills in this area. Physiotherapists are the healthcare providers who probably see the greatest number of patients with WAD and, by virtue of the health system set-up, spend the most time with these individuals. Physical therapists are therefore well placed to take on a coordination or 'gatekeeper' role in the management of WAD, and research into health services models that include physiotherapists in such a role is also needed.

Conclusion

Whiplash is a complex, heterogeneous, intriguing condition involving both physical (motor and sensory) disturbances and psychological distress. It is also one of the most frustrating conditions for clinicians to manage. It would appear that the quest to understand WAD better has only just begun and the results from recent research efforts have paved the way for further directions for research. As new knowledge emerges, the clinical assessment of the condition will become more informed and this will translate to improved outcomes for injured people.

References

Bennett M, Smith BH, Torrance N, et al. 2005. The S-LANSS score for identifying pain of predominantly neuropathic origin: validation for use in clinical and postal research. J Pain 6: 149–158.

Bennett M, Attal N, Backonja MM, et al. 2007. Using screening tools to identify neuropathic pain. Pain 127: 199–203.

Buitenhuis J, Spanje, J, Fidler V. 2003. Recovery from acute whiplash: the role of coping styles. Spine 28: 896–901.

Buitenhuis J, de Jong PJ, Jaspers JP, et al. 2006. Relationship between post-traumatic stress disorder symptoms and the course of whiplash complaints. J Psychosom Res 61: 681–689.

Carroll L, Cassidy D, Cote P. 2006. The role of pain coping strategies in prognosis after whiplash injury: passive coping predicts slowed recovery. Pain 124: 18–26.

Carroll L, Holm LW, Hogg-Johnson S, et al. 2008. Course and prognostic factors for neck pain in whiplash-associated disorders (WAD): results of the Bone and Joint Decade 2000–2010 Task Force on Neck Pain and Its Associated Disorders. Spine 33: 583–592.

Chien A, Eliav E, Sterling M. 2008. Whiplash (Grade II) and cervical radiculopathy share a similar sensory presentation: an investigation using quantitative sensory testing. Clin J Pain 24: 595–603.

Chien A, Eliav E, Sterling M. 2009. Hypoaesthesia occurs with sensory hypersensitivity in chronic whiplash – further evidence of a neuropathic condition. Man Ther 14: 138–146.

Chien A, Eliav E, Sterling M. 2010. Sensory hypoaesthesia is a feature of chronic whiplash but not chronic idiopathic neck pain. Man Ther 15: 48–53.

Crouch R, Whitewick R, Clancy M, et al. 2006. Whiplash associated disorder: incidence and natural history over the first. Emerg Med J 23: 114–118.

Curatolo M, Arendt-Nielsen L, Petersen-Felix S. 2004. Evidence, mechanisms and clinical implications of central hypersensitivity in chronic pain after whiplash injury. Clin J Pain 20: 469–476.

Curatolo M, Bogduk N, Ivancic PC, et al. 2011. The role of tissue damage in whiplash associated disorders. Spine 36: S309–S315.

Cusick J, Pintar F, Yoganandan N. 2001. Whiplash syndrome: kinematic factors influencing pain patterns. Spine 26: 1252–1258.

Daenen L, Nijs J, Raadsen B, et al. 2013. Cervical motor dysfunction and its predictive value for long-term recovery in patients with acute whiplash-associated disorders: a systematic review. Man Ther 45: 113–122.
Dall'Alba P, Sterling M, Treleaven JM, et al. 2001. Cervical range of motion discriminates between asymptomatic and whiplash subjects. Spine 26: 2090–2094.
Elliott J, Jull G, Noteboom JT, et al. 2006. Fatty infiltration in the cervical extensor muscles in persistent whiplash associated disorders: an MRI analysis. Spine 31: E847–E851.
Elliott JM, Noteboom JT, Flynn TW, et al. 2009a. Characterization of acute and chronic whiplash-associated disorders. J Orthop Sports Phys Ther 39: 312–323
Elliott J, Terling M, Noteboom JT, et al. 2009b. The clinical presentation of chronic whiplash and the relationship to findings of MRI fatty infiltrates in the cervical extensor musculature: a preliminary investigation. Eur Spine J 18: 1371–1378.
Elliott J, O'Leary S, Sterling M, et al. 2010. MRI findings of fatty infiltrate in the cervical flexors in chronic whiplash. Spine 35: 948–954.
Elliott J, Pedler A, Jull G, et al. 2014. Differential changes in muscle composition exist in traumatic and non-traumatic neck pain. Spine 39: 39–47.
Foa E, Cashman L, Jaycox L, et al. 1997. The validation of a self-report measure of posttraumatic stress disorder: the posttraumatic diagnostic scale. Psychol Assessment 9: 445–451.
Goldsmith R, Wright C, Bell SF, et al. 2012. Cold hyperalgesia as a prognostic factor in whiplash associated disorders: a systematic review. Man Ther 17: 402–410.
Hill J, Whitehurst DH, Lewis M, et al. 2011. Comparison of stratified primary care management for low back pain with current best practice (STarT Back): a randomised controlled trial. Lancet 378: 1560–1571.
Horowitz M, Wilner N, Alvarez W. 1979. Impact of Events Scale: a measure of subjective stress. Psychosom Med 41: 209–218.
Hunt M, Keefe FJ, Bryant C, et al. 2013. A physiotherapist-delivered, combined exercise and pain coping skills training intervention for individuals with knee osteoarthritis: a pilot study. Knee 20: 106–112.
Jensen T, Baron R. 2003. Translation of symptoms and signs into mechanisms in neuropathic pain. Pain 102: 1–8.
Jull G, Kristjansson E, Dall'Alba P. 2004. Impairment in the cervical flexors: a comparison of whiplash and insidious onset neck pain patients. Man Ther 9: 89–94.
Jull G, Sterling M, Kenardy J, et al. 2007. Does the presence of sensory hypersensitivity influence outcomes of physical rehabilitation for chronic whiplash? A preliminary RCT. Pain 129: 28–34.
Jull G, Sterling M, Falla D, et al. 2008. Whiplash, headache and neck pain: research based directions for physical therapies. Edinburgh: Elsevier.
Jull G, Kenardy J, Hendrikz J, et al. 2013. Management of acute whiplash: a randomized controlled trial of multidisciplinary stratified treatments. Pain 154: 1798–1806.
Kamper S, Rebbeck TJ, Maher CG, et al. 2008. Course and prognostic factors of whiplash: a systematic review and meta-analysis. Pain 138: 617–629.
Kasch H, Stengaard-Pedersen K, Arendt-Nielsen L, et al. 2001. Headache, neck pain and neck mobility after acute whiplash injury. Spine 26: 1246–1251.
Kasch H, Qerama E, Bach FW, et al. 2005. Reduced cold pressor pain tolerance in non-recovered whiplash patients: a 1 year prospective study. Eur J Pain 9: 561–569.
Kivioja J, Jensen I, Lindgren U. 2005. Early coping strategies do not influence the prognosis after whiplash injuries. Injury 36: 935–940.
Koelbaek-Johansen M, Graven-Nielsen T, Schou Olesen A, et al. 1999. Muscular hyperalgesia and referred pain in chronic whiplash syndrome. Pain 83: 229–234.
Kongsted A, Bendix T, Qerama E, et al. 2008. Acute stress response and recovery after whiplash injuries. A one year prospective study. Eur J Pain 12: 455–463.
Lamb S, Gates S, Williams MA, et al. 2013. Emergency department treatments and physiotherapy for acute whiplash: a pragmatic, two-step, randomised controlled trial. Lancet 381: 546–556.
Lim E, Sterling M, Stone A, et al. 2011. Central hyperexcitability as measured with nociceptive flexor reflex threshold in chronic musculoskeletal pain: a systematic review. Pain 152: 1811–1820.
Lord S, Barnsley L, Wallis BJ, et al. 1996. Chronic cervical zygapophyseal joint pain after whiplash: a placebo-controlled prevalence study. Spine 21: 1737–1743.
MAIC. 2012. Annual report 2011–2012. Brisbane: MAIC. Online. Available: http://www.maic.qld.gov.au/forms-publications-stats/pdfs/2012-13_MAIC_Annual_Report.pdf.
Maxwell S, Sterling M. 2012. An investigation of the use of a numeric pain rating scale with ice application to the neck to determine cold hyperalgesia. Man Ther 18: 172–174.
McLean S, Clauw DJ, Abelson JL, et al. 2005. The development of persistent pain and psychological morbidity after motor vehicle collision: integrating the potential role of stress response systems into a biopsychosocial model. Psychosom Med 67: 783–790.
McLean S, Diatchenko L, Lee YM, et al. 2011. Catechol O-methyltransferase haplotype predicts immediate musculoskeletal neck pain and psychological symptoms after motor vehicle collision. J Pain 12: 101–107.
Michaleff Z, Maher C, Sterling M, et al. 2014. Comprehensive physiotherapy exercise program or advice alone for chronic whiplash (PROMISE): a pragmatic randomised controlled trial (ACTRN12609000825257). Lancet 384(9938): 133–141. doi: 10.1016/S0140-6736(14)60457-8.
Nederhand M, Hermens HJ, Ijzerman MJ, et al. 2002. Cervical muscle dysfunction in chronic whiplash associated disorder grade 2: the relevance of trauma. Spine 27: 1056–1061.
Ng TS, Pedler A, Vicenzino B, et al. 2014. Less efficacious conditioned pain modulation and sensory hypersensitivity in chronic whiplash-associated disorders in Singapore. Clin J Pain 30(5): 436–442. doi: 10.1097/AJP.0b013e3182a03940.
Passatore M, Roatta S. 2006. Influence of sympathetic nervous system on sensorimotor function: whiplash associated disorders (WAD) as a model. Eur J Appl Physiol 98: 423–449.
Ritchie C, Hendrizk J, Kenardy J, et al. 2013. Derivation of a clinical prediction rule to identify both chronic moderate / severe disability and full recovery following whiplash injury. Pain 154: 2198–2206.
Rivest K, Coté JN, Dumas JP, et al. 2010. Relationships between pain thresholds, catastrophizing and gender in acute whiplash injury. Man Ther 15: 154–159.
Scott D, Jull G, Sterling M. 2005. Widespread sensory hypersensitivity is a feature of chronic whiplash-associated disorder but not chronic idiopathic neck pain. Clin J Pain 21: 175–181.
Smith A, Jull G, Schneider G, et al. 2014. Cervical radiofrequency neurotomy reduces central hyper-excitability and improves neck movement in individuals with chronic whiplash. Pain Med 15: 128–141.
Spearing N, Connelly L. 2011. Is compensation 'bad for health'? A systematic meta-review. Injury 42: 15–24.
Spearing N, Connelly LB, Gargett S, et al. 2012. Does compensation have a negative effect on health after whiplash? Pain 153: 1274–1282.
Spitzer W, Skovron ML, Salmi LR, et al. 1995. Scientific monograph of Quebec Task Force on whiplash associated disorders: redefining 'whiplash' and its management. Spine 20: 1–73.
Sterling M. 2004. A proposed new classification system for whiplash associate disorders – implications for assessment and management. Man Ther 9: 60–70.
Sterling M. 2006. Sensory hypersensitivity and psychological distress following whiplash injury: Is there a relationship? In: Australian Pain Society Annual Scientific Meeting. Melbourne. [Verbal presentation.]
Sterling M, Kenardy J. 2006. The relationship between sensory and sympathetic nervous system changes and acute posttraumatic stress following whiplash injury: a prospective study. J Psychosom Res 60: 387–393.
Sterling M, Pedler A. 2009. A neuropathic pain component is common in acute whiplash and associated with a more complex clinical presentation. Man Ther 14: 173–179.
Sterling M, Jull G, Vicenzino B, et al. 2003a. Sensory hypersensitivity occurs soon after whiplash injury and is associated with poor recovery. Pain 104: 509–517.
Sterling M, Jull G, Vicenzino B, et al. 2003b. Development of motor system dysfunction following whiplash injury. Pain 103: 65–73.
Sterling M, Kenardy J, Jull G, et al. 2003c. The development of psychological changes following whiplash injury. Pain 106: 481–489.
Sterling M, Jull G, Vicenzino B, et al. 2005. Physical and psychological factors predict outcome following whiplash injury. Pain 114: 141–148.
Sterling M, Jull G, Kenardy J. 2006. Physical and psychological predictors of outcome following whiplash injury maintain predictive capacity at long term follow-up. Pain 122: 102–108.
Sterling M, Hodkinson E, Pettiford C, et al. 2008. Psychologic factors are related to some sensory pain thresholds but not nociceptive flexion reflex threshold in chronic whiplash. Clin J Pain. 24: 124–130.
Sterling M, Hendrikz J, Kenardy J. 2010. Developmental trajectories of pain / disability and PTSD symptoms following whiplash injury. Pain 150: 22–28.
Sterling M, Carroll LJ, Kasch H, et al. 2011a. Prognosis after whiplash injury: where to from here? Discussion paper 4. Spine 36: S330–S334.

Sterling M, Hendrikz J, Kenardy J, 2011b. Similar factors predict disability and PTSD trajectories following whiplash injury. Pain 152: 1272–1278.
Sterling M, McLean SA, Sullivan MJ, et al. 2011c. Potential processes involved in the initiation and maintenance of whiplash associated disorders (WAD). Spine 36: S322–S329.
Sterling M, Hendrikz J, Kenardy J, et al. 2012. Assessment and validation of prognostic models for poor functional recovery 12 months after whiplash injury: a multicentre inception cohort study. Pain 153: 1727–1734.
Stewart M, Maher CG, Refshauge KM, et al. 2007. Randomised controlled trial of exercise for chronic whiplash associated disorders. Pain 128: 59–68.
Stone A, Vicenzino B, Lim EC, et al. 2012. Measures of central hyperexcitability in chronic whiplash associated disorder – a systematic review and meta-analysis. Man Ther 18: 111-117.
Sturzenegger M, Radanov B, Stefano GD. 1995. The effect of accident mechanisms and initial findings on the long-term course of whiplash injury. J Neurol 242: 443–449.
Teasell R, McClure JA, Walton D, et al. 2010. A research synthesis of therapeutic interventions for whiplash-associated disorder (WAD): part 2 – interventions for acute WAD. Pain Res Manage 15: 295–304.
Treleaven J, Jull G, Sterling M. 2003. Dizziness and unsteadiness following whiplash injury – characteristic features and relationship with cervical joint position error. J Rehabil 34: 1–8.
Treleaven J, Jull G, Low Choy N. 2005a. Standing balance in persistent whiplash: a comparison between subjects with and without dizziness. J Rehabil Med 37: 224–229.
Treleaven J, Jull G, Low Choy N. 2005b. Smooth pursuit neck torsion test in whiplash associated disorders: relationship to self-reports of neck pain and disability, dizziness and anxiety. J Rehabil Med 37: 219–223.
Van Oosterwijck J, Nijs J, Meeus M, et al. 2013. Evidence for central sensitization in chronic whiplash: a systematic literature review. Eur J Pain 17: 299–312.
Vlaeyen J, Kole-Snijders A, Boeren R, 1995. Fear of movement / reinjury in chronic low back pain patients and its relation to behavioural performance. Pain 62: 363–372.
Walton D, Pretty J, MacDermid JC, et al. 2009. Risk factors for persistent problems following whiplash injury: results of a systematic review and meta-analysis. J Orthop Sports Phys Ther 39: 334–350
Walton D, MacDermid JC, Nielson W, et al. 2011. Pressure pain threshold testing demonstrates predictive ability in people with acute whiplash. J Orthop Sports Phys Ther 41: 658–665.
Walton D, Carroll LJ, Kasch H, et al. 2013a. An overview of systematic reviews on prognostic factors in neck pain: results from the International Collaboration on Neck Pain (ICON) project. Open Orthop J 7: 494–505.
Walton D, MacDermid JC, Giorgianni AA, et al. 2013b. Risk factors for persistent problems following acute whiplash injury: update of a systematic review and meta-analysis. J Orthop Sports Phys Ther 43: 31–43.
Wenzel H, Haug TT, Mykletun A, et al. 2002. A population study of anxiety and depression among persons who report whiplash traumas. J Psychosom Res 53: 831.
Williamson E, Williams M, Gates S, et al. 2008. A systematic review of psychological factors and the development of late whiplash syndrome. Pain 135: 20–30.
Winkelstein BA, Nightingale RW, Richardson WJ, et al. 2000. The cervical facet capsule and its role in whiplash injury. Spine 25: 1238–1246.
Woodhouse A, Vasseljen O. 2008. Altered motor control patterns in whiplash and chronic neck pain. BMC Musculoskelet Dis 9: 90.
Yunus M. 2007. Fibromyalgia and overlapping disorders: the unifying concept of central sensitivity syndromes. Semin Arthritis Rheum 36: 339–356.

11 Chapter

Differential Diagnosis and Treatment of Cervical Myelopathy, Cervical Radiculopathy and Cervical Myeloradiculopathy

Chad Cook, Amy Cook

CHAPTER CONTENTS

Introduction 118
Review of proposed pathology and patho-biomechanics 119
Clinical signs and symptoms 119
  Myelopathy 119
  Radiculopathy 120
  Myeloradiculopathy 120
Current best evidence with regard to diagnosis 120
  Cervical myelopathy 120
  Cervical radiculopathy 122
  Cervical myeloradiculopathy 124
  Imaging 124
  Nerve condition responses 125
Essential aspects of differential diagnosis 126
Current best evidence with regard to prognosis 126
Current best evidence with regard to treatment 127
  Conservative approaches 127
  Surgical approaches 128

Introduction

Cervical spine pain is a common musculoskeletal complaint affecting 66–70% of individuals within their lifetime (Anderson et al 1993), with 54% having experienced symptoms within the previous 6 months (Côté et al 1998). Cervical spine pain can significantly affect physical and social function (Brown et al 2009), with correspondingly high levels of healthcare usage and costs (Brattberg et al 1989) and up to 5% of individuals indicating high disability (Côté et al 1998). Cervical spine pain is more prevalent in individuals who are educated, who have a history of injury or trauma, or who suffer from consistent headaches (Brown et al 2009).

Cervical spine pain can originate from a tumour, injurious event, infection, inflammatory disorder, metabolic condition and / or degeneration (Ahn et al 2007; Binder 2007). The most common cause is degeneration – often termed cervical spondylosis. This is caused by degeneration of tissues such as the cervical disc and cartilaginous end plates, osteophytes along the vertebral body, facets and uncovertebral joints, and ossification or thickening of the ligamentum flavum and posterior longitudinal ligament (Rao & Fehlings 1999; McCormick et al 2003).

Two specific diagnoses associated with degenerative changes in the cervical spine are: (1) cervical myelopathy and (2) cervical radiculopathy. Both conditions involve debilitating neurological symptoms that may progress toward disability if inadequately treated (McCormick et al 2003). In severe cases, radiculopathic and myelopathic changes can occur simultaneously, resulting in myeloradiculopathy. Cervical myeloradiculopathy is a major management challenge and often leads to significant movement disorders (Wong et al 2004).

It has been purported that myelopathy is present in 90% of individuals by the seventh decade of life (Dvorak 1998) and is recognized as the most common form of spinal cord dysfunction in individuals over the age of 55 (Brown et al 2009). Cervical myelopathy most commonly affects males (Montgomery & Brower 1992) and those of Asian descent (Jayakumar et al 1996). It is believed that a large percentage of elderly patients have mild cervical myelopathy that often goes unnoticed, as the signs and symptoms are frequently attributed to a normal ageing process (Brown et al 1991, 2009). A delayed diagnosis of cervical myelopathy is frequent among primary care physicians (Behrbalk et al 2013) and other first-line practitioners.

Cervical radiculopathy is defined as an abnormality of a nerve root, which originates in the cervical spine (Polston 2007). It has a purported prevalence of 3.3 cases per 1000 people (Wainner et al 2003) to 83.2 per 100 000 (Polston 2007), affecting men more frequently than women (Radhakrishnan et al 1994). The condition has a peak annual incidence of 2.1 cases per 1000, and occurs most commonly in the fourth and fifth decades of life (Wainner & Gill 2000). The seventh (60%) and the sixth (25%) cervical nerve roots are the most common regions affected (Malanga 1997).

The natural history of myeloradiculopathy is unclear – the signs and symptoms are inconsistent and the pathophysiological mechanisms are multifactorial in nature. The prevalence of myeloradiculopathy is unknown – although patients with movement disorders such as cerebral palsy, torticollis and Tourette syndrome demonstrate accelerated propensity for spondylosis and myeloradiculopathy (Wong et al 2004). Infectious conditions such as schistosomiasis are the most-investigated disease processes associated with myeloradiculopathy in the literature.

Cervical myelopathy, cervical radiculopathy and cervical myeloradiculopathy may cause significant pain and debilitation and are the focus of this chapter. In particular, we plan to focus on correct diagnosis, prognosis and currently recommended treatment of each condition.

Review of Proposed Pathology and Patho-Biomechanics

Myelopathy, radiculopathy and myeloradiculopathy involve both structural and movement-related abnormalities. Progressive degenerative changes result structurally in disc height losses and reduction of space in the spinal canal and intervertebral foramina. Structural changes to the intervertebral discs, ligaments and capsule lead to viscoelastic losses and movement abnormalities (Pope 2001). In particular, flexion–extension movements may cause a variety of neurological symptoms in severe degenerated conditions (Wilson et al 1991). During extension, the spinal canal shortens and narrows because of infolding of ligaments. The ligamentous infolding causes dorsolateral encroachment in the canal. In addition, the disc may bulge posteriorly in selected situations, further reducing space dorsolaterally. These structural changes may lead to kinetic changes such as decreased movement, compression of dorsolateral nerve roots or nerve root ganglia, compression of the spinal cord and pain (Pope 2001).

Cervical spine myelopathy is hallmarked by the stenotic encroachment of the cervical spinal cord and corresponding neurological changes (Brown et al 2009). This encroachment may lead to structural and vascular changes and originates from sagittal narrowing of the spinal canal. The narrowing may cause compression of the spinal cord and often originates from: (1) osteophytes secondary to degeneration of intervertebral joints, (2) stiffening of connective tissues such as the ligamentum flavum at the dorsal aspect of the spinal canal, which can impinge on the cord by 'buckling' when the spine is extended, (3) degeneration of intervertebral discs together with subsequent bony changes, and (4) other degenerative connective tissue changes (Wong et al 2004). Non-degenerative, structural-based conditions may be associated with syringomyelia, an arachnoid cyst, a tumour or epidural lipomatosis (Durrant & True 2002).

Dynamic movements of the spinal cord are regulated by the spinal column and the anchoring elements of the spinal cord. The primary anchoring elements are the dentate ligaments and the filum terminale (Durrant & True 2002). In normal subjects, length changes of the spinal cord range from 4.5 to 7.5 cm, with flexion increasing tension in the spinal cord and extension decreasing tension (Breig 1978). Spinal cord compression occurs from a number of mechanisms, most notably the friction that is present from degenerative changes during movements of extension and flexion. Ventral osteophytes can prevent movement of the spinal cord upwards and downwards during physiological motions (Bartels et al 2007). Furthermore, thickening of tissues and bony changes, which results in a spondylitic bar, increases the friction placed upon the spinal cord during movements and causes permanent damage (Bartels et al 2007).

Cervical radiculopathy is caused by a cascade of events that leads to nerve root distortion, intraneural oedema, impaired circulation and focal nerve ischaemia, a localized inflammatory response and altered nerve conduction (Truumees & Herkowitz 2000). The localized inflammatory response is stimulated by chemical pain mediators within the disc, which may incite the production of inflammatory cytokines, substance P, bradykinin, tumour necrosis factor-α and prostaglandins (Albert & Murrell 1999; Rhee et al 2007). These chemical pain mediators are not typically present in chronic disc lesions (Durrant & True 2002). Along with the production of chemicals, the membrane surrounding the dorsal root ganglion, which is more permeable allowing a local inflammatory response, may contribute to cervical radiculopathy (Rao & Fehlings 1999).

The most common compressive causes of cervical radiculopathy are disc herniation and degenerative spine components such as osteophytes, facet joint hypertrophy and ligament hypertrophy (Truumees & Herkowitz 2000). Disc herniation occurs when nuclear material from an acute soft disc herniation impinges on a nerve root either posterolaterally or intraforaminally (Rhee et al 2007). The degenerative causes are associated with a loss of disc height and a 'hard disc' bulging with resultant compressive elements such as the ligaments (Albert & Murrell 1999) and osteophytes (Rhee et al 2007). Location-wise, anterior causes (soft or hard disc herniation and osteophytes from the uncinate processes) are the most common cause of radicular symptoms (Rhee et al 2007). Other causes include ischaemia, trauma, neoplastic infiltration, spinal infections, post-radiation, immune-mediated diseases, lipoma and congenital disorders (Truumees & Herkowitz 2000).

Cervical myeloradiculopathy is believed to occur during chronic spondylosis and repetitive compressive damage to the cervical spinal cord and roots, but may also occur acutely upon a flexion / extension injury (Lewis et al 2008). Compression may result from anterior spondylotic spurs, posterior infolding of ligaments, or both (Frank 1993). Changes may involve demyelination, vascular compromise and inflammation of the nerve roots.

Clinical Signs and Symptoms

Myelopathy

Myelopathy is characterized by a variable distribution pattern (Brown et al 2009) and may involve clinical findings in the lower extremities first, with subsequent gait-related changes, weaknesses of the legs and spasticity (Bartels et al 2007; Harrop et al 2007). Gait disturbances are associated with upper motor neuron changes involving dysfunctional corticospinal and spinocerebellar tracts. Later, lower motor neuron findings in the upper extremities may occur, such as loss of strength, atrophy and difficulty in fine finger movements (Cook et al 2007, 2009; Harrop et al 2007).

Additional signs and symptoms of cervical myelopathy manifest as pain in the cervical, upper quarter region or shoulder, widespread numbness, paraesthesia, and sensory and ataxic changes of the lower extremities (Polston 2007). Findings may include tetraspasticity (Dvorak 1998), gait-related clumsiness (Dvorak 1998), spasticity, hyper-reflexia (Crandall & Batzdorf 1966) and the presence of primitive reflexes (Hawkes 2002). Other clinical findings indicative of progressive decline include acquired spastic paraparesis (Hawkes 2002), tetraparesis and paraparesis (Montgomery & Brower 1992). Because the signs and symptoms are often sequential, weakness and stiffness of the legs (Adams & Victor 1999) typically precede pain and the occasional findings of bowel and bladder changes (Thongtrangan et al 2004).

There is a distinct possibility of mixed presentation of signs and symptoms with myelopathy. Reflexes and sensibility changes may actually be depressed at the level of compression (C5–C8), with hyper-reflexia at the levels below the lesion (Brown et al 2009). In addition, uncommon symptoms may be present with myelopathic conditions, including restless legs secondary to loss of descending inhibition of the corticospinal tract, nausea, dizziness and dysphagia, which can occur from compression of vertebral artery (Brown et al 2009).

Radiculopathy

For cervical radiculopathy, neurological symptoms may lead to pain, motor weakness or sensory deficits along the affected nerve root (Rao & Fehlings 1999; Polston 2007; Rhee et al 2007). Depending on the nerve root affected, symptoms may exist concurrently in the neck, shoulder, upper arm and forearm (Polston 2007). Often, pain and sensibility changes are not consistent and may result in a dull ache to a severe burning pain in the neck and arm. Pain is typically noted in the medial border of the scapula and shoulder, which can progress down the ipsilateral arm and hand along the sensory distribution of the involved nerve root (Wolff & Levine 2002). The pain may not be localized, however, because multiple nerve roots can cause similar distribution patterns (Ellenberg et al 1994).

Motor weakness associated with radiculopathy may provide a variety of clinical scenarios and is associated with specific nerve root levels (Polston 2007). Specific nerve root weakness typically presents in the following patterns: scapular weakness with C4; shoulder abduction or forearm flexion weakness with C5; wrist extension / supination with C6; triceps or wrist flexion / pronation with C7; and finger flexors / interossei with C8 (Tsao et al 2003). Another study (Tsao et al 2003) noted that motor weakness, often with fasciculations, is present in 61% to 68% of patients. Advanced cervical radiculopathy cases may present with muscle wasting and fasciculations (Polston 2007). Henderson and colleagues (1983) noted that triceps weakness due to C7 radiculopathy was present in 37% of the 846 subjects, whereas biceps weakness was present in 28%.

Sensibility changes (sensation variations) of the affected nerve roots may help to localize the level of the lesion. C4 nerve root distribution tends to affect the shoulder and upper arm, C5 nerve root distribution the lateral aspect of the arm, C6 nerve root distribution the lateral aspect of the forearm, hand and thumb, C7 nerve root distribution the dorsal lateral forearm and third digit, and C8 nerve root distribution the medial forearm, hand and fourth and fifth digits (Chien et al 2008).

Cervical radiculopathy typically presents with diminished deep tendon reflexes (muscle stretch reflex). Such reflexes are an involuntary response, which offers an objective assessment of neurological impairment (Durrant & True 2002). Loss of deep tendon reflexes is usually said to be the most reliable clinical finding (Marshall & Little 2002) and has been noted in 70% of the cases (Tsao et al 2003). Generally, the decline in reflexes follows a predictable radicular pattern.

Myeloradiculopathy

The signs and symptoms of cervical myeloradiculopathy lead to a complex clinical presentation (Baba et al 1998). In most cases, the presentation of myeloradiculopathy involves both the cardinal signs and the symptoms of the two separate diseases. For example, a common presentation comprises radicular symptoms in the arm (pain and weakness) and myelopathic symptoms in the legs (gait disturbances, loss of position and vibratory sense, and spasticity) (Frank 1993).

The challenges occur when clinical signs and symptoms overlap. In these selected cases, which typically involve highly affected, chronic spondylitic changes, differentiation of the condition is less probable.

Current Best Evidence with Regard to Diagnosis

Cervical myelopathy

Patient history

In most cases, myelopathic changes are slow and progressive (Masdeu et al 1997). Initial symptoms are typically vague and are often mistaken as changes associated with 'old age'. Often, patients will indicate problems after a period of rest or inactivity (Bednarik et al 2004). Gait problems are the first symptoms associated with myelopathy but it is often the motor changes (such as spasticity, weakness and clumsiness of the arms and hands) that warrant the carrying out of work-up (Masdeu et al 1997; Bednarik et al 2004). Twenty to sixty-two per cent of individuals with cervical myelopathy will deteriorate by 3–6 years, with average functional declines of 8% by 1 year and 23% by 4 years (Fehlings et al 2013).

Myelopathic changes occur either after a prolonged bout of spondylitic changes or after trauma in patients with relatively recent degenerative changes. Most patients are older, have experienced range-of-motion (ROM) limitations or pain with selected positions such as end-range rotation and extension, and have routinely had bouts of radiculopathy in the past (Bednarik et al 2004). In fact, the strongest predictor of future myelopathy is a history of radiculopathy (Bednarik et al 2004).

Sensory changes are inconsistent but generally occur later more often than early, and in the upper extremities more than the lower extremities (Masdeu et al 1997). Initial symptoms in milder cases can start with hand clumsiness or numbness, which may be unilateral at first, before gait abnormalities are noted (Polston 2007). Hand clumsiness or numbness involves less sensory loss than motor dysfunction and is, in essence, an apraxia of the distal upper extremities and hands (Good et al 1984). Diminished vibration sense is often seen in the lower extremities (Masdeu et al 1997).

Other symptoms may include decreased appreciation of pain, hot or cold, decreased response to sharp or dull pain, and restless legs (Brown et al 2009). Long-term cases may involve wasting or fasciculation of the biceps (Harrop et al 2007). In very rare cases, bowel and bladder disturbances may occur; presence of urinary retention, dribbling incontinence or fecal incontinence should raise concern of a condition other than myelopathy such as cauda equina syndrome (Masdeu et al 1997).

Outcome measures

There are a number of clinician-scored outcome measures for myelopathy represented in the literature. The Nurick score comprises five definitive explanations of the effects of the condition and is scored from 0 to 5 (0 representing root involvement but no evidence of spinal cord disease, and 5 representing chair-bound or bedridden status). However, it suffers from a lack of responsiveness as each grade reflects substantial jumps in clinical condition (Nurick 1972).

The most-used score appears to be the Japanese Orthopaedic Association (JOA) score, which is effective at measuring changes in patients' conditions (Vitzhum & Dalitz 2007). The JOA is a disease-specific, physician-oriented scale designed to assess the neurological status of a patient that allows surgeons to measure pre- and post-intervention changes. The scale involves a number of constructs including scoring of feeding, upper extremity shoulder and elbow function, lower extremity gait capabilities, sensory involvements, and bowel and bladder control (Dalitz & Vitzhum 2008).

The European Myelopathy Score (EMS) is a disease-specific, physician-oriented scale that involves a number of constructs including gait function, walking dysfunction, climbing stairs, bladder and bowel function, handwriting, eating, dressing, and activities associated with sensory loss and proprioception (Vitzhum & Dalitz 2007). The scale is more sensitive to change than the JOA and the Nurick scores, but is not routinely used in clinical practice.

Physical examination

Observation

Diagnosis of myelopathy is challenging, particularly in the early stages of the condition, as symptoms may present variously as hyper-reflexia (MacFadyen 1984; Polston 2007), clumsiness in gait (Matsuda et al 1991; Bednarik et al 2004), neck stiffness (Montgomery & Brower 1992; Chiles et al 1999), shoulder pain (Lev et al 2001), paraesthesia in one or both arms or hands (Good et al 1984) or radiculopathic signs (Nurick 1972; Montgomery & Brower 1992).

Active and passive movements

Both active and passive neck movements are often limited – specifically rotation, side-flexion and extension. ROM loss in the upper extremity is found inconsistently. Symptoms may or may not be reproduced during movements. In some cases, extension triggers neurological symptoms down the thoracic spine, but this condition typically occurs only in patients with chronic spondylar changes.

Gait symptoms associated with myelopathy are slow and progressive. These may involve difficulty in initiating movements, walking briskly and a tendency to trip (Masdeu et al 1997). Other gait changes include development of paraparesis, described as heaviness of legs, trembling and cramping of thigh and calf muscles, and difficulty in negotiating steps, curbs and getting in and out of vehicles (Masdeu et al 1997).

On some occasions, symptoms may include hyper-reflexia, which in severe cases may involve bilateral clonus and extensor plantar reflexes. Pathological reflexes are generally present only in patients with long-standing, chronic degenerative conditions (Brown et al 2009). Upper extremity reflex changes are less consistent and often depend on the site of structural impairment (Masdeu et al 1997). Higher level cervical involvement can cause hyper-reflexia throughout the upper and lower extremities. Mid or lower levels of cervical involvement may result in hyporeflexia (radicular symptoms) at levels above the site of the injury and hyper-reflexia below these levels.

Clinical tests such as single leg stance, tandem walking and basic coordination exercises will be challenges to patients with myelopathy. Coordination testing such as nose-to-hand tests, braiding, Frenkel's test and arm rolling are often poorly performed in patients with late-stage myelopathy. Patients may overshoot targets, demonstrate poor dexterity during activities and struggle with fine motor tasks.

Confirmation tests

The clinical examination for myelopathy includes the use of Hoffmann's test (Emery et al 1998; Cook et al 2007, 2009), deep tendon reflex testing (Denno & Meadows 1991; Cook et al 2007, 2009), inverted supinator sign (Estanol & Marin 1976), suprapatellar quadriceps reflex testing (de Freitas & Andre 2005), hand withdrawal reflex testing (Denno & Meadows 1991), Babinski sign (Ghosh & Pradhan 1998) and clonus (Young 2000). Nearly all of these tests are specific (as opposed to sensitive) and are useful for ruling in a suspected condition rather than ruling out the condition. Despite the fact that most of these tests are routinely used to screen for myelopathy, the inherent diagnostic accuracy of each test limits its effectiveness for screening.

Hoffmann's test or 'sign' consists of involuntary flexion of a varied combination of the neighbouring fingers and / or thumb, and is commonly used to detect an upper motor neuron dysfunction (Emery et al 1998). The test is performed by stabilizing the middle finger proximal to the distal interphalangeal joint and striking its fingernail with the opposite hand. A number of studies have analysed the sensitivity and specificity of the test, and have demonstrated that it is generally a specific test, having yielded sensitivity values ranging from 25% to 68% (Glaser et al 2001; Houten & Noce 2008; Cook et al 2009) (Fig. 11.1).

The **inverted supinator sign** is a C7 response during a deep tendon reflex assessment of C6 (brachioradialis). The test is performed in the same fashion as a brachioradialis deep tendon reflex test and the response for a pathological finding involves finger flexion and / or elbow extension, as against a

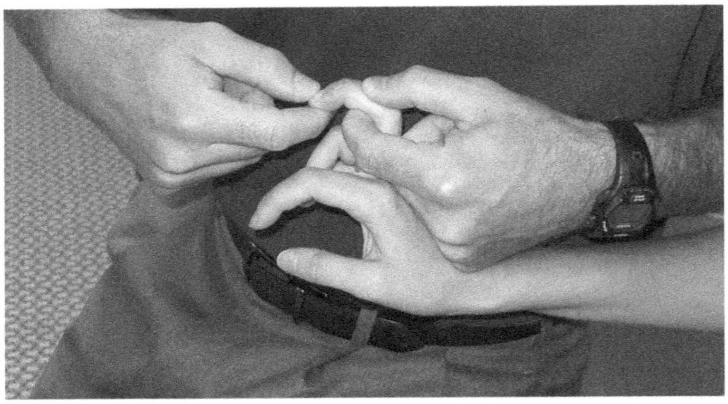

Figure 11.1 **Hoffman's test.**

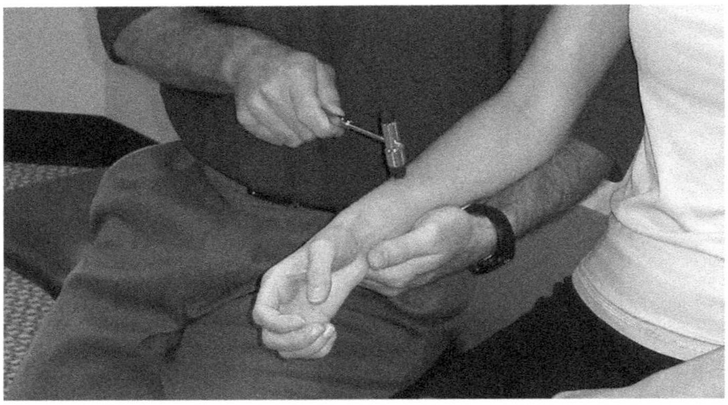

Figure 11.2 **Inverted supinator sign.**

normal response of wrist pronation and / or elbow flexion. To our knowledge, the test has been investigated only once and has demonstrated a sensitivity of 61% and specificity of 78% (Cook et al 2009) (Fig. 11.2).

The **Babinski test** involves the elicitation of an extensor toe sign during stroking of the plantar aspect of the foot. The test is also more specific than sensitive, demonstrating a sensitivity of 33% (Houten & Noce 2008) and of 24% in two more recent studies (Cook et al 2009). Cook et al (2009) found the Babinski sign to have the best diagnostic value of all the confirmation tests, providing a positive likelihood ratio (+LR) of 4.0 (1.1–16.6).

A finding of repetitive beats of three or more after striking the anterior aspect of the patient's foot whilst sitting is associated with a positive finding of clonus. Clonus has been investigated in two studies; however, both of these have demonstrated poor sensitivity (10% in Houten & Noce 2008, and 14% in Cook et al 2009).

A clinical prediction rule consisting of the Hoffmann's test, Babinski's sign, the inverted supinator sign, age >45 years and any notable gait abnormality was associated with a diagnosis of cervical spine myelopathy (Cook et al 2010). If none of the symptoms were present, the post-test likelihood of the condition was less than 9%. If three of the five variables were present, the post-test likelihood of the condition increased to 94%. At present, however, this clinical prediction rule has not been validated independently.

Cervical radiculopathy

Patient history

It is important to determine the individual's main complaint – for example, numbness, weakness, or location of symptoms (Wolff & Levine 2002). If pain is a complaint then a pain drawing is beneficial to establish its pattern and location. A pain drawing allows the clinician to determine whether the pain radiates and, if so, the distribution of the symptoms (Honet & Puri 1976). In addition to identifying the main complaint, it is important to isolate any activities or head movements that trigger the concordant symptoms. One must also check for presence of concomitant symptoms such as gait changes, or bowel, bladder or lower extremity conditions that are suggestive of myelopathy, and address whether there were any similar episodes in the past and whether any treatment was provided for the present and / or past episodes. Identification of the demographic and social history including age, sex, stress, occupation, recreational activities and nicotine usage is suggested (Honet & Puri 1976).

Outcome measures

There are no specific outcome measures for cervical radiculopathy. The Neck Disability Index (NDI) is the most frequently used functional outcome tool for cervical-related disabilities. This outcome assessment tool was created by modifying the Oswestry Disability Index and is extremely reliable. The NDI determines the extent of disability and is designed to measure activity limitations due to neck pain and disability (Pietrobon et al 2002). It has been used regularly in previous studies that have investigated functional status (Smith 1979).

A visual analogue scale (VAS) or a numeric analogue scale is a common scale used to quantify pain and has historically been used as an outcome tool (Downie et al 1978; Langley & Sheppeard 1985). The VAS for pain in the cervical spine does have a test–retest reliability of 0.95 to 0.97 (McCormick et al 2003) and MCID (minimal clinically important difference) of 12±3 mm (Kelly et al 2005). The VAS involves quantification of pain on a numbered line (i.e. rating the level of pain he / she is currently experiencing as 0–100: 0 indicates no pain and 100 indicates the worst pain imaginable). The scale is easy to administer, but lacks any dimensionality other than intensity (Szpalski & Gunzburg 2001).

Physical examination

Observation

Patients with cervical radiculopathy will often hold their head away from the affected side and avoid rotation to that side (Wolff & Levine 2002). In some cases, patients may cradle their affected arm or place it behind or on top of their head to reduce the tension on the nerve root (Davidson et al 1981).

Active and passive movements

All planes of motion of the cervical spine should be assessed with active and passive movements. The active ROM is typically decreased, and specifically rotation to the affected side (Wainner et al 2003) and extension. ROM assessment is typically reliable and is considered a useful clinical measure (Fletcher & Bandy 2008). Responses to look for include any movements associated with the pain / symptoms noted during the history portion of the exam.

Confirmation tests

Neurological testing

Dermatome testing involves examination of motor function, sensibility changes and deep tendon reflex modifications along a nerve root distribution. Cervical nerve roots exit above their correspondingly numbered pedicles (e.g. C6 exits between C5 and C6 vertebrae) with the exception of the C8 nerve root, which exits above T1. With infrequent exceptions, disc herniation or some other space-offending structure at a specific site (e.g. C4–C5) will affect the nerve root from that site (Rhee et al 2007).

For two primary reasons, it is important to note that the absence of radiating symptoms in a dermatomal distribution does not rule out the presence of nerve root compression (Rhee et al 2007). First, the presence of upper trapezius or interscapular pain may be the extent of the symptoms for that patient (Rhee et al 2007); as the condition progresses, symptoms may or may not migrate to the upper arm. Secondly, the clinical tests associated with motor testing, sensibility testing and deep tendon reflex testing have routinely demonstrated very low sensitivity values, which suggests that the clinical findings may be below the threshold of these particular tests (Cook & Hegedus 2008). The most common nerve roots affected are C5, C6, C7, C8 and T1. Specific nerve roots may demonstrate predictable patterns of motor functional losses, sensory changes or reflex changes.

A manual muscle test is performed to identify minimal weakness along a myotome distribution to determine a local nerve root involvement. According to Yoss et al (1958), a manual muscle test offers greater specificity than either reflex or sensory testing, and single-root-level involvement can be diagnosed clinically 75–80% of the time. The manual muscle tests may best be initiated in a gravity-induced position, with testing of the uninvolved limb first in order to compare both sides. The clinician should look for subtle changes and apply the force proximal to the next distal joint (Ellenberg et al 1994; Malanga 1997). The following grading of 0 to 5 is recommended: 0 / 5 no movement; 3 / 5 antigravity; 5 / 5 normal (Honet & Puri 1976).

The grading of deep tendon reflexes (DTR) ranges from 0 (absent) to 4 (clonus, very brisk). Reflex abnormality is found primarily from nerve root involvement of C5 through to C8 (Polston 2007; Chien et al 2008). The DTR is tested with the muscle of the tendon relaxed and the clinician applying a slight stretch to the tendon, followed by tapping the tendon with a reflex hammer. Reflex abnormality of the deltoid, biceps and brachioradialis is noted from C5 and C6 involvement, the triceps from C7, and the finger flexors from C8 (Honet & Puri 1976).

Provocation tests

There are only a few provocation tests that are typically performed when assessing for cervical radiculopathy. **Spurling's sign** combines the motions of cervical lateral bending and compression, which reduces space within the foraminal area (Tsao et al 2003). The test is considered positive if symptoms of radicular pain are either reproduced or worsen. According to Honet et al (1976), Spurling's sign demonstrates high specificity and low sensitivity for cervical radiculopathy (Cook & Hegedus 2008) (Fig. 11.3).

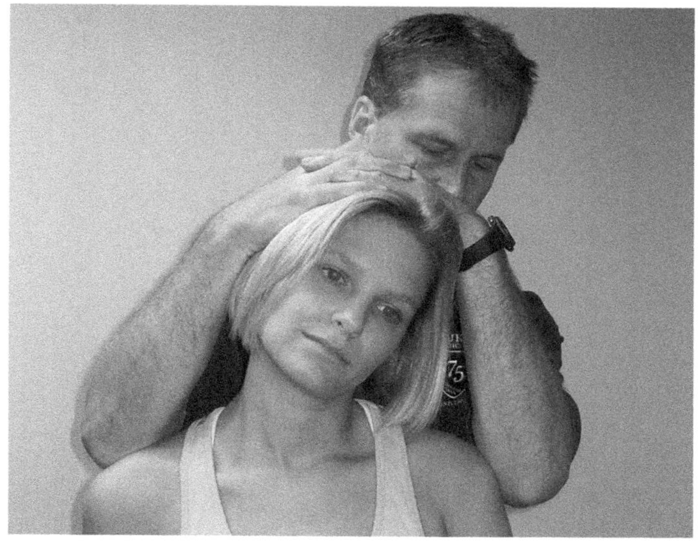

Figure 11.3 Spurling's sign.

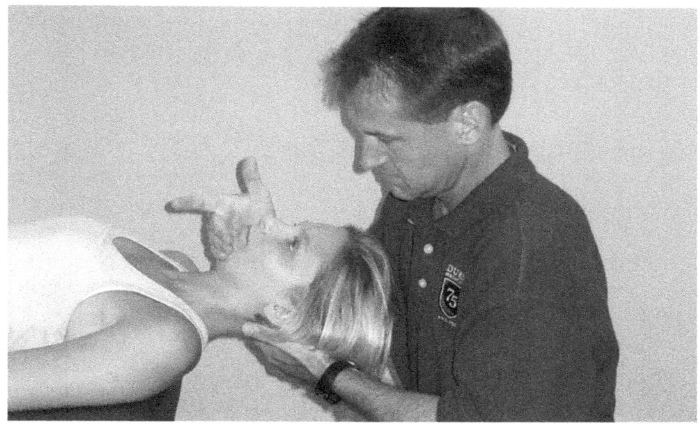

Figure 11.4 Cervical distraction test.

The **cervical distraction test** is another test offered for cervical radiculopathy assessment. The test is performed with the patient supine and the clinician supporting the head with a chin cradle grip. The clinician applies a traction force to the cervical area. If symptoms are reduced with this test, it is considered positive. Viikari Junatura et al (2000) noted a specificity of 100, with a QUADAS score of 11 for ruling in cervical radiculopathy (Fig. 11.4).

Another test to consider is the **upper limb tension sign** (ULTT). According to Cook and Hegedus (2008), this test is excellent as a screening test for ruling out cervical radiculopathy. The test is performed with the patient supine, the forearm supinated, and the wrist and fingers extended. Ulnar deviation is applied. If no symptoms are reproduced the clinician then extends the elbow. If symptoms are still not reproduced then lateral flexion of the cervical spine is performed. Reproduction of concordant, asymmetric symptoms in the distal area denotes a positive test (Fig. 11.5).

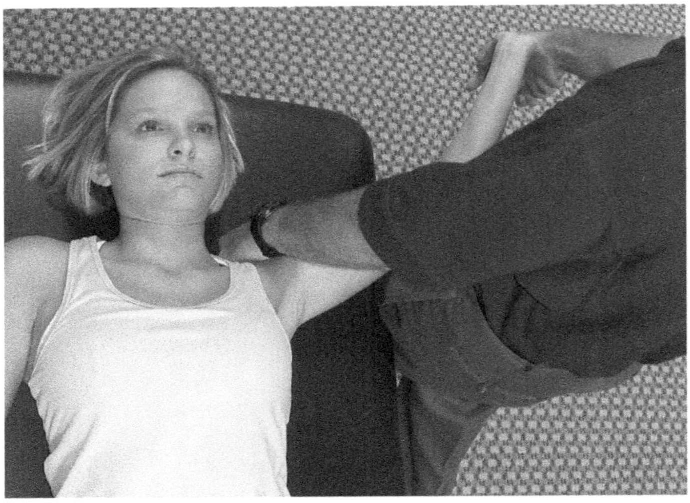

Figure 11.5 Upper limb tension sign.

Wainner et al (2003) developed a clinical prediction rule for ruling in cervical radiculopathy. The combined tests include Spurling's, ROM <60°, the cervical distraction test and ULTT. When all four tests are positive the specificity was 99%, with an LR+ of 30.0 (QUADAS=10).

Cervical myeloradiculopathy

Patient history

The most common reports of symptoms include subtle neck pain, radiculitis and radicular pain in the arms, and trouble with gait or coordination of the lower extremities. Electrophysiological evidence of cervical radiculopathy and radiographic evidence of cervical myelopathy have been shown to predict future disease progression and may warrant surgical intervention (Fehlings et al 2013). In chronic conditions, patients may also indicate difficulty with upper extremity coordination activities. Most of the reported signs and symptoms are analogous to concomitant myelopathy and radiculopathy. Other than infectious conditions, most myeloradiculopathic symptoms are insidious, progressive and have a chronic presentation.

Physical examination

Positive findings may occur with stenotic movements of rotation, side-flexion and extension. Most patients will exhibit problems with gait examination but typically only during higher level gait changes such as single-legged stance, tandem walking and Romberg positions. Coordination losses may be prevalent in the lower and, potentially, upper extremities, with sensation changes most common in the upper extremities.

Outcome measures

There are no exclusive outcome measures for myeloradiculopathy, thus the same tools used for measurement of myelopathy (e.g. Nurick scale, JOA score and EMS) and radiculopathy (NDI and VAS) are used to evaluate changes in patients' conditions.

Confirmation tests

There are no dedicated clinical tests designed to identify myeloradiculopathy. Typically, the same tests used to confirm myelopathy (e.g. Hoffmann's test, inverted supinator sign) and radiculopathy (Spurling's sign, cervical distraction test) are used in the clinical confirmation phase.

Imaging

Plain film radiograph

Plain film radiography is useful in identifying stenosis and the extensiveness of degenerative joint disease (Brown et al 2009). In addition, radiography is used to determine canal stenosis and, at present, 13 mm or less of anterior–posterior (sagittal diameter) width is considered a risk factor in the development of myelopathy (Brown et al 2009). Nevertheless, smaller patients may have decreased diameters and hence this value may not be as useful as a ratio measure (Brown et al 2009). Radiographs are often used to determine the extent of degeneration.

Magnetic resonance imaging and computed tomography scan

Magnetic resonance imaging (MRI) is considered the best imaging method for myelopathy because it expresses the amount of compression placed on the spinal cord (Fukushima et al 1991), and demonstrates relatively high levels of sensitivity (79–95%) and specificity (82–8%) (LR+ 4.39 to 7.92; LR– 0.06 to 0.27) in identifying selected abnormalities such as space-occupying tumours (Fujiwara et al 1989), disc herniation (Yousem et al 1992) and ligamentous ossification (Mizuno et al 2001). The MRI provides the ability to rule out a tumour or syrinx (fluid-filled cavity that develops in the spinal cord) and detailed views of the spinal cord, intervertebral disc, vertebral osteophytes and ligaments – all structures that potentially compress the spinal cord (Gross & Benzel 1999). Furthermore, MRI findings have been shown to correlate with preoperative severity of cervical compressive myelopathy and prognosis after surgery (Ono 1977; Yousem et al 1992). Patients with advanced cord changes often demonstrate poor outcomes after surgery and those with only minor compression tend to demonstrate fair recovery or retardation of progression of symptoms (Yoshimatsu et al 2001).

Changes associated with myelopathy may lead to anterior–posterior width reduction of the spinal cord, cross-sectional evidence of cord compression, or obliteration of the subarachnoid space (Fukushima et al 1991). At present, there are no definitive objective findings on MRI consistently described by radiologists that are reflective of myelopathy, with the exception of myelomalacia, which is identified through changes in signal intensity to the cord. Such changes have been described as the most appropriate 'gold standard' for confirmation of a spinal cord compression myelopathy (Fukushima et al 1991), but are also present only in advanced chronic cases (Fig. 11.6).

MRI findings are not conclusively indicative of cervical myelopathy (Bednarik et al 2004). Cord-related changes and subsequent symptoms from cervical myelopathy overlap with other types of intrinsic myelopathy, such as multiple

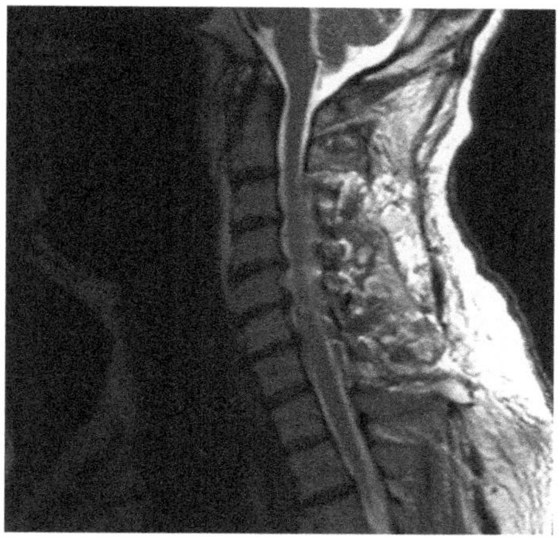

Figure 11.6 MRI changes reflecting cord compression and myelomalacia.

sclerosis, syrinx and amyotrophic lateral sclerosis. Careful screening of the MRI, including the presence of T2-weighted changes, is crucial to show clear, relevant spinal cord compression (Jeffreys 2007). False positives are common because cord compression alone does not directly equate to clinical signs and symptoms (Estanol & Marin 1976). Diagnosis is usually made from a detailed history of progressive patient symptoms, weakness and hyper-reflexia on examination, and clear compression of the spinal cord at an appropriate symptomatic level on the MRI scan, with or without T2 changes. Since T2 MRI changes usually do not abate with surgery (Wada et al 1999), these changes are indicative more of damage than of reversible ischaemia. A dedicated criterion standard such as the singular use of an MRI scan used to determine myelopathy does not exist (Sung & Wang 2001).

The MRI has demonstrated superiority in identification of a herniated nucleus pulposus (Wilmink 2001) and structural changes from spondylosis (Wilmink 2001). It has demonstrated comparable findings with myelography and cervical radiculopathy myelography (Larsson et al 1989), but may exhibit limitations in identifying the extent of root compression (Barlett et al 1996).

It is difficult to differentiate a soft and a hard disc herniation through imaging methods (Rhee et al 2007). Specificity of the MRI for nerve root compression is suspect; however, it identifies abnormal findings in 10% of subjects who were asymptomatic (Boden et al 1990). Sensitivity of an MRI is very good (Birchall et al 2003). Significant compression can occur before changes are seen clinically (Birchall et al 2003).

As a whole, the most compelling findings are associated with complete occlusion of the entrance to the intervertebral foreman by a laterally migrated mass on MRI, followed by narrowing of a foramen by osteophytes (which may cause nerve root swelling). The poorest association includes disc herniation because the nerve root can often move out of the way of the offending intruder (Birchall et al 2003).

Computed tomography (CT) is less commonly used in assessment of the extent of degeneration of the cervical spine. Although it is less costly, faster and more reliable, it does have significant limitations in detection of both cervical radiculopathy and myelopathy. The inherent low-contrast resolution during assessment of soft tissue obviates the need for a CT myelography, which is troublesome when dealing with small disc herniation or limited intrusion into the intervertebral foramina (Maigne & Deligne 1994).

Nerve condition responses

Aside from MRI, a neuromuscular test such as an electromyogram / electroneurogram (EMG / ENG) is often used to differentiate cervical myelopathy from carpal tunnel syndrome, or other peripheral nerve problems. Since cervical myelopathy is an upper motor neuron syndrome, the EMG is expected to display a normal finding unless there are intervening root or peripheral nerve problems. Kang and Fan (1995) reported normal results for EMG in 100% of patients diagnosed with cervical myelopathy. Evoked potentials have demonstrated the greatest assistance with the diagnosis of cervical myelopathy. Motor evoked potentials have a reported 70% sensitivity in the upper extremity muscles and 95% sensitivity in muscles of the lower extremity for the diagnosis of cervical myelopathy (De Mattei et al 1993). From an electrodiagnostic standpoint, the use of sensory evoked potentials (SEP) has demonstrated superior diagnostic ability, as Kang and Fan (1995) reported abnormal SEP in 19 of 20 patients diagnosed with cervical myelopathy.

Tests of nerve condition responses such as EMG and nerve conduction studies (often abbreviated to NCV, V standing for velocity) are occasionally used to differentiate radiculopathy for peripheral entrapment disorders (Rhee et al 2007). Because of limitations in nerve condition testing, the MRI has supplanted nerve condition responses as the tool of choice (Polston 2007). For example, of the cervical spinal nerves, only C4–C8 have limb representation that allows differentiation (Truumees & Herkowitz 2000). In addition, results of the tests may vary considerably depending on the age of the lesion, the segmental level analysed and the diagnostic application of the test (Polston 2007).

EMG is an electrical recording of muscle activity and involves insertion of a fine needle into the tested muscle. In order to diagnose with EMG, the reading must be abnormal for two or more different muscles and peripheral nerves from the same nerve root (Durrant & True 2002). The EMG is considered a useful diagnostic tool for cervical radiculopathy (Durrant & True 2002). Two recordings are taken, one at rest and one during a contraction. A normal response involves only brief EMG activity during needle insertion, then no activity when the muscle is at rest. During contraction, motor unit action potentials that reflect electrical activity within the muscle appear on the recording screen, with corresponding increases as more muscle fibres are solicited.

Abnormal responses exhibit electrical activity at rest, alterations in the pattern of firing activity, and decreases in amplitude and duration of the spikes on the recording screen. The findings may demonstrate contractions of other muscles (compensatory) and poor recruitment in nerve-related disorders such as radiculopathy. Concentric needle EMG testing has demonstrated sensitivities of 50–93% and appears to be the best and most widely accepted method of electrodiagnostic testing (Prahlow & Buschbacher 2003).

An NCV consists of stimulation of the nerve and recording of the evoked potential, either from the muscles or from the nerve (to study the sensory response). NCV assesses the extent of axonal loss of large myelinated nerve fibre (Cook

Table 11.1 Differentiation of referred pain characteristics

Characteristic	Radiculopathy	Myelopathy	Somatic referred pain	Visceral pain
Axial distribution	+	+	+	+
Upper extremity muscle weakness	+	+	–	–
Lower extremity muscle weakness	+	+	–	–
Upper extremity sensory disturbance	+	+	–	–
Lower extremity sensory disturbance	+	+	–	–
Clumsiness	–	+	–	–
Gait disturbance	+ or –	+	–	–
Spurling's sign	+	–	+ or –	–
Sensory deficit	+ or –	+ or –	–	–
Loss of vibratory sense	–	Yes (LE)	–	–
Tendon reflex changes	Diminished + or –	Increased	–	–
Muscle wasting	Unilateral + or –	Bilateral	–	–
Babinski sign	–	+	–	–
Hoffman's sign	–	+	–	–
Muscle tone	Normal	Increased	Normal	Normal
Limb tension test	+	+ or –	–	–

LE = lateral epicondylitis.

et al 2009). The test involves measurement of the time delay between stimulation and response at two stimulation sites with a calculation of the distance between the sites (Smith 1979).

The two late responses most commonly analysed include the H-reflex and the F-wave. The H-reflex (Hoffmann's reflex) assesses an afferent 1a sensory nerve and an efferent alpha motor nerve. The F-wave analyses motor nerves only and is often normal in patients who have suspected radiculopathy. Because of a propensity for poor sensitivity, NCV tests should never be used in isolation (Rhee et al 2007).

Selective diagnostic nerve root block (SNRB) is a test to identify whether a specific nerve root is causing the patient's pain. The test is considered both sensitive and specific for radiculopathy (Malanga 1997).

Essential Aspects of Differential Diagnosis

Two definitive elements of differential diagnosis are necessary. First, one must rule out the presence of red flags such as fever, chills, history of cancer, intravenous drug use and other sinister conditions. Secondly, infectious conditions such as schistosomiasis will generally have a rapid onset (which is uncharacteristic of spondylotic causes) and may progress more rapidly towards debilitation. Cervical myelopathy requires differentiation from a number of other conditions including amyotrophic lateral sclerosis, multiple sclerosis, spinal cord tumours and cerebrovascular disease (Brown et al 2009). In some cases, viral diseases can cause spinal cord degeneration. The most difficult differential diagnosis is when both radicular and myelopathic changes are present (Table 11.1).

Current Best Evidence with Regard to Prognosis

Prognosis for myelopathy and myeloradiculopathy without surgical intervention is mixed. It is generally assumed that the condition, which is a progressive degenerative process, will result in continuing worse outcomes over time; however, a number of subjects with mild cases of cord compression who do not receive prophylactic surgery do not decline and maintain their current level of function (Matsumoto et al 2000). Two recent clinical prediction rules have suggested that shorter duration of symptoms, non-smoking, absence of psychological comorbidity, younger age, a Nurick grade of 2 or less, and gait abnormality at baseline are all associated with positive outcomes at 1 year (Pumberger et al 2013; Tetreault et al 2013).

There is limited research on the prognosis of cervical radiculopathy. Most authors indicate that about two-thirds of cervical radiculopathy conditions resolve with conservative care (Lees & Turner 1963). Some authors note that, due to the benign course of cervical radiculopathy, in which up to 75% recovery naturally, conservative care is the recommended initial treatment (Polston 2007). A long-term follow-up study of 51 subjects with cervical radiculopathy who were treated conservatively showed that 45% had one episode of pain and 30% had mild symptoms (Lees & Turner 1963).

Current Best Evidence with Regard to Treatment

Conservative approaches

Myelopathy

Conservative management including treatment of pain, of gait impairments, limb mobility, and reduction of risk of falls may be appropriate for a number of patients because myelopathy may exhibit only minor impairment with no progression (Matsumoto et al 2000). Initially, immobilization of the cervical spine with a collar is used to stabilize the spine in neutral or slight flexion. Although some evidence exists for the effective treatment of early myelopathic changes via conservative physical therapy interventions (i.e. traction and thoracic manipulation) (Browder et al 2004; Murphy et al 2006), conclusive evidence for the effectiveness of surgical intervention for myelopathy suggests that surgery should be pursued when symptoms are progressive and destructive (Fujiwara et al 1989). Conservative care has been shown to be beneficial in 30–50% of patients (McCormick et al 2003); however, there is a paucity of evidence to support most conservative approaches for myelopathy and future research is definitely needed (Rhee et al 2013).

Treatment after surgical intervention may include strengthening of weakened areas, gait training and proprioceptive exercises. At present, there is no literature that either supports or refutes the use of conservative rehabilitation after surgical management of myelopathy.

Radiculopathy

A stepwise approach addressing predominant signs and symptoms of cervical radiculopathy is often used. Typically, during the acute stage of cervical radiculopathy the treatment should aim at reducing inflammation and pain, at educating the patient and at avoiding increasing any neurological deficits. Treatment for inflammation and pain may include ice, heat, non-steroidal anti-inflammatory drugs (NSAIDs), analgesics, rest, possible immobilization and traction.

A derivation clinical prediction rule has been developed that outlined patients with neck pain who were most likely to benefit from a concomitant programme of cervical traction and exercise (Raney et al 2009). The study identified: (1) a positive abduction test, (2) peripheralization of symptoms, (3) a positive upper limb tension test, (4) a positive neck distraction test and (5) age >55 years. Although the authors reported an increase in post-test probability of improvement to 94.8% when four of these five variables were present, the findings should be interpreted with caution as they demonstrated very wide confidence intervals (2.5–227.9).

There is no evidence that immobilization via a cervical collar / brace will reduce the duration or severity of cervical radiculopathy (Naylor 1979). If immobilization is employed, the time-frame should be limited to 1–2 weeks owing to the negative effects from long-term immobilization. Limited evidence is available to support traction as an early intervention. A recent randomized clinical trial by Young et al (2009) reported no significant differences between two patient groups classified with cervical radiculopathy when evaluating the effectiveness of mechanical cervical traction. Jensen and Harms-Ringdahl (2007) found that, when comparing acute and chronic neck pain interventions, ROM had the strongest evidence in terms of reducing pain in the acute phase, and combined physical agents for acute and chronic pain reduction.

Patient education should address the cause of the pain, and activity modification to improve or reduce further progression of symptoms advancement. Patients showed reduction in pain and increased satisfaction when instructed on an individual home exercise programme compared with written information (Jensen & Harms-Ringdahl 2007). Patients should have a home programme of stretching and strengthening once the radiculopathy symptoms have resolved.

During subacute management, physical therapy is typically prescribed. The literature to date has not verified the long-term benefits of modalities such as heat, ice, massage, ultrasound and electrical stimulation, although these have been shown to have some benefit in uncontrolled studies (Rhee et al 2007). Once the patient's pain and inflammation are reduced, a progression by physical therapy to address ROM, flexibility and strength should be initiated. Strengthening exercises include isometrics of the cervical muscles and isotonics for stabilization of the scapular region, which includes the trapezius, rhomboids, serratus anterior and latissimus dorsi muscles (Malanga 1997). Progression to resistive exercises is appropriate so long as the patient's symptoms are not aggravated. The literature also encourages continued aerobic exercise throughout the course of rehabilitation to reduce overall deconditioning (Malanga 1997; Tsao et al 2003). Nerve-gliding exercises have been shown to be more effective than a control group for short-term improvements and should be considered as a conservative care option (Nee et al 2012). Also, absence of neuropathic pain, older age and lower deficits in median nerve neurodynamic test range of motion predict successful outcomes (Nee et al 2013).

Steroid injection is a common intervention in patients with cervical radiculopathy for reduction of inflammation although there have been only a few randomized clinical trials to support the efficacy of the approach (Polston 2007). These injections are often offered when a patient is not responding to a course of conservative treatment including medications, rest and physical therapy. The studies that have been performed show a positive outcome of up to 60% for long-term relief (Malanga 1997).

Overall, there is low-quality evidence suggesting quicker return to outcomes for surgery compared with a conservative approach; however, it is worth noting that the studies suggesting such benefit have a high risk of bias (van Middelkoop et al 2013).

Myeloradiculopathy

At present, conservative treatment for myeloradiculopathy includes palliative care, gait training by physical therapists, and ROM and strengthening exercises to retard the progression of the degenerative changes. However, there is a dearth of evidence to support conservative care for this condition as most patients do receive surgical intervention.

Surgical approaches

Surgical approaches are aimed at removing the offending compressive disorders from the nerve and decompressing the cord to allow the cord to move without friction and further damage (Frank 1993). In order to decide which surgical approach to use, surgeons must consider the lesion location (Witwer & Trost 2007), the number of levels involved (Witwer & Trost 2007), the specific pathology (Witwer & Trost 2007), the patient's age, neurological function and cervical alignment (Heller et al 2001) and radiographic imaging (Witwer & Trost 2007) as well as an individual surgeon's familiarity with the technique (Heller et al 2001).

Surgical treatment has been shown to retard the effects of cervical myelopathy when it is caught quickly (Fujiwara et al 1989). A number of factors can influence the outcome of surgery, most notably: chronicity of symptoms (Matsumoto et al 2000), whether radiculopathy is also present with myelopathy (Shamji et al 2009), and the person's age and integrity of their spine (Fujiwara et al 1989). In addition, the type of surgical approach is often selected based on the symptoms at hand. All surgeries involve some element of decompression of the spinal canal and may involve an anterior or posterior approach (McCormick et al 2003). At present, a series of trials have failed to prove the superiority of one over the other, although short-term complications are higher in patients who receive posterior approaches (Cybulski & D'Angelo 1988).

It is important to note that, on some occasions, continued neurological deterioration can occur after surgery secondary to ischaemia (Smith-Hammond et al 2004). This condition is a diagnosis of exclusion (once haematoma and dislocation are ruled out) and has a gradual but damaging progression.

Anterior approaches

Anterior surgery is performed for unilateral or bilateral radiculopathy or myelopathy when there is a single dominant level, or in the face of kyphosis. Anterior fusion is considerably more common, but is associated with increases in operative time and use of instrumentation (Iwasaki et al 2007).

Generally, anterior decompression and fusion is performed when one or two levels of cervical myelopathy are present (Cybulski & D'Angelo 1988). The approach generally involves an anterior osteophytectomy and removal of the vertebral bodies. One significant benefit of this approach is that further formation of anterior and posterior bony spurs should be prevented, spurs present may actually regress and, as the segment is distracted during the surgery, the buckling of the ligamentum flavum is improved (Masaki et al 2007).

The procedure involves a transverse (one or two levels) or vertical (multiple levels) anterior approach following the anterior border of the sternocleidomastoid muscle. The discs are removed and replaced, typically with a bone intradisc transplant. In most cases, anterior plating is provided to reduce the risk of non-union. The approach is considered useful when addressing the vascular elements associated with myelopathy and it may result in less scar formation than that seen with a posterior approach (Masaki et al 2007).

The success rate for anterior decompression and fusion is very high (90%) (Masaki et al 2007) and complications are generally low (Cybulski & D'Angelo 1988). Many have promoted the use of anterior fusion, indicating that it results in fewer complications, vascular damage and less osteophyte growth than either laminectomy or laminoplasty (Masaki et al 2007). Furthermore, an anterior approach may be preferred over a posterior approach such as laminoplasty when ossification of the posterior longitudinal ligament is prevalent (Glaser et al 2001). However, physician preference and skill-set probably dictate the selection of the surgical method to a greater extent than do patient presentation and published outcomes.

Posterior approaches

Posterior surgery is preferred in cases of deformity, in multisegmental and dorsal pathology (Witwer & Trost 2007) and in severe myelopathy as it more completely decompresses the entire relevant cervical spine, but is not preferred when there is a single dominant level or in kyphosis (Iwasaki et al 2007). When multiple levels are involved, partial removal of two or more vertebral bodies, plus removal of the posterior longitudinal ligament and any remaining spurs, may be necessary. Anterior approaches are not warranted when radicular symptoms are predominant.

There are two primary posterior approaches to myelopathy: (1) laminectomy with fusion and (2) laminoplasty. Posterior laminectomy and fusion is indicated when cervical stenosis causes lower extremity and / or upper extremity loss of function. Complications have included nerve damage, lack of fusion, high levels of blood loss during surgery, insufficient decompression, and infection (Epstein 2003). A laminoplasty is indicated in cases of cervical stenosis, which has originated from posterior longitudinal ligament ossification, buckling of the ligamentum flavum or structural changes within the spinal canal. The most common complications reported have included loss of ROM, inadequate decompression, and loss of sagittal alignment (Epstein 2002). The surgical approach involves decompression of the spinal cord posteriorly by enlarging the spinal canal but retaining the laminae. A laminoplasty is not considered superior to an anterior or posterior approach because it decompresses less space.

A laminoplasty involves one of two methods, the most common being an open-door laminoplasty. A cervical open-door laminoplasty expands the diameter of the spinal canal, decompressing the nerves and spinal cord. This surgery is typically performed in about 2 h. During a cervical laminoplasty, an incision is performed in the back of the neck. The posterior portion of the bony spinal canal, or lamina, will be elevated. A portion of the thickened ligament will also be removed. The spinal canal diameter will be widened, decompressing the spinal cord and nerves. The lamina will then be held in the open position using titanium miniplates.

A laminectomy and fusion approach generally involves posterior unilateral or bilateral removal of the lamina and a partial facetectomy. Candidates are patients who have adequate preservation of the cervical lordosis (minimum of 10°) (Epstein 2002). Often, the decompression represents two segments above and below and is much more extensive than an anterior decompression. The procedure typically involves a posterior midline incision and dissection of the paracervical muscles from the spinous processes between C2 and T1 (Heller et al 2001). The laminectomy requires removal of either moderate or large amounts of the facets, furthering the likelihood of instability after surgery unless fusion is employed concurrently.

To our knowledge, there is only one study (Kaminsky et al 2004) that has retrospectively analysed outcomes for patients with myelopathy and radiculopathy, and one study (Herkowitz 1988) that retrospectively compared anterior cervical fusion, posterior fusion and laminectomy, and laminoplasty. A third study (Nakano et al 1988) has analysed outcomes for patients with myeloradiculopathy. However, no studies to date have prospectively randomly assigned comparable patients with myelopathy so as to compare outcomes after laminoplasty or laminectomy and fusion.

References

Adams R, Victor M. 1999. Diseases of the spinal cord, peripheral nerve and muscle. In: Adam RD, Victor M (eds) Principles of neurology, 5th edn. New York: McGraw-Hill, pp 1100–1101.

Ahn NU, Ahn UM, Ipsen B, et al. 2007. Mechanical neck pain and cervicogenic headache. Neurosurgery 60 (Suppl 1): S21–S27.

Albert TJ, Murrell SE. 1999. Surgical management of cervical radiculopathy. J Am Acad Orthop Surgeons 7: 368–376.

Anderson HI, Ejlertsson G, Leden I, et al. 1993. Chronic pain in a geographically defined population: studies of differences in age, gender, social class and pain localisation. Clin J Pain 9: 174–182.

Baba H, Maezawa Y, Uchida K, et al. 1998. Cervical myeloradiculopathy with entrapment neuropathy: a study based on the double crush. Spinal Cord 36: 399–404.

Barlett RJ, Hill CA, Devlin R, et al. 1996. Two-dimensional MRI at 1.5 and 0.5 T versus CT myelography in the diagnosis of cervical radiculopathy. Neuroradiology 38: 142–147.

Bartels RH, Verbeek ALM, Grotenhuis JA. 2007. Design of Lamifuse: a randomized, multi-centre controlled trial comparing laminectomy without or with dorsal fusion for cervical myeloradiculopathy. BMC Musculoskel Dis 8: 111.

Bednarik J, Kadanak Z, Dusek L, et al. 2004. Presymptomatic spondylotic cervical cord compression. Spine 29: 2260–2269.

Behrbalk E, Salame K, Regev G, et al. 2013. Delayed diagnosis of cervical spondylotic myelopathy by primary care physicians. Neurosurg Focus 35: E1.

Binder AI. 2007. Cervical spondylosis and neck pain. BMJ 334: 527–531.

Birchall D, Connelly D, Walker L, et al. 2003. Evaluation of magnetic resonance myelography in the investigation of cervical spondylotic radiculopathy. Br J Radiol 76: 525–531.

Boden SD, McCowin PR, Davis DO, et al. 1990. Abnormal magnetic-resonance scans of the cervical spine in asymptomatic subjects: a prospective investigation. J Bone Joint Surg 72: 1178–1184.

Brattberg G, Thorslund M, Wikman A. 1989. The prevalence of pain in a general population: the results of a postal survey in a county of Sweden. Pain 37: 215–222.

Breig A. 1978. Adverse mechanical tension in the central nervous system: an analysis of cause and effect, relief by functional neurosurgery. Stockholm: John Wiley.

Browder DA, Erhard RE, Piva SR. 2004. Intermittent cervical traction and thoracic manipulation for management of mild cervical compressive myelopathy attributed to cervical herniated disc: a case series. J Orthop Sports Phys Ther 34: 701–712.

Brown PJ, Marino RJ, Herbison GJ, et al. 1991. The 72-hour examination as a predictor of recovery in motor complete quadriplegia. Arch Phys Med Rehabil 72: 546–548.

Brown S, Guthmann R, Hitchcock K, et al. 2009. Clinical inquiries: which treatments are effective for cervical radiculopathy? J Fam Pract 58: 97–99.

Chien A, Eliav E, Sterling M. 2008. Whiplash (grade II) and cervical radiculopathy share a similar sensory presentation: an investigation using quantitative sensory testing. Clin J Pain 24: 595–603.

Chiles BW 3rd, Leonard MA Choudhri HF, et al. 1999. Cervical spondylotic myelopathy: patterns of neurological deficit and recovery after anterior cervical decompression. Neurosurgery 44:762–769.

Cook C, Hegedus E. 2008. Orthopedic physical examination tests: an evidence based approach. Upper Saddle River, NJ: Prentice Hall.

Cook CE, Hegedus E, Pietrobon R, et al. 2007. A pragmatic neurological screen for patients with suspected cord compressive myelopathy. Phys Ther 87: 1233–1242.

Cook C, Roman M, Stewart K, et al. 2009. Reliability and diagnostic accuracy of clinical special tests for myelopathy in patients seen for cervical dysfunction. J Orthop Sports Phys Ther 39: 172–178.

Cook C, Brown C, Isaacs R, et al. 2010. Clustered clinical findings for diagnosis of cervical spine myelopathy. J Man Manip Ther 18:175–180.

Côté P, Cassidy L, Carroll L. 1998. The Saskatchewan Health and Back Pain Survey: the prevalence of neck pain and related disability in Saskatchewan adults. Spine 23: 1689–1698.

Crandall PH, Batzdorf U. 1966. Cervical spondylotic myelopathy. J Neurosurg 25: 57–66.

Cybulski GR, D'Angelo CM. 1988. Neurological deterioration after laminectomy for spondylotic cervical myeloradiculopathy: the putative role of spinal cord ischaemia. J Neurol Neurosurg Psychiatry 51: 717–718.

Dalitz K, Vitzthum HE. 2008. Evaluation of five scoring systems for cervical spondylogenic myelopathy. Spine J. [Epub ahead of print.]

Davidson R, Dunn E, Metzmaker J. 1981. The shoulder abduction test in the diagnosis of radicular pain in cervical extradural compression monoradiculopathies. Spine 6: 441–445.

De Freitas GR, Andre C. 2005. Absence of the Babinski sign in brain death: a prospective study of 144 cases. J Neurol 252: 106–107.

De Mattei M, Paschero B, Sciarretta A, et al. 1993. Usefulness of motor evoked potentials in compressive myelopathy. Electromyogr Clin Neurophysiol 33: 205–216.

Denno JJ, Meadows GR. 1991. Early diagnosis of cervical spondylotic myelopathy: a useful clinical sign. Spine 16: 1353–1355.

Downie WW, Leatham PA, Rhind VM, et al. 1978. Studies with pain rating scales. Ann Rheum Dis 37: 378–381.

Durrant DH, True JM. 2002. Myleopathy, radiculopathy, and peripheral entrapment syndromes. London: CRC.

Dvorak J. 1998. Epidemiology, physical examination, and neurodiagnostics. Spine 23: 2663–2673.

Ellenberg MR, Honet JC, Treanor WJ. 1994. Cervical radiculopathy. Arch Phys Med Rehabil 75: 342–352.

Emery SE, Bohlman HH, Bolesta MJ. 1998. Anterior cervical decompression and arthrodesis for the treatment of cervical spondylotic myelopathy: two to seventeen-year follow-up. J Bone Joint Surg 80A: 941–951.

Epstein N. 2002. Posterior approaches in the management of cervical spondylosis and ossification of the posterior longitudinal ligament. Surg Neurol 58: 194–208.

Epstein N. 2003. Laminectomy for cervical myelopathy. Spinal Cord 41: 317–327.

Estanol BV, Marin OS. 1976. Mechanism of the inverted supinator reflex: a clinical and neurophysiological study. J Neurol Neurosurg Psychiatry 39: 905–908.

Fehlings MG, Wilson JR, Yoon SR, et al. 2013. Symptomatic progression of cervical myelopathy and the role of nonsurgical management: a consensus statement. Spine 38: S19–S20.

Fletcher JP, Bandy WD. 2008. Intrarater reliability of CROM measurement of cervical spine active range of motion in persons with and without neck pain. J Orthop Sports Phys Ther 38: 640–645.

Frank E. 1993. Approaches to myeloradiculopathy. Western J Med 158: 71–72.

Fujiwara K, Yonenobu K, Ebara S, et al. 1989. The prognosis of surgery for cervical compression myelopathy – an analysis of the factors involved. J Bone Joint Surg (Br) 71: 393–398.

Fukushima T, Ikata T, Taoka Y, et al. 1991. Magnetic resonance imaging study on spinal cord plasticity in patients with cervical compression myelopathy. Spine 16: S534–S538.

Ghosh D, Pradhan S. 1998. 'Extensor toe sign' by various methods in spastic children with cerebral palsy. J Child Neurol 13: 216–220.

Glaser JA, Cure JK, Bailey KL, et al. 2001. Cervical spinal cord compression and the Hoffmann sign. Iowa Orthop J 21:49–52.

Good DC, Couch JR, Wacaser L. 1984. 'Numb, clumsy hands' and high cervical spondylosis. Surg Neurol 22: 285–291.

Gross J, Benzel E. 1999. In: Camins MD (ed) Techniques in neurosurgery. Philadelphia: Lippincott Williams & Wilkins, pp 162–176.

Harrop JS, Hanna A, Silva MT, et al. 2007. Neurological manifestations of cervical spondylosis: an overview of signs, symptoms, and pathophysiology. Neurosurgery 60: S14–S20.

Hawkes C. 2002. Smart handles and red flags in neurological diagnosis. Hosp Med 63: 732–742.

Heller JG, Edwards C, Murakami H, et al. 2001. Laminoplasty versus laminectomy and fusion for multilevel cervical myelopathy. Spine 26: 1330–1336.

Henderson CM, Hennessy RG, Shuey HM Jr, et al. 1983. Posterior–lateral foraminotomy as an exclusive operative technique for cervical radiculopathy: a review of 846 consecutively operated cases. Neurosurgery 13: 504–512.
Herkowitz HN. 1988. A comparison of anterior cervical fusion, cervical laminectomy, and cervical laminoplasty for the surgical management of multiple level spondylotic radiculopathy. Spine 13: 774–780.
Honet JC, Puri K. 1976. Cervical radiculitis: treatment and results in 82 patients. Arch Phys Med Rehabil 57: 12–16.
Houten JK, Noce LA. 2008. Clinical signs of cervical myelopathy and the Hoffmann sign. J Neurosurg Spine 9: 237–242.
Iwasaki M, Okuda S, Miyauchi A, et al. 2007. Surgical strategy for cervical myelopathy due to ossification of the posterior longitudinal ligament. Part 2: advantages of anterior decompression and fusion over laminoplasty. Spine 32: 654–660.
Jayakumar PN, Kolluri VR, Vasudev MK, et al. 1996. Ossification of the posterior longitudinal ligament of the cervical spine in Asian Indians: a multiracial comparison. Clin Neurol Neurosurg 98: 142–148.
Jeffreys E. 2007. Disorders of the cervical spine. London: Butterworth.
Jensen I, Harms-Ringdahl K. 2007. Strategies for prevention and management of musculoskeletal conditions: neck pain. Best Pract Res Clin Rheumatol 21: 93–108.
Kaminsky SB, Clark CR, Traynelis VC. 2004. Operative treatment of cervical spondylotic myelopathy and radiculopathy: a comparison of laminectomy and laminoplasty at five year average follow up. Iowa Orthop J 24: 95–105.
Kang DX, Fan DS. 1995. The electrophysiological study of differential diagnosis between amyotrophic lateral sclerosis and cervical spondylotic myelopathy. Electromyogr Clin Neurophysiol 35: 231–238.
Kelly KG, Cook T, Backonja MM. 2005. Pain ratings at the thresholds are necessary for interpretation of quantitative sensory testing. Muscle Nerve 32: 179–184.
Langley GB, Sheppeard H. 1985. The visual analogue scale: its use in pain measurement. Rheumatol Int 5: 145–148.
Larsson EM, Holtås S, Cronqvist S, et al. 1989. Comparison of myelography, CT myelography and magnetic resonance imaging in cervical spondylosis and disk herniation: pre- and postoperative findings. Acta Radiol 30: 233–239.
Lees F, Turner JW. 1963. Natural history and prognosis of cervical spondylosis. BMJ 2: 1607–1610.
Lev N, Maimon S, Rappaport ZH, et al. 2001 Spinal dural arteriovenous fistulae: a diagnostic challenge. Israel Med Assoc J 3: 492–496.
Lewis PB, Rue JP, Byrne R, et al. 2008. Cervical syrinx as a cause of shoulder pain in 2 athletes. Am J Sports Med 36: 169–172.
MacFadyen DJ. 1984. Posterior column dysfunction in cervical spondylotic myelopathy. Can J Neurol Sci 11: 365–370.
Maigne JY, Deligne L. 1994. Computed tomographic follow-up study of 21 cases of nonoperatively treated cervical intervertebral soft disc herniation. Spine 19: 189–191.
Malanga GA. 1997. The diagnosis and treatment of cervical radiculopathy. Med Sci Sports Exerc 29: S236–S245.
Marshall GL, Little JW. 2002. Deep tendon reflexes: a study of quantitative methods. J Spinal Cord Med 25: 94–99.
Masaki T, Yamazaki M, Okawa A, et al. 2007. An analysis of factors causing poor surgical outcome in patients with cervical myelopathy due to ossification of the posterior longitudinal ligament: anterior decompression with spinal fusion versus laminoplasty. J Spinal Dis Tech 20: 7–13.
Masdeu JC, Sudarsky L, Wolfson L. 1997. Gait disorders of aging: falls and therapeutic strategies. Philadelphia: Lippincott-Raven.
Matsuda Y, Miyazaki K, Tada K, et al. 1991. Increased MR signal intensity due to cervical myelopathy: analysis of 29 surgical cases. J Neurosurg 74: 887–892.
Matsumoto M, Toyama Y, Ishikawa M, et al. 2000. Increased signal intensity of the spinal cord on magnetic resonance images in cervical compressive myelopathy: does it predict the outcome of conservative treatment? Spine 25: 677–682.
McCormick WE, Steinmetz MP, Benzel EC. 2003. Cervical spondylotic myelopathy: make the difficult diagnosis, then refer for surgery. Cleve Clin J Med 70: 899–904.
Mizuno J, Nakagawa H, Hashizume Y. 2001. Analysis of hypertrophy of the posterior longitudinal ligament of the cervical spine, on the basis of clinical and experimental studies. Neurosurgery 49: 1091–1098.
Montgomery DM, Brower RS. 1992. Cervical spondylotic myelopathy: clinical syndrome and natural history. Orthop Clin North Am 23: 487–493.
Murphy DR, Hurwitz EL, Gregory AA. 2006. Manipulation in the presence of cervical spinal cord compression: a case series. J Manipul Physiol Ther 29: 236–244.
Nakano N, Nakano T, Nakano K. 1988. Comparison of the results of laminectomy and open-door laminoplasty for cervical spondylotic myeloradiculopathy and ossification of the posterior longitudinal ligament. Spine 13: 792–794.
Naylor A. 1979. Factors in the development of the spinal stenosis syndrome. J Bone Joint Surg (Br) 61B: 306–309.
Nee RJ, Vicenzino B, Jull GA, et al. 2012. Neural tissue management provides immediate clinically relevant benefits without harmful effects for patients with nerve-related neck and arm pain: a randomized trial. J Physiother 58: 23–31.
Nee RJ, Vicenzino B, Jull GA, et al. 2013. Baseline characteristics of patients with nerve-related neck and arm pain predict the likely response to neural tissue management. J Orthop Sports Phys Ther 43: 379–391.
Nurick S. 1972. The natural history and the results of surgical treatment of the spinal cord disorder associated with cervical spondylosis. Brain 95(1):101–108.
Ono K. 1977. Cervical myelopathy secondary to multiple spondylotic protrusions: a clinicopathologic study. Spine 2: 125.
Pietrobon R, Coeytaux RR, Carey TS, et al. 2002. Standard scales for measurement of functional outcome for cervical pain or dysfunction: a systematic review. Spine 7: 515–522.
Polston DW. 2007. Cervical radiculopathy. Neurol Clin 25: 373–385.
Pope MH. 2001. Cervical spine biomechanics. In: Szpalski M, Gunzburg R (eds) The degenerative cervical spine. Philadelphia: Lippincott Williams & Wilkins, pp 143–149.
Prahlow ND, Buschbacher RM. 2003. An introduction to electromyography: an invited review. J Long Term Eff Med Implants 13: 289–307.
Pumberger M, Froemel D, Aichmair A, et al. 2013. Clinical predictors of surgical outcome in cervical spondylotic myelopathy: an analysis of 248 patients. Bone Joint J 95B: 966–971.
Radhakrishnan K, Litchy WJ, O'Fallon WM, et al. 1994. Epidemiology of cervical radiculopathy: a population-based study from Rochester, Minnesota, 1976 through 1990. Brain 117: 325–335.
Raney NH, Petersen EJ, Smith T, et al. 2009. Development of a clinical prediction rule to identify patients with neck pain likely to benefit from cervical traction and exercise. Eur J Spine 18: 382–391.
Rao S, Fehlings MG. 1999. The optimal radiologic method of assessing spinal cord compromise and cord compression in patients with cervical spinal cord injury: Part 1: an evidence based analysis of the published literature. Spine 24: 598–604.
Rhee JM, Yoon T, Riew KD. 2007. Cervical radiculopathy. J Am Acad Orthop Surg 15: 486–494.
Rhee JM, Shamji M, Erwin W, et al. 2013. Nonoperative management of cervical myelopathy: a systematic review. Spine 38: S55–S67.
Shamji MF, Cook C, Pietrobon R, et al. 2009. Impact of surgical approach on complication and resource utilization of cervical spine fusion: a nationwide perspective to the surgical treatment of diffuse cervical spondylosis. Spine J 9: 31–38.
Smith MS. 1979. Babinski sign – abduction also counts. JAMA 242: 1849–1850.
Smith-Hammond CA, New KC, Pietrobon R, et al. 2004. Prospective analysis of incidence and risk factors of dysphagia in spine surgery patients: comparison of anterior cervical, posterior cervical, and lumbar procedures. Spine 29: 1441–1446.
Sung RD, Wang JC. 2001. Correlation between a positive Hoffmann's reflex and cervical pathology in asymptomatic individuals. Spine 26: 67–70.
Szpalski M, Gunzburg R. 2001. The degenerative cervical spine. Philadelphia: Lippincott Williams & Wilkins.
Tetreault LA, Kopjar B, Vaccaro A, et al. 2013. A clinical prediction model to determine outcomes in patients with cervical spondylotic myelopathy undergoing surgical treatment: data from the prospective, multi-center AOSpine North America Study. J Bone Joint Surg (Am) 95: 1659–1666.
Thongtrangan I, Le H, Park J, et al. 2004. Cauda equina syndrome in patients with low lumbar fractures. Neurosurg Focus 16: E6.
Truumees E, Herkowitz HN. 2000. Cervical spondylotic myelopathy and radiculopathy. Instr Course Lect 49: 339–360.
Tsao BE, Levin KH, Bodner RA. 2003. Comparison of surgical and electrodiagnostic findings in single root lumbosacral radiculopathies. Muscle Nerve 27: 60–64.
van Middelkoop M, Rubinstein SM, Ostelo R, et al. 2013. Surgery versus conservative care for neck pain: a systematic review. Eur Spine J 22: 87–95.

Viikari Junatura E, Takala E, Riihimaki H, et al. 2000. Predictive validity of signs and symptoms in the neck and shoulders. J Clin Epidemiol 53: 800–808.
Vitzhum HE, Dalitz K. 2007. Analysis of five specific scores for cervical spondylogenic myelopathy. Eur Spine J 16: 2096–2103.
Wada E, Yonenobu K, Suzuki S, et al. 1999. Can intramedullary signal change on magnetic resonance imaging predict surgical outcome in cervical spondylotic myelopathy? Spine 24: 455–461.
Wainner RS, Fritz JM, Irrgang J, et al. 2003. Reliability and diagnostic accuracy of the clinical examination and patient self-report measures for cervical radiculopathy. Spine 28: 52–62.
Wainner RS, Gill H. 2000. Diagnosis and nonoperative management of cervical radiculopathy. J Orthop Sports Phys Ther 30: 728–744.
Wilmink JT. 2001. Cervical imaging: dynamic aspects and clinical significance. In: Szpalski M, Gunzburg R (eds) The degenerative cervical spine. Philadelphia: Lippincott Williams & Wilkins.
Wilson DW, Pezzuti RT, Place JN. 1991. Magnetic resonance imaging in the preoperative evaluation of cervical radiculopathy. Neurosurgery 28: 175–179.
Witwer BP, Trost GR. 2007. Cervical spondylosis: ventral or dorsal surgery. Neurosurgery 60: S130–S136.
Wolff MW, Levine LA. 2002. Cervical radiculopathies: conservative approaches to management. Phys Med Rehabil Clin North Am 13: 589–608.
Wong TM, Leung HB, Wong WC. 2004. Correlation between magnetic resonance imaging and radiographic measurement of cervical spine in cervical myelopathic patients. J Orthop Surg 12: 239–242.
Yoshimatsu H, Nagata K, Goto H, et al. 2001. Conservative treatment for cervical spondylotic myelopathy: prediction of treatment effects by multivariate analysis. Spine J 1: 269–273.
Yoss RE, Corbin KB, MacCarty CS, et al. 1958. Significance of symptoms and signs in localization of involved root in cervical disk protrusion. Neurology 7: 673–685.
Young IA, Michener LA, Cleland JA, et al. 2009. Manual therapy, exercise, and traction for patients with cervical radiculopathy: a randomized clinical trial. Phys Ther 89: 632–642.
Young WF. 2000. Cervical spondylotic myelopathy: a common cause of spinal cord dysfunction in older persons. Am Family Phys 62: 1064–1070.
Yousem DM, Atlas SW, Hackney DB, et al. 1992. Cervical spine disc herniation: comparison of CT and 3DFT gradient echo MR scans. J Comp Assist Tomogr 16: 345–351.

12 Chapter

Thoracic Outlet Syndrome

Susan W. Stralka

CHAPTER CONTENTS

Overview and history of thoracic outlet syndrome 132
Pathoanatomical causes of thoracic outlet syndrome 132
Functional causes of thoracic outlet syndrome 133
Entrapment sites 133
Aetiology of thoracic outlet syndrome 134
Clinical symptoms of thoracic outlet syndrome 134
Neurological symptoms 135
Arterial symptoms 135
Venous symptoms 135
Sympathetic-mediated pain in thoracic outlet syndrome 136
Diagnosing thoracic outlet syndrome 136
Differential diagnosis 136
Provocative test – used in diagnosis of thoracic outlet syndrome 136
Imaging assessment of thoracic outlet syndrome 138
Clinical treatment and management of thoracic outlet syndrome 138
Therapy evaluation of thoracic outlet syndrome 138
Breathing patterns 138
Muscle imbalance 138
Joint stiffness 139
Neurogenic pain 139
Intervention for thoracic outlet syndrome 139
Conclusion 140

Overview and History of Thoracic Outlet Syndrome

Thoracic outlet syndrome (TOS) is a broad term used to describe upper extremity symptoms. These symptoms are related to compression or tension of the brachial plexus, the subclavian artery and subclavian vein in an area located above the first rib and behind the clavicle. Often, one patient may be seen by numerous specialists before this syndrome is identified. The anterior scalene muscle, the middle scalene muscle and the first rib border the thoracic outlet. Pathological or dysfunction related to these structures as well as the clavicle bone, pectoralis minor, omohyoid, subclavius, scalene minimus, cervical rib or transverse process of C7 have been associated with TOS (Mackinnon et al 1996). These neurovascular structures in their course from the interscalene triangle to the axilla are covered with a fascial sheath that is part of the deep cervical fascia, which can become problematic (Atasoy 2004). Fibrous bands, both congenital and acquired, also restrict movements of the clavicle and first rib. The term 'TOS' does not specify the compressing agent and does not identify the structure being compressed. Therefore this syndrome should be differentiated by using the terms arterial TOS (ATOS), venous TOS (VTOS) or neurogenic TOS (NTOS).

Peet first used the term 'thoracic outlet syndrome' in 1956 and indicated that compression of neurovascular structures occurs in the interscalene triangle causing cervical–brachial pain, numbness and other disorders of the upper extremity; he used this term to group them under one name representing a single common element of neurovascular structures (Samarasam et al 2004). It was not until 1958 that Robb proposed the term 'thoracic outlet compression syndrome'. The clinical signs are variable owing to the variety of tissue that can be involved, as well as the compression or entrapment area (Fig. 12.1). Today TOS is classified according to the three areas: the brachial plexus (NTOS), which comprises 90% or more of cases, the subclavian vein (VTOS), which occurs in 6–7%, and the subclavian artery (ATOS), which occurs in 3–4% (Sanders et al 2008).

Compression of the vascular system is easier to identify and presents more urgently in arterial or venous thrombosis than do symptoms in NTOS (Fugate et al 2009). The main controversy in patients with the last syndrome (NTOS) relates to diagnosis. Neurological-type complaints such as paraesthesia, numbness and pain must be based on interpretation of the history, symptoms or clinical examination. These symptoms make the NTOS somewhat of an enigma as some healthcare professionals tend to overdiagnose it whereas others underdiagnose it, with or without correlating the clinical signs and symptoms.

Pathoanatomical Causes of Thoracic Outlet Syndrome

The thoracic outlet region includes three major areas in which compression can occur: the interscalene space or triangle, the costoclavicular space and the subpectoralis minor space. Other causes are congenital bony structures, fibromuscular anomalies, postural deviations and muscle imbalances. It has been reported that subjects who have congenital bony or

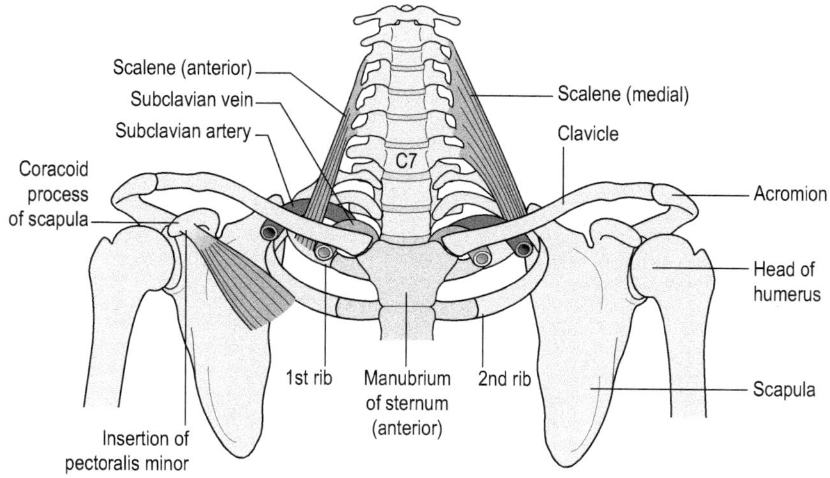

Figure 12.1 Anatomy of the thoracic outlet area.

fibromuscular variations in the thoracic outlet region and experience some type of trauma are at risk of developing TOS. Trauma can result in muscle spasm, inflammation and fibrosis, which further narrow the spaces and results in compression of the neurovascular structure (Atasoy 2004).

The incidence of a cervical rib is less than 1% and may be bilateral. The cervical rib size varies from a bony exostosis to a full-grown cervical rib with ligamentous cartilaginous or bony attachment to the first rib. The female: male ratio is 2:1 (Atasoy 2004). A cervical rib or other rib anomalies cause the brachial plexus to be pulled against the fascial bands and C8–T1 symptoms can develop. A cervical rib, along with forward shoulders and poor posture, can cause pressure on the plexus and the vessels. Following a fracture of the first rib, excess callous formation can occur creating a narrow space, and leading to pressure on the brachial plexus and subclavian vessels.

Functional causes of thoracic outlet syndrome

Poor posture, abnormal breathing patterns, cervical or thoracic dysfunctions, muscle imbalances and shoulder pathologies are commonly seen in TOS (medifocus.com 2009). Abnormal posture in which the head and shoulders are held in a forward position along with arm elevation greater than 90° may cause neurovascular consequences. Over time, shortening of various neck musculatures may occur, which in turn causes posterior shoulder girdle weakness. The longus and longissimus cervicis, upper and middle rhomboids and lower trapezius become weakened. To compensate for the forward orientation of the glenoid fossa of the humerus, the serratus anterior muscle becomes shortened by abduction of the scapula. This scenario causes lengthening of the lower and middle trapezius in supporting the scapula, causing a mechanical disadvantage and early fatigue. These alterations result in the upper trapezius, rhomboids major and minor muscles, along with the levator scapulae, having to function as accessory muscles to elevate the shoulder and arm.

The entire cycle continues to cause weakness in some muscles and shortening of other muscles. Other functional causes, such as abduction over 110°, put tension on the median nerve and cause the ancillary artery to be compressed in the bicipital groove. In the axilla, compression can be caused by a fibrous extension of the latissimus dorsi and pectoralis major muscles as they insert in the bicipital groove. With arm abduction or external rotation, the neurovascular bundle is compressed under the arch, producing symptoms. There are histopathological changes that occur to a nerve undergoing chronic compression, which takes place in TOS. A thorough history, comprehensive physical examination and specific provocation test can identify the structure causing compromise as well as to help to determine muscle weakness and tightness.

Entrapment sites

Interscalene space triangle

The neurovascular bundle that includes the brachial plexus trunks and subclavian vessels runs from the base of the neck towards the axilla and the arm. The first narrowing area is the most proximal and is named the interscalene triangle. This triangle is bordered by the anterior scalene muscle anteriorly, the middle scalene muscle posteriorly, and inferiorly along with the base by the medial surface of the first rib (Atasoy 2004) (Fig. 12.2).

The scalene minimus muscle, which is found in only 30–50% of TOS cases, is located between the subclavian artery and the T1 root of the brachial plexus, which can be a source of compression. The anterior and middle scalene muscles are respiratory muscles, which elevate the first rib as well as slightly flex and rotate the neck. The insertion of these muscles in the first rib overlaps and causes a V formation. This overlapping creates a narrow space, which elevates the position of the subclavian artery and the brachial plexus. It has been noted that in some cases the middle scalene muscle inserts along the full length of the first rib, creating a narrow space through which the neurovascular structures must pass. When there is overlapping of the scalene muscle, there is also a prominent transverse process of the C7 process and the cervical rib. This has often been described as a U or sling formation by these muscles, which may cause elevation and pressure from the structures below. At the proximal portion of the triangle, the scalene muscles may overlap, which again causes

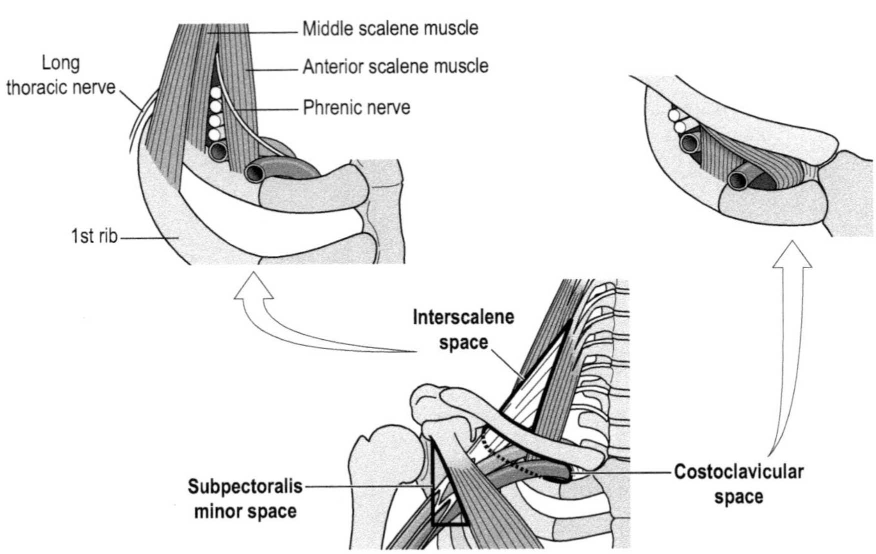

Figure 12.2 Three potential spaces in the thoracic outlet area that can be responsible for TOS.

a decrease in the opening and hence pressure from the brachial plexus above. It has been noted that, at times, a thick fibrous coverage of the plexus extending from the scalene sheath can cause adhesions and pressure on the plexus. The scalene muscles can scar or hypertrophy with trauma or repetitive motion that further contributes to compression. Some researchers have found atrophy of type II muscle fibres, predominance of type I fibres and a 25% increase in connective tissue in the scalene muscles (Sanders 1990) following injury.

Costoclavicular space

The costoclavicular space is a triangular area bordered anteriorly by the middle third of the clavicle, posteromedially by the first rib, and posterolaterally by the upper border of the scapula (Talu 2005). The subclavian artery, vein and brachial plexus all pass through the costoclavicular space (see Fig. 12.2). Compression of the brachial plexus and the subclavian artery and vein can occur as the result of congenital abnormalities, trauma to the first rib or clavicle, and structural changes in the subclavian muscle or the costocoracoid ligament.

Compression can occur if the clavicle or first rib is fractured followed by a haematoma occurring at the fracture site resulting in excessive scar tissue and callus build-up. As mentioned earlier, persons with forward shoulders, which represents poor posture or a disabling illness, may develop narrowing of the costoclavicular space, which has been shown to lead to TOS symptoms. With shoulder abduction, the scapula and coracoid move downwards, which causes traction on the subclavius muscle and costocoracoid ligament, adding additional pressure on the neurovascular structures. The clavicle, during shoulder abduction, moves backwards and upwards 30–35° at the sternoclavicular joint, which may add to the narrowing to the costoclavicular space.

Subpectoralis minor space

The subpectoralis minor space is located just below the coracoid process and under the pectoralis minor muscle insertion to this process (see Fig. 12.2). The pectoralis minor runs from the third to the fifth ribs over the thorax and ends at the coracoid process. This muscle is completely covered by the pectoralis major muscle. With shortening, the pectoralis minor can lead to a narrowing in the subpectoralis minor space, increasing pressure on the blood vessels and brachial plexus. The tight pectoralis minor muscle may also compress the neurovascular structures during hyperabduction. Wright termed this syndrome **hyperabduction syndrome**, which closes down the costoclavicular space due to the up-and-down motion of the clavicle (Beyer & Wright 1951).

Aetiology of Thoracic Outlet Syndrome

TOS is 3–4 times as frequent in women as in men between the ages of 20 and 50 years (Brismée et al 2004). It is speculated that females have less-developed muscles, a greater tendency for drooping shoulders owing to additional breast tissue, a narrowed thoracic outlet and an anatomical lower sternum – all changing the angle between scalene muscles. This may be one reason why females are more prone to developing this syndrome (Hursh & Thanki 1985); another could be an increase in hormones that cause laxity, as a result of which there is superior subluxation of the first rib (Brismee et al 2004) (Table 12.1). Common symptoms collected from 17 reports are listed in Table 12.2 (Sanders & Haug 1991).

Clinical Symptoms of Thoracic Outlet Syndrome

The term 'vascular TOS' is non-specific and it does not imply neurogenic, arterial or venous compression; nor does it address which structure is involved. Historically, symptoms and physical findings are more specific (Sanders et al 2008); patients typically complain of pain in the subscapular, scapular, cervical and cervical thoracic regions and of occipital headaches. Paraesthesia and numbness may be present in the

Table 12.1 Conditions causing nerve trauma

Aetiology	%
Neck trauma	86
Rear-end motor vehicle accident	32
Side- or front-end motor vehicle accident	24
Work injury, including repetitive strain injuries	22
Other neck trauma	8
Cervical or anomalous first rib	2
Unknown or spontaneous	12

Table 12.2 Symptoms from nerve irritation

Symptoms	%
Neck pain	92
Shoulder pain	70
Arm pain	80
Paraesthesia	95
All five fingers	46
Fingers 1–3	30
Fingers 4–5	14
No paraesthesia	10
(Modified from Sanders & Haug 1991.)	

entire hand region or parts of it. Often the symptoms are exacerbated when the person uses the arms in an elevated position and there is a heavy, tired, aching sensation along with numbness or paraesthesia.

Common clinical presentations of TOS include:

- numbness / tingling that often occurs in the ring and small fingers but can encompass the entire hand
- paraesthesiae occurring at night and / or during daily activities
- vague pain in the uninvolved extremity, which can occur in hand, elbow, shoulder and / or cervical spine
- subjective complaints of hand / arm weakness, especially with arms raised overhead
- subjective complaints of swelling in the absence of true swelling
- the common symptoms collected from the 17 reports listed in Table 12.2.

Neurological symptoms

TOS symptoms may develop spontaneously or following injury in the neck and / or shoulder region. A list of conditions causing nerve trauma is given in Table 12.1. Basic concepts of TOS are a mechanical predisposition (Brantigan & Roos 2004); symptoms are primarily caused by neurological structural anomalies. Trauma may precipitate the neurological type of TOS in certain susceptible individuals. The upper plexus includes symptoms involving the C5, C6 and C7, whereas the lower plexus principally involves the C8–T1 levels.

When the upper plexus is involved, there is pain in the side of the neck and this pain may radiate to the ear and face. Headaches are not uncommon when the upper plexus is involved. Some patients state that on the affected side there is a 'stuffy ear'. Often the pain radiates from the ear posteriorly to the rhomboids and anteriorly over the clavicle and pectoralis regions. The pain may move laterally to the trapezius and deltoid muscles and down the C5–C6 radial nerve area. Lower plexus patients have symptoms that present in the anterior or posterior shoulder region and radiate down the ulnar side of the forearm into the hand, the ring and small fingers, as well as muscle tenderness with trigger points that can be located in the supraclavicular and infraclavicular areas. Headaches may be disabling and can increase with arm activity. At times, the pain with lower plexus involvement mimics the pain associated with cardiac angina.

Injury or repetitive stresses causing chronic muscle spasm may precipitate the syndrome. A common problem is hyperextension–flexion or whiplash injury of the neck. The TOS symptom may show up immediately, or may be delayed for weeks or months. Cervical and shoulder sprain symptoms usually occur immediately after the whiplash with persisting symptoms of neck and shoulder pain and stiffness before being diagnosed as TOS (Brantigan & Roos 2004). As the whiplash symptoms gradually improve over time, the post-traumatic TOS involving the brachial plexus worsens.

Arterial symptoms

Symptoms of ATOS usually develop spontaneously and are unrelated to trauma or work. These patients often have true claudication of the arm, particularly when the arm is elevated. These arterial symptoms occur from compression of the subclavian artery in the area of the first rib. Arterial symptoms differ from the whole-arm numbness and heaviness that persists when the arm is elevated in patients with neurological TOS, as well as presenting with very little shoulder or neck symptoms. In patients with arterial symptoms, a cervical rib or an enlarged transverse process of C7 may be causing the problem.

Physical findings are those of arterial occlusion: loss of pulses at rest, perhaps colour changes and ischaemic finger tips as well as coldness, paraesthesia and fatigue. Arterial symptoms include digital and hand ischaemic symptoms (coldness, pallor, paraesthesia and fatigue of the arm). In the supraclavicular area, there is sometimes a tender lump, bony prominence or even pulsation of the subclavian artery. Arterial TOS accounts for less than 5% of TOS and typically results from long-term intermittent vascular compression. A cervical X-ray is used as a screening test to rule out ATOS (Brantigan & Roos 2004).

Venous symptoms

The VTOS comprises only 2–3% of all TOS patients. Venous symptoms may be preceded by excessive activity using the upper extremity. The precipitating factor that leads to thrombosis is typically excessive arm activity such as throwing a baseball, swimming, weightlifting or working with arms elevated. Swelling, oedema, cyanosis and arm discomfort, which is aggravated with exercise, along with distended superficial veins, shoulder and chest wall, are common venous symptoms.

It is not uncommon to have a subclavian vein thrombosis at the first-rib level. When this occurs, there is a sudden onset of dusky cyanosis, oedema and extreme limb discomfort. It is important to diagnose this immediately and surgical decompression is necessary so that the symptoms do not become chronic. Physicians who diagnose only the vascular forms of TOS are misdiagnosing the vast majority of patients who have non-vascular TOS (Brantigan & Roos 2004).

Sympathetic-mediated Pain in Thoracic Outlet Syndrome

Some of the painful symptoms in individuals with NTOS may be due to overlapping signs and symptoms of complex regional pain syndrome (CRPS) (Kaymak & Ozcakar 2004). In NTOS, the coldness and colour changes may not be caused by ischaemia due to obstruction of the subclavian vessels, but due to an overactive sympathetic nervous system (SNS). Allodynia, hyperalgesia, prolonged periods of red or blue hand, persistent oedema, excessive warmth and sweating changes are often present.

Sympathetic-mediated pain may be related to a direct injury to the sympathetic axons in the cords or trunks of the brachial plexus as well as an activation of the somatosympathetic reflex in which a somatic root injury will activate the sympathetic system over several ascending and descending dermatomes (Schwartzman 1987; Casey et al 2003). Anatomically, the SNS fibres run on the circumference of the nerve root of C8, T1 and lower trunk of the brachial plexus. When the nerves are compressed the sympathetic fibres are activated, producing Raynaud's phenomenon. This may explain how coldness and colour changes are frequently seen with both NTOS and ATOS.

Often, clinicians use the term 'compressor' or 'releaser' to categorize symptoms. The term **compressor** is used to evaluate patients who complain of symptoms when performing overhead activities. These patients have no paraesthesia at night unless the arm is overhead or their occupation requires overhead work for long periods. This compression occurs when the arm is raised overhead, which then causes the brachial plexus to turn over the first rib then under the clavicle at the costoclavicular space. When the patient lowers the arm, the compression on the blood supply to the nerve is off and the symptoms decrease. The Roos test is often positive when a patient has what is commonly called compressor TOS.

The term **releaser** is used to identify patients who experience symptoms primarily at night, who work in more sedentary jobs, or who may have poor posture along with large or heavy upper extremities. The term **release phenomenon** means the brachial plexus is being pulled down, then venous pooling occurs around the nerve, which inhibits blood flow to the peripheral nerve. Gravity has an effect when sitting and standing, which places tension on the nerve. When the patient lies down, the tension is gradually released and the blood flow returns to the nerves. As reported by Liu (personal communication), it takes 4–6 hours after the removal of compression for the blood flow to return to the nerve. This may explain why a patient aches at the same time every night with paraesthesia or pain. Lundborg (1970) believes this occurrence at night is due to the axons firing and so patients experience paraesthesia.

Women report the release phenomenon more often than men owing to the weight of the breasts pulling on their bra straps and / or kyphotic posture. The bra straps are capable of creating compression of the brachial plexus, while the kyphotic posture, in which there is an increase of the shoulder girdle, causes increased tension of the brachial plexus and closes down the thoracic outlet. Brismée et al (2004) found that women were found to report symptoms associated with the release phenomenon about twice as often as men.

Diagnosing Thoracic Outlet Syndrome

The diagnosis of TOS is essentially based on history and clinical examination. In order to diagnose accurately, the clinical presentation must be evaluated as either neurogenic or vascular. Neurogenic presentation is linked to compression of the brachial plexus and vascular to compression of the subclavian vessels. TOS manifestations are varied and there is no single definitive test. Common symptoms experienced with TOS include paraesthesia, numbness, pain and burning. Advanced symptoms include muscle weakness, especially in the ulnar nerve distribution.

Diagnosis is based on a total clinical picture that comprises a careful meticulous history, review of medical records and clinical examination. For NTOS, the examination also includes tenderness over the scalene muscles, trapezius muscle and anterior chest wall, a positive Tinel's sign over the brachial plexus in the neck, reduced sensation to very light touch in the fingers and a positive response to several provocative manoeuvres that put stress on the plexus to elicit symptoms. A list of these manoeuvres and incidence of positive responses is seen in the symptoms in Table 12.2.

Differential diagnosis

To have a precise diagnosis, it must be made by history, physical examination, provocative tests and, if needed, ultrasound, radiological evaluation and / or electrodiagnostic evaluation (Brantigan & Roos 2004). There are multiple diagnoses to consider in the differential diagnosis of TOS. Consideration must be given to musculoskeletal pathology that could mimic a TOS presentation. Cervical radiculopathy as well as ulnar neuropathy may present with similar symptoms as TOS, including hypothenar and / or intrinsic wasting (Box 12.1).

Provocative test – used in diagnosis of thoracic outlet syndrome

The physical examination as well as the other tests must be done so as to avoid exacerbating symptoms. Clinicians rely on clinical tests for alteration of radial pulse. A few of these tests are listed below (for all tests, the patient is in a seated position and the examiner palpates the radial pulse):

Box 12.1 Differential diagnosis of thoracic outlet syndrome

- Cervical disc disease
- Cervical facet disease, spondylosis
- Malignancies (Pancoast tumour, local tumours, e.g. nerve sheath tumours, spinal cord tumours)
- Peripheral nerve entrapments (ulnar and/or median nerve entrapment)
- Brachial plexitis
- Shoulder pathology
- Muscular spasms, fibromyalgia
- Neurological disorders (multiple sclerosis)
- Chest pain, angina
- Vasculitis
- Vasospastic disorder (Raynaud disease)
- Neuropathic syndromes of upper extremity (CRPS I, II)
- Thoracic 4 (T4) syndrome
- Sympathetic-mediated pain
- Dull pain, discomfort, aching with tightness in mid-thoracic area

- **Adson test:** The patient is asked to rotate the head and elevate the chin towards the affected side. If the radial pulse on that side is absent or decreased then the test is positive, showing that the vascular component of the neurovascular bundle is compressed by the scalene anterior muscle or cervical rib. This test has shown a sensitivity of 79% and specificity of 76% (Gillard et al 2001).
- **Wright's test:** The patient's arm is hyperabducted. If there is a decrease or absence of a pulse on one side then the test is positive, showing that the axillary artery is compressed by the pectoralis minor muscle or coracoid process due to stretching of the neurovascular bundle. Gillard et al (2001) found a sensitivity of 70% and specificity of 53% for pulse abolition.

Patients with intermittent symptoms that are associated with specific movements or positions of the upper quadrant, which increases or decreases the compression and tension of neural structures, will need to utilize these tests below:

- **Roos test:** The patient has arms at 90° abduction and the therapist puts downwards pressure on the scapula as the patient opens and closes the fingers. If the TOS symptoms are reproduced within 90 seconds, the test is positive.
- **Cyriax release test:** The patient can be sitting or standing with arms supported or resting on a pillow with forearms at neutral for a period of at least 3 minutes – as symptoms such as paraesthesia and numbness may not occur instantly. This position passively elevates the shoulder girdle bilaterally with the patient's trunk positioned posteriorly to assure shoulder girdle end range. A positive test is when a release phenomenon occurs, including reproduction of symptoms. One theory suggests that paraesthesia is the most common symptom for those individuals with a release phenomenon followed by numbness and occasionally pain. According to Cyriax (1978), paraesthesia and numbness appear when a nerve trunk or cord is first compressed, followed by a return of normal sensation. After pressure is released from the plexus, these symptoms reoccur latently. This outcome is different from the phenomenon associated with nerve root compression, which produces persistent symptoms until the root pressure is released (Cyriax 1978; Brismée et al 2004). Brismée et al (2004) showed that a 1-minute modified Cyriax release test is the optimal time limit to maximize the specificity of the test (specificity of 97%).
- **Costoclavicular test:** This test may be used for both neurological and vascular compromise. The patient brings his shoulders posteriorly and hyperflexes his chin. A decrease in symptoms means that the test is positive and that the neurogenic component of the neurovascular bundle is compressed. This test has shown a specificity ranging from 53% to 100% depending on the assessment of vascular changes or pain respectively (Ryan & Jensen 1995; Nord et al 2008).
- **Elevated first-rib test:** For right first-rib elevation, patients will demonstrate a significant loss of right lateral flexion, with hard end-fill in the position of left rotation indicating an elevated hypomobile first rib on the involved side. The second phase of the test consists of passively rotating the neck to the symptomatic side to end range, followed by lateral flexion of the neck to the opposite side. This test is considered positive when there is a decrease of lateral flexion and a hard end-fill on the effected side compared with the contralateral side.
- **Upper limb neurodynamics testing:** This test is used to rule out neurogenic pain and to provoke symptoms. Neural tissue assessment can be assessed by active movement dysfunction, passive movement dysfunction, adverse response to neural tissue provocation test, hyperalgesic response to palpation of nerve trunks, hyperalgesic responses to palpation of related cutaneous tissue and evidence of related local pathology (Hall & Elvey 1999). (For this topic see Ch 64.)

The study by Sanders et al (2008) reported on 50 patients with positive provocative testing (Table 12.3). Gillard et al (2001) showed that a cluster of two provocative tests displayed the highest sensitivity (90%), whereas a cluster of five provocative tests increased the specificity to 84%.

Table 12.3 **Positive physical findings**

Positive physical findings – 50 patients	%
Upper limb tension test (ULTT)	98
90° abduction in external rotation	100
Scalene muscle tenderness	94
Scalene pressure yields radiating symptoms	92
Neck rotation to opposite side	90
Head tilt to opposite side	90
Sensation to light touch	68

(Modified from Sanders et al 2008.)

Imaging assessment of thoracic outlet syndrome

TOS presents a challenge to diagnosticians and controversy exists regarding what test and imaging assessment should be used for diagnosis. Unfortunately, many physicians doubt the diagnosis of the pathology because it cannot be radiographically or electrophysiologically determined. One school of thought suggests that patients must demonstrate true neurological signs to be diagnosed with TOS and be confirmed by electromyography or nerve conduction velocity for brachial plexus compression and / or Doppler studies for vascular compromise as well as radiography to rule out cervical rib.

Another school of thought would diagnose TOS by the interpretation of the history, symptoms and clinical examination. Clinical testing of TOS has been highly debated in literature and no single test or questionnaire is universally accepted for its diagnosis (Mackinnon & Novak 2002).

Clinical diagnosis can be assisted by the use of imaging to demonstrate the nature and location of the structure undergoing compression and the structure producing compression, but this is not always necessary. The first radiographic procedure should be a cervical plain radiography to assess for bone abnormalities as well as to differentiate the diagnosis. Computed tomography (CT) and angiography or magnetic resonance imaging (MRI) should be performed with postural manoeuvres in order to show the compression dynamically (Demondion et al 2006).

Clinical Treatment and Management of Thoracic Outlet Syndrome

Conservative treatment is indicated in patients unless there is significant neural loss or vascular compromise (Leffert 1991). The focus for conservative treatment is to decrease extrinsic pressure, reducing intrinsic irritation. The goal is to decrease pressure on the neurovascular bundle and give patients the tools to manage their TOS. Conservative management of TOS consists of (in no particular order): restoring normal breathing patterns, reducing inflammation, decreasing muscle tension, elongating tight muscles, strengthening weak musculature, maintaining neural excursion and mobile joints, improving posture and body mechanics, and restoring muscle balance (Watson et al 2009).

Therapy evaluation of thoracic outlet syndrome

The subjective history examination is most helpful to understand patients' perception of the symptoms and duration of time or chronicity of the symptoms. The diagnosis and effective treatment of patients presenting with TOS is challenging owing to its being a syndrome involving many pain sources. Provocation and specific functional tests provide information to design an orthopaedic manual therapy management programme as well as address other dysfunctions. TOS can cause pain in the cervical and thoracic area and specific muscle groups, and paraesthesia and numbness in the upper extremity. It is important to identify the structure causing the symptoms and to identify areas of hypomobility or hypermobility. The provocation tests are important to assist in isolating the pain generators and the mobility testing determines areas of segmental dysfunction. It is this author's experience that identifying the abnormalities in the following areas and designing a treatment programme around these abnormalities will assist in successful outcomes.

Breathing patterns

Analysing the patient's breathing pattern cannot be understated. Patients with TOS tend to breath with their upper thorax without any abdominal movement. When this occurs the accessory muscles, particularly the scalene, elevate the first rib causing narrowing of the thoracic outlet. When examining a patient who uses the accessory respiratory muscle, as opposed to diaphragmatic breathing, it is not uncommon to find a decrease in hand temperature and decrease in blood flow because of abnormal sympathetic tone or vascular compromise. The sympathetic nervous system uses this normal protective response of vasal restriction that alters blood flow. It is important to change the breathing pattern to a more relaxed diaphragmatic breathing that allows for opening in the thoracic outlet and reduces muscle tension. The abnormal breathing pattern of not using the diaphragm perpetuates a vicious cycle of pain, spasm and congestion. The key to teaching is to ask the patient to lie supine with both hands placed on the upper abdomen and lower rib cage. The abdomen lifts with respiration and lowers with expiration. Observing hand movement will determine whether breathing is done correctly. The scalene, in abnormal breathing, tends to contract through the full inspiratory phase. This maintains the elevation of the first rib, which in turn will compromise the space for the subclavian vein to remain uncompressed.

By performing relaxed repeated breathing patterns, there is a decrease in muscle tension. Imbalances in the pressure gradients with TOS cause an increase in tunnel pressure, which results in venous stasis and hypoxia. If this hypoxia continues the oedema around the nerve, as well as fibroblastic changes, can cause scarring. Edgelow (2004) uses an analogy to describe this situation as a river flowing into a lake and a river flowing out of the lake, in which the inflow equals the outflow. In this state, the volume of the lake is constant, the oxygen content is high, and the pollution content is low. Should there be an obstruction affecting the outflow, then the volume of the lake would increase, the oxygen content would decrease and the pollution would increase.

Muscle imbalance

Muscle imbalance is a major source of symptoms in patients with TOS. Abnormal postures such as forward-held head, rounded shoulders and protracted shoulders are damaging postures for the scapular and neck muscles and should be addressed immediately. It is important to make sure that the scalene muscles, which elevate the first rib, are not tense. If the scapula muscles are weak, then an abnormal scapular movement pattern will result in weakness in the middle and lower trapezius and serratus anterior muscles. The scalene can overwork, causing more entrapment. An evaluation of posture should include evaluating multiple joint and scapula movements. It is important to assist the scapula position at rest and see whether the scapula is depressed and downwardly rotated, which can be a contributing factor to TOS. In the above example, the scapula would be lower than T2–T7 and the slope of the shoulders would be increased, which would make the neck appear longer. With scapula depression during overhead reaching, there are changes occurring at the acromioclavicular (AC) joint especially with large and heavy arms. The AC joint, usually at the end range, will show creases that increase in overhead activities. A downwardly rotated scapula can be identified because its inferior angle is closer to the spine than the superior angle. Another way to assess scapula downward rotation is evaluating movement into flexion and abduction; this movement normally causes signs of pulling or pain located in the teres major and latissimus dorsi region (Sahrmann 2002).

Joint stiffness

The brachial plexus can be compressed with joint stiffness or capsular tightness. Several authors have proposed mobilization of the cervical, thoracic, sternoclavicular, AC and costotransverse joints to improve joint stiffness or hypomobility, range of motion and capsular tightness in upper quadrant conditions (Brismée et al 2005; Vanti et al 2007). Manual therapy techniques aimed at the joints, soft tissue and neural structure of the upper quadrant including the cervical and thoracic spine have been successful in treatment. Research has shown that thoracic mobilization, especially at the T4 area, is helpful to provide an inhibitory influence on the SNS and causes immediate post-treatment pain relief (Yip-Menck et al 2000). Thoracic mobilization has proven effective in improving posture, hand and skin temperature as well as pain in TOS (see Ch 13). The study by Stralka (2000), using grade III oscillation movement posterior-anterior at T4 level, showed similarities in increased hand and skin temperature. Taskaynatan et al (2007) reported that inclusion of mechanical cervical traction reduced complaints of numbness in patients with TOS.

Evidence exists that thoracic joint mobilization decreases pain (Colachis et al 1966; Saal et al 1966; Browder et al 2004) and it has been theorized that biomechanical disturbances of the thoracic spine can contribute to cervical disorders (Greenman 1996; Norlander et al 1997; Browder et al 2004; Gross et al 2004). When the SNS responds there is a normal protective response of vasoconstriction that alters blood flow. Automatic improper breathing patterns along with pain, stress and anxiety can cause SNS activity that maintains a cycle of pain, tension and dysfunction. The involvement of the SNS by researchers is controversial – but my experience has shown that, by changing the sympathetic activity, there can be a positive influence on the patients' symptoms.

Neurogenic pain

It is the author's experience that upper limb nerve tension testing provocative manoeuvres along with clinical examination are extremely helpful in identifying NTOS. Neural mobility is an important part of a successful outcome. The provocation testing will reveal whether the patient is a releaser or a compressor, and this is useful in educating the patient as to which positions of comfort will decrease symptoms. The upper limb nerve tension testing is useful for identifying the area of specific brachial plexus entrapments. With TOS, the lower trunk / medial cord (C7–T1) is most commonly involved. The upper limb nerve tension testing and Tinel's test often locate the neurogenic irritability both proximal and distal, which is commonly referred to as a double-crush syndrome (Plewa & Delinger 1998). These tests should not aggravate the symptoms (see Ch 65).

Reproduction of radiating neurogenic arm pain with paraesthesia is a positive response. When this test is positive, it is an indicator of compression against the nerve roots or brachial plexus.

Intervention for thoracic outlet syndrome

There are many schools of thought contributing to the therapy and management of TOS. Peter Edgelow, a physiotherapist, utilizes three concepts that are the guiding principles for effective treatment of neurovascular entrapment, which are built on the fundamental idea that entrapment occurs as a consequence of trauma affecting the nerve or vascular system (Edgelow 2004). His first concept is patient empowerment, which means patients must be responsible and in control of their own care in order for treatment to be long lasting. The importance of treating the whole person cannot be underestimated and is supported by this author. The most successful outcomes are obtained with application of a multifactorial approach starting with patients being empowered to take care of their own problems by understanding both their TOS dilemma as well as the treatment solution. In treatment, it is important to gain patients' trust, stay in contact with them and make sure they understand their problem. The impact of having this long-lasting pain syndrome without correctly being diagnosed as TOS is that individuals feel they are losing control of their life. Restoring the feeling of 'being in control' has a positive impact on the individual. However, it has been my experience that there is no quick fix in treating patients with TOS; that is why patients must understand the length of the programme and be diligent with the exercise programmes. It is also important for the patient to understand the risks and rewards in paying close attention to symptoms; understanding the problem and the solution reinstates control in the patient's life. Edgelow (2004) also suggests that individual risk factors, health habits, daily living demands and belief systems that can be controlled are important for the treatment of TOS.

The second concept is that neurovascular entrapment is a problem of stenosis. Stenosis should not be thought of as a rigid narrowing of an anatomical part, but rather a series of events and circumstances. These events may result in irreversible narrowing. The stenosis caused by the presence of a cervical rib or dysfunction of the scalene may be irreversible, but the stenosis due to abnormal breathing patterns and abnormal posture can be reversed (Edgelow 2004).

The third concept Edgelow stresses is that of fluid dynamics. As structural and fluid changes cause restriction in the size of the thoracic outlet, they also cause changes in the pressure gradient, which also affects the local neural circulation and the venous and lymphatic return to the entire upper extremity.

Conclusion

Communication between the referring physician and physical therapist is a necessity to assure positive outcomes. Many authors combine treatment of soft tissues and joints with neural tissue treatment (Edgelow 2004). This management includes posture correction, treatment of affected structures – including nerve excursions, muscular and articular structures – as well as addressing the emotional component, which is necessary for successful outcomes.

The goal of treatment is to teach the patient to open up the space between the clavicle and first rib by stretching tight muscles, strengthening weak musculature, decreasing nerve tension in the upper quadrant, improving temperature differences in the hand, improving diaphragmatic breathing and increasing spinal mobility in the cervical–thoracic area. A clear understanding and interpretation of the provocative test are necessary for successful outcomes. Patients must realize that a period of 6 months or longer may be necessary to make a lasting effect on their symptoms.

As we manage patients, I have found that they may perform stretching exercises without using proper techniques. Most patients do not understand that lateral flexion without stabilizing the first rib continues to add additional compression and tension in the scalene muscles. They must be instructed in lateral flexion with slight rotation along with using a towel or a strap to hold the rib in a caudal position.

A total-wellness concept of good eating habits and aerobic conditioning should also be followed. Many TOS patients are in poor aerobic condition, which results in decreased respiratory function and overuse of the scalene, trapezius and sternocleidomastoid muscles. Postural correction, including spinal extension, will allow better chest expansion with inspiration resulting in diaphragmatic excursion and will decrease the usage of the accessory respiratory muscles (Mackinnon & Novak 2002).

Clinical experience has shown that, by identifying the mechanical origin of symptoms, a successful treatment programme consisting of symptom alleviation is most helpful, along with empowering patients to be in charge of their own symptoms. Educating the patient in proper posture and breathing patterns both at work and at leisure is the cornerstone for designing a treatment programme. Physical therapy that addresses postural abnormalities, neural mobility, joint mobility and muscle imbalances is effective in relieving symptoms of TOS.

References

Atasoy E. 2004. Thoracic outlet syndrome: anatomy. Hand Clin 20: 7–14.

Beyer JA, Wright IS. 1951. The hyperabduction syndrome: with special reference to its relationship to Raynaud's syndrome. Circulation 4: 161–172.

Brantigan CO, Roos DB. 2004. Diagnosing thoracic outlet syndrome. Hand Clin 20: 17–36.

Brismée JM, Gilbert K, Isom K, et al. 2004. Rate of false positive using the Cyriax release test for thoracic outlet syndrome in an asymptomatic population. J Man Manip Ther 12: 73–81.

Brismée JM, Phelps V, Sizer PS. 2005. Differential diagnosis and treatment of chronic neck and upper trapezius pain and upper extremity paresthesia: a case study involving the management of an elevated first rib and uncovertebral joint dysfunction. J Man Manip Ther 13: 79–90.

Browder DA, Erhard RE, Piva SR. 2004. Intermittent cervical traction and thoracic manipulation for management of mild cervical compressive myelopathy attributed to cervical herniated disc: a case series. J Orthop Sports Phys Ther 34: 701–712.

Casey RG, Richards S, O'Donahoe M. 2003. Exercise induced clinical ischaemia of the upper limb secondary to a cervical rib. Br J Sports Med 37: 455–456.

Colachis SC, Strohm BR. 1966. Effect of duration of intermittent cervical traction on vertebral separation. Arch Phys Med Rehabil 47: 353–359.

Cyriax J. 1978. Textbook of orthopedic medicine: diagnosis of soft tissue lesions, 7th edn. Vol 1. London: Baillière Tindall.

Demondion X, Herbinet P, Van Sint Jan S. 2006. Imaging assessment of thoracic outlet syndrome. Radiographics 26: 1735–1750.

Edgelow PL. 2004. Neurovascular consequences of cumulative trauma disorders affecting the thoracic outlet: a patient-centered treatment approach. Neurological considerations. In: Donatelli RA (ed) Physical therapy of the shoulder, 4th edn. Edinburgh: Churchill Livingstone, pp 205–238.

Fugate MW, Rotellini-Coltvet L, Freischlag JA. 2009. Current management of thoracic outlet syndrome. Curr Treat Options Cardiovasc Med 11: 176–183.

Gillard J, Perez-Cousin M, Hachulla E, et al. 2001. Diagnosing thoracic outlet syndrome: contribution of provocative tests, ultrasonography, electrophysiology, and helical computed tomography in 48 patients. Joint Bone Spine 68: 416–424.

Greenman PE. 1996. Principles of manual medicine. Philadelphia: Lippincott Williams & Wilkins.

Gross AR, Hoving JL, Haines TA, et al. 2004. Manipulation and mobilization for mechanical neck disorders. Cochrane Database Syst Rev 1: CD004249. (Update in Cochrane Database Syst Rev. 2010. (1): CD004249.)

Hall TM, Elvey RL. 1999. Nerve trunk pain: physical diagnosis and treatment. Man Ther 4: 63–73.

Hursh LF, Thanki A. 1985. The TOS. Postgrad Med 77: 197–199.

Kaymak B, Ozcakar L. 2004. Complex regional pain syndrome in thoracic outlet syndrome. Br J Sports Med 38: 364–368.

Leffert RD. 1991. Thoracic outlet syndrome. In: R Tubiana R (ed) The hand, 4th edn. Philadelphia: WB Saunders, pp 343–351.

Lundborg G. 1970. Iscli nerve injury. Scand J Plast Reconstr Surg Hand Surg 65: 1–113.

Mackinnon SE, Novak CB. 2002. Thoracic outlet syndrome. Curr Probl Surg 39: 1070–1145.

Mackinnon SE, Patterson GA, Novak CB. 1996. Thoracic outlet syndrome: a current overview. Semin Thoracic Cardiovasc Surg 8(2): 176–182.

medifocus.com. 2009 (updated 7 Aug 2014). Thoracic outlet syndrome: a comprehensive guide to symptoms, treatment, research, and support. MediFocus Guide RT017. Online. Available: http://www.medifocus.com/2009/landingp2.php?gid=RT017&?a=a (accessed 24 Nov 2014).

Nord KM, Kappor P, Fisher J, et al. 2008. False positive rate of thoracic outlet syndrome diagnostic maneuvers. Electromyogr Clin Neurophysiol 48: 67–74.

Norlander S, Gustavsson BA, Lindell J, et al. 1997. Reduced mobility in the cervico-thoracic motion segment – a risk factor for musculoskeletal neck–shoulder pain: a two-year prospective follow-up study. Scand J Rehabil Med 29: 167–174.

Plewa M, Delinger M. 1998. The false-positive rate of thoracic outlet syndrome shoulder maneuvers in healthy subjects. Acad Emerg Med 5: 337–342.

Ryan GM, Jensen C. 1995. Thoracic outlet syndrome: provocative examination maneuvers in a typical population. J Shoulder Elbow Surg 4: 113–117.

Saal JS, Saal JA, Yurth EF. 1996. Nonoperative management of herniated cervical intervertebral disc with radiculopathy. Spine 21: 1877–1883.

Sahrmann SA. 2002. Diagnosis and treatment of movement impairment syndromes. St Louis: CV Mosby, pp 193–261.

Samarasam I, Sadhu D, Agarwal S, et al. 2004. Surgical management of thoracic outlet syndrome: a 10-year experience. J Surg 74: 450–454.

Sanders RJ. 1990. Scalene muscle abnormalities in traumatic thoracic outlet syndrome. Am J Surg 159: 231–236.

Sanders RJ, Haug CE. 1991. Thoracic outlet syndrome: a common sequela of neck injuries. Philadelphia: Lippincott Williams & Wilkins, pp 26–73.

Sanders RJ, Hammond SL, Rao NM. 2008. Thoracic outlet syndrome: a review. Neurologist 14: 365–373.

Schwartzman RJ. 1987. Clinical syndromes of RSD and TOS. Philadelphia: Greater Philadelphia Pain Society.

Stralka SW. 2000. Effects of mobilization of fourth thoracic vertebra on pain and hand skin temperature in adult women with complex regional pain syndrome. Memphis: University of Tennessee. [Thesis.]

Talu GK. 2005. Thoracic outlet syndrome: a review. Agri 17: 5–9.
Taskaynatan MA, Balaban B, Yasar E, et al. 2007. Cervical traction in conservative management of thoracic outlet syndrome. J Musculoskeket Pain 15: 89–94.
Vanti C, Natalini L, Romeo A, et al. 2007. Conservative treatment of thoracic outlet syndrome. A review of the literature. Eura Medicophys 43: 55–70.
Watson LA, Pizzari T, Balster S. 2009. Thoracic outlet syndrome part 1: clinical manifestations, differentiation and treatment pathways. Man Ther 14: 586–595.
Yip-Menck J, Mais S, Kulig K. 2000. Consideration of thoracic spine dysfunction in upper extremity complex regional pain syndrome type I: a case report. J Orthop Sports Phys Ther 30: 401–409.

13 Chapter

Thoracic Spine Manipulation

William Egan, Paul E. Glynn, Joshua A. Cleland

CHAPTER CONTENTS

Introduction	142
Regional interdependence of the thoracic spine, rib cage and the upper quarter	143
Biomechanical relationship between the thoracic spine and upper quarter	143
Pain referral patterns of the thoracic spine	143
Association between thoracic spine impairments and upper quarter pain syndromes	143
Evidence for manual therapy management of the thoracic spine and rib cage in upper quarter pain syndromes	144
Examination and screening of the thoracic spine and rib cage in patients with upper quarter musculoskeletal pain	148
Postural screen of the thoracic spine and rib cage	148
Thoracic spine active range of motion	149
Mobility testing of the first rib	149
Segmental mobility testing of the thoracic spine and rib cage	149
Interpretation of the examination and reassessment	149
Manual therapy interventions for the thoracic spine and rib cage	150
Seated upper thoracic thrust manipulation	150
Seated mid-thoracic thrust manipulation	151
Prone upper thoracic thrust manipulation	151
Prone mid-thoracic thrust and non-thrust manipulation	151
Supine upper and mid-thoracic thrust manipulation	152
Seated first-rib thrust and non-thrust manipulation	153
Supine first-rib thrust and non-thrust manipulation	154
Prone or side-lying ribs non-thrust manipulation	154
Supine ribs thrust manipulation	154
Exercise interventions to augment the manual therapy techniques	154
Conclusion	155

Introduction

For individuals with upper quarter musculoskeletal disorders, the thoracic spine is infrequently the primary source of symptoms. However, taking into account the concept of regional interdependence, the thoracic spine and rib cage can play a significant role in the perpetuation and management of upper quarter pain (Wainner et al 2007; Sueki et al 2013). For instance, a 45-year-old female presents to your clinic with mechanical neck pain. Her pain is of recent onset, occurring insidiously within the last 2 weeks, and she denies any symptoms radiating to the upper extremity below the shoulder. After a clinical examination that identified no signs of serious disease or contraindications, you elect to perform thrust manipulation targeting her upper and mid thoracic spine. You also instruct her on mobility exercises for her cervical spine as well as deep neck flexor retraining. The patient returns 3 days later and reports a 3-point reduction on the Numerical Rating of Pain Scale (NRPS) and a 25% decrease on the Neck Disability Index (NDI).

You also examine a 37-year-old male with right shoulder pain; signs and symptoms are consistent with subacromial impingement syndrome as well as mobility impairments of his thoracic spine and rib cage. You perform a thrust manipulation of the patient's upper and mid thoracic spine in addition to non-thrust mobilization of the patient's rib cage. Immediately following the manipulation the patient reports a 50% decrease in resting pain and his pain-free active shoulder elevation is increased by 10°. You instruct the patient in thoracic extension mobility exercises as well as strengthening exercises for the lower trapezius and serratus anterior muscles. Upon return to the clinic 5 days later, the patient's score on the Shoulder Pain and Disability Index (SPADI) is decreased by 25%. These two hypothetical clinical scenarios are based on the findings from recent clinical trials (Bergman et al 2004; González-Iglesias et al 2009b). Therefore, addressing impairments in the thoracic region can lead to improvements in pain and disability in patients with different upper quarter musculoskeletal disorders including the neck, shoulder and elbow regions.

In the management of patients with upper quarter disorders the thoracic spine has traditionally been overlooked. However, there is evidence suggesting a strong biomechanical relationship between the thoracic spine, rib cage and the upper quarter (Sobel et al 1996; Kebaetse et al 1999; Theodoridis & Ruston 2002; Crosbie et al 2008). Further, studies have shown that manual therapy treatment directed towards the thoracic spine can have a positive impact on the outcomes of individuals with disorders of the upper extremity and cervical spine (Winters et al 1997; Bergman et al 2004; Young et al 2009; Huisman et al 2013). This chapter covers anatomical- and biomechanical-related aspects of the thoracic spine, scientific and clinical evidence for the relevance of the thoracic spine for upper quarter pain syndromes, thoracic spine and rib cage exploration and manipulative interventions.

Regional Interdependence of the Thoracic Spine, Rib Cage and the Upper Quarter

Biomechanical relationship between the thoracic spine and upper quarter

The structure and function of the thoracic spine and rib cage create a symbiotic relationship with the cervical spine and upper extremity. The thoracic column serves as the base of support for the cervical spine and is intimately involved with the neck at the region of the cervicothoracic junction. Stiffness and movement impairments of the cervicothoracic junction are common findings in patients with primary complaints of neck pain, headaches or upper extremity pain syndromes (Sobel et al 1997; Piva et al 2006; Cleland et al 2007a; Berglund et al 2008). The posture of the thoracic spine has been shown to influence the posture of cervical spine and upper extremity (Kebaetse et al 1999). For instance, an increase in the thoracic kyphosis, which is common in the typical office worker, is associated with a forward head posture as well as an abducted and anteriorly tipped scapular position. To achieve full functional movement of the cervical spine and upper extremities, concomitant motion of the thoracic spine and rib cage and an erect, neutral thoracic posture are required. For example, full upper extremity elevation is accompanied by thoracic extension and ipsilateral side-bending (Theodoridis & Ruston 2002). Theoretically this would also require external rotation of the ipsilateral ribs, which has been associated with thoracic spine extension (Cropper 1996). It has been shown that a slouched or flexed thoracic posture leads to decreased scapular posterior tipping during maximum glenohumeral abduction motion and decreased abduction force at 90° of abduction compared with an erect thoracic posture (Kebaetse et al 1999). Key postural muscles span from the thoracic spine to scapular regions. These muscles include the middle and lower portions of the trapezius and the serratus anterior. Postural or movement impairments in the thoracic region could play a role in dysfunction of these muscles and therefore have a direct influence on movement impairments and pain in the cervical and upper extremity regions. Two studies found that lower trapezius muscle strength increased after either thrust manipulation or non-thrust mobilization targeting the mid to lower thoracic spine (Liebler et al 2001; Cleland et al 2004a). Although both of these studies involved asymptomatic subjects and measured immediate changes in strength only, they suggested a clinically significant relationship between the thoracic spine and the lower trapezius muscle.

Pain referral patterns of the thoracic spine

It is uncommon for the thoracic spine to cause referred pain to the cervical or upper extremity regions. The cervical spine and upper extremities do not receive direct innervation from the thoracic roots, with the exception of the first thoracic nerve root. However, the sympathetic nervous system via the sympathetic chain, running anterior to the costovertebral joints, can have a systemic effect and contribute to symptoms in the neck and upper extremities. A clinical syndrome referred to as the 'T4 syndrome' has been described as a constellation of signs and symptoms associated with stiffness of the upper to mid thoracic region (Conroy & Schneiders 2005). Typical signs and symptoms include headaches, neck pain and arm pain, and bilateral 'stoking glove' paraesthesiae. It is thought that these signs and symptoms could be resulting in part from dysfunction of the thoracic spine and its influence on the sympathetic nervous system.

Furthermore, a published case report described a decrease in symptoms in a patient with upper extremity complex regional pain syndrome after a thrust manipulation directed to the upper thoracic spine (Menck et al 2000). In pain-mapping studies of the thoracic spine facet joints and costotransverse joints, local pain adjacent to the injected site is most commonly reported (Dreyfuss et al 1994; Fukui et al 1997; Young et al 2008). Subjects in these studies have not reported referred pain into the neck or the upper extremity regions. Given the lack of a neuroanatomical relationship with the cervical spine or upper extremities, this is not surprising. Patients with symptomatic thoracic disc herniation typically report thoracic spine and chest wall pain and do not report neck or arm pain (Wood et al 1999). With the exception of symptoms originating from the upper two thoracic segments and the thoracic sympathetic chain, the thoracic spine as a direct source of referred pain or symptoms to the cervical spine or upper extremity regions is unlikely.

Association between thoracic spine impairments and upper quarter pain syndromes

Postural impairments and movement dysfunctions of the thoracic spine have been found in patients with upper quarter musculoskeletal disorders. In a series of studies, Norlander et al (1996, 1997) found that movement dysfunction of the upper thoracic spine was associated with upper quarter symptoms in a group of laundry workers. In their initial study and 2-year follow-up, Norlander et al (1996, 1997) found that a decrease in forward flexion mobility of C7–T1, compared with T1–T2, predicted complaints of neck and shoulder pain. They referred to this finding as an 'inverse C7–T1 relationship', because in healthy subjects they found that C7–T1 had greater flexion mobility than T1–T2. In a third study, Norlander and Nordgren (1998) found that a reduction in forward flexion mobility of C7–T1 and T1–T2 was associated with a threefold increase in complaints of neck pain, headaches, shoulder pain and bilateral hand weakness in a group of electrical and laundry workers. These authors hypothesized that sensory input from joint receptors of the dysfunctional thoracic segments could potentially contribute to the neck and shoulder symptoms. Further research is required to make definitive conclusions.

Movement dysfunction of the thoracic spine, rib cage and shoulder girdle has been associated with patients reporting shoulder pain in primary care practices. In a 12–18-month follow-up of patients with shoulder complaints, Winters et al (1999) found that patients who reported that their shoulder pain was not 'cured' were more likely to have pain or limited mobility of the shoulder girdle. These authors defined the shoulder girdle as the cervical and upper thoracic spine, or upper ribs. This was in comparison to patients diagnosed with a synovial disorder originating from the glenohumeral, acromioclavicular or subacromial joints without dysfunction of the shoulder girdle. In another study, it was shown that patients presenting with shoulder girdle disorders responded well to manipulative therapy targeting impairments in this region, whereas patients with synovial disorders responded best to steroid injection (Winters et al 1997).

Lateral elbow pain, a common upper extremity musculoskeletal disorder, has been associated with several impairments. Amongst these are pain and mobility restrictions of the cervical and thoracic spine. One study found that subjects with lateral elbow pain had significantly higher frequency of positive responses with spring testing over the T1–T7 regions compared with subjects without elbow pain (Berglund et al 2008). However, definitive conclusions could not be drawn about the association between pain with thoracic spring testing and lateral elbow pain in this study, and this finding may be attributed to the phenomenon of central sensitization of pain. Nevertheless, assessment and management of thoracic spine impairments in patients with elbow pain is the consideration in the clinic. In a small pilot study and a larger retrospective study, Cleland et al (2004b, 2005a) found that patients who received manual therapy procedures targeting the cervical and thoracic region in addition to treatment of the elbow achieved more favourable outcomes than did those patients who received management of the elbow only.

Evidence for Manual Therapy Management of the Thoracic Spine and Rib Cage in Upper Quarter Pain Syndromes

Due to the relatively small number of patients with primary complaints of thoracic spine and chest wall pain, there is only low-quality evidence supporting the use of manual therapy procedures in the management of thoracic spine and chest wall pain. In a pilot study, Schiller (2001) found that patients with mechanical thoracic spine pain showed a significantly greater reduction in pain scores after six treatments of manipulative therapy targeting the thoracic spine compared with a placebo control group. Techniques utilized in the study were short lever thrusts with direct contact on the transverse processes. In a case report Kelley and Whitney (2006) described the immediate relief of right lower chest wall pain after a non-thrust manipulation of the mid thoracic spine in an adolescent athlete. Fruth (2006) reported a case of a patient with right upper thoracic pain that was resolved after seven physical therapy visits including non-thrust manipulation of the ribs, ischaemic compression of trigger points and therapeutic exercise. In a retrospective review of 73 patients reporting to a rheumatology clinic with a primary complaint of thoracic spine pain, Bruckner et al (1987) reported that the majority of the patients were either pain free (77%) or noted slight improvement (15%) after postural advice and manipulative treatment of the thoracic spine. The majority of patients (75%) in this retrospective review reported mid-thoracic pain and about half also complained of anterior chest wall pain. Patients with chest wall pain should receive a differential diagnosis to rule out cardiac and visceral disorders. Musculoskeletal pain involving the thoracic spine can potentially cause pseudoanginal or pseudovisceral pain.

There have been two reports in the literature concerning patients with anterior chest or abdominal pain who have been worked up for cardiac and visceral disorders with negative findings (Hamberg & Lindahl 1981; Benhamou et al 1993). These patients were found to have mechanical thoracic pain that responded to either manipulation of the thoracic spine or injection of the costovertebral joints. Another study identified historical questions that assist the clinician in determining the source of a patient's abdominal pain as being musculoskeletal in origin (Sparkes et al 2003). For abdominal pain to be considered of musculoskeletal origin, the patient should answer yes to two questions and no to one question. This leads to a positive likelihood ratio of 4.2 that the patient's pain is of musculoskeletal origin.

The 'yes' questions are:

- Does coughing, sneezing, or taking a deep breath make your pain feel worse?
- Do activities such as bending, sitting, lifting, twisting, or turning over in bed make your pain feel worse?

The 'no' question is:

- Has there been any change in your bowel habits since the start of your symptoms?

There has been a recent emergence in the literature of studies investigating the effect of manual therapy procedures targeting the thoracic spine in patients with neck disorders. Given the small risk of serious adverse events associated with cervical thrust manipulation, some authors advocate thoracic thrust manipulation as a safe alternative to cervical manipulation especially in the presence of severe symptoms or radiculopathy, or post whiplash (Piva et al 2000; Pho & Godges 2004; Childs et al 2005). There are a few studies showing that patients with mechanical neck pain benefit from thrust manipulation of the thoracic spine. These include two case series, nine randomized clinical trials, a preliminary clinical prediction rule study and two systematic reviews (Savolainen et al 2004; Cleland et al 2005b, 2007a, 2007c, 2010; Fernández-de-las-Peñas et al 2007; Krauss et al 2008; González-Iglesias et al 2009a, 2009b; Cross et al 2011; Lau et al 2011; Puentedura & Landers 2011; Huisman et al 2013; Masaracchio et al 2013). These studies are of varying quality, and some of the evidence is conflicting, but in sum provide substantial evidence that patients with mechanical neck pain can experience clinically meaningful improvement in pain and disability following thrust manipulation of the thoracic spine. It is important to note, however, that in several of the studies the thoracic spine manipulation was augmented by a therapeutic exercise programme. In these studies various techniques were utilized including seated, prone and supine thrusts targeting both the mid and upper thoracic spine. Table 13.1 provides an overview of these studies involving patients with mechanical neck pain.

Neck pain after a whiplash injury is very common. There has been one randomized clinical trial and one case report concerning manipulation of the thoracic spine in patients with neck pain after a whiplash injury. In a two-part study,

Table 13.1 **Overview of studies involving thoracic spine manipulation for patients with mechanical neck pain**

Author year	Study design	Subjects	Interventions	Outcomes
Cleland et al 2005b	RCT	36 patients with mechanical neck pain	Supine thoracic thrust manipulation vs placebo.	Immediate clinically significant reduction in neck pain following thrust compared with placebo.
Cleland et al 2007c	RCT	60 patients with mechanical neck pain	6 sessions of thoracic thrust manipulation and exercise vs non-thrust manipulation and exercise.	At the completion of 6 sessions the thrust group achieved clinically significant more reduction in pain and disability as measured by the NDI compared with the non-thrust group.
Cleland et al 2007a	Prospective cohort study	78 patients with mechanical neck pain	All subjects received up to 2 sessions of thoracic thrust manipulation targeting both the mid and upper thoracic spine and ROM exercise for the cervical spine. Patients achieving at least 3 of 6 variables have a positive likelihood ratio of 5.5 for a successful outcome with the intervention.	The following variables comprised the clinical prediction rule for patients who would achieve clinically meaningful improvement on the Global Rating of Change scale: 1. Symptoms < 30 days 2. No symptoms below the shoulder 3. Looking up does not aggravate symptoms 4. FABQPA score < 12 5. Diminished upper thoracic spine kyphosis 6. Cervical extension ROM < 30°.
Cleland et al 2010	RCT	140 patients with mechanical neck pain. Half of the patients in each group met 3 of the variables for the above-mentioned CPR.	2 sessions of thoracic spine manipulation and cervical range of motion exercise followed by 3 sessions of cervical strengthening and stretching exercises, vs 5 sessions of cervical strengthening and stretching exercise.	There was a clinically meaningful difference in disability at short- and long-term follow-up and pain at short-term follow-up favouring thoracic spine manipulation combined with exercise compared with exercise alone. Status on the above-mentioned CPR did not affect the outcome within either group.
Cross et al 2011	Systematic review	6 RCTs involving patients with mechanical neck pain	In all 6 studies the experimental group received thoracic spine manipulation. Note: All six of these studies are included in this table.	Effect sizes for pain in favour of thoracic spine manipulation varied from small to large across studies. Effect sizes for patient reported neck disability questionnaires in favour of thoracic manipulation were moderate to large.
Fernández-de-las-Peñas et al 2007	Case Series	7 patients with mechanical neck pain	All patients received a single thrust manipulation in sitting targeting the upper thoracic spine.	All patients achieved an immediate reduction in resting pain and improved cervical range of motion following the manipulation.
Flynn et al 2001	Case series	26 patients with neck pain	All patients received thrust manipulation targeting hypomobile segments including the upper and mid thoracic spine and rib cage.	Immediately post intervention, patients experienced a clinically meaningful improvement in cervical ROM and a reduction in resting pain.
González-Iglesias et al 2009a	RCT	45 patients with mechanical neck pain	6 sessions of TENS, exercise and massage vs the same programme plus thoracic spine thrust manipulation in sitting 1×/week ×3 weeks.	Patients in the manipulation group achieved a clinically significant greater reduction in pain and disability scores and increased cervical range of motion compared with the non-manipulation group at the completion of the intervention.

Continued

Table 13.1 **Overview of studies involving thoracic spine manipulation for patients with mechanical neck pain—cont'd**

Author year	Study design	Subjects	Interventions	Outcomes
González-Iglesias et al 2009b	RCT	45 patients with mechanical neck pain	5 sessions on electrothermal therapy vs the same treatment plus a seated thoracic thrust manipulation 1×/week × 3 weeks.	Patients in the manipulation group achieved a clinically significant greater reduction in pain and disability scores than the non-manipulation group at the end of the intervention, and at 2-week follow-up. The manipulation group continued show a clinically meaningful improvement in pain compared with the non-manipulation group at the 4-week follow-up.
Huisman et al 2013	Systematic review	10 RCTs involving 677 patients with mechanical neck pain	In all 10 studies the experimental group received thoracic spine manipulation. Note: All 10 of these studies are included in this table.	8 of the 10 studies reported a clinically significant reduction in pain and disability with thoracic spine manipulation. There is insufficient evidence to state that thoracic spine manipulation is superior to control interventions at this time.
Krauss et al 2008	RCT	22 patients with mechanical neck pain	Thoracic thrust manipulation to the T1–T4 segments in supine vs a control group	The thoracic manipulation group reported a clinically meaningful increase in right and left cervical rotation range of motion and a decrease in pain with right cervical rotation compared with the control group.
Lau et al 2011	RCT	120 patients with chronic neck pain	8 sessions of thoracic spine manipulation, infrared radiation therapy, exercise, and education vs 8 sessions of infrared radiation therapy and education alone.	The thoracic manipulation and exercise group reported a clinically meaningful difference in neck pain and disability compared with the control group at 6-month follow-up.
Masaracchio et al 2013	RCT	64 patients with mechanical neck pain	2 sessions of thoracic spine thrust manipulation, cervical spine non-thrust manipulation, and cervical range of motion exercise vs 2 sessions of cervical spine non-thrust manipulation and exercise.	The thoracic spine manipulation and cervical non-thrust manipulation group reported a clinically meaningful difference in neck pain and disability at 1-week follow up compared with the cervical non-thrust manipulation group.
Puentedura et al 2011	RCT	24 patients with neck pain who met at least 4 out of the 6 variables on the thoracic spine manipulation CPR	2 sessions of thoracic spine manipulation and range of motion exercise followed by 3 sessions of cervical strengthening and stretching exercise vs 2 sessions of cervical spine manipulation and range of motion exercise followed by 3 sessions of cervical strengthening and stretching exercise.	The cervical spine manipulation and exercise group reported a clinically meaningful difference in neck pain and disability at short- and long-term follow-up compared with the thoracic spine manipulation group.
Savolainen et al 2004	RCT	75 subjects with mechanical neck pain	4 sessions of thoracic manipulation vs instruction in an exercise programme.	Subjects in the manipulation group reported a significantly lower level of worst perceivable pain at 12-month follow-up.
Sillevas et al 2010	RCT	100 patients with chronic neck pain	1 session of thoracic spine manipulation vs placebo.	No within or between group differences in pain or sympathetic nervous system activity at immediate follow-up.

RCT=randomized controlled trial; ROM=range of motion; CPR=clinical prediction rule; NDI=neck disability index; TENS=transcutaneous nerve stimulation.

Fernández-de-las-Peñas et al (2004) first compared the incidence of thoracic spine dysfunction in patients suffering mechanical neck pain with those who had neck pain from a whiplash. Thoracic spine dysfunction was identified by palpation for asymmetry in thoracic flexion and pain, or hypomobility associated with spring testing of the thoracic spine; based on these criteria, 69% of patients with whiplash had thoracic joint dysfunction compared with 13% who had mechanical neck pain. In the second part of the study, 88 patients with whiplash were randomized to receive either 15 sessions of physiotherapy consisting of electrothermal modalities, ultrasound, massage and exercise or the same physiotherapy with the addition of two sessions of thoracic manipulation. The manipulation technique utilized was a supine thrust technique targeting the T4–T5 segment. At the completion of the study, the group receiving the thoracic manipulation experienced significantly greater reduction in neck pain, measured on a visual analogue scale (VAS), compared with the physiotherapy group.

Pho and Godges (2004) presented a case report of a patient with neck pain after a whiplash injury. Initial management of the patient included thoracic spine thrust and non-thrust manipulation during the first two treatment sessions as the cervical spine was deemed too irritable for assessment and treatment in the initial stages. The patient experienced a full resolution of symptoms, disability and range-of-motion deficits after four sessions of physical therapy. There is emerging evidence that thrust and non-thrust manipulation of the thoracic spine comprise an integral part of multimodal approaches in the management of patients with cervical radiculopathy. Cleland et al (2005c) and Waldrop (2006) published case series of patients diagnosed with cervical radiculopathy using a similar multimodal interventional approach. Interventions included thrust manipulation of the thoracic spine, non-thrust manipulation of the cervical spine, intermittent traction and therapeutic exercise. In both case series, the majority of patients experienced a clinically meaningful reduction in pain and disability at the end of the physical therapy intervention and at medium-term follow-up. In a prospective cohort study involving patients with cervical radiculopathy, Cleland et al (2007b) identified variables that predicted short-term success with physical therapy management. Success was defined as surpassing the minimally clinically important difference on the NDI, the Patient Specific Functional Scale, the NRPS, and the Global Rating of Change (GRC) scale. The predictor variables were age <54, looking down does not worsen symptoms, the dominant arm is not affected, and the patient received multimodal therapy including cervical traction, manual therapy that typically included thoracic spine manipulation, and deep neck flexor strengthening during at least 50% of the visits. Patients meeting three of these four variables had a positive likelihood ratio of 5.2 for success. In a high-quality randomized controlled trial, Young et al (2009) compared a multimodal approach including thoracic spine thrust manipulation, cervical non-thrust manipulation and therapeutic exercises with and without mechanical cervical traction in patients with cervical radiculopathy. Patients received an average of two treatment sessions per week for 4 weeks. Therapists were required to include at least one manual therapy intervention targeting both the mid and upper thoracic spine during each visit. Thrust techniques were conducted in sitting, supine and prone. Both groups experienced a clinically meaningful decrease in pain and disability at 2 and 4 weeks, with no differences between the groups.

In addition to cervical radiculopathy there is some evidence that thrust manipulation of the thoracic spine can assist with the management of patients with mild, grade I cervical compressive myelopathy. In a case series involving seven patients, Browder et al (2004) reported that a multimodal management programme of thoracic spine thrust manipulation and intermittent mechanical cervical traction resulted in a clinically meaningful reduction in pain and disability in all patients with an average of nine treatment sessions. Although it is difficult to parcel out the individual effects of thoracic spine manipulation from these studies, it was included in all of them and probably plays an integral part of the multimodal management of patients with cervical radiculopathy. In the authors' experience, most patients with cervical radiculopathy report significant relief of symptoms, especially in the scapular region, and improvement in cervical range of motion immediately following thoracic thrust manipulation.

Patients with cervicogenic headache form a clinically important subgroup for the clinician specializing in musculoskeletal disorders. Conservative management involving manual therapy and exercise has been shown to produce clinically meaningful benefits for patients in this subgroup (Jull et al 2002). Postural and mobility impairments involving the thoracic region can play a role in the perpetuation of these headaches. Furthermore, thrust and non-thrust manipulation of the thoracic spine could cause a reduction in headache pain by alternating the tension of multisegmental muscle spanning from the thoracic to the upper cervical region. In the randomized trial conducted by Jull et al (2002), patients receiving manual therapy, exercise or a combination of the two achieved a clinically meaningful reduction in headache frequency and intensity. Manual therapy procedures were selected by the clinician and included both thrust and non-thrust manipulations of the cervical and upper thoracic spine based on the patient's impairments, signs and symptoms. The exercise programme included postural, motor control and endurance exercises targeting the deep cervical flexors and scapular stabilizing muscles. In a case report of a patient with a headache, Viti and Paris (2000) reported a reduction in the patient's headache pain 4 days following a thrust manipulation of the upper thoracic spine. Previous management of the patient's impairments of the upper cervical region over five visits had failed to produce a change in symptoms. Preliminary evidence suggests that thrust and non-thrust manipulation of the thoracic spine can play a role in the multimodal management of patients with cervicogenic headache; however, additional high-quality research is required to investigate this hypothesis further.

As mentioned above, the thoracic spine is intimately involved with the shoulder region owing to the concomitant motion of the thoracic spine during movements of the shoulder. Additionally a neutral, erect posture is required for full range of motion of the shoulder. Three high-quality studies have investigated the use of thrust and non-thrust manipulation of the thoracic region in patients with shoulder disorders (Winters et al 1997; Bang & Deyle 2000; Bergman et al 2004). In two separate randomized clinical trials, Winters et al (1997) and Bergman et al (2004) both reported that manipulative therapy targeting the cervical spine, upper thoracic spine and upper rib cage led to a clinically meaningful reduction in pain and disability, at short- and medium-term follow-up, in patients suffering shoulder pain with signs and symptoms of shoulder girdle dysfunction. Comparison groups included non-manipulative physiotherapy, usual medical care, or steroid injection. Patients in both studies received up to six sessions of manipulative therapy provided by experienced manual physical therapists. Bang and Deyle (2000) compared exercise alone with exercise with manual therapy in patients with subacromial impingement syndrome. Patients in both groups received six sessions of treatment. At the completion of the study, patients in the manual therapy group experienced a clinically meaningful reduction in pain, disability and improvement in strength compared with the exercise group. Manual therapy included both thrust and non-thrust manipulation of the glenohumeral joint, clavicle, cervical spine, thoracic spine and rib cage.

These three studies provide evidence that manual therapy management of the thoracic spine, as part of a multimodal treatment programme, can lead to positive outcomes for patients with shoulder pain. However, it is unclear how much manual therapy of the thoracic spine, in isolation, contributes to the outcome. Boyles et al (2009) addressed this question in a prospective case series of 54 patients with shoulder impingement syndrome. They reported that pain, disability and global rating of change were improved 48 hours after performing thrust manipulation of the upper and mid thoracic spine and rib cage. Seated thrust techniques were utilized to manipulate the thoracic spine and a supine technique was used to manipulation the ribs. Although it is unlikely that the thoracic and rib joints can directly refer pain to the shoulder region, Boyle (1999) reported that two patients' shoulder symptoms were completely resolved after non-thrust manipulation of the ipsilateral second rib.

Mintken et al (2010) reported the results of a clinical prediction rule derivation study involving thoracic spine manipulation for patients with shoulder pain. In this study, 80 patients with a variety of shoulder disorders, excluding those with contraindications to thoracic spine thrust manipulation, received up two sessions of thoracic spine thrust manipulation, cervical non-thrust manipulation and spinal mobility exercises. A rating of at least +4 on the 15-point GRC scale was used as the marker for success. Based on this criterion, 61% of the patient population had a successful outcome with up to two sessions of the aforementioned intervention programme. Using stepwise logistic regression, the authors derived five variables that were predictive of success with the intervention programme: pain-free shoulder flexion range of motion $<127°$, shoulder internal rotation at 90° of abduction $<53°$, a negative Neer test, not taking medications for pain, and duration of symptoms <90 days. Patients meeting at least three of these five variables had a positive likelihood ratio of 5.4 for a successful outcome, which translates into an 89% post-test probability of success. This single-arm trial has limitations and the clinical prediction rule is awaiting derivation with a randomized controlled trial. However, this study adds to the evidence that thoracic spine manipulation, as part of a multimodal intervention package, can lead to decreased pain and disability for patients with shoulder pain.

To investigate further the potential mechanisms behind decreased pain and improved mobility associated with thoracic manipulation for subjects with shoulder pain, Muth et al (2012) completed a laboratory-based study. The researchers used surface electromyography and an electromagnetic tracking device to measure scapular muscle activity and kinematics pre and post thoracic spine manipulation, in 30 patients aged 18–45 years who had signs of rotator cuff tendinopathy. Post manipulation there were no significant differences in scapular muscle activity or kinematics, with the exception of a small increase in middle trapezius muscle activity and a small decrease in scapular upward rotation. However, immediately after manipulation, subjects reported a significant decrease in pain with provocative shoulder testing and active shoulder elevation. Subjects also reported a clinically significant improvement in shoulder function via standardized self-reported questionnaires at 7–10 days post manipulation. The authors concluded that thoracic spine manipulation leads to an immediate improvement in shoulder function and decreased pain, but these findings are not explained by a change in scapular muscle activity or kinematics.

As described above, mobility impairments and tenderness of the thoracic spine are common in patients reporting lateral elbow pain (Berglund et al 2008). Manual therapy management of the cervicothoracic spine, in addition to local treatment directed to the elbow, has been shown to lead to improved outcomes in fewer visits, compared with local treatment of the elbow alone (Cleland et al 2004b, 2005a).

Examination and Screening of the Thoracic Spine and Rib Cage in Patients with Upper Quarter Musculoskeletal Pain

A full comprehensive musculoskeletal examination involving medical screening, patient history and a physical examination should be undertaken for all patients with upper quarter region complaints. What follows are the selected examination procedures that assist with identifying impairments that would be amenable to manipulation of the thoracic spine and rib cage. The reader is referred to other chapters of this book for other examination procedures. The examination is described by the patient's position.

Postural screen of the thoracic spine and rib cage

The examination of the thoracic spine begins with a postural screen aiming to identify regions of the thoracic spine that deviate from what is considered a normal, smooth thoracic kyphosis. Areas of increased or decreased kyphosis involving the upper, mid and lower thoracic regions can be recorded. Observation for thoracic postural deviation in this fashion has fair-to-moderate reliability (Cleland et al 2006). For the clinical prediction rule developed by Cleland et al (2007a), a reduction in the upper thoracic kyphosis emerged as a predictor variable for success with thoracic manipulation in patients with mechanical neck pain. The examiner can palpate for alterations in the normal thoracic curvature by running his or her fingers along either side of the thoracic spine in the region of the paraspinal muscles. Areas of altered soft tissue tension and tenderness suggestive of underlying segmental dysfunction can be detected. Additionally, the examiner can palpate the rib angles for tenderness by having the patient place his or her ipsilateral hand on the opposite shoulder to abduct the scapula out of the way. Tenderness of the rib angle is suggestive of underlying dysfunction of the rib (Flynn et al 2001).

Thoracic spine active range of motion

Active mobility testing of the thoracic spine in sitting commences with testing the patient's active range of motion in cardinal planes. Overpressure is applied if the motion is not pain provoking. Range of motion can be recorded using a bubble inclinometer over selected thoracic levels. The inclinometer is placed in the sagittal plane for flexion / extension and in the frontal plane for side-bending (Molina et al 2000). Seated active thoracic rotation followed by clinician overpressure can serve as a clinically efficient screen of thoracic spine. Pain and a visual gross judgement of range of motion can be recorded quickly with this test.

Mobility testing of the first rib

Screening for elevation of the first rib is completed in sitting with the examiner palpating the relative height of the first rib. The first rib is found and palpated by standing behind the patient and pulling back the upper trapezius muscle. The clinician can then rest his or her fingers on the posterior superior aspect of the first rib and make a visual judgement of the relative height of the first rib. The cervical rotation lateral flexion test (CRLF) advocated by Lindgren et al (1989) can also be performed to screen for elevation of the first rib. During this test the cervical spine is passively rotated to the contralateral side and then maximally side-bent in the sagittal plane. A reduction in side-bending mobility is suggestive of an elevated first rib on the side opposite from that to which the cervical spine was rotated.

Mobility testing of the first rib with the patient in supine is undertaken by the clinician applying a caudal glide to the posterior, superior aspect of the first rib using the palmar side of the second metacarpal phalangeal joint. Mobility or pain is recorded and is suggestive of dysfunction of the first rib. The clinician can also screen the first rib during inspiration and expiration by palpating the anterior aspect underneath the medial clavicle. A relative reduction in the excursion of motion during inspiration and expiration is suggestive of hypomobility of the first rib.

Segmental mobility testing of the thoracic spine and rib cage

The remaining ribs can be screened in a similar fashion and, conventionally, they are examined in groups of three to four dividing the rib cage into the upper, mid and lower regions. The clinician can also perform passive accessory mobility of the anterior ribs by springing in an anterior to posterior direction over the costosternal joints utilizing the thumbs (Maitland et al 2001). The clinician records the presence or absence of pain and notes whether the mobility is normal, hypomobile or hypermobile for each rib (Heiderscheit & Boissonnault 2008).

Segmental mobility testing of the thoracic spine, utilizing posterior to anterior spring testing, is conducted with the patient prone. The clinician screens the thoracic spine for mobility and pain by applying his or her hypothenar eminence to the thoracic spinous process and producing a graded posterior-to-anterior force. The examiner records the presence or absence of pain and notes whether the mobility is normal, hypomobile or hypermobile for each thoracic segment (Cleland et al 2006; Heiderscheit & Boissonnault 2008). The clinician can spring unilaterally over the thoracic transverse processes in a similar fashion. The ribs are also screened for mobility and pain. Using a crossed-hands technique, the clinician stabilizes the opposite side of the thoracic spine with his or her hypothenar eminence lateral to the spinous process and springs over each rib angle, utilizing the hypothenar eminence of the opposite hand. Segmental mobility testing of the thoracic spine has poor-to-fair inter-rater reliability for assessment of both pain and mobility in patients with neck pain (Cleland et al 2006). In two studies involving subjects without symptoms, reliability of segmental mobility testing of the thoracic spine and ribs improved when an expanded definition of agreement was utilized (Christensen et al 2002; Heiderscheit & Boissonnault 2008); due to the potential inaccuracy of identifying a specific thoracic spinal level, these authors allowed for mobility agreement within and between raters to within ±1 vertebral level.

Interpretation of the examination and reassessment

Using a compilation of the above examination procedures, the clinician can make a reasonable clinical judgement regarding the presence / absence of thoracic spine mobility impairments. Mobility impairments of the thoracic spine and rib cage are common clinically, both in patients with upper quarter musculoskeletal pain and also in those without symptoms (Heiderscheit & Boissonnault 2008). Similar to other spinal regions, thoracic spine mobility becomes reduced with increasing age (Edmondston & Singer 1997). Previous experts in manipulative therapy have described a detailed examination scheme in attempts to identify the segment and the direction of specific mobility impairments of the thoracic spine and rib cage. Following these biomechanical diagnoses, a manipulative procedure is then selected that matches the specified movement dysfunction. As stated above, reliability of segmental mobility testing of the thoracic spine and rib cage is fair. Additionally, research has shown that examination and manual therapy intervention procedures affect a region of the spine rather than a specific segment (Powers et al 2003; Ross et al 2004). We therefore propose a pragmatic examination process based on recent evidence. For example, to identify mobility impairments of a region of the thoracic spine, the examiner should find increased or decreased thoracic kyphosis in that region, limited active range of motion, soft tissue hypertonicity or tenderness, and hypomobility with spring testing. This examination scheme is also applied to the rib cage. Tenderness over the rib angle, reduced excursion during respiration and hypomobility with spring testing over the anterior or posterior aspect of the rib all suggest a mobility impairment of the rib. To identify a mobility impairment of the first rib, the examiner could use a combination of reduced mobility with spring testing, reduced excursion during respiration, tenderness over the rib angle, the presence of perceived superior elevation of the rib and a positive CRLF test. To identify the thoracic spine as a pain generator or source of the patient's symptoms, the patient's familiar symptoms should be reproduced with examination procedures. For example, in the case report by Boyle (1999) the clinician reproduced the patient's familiar shoulder pain with posterior to anterior spring over the shaft of the ipsilateral second rib.

Often clinicians apply manual therapy procedures to an asymptomatic region of the thoracic spine in patients with neck or upper extremity disorders. Therefore, we recommend that the clinician bases the success or value of a particular technique on the effect it has on functional movement of the region of symptoms. For example, following manipulation of the thoracic spine, the clinician can then reassess the pain and range of motion associated with shoulder elevation in a patient with subacromial impingement syndrome. Likewise, pain-free grip strength could be retested after thoracic or rib thrust manipulation for a patient with lateral elbow pain. For patients with primary complaint of thoracic spine pain, functional reassessment procedures involving the thoracic spine, such as seated trunk rotation, are utilized.

Manual Therapy Interventions for the Thoracic Spine and Rib Cage

Complications from thrust or non-thrust manipulation of the thoracic spine are rare. As part of a comprehensive examination, a patient should be screened for conditions that require medical referral or contraindicate manipulation. Typical contraindications for manipulation in the thoracic region would include bone weakness or demineralization resulting from neoplasms, trauma, infection or metabolic conditions (osteoporosis). The presence of signs of central cord compression, suggesting a possible massive thoracic disc herniation, also contraindicates manipulation until diagnostic imaging is obtained. When deciding whether an individual patient would benefit from thoracic manipulation, it is helpful to consider the inclusion and exclusion criteria of clinical trials involving thoracic manipulation. For example, several trials had an age limit of 18–60 (Cleland et al 2005b, 2007a, 2007c, 2010; Masaracchio et al 2013) whereas in others the limit was 18–45 (González-Iglesias et al 2009a, 2009b). With proper patient screening, thoracic spine manipulation is inherently safe provided the clinician is properly trained in the techniques and avoids the unnecessary use of excessive force or amplitude. Minor side effects of temporary soreness are common after manipulation, so it is helpful to warn patients so that they are not alarmed (Cleland et al 2007c).

Biomechanical theories abound to explain the mechanisms by which spinal manipulation produces clinically important reduction in pain and disability. Specifically for the thoracic spine, it is thought that an improvement in mobility in the thoracic region following manipulation allows for enhanced pain-free mobility of the cervical or upper extremity region. It has also been proposed that improving mobility in the thoracic spine will take stress off of adjacent, hypermobile cervical spine or shoulder joints. However, evidence is emerging that mechanisms behind the effects of manual therapy procedures have a predominantly neurophysiological component (Bialosky et al 2009). Analgesic effects after manipulation are thought to occur at the peripheral, spinal cord and central nervous system levels. Effects include a reduction in reflexive muscular activity surrounding the spinal region manipulated, inhibition of pain production through gaiting mechanisms and activation of endogenous opioids, and alteration of pain processing in the brain. Non-specific effects involving a placebo response and patients' expectations of the treatment probably play a role in the effects of manual therapy (Bialosky et al 2008). With this in mind, clinicians can select particular manipulative techniques based on patient comfort, clinician experience and skill, and evidence from high-quality research as opposed to selecting a procedure that matches a particular biomechanical lesion. Descriptions of manual techniques for both the thoracic spine and ribs follow; techniques for this chapter were selected based on what has been utilized in published clinical trials and the authors' clinical experience. For a comprehensive description of other thoracic spine manipulation techniques, readers are referred to other texts (Flynn et al 2001; Maitland et al 2001; Gibbons & Tehan 2006). In keeping with the recent recommendations for manual therapy terminology, all procedures will be referred to as manipulations (Mintken et al 2008). Thrust manipulation will refer to those techniques involving a quick or high-velocity thrust. Non-thrust manipulations are techniques applied with lower velocity in a graded fashion.

Seated upper thoracic thrust manipulation

The patient sits on a treatment table with his or her hands clasped behind the neck, and as low down on the cervical spine as possible (Fig. 13.1). The clinician stands behind the patient, loops the hands through the patient's arms and places the hands clasped over the patient's hands. The clinician then leans backwards to take up slack in a superior direction. A thrust is delivered by the clinician thrusting upwards towards the ceiling in an attempt to create a distraction force in the patient's upper thoracic region. The thrust should be generated by the clinician's legs. Care is taken with this procedure

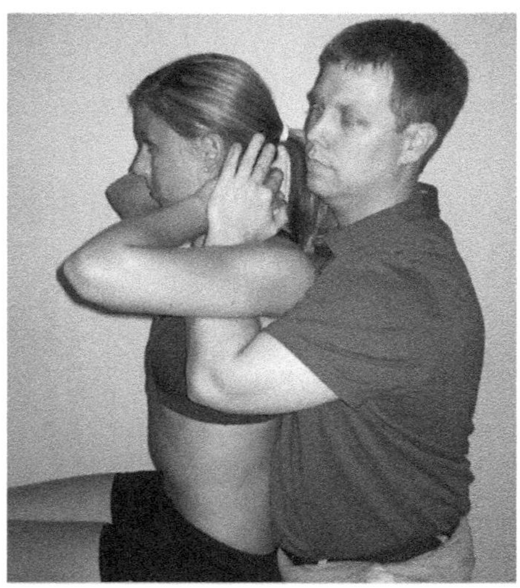

Figure 13.1 Seated upper thoracic thrust manipulation.

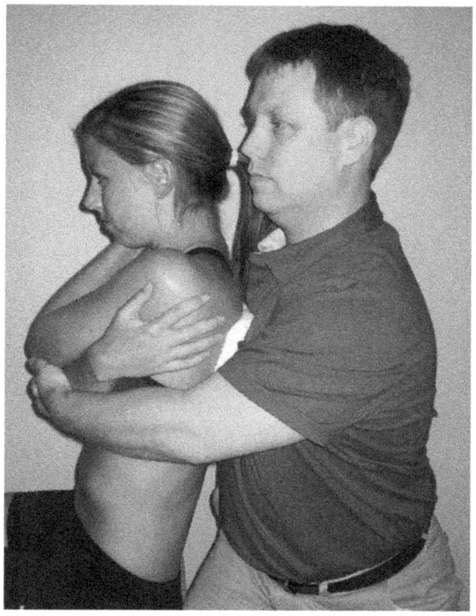

Figure 13.2 **Seated mid-thoracic thrust manipulation.**

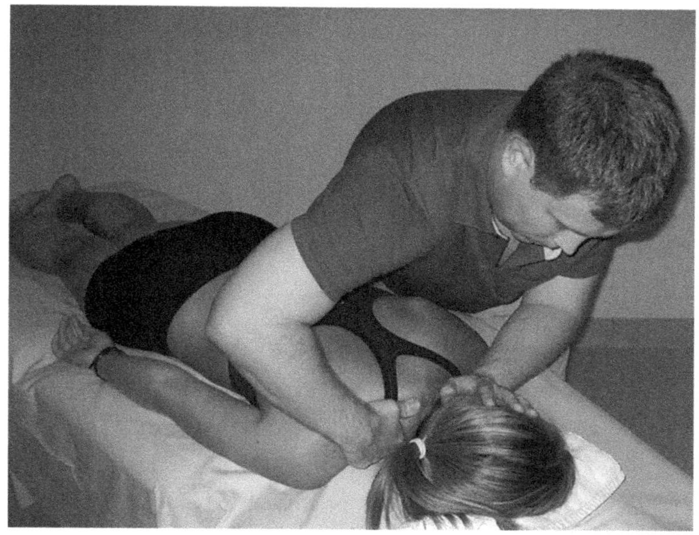

Figure 13.3 **Prone upper thoracic thrust manipulation.**

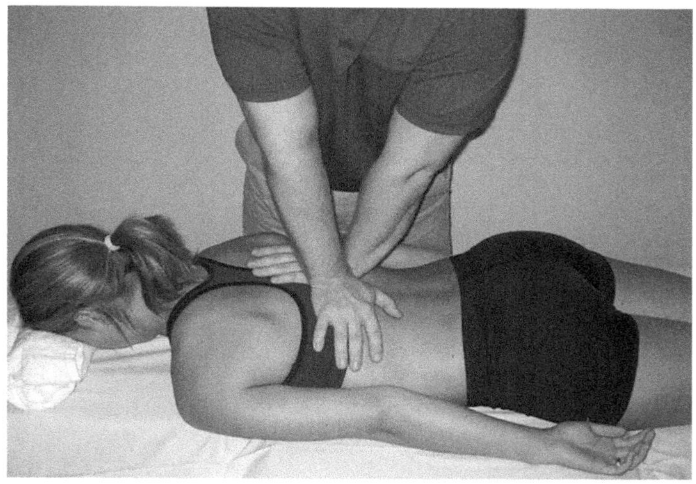

Figure 13.4 **Prone mid-thoracic thrust and non-thrust manipulation.**

not to strain to the patient's shoulder girdle. If the patient experiences shoulder discomfort or is unable to attain the position with his or her arms then this technique is abandoned.

Seated mid-thoracic thrust manipulation

The patient sits on the treatment table with his or her arms across the body with the hands grasping the opposite posterior shoulder region (Fig. 13.2). Clinical experience suggests that the most comfortable position is with the elbows in parallel; this also allows for the clinician to attempt the technique on a larger patient. The clinician applies the sternum to the patient's mid-thoracic spine. Alternatively a rolled towel can be placed horizontally on the caudal vertebra of the segment of interest between the patient and the clinician in an attempt to be segment specific. The clinician reaches round the patient and grasps the patient's lower elbow. If possible the clinician interlocks the hands. The clinician takes up slack by adducting the arms, retracting the shoulder girdle, and pushing the chest towards the patient's thoracic spine. A high-velocity thrust is performed by the clinician thrusting through the patient's arms in an anterior-to-posterior direction whilst keeping the chest pushed forwards. Some clinicians attempt to produce a distractive force by lifting the patient during this procedure, although with a larger patient this could potentially injure the clinician. If the clinician cannot reasonably reach his or her arms around the patient, another technique should be selected.

Prone upper thoracic thrust manipulation

With the patient lying prone, the clinician stands to one side of the patient. The clinician rotates the patient's head and neck to the opposite side (Fig. 13.3). The clinician then applies either the thumb or pisiform to the lateral aspect of the spinous process of the caudal vertebra of the segment of interest. Slack is taken up by the clinician applying the other hand to the patient's head and gently applying further rotation, contralateral side-bending and extension until the spinous process of the segment begins to first move. The clinician delivers the thrust to the spinous process by translating it across the table in an attempt to 'gap' the joint on the opposite side. During the thrust the clinician maintains the patient's head and neck position with the opposite hand. Care is taken to avoid thrusting through the patient's head and neck. If the patient experiences pain in the cervical region during the technique it can be attempted from the other side with the cervical spine rotated in the opposite direction, or another technique should be selected.

Prone mid-thoracic thrust and non-thrust manipulation

With the patient prone the examiner applies the hypothenar eminences just lateral to the spinous processes over the mid-thoracic region (Fig. 13.4). Slack is taken up by the examiner slightly twisting his or her hands in order to obtain a soft tissue or skin lock. From this position, graded non-thrust manipulations or a thrust manipulation can be delivered in a posterior-to-anterior direction towards the table. The thrust can deliver after the patient exhales. Care is taken to avoid producing excessive force or amplitude with this procedure. The clinician should ensure that the contact is just lateral to the spinous process so as to avoid injury to the patient's ribs. The clinician should adjust the angle of the hand placement, based on the contour of the patient's kyphosis, in order to remain perpendicular to the spine.

Supine upper and mid-thoracic thrust manipulation

With the patient supine the clinician instructs the patient to roll to his or her side. The clinician places one hand on the caudal vertebra of the segment of interest in the upper or mid thoracic region. The clinician's hand then serves as the fulcrum for the manipulation. A number of hand-holds are possible, including either a pistol grip or an open-hand technique. With the pistol grip the transverse processes of the thoracic segment are stabilized by the clinician's hypothenar eminence and second metacarpophalangeal joint with the spinous process in between (Fig. 13.5). With the open-hand technique, the clinician applies his thenar eminence to one side of the thoracic spine just lateral to the spinous process (Fig. 13.6). The clinician then rolls the patient back to the fully supine position whilst maintaining the hand position. The patient is instructed to either clasp his or her hands behind the neck (Fig. 13.7) or cross the arms across the chest with the elbows parallel (Fig. 13.8). Patient arm positioning is based on patient and clinician preference. Some patients prefer the hands clasped behind the neck to avoid pressure on the chest or breast tissue. Others report discomfort in the cervical region or are unable to obtain this position owing to inflexibility of the upper extremities. From this position, the clinician uses the other hand to flex or extend the patient down the region of interest so pressure is felt just over the clinician's bottom hand serving as the fulcrum. This is accomplished by the clinician either cradling the patient's head and neck (Fig. 13.9) or using the patient's arm (Fig. 13.10).

Clinical experience suggests that extension is usually utilized in the upper thoracic region from T1 to T3, whereas

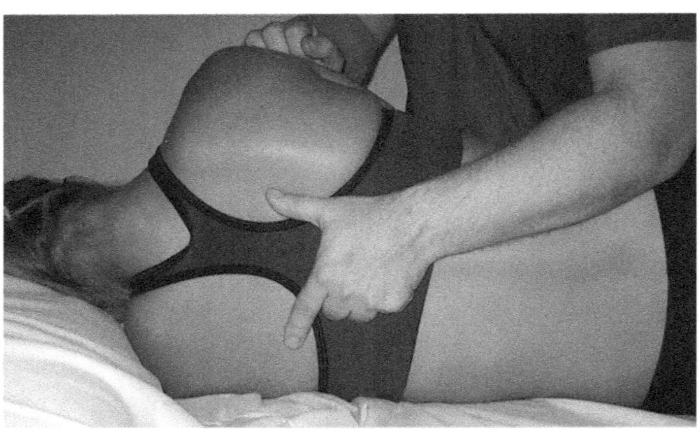

Figure 13.5 Pistol grip for supine upper and mid-thoracic thrust manipulation.

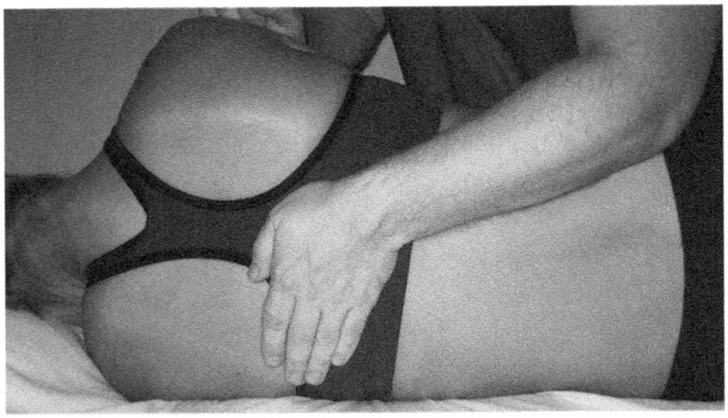

Figure 13.6 Open hand for supine upper and mid-thoracic thrust manipulation.

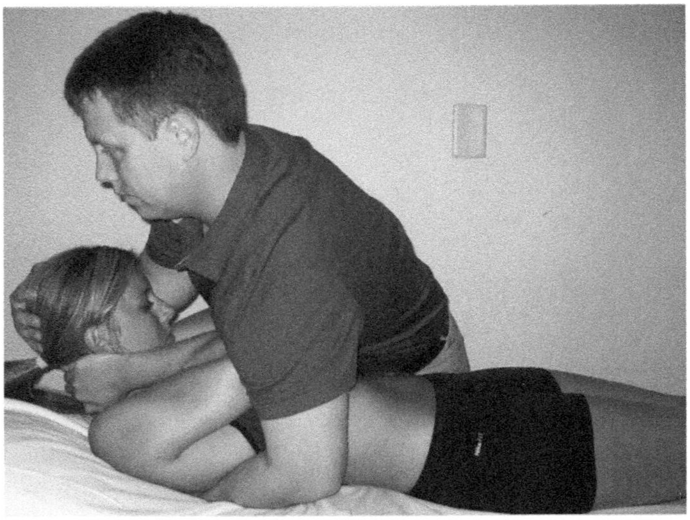

Figure 13.7 Supine upper and mid-thoracic thrust manipulation with hands behind the neck.

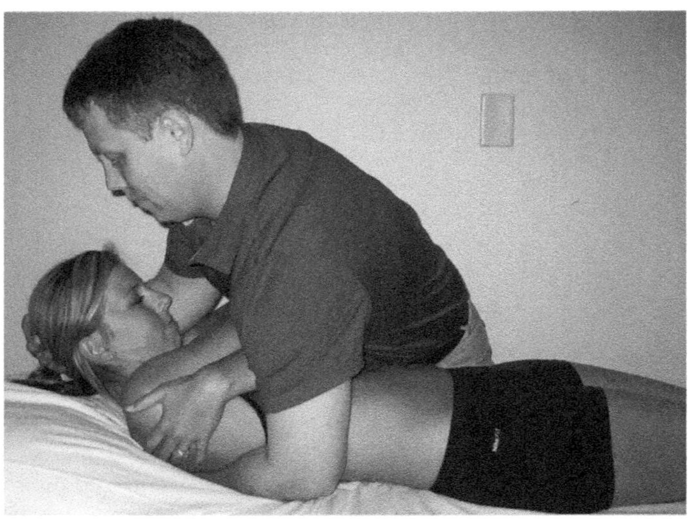

Figure 13.8 Supine upper and mid-thoracic thrust manipulation with arms across the chest.

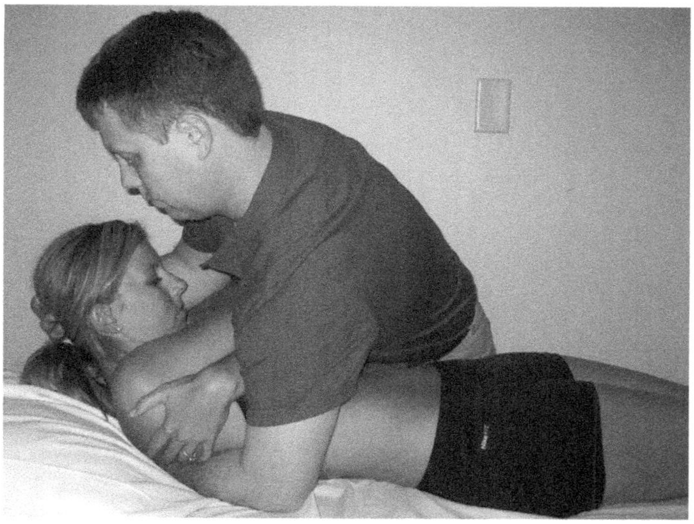

Figure 13.9 Supine upper and mid-thoracic thrust manipulation with head flexion.

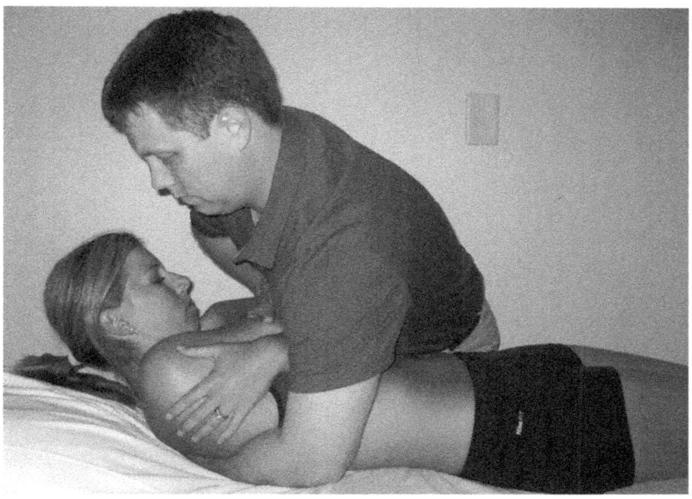

Figure 13.10 Supine upper and mid-thoracic thrust manipulation with hand flexion.

flexion is usually utilized in the mid thoracic region (T4–T9). The clinician then takes up the slack by applying an anterior-to-posterior and slightly cranial force through the patient's arms and towards the fulcrum on the table. A thrust is delivered by the clinician through the patient's arms and towards the table. The thrust can be delivered after patient exhalation. Care is taken to avoid producing excessive force or amplitude with this technique. If the patient experiences pain in the shoulder the technique can be modified so that one of the patient's arms is crossed over the chest while the painful shoulder is left comfortably on the table (Fig. 13.11).

Seated first-rib thrust and non-thrust manipulation

The patient sits on the table and the clinician stands behind the patient with one foot on the table and the knee in the

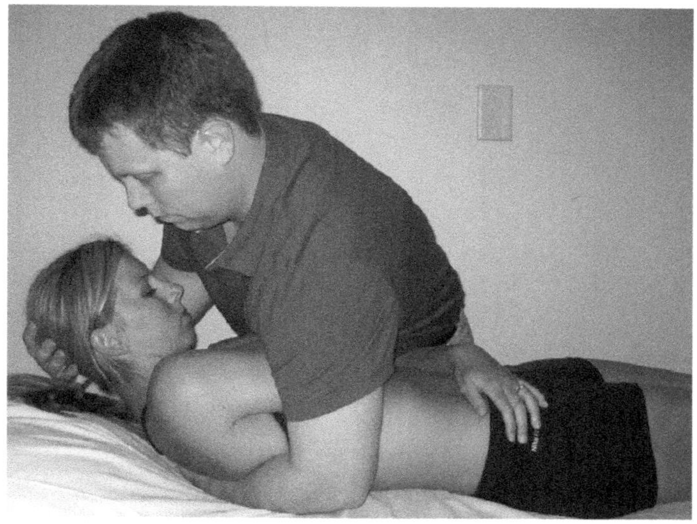

Figure 13.11 Supine upper and mid-thoracic thrust manipulation adapted for patients with painful shoulder.

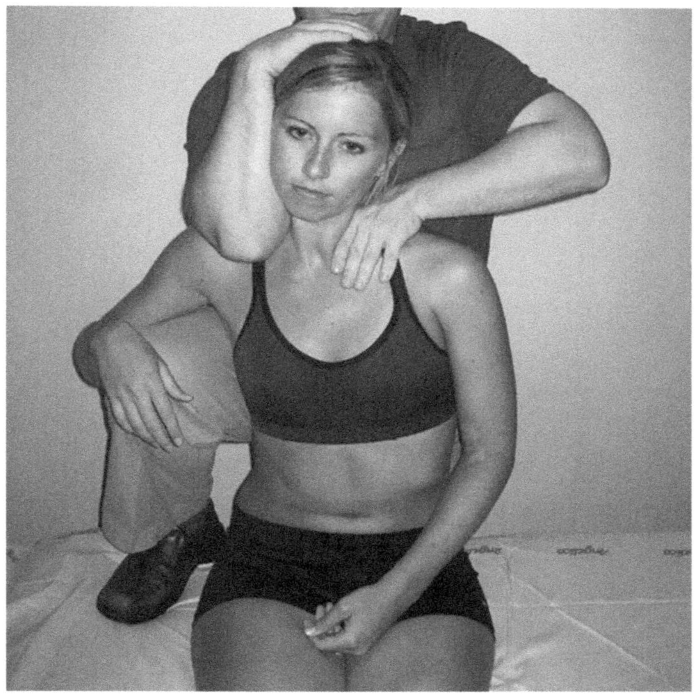

Figure 13.12 Seated first-rib thrust and non-thrust manipulation.

patient's axilla on the side opposite that of the manipulation (Fig. 13.12). The clinician applies the chest to the patient's thoracic region and places the forearm along the patient's head and cervical region, again on the opposite side. The clinician contacts the posterior, superior aspect of the patient's first rib with either the palmar aspect of the second metacarpophalangeal joint or the hypothenar eminence. The clinician, using the whole body, translates the patient towards the knee to produce side-bending of the cervical and thoracic region towards the side to be manipulated. This places the patient's scalene muscles on slack and brings the first rib towards the clinician's thrusting hand. Further localization is achieved by the clinician slightly retracting the patient's cervical spine and

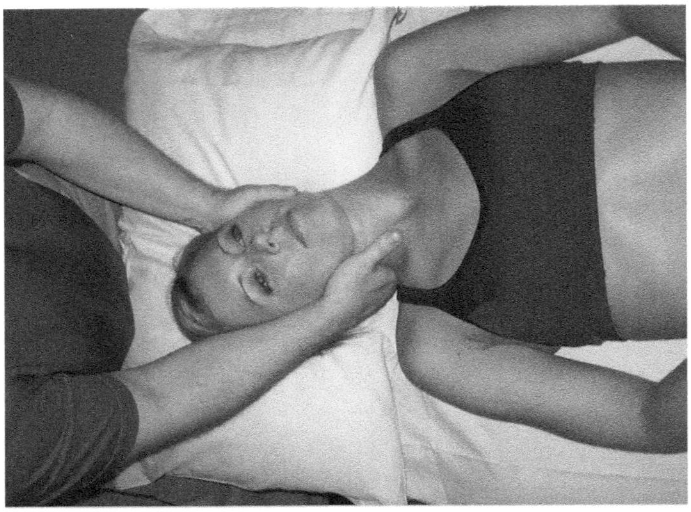

Figure 13.13 **Supine first-rib thrust and non-thrust manipulation.**

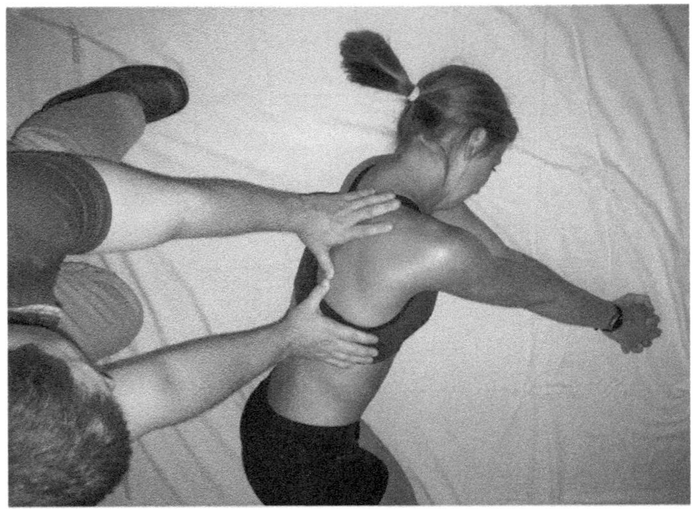

Figure 13.14 **Side-lying ribs non-thrust manipulation.**

rotating it to the opposite side. The clinician can then deliver graded non-thrust manipulations, or a thrust in a caudal and medial direction. Care is taken not to compress the patient's cervical spine with the non-thrusting hand.

Supine first-rib thrust and non-thrust manipulation

With the patient supine, the clinician contacts the posterior, superior aspect of the patient's first rib with the palmar aspect of the second metacarpophalangeal joint (Fig. 13.13). With the opposite hand the clinician then side-bends the patient's neck towards the side to be manipulated so as to put the scalene muscles on slack. The clinician performs graded non-thrust manipulation or a thrust in a caudal and medial direction; the thrust can be performed after patient exhalation.

Prone or side-lying ribs non-thrust manipulation

To perform non-thrust manipulation of the ribs, the clinician can contact either the rib angle in prone or the costosternal joints in supine, and apply non-thrust mobilizations. These non-thrust manipulations can also be performed in side-lying with the patient's trunk rotated to either side in order to improve thoracic spine rotation (Fig. 13.14).

Supine ribs thrust manipulation

This technique is almost identical to the supine thoracic thrust manipulation. To manipulate the rib, the clinician stands on the opposite side of the rib to be manipulated. The clinician instructs the patient to roll to one side and contacts the rib just lateral to the transverse process with the thenar eminence (Fig. 13.15). The patient is rolled back into the supine position. The patient is then instructed to either clasp the hands behind the neck or place the arms across the chest. The clinician then flexes or extends the patient's trunk to localize the force towards the rib. The clinician delivers a thrust to the rib

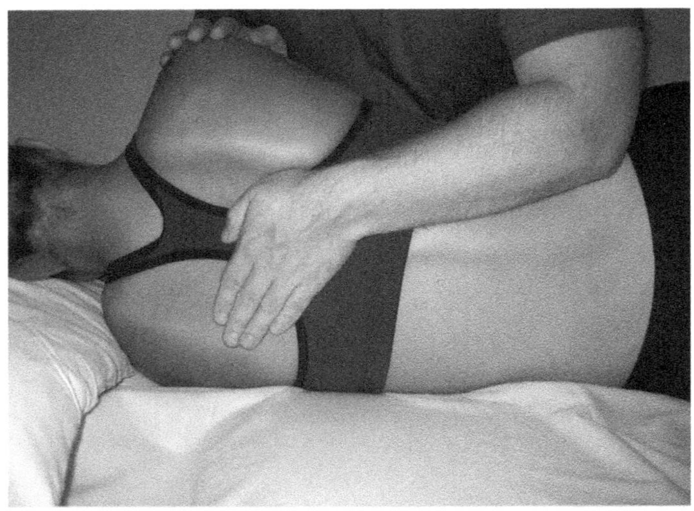

Figure 13.15 **Contact for supine ribs thrust manipulation.**

through the patient's arms and towards the table. The thrust can be delivered after patient exhalation. Care is taken to avoid using excessive amplitude or force. This technique tends to be less comfortable than the supine thoracic thrust so it is best to perform it quickly so that pressure is not applied to the patient's rib for a long period of time.

Exercise interventions to augment the manual therapy techniques

Typically both thoracic thrust and non-thrust manipulations are augmented by patient self-mobilization exercises. In the authors' clinical experience, it is advantageous to follow manual therapy procedures immediately with active exercise. It has been suggested that manual therapy provides a window of opportunity after which exercise is facilitated (Raney et al 2007). The reader is directed to other chapters of this book for upper quarter strengthening and stretching exercises and for mobility exercises involving other upper quarter regions. The following text describes exercises to improve thoracic spine and rib cage mobility.

For the patient who lacks extension range of motion, an extension mobilization exercise can be utilized. The patient is instructed to clasp the hands behind the neck in order to stabilize the cervical spine. A fulcrum is placed in the region to be mobilized and the patient performs thoracic extension over the fulcrum. Several objects can be utilized as a fulcrum, including the arm of a couch, the back of a chair, a foam roller, a rolled towel or a mobilization wedge.

For the patient lacking thoracic spine flexion, a 'flexion mobilization' exercise is utilized. This can be accomplished in either quadruped or with the patient's hands on the wall in a push-up position. The patient is instructed to flex the cervical and thoracic spine and protract the scapulae. This exercise has the added benefit of activating the serratus anterior muscles.

Patients with rib mobility restrictions can be instructed in the 'barrel hug' exercise. With the patient seated, the clinician instructs the patient to pretend that he / she is holding onto a large barrel, which produces thoracic flexion and shoulder girdle protraction. The patient is then instructed to side-bend and rotate the trunk away from the side of the hypomobile rib. The patient can be instructed to perform this during full exhalation.

The 'side-lying arm sweep' exercise can be used for general thoracic spine and rib cage mobility. The patient lies on one side and, starting with the arm overhead, sweeps the arm downwards towards the legs and the back, up and around to the starting position. The patient can pause in areas where stiffness or a stretching sensation is felt and oscillate the shoulder girdle into protraction / retraction and trunk into rotation.

First-rib hypomobility is addressed by the patient applying a downward pressure to the rib with a rolled towel or sheet. The sheet or towel is looped over the patient's shoulder and onto the first rib. The patient is instructed to drop the ipsilateral shoulder down and side-bend the cervical spine towards the rib to put the scalene muscles on slack. Using the towel, the patient can apply a mobilization to the rib in a caudal direction.

Conclusion

In patients with upper quarter musculoskeletal disorders, the thoracic spine and rib cage may play a significant role. The thoracic spine and rib cage are biomechanically linked to the cervical spine and upper extremity. Mobility impairments of the thoracic spine and rib cage are common in patients with upper quarter disorders. Evidence has shown that manual therapy interventions targeting the thoracic spine and rib cage can lead to positive outcomes in patients with a variety of upper quarter musculoskeletal disorders. Utilizing the concept of regional interdependence, the clinician should screen the thoracic spine and rib cage and address impairments found in patients presenting with neck, shoulder and elbow disorders. Thoracic spine manual therapy procedures are rarely used in isolation, but instead comprise part of a comprehensive, multimodal treatment programme utilizing manual therapy for other upper quarter regions, exercise and patient education. Future research will assist the clinician in identifying patients who will benefit from thoracic manipulation and also in determining the optimal dosage of manipulation.

References

Bang MD, Deyle GD. 2000. Comparison of supervised exercise with and without manual physical therapy for patients with shoulder impingement syndrome. J Orthop Sports Phys Ther 30: 126–137.

Benhamou CL, Roux C, Tourliere D, et al. 1993. Pseudovisceral pain referred from costovertebral arthropathies: twenty-eight cases. Spine 18: 790–795.

Berglund KM, Persson BH, Denison E. 2008. Prevalence of pain and dysfunction in the cervical and thoracic spine in persons with and without lateral elbow pain. Man Ther 13: 295–299.

Bergman GJ, Winters JC, Groenier KH, et al. 2004. Manipulative therapy in addition to usual medical care for patients with shoulder dysfunction and pain: a randomized, controlled trial. Ann Intern Med 141: 432–439.

Bialosky JE, Bishop MD, Robinson ME, et al. 2008. The influence of expectation on spinal manipulation induced hypoalgesia: an experimental study in normal subjects. BMC Musculoskelet Disord 9: 19.

Bialosky JE, Bishop MD, Price DD, et al. 2009. The mechanisms of manual therapy in the treatment of musculoskeletal pain: a comprehensive model. Man Ther 14: 531–538.

Boyle JJ. 1999. Is the pain and dysfunction of shoulder impingement lesion really second rib syndrome in disguise? Two case reports. Man Ther 4: 44–48.

Boyles RE, Ritland BM, Miracle BM, et al. 2009. The short-term effects of thoracic spine thrust manipulation on patients with shoulder impingement syndrome. Man Ther 14: 375–380.

Browder DA, Erhard RE, Piva SR. 2004. Intermittent cervical traction and thoracic manipulation for management of mild cervical compressive myelopathy attributed to cervical herniated disc: a case series. J Orthop Sports Phys Ther 34: 701–712.

Bruckner FE, Allard SA, Moussa NA. 1987. Benign thoracic pain. J R Soc Med 80: 286–289.

Childs JD, Flynn T, Fritz J, et al. 2005. Screening for vertebrobasilar insufficiency in patients with neck pain: manual therapy decision-making in the presence of uncertainty. J Orthop Sports Phys Ther 35: 300–306.

Christensen HW, Vach W, Vach K, et al. 2002. Palpation of the upper thoracic spine: an observer reliability study. J Manipulative Physiol Ther 25: 285–292.

Cleland JA, Selleck BS, Stowel TEA. 2004a. Short-term effects of thoracic manipulation on lower trapezius muscle strength. J Man Manip Ther 12: 82–90.

Cleland JA, Whitman JM, Fritz JM. 2004b. Effectiveness of manual physical therapy to the cervical spine in the management of lateral epicondylalgia: a retrospective analysis. J Orthop Sports Phys Ther 34: 713–722.

Cleland JA, Flynn TW, Palmer J. 2005a. Incorporation of manual therapy directed at the cervico-thoracic spine in patients with lateral epicondylalgia: a pilot clinical trial. J Man Manip Ther 13: 143–151.

Cleland JA, Childs JD, McRae M, et al. 2005b. Immediate effects of thoracic manipulation in patients with neck pain: a randomized clinical trial. Man Ther 10: 127–135.

Cleland JA, Whitman JM, Fritz JM, et al. 2005c. Manual physical therapy, cervical traction, and strengthening exercises in patients with cervical radiculopathy: a case series. J Orthop Sports Phys Ther 35: 802–811.

Cleland JA, Childs JD, Fritz JM, et al. 2006. Inter-rater reliability of the history and physical examination in patients with mechanical neck pain. Arch Phys Med Rehabil 87: 1388–1395.

Cleland JA, Childs JD, Fritz JM, et al. 2007a. Development of a clinical prediction rule for guiding treatment of a subgroup of patients with neck pain: use of thoracic spine manipulation, exercise, and patient education. Phys Ther 87: 9–23.

Cleland JA, Fritz JM, Whitman JM, et al. 2007b. Predictors of short-term outcome in people with a clinical diagnosis of cervical radiculopathy. Phys Ther 87: 1619–1632.

Cleland JA, Glynn P, Whitman JM, et al. 2007c. Short-term effects of thrust versus non-thrust mobilization / manipulation directed at the thoracic spine in patients with neck pain: a randomized clinical trial. Phys Ther 87: 431–440.

Cleland JA, Mintken PE, Carpenter K, et al. 2010. Examination of a clinical prediction rule to identify patients with neck pain likely to benefit from thoracic spine thrust manipulation and a general cervical range of motion exercise: multi-center randomized clinical trial. Phys Ther 90: 1239–1250.

Conroy JL, Schneiders AG. 2005. The T4 syndrome. Man Ther 10: 292–296.

Cropper JR. 1996. Regional anatomy and biomechanics. In: Flynn TW (ed) The thoracic spine and ribcage. Boston: Butterworth-Heinemann, pp 3–30.

Crosbie J, Kilbreath SL, Hollmann L, et al. 2008. Scapulo-humeral rhythm and associated spinal motion. Clin Biomech 23: 184–192.

Cross KM, Keunze C, Grindstaff T, et al. 2011. Thoracic spine thrust manipulation improves pain, range of motion, self-reported function in patients with mechanical neck pain: a systematic review. J Orthop Sports Phys Ther 41: 633–642.

Dreyfuss P, Tibiletti C, Dreyer SJ. 1994. Thoracic zygapophyseal joint pain patterns. A study in normal volunteers. Spine 19: 807–811.

Edmondston SJ, Singer KP. 1997. Thoracic spine: anatomical and biomechanical considerations for manual therapy. Man Ther 2: 132–143.

Fernández-de-las-Peñas C, Fernández-Carnero J, Fernández AP, et al. 2004. Dorsal manipulation in whiplash injury treatment: a randomized controlled trial. J Whiplash Relat Disord 3: 55–72.

Fernández-de-las-Peñas C, Palomeque-del-Cerro L, Rodriguez-Blanco C, et al. 2007. Changes in neck pain and active range of motion after a single thoracic spine manipulation in subjects presenting with mechanical neck pain: a case series. J Manipulative Physiol Ther 30: 312–320.

Flynn T, Whitman J, Magel J. 2001. Orthopaedic manual physical therapy management of the cervical-thoracic spine and ribcage. Louisville, KY: Evidence in Motion.

Fruth SJ. 2006. Differential diagnosis and treatment in a patient with posterior upper thoracic pain. Phys Ther 86: 254–268.

Fukui S, Ohseto K, Shiotani M. 1997. Patterns of pain induced by distending the thoracic zygapophyseal joints. Reg Anesth 22: 332–336.

Gibbons P, Tehan P, 2006. Manipulation of the spine thorax and pelvis, 2nd edn. Edinburgh: Churchill Livingstone.

González-Iglesias J, Fernández-de-las-Peñas C , Cleland JA, et al. 2009a. Inclusion of thoracic spine thrust manipulation into an electro-therapy / thermal program for the management of patients with acute mechanical neck pain: a randomized clinical trial. Man Ther 14: 306–313.

González-Iglesias J, Fernández-de-las-Peñas C, Cleland JA, et al. 2009b. Thoracic spine manipulation for the management of patients with neck pain: a randomized clinical trial. J Orthop Sports Phys Ther 39: 20–27.

Hamberg J, Lindahl O. 1981. Angina pectoris symptoms caused by thoracic spine disorders: clinical examination and treatment. Acta Med Scand 644: S84–86.

Heiderscheit B, Boissonnault W. 2008. Reliability of joint mobility and pain assessment of the thoracic spine and rib cage in asymptomatic individuals. J Man Manip Ther 16: 210–216.

Huisman PA, Speksnijder CM, de Wijer A. 2013. The effects of thoracic spine manipulation in individuals with non-specific neck pain: a systematic review. Disabil Rehabil 35: 1677–1685.

Jull G, Trott P, Potter H, et al. 2002. A randomized controlled trial of exercise and manipulative therapy for cervicogenic headache. Spine 27:1835–1843.

Kebaetse M, McClure P, Pratt NA. 1999. Thoracic position effect on shoulder range of motion, strength, and three-dimensional scapular kinematics. Arch Phys Med Rehabil 80: 945–950.

Kelley JL, Whitney SL. 2006. The use of non-thrust manipulation in an adolescent for the treatment of thoracic pain and rib dysfunction: a case report. J Orthop Sports Phys Ther 36: 887–892.

Krauss J, Creighton D, Ely JD, et al. 2008. The immediate effects of upper thoracic translatoric spinal manipulation on cervical pain and range of motion: a randomized clinical trial. J Man Manip Ther 16: 93–99.

Lau HM, Wing Chiu TT, Lam TH. 2011. The effectiveness of thoracic manipulation on patients with chronic mechanical neck pain – a randomized controlled trial. Man Ther 16: 141–147. doi: 10.1016/j.math.2010.08.003.

Liebler EJ, Tufano-Coors L, Douris P, et al. 2001. The effect of thoracic spine mobilization on lower trapezius strength testing. J Man Manip Ther 9: 207–212.

Lindgren KA, Leino E, Manninen H. 1989. Cineradiography of the hypomobile first rib. Arch Phys Med Rehabil 70: 408–409.

Maitland GD, Banks K, English K, et al. 2001. Maitland's vertebral manipulation, 6th edn. London: Butterworth.

Masaracchio M, Cleland J, Hellman M, et al. 2013. Short-term combined effects of thoracic thrust manipulation and cervical non-thrust manipulation in individuals with mechanical neck pain: a randomized clinical trial. J Orthop Sports Phys Ther 43: 118–127.

Menck JY, Requejo SM, Kulig K. 2000. Thoracic spine dysfunction in upper extremity complex regional pain syndrome type I. J Orthop Sports Phys Ther 30: 401–409.

Mintken PE, Cleland JA, Carpenter KJ, et al. 2010. Some factors predict successful short-term outcomes in individuals with shoulder pain receiving cervicothoracic manipulation: a single-arm trial. Phys Ther 90: 26–42.

Mintken PE, DeRosa C, Littl T, et al; American Academy of Orthopaedic Manual Physical Therapists. 2008. AAOMPT clinical guidelines: a model for standardizing manipulation terminology in physical therapy practice. J Orthop Sports Phys Ther 38: A1–A6.

Molina C, Robbins D, Roberts H, et al. 2000. Reliability and validity of single inclinometer measurements for thoracic spine range of motion (abstract). J Man Manip Ther 8: 143.

Muth S, Barbe MR, Lauer R, et al. 2012. The effects of thoracic spine manipulation in subjects with rotator cuff tendinopathy. J Orthop Sports Phys Ther 42: 1005–1016.

Norlander S, Nordgren B. 1998. Clinical symptoms related to musculoskeletal neck–shoulder pain and mobility in the cervico-thoracic spine. Scand J Rehabil Med 30: 243–251.

Norlander S, Aste-Norlander U, Nordgren B, et al. 1996. Mobility in the cervico-thoracic motion segment: an indicative factor of musculo-skeletal neck-shoulder pain. Scand J Rehabil Med 28: 183–192.

Norlander S, Gustavsson BA, Lindell J, et al. 1997. Reduced mobility in the cervico-thoracic motion segment – a risk factor for musculoskeletal neck–shoulder pain: a two-year prospective follow-up study. Scand J Rehabil Med 29: 167–174.

Pho C, Godges J. 2004. Management of whiplash-associated disorder addressing thoracic and cervical spine impairments: a case report. J Orthop Sports Phys Ther 34: 511–519.

Piva SR, Erhard RE, Al-Hugail M. 2000. Cervical radiculopathy: a case problem using a decision-making algorithm. J Orthop Sports Phys Ther 30: 745–754.

Piva SR, Erhard RE, Childs JD, et al. 2006. Inter-tester reliability of passive inter-vertebral and active movements of the cervical spine. Man Ther 11: 321–330.

Powers CM, Kulig K, Harrison J, et al. 2003. Segmental mobility of the lumbar spine during a posterior to anterior mobilization: assessment using dynamic MRI. Clin Biomech 1: 80–83.

Puentedura EJ, Landers EJ, Cleland JA, et al. 2011. Thoracic spine thrust manipulation versus cervical spine thrust manipulation in patients with acute neck pain: a randomized clinical trial. J Orthop Sports Phys Ther 41: 208–220.

Raney NH, Teyhen NH, Childs JD. 2007. Observed changes in lateral abdominal muscle thickness after spinal manipulation: a case series using rehabilitative ultrasound imaging. J Orthop Sports Phys Ther 37: 472–479.

Ross JK, Bereznick DE, McGill SM. 2004. Determining cavitation location during lumbar and thoracic spinal manipulation: is spinal manipulation accurate and specific? Spine 29: 1452–1457.

Savolainen A, Ahlberg J, Nummila H, et al. 2004. Active or passive treatment for neck–shoulder pain in occupational health care? A randomized controlled trial. Occup Med 54: 422–424.

Schiller L. 2001. Effectiveness of spinal manipulative therapy in the treatment of mechanical thoracic spine pain: a pilot randomized clinical trial. J Manipulative Physiol Ther 24: 394–401.

Sillevas R, Cleland J, Hellman M, et al. 2010. Immediate effects of a thoracic spine thrust manipulation on the autonomic nervous system: a randomized clinical trial. J Man Manip Ther 18: 181–190.

Sobel JS, Kremer I, Winters JC, et al. 1996. The influence of the mobility in the cervicothoracic spine and the upper ribs (shoulder girdle) on the mobility of the scapulohumeral joint. J Manipulative Physiol Ther 19: 469–474.

Sobel JS, Winters JC, Groenier K, et al. 1997. Physical examination of the cervical spine and shoulder girdle in patients with shoulder complaints. J Manipulative Physiol Ther 20: 257–262.

Sparkes V, Prevost AT, Hunter JO. 2003. Derivation and identification of questions that act as predictors of abdominal pain of musculoskeletal origin. Eur J Gastroenterol Hepatol 15: 1021–1027.

Sueki DG, Cleland JA, Wainner RW. 2013. A regional interdependence model of musculoskeleral dysfunction: research, mechanisms, and clinical implications. J Man Manip Ther 21: 90–102.

Theodoridis D, Ruston S. 2002. The effect of shoulder movements on thoracic spine 3D motion. Clin. Biomech 17: 418–421.

Viti JA, Paris SV. 2000. The use of upper thoracic manipulation in a patient with headache. J Man Manip Ther 8: 25–28.

Wainner RS, Whitman J, Cleland JA, et al. 2007. Regional interdependence: a musculoskeletal examination model whose time has come. J Orthop Sports Phys Ther 37: 658–660.

Waldrop MA. 2006. Diagnosis and treatment of cervical radiculopathy using a clinical prediction rule and a multimodal intervention approach: a case series. J Orthop Sports Phys Ther 36: 152–159.

Winters JC, Jorritsma W, Groenier KH, et al. 1999. Treatment of shoulder complaints in general practice: long term results of a randomised, single blind study comparing physiotherapy, manipulation, and corticosteroid injection. BMJ 318: 1395–1396.

Winters JC, Sobel JS, Groenier KH, et al. 1997. Comparison of physiotherapy, manipulation, and corticosteroid injection for treating shoulder complaints in general practice: randomised, single blind study. BMJ 314: 1320–1325.

Wood KB, Schellhas KP, Garvey TA, et al. 1999. Thoracic discography in healthy individuals. A controlled prospective study of magnetic resonance imaging and discography in asymptomatic and symptomatic individuals. Spine 24: 1548–1555.

Young BA, Gill HE, Wainner RS, et al. 2008. Thoracic costotransverse joint pain patterns: a study in normal volunteers. BMC Musculoskelet Disord 9: 140.

Young IA, Michener LA, Cleland JA, et al. 2009. Manual therapy, exercise, and traction for patients with cervical radiculopathy: a randomized clinical trial. Phys Ther 89: 632–642.

14 Chapter

Joint Mobilization and Manipulation of the Cervical Spine

John R. Krauss, Douglas S. Creighton, Joshua A. Cleland, César Fernández-de-las-Peñas

CHAPTER CONTENTS

Introduction 158
Evidence for cervical manipulation and mobilization 158
Hypothesized mechanisms of effect 159
Specificity of manipulation and mobilization 159
Selecting patients for cervical manipulation and mobilization 160
Adverse reactions to cervical manipulation and mobilization 160
Translatoric spinal manipulation and mobilization 161
Translatoric traction techniques 161
Translatoric articular/facet separation techniques 162
Translatoric facet-gliding techniques 165
Posterior–anterior cervical mobilization 168
Posterior–anterior unilateral upper cervical spine mobilization 168
Posterior–anterior unilateral mid-cervical spine mobilization 168
Transverse unilateral mid-cervical spine mobilization 169
Cervical spine manipulative procedures 169
C2–C6 separation of zygapophyseal articular joint: manipulation in rotation 169
Atlanto-axial separation of zygapophyseal articular joint: upper cervical spine manipulation 170
Conclusion 170

Introduction

It is estimated that 18–250 million manipulations are performed in the United States each year (Shekelle & Coulter 1997; Licht et al 2003), with over 2 million cervical manipulations performed on the cervical spine in Britain and Scotland alone (Thiel & Bolton 2004). The technique of manipulation and mobilization of the spine was documented as far back as 400 BCE (Sigerist 1951) and it continues to be used by modern medical professionals, including physical therapists, chiropractors and osteopaths, in the treatment of neck and head pain. However, despite the long history and continued use of these manual therapy interventions, there remains debate surrounding the safety and efficacy of cervical spine manipulative treatment.

Evidence for Cervical Manipulation and Mobilization

There is considerable evidence suggesting that manipulation and mobilization are effective in immediately improving the cervical range of motion, decreasing neck pain and improving function when applied to the cervical (Pikula 1999; Martinez-Segura et al 2006; Puentedura et al 2012b; Saavedra-Hernández et al 2013) and thoracic (Cleland et al 2005, 2007a, 2010; Krauss et al 2008; González-Iglesias et al 2009; Saavedra-Hernández et al 2013) spine. Furthermore, other studies support the effectiveness of cervical spine manipulation / mobilization for decreasing symptoms in the shoulder (McClatchie et al 2009) and the elbow (Cleland et al 2004). In a retrospective case audit of 112 cases, Cleland et al (2004) showed that significantly fewer treatments were required for those patients with lateral epicondylalgia who received additional manual therapy to the cervical spine.

It should be noted that, whereas there is considerable evidence supporting thoracic manipulation for neck pain (Cleland et al 2005, 2007a, 2010; Krauss et al 2008; González-Iglesias et al 2009; Saavedra-Hernández et al 2013), clinicians must also consider the added benefit of incorporating cervical spine manipulation into a multimodal treatment approach. Puentedura et al (2011) compared the effects of cervical spine manipulation with thoracic spine manipulation for the management of a group of patients with mechanical neck pain who met four out of six of the clinical prediction rule criteria for thoracic spine trust manipulation based on Cleland et al (2007a). The results found that the group receiving cervical spine manipulation experienced greater improvements in pain and function at both the short- and long-term follow-ups. Saavedra-Hernández et al (2013) reported that, in patients with chronic mechanical neck pain, the inclusion of cervical manipulation into a multimodal manipulative intervention leads to a greater reduction in disability than the application of cervical spine manipulation alone. In addition, a number of studies have indicated that single applications of cervical or thoracic manipulation are more effective than single applications of mobilization in immediately reducing cervical pain and increasing range of motion and function (Martinez-Segura et al 2006; Cleland et al 2007b; Dunning et al 2012). In contrast, other studies found that applications of either treatment appear to yield similar results in terms of effects (Cassidy et al 1992; Hurwitz et al 2002; Leaver et al 2010).

In the management of chronic neck pain (pain lasting more than 6 months), multimodal intervention combining manipulation or mobilization with exercise, or cervical with thoracic manipulations, results in superior outcomes compared with using either therapy in isolation (Gross et al 2002a, 2002b, 2004; Dunning et al 2012; Saavedra-Hernández et al 2013; Vincent et al 2013). Finally, the early use of mobilization and manipulation in the management of acute neck disorders appears to be associated with better outcomes than when these treatments are delayed (Boissonnault & Badke 2008).

Hypothesized Mechanisms of Effect

Historically, several potential mechanisms have been hypothesized to account for the outcomes associated with manipulation and mobilization. Biomechanical effects have been speculated to occur, due to one or more of the following mechanisms: (1) release of entrapped synovial folds or plica, (2) relaxation of hypertonic muscle by sudden stretching, (3) disruption of articular or periarticular adhesions, (4) restoration of the proper mid-position at rest and (5) restoration of normal physiological range of motion in joints that are 'stuck' in an end-range position (Shekelle 1994; Evans 2002). Anatomical structures (Bogduk & Jull 1985; Giles & Taylor 1987; Mercer & Bogduk 1993) and biomechanical mechanisms (Palfrey & Newton 1970; Semlak & Ferguson 1970) have been identified that partially support mechanisms 1–3; however, supportive evidence for mechanisms 4–5 is still lacking (Gal et al 1995, 1997; Evans 2002).

One event that has been hypothesized to account for some of the biomechanical mechanisms associated with the positive results of spinal manipulation and mobilization is the formation and release of gas bubbles within the synovial fluid during manipulation. This event generates a 'cracking, popping or clicking' noise, termed a **cavitation,** and has been viewed as a sign that the manipulation was applied correctly (Evans & Breen 2006). However, several studies suggest that improvement in pain and range of motion following manipulation may not be dependent on the generation of joint cavitation (Herzog et al 1995; Flynn et al 2003, 2006; Ross et al 2004).

It has been also suggested that the biomechanical effects of manipulation may be only partially responsible for the patient improvements associated with manual therapy techniques directed at the neck (Bialosky et al 2009b). Neurophysiological effects are probably contributing to the overall effect of manual therapy and can be further classified as peripheral, spinal and supraspinal mechanisms (Sterling et al 2001; Bialosky et al 2009b). Peripheral mechanisms are associated with reduction of blood and serum levels of cytokines, and changes in levels of β-endorphin, *N*-palmitoylethanolamide, anandamide, serotonin, endogenous cannabinoids and substance P (McPartland et al 2005; Teodorczyk-Injeyan et al 2006; Degenhardt et al 2007).

In addition to peripheral nervous system mechanisms, manipulation and mobilization have been proposed to impact on spinal cord mechanisms (Pickar & Wheeler 2001; Malisza et al 2003a, 2003b; Boal & Gillette 2004). For example, it has been shown that cervical spine manipulation exerts a hypoalgesic effect and can result in increased pain pressure thresholds at the neck and elbow in both healthy subjects (Fernández-de-las-Peñas et al 2007, 2008) and individuals with lateral elbow pain (Fernández-Carnero et al 2008). Additionally, healthy individuals and patients with low back pain have exhibited increased tolerance to thermal stimuli following a lumbopelvic manipulation (Bialosky et al 2009a).

Changes in dorsal horn activation in the spinal cord (Malisza et al 2003a), an endogenous opioid response (Vernon et al 1986) and improved psychological outcomes (Williams et al 2007) have also been associated with joint mobilization and manipulation. Lastly, manipulation and mobilization may reduce spinal cord responses through activation of supraspinal descending pain inhibition through the anterior cingular cortex, amygdala, periaqueductal grey and rostral ventromedial medulla (Hsieh et al 1995; Vogt et al 1996; Derbyshire et al 1997; Iadarola et al 1998; Peyron et al 2000; Pickar 2002; Moulton et al 2005; Guo et al 2006; Bee & Dickenson 2007; Oshiro et al 2007; Staud et al 2007).

Specificity of Manipulation and Mobilization

Based on the available literature, it is likely that both biomechanical and neurophysiological mechanisms account for the principle outcomes (pain reduction and motion improvement) associated with mobilization and manipulation (Bialosky et al 2009b). Accepting this notion, the question has been raised of whether manual therapy techniques need be, and can be, specific in terms of the movements and outcomes generated in the spine during treatment (Cleland & Childs 2005; Flynn 2006; Aquino et al 2009; Schomacher 2009). Studies have examined the effects of manipulative techniques using centrally applied posterior to anterior pressures (central PAs) on the spinous processes in the lumbar and cervical spines (Powers et al 2003; Kulig et al 2004; Lee et al 2005). These authors concluded that the greatest motion was generated at the point of contact. They also concluded that motion was generated at segments both cranial and caudal to the point of contact. Outcomes studies using the same mobilization technique concluded that there was no difference in levels of pain based on whether the most painful segment was treated or whether a randomly selected segment was treated (Beneck et al 2005; Landel et al 2008; Aquino et al 2009). When evaluating the outcomes-based studies that used the central PA technique, only some of the studies indicated the amount of force used during mobilization (Maitland grade IV) (Beneck et al 2005; Hengeveld et al 2005; Landel et al 2008); the other left the decision of force to the discretion of the therapist, which was not specified (Aquino et al 2009). Finally, the outcomes that were reported were immediate in nature and provide no insight into the implications of repeated applications of these techniques in terms of both positive effects and adverse responses.

Caution should be used therefore when generalizing the results of these studies to all mobilization and manipulation techniques. Although these studies provide valuable insights into the inter-relationship of movement between vertebrae when a single central force is applied to the spine in a mid-position, they examine only one technique. In addition, the technique makes no attempt to stabilize adjacent spinal levels, leaving the degree of specificity in question. It has been speculated that poorly localized and overly forceful manipulations may provoke adverse responses when applied through degenerative spinal segments (Assendelft et al 1996; Murphy 2006; Murphy et al 2006). For example, rotational manipulation of the cervical spine has been associated with increased risk of carotid or vertebral artery dissection (Assendelft et al 1996; Smith et al 2003). However, recent studies debate this assertion (Herzog et al 2012; Thomas et al 2013; Quesnele et al 2014). Thomas et al (2013) concluded that end-range rotational techniques do not alter blood flow to the brain any more than other manual therapy techniques. To date no studies have directly compared the implications of attempting to stabilize an adjacent segment or not during a manipulation on either outcomes or adverse events.

It seems reasonable that, in order to minimize the risk of adverse events hypothesized to be associated with spinal manipulation, it is necessary to screen individuals carefully when using manual therapy techniques. Additionally, there seems to be a general consensus amongst the majority of member organizations belonging to the International Federation of Orthopaedic Manipulative Physical Therapists (IFOMPT) regarding the need to reduce the use of rotation forces during manipulation of the cervical spine (Carlesso & Rivett 2011).

Selecting Patients for Cervical Manipulation and Mobilization

Selection of patients who respond positively to manipulation and who will not experience adverse responses has traditionally been attempted through the use of a comprehensive history and physical exam and the use of premanipulative testing such as the vertebral artery test (Carlesso & Rivett 2011). The literature suggests that serious adverse events may be partially prevented through adequate screening for absolute contraindications and manipulative 'red flags' (Childs et al 2005; Puentedura et al 2012a). Absolute contraindications to cervical manipulation include acute fractures, dislocations, ligamentous ruptures, instability, infection, tumours, acute myelopathy, acute soft tissue injury, osteoporosis, ankylosing spondylitis, rheumatoid arthritis, vascular disease, vertebral artery abnormalities, connective tissue disease and anticoagulant therapy (Puentedura et al 2012a). Relative contraindications to cervical manipulation include previous diagnosis of vertebrobasilar insufficiency, facial / intraoral anaesthesia / paraesthesia, visual disturbances, dizziness / vertigo, blurred vision, diplopia, nausea, tinnitus, drop attacks, dysarthria, dysphagia and no change or worsening of symptoms after multiple manipulations (Puentedura et al 2012a). Unfortunately, although adequate screening may reduce the risk of serious adverse events it does not eliminate it (Puentedura et al 2012a), nor do tests and measures such as the vertebral artery test appear to predict accurately the responses of these vascular structures to rotational manipulation (Arnold et al 2004; Thiel & Rix 2005).

Other attempts to improve patient selection include the use of clinical predication rules (CPRs) that, in general, attempt to match patient characteristics to patient interventions (Childs & Cleland 2006). In terms of manipulation, efforts in this area have resulted in CPRs that identify individual characteristics (e.g. number of days since onset of symptoms and joint hypomobility) and conditions (acute neck pain, cervicogenic headaches and radiculopathy) that respond favourably to manipulation in the lumbar, thoracic and cervical spines (Flynn et al 2002; Childs et al 2004; Cleland et al 2006, 2007a, 2007c; Fleming et al 2007; Puentedura et al 2012b). Although CPRs provide valuable insight into the connection between examination findings and treatment response, studies performed for neck-related conditions have yet to be validated. In fact, Cleland et al (2010) attempted to validate the CPR for manipulating the thoracic spine for individuals with mechanical neck pain; however, the results showed that the original CPR (Cleland et al 2007a) was not found to be valid in the new group of patients. Therefore, it has been recommended that further research is necessary before these CPRs can be generally applied with confidence (Hancock et al 2007; May & Resendale 2009).

In contrast to relying solely on screening for contraindications and red flags or selecting patients who match a prefabricated manipulative technique, the authors suggest a more clinically pragmatic approach of designing / tailoring the manipulative technique to each patient's specific movement impairment. The main principle behind this approach is the notion that manual stabilization, segmental pre-positioning and the direction of force used during manipulation or mobilization impact the amount of force and direction of movement generated within the treatment segment and the surrounding spinal levels (Krauss et al 2006). The specific forces used during treatment are disc traction, facet separation or facet gliding as either sustained stretches (mobilizations) or impulses (manipulations). The selection of the specific type of cervical technique (disc traction, facet separation or facet gliding) and the degree to which manual stabilization and pre-positioning of non-treatment segments are used depends on: (1) the amount and type of motion restriction (tissue resistance), (2) the number of restricted spinal levels, (3) symptom duration and intensity, (4) the degree of anatomical and pathomechanical changes at both the treatment segment and the adjacent spinal segments and (5) the degree to which it is allowed to produce / reproduce the patient's symptoms (Maitland et al 2005). Evidence supports the influence of pre-positioning and manual stabilization in reducing movement in adjacent spinal levels for the upper cervical spine (Cattrysse et al 2007a, 2007b). In addition, there is also limited evidence that techniques using these principles can be applied without adverse response to patients with degenerative spinal conditions (Creighton et al 2005; Kondratek et al 2006).

Adverse Reactions to Cervical Manipulation and Mobilization

When considering the issue of safety, adverse reactions associated with manipulation and mobilization range from minor and self-limiting injuries such as headaches, stiffness and limitations in motion (Senstad et al 1996; Lebouef-Yde et al 1997; Cagnie et al 2004; Hurwitz et al 2005) to serious injuries including permanent neurological deficits, dissection of a carotid or vertebral artery, and death (Di Fabio 1999; Ernst 2002; Haldeman et al 2002; Licht et al 2003; Oppenheim et al 2005). Additional adverse responses potentially associated with cervical spine manipulation include worsening of pre-existing disc herniation, acute disc herniation resulting in both radiculopathy and myelopathy and, in patients with cervical spondylotic changes, worsening of both radiculopathy and myelopathic disturbances (Lee et al 1995; Padua et al 1996; Malone et al 2002; Tseng et al 2002). Evidence from the scientific literature suggests that adverse reactions are more likely following spinal manipulation than mobilization and they occur in the cervical spine more often than in other spinal regions (Senstad et al 1996; Lebouef-Yde et al 1997; Hurwitz et al 2005). An estimated 35–65% of patients report minor side effects following their first manipulation (Senstad et al 1996; Lebouef-Yde et al 1997; Cagnie et al 2004; Hurwitz et al 2005). In general, it appears that minor adverse responses occur at a higher rate (one incident for every 476–1573 manipulations) (Di Fabio 1999) compared with serious adverse responses, which occur at an estimated rate of 1 incident per 20 000–3 000 000 manipulations (Hurwitz et al 1996; Lebouef-Yde et al 1997; Shekelle & Coulter 1997; Di Fabio 1999; Gross et al 2002a; Haldeman et al 2002; Licht et al 2003; Oppenheim et al 2005).

The actual number of adverse responses to cervical manipulation is difficult to estimate owing to factors such as practitioner under-reporting, failure to follow up patients who do not return for treatment after receiving spinal joint manipulation, and the potential delay in symptom onset following manipulation (Assendelft et al 1996; Di Fabio 1999; Norris et al 2000; Ernst 2002; Oppenheim et al 2005; Carlesso et al 2010a). With the exception of the most severe cases, the classification of adverse responses within the literature has lacked clear and consistent nomenclature, especially regarding loss of function and follow-up treatment (Carlesso et al 2010b). To address this, Carnes et al (2010) suggest a three-layered pragmatic approach to the qualification of adverse events that includes the duration, severity, description, treatment and functional implications of the adverse response to manipulation. Using these qualifiers, major, moderate and minor adverse events would be described as follows: (1) major adverse events are medium to long term in duration, moderate to severe in severity, described as unacceptable by the patient and require further treatment for resolution; (2) moderate adverse events are the same as major adverse events in all respects except that they are moderate in severity; and (3) mild adverse events are of short duration, mild in severity, self-limiting and require no further treatment (Carnes et al 2010).

Although serious adverse events have been associated with cervical manipulation, a cause-and-effect relationship cannot be directly inferred. A study by Cassidy et al (2008) reviewed 818 cases of vertebral artery strokes admitted to hospitals in Ontario, Canada, between 1993 and 2002. The authors found that the risk of patients having a spontaneous vertebrobasilar artery stroke associated with chiropractic visits is the same as that for patients seeing their primary care physician for reports of neck and head pain. In fact, it has been reported that individuals presenting with a vertebral artery dissection typically experience head and neck pain in a similar distribution to that of mechanical neck pain (Kerry & Taylor 2006) Therefore careful screening of subjects with neck and head pain is essential in an attempt to determine whether symptoms may potentially be vascular in nature or if the patient is presenting with mechanical neck pain. Kerry and Taylor (2006) have described common symptoms that individuals with vertebrobasilar insufficiency may experience, such as dizziness, drop attacks, diplopia, dysarthria, dysphagia, ataxia, nausea, numbness and nystagmus. Puentedura et al (2012a) reviewed 134 case reports of patients who had experienced an adverse event associated with a cervical spine manipulation. The findings indicated that if proper screening of red flags and contraindications were performed then 44.8% of those adverse events would have potentially been prevented.

Translatoric Cervical Manipulation and Mobilization

The techniques presented in this section were co-developed by Freddy Kaltenborn (PT, OMT) and Olaf Evjenth (PT, OMT) of Norway. The emphasis of these techniques is an attempt to avoid moderate to severe adverse responses (Carnes et al 2010) and to try to maximize outcomes in terms of pain, mobility and disability. Interestingly, the challenges Kaltenborn and Evjenth faced as they began developing these techniques in 1970 continues to be reflected today in terms of adverse responses, mechanisms of effect, specificity and outcomes (Krauss et al 2006; Kaltenborn 2008). For the purposes of this section we use terminology consistent with an international perspective where: (1) manipulation is defined as a high-velocity low-amplitude movement delivered at the end of available restricted joint motion and within the normal anatomical range of joint motion, and (2) mobilization is defined as a low-velocity varying amplitude (static holding, low or moderate amplitude) movement delivered at various points in the joints restricted range of motion or at the end of the available restricted joint motion and within the normal anatomical range of joint motion. More specifically, mobilization forces are applied within the available range of joint motion in a static or oscillatory manner when pain and / or orthopaedic conditions associated with tissue weakness and loss of structural stability of a motion segment are present (Miyazaki et al 2008). In contrast, manipulation, and sometimes mobilization, is applied at the end of available joint motion when pain and / or orthopaedic conditions associated with tissue tightness are present.

Techniques presented in this section of the chapter are grouped according to type and described using the American Academy of Orthopedic Manual Physical Therapy's (AAOMPT) recommended standardized terminology, which includes: (1) the rate of application, (2) location in range of available movement, (3) direction of force, (4) target of force, (5) relative structural movement and (6) patient position (Mintken et al 2008). Additional insights regarding the use of the techniques and errors to avoid are also provided.

Translatoric traction techniques

Translatoric traction techniques are used to unload / decompress the disc joint and intervertebral foramen contents

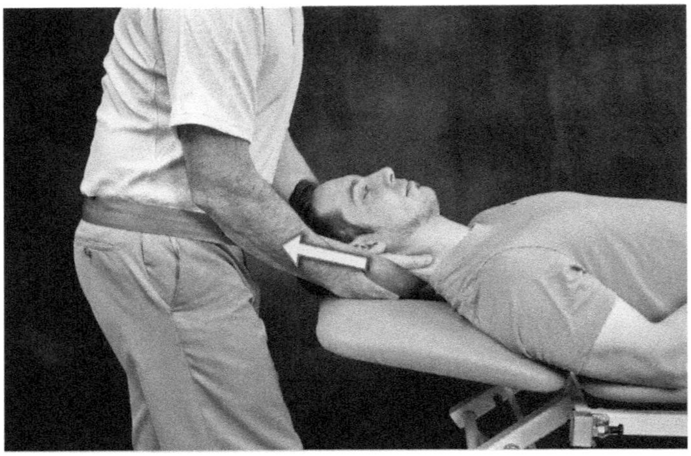

Figure 14.1 **C2–C7 disc traction in supine.**

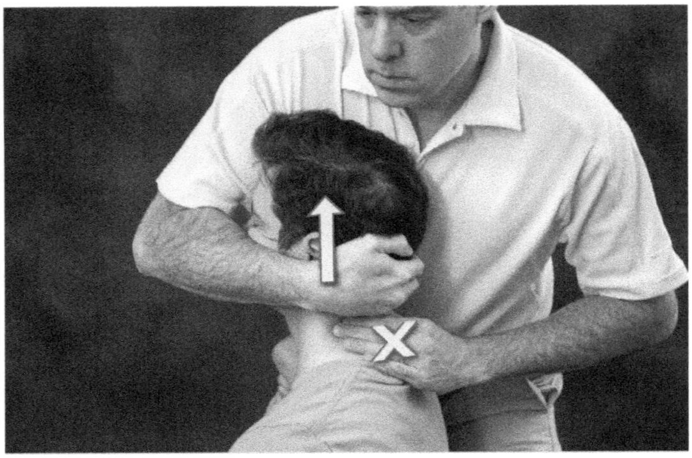

Figure 14.2 **C2–C7 disc traction seated.**

(nerves, arteries, veins and lymphatics). Disc traction manipulations are performed at a right angle to the disc joint in what is essentially a cranially directed force. During disc traction, bilaterally applied manipulative forces are used in an attempt to generate equal movement / traction of all parts of the intervertebral joint.

C2–C7 disc traction in supine (Fig. 14.1)

The patient is supine in a position of greatest comfort where signs and symptoms are most minimal. The therapist stands facing the top of the patient's head. The therapist's left and right hands contact the posterior surface of the transverse processes, lamina, inferior articular processes and spinous process of the cranial vertebra in the treatment segment. A belt may be placed around the therapist's waist and over the therapist's hands to assist in the generation of traction forces. The slack in the treatment segment is taken up in a cranial direction with both hands and the manipulation or mobilization is delivered using the same direction of motion.

Specificity: Generally low; degree to which traction occurs in the spinal segments caudal to the point of contact is dependent on factors such as amount of force used and the amount of motion available at each spinal segment.

Note: In cases of cervical nerve irritation secondary to disc degeneration, the authors recommend disc traction mobilization and manipulation. If radicular irritation is not stable – in other words the radicular discomfort is severe and variable – generally we recommend oscillatory disc traction mobilization. Above all, we feel that success in terms of immediate radicular symptom reduction with manual disc traction is often a matter of positioning as opposed to a matter of manipulative speed or force. We attempt to position the patient's affected segments using a combination of flexion, side-bending and rotation such that the patient's symptoms decrease prior to the beginning application of the disc traction mobilization procedure. Finally, the cranial vertebra of the involved segment must be used in order to try to decompress the irritated nerve root.

C2–C7 disc traction seated (Fig. 14.2)

The patient is sitting in a position of greatest comfort where signs and symptoms are most minimal. The therapist stands in front of and to the right of the patient. The therapist's right hand contacts the left side of the inferior articular process and lamina of the cranial vertebra in the treatment segment. The right side of the therapist's chest is placed against the right side of the patient's head. The therapist's left hand contacts the bilateral laminae of the caudal vertebra. The slack in the treatment segment is taken up in a cranial direction with the right hand and chest. The therapist's left hand presses in a caudal direction as the slack is taken up. The manipulation or mobilization force is directed cranially.

Specificity: This technique seems to be more specific than the supine version because of manual stabilization of the caudal vertebrae; however, this is still considered a lower specificity technique.

Note: We often use seated disc traction mobilization and manipulation in patients who present with single or multisegment hypomobility, which is more commonly seen in older patients with late-grade disc degeneration (Miyazaki et al 2008). Patients who are less symptomatic – in other words more 'stiffness (resistance) dominant' – may benefit from the increased specificity and resultant increased manipulative force that this technique facilitates. Note in Figure 14.2 how the non-manipulating hand manually stabilizes the caudal vertebra in a ventral and caudal direction prior to applying a cranially directed mobilization or manipulation.

Translatoric articular / facet separation techniques

The biomechanical objective of translatoric articular / facet separation techniques is to unload or decompress the articular surfaces of the occipito-atlanto (OA) and atlanto-axial (AA) joints and the facet joints in the lower cervical spine. Obviously, any articular / facet separation technique will induce some of the potential neurophysiological mechanisms briefly discussed earlier in this chapter.

Techniques grouped in this category generate separation of the articular surfaces (OA and AA articulations and C2–C7 facets), which is different from disc traction in that separation of all points of the articular surface is not equal. This is due in part to the use of unilaterally generated impulses in addition to the orientation of the facet surfaces. In the upper cervical spine, as the articular surfaces of the joints are positioned

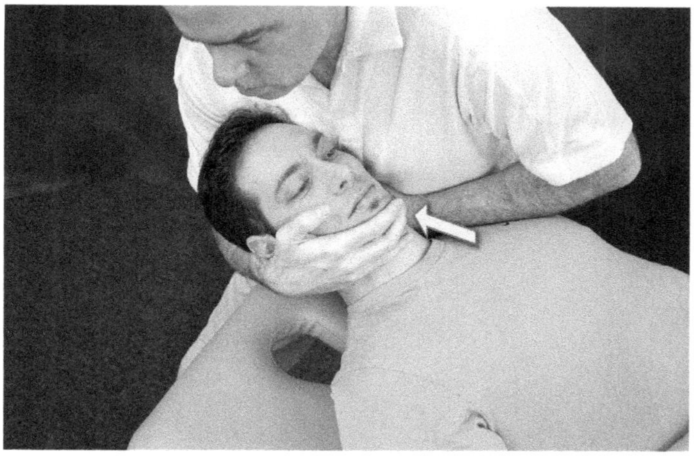

Figure 14.3 Occipito-atlanto separation in supine.

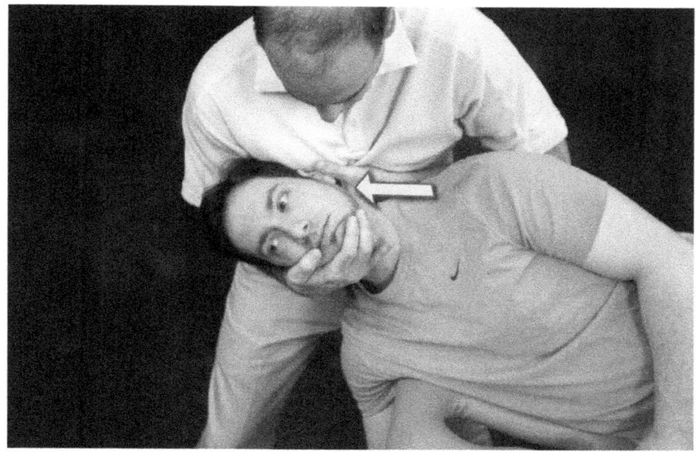

Figure 14.4 Atlanto-axial separation in side-lying.

in the transverse plane, the manipulation is directed cranially and slightly medially to maintain bony contact. In the lower cervical spine, the facet joints are oriented approximately 45° from the horizontal. To generate the greatest amount of facet separation in the lower cervical spine the treatment segment is positioned in opposite side-bending and rotation and the manipulation is directed in a ventral, medial and caudal direction. If applying this technique with a thrust, the position of the segment and the cervical facet joint should be such that the facet is in its most loosely packed position for separation.

Occipito-atlanto separation in supine (Fig. 14.3)

The patient is positioned supine with slight left side-bending, right rotation and dorsal flexion of the occiput on the atlas. The therapist is positioned to the left of the patient's head, neck and shoulder. The therapist's right hand and forearm are positioned behind the patient's head and against the right side of the patient's face. The therapist's left hand contacts the inferior edge of the patient's left mastoid process. The slack between occiput and atlas is taken up in a cranial direction by the therapist's right hand and chest. The manipulation / mobilization is delivered by the left hand in a cranial direction.

Specificity: This is typically an articulation that responds with a cavitation when the technique is performed with the correct speed and pre-positioning. No attempt is made to stabilize caudally so movement will occur below the point of contact.

Note: The authors feel that loosening the OA joint is often necessary in cases of upper cervical motion impairment. A few degrees of coupled side-bending and rotation are available at the C0 / C1 segment, but given the ligamentous connection (alar ligament) between the lateral masses of the occiput and the dens process of C2, improvement of mobility at C0 / C1 can in some cases also improve coupled rotation at the C2 motion segment. Improvement of coupled rotation at either the C0 / C1 segment or the C2 / C3 segment can often improve upper cervical spine coupled rotation. Anecdotally, in patients where arthritic degeneration has resulted in capsular shortening at the OA joint and in patients who report an increase in occipital pain with active and passive upper cervical motion, the authors have found good reduction in occipital pain referral after the application of OA traction manipulation.

Atlanto-axial separation in side-lying (Fig. 14.4)

The patient is positioned in side-lying with slight right side-bending, left rotation and dorsal flexion of the atlas on the axis. The therapist is positioned behind the patient's head, neck and upper torso. The therapist's right hand and forearm are positioned under the right side of the patient's head with the index and middle fingers cupped around the patient's chin. The therapist's left hand contacts the inferior edge of the patient's transverse process and posterior arch of atlas. The slack between atlas and axis is taken up in a cranial direction by the therapist's right hand and chest. The manipulation or mobilization is delivered by the left hand in a cranial direction.

Specificity: Generally low; the degree to which traction occurs in the spinal segments caudal to the point of contact is dependent on factors such as amount of force used and the amount of motion available at each spinal segment.

Note: We feel that rotational pre-positioning to the upper cervical segments using a slow movement that the patient can stop is a safe and acceptable way to take up available capsule–ligamentous slack. Consistent with the teaching of the majority of member organizations of IFOMPT, some authors of this chapter discourage the use of high-velocity rotational manipulation of the atlas on the axis (Carlesso & Rivett 2011). Rather, after slow rotational pre-positioning of the upper cervical region, the authors recommend short-amplitude translational movements in a cranial direction of the atlas on the axis as seen in Figure 14.4. Additionally the authors rarely find significant capsular restriction of the lateral AA joint (Lakshmanan et al 2005).

C2–C7 facet separation seated version 1 (Fig. 14.5)

With the patient seated, the patient's cervical spine down through the treatment segment is positioned in right side-bending and left rotation. The therapist stands to the left of the patient. The therapist's left hand supports the right

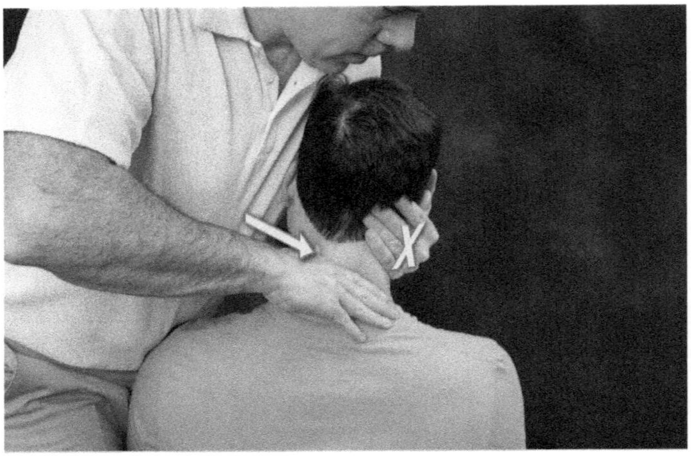

Figure 14.5 **C2–C7 facet separation seated version 1.**

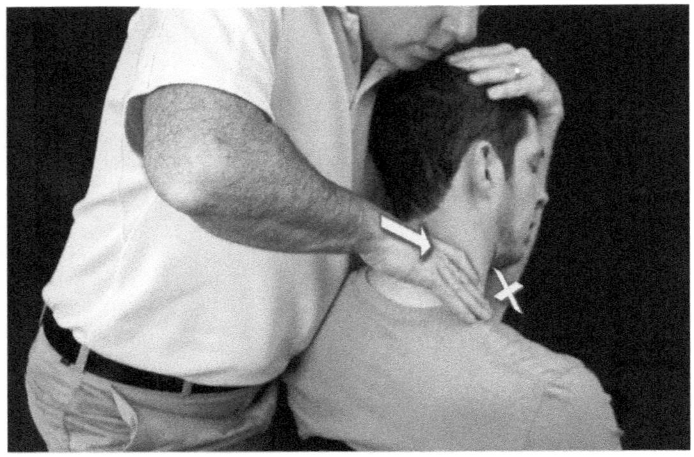

Figure 14.6 **C2–C7 facet separation seated version 2.**

posterior edge of the transverse process, articular process and lamina of the cranial vertebra in the treatment segment. The therapist's right thumb contacts the lamina and superior articular process of the caudal vertebra in the treatment segment. The slack in the treatment segment is taken up through pre-positioning in right side-bending and left rotation and by applying a slight cranial force on the cervical spine with the left hand and shoulder. The manipulation is delivered by the therapist's right thumb in a ventral, medial and caudal direction.

Specificity: This technique is more specific than others in terms of the motion generated at the treatment segment and the direct manual contact point on the inferior facet. In addition, the pre-positioning and support of the cranial vertebra may reduce motion in segments cranial to the treatment segment. Movement of the caudal segments may occur towards a mid-position.

Note: In complicated cervical presentations (e.g. mid to lower cervical disc degeneration with symptomatic hypermobility or radicular irritation (Dai 1998)), this version of facet joint distraction can allow for simultaneous application of manual traction. This is applied with the therapist's non-manipulating hand and the chest while the therapist's thumb applies a specific facet joint distraction to the hypomobile level. Application of a sustained manual traction takes up ligamentous slack and prevents excessive angular and translational movement at degenerated hypermobile cervical segments or segments with discogenic or spondylotic irritation.

C2–C7 facet separation seated version 2 (Fig. 14.6)

With the patient seated, the patient's cervical spine down through the treatment segment is positioned in left side-bending and right rotation. The therapist stands to the left of the patient. The therapist's left forearm is placed against the left side of the patient's face and neck supporting the head position. The radial border of the therapist's right second metacarpophalangeal (MCP) joint contacts the lamina and superior articular process of the caudal vertebra in the treatment segment. The slack in the treatment segment is taken up through pre-positioning in left side-bending and right rotation. The manipulation or mobilization is delivered by the radial border of the therapist's right hand in a ventral, medial and caudal direction.

Specificity: This technique also seems to be specific in terms of the motion generated at the treatment segment and the direct manual contact point on the inferior facet. In addition, the pre-positioning and support of the cranial vertebra could reduce motion in segments cranial to the treatment segment. Movement of the caudal segments may occur towards a mid-position.

Note: The authors often apply this version of facet distraction in the more 'stiffness-dominant' patients. A case report found that this version of facet distraction was useful when applied below a degenerated hypermobile mid to lower (C4–C6) cervical segment (Kondratek et al 2006). However, care should be taken when applying this technique above a symptomatically degenerated hypermobile segment, given the compressive load caused by the caudal force component of this technique. The authors have also found that this manual intervention does not significantly change vertebral artery flow velocity or lumen diameter (Creighton et al 2011).

C2–C7 facet separation in supine contralateral gap (Fig. 14.7)

With the patient supine, the patient's cervical spine down through the treatment segment is positioned in left side-bending and right rotation. The therapist stands to the left of the patient's head, neck and shoulder. The therapist's right forearm is placed against the right side of the patient's face supporting the head position. The radial border of the therapist's left second MCP joint contacts the left inferior and superior articular processes of the treatment segment. The slack in the treatment segment is taken up through pre-positioning in left side-bending and right rotation. The mobilization / manipulation is delivered by the radial border of the therapist's left hand in a medial, slightly cranial and slightly dorsal direction.

Specificity: This technique is considered moderately specific in terms of the motion generated at the treatment segment. Specificity is enhanced by taking up soft tissue slack in the treatment segment through pre-positioning in side-bending and rotation. Impulses that are too long or movement of the support hand and therapist's body may generate unwanted movement in the spinal segments cranial and caudal to the treatment segment.

Note: The authors often apply this mobilization / manipulation technique in patients who demonstrate facet joint hypomobility and overlying soft tissue tenderness on the same side. Figure 14.7 shows how the right facet joint is separated using a manual contact and manipulative force applied on the left side of the neck.

C7 facet separation in supine (Fig. 14.8)

With the patient supine, the patient's C7 spinal segment is positioned in slight left side-bending and right rotation. A large mobilization wedge (Norsk wedge pictured) is placed under the upper thoracic spine with the base facing cranial and positioned under T1. The therapist stands to the left of the patient's shoulder. The ulnar border of the therapist's left hand presses in the direction of the anterior surface of the patient's right transverse process of C7. The therapist's right hand is placed over the left to support the contact and wrist and hand position. The slack in the treatment segment is taken up through pre-positioning. The manipulation or mobilization is delivered by the ulnar border of the therapist's left hand in a dorsal, lateral and cranial direction.

Specificity: Due to the contact on C7 and the firm stabilization provided by the wedge, this technique is considered moderately specific.

Note: In patients with hypomobile C7 / T1 segments, the authors of this chapter have found that this mobilization / manipulation technique provides a good stretch to the periarticular structures at the C7 / T1 articulation.

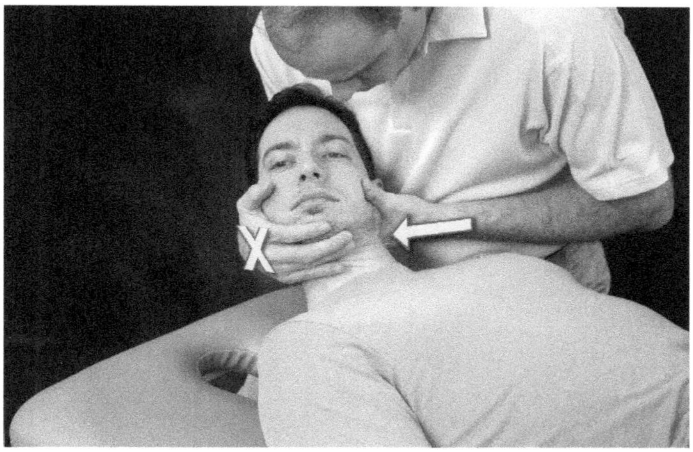

Figure 14.7 C2–C7 facet separation in supine contralateral gap.

Translatoric facet-gliding techniques

Translatoric facet-gliding techniques are directed parallel to the articular surfaces in the upper and lower cervical spines. In the upper cervical spine the manipulative force is principally directed in a ventral and dorsal direction. In the lower cervical spine (C2–C7) the force directions are ventral, medial and cranial and dorsal. The decision regarding the direction of movement used for gliding techniques is determined by the direction of restricted motion. More specifically, dorsal gliding at the OA joint is used when ventral flexion of the joint is restricted, and ventral gliding at the OA joint is used when dorsal flexion is restricted. In the lower cervical spine, ventral cranial gliding is used when ventral flexion is limited, or in the case of a right unilateral restriction when ventral flexion and left side-bending and left rotation are restricted. Dorsal caudal gliding is used when dorsal flexion is restricted, or in the case of right unilateral restrictions when dorsal flexion and right side-bending and rotation are restricted. During these techniques it is important that the compression forces are avoided during gliding. This is accomplished by applying a small amount of (Kaltenborn grade 1) traction to the joint prior to gliding.

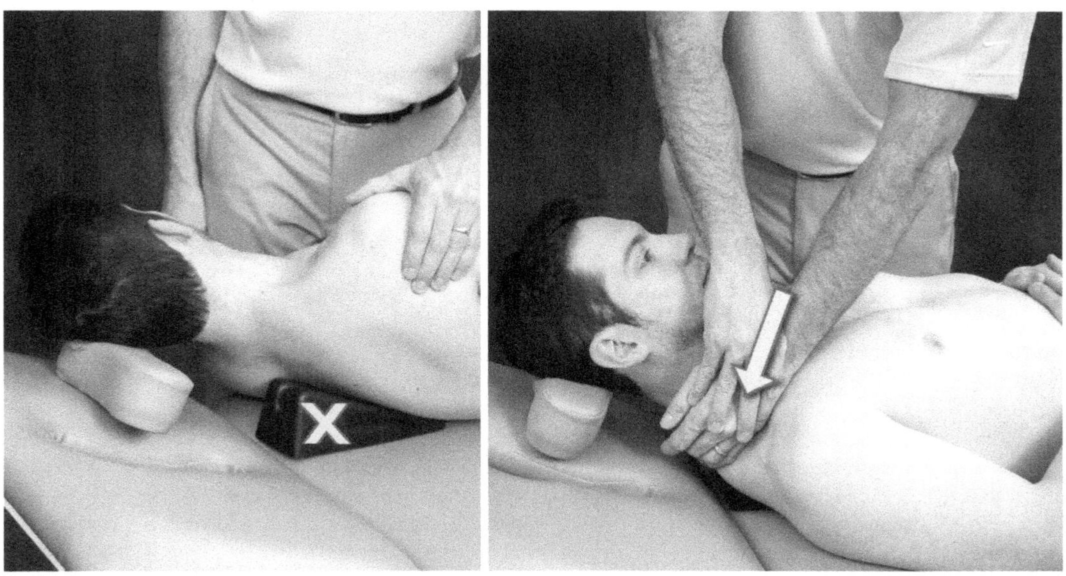

Figure 14.8 C7 facet separation in supine.

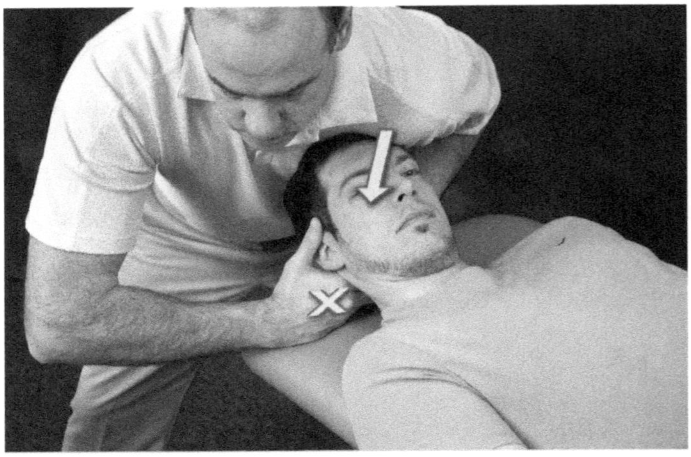

Figure 14.9 **Occipito-atlanto unilateral dorsal glide in supine.**

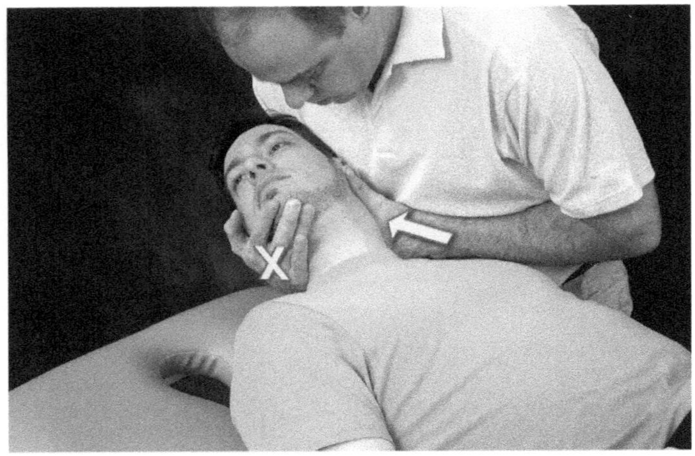

Figure 14.10 **C2–C6 facet ventral-cranial glide in supine.**

Occipito-atlanto unilateral dorsal glide in supine (Fig. 14.9)

The patient is positioned in supine with slight ventral flexion of the occiput on the atlas. The therapist stands facing the head of the patient. The therapist's left hand is placed posteriorly under the patient's occiput. The therapist's left shoulder is positioned anteriorly on the patient's forehead superior to the patient's left eye. The therapist's right hand contacts and stabilizes the right transverse process and posterior arch of atlas with the MCP and radial border of their index finger. The slack in the right OA joint is taken up by applying a dorsal and medial pressure with the therapist's left shoulder in the direction of the stabilizing hand. The mobilization force is applied in a dorsal and medial direction by the therapist's left shoulder.

Specificity: This technique can be considered specific due to segmental pre-positioning and the firm stabilization provided to the atlas by the therapist's hand positioned between the posterior arch of atlas and the treatment table.

Note: We have found that the occiput dorsal mobilization technique often reduces complaints of upper cervical pain and improves upper cervical flexion. This improved motion gives patients with postural impairments an improved ability to bring their eyes into a more horizontal position.

C2–C6 facet ventral-cranial glide in supine (Fig. 14.10)

The patient is positioned supine with the lower cervical spine in left side-bending, right rotation and slight ventral flexion. The treatment segment is positioned in right side-bending, right rotation and slight ventral flexion. The therapist is positioned to the left of the patient's head, neck and left shoulder. The therapist's right hand and forearm are positioned under the right side of the patient's head with the ulnar side of the hand contacting the right inferior articular process, lamina and spinous process of the cranial vertebra in the treatment segment. The slack in the treatment segment is taken up during pre-positioning. The manipulation is applied by the therapist's left hand in a ventral, medial and cranial direction.

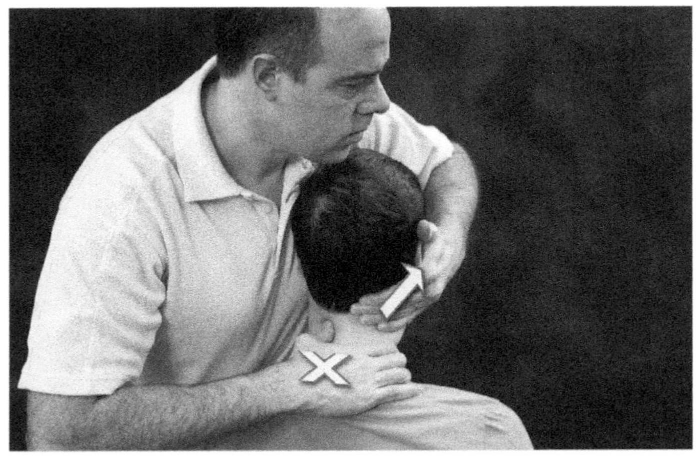

Figure 14.11 **C2–C6 facet ventral-cranial glide seated.**

Specificity: Due to the use of spinal locking and manual reinforcement this technique seems to be specific. When applied correctly this technique typically generates a cavitation.

Note: Loosening coupled rotation and side-bending at the C2 segment may assist in improving rotation of the dens within its osteoligamentous ring. This improves the ligamentous tensioning mechanism between the alar ligament and the occiput. As a result, improved coupled rotation at the C2 segment may enhance coupled motion at the OA segment.

C2–C6 facet ventral-cranial glide seated (Fig. 14.11)

The patient is seated with the lower cervical spine in right side-bending, left rotation and slight ventral flexion. The treatment segment is positioned in left side-bending, left rotation and slight ventral flexion. The therapist is positioned to the left of the patient's head, neck and left shoulder. The radial border of the therapist's left hand contacts the right inferior articular process of the cranial vertebra in the treatment segment. The therapist's right thumb presses ventrally and medially against the left side of the caudal vertebra's lamina.

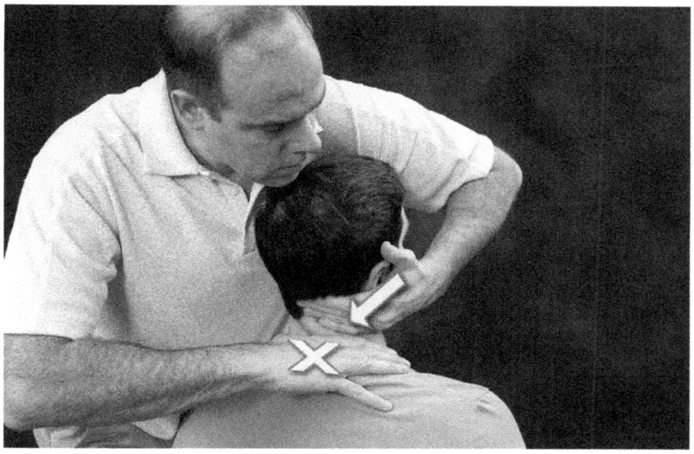

Figure 14.12 C2–C6 facet dorsal-caudal glide seated.

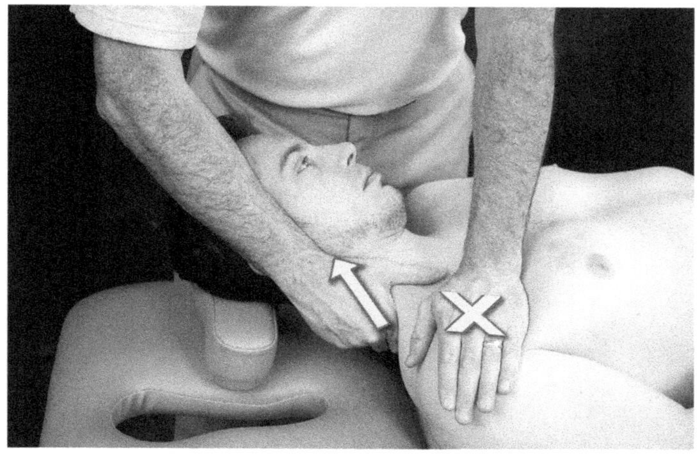

Figure 14.13 C7 facet ventral-cranial glide in supine.

Slack in the treatment segment is taken up during pre-positioning. The manipulation is applied by the therapist's left hand in a ventral, medial and cranial direction.

Specificity: Due to the use of spinal locking and manual reinforcement this technique can be specific.

Note: When manipulating the C2 segment, care must be taken that the manipulating hand is not placed on the atlas.

C2–C6 facet dorsal-caudal glide seated (Fig. 14.12)

The patient is seated with the lower cervical spine in left side-bending, right rotation and slight extension. The treatment segment is positioned in right side-bending, right rotation and dorsal flexion. The therapist is positioned to the left of the patient's head, neck and left shoulder. The radial border of the therapist's left hand contacts the right inferior articular process of the cranial vertebra in the treatment segment. The therapist's left thumb presses ventrally and medially against the left side of the caudal vertebra's lamina. The slack in the treatment segment is taken up during pre-positioning. The manipulation is applied by the therapist's left hand in a dorsal, medial and caudal direction.

Specificity: This technique can be specific due to spinal pre-positioning and manual stabilization; however, some movement may occur above and below the treatment segment.

Note: This mobilization appears to be effective in improving cervical rotation restriction but may increase cervical symptoms from an infra-adjacent segment that is compression sensitive (e.g. irritated nerve root). If this is encountered, the authors recommend the addition of a cranially directed traction force applied to the patient's head by the practitioner's chest during the mobilization procedure.

C7 facet ventral-cranial glide in supine (Fig. 14.13)

The patient is positioned supine with the C7 in left side-bending, left rotation and slight flexion. The therapist is positioned to the left of the patient's head, neck and left shoulder. The radial border of the therapist's right hand contacts the right inferior articular process of C7. The therapist's left hand presses dorsally on the patient's right shoulder to stabilize T1. The slack in the treatment segment is taken up during pre-positioning. The manipulation is applied by the therapist's right hand in a ventral, medial and cranial direction.

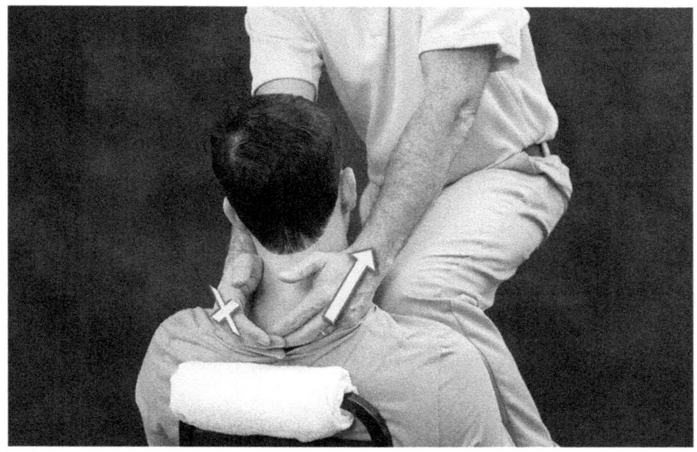

Figure 14.14 C7 facet ventral-cranial glide seated.

Specificity: Some movement may occur in the spinal segments cranial to C7; however, very little motion should occur in the spinal segments below.

Note: In patients with hypomobile C7 / T1 segments, the authors of this chapter have found that this mobilization / manipulation technique provides a good stretch to the periarticular structures at the C7 / T1 articulation.

C7 facet ventral-cranial glide seated (Fig. 14.14)

The patient is seated with the C7 in slight left side-bending, left rotation and slight flexion. The therapist is positioned in front of the patient with his left knee positioned anteriorly contacting the patient's right shoulder and chest. The ulnar border of the therapist left hand contacts the posterior surface of the transverse process of C7 on the right. The ulnar border of the therapist's right hand contacts the left posterior laminae and facets of C7 and T1. The slack in the treatment segment is taken up during pre-positioning. The manipulation is applied by the therapist's left hand in a ventral, medial and cranial direction.

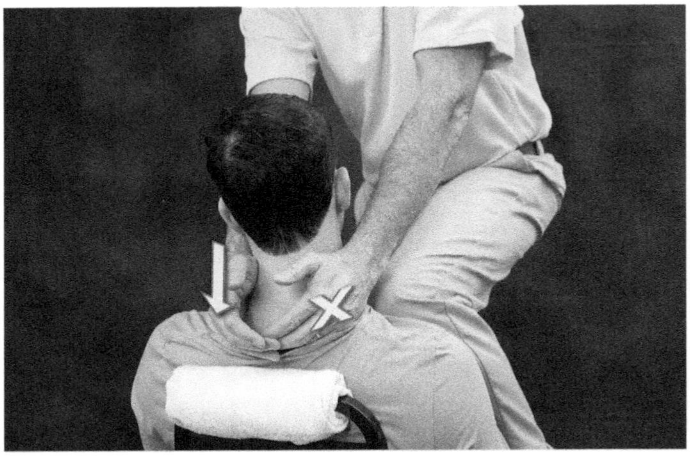

Figure 14.15 C7 facet dorsal-caudal glide seated.

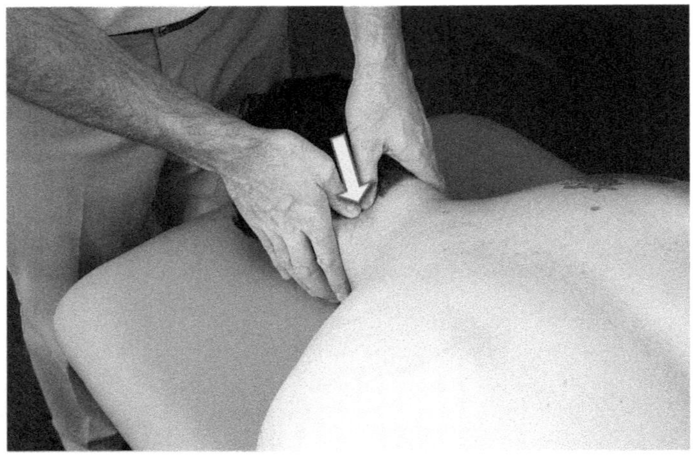

Figure 14.16 Posterior–anterior unilateral upper cervical spine mobilization.

Specificity: Little movement should occur above or below the treatment segment.

Note: Patients whose cervical conditions are less painful and more dominated by stiffness, or who perhaps present only with cervical discomfort closer to the end range of an active cervical movement, often respond well to this technique.

C7 facet dorsal-caudal glide seated (Fig. 14.15)

The patient is seated with the C7 in slight left side-bending, left rotation and dorsal flexion. The therapist is positioned in front of the patient with his left knee positioned anteriorly contacting the patient's right shoulder and chest. The ulnar border of the therapist right hand contacts the posterior surface of the transverse process of C7 on the left. The ulnar border of the therapist's left hand contacts the right posterior laminae and facets of C7 and T1. The slack in the treatment segment is taken up during pre-positioning. The manipulation is applied by the therapist's right hand in a dorsal, medial and caudal direction.

Specificity: Little movement should occur above or below the treatment segment.

Note: Patients whose cervical conditions are less painful and more dominated by stiffness, or who perhaps present only with cervical discomfort closer to the end range of an active cervical movement, often respond well to this technique.

Posterior–anterior Cervical Mobilization

Posterior–anterior cervical joint mobilization can be used as an assessment or treatment method (Maitland et al 2005). When selecting the technique, the therapist has to make the following important decisions: (a) to what degree it is allowed to produce / reproduce the patient's symptoms and (b) to what degree it is necessary to mobilize into tissue resistance. Maitland et al (2005) performed treatment techniques in an oscillatory manner. These oscillations can be performed with different amplitudes in different positions in the range of movement (readers are referred to the textbook *Maitland's vertebral manipulation* (Maitland et al 2005) for further information on the Maitland approach). In the current section we will describe the most common posterior–anterior joint mobilization targeted to the cervical spine.

Posterior–anterior unilateral upper cervical spine mobilization (Fig. 14.16)

The patient is prone with the cervical spine in a neutral position. The pads of the therapist's left and right thumbs contact over the posterior–lateral aspect of atlas (C1) in line with the OA (C0–C1) joint on the targeted side. The therapist's arms and thumbs are directed slightly medially and cranially. The remaining portions of the therapist's hands remain relaxed and in contact with the left and right sides of the upper neck. Oscillatory pressure is directed through the thumbs in a posterior–anterior direction on C1. When performed correctly a small extension movement of the head will occur without any rotation or side-bending.

Note: This technique may be used for the treatment of cervicogenic headache. If headache pain is present with pressure at C1, the oscillatory amplitude and starting depth may cause slight discomfort during its application. However, the headache symptoms should gradually ease and not worsen as treatment progresses.

Posterior–anterior unilateral mid-cervical spine mobilization (Fig. 14.17)

The patient is prone with the cervical spine in a neutral position. The pads of the therapist's left and right thumbs contact over the articular process (mid-cervical segment illustrated). The therapist's arms and thumbs are directed slightly medially (approximately 30°). The remaining portions of the therapist's hands remain relaxed and in contact with the left and right sides of the upper neck. Oscillatory pressure is directed through the thumbs in a posterior–anterior direction on the treatment articulation. When performed correctly a small extension movement of the head will occur without any rotation or side-bending.

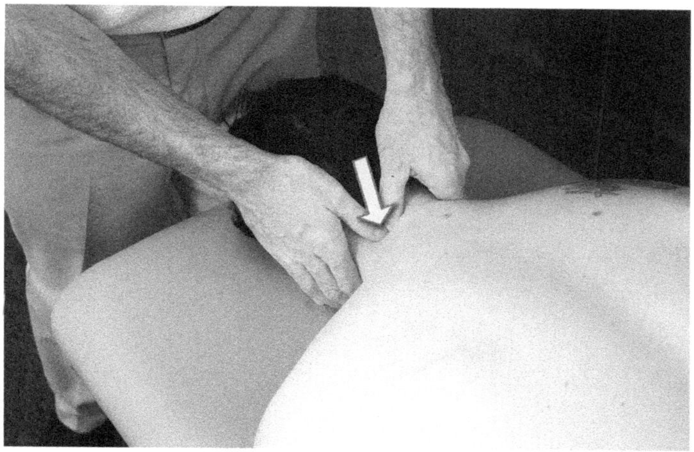

Figure 14.17 **Posterior–anterior unilateral mid-cervical spine mobilization.**

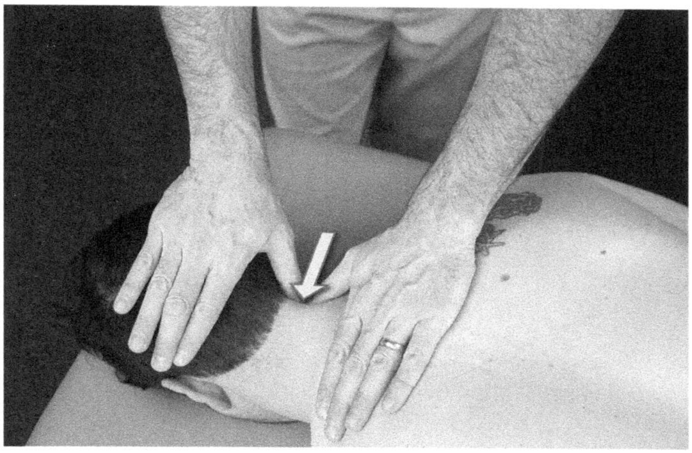

Figure 14.18 **Transverse unilateral mid-cervical spine mobilization.**

Note: Care should be taken when applying this technique adjacent to a spinal segment with reactive hypermobility or radiculopathy. If these conditions are present then either the oscillatory amplitude or starting depth of movement should be adjusted to avoid provocation of neurogenic symptoms.

Transverse unilateral mid-cervical spine mobilization (Fig. 14.18)

The patient is prone with the cervical spine in slight extension and neutral side-bending and rotation. The therapist stands on the side of the patient. The pads of his left and right thumbs contact the right side of the spinous process / lamina (mid-cervical segment illustrated). The therapist's arms and thumbs are directed medially. The remaining portions of the therapist's hands remain relaxed and in contact with the dorsal skull and upper thoracic spine. Oscillatory pressure is directed through the thumbs in a lateral to medial direction on the spinous process. When performed correctly a small side-bending and rotation movement of the neck will occur without any flexion or extension.

Note: Because the spinous process contact used in this technique can easily generate movement, only very gentle and small oscillations should be used. In addition, care should be taken to avoid discomfort due to thumb tip pressure. This technique is most indicated for patients experiencing unilateral cervical symptoms.

Cervical Spine Manipulative Procedures

There are numerous factors that may help determine the suitability of the patient to receive cervical joint manipulation. These factors depend on both the patient and the clinician. In determining whether spinal manipulation should be the appropriate intervention for a patient, it is generally recommended that the clinician assesses joint glide and end feel at the end of the available passive range in the segment identified as dysfunctional, for detection of a firm end feel that arrives slightly early in the passive range of motion (Krauss et al 2006; Pettman 2006). There is little evidence, however, to guide the clinician with regard to the validity of assessing end feel as an indicator for joint manipulation. Therefore, proper clinical reasoning should determine whether this intervention is the most appropriate for a particular individual at any moment during the treatment.

There are three important components of the spinal manipulation requiring consideration: velocity, amplitude and force. It has been argued that the term 'high-velocity' may be a misnomer, since the technique starts at zero velocity, and it has therefore been referred to by several authors as a 'high-acceleration' rather than a 'high-velocity' technique (Pettman 2006). Secondly, keeping the amplitude low minimizes the potential risk of damage to the joint complex and its surrounding tissues, particularly manipulations targeted to the upper cervical spine. Thirdly, the magnitude of the force is also important. If adequate localization and accumulative tension of the movable barrier is achieved, little force is required for successful technique. Some factors that may be associated with poor outcomes with cervical joint manipulation are listed in Box 14.1 (Krauss et al 2006).

C2–C6 separation of zygapophyseal articular joint: manipulation in rotation (Fig. 14.19)

The patient is supine with the cervical spine in a neutral position. The MCP joint of the index finger of the therapist makes contact over the posterior–lateral aspect of the articular process of the cranial vertebra in the treatment segment. The therapist cradles the patient's head with the other hand. The cervical spine is slightly flexed down to the targeted segment. Gentle ipsilateral side-flexion and contralateral rotation to the targeted side are introduced until slight tension is perceived in the tissues at the contact point. A high-velocity low-amplitude cervical spine manipulation is directed upwards and medially in the direction of the subject's contralateral eye.

Note: Do not combine rotation and side-bending in the manipulative force, because this may increase the friction at the joint surfaces and tension in the periarticular structures, which may cause the operator to increase the force of the thrust to overcome this resistance.

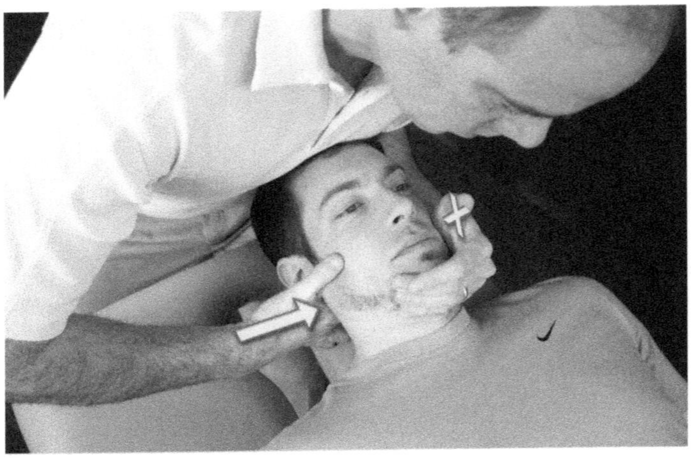

Figure 14.19 C2–C6 separation of zygapophyseal articular joint: manipulation in rotation.

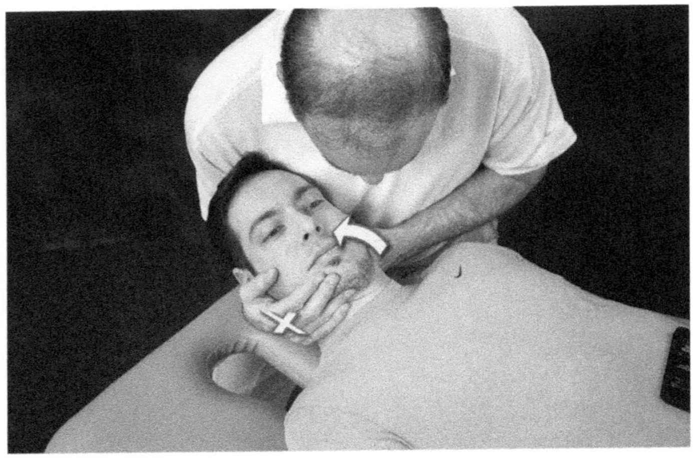

Figure 14.20 Atlanto-axial separation of zygapophyseal articular joint: upper cervical spine manipulation.

Box 14.1 Factors associated with poor outcomes with cervical joint manipulation

Clinician-related factors

- Inadequate clinical training and experience
- Inadequate patient physical examination
- Diagnostic error
- Poor choice of manipulative procedures
- Incorrect patient positioning during technique
- Poorly applied technique
- Excessive manipulative force or amplitude
- Lack of interpersonal and communication skills

Patient-related factors

- Personal expectations of the patient
- Prior experiences with previous clinicians (mostly bad)
- Emotional, psychological and behavioural factors
- Patient fear and apprehension
- Too much pain in too many directions of spinal motion
- Congenital abnormalities
- Multiple medical comorbidities

Atlanto-axial separation of zygapophyseal articular joint: upper cervical spine manipulation (Fig. 14.20)

The patient is supine with the cervical spine in a neutral position. The MCP joint of the index finger of the therapist contacts over the posterior–lateral aspect of the articular process of the AA (C1–C2) joint in the targeted side. The therapist grasps the patient's chin with the other hand and uses the forearm to support the patient's head. The cervical spine is flexed approximately over the targeted segment. Gentle contralateral rotation to the targeted side is introduced until slight tension is perceived in the tissues at the contact point (AA joint). A lateral glide of the AA joint is slightly introduced to increase the tension. A high-velocity low-amplitude upper cervical spine manipulation is executed horizontally in the direction of the subject's contralateral eye.

Note: It is important to note that the upper cervical spine manipulation is not executed by increasing the rotation of the cervical spine, which is a dangerous movement for the vertebral artery. The impulse is applied in the lateral glide of the AA joint.

Conclusion

In summary, recent years have seen great advances in our understanding of the factors associated with successful management of neck and arm pain through the use of mobilization and manipulation of the cervical spine. However, questions and challenges still remain unanswered and require continued open discussion by all practitioners of these interventions. Advancement in our understanding of the possibilities and pitfalls of the clinical practice of cervical mobilization and manipulation requires continued careful examination of practitioners' beliefs, whether they are based on emerging literature or expert opinion.

References

Aquino RL, Caires PM, Furtado FC, et al. 2009. Applying joint mobilization at different cervical vertebral levels does not influence immediate pain reduction in patients with chronic neck pain: a randomized clinical trial. J Man Manip Ther 17: 95–100.

Arnold C, Bourassa R, Langer T, et al. 2004. Doppler studies evaluating the effect of a physical therapy screening protocol on vertebral artery blood flow. Man Ther 9: 13–21.

Assendelft WJ, Bouter LM, Knipschild PG. 1996. Complications of spinal manipulation: a comprehensive review of the literature. J Fam Pract 42: 475–480.

Bee LA, Dickenson AH. 2007. Rostral ventromedial medulla control of spinal sensory processing in normal and pathophysiological states. Neuroscience 147: 786–793.

Beneck G, Kulig K, Landel R, et al. 2005. The relationship between lumbar segmental motion and pain response produced by a posterior–to-anterior force in persons with nonspecific low back pain. J Orthop Sports Phys Ther 35: 203–209.

Bialosky JE, Bishop MD, Robinson ME, et al. 2009a. Spinal manipulative therapy has an immediate effect on thermal pain sensitivity in people with low back pain: a randomized controlled trial. Phys Ther 89: 1292–303.

Bialosky JE, Bishop MD, Price DD, et al. 2009b. The mechanisms of manual therapy in the treatment of musculoskeletal pain: a comprehensive model. Man Ther 14: 531–538.

Boal RW, Gillette RG. 2004. Central neuronal plasticity, low back pain and spinal manipulative therapy. J Manipulative Physiol Ther 27: 314–326.

Bogduk N, Jull G. 1985. The theoretical pathology of acute locked back: a basis for manipulative therapy. Man Med 1: 78–82.

Boissonnault WG, Badke MB. 2008. Influence of acuity on physical therapy outcomes for patients with cervical disorders. Arch Phys Med Rehabil 89: 81–86.

Cagnie B, Vinck E, Beernaert A, et al. 2004. How common are side effects of spinal manipulation and can these side effects be predicted? Man Ther 9: 151–156.

Carlesso L, Rivett D. 2011. Manipulative practice in the cervical spine: a survey of IFOMPT member countries. J Man Manip Ther 19: 66–70.

Carlesso LC, Gross AR, Santaguida PL, et al. 2010a. Adverse events associated with the use of cervical manipulation and mobilization for the treatment of neck pain in adults: a systematic review. Man Ther 15: 434–444.

Carlesso LC, Macdermid JC, Santaguida LP. 2010b. Standardization of adverse event terminology and reporting in orthopaedic physical therapy: application to the cervical spine. J Orthop Sports Phys Ther 40: 455–463.

Carnes D, Mullinger B, Underwood M. 2010. Defining adverse events in manual therapies: a modified Delphi consensus study. Man Ther 15: 2–6.

Cassidy JD, Boyle E, Côté P, et al. 2008. Risk of vertebrobasilar stroke and chiropractic care: results of a population-based case-control and case-crossover study. Spine 33: S176–S183.

Cassidy JD, Lopes AA, Yong-Hing K. 1992. The immediate effect of manipulation versus mobilization on pain and range of motion in the cervical spine: a randomized controlled trial. J Manipulative Physiol Ther 15: 570–575.

Cattrysse E, Baeyens JP, Clarys JP, et al. 2007a. Manual fixation versus locking during upper cervical segmental mobilization. Part 1: an in vitro three-dimensional arthrokinematic analysis of manual flexion-extension mobilization of the atlanto-occipital joint. Man Ther 12: 342–352.

Cattrysse E, Baeyens JP, Clarys JP, et al. 2007b. Manual fixation versus locking during upper cervical segmental mobilization. Part 2: an in vitro three-dimensional arthrokinematic analysis of manual axial rotation and lateral bending mobilization of the atlanto-axial joint. Man Ther 12: 353–362.

Childs JD, Cleland JA. 2006. Development and application of clinical prediction rules to improve decision making in physical therapist practice. Phys Ther 86: 122–131.

Childs JD, Fritz JM, Flynn TW, et al. 2004. A clinical prediction rule to identify patients with low back pain most likely to benefit from spinal manipulation: a validation study. Ann Intern Med 141: 920–928.

Childs JD, Flynn TW, Fritz JM, et al. 2005. Screening for vertebrobasilar insufficiency in patients with neck pain: manual therapy decision-making in the presence of uncertainty. J Orthop Sports Phys Ther 35: 300–306.

Cleland JA, Childs JD. 2005. Does manual therapy technique matter? Orthop Division Rev Sept / Oct: 27–28.

Cleland JA, Whitman JM, Fritz JM. 2004. Effectiveness of manual physical therapy to the cervical spine in the management of lateral epicondylalgia: a retrospective analysis. J Orthop Sports Phys Ther 34: 713–722.

Cleland JA, Childs JD, McRae M, et al. 2005. Immediate effects of thoracic manipulation in patients with neck pain: a randomized clinical trial. Man Ther 10: 127–135.

Cleland JA, Fritz JM, Whitman JM, et al. 2006. The use of a lumbar spine manipulation technique by physical therapists in patients who satisfy a clinical prediction rule: a case series. J Orthop Sports Phys Ther 36: 209–214.

Cleland JA, Childs JD, Fritz JM, et al. 2007a. Development of a clinical prediction rule for guiding treatment of a subgroup of patients with neck pain: use of thoracic spine manipulation, exercise, and patient education. Phys Ther 87: 9–23.

Cleland JA, Glynn P, Whitman JM, et al. 2007b. Short-term effects of thrust versus nonthrust mobilization / manipulation directed at the thoracic spine in patients with neck pain: a randomized clinical trial. Phys Ther 87: 431–440.

Cleland JA, Fritz JM, Whitman J, et al. 2007c. Predictors of short-term outcome in people with a clinical diagnosis of cervical radiculopathy. Phys Ther 87: 1619–1632.

Cleland JA, Mintken PE, Carpenter K, et al. 2010. Examination of a clinical prediction rule to identify patients with neck pain likely to benefit from thoracic spine thrust manipulation and a general cervical range of motion exercise: multi-center randomized clinical trial. Phys Ther 90: 1239–50.

Creighton D, Viti J, Krauss J. 2005. Use of translatoric mobilization in a patient with cervical spondylotic degeneration: a case report. J Man Manip Ther 13: 12–26.

Creighton D, Kondratek M, Krauss J, et al. 2011. Ultrasound analysis of the vertebral artery during non-thrust cervical translatoric spinal manipulation. J Man Manip Ther 19: 84–90.

Dai L. 1998. Disc degeneration and cervical instability. Correlation of magnetic resonance imaging with radiography. Spine 23: 1734–1738.

Degenhardt BF, Darmani NA, Johnson JC, et al. 2007. Role of osteopathic manipulative treatment in altering pain biomarkers: a pilot study. J Am Osteopath Assoc 107: 387–400.

Derbyshire SW, Jones AK, Gyulai F, et al. 1997. Pain processing during three levels of noxious stimulation produces differential patterns of central activity. Pain 73: 431–445.

Di Fabio RP. 1999. Manipulation of the cervical spine: risks and benefits. Phys Ther 79: 50–65.

Dunning JR, Cleland JA, Waldrop MA, et al. 2012. Upper cervical and upper thoracic thrust manipulation versus nonthrust mobilization in patients with mechanical neck pain: a multicenter randomized clinical trial. J Orthop Sports Phys Ther 42: 5–18.

Ernst E. 2002. Manipulation of the cervical spine: a systematic review of case reports of serious adverse events. Med J Aust 176(8): 376–380.

Evans DW. 2002. Mechanisms and effects of spinal high-velocity, low-amplitude thrust manipulation: previous theories. J Manipulative Physiol Ther 25: 251–262.

Evans DW, Breen AC. 2006. A biomechanical model for mechanically efficient cavitation production during spinal manipulation: prethrust position and the neutral zone. J Manipulative Physiol Ther 29: 72–82.

Fernández-Carnero J, Fernández-de-las-Peñas C, Cleland JA. 2008. Immediate hypoalgesic and motor effects after a single cervical spine manipulation in subjects with lateral epicondylalgia. J Manipulative Physiol Ther 31: 675–681.

Fernández-de-las-Peñas C, Alonso-Blanco C, Cleland JA, et al. 2008. Changes in pressure pain thresholds over C5–C6 zygapophyseal joint after a cervicothoracic junction manipulation in healthy subjects. J Manipulative Physiol Ther 31: 332–7

Fernández-de-las-Peñas C, Pérez-de-Heredia M, Brea-Rivero M, et al. 2007. Immediate effects on pressure pain threshold following a single cervical spine manipulation in healthy subjects. J Orthop Sports Phys Ther 37: 325–329.

Fleming R, Forsythe S, Cook C. 2007. Influential variables associated with outcomes in patients with cervicogenic headache. J Man Manip Ther 15: 155–164.

Flynn T, Fritz J, Whitman J, et al. 2002. A clinical prediction rule for classifying patients with low back pain who demonstrate short-term improvement with spinal manipulation. Spine 27: 2835–2843.

Flynn TW. 2006. There's more than one way to manipulate a spine. J Orthop Sports Phys Ther 36: 198–199.

Flynn TW, Fritz JM, Wainner R, et al. 2003. The audible pop is not necessary for successful spinal high-velocity thrust manipulation in individuals with low back pain. Arch Phys Med Rehabil 84: 1057–1060.

Flynn TW, Childs JD, Fritz JM. 2006. The audible pop from high-velocity thrust manipulation and outcome in individuals with low back pain. J Manipulative Physiol Ther 29: 40–45.

Gal JM, Herzog W, Kawchuk GN, et al. 1995. Forces and relative vertebral movements during SMT to unembalmed post-rigor human cadavers: peculiarities associated with joint cavitation. J Manipulative Physiol Ther 18: 4–9.

Gal JM, Herzog W, Kawchuk GN, et al. 1997. Movements of vertebrae during manipulative thrusts to unembalmed human cadavers. J Manipulative Physiol Ther 20: 30–40.

Giles LG, Taylor JR. 1987. Human zygapophyseal joint capsule and synovial fold innervation. Br J Rheumatol 26: 93–98.

González-Iglesias J, Fernández-de-las-Peñas C, Cleland JA, et al. 2009. Thoracic spine manipulation for the management of patients with neck pain: a randomized clinical trial. J Orthop Sports Phys Ther 39: 20–27.

Gross AR, Hoving JL, Haines TA, et al. 2004. A Cochrane review of manipulation and mobilization for mechanical neck disorders. Spine 29: 1541–1548.

Gross AR, Kay TM, Kennedy C, et al. 2002a. Clinical practice guideline on the use of manipulation or mobilization in the treatment of adults with mechanical neck disorders. Man Ther 7: 193–205.

Gross AR, Kay TM, Hondras M, et al. 2002b. Manual therapy for mechanical neck disorders: a systematic review. Man Ther 7: 131–149.

Guo W, Robbins MT, Wei F, et al. 2006. Supraspinal brain-derived neurotrophic factor signaling: a novel mechanism for descending pain facilitation. J Neurosci 26: 126–137.

Haldeman S, Kohlbeck FJ, McGregor M. 2002. Unpredictability of cerebrovascular ischemia associated with cervical spine manipulation. Spine 27: 49–55.

Hancock MJ, Maher CG, Latimer J, et al. 2007. Assessment of diclofenac or spinal manipulative therapy, or both, in addition to recommended first-line treatment for acute low back pain: a randomised controlled trial. Lancet 370: 1638–1643.

Hengeveld E, Banks K, Maitland GD. 2005. Maitland's vertebral manipulation. Oxford: Elsevier Butterworth-Heinemann.

Herzog W, Conway PJ, Zhang YT, et al. 1995. Reflex responses associated with manipulative treatments on the thoracic spine: a pilot study. J Manipulative Physiol Ther 18: 233–236.

Herzog W, Leonard TR, Symons B, et al. 2012. Vertebral artery strains during high-speed, low amplitude cervical spinal manipulation. J Electromyogr Kinesiol 22: 740–746.

Hsieh JC, Belfrage M, Stone-Elander S, et al. 1995. Central representation of chronic ongoing neuropathic pain studied by positron emission tomography. Pain 63: 225–236.

Hurwitz EL, Aker PD, Adams AH, et al. 1996. Manipulation and mobilization of the cervical spine. Spine 21: 1746–1759.

Hurwitz EL, Morgenstern H, Harber P, et al. 2002. A randomized trial of chiropractic manipulation and mobilization for patients with neck pain: clinical outcomes from the UCLA neck-pain study. Am J Public Health 92: 1634–1641.

Hurwitz EL, Morgenstern H, Vassilaki M, et al. 2005. Frequency and clinical predictors of adverse reactions to chiropractic care in the UCLA neck pain study. Spine 30: 1477–1484.

Iadarola M, Berman K, Zeffiro T, et al. 1998. Neural activation during acute capsaicin-evoked pain and allodynia assessed with PET. Brain 121: 931–947.

Kaltenborn F. 2008. Traction-manipulation of the extremities and spine. Oslo: Norli.

Kerry R, Taylor AJ. 2006. Cervical arterial dysfunction assessment and manual therapy. Man Ther 11: 243–53.

Kondratek M, Creighton D, Krauss J. 2006. Use of translatoric mobilization in a patient with cervicogenic dizziness and motion restriction: a case report. J Man Manip Ther 14: 140–151.

Krauss J, Evjenth O, Creighton DS. 2006. Translatoric spinal manipulation for physical therapists. Lakeview: Media LLC Publications.

Krauss J, Creighton D, Ely JD, et al. 2008. The immediate effects of upper thoracic translatoric spinal manipulation on cervical pain and range of motion: a randomized clinical trial. J Man Manip Ther 16: 93–99.

Kulig K, Landel R, Powers CM. 2004. Assessment of lumbar spine kinematics using dynamic MRI: a proposed mechanism of sagittal plane motion induced by manual posterior-to-anterior mobilization. J Orthop Sports Phys Ther 34: 57–64.

Lakshmanan P, Jones A, Howes J, et al. 2005. CT evaluation of the pattern of odontoid fractures in the elderly – relationship to upper cervical spine osteoarthritis. Eur Spine J 14: 78–83.

Landel R, Kulig K, Fredericson M, et al. 2008. Intertester reliability and validity of motion assessments during lumbar spine accessory motion testing. Phys Ther 88: 43–49.

Leaver AM, Maher CG, Herbert RD, et al. 2010. A randomized controlled trial comparing manipulation with mobilization for recent onset neck pain. Arch Phys Med Rehabil 91: 1313–1318.

Lebouef-Yde C, Hennius B, Rudberg E, et al. 1997. Side effects of chiropractic treatment: a prospective study. J Manipulative Physiol Ther 20: 223–228.

Lee KP, Carlini WG, McCormick G, et al. 1995. Neurologic complications following chiropractic manipulation: a survey of California neurologists. Neurology 45: 1213–1215.

Lee RY, McGregor AH, Bull AM, et al. 2005. Dynamic response of the cervical spine to posteroanterior mobilisation. Clin Biomech 20: 228–231.

Licht PB, Christensen HW, Hoilund-Carlsen PF. 2003. Is cervical spinal manipulation dangerous? J Manipulative Physiol Ther 26: 48–52.

Maitland GD, Hengeveld E, Banks K, et al. 2005. Maitland's vertebral manipulation, 7th edn. New York: Elsevier Butterworth-Heinemann.

Malisza KL, Stroman PW, Turner A, et al. 2003a. Functional MRI of the rat lumbar spinal cord involving painful stimulation and the effect of peripheral joint mobilization. J Magn Reson Imaging 18: 152–159.

Malisza KL, Gregorash L, Turner A, et al. 2003b. Functional MRI involving painful stimulation of the ankle and the effect of physiotherapy joint mobilization. Magn Reson Imaging 21: 489–496.

Malone DG, Baldwin NG, Tomecek FJ, et al. 2002. Complications of cervical spine manipulation therapy: 5-year retrospective study in a single-group practice. Neurosurg Focus 13: ecp1.

Martinez-Segura R, Fernández-de-las-Peñas C, Ruiz-Saez M, et al. 2006. Immediate effects on neck pain and active range of motion after a single cervical high-velocity low-amplitude manipulation in subjects presenting with mechanical neck pain: a randomized controlled trial. J Manipulative Physiol Ther 29: 511–517.

May S, Resendale R. 2009. Prescriptive clinical predication rules in back pain research: a systematic review. J Man Manip Ther 17: 36–45.

McClatchie L, Laprade J, Martin S, et al. 2009. Mobilizations of the asymptomatic cervical spine can reduce signs of shoulder dysfunction in adults. Man Ther 14: 369–374.

McPartland JM, Giuffrida A, King J, et al. 2005. Cannabimimetic effects of osteopathic manipulative treatment. J Am Osteopathic Assoc 105: 283–291.

Mercer S, Bogduk N. 1993. Intra-articular inclusions of the cervical synovial joints. Br J Rheumatol 32: 705–710.

Mintken PE, DeRosa C, Little T, et al. 2008. AAOMPT clinical guidelines: a model for standardizing manipulation terminology in physical therapy practice. J Orthop Sports Phys Ther 38: A1–A6.

Miyazaki M, Hong SW, Yoon SH, et al. 2008. Kinematic analysis of the relationship between the grade of disc degeneration and motion unit of the cervical spine. Spine 33: 187–193.

Moulton EA, Keaser ML, Gullapalli RP, et al. 2005. Regional intensive and temporal patterns of functional MRI activation distinguishing noxious and innocuous contact heat. J Neurophysiol 93: 2183–2193.

Murphy DR. 2006. Herniated disc with radiculopathy following cervical manipulation: nonsurgical management. Spine J 6: 459–463.

Murphy DR, Hurwitz EL, Gregory AA. 2006. Manipulation in the presence of cervical spinal cord compression: a case series. J Manipulative Physiol Ther 29: 236–244.

Norris JW, Beletsky V, Nadareishvili ZG. 2000. Sudden neck movement and cervical artery dissection. The Canadian Stroke Consortium. CMAJ 163: 38–40.

Oppenheim JS, Spitzer DE, Segal D. 2005. Nonvascular complications following spinal manipulation. Spine J 5: 660–667.

Oshiro Y, Quevedo AS, McHaffie JG, et al. 2007. Brain mechanisms supporting spatial discrimination of pain. J Neurosci 27: 3388–3394.

Padua L, Padua R, LoMonaco M, et al. 1996. Radiculomedullary complications of cervical spinal manipulation. Spinal Cord 34: 488–492.

Palfrey AJ, Newton M. 1970. The viscosity of synovial fluid at high shear rates. J Anat 106: 404.

Pettman E. 2006. Manipulative thrust techniques: an evidence-based approach. Abbotsford, Canada: Aphema Publishing.

Peyron R, Laurent B, García-Larrea L. 2000. Functional imaging of brain responses to pain: a review and meta-analysis. Clin Neurophysiol 30: 263–288.

Pickar JG. 2002. Neurophysiological effects of spinal manipulation. Spine J 2: 357–371.

Pickar JG, Wheeler JD. 2001. Response of muscle proprioceptors to spinal manipulative-like loads in the anesthetized cat. J Manipulative Physiol Ther 24: 2–11.

Pikula JR. 1999. The effect of spinal manipulative therapy (SMT) on pain reduction and range of motion in patients with acute unilateral neck pain: a pilot study. J Can Chiropr Assoc 43: 111–119.

Powers CM, Kulig K, Harrison J, et al. 2003. Segmental mobility of the lumbar spine during a posterior to anterior mobilization: assessment using dynamic MRI. Clin Biomech 18: 80–83.

Puentedura EJ, Landers MR, Cleland JA, et al. 2011. Thoracic spine thrust manipulation versus cervical spine thrust manipulation in patients with acute neck pain: a randomized clinical trial. J Orthop Sports Phys Ther 41: 208–220.

Puentedura EJ, March J, Anders J, et al. 2012a. Safety of cervical spine manipulation: are adverse events preventable and are manipulations being performed appropriately? A review of 134 case reports. J Man Manip Ther 20: 66–74.

Puentedura EJ, Cleland JA, Landers MR, et al. 2012b Development of a clinical prediction rule to identify patients with neck pain likely to benefit from thrust joint manipulation to the cervical spine. J Orthop Sports Phys Ther 42: 577–592.

Quesnele JJ, Triano JJ, Noseworthy MD, et al. 2014. Changes in vertebral artery blood flow following various head positions and cervical spine manipulation. J Manipulative Physiol Ther 37: 22–31.

Ross JK, Bereznick DE, McGill SM. 2004. Determining cavitation location during lumbar and thoracic spinal manipulation: is spinal manipulation accurate and specific? Spine 29: 1452–1457.

Saavedra-Hernández M, Arroyo-Morales M, Cantarero-Villanueva I, et al. 2013. Short-term effects of spinal thrust joint manipulation in patients with chronic neck pain: a randomized clinical trial. Clin Rehabil 27: 504–512.

Schomacher J. 2009. The effect of analgesic mobilization technique when applied at symptomatic or asymptomatic levels of the cervical spine in subjects with neck pain: a randomized controlled trial. J Man Manip Ther 17: 101–108.

Semlak K, Ferguson AB. 1970. Joint stability maintained by atmospheric pressure: an experimental study. Clin Orthop Relat Res 68: 294–300.

Senstad O, Lebouef-Yde C, Borchgrevink C. 1996. Predictors of side effects to spinal manipulative therapy. J Manipulative Physiol Ther 19: 441–445.

Shekelle PG. 1994. Spinal manipulation. Spine 19: 858–861.

Shekelle PG, Coulter I. 1997. Cervical spine manipulation: summary report of a systematic review of the literature and a multidisciplinary expert panel. J Spinal Disord 10: 223–228.

Sigerist HE. 1951. A history of medicine, Vol. I: Primitive and archaic medicine. New York: Oxford University Press.

Smith WS, Johnston SC, Skalabrin EJ, et al. 2003. Spinal manipulative therapy is an independent risk factor for vertebral artery dissection. Neurology 60: 1424–1428.

Staud R, Craggs JG, Robinson EM, et al. 2007. Brain activity related to temporal summation of C-fiber evoked pain. Pain 129: 130–142.

Sterling M, Jull G, Wright A. 2001. Cervical mobilisation: concurrent effects on pain, sympathetic nervous system activity and motor activity. Man Ther 6: 72–81.

Teodorczyk-Injeyan JA, Injeyan H, Ruegg R. 2006. Spinal manipulative therapy reduces inflammatory cytokines but not substance P production in normal subjects. J Manipulative Physiol Ther 29: 14–21.

Thiel H, Bolton J. 2004. Estimate of the number of treatment visits involving cervical spine manipulation carried out by members of the British and Scottish Chiropractor Associations over a one-year period. Clin Chiropr 7: 163–167.

Thiel H, Rix G. 2005. Is it time to stop functional pre-manipulation testing of the cervical spine? Man Ther 10: 154–158.

Thomas LC, Rivett DA, Bateman G, et al. 2013. Effect of selected manual therapy interventions for mechanical neck pain on vertebral and internal carotid arterial blood flow and cerebral inflow. Phys Ther 93: 1563–1574.

Tseng SH, Lin SM, Chen Y, et al. 2002. Ruptured cervical disc after spinal manipulation therapy: report of two cases. Spine 27: E80–E82.

Vernon H, Dhami M, Howley T, et al. 1986. Spinal manipulation and beta-endorphin: a controlled study of the effect of a spinal manipulation on plasma beta-endorphin levels in normal males. J Manipulative Physiol Ther 9: 115–123.

Vincent K, Maigne JY, Fischhoff C, et al. 2013. Systematic review of manual therapies for nonspecific neck pain. Joint Bone Spine 80: 508–515.

Vogt BA, Derbyshire S, Jones AK. 1996. Pain processing in four regions of human cingulate cortex localized with co-registered PET and MR imaging. Eur J Neurosci 8: 1461–1473.

Williams NH, Hendry M, Lewis R, et al. 2007. Psychological response in spinal manipulation (PRISM): a systematic review of psychological outcomes in randomised controlled trials. Complement Ther Med 15: 271–283.

15 Chapter

Therapeutic Exercise for Mechanical Neck Pain

Carol Kennedy

CHAPTER CONTENTS

Introduction	174
Exercises for motor function	175
Recruitment	175
Strength and endurance	176
Side-flexion/rotation exercises for asymmetric weakness	179
Motor control	180
Mobility exercises	182
Generalized active range of motion	182
Articular/self-mobilization	183
Myofascial extensibility	184
Neurodynamics	185
Postural correction exercises	185
Muscle imbalance	185
Articular system	186
Neuromeningeal system	186
Posture corrections	186
Somatosensory dysfunction	186

Introduction

The use of specific therapeutic exercise as an adjunct to manual therapy treatment has been a major emphasis of physiotherapy in recent years as part of the multimodal approach to management of acute and chronic mechanical neck pain (MNP). It can be challenging to develop a comprehensive exercise programme, attempting to address the many factors involved, yet not overload or irritate the neck.

In a systematic review of the conservative management of MNP, Gross et al (2007) found strong evidence of benefit for long-term pain reduction, improved function and positive global perceived benefit for a combination of manual therapy and exercise for subacute and chronic mechanical neck disorders. There was also moderate evidence for long-term improved function for neck-strengthening and stretching exercises in chronic subjects. For the use of vertigo exercises, there was moderate evidence for high global perceived effect. Sarig-Bahat (2003), in a review of the use of exercise alone, concluded that there was strong evidence supporting the effectiveness of dynamic resisted strengthening and proprioceptive exercises. There was also moderate evidence to support the use of early mobility exercises for acute whiplash-associated disorder (WAD). Several studies (Jull et al 2002; Ylinen et al 2006; Walker et al 2008) have shown improvements to be maintained over the long term of 1 to 3 years, even though continuation of home exercises following the initial training was inconsistent (Ylinen et al 2007a).

An updated Cochrane Review has recently concluded that there is moderate-quality evidence supporting combined specific cervical and scapular–thoracic stretching and strengthening for pain relief post treatment and at intermediate follow-up, and improved function in both the short term and the intermediate term for chronic neck pain (Kay et al 2012). Low- to moderate-quality evidence shows no benefit of upper extremity or general exercise programmes alone. Low- to moderate-quality evidence supports self-mobilization and low-load neck and scapular endurance exercises in reducing pain, improving function and global perceived effect in the long term for cervicogenic headache. Low-quality evidence supports neck-strengthening exercise programmes in acute cervical radiculopathy for pain relief in the short term. Moderate-quality evidence demonstrates that patients are very satisfied with their care when treated with therapeutic exercise (Kay et al 2012).

Supervised exercise programmes have been found to be more effective than either home exercise or exercise advice in improving self-efficacy, fear of movement/re-injury and pain disability (Taimela et al 2000; Bunketorp et al 2006). In their qualitative study, Escolar-Reina et al (2010) found that patients were more likely to adhere to their home exercise programme in the following circumstances: the exercises were not too time consuming or disruptive to their daily routine, they were not too complex, they had received adequate feedback and supervision when learning the exercises, and the therapist style and exercise experience had been positive.

Conley et al (1997) demonstrated that exercises focusing on the upper extremity did not result in hypertrophy of the cervical musculature; strengthening had to be directed specifically to the neck.

Although it is clear that cervical exercise programmes are an effective component in the management of neck pain, the type of exercise that is most effective has not yet been determined. Various programmes of low-load craniocervical flexion (CCF) exercises, higher load head-lift exercises and resisted static and dynamic exercises have all been found to be effective in terms of reducing pain and improving function, but one is not necessarily superior to the others (Jordan et al 1998; Randlov et al 1998; Bronfort et al 2001; Jull 2000; Falla et al 2006; Vassiliou et al 2006). Higher loaded exercises do seem to be more effective in increasing overall strength and decreasing fatigability (Falla et al 2006; Ylinen et al 2006). The lower load exercise has been shown to be superior for postural control (Falla et al 2007a) and normalizing patterning during craniocervical flexion. The higher load programmes have not been tested in groups with higher pain levels and may not be appropriate for that patient population. Gains made with an exercise appear to be directly linked to the mode of that exercise. O'Leary et al (2012) compared a coordination (the CCF nod task with the pressure biofeedback unit) and endurance (isometric flexor endurance training) exercise group with a mobility control group over 10 weeks. All three groups achieved improvement in pain and disability, but each group improved predominately in the motor performance of their assigned mode of exercise, with only minimal change in the other domains. It is important to consider this and include various modes of exercise when designing comprehensive cervical rehabilitation programmes.

This chapter describes various therapeutic exercise interventions for the common impairments seen in patients with mechanical neck pain.

Exercises for Motor Function

Abnormal recruitment patterning of the anterior cervical muscles occurs in subjects with neck pain, with a tendency towards overdominance of the superficial muscle groups and inhibition of the deep spinal stabilizers (Jull 2000; Sterling et al 2003, 2004; Falla et al 2004a; Jull et al 2004, 2007a). This impaired recruitment pattern appears to be more directly linked to neck pain and its intensity than to the chronicity or degree of disability (Cagnie et al 2011a; O'Leary et al 2011). Subjects with neck pain also demonstrate abnormalities in extensor muscle recruitment and patterning, with excessive superficial activity and inhibition of the deeper layers and delayed relaxation times (Cagnie et al 2011b; Elliott et al 2010a; Schomaker & Falla 2013). In low-load situations this imbalance is more apparent, although there is also true weakness and lack of endurance of both deep and superficial muscle groups (Falla et al 2003; O'Leary et al 2007). A timing delay of the neck stabilizers occurs during arm motion, most noticeably the deep neck flexors (DNF), compromising spinal control during upper extremity function (Falla et al 2004b). Studies have shown a tendency towards overactivity in the upper trapezius muscle (UFT) and anterior superficial neck muscles during repetitive arm activities and head lift, with prolonged relaxation times post activity (Nederhand et al 2000, 2002; Falla et al 2004c; Szeto et al 2005). On imaging, subjects with neck pain or headache exhibit atrophy and histological changes of the deep neck flexor and extensor muscles at the effected segment (Hallgren et al 1994; Uhlig et al 1995; Kristjansson 2004; Elliott et al 2006, 2008a, 2008b, 2009, 2010b, 2011; Fernández-de-las-Peñas et al 2007, 2008). Changes appear to be more profound in subjects with traumatic (WAD) as compared with insidious onset neck pain.

Clinically then, it seems important to begin motor retraining in mechanical neck pain patients by focusing on the ability to recruit and isolate the deep neck flexors and extensors in low-load situations. Prolonged holds emphasize the endurance function. During any upper extremity exercises, a preset DNF recruitment nod to neutral could potentially help retrain the timing impairment. It is important to encourage complete relaxation of all muscle groups, particularly superficial ones, following exercise and activity. Progression onto higher load exercises will then regain strength of the full synergy, but one must ensure that there is contribution from the deeper muscle groups. Depending on the patient's occupation and activities, this may require additional load beyond the weight of the head.

Recruitment

Deep neck flexors

The basic exercise used to retrain the DNF is the head nod of CCF. Although longus capitus and colli muscles are often considered together as the DNF, Cagnie et al (2008) showed that the longus capitus is the primary muscle during this motion. The patient is instructed in the proper technique of CCF. Through palpation of the anterior neck both the sternocleidomastoid (SCM) and anterior / middle scalene are monitored, nodding as far into range as possible without activating these muscles. If the cervical extensors are particularly tight, the superficial flexors will contract early to overcome the resistance, making it more effective to lengthen those first to allow a freer nod motion. Unwanted hyoid muscle activity is minimized by having the tongue rest in the roof of the mouth, with the jaw relaxed. The head must remain in contact with the surface, but retraction avoided. Cues such as 'slide the back of your head up the surface' or 'look down with your eyes as you initiate the nod' may help the patient recruit the deep muscles in isolation. The nod should be held for a count of 10 and repeated 10 times, twice daily (Jull et al 2002). The argument could be made that to truly learn and solidify a new movement pattern, some form of this exercise and any other motor pattern retraining exercises should be repeated multiple times a day, even if for just a few repetitions.

DNF recruitment and isolation can be performed either in supine or up against the wall. Theoretically the wall position is easier because of gravity-assist, but some patients will relax the superficial muscles more effectively in lying and patients with poor posture are often better supported in that position. In standing, the head must remain in contact with the wall throughout the exercise to ensure the use of the flexors, rather than eccentric extensor activity (Fig. 15.1). In supine position, the use of a towel roll helps to support the normal lordosis of the cervical spine. However, some patients find the roll uncomfortable or will tend to press back against it using retraction instead of the correct CCF motion. Pillow support tends to be easier than none. Clinical reasoning should be utilized to determine which option is optimal for any given patient.

In patients with longstanding bracing patterns of their neck, the SCM and scalene muscles often become so facilitated that they are used as primary muscles of respiration. Downtraining may start with diaphragmatic breathing exercises,

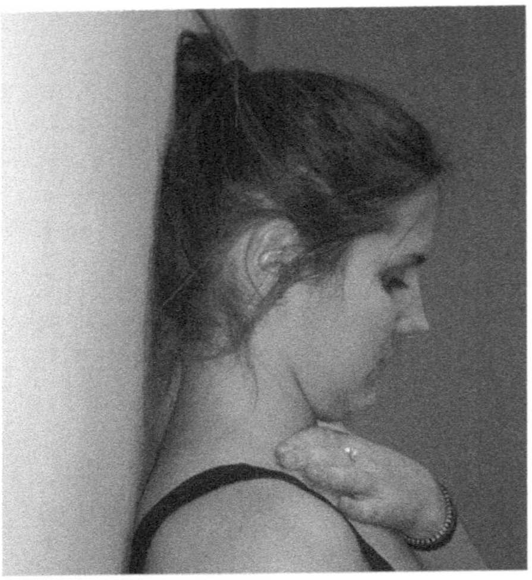

Figure 15.1 Wall slide deep neck flexor recruitment exercise. Keeping the head in contact with the wall, the head is nodded as far as possible without any activity in the superficial muscles, palpated at the anterior neck.

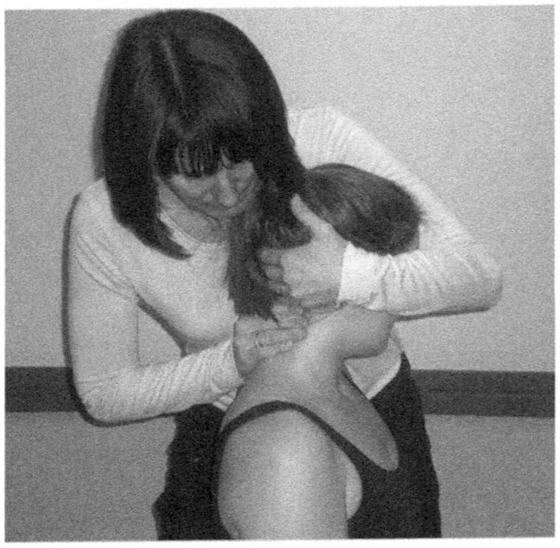

Figure 15.2 Muscle energy recruitment technique. Recruitment of the right C2/3 multifidus muscle is achieved by utilizing a muscle energy type technique.

encouraging lateral costal motion whilst monitoring the SCM and scalene to reduce their excessive activity.

Deep neck extensors

Isolated recruitment of a segmental muscle is difficult, but a 'muscle energy' type technique or electrical muscle stimulation may help teach the patient to feel the desired localized contraction of multifidus or a posterior suboccipital muscle (Fig. 15.2). The patient can then practise an auto-resisted isometric or concentric contraction at the affected level (Fig. 15.3). Resistance must be light to encourage deep rather than superficial muscle contraction. In supine, a towel roll under the neck may help the patient perform a unilateral extension quadrant motion to facilitate multifidus contraction. Schomaker et al (2012) found that resistance applied at the vertebral arch of C2 was more effective in preferentially recruiting deeper rather than superficial extensors, compared with pressure at the occiput or C5.

Another method to recruit the DNF is to use a segmental extension motion from a slump position starting in the thorax

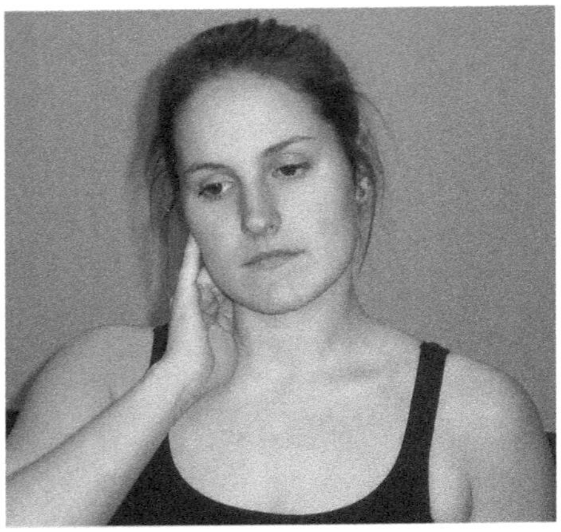

Figure 15.3 Auto-resisted deep neck extensor muscle exercise. The patient is taught to resist extension/side-flexion at the affected level to recruit the multifidus muscle segmentally.

and moving cranially (Fig. 15.4A–C). If the chin is kept tucked initially, the superficial muscles will be less active during this motion (Mayoux-Benhamou et al 1997). As motion is performed segmentally, focus is on the deeper muscle layers. The motion must also be kept fluid and relaxed, as bracing will only encourage the rigidity that is so often seen in patients with chronic neck pain.

Strength and endurance

As stated previously, although both low-load (CCF nod) and higher load (head-lift) exercises appear equally effective in reducing pain and disability, higher load exercise using added resistance may be more effective in regaining full strength and endurance. Therefore, to optimize return of normal neck muscle function, higher load exercise progressions should be included at some point in the rehabilitation programme. However, in cases of more severe neck pain, higher load exercises, if done too early, tend to exacerbate the pain, which would further inhibit normal muscle function. In those patients with longstanding protective bracing and rigidity, it would seem counterintuitive to add higher loads, which encourage even more superficial muscle activation. On the other hand, patients with low-intensity neck pain and generalized muscle weakness would tolerate and benefit from fairly rapid progression to higher load exercises as long as they demonstrate appropriate muscle balance. As the deep musculature should contract to stabilize the spine prior to any loading, initiating and maintaining a DNF nod throughout the higher loaded exercises would encourage optimal patterning.

Higher load flexor progressions

Auto-resisted exercises can be graded and are lower load than head-lift exercises. The use of hands or a ball under the chin to resist an isometric or concentric contraction encourages the CCF pattern. An isometric holding contraction can be progressed in sitting by having the patient nod to cervical neutral and maintain this as they lean back at the hips to add gravity resistance. This can be further progressed by performing the sit-back on an exercise ball, moving farther back

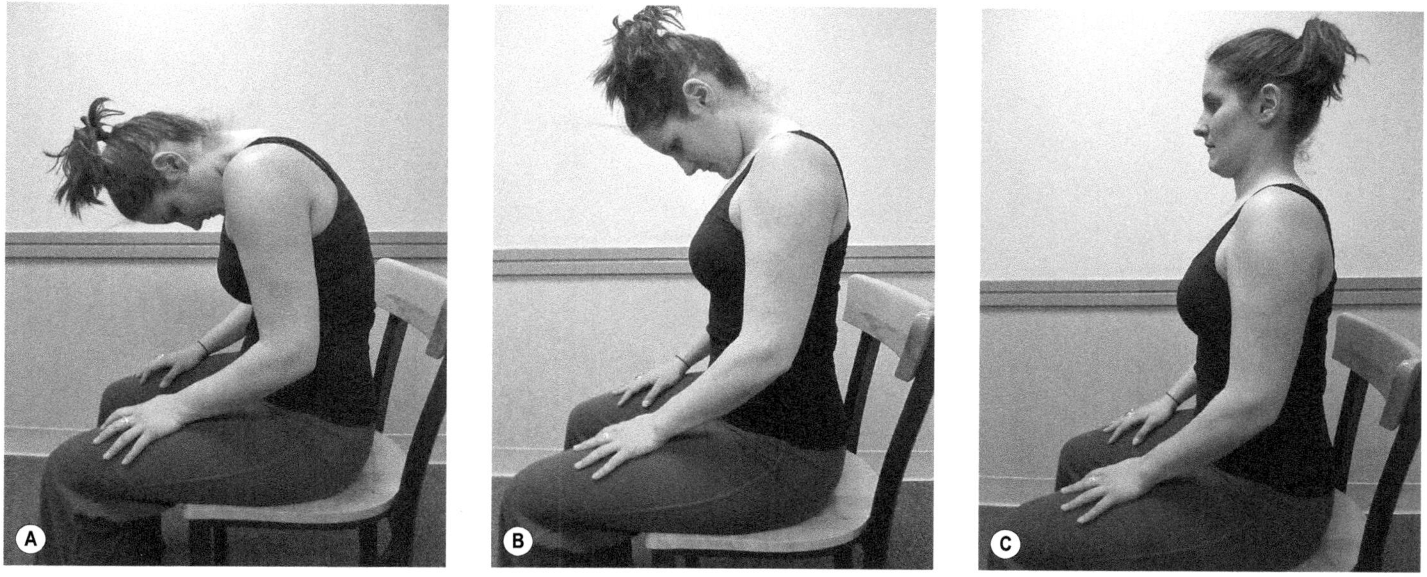

Figure 15.4 Segmental extension from slump: (**A**) Starting in a flexed slump position, segmental extension proceeds from the mid-thoracic spine cranially. (**B**) Once the thorax is in neutral, segmental extension continues from the lower cervical spine to the craniovertebral region. (**C**) In the erect position, the nod is released to the neutral neck position.

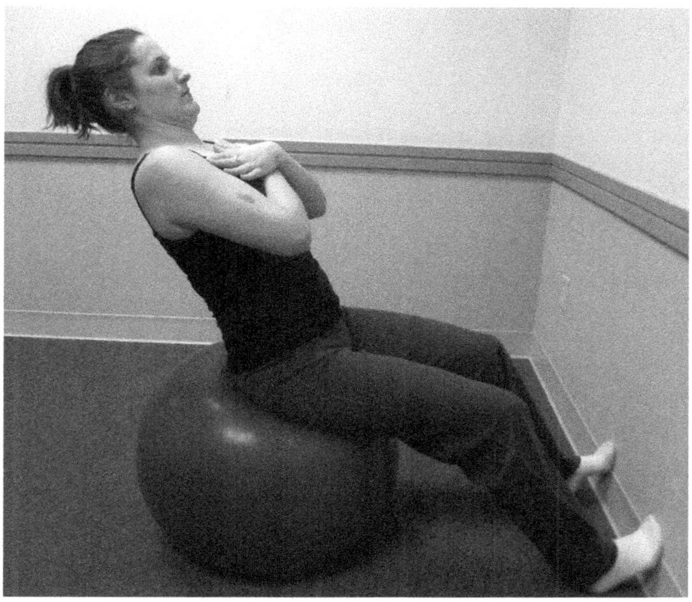

Figure 15.5 Sit-back flexor strength progression. The patient can increase loading for the cervical flexors doing sit-back exercises on the ball, maintaining a neutral deep neck flexor nod.

into range and holding for progressively longer periods of time (Fig. 15.5).

A nod lift-off motion can be performed on an incline (Fig. 15.6). The patient uses a nod motion to lift the head just off the surface to a neutral position. Endurance can be emphasized by progressively increasing the hold time and the exercise made more difficult by gradually reducing the angle of the incline.

Theraband® can be used to add resistance. As an isometric exercise in sitting, the patient adopts a cervical-neutral nod with the band around the forehead and, while maintaining

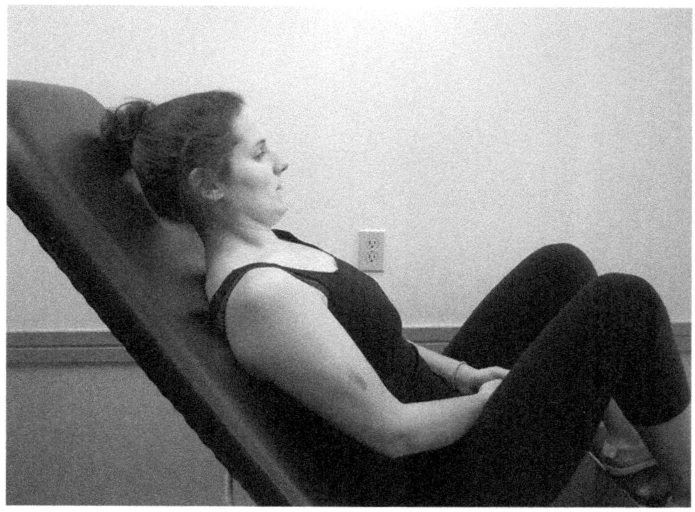

Figure 15.6 Nod lift-off on an incline. The patient lifts the head off the incline using a deep neck flexor nod action, holding a cervical-neutral posture.

neutral, leans forwards at the hips to add resistance (Fig. 15.7). Alternatively, the band can be used to resist a through-range isotonic exercise, ensuring that forward translation is controlled. In standing, lunges can be used to increase the tension in the band, with the patient maintaining a neutral nod position throughout the step forward and then back to the start position. Because of the higher balance challenge, there is a degree of perturbation imparted to the head and neck, which demands a higher degree of dynamic stabilization (Fig. 15.8).

In supine, a head-lift exercise can be performed in two different ways. As an isometric contraction, the patient maintains a neutral nod and lifts the head off the surface, holding for progressively longer periods of time. Another option is an isotonic segmental flexion curl-up exercise, continuing the nod through to inner range (Fig. 15.9). In an MRI study,

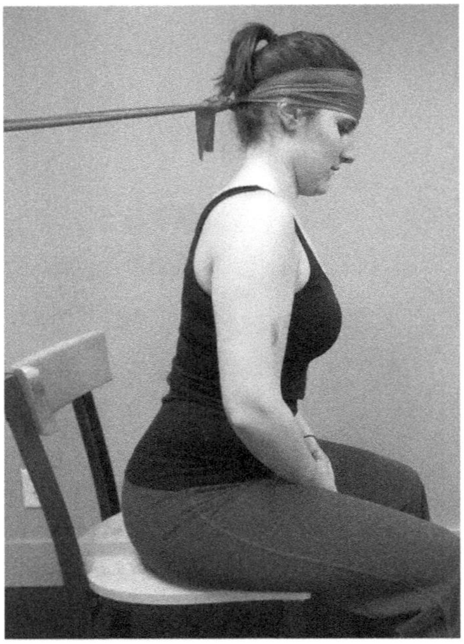

Figure 15.7 Elastic band resisted flexors. Maintaining a cervical nod, the body is leaned forwards at the hips to increase the tension in the band to strengthen the cervical flexor synergy.

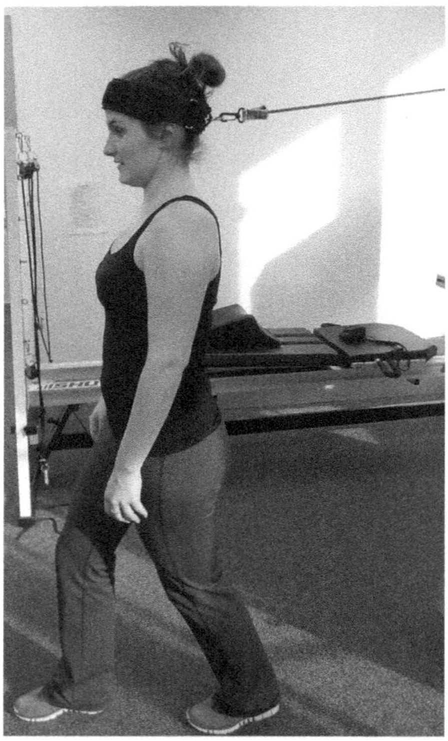

Figure 15.8 Elastic band forward lunge. Maintaining cervical neutral, a forward lunge motion is performed applying a flexor strength load with a perturbation.

Cagnie et al (2008) showed that the longus capitus and colli along with the SCM were all more active with this second exercise, with relatively greater contribution from the DNF in the curl-up exercise than in the neutral nod-lift option. It may be beneficial to use a towel roll as a fulcrum under the neck to encourage the curl-up action.

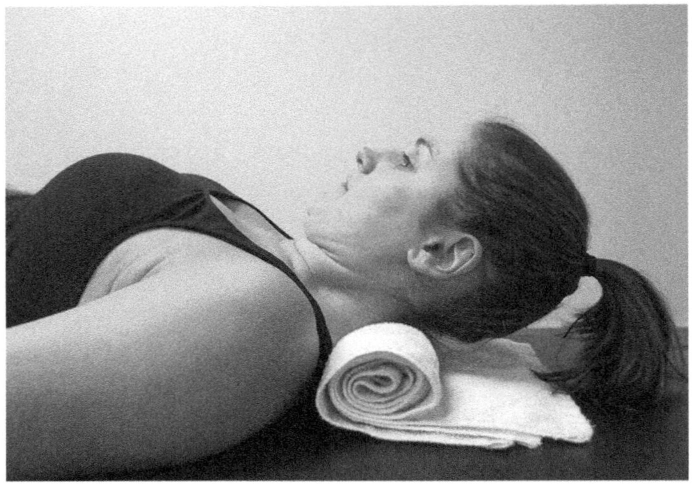

Figure 15.9 Curl-up head lift. The patient initiates the exercise with a craniocervical flexion motion and continues to flex through to inner range. The towel roll can facilitate the segmental nature of the motion.

Higher load extensor progressions

DNF strengthening can be progressed by increasing the load effect of gravity in four-point kneeling (4PK). The start position is with the head dropped into full flexion and the back sagged (Fig. 15.10A). The patient is first instructed to find neutral lumbopelvic posture. Then he or she is taught to obtain a neutral thorax by pressing up through the arms to a *slight* kyphosis, not overflexing (Fig. 15.10B). Keeping the chin tucked initially, and starting at the lower cervical spine, the head is brought in line with the trunk through segmental extension. The chin tuck is relaxed slightly at the end of the motion to ensure that a neutral cervical lordosis is obtained rather than over-retraction, with the plane of the face parallel to the floor (Fig. 15.10C). This position is held for the count of 10 seconds. By reversing the motion, starting with segmental flexion at the upper cervical spine until the head is hanging in full flexion, eccentric loading of the cervical extensors occurs. For less loading, the position is modified to a forward lean at either the wall or a counter. If the patient is unable to tolerate the load through the wrists, the prone on-elbows position may be used, or the patient can lie just over the end of the bed and perform only the cervical component of the motion. Once a patient can accomplish this motion, the exercise is progressed into hyperextension, controlling any collapse of the mid-cervical spine into anterior translation. Adding pure rotation in the neutral 4PK position will focus on retraining the posterior suboccipitals as the upper cervical spine is responsible for the majority of cervical spine rotation (Fig. 15.11).

An alternative exercise can be done prone over an exercise ball (Fig. 15.12). The head is brought up into cervical neutral, the arms lifted using the scapular stabilizers, and then the trunk is lifted off the ball into thoracic extension. This incorporates the essential interaction between the head, neck, shoulder girdle and thoracic spine.

Elastic band resistance can be used to obtain a graded increase in load in the 4PK position. Alternatively, in sitting, the patient adopts a cervical-neutral nod with the band around the back of the head, and while maintaining neutral, leans

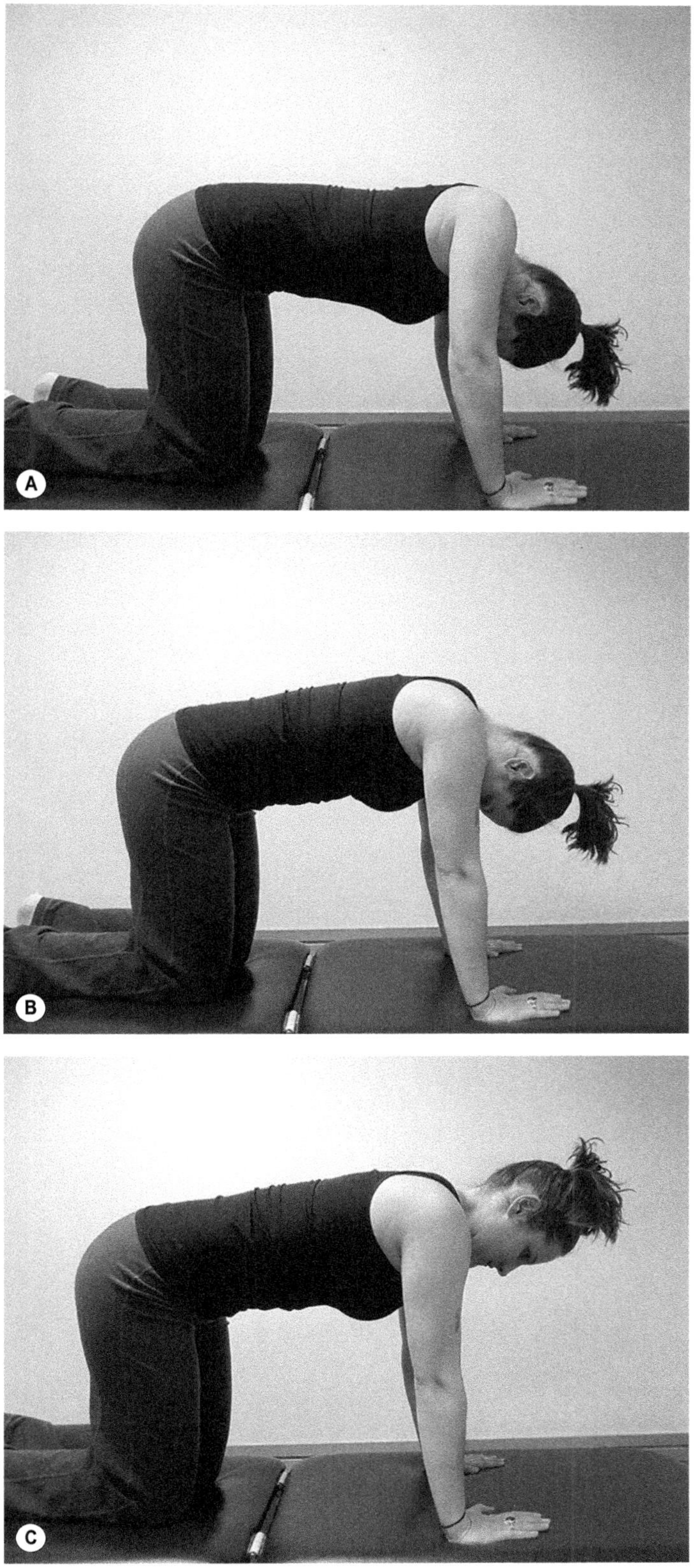

Figure 15.10 **Segmental extension in four-point kneeling:** (**A**) The exercise starts with the head hanging into flexion and the thorax sagged between the scapulae. (**B**) Lumbosacral neutral is found and then thoracic neutral achieved by pressing up through the arms. (**C**) Subsequently the cervical spine is extended segmentally starting at the cervicothoracic junction until the head and neck reach neutral.

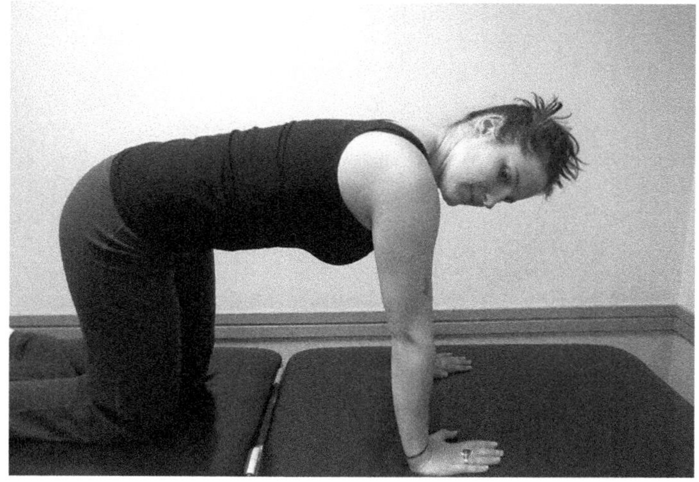

Figure 15.11 **Pure rotation in neutral four-point kneeling.** Pure rotation is added, ensuring no compensatory side-flexion/extension, to challenge the posterior suboccipital muscles, practise motor control and address asymmetrical muscle weakness.

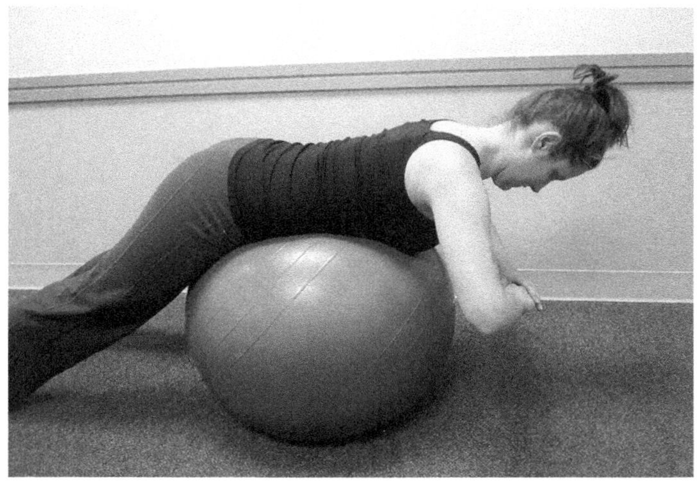

Figure 15.12 **Integrated extension.** Prone on a ball, the head and neck are brought up into cervical neutral, the arms lifted off the ball to activate the scapular stabilizers, and then the sternum lifted off the ball to recruit the thoracic extensors.

backwards at the hips to add resistance. A backward lunge in the standing position, again maintaining the cervical-neutral nod position, is another option, which adds a further perturbation challenge. The patient could also hold the band in front and resist a retraction motion to neutral (Fig. 15.13). Clinical reasoning should be used to determine which of these exercises would optimally address a patient's specific dysfunction.

Side-flexion/rotation exercises for asymmetric weakness

In many patients with unilateral dominant symptoms, atrophy and weakness will be more profound on that side. Although the previously described exercises often regain strength bilaterally, there may be certain situations where loading asymmetrically through rotation and side-flexion may be more appropriate. Many of these exercises would also be considered motion control exercises.

Using a foam wedge pillow, the slope can act as resistance when the head is placed in an offset position. The patient is instructed to maintain a preset DNF nod throughout the exercise (Fig. 15.14A). In the right offset position, the head is slowly lowered down the slope into right rotation, utilizing eccentric control of the muscles on the left side of the neck (Fig. 15.14B). The motion is then reversed, using the left muscles concentrically to bring the head back to the start position and continue up the slope into full left rotation. The head is then returned to neutral and the nod relaxed before repeating.

Pure rotation performed in either the 4PK position or the nod lift-off on the incline will add asymmetric load to the flexors or extensors respectively (Fig. 15.15, see also 15.11). The patient is instructed to avoid the common compensations of either side-flexion or craniovertebral extension, particularly towards the end of range. Diagonal motion into a flexion quadrant during a supine curl-up exercise, or an extension quadrant in 4PK will also bias the load unilaterally.

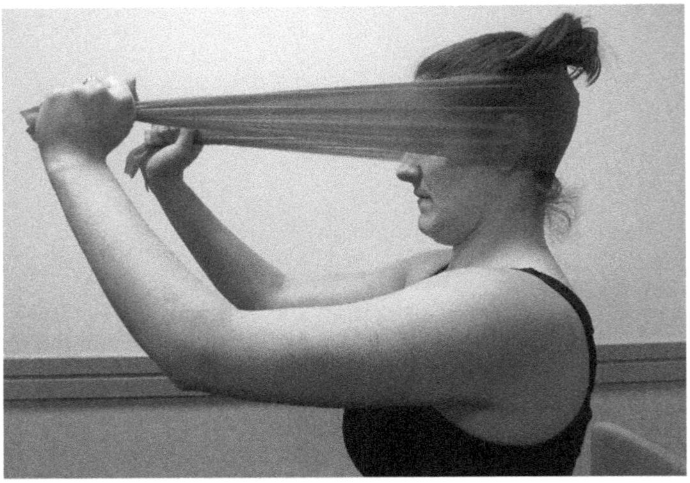

Figure 15.13 Band retraction. The band is held looped around the back of the head to apply resistance to a nod/retract motion to strengthen the cervical extensors.

Isometrics can be performed into the weak rotation or side-flexion. Wall support and a preset nod will help prevent unwanted translation. An elastic band can be used as resistance for isometric or isotonic exercise into side-flexion or rotation, and sideways or diagonal forward or backward lunges can also be used to provide an asymmetric load.

The weight of the head can be used as load in a side-lying position, with or without a pillow or towel roll under the neck to act as a fulcrum. Once again, the preset nod is performed prior to tilting the head up into side-flexion, emphasizing the angular motion rather than translation.

Motor control

For upper quadrant function, it is necessary to have the ability to maintain cervical neutral during upper limb motion and loading. Deep and superficial muscle balance, timing, as well as relaxation post activity need to be addressed. Falla et al (2008) found that neither low nor higher load flexor exercise programmes resulted in improvement of the muscle recruitment timing abnormalities during arm lift, so perhaps this needs to be practised as a specific functional exercise. It is also important to have segmental control during head and neck movements, as many daily activities require a mobile neck.

Cervical neutral during limb load

Clinical reasoning must be applied to each patient presentation to determine which arm movements, in which positions, with which load, are best suited for that patient at that stage of rehabilitation. The patient must be cued on how both to achieve optimal posture and to use a preset DNF nod to activate the stabilizers prior to any limb-load motion. The patient may be asked to release and reset this nod prior to each repetition to focus on the timing pattern, or if endurance is the goal then the nodded, cervical-neutral position should be held throughout all repetitions for each set of the exercise.

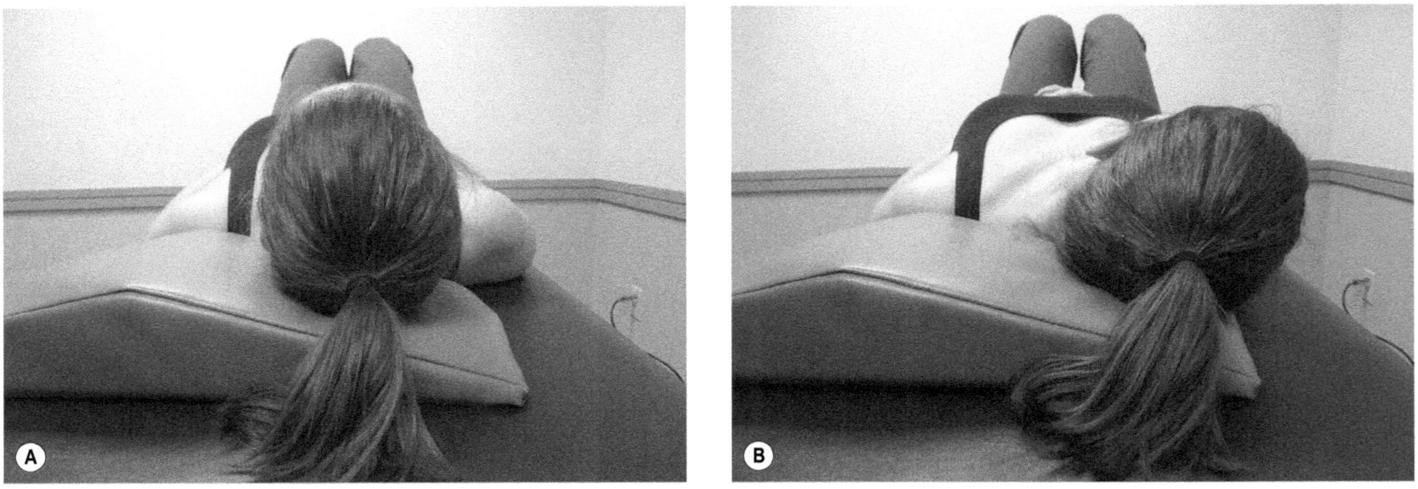

Figure 15.14 Wedge pillow offset: (**A**) The head is placed in the right offset position on the wedge pillow. (**B**) Maintaining a deep neck flexor nod throughout, the head is slowly rotated down the slope, working the left-sided muscles eccentrically. The exercise is completed by returning the head back up the slope continuing to full left rotation and then back to neutral.

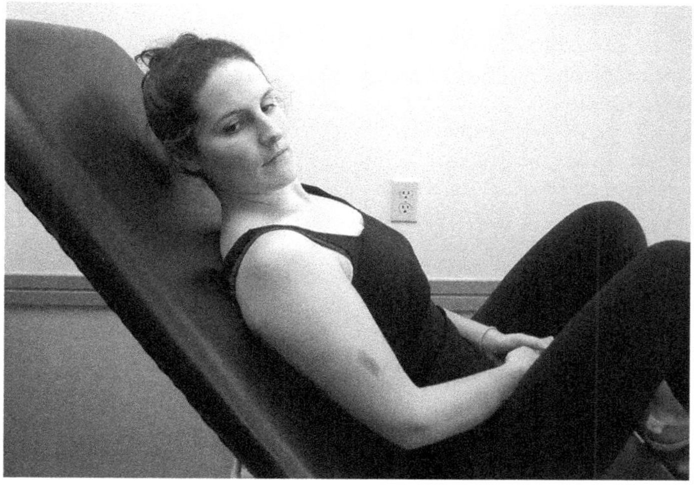

Figure 15.15 Pure rotation in nod lift-off. Pure rotation is added to the nod lift-off exercise on an incline to increase the loading, target asymmetric weakness and practise higher load spinal motor control.

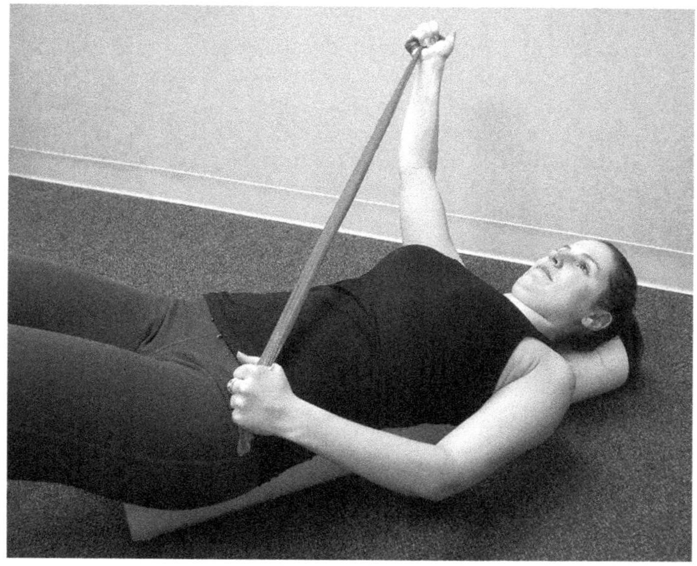

Figure 15.16 Motor control with limb load. Positioned on a foam roll, a deep neck flexor nod is maintained whilst strengthening the lower trapezius muscle to improve both spinal and scapular control.

- **Positions:** In a patient with an irritable neck and poor motor control, arm movements may be performed with the patient in supine on a mat before progressing to a full or half foam roll. In the lying position, gravity along with head contact on the surface helps to prevent the tendency to protrude the head during overhead limb motion. When progressing into sitting and then standing, support against the wall can give feedback of head position. Sitting can be progressed to unsupported sitting on a ball, and standing progressed to standing on a wobble board. The 4PK position particularly challenges control of the anterior head drift so commonly seen with the forward head posture (FHP), and is similar to the loads experienced by those who lean forwards for their occupation or activities.
- **Arm motions:** Arm movements are chosen starting with those that are the least provocative, and progressing to those that challenge spinal control. Bilateral flexion stresses anterior translation in the neck, whereas unilateral flexion or abduction stresses lateral translation. Starting with movements below shoulder level is less of a challenge. Reciprocal movements of the arms create a perturbation at the neck that increases as the speed of movement increases. Often there is an associated muscle imbalance at the shoulder girdle that needs to be addressed and then these arm motions are used to improve the scapular resting position, muscle balance and control, and simultaneously challenge maintenance of cervical neutral. If before each arm movement the patient is reminded to perform a preset DNF nod, both the timing and motor control are emphasized. Care must be taken to ensure that these shoulder girdle exercises are not at too high a level for the patient to maintain cervical neutral. Often the focus is on down-training those muscles that are overactive, as much as true strengthening of the weak muscles.
- **Resistance:** Weight may be added to the limb motions through free weights, elastic tubing and pulleys. Initially keeping weights low and emphasizing proper movement patterns will do more for motor control than the strengthening effect of higher loads. It is most efficient if the resisted exercises are focused on strengthening those scapular stabilizers required to improve shoulder girdle function (Fig. 15.16).

Segmental control during neck motion

The neutral zone is that portion of the range of motion in which there is minimal resistance to movement by the inert stabilizing structures of the spine (Panjabi 1992). The joints of the cervical spine, particularly the craniovertebral joints, have a large neutral zone compared with other regions of the spine. Motion within this portion of the range relies heavily on the dynamic control of the stabilizing musculature.

Some segmental motor control exercises are low load and can be integrated into the exercise programme at the early stages of rehabilitation. Using the foam wedge pillow with the head starting on the peak allows controlled non-weight-bearing motion. The patient begins the exercise by performing the DNF preset nod and then controls the neck motion as the head moves down the slope in one direction, back to the peak and then to the opposite side. As described previously for strengthening, the offset position would add a further load to challenge the motor control (see Fig. 15.14).

Pure eye-level rotation and pure side-flexion can be practised through the maximal range that can be performed without losing controlled uniplanar motion. They can be done at the wall, keeping the head in contact with it to give feedback for the maintenance of cervical neutral. For side-flexion, mirror feedback can also be added. For rotation a laser pointer headband can be used, as scribing a horizontal line during rotation will ensure the eye-level pure rotation pattern. Higher load pure rotation exercises can be done in both the incline nod lift-off and 4PK positions (see Figs 15.11, 15.15). This ensures that these positions are being maintained without rigidity, as the neck is still free to move.

Controlled flexion / extension has been previously described as a segmental motion from a slump position up to neutral and returning to flexion. This can be performed initially in sitting and then progressed to 4PK (see Figs 15.4, 15.10). Controlled hyperextension can be practised in sitting or 4PK, ensuring that there is no collapse into anterior translation during the motion (Fig. 15.17). Controlled hyperextension in the seated lean-back position is a further challenge to the flexor group and is a useful exercise for patients who need to work looking overhead. It is important to control any tendency to collapse in the mid-cervical spine, and also to initiate the return with a nodding pattern (Fig. 15.18A–C).

Mobility Exercises

Reduced cervical spine mobility is a feature of individuals with neck pain (Dall'Alba et al 2001; Dumas et al 2001; Kasch et al 2001; Ogince et al 2007). Potential sources of this mobility impairment include the joint structures, myofascial extensibility or abnormal tension within the neuromeningeal system. Pain and fear avoidance may play a role in limiting a patient's willingness to move actively. Cervical mobility may also be affected by the starting position of the shoulder girdle. If retesting the cervical active range of motion with the scapula position corrected immediately results in increased range, then motor control around the shoulder needs to be addressed. As a multimodal approach including both manual therapy and exercise is the most effective in managing neck pain (Gross et al 2007), motion regained by manual therapy should be maintained with specific exercise.

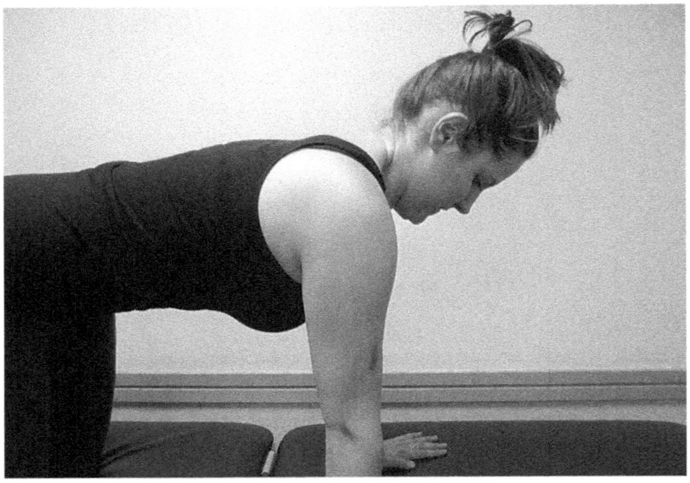

Figure 15.17 Spinal motion control in four-point kneeling. Hyperextension is practised in 4PK controlling for collapse into anterior translation.

Generalized active range of motion

Even in the earliest stages of acute WAD, patients can be instructed in active pain-free mobility exercises. Initially these movements may be performed non-weight-bearing in supine with pillow support. A foam wedge pillow can be used to assist the motion down the slope of the wedge. This exercise does tend to combine ipsilateral side-bending and rotation with slight extension. If there is a concern regarding foraminal compression, the exercise should be modified, perhaps restricting the movement to the side opposite on which the symptoms occur so as to encourage 'opening' of the intervertebral foramen.

In a series of studies, Rosenfeld et al (2000, 2003, 2006) found that WAD subjects who performed repeated cervical rotation 10 times per hour had less pain, less sick time and a better range of motion at 3 years than controls, and more so if the movements were started early on in treatment (within 96 hours) rather than later (>2 weeks).

Movement may start uniplanar, but combined movements into the flexion ovoid of motion will bias lengthening of structures unilaterally. When attempting to regain a loss of extension, consideration must be given to the effects on vascular and neurological tissues, particularly in the extension quadrant. Often the problem with extension range is compression pain rather than decreased length, and perhaps here a motor

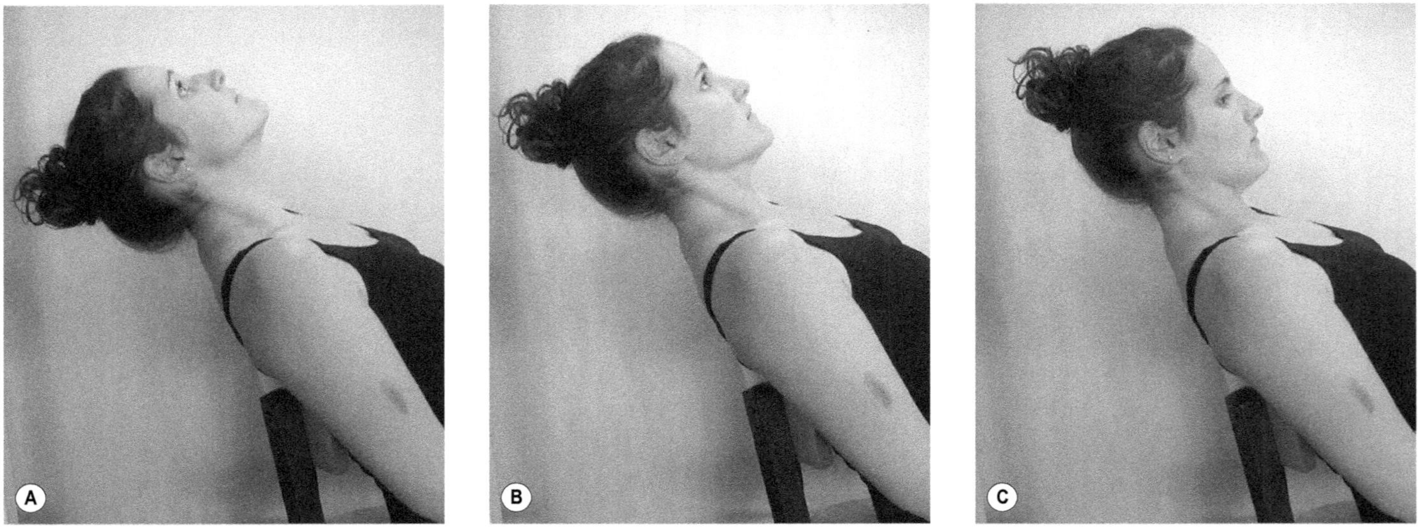

Figure 15.18 Controlled extension pattern in lean-back: (**A**) The head is taken back into extension as far as can be controlled and is pain free. (**B**) Return from end of range is initiated with a nod motion. (**C**) The head is brought back into a full craniovertebral nod position.

control approach would be more appropriate. Segmental joint restrictions of extension can be addressed with the localized self-mobilization exercises described below.

Although the focus here is on mobility, practising correct movement patterns should be emphasized from the start. Integration of mobility exercises with motor control will achieve greater success in obtaining pain-free functional movement.

Articular / self-mobilization

Segmental mobility restrictions are best treated with manual therapy with specific self-mobilization exercises to maintain the range gained. The patient can be taught to localize the motion to the involved segment with his or her fingers or the edge of a towel. An atlanto-axial (AA) towel rotation mobilization exercise has been found to be effective in the treatment of cervicogenic headaches (Hall et al 2007). The following are instructions for segmental self-mobilization exercises (Fig. 15.19):

Craniovertebral region

Occipito-atlanto (OA) flexion (bilateral / unilateral):

- Sit tall in a chair.
- Stabilize the neck by placing clasped hands just under the skull, being careful not to pull the neck forwards.
- Nod the head on the neck, tucking the chin back, lifting the skull at the back (Fig. 15.19A).
- To bias to one side, tilt the head away from the stiff side and rotate the chin towards the armpit on that stiff side (Fig. 15.19B).

OA extension (unilateral):

- Sit tall in a chair.
- Stabilize the neck by placing clasped hands around the neck holding back, just under the angle of the jaw on the stiff side.
- Tip the head towards the stiff side, rotating away and poking the chin forwards and towards the opposite elbow (Fig. 15.19C).

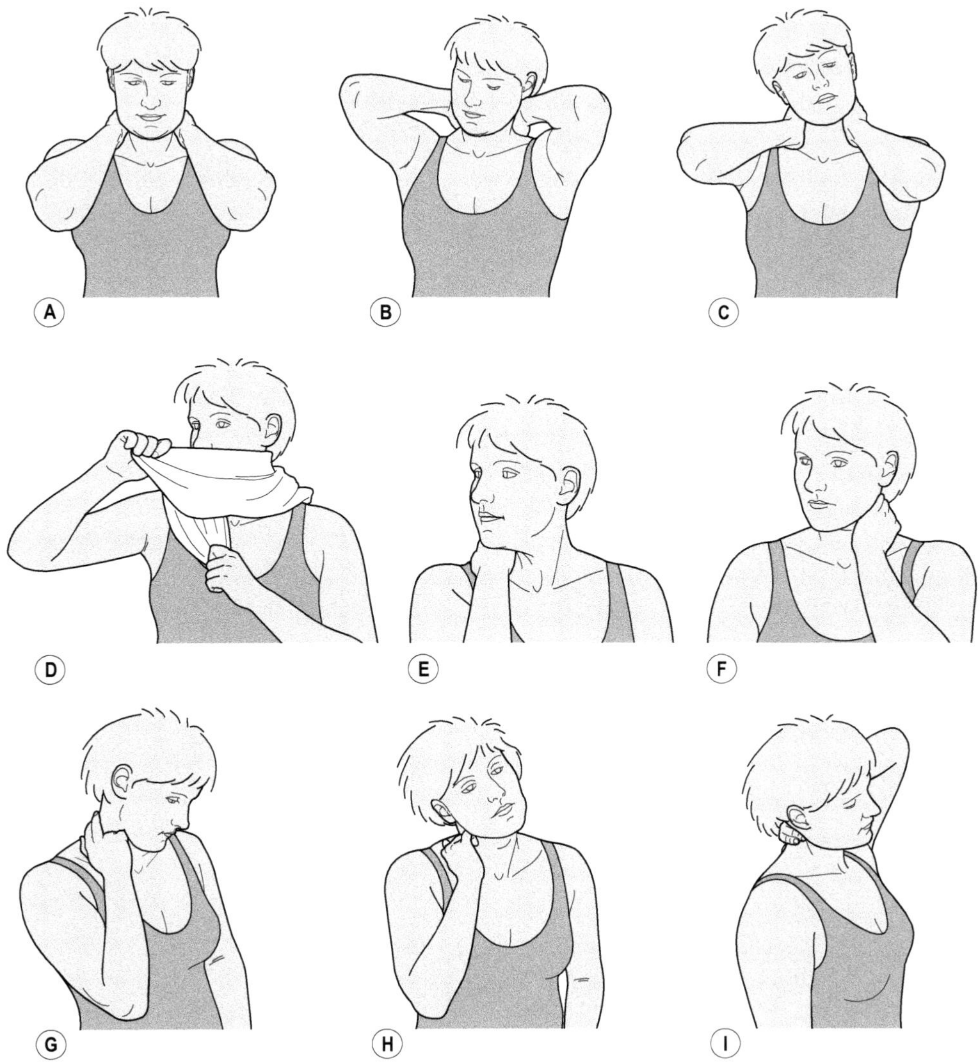

Figure 15.19 Self-mobilization exercises: (**A**) Bilateral OA flexion. (**B**) Unilateral OA flexion. (**C**) Unilateral OA extension. (**D**) AA right rotation. (**E**) Bias right lateral AA joint. (**F**) Bias left lateral AA joint. (**G**) Mid-cervical unilateral flexion. (**H**) Unilateral extension. (**I**) Left lateral glide.

AA joint rotation (right rotation restriction):

- Sit tall in a chair.
- Stabilize the neck by placing clasped hands behind the neck with little fingers at the large bump at the top of the neck below the skull, being careful not to pull the neck forwards.
- Turn the head into pure right rotation, keeping the eyes level and not allowing any tilt or chin poke.
- To bias to right joint:
  - tuck the chin into a bit of flexion before rotating
  - hold the neck forward with right hand behind neck on the right side (Fig. 15.19E).
- To bias to left joint:
  - tip chin up slightly before rotating
  - hold the neck backward with left hand slightly in front of neck on the left side (Fig. 15.19F).
- A towel can also be used to stabilize and overpress the rotation motion (Fig. 15.19D).

Mid-cervical spine

- Use one hand to find the stiff joint (thick, tender spot at back / side of neck).
- Stabilize the bottom bone of that joint by pushing in gently with the fingers.
- A towel can be used to fixate the joint and apply overpressure.
- For flexion:
  - nod the head into flexion, tilt and rotate away from the stiff joint
  - a tug should be felt at the stiff joint (Fig. 15.19G).
- For extension:
  - tip the head back, side bend and rotate towards the stiff joint
  - use pressure up and in with fingers to focus the motion to the stiff joint
  - the whole of the head and neck should not have to go into extension (Fig. 15.19H).
- For left lateral glide right side-flexion:
  - the left hand reaches around from the opposite side to pull the top bone across into left lateral glide as the head is tipped towards the stiff right side (Fig. 15.19I)

  or
  - as the head is tilted towards the right, the top bone is pushed laterally to the left to encourage the lateral glide required for side-bending.

Myofascial extensibility

Individuals with neck pain, particularly cervicogenic headache, have a higher incidence of muscle tightness than do controls (Zito et al 2006; Jull et al 2007a). Stretching exercises have been found to be effective in reducing neck pain in some populations (Gross et al 2007; Ylinen et al 2007b). For individuals with WAD, excessive activity and prolonged relaxation times have been found for several muscle groups. In these cases, a focus on motor patterning and relaxation following activity may be more valuable than stretching. The resting position of the scapula may place a muscle in a lengthened position, making it feel tight to the patient even though it is not short. Probably as a protective mechanism, UFT has been found to be tighter in subjects with adverse tension in the neuromeningeal system (Edgar et al 1994) and so this should be addressed prior to any lengthening exercises for the UFT.

Muscles that tend to tighten are the posterior suboccipitals, long cervical extensors, anterior and middle scalene, SCM, levator scapula and upper trapezius (Janda 1994). Length tests are well described elsewhere (Kendall & McCreary 1983), and these should be used to confirm true muscle shortening before instituting a stretching programme. The effects of a specific muscle-lengthening exercise on either stiff or hypermobile joints should also be considered, and the exercises modified as indicated. To elongate tissue, the exercise should be performed as a prolonged hold for 20–30 seconds, and repeated 3–5 times.

In patients with tight cervical extensors, there is often a region of relative flexibility in the upper or mid-thoracic spine. Performing the lengthening exercise at the wall with the thoracic spine in contact with the wall or towel roll will focus the stretch to the upper and mid-cervical regions. For the suboccipital group, the nod motion is the focus, and a fist placed under the chin may improve the localization as a passive stretch is added (Fig. 15.20). As the long extensors attach at the base of the skull, this nod must be maintained as the head is dropped further forwards to lengthen the rest of the long cervical extensors (Fig. 15.21). Tilting the head to the right or left is indicated for asymmetric tightness.

As the scalene muscles tend to be overdominant in patients with neck pain, active lengthening with a focus on 'letting go' may be the most appropriate approach. When performed at the wall in a neutral preset DNF nod, the tendency to collapse into extension during lengthening is minimized (Fig. 15.22). For the middle scalene, pure side-flexion is performed. For the anterior scalene, adding rotation towards the stiff side localizes stretch to that portion of the muscle. Either manually stabilizing the first rib or breathing out will prevent the rib from elevating as the muscle is lengthened. If the muscle is

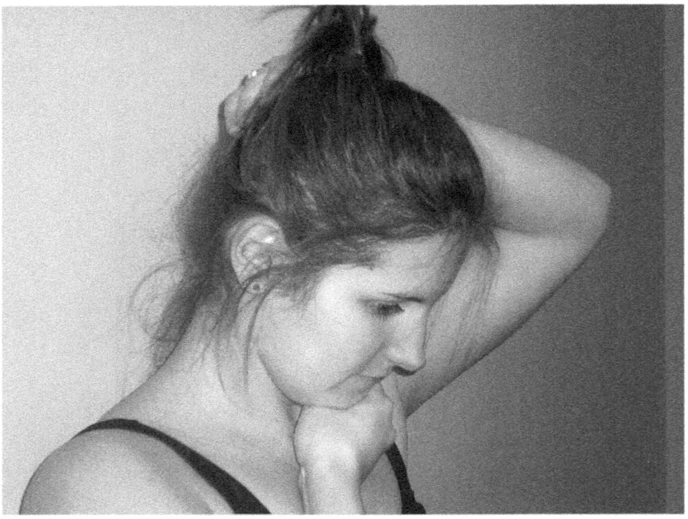

Figure 15.20 Suboccipital lengthening exercise. Standing at the wall, using a nod motion and a fist under the chin helps to focus the stretch to the suboccipital muscles.

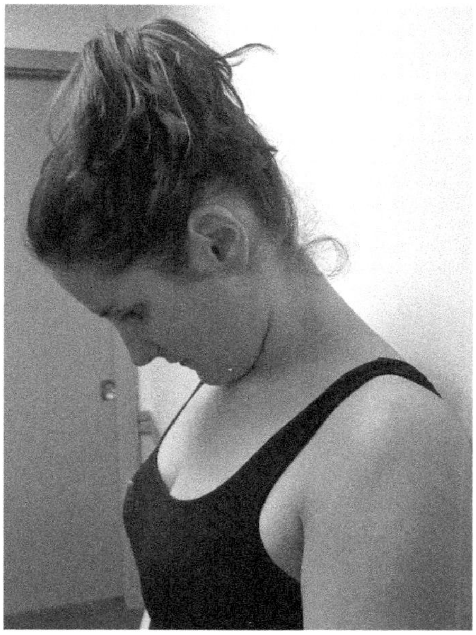

Figure 15.21 Cervical extensor lengthening exercise. Maintaining the thorax against the wall and keeping a chin tuck position helps focus the stretch to the long cervical extensors.

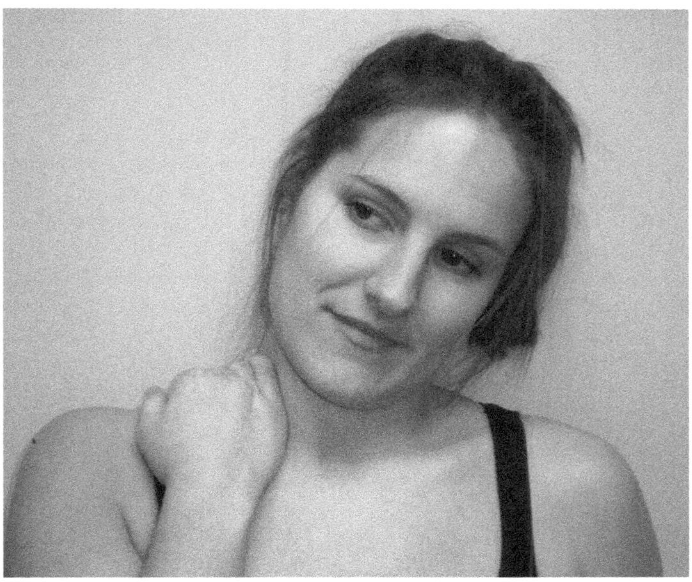

Figure 15.22 Scalene medius lengthening exercise. Standing at the wall and maintaining a chin nod helps prevent collapse into extension while lengthening the scalene as a group into pure side-flexion. The first rib is fixated on the stiff side. To bias to the anterior scalene, the head can be rotated slightly to the stiff side.

truly short, the patient may use the opposite hand to increase the stretch passively.

The SCM also has a tendency towards overactivity but often regains its normal length by focusing on DNF recruitment. The muscle can be lengthened by side-flexion away, rotation towards, and extension of the head on the trunk with the chin held tucked.

To stretch the levator scapula, the neck must be flexed, side-flexed and rotated away. There are two bands described in the literature (Behrsin & Maguire 1986; Diener 1998). The vertical band is lengthened further by adding upward rotation and depression of the scapula with the arm overhead. The horizontal fibres may be more effectively lengthened by depression and downward rotation with the arm behind the back.

The UFT are lengthened by dropping the head into flexion, side-flexing away and rotating towards the stiff side. The scapula is depressed and downwardly rotated by reaching the hand down behind the back.

Neurodynamics

Adverse tension in the neuromeningeal system can affect cervical spine mobility. The assessment and interventions focused on this component are dealt with in Chapter 65 of this book.

Postural Correction Exercises

The optimal posture is that of cervical neutral, where the head is located directly above the shoulders and trunk. The craniovertebral region is in relative flexion and the mid-cervical spine maintains a slightly lordotic position, with the plane of the face being vertical. A slightly kyphotic curve is considered neutral for the thoracic spine. The most common postural impairment of the cervical spine is the FHP.

FHP has historically been associated with an increased likelihood of neck pain, although the research is inconsistent (Watson & Trott 1993; Treleaven et al 1994; Michaelson et al 2003; Yip et al 2008). Harman et al (2005) found that a postural correction exercise programme resulted in significant improvement in static measures of FHP. Falla et al (2007a) investigated the ability to maintain erect posture over time whilst completing a computer-type task. There was an increase in thoracic flexion and forward drift of the head over time in subjects with neck pain compared with controls, which showed a similar but lesser tendency. Low-load CCF training or higher load strength exercise both resulted in improved control of the thoracic posture, but only the CCF training group showed improvement in cervical posture. Both groups showed a similar decrease in pain and disability. Activation of the DNF is higher in subjects instructed in lumbopelvic postural correction with verbal and handling cues than in those subjects merely told to 'sit straight', which suggests that specific postural instruction is important (Falla et al 2007b).

Patients must be individually assessed to determine the cause of their FHP and therefore the focus of their specific postural correction. The following areas need to be addressed with exercise intervention, much of which has already been discussed in previous sections of this chapter.

Muscle imbalance

The following muscles tend to weaken and require recruitment, strength or endurance exercises: deep neck flexors and extensors, scapular stabilizers and upper thoracic extensors. With FHP, the following muscles tend to tighten and require lengthening exercises: cervical extensors (suboccipital and long superficial extensors), scalene, upper trapezius, levator scapula, and pectoralis major and minor.

Articular system

The following regions tend to become hypomobile and require mobility exercises to regain range: upper cervical flexion, cervicothoracic extension, and upper and mid-thoracic extension; patients with lordotic upper thoracic spines must regain flexion to a neutral kyphosis.

Neuromeningeal system

Adverse tension in the neuromeningeal system may also contribute to postural abnormalities in the upper quadrant and must be assessed and addressed depending on the specific dysfunctions found (see Ch 65).

Posture corrections

Depending on exactly which mechanisms have caused the impaired posture, specific cues can be used to teach patients how to attain a more optimal resting position. This can be reinforced throughout their exercise programme. Often after cuing a neutral lumbopelvic lordosis and a sternal lift, the head automatically comes back in line with the trunk. Depending on how the head has drifted forwards, varying degrees of retraction, occipital lift or nod can be added. Pearson and Walmsley (1995) showed that repeated retractions in asymptomatic subjects improved cervical resting posture. Care must be taken to avoid over-retraction, however. It is also important to educate the patient on neutral scapular positioning. The patient can practise these corrections in multiple positions, many times a day (Fig. 15.23).

The DNF nod exercise can be utilized to address many of the dysfunctions seen with postural impairment and when done at the wall can also improve proprioceptive awareness. It will mobilize craniovertebral flexion, lengthen the tight posterior structures and begin to recruit the DNF shown to improve the ability to prevent forward drift of the head. The segmental extension from a slump position in sitting and 4PK is also an effective exercise to control FHP. Often thoracic extension mobility must be regained, and then the muscles that help maintain optimal thoracic and shoulder girdle posture must be re-educated and strengthened. Alternatively, those patients with a flattened or lordotic upper thoracic spine and excessive bracing of the long, superficial thoracic extensors must learn to relax by dropping the sternum down slightly to regain a neutral kyphotic spine.

The patient then practises the maintenance of optimal posture while incorporating arm movements, initially unloaded but then adding free weights, tubing or pulleys. Progression to an unstable base will increase the challenge and also assist in balance control. Using movements and positions required for work or sport will help carry over the postural control to functional activity. These types of exercises and their progressions have been described in the motor control section of this chapter (see Fig. 15.16).

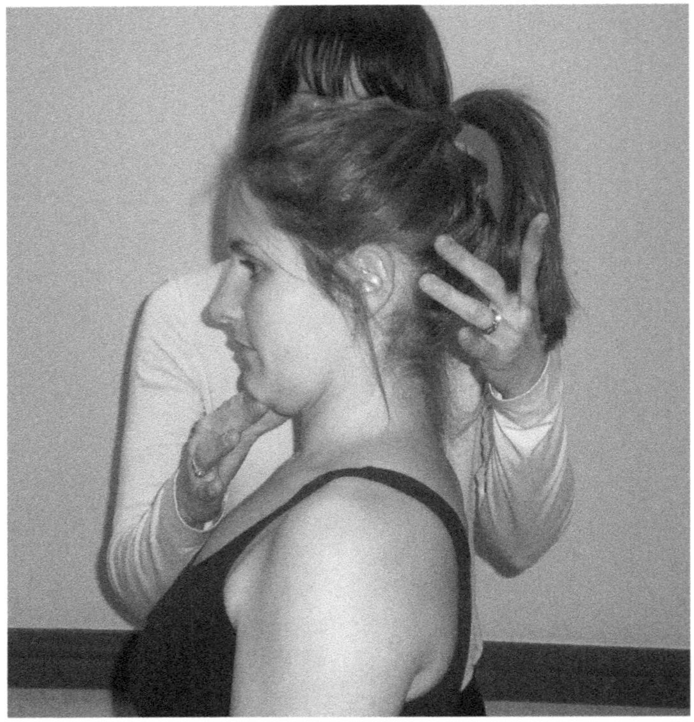

Figure 15.23 Postural cueing. Physical and verbal cues are used to assist the patient to find both lumbosacral and thoracic neutral. Any further correction required for the head and neck is achieved through a combination of nod, occipital lift and retraction as needed.

Somatosensory Dysfunction

Subjects with neck pain, particularly those with WAD and symptoms of dizziness, exhibit impairments of balance, kinaesthetic awareness, eye movement control and eye–head coordination (Revel et al 1991; Heikkila & Astrom 1996; Loudon et al 1997; Treleaven et al 2003, 2005a, 2005b, 2006, 2011; Kristjansson & Falla 2009). This has been described in detail earlier in the text and the reader is directed to Chapter 10 for further information.

Specific exercises focusing on sensorimotor control can be used to improve these impairments, and have also been found to improve pain, mobility and disability as a secondary gain (Revel et al 1994; Hansson et al 2006; Jull et al 2007b). Manual therapy also improves sensorimotor function and so should be included with exercise for optimal management of this patient subgroup (Karlberg et al 1996; Palmgren et al 2006; Reid et al 2008).

Balance retraining can be progressed through various levels of challenge, starting with narrowed or tandem stance on a firm surface with eyes open, and progressing at the other end of the continuum to single-leg stance on an unstable surface with eyes closed. Physiotherapists are familiar with the multitude of options that can be employed to retrain balance, and should use clinical reasoning to develop a progressive exercise programme suited to the needs of the specific patient.

Kinaesthetic awareness can be trained in several ways. Recruitment exercises for the posterior suboccipital muscles such as pure rotation in 4PK may be useful as these muscles have substantial proprioceptive input. Using the pressure biofeedback cuff, patients can practise nodding to specific points in range with their eyes closed, then checking and correcting the position on the gauge once they open their eyes. Head repositioning to neutral or specific points in range can be

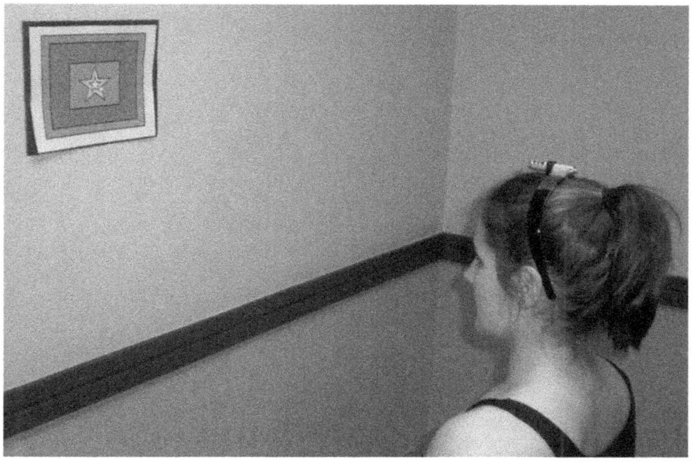

Figure 15.24 Kinaesthetic awareness and eye movement control. Tracing a figure with a laser pointer attached to the head facilitates both position sense and eye/head control.

practised with a laser pointer and target. However, a recent study showed that repositioning of the trunk under the head was a more sensitive test and this may have future implications for both testing and retraining kinaesthetic awareness (Chen & Treleaven, 2013). Tracing a figure with the pointer would combine eye / head control with position sense (Fig. 15.24).

Eye movement control exercises include, for example, following a moving target, gaze fixation whilst moving the head, as well as eye / head coordination movements.

Several components of sensorimotor function can be combined in a single exercise to increase the challenge and assist in carry-over to more functional activities. For example, the patient can practise gaze fixation or eye movement control whilst tandem walking and changing directions.

References

Behrsin J, Maguire K. 1986. Levator scapula action during shoulder movement: a possible mechanism for shoulder pain of cervical origin. Aust J Physiother 32: 101–106.

Bronfort G, Evans R, Nelson B, et al. 2001. A randomized clinical trial of exercise and spinal manipulation for patients with chronic neck pain. Spine 26: 788–797.

Bunketorp L, Carlsson L, Stener-Victorin E. 2006. The effectiveness of a supervised physical training model tailored to the individual needs of patients with whiplash-associated disorder: a randomized controlled trial. Clin Rehabil 20: 201–217.

Cagnie B, Dickx N, Peeters I, et al. 2008. The use of functional MRI to evaluate cervical flexor activity during different cervical flexion exercises. J Appl Physiol 104: 230–235.

Cagnie B, Dirks R, Schouten R, et al. 2011a. Functional reorganization of cervical flexor activity because of induced muscle pain evaluated by muscle functional magnetic resonance imaging. Man Ther 16: 470–475.

Cagnie B, O'Leary S, Elliott J, et al. 2011b. Pain-induced changes in the activity of the cervical extensor muscles evaluated by functional magnetic resonance imaging. Clin J Pain 27: 392–397.

Chen X, Treleaven J. 2013. The effect of neck torsion on joint position error in subjects with chronic neck pain. Man Ther 18:562–567.

Conley MS, Stone MH, Nimmons M, et al. 1997. Specificity of resistance training responses in neck muscle size and strength. Eur J Appl Physiol Occup Physiol 75: 443–448.

Dall'Alba PT, Sterling M, Treleaven J, et al. 2001. Cervical range of motion discriminates between asymptomatic persons and those with whiplash. Spine 26: 2090–2094.

Diener I. 1998. The effect of levator scapula tightness on the cervical spine: proposal of another length test. J Man Manip Ther 6: 78–86.

Dumas JP, Arsenault AB, Boudreau G, et al. 2001. Physical impairments in cervicogenic headache: traumatic vs nontraumatic onset. Cephalalgia 21: 884–893.

Edgar D, Jull G, Sutton S. 1994. The relationship between upper trapezius muscle length and upper quadrant neural tissue extensibility. Aust J Physiother 40: 99–103.

Elliott J, Jull G, Noteboom J, et al. 2006. Fatty infiltration in the cervical extensor muscles in persistent whiplash-associated disorders: a magnetic resonance imaging analysis. Spine 31: 847–855.

Elliott J, Jull G, Noteboom J, et al. 2008a. MRI study of the cross sectional area for the cervical extensor musculature in patients with persistent whiplash associated disorders (WAD). Man Ther 13: 258–265.

Elliott J, Sterling M, Noteboom J, et al. 2008b. Fatty infiltrate in the cervical extensor muscles is not a feature of chronic, insidious-onset neck pain. Clin Radiol 63: 681–687.

Elliott J, Sterling M, Noteboom J, et al. 2009. The clinical presentation of chronic whiplash and the relationship to findings of MRI fatty infiltrates in the cervical extensor musculature: a preliminary investigation. Eur Spine J 18: 1371–1378.

Elliott JM, O'Leary S, Sterling M, et al. 2010a. Magnetic resonance imaging findings of fatty infiltrate in the cervical flexors in chronic whiplash. Spine 35: 948–954.

Elliott JM, O'Leary S, Cagnie B, et al. 2010b. Craniocervical orientation affects muscle activation when exercising the cervical extensors in healthy subjects. Arch Phys Med Rehabil 91: 1418–1422.

Elliott J, Pedler JA, Kenardy J, et al. 2011. The temporal development of fatty infiltrates in the neck muscles following whiplash injury: an association with pain and posttraumatic stress. PLoS ONE 6: e21194.

Escolar-Reina P, Medina-Mirapeix F, Gascón-Cánovas J, et al. 2010. How do care-provider and home exercise program characteristics affect patient adherence in chronic neck and back pain: a qualitative study. BMC Health Services Res 10: 60.

Falla D, Rainoldi A, Merletti R, et al. 2003. Myoelectric manifestations of sternocleidomastoid and anterior scalene muscle fatigue in chronic neck pain patients. Clin Neurophysiol 114: 488–495.

Falla D, Jull G, Hodges P, et al. 2004a. Patients with neck pain demonstrate reduced electromyographic activity of the deep cervical flexor muscles during performance of the craniocervical flexion test. Spine 29: 2108–2114.

Falla D, Jull G, Hodges P. 2004b. Feedforward activity of the cervical flexor muscles during voluntary arm movements is delayed in chronic neck pain. Exp Brain Res 157: 43–48.

Falla D, Bilenkij G, Jull G, 2004c. Patients with chronic neck pain demonstrate altered patterns of muscle activity during performance of an upper limb task. Spine 29: 1436–1440.

Falla D, Jull G, Hodges P, et al. 2006. An endurance-strength training regime is effective in reducing myoelectric manifestations of cervical flexor muscle fatigue in females with chronic neck pain. Clin Neurophysiol 117: 828–837.

Falla D, Jull G, Russell T, et al. 2007a. Effect of neck exercise on sitting posture in patients with chronic neck pain. Phys Ther 87: 408–417.

Falla D, O'Leary S, Fagan A, et al. 2007b. Recruitment of the deep cervical flexors during a postural-correction exercise performed in sitting. Man Ther 12: 139–143.

Falla D, Jull G, Hodges P, et al. 2008. Training the cervical muscles with prescribed motor tasks does not change muscle activation during a functional activity. Man Ther 13: 507–512.

Fernández-de-las-Peñas C, Bueno A, Ferrando J, et al. 2007. Magnetic resonance imaging study of the morphology of the cervical extensor muscles in chronic tension-type headache. Cephalalgia 27: 355–362.

Fernández-de-las-Peñas C, Alber-Sanchis C, Buil M, et al. 2008. Cross-sectional area of the cervical multifidus muscle in females with chronic bilateral neck pain compared to controls. J Orthop Sports Phys Ther 38: 175–180.

Gross AR, Goldsmith C, Hoving J, et al. 2007. Conservative management of mechanical neck disorders: a systematic review. J Rheumatol 34: 1083–1102.

Hall T, Chan H, Christensen L, et al. 2007. Efficacy of a C1-2 self sustained natural apophyseal glide (Snag) in the management of cervicogenic headache. J Orthop Sports Phys Ther 37: 100–107.

Hallgren RC, Greenman PE, Rechtien JJ. 1994. Atrophy of suboccipital muscles in patients with chronic pain: a pilot study. J Am Osteopath Assoc 94: 1032–1038.

Hansson EE, Nils-Ove Månsson A, Karin AM, et al. 2006. Dizziness among patients with whiplash-associated disorder: a randomized controlled trial. J Rehabil Med 38: 387–390.
Harman K, Hubley-Kozey CL, Butler H. 2005. Effectiveness of an exercise program to improve head forward posture in normal adults: a randomized controlled 10 week trial. J Man Manip Ther 13: 163–176.
Heikkila H, Astrom PG. 1996. Cervicocephalic kinesthetic sensibility in patients with whiplash injury. Scand J Rehabil Med 28: 133–138.
Janda V. 1994. Muscles and motor control in cervicogenic disorders: assessment and management. In: Grant R (ed) Physical therapy for the cervical and thoracic spine. Melbourne: Churchill Livingstone, p 195.
Jordan A, Bendix T, Nielsen H, et al. 1998. Intensive training, physiotherapy, or manipulation for patients with chronic neck pain. A prospective, single-blinded, randomized clinical trial. Spine 23: 311–318.
Jull G. 2000. Deep neck flexor dysfunction in whiplash. J Musculoskelet Pain 8: 143–154.
Jull G, Trott P, Potter H, et al. 2002. A randomized controlled trial of exercise and manipulative therapy for cervicogenic headache. Spine 27: 1835–1843.
Jull G, Kristjansson E, Dall'Alba P. 2004. Impairment in the cervical flexors: a comparison of whiplash and insidious onset neck pain patients. Man Ther 9: 89–94.
Jull G, Amiri M, Bullock-Saxton J, et al. 2007a. Cervical musculoskeletal impairment in frequent intermittent headache. Part 1: subjects with single headaches. Cephalalgia 27: 793–802.
Jull G, Falla D, Treleaven J, et al. 2007b. Retraining cervical joint position sense: the effect of two exercise regimes. J Orthop Res 25: 404–412.
Karlberg M, Magnusson M, Malmstrom E, et al. 1996. Postural and symptomatic improvement after physiotherapy in patients with dizziness of suspected cervical origin. Arch Phys Med Rehabil 77: 874–882.
Kasch H, Stengaard-Pedersen K, Arendt-Nielsen L, et al. 2001. Headache, neck pain and neck mobility after acute whiplash injury. Spine 26: 1246–1251.
Kay T, Gross A, Goldsmith C, et al. 2012. Exercises for mechanical neck disorders. Cochrane Database Syst Rev 8: CD004250.
Kendall FP, McCreary EK. 1983. Muscles, testing and function, 3rd edn. Baltimore: Williams & Wilkins.
Kristjansson E. 2004. Reliability of ultrasonography for the cervical multifidus muscle in asymptomatic and symptomatic subjects. Man Ther 9: 83–88.
Kristjansson E, Falla D. 2009. Sensorimotor function and dizziness in neck pain: implications for assessment and management. J Orthop Sports Phys Ther 39: 364–377.
Loudon JK, Ruhl M, Field E. 1997. Ability to reproduce head position after whiplash injury. Spine 22: 865–868.
Mayoux-Benhamou MA, Revel M, Vallee C. 1997. Selective electromyography of dorsal neck muscles in humans. Exp Brain Res 113: 353–360.
Michaelson P, Michaelson M, Jaric S, et al. 2003. Vertical posture and head stability in patients with chronic neck. J Rehabil Med 35: 229–235.
Nederhand MJ, Ijerman MJ, Hermens HJ, et al. 2000. Cervical muscle dysfunction in the chronic whiplash associated disorder grade II (WAD-II). Spine 25: 1938–1943.
Nederhand MJ, Hermens HJ, IJerman MJ, et al. 2002. Cervical muscle dysfunction in chronic whiplash-associated disorder grade 2. Spine 27: 1056–1061.
Ogince M, Hall T, Robinson K, et al. 2007. The diagnostic validity of the cervical flexion-rotation test in C1 / 2-related cervicogenic headache. Man Ther 12: 256–262.
O'Leary S, Jull G, Kim M, et al. 2007. Cranio-cervical flexor muscle impairment at maximal, moderate and low loads is a feature of neck pain. Man Ther 12: 34–39.
O'Leary S, Falla D, Jull G. 2011. The relationship between superficial muscle activity during the cranio-cervical flexion test and clinical features in patients with chronic neck pain. Man Ther 16: 452–455.
O'Leary S, Jull G, Kim M, et al. 2012. Training mode-dependent changes in motor performance in neck pain. Arch Phys Med Rehabil 93: 1225–1233.
Palmgren PJ, Sandstrom PJ, Lundqvist FJ, et al. 2006. Improvement after chiropractic care in cervicogenic kinesthetic sensibility and subjective pain intensity in patients with nontraumatic neck pain. J Manipulative Physiol Ther 29: 100–106.
Panjabi M. 1992. The stabilizing system of the spine. Part 1: Function, adaptation, and enhancement. Part 2: Neutral zone and instability hypothesis. J Spinal Disord 5: 383–397.
Pearson N, Walmsley R. 1995. Trial into the effects of repeated neck retractions in normal subjects. Spine 20: 1245–1250.
Randlov A, Ostergaaed M, Manniche C, et al. 1998. Intensive dynamic training for females with chronic neck / shoulder pain. A randomized controlled trial. Clin Rehabil 12: 200–210.
Reid S, Rivett D, Katekar M, et al. 2008. Sustained natural apophyseal glides (SNAGs) are an effective treatment for cervicogenic dizziness. Man Ther 13: 357–366.
Revel M, Andre-Deshays C, Minguet M. 1991. Cervicocephalic kinesthetic sensibility in patients with cervical pain. Arch Phys Med 72: 288–291.
Revel M, Minguet M, Gergoy P, et al. 1994. Changes in cervicocephalic kinesthesia after a proprioceptive rehabilitation program in patients with neck pain. Arch Phys Med Rehabil 75: 895–899.
Rosenfeld M, Gunnarsson R, Borenstein P. 2000. Early intervention in whiplash-associated disorders. Spine 25: 1782–1787.
Rosenfeld M, Seferiadis A, Carlsson J, et al. 2003. Active intervention in patients with whiplash-associated disorders improves long term prognosis. Spine 28: 2491–2498.
Rosenfeld M, Seferiadis A, Gunnarsson R. 2006. Active involvement and intervention in patients exposed to whiplash trauma in automobile crashes reduces costs. Spine 31: 1799–1804.
Sarig-Bahat H. 2003. Evidence for exercise therapy in mechanical neck disorders. Man Ther 8: 10–20.
Schomaker J, Falla D. 2013. Function and structure of the deep cervical extensor muscles in patients with neck pain. Man Ther 18: 360–366.
Schomaker J, Petzke F, Falla D. 2012. Localised resistance selectively activates the semispinalis cervicis muscle in patients with neck pain. Man Ther 17: 544–548.
Sterling M, Jull G, Vicenzino B, et al. 2003. Development of motor dysfunction following whiplash injury. Pain 103: 65–73.
Sterling M, Jull G, Vicenzino B, et al. 2004. Characterization of acute whiplash associated disorders. Spine 29: 182–188.
Szeto G, Straker L, O'Sullivan P. 2005. A comparison of symptomatic and asymptomatic office workers performing monotonous keyboard work. Man Ther 10: 270–291.
Taimela S, Takala EP, Asklof T, et al. 2000. Active treatment of chronic neck pain: a prospective randomized intervention. Spine 25: 1021–1027.
Treleaven J, Jull G, Atkinson L. 1994. Cervical musculoskeletal dysfunction in post-concussional headache. Cephalalgia 14: 273–279.
Treleaven J, Jull G, Grip H. 2011. Head eye co-ordination and gaze stability in subjects with persistent whiplash associated disorders. Man Ther 16: 252–257.
Treleaven J, Jull G, LowChoy N. 2003. Dizziness and unsteadiness following whiplash injury: characteristic features and relationship with cervical joint position error. J Rehabil Med 35: 36–43.
Treleaven J, Jull G, LowChoy N. 2005a. Standing balance in persistent whiplash: a comparison between subjects with dizziness and without dizziness. J Rehabil Med 37: 224–229.
Treleaven J, Jull G, LowChoy N. 2005b. Smooth pursuit neck torsion test in whiplash associated disorders: relationship to self-reports of neck pain and disability, dizziness and anxiety. J Rehabil Med 37: 219–223.
Treleaven J, Jull G, LowChoy N. 2006. The relationship of cervical joint position error to balance and eye movement disorders in persistent whiplash. Man Ther 11: 99–106.
Uhlig Y, Weber B, Grob D, et al. 1995. Fibre composition and fibre transformation in neck muscles of patients with dysfunction of the cervical spine. J Orthop Res 13: 240–249.
Vassiliou T, Kaluza G, Putzke C, et al. 2006. Physical therapy and active exercises – an adequate treatment for prevention of late whiplash syndrome? Pain 124: 69–76.
Walker M, Boyles R, Young B, et al. 2008. The effectiveness of manual physical therapy and exercise for mechanical neck pain. Spine 33: 2371–2378.
Watson D, Trott P. 1993. Cervical headache: an investigation of natural head posture and upper cervical flexor muscle performance. Cephalalgia 13: 272–282.
Yip C, Chiu T, Poon A. 2008. The relationship between head posture and severity and disability of patients with neck pain. Man Ther 13: 148–154.
Ylinen J, Häkkinen A, Takala E, et al. 2006. Effects of neck muscle strengthening in women with chronic neck pain: one year follow-up study. J Strength Cond Res 20: 6–13.
Ylinen J, Häkkinen A, Takala E, et al. 2007a. Neck muscle training in the treatment of chronic neck pain: a three-year follow-up. Eura Medicophys 43: 161–169.
Ylinen J, Häkkinen A, Takala E, et al. 2007b. Stretching exercises vs manual therapy in treatment of chronic neck pain: a randomized controlled cross-over trial. J Rehabil Med 39: 126–132.
Zito G, Jull G, Story I. 2006. Clinical tests of musculoskeletal dysfunction in the diagnosis of cervicogenic headache. Man Ther 11: 118–129.

PART 3

Lumbar Spine Pain Syndromes

16 Mechanical Low Back Pain — 191
Scott Burns, Edward Foresman, Stephenie Kraycsir and Joshua A. Cleland

17 Lumbar Radiculopathy — 199
Chad Cook and Mark Wilhelm

18 Lumbar Spine Instability — 210
Bryan S. Dennison and Michael H. Leal

19 Lumbar Spine in Lower Extremity Pain Syndromes — 221
Scott Burns, Paul E. Glynn, Edgar Savidge and Joshua A. Cleland

20 The Contribution of the Pelvic Floor Muscles to Pelvic Pain — 226
Ruth Jones

21 Chronic Low Back Pain — 236
Mark D. Bishop, Joel E. Bialosky and Charles W. Gay

22 Joint Mobilization and Manipulation of the Lumbar Spine — 245
Emilio J. Puentedura

23 Therapeutic Exercise for Mechanical Low Back Pain — 255
Carol Kennedy and Lenerdene Levesque

24 Sacroiliac Joint as a Source of Pain: Diagnosis and Management — 274
Kenneth E. Learman

Chapter 16

Mechanical Low Back Pain

Scott Burns, Edward Foresman, Stephenie Kraycsir, Joshua A. Cleland

CHAPTER CONTENTS

Introduction	191
Screening	191
Staging process	192
Stage I	192
Stage II and III individuals	197
Conclusion	197

Introduction

Low back pain (LBP) is a very common and costly diagnosis worldwide (Dagenais et al 2008; Itoh et al 2013). In the United States, it has been reported that within the last 3 months 26–31% of adults have experienced an episode of LBP lasting at least 1 day (Deyo et al 2006; Strine & Hootman 2007). In a cross-sectional epidemiological study in Spain, approximately 20% of people experienced a significant episode of LBP (Fernández-de-las-Peñas et al 2011). In Japan, a steady increase in cost of care for work-related low back injuries was observed from 2002 to 2011 (Itoh et al 2013).

Mechanical LBP was the fifth most common reason that patients sought care from their physicians (Hart et al 1995). In the United States, the number of physician visits related to LBP increased from an estimated 15 million to 34 million from 1995 to 2007 (Hart et al 1995; Deyo et al 2006). Itoh et al (2013) also showed a similar increase in prevalence in Japanese work-related low back injuries.

Rehabilitation professionals, including chiropractic, manual therapy and massage professionals, are commonly utilized in the treatment of LBP. However, the cost associated with these interventions is highly variable and has yielded mixed results. Dagenais et al (2008) have reported that rehabilitation professionals, including chiropractors and physical therapists, accounted for approximately 3–61% of direct medical costs associated with the management of LBP. Overall, there is an increase in patients seeking care for their LBP and the costs associated with their care; however, optimal management of these individuals continues to be elusive.

Several clinical practice guidelines outline various therapeutic approaches when it comes to managing a patient with LBP (Koes et al 2001; Staal et al 2003; Airaksinen et al 2006; Delitto et al 2012). Although there is no universal approach to treatment of individuals with LBP, the treatment-based classification system offers a simple and non-complex approach to the management of these patients. The aim of the treatment-based classification approach is to identify a patient that is likely to respond to a particular intervention early in the course of care to optimize the outcomes. The treatment-based classification approach may be applied to varying LBP conditions, but acute, mechanical LBP may be the most appropriate. The treatment-based classification approach has shown sufficient reliability for clinical use, but it has some limitations (Stanton et al 2011).

The treatment-based classification system for LBP attempts first to place a patient into a stage based on disability and duration of symptoms (see Table 16.2). Stage I generally captures patients with acute LBP who have higher pain and disability scores. In stage I, there are clinical characteristics that assist in allocating patients into one of four separate treatment subgroups as a strategy to improve patient outcomes (Delitto et al 1995; Brennan et al 2006). These subgroups include: manipulation, specific exercise, stabilization and traction.

In this chapter, we will focus on the application of stage I evaluation and intervention for individuals with mechanical LBP only. We will outline the treatment-based classification staging process as well as review the specific examination and intervention techniques. Specific conditions such as lumbar radiculopathy or spinal stenosis will be covered in other chapters of this textbook.

Screening

The first step in using the treatment-based classification system for LBP is to determine whether the patient is appropriate for conservative care. A clinician must perform a careful historical examination and physical examination to establish whether the patient has any red flag indicators for referral. Red flags are considered clinical findings that may indicate a serious pathology is present (Delitto et al 2012). Serious pathologies that a clinician may encounter during evaluation of LBP include: neoplastic conditions, spinal fracture, infection, cauda equina syndrome and ankylosing spondylitis (Table 16.1).

Henschke et al (2009) demonstrated, in an inception cohort of 1172 patients receiving primary care for acute LBP, that 11 cases (0.9%) were of serious pathology. The most common

Table 16.1 **Common red flag conditions for individuals presenting with lumbar spine complaints**

Neoplastic conditions	Spinal fractures	Spinal infection	Cauda equina syndrome	Ankylosing spondylitis
Prior history of cancer Age over 50 years Unexplained weight loss Symptoms are unrelieved with bed rest	Major trauma, secondary to direct blow to spine, sports injury, motor vehicle accident, or a fall from a height Compression fracture (particularly in older adults) Minor trauma or strenuous lifting in older or potentially osteoporotic athletes Prolonged corticosteroid use	Recent fever and chills Recent bacterial infection or a history of IV drug abuse History of immune suppression (from steroid use, transplant, or disease process)	Serious and/or progressive neurological deficit of bilateral lower extremities Recent onset of bladder dysfunction, such as urinary retention, increased frequency or overflow incontinence Groin region anaesthesia	Male>female Get out of bed at night secondary to pain Stiffness in the morning Age at onset <35 years No relief when lying down Relief with exercise and activity

serious pathology was spinal fracture, which accounted for 8 of the 11 cases. The authors state that patients with an age >70 years, prolonged use of corticosteroids and/or significant trauma may be at greater risk for spinal fractures. Malignancy may also be an important red flag condition to screen in patients with LBP, with it accounting for approximately 0.7% (Deyo & Diehl 1988). Several historical questions may be useful to determine the risk of malignancy including age >50 years, previous history of cancer, unexplained weight loss, failure to improve with 1 month of conservative care and no relief with bed rest. A previous history of cancer was most predictive of current malignancy (Deyo et al 1992).

Medical questionnaires are often used in screening of red flags in the treatment of mechanical LBP to identify symptom presentation such as onset of symptoms, progression, nature, pattern of behaviour in a 24-hour period, and specific movements or positions that affect symptoms (Delitto et al 2012). Additionally, the clinician should also be conscious of psychosocial factors the patient exhibits because they may contribute to the patient's persistent pain and disability. Psychosocial variables may be identified using specific outcome measures such as the Fear-avoidance Beliefs Questionnaire, Subgroups for Targeted Treatment (STarT) Back Screening Tool, Pain Catastrophizing Scale, etc.

Other important outcome measures used in the management of LBP include the Oswestry Disability Index and Roland Morris Disability Questionnaire. These outcomes can help the clinician to identify the patient baseline status in regard to pain, function and disability. (For additional information regarding the physical examination see Ch 5.)

Staging Process

The next step in using the treatment-based classification system for treatment of mechanical LBP is to classify patients into one of three stages according to severity of symptoms by using to their activity level and disability score from the Oswestry Disability Index (Delitto et al 1995). Stage I includes patients with acute onset where pain and disability ratings are highest. Stage II includes patients with subacute pain and pain and disability ratings have begun to decrease and the patient is beginning to return to daily routines. Patients in stage III have relatively little pain or disability, but require physical conditioning to return to great physical demands (Delitto et al 1995; Fritz et al 2007) (Table 16.2).

Table 16.2 **Staging process for the treatment-based classification algorithm**

	Stage I	Stage II	Stage III
Functional capacity	Unable to: • stand ≥15 minutes • sit ≥30 minutes • walk ≥¼ mile (400 m)	Exceeds all criteria of stage I Difficulty with basic functional activities of daily living (ADLs) (e.g. vacuuming, lifting)	Able to perform basic functional ADLs Cannot participate fully in sport
Modified Oswestry Disability Score	≥20%	≤20%	≤20%

Stage I

Stage I addresses four common rehabilitation strategies that are commonly implemented for patients with acute LBP including manipulation, directional preference exercise, stabilization exercise and traction. Each subgroup has specific tests and measures, which assist the clinician in identifying the appropriate subgroup(s) (Table 16.3).

Directional preference exercise and spinal manipulation may be the most commonly used in the treatment of patients with acute LBP. George and Delitto (2005) found that, of 131 participants with acute LBP, 38.9% were classified for specific

Table 16.3 Stage I subgroups and criteria

Manipulation	Specific exercise	Traction	Stabilization
No symptoms distal to the knee Acute onset ≤16 days Fear-avoidance Beliefs Questionnaire – work subscale ≤19 Lumbar hypomobility of at least one segment One hip passive internal rotation ≥35° (measured in prone)	**Extension** Symptoms distal to the buttock Directional preference for extension Symptoms peripheralize with flexion Centralization with extension **Flexion** Age ≥50 years Directional preference for flexion Evidence of spinal stenosis on imaging **Lateral shift** Visible frontal plane deviation Directional preference for lateral translational movements	Presence of leg symptoms Signs of nerve root compression (myotomal, dermatomal or reflex abnormalities) Peripheralization with extension Positive crossed straight leg raise	Age ≤40 years Straight leg raise ≥91° Aberrant motions Positive prone instability test

exercise, 32.1% for manipulation, 21.4% for stabilization and 7.6% for traction.

This subgrouping strategy is a simplistic method used to guide the clinician in providing an appropriate intervention to a patient with acute LBP. However, this system is not perfect. Often times, patients may be categorized into multiple subgroups, which will complicate the decision making of the clinician. On the other hand, some patients may not be classifiable within this framework. Stanton et al (2011) reported that approximately 50% of individuals with LBP were categorized into a single subgroup, 25% fitted more than one subgroup and 25% did not fit any subgroup. It is important to realize the limitations of the treatment-based classification approach and that it is a dynamic and fluid categorization process requiring the constant assessment of the provider.

Spinal manipulation group

Manipulation refers to performing a high-velocity, low-amplitude thrust procedure to a patient's lumbar spine. It is important to realize that spinal manipulation for the purposes of this chapter does not include non-thrust oscillatory mobilizations that are also commonly performed in rehabilitation settings and are referred to as spinal mobilization.

Flynn et al (2002) completed a derivation study to identify patient characteristics that were likely to lead to dramatic success using spinal manipulation. Five predictor variables were identified: short duration of symptoms (<16 days), no symptoms distal to the knee, a Fear-avoidance Beliefs Questionnaire work subscale score <19, at least one hip with >35° internal rotation range of motion and hypomobility of one lumbar segment. In that derivation trial, a supine lumbopelvic manipulation (see Fig. 16.1) was performed and a basic mobility home exercise was prescribed. The patients returned 48 hours later to determine whether dramatic success was achieved. In this study a 50% reduction of the Oswestry Disability Index was the indicator of success. If patients failed to meet this criterion on the 48-hour follow-up the same manipulation technique was applied and the patient returned 2 days later. Flynn et al (2002) determined that patients with four out of the five predictor variables had a 95% chance of achieving the rapid improvement in disability rating. A validation study examining these predictor variables was performed and confirmed that the five variables did indeed identify a subgroup of patients who are more likely to respond to the manipulation. From that follow-up study, the authors identified the 'two-factor' rule: patients without symptoms below the knee and onset of ≤16 days had a 91% chance of experiencing significant disability and pain reduction within 48 hours after lumbar thrust manipulation (Childs et al 2004).

If the supine lumbopelvic thrust manipulation is not possible with a particular patient secondary to discomfort, an alternative technique has been shown to be equally effective. This is a neutral side-lying lumbar technique (see Fig. 16.2). Non-thrust oscillatory mobilization techniques may also be implemented; however, there appears to be a significant difference if a subgroup of patients receive the high-velocity, low-amplitude thrust manipulation (Cleland et al 2006).

In order to apply this manipulative technique to a patient in the clinical setting, the clinician needs to ensure a solid understanding of the tests and measures used to identify potential responders. Additionally, in these studies subjects were between the ages of 18 and 60 years with a chief complaint of LBP with or without leg symptoms. Subjects were excluded if they exhibited any sign of nerve root compression, had had surgery to the lumbar spine, were currently pregnant or had a history of osteoporosis.

In order to identify accurately those patients who may fit into this subgroup, it is important to perform the predictor variables in a similar fashion that was performed in the studies. Using a bubble inclinometer on the lateral aspect of the fibula, internal rotation range of motion of the hip is performed with the patient in the prone position and the knee passively flexed to 90°. The clinician passively internally rotates the limb until the visual observation of pelvic movement occurs or passive end feel of the hip joint is reached. Mobility of the lumbar spine is assessed using posterior–anterior spring testing at each lumbar level. The clinician will determine the presence / absence of pain and mobility at each segmental level (Flynn et al 2002).

Many different manipulation and mobilization techniques have been described, but there is presently no evidence for the superiority of one approach over another. In fact, emerging evidence suggests that the choice of technique may not be as important as was previously thought (Chiradejnant et al 2003; Cleland et al 2009). The correct identification of the

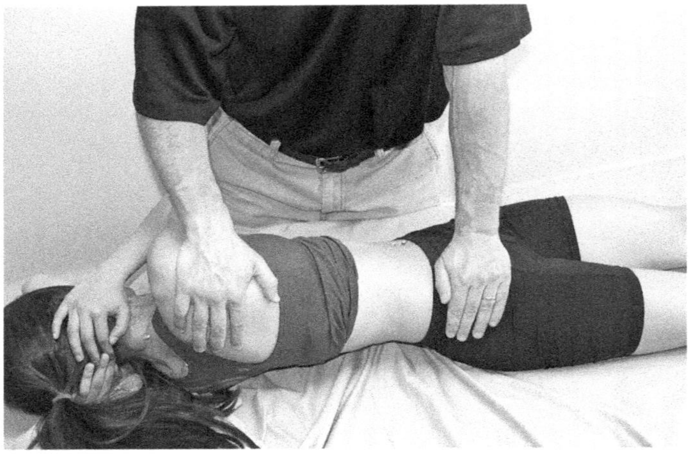

Figure 16.1 Lumbopelvic manipulation performed with the patient supine.

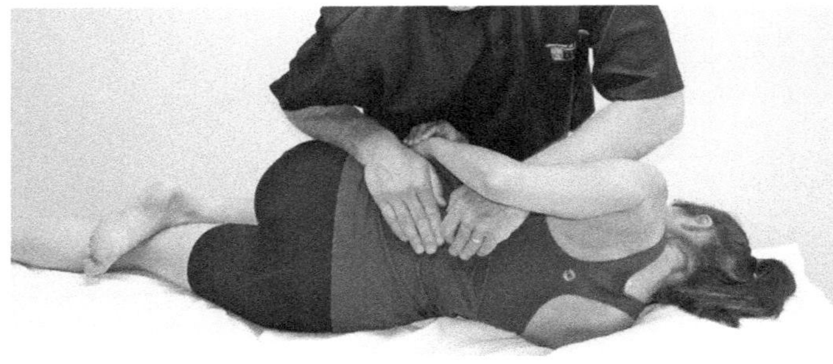

Figure 16.2 Lumbar spine manipulation performed with the patient side-lying.

patient who actually needs manipulation is likely to be more important than the particular technique chosen by the therapist. Part of the explanation for the lack of importance of the specific technique may be that manipulation procedures are less specific than was previously thought. Beffa and Mathews (2004) examined the relationship between manipulation techniques targeted at specific spinal levels and the spinal levels actually producing a cavitation during the technique. The authors reported no significant correlation between the spinal levels producing the cavitation sounds and the spinal levels targeted by the technique.

It is important to note that manipulation, or any manual therapy, is not commonly utilized in isolation. Typically physical therapists may instruct a patient in other therapeutic activities including mobility, flexibility and strengthening exercises. Here we describe two spinal manipulative techniques commonly used for mechanical LBP, but readers are referred to Chapter 22 for additional information regarding manipulation techniques of the lumbar spine.

Manipulation performed with the patient supine (Fig. 16.1)

The supine lumbar manipulation technique was utilized in the derivation (Flynn et al 2002) and validation study (Childs et al 2004). The technique is performed with patients in supine and the clinician on the side opposite to their symptoms. The patient is asked to interlace the fingers behind the head. The clinician creates ipsilateral side-bending of the lumbar spine by moving the lower extremities toward the side of symptoms. The upper body of the patient is side-bent towards the side of symptoms and contralaterally rotated. The clinician contacts the involved anterior superior iliac spine of the patient whilst contralaterally rotating the patient's upper body. The clinician provides an anterior-to-posterior force through the pelvis. If the patient is uncomfortable or unable to relax during the set-up of the procedure, it is advised to select an alternative technique.

Manipulation performed with the patient side-lying (Fig. 16.2)

The side-lying neutral lumbar manipulation is commonly used in rehabilitation settings. In this procedure, the clinician will attempt to target a particular lumbar segment that was identified as being hypomobile and / or painful during physical examination. As described above, it may be challenging to direct the manipulative force at a particular segment but, in fact, it may move the entire lumbar region.

The clinician should place the patient in the side-lying position with the painful side up. The clinician begins by flexing the top leg until motion is palpated at the targeted lumbar level. The next step is to rotate the patient's trunk down to the targeted level. Once this position is achieved, the clinician should determine the patient's comfort level and proceed only if the patient is able to tolerate the position. The clinician will stabilize the torso with one forearm, while the caudal forearm will rotate the pelvis toward the clinician. During this time, the clinician is attempting to engage the hypomobile segment. Once engaged, the clinician may elect to deliver a high-velocity, short-amplitude thrust through the pelvis.

Specific exercise group

Patients appropriate for the specific exercise subgroup of the treatment-based classification demonstrate a directional preference for movement during the examination, which is an improvement in symptoms or range of motion in response to a specific single or repeated trunk movements and positioning techniques (Werneke et al 2011). There are three common categories of directional preference in this subgroup including extension, flexion and lateral shift. Directional preference may just indicate a position or motion improving symptoms; however, centralization of symptoms may also be noted during the examination. Centralization is when referred spinal symptoms are progressively abolished in a distal-to-proximal direction in response to deliberate application of movements or postures, and it is crucial in identifying individuals likely to benefit from specific exercise programmes (Werneke & Hart 2001; Aina et al 2004; Werneke et al 2008).

Utilizing the treatment-based classification approach, the clinician assesses for a directional preference in weight-bearing or non-weight-bearing positions for a particular direction of movement of the lumbar spine with the main goal of centralization of symptoms (Browder et al 2007). Matching the individual to the appropriate directional preference category is of particular importance as it has been reported that 84% of individuals matched to the appropriate direction of exercise had significant reductions in pain and disability within the first 2 weeks of treatment (Long et al 2008).

Dosage of directional preference exercises is variable; however, Browder et al (2007) instructed subjects to perform one set of 10 repetitions frequently throughout the day. Posture education may also be important for instructing patients in activities or positions that may alter their symptoms. Here we briefly summarize treatment considerations for specific exercise-oriented classification.

Flexion-oriented exercises

A directional preference for flexion is most common in older adult populations (age >50 years) typically with imaging evidence or a medical diagnosis of lumbar spinal stenosis (Fritz et al 2007). Patients who have lumbar stenosis are likely to report pain with walking or extension of lumbar spine, or bilateral lower extremity symptoms, and their symptoms are relieved with sitting.

Patients in a flexion-oriented specific exercise classification may benefit from performing repeated end-range flexion exercises. Flexion exercises are usually easiest to perform with the patient in the supine or quadruped positions. The posterior pelvic tilt or single / double knee to chest exercise may be good exercises to promote flexion of the lumbar spine. Exercises should be dosed according to patient response and performed frequently throughout the day as part of a home exercise programme.

Patients in the flexion-oriented specific exercise classification tend to be older, with degenerative joint changes, and stiffness of the lumbar spine and hip joints. If stiffness is detected in the lumbar spine with passive accessory mobility testing, mobilizations may be performed. Prone posterior-to-anterior mobilization is useful for many patients, with the lumbar spine positioned in some flexion with the aid of pillows placed under the abdomen to avoid peripheralization of symptoms due to excessive extension. The clinician performs the mobilization by contacting the lumbar spinous process with the hypothenar eminence of the hand and performing oscillatory mobilizations. The clinician should be mindful to avoid any worsening of patients' symptoms.

Additionally, case studies involving patients with lumbar stenosis have advocated intervention strategies including mobilization or manipulation for the lumbar spine and / or hip joint, general lower extremity strengthening exercise, neural mobilizations and a walking programme possibly facilitated with body weight-supported treadmill ambulation (Murphy et al 2006; Whitman et al 2006).

Extension-oriented exercises

Extension-oriented exercises or McKenzie exercises have been recommended as a potential intervention for individuals with pain radiating below the knee (Bach & Holten 2009). Approximately 40–56% of individuals with acute LBP with radicular symptoms will achieve centralization with extension-oriented exercises (Aina et al 2004). When performing extension-oriented exercises, the clinician is attempting to determine the presence of directional preference and / or centralization.

Extension-oriented exercises programmes can be prescribed in a variety of ways. In the beginning, the extension-oriented exercises should be completed using patient-generated forces only. This may include exercises such as prone lying, prone on elbows and prone press-ups. These exercises have demonstrated superior short-term outcomes compared with non-steroidal anti-inflammatories (NSAIDs) or educational booklets (Busanich & Verscheure 2006). Education should be also provided to the patient to avoid positions that aggravate or peripheralize the symptoms. (Readers are referred to Ch 7 for additional information regarding the McKenzie method applied to the spine.)

Joint mobilization to promote extension

Depending on the patient symptom response, the clinician may elect to provide a manual force to promote additional relief of symptoms or centralization. A common manual force may be posterior–anterior lumbar mobilizations in the prone or extended position. The patient may be progressively positioned into more extension by having the patient prone on the elbows or performing a prone press-up whilst the mobilizations are delivered. Research suggests that the specific choice of a mobilization technique is not important for achieving pain relief – only that the mobilization is being performed in the lower lumbar spine instead of the upper lumbar spine (Chiradejnant et al 2003).

Lateral shift exercises

Individuals with lateral deviation or shift of the lumbar spine have been associated with poor prognosis (Porter & Miller 1986) especially when this is present with a crossed straight leg raise (Khuffash & Porter 1989). Lateral deviation or a lateral lumbar shift is a common presentation in the treatment of LBP and has been thought to be associated with disc pathology, but the exact mechanism is unknown (Laslett 2009). McKenzie (1981) defines a lateral lumbar shift as lateral displacement of the patient's trunk in relation to the pelvis and is clinically relevant if side-glide tests change patient reporting of pain intensity or location.

Patients with a lateral shift deformity who are able to centralize their symptoms with pelvic translocation movement testing in standing are treated with weight-bearing shift correction exercises. The patient should be taught to perform the pelvic translocation movement in the direction that produced the centralization during the examination. The extension-oriented exercises described for the extension specific exercise classification may also be helpful once the visible shift has been reduced.

If a patient's symptoms peripheralize with weight-bearing pelvic translocation movements, the clinician may opt to try non-weight-bearing exercises. These exercises commence with the patient in prone and the clinician attempts to translate the pelvis to correct the shift. Positioning the table into some flexion or the use of pillows under the abdomen may be necessary in order to reduce pain and avoid peripheralization of symptoms, if the patient is uncomfortable in prone. Once the lateral shift appears to be reduced, the clinician may opt to begin extension-oriented exercises with or without manual therapy interventions.

Stabilization group

Patients with lumbar segmental instability have been proposed as a unique subgroup of patients with LBP; however, there have been conflicting studies regarding criteria to define this condition (O'Sullivan 2000; Hicks et al 2003). A clinical prediction rule was defined by Hicks et al (2005) for patients who would be successful, with a stabilization classification for treatment and include: age <40 years, positive prone instability test, presence of aberrant movements and a passive straight leg raise test >91°. If three of four variables were positive the likelihood of success using this particular stabilization programme would be improved.

Examination items

The prone instability test has patients supporting their torso at the end of the table with their feet on the floor. The examiner applies a posterior–anterior force on each lumbar segment, assessing for pain reproduction. If pain reproduction is noted, the patient is asked to lift the feet from the ground and the posterior–anterior pressure is reapplied. If pain is elicited this would indicate a positive test (Schneider et al 2008).

During supine passive straight leg raise test, the examiner passively flexes the hip with the knee extended until the examiner feels resistance, and hence range of motion is recorded (Hicks et al 2005). Aberrant movements are clinical signs of lumbar segmental instability and include: painful arc during flexion or upon return to extension, an instability catch, Gower sign or 'thigh climbing', and reversal of lumbopelvic rhythm (Hicks et al 2003). (For operational definitions of these conditions, see the study by Hicks et al (2003).)

Intervention

Hicks et al (2005) designed a comprehensive spine stabilization programme to challenge the transversus abdominis, erector spinae, multifidus and quadratus lumborum muscles. In their programme, repeated submaximal efforts were encouraged in order to imitate the typical function of these muscle groups in spine stabilization. Additionally, exercise selection should be based upon the patient's functional demands and progression of exercises should be dependent on the response and tolerance of the patient. In this study, 54 subjects completed the 16-session supervised exercise programme. Approximately 33% of subjects experienced a 50% or greater reduction in disability. On the contrary, 28% of subjects experienced no change or worsening in symptoms.

Patients in the stabilization classification should be educated to avoid end-range movements of the lumbar spine in order to avoid positions that may overload the passive stabilizing structures of the spine. Lifting even light loads from a position of near-end-range lumbar spinal flexion should be avoided because of the potentially damaging forces created in the ligaments and intervertebral discs of the spine by such movements (McGill 1988).

Although the literature supports the usefulness of active, strengthening exercise programmes, studies comparing different stabilization strengthening routines have generally not found any differences when used in fairly heterogeneous groups of patients (Danneels et al 2001; Koumantakis et al 2005).

One potential approach to identifying an appropriate exercise routine is to identify exercises that optimally challenge important stabilizing muscles without imposing any potentially dangerous loads on the spine. The transversus abdominis muscle is often a favourite target during rehabilitation of patients with LBP. Training the transversus abdominis may be initiated by teaching the patient the abdominal-bracing manoeuvre (Richardson & Jull 1995) by drawing the navel up towards the head and in towards the spine so that the stomach flattens but the spine remains in its neutral position. Research has shown that the abdominal-bracing manoeuvre will activate the transversus abdominis to a greater extent than a traditional pelvic tilt exercise, in which the patient is instructed to flatten the spine (Urquhart et al 2005). The clinician will need to instruct the patient to avoid engaging superficial musculature such as the rectus abdominis. Once the patient can perform the abdominal-bracing manoeuvre properly, more-challenging activities can be added, such as bridging or marching in hook-lying. It is recommended that abdominal bracing should be combined with other aspects of the stabilization programme, and eventually be incorporated into more functional positions and postures that would challenge each individual patient in his or her everyday activities.

The oblique abdominal muscles can be exercised effectively with the horizontal side support exercise or side plank. This exercise produces high levels of electromyographic (EMG) activity in the oblique abdominals with low compression forces (Kavcic et al 2004). To perform the horizontal side support exercise, the patient is side-lying with the knees bent or straight whilst the torso is supported on the forearm. The patient then lifts the pelvis from the table and places the spine in a neutral position. The patient should perform the side support exercise for progressively longer sustained periods of time and higher repetitions. If asymmetry exists, it should be a goal to achieve equality in strength and endurance between sides.

Strengthening of the erector spinae muscles may be important because these are the primary source of extension torque for lifting tasks. The erector spinae muscles produce the extensor force needed for lifting, whereas the segmental extensors, primarily the multifidus muscles, provide stabilization of individual lumbar motion segments. Current evidence suggests that the multifidus tends to atrophy in patients with chronic LBP, and failure to regain normal morphology and endurance of multifidus and erector spinae muscles may be a risk factor for recurrence of LBP (Danneels et al 2001; Koumantakis et al 2005). Research has further shown that the multifidus muscles do not automatically recover full strength and endurance after the first episode of LBP, unless specific exercises are performed (Hides et al 1996). These findings emphasize the need for clinicians to focus attention on rehabilitation of the extensor musculature, with a particular focus on regaining endurance and strength of the multifidus muscles.

The erector spinae and multifidus muscles can be trained using extension exercises. Caution must be employed, however, because extension exercises also tend to produce high levels of compression on the lumbar spine, which may not be tolerated by all patients. A relatively safe patient position from which to begin an extension exercise programme is quadruped. Whilst in the quadruped position, the patient may be asked to extend one leg or one arm to a horizontal position whilst maintaining the abdominal bracing. Raising the opposite arm and leg simultaneously offers more efficient training of the multifidus and erector spinae muscles with sufficient muscle EMG activity levels, while maintaining safe levels of lumbar compression (Kavcic et al 2004). Bridging exercises performed from a supine or hook-lying position while maintaining abdominal bracing also provide a relatively safe and effective method for activating the multifidus and erector spinae muscles. Having the patient extend one leg from the bridge position requires slightly greater lumbar extensor muscle activity (Kavcic et al 2004).

Traction group

There is conflicting evidence for the efficacy of intermittent mechanical lumbar traction for patients with LBP (Delitto et al 2012). It has been proposed that sciatica is a primary factor for traction being beneficial in individuals with LBP. The subgroup of patients that will benefit from mechanical traction has been reported by Fritz et al (2007) in a randomized clinical trial of 64 subjects to include: presence of sciatica, signs of nerve root compression, peripheralization of symptoms with extension movements, and a positive crossed straight leg raise test.

Individuals with mechanical LBP and who fit this subgroup often exhibit signs of nerve root compression including myotomal, dermatomal and / or deep tendon reflex abnormalities. A crossed straight leg raise is performed identically to the straight leg raise test except that the opposite extremity is raised. It is a positive test if pain is reproduced in the involved extremity.

Mechanical traction is most often performed with the patient prone, but may also be performed in supine position. If the patient is supine, flexing the hips and knees will tend to place the lumbar spine into more flexion – a position that may be more appropriate and comfortable for older patients with imaging findings suggesting lumbar spinal stenosis. The goal of treatment with mechanical traction is to centralize the patient's symptoms and permit the patient to progress into another classification, most often a specific exercise classification. Patients within the traction classification should be monitored closely. If reassessment shows that the patient is able to centralize symptoms with active movements, progression to a specific exercise classification would be indicated. If the patient's symptoms and signs of nerve root compression continue to worsen, referral for injections, medication or other treatment options such as surgery may be warranted.

In the randomized clinical trial performed by Fritz et al (2007), 91% of the individuals who demonstrated peripheralization with extension achieved a 50% decrease in their modified Oswestry Disability Index scores with the addition of mechanical traction. Additionally, they experienced an average improvement of 29 points compared with 13 in the extension-oriented exercise-only group (Fritz et al 2007). Static traction was applied for 12 minutes at an intensity of 40–60% of the patient's body weight based on tolerance and symptom response. After completing the traction, the subjects remained prone for at least 2 minutes, and then performed a set of prone press-ups before returning to weight-bearing. This treatment was applied for a maximum of 12 sessions over a 6-week time frame (4 sessions per week for the first 2 weeks, then once a week in weeks 3–6).

Stage II and III individuals

The appropriate management of the individual who is in stage II or III of the treatment-based classification is not clear. Most commonly, subjects in these stages are managed using an impairment-based approach. The clinician will target impairments in flexibility, strength, endurance and joint mobility with interventions. Evans et al (2010) observed that individuals had impairments in strength, flexibility and neuromuscular control of muscles surrounding the hip and pelvis region. These findings may indicate potential areas to target with intervention programmes.

Impairments may be readily apparent in the local areas, but may also be present in adjacent regions. Impairments in adjacent regions may also contribute to the primary complaint of LBP and should be examined by the clinician (Whitman et al 2006; Wainner et al 2007; Burns et al 2010).

Another significant component of the management of individuals in stage II or III includes issuance of a home exercise programme aimed at reducing the recurrence of LBP. A comprehensive home exercise programme that targets identified musculoskeletal impairments and incorporates task-specific exercises is preferred (Delitto et al 1995; George & Delitto 2002). The clinician may choose to blend exercises that focus on neuromuscular control, strength, endurance and mobility. With all exercise programmes, education regarding adherence, proper progression and avoidance of overtraining is essential. In the acute LBP population, advice and education appears beneficial, but there is conflicting evidence regarding the influence of education on the recurrence of LBP (Liddle et al 2007).

Conclusion

The treatment-based classification approach has sufficient reliability for use within clinical practice settings and may assist providers in appropriately matching patients with LBP to a particular intervention with the intent of maximizing patient outcomes. This is one emerging approach to the management of mechanical LBP; however, a plethora of management models exists and usage will be at the discretion of the individual provider.

References

Aina A, May S, Clare H. 2004. The centralization phenomenon of spinal symptoms – a systematic review. Man Ther 9: 134–143.

Airaksinen O, Brox J, Cedraschi C. 2006. European guidelines for the management of chronic non-specific low back pain. Eur Spine J 15: S192–300.

Bach S, Holten K. 2009. Guideline update: what's the best approach to acute low back pain? J Fam Pract 58: E1.

Beffa R, Mathews R. 2004. Does the adjustment cavitate the targeted joint? An investigation into the location of cavitation sounds. J Manipul Physiol Ther 27: e2.

Brennan G, Fritz J, Hunter S, et al. 2006. Identifying subgroups of patients with acute / sub-acute non-specific low back pain. Spine 31: 623–631.

Browder D, Childs J, Cleland J, et al. 2007. Effectiveness of an extension-oriented treatment approach in a subgroup of subjects with low back pain: a randomized clinical trial. Phys Ther 87: 1608–1618.

Burns S, Mintken P, Austin G. 2010. Clinical decision making in a patient with secondary hip–spine syndrome. Physiother Theory Prac 25: 384–397.

Busanich B, Verscheure S. 2006. Does McKenzie therapy improve outcomes for back pain? J Athl Train 41: 117–119.

Childs J, Fritz J, Flynn T, et al. 2004. A clinical prediction rule to identify patients likely to benefit from spinal manipulation: a validation study. Ann Int Med 141: 920–928.

Chiradejnant A, Maher C, Latimer J, et al. 2003. Efficacy of 'therapist-selected' versus 'randomly selected' mobilisation techniques for the treatment of low back pain. Aust J Physiother 49: 233–241.

Cleland J, Fritz J, Childs J, et al. 2006. Comparison of the effectiveness of three manual physical therapy techniques in a subgroup of patients with low back pain who satisfy a clinical prediction rule: study protocol of a randomized clinical trial. BMC Musculoskel Dis 7: 1–9.

Cleland JA, Fritz JM, Kulig K, et al. 2009. Comparison of the effectiveness of three manual physical therapy techniques in a subgroup of patients with

low back pain who satisfy a clinical prediction rule: a randomized clinical trial. Spine 34: 2720–2729.
Dagenais S, Caro J, Haldeman S. 2008. A systematic review of low back pain cost of illness students in the United States and internationally. Spine 8: 8–20.
Danneels L, Vanderstraeten G, Cambier D. 2001. Effects of three different training modalities on the cross sectional area of the lumbar multifidus muscle in patients with chronic low back pain. Br J Sports Med 35: 186–191.
Delitto A, Erhard R, Bowling R. 1995. A treatment-based classification approach to low back syndrome: identifying and staging patients for conservative treatment. Phys Ther 75: 470–485.
Delitto A, George S, Van Dillen L, et al.; Orthopaedic Section of the American Physical Therapy Association. 2012. Low back pain. J Orthop Sports Phys Ther 42(4): A1–57. doi: 10.2519/jospt.2012.0301.
Deyo R, Diehl A. 1988. Cancer as a cause of back pain: frequency, clinical presentation, and diagnostic strategies. J General Int Med 3:230–238.
Deyo R, Rainville J, Kent D. 1992. What can the history and physical examination tell us about low back pain? JAMA 268: 760–765.
Deyo R, Mirza S, Martin B. 2006. Back pain prevalence and visit rates: estimates from U.S. national surveys, 2002. Spine 31: 2724–2727.
Evans K, Cady K, Dobson A, et al. 2010. Results of a musculoskeletal preparticipation screening programme in BUCS Super 8 Rugby League players. Br J Sports Med 44: i5.
Fernández-de-las-Peñas C, Hernandez-Barrera V, Alonso-Blacno C, et al. 2011. Prevalence of neck and low back pain in community-dwelling adults in Spain: a population based national study. Spine 36: E213–E219.
Flynn T, Fritz J, Whitman J, et al. 2002. A clinical prediction rule for classifying patients with low back pain who demonstrate short-term improvement with spinal manipulation. Spine 27: 2835–2843.
Fritz J, Lindsay W, Matheson J. 2007. Is there a subgroup of patients with low back pain likely to benefit from mechanical traction? Results of a randomized clinical trial and subgrouping analysis. Spine 32: E793–E800.
George S, Delitto A. 2002. Management of the athlete with low back pain. Clin J Sports Med 21: 105–120.
George S, Delitto A. 2005. Clinical examination variables discriminate among treatment-based classification groups: a study of construct validity in patients with acute low back pain. Phys Ther 85: 306–314.
Hart L, Deyo R, Cherkin D. 1995. Physician office visits for low back pain: frequency, clinical evaluation, and treatment patterns from a U.S. national survey. Spine 20: 11–19.
Henschke N, Maher C, Refshauge K. 2009. Prevalence of and screening for serious pathology in patients presenting to primary care settings with acute low back pain. Arthritis Rheum 60: 3072–3080.
Hicks G, Fritz J, Delitto A, et al. 2003. Inter-rater reliability of clinical examination measures for identification of lumbar segmental instability. Arch Phys Med Rehabil 84: 1858–1864.
Hicks G, Fritz J, Delitto A, et al. 2005. Preliminary development of a clinical prediction rule for determining which patients with low back pain will respond to a stabilization exercise program. Arch Phys Med Rehabil 86: 1753–1762.
Hides J, Richardson C, Jull G. 1996. Multifidus muscle recovery is not automatic after resolution of acute, first episode low back pain. Spine 21: 2763–2769.
Itoh H, Kitamura F, Yokoyama K. 2013. Estimates of annual medical costs of work-related low back pain in Japan. Ind Health 51: 524–529.
Kavcic N, Grenier S, McGill S. 2004. Quantifying tissue loads and spine stability while performing commonly prescribed low back stabilization exercises. Spine 29: 2319–2329.
Khuffash B, Porter R. 1989. Cross leg pain and trunk list. Spine 14: 602–603.
Koes B, van Tulder M, Ostelo R, et al. 2001. Clinical guidelines for the management of low back pain in primary care: an international comparison. Spine 26: 2504–2513.
Koumantakis G, Watson P, Oldham J. 2005. Trunk muscle stabilization training plus general exercise versus general exercise only: randomized controlled trial of patients with recurrent low back pain. Phys Ther 85: 209–225.
Laslett M. 2009. Manual correction of an acute lumbar lateral shift: maintenance of correction and rehabilitation: a case report with video. J Manual Manipul Ther 17: 78–85.
Liddle S, Gracey J, Baxter G. 2007. Advice for the management of low back pain: a systematic review of randomised controlled trials. Man Ther 12: 310–327.
Long A, May S, Fung T. 2008. Specific directional exercises for patients with low back pain: a case series. Physiother Can 60: 307–317.
McGill S. 1988. Estimation of force and extensor movement contributions of the disc and ligaments. Spine 13: 1395–1402.
McKenzie R. 1981. The lumbar spine: Mechanical Diagnosis and Therapy. Waikanae, NZ: Spinal Publications.
Murphy D, Hurwitz E, Gregory A, et al. 2006. A non-surgical approach to the management of lumbar spinal stenosis: a prospective observational cohort study. BMC Musculoskel Dis 7: 1–8.
O'Sullivan P. 2000. Lumbar segmental instability: clinical presentation and specific stabilizing exercise management. Man Ther 5: 2–12.
Porter R, Miller C. 1986. Back pain and trunk list. Spine 11: 596–600.
Richardson C, Jull G. 1995. Muscle control–pain control: what exercises would you prescribe? Man Ther 1:2–10.
Schneider M, Erhard R, Brach J, et al. 2008. Spinal palpation for lumbar segmental mobility and pain provocation: an interexaminer reliability study. J Manipul Physiol Ther 31: 465–473.
Staal J, Hlobil H, van Tulder M. 2003. Occupational health guidelines for the management of low back pain: an international comparison. Occup Environ Med 60: 618–626.
Stanton T, Fritz J, Hancock M, et al. 2011. Evaluation of treatment-based classification algorithm for low back pain: a cross sectional study. Phys Ther 91: 496–509.
Strine T, Hootman J. 2007. US national prevalence and correlates of low back and neck pain among adults. Arthritis Rheum 57: 656–665.
Urquhart D, Hodges P, Allen T, et al. 2005. Abdominal muscle recruitment during a range of voluntary exercises. Man Ther 10: 144–153.
Wainner R, Whitman J, Cleland J, et al. 2007. Regional interdependence: a musculoskeletal examination model whose time has come. J Orthop Sports Phys Ther 37: 658–660.
Werneke M, Hart D. 2001. Centralization phenomenon as a prognostic factor for chronic low back pain and disability. Spine 26: 758–764.
Werneke M, Hart D, Resnik L, et al. 2008. Centralization: prevalence and effect on treatment outcomes using a standardized operational definition and measurement method. J Orthop Sports Phys Ther 38: 116–125.
Werneke M, Hart D, Cutrone G, et al. 2011. Association between directional preference and centralization in patients with low back pain. J Orthop Sports Phys Ther 41: 22–31.
Whitman J, Flynn T, Childs J, et al. 2006. A comparison between two physical therapy treatment programs for patients with lumbar spinal stenosis: a randomized clinical trial. Spine 31: 2541–2549.

Chapter 17

Lumbar Radiculopathy

Chad Cook, Mark Wilhelm

CHAPTER CONTENTS

Aetiology and background	199
Prevalence	199
Definitions	199
Natural history	200
Clinical signs and symptoms	200
Anatomy and pathogenesis of lumbar radiculopathy	200
Anatomy	200
Pathogenesis	201
Essential aspects of differential diagnosis	201
An evidence-based clinical examination	201
Patient history	201
Physical examination	202
Provocation tests	202
Outcome measures	204
Imaging	204
Nerve condition responses	204
Current best evidence with regard to treatment	205
Conservative approaches	205
Injection	207
Surgical approaches	207

Aetiology and Background

Prevalence

Low back pain (LBP) is a common, disabling disorder that places a burden both on individuals and on society, with associated loss of work and medical costs (van Tulder et al 1995; Assendelft et al 2004). Studies of LBP have proposed point prevalences between 6% and 33% and 1-year prevalences between 22% and 65% (Loney & Stratford 1999; Walker 2000; Dagenais et al 2010). The lifetime prevalence of LBP has been estimated at approximately 84% (Airaksinen et al 2006). In the United States of America (USA) alone, treatments for LBP cost over $50 billion annually, whereas indirect costs for LBP are estimated at $7.4–19.8 billion; incremental costs for LBP exceed $26 billion a year (Liledahl et al 2010). Combined annual estimates in the USA have exceeded $90 billion in total costs (Foster 2011).

Definitions

Low back disorders are best divided by their mechanical and non-mechanical origins, with the relatively rare non-mechanical origins consisting of: (1) neoplasias, such as multiple myeloma, lymphoma / leukaemia, and breast, lung, prostate, kidney, spinal cord, vertebral and retroperitoneal tumours; (2) infections, such as osteomyelitis, septic discitis, paraspinous abscess, epidural abscess and shingles; (3) inflammatory arthritis, including ankylosing spondylitis, psoriatic spondylitis, Reiter's syndrome, and Scheuermann's and Paget diseases; (4) visceral, which may include symptoms originating from an aortic aneurysm, prostatitis, endometriosis, nephrolithiasis, pyelonephritis, perinephric abscess, pancreatitis, cholecystitis, or a penetrating ulcer (Jarvik & Deyo 2002). Mechanical origins of LBP are further divided into conditions such as anatomically oriented LBP and low-back-related leg pain. Lumbar radiculopathy is considered the most common form of neuropathic pain (Dworkin et al 2007).

Lumbar radiculopathy is a subclassification of LBP that is often characterized by a radiating pain in one or more lumbar dermatomes that may or may not be accompanied by other radicular irritation symptoms (Van Boxem et al 2010). In the literature, the terms 'radicular pain', 'sciatica' and 'radiculopathy' are also often used interchangeably (Van Boxem et al 2010), despite the fact that these terms do not necessarily describe the same conditions. By definition, **radicular pain** is a symptom that involves a region beyond the spine, and it is very possible that the radicular pain does not originate within the low back. **Sciatica** is also considered a symptom rather than a diagnosis (Konstantinou & Dunn 2008), and it characteristically involves radiating leg pain that follows a dermatomal pattern (Koes et al 2007) along the distribution of the sciatic nerve (Stafford et al 2007). Although sciatica may also not originate in the low back, it is thought that 90% of cases of sciatica are caused by a lumbar herniated disc (Koes et al 2007). **Lumbar radiculopathy** is objective loss of sensory and / or motor function as a result of conduction block of one or more lumbar nerves. Symptoms may include numbness, motor loss, muscle wasting, weakness, and loss of reflexes (Govind 2004), and lumbar radiculopathy can be diagnosed with one or all of these symptoms. Causally, for this book chapter, lumbar radiculopathy will be considered as pain radiating into one or more dermatomes caused by nerve root irritation / inflammation and / or compression. Lumbar radiculopathy may have radicular pain and may also be described as sciatica; however, not all radicular pain or sciatica is radiculopathy.

Natural history

In the general population, the annual prevalence of lumbar radiculopathy has been reported as from 9.9% to 25%, whereas the point prevalence is reported at 4.6% to 13.4% and lifetime prevalence is estimated at 1.2% to 43% (Konstantinou & Dunn 2008). The most frequent region for lumbar radiculopathy is L5 (Hsu et al 2011). Cook et al (2013) recently captured risk factors for first-time incidence of lumbar radicular pain. Preventable and modifiable risk factors included smoking, obesity and a number of occupational factors. Caution must be used, however, since these factors are also associated with a myriad of other potentially contributing elements such as unhealthy lifestyle choices or lower socioeconomic status. Furthermore, radicular symptoms were poorly operationally defined across studies.

Most cases of radiculopathy are self-limiting, and symptoms resolve over the course of weeks to months (Casey 2011). Once acquired, symptoms associated with lumbar radiculopathy often resolve within 2–4 weeks with or without treatment (van Tulder et al 2010). The few whose symptoms do not resolve report higher levels of disability, loss of function, and pain than do LBP-only individuals (Goode et al 2011). Weber (1993) reported that pain completely or partially resolves in 60% of the patients within 12 weeks of onset, but also identified about 30% of the patients who still had symptoms after 3 months to 1 year. Older subjects with lumbar stenosis generally have a poorer overall outcome (Van Boxem et al 2010).

Clinical signs and symptoms

There are a number of signs and symptoms associated with lumbar radiculopathy. Symptoms include definitions of pain affiliated along dermatomes. Dermatomes are defined as an area of skin supplied with afferent nerve fibres by a single posterior spinal root. Symptoms include pain, numbness and tingling in the legs, and corresponding LBP. The most common descriptors for pain include periodic bouts of attacks and, when present, burning and prickling sensations (Mahn et al 2011). Symptoms can also be categorized by location and severity. Hsu et al (2011) describe lumbar radiculopathy from the least severe to the most severe (Table 17.1).

Signs include identifiable objective findings affiliated with myotomes. Myotomes are defined as a group of muscles innervated by a single spinal nerve. Signs may include weakness and potential wasting of muscles, and diminished reflexes, generally along the L4, L5 or myotome pattern (Lee-Robinson & Lee 2010). Deep tendon reflexes are an involuntary response, which offers an objective assessment for neurological impairment (Durrant & True 2002). Loss of deep tendon reflexes is usually said to be the most robust clinical finding associated with lumbar radiculopathy (Marshall & Little 2002). Reflex loss may occur at the Achilles tendon (an S1 problem), at the knee extensors (primarily L4 but also L2 and L3) or less commonly at the hamstrings (L4–S2).

Table 17.1 **Description of lumbar radiculopathy by severity**

Severity level	Description	Sensory and motor involvement
Mild	Pure sensory/painful radicular pattern, characterized by radicular pain and a segmental pattern of sensory dysfunction but no other neurological deficits	No
Moderate	Mild motor deficit pattern, characterized by radicular pain, sensory dysfunction and mild non-progressive segmental motor weakness and/or reflex change	Yes
Severe	Marked motor deficit pattern, characterized by radicular pain and sensory dysfunction with severe or worsening motor deficits	Yes

Anatomy and Pathogenesis of Lumbar Radiculopathy

Anatomy

A quick review of the anatomy of the lumbar spine may improve the understanding of the pathogenesis of lumbar radiculopathy. The lumbar spine consists of five lumbar vertebrae, five corresponding intervertebral discs, 12 facet joints (T12–L1 to L5–S1) and multiple ligaments, and muscular and neurological contributions. The design of the lumbar spine allows viscoelastic motion, energy absorbance and movements with six degrees of freedom. These functions depend on muscular, bone and ligamentous components for mechanical tasks (Bogduk 1997).

Lumbar vertebrae can be divided into three sections from anterior to posterior. The anterior portion is the vertebral body, which is essentially flat on the superior and inferior surfaces and provides contact points for the intervertebral disc (Bogduk 1997). The middle section in the lumbar spine includes the pedicles, which are strong posterior projections. The posterior portion of the vertebrae includes the inferior and superior articular processes, the spinous process and the transverse processes.

The vertebral (spinal) canal and the intervertebral foramen are surrounded by a number of anatomical structures. The anterior wall of the vertebral canal is formed by the posterior surfaces of the lumbar vertebra and the posterior wall is formed by the lamina and ligamenta flava of the same vertebra (Bogduk 1997). Laterally, the facets provide a partial barrier. The intervertebral foramen is surrounded by the disc anteriorly, the pedicle inferiorly and superiorly, and by the zygapophyseal joints posteriorly (Bogduk 1997). Structural damage or a space-occupying lesion in any of these regions may increase the risk of developing lumbar radiculopathy.

Clinical presentations of lumbar radiculopathy vary according to the level of nerve root or roots involved. All lumbar and sacral spinal nerve roots originate at the T10 to L1 vertebral level, where the spinal cord ends at the conus medullaris. The roots then course down through the spinal canal, forming the cauda equina, until each root exits at its respective intervertebral foramen. All lumbar nerve roots exit the spinal canal at the neural foramina below their respective vertebrae. For example, the L5 nerve roots exit via the neural foramina at the L5 / S1 disc space level. Thus, posterolateral disc herniation of the L3 / L4 disc usually compresses the L4 nerve root, whereas a posterolateral disc herniation of the L4 / L5 disc typically compresses the L5 nerve root.

Each spinal nerve arises from a ventral and a dorsal nerve root, which meet to form the spinal nerve in the intervertebral foramen (Bogduk 1997). Dorsal root ganglia tend to be located within the neural foramina, and not the spinal canal. However, at the low lumbar levels there is a tendency for dorsal root ganglia to reside proximal to the neural foramina, within the spinal canal (Hsu et al 2011). Each dorsal root communicates to a dorsal root ganglion that contains the cell bodies of the sensory fibres of the dorsal roots. The dorsal root transmits sensory fibres whereas the ventral root primarily transmits motor fibres (Bogduk 1983). Each spinal nerve exits the intervertebral foramen with dural structures, an extension of the dura mater and arachnoid mater, which is commonly referred to as the dural sleeve (Bogduk 1983). In the intervertebral foramen, the amount of space is extremely limited – thus the structures in this region are predisposed to problems associated with space-occupying lesions.

Pathogenesis

Lumbar radiculopathy may have both mechanical and non-mechanical origins. Mechanically, lumbar radiculopathy is most commonly associated with a lumbar disc herniation, but it can also be associated with spondylolisthesis, spondylolysis or lumbar stenosis. Non-mechanical contributors may be synovial cysts, infection, tumours and / or vascular abnormalities (Govind 2004). Space-invading lesions are typically the initial ingredients in the development of lumbar radiculopathy.

In 1934, Mixter and Barr (1934) first implicated the role of a lumbar disc herniation as the cause of several lumbar radicular pain syndromes. Their implicit principle had been a preponderate assumption that compression of neural elements was the sole aetiological factor leading to the manifestation of symptoms (DePalma et al 2005). Subsequent knowledge has shown, however, that mechanical influence is not the sole aetiological factor.

Herniated lumbar discs cause mechanical and chemical irritation of the nerve roots leading to complaints of radiculopathy (Bruggeman & Decker 2011). For lumbar radiculopathy to be present there must be: (1) mechanical stimulation, typically through compression or tension, and (2) a chemically mediated non-cellular inflammatory reaction, which might occur through a disc rupture. Nerve roots subjected to sustained compression or tension for extended periods may become sensitized to mechanical stimulation. Long-term contributions of mechanical / chemical irritation may lead to vascular changes of the nerve including focal demyelination, intraneural oedema, impaired microcirculation, Wallerian degeneration and, potentially, partial axonal damage (Govind 2004).

There are findings supporting that mechanical stimulation is not the only element responsible for lumbar radiculopathy. There is little correlation between the severity of lumbar radiculopathy and the size of the space-occupying lesion (DePalma et al 2005), specifically a lumbar disc herniation, which is measureable using magnetic resonance imaging (MRI). Large disc herniations may cause no symptoms (Halperin et al 1982; Wiesel et al 1984). In some cases, individuals have resolved symptoms despite the retained presence of a notable mass (Govind 2004). Furthermore, a number of studies (Rydevik et al 1984; Ozaktay et al 1995; Nygaard et al 1997) have reported the benefit of hydrocortisone injections for intervertebral-disc-associated lumbar radiculopathy. Conservative treatment is often effective, despite non-resolution of the disc herniation (Mulleman et al 2006). Indeed, since the early 1950s, a growing body of evidence has supported the clinical utility of transforaminal, or selective nerve root, injections of anaesthetic or corticosteroids.

Essential Aspects of Differential Diagnosis

Lumbar radiculopathy is a clinical diagnosis that uses imaging for confirmation. In the majority of cases, a herniated disc is the offending compressive disorder with other mechanical conditions such as spondylolisthesis, spondylolysis or lumbar stenosis. Competing diagnoses may include cauda equina syndrome (CES), infectious conditions, synovial cysts, tumour and / or vascular abnormalities (Govind 2004). As a clinical diagnosis, immediate imaging is not recommended if the diagnosis can be made early. Hsu et al (2011) recommend immediate imaging for radiculopathy with urinary retention, saddle anaesthesia, bilateral neurological symptoms or signs, suspected neoplasm and suspected epidural abscess. If infection is suspected, a lumbar puncture and cerebrospinal fluid analysis are warranted. As with all conditions that originate at the low back, a strong and detailed clinical examination is necessary for proper treatment decision making.

An Evidence-based Clinical Examination

Patient history

It is important to determine the main complaint (e.g. numbness, weakness, location of symptoms) of the subject (Wolff & Levine 2002). Pain and sensory symptoms such as paraesthesia, dysaesthesia, hyperaesthesia or anaesthesia that involve a specific lumbar dermatome are suggestive of a diagnosis of lumbar radiculopathy (Hsu et al 2011). Pain that worsens during forward-bending or straightening of the leg at the knee may be associated with lumbar radiculopathy. Pain that worsens during bowel straining (the Valsalva manoeuvre) may be associated with lumbar herniated disc and subsequent radiculopathy. Bowel / bladder symptoms (new urinary retention or incontinence) with LBP, bilateral sciatica, saddle hypo-aesthesia or anaesthesia, motor weakness of the lower extremities, impairment of anal, bulbocavernosus, medioplantar and Achilles tendon reflexes bilaterally, rectal and bladder sphincter dysfunction as well as sexual impotence all suggest CES, and so demand immediate work-up (Orendácová et al 2001).

Muscle weakness is less commonly a complaint of individuals with lumbar radiculopathy. Certainly, weakness at specific muscles within lumbar myotomes should also raise suspicion for the diagnosis of lumbar radiculopathy. Complaints of weakness may be specific to functional difficulties such as walking with smooth coordination, difficulty in getting up from a chair, or dragging one's foot during the swing phase of gait.

If pain is a complaint, a pain drawing is beneficial to establish a pattern and location of the pain. A pain drawing allows one to determine whether the pain radiates and, if so, the distribution of the symptoms (Honet & Puri 1976). It is also important to isolate activities or specific lumbar movements that trigger the concordant symptoms. These findings may help develop an educational plan for pain relief but may also provide important information that can be used to direct treatment.

General findings such as duration of symptoms, history of LBP, history of smoking and obesity, and a number of occupational factors (e.g. heavy work load, disdain towards supervisor or job, etc.) are risk factors for the development of lumbar radiculopathy, but have also been shown to be prognostic factors for delayed outcome (Cook 2012a, Cook et al 2013).

Physical examination

Observation

Although a 'flattened' low back posture has been clinically affiliated with lumbar radiculopathy, there is no evidence to support this within the literature. The presence of muscle wasting along myotomal patterns is related to long-term, severe radiculopathy. Those with severe lumbar radiculopathy may stand with their affected limb in knee flexion to reduce the tension that may occur with an extended knee. On occasions where a herniated lumbar disc is present as the cause of radiculopathy, the patient's posture and gait should be examined for lateral list (Humphreys & Eck 1999). An acquired scoliosis may occur as well as a mechanism to reduce nerve tension or foramen compression.

Active and passive movements

All planes of motion of the lumbar spine should be assessed with active and passive movements. Responses to look for are any movements that are associated with the pain / symptoms noted during the history portion of the exam. Often, forward trunk flexion is accompanied by peripheralization of symptoms towards the legs or buttocks. Repeated movement into flexion often worsens the nature of the symptoms. Extension may originally present with sharp LBP but may also diminish the radicular symptoms with repeated movements.

Neurological testing

Neurological testing involves examination of motor function, sensibility changes and deep tendon reflex modifications along a nerve root distribution. It is important to note that absence of radiating symptoms in a dermatomal distribution does not rule out the presence of nerve root compression because this finding has low sensitivity (Rhee et al 2007).

A manual muscle test is performed to identify minimal weakness along a myotome distribution to determine a local nerve root involvement. The following grading of 0 to 5 is recommended: 0 / 5 no movement, 3 / 5 antigravity and 5 / 5 normal (Honet & Puri 1976). Cook and Hegedus (2012) report the values from a number of studies that have addressed manual muscle testing and *all* found higher specificity values than sensitivity values. Sensibility testing involves assessment of changes in patient reports of sensation along dermatomes. Typically, testing measures are confined to assessment of light touch, whether or not one can feel a pin-prick, or differentiate hot from cold. The grading of deep tendon reflexes is from 0 (absent) to 4 (clonus, very brisk). Deep tendon reflexes should be assessed at both the quadriceps (L2 / L3 / L4) and Achilles (S1) tendons. Unfortunately, there is no reliable reflex to assess L5, the most common root compressed in mechanical lumbar radiculopathy. As with manual muscle testing and sensibility testing, the sensitivity of these tests is low and the reliability depends on the skill level of the clinician performing the testing.

All neurological testing is based on the assumption of the regularity of dermatomes and myotomes. Although lumbar radiculopathy requires clinical confirmation of pain along a dermatome, weaknesses along myotomes or some combination of these characteristics, variability exists within subjects regarding myotome and dermatome patterns (Lee et al 2008). Areas of overlap of sensory regions are called non-autonomous zones: areas in which nerves may supply sensation. Autonomous zones are areas in which individual or dedicated nerve roots supply sensation. Foerster (1933) identified the most exclusive of these: the sole of the foot (S1), the dorsum of the foot (L5), the medial calf (L4), and the anterior thigh (L2 and L3). Table 17.2 defines the areas of pain through sensibility testing, whereas Table 17.3 describes expected muscle weaknesses captured through myotomal testing.

Provocation tests

Straight leg raise

The straight leg raise (SLR) is the common provocation test used when differentially diagnosing lumbar radiculopathy. The SLR was first operationally described in 1864 by Dr Charles Lasègue, but it was his student, Forst, who used the test to describe present-day radiculopathy (Scaia et al 2012). Although the test is sometimes performed variably, the classical performance involves the patient lying horizontally in supine position on an examiner's table. The knee remains fully extended, while the examiner raises the patient's leg slowly off the table (while supporting the knee with one hand to maintain full extension). The examiner continues to raise the leg until the maximum flexion of the hip is reached or until the patient reports the onset of leg pain (or symptom provocation) in the involved extremity (Scaia et al 2012). Other methods of performance include measurement of differences in the angle at the hip in which the SLR is reached (in comparison with the other leg).

Table 17.2 Dermatomal regions of pain for lumbar radiculopathy

Region	Anatomical description	Testing	Frequency
L1	Symptoms on presentation generally involve pain, paraesthesia, and sensory loss in the inguinal region	Sensibility testing near the inguinal region	Not common
L2–L3	Sensation may be reduced over the anterior thigh	Sensibility testing at the anterior thigh above the knee	Uncommon
L3–L4	Sensation may be reduced at the medial aspect of the lower leg at and below the knee	Sensibility testing at the medial knee and lower medial leg	Common
L5	Back pain that radiates down the lateral aspect of the leg into the foot; sensation changes laterally	Sensibility testing at the lateral aspect of the lower leg	Very common

Table 17.3 Myotomal regions and findings for lumbar radiculopathy

Region	Anatomical description	Testing	Frequency
L1	Rarely, minor hip flexion weakness is present	Hip flexor manual muscle testing	Not common
L2–L3	Some hip flexion and knee extension weakness	Hip flexor testing in supine with knee extended	Uncommon
L3–L4	Knee extension weakness	Knee extension testing in sitting	Common
L5	Strength can be reduced in foot dorsiflexion, toe extension, foot inversion and foot eversion; weakness of leg abduction may also be evident in severe cases	Strength testing of ankle dorsiflexion and hip abduction	Very common

In surgical populations the SLR is associated with a disc herniation in most studies and it has demonstrated high sensitivity (pooled estimate 0.92, 95% CI 0.87–0.95) with widely varying specificity (0.10–1.00, pooled estimate 0.28, 95% CI 0.18–0.40) (van der Windt et al 2010). Because what constitutes a positive test has varied so significantly within the literature, Scaia et al (2012) evaluated the diagnostic accuracy of the pain-provocation-based SLR only and found variations in sensitivity and specificity. If the test is truly more sensitive than specific, it should be used to rule out lumbar radiculopathy.

Bowstring sign

The bowstring sign is a variation of the SLR in which an end manoeuvre is used to differentiate whether nerve tension is the cause of the symptom. The examiner raises the patient's extended leg (at the knee) on the symptomatic side with the foot fully dorsiflexed. The leg raise continues until the patient reports pain. The bowstring sign refers to the relief of radicular pain when the knee is flexed during a positive straight leg raise (Hsu et al 2011).

Crossed straight leg raise

The crossed SLR test (which is also known as the well leg raise test) is performed in a similar fashion to the SLR test, except that the opposite limb to the affected leg is the one that is raised. The knee remains fully extended while the examiner raises the patient's leg slowly off the table (while supporting the knee with one hand to maintain full extension). The examiner continues to raise the leg until the maximum flexion of the hip is reached or until the patient reports the onset of leg pain (or symptom provocation) in the involved extremity (Cook & Hegedus 2012). A Cochrane review (van der Windt et al 2010) reported high specificity (pooled estimate 0.90, 95%CI 0.85–0.94) with consistently low sensitivity (pooled estimate 0.28, 95% CI 0.22–0.35), which suggests that a positive finding should rule in the diagnosis of lumbar radiculopathy – although a negative finding is unlikely to rule it out.

Slump sit test

Cook and Hegedus (2012) describe the slump sit test as follows. The patient sits straight with the arms behind the back, the legs together and the posterior aspect of the knees against the edge of the treatment table. The patient then slumps as far as possible, producing full trunk flexion; the examiner applies firm overpressure into flexion to the patient's back, being careful to keep the sacrum vertical. While maintaining full spinal flexion with overpressure, the examiner either asks the patient to extend the knee or passively extends it. The examiner moves the foot into dorsiflexion while maintaining knee extension. Neck flexion is then added to assess symptoms. Neck flexion is released to see whether symptoms abate. A positive test is concordant reproduction of symptoms, sensitization and asymmetry findings. Although not nearly as well investigated as the SLR, the test appears to have similar diagnostic accuracy – demonstrating greater sensitivity than specificity.

Femoral nerve tension test

The femoral nerve tension test is performed by placing the patient prone on the table and passively extending the hip and leg straight up off of the plane of the table (Hsu et al 2011). Theoretically, this procedure places tension on the upper lumbar nerve roots (L2, L3 and L4) although it is likely that the test is primarily useful during assessment of a far lateral disc herniation. Its diagnostic accuracy has been studied only once, and was found to demonstrate high sensitivity for extreme lateral disc herniation (Cook & Hegedus 2012).

Outcome measures

Functional outcome scales are characterized by their properties of reliability, validity and responsiveness to clinical changes. These properties ensure that data are collected and interpreted in a systematic and reproducible way, allowing comparison between different patient populations (Pietrobon et al 2002). Functional outcome scales allow clinicians to develop a baseline level of disability for patients and help to quantify the patient's condition for better overall understanding.

There are no specific outcomes measures for lumbar radiculopathy. However, two commonly used outcome instrument scales for LBP that are appropriate for lumbar radiculopathy are the Roland Morris Disability Questionnaire (RMQ) and the Oswestry Disability Index (ODI). Both are considered region-specific questionnaires (each focuses on one area of the body) and have been well documented in the literature.

The ODI is a multidimensional scale and has been used to document changes in muscle activity, pain and psychological factors and work status (Taylor et al 1999). The ODI has been used to evaluate pre- and post-surgical outcomes, as well as a benchmark for determination of treatment effectiveness. Four versions of the ODI are available in English and nine in other languages. The data for the ODI provide both validation and standards for other users and indicate the power of the instrument for detecting change in sample populations (White & Velozo 2002).

The RMQ is a one-dimensional scale and is a useful short functional disability questionnaire that focuses on activity intolerances related to the impairment associated with LBP. The RMQ was originally developed from the Sickness Impact Profile (SIP) although the RMQ is much simpler, quicker and easier to use (Taylor et al 1999). As with the ODI, the RMQ has been used in all forms of outcome investigation including research. Like most valuable outcome instruments, it is particularly responsive to change in acute populations with LBP (Bombardier 2000).

Although not considered a functional outcomes measure, report of pain is frequently used to measure change associated with an intervention. Pain severity outlines the self-reported value of 'how much the pain hurts' versus pain affect, which reflects a mental status affect associated with continuous pain (Bombardier 2000). Two examples of measures associated with pain severity include the visual analogue scale (VAS) and the numeric pain rate scale (NPRS).

Imaging

There are a number of imaging methods used to confirm the presence of lumbar radiculopathy. Because lumbar radiculopathy is a clinical diagnosis, a detailed clinical examination should always occur prior to the use of imaging. Imaging is substantially overused for patients with LBP and should be considered only after a 30-day period and failure to respond to conservative care (van Tulder et al 2006; Chou et al 2009).

Plain film radiograph

Plain film radiography is useful in identifying stenosis and the extensiveness of degenerative joint disease (Brown et al 2009). Radiographs can show narrowing in the openings and, on rare occasions, signs of infection, but fail to provide an accurate view of soft tissue. In addition, they use ionizing radiation that can damage the body and could potentially cause cancer. Consequently, plain radiographs are not recommended in the work-up of lumbar radiculopathy unless there is a need to evaluate for infection, fracture, malignancy, extensiveness of degenerative changes, disc space narrowing or type of prior surgery (Hsu et al 2011).

Magnetic resonance imaging

A magnetic resonance image does not use ionizing radiation, has good visualizing capacities, especially of the soft tissues, and is considered the most useful method for the detection of sinister disorders such as spinal infections and spinal metastases (Wassenaar et al 2012). MRI has demonstrated superiority in identification of a herniated nucleus pulposus (Wilmink 2001; Wassenaar et al 2012) and structural changes associated with degeneration such as stenosis (Wilmink 2001). It has also been identified as useful for assessing nerve root compression (Wassenaar et al 2012).

Wassenaar et al (2012) recently evaluated the diagnostic accuracy of MRI for a herniated disc, nerve root compression and stenosis. For identification of a herniated disc, MRI has a pooled summary estimate of sensitivity and specificity of 75% (95% CI 65–83%) and 77% (95% CI 61–88%) respectively. This provides a positive likelihood ratio of 3.30 (95% CI 1.76–6.21) and a negative likelihood ratio of 0.33 (95% CI 0.21–0.50). For the two studies that evaluated nerve root compression, the results demonstrated a range of sensitivity from 81% to 92% and a range of specificity from 52% to 100%. For lumbar stenosis, the MRI showed high sensitivities of 87% and 96% coupled with lower specificities of 68% and 75%. These results suggest that errors in diagnoses are possible using MRI, especially since specificity values are not very strong.

Computed tomography scan

Computed tomography (CT) is less commonly used in assessment of the extent of degeneration of the lumbar spine. A CT scan can assess osseous structures better than either plain radiography or MRI; however, CT alone is unable to visualize nerve roots, so it is not helpful in the direct imaging of a radicular process (Hsu et al 2011). For identifying a lumbar disc herniation, CT has a similar pooled summary estimate of diagnostic accuracy with a sensitivity of 77.4% and specificity of 73.7%, compared with a reference standard of surgical findings (van Rijn et al 2012). These values are markedly similar to MRI.

Nerve condition responses

The most commonly used nerve condition responses for testing lumbar radiculopathy are electromyography (EMG) and nerve conduction studies (NCS). The two tests are generally used in combination. Both NCS and EMG have higher diagnostic utility for lumbar radiculopathy when neurological weakness has been present for at least 3 weeks, which is also why these tests are ordered for individuals with persistent unexplained symptoms (Hsu et al 2011). In addition, the tests are not nearly as useful if the severity or radiculopathy is confined to pain or sensory loss only (Hsu et al 2011).

Tests such as EMG and NCS are occasionally used to differentiate radiculopathy for peripheral entrapment disorders (Rhee et al 2007). Yet differentiating peripheral neuropathy and lumbar radiculopathy in patients with lumbar stenosis using EMG and routine NCS is clinically challenging, because peripheral entrapment and low back disorders may be present simultaneously in older patients (Plastaras 2003). EMG is an electrical recording of muscle activity and involves insertion of a fine needle into the tested muscle. In order to diagnose with an EMG, the reading must be abnormal for two or more different muscles and peripheral nerves from the same nerve root (Durrant & True 2002). Two recordings are taken, one at rest and one during a contraction. A normal response involves only brief EMG activity during needle insertion, then no activity when the muscle is at rest. During contraction, motor unit action potentials that reflect electrical activity within the muscle appear on the recording screen, with corresponding increases as more muscle fibres are solicited.

A nerve conduction velocity (NCV) test consists of stimulation of the nerve and recording of the evoked potential, either from the muscles or from the nerve (to study the sensory response). NCV assesses the extent of axonal loss of large myelinated nerve fibres (Cook et al 2009). The test involves measurement of the time delay between stimulation and response at two stimulation sites with a calculation of the distance of the sites (Smith 1979).

The two late responses most commonly analysed are the H-reflex and the F-wave. The H-reflex (Hoffmann's reflex) assesses an afferent 1a sensory nerve and an efferent alpha motor nerve. H-reflex testing tends to be more specific than sensitive (Cho et al 2010). The American Association of Neuromuscular and Electrodiagnostic Medicine concluded that peripheral limb EMG H-reflex testing is recommended for diagnosis of lumbar radiculopathy (Hsu et al 2011). The F-wave analyses motor nerves only and is often normal in patients who have suspected radiculopathy. F-wave studies have demonstrated poor sensitivity (Cho et al 2010) and because of this should never be used in isolation (Rhee et al 2007).

Current Best Evidence with Regard to Treatment

Conservative approaches

A bout of conservative care is recommended prior to interventions such as surgery or injection therapy. Typically, during the acute stage of lumbar radiculopathy the treatment should aim at reducing inflammation and pain, patient education and avoidance of increasing any neurological deficits. Treatment for inflammation and pain may include ice, heat, non-steroidal anti-inflammatory drugs (NSAIDs), analgesics, rest and traction. A combination of approaches is generally provided in clinical practice.

Hahne et al (2010) evaluated the benefit of multiple treatment options associated with lumbar radiculopathy. Within their review, they identified that there is moderate evidence that stabilization exercises are better than no treatment at short-term follow-up. Kennedy and Noh (2011) also recommended core stabilization exercises to correct possible alterations to spine biomechanics as a result of lumbosacral radiculopathy. Prior to these two studies, Murphy et al (2009) had found that lumbar stabilization exercises were beneficial when included as part of a multimodal treatment approach for individuals with lumbar radiculopathy secondary to a herniated disc as confirmed by MRI. In that study, the need for lumbar stabilization exercises was based on the result of three tests: (1) the hip extension test, (2) the segmental instability test and (3) the active SLR test.

Hahne et al (2010) also reported that manipulation was better than sham manipulation at short-term and intermediate-term follow-up for people with acute lumbar disc herniation and radiculopathy who had an intact annulus. The manipulation techniques used in the three trials were different but consisted of versions of soft tissue manipulation or massage along with high-velocity rotational thrusts (Fig. 17.1). A high-velocity, rotational lumbar spine thrust is theorized to isolate a given segment to improve movement and to relieve pain. The actual benefits beyond the clinical effects reported, which are associated with this technique for patients with radiculopathy, are only speculative.

The authors also reported that no difference exists between traction, laser and ultrasound at short- and intermediate-term follow-up (Hahne et al 2010). One study included in the review provided moderate evidence that the addition of mechanical traction to electrotherapy methods (hot pack, ultrasound and diadynamic currents) and medication (ibuprofen, mephenoxalone and paracetamol) reduce the risk of radiculopathy at short-term follow-up, but provide no additional short-term benefit for pain intensity or risk of having LBP (Ozturk et al 2006). A Cochrane systematic review assessing the use of traction for treatment of LBP with and without

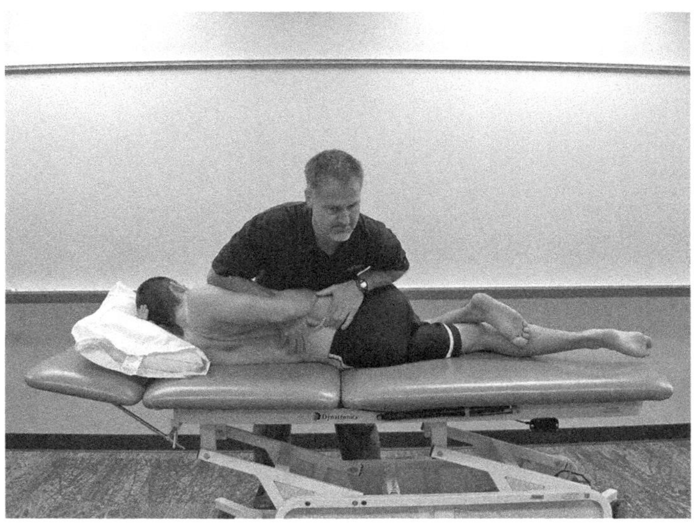

Figure 17.1 A high-velocity, rotational lumbar spine thrust manipulation.

sciatica concluded that, whereas there were a few low-quality papers reporting positive results, the majority of current literature suggests that traction may not be effective and that using traction as a stand-alone treatment is not supported by the current evidence (Clarke et al 2007).

Traction can be performed using different methods, including mechanically applied approaches and manually applied approaches by either the treating physical therapist or the patient (autotraction) (Clarke et al 2007; Hahne et al 2010). Whereas most of the studies included in the systematic review by Clarke et al (2007) assessed the effect of mechanical traction, there were a number of studies describing a wide variety of autotraction techniques and two studies that used manual traction by the clinician. These last two studies used a supine method during which a manual traction force was produced by the clinician's body and transferred to the patient through a harness fixed around the patient, which then provided the distracting force (Clarke et al 2007). Neither of these two studies was able to demonstrate a significant difference between this technique and other traction techniques, or a comparison intervention of isometric exercises (Clarke et al 2007). Cook (2012b) advocates the use of manual traction techniques in order to direct the distraction force more easily to the appropriate region. These manual traction methods may include side-lying gapping procedures designed to decompress the targeted segment (Fig. 17.2) and supine methods, which provide a gentler decompression procedure (Cook 2012b).

Fritz et al (2007) identified a subgroup of patients who are more likely to benefit from mechanical traction. The baseline characteristics associated with greater improvement with mechanical traction were: presence of leg symptoms, signs of nerve root compression and either peripheralization with extension movements or a positive crossed straight leg raise (Fritz et al 2007). Mechanical traction was combined with extension-oriented treatment and compared with extension-oriented treatment alone. Mechanical traction was administered for a 2-week period while the extension-oriented treatment was continued for an additional 4 weeks. At the 2-week assessment, patients in the mechanical traction group demonstrated significantly more improvement than those receiving extension-oriented treatment alone. At the 6-week follow-up, however, there was no significant difference between the two groups – both demonstrating significant improvement over baseline measurements (Fritz et al 2007).

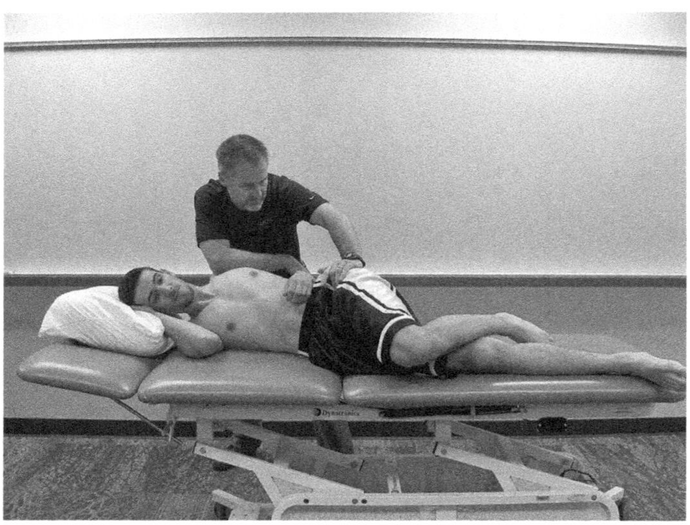

Figure 17.2 Side-lying manual traction technique.

Much of the available research assessing the utility of traction seems to suffer from poor research design in general, which can lead to confusion over the effectiveness of the technique (Krause et al 2000). Many of the studies included in the systematic review by Clarke et al (2007) used low-dose traction as a sham intervention, although it has been shown that a similar low-dose sham traction force showed an improvement of 50% in a population with non-specific LBP (Beurskens et al 1997). An effect of this size shown by a comparative sham intervention may minimize the stated effect of the original intervention (Krause et al 2000).

Mechanically oriented lumbar radiculopathy may benefit from various lumbar-related movements. During the mechanical portion of the assessment, particular directions of lumbar movement may be identified as: (1) improving symptoms (centralizing), (2) making symptoms worse (peripheralizing) or (3) no change in symptoms. Centralization is characterized by symptoms that are progressively abolished in a distal-to-proximal pattern during end-range lumbar movement tests (McKenzie & May 2003). If a patient's symptoms are found to centralize upon end-range movements during examination, these end-range loading movements, which are commonly referred to as directional preference, may be used as treatment options (McKenzie & May 2003, see also Ch 7). Several studies have reported some subjects experiencing an increase in localized LBP while concurrently experiencing centralization of radiating symptoms; this does not preclude the possibility of further centralization from continued end-range exercises and should not rule out repeated end-range exercises as a treatment option (Kopp et al 1986; Murphy et al 2009).

The most common movement directions for centralization are end-range extension, right or left side glide, and flexion (Murphy et al 2009). Between 42% and 61% of patients with lumbar radiculopathy secondary to a herniated disc were found to have symptoms that centralize with end-range movements (Kopp et al 1986; Alexander et al 1992; Murphy et al 2009). Only one of these studies (Murphy et al 2009) assessed directions other than extension as a possible source of centralization whereas the others (Kopp et al 1986; Alexander et al 1992) assessed only centralization as a result of extension. If all movement directions were assessed as potential centralizing movements then the percentage of patients who centralized with passive end-range movements might be closer to the upper range reported earlier (Wetzel & Donelson 2003; Murphy et al 2009). Repeated end-range movements in lying or standing have shown to be more beneficial in patients with acute radiculopathy secondary to disc herniation who also have an intact annulus (Kopp et al 1986). A recent study by Werneke et al (2008) in patients with radiating LBP suggested that symptoms were more likely to centralize for patients with acute symptoms (less than 21 days duration) and for patients aged between 18 and 44 years. Additionally, centralization appears more likely to occur in patients who have less distally radiating symptoms, but the time to complete centralization of symptoms did not correlate with radiating distance (Sufka et al 1998). Patients who have centralization of pain as a result of end-range movements in any direction have been shown to be associated with more favourable short-term and long-term outcomes than those who do not centralize (Sufka et al 1998; Werneke et al 2008; Murphy et al 2009). In contrast, those who have peripheralization of symptoms, which occurs in only a small portion of the population, appear to be associated with a more negative outcome (Murphy et al 2009).

Injection

Epidural steroid injections are frequently used during the treatment of lumbar radiculopathy. Despite the conflicting evidence of their benefit, epidural steroid injections for older Americans have increased dramatically over the last several years (Argoff & Sims-O'Neill 2009). In 1999, nearly 50 million dollars were spent on lumbar epidural steroid injections.

The premise behind epidural steroid injections is based on the recognition that inflammatory mediators affect the nerve root during lumbar radiculopathy and that steroids decrease swelling in the localized, targeted region. The first reported treatment was in 1952 (DePalma et al 2005). A year later, Lievre et al published the results of a series of patients treated with periradicular steroid injections (DePalma et al 2005).

There are two primary forms of epidural steroid injections, which unfortunately are often considered universal. The interlaminar (or translaminar) epidural injection involves injectant targeted between the lamina of the offending site. It requires relatively large volumes of the injectant for delivering steroids to the target site; this has the risk of an extra-epidural and intravascular needle placement. Transforaminal epidural injections are targeted near the nerve root in the intervertebral foramen. A transforaminal epidural steroid injection uses a small volume of local anaesthetic to anaesthetize the spinal nerve, but it will also partially anaesthetize the dura, the posterior longitudinal ligament, the intervertebral disc and the facet joint. A fluoroscopy-guided approach is commonly used to improve the location of the treatment.

The International Spinal Injection Society (ISIS) recommends the utilization of the nomenclature based on the precise anatomical descriptors – that is, transforaminal and interlaminar for the description of epidural injections (Sung 2006). As with all non-conservative treatments, there are risks. These risks include a small risk of infection, dural puncture (which can lead to headaches), bleeding and, although extremely rare, nerve damage.

There is some evidence that transforaminal injections are superior to placebo injections and even stronger evidence that these injections should be used as surgery-sparing interventions. Strong evidence exists for interlaminar epidural steroid injection for short-term relief and limited evidence for long-term relief in management of lumbar radiculopathy (Boswell et al 2007). There is also good evidence that transforaminal injections are more effective than interlaminar injections (Roberts et al 2009). Despite these positive findings, injection therapy is not recommended by most guidelines for treatment of LBP (Koes et al 2010).

Surgical approaches

Surgical approaches are aimed at removing the offending compressive structures from the nerve (Frank 1993). In the United States, the increase in spinal surgery as a treatment of choice for lumbar radiculopathy has increased significantly over the last several years. The most commonly used surgical approaches involve a form of decompression surgery, or fusion and decompression.

The posterior lumbar discectomy, hemilaminotomy and foraminotomy was the most commonly performed decompressive procedure of the lumbar spine in the early 2000s (Storm et al 2002), but the use of spinal fusion in combination with decompression, specifically complex spinal fusion, has increased dramatically in recent years. Between 1998 and 2008, the annual number of spinal fusion discharges for treatment of lumbar radiculopathy or other related conditions increased 2.4-fold, or by approximately 137% (Rajaee et al 2012). The number of reported discharges with spinal fusion increased correspondingly from 174 223 in 1998 to 413 171 in 2008 (Rajaee et al 2012). For older adults with stenosis, overall surgical rates declined slightly between 2002 and 2007, but the rate of complex fusion procedures increased 15-fold, from 1.3 to 19.9 per 100 000 beneficiaries. Complex fusions harbour greater risks with surgery – 5.6% experiencing life-threatening complications versus 2.3% with decompression alone (Deyo et al 2010). Certainly, with risks such as these, careful patient selection is the key to successful surgical intervention.

Determining who is a surgical candidate for lumbar radiculopathy is no easy task. Generally, patients with lumbar radiculopathy also present with a variety of comorbidities as well as misconceptions about the benefit and risks associated with surgery. In addition, because lumbar radiculopathy often has a favourable prognosis, identification of those with true neurological problems that have not responded to conservative treatment is warranted. It is crucial to determine the extent of the disability and this is best identified through patient-report measures or through a careful patient history. Imaging may be useful to help verify the presence or absence of a pathological condition and the offending anatomical location (Storm et al 2002).

The L4–L5 and L5–S1 levels are responsible for greater than 95% of lumbar disc herniations, with L5–S1 herniations occurring slightly more frequently. Much less common are herniations at the L1–L2, L2–L3 and L3–L4 levels, which account for less than 5% of herniations (Patten 1995). Surgery must be considered immediately if CES is suspected as this condition is a spinal emergency; CES occurs in approximately 2% of cases of herniated lumbar discs (Gitelman et al 2008). In this syndrome, patients experience a combination of saddle anaesthesia, abnormal lower extremity reflexes, and neurogenic bowel or bladder symptoms (Bruggeman & Decker 2011).

Potential surgical candidates need to know the risk associated with surgery as well. Life-threatening risks are especially prevalent with complex spinal fusion; however, other risks such as soft tissue infection (0.4–2%), meningitis, discitis, osteomyelitis, bleeding, arachnoiditis, nerve root injury (<1%), permanent numbness, weakness or paralysis, bladder or bowel dysfunction, sexual dysfunction, dural tears with cerebrospinal fluid leak and pseudomeningocoele formation, deep venous thrombosis, delayed spinal instability and fusion failure and pseudoarthrosis formation, and anaesthetic risks (including death) are all possible (Abramovitz 1993). There is no such thing as 'minor' lumbar spine surgery, and therefore the risks must always be weighed against the potential rewards.

So far, the rewards associated with surgery (in the absence of CES) appear to be short term only. For radiculopathy with herniated lumbar disc, there is good evidence that standard open discectomy and microdiscectomy are moderately superior to non-surgical therapy (a non-standardized conservative approach) for improvement in pain and function through 2 to 3 months. For symptomatic spinal stenosis with or without degenerative spondylolisthesis, there is good evidence that decompressive surgery is moderately superior to non-surgical therapy (a non-standardized conservative approach) through 1 to 2 years. On average, both groups – conservative and surgical – experience improvement with or without surgery, and the benefits associated with surgery decrease with long-term follow-up (Chou et al 2009).

References

Abramovitz JN. 1993. Complications of surgery for discogenic disease of the spine. Neurosurg Clin North Am 4: 167–176.
Airaksinen O, Brox JI, Cedraschi C, et al. 2006. European guidelines for the management of chronic nonspecific low back pain. Eur Spine J 15: S192–300.
Alexander AH, Jones AM, Resenbaum DH Jr. 1992. Nonoperative management of herniated nucleus pulposus: patient selection by the extension sign. Long-term follow-up. Orthop Rev 21: 181–188.
Argoff CE, Sims-O'Neill C. 2009. Epidural steroid injections are useful for the treatment of low back pain and radicular symptoms: con. Curr Pain Headache Rep 13: 35–38.
Assendelft WJJ, Morton SC, Yu EI, et al. 2004. Spinal manipulative therapy for low back pain: a meta-analysis of effectiveness relative to other therapies. Ann Int Med 138: 871–881.
Beurskens AJ, de Vet HC, Koke AJ, et al. 1997. Efficacy of traction for nonspecific low back pain. 12-week and 60 month results of a randomized clinical trial. Spine 22: 2756–2762.
Bogduk N. 1983. The innervation of the lumbar spine. Spine 8: 286–293.
Bogduk N 1997. Clinical anatomy of the lumbar spine and sacrum, 3rd edn. New York: Churchill Livingstone.
Bombardier C. 2000. Outcome assessments in the evaluation of treatment of spinal disorders. Spine 25: 3100–3103.
Boswell MV, Trescot AM, Datta S, et al. 2007. Interventional techniques: evidence-based practice guidelines in the management of chronic spinal pain. Pain Phys 10: 107–111.
Brown S, Guthmann R, Hitchcock K, et al. 2009. Clinical inquiries: which treatments are effective for cervical radiculopathy? J Fam Pract 58: 97–99.
Bruggeman AJ, Decker RC. 2011. Surgical treatment and outcomes of lumbar radiculopathy. Phys Med Rehabil Clin North Am 22: 161–177.
Casey E 2011 Natural history of radiculopathy. Phys Med Rehabil Clin North Am 22: 1–5.
Cho SC, Ferrante MA, Levin KH, et al. 2010. Utility of electrodiagnostic testing in evaluating patients with lumbosacral radiculopathy: an evidence-based review. Muscle Nerve 42: 276–282.
Chou R, Fu R, Carrino JA, et al. 2009 Imaging strategies for low-back pain: systematic review and meta-analysis. Lancet 373: 463–472.
Clarke JA, van Tulder MW, Blomberg SEI, et al. 2007. Traction for low-back pain with or without sciatica. Cochrane Database System Rev 2: CD003010.
Cook CE. 2012a. Risk factor associated with first time incidence sciatica. Ohio Physical Therapy Conference, Columbus, OH. [Poster presentation.]
Cook CE. 2012b. Manual therapy of the lumbar spine. In: Cook CE. Orthopedic manual therapy: an evidence based approach, 2nd edn. Upper Saddle River: NJ Prentice Hall, pp 290–291.
Cook C, Hegedus E. 2012. Orthopedic physical examination tests: an evidence based approach, 2nd edn. Upper Saddle River: NJ Prentice Hall.
Cook C, Roman M, Stewart K, et al. 2009. Reliability and diagnostic accuracy of clinical special tests for myelopathy in patients seen for cervical dysfunction. J Orthop Sports Phys Ther 39: 172–178.
Cook CE, Learman KE, O'Halloran BJ, et al. 2013. Which prognostic factors for low back pain are generic predictors of outcome across a range of recovery domains? Phys Ther 93: 32–40.
Dagenais S, Gay RE, Tricco AC, et al. 2010. NASS contemporary concepts in spine care: spinal manipulation therapy for acute low back pain. Spine J 10: 918–940.
DePalma MJ, Bhargava A, Slipman CW. 2005. A critical appraisal of the evidence for selective nerve root injection in the treatment of lumbosacral radiculopathy. Arch Phys Med Rehabil 86: 1477–1483.
Deyo RA, Mirza SK, Martin BI, et al. 2010. Trends, major medical complications, and charges associated with surgery for lumbar spinal stenosis in older adults. JAMA 303: 1259–1265.
Durrant DH, True JM. 2002. Myleopathy, radiculopathy, and peripheral entrapment syndromes. London: CRC.
Dworkin RH, O'Connor AB, Backonja M, et al. 2007. Pharmacologic management of neuropathic pain: evidence based recommendations. Pain 132: 237–251.
Foerster O. 1933. The dermatomes in man. Brain 56: 1.
Foster N. 2011. Barriers and progress in the treatment of low back pain. BMC Med 9: 108.
Frank E. 1993. Approaches to myeloradiculopathy. Western J Med 158: 71–72.
Fritz JM, Lindsay W, Matheson JW, et al. 2007. Is there a subgroup of patients with low back pain likely to benefit from mechanical traction? Results of a randomized clinical trial and subgrouping analysis. Spine 32: E793–E800.
Gitelman A, Hishmeh S, Morelli BN, et al. 2008. Cauda equina syndrome: a comprehensive review. Am J Orthop 37: 556–562.
Goode A, Cook C, Brown C, et al. 2011. Differences in comorbidities on low back pain and low back related leg pain. Pain Pract 11: 42–47.
Govind J. 2004. Lumbar radicular pain. Aust Family Phys 33: 409–412.
Hahne AJ, Ford JJ, McMeeken JM. 2010. Conservative management of lumbar disc herniation with associated radiculopathy: a systematic review. Spine 35: E488–E504.
Halperin N, Agasi M, Hendel D. 1982. Painless root compression following disc extrusion. Arch Orthop Trauma Surg 101: 63–66.
Honet JC, Puri K. 1976. Cervical radiculitis: treatment and results in 82 patients. Arch Phys Med Rehabil 57: 12–16.
Hsu PS, Shefner JM, Dashe JF, et al. 2011. Lumbosacral radiculopathy: pathophysiology, clinical features, and diagnosis. UptoDate 19: 1.
Humphreys SC, Eck JC. 1999. Clinical evaluation and treatment options for herniated lumbar disc. Am Family Phys 59: 575–88.
Jarvik J, Deyo R. 2002. Diagnostic evaluation of low back pain with emphasis on imaging. Ann Int Med 137: 586–597.
Kennedy DJ, Noh MY. 2011. The role of core stabilization in lumbosacral radiculopathy. Phys Med Rehabil Clin North Am 22: 91–103.
Koes BW, van Tulder MW, Peul WC. 2007. Diagnosis and treatment of sciatica. BMJ 334: 1313–1317.
Koes BW, van Tulder M, Lin CW, et al. 2010. An updated overview of clinical guidelines for the management of non-specific low back pain in primary care. Eur Spine J 19: 2075–2094.
Konstantinou K, Dunn KM. 2008. Sciatica: review of epidemiological studies and prevalence estimates. Spine 33: 2464–2472.
Kopp JR, Alexander AH, Turocy RH, et al. 1986. The use of lumbar extension in the evaluation and treatment of patients with acute herniated nucleus pulposus. A preliminary report. Clin Orthop Relat Res 202: 211–218.
Krause M, Refshauge M, Dessen M, et al. 2000. Lumbar spine traction: evaluation of effects and recommended application for treatment. Man Ther 5: 72–81.
Lee MW, McPhee RW, Stringer MD. 2008. An evidence-based approach to human dermatomes. Clin Anat 21: 363–373.
Lee-Robinson A, Lee AT. 2010. Stepping up toe extension and flexion strength testing: a new method to record additional weakness. Am J Phy Med Rehabil 89: 598–600.
Liledahl R, Finch M, Axene D, et al. 2010. Cost of care for common back pain conditions initiated with chiropractic doctor vs. medical doctor / doctor of osteopathy as first physical: experience of one Tennessee-based general health insurer. J Manipul Physiol Ther 33: 640–643.
Loney PL, Stratford PW. 1999. The prevalence of low back pain in adults: a methodological review of the literature. Phys Ther 79: 384–396.
Mahn F, Hüllemann P, Gockel U, et al. 2011. Sensory symptom profiles and co-morbidities in painful radiculopathy. PLoS ONE 6: e18018.
Marshall GL, Little JW. 2002. Deep tendon reflexes: a study of quantitative methods. J Spinal Cord Med 25: 94–99.
McKenzie RA, May S. 2003. The lumbar spine: mechanical diagnosis and therapy, 2nd edn. Waikenae, NZ: Spinal Publications.
Mixter WJ, Barr JS. 1934. Rupture of the intervertebral disc with involvement of the spinal cord. N Engl J Med 211: 210.
Mulleman D, Mammou S, Griffoul I, et al. 2006. Pathophysiology of disk-related sciatica. I. Evidence supporting a chemical component. Joint Bone Spine 73: 151–158.
Murphy DR, Hurwitz EL, McGovern EE. 2009. A nonsurgical approach to the management of patients with lumbar radiculopathy secondary to

herniated disk: a prospective observational cohort study with follow-up. J Manipul Physiol Ther 32: 723–733.
Nygaard OP, Mellgren SI, Osterud B. 1997. The inflammatory properties of contained and noncontained lumbar disc herniation. Spine 22: 2484–2488.
Orendácová J, Cízková D, Kafka J, et al. 2001. Cauda equina syndrome. Progr Neurobiol 64: 613–637.
Ozaktay AC, Cavanaugh J, Blagoev D, et al. 1995. Phospholipase A2-induced electrophysiologic and histologic changes in rabbit dorsal lumbar spine tissues. Spine 20: 2659–2668.
Ozturk B, Gunduz OH, Ozoran K, et al. 2006. Effect of continuous lumbar traction on the size of herniated disc material in lumbar disc herniation. Rheumatol Int 26: 622–626.
Patten J. 1995. Spinal cord in relation to the vertebral column. In: Patten J. Neurological differential diagnosis, 2nd edn. Berlin: Springer-Verlag, Ch 15, pp 247–281.
Pietrobon R, Coeytaux R, Carey T, et al. 2002. Standard scales for measurement of functional outcome for cervical pain or dysfunction. Spine 27: 515–522.
Plastaras CT. 2003. Electrodiagnostic challenges in the evaluation of lumbar spinal stenosis. Phys Med Rehabil Clin North Am 14: 57–69.
Rajaee SS, Bae HW, Kanim LE, et al. 2012. Spinal fusion in the United States: analysis of trends from 1998 to 2008. Spine 37: 67–76.
Rhee JM, Yoon T, Riew KD. 2007. Cervical radiculopathy. J Am Acad Orthop Surg 15: 486–494.
Roberts ST, Willick SE, Rho ME, et al. 2009. Efficacy of lumbosacral transforaminal epidural steroid injections: a systematic review. PM R 1: 657–668.
Rydevik B, Brown MD, Lundborg G. 1984. Pathoanatomy and pathophysiology of nerve root compression. Spine 9: 7–15.
Scaia V, Baxter D, Cook C. 2012. The pain provocation-based straight leg raise test for diagnosis of lumbar disc herniation, lumbar radiculopathy, and / or sciatica: a systematic review of clinical utility. J Back Musculoskelet Rehabil 25(4):215–223.
Smith MS. 1979. Babinski sign – abduction also counts. JAMA 242: 1849–1850.
Stafford MA, Peng P, Hill DA. 2007. Sciatica: a review of history, epidemiology, pathogenesis, and the role of epidural steroid injection in management. Br J Anaesthes 99: 461–473.
Storm PB, Chou D, Tamargo RJ. 2002. Surgical management of cervical and lumbosacral radiculopathies: indications and outcomes. Phys Med Rehabil Clin N Am 13: 735–759.
Sufka A, Hauger B, Trenary M, et al. 1998. Centralization of low back pain and perceived functional outcome. J Orthop Sports Phys Ther 27: 205–212.
Sung MS. 2006. Epidural steroid injection for lumbosacral radiculopathy. Kor J Radiol 7: 77–79.
Taylor S, Taylor AE, Foy MA. 1999. Responsiveness of common outcome measures of patients with low back pain. Spine 24: 1805–1812.
Van Boxem, K, Cheng J, Patijn J, et al. 2010. Lumbosacral radicular pain. Pain Pract 10: 339–358.
van der Windt DA, Simons E, Riphagen II, et al. 2010. Physical examination for lumbar radiculopathy due to disc herniation in patients with low-back pain. Cochrane Database Syst Rev 2: CD007431.
van Rijn RM, Wassenaar M, Verhagen AP, et al. 2012. Computed tomography for the diagnosis of lumbar spinal pathology in adult patients with low back pain or sciatica: a diagnostic systematic review. Eur Spine J 21: 228–239.
van Tulder MW, Koes BW, Bouter LM. 1995. A cost-of-illness study of back pain in the Netherlands. Pain 62: 233–240.
van Tulder M, Becker A, Bekkering T, et al. 2006. European guidelines for the management of acute nonspecific low back pain in primary care. Eur Spine J 15: S169–S191.
van Tulder M, Peul W, Koes B. 2010. Sciatica: what the rheumatologist needs to know. Nat Rev Rheumatol 6: 139–145.
Walker BF. 2000. The prevalence of low back pain: a systematic review of the literature from 1966 to 1998. J Spinal Dis 13: 205–217.
Wassenaar M, van Rijn RM, van Tulder MW, et al. 2012. Magnetic resonance imaging for diagnosing lumbar spinal pathology in adult patients with low back pain or sciatica: a diagnostic systematic review. Eur Spine J 21: 220–227.
Weber H. 1993. The natural course of disc herniation. Acta Orthop Scand Suppl 251: 19–20.
Werneke MW, Hart DL, Resnik L, et al. 2008. Centralization: prevalence and effect on treatment outcomes using a standardized operational definition and measurement method. J Orthop Sports Phys Ther 38: 116–125.
Wetzel FT, Donelson R. 2003. The role of repeated end-range / pain response assessment in the management of symptomatic lumbar discs. Spine J 3: 146–154.
White LJ, Velozo CA. 2002. The use of Rasch measurement to improve the Oswestry classification scheme. Arch Phys Med Rehabil 83: 822–831.
Wiesel SW, Tsourmas N, Feffer HL, et al. 1984. A study of computer-assisted tomography: I. The incidence of positive CAT scans in asymptomatic group of patients. Spine 9: 549–551.
Wilmink JT. 2001. Cervical imaging: dynamic aspects and clinical significance. In: Szpalski M, Gunzburg R (eds) The degenerative cervical spine. Philadelphia: Lippincott Williams & Wilkins.
Wolff MW, Levine LA. 2002. Cervical radiculopathies: conservative approaches to management. Phys Med Rehabil Clin North Am 13: 589–608.

18 Chapter

Lumbar Spine Instability

Bryan S. Dennison, Michael H. Leal

CHAPTER CONTENTS

Historical appreciation of low back pain 210
Guideline adherence and practice variability 211
Diagnostic challenge of low back pain 211
The treatment-based classification system 212
Research investigating the treatment-based classification system 213
The treatment-based classification system: focus on the stabilization subgroup 213
Clinical management of lumbar spine instability 214
First level of classification and the patient interview 214
Self-reported symptoms and clinician pattern recognition 214
Second level of classification: physical examination 215
Evidence for physical examination findings 216
Sequencing of the physical examination 216
Proposed clinical examination for lumbar spine instability 216
Screening tests 216
Confirmatory tests 217
Clinical prediction rules in the treatment-based classification system 218
Conclusion 219

Historical Appreciation of Low Back Pain

The diagnosis and management of low back pain has affected the world for centuries – seemingly reaching back to the beginning of time itself. The Edwin Smith papyrus is the oldest surviving manuscript, dating back to at least the 17th century BC, describing scientific observation of signs and symptoms of spine injuries, classifications of spine injuries, hypotheses on mechanisms of spine injuries and suggested treatment for these injuries (van Middendorp et al 2010). It is interesting to observe, when looking at the descriptions of the spine injuries from the Edwin Smith papyrus, how familiar the ancient spine injuries are to modern-day spine injuries encountered in primary or emergency care today. In light of this, the great researcher and physician, Gordon Waddell, questioned whether anything has really changed, over thousands of years, with regards to back pain (Waddell 1995). He did acknowledge the progressive change in the *understanding* and *management* of low back pain that has occurred over the years. But this progress is suspect with regards to any appreciable influence our current understanding and management have had on *improving* the prevalence or disastrous effects of low back pain (Martin et al 2008). In 1995, Waddell classically noted that 'Low back pain is a twentieth-century health care disaster.' He went on to encourage the healthcare community as a whole to change its approach to managing this condition (Waddell 1995). Nine years later, in 2004, the ultimate management of low back pain had not improved. Waddell once again recognized the ongoing dilemma of low back pain and the lack of improvement in managing this condition. He noted 'Back pain was a 20th-century medical disaster and the legacy reverberates into the new millennium' (Waddell 2004). Moving ahead into the 'new millennium', low back pain continues to plague the modern world as Waddell noted. The Global Burden of Disease (GBD) Study 2010 sought to investigate the worldwide effects of low back pain. For the study, low back pain was operationally defined as follows: 'Activity-limiting low back pain (+/− pain referred into one or both lower limbs) that lasts for at least 1 day. The 'low back' is defined as the 'area on the posterior aspect of the body from the lower margin of the twelfth ribs to the lower gluteal fold' (Hoy et al 2010). The results of the GBD study, using the operational definition above, concluded that low back pain is now recognized as the global 'leading cause of disability in both developed and developing countries', trumping 290 other diseases and injuries that were evaluated in the GBD study (Buchbinder et al 2013). In addition to its rise to the top billing as the 'leading cause of disability' in 2010, low back pain also jumped from the 12th-ranking global contributor to disability-adjusted life years (DALYs) in 1990, to the 7th-ranking global contributor to DALYs in 2010 (http://www.healthmetricsandevaluation.org/gbd/visualizations/gbd-arrow-diagram) (Table 18.1). Adding to the societal impacts of ongoing, but increasing, disability and increasing prevalence, there has also been an increasing economic burden associated with low back pain as costs associated with managing the condition have risen. In the United States alone there was a 65% increase in costs associated with managing spinal pain (neck and low back) from 1997 to 2005. The estimated increase in costs for neck and low back pain in 2005 alone totalled 85.9 billion dollars. This was a substantial increase in costs from 1984 and 1994 (Martin et al 2008, Fig. 18.1).

Table 18.1 **Top global rankings of diseases and injuries with respect to disability-adjusted life years**

1990	2010
1. Lower respiratory infections	1. Ischaemic heart disease
2. Diarrhoeal diseases	2. Lower respiratory infections
3. Preterm birth complications	3. Stroke
4. Ischaemic heart disease	4. Diarrhoeal diseases
5. Stroke	5. HIV/AIDS
6. COPD	6. Malaria
7. Malaria	7. **Low back pain**
8. Tuberculosis	8. Preterm birth complications
9. Protein-energy malnutrition	9. COPD
10. Neonatal encephalopathy	10. Road injury
11. Road injury	11. Neonatal encephalopathy
12. **Low back pain**	12. Protein-energy malnutrition

Table adapted from IHMW website http://www.healthmetricsandevaluation.org/. Note that, in 2010, the rankings are shown only for the corresponding diseases/injuries noted in 1990. COPD = chronic obstructive pulmonary disease.

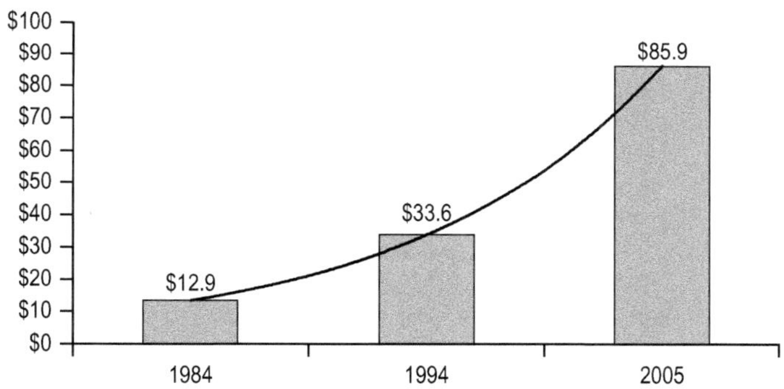

Figure 18.1 Spine-related medical expenditures. (Adapted from Martin et al 2008.) Note that the data are expressed in billions of dollars.

Disappointingly, increased costs, advances in understanding and technology associated with managing low back pain have not resulted in equal decreases in reported low-back-related disability over time (Martin et al 2008; Deyo 2011).

Guideline Adherence and Practice Variability

Recognizing the ongoing challenge of low back pain on a global scale, physical therapists have directed research efforts to direct care more effectively and accurately to individuals with low back pain. One of the hypothesized challenges to efficiently managing low back pain is the presence of practice variability and a lack of adherence to clinical practice guidelines among healthcare providers. Traditionally, the patient was the centre of the adherence discussion if suboptimal outcomes were associated with patient non-adherence to the provider's suggested management recommendations (Osterberg & Blaschke 2005). This myopic view of adherence, focusing only on the patient's role, has changed due to the increasing use of medical clinical practice guidelines in the 1990s. The increasing use of these guidelines in medicine has broadened the discussion of adherence, moving beyond narrowly focused analyses of patient behaviour to include healthcare provider behaviour (Cabana & Kiyoshi-Teo 2010). Discussions on adherence now appreciate the collaborative interaction between patients and healthcare providers. Analysis of healthcare provider adherence to practice guidelines in the clinical setting has revealed that healthcare providers were not much better than patients when it came to adherence (Cabana 2010). Specifically to low back pain, physicians (Bishop & Wing 2006; Feuerstein et al 2006; Williams et al 2010; Ivanova et al 2011) and physical therapists (Bekkering et al 2005; Delitto 2005; Strand et al 2005; Swinkels et al 2005; Feuerstein et al 2006; Fritz et al 2007b) alike exhibit deficiencies in adhering to low back clinical practice guidelines. The lack of compliance with clinical practice guidelines provides ample opportunity for the possibility of variation in clinical practice (Deyo 1986) and resultant adverse risks (Williams et al 2010). It is recognized that variability in practice is associated with suboptimal outcomes (Feuerstein et al 2006). Conversely, the use of clinical practice guidelines is associated with superior outcomes and improved cost management (McGuirk et al 2001; Brennan et al 2006; Fritz et al 2007b, 2008; Cabana 2010). The publication of practice guidelines is not sufficient to ensure clinical incorporation (Gross et al 2001). Multifactorial challenges exist in implementing clinical practice guidelines into current practice (Table 18.2).

Table 18.2 **Barriers to guideline adherence**

Cabana et al (1999)	Competing practice demands The limited time to apply an increasing number of guideline recommendations
Deyo (2011)	Clinician unawareness of newer guidelines and evidence A paucity of definitive evidence for or against certain practices Emergence of local practice styles Medicolegal concerns Inconsistent, sometimes contradictory, expert recommendations

Diagnostic Challenge of Low Back Pain

In an effort to maximize outcomes and reduce costs associated with the global challenge of low back pain, physical therapists have made efforts to decrease practice variability by establishing evaluation and treatment system guidelines that can better inform and guide physical therapy management strategies for low back pain. One such effort has been the development of a treatment-based classification system for low back pain (Delitto et al 1995). The basis for the development of the treatment-based classification system was the recognized failure of a diagnostic, pathoanatomical model to explain with accuracy and successfully treat individuals with low back pain. The diagnostic enigma of low back pain drove the development of the treatment-based classification systems. Due to the complex nature of low back symptoms, pathoanatomically based clinical examination and diagnostic testing had not proven useful means for determining the exact cause of low-back-related symptoms (White & Gordon 1982; Cook & Hegedus 2011). It has been suggested that between 85% and 95% of patients with low back pain cannot be given an exact diagnosis (White & Gordon 1982; Waddell 2005). To complicate the diagnostic process for low back pain further, it is recognized that low back pain rarely occurs in isolation (Hagen et al 2006; Hartvigsen et al 2013). In fact, patients presenting with a complaint of primary musculoskeletal pain in a specific region also report comorbidities and additional musculoskeletal pain in other regions of their body. This is especially true for patients with low back pain (Natvig et al 2001; Hagen et al 2006). The presence of widespread pain phenomenon adds to the clinical challenge of determining an exact diagnosis for patients presenting with low back pain and presents prognostic implications which challenge the patient's outcome (Croft 2009). Low back pain research to date has largely focused on narrowly defined inclusion criteria focusing, at best, on regionally defined symptoms of low back pain or single pain sites (i.e. low back region with or without referral into one or both of the extremities). Very little attention, beyond prognostic implications, is given to considering the potential role of the presence of multisite musculoskeletal pain and / or the presence of other patient comorbidities. These issues have confounded the diagnostic process for patients with complaints of low back pain. When seeking care, patients with low back pain present to a healthcare provider with symptoms that are assessed in light of predefined diagnoses (Tschudi-Madsen et al 2011). When no predefined diagnosis matches the symptom presentation(s), these patients are given the label of mechanical (White & Gordon 1982; Deyo 1986) or non-specific low back pain (Coste et al 1991). Non-specific low back pain has been defined as 'back pain complaints occurring without identifiable specific anatomical or neuro-physiological causative factors' by the International Association for the Study of Pain Task Force on Pain in the Workplace in 1995 (Zusman 1997). This definition describes symptoms of low back pain, or describes low back pain in terms of a syndrome, but is not in and of itself a diagnosis (Cedraschi et al 1999). Basically, what has been given the diagnostic label 'non-specific low back pain' is nothing more than the determination that no other diagnoses are being considered (Frank 1993). But this diagnostic label has done nothing to assist healthcare providers in effectively and efficiently managing low back pain. Specifically in physical therapy practice, accurate diagnoses are useful at times in clinical practice to assist with intervention decision making when a specific diagnosis is not able to be confidently determined, and the ability to direct specific care is a challenge for the physical therapist. As such clinicians are left to rely on the presence of signs, symptoms and pattern recognition to begin generating hypotheses of how best to direct care (Delitto et al 1995). The development of the treatment-based classification system was an attempt to improve the assessment and management of individuals with low back pain. To this end, the treatment-based classification system sought to identify, a priori, patients with clinical presentations who will respond to targeted interventions without having to rely on pathoanatomical diagnostic labels.

Not all patients with low back pain will respond to the same type of intervention; thus subgrouping individuals with low back pain may result in more efficient and optimal treatment strategies (Kent & Keating 2004). To the practising clinician, this approach seems glaringly obvious. But low back pain research has not traditionally taken this approach when investigating low back pain management strategies. Rather, it has viewed low back pain as a homogeneous entity and directed treatment towards this entity as a whole (Malmivaara et al 1995). The study results have been a washout, with no further insight gained into progressing the management of patients with low back pain (Riddle 1998). The treatment-based classification system proposed by Delitto et al (1995) viewed low back pain, in contrast, as a heterogeneous entity and sought to identify unique homogeneous subgroups within the low back pain population. These homogeneous subgroups would then receive targeted interventions.

The Treatment-Based Classification System

The original Delitto classification was intended to target patients with acute low back pain or acute exacerbations of low back pain (Fritz et al 2007a). Delitto et al (1995) defined acuteness operationally, based on the severity of the presentation and not an arbitrarily selected number of days since onset of the low back symptoms (Delitto et al 1995; Fritz & George 2000). The original treatment-based classification system described seven different classifications for those patients presenting with low back pain. In 2000 these seven classifications were streamlined into four classifications, based on treatment similarities (Fritz & George 2000). The classification algorithm remained unchanged until 2006 when it was updated and modified again (Brennan et al 2006). This modification added additional components to the algorithm to assist clinicians in identifying subgroups with definitive classifications. In addition, the update added further decision-making aids to assist the clinician when a patient presented with an unclear classification. The modified algorithm would guide the clinician in determining the subgroup which 'best fitted' the patient. As the current body of knowledge increased at the time, the 2006 update also added a hierarchical structure to the algorithm (Brennan et al 2006). However, this modification did not (unlike the 2000 version) include a traction subgroup as the study excluded patients with signs of nerve root compression. In addition, the current state of evidence at that time did not provide clinicians with confidence to identify accurately a subgroup of individuals with low back pain who were likely to respond to lumbar mechanical traction (Fritz et al 2007a). Finally, Stanton et al (2011) presented an algorithm that once more included the traction subgroup; they termed this algorithm a 'comprehensive algorithm' owing to the completeness of the algorithm in including all of the classification subgroups plus additional decision-making aids for patients with clear and unclear subgroup presentations. Table 18.3 shows the evolution of the treatment-based classification algorithm over time.

Table 18.3 Treatment-based classification algorithm evolution over time

	Delitto et al (1995)	Fritz & George (2000)	Brennan et al (2006)	Stanton et al (2011)
Classification subgroup	Immobilization	Immobilization	Stabilization	Stabilization
	Lumbar mobilization	Mobilization	Manipulation	Manipulation
	Sacroiliac mobilization			
	Extension syndrome	Specific exercise	Specific exercise	Specific exercise
	Flexion syndrome			
	Lateral shift			
	Traction	Traction	Traction*	Traction
			Unclear classification criteria – not including traction**	Unclear classification criteria – including traction

*Traction was not included in this algorithm as patients with signs of nerve root compression were excluded.
**The first classification algorithm to include decision-making assistance for when a patient does not meet a specific subgroup. The algorithm suggests that the clinician identifies which subgroup the patient fits best.

Research Investigating the Treatment-based Classification System

There has been a plethora of research evaluating the treatment-based classification model. Practice models should be re-evaluated as new evidence emerges (Fritz et al 2006; Apeldoorn et al 2010). Riddle (1998) evaluated the original model by Delitto et al (1995) and found that many of the system criteria lacked reliability and validity. The modified algorithm by Brennan et al (2006) further assessed the reliability of the treatment-based classification examination items and the influence of experience in users of the model (Fritz et al 2006). The majority of the individual examination items from the algorithm were found to have good reliability. When judgements of centralization using repeated or sustained extension movements were analysed, the inter-rater reliability was fair. The same was true for judgements of aberrant movements. When examining the influence of clinician experience and the classification system, Fritz et al (2006) found that the modified algorithm could be used reliably by physical therapist practitioners regardless of the number of years of practice experience or experience in using the classification system. The results pertaining to clinician experience are similar to the findings of Henry et al (2012), which showed good inter-rater reliability for novice judgement in applying the algorithm as described by Fritz et al in 2006. The classification system has been show to improve the outcomes for patients treated using this approach (Brennan et al 2006). The algorithm was further labelled the 'comprehensive algorithm' in 2011; when it was evaluated, this further-refined algorithm demonstrated moderate reliability – this level of reliability can provide a reasonable level of confidence to the practising clinician for incorporating the comprehensive algorithm into clinical practice (Stanton et al 2011). As originally proposed by Delitto et al (1995), the classification system does seem better suited for patients with acute symptoms. Apeldoorn et al (2012a) evaluated the algorithm put forth by Brennan et al in 2006 against a population of individuals in Amsterdam with a current complaint of low back pain greater than 6 weeks. Their intent was to assess the utility of the modified Delitto classification in a population of patients with longer-term pain states (subacute and chronic). Their results suggested that the classification system does not improve outcomes for individuals with time-based categorized subacute (6–12 weeks) and chronic (>12 weeks) low back pain (Apeldoorn et al 2012a). Furthermore, a cost analysis revealed that the classification approach for subacute and chronic low back pain was not cost effective compared with an equal population of patients managed usually with physical therapy (Apeldoorn et al 2012b).

The Treatment-based Classification System: Focus on the Stabilization Subgroup

The authors of this chapter realize there is ongoing debate over the utility of the treatment-based classification system. That debate is beyond the scope of this chapter. Treating clinicians assess their patients as best they can to determine a treatment direction, and it is our hope that we can present an evidence-informed framework, using the treatment-based classification model, that will allow treating clinicians to proceed with confidence when managing patients with clinical presentations that seem ideally matched to stabilization interventions. We understand that there are other classification systems available; however, research to date suggests that the treatment-based classification system is ideal for assessing and managing patients with acute low back pain. We appreciate the limitations of the treatment-based classification system – specifically the bias towards predominantly regionally defined low back pain without anything more than prognostic appreciation for multisite pain presentations and other comorbidities – but also, in spite of this limitation, that patients with low back pain complaints can present with predominantly 'localized low back pain' symptoms (Natvig et al 2001), although this is not the norm (Kamaleri et al 2008). The emerging evidence indicates that the treatment-based classification system is a useful management tool in this specific subgroup (i.e. patients presenting with localized low back pain), and also that patient-related outcomes and costs associated with the treatment-based classification system improve when the model is used in clinical practice. In keeping with the originally targeted population, and the recent evidence suggesting the reliability of the classification system in individuals with acute low back pain (Henry et al 2012; Stanton et al 2011), in this chapter we will focus on patients presenting with acute low back symptoms who would be classified into the stabilization category with suspected lumbar spine instability.

Clinical Management of Lumbar Spine Instability

Current best evidence has advocated a treatment-based classification approach for the overall management of patients with low back pain. Emphasis has been placed on matching the patient to optimal interventions based on the identification of signs and symptoms collected during the patient interview and physical examination (Delitto et al 1995; Fritz & George 2000; Fritz et al 2003; Brennan et al 2006; Werneke et al 2009). The clinical decision-making process involved in applying this treatment-based classification strategy comprises two distinct levels. The first level requires that the therapist determine whether the patient is appropriate for physical therapy services through a comprehensive medical screen including a red flag assessment. This initial step is accomplished via a comprehensive patient interview. The second level of the classification schema involves directing the patient to their matched intervention(s) or subgroup based on presenting signs and symptoms as well as their respective physical examination findings (Fritz & George 2000; Fritz et al 2003).

First level of classification and the patient interview

Step one of this classification approach begins with a comprehensive review of the patient's medical history and a medical screen encompassing a review of both general health and specific systems (Boissonnault 2005). General health questions should be asked of all patients inquiring about the following: (1) fatigue, (2) malaise, (3) weakness, (4) unexplained weight loss / gain, (5) nausea, (6) paraesthesia or numbness, (7) dizziness or lightheadedness, (8) change in mentation or cognition, and (9) chills, sweats or fever. Specific questions about the mechanism of injury or history of a traumatic event can be a potential indicator for spinal fracture. The thoracolumbar area of the spine has been reported as the most common location where fractures occur. These are usually the result of motor vehicle collisions, blunt force trauma, as well as accidents and falls. Many of these fractures (40–80%) are considered biomechanically unstable (Wood et al 2014). As part of the red flag assessment, it is essential for clinicians to note any complaints of weakness, sensation changes or motor loss as such symptoms would guide them to performing full motor and sensory examination and potential referral for additional imaging or emergency services. It is critical to understand that lumbar spine instability could be caused by the trauma or is a secondary effect of the event. Should this be suspected, an appropriate referral would need to be made to clear the individual medically before initiating physical therapy services. (See Ch 4 for further information on history taking.)

Patient self-administered questionnaires can assist with this data collection as well. These tools have been shown to be accurate for reporting important health history information and in assisting the clinician to decide whether or not to proceed further to the second level of classification (Pecoraro et al 1979; Boissonnault 2005). A specific system screen (cardiovascular, pulmonary, gastrointestinal, urogenital, endocrine, nervous, integumentary systems) follows based on the initial information gathered from the general health questions review including the body chart and self-administered questionnaires. The patient interview is a key component in attempting to recognize serious spinal pathology that may warrant additional concern including appropriate medical follow-up with a primary care practitioner (Greene 2001; Greenhalgh & Selfe 2009). The patient interview also drives the overall planning process for the objective examination and progression to the second stage of care and intervention application. For patients with suspected lumbar spine instability any recent imagining procedures may be of importance to the practitioner, as well as the specific views that were taken. Although radiographic findings are considered to be the most quantifiable measure for the differential diagnosis of lumbar spine instability, recent literature has investigated potential physical examination tests to assist the clinician in their differential diagnosis process in the absence of radiographs (Alqarni et al 2011). This is a crucial component to the patient-centred care model where the use of clinical tests to identify hypothesized lumbar spine instability would provide a decreased exposure to radiation, improve access to healthcare and decrease costs associated with diagnostic imaging procedures.

Self-reported symptoms and clinician pattern recognition

Specific self-reported symptoms, as well as examination findings, have been shown to be beneficial to the clinician with regard to their clinical decision-making process and improving probability estimates for the differential diagnosis of lumbar spine instability. Patient self-reports of recurrent locking, catching or giving way of the low back during active motions have historically been a patient history item that clinicians would use to hypothesize the probability of lumbar spine instability (Fritz et al 1998). Furthermore, studies have also looked at the duration of symptoms, age of the patient, as well as fear-avoidance behaviour and decreased willingness to move as potential variables for indicating individuals who would benefit from a stabilization programme (Hicks et al 2005). A Delphi study conducted by Cook et al (2006) looked at 168 expert physical therapists' consensus regarding specific subjective and objective examination data for the proper identification of lumbar spine instability. Physical therapists in this study were either board certified in orthopaedics by the American Physical Therapy Association (APTA) or Fellows of the American Academy of Orthopaedic Manual Physical Therapists (AAOMPT). Common self-reported complaints included the following: pain with unsupported sitting, increasing pain with sustained positions, a history of painful catching or locking sensation during spinal

Box 18.1 Three most common patient interview findings reported by experts* to be most likely and least likely to be related to lumbar spine clinical instability

Findings *most likely* to be related to lumbar spine clinical instability

- Reports feelings of 'giving way' or back 'giving out'
- Self-manipulator who feels the need to frequently crack or pop the back
- Frequent bouts or episodes of symptoms

Findings *least likely* to be related to lumbar spine clinical instability

- Pain through range of motion (i.e. through range pain)
- Intolerance of prone position
- Spine instability does not exist

(Adapted from Cook et al 2006.)
*168 physical therapists identified as Orthopaedic Clinical Specialists (OCS) or Fellows of the American Academy of Orthopaedic Manual Physical Therapists.

Box 18.2 Three most common objective factors reported by experts* to be most likely and least likely to be related to lumbar spine clinical instability

Objective factors *most likely* to be related to lumbar spine clinical instability

- Poor lumbopelvic control, including segmental hinging or pivoting with movement, as well as poor proprioceptive function
- Poor coordination/neuromuscular control, including juddering or shaking
- Decreased strength and endurance of local muscles at level of segmental instability

Objective factors *least likely* to be related to lumbar spine clinical instability

- Non-objectifiable: segmental instability cannot be objectified in the clinic
- Unresponsiveness to treatment, including manual techniques and exercise
- Segmental instability does not exist

(Adapted from Cook et al 2006.)
*168 physical therapists identified as Orthopaedic Clinical Specialists (OCS) or Fellows of the American Academy of Orthopaedic Manual Physical Therapists.

movement, pain returning from spinal flexion, pain with sudden or trivial activities, and pain with transitional activities. The three *most* common agreed-upon patient findings suggesting lumbar spine clinical instability noted by the experts, as well as the three most common agreed-upon patient interview findings *least* likely related to lumbar spine clinical instability, are listed in Box 18.1. The experts were also asked the same question regarding the objective examination and what factors were reported the most and the least related to lumbar spine clinical instability. The three most common objective factors reported by experts as *most* related to lumbar spine instability, as well as the three most common objective findings *least* likely to be related with lumbar spine clinical instability, are listed in Box 18.2.

Second level of classification: physical examination

After a thorough and comprehensive patient interview has been completed, the list of potential diagnoses is then refined. The classification process continues with the physical examination to investigate further the list of the examiner's potential hypotheses. The physical examination can include elements of patient observation, active spinal motion testing, palpation, muscle length, muscle strength, passive physiological and accessory motion testing, as well as special tests. Special tests and physical examination findings assist the clinician in clinical decision making in a broader context as either confirmatory or screening tests. Findings of the physical examination tests are then used to retain, modify, rule in or rule out previously hypothesized conditions. It is important to note that most clinicians will not make a decision based on a single test finding and will use tests in a cluster to strengthen the probability that a patient has a specific musculoskeletal disorder (Cook & Hegedus 2011).

Diagnostic and screening tests require the use of a reference standard to determine their overall accuracy. The accuracy of a clinical special test is defined as the measurement of agreement between the reference standard and the clinical test (Fritz & Wainner 2001). The reference standard is considered the closest description of the actual disorder being present. In diagnostic studies the results of the reference standard are compared against the clinical test in question to determine the percentage of individuals correctly identified or diagnosed with the disorder. Physical examination tests can never absolutely rule in (confirmatory) or rule out (exclude) the presence of a suspected disease and or pathology. Clinical and special tests, though, can be used to assist the examiner in altering the probability or estimate that the patient has a specific musculoskeletal disorder. Diagnostic accuracy statistics such as sensitivity, specificity and likelihood ratios (LRs) can assist the clinician in choosing the most applicable test to refine their clinical decision-making process (Jaeschke et al 1994). (See Ch 5 for further details on psychometric data of physical examination procedures.)

Achieving a reference standard for the clinical diagnosis of lumbar spine instability is difficult for three key reasons: (1) there is little evidence correlating the pathophysiology of spinal instability with patient's self-reported symptoms of pain and/or disability, (2) radiographic measurements may contain errors during movement of less than 5 mm, which are frequently reported with lumbar spine instability cases, and (3) 'normal' spine motion has yet to be defined (Cook et al 2006). This is especially important with regards to individuals who show variable segmental mobility in their spine yet are asymptomatic and functioning without any difficulties. Despite these issues, practitioners have reported a consensus of similar patient interview answers and comments as well as physical examination findings that they would typically see in patients with lumbar spine instability, as mentioned previously in this chapter.

Evidence for physical examination findings

With regards to the physical examination and evidence to support its components, Hicks et al (2003) looked at a barrage of clinical examination measures that were proposed to identify the reliability component of special tests looking at lumbar spine instability. The results of this study agreed with previous findings regarding the difficulty with segmental mobility assessment in terms of the lack of reliability. Other tests investigated included the prone instability test and aberrant motions with range-of-motion testing, which demonstrated higher levels of inter-rater reliability (agreement beyond chance between examiners). Additional examination measures such as the Beighton Ligamentous Laxity Scale showed high reliability for generalized ligamentous laxity. Because these clinical tests and measures have a high level of reliability, clinicians can expect to achieve similar results when performing them in the clinic. Fritz et al (2005) had also looked at the diagnostic utility of clinical tests for radiographic instability. Flexion–extension radiographic findings for 49 individuals with low back pain were used as a reference standard. If imaging findings revealed specifically either two segments with rotational / translational instability or one segment with both rotational and translational instability, this was considered positive as a reference standard for instability. The authors found that two clinical predictor variables – a lack of hypomobility of the lumbar spine through passive accessory motion testing and lumbar flexion greater than 53° – provided a substantial shift in post-test probability for the diagnostic accuracy of lumbar spine instability.

Sequencing of the physical examination

Given the difficulty with finding an optimal confirmatory or screening test with satisfactory diagnostic accuracy statistics, it is imperative for the physical examination process to follow an organized and reproducible methodology. Typical formats may focus on patient positioning as the determinant for which tests should be performed, and at what point during the examination process they occur. An example would be the standing, sitting, supine and then prone sequencing. Other approaches may look at active movement followed by passive movement, palpation and other examination tests (i.e. neurological examination, motor strength, motor control, palpation and special tests). It has been suggested that many special tests used in the differential diagnosis process for lumbar spine instability can be broken down into two large subgroups; this would include a series of passive tests followed then by active tests. Passive tests would include the following: passive accessory intervertebral motion (PAIVM), passive physiological intervertebral motion (PPIVM), the prone instability test (PIT) and the prone lumbar extension test (PLE). Active tests may include observation of an instability catch or hinge in returning from spinal flexion, as well as functional signs that reproduce the patient's symptoms such as going from sit to stand or any other transitional positions.

In order to optimize the objective examination process, physical tests and measures that specifically look at screening and diagnostic clarification should occur at specific times

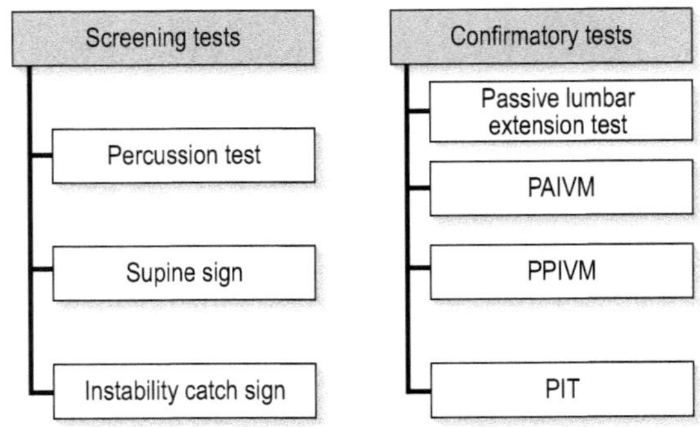

Abbreviations: PAIVM, passive accessory intervertebral motion; PPIVM, passive physiological intervertebral motion; PIT, prone instability test

Figure 18.2 Proposed lumbar spine instability physical examination items.

during the physical examination. With regards to sequencing the examination, it has been recommended that screening tests are typically performed at the beginning of the examination and confirmatory tests are performed towards the end of the examination. The purpose of specific screening tests and measures is to assist the examiner in ruling out potential diagnosis, whereas the purpose of confirmatory tests is to validate or differentiate between the remaining competing diagnoses. An added benefit to this sequencing is that it helps reduce not only misuse bias (i.e. using a low –LR test or high-sensitivity test last) but also the **recency effect**, which occurs when the examiner weighs current events as more important than earlier events (Cook 2010). This happens commonly when a majority of special tests are performed towards the end of the examination and therefore the examiner holds those tests as being more 'truthful' than those performed earlier. Placing tests that are highly sensitive and help rule out potential diagnoses that may be of serious nature first is a step towards reducing these types of biases. In keeping with the recommended sequencing, the physical examination tests and measures have been listed in order of screening tests first followed by confirmatory tests. The authors propose the following clinical examination model for the examination of lumbar spine instability below, as well as the entire format detailed in Figure 18.2. The format for each clinical test is the description followed by the diagnostic accuracy, concluding with a clinical summary.

Proposed Clinical Examination for Lumbar Spine Instability

Screening tests

The initial three screening tests for potential lumbar spine fracture and lumbar spine instability are reported in either a standing (percussion test and instability catch sign) or a supine position (supine sign). Most patient examinations include a standing and/or supine component based on the patient's presentation and tissue irritability. These two positions therefore would be appropriate and realistic for a day one assessment of the patient.

Percussion test

The percussion test as described by Langdon et al (2010) is performed with the patient standing. The examiner stands behind and off to the side of the patient. A force is then given at each spinal level with a closed fist. Multiple levels can be assessed by going up and down the spine. A test is positive when the patient reports a sharp or sudden pain. This test was shown to be highly sensitive (88%), as well as having a strong +LR of 8.8 and –LR of 0.14.

Clinical summary: The percussion test can be used as an initial screen for potential compression fractures, especially for patients who may not be able to adopt a supine position.

Supine sign

The supine sign, also described by Langdon et al (2010), is performed with the patient in a supine position. The patient is asked to lie supine with only one pillow and with the legs straight. The sign is positive when the patient is unable to lie supine because of severe pain in their spine. Statistically this test was both sensitive (81%) and specific (93%) with a +LR of 11.6 and –LR of 0.20.

Clinical summary: Despite having a strong +LR, this test is easy to perform and can be done early on in the examination process. Given its sensitivity (81%), this test should be used in combination with the instability catch sign.

Instability catch sign

The instability catch sign, reported by Kasai et al (2006), is performed with the patient starting in a standing position. The patient is then asked to flex forward as if going to touch the toes and then return to an erect position. The test is positive test if the patient cannot return to an erect standing position. This test is highly sensitive (85.7%) in nature, with a –LR of 0.31.

Clinical summary: This is an ideal screening test as part of the examination process. The physical examination should include an assessment of active spinal motion, and during that assessment the examiner can record this finding quite easily.

Confirmatory tests

The confirmatory or diagnostic tests listed in this section have been reviewed from the body of literature on lumbar spine instability and the diagnostic capability assessment of these special tests is reported. Positive likelihood ratios have been provided to demonstrate the probability assessment that one may have with a positive test finding.

Passive lumbar extension test

The passive lumbar extension test, as described by Kasai et al (2006), was designed to look at hypothesized structural instability of the spine. The patient is placed in a prone position while the examiner lifts both extremities into extension to a height of approximately 30 cm while keeping the knees extended. A small pull on the legs is applied as the legs are elevated. The test is positive test if patients report a strong pain sensation, a very heavy feeling, or a feeling that their low back was going to come off that resolves upon returning to the starting position. This test was found to be both highly sensitive and specific, with a +LR of 8.8 and –LR of 0.2.

Clinical summary: This test is a useful confirmatory test for improving one's probability of hypothesized structural instability of the spine as well as being a lumbar spine instability screening test (84.2% sensitive). This can include potential biomedical issues such as canal stenosis, spondylolisthesis and degenerative scoliosis.

Passive accessory intervertebral motion

PAIVM was initially investigated as a potential diagnostic tool or confirmatory test for radiographic instability (Fritz et al 2005). The patient is positioned in prone and the examiner applies a posterior–anterior force on the spinous process using a thumb pad to thumb pad grip or the hypothenar eminence. Pressure is applied perpendicular to the spinous process of the lumbar segment. The examiner judges the mobility of the segment as normal, hypermobile or hypomobile. The presence of pain is recorded as present or absent. Lack of hypomobility with intervertebral testing was found to be the best individual test for instability, with a +LR of 9.0. When both this finding and lumbar spine flexion were >53°, a +LR of 12.8 was achieved.

Clinical summary: PAIVMs are useful confirmatory tests for radiographic instability especially if there is a lack of hypomobility present and spinal flexion >53°.

Passive physiological intervertebral movements for extension and flexion

The PPIVM described by Abbott et al (2005) looked at the ability of selected manual tests to detect abnormal sagittal planar motion derived from flexion extension radiographs. For the extension PPIVM, the patient is first positioned in side-lying. The examiner than palpates the interspinous space between two adjacent spinous processes. Keeping one finger there, the other hand grasps the patient's uppermost flexed leg and moves the lumbar spine from neutral to extension using the lower extremity. A positive test is identified by detection of excessive movement during examination. For flexion PPVIM, the hand placement and position of the patient are exactly the same as in extension, except that the examiner moves the uppermost extremity from neutral to flexion. A positive test is identified by detection of excessive movement during examination. For PPIVM testing, the authors used a five-point ordinal scale with 0 and 1 indicating hypomobility, normal mobility scoring a 2, while 3 and 4 were considered hypermobile. In both flexion and extension, a grade of 4 was considered positive for lumbar spine instability. Both PPIVMs were specific for the diagnosis of both rotational and translational lumbar spine instability, but showed poor sensitivity. Extension PPIVMs that scored a grade 4 had a +LR of 8.4 and 7.1 for rotational and translational instability, while flexion PPIVMs scored a +LR of 4.1 and 8.7.

Clinical summary: PPIVMs in this case are useful confirmatory tests, with extension-oriented PPIVMs yielding slightly improved diagnostic capabilities over their flexion counterpart.

Prone instability test

The PIT, described by Hicks et al (2003), is a pain provocation test. The patient is positioned prone on a table with the torso and legs hanging off the edge of the table and feet resting on the floor. The examiner then performs a posterior–anterior intervertebral manoeuvre. The patient is asked to report any provocation of pain. The patient then lifts the heels off the ground, and the examiner performs the posterior–anterior intervertebral manoeuvre once again. The patient may be hand-holding the table to help maintain position during the test. A positive test occurs when the pain is provoked during the first part of the test but disappears when the test is repeated with the legs off the floor. A systematic review by Alqarni et al (2011) looked at a barrage of clinical tests for diagnostic accuracy for lumbar spine instability. Their data showed this test to have a +LR of 1.4 and a −LR of 0.7. These values demonstrate only small to very small and sometimes rarely important change regarding probability shifts. This test appears to have little diagnostic accuracy value in isolation. For an intervention perspective, though, it was found to be a key variable in the clinical predication rule for patients who would benefit from a lumbar stabilization programme for low back pain (Hicks et al 2005). This was interesting in that the single-item likelihood value of this test in that cluster was a +LR of 1.7, but, as a predictor for those patients who would not respond well to a lumbar stabilization programme if this test was negative, the +LR was 5.0. The only other item that was found to be more predictive for patients who would respond poorly to a lumbar spine stabilization programme was the lack of lumbar hypermobility with spring testing (+LR 9.2).

Clinical summary: Although this test has poor diagnostic accuracy as a stand-alone test item for improving the diagnostic probability of lumbar spine instability, it is part of a cluster of four tests in which if three or more are positive then the patient would have a +LR of 4.0 that they would benefit from a lumbar spine stabilization exercise approach. This test would have a + LR of 5.0 if found negative (i.e. pain does not go away while the posterior–anterior manoeuvre is applied and the feet are up in the air), indicating that they would not respond well to a lumbar spinal stabilization exercise programme.

Clinical prediction rules in the treatment-based classification system

Clinical prediction rules (CPRs) have been developed to provide physical therapists with an evidence-based tool to assist in patient management and to improve clinical decision making. They are used to assist the clinician in establishing a diagnosis or prognosis, as well as determining which patients may benefit from a particular intervention approach. Despite the current implementation and widespread popularity, the application of CPRs in the clinical settings is not without limitations. CPRs require an evidence-based review and in-depth analysis prior to their implementation into the clinical setting. They follow a typical pattern of development, starting from a derivation component, moving to a validation stage and ending with an impact analysis (Glynn & Weisbach 2011). Each stage builds upon the preceding ones as this continuum of quality and validity are improved upon for clinical use.

With regards to lumbar spine instability, there is one CPR currently that has been established for the intervention aspect in that patient population. Hicks et al (2005) completed a preliminary development of a CPR for determining which patients with low back pain would respond to a stabilization programme. The findings would be integrated into the evolving classification system as the criteria for the stabilization category. The prediction rule was able to determine which variables predicted not only success but also failure for individuals instructed in a stabilization exercise programme. The stabilization programme was scheduled twice a week for 8 weeks under the supervision of a physical therapist. These patients were also given a home exercise programme to perform daily and were asked to complete a compliance log for home exercises to verify that they had completed those tasks. The exercise programme was based on current best evidence and focused on stabilizing motor patterns of both global and local musculature. Repeated submaximal efforts were performed and exercises were progressed by the therapist by criteria that they were given. A description of that exercise protocol with criteria for progression can be found in Table 18.4. Results showed that four predictor variables were identified for a patient to benefit from a lumbar spine stabilization exercise programme: positive PIT, aberrant movements present, average straight leg raise >91° and age >40 years old. Regarding aberrant movements, these movements would include any the following descriptions: an instability catch, a painful arc of motion, and patients climbing up their thighs with their hands to assist them 'thigh climbing' (which has also been described as Gowers' sign or a reversal of the lumbopelvic rhythm). If three out of four of the success predictor variables were present (+LR 4.0) there was a small but sometimes meaningful increase in the probability that the patient would experience at least 50% improvement in function after 8 weeks of lumbar stabilization. Chapter 23 explains the different exercises for patients with lumbar spine instability.

The four variables that were identified that indicated which patients would probably fail with a stabilization treatment were: negative PIT, aberrant movements absent, Fear-avoidance Beliefs Questionnaire physical activity subscale score >9 and no hypermobility with lumbar spring testing. If at least two of the four non-success predictor variables were present (+LR 6.3) there was a moderate shift in probability that the patient would not improve with lumbar stabilization. In both cases, outcomes were based on pain and self-reported questionnaires looking at disability level (Oswestry Disability Index) and fear avoidance (Fear-avoidance Beliefs Questionnaire). Recently Rabin et al (2014) performed a randomized controlled validation study of the preliminary CPR. They found that, although they could not validate the CPR because of the small sample size and its low relative power, a modified CPR of aberrant motions and a positive PIT yielded a strong predictive capability for those patients that would benefit from a lumbar spine stabilization programme. The authors note that, because these findings are under a post-hoc analysis, the next step would be to include this modified CPR in a formal research design model.

Table 18.4 **Stabilization exercises with criteria for progression of each exercise**

Primary muscle group	Exercises	Criteria for progression
Transversus abdominis	Abdominal bracing	30 reps with 8 s hold
	Bracing with heel slide	20 reps per leg with 4 s hold
	Bracing with leg lifts	20 reps per leg with 4 s hold
	Bracing with bridging	30 reps with 8 s hold, then progress to 1 leg
	Bracing in standing	30 reps with 8 s hold
	Bracing with standing row exercise	20 reps per side with 6 s hold
	Bracing with walking	20 reps per side with 6 s hold
Erector spinae/multifidus	Quadruped arm lifts with bracing	30 reps with 8 s hold on each side
	Quadruped leg lifts with bracing	30 reps with 8 s hold on each side
	Quadruped alternate arm and leg lifts with bracing	30 reps with 8 s hold on each side
Quadratus lumborum	Side support with knees flexed	30 reps with 8 s hold on each side
	Side support with knees extended	30 reps with 8 s hold on each side
Oblique abdominals	Side support with knees flexed	30 reps with 8 s hold on each side
	Side support with knees extended	30 reps with 8 s hold on each side

(Table based on Hicks et al 2005.)

Conclusion

Based on current best evidence, clinicians are encouraged to consider the clinical utility of the tests noted above in their clinical decision-making framework. Using specific tests with diagnostic accuracy assists clinicians in classifying patients with lumbar spine instability who can be matched to the stabilization subgroup. In addition, tests with adequate diagnostic utility can assist in the exclusion of more serious and sinister conditions such as frank instability or potential vertebral fractures. It is important to point out that these tests individually or in a cluster of tests are probably more extensive than just a diagnostic tool. They can assist in driving treatment decisions as well as noting changes both within and between clinic sessions. The development of classification systems is dynamic: evolving evidence will further inform the development and utility of the classification system, which will assist clinicians in providing an even better quality of care for their patients with acute low back pain. We look forward to these future developments.

References

Abbott JH, Fritz JM, McCane B, et al. 2005. Lumbar segmental instability: a criterion-related validity study of manual therapy assessment. BMC Musculoskel Dis 6: 56.

Alqarni A, Schneiders AG, Hendrick PA. 2011. Clinical tests to diagnose lumbar segmental instability: a systematic review. J Orthop Sports Phys Ther 41: 130–140.

Apeldoorn AT, Ostelo RW, van Helvoirt H, et al. 2010. The cost-effectiveness of a treatment-based classification system for low back pain: design of a randomized controlled trial and economic evaluation. BMC Musculoskel Dis 11: 58–70.

Apeldoorn AT, Ostelo R, van Helvoirt H, et al. 2012a. A randomized controlled trial on the effectiveness of a classification-based system for sub-acute and chronic low back pain. Spine 37:1347–1356.

Apeldoorn AT, Bosmans JE, Ostelo RW, et al. 2012b. Cost-effectiveness of a classification-based system for sub-acute and chronic low back pain. Eur Spine J 21: 1290–1300.

Bekkering GE, van Tulder M, Hendriks E, et al. 2005. Implementation of clinical guidelines on physical therapy for patients with low back pain: randomized trial comparing patient outcomes after a standard and active implementation strategy. Phys Ther 85: 544–555.

Bishop PB, Wing PC. 2006. Knowledge transfer in family physicians managing patients with acute low back pain: a prospective randomized control trial. Spine J 6: 282–288.

Boissonnault WG. 2005. Primary care for the physical therapist examination and triage. St Louis: Elsevier Saunders, pp 53–104.

Brennan GP, Fritz JM, Hunter SJ, et al. 2006. Identifying subgroups of patients with acute / subacute 'nonspecific' low back pain: results of a randomized clinical trial. Spine 31: 623–631.

Buchbinder R, Fiona MB, Lyn MM, et al. 2013. Placing the global burden of low back pain in context. Best Pract Res Clin Rhematol 27: 575–589.

Cabana MD. 2010. Adherence, not just for patients: comment on 'low back pain and best practice care'. Arch Int Med 170: 277–278.

Cabana MD, Kiyoshi-Teo H. 2010. The broader picture on guideline adherence. J Parenteral Enteral Nutr 34: 593–594.

Cabana MD, Rand CS, Powe NR, et al. 1999. Why don't physicians follow clinical practice guidelines? A framework for improvement. JAMA 282: 1458–1465.

Cedraschi C, Robert J, Goerg D, et al. 1999. Is chronic non-specific low back pain chronic? Definitions of a problem and problems of a definition. Br J Gen Pract 49: 358–362.

Cook C. 2010. The lost art of the clinical examination: an overemphasis on clinical special tests. J Man Manipul Ther 18: 3–4.

Cook C, Hegedus E. 2011. Diagnostic utility of clinical tests for spinal dysfunction. Man Ther 16:21–25.

Cook C, Brismee JM, Sizer P. 2006. Subjective and objective descriptors of clinical lumbar spine instability. Man Ther 11: 11–21.

Coste J, Spira A, Ducimetiere P, et al. 1991. Clinical and psychological diversity of non-specific low-back pain: a new approach towards the classification of clinical subgroups. J Clin Epidemiol 44:1233–1245.

Croft P. 2009. The question is not 'have you got it'? but 'how much of it have you got'? Pain 141: 6–7.

Delitto A. 2005. Research in low back pain: time to stop seeking the elusive 'magic bullet'. Phys Ther 85: 206–208.

Delitto A, Erhard RE, Bowling RW. 1995. A treatment-based classification approach to low back syndrome: identifying and staging patients for conservative treatment. Phys Ther 75: 470–485.

Deyo RA. 1986. Early diagnostic evaluation of low back pain. J Gen Int Med 1: 328–338.

Deyo RA. 2011. Managing patients with back pain: putting money where our mouths are not. Spine J 11: 633–635.

Feuerstein M, Hartzell M, Rogers HL, et al. 2006. Evidence-based practice for acute low back pain in primary care: patient outcomes and cost of care. Pain 124: 140–149.

Frank A. 1993. Low back pain. BMJ 306: 901–909.

Fritz JM, George S. 2000. The use of a classification approach to identify subgroups of patients with acute low back pain. Interrater reliability and short-term treatment outcomes. Spine 25:106–114.

Fritz JM, Wainner RS. 2001. Examining diagnostic tests: an evidence-based perspective. Phys Ther 9: 1546–1564.
Fritz J, Erhard RE, Hagen BF. 1998. Segmental instability of the lumbar spine. Phys Ther 78: 889–896.
Fritz JM, Delitto A, Erhard RE. 2003. Comparison of classification-based physical therapy based on clinical practice guidelines for patients with acute low back pain: a randomized clinical trial. Spine 28: 1363–1371.
Fritz JM, Piva SR, Childs JD. 2005. Accuracy of the clinical examination to predict radiographic instability of the lumbar spine. Eur Spine J 14: 743–750.
Fritz JM, Brennan GP, Clifford SN, et al. 2006. An examination of the reliability of a classification algorithm for subgrouping patients with low back pain. Spine 31: 77–82.
Fritz JM, Cleland JA, Childs JD. 2007a. Sub-grouping patients with low back pain: evolution of a classification approach to physical therapy. J Orthop Sports Phys Ther 37: 290–302.
Fritz JM, Cleland JA, Brennan GP. 2007b. Does adherence to the guideline recommendation for active treatments improve the quality of care for patients with acute low back pain delivered by physical therapists? Medical Care 45: 973–980.
Fritz JM, Cleland JA, Speckman M, et al. 2008. Physical therapy for acute low back pain: associations with subsequent healthcare costs. Spine 33: 1800–1805.
Glynn P, Weisbach C. 2011. Clinical prediction rules: a physical therapy reference manual. Sudbury MA: Jones and Bartlett.
Greene G. 2001. 'Red flags': essential factors in recognizing serious spinal pathology. Man Ther 6: 253–255.
Greenhalgh S, Selfe J. 2009. A qualitative investigation of red flags for serious spinal pathology. Physiotherapy 95: 224–227.
Gross PA, Greenfield S, Cretin S, et al. 2001. Optimal methods for guideline implementation: conclusions from Leeds Castle meeting. Med Care 39: II85–II92.
Hagen EM, Svensen E, Eriksen HR, et al. 2006. Comorbid subjective health complaints in low back pain. Spine 31: 1491–1495
Hartvigsen J, Natvig B, Ferreira M. 2013. Is it all about a pain in the back? Best Pract Res Clin Rheumatol 27: 613–623
Henry SM, Fritz JM, Trombley AR, et al. 2012. Reliability of a treatment-based classification system for subgrouping people with low back pain. J Orthop Sports Phys Ther 42: 797–805.
Hicks GE, Fritz JM, Delitto AD, et al. 2003. Inter-rater reliability of clinical examination measures for identification of lumbar segmental instability. Arch Phys Med Rehabil 84: 1858–1864.
Hicks GE, Fritz JM, Delitto A, et al. 2005. Preliminary development of a clinical prediction rule for determining which patients with low back pain will respond to a stabilization exercise program. Arch Phys Med Rehabil 86: 1753–1762.
Hoy D, March L, Brooks P, et al. 2010. Measuring the global burden of low back pain. Best Pract Res Clin Rheumatol 24: 155–165.
Ivanova JI, Birnbaum HG, Schiller M, et al. 2011. Real-world practice patterns, health-care utilization, and costs in patients with low back pain: the long road to guideline-concordant care. Spine J 11: 622–632.
Jaeschke R, Guyatt GH, Sackett DL. 1994. Users' guides to the medical literature. III. How to use an article about a diagnostic test. B. What are the results and will they help me in caring for my patients? JAMA 271: 703–707.
Kamaleri Y, Natvig B, Ihlebaek CM, et al. 2008. Localized or widespread musculoskeletal pain: does it matter? Pain 138: 41–46.
Kasai Y, Morishita K, Kawakita E, et al. 2006. A new evaluation for lumbar spine instability: passive lumbar extension test. Phys Ther 86: 1661–1667.
Kent P, Keating J. 2004. Do primary-care clinicians think that nonspecific low back pain is one condition? Spine 29: 1022–1031.
Langdon J, Way A, Heaton S, et al. 2010. Vertebral compression fractures – new clinical signs to aid diagnosis. Ann R Coll Surg Engl 92: 163–166.
Malmivaara A, Häkkinen U, Aro T, et al. 1995. The treatment of acute low back pain – bed rest, exercises, or ordinary activity? N Engl J Med 332: 351–355.
Martin BI, Deyo RA, Mirza SK, et al. 2008. Expenditures and health status among adults with back and neck problems. JAMA 299: 656–664.
McGuirk B, King W, Govind J, et al. 2001. Safety, efficacy, and cost effectiveness of evidence-based guidelines for the management of acute low back pain in primary care. Spine 26: 2615–2622.
Natvig B, Bruusgaard D, Eriksen W. 2001. Localized low back pain and low back pain as part of widespread musculoskeletal pain: two different disorders? A cross-sectional population study. J Rehabil Med 33: 21–25.
Osterberg L, Blaschke T. 2005. Adherence to medication. N Engl J Med 353: 487–497.
Pecoraro RE, Inui TS, Chen MS, et al. 1979. Validity and reliability of a self-administered health history questionnaire. Public Health Rep 94: 231–238.
Rabin A, Shashua A, Pizem K, et al. 2014. A clinical prediction rule to identify patients with low back pain who are likely to experience short-term success following lumbar stabilization exercises: a randomized controlled validity study. J Orthop Sports Phys Ther 44: 6–B13.
Riddle DL. 1998. Classification and low back pain: a review of the literature and critical analysis of selected systems. Phys Ther 78:708–737.
Stanton TR, Fritz JM, Hancock MJ, et al. 2011. Evaluation of a treatment-based classification algorithm for low back pain: a cross-sectional study. Phys Ther 91: 496–509.
Strand LI, Kvale A, Råheim M, et al. 2005. Do Norwegian manual therapists provide management for patients with acute low back pain in accordance with clinical guidelines? Man Ther 10: 38–43.
Swinkels IC, van den Ende CH, van den Bosch W, et al. 2005. Physiotherapy management of low back pain: does practice match the Dutch guidelines? Aust J Physiother 51: 35–41.
Tschudi-Madsen H, Kjeldsberg M, Natvig B, et al. 2011. A strong association between non-musculoskeletal symptoms and musculoskeletal pain symptoms: results from a population study. BMC Musculoskel Dis 12: 285–293.
van Middendorp JJ, Sanchez GM, Burridge AL. 2010. The Edwin Smith papyrus: a clinical reappraisal of the oldest known document on spinal injuries. Eur Spine J 19: 1815–1823.
Waddell G. 1995. Modern management of spinal disorders. J Manipul Physiol Ther 18: 590–596.
Waddell G. 2004. The back pain revolution. London: Churchill Livingstone.
Waddell G. 2005. Subgroups within 'nonspecific' low back pain. J Rheumatol 32: 395–396.
Werneke MW, Hart DL, George SZ, et al. 2009. Clinical outcomes for patients classified by fear-avoidance beliefs and centralization phenomenon. Arch Phys Med Rehabil 90: 768–777.
White AA, Gordon SL. 1982. Synopsis: workshop on idiopathic low-back pain. Spine 7: 141–149.
Williams CM, Maher CG, Hancock MJ, et al. 2010. Low back pain and best practice care: a survey of general practice physicians. Arch Int Med 170: 271–277.
Wood KB, Li W, Lebi DS, et al. 2014. Management of thoracolumbar spine fractures. Spine J 14: 145–164.
Zusman M. 1997. Instigators of activity intolerance. Man Ther 2:75–86.

Chapter 19

Lumbar Spine in Lower Extremity Pain Syndromes

Scott Burns, Paul E. Glynn, Edgar Savidge, Joshua A. Cleland

CHAPTER CONTENTS

Introduction 221
Lumbar spine treatment for hip disorders 221
Lumbar spine treatment for knee disorders 222
Lumbar spine treatment for foot and ankle disorders 223
Lumbar spine treatment for lower extremity neurodynamics 223
Conclusion 223

Introduction

The term 'regional interdependence' is used to describe the relationship between impairments in adjacent regions of the body and patients' primary location of symptoms (Wainner et al 2007). Most clinicians examine adjacent anatomical regions in search of related impairments; however, more emerging research may indicate a need to consider more remote regions (Suter et al 1999; Bang & Deyle 2000; Lowry et al 2008). The influence of manual therapy applied centrally to the spine on the local and distal musculature has been studied throughout the body. In a prospective cohort study, Suter and McMorland (2002) demonstrated the immediate, bilateral, significant reduction in biceps inhibition and increase in biceps torque after a mid-cervical spine thrust manipulation. Dunning and Rushton (2009) performed a cohort study on 54 asymptomatic individuals. Participants were allocated to sham cervical manipulation, cervical manipulation or control group. The individuals receiving the mid-cervical thrust manipulation demonstrated a significant increase in their bilateral biceps EMG (electromyographic) activity compared with the other two treatment groups (Dunning & Rushton 2009). Manual therapy directed at the thoracic spine has also demonstrated the ability to influence adjacent areas, such as the cervical spine (Cleland et al 2007, 2010; Gonzalez-Iglesias et al 2009a, 2009b; Lau et al 2011) and shoulder (Bang & Deyle 2000; Bergman et al 2004; Boyles et al 2009; Mintken et al 2010), as well as local musculature including the lower trapezius (Liebler et al 2001; Cleland et al 2004).

As noted, the research demonstrating the effect of a regional interdependence approach to care has been conducted throughout the body; however, this chapter will focus on research pertaining to the lumbar spine and its effect on the lower extremities. It will discuss the regional interdependence concepts for the hip, knee, foot / ankle and the role of the lumbar spine with respect to neurodynamics.

Lumbar Spine Treatment for Hip Disorders

Due to the anatomical proximity and shared musculature of the lumbar spine and the hip, much effort has been given to identifying the therapeutic relationship between these two areas. The term 'hip–spine syndrome' was originally proposed by Offierski and McNab (1983) to describe the influence of the pathological hip joint on the lumbar spine. Research has indicated that decreased hip range of motion and / or decreased hip muscle endurance may contribute to low back pain and thus should be noted by the examining therapist (Reiman et al 2009). In a case study by Burns et al (2010) an impairment-based treatment approach including manual therapy and exercise, targeted to the hip region, was successful in resolving their patients' hip as well as low back symptoms in four visits. Symptom relief continued at the long-term follow-up points of 3 and 6 months. In a follow-up case series, Burns et al (2011) took eight subjects with chronic low back pain and provided manual therapy and exercises directed at the hip area. Treatment was provided for three sessions over a 1-week time span. Approximately 62% of individuals reported with at least a 'moderately better' rating of perceived improvement, and 25% reduction in modified Oswestry Disability Index scores was noted. Although the body of literature indicating the influence of hip treatment on the lumbar spine continues to grow, the effect of lumbar spine treatment on hip conditions has not been well studied in isolation.

Herzog et al (1999) studied the immediate EMG response to lumbar and sacroiliac thrust manipulation on the gluteal muscles of 10 asymptomatic individuals. They found a three-fold increase in baseline EMG value in 80% of the subjects immediately after the thrust manipulation. Chilibek et al (2011) evaluated the effect of lumbopelvic thrust manipulation on the relative lower extremity strength differences in healthy subjects. Fifty subjects with at least a 15% side-to-side lower extremity strength difference were randomized to receive side-lying lumbopelvic manipulation or a placebo in which only the set-up was applied. Results indicated a significant change in relative strength difference of hip flexion in the treatment group compared with the control group. Furthermore, hip abduction strength increased in the weaker limb immediately post-manipulation, suggesting decreased inhibition.

Lumbar Spine Treatment for Knee Disorders

Although the pathoanatomical influence of the lumbar spine on the knee joint is plausible through the osteokinematic connection of the pelvis, the more likely explanation for the connection of these areas lies in the ability of the lumbar spine to affect the nervous system directly. The contractile tissue surrounding the knee joint is innervated by the femoral and sciatic nerves, both of which exit the spine in the lumbar region. Through the manual treatment of the lumbar spine, a neurophysiological effect is created via the aforementioned nerves subsequently influencing the contractile tissue, movement and pain patterns at the knee. The research surrounding this theory has been expanding over the past decade. Suter et al (1999) performed a small prospective cohort study of 18 individuals with anterior knee pain. Subjects were measured before and after side-lying lumbopelvic thrust manipulation to determine the influence of the manipulation on knee extensor muscle strength and inhibition. Results indicated a statistically significant reduction in muscle inhibition, as well as a significant increase in muscle torque, after the thrust manipulation. Suter et al (2000) followed up this study by performing a randomized trial in which 28 individuals were randomized to receive either just an evaluation or an evaluation followed by a lumbar spine manipulation. Quadriceps muscle inhibition and strength were measured before the examination as well as immediately after the exam or manipulation in both groups. Results again demonstrated a significant reduction in muscle inhibition as well as an increase in quadriceps strength; however, this did not reach the level of statistical significance. To evaluate further the neurophysiological effect of lumbar manipulation versus arthrokinematic inhibition at the knee joint, Hillerman et al (2006) compared the effect of side-lying lumbopelvic manipulation and tibiofemoral distraction manipulation on quadriceps strength. A convenience sample of 20 subjects with patellofemoral pain syndrome (PFPS) was assigned to receive either a lumbopelvic or a tibiofemoral thrust manipulation. Maximum voluntary quadriceps contraction was measured before and immediately after manipulation. The results indicated that only the group receiving lumbopelvic manipulation showed a statistically significant increase in quadriceps strength.

Although the previous studies demonstrated an increase in quadriceps function after lumbopelvic manipulation in patients with patellofemoral knee pain (Suter et al 1999, 2000; Hillerman et al 2006), it was unclear which patients would most be likely to benefit from these interventions. Iverson et al (2008) designed a prospective cohort / predictive study to investigate the effect of spinal manipulation on pain and overall functional change in individuals with PFPS. Forty-nine subjects were examined and treated with a supine lumbopelvic thrust manipulation. Immediately after manipulation, they rated their pain with the three functional lower extremity tests using the Numeric(al) Pain Rating Scale (NRPS). Subjects also rated their overall functional change using the Global Rating of Change (GRC / GROC) scale. Of the 49 subjects completing the study, 45% were classified as 'treatment success' based on a 50% or greater change in pain or a four-point positive change on the GRC. Logistic regression analysis of predictive variables identified a test item cluster of five variables that predicted successful outcome with manipulation. These variables included: a side-to-side difference in hip internal rotation >14°, ankle dorsiflexion with the knee flexed >16°, a navicular drop >3 mm, and subjectively describing squatting as the most painful activity. Of the five predictive variables, a side-to-side difference of prone hip internal rotation >14° was the most predictive of treatment success, increasing the post-test probability of treatment success to 80% (+LR 4.9). If three out of five variables were present, this increased the post-test probability of success to 94%.

Although spinal thrust manipulation has been shown to have an immediate effect on quadriceps function (Suter et al 1999, 2000; Hillerman et al 2006) and in certain cases on symptomatic and functional improvement (Iverson et al 2008), more-recent research indicates that the effect may of short duration. Grindstaff et al (2009) compared the effect of lumbar spinal manipulation, lumbar passive range of motion and prone extension on quadriceps function across time. Forty-two healthy subjects were randomized to receive one of the three interventions. Quadriceps force output and percentage activation were measured before and after intervention for all subjects. Whereas secondary analysis supported previous research indicating an immediate increase in quadriceps force and activation, there was no significant change in quadriceps function after 20 minutes. Grindstaff et al (2012) performed a similar study using subjects with PFPS. In contrast to previous research, this failed to show any significant change in quadriceps function after intervention. Given the breadth of research indicating the immediate effect of lumbar manual therapy on quadriceps function and symptoms, clinicians should consider the post-manipulation phase as an opportunity to enhance muscle function and patient comfort through the combined effect of therapeutic exercise.

In fact, the combination of lumbar spine manual therapy and therapeutic exercise has been shown to be an effective treatment strategy beyond the diagnosis of knee osteoarthritis (Deyle et al 2000, 2005). Deyle et al (2005) compared manual therapy and exercise with sham ultrasound in subjects with knee osteoarthritis. Subjects in the treatment group received manual therapy focused on the lumbar spine, hip, knee and ankle based on examination findings together with therapeutic exercise to address knee range of motion and strength 2–3× / week for 4 weeks, while subjects in the control group received sham ultrasound at the knee. Results indicated that the treatment group had significantly improved patient-perceived pain, stiffness and function as well as 6-minute walk-time at 8 weeks, which persisted at 1 year. Furthermore, a smaller percentage of patients in the treatment group required injection or surgery at 1 year compared with the control group. In a follow-up study, Deyle et al (2005) compared a similar manual therapy plus exercise programme in the clinic plus a home exercise reinforcement programme with a home programme in isolation in patients with osteoarthritis. They found that patients treated with the impairment-based manual therapy to the lower extremity and lumbar spine combined with exercise had significantly greater improvement in pain, stiffness and patient-reported function at 4 and 8 weeks compared with the home programme in isolation. Although these differences were not sustained at 1 year follow-up, the use of manual therapy and supervised therapeutic exercise produced greater short-term (<8 weeks) benefits.

A multimodal treatment approach incorporating the entire kinetic chain for patients with knee disorders is further supported in a case series by Lowry et al (2008). Five patients with PFPS were treated with a combination of manual therapy directed at the lumbopelvic region and entire lower quarter, exercise, taping and orthotics. Treatments were administered in an impairment-based model and four out of five patients demonstrated significant improvement in pain and function. This case series supports previous research indicating the use of manual therapy at the lumbar spine and lower quadrant with exercise, and highlights the importance of considering the entire kinetic chain in the management of knee disorders.

Lumbar Spine Treatment for Foot and Ankle Disorders

In contrast to the knee, there are currently no known studies on manual therapy to the lumbar spine on subjective, objective or functional changes to the foot and ankle. However, there is evidence indicating that manual therapy applied to the lumbar spine influences the neurophysiology of the foot and ankle, measured by skin conductance and alteration of the H-reflex or α-motor-neuron excitability (Dishman & Bulbulia 2000; Dishman et al 2002; Perry & Green 2008; Perry et al 2011). Dishman et al (2002) compared the effect of thrust with that of non-thrust lumbar spine mobilization on the α-motor-neuron excitability of the gastrocnemius muscle. Seventeen subjects were randomized to receive either a thrust or a non-thrust mobilization and the change in amplitude of the Hoffman reflex (H-reflex) of the gastrocnemius was recorded. Results indicated that both interventions caused a significant decrease in amplitude, suggesting a decrease in motor-neuron excitability. In a follow-up study, Dishman et al (2002) demonstrated similar results comparing lumbar and cervical manipulation on gastrocnemius motor-neuron excitability. In 36 healthy adults, they demonstrated that lumbar spine thrust manipulation created a transient decrease in motor-neuron excitability in the calf, which lasted less than 60 seconds. Perry and Green (2008) investigated the effect of lumbar mobilization on the sympathetic nervous system in the lower extremity by measuring skin conductance on the dorsum of the foot. Forty-five healthy adults were randomized to receive grade III unilateral posterior–anterior (PA) glide at the lumbar spine, a placebo PA glide, or a position only as a control group. They demonstrated a significant change in skin conductance with the mobilization group, whereas the placebo and control groups showed no change in conductance. In a follow-up study, Perry et al (2011) compared lumbar manipulation versus lumbar extension exercises on skin conductance as a measure of sympathetic nervous system activity. Skin conductance at the plantar aspect of the foot was recorded before and after intervention in a group of 50 healthy subjects randomized to receive lumbar manipulation or extension exercises. Both groups exhibited a significant change in skin conductance with a significant greater change in the manipulation group (76% change) than in the extension exercise group (36% change). Given the neurophysiological effect of lumbar manipulation at the lower leg, and the effect on pain, strength, muscle length and function at the hip and knee, it is plausible that a similar effect would be seen at the foot and ankle. Clinical research is needed to investigate the effect of manual therapies applied to the lumbar spine on pain, strength and functional outcome in patients with foot and ankle disorders. Table 19.1 provides a summary of key articles associated with regional interdependence of the lower extremity.

Lumbar Spine Treatment for Lower Extremity Neurodynamics

Butler (2000) has described the integration of morphological, biomechanical and physiological functions as neurodynamics, and impairment in this system can impact on resting muscle length, strength and pain. It has been suggested that manual treatment of the lower back may influence afferent and efferent pathways and alter lower extremity neurodynamics and play a role in restoring movement and function. Cibulka et al (1986) studied the effect of sacroiliac manipulation on resting hamstring length in 20 subjects diagnosed with hamstring strain. Patients in the treatment group treated with a supine lumbopelvic manipulation demonstrated a significant increase in hamstring length compared with those in the control group. Szlezak et al (2011) found a similar result on hamstring length measured with a straight leg raise. Thirty-six healthy individuals were randomized to a mobilization group, stretching group and control group. The researchers found that those in the mobilization group receiving unilateral PA mobilization to the lumbar spine had an increase in resting straight leg raise excursion compared with those in the control or stretching groups. Hip and knee dysfunction can be a result of, and can contribute to, hypertonicity in the hamstring as a protective mechanism, and treatment of the lumbar spine could be considered with these disorders. (Additional information regarding neurodynamics may be found in Chs 64 and 65.)

Conclusion

There is clearly a role of the lumbar spine in many regions of the lower extremity; however, much remains unknown with regards to the distinct role of interventions targeting adjacent regions. Currently most of the regional interdependence research has examined immediate impairment-based outcomes (Cibulka et al 1986; Herzog et al 1999; Suter et al 2000; Hillerman et al 2006; Chilibek et al 2011; Perry et al 2011); however, more recent studies have begun to investigate the functional outcomes associated with treating patients within a regional interdependence framework (Deyle et al 2000, 2005; Lowry et al 2008; Burns et al 2010, 2011).

Table 19.1 **Key articles for lower extremity regional interdependence**

Author (year)	Study design	Sample size	Patient population	Interventions	Key findings/results
Hip					
Herzog et al (1999)	Case series	*n*=10 (asymptomatic males)	Asymptomatic	Spinal manipulation throughout entire spine	80% of subjects experiences a threefold increase in gluteal EMG
Chilibek et al (2011)	RCT	*n*=50	>15% strength deficits between leg	Lumbar manipulation	Increase in hip flexion strength Increase in hip abduction strength
Cibulka et al (1986)	RCT	*n*=20	Hamstring strain	Sacroiliac joint thrust manipulation	Increase muscle peak torque of hamstrings
Knee					
Suter et al (1999)		*n*=18 (14 unilateral; 4 bilateral)	Anterior knee pain	Side-lying sacroiliac joint thrust manipulation	Immediate increased knee extensor torque and decreased knee extensor inhibition
Suter et al (2000)	RCT	*n*=28 (23 symptomatic; 5 asymptomatic)	Anterior knee pain	Side-lying sacroiliac joint thrust manipulation	Immediate decreased knee extensor inhibition
Hillerman et al (2006)	RCT	*n*=20	Asymptomatic	Sacroiliac manipulation vs tibiofemoral mobilization	Sacroiliac joint manipulation group had increased quadriceps muscle strength
Iverson et al (2008)	Prospective cohort	*n*=49	Patellofemoral pain syndrome	Supine lumbopelvic manipulation	45% of patients had a +4 or greater rating on the GROC Test-item cluster identification
Grindstaff et al (2009)	RCT	*n*=42	Asymptomatic individuals	Lumbar manipulation, lumbar passive range of motion or extension exercise	Immediate increase in quadriceps force output with manipulation – lasted 20 minutes
Grindstaff et al (2012)	RCT	*n*=48	Patellofemoral pain syndrome	Lumbar manipulation, lumbar passive range of motion or extension exercise	No change in quadriceps activation or force output
Lowry et al (2008)	Case series	*n*=5	Patellofemoral pain syndrome	Impairment-based manual therapy to entire lower quarter, exercise, taping and orthotics	80% of subjects had improved pain and function
Deyle et al (2000)	RCT	*n*=83	Knee osteoarthritis	Impairment-based manual therapy to the lower extremity vs sham ultrasound	Improved pain, stiffness, function and 6-minute walk-test scores favouring manual therapy group
Deyle et al (2005)	RCT	*n*=134	Knee osteoarthritis	Impairment based manual therapy to the lower extremity vs home exercise programme	Improved pain, stiffness, function and 6-minute walk-test scores favouring manual therapy group (at 4 and 8 weeks) Groups were equal at 1 year
Ankle/Foot					
Dishman et al (2000)	RCT	*n*=17	Asymptomatic	Thrust vs non-thrust lumbar manipulation	Decreased motor neuron excitability of the gastrocnemius
Perry et al (2011)	RCT	*n*=50	Asymptomatic	Lumbar manipulation vs extension exercises	Skin conductance was increased in the manipulation > exercise group

EMG=electromyographic, RCT=randomized controlled trial, GROC=global rate of change.

The majority of the current research has focused on the buttock, hip, thigh and knee, while there is a relative lack of articles discussing the relationship of the lumbar spine in ankle / foot disorders. In the upper extremity, some research has been conducted examining the effects of cervicothoracic treatment in distal upper extremity conditions such as carpal tunnel syndrome, so it is also possible to foresee a potential association between the lumbar spine and distal lower extremity conditions (Davis et al 1998).

Although the evidence supporting a direct, causal relationship may be lacking, the current evidence may compel the clinician to examine and potentially intervene on regions adjacent to and / or remote from a patient's primary location of sensory symptoms. Implementation of an impairment-based approach to interventions with continuous reassessment of the patient's response to treatments may lead to superior outcomes. Additionally, this methodology may assist the clinician in identification and implementation of a plan of care that is individually tailored to the patient and increase the probability of a successful outcome.

References

Bang M, Deyle G. 2000. Comparison of supervised exercise with and without manual physical therapy for patients with shoulder impingement syndrome. J Orthop Sport Phys Ther 30: 126–137.

Bergman G, Winters J, Groenier K, et al. 2004. Manipulative therapy in addition to usual medical care for patients with shoulder dysfunction and pain. Ann Intern Med 141: 432–439.

Boyles R, Ritland B, Miracle B, et al. 2009. The short-term effects of thoracic spine thrust manipulation on patients with shoulder impingement syndrome. Man Ther 14: 375–380.

Burns S, Mintken P, Austin G. 2010. Clinical decision making in a patient with secondary in a patient with secondary hip–spine syndrome. Physiother Theory Pract 27: 384–397.

Burns S, Mintken P, Austin G, et al. 2011. Short-term response of hip mobilizations and exercise in individuals with chronic low back pain: a case series. J Man Manip Ther 19: 100–107.

Butler D. 2000. The sensitive nervous system. Adelaide, Australia: Noigroup Publications.

Chilibek P, Cornish S, Schulte A, et al. 2011. The effect of spinal manipulation on imbalances in leg strength. J Can Chiropract Assoc 55: 183–192.

Cibulka MT, Rose SJ, Delitto A, et al. 1986. Hamstring muscle strain treated by mobilizing the sacroiliac joint. Phys Ther 66: 1220–1223.

Cleland J, Selleck B, Stowell T, et al. 2004. Short-term effects of thoracic manipulation on lower trapezius muscle strength. J Manual Manipul Ther 12: 82–90.

Cleland J, Glynn P, Whitman J, et al. 2007. Short-term effects of thrust vs. non-thrust mobilization / manipulation directed at the thoracic spine in patients with neck pain: a randomized clinical trial. Phys Ther 87: 431–440.

Cleland J, Mintken P, Carpenter K, et al. 2010. Examination of a clinical prediction rule to identify patients with neck pain likely to benefit from thoracic spine thrust manipulation and a general cervical range of motion exercise: multi-center randomized clinical trial. J Orthop Sport Phys Ther 90: 1239–1250.

Davis P, Hulbert J, Kassak K, et al. 1998. Comparative efficacy of conservative medical and chiropractic treatments for carpal tunnel syndrome: a randomized clinical trial. J Manip Physiol Ther 21: 317–326.

Deyle G, Henderson N, Matekel R, et al. 2000. Effectiveness of manual physical therapy and exercise in osteoarthritis of the knee. Ann Int Med 132: 173–181.

Deyle G, Allison S, Matkel R, et al. 2005. Physical therapy treatment effectiveness for osteoarthritis of the knee: a randomized comparison of supervised clinical exercise and manual therapy procedures versus a home exercise program. Phys Ther 85: 1301–1317.

Dishman D, Bulbulia R. 2000. Spinal reflex attenuation associated with spinal manipulation. Spine 25: 2519–2525.

Dishman D, Cunningham B, Burke J. 2002. Comparison of tibial nerve H-reflex excitability after cervical and lumbar spine manipulation. J Manipul Physiol Ther 25: 318–325.

Dunning J, Rushton A. 2009. The effects of cervical high-velocity low-amplitude thrust manipulation on resting electromyographic activity of the biceps brachii muscle. Man Ther 14:508–513.

González-Iglesias J, Fernández-de-las-Peñas C, Cleland J, et al. 2009a. Thoracic spine manipulation for patients with neck pain: a randomized clinical trial. J Orthop Sport Phys Ther 39: 20–27.

González-Iglesias J, Fernández-de-las-Peñas C, Cleland J, et al. 2009b. Inclusion of thoracic spine thrust manipulation into an electro-therapy / thermal program for the management of patients with acute mechanical neck pain: a randomized clinical trial. Man Ther 14: 306–313.

Grindstaff T, Hertel J, Beazell J, et al. 2009. Effects of a lumbopelvic joint manipulation on quadriceps activation and strength in healthy individuals. Man Ther 14: 415–420.

Grindstaff T, Hertel J, Beazell J, et al. 2012. Lumbo-pelvic joint manipulation and quadriceps activation of people with patellofemoral pain syndrome. J Athletic Train 47: 24–31.

Herzog W, Scheele D, Conway PJ. 1999. Electromyography responses of back and limb muscles associated with spinal manipulative therapy. Spine 24: 146–152.

Hillerman B, Gomes A, Korporaal C, et al. 2006. A pilot study comparing the effects of spinal manipulative therapy with those of extra-spinal manipulative therapy on quadriceps muscle strength. J Manipul Physiol Ther 29: 145–149.

Iverson C, Sutlive T, Crowell M, et al. 2008. Lumbopelvic manipulation for the treatment of patients with patellofemoral pain syndrome: development of a clinical prediction rule. J Orthop Sports Phys Ther 38: 297–312.

Lau H, Chiu T, Lam T. 2011. The effectiveness of thoracic manipulation on patients with chronic mechanical neck pain: a randomized controlled trial. Man Ther 16: 141–147.

Liebler EJ, Tfano-Coors L, Douris P, et al. 2001. The effect of thoracic spine mobilization on lower trapezius strength testing. J Manual Manipul Ther 9: 207–212.

Lowry C, Cleland J, Dyke K. 2008. Management of patients with patellofemoral pain syndrome using a multimodal approach: a case series. J Orthop Sports Phys Ther 38: 691–702.

Mintken P, Cleland J, Carpenter K, et al. 2010. Some factors predict successful short-term outcomes in individuals with shoulder pain receiving cervicothoracic manipulation: a single-arm trial. Phys Ther 90: 26–42.

Offierski C, McNab I. 1983. Hip–spine syndrome. Spine 8: 316–321.

Perry J, Green A. 2008. An investigation into the effects of a unilaterally applied lumbar mobilization technique on peripheral sympathetic nervous system activity in the lower limbs. Man Ther 13: 492–499.

Perry J, Green A, Singh S, et al. 2011. A preliminary investigation into the magnitude of effect of lumbar extension exercises and a segmental rotatory manipulation on sympathetic nervous system activity. Man Ther 16: 190–195.

Reiman M, Weisbach PC, Glynn P. 2009. The hips influence on low back pain: a distal link to a proximal problem. J Sports Rehabil 18: 24–32.

Suter E, McMorland G. 2002. Decrease in elbow flexor inhibition after cervical spine manipulation in patients with chronic neck pain. Clin Biomech 17: 541–544.

Suter E, McMorland G, Herzog W, et al. 1999. Decrease in quadriceps inhibition after sacroiliac joint manipulation in patients with anterior knee pain. J Manipul Physiol Ther 22:149–153.

Suter E, McMorland G, Herzog W, et al. 2000. Conservative lower back treatment reduces inhibition in knee-extensor muscles: a randomized controlled trial. J Manipulative Physiol Ther 23: 76–80.

Szlezak A, Georgilopoulos P, Bullock-Saxton J, et al. 2011. The immediate effect of unilateral Z-joint mobilization on neurodynamics: a randomized controlled study. Man Ther 16: 609–613.

Wainner R, Whitman J, Cleland J, et al. 2007. Regional interdependence: a musculoskeletal examination model whose time has come. J Orthop Sports Phys Ther 37: 658–660.

20 Chapter

The Contribution of the Pelvic Floor Muscles to Pelvic Pain

Ruth Jones

CHAPTER CONTENTS

Introduction 226
Anatomy and neural control 226
Pelvic floor muscles and lumbopelvic pain 227
Chronic pelvic pain 227
Conservative management of chronic pelvic pain 228
A clinical-reasoned approach for conservative management of chronic pelvic pain 230
Understanding current pain science 230
Movement system dysfunction 230
Pelvic floor muscle function 230
Case reports 232
Conclusion 233

Introduction

The pelvic floor is a fascinating, intricate structure, which by virtue of its anatomical position is a challenging, understudied region of the body (Ashton-Miller & DeLancey 2007). The pelvic floor is essential for continence, pelvic organ support, sexual activity, conception, fertility and vaginal delivery (DeLancey 1990, 2005; Howard et al 2000; Herschorn 2004; Baytur et al 2005). There is also increasing evidence that the pelvic floor muscles contribute to respiration (Hodges et al 2007), spinal stability, and containment of intra-abdominal pressure (IAP) (Hemborg et al 1985; Pool-Goudzwaard et al 2004; Smith et al 2008). The physiological mechanisms by which these muscles perform these roles are not clearly understood yet, which is predominately due to a lack of suitable instrumentation.

Pelvic floor dysfunction is a significant problem for both women and men and encompasses both urinary and faecal incontinence, pelvic organ prolapse (POP) and pelvic pain (Martins et al 2007), with estimates in the USA indicating that between 21% and 26% of American women have at least one pelvic floor disorder, with the greatest percentage experiencing urinary incontinence (Nygaard et al 2008). Pelvic floor dysfunction affects up to 400 000 American women so severely that they require surgery, and 30% of those will require further surgery (Olsen et al 1997; Boyles et al 2003). The exact mechanisms for the development of pelvic floor disorders remain controversial; however, a combination of neuropathic changes and muscle, fascial or connective tissue damage is most likely to be responsible (Shafik et al 2005; Ashton-Miller & DeLancey 2007; Petros 2007; Smith et al 2007).

Anatomy and Neural Control

As the pelvic floor muscles form the inferior aspect of the lumbopelvic cylinder (LPC) and IAP is generated by coactivation of the pelvic floor muscles, the diaphragm and the abdominal muscles (Hemborg et al 1985; Hodges & Gandevia 2000), this implies that coordinated coactivation of the muscles of the LPC is necessary in order to balance the functional demands of continence, respiration and lumbopelvic stability (Hemborg et al 1985; Hodges & Gandevia 2000; Pool-Goudzwaard et al 2004; Hodges et al 2007). As the support mechanisms of the pelvic floor are responsible for the maintenance of continence and prevention of POP during increases in IAP (Ashton-Miller & DeLancey 2007), functionally the pelvic floor has the dual role of allowing the passage of urine and faeces at the appropriate time, whilst also preventing incontinence. Therefore, given the multipurpose role of the pelvic floor muscles, the motor control challenge of these muscles is significant and the efficiency of them will not only rely upon the anatomical integrity of the pelvic floor, but also depend on the central nervous system (CNS) response to satisfy hierarchical demands of function.

There is a constant low level of muscle activity in the LPC muscles and increased activity when the CNS can predict timing of increased demand / load, such as occurs in coughing, lifting or limb movements (Constantinou & Govan 1982; Moseley et al 2002; Barbic et al 2003). The CNS must therefore interpret the multiple afferent inputs and generate a coordinated response so that muscle activity occurs at the right time, with the appropriate level of contraction.

The pelvic floor muscles are composed of smooth and striated muscle fibres (Shafik et al 2002), approximately two-thirds of which are type I (Gosling et al 1981) – reflecting the need for endurance in a continuous supportive function (Shafik et al 2003). It is thought that the pelvic floor muscles predominantly contract or relax en masse (Shafik 1998) yet, due to the separate though identical innervation of each individual muscle, there may also exist the capacity for voluntary selective activity by which an individual muscle might behave independently from the others (Shafik 1998; Kenton & Brubaker 2002). There are different opinions regarding the exact innervation of the pelvic floor muscles; however, there is consensus that the nerve supply is from the pudendal nerve with direct branches from the sacral nerves S3–S4 (Shafik 2000; Guaderrama et al 2005; Grigorescu et al 2008). The pudendal nerve carries motor, sensory and autonomic fibres; consequently both afferent and efferent pathways can be affected by its injury (Gray et al 1995). The posterior femoral cutaneous nerve (S1–S3 / 4) gives rise to the inferior cluneal and perineal branches and has also been implicated in chronic pelvic pain (CPP) (Darnis et al 2008; Tubbs et al 2009).

Neural control of the pelvic organs is affected by a coordination of somatic and autonomic motor nervous systems, and sensory information and feedback are supplied by both visceral and somatic sensory fibre systems (Enck & Vodusek 2006). The somatic innervation is largely from the lumbar, sacral and coccygeal plexuses. The pelvic sympathetic innervation produces vasomotor effects, inhibits peristaltic contraction of the rectum and stimulates contraction of the internal genitals during orgasm, producing ejaculation in males (Pattern & Hughes 2008). Parasympathetic innervation causes contraction of the bladder and rectum for micturition and defecation, and clitoral or penile erection (Pattern & Hughes 2008). The pelvic visceral afferents travel with the parasympathetic fibres to the spinal ganglia (S2–S4). Nociceptive visceral afferents from the prostate, seminal vesicles, vagina, cervix, distal sigmoid colon and rectum follow parasympathetic fibres to the spinal ganglia. Nociceptive visceral afferents from the bladder, ovaries and uterus travel with the sympathetic fibres to the inferior thoracic and superior lumbar spinal ganglia (Pattern & Hughes 2008). The autonomic nerves help to control micturition, defecation and sexual intercourse. The sympathetic nerves arise from the lumbar splanchnic nerves and the parasympathetic nerves from the pelvic splanchnic nerves. Therefore, due to the intimate and similar anatomical innervations between the pelvic floor and pelvic organs (a viscera–somatic relationship), when evaluating the patient with pelvic floor pain it is important to consider the lumbosacral plexus, the individual peripheral nerves and the sympathetic chain.

Pelvic Floor Muscles and Lumbopelvic pain

Women with incontinence, respiratory disorders and gastrointestinal symptoms have increased risk for the development of lumbopelvic pain (Smith et al 2009). Additional evidence exists connecting diaphragmatic and breathing pattern disorders with various forms of pelvic girdle dysfunction (O'Sullivan et al 2002; O'Sullivan & Beales 2007) as well as with CPP and associated symptoms, such as stress incontinence (Smith et al 2006, 2007; Hodges et al 2007; O'Sullivan & Beales 2007). It is also suggested that there is a connection between sacroiliac joint (SIJ) stability and respiratory and pelvic floor function, particularly in women (Hodges et al 2007). The development of low back pain during pregnancy (PLBP) increases the odds of developing pelvic floor disorder complaints, especially there was a negative active straight leg raise test (Pool-Goudzwaard et al 2004). In one study of patients with PLBP, pelvic floor activity had higher resting tone and shorter endurance time (Pool-Goudzwaard et al 2004); 52% had a combination of low back pain and pelvic floor dysfunction and 82% of these stated that their complaints started with low back pain prior to the pelvic floor dysfunction. More recently, pelvic floor muscle dysfunction as measured by ultrasound has also been found to be present in men suffering from CPP; the anorectal angle at rest was more acute in urological chronic pelvic pain syndrome (UCPPS) than controls and this angle was correlated with pain, sexual dysfunction and anxiety (Davis et al 2011). Furthermore, there was less upward movement of the pelvic floor muscles during contraction, and reduced contractile endurance in CPP men above normal individuals.

As stated, there is evidence of a different response of the pelvic floor muscles to lumbopelvic pain – that is, either increased or decreased activity (O'Sullivan et al 2002; Pool-Goudzwaard et al 2004; Davis et al 2011). O'Sullivan and Beales (2007) suggested that such changes may represent a response to a pain disorder (i.e. it may be adaptive), or might promote abnormal tissue strain and therefore be seen to be 'maladaptive', or provocative of subsequent pain disorders. Maladaptive changes might in turn lead to a deficit in motor control or increased motor activation resulting in a mechanism for ongoing peripheral pain sensitization, leading to chronic pain involving the pelvis and pelvic floor structures (O'Sullivan 2005; Smith et al 2009).

In summary, it is understood that, in the presence of postural changes, respiratory demands, lumbopelvic pain and stress incontinence, the function of the LPC muscles can be altered (Hemborg et al 1985; Hides et al 1996; Hodges & Richardson 1996, 1998; Hodges & Gandevia 2000; Moseley et al 2002; O'Sullivan et al 2002; Jones et al 2006; Hodges et al 2007; Dickx et al 2008). There is evidence that skilled voluntary activation of those relevant muscles with altered motor recruitment can reduce pain, disability and recurrence rate for musculoskeletal conditions (Hides et al 2001; Cowan et al 2003; Ferreira et al 2006), restore motor coordination including automatic postural adjustments (Cowan et al 2003; Tsao & Hodges 2007, 2008) and reverse cortical reorganization in people with recurrent pain (Tsao et al 2010). These findings suggest that the muscles of the LPC should be evaluated and rehabilitated in patients with CPP. To date, however, no scientific trial has evaluated this clinical approach for the pelvic floor muscles in this subgroup of pain patients.

Chronic Pelvic Pain

Chronic pelvic pain (CPP) is non-malignant pain perceived in structures related to the pelvis of either men or women. In the case of documented nociceptive pain that becomes chronic, pain must have been continuous or recurrent for at least 6 months. If non-acute and central sensitization pain mechanisms are well documented, then the pain may be regarded as chronic, irrespective of the time period (Fall et al 2010). CPP is then subdivided into those conditions with well-defined classical pathology, such as infection and cancer, and those where no obvious pathology is found. Chronic pelvic pain syndrome (CPPS) is the occurrence of CPP where there is no proven infection or other obvious local pathology that may account for the pain; it is often associated with symptoms suggestive of lower urinary tract, sexual, bowel or gynaecological dysfunction and has negative cognitive, behavioural, sexual and emotional consequences (Fall et al 2010).

Howard (2003) suggests that approximately 15–20% of women aged 18 to 50 years have experienced CPP lasting for more than 1 year, and an 8% prevalence rate for CPPS has been estimated in the US male population (Anderson 2008). However, overall prevalence rates of CPP are likely to be underdiagnosed, partly as a result of the lack of agreed-upon definitions and subsequent difficulty in categorizing CPP (Fall et al 2010).

Due to the sensitisation processes involved in CPP (Fall et al 2010), persistent pain is associated with changes in the CNS that may maintain the perception of pain in the absence of acute injury, so that the pelvic floor muscles may become hyperalgesic, and contain multiple active trigger points. This process may lead to organs becoming sensitive, for example the uterus in dyspareunia and dysmenorrhoea, or the bowel in irritable bowel syndrome (IBS). Men with chronic prostatitis have more generalized pain sensitivity (Berger et al 2007), and current thinking suggests that if there has been infection or trauma this results in neurogenic inflammation in peripheral tissues and the CNS (Pontari & Ruggieri 2008).

The symptoms of CPP / CPPS appear to result from interplay between psychological factors and dysfunction in the immune, neurological and endocrine systems (Pontari & Ruggieri 2008). It therefore seems that therapeutic approaches should adopt treatment strategies that take account of these multiple interacting factors.

Conservative Management of Chronic Pelvic Pain

Many investigators believe that the source of pain and dysfunction in men and women with CPP, including chronic testicular pain, relates to chronic tension in myofascial tissue in and around the pelvic floor (Anderson et al 2005, 2009; Curtis Nickel et al 2007; Planken et al 2010). The pathogenic mechanisms associated with the development of pelvic genitourinary symptoms are unknown as it remains difficult to explain the role of painful pelvic floor tissues – particularly as, up until recently, studies of pelvic floor muscle function have focused on the evaluation of the strength and endurance of voluntarily initiated contractions (Laycock et al 2001; Bø & Finckenhagen 2003; Dumoulin et al 2003) rather than issues of motor control. Classically, trigger points in the pelvic floor muscles have been documented as referring symptoms to the lumbar spine, posterior thigh, coccyx, abdomen, perineum, groin, testicles, penis and vulva (Anderson et al 2009) (Fig. 20.1). Specifically the obturator internus muscle (Fig. 20.2) is reported to refer most commonly to the abdomen and groin, and to be responsible for a sensation as if there is something inside the rectum or vagina (like a golf ball). Also the coccygeus / ischiococcygeus is reported to refer to the coccyx and gluteal region and to be responsible for pain occurring pre- / post-bowel movement and / or full-bowel sensations and discomfort. The pubococcygeus is reported to be the most important for male pelvic pain; it can refer to the tip of the penis, the bladder and urethra, and can mimic the sensation

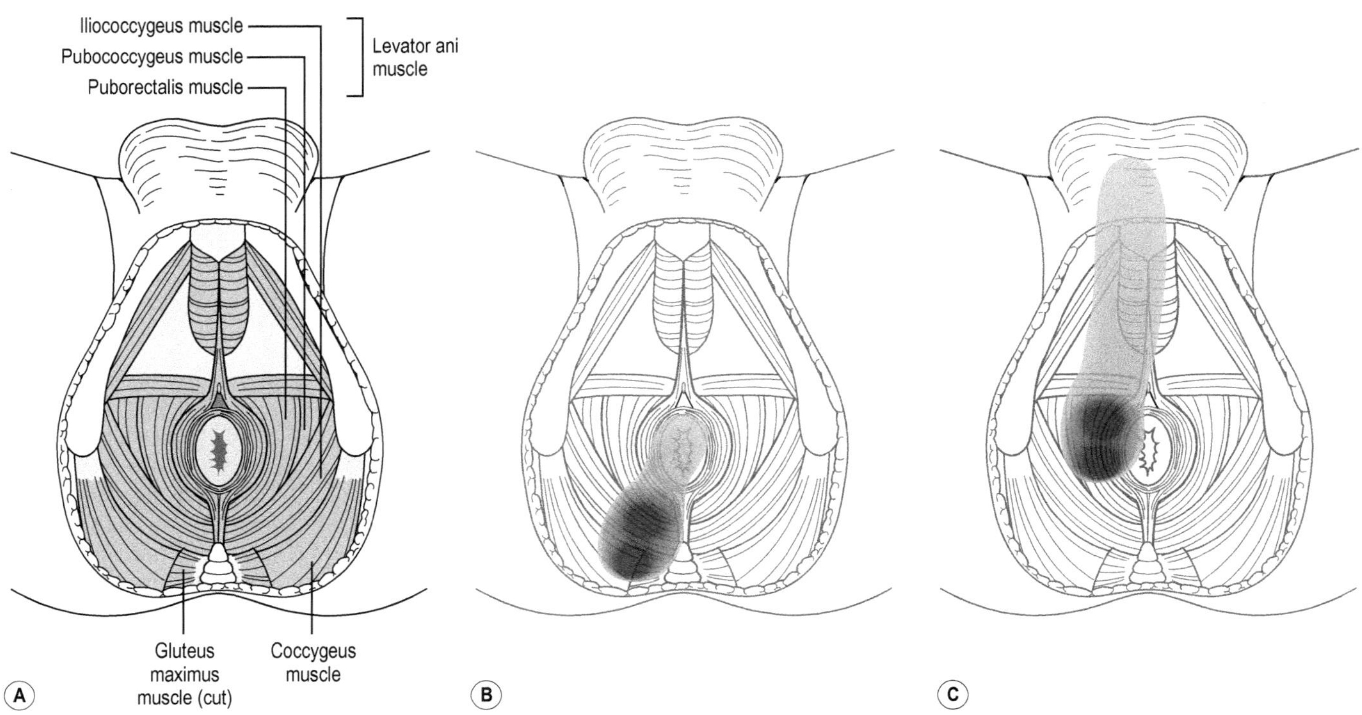

Figure 20.1 The pelvic floor muscles: (**A**) Scheme of muscles. (**B**) Referred pain from coccygeus or iliococcygeus muscle trigger points. (**C**) Referred pain from pubococcygeus or levator ani muscle trigger points. (Reproduced from Chaitow L, Lovegrove Jones R (eds). 2012. Chronic pelvic pain and dysfunction: practical physical medicine. London: Elsevier Churchill Livingstone, with permission. Picture from the same author.)

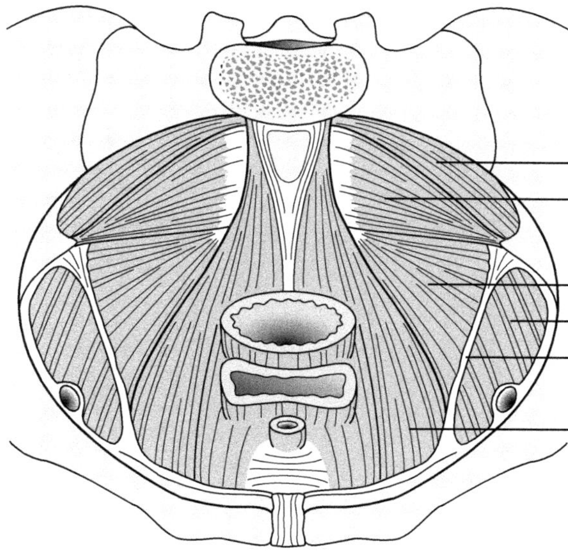

Figure 20.2 Scheme of the pelvic floor musculature. (Reproduced from Chaitow L, Lovegrove Jones R (eds). 2012. Chronic pelvic pain and dysfunction: practical physical medicine. London: Elsevier Churchill Livingstone, with permission. Picture from the same author.)

of pressure or fullness of the prostate. The iliococcygeus can also refer to the lateral abdominal wall, the perineum and anal sphincter, and to be responsible for a sensation of prostate fullness and pain (Anderson et al 2009).

It is thought that there are general reasons why a person may develop excessive tension in the myofascial tissue of the pelvic floor – such as straining, habitual tightening, trauma and inflammation – and therefore potentially develop active trigger points. Other reasons that have been suggested include childbirth trauma, recurrent urinary tract infection, digestive tract disorders, IBS, prolapse, pelvic surgery, constipation, defecation dysfunction, haemorrhoids / fistulae / fissures, sexual abuse, pelvic inflammatory disease / endometriosis, scar tissue / adhesions, and trauma to the coccyx or other pelvic trauma (Carter 2000; Tu et al 2006; Fitzgerald et al 2009). Studies using trigger point release of the pelvic floor have shown improvement in symptoms of interstitial cystitis (Weiss 2001; Doggweiler-Wiygul & Wiygul 2002), altered libido, ejaculatory, penile and erectile pain, urinary symptoms, and ejaculatory dysfunction in men with CPP (Anderson et al 2006, 2009, 2011). Trigger point deactivation of the levator ani by injection was also shown to be of significant value in the management of patients with CPP (Langford et al 2007).

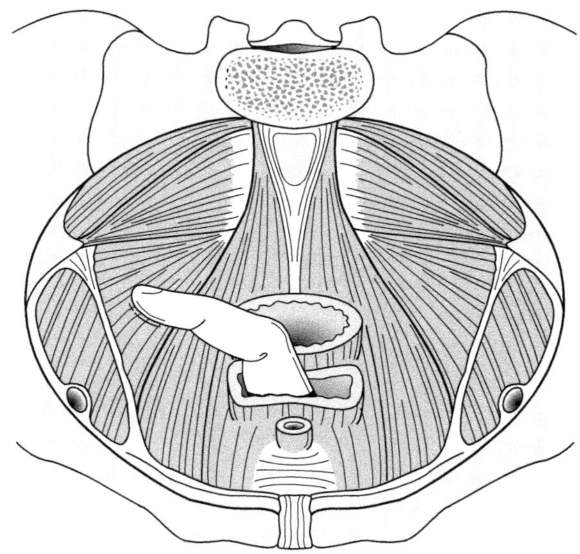

Figure 20.3 Scheme of the internal technique for trigger point treatment. (Reproduced from Chaitow L, Lovegrove Jones R (eds). 2012. Chronic pelvic pain and dysfunction: practical physical medicine. London: Elsevier Churchill Livingstone, with permission. Picture from the same author.)

A multicentre study has demonstrated the feasibility of performing clinical therapeutic trials utilizing muscle and connective tissue physiotherapy to treat urological CPPS (Fitzgerald et al 2009). A comparison group of patients were randomized to receive either total-body traditional Western massage with no myofascial release or internal pelvic therapy. Those who were randomized to the myofascial therapy group underwent connective tissue manipulation to all body wall tissues (see Fig. 20.2) of the abdominal wall, back, buttocks and thighs as well as internal pelvic floor muscles clinically found to contain connective tissue abnormalities and / or trigger point release to painful myofascial trigger points (Fig. 20.3). This was done until a change was noted in the treated tissue. Manual techniques such as trigger point release with or without active contraction or reciprocal inhibition, manual stretching of the trigger point region were used on the identified trigger points. A secondary outcome of the study revealed good patient response to the internal and external physical therapy as compared with generalized external Western massage only (57% versus 28% respectively). This form of therapy was expanded to a larger trial in women suffering from interstitial cystitis or painful bladder syndrome; the global response assessment response rate was 26% in the global therapeutic massage group and 59% in the myofascial physical therapy group (Fitzgerald et al 2012).

A Clinical-reasoned Approach for Conservative Management of Chronic Pelvic Pain

In the management of a patient with pelvic pain it would be convenient to focus solely on the end organ that is perceived to be 'at fault'. However, the human body operates as a system, and is modulated by several factors from somatic, physiological, cognitive, emotional, psychological and social domains, all of which have the potential to influence nociception (Moseley 2008; Fall et al 2010). Each component of the movement system is likely to influence distal and proximal regions; therefore, when assessing (and treating) a patient with pelvic pain, as clinicians we need to adopt a holistic clinically reasoned approach so as to identify the particular influences that have caused, maintained and / or exacerbated a patient's condition, whilst reminding ourselves that any dysfunction observed may not be even relevant to the presenting condition and will also be influenced by the therapist's perspective and different belief systems. The following section describes the systematic approach that the author of the chapter uses, which takes into account these multiple factors.

Understanding current pain science

It is important to understand the patient's pain perception and beliefs and link this to current pain science. This is especially important with patients complaining of chronic pain as many patients still equate pain with damage and avoid activities, such as sitting, that 'hurt'. For example, many patients with CPP believe that they have pudendal nerve entrapment (PNE) and believe that sitting compresses the pudendal nerve, as indicated by increasing pain, and therefore will often only sit with 'cut-out' cushions and avoid 'hard' chairs. The clinician explaining how multiple factors contribute to the pain experience is an important way of reducing the threat associated with pelvic pain. A '10 points to pain™' model is one concept that a number of patients and clinicians have found useful (Jones 2003, unpublished) (Fig. 20.4). It is an easy way to demonstrate that pain can develop for many different reasons and works on the premise that pain is rarely the result of one single incident, but normally stems from a range of different issues or *a whole lifestyle* that contributes to the 10 points and painful state. In this way, the patient and therapist can move away from the solely structural pathological model to one that considers, for example, the brain in pain, the patient's beliefs about their pain and nutritional issues, in addition to any pathology or motor control issues.

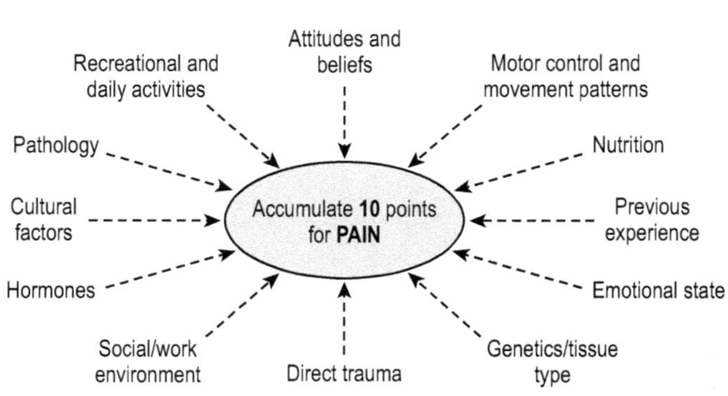

Figure 20.4 Accumulate 10 points to pain: some factors that appear to influence the accumulation of a pain experience. (Adapted from Jones 2003.)

Movement system dysfunction

Various classifications for the analysis of movement and the subclassification of movement dysfunction have been proposed (McGill 2002; Sahrmann 2002; McKenzie & May 2003; O'Sullivan 2005) and in some instances are gaining good evidence of validity and reliability (Van Dillen et al 1998, 2003; Dankaerts et al 2006; Harris-Hayes & Van Dillen, 2009). The musculoskeletal factors that need to be considered include the passive and active stiffness of the lumbopelvic spine and hips, which will be influenced by muscle and fascial systems, all under neuronal control. Assessment of the neural system is therefore critical, particularly neural mobility (Hall et al 1998; Walsh et al 2009). Structural differences such as bony variation of the pelvis and femur, imbalances of strength, length, timing and magnitude of recruitment of the trunk and hip muscles will also need to be assessed during test movements, as well as specific functional activities where possible.

Pelvic floor muscle function

Indications that there may be a pelvic floor component to the patient presenting with pelvic pain are clinically revealed by use of validated questionnaires, such as the NIH-Chronic Prostatitis Symptom Index (NIH-CPSI) for males (Fig. 20.5) and the version adapted for females (Fig. 20.6) (Litwin 2002). There is strong evidence to suggest that questionnaires are a powerful tool to indicate UCPPS (Anderson 2011). In investigating pelvic floor muscle function, it is important for the therapist to evaluate:

1. The resting activity of the pelvic floor muscles, to see whether there is over- / underactivity
2. The voluntary activation of the pelvic floor muscles including power, endurance and direction of contraction
3. The ability of the pelvic floor muscles to release to their resting position
4. Structural dysfunction, such as prolapse
5. Neural integrity, for example the pudendal nerve for signs of irritability (positive Tinel's sign)
6. Any active trigger points within the pelvic floor muscles.

Active trigger points are particularly helpful if they are found to reproduce the patient's symptoms; however, these do not have to be limited to those that refer only to these particular areas. It is important that the clinician explain to patients with CPP that many areas may be hyperalgesic and not relevant to the presenting condition, thereby reducing the threat associated with the pain experienced. Clinical experience has been that men without pelvic pain on palpation of a point close to the prostate, near the pubic symphysis, have no referral to the penis, whereas men with CPP have referred symptoms to the shaft or tip of the penis. This is a positive

NIH-Chronic Prostatitis Symptom Index (NIH-CPSI) (for males)

Center for Urologic and Pelvic Pain

Name: ______________________
Date: ______________________

Pain or Discomfort

1. In the last week, have you experienced any pain or discomfort in the following areas?

	Yes	No
a. Area between rectum and testicles (perineum)	1	0
b. Testicles	1	0
c. Tip of the penis (not related to urination)	1	0
d. Below your waist, in your pubic or bladder area	1	0

2. In the last week, have you experienced:

	Yes	No
a. Pain or burning during urination?	1	0
b. Pain or discomfort during or after sexual climax (ejaculation)?	1	0

3. How often have you had pain or discomfort in any of these areas over the last week?
 0 Never
 1 Rarely
 2 Sometimes
 3 Often
 4 Usually
 5 Always

4. Which number best describes your AVERAGE pain or discomfort on the days that you had it, over the last week?
0 1 2 3 4 5 6 7 8 9 10
NO PAIN — PAIN AS BAD AS YOU CAN IMAGINE

Urination

5. How often have you had a sensation of not emptying your bladder completely after you finished urinating, over the last week?
 0 Not at all
 1 Less than 1 time in 5
 2 Less than half the time
 3 About half the time
 4 More than half the time
 5 Almost always

6. How often have you had to urinate again less than two hours after you finished urinating, over the last week?
 0 Not at all
 1 Less than 1 time in 5
 2 Less than half the time
 3 About half the time
 4 More than half the time
 5 Almost always

Impact of Symptoms

7. How much have your symptoms kept you from doing the kinds of things you would usually do, over the last week?
 0 None
 1 Only a little
 2 Some
 3 A lot

8. How much did you think about your symptoms, over the last week?
 0 None
 1 Only a little
 2 Some
 3 A lot

Quality of Life

9. If you were to spend the rest of your life with your symptoms just the way they have been during the last week, how would you feel about that?
 0 Delighted
 1 Pleased
 2 Mostly satisfied
 3 Mixed (about equally satisfied and dissatisfied)
 4 Mostly dissatisfied
 5 Unhappy
 6 Terrible

Scoring the NIH-Chronic Prostatitis Symptom Index Domains
Pain: Total of items 1a, 1b, 1c,1d, 2a, 2b, 3, and 4 =____
Urinary Symptoms: Total of items 5 and 6 =____
Quality of Life & Impact: Total of items 7, 8, and 9 =____

Figure 20.5 NIH-Chronic Prostatitis Symptom Index (NIH-CPSI) (for males). (Adapted from Litwin et al. 1999. J Urol 162: 369–375.)

diagnostic test called the 'sign of the penis' (SOP) (Jones 2014, unpublished) and as their symptoms clear the SOP becomes negative.

If active trigger points are found, patients (or their partners) can practise self-management using a variety of methods such as internal pelvic trigger point wand (Fig. 20.7) (Anderson et al 2011), which in this clinician's experience helps to speed recovery. In addition to self-release, many patients need to be advised to check frequently whether they are unconsciously contracting their pelvic floor, either directly or by co-contracting via their abdominal muscles. A clinically useful technique involves teaching the patient to breathe into the abdomen whilst simultaneously relaxing the abdomen and pelvic floor (Whelan 2012).

Female NIH-Chronic Prostatitis Symptom Index (NIH-CPSI)

Center for Urologic and Pelvic Pain

Name: ______________________________
Date: ______________________________

Pain or Discomfort

1. In the last week, have you experienced any pain or discomfort in the following areas?

	Yes	No
a. Area between rectum and vagina (perineum)	1	0
b. Labia	1	0
c. Clitoris (not related to urination)	1	0
d. Below your waist in your pubic area	1	0
e. Below your waist in your rectal area	1	0

2. In the last week, have you experienced:

	Yes	No
a. Pain or burning during urination?	1	0
b. Pain or discomfort during or after sexual climax?	1	0

3. How often have you had pain or discomfort in any of these areas over the last week?

0 Never
1 Rarely
2 Sometimes
3 Often
4 Usually
5 Always

4. Which number best describes your AVERAGE pain or discomfort on the days that you had it, over the last week?

0 1 2 3 4 5 6 7 8 9 10
NO PAIN — PAIN AS BAD AS YOU CAN IMAGINE

Urination

5. How often have you had a sensation of not emptying your bladder completely after you finished urinating, over the last week?

0 Not at all
1 Less than 1 time in 5
2 Less than half the time
3 About half the time
4 More than half the time
5 Almost always or always

6. How often have you had to urinate again less than two hours after you finished urinating, over the last week?

0 Not at all
1 Less than 1 time in 5
2 Less than half the time
3 About half the time
4 More than half the time
5 Almost always

Impact of Symptoms

7. How much have your symptoms kept you from doing the kinds of things you would usually do, over the last week?

0 None
1 Only a little
2 Some
3 A lot

8. How much did you think about your symptoms, over the last week?

0 None
1 Only a little
2 Some
3 A lot

Quality of Life

9. If you were to spend the rest of your life with your symptoms just the way they have been during the last week, how would you feel about that?

0 Delighted
1 Pleased
2 Mostly satisfied
3 Mixed (about equally satisfied and dissatisfied)
4 Mostly dissatisfied
5 Unhappy
6 Terrible

Scoring the NIH-Chronic Prostatitis Symptom Index Domains

Pain: Total of items 1a, 1b, 1c, 1d, 1e, 2a, 2b, 3, and 4 =____
Urinary Symptoms: Total of items 5 and 6 =____
Quality of Life Impact: Total of items 7, 8, and 9 =____

Figure 20.6 Female NIH-Chronic Prostatitis Symptom Index (NIH-CPSI). (Adapted from Litwin et al. 1999. J Urol 162: 369–375.)

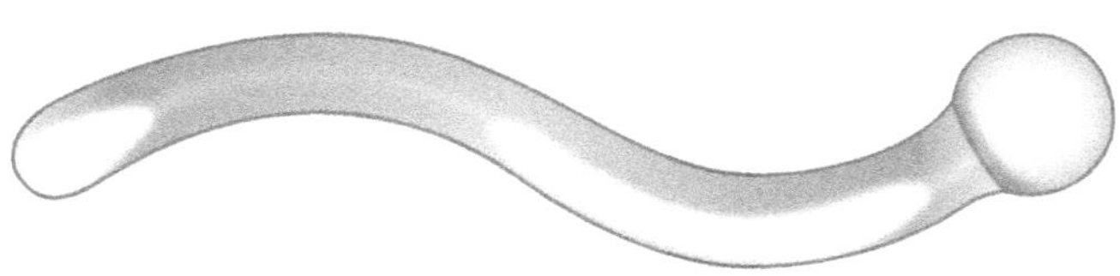

Figure 20.7 Internal pelvic trigger point wand.

Case Reports

Finally, to illustrate the complexity of the clinician evaluating a patient with CPP, consider the following short case histories with discussion afterwards.

Case report 1

A 50-year-old woman complained of a 5-year history of pelvic pain, posterior thigh pain and 'lumpy' intravaginal pain with dyspareunia, and consequently had avoided having penetrative sex with her husband. Active straight leg raise was technically negative, but she held her breath during the test. Palpation of L5 / S1 reproduced the lumpy intravaginal pain. The slump test was positive and reproduced her posterior thigh pain, and she also exhibited movement system dysfunction in her lumbar spine, moving excessively into extension and rotation. At the time the clinician had not learnt to evaluate the pelvic floor muscles and concluded that she had a L5 / S1 joint dysfunction, with no signs of instability but with concurrent neural involvement. Treatment consisted of five sessions of manual therapy to the thoracic, lumbar and SIJ with neural tissue mobilization, plus a specific home exercise programme to optimize her movement system balance. She was pain free on discharge, but had not resumed sexual intercourse as she said that she was not 'interested'.

Two years later, she returned to clinic having had a return of the lumpy intravaginal pain. There had been no specific physical event; however, her husband had died and she was extremely distressed, believing she had not been a 'good' wife as they had not resumed sexual intercourse. On physical assessment it was possible to reproduce her intravaginal pain both with palpation of L5 / S1 and by palpation of her pelvic floor muscles.

Case report 2

A 30-year-old football player complaining of longstanding bilateral groin pain with 'gapping' sensations at the symphysis pubis came for treatment. He stated that there had been a gradual onset of anterior abdominal wall pain with running, which had increased in intensity over some weeks. He had been diagnosed with chronic left-sided osteitis pubis, with a magnetic resonance imaging scan indicating some bone marrow oedema margins of the symphysis pubis. He had been treated surgically 8 months post injury but was not making any progress, and was subsequently diagnosed with an inguinal hernia, then a labral hip tear, and treated surgically again with no effect. Symptoms were aggravated by running, hip abduction, gluteal clenching and, on closer questioning, he revealed he also had concurrent perineal pain. An NIH-CPSI form revealed signs of urinary dysfunction (and urinary frequency), which he thought was normal. Palpation of active pelvic floor muscle trigger points near the insertion of the pubococcygeus muscle reproduced rectal / obturator pain and a 'gapping' sensation at the symphysis pubis. There was a negative Tinel's sign on the pudendal nerve; also muscle strength grade 3 (modified Oxford scale) and endurance reduced the symptoms. After five treatments of trigger point release to the pelvic floor muscles, the player was back to full-time football with no symptom recurrence.

Case report 3

A 24-year-old female complaining of vulval pain had been diagnosed with pudendal nerve entrapment with positive EMG findings. Her aggravating factors were walking, particularly up hill, and bending, and pain was eased by ice and lying on her side. Palpation of her symphysis pubis reproduced her vulval pain and an active straight leg raise test was positive. Treatment consisted of movement system balance corrective exercises and use of a sacral belt. Three months later she successfully managed to climb Mount Kilimanjaro without pain.

Conclusion

In summary, the role of the therapist is to identify and correct the movement system dysfunction relating to the presenting condition. However, as most treatment options for pelvic pain are currently empirical, there is a great requirement for careful clinical reasoning when approaching the management of a patient with pelvic pain. This chapter presents evidence to allow consideration of the pelvic floor muscle movement system dysfunction as a potential contributor to pelvic pain and other related presenting disorders. Possible aids to assessment and treatment are discussed.

References

Anderson RU. 2008. Commentary on the mechanisms in prostatitis / chronic pelvic pain syndrome. J Urol 179: S68.

Anderson RU. 2011. Chronic prostatitis / chronic pelvic pain: is there a psychosocial component? Can Urol Assoc J 5: 333–334.

Anderson RU, Wise D, Sawyer T, et al. 2005. Integration of myofascial trigger point release and paradoxical relaxation training treatment of chronic pelvic pain in men. J Urol 174: 155–160.

Anderson RU, Wise D, Sawyer T, et al. 2006. Sexual dysfunction in men with chronic prostatitis / chronic pelvic pain syndrome: improvement after trigger point release and paradoxical relaxation training. J Urol 176: 1534–1539.

Anderson RU, Sawyer T, Wise D, et al. 2009. Painful myofascial trigger points and pain sites in men with chronic prostatitis / chronic pelvic pain syndrome. J Urol 182: 2753–2758.

Anderson RU, Wise D, Sawyer T, et al. 2011. 6-day intensive treatment protocol for refractory chronic prostatitis / chronic pelvic pain syndrome using myofascial release and paradoxical relaxation training. J Urol 185: 1294–1299.

Ashton-Miller JA, DeLancey JO. 2007. Functional anatomy of the female pelvic floor. Ann N Y Acad Sci 1101: 266–296.

Barbic M, Kralj B, Cor A. 2003. Compliance of the bladder neck supporting structures: importance of activity pattern of levator ani muscle and content of elastic fibers of endopelvic fascia. Neurouro. Urodyn 22: 269–276.

Baytur YB, Deveci A, Uyar Y, et al. 2005. Mode of delivery and pelvic floor muscle strength and sexual function after childbirth. Int J Gynaecol Obstet 88: 276–280.

Berger RE, Ciol MA, Rothman I, et al. 2007. Pelvic tenderness is not limited to the prostate in chronic prostatitis / chronic pelvic pain syndrome (CPPS) type IIIA and IIIB: comparison of men with and without CP / CPPS. BMC Urol 7: 17.

Bø K, Finckenhagen HB. 2003. Is there any difference in measurement of pelvic floor muscle strength in supine and standing position? Acta Obstet Gynecol Scand 82: 1120–1124.

Boyles SH, Weber AM, Meyn L. 2003. Procedures for urinary incontinence in the United States, 1979–1997. Am J Obstet Gynecol 189: 70–75.

Carter JE 2000 Abdominal wall and pelvic myofascial trigger points. In: Howard FM (ed) Pelvic pain. Philadelphia: Lippincott Williams & Wilkins, pp 314–358.

Chaitow L, Lovegrove Jones R (eds). 2012. Chronic pelvic pain and dysfunction: practical physical medicine. London: Elsevier Churchill Livingstone.

Constantinou CE, Govan DE. 1982. Spatial distribution and timing of transmitted and reflexly generated urethral pressures in healthy women. J Urol 127: 964–969.

Cowan SM, Bennell KL, Hodges PW, et al. 2003. Simultaneous feedforward recruitment of the vasti in untrained postural tasks can be restored by physical therapy. J Orthop Res 21: 553–558.

Curtis Nickel J, Baranowski AP, Pontari M, et al. 2007. Management of men diagnosed with chronic prostatitis / chronic pelvic pain syndrome who have failed traditional management. Rev Urol 9: 63–72.

Dankaerts W, O'Sullivan PB, Straker LM, et al. 2006. The inter-examiner reliability of a classification method for non-specific chronic low back pain patients with motor control impairment. Man Ther 11: 28–39

Darnis B, Robert R, Labat JJ, et al. 2008. Perineal pain and inferior cluneal nerves: anatomy and surgery. Surg Radiol Anat 30: 177–183.

Davis SN, Morin M, Binik YM, et al. 2011. Use of pelvic floor ultrasound to assess pelvic floor muscle function in Urological Chronic Pelvic Pain Syndrome in men. J Sex Med 11: 3173–3180. doi:10.1111/j.1743-6109.2011.02452.x.

DeLancey JO 1990. Anatomy and physiology of urinary continence. Clin Obstet Gynecol 33: 298–307.

DeLancey JO 2005. The hidden epidemic of pelvic floor dysfunction: achievable goals for improved prevention and treatment. Am J Obstet Gynecol 192: 1488–1495.

Dickx N, Cagnie B, Achten E, et al. 2008. Changes in lumbar muscle activity because of induced muscle pain evaluated by muscle functional magnetic resonance imaging. Spine 33: E983–E989.

Doggweiler-Wiygul R, Wiygul JP. 2002. Interstitial cystitis, pelvic pain, and the relationship to myofascial pain and dysfunction: a report on four patients. World J Urol 20: 310–314.

Dumoulin C, Bourbonnais D, Lemieux MC. 2003. Development of a dynamometer for measuring the isometric force of the pelvic floor musculature. Neurourol Urodyn 22: 648–653.

Enck P, Vodusek DB. 2006. Electromyography of pelvic floor muscles. J Electromyogr Kines 16: 568–577.

Fall M, Baranowski AP, Elneil S, et al. 2010. EAU guidelines on chronic pelvic pain. Eur Urol 57: 35–48.

Ferreira PH, Ferreira ML, Maher CG, et al. 2006. Specific stabilisation exercise for spinal and pelvic pain: a systematic review. Aust J Physiother 52: 79–88.

FitzGerald MP, Anderson RU, Potts J, et al. 2009. Randomized multicenter feasibility trial of myofascial physical therapy for the treatment of urological chronic pelvic pain syndromes. J Urol 82: 570–580.

FitzGerald MP, Payne CK, Lukacz ES, et al. 2012. Randomized multicenter clinical trial of myofascial physical therapy in women with interstitial cystitis / painful bladder syndrome and pelvic floor tenderness. Urol 187: 2113–2118.

Gosling JA, Dixon JS, Critchley HO, et al. 1981. A comparative study of the human external sphincter and periurethral levator ani muscles. Br J Urol 53: 35–41.

Gray H, Williams PL, Bannister LH. 1995. Gray's anatomy: the anatomical basis of medicine and surgery, 38th edn. New York: Churchill Livingstone.

Grigorescu BA, Lazarou G, Olson TR, et al. 2008. Innervation of the levator ani muscles: description of the nerve branches to the pubococcygeus, iliococcygeus, and puborectalis muscles. Int Urogynecol J 19: 107–116.

Guaderrama NM, Liu J, Nager CW, et al. 2005. Evidence for the innervation of pelvic floor muscles by the pudendal nerve. Obstet Gynecol 106: 774–781.

Hall T, Zusman M, Elvey R. 1998. Adverse mechanical tension in the nervous system? Analysis of straight leg raise. Man Ther 3: 140–146.

Harris-Hayes M, Van Dillen LR. 2009. The inter-tester reliability of physical therapists classifying low back pain problems based on the movement system impairment classification system. PM R 1:117–126. doi:10.1016/j.pmrj.2008.08.001.

Hemborg B, Moritz U, Lowing H. 1985. Intra-abdominal pressure and trunk muscle activity during lifting. IV. The causal factors of the intra-abdominal pressure rise. Scand J Rehabil Med 17: 25–38.

Herschorn S. 2004. Female pelvic floor anatomy: the pelvic floor, supporting structures, and pelvic organs. Rev Urol 6: S2–S10.

Hides JA, Jull GA, Richardson CA. 2001. Long-term effects of specific stabilizing exercises for first episode low back pain. Spine 26: E243–E248.

Hides JA, Richardson CA, Jull GA. 1996. Multifidus muscle recovery is not automatic after resolution of acute, first-episode low back pain. Spine 21: 2763–2769.

Hodges PW, Gandevia S. 2000. Changes in intra-abdominal pressure during postural and respiratory activation of the human diaphragm. J Appl Physiol 89: 967–976.

Hodges PW, Richardson CA. 1996. Inefficient muscular stabilization of the lumbar spine associated with low back pain: a motor control evaluation of transversus abdominis. Spine 21: 2640–2650.

Hodges PW, Richardson CA. 1998. Delayed postural contraction of transversus abdominis in low back pain associated with movement of the lower limb. J Spinal Disord 11: 46–56.

Hodges PW, Sapsford R, Pengel LH. 2007. Postural and respiratory functions of the pelvic floor muscles. Neurourol Urodyn 26: 362–371.

Howard D, Miller JM, DeLancey JO, et al. 2000. Differential effects of cough, valsalva, and continence status on vesical neck movement. Obstet Gynecol 95: 535–540.

Howard FM. 2003. Chronic pelvic pain. Obstet Gynecol 101: 594–611.

Jones RC, 2003. The back detective. [Course notes and book in preparation.]

Jones RC, 2014. The back detective. [Course notes and book in preparation.]

Jones RC, Peng Q, Shishido K, et al. 2006. 2D ultrasound imaging and motion tracking of pelvic floor muscle activity during abdominal manoeuvres in stress urinary incontinent women [abstract]. Neurourol Urodyn 25: S72.

Kenton K, Brubaker L. 2002. Relationship between levator ani contraction and motor unit activation in the urethral sphincter. Am J Obstet Gynecol 187: 403–406.

Langford CF, Udvari Nagy S, Ghoniem GM. 2007. Levator ani trigger point injections: an underutilized treatment for chronic pelvic pain. Neurourol Urodyn 26: 59–62

Laycock J, Brown J, Cusack C, et al. 2001. Pelvic floor reeducation for stress incontinence: comparing three methods. Br J Community Nurs 6: 230–237.

Litwin MS. 2002. A review of the development and validation of the National Institutes of Health Chronic Prostatitis Symptom Index. Urology 60: S14–S18.

Litwin MS, McNaughton-Collins M, Fowler FJ Jr, et al. 1999. The National Institutes of Health Chronic Prostatitis Symptom Index: development and validation of a new outcome measure. Chronic Prostatitis Collaborative Research Network. J Urol 162(2): 369–375.

Martins JAC, Pato MPM, Pires EB, et al. 2007. Finite element studies of the deformation of the pelvic floor. Ann N Y Acad Sci 1101: 316–334.

McGill S. 2002. Low back disorders: evidence-based prevention and rehabilitation. Champaign, IL: Human Kinetics.

McKenzie R, May S. 2003. The lumbar spine: mechanical diagnosis and therapy, 2nd edn. Waikanae: Spinal Publications.

Moseley GL. 2008. Pain, brain imaging and physiotherapy: opportunity is knocking. Man Ther 13: 475–477.

Moseley GL, Hodges PW, Gandevia SC. 2002. Deep and superficial fibers of the lumbar multifidus muscle are differentially active during voluntary arm movements. Spine 27: E29–E36.

Nygaard I, Barber MD, Burgio KL, et al. 2008. Prevalence of symptomatic pelvic floor disorders in US women. JAMA 300: 1311–1316.

Olsen AL, Smith VJ, Bergstrom JO, et al. 1997. Epidemiology of surgically managed pelvic organ prolapse and urinary incontinence. Obstet Gynecol 89: 501–506.

O'Sullivan P. 2005. Diagnosis and classification of chronic low back pain disorders: maladaptive movement and motor control impairments as underlying mechanism. Man Ther 10: 242–255.

O'Sullivan PB, Beales DJ. 2007. Changes in pelvic floor and diaphragm kinematics and respiratory patterns in subjects with sacroiliac joint pain following a motor learning intervention: a case series. Man Ther 12: 209–218.

O'Sullivan PB, Beales DJ, Beetham JA, et al. 2002. Altered motor control strategies in subjects with sacroiliac joint pain during the active straight-leg-raise test. Spine 27: E1–E8.

Pattern D, Hughes J. 2008. Anatomy of the urogenital pain systems. In: Baranowski AP, Abrams P, Magnus F (eds) Urogenital pain in clinical practice. Boca Raton, FL: CRC / Informa Healthcare, pp 23–43.

Petros PE. 2007. The anatomy and dynamics of pelvic floor function and dysfunction. In: Petros PE (ed) The female pelvic floor: function, dysfunction and management according to the integral theory, 2nd edn. Würzburg: Springer Medizin Verlag, Ch 2, pp 17–76.

Planken E, Voorham-van der Zalm PJ, Lycklama A, et al. 2010. Chronic testicular pain as a symptom of pelvic floor dysfunction. J Urol 183: 177–181.

Pontari MA, Ruggieri MR. 2008. Mechanisms in prostatitis / chronic pelvic pain syndrome. J Urol 179: S61–S67.

Pool-Goudzwaard A, van Dijke GH, van GM, et al. 2004. Contribution of pelvic floor muscles to stiffness of the pelvic ring. Clin Biomech 19: 564–571.

Sahrmann SA. 2002. Diagnosis and treatment of movement impairment syndromes. Maryland Heights, MO: CV Mosby Elsevier.

Shafik A. 1998. A new concept of the anatomy of the anal sphincter mechanism and the physiology of defecation: mass contraction of the pelvic floor muscles. Int Urogynecol J Pelvic Floor Dysfunct 9: 28–32.

Shafik A. 2000. Neuronal innervation of urethral and anal sphincters: surgical anatomy and clinical implications. Curr Opin Obstet Gynecol 12: 387–398.
Shafik A, Asaad S, Doss S. 2002. The histomorphologic structure of the levator ani muscle and its functional significance. Int Urogynecol J 13: 116–124.
Shafik A, Doss S, Asaad S. 2003. Etiology of the resting myoelectric activity of the levator ani muscle: physioanatomic study with a new theory. World J Surg 27: 309–314.
Shafik A, Ahmed I, Shafik AA, et al. 2005. Surgical anatomy of the perineal muscles and their role in perineal disorders. Anat Sci Int 80: 167–171.
Smith MD, Russell A, Hodges PW. 2006. Disorders of breathing and continence have a stronger association with back pain than obesity and physical activity. Aust J Physiother 52: 11–16.
Smith MD, Coppieters MW, Hodges PW. 2007. Postural response of the pelvic floor and abdominal muscles in women with and without incontinence. Neurourol Urodyn 26: 377–385.
Smith MD, Russell A, Hodges PW. 2008. Is there a relationship between parity, pregnancy, back pain and incontinence? Int Urogynecol J 19: 205–211.
Smith MD, Russell A, Hodges P. 2009. Do incontinence, breathing difficulties and gastrointestinal symptoms increase the risk of future back pain? J Pain 10: 876–886.
Tsao H, Hodges PW. 2007. Immediate changes in feedforward postural adjustments following voluntary motor training. Exp Brain Res 181: 537–546.
Tsao H, Hodges PW. 2008. Persistence of improvements in postural strategies following motor control training in people with recurrent low back pain. J Electromyogr Kinesiol 18: 559–567.
Tsao H, Druitt TR, Schollum TM, et al. 2010. Motor training of the lumbar paraspinal muscles induces immediate changes in motor coordination in patients with recurrent low back pain. J Pain 11: 1120–1128.
Tu FF, As-Sanie S, Steege JF. 2006. Prevalence of pelvic musculoskeletal disorders in a female chronic pelvic pain clinic. J Reprod Med 51: 185–189.
Tubbs R, Miller J, Loukas M, et al. 2009. Surgical and anatomical landmarks for the perineal branch of the posterior femoral cutaneous nerve: implications in perineal pain syndromes. J Neurosurg 111: 332–335.
Van Dillen LR, Sahrmann SA, Norton BJ, et al. 1998. Reliability of physical examination items used for classification of patients with low back pain. Phys Ther 78: 979–988.
Van Dillen LR, Sahrmann SA, Norton BJ, et al. 2003. Movement system impairment-based categories for low back pain: stage 1 validation. J Orthop Sports Phys Ther 33: 126–142.
Walsh J, Ther M, Hall T. 2009. Agreement and correlation between the straight leg raise and slump tests in subjects with leg pain. J Manipulative Physiol Ther 32: 184–192.
Weiss JM. 2001. Pelvic floor myofascial trigger points: manual therapy for interstitial cystitis and the urgency-frequency syndrome. J Urol 166: 2226–2231.
Whelan M 2012. Practical anatomy, examination, palpation and manual therapy release techniques for the pelvic floor. In: Chaitow L, Lovegrove Jones R (eds) Chronic pelvic pain and dysfunction: practical physical medicine. London: Elsevier Churchill Livingstone, pp 311–338.

21 Chapter

Chronic Low Back Pain

Mark D. Bishop, Joel E. Bialosky, Charles W. Gay

CHAPTER CONTENTS

Introduction	236
Acute versus chronic low back pain	236
Altered nociceptive transmission in chronic low back pain	237
Neuroimaging in chronic low back pain	237
Manual interventions for chronic low back pain	239
Joint-biased manual therapies	239
Soft-tissue-biased manual therapies	240
Nerve-biased manual therapies	240
Factors associated with efficacy of interventions in chronic low back pain	241
Expectation	241
Patient preference	241
Patient–clinician relationship	242
Conclusion	242

Introduction

Low back pain is defined as pain, stiffness or discomfort primarily located below the 12th rib and above the inferior gluteal fold. There may or may not be leg pain, or sciatica, associated with low back pain. The taxonomy used describes an episode of pain including terms related to the temporal duration of the pain such as acute, subacute and chronic pain as well to the fluctuations in the intensity of the pain – recurrent and transient, for example (Von Korff & Saunders 1996).

Of particular interest in this chapter is chronic, constant low back pain, hereafter called chronic low back pain (cLBP). The primary description of cLBP is related to the temporal duration of the painful episode. For example, international health organizations such as the International Association for the Study of Pain (IASP 1986) and the World Health Organization (WHO) define chronic pain as pain that has persisted beyond normal tissue healing time (National Research Council of the National Academies 2008). The premise behind this definition is that, whatever the original insult to a peripheral tissue, it has mainly resolved. The IASP suggests that this resolution should have occurred after approximately 3 months, a length of time commonly used by other organizations such as the American Academy of Family Practitioners and Agency for Quality Healthcare. However, different groups have suggested as short a time as 7 weeks or as long as 6 months of pain is required to indicate the presence of cLBP (Van den Hoogen et al 1998; Andersson 1999; Walker 2000). Alternative definitions also may include criteria for the number of days that pain is experienced; for example, Von Korff and Saunders (1996) suggested that pain should be present for more than half the days within a 12-month period in either single or multiple episodes.

The result of these varied definitions regarding what actually constitutes cLBP is that studies of the prevalence of cLBP are difficult to compare. In such a way, using the criterion of 'pain lasting 6 months or more' epidemiological studies found a prevalence of 15%. Shorter lengths of time result in a more variable estimate of prevalence ranging from 4% to 24% (Juniper et al 2009). Despite this variation, cLBP remains a significant social and economic burden on healthcare systems worldwide and there is evidence that the prevalence is rising. For example, in the United States of America it was estimated that between 1992 and 2006 the prevalence of low back pain increased by 162%. This increase was driven by increases of 219% in the 45–54-year age group (Freburger et al 2009).

Acute versus Chronic Low Back Pain

A fundamental issue surrounding low back pain, both acute and chronic, is whether it is a symptom or a disease. It might suffice to say that, in general, acute low back pain is considered a symptom, and use of diagnostic studies to identify an underlying spinal pathology is not recommended, for two primary reasons: (1) most acute back pain episodes resolve over time, and (2) cross-sectional data and longitudinal studies have found poor associations between clinical outcomes and the presence of spinal pathology (Deyo 2002). The majority of clinical practice guidelines for low back pain endorse approaches where most patients (~90%) do not receive a pathoanatomical diagnosis, but instead receive the label 'non-specific low back pain'.

In contrast, chronic pain is argued to be a brain disease (Sullivan et al 2013); for example, the National Research Council of the National Academies (2008) stated, that regardless of where the initial injury occurred, including the lumbar spine, the functional, structural and chemical changes in the brain associated with chronic pain place it into the realm of disease state. Furthermore, a summary point in a report from the Institute of Medicine (2011, p 39) states 'chronic pain can be a disease itself'. A final example that exemplifies the current state of affairs comes from the website of the European Federation of the International Association for the Study of Pain (IASP), which states that, although acute pain may reasonably be considered a symptom of disease or injury, chronic and recurrent pain is a specific healthcare problem – a disease in its own right (http://www.efic.org/index.asp?sub=724B97A2EjBu1C).

The pathophysiology of cLBP remains poorly understood. As pointed out earlier, chronology is used to distinguish acute from chronic stages; however, the exact point when back pain moves from an acute (symptom) to a chronic (disease) stage looks less likely to be a simple matter of time. The lack of a developmental perspective in cLBP creates a chasm in the understanding of biological changes taking place between acute and chronic pain stages. Thus, the targeting of biological changes to prevent the 'chronification' of acute low back pain remains an unattainable goal. In the following sections, we will discuss insights and discoveries from two fields of research being applied to cLBP: quantitative sensory testing (QST) and neuroimaging. These fields have shed some light onto neurobiological differences that exist in individuals with persistent pain compared with individuals who are not experiencing pain. Further research is needed to determine whether these differences are indeed changes that evolve and contribute to pain persistence.

Altered Nociceptive Transmission in Chronic Low Back Pain

Quantitative sensory testing is the application of a quantifiable amount of a sensory modality to different tissues of the body, such as skin, muscle and viscera (Arendt-Nielsen & Yarnitsky 2009; Arendt-Nielsen & Graven-Nielsen 2011). Different sensory modalities can be used, such as thermal, mechanical, chemical, electrical and ischaemia. Pain sensitivity testing is a subcategory of QST, and records a psychophysical response to a quantifiable amount of stimulus. Psychophysical responses include the minimal amount of a stimulus to generate pain (threshold) the maximum amount of stimulus that is tolerable (tolerance) and / or the change in perceived intensity of pain to repeated stimulations (temporal summation) or multiple locations of stimulation (spatial summation).

Pain sensitivity tests can distinguish groups of patients with cLBP from groups of pain-free subjects. Patients with cLBP display increased sensitivity to stimulation of lumbar tissues (Clauw et al 1999; Kobayashi et al 2009; Blumenstiel et al 2011) and tissues distant from the site of pain – that is, the leg or the thumb (Giesecke et al 2004; O'Neill et al 2007). The rationale behind performing pain sensitivity tests in remote locations (i.e. outside the primary painful area) is that pain hypersensitivity detected after stimulation of healthy tissue is considered a consequence of alterations in central processing (Curatolo 2011). The increased sensitivity over both the lumbar spine and remote locations suggest cLBP is associated with widespread central hypersensitivity, which is abnormal central nervous system (CNS) processing of pain (Latremoliere & Woolf 2009). As measures of discrimination, several pain sensitivity tests have fair receiver-operating characteristics (ROC) and likelihood ratios. Those tests that may be useful include: pressure pain threshold at the site of most severe pain (fitted area under the ROC, 0.87), electrical stimulation pain threshold (ROC 0.87), pressure pain tolerance at the site of most severe pain (ROC 0.81), pressure pain threshold at remote (suprascapular) region (ROC 0.80) and temporal summation of pain (ROC 0.80) (Neziri et al 2012).

QST can also assess kinaesthesia (e.g. body awareness). For kinaesthesia, psychophysical responses are recorded to quantifiable amounts of stimulus, but these responses are not related to the perception of pain. Examples include the amount of vibration or pressure that is first perceivable (detection threshold), the minimum distance at which two separate stimuli can be identified (two-point discrimination) and the percentage agreement between the locations of a stimulus with reference to a marked body chart (localization).

People with cLBP have been shown to exhibit higher detection thresholds in the low back compared with a pain-free population (Blumenstiel et al 2011; Puta et al 2013). In locations remote from the low back, some have found higher detection thresholds (Puta et al 2013), whereas others have found no differences between healthy controls and cLBP (Blumenstiel et al 2011). For two-point discrimination, cLBP patients have been shown to require larger distances to perceive two stimuli being applied to the lumber spine as being distinct, compared with healthy controls (Wand et al 2010). In addition, cLBP patients are more likely to mislocalize sensory information delivered to the back than pain-free controls (Wand et al 2013). Although these sensory tests have been able to distinguish cLBP patients from healthy controls, none of the investigations found a relationship between the sensory tests and clinical profiles (Wand et al 2010, 2013; Blumenstiel et al 2011; Puta et al 2013).

Another subcategory of QST comprises electrophysiological reflexive tests, such as the nociceptive withdrawal reflex (NWR) and reflex receptive fields (RRF). These tests are used to assess nociceptive hyperexcitability. Decreases in the amount of stimulus to induce a withdrawal reflex and enlargement of the RRF are indicative of spinal cord hyperexcitability. The spinal hyperexcitability could be a consequence of an increased number of responsive spinal neurons or an expansion of the receptive fields of spinal neurons as a result of increased synaptic sensitivity.

Patients with cLBP display lower NWR thresholds to single and repeated electrical stimulation (Biurrun Manresa et al 2013). The discriminative ability of the single electrical stimulation reflex threshold is adequate, with an ROC of 0.83 (Neziri et al 2012). Compared with pain-free volunteers, patients with cLBP have demonstrated enlarged RRF in areas distant from the site of expected tissue damage, which indicates widespread spinal hyperexcitability (Biurrun Manresa et al 2013). An unexpected result is that patients with acute lower back pain demonstrate similar NWR and RFR differences compared with pain-free volunteers and no differences compared with patients with cLBP (Biurrun Manresa et al 2013).

Neuroimaging in Chronic Low Back Pain

Research from the field of neuroscience has provided evidence that subtle neurobiological differences exist between people with cLBP and pain-free volunteers. Neurobiology includes the study of the nervous system and how it is organized into functional circuits that process information and mediate behaviour. Differences in neurobiology between cLBP populations and pain-free volunteers have been investigated with advanced neuroimaging techniques such as magnetic resonance imaging (MRI) (Grachev et al 2000, 2002; Apkarian et al 2004; Giesecke et al 2004; Kobayashi et al 2009; Baliki et al 2011), positron emission tomography (PET) (Derbyshire et al 2002), magnetoencephalography (MEG) (Flor et al 1997) and a combination of transcranial magnetic stimulation (TMS) and intramuscular fine-wire electromyography (EMG) (Tsao et al 2008). These techniques have demonstrated differences in both cortical structure and function between cLBP populations and pain-free controls.

Differences in cortical structure have been assessed using MRI with two outcome measures: voxel-based morphometry (VBM) and diffusion tensor imaging (DTI). VBM estimates cortical and subcortical grey matter (GM) thickness and volume by parcellating structural MRI images; whereas DTI estimates fractional anisotrophy (FA), which is derived from a combination of intravoxel isotropy and intervoxel structural similarity. Using FA, a probability of movement is estimated and information on white matter (WM) tracts and structural connectivity is inferred (Basser & Pierpaoli 2011).

When comparing populations suffering cLBP with pain-free volunteers, structural differences have been found. Using VBM, both global (whole-brain) (Apkarian et al 2004) and regional (brain regions) (Apkarian et al 2004; Seminowicz et al 2011) GM differences have been found. In general, cLBP subjects show a decreased global GM volume (Apkarian et al 2004). Regional approaches in cLBP subjects have shown GM reductions in the left dorsal lateral prefrontal cortex, bilateral anterior insula, left frontal operculum, left posterior insula, left primary somatosensory cortex, left medial temporal lobe, bilateral thalami and right anterior cingulate cortex compared with age-matched control subjects (Apkarian et al 2004; Seminowicz et al 2011). DTI has also shown differences in the structural integrity of WM within regions of the superior and inferior longitudinal fasciculus and regions of the anterior and posterior cingulate cortices (Mansour et al 2013). These differences were found when comparing a group of 46 subacute low back pain subjects; in the cohort who continued to experience low back pain 1 year later, there were lower FA values in those regions of WM previously identified. However, the range of FA values in healthy controls includes both of the FA values in the subacute population. The extent to which the structural integrity of these WM regions predisposes individuals to a greater risk of chronicity needs further research.

Differences in cortical function have been assessed using MEG, a combination of TMS and intramuscular fine-wire EMG and functional MRI (fMRI). MEG has been used to assess the cortical representation of body areas in the primary somatosensory cortex. Using MEG, Flor et al (1997) showed that the cortical representation of the lumbar spine was shifted medially in cLBP subjects compared with that in pain-free volunteers. Using a combination of TMS and EMG, Tsao et al (2008) assessed the cortical representation (volume and centre of gravity) of the transverse abdominis muscle within the motor cortex in cLBP subjects. They found that cortical representation was larger (volume) and shifted posteriorly and laterally (centre of gravity) in cLBP subjects compared with pain-free volunteers. Researchers have speculated that these shifts in sensory and motor representations are representative of cortical reorganization – that is, neuroplasticity (Flor et al 1997; Tsao et al 2008).

Functional MRI has also been used to investigate differences in cortical function. fMRI measures the blood-oxygenation-level-dependent (BOLD) signal. This signal can be used to estimate cortical function, as neuronal activity is associated with local changes in cerebral blood flow, blood volume and blood oxygenation, termed the dynamic response (Kwong et al 1992). The haemodynamic response generates a typical change in the BOLD signal, the key link being the difference in magnetic properties between the oxygen-rich and oxygen-poor blood (Kwong et al 1992; Miezin et al 2000; Logothetis 2002).

To investigate cortical function, two analytical approaches are commonly used with fMRI BOLD signals. The first approach uses the timing of events to estimate whereabouts in the brain a haemodynamic response is occurring. To assess cortical regions involved in the processing and modulation of the pain experience, the event is typically the application of a noxious stimulus. An alternative approach is to take the time series of the BOLD signal from a cortical region and estimate the correlation (functional connectivity) with that in other cortical regions. This approach estimates the relationship of BOLD signal fluctuations between spatially distinct brain regions while at rest or during a task. Both approaches have been used in cLBP populations.

Using the first approach mentioned above, researchers have tailored the noxious stimulus in two different ways. The first method tailors the intensity of the stimulus to create equal sensations across subjects. The second method uses a standard amount of stimulus across subjects, which inevitably creates differences in the perceived intensity and unpleasantness. Tailoring the intensity of the stimulus to create equal sensations results in similar haemodynamic responses in activated brain regions between cLBP subjects and pain-free subjects; however, for the cLBP subjects the average stimulus intensity was significantly lower. When a standard stimulus was applied to all subjects, a greater haemodynamic response was seen in the brain regions of cLBP subjects compared with pain-free controls. In cLBP subjects, an increased BOLD signal was reported in the contralateral primary somatosensory cortex, secondary somatosensory cortex, inferior partial lobe, insula, anterior cingulate cortex and the ipsilateral secondary somatosensory cortex and cerebellum (Giesecke et al 2004; Gracely et al 2004; Kobayashi et al 2009). Researchers concluded that the augmented cortical activity is representative of sensitization of brain regions involved in nociception processing and modulation.

Using the second approach, researchers have found functional connectivity differences between cLBP subjects and pain-free controls during a cognitive task and at rest (Baliki et al 2008; Tagliazucchi et al 2010). During a cognitive task, cLBP subjects had less deactivation of the default mode network (DMN); in these individuals a region of the DMN, the medial prefrontal cortex, showed increased connectivity with brain regions that were active during the cognitive task compared with the control group (Baliki et al 2008). In another study, cLBP subjects at rest showed greater connectivity between the same DMN and the insular cortex bilaterally (Tagliazucchi et al 2010). Researchers have suggested these findings are representative of altered cortical function in subjects with cLBP.

Although there is clear evidence that brain function, structure and chemistry are amiss in people with cLBP, the extent to which they are modifiable to treatment is directly relevant for clinician-scientists. In cLBP subjects, brain structure has been shown to change and be more reflective of pain-free control subjects following successful pharmacological, injection and surgical interventions (Seminowicz et al 2011; Younger et al 2011); however, in those subjects where no improvement was seen, no change in structure was found. Functional brain changes have also been shown to recover in subjects after a therapeutic intervention. Sensory and motor representations in the cortex have been shown to shift following a course of specialized sensory discrimination and motor training; these interventions induce changes such that the cortical representations become more like those of pain-free controls (Flor & Diers 2009; Tsao et al 2010; Moseley & Flor 2012). Lastly, the haemodynamic response to noxious stimulus has been shown to change in cortical regions over time following a behavioural intervention (Jensen et al 2012). Thus, it can be stated that differences in brain structure and function identified in cLBP patients are reversible (i.e. do not reflect irreversible brain damage) and that the structural and functional differences appear to normalize when an individual's pain experience is adequately treated.

The transition of back pain from acute (symptom) to chronic (disease) stages remains poorly understood, and is an interesting research area that will hopefully be fruitful. However, taken together, the results from the fields of QST and neuroimaging provide a growing body of evidence suggesting that abnormalities of the nervous system are salient features of cLBP. Thus, classification of back pain by time alone appears overly simplistic and reliance on this approach appears to be a consequence of inadequate pathophysiological information. It is plausible that altered self-perception is maladaptive and contributes to the maintenance of cLBP, and may hence be a target for treatment.

Manual Interventions for Chronic Low Back Pain

In the United States, The National Center for Complementary and Alternative Medicine (NCCAM) has established categories for many non-pharmacological and non-surgical interventions for cLBP including mind–body medicine and manipulative and body-based interventions. Mind–body interventions pertinent in the context of the manual therapies are discussed in more detail in Chapter 6, whereas different spinal joint manipulation and mobilization interventions are described in Chapter 22; therefore, the focus of this chapter will be application of manipulative and body-based interventions by practitioners of manual therapies. Manual therapies include techniques that focus primarily on the structures and systems of the body, including the bones and joints (joint biased), the soft tissues (soft tissue biased), and the neurovascular system (nerve biased).

Joint-biased manual therapies

Joint-biased interventions include treatments such as spinal manipulation and mobilization applied either manually by practitioners or with the assistance of devices. These techniques provide passive movement of joints beyond their normal range of motion in the case of spinal manipulation and within its normal range of motion for spinal joint mobilization. In the United States of America, it is estimated that approximately 8.6% of the population see a practitioner providing this form of manual therapy, spending a total close to $3.9 billion annually (Nahin et al 2009); in fact, the most common condition or complaint for these visits was low back pain (17.8%). Lin et al (2011) found evidence supporting the cost effectiveness of spinal joint manipulation for cLBP.

Several large systematic reviews and meta-analyses have been performed of the effectiveness of manual therapies used to treat individuals with cLBP (Chou et al 2007; Rubinstein et al 2010; van Middelkoop et al 2011). One review for the Cochrane group, for example, focused on joint-biased techniques (Rubinstein et al 2011). The review group identified 26 clinical trials of sufficient quality to be included in the meta-analyses. (Meta-analysis is a method that allows the results of multiple studies to be combined to increase the statistical power to find real effects.) In this review the analyses included studies that used high-velocity low-amplitude techniques and low-amplitude low-velocity oscillation techniques to manage cLBP (Rubinstein et al 2011). The results of this meta-analysis indicated there was high-quality evidence that joint-biased techniques used alone have a short-term effect (1-month follow-up) on both pain relief and functional status compared with sham interventions and other therapeutic modalities. The mean difference (MD) between changes in pain for the joint-biased technique and the change in pain for the other interventions was −4.16 (95% CI −6.97 to −1.36). This indicates that for the joint-biased technique the average reduction in pain was 4.16 greater than with the other interventions (Rubinstein et al 2011). Mean differences are used when all the studies included in the meta-analysis use the same measurement, in this case for pain intensity. When different scales are used (e.g. the Oswestry Disability Index or the Roland Morris Disability Scale for disability), standardized mean differences are calculated (SMD) instead for meta-analysis purposes. For functional status, the SMD in the above review was −0.22 (95% CI −0.36 to −0.07) when compared with other interventions, indicating that the joint-biased techniques showed a 0.22 standard deviation improvement compared with the other interventions (Rubinstein et al 2011).

For pain, when a joint-biased technique was used alone, statistically significantly better pain relief was noted compared with other interventions at follow-up periods of both 1 and 6 months (MD −2.76, 95% CI −5.19 to −0.32 and MD −3.07, 95% CI −5.42 to −0.71, respectively). For functional status, there was high-quality evidence that joint-biased techniques alone provide statistically significantly better functional improvement at 1-month than do other interventions (SMD −0.17, 95% CI −0.29 to −0.06); however, this benefit is not apparent 3 and 6 months later. There was varying quality of evidence that a joint-biased technique has a significant short-term effect on pain relief and functional status when added to another intervention. However, there is little evidence that specific joint-biased techniques are superior to sham manual therapies when used in patients with cLBP in the long term (Rubinstein et al 2011).

Many readers may argue that the specifics of the techniques (thrust versus oscillation) should be considered because these categories of technique are theorized to effect change in pain through different mechanisms (Pickar 2002; Triano 2001). However, mechanistic theories of action alone cannot explain clinical improvement in patients with cLBP and more recent literature has focused on the neurological system (George et al 2006; Bialosky et al 2009). Specific analyses were also performed in the review to address the extent to which the type of technique (thrust or oscillatory mobilization) or type of practitioner might have modified the effects detected. However, those analyses showed that the technique or the practitioner had no influence on the pooled effects calculated, indicating similar effects both when comparing techniques and when comparing providers (Rubinstein et al 2011).

Williams et al (2007) completed a separate meta-analysis of trials that focused on the effect of joint-biased interventions on psychological factors such as depression, anxiety, self-efficacy and fear-avoidance beliefs as the outcomes of treatment. These authors reported that treatment with joint-biased techniques resulted in superior outcomes compared with a 'verbal intervention' (predominantly education interventions) at both short-term (SMD −0.33, 95% CI −0.47 to −0.19) and longer-term follow-up periods (SMD −0.27, 95% CI −0.40 to −0.14). Joint-biased interventions were also superior to simple exercises and to acupuncture (SMD −0.13, 95% CI −0.24 to −0.01 at 1–5 months and SMD −0.11, 95% CI −0.25 to −0.02 at 6–12 months) (Williams et al 2007). Similar to pain and functional status outcomes, there was no difference between the effects of joint-biased interventions and sham interventions when compared directly (Williams et al 2007).

It should be noted that all these reported effects were noted across heterogeneous groups of participants. Subgrouping of patients, to match treatments to patient signs and symptoms, is indicated to be an important factor to consider in acute low back pain episodes (Childs et al 2004). Whether this is also the case in cLBP has not been established; however, recent work by Cook et al (2013) would suggest that it is not. In summary, joint-biased techniques provide greater pain relief and better improvements in function than other therapeutic modalities and other interventions in the short term, suggesting faster rates of recovery in patients with cLBP.

Soft-tissue-biased manual therapies

Soft-tissue-biased therapies include techniques such as Swedish massage, deep tissue massage, trigger point therapy, shiatsu massage and various forms of myofascial treatments. These therapies are often manually applied, but can also be performed with instruments. In the United States approximately 8.3% of the population will see a practitioner who provides a soft-tissue-biased intervention, spending close to $4.2 billion annually (Nahin et al 2009). The most common condition / complaint for these visits is low back pain (17.3%).

A systematic review developed Ottawa Panel evidence-based clinical practice guidelines on therapeutic massage for low back pain (Brosseau et al 2012). The interventions considered included muscle-biased manual therapies (Swedish massage, fascial or connective tissue release techniques, cross-fibre friction and myofascial trigger point techniques). The included studies had to compare muscle-biased manual therapies with a control group that received no intervention, placebo (sham laser treatment), usual care, self-care education, relaxation therapy, sham manual therapy or exercise. In this review there were no direct comparisons of muscle-biased manual therapies to joint-biased techniques (Brosseau et al 2012). The Ottawa Panel was able to demonstrate that muscle-biased manual therapies were effective at providing short-term improvement of cLBP symptoms and decreasing disability immediately post treatment, and short-term relief when muscle-biased manual therapy was combined with therapeutic exercise and education. In fact, this conclusion was previously suggested by the Cochrane systematic review that concluded massage can be beneficial in the management of non-specific low back pain (Furlan et al 2008).

Cherkin et al (2011) investigated structural massage (myofascial, neuromuscular and other soft tissue techniques) compared with usual care (no massage interventions) and demonstrated clinically important benefits, with decreases in both disability and symptom bothersomeness. The strongest evidence of benefit was at the end of treatment at 10 weeks (MD −2.5, 95% CI −3.56 to −1.44), with little evidence of longer-term benefits at 16 or 42 weeks after the intervention. When relaxation massage (effleurage, petrissage, circular friction, vibration, rocking and jostling, and holding) was compared with control (usual care), clinically important benefits were demonstrated at 10 weeks for improved symptoms (symptom bothersomeness score) and decreased disability was demonstrated at 10, 16 and 42 weeks after treatment.

Little et al (2008) investigated therapeutic massage techniques (practitioners could choose from effleurage, kneading, petrissage, percussion, and neuromuscular trigger point release) versus normal care (no massage). This study demonstrated clinically important benefits in terms of decreased disability at 12 weeks but not at 40 weeks. Preyde (2000) compared soft-tissue manipulation with sham laser treatment in patients with subacute low back pain. This author showed there were clinically important benefits demonstrated for the improvement of pain intensity and quality, and decreased disability, in subjects treated with the soft tissue techniques. This study also compared comprehensive massage therapy (massage, remedial exercise and posture education) to exercise and posture education. There were also clinically important benefits demonstrated for the improvement of pain and quality, and decreased disability. Readers can find several soft-tissue biased interventions targeted to myofascial trigger points in Chapter 60. In summary, soft-tissue-biased manual therapies provide greater benefits to patients with cLBP compared with usual care and postural exercises.

Nerve-biased manual therapies

Nerve-biased techniques use passive, active or a combined movement of the spine and / or extremities within their normal range of motion, in ways to elongate, slide, glide, stretch or tension neural structures. These techniques are often referred to as neural mobilization. Unlike muscle- and joint-biased therapies, where professions are somewhat linked with those treatments (massage therapists for soft tissue biased and chiropractors for joint biased), nerve-biased therapies are often incorporated along with other manual therapies. As such there is a lack of data on the usage of or expenditures on nerve-biased therapies. (Readers are referred to Chs 64 and 65 for more details on clinical neurodynamic applications.)

No systematic reviews or meta-analyses related to nerve-biased interventions for cLBP have been identified. Cleland et al (2006) found that the addition of slump stretching (a form of neural mobilization) to a treatment regimen of spinal mobilization and exercise twice per week for 3 weeks in patients with non-radicular low back pain and mild to moderate neural mechanosensitivity (n=16) produced greater improvements at the end of the treatment in disability, pain reduction and centralization of symptoms compared with patients who did not receive neural mobilization (n=14). A recent study by Schäfer et al (2011) indicated that, in patients with peripheral nerve sensitization, neural mobilizations (sliding techniques) may provide benefit in reducing pain and disability, compared with other patients with back and leg pain. Using a similar study design as Cleland et al (2006) but a larger sample (n=60), Nagrale et al (2012) found that the addition of slump stretching to a regimen of spinal mobilization and exercise for patients with non-radicular low back pain with duration >3 months resulted in greater improvement at 3 and 6 weeks in disability, pain reduction and fear-avoidance belief attenuation compared with patients receiving only spinal mobilization and exercise.

Factors Associated with Efficacy of Interventions in Chronic Low Back Pain

Studies investigating the effectiveness of interventions for individuals experiencing cLBP often conclude that treatment is better than no treatment; however, the effects of individual interventions have not been distinguished (Chou et al 2007) and are associated with small-to-moderate effect sizes (Keller et al 2007; Machado et al 2009). This is consistent with the research presented above. Specifically in manual therapy studies, similar clinical outcomes are observed in response to differing techniques (Kent et al 2005) and variable physical parameters of the same technique (Hessell et al 1990; Ngan et al 2005). Collectively, these findings suggest that the treatment process may be more important than the specific manual therapy intervention for individuals experiencing cLBP.

Factors related to the treatment process include individual preference, expectation of treatment effectiveness, and the relationship between patient and healthcare provider (Preference Collaborative Review Group 2008). These factors are all influential in the effectiveness of all interventions for pain. For example, pain medication is significantly more effective when provided by a healthcare provider who is visible to a patient than when the patient is unaware that he or she is receiving the medication (Colloca et al 2004). Treatment contextual factors may be manipulated to influence clinical outcomes; specifically, pain reduction in response to placebo is significantly enhanced when individuals are instructed to expect pain relief (Vase et al 2009, Kaptchuk et al 2008a) or when accompanied by an augmented interaction with the treating healthcare provider (Kaptchuk et al 2008b). Furthermore, the analgesic effect of a medication may be abolished when an individual expects more pain (Bingel et al 2011). The following sections will review the literature related to specific contextual factors with the potential to influence treatment responses to interventions for individuals presenting with cLBP.

Expectation

Expectation is what a patient believes will occur and is prognostic for LBP-related outcomes. For example, systematic reviews have concluded expectations are predictive of work-related outcomes (Iles et al 2008) and functional outcomes (Iles et al 2009) in individuals with non-chronic LBP. Specific to cLBP, expectations are predictive of missed work time (Kuijer et al 2006) and response to conservative interventions (Goossens et al 2005; Linde et al 2007; Smeets et al 2008). Expectation may also mediate outcomes of specific interventions. Kalauokalani et al (2001) randomly assigned 135 individuals with cLBP to receive either acupuncture or massage. Group-related differences were not observed in the primary outcome related to function; however, participants with greater expectation for acupuncture who received acupuncture exhibited significantly better outcomes than those with higher expectation for massage who received acupuncture and vice versa. The placebo literature suggests these types of expectations may be manipulated to influence pain. The effect size of placebo analgesia is small in placebo control studies in which participants are told to expect a 50% chance of receiving a placebo – that is, 'you are going to receive the active treatment or a placebo' (Vase et al 2009). In contrast, placebo analgesia is much larger in studies of placebo in which an instructional set aimed at enhancing expectation is used (Vase et al 2009); for example, saline provided along with the instructional set, 'the agent you have just been given is known to significantly reduce pain in some patients', was as effective as lidocaine in reducing pain sensitivity in participants with irritable bowel syndrome (Vase et al 2003). Collectively, this body of literature suggests that expectation is a prognostic factor for cLBP, may mediate the results of treatment for cLBP and is perhaps a treatment target itself for enhancing the effectiveness of rehabilitation interventions.

Patient preference

Patient preferences are closely related to expectations (Lurie et al 2008; Sherman et al 2010), and preference for a given intervention enhances the likelihood of success in response to that intervention. A systematic review and meta-analysis concluded that better outcomes occurred in individuals receiving a preferred treatment than in those with no preference and in those not receiving their preferred treatment (Preference Collaborative Review Group 2008). However, individual studies have not consistently determined preference as influential in clinical outcomes for subjects with low back pain. Donaldson et al (2013) randomly assigned 149 patients with low back pain to receive either thrust manipulation with exercise or non-thrust manipulation with exercise. Participant preference for thrust or non-thrust manipulation was not associated with any of the studied outcomes. Generally, the literature suggests that patient preference is a similar construct to expectation. Although not investigated as extensively, patient preference is associated with outcomes related to musculoskeletal pain; however, it is not consistently associated with outcomes related to low back pain.

Patient–clinician relationship

The relationship between the patient and healthcare provider may also influence clinical outcomes (Di Blasi et al 2001; Hall et al 2010). For example, in one study 200 primary care patients presenting with symptoms without signs were randomly assigned to receive a positive consultation (physician provided a diagnosis and assurance of rapid improvement) or a negative consultation (physician expressed uncertainty as to the diagnosis and uncertainty as to the likely response to treatment). Sixty-four per cent of the participants receiving the positive consultation were better in 2 weeks, whereas only 39% of participants receiving the negative consultation were better within the same time (Thomas 1987). Similarly, a systematic review concluded 'Physicians who adopt a warm, friendly, and reassuring manner are more effective than those who keep consultations formal and do not offer reassurance' (Di Blasi et al 2001). The placebo literature suggests that the clinician–patient relationship may be manipulated so as to enhance clinical outcomes. A study of 262 individuals with irritable bowel syndrome randomly assigned participants to a waiting list, placebo acupuncture with limited clinician–patient interaction, and a waiting list with augmented patient–clinician interaction (Kaptchuk et al 2008a). The augmented interaction consisted of several questions related to symptoms, interference with daily activities and relationships, and the patient's understanding of the condition. The augmented interaction was provided in a warm manner with active listening and expression of empathy by the healthcare provider along with communication of confidence in the patient's likelihood of benefiting from the intervention. Participants receiving the placebo with augmented interaction demonstrated significantly better clinical outcomes at 3 weeks than those on the waiting list and those receiving the placebo with limited interaction (Kaptchuk et al 2008b). In a study of low back pain, the relationship between the physical therapist and the patient as measured at the second treatment session was predictive of the clinical outcome at 8 weeks (Ferreira et al 2013). Furthermore, the clinical efficacy of interferential electrical stimulation is significantly greater when provided with an augmented interaction than when provided with limited clinician–patient interaction. Collectively, this body of scientific literature suggests that the patient–clinician interaction affects clinical outcomes and may be manipulated to enhance the effectiveness of interventions for pain.

Conclusion

As mentioned previously, low back pain is a heterogeneous condition often lacking an identifiable anatomical basis (Deyo 2002). Subsequently, a pathoanatomical diagnosis is generally not helpful for directing treatment, necessitating treatment approaches focused upon identifying those individuals likely to respond positively to a particular intervention (Deyo et al 2009). Also relatively small effect sizes are associated with treatments for cLBP (Keller et al 2007; Machado et al 2009) and so there is uncertainty about which intervention is best for which patient with cLBP. As indicated above, manual therapies targeting different tissues may have similar overall effects when compared with inert interventions, but no one outperforms the others. In other words, choosing to perform a manual therapy for a patient with cLBP provides better outcomes than not performing any manual therapy; however, the particular therapy chosen may not be as important. In addition, consideration and management of treatment contextual factors are warranted, such as the patient's preference and expectations for the interventions provided, and the therapeutic relationship between patient and therapist. Consideration of these factors may both enhance outcomes to specific interventions and aid in determining the best intervention for a given patient.

References

Andersson GB. 1999. Epidemiological features of chronic low-back pain. Lancet 354: 581–585.

Apkarian AV, Sosa Y, Sonty S, et al. 2004. Chronic back pain is associated with decreased prefrontal and thalamic gray matter density. J Neurosci 24: 10410–10415.

Arendt-Nielsen L, Graven-Nielsen T. 2011. Translational musculoskeletal pain research. Best Pract Res Clin Rheumatol 25: 209–226.

Arendt-Nielsen L, Yarnitsky D. 2009. Experimental and clinical applications of quantitative sensory testing applied to skin, muscles and viscera. J Pain 10: 556–572.

Baliki MN, Geha PY, Apkarian AV, et al. 2008. Beyond feeling: chronic pain hurts the brain, disrupting the default-mode network dynamics. J Neurosci 28: 1398–1403.

Baliki MN, Baria AT, Apkarian AV. 2011. The cortical rhythms of chronic back pain. J Neurosci 31: 13981–13990.

Basser PJ, Pierpaoli C. 2011. Microstructural and physiological features of tissues elucidated by quantitative-diffusion-tensor MRI. J Magn Reson 213: 560–570.

Bialosky JE, Bishop MD, Robinson ME, et al. 2009. Spinal manipulative therapy has an immediate effect on thermal pain sensitivity in people with low back pain: a randomized controlled trial. Phys Ther 89: 1292–1303.

Bingel U, Wanigasekera V, Wiech K, et al. 2011. The effect of treatment expectation on drug efficacy: imaging the analgesic benefit of the opioid remifentanil. Sci Transl Med 3: 70ra14. doi:10.1126/scitranslmed.3001244.

Biurrun Manresa JA, Neziri AY, Curatolo M, et al. 2013. Reflex receptive fields are enlarged in patients with musculoskeletal low back and neck pain. Pain 154: 1318–1324.

Blumenstiel K, Gerhardt A, Rolke R, et al. 2011. Quantitative sensory testing profiles in chronic back pain are distinct from those in fibromyalgia. Clin J Pain 27: 682–690.

Brosseau L, Wells GA, Poitras S, et al. 2012. Ottawa Panel evidence-based clinical practice guidelines on therapeutic massage for low back pain. J Bodyw Mov Ther 16: 424–455.

Cherkin DC, Sherman KJ, Kahn J, et al. 2011. A comparison of the effects of 2 types of massage and usual care on chronic low back pain: a randomized, controlled trial. Ann Intern Med 155: 1–9.

Childs JD, Fritz JM, Flynn TW, et al. 2004. A clinical prediction rule to identify patients with low back pain most likely to benefit from spinal manipulation: a validation study. Ann Intern Med 141: 920–928.

Chou R, Huffman LH; American Pain Society; American College of Physicians. 2007. Non-pharmacologic therapies for acute and chronic low back pain: a review of the evidence for an American Pain Society / American College of Physicians clinical practice guideline. Ann Intern Med 147: 492–504.

Clauw DJ, Williams D, Lauerman W, et al. 1999. Pain sensitivity as a correlate of clinical status in individuals with chronic low back pain. Spine 24: 2035–2041.

Cleland JA, Childs JD, Palmer JA, et al. 2006. Slump stretching in the management of non-radicular low back pain: a pilot clinical trial. Man Ther 11: 2792–2796.

Colloca L, Lopiano L, Lanotte M, et al. 2004. Overt versus covert treatment for pain, anxiety, and Parkinson's disease. Lancet Neurol 3: 679–684.

Cook CE, Learman KE, O'Halloran BJ, et al. 2013. Which prognostic factors for low back pain are generic predictors of outcome across a range of recovery domains? Phys Ther 93: 32–40.

Curatolo M. 2011. Diagnosis of altered central pain processing. Spine 36: S200–S204.
Derbyshire SWG, Jones AKP, Creed F, et al. 2002. Cerebral responses to noxious thermal stimulation in chronic low back pain patients and normal controls. Neuroimage 16: 158–168.
Deyo RA. 2002. Diagnostic evaluation of LBP: reaching a specific diagnosis is often impossible: Arch Intern Med 162: 1444–1447.
Deyo RA, Mirza SK, Turner JA, et al. 2009. Overtreating chronic back pain: time to back off? J Am Board Fam Med 22: 62–68.
Di Blasi Z, Harkness E, Ernst E, et al. 2001. Influence of context effects on health outcomes: a systematic review. Lancet 357: 757–762.
Donaldson M, Learman K, O'Halloran B, et al. 2013. The role of patients' expectation of appropriate initial manual therapy treatment in outcomes for patients with low back pain. J Manipulative Physiol Ther 36: 276–283.
Ferreira PH, Ferreira ML, Maher CG, et al. 2013. The therapeutic alliance between clinicians and patients predicts outcome in chronic low back pain. Phys Ther 93: 470–478.
Flor H, Diers M. 2009. Sensorimotor training and cortical reorganization. Neurorehabilitation 25: 19–27.
Flor H, Braun C, Elbert T, et al. 1997. Extensive reorganization of primary somatosensory cortex in chronic back pain patients. Neurosci Lett 224: 5–8.
Freburger JK, Holmes GM, Agans RP, et al. 2009. The rising prevalence of chronic low back pain. Arch Intern Med 169: 251–258.
Furlan AD, Imamura M, Dryden T, et al. 2008. Massage for low-back pain. Cochrane Database Syst Rev 4: CD001929.
George SZ, Bishop MD, Bialosky JE, et al. 2006. Immediate effects of spinal manipulation on thermal pain sensitivity: an experimental study. BMC Musculoskelet Disord 7: 68.
Giesecke T, Gracely RH, Grant MA, et al. 2004. Evidence of augmented central pain processing in idiopathic chronic low back pain. Arthritis Rheum 50: 613–623.
Goossens ME, Vlaeyen JW, Hidding A, et al. 2005. Treatment expectancy affects the outcome of cognitive-behavioral interventions in chronic pain. Clin J Pain 21: 18–26.
Gracely RH, Geisser ME, Giesecke T, et al. 2004. Pain catastrophizing and neural responses to pain among persons with fibromyalgia. Brain 127: 835–843.
Grachev ID, Fredrickson BE, Apkarian AV. 2000. Abnormal brain chemistry in chronic back pain: an in vivo proton magnetic resonance spectroscopy study. Pain 89: 7–18.
Grachev ID, Fredrickson BE, Apkarian AV. 2002. Brain chemistry reflects dual states of pain and anxiety in chronic low back pain. J Neural Trans 109: 1309–1334.
Hall AM, Ferreira PH, Maher CG, et al. 2010. The influence of the therapist–patient relationship on treatment outcome in physical rehabilitation: a systematic review. Phys Ther 90: 1099–1110.
Hessell BW, Herzog W, Conway PJ, et al. 1990. Experimental measurement of the force exerted during spinal manipulation using the Thompson technique. J Manipulative Physiol Ther 13: 448–453.
Institute of Medicine of the National Academies. 2011. Relieving pain in America: a blueprint for transforming prevention, care, education, and research. Washington, DC: IOM, p 39.
IASP: International Association for the Study of Pain. 1986. Classification of chronic pain. Descriptions of chronic pain syndromes and definitions of pain terms. Prepared by the International Association for the Study of Pain, Subcommittee on Taxonomy. Pain 3: S1–S226.
Iles RA, Davidson M, Taylor NF. 2008. Psychosocial predictors of failure to return to work in non-chronic non-specific low back pain: a systematic review. Occup Environ Med 65: 507–517.
Iles RA, Davidson M, Taylor NF, et al. 2009. Systematic review of the ability of recovery expectations to predict outcomes in non-chronic non-specific low back pain. J Occup Rehabil 19: 25–40.
Jensen KB, Kosek E, Wicksell R, et al. 2012. Cognitive behavioral therapy increases pain-evoked activation of the prefrontal cortex in patients with fibromyalgia. Pain 153: 1495–1503.
Juniper M, Le TK, Mladsi D. 2009. The epidemiology, economic burden, and pharmacological treatment of chronic low back pain in France, Germany, Italy, Spain and the UK: a literature-based review. Expert Opin Pharmacother 10: 2581–2592.
Kalauokalani D, Cherkin DC, Sherman KJ, et al. 2001. Lessons from a trial of acupuncture and massage for low back pain: patient expectations and treatment effects. Spine 26: 1418–1424.
Kaptchuk TJ, Kelley JM, Deykin A, et al. 2008a. Do 'placebo responders' exist? Contemp Clin Trials 29: 587–595.
Kaptchuk TJ, Kelley JM, Conboy LA, et al. 2008b. Components of placebo effect: randomised controlled trial in patients with irritable bowel syndrome. BMJ 336: 999–1003.
Keller A, Hayden J, Bombardier C, et al. 2007. Effect sizes of non-surgical treatments of non-specific low-back pain. Eur Spine J 16: 1776–1788.
Kent P, Marks D, Pearson W, et al. 2005. Does clinician treatment choice improve the outcomes of manual therapy for nonspecific low back pain? A meta-analysis. J Manipulative Physiol Ther 28: 312–322.
Kobayashi Y, Kurata J, Sekiguchi M, et al. 2009. Augmented cerebral activation by lumbar mechanical stimulus in chronic low back pain patients: an fMRI study. Spine 34: 2431–2436.
Kuijer W, Brouwer S, Preuper HR, et al. 2006. Work status and chronic low back pain: exploring the International Classification of Functioning, Disability and Health. Disabil Rehabil 28: 379–388.
Kwong KK, Belliveau JW, Chesler DA, et al. 1992. Dynamic magnetic resonance imaging of human brain activity during primary sensory stimulation. Proc Natl Acad Sci USA 89: 5675–5679.
Latremoliere A, Woolf CJ. 2009. Central sensitization: a generator of pain hypersensitivity by central neural plasticity. J Pain 10: 895–926.
Lin CW, Haas M, Maher CG, et al. 2011. Cost-effectiveness of guideline-endorsed treatments for low back pain: a systematic review. Eur Spine J 20: 1024–1038.
Linde K, Witt CM, Streng A, et al. 2007. The impact of patient expectations on outcomes in four randomized controlled trials of acupuncture in patients with chronic pain. Pain 128: 264–271.
Little P, Lewith G, Webley F, et al. 2008. Randomised controlled trial of Alexander technique lessons, exercise, and massage (ATEAM) for chronic and recurrent back pain. BMJ 337: A884.
Logothetis NK. 2002. The neural basis of the blood-oxygen-level-dependent functional magnetic resonance imaging signal. Philos Trans R Soc Lond B Biol Sci 357: 1003–1037.
Lurie JD, Berven SH, Gibson-Chambers J, et al. 2008. Patient preferences and expectations for care: determinants in patients with lumbar intervertebral disc herniation. Spine 33: 2663–2668.
Machado LA, Kamper SJ, Herbert RD, et al. 2009. Analgesic effects of treatments for non-specific low back pain: a meta-analysis of placebo-controlled randomized trials. Rheumatology 48: 520–527.
Mansour AR, Baliki MN, Huang L, et al. 2013. Brain white matter structural properties predict transition to chronic pain. Pain 154: 2160–2168.
Miezin FM, Maccotta L, Ollinger JM, et al. 2000. Characterizing the hemodynamic response: effects of presentation rate, sampling procedure, and the possibility of ordering brain activity based on relative timing. Neuroimage 11: 735–759.
Moseley GL, Flor H. 2012. Targeting cortical representations in the treatment of chronic pain: a review. Neurorehabil Neural Repair 26: 646–652.
Nagrale AV, Patil SP, Gandhi RA, et al. 2012. Effect of slump stretching versus lumbar mobilization with exercise in subjects with non-radicular low back pain: a randomized clinical trial. J Man Manip Ther 20: 35–42.
Nahin RL, Barnes PM, Stussman BJ, et al. 2009. Costs of complementary and alternative medicine (CAM) and frequency of visits to CAM practitioners: United States, 2007. Natl Health Stat Report 18: 1–14.
National Research Council of the National Academies. 2008. Emerging cognitive neuroscience and related technologies. Washington, DC: National Academies Press.
Neziri AY, Curatolo M, Limacher A, et al. 2012. Ranking of parameters of pain hypersensitivity according to their discriminative ability in chronic low back pain. Pain 153: 2083–2091.
Ngan JM, Chow DH, Holmes AD. 2005. The kinematics and intra- and inter-therapist consistencies of lower cervical rotational manipulation. Med Eng Phys 27: 395–401.
O'Neill S, Manniche C, Graven-Nielsen T, et al. 2007. Generalized deep-tissue hyperalgesia in patients with chronic low-back pain. Eur J Pain 11: 415–420.
Pickar JG. 2002. Neurophysiological effects of spinal manipulation. Spine J 2: 357–371.
Preference Collaborative Review Group. 2008. Patients' preferences within randomised trials: systematic review and patient level meta-analysis. BMJ 337: A1864.
Preyde M. 2000. Effectiveness of massage therapy for sub-acute low-back pain: a randomized controlled trial. CMAJ 162: 1815–1820.
Puta C, Schulz B, Schoeler S, et al. 2013. Somatosensory abnormalities for painful and innocuous stimuli at the back and at a site distinct from the region of pain in chronic back pain patients. PLoS One 8: e58885.
Rubinstein SM, van Middelkoop M, Assendelft WJ, et al. 2011. Spinal manipulative therapy for chronic low-back pain: an update of a Cochrane review. Spine 36: E825–E846.

Rubinstein SM, van Middelkoop M, Kuijpers T, et al. 2010. A systematic review on the effectiveness of complementary and alternative medicine for chronic non-specific low back pain. Eur J Spine 19: 1213–1228.

Schäfer A, Hall T, Müller G, et al. 2011. Outcomes differ between subgroups of patients with low back and leg pain following neural manual therapy: a prospective cohort study. Eur Spine J 20: 482–490.

Seminowicz DA, Wideman TH, Naso L, et al. 2011. Effective treatment of chronic low back pain in humans reverses abnormal brain anatomy and function. J Neurosci 31: 7540–7550.

Sherman KJ, Cherkin DC, Ichikawa L, et al. 2010. Treatment expectations and preferences as predictors of outcome of acupuncture for chronic back pain. Spine 35: 1471–1477.

Smeets RJ, Beelen S, Goossens ME, et al. 2008. Treatment expectancy and credibility are associated with the outcome of both physical and cognitive-behavioral treatment in chronic low back pain. Clin J Pain 24: 305–315.

Sullivan MD, Cahana A, Derbyshire S, et al. 2013. What does it mean to call chronic pain a brain disease? J Pain 14: 317–322.

Tagliazucchi E, Balenzuela P, Fraiman D, et al. 2010. Brain resting state is disrupted in chronic back pain patients. Neurosci Lett 485: 26–31.

Thomas KB. 1987. General practice consultations: is there any point in being positive? BMJ 294: 1200–1202.

Triano JJ. 2001. Biomechanics of spinal manipulative therapy. Spine J 1: 121–130.

Tsao H, Galea MP, Hodges PW. 2008. Reorganization of the motor cortex is associated with postural control deficits in recurrent low back pain. Brain 131: 2161–2171.

Tsao H, Galea MP, Hodges PW. 2010. Driving plasticity in the motor cortex in recurrent low back pain. Eur J Pain 14(8): 832–839.

Van den Hoogen HJ, Koes BW, van Eijk JT, et al. 1998. On the course of low back pain in general practice: a one year follow up study. Ann Rheum Dis 57: 13–19.

van Middelkoop M, Rubinstein SM, Kuijpers T, et al. 2011. A systematic review on the effectiveness of physical and rehabilitation interventions for chronic non-specific low back pain. Eur Spine J 20: 19–39.

Vase L, Robinson ME, Verne G, et al. 2003. The contributions of suggestion, desire, and expectation to placebo effects in irritable bowel syndrome patients: an empirical investigation. Pain 105: 17–25.

Vase L, Petersen GL, Riley JL 3rd, et al. 2009. Factors contributing to large analgesic effects in placebo mechanism studies conducted between 2002 and 2007. Pain 145: 36–44.

Von Korff M, Saunders K. 1996. The course of back pain in primary care. Spine 21: 2833–2837.

Walker BF. 2000. The prevalence of low back pain: a systematic review of the literature from 1966 to 1998. J Spinal Disord 13: 205–217.

Wand BM, Di Pietro F, George P, et al. 2010. Tactile thresholds are preserved yet complex sensory function is impaired over the lumbar spine of chronic non-specific low back pain patients: a preliminary investigation. Physiotherapy 96: 317–323.

Wand BM, Keeves J, Bourgoin C, et al. 2013. Mislocalization of sensory information in people with chronic low back pain: a preliminary investigation. Clin J Pain 29: 737–743.

Williams NH, Hendry M, Lewis R, et al. 2007. Psychological response in spinal manipulation (PRISM): a systematic review of psychological outcomes in randomised controlled trials. Complement Ther Med 15: 271–283.

Younger JW, Chu LF, D'Arcy NT, et al. 2011. Prescription opioid analgesics rapidly change the human brain. Pain 152: 1803–1810.

Chapter 22

Joint Mobilization and Manipulation of the Lumbar Spine

Emilio J. Puentedura

CHAPTER CONTENTS

Towards standardizing nomenclature	245
Evidence for spinal manipulative therapy	246
Clinical prediction rules	246
The audible pop	248
Spinal positioning and locking	248
Safety and manipulative techniques	249
Contraindications and precautions	249
Spinal mobilization and manipulation techniques	250
Central posterior-to-anterior mobilization	250
Unilateral posterior-to-anterior mobilization	250
Lumbar rotation mobilization: grades I–IV	251
Lumbopelvic regional manipulation	251
Lumbar rotation in neutral or extension manipulation	252
Lumbar rotation in flexion manipulation	252
Conclusion	253

Towards Standardizing Nomenclature

Spinal manipulative therapy (SMT) has a very rich and diverse history. It has long been practised by a wide variety of clinicians including physical therapists, physicians, osteopathic physicians, chiropractors, and even massage therapists and laypersons. The problem is that there are many and varied definitions for the term 'spinal manipulative therapy'. To some extent, the definitions used have depended upon the practitioner applying the technique: the chiropractic profession has traditionally called it 'spinal adjustment', the osteopathic profession has used the term 'high-velocity low-amplitude (HVLA) thrust manipulation', and physical therapists have called it either 'spinal manipulation' or 'grade V spinal mobilization'. Descriptions of the actual SMT techniques performed by the various professions have also been extremely diverse and often based upon each individual profession's theoretical constructs and schemata.

This confusion surrounding manipulation terminology led to a call for a more standardized nomenclature in the physical therapy profession, and in 2008 the American Academy of Orthopedic Manual Physical Therapists (AAOMPT) formed a task force to develop a model for standardizing manipulation terminology in physical therapy practice (Mintken et al 2008). The task force proposed that orthopaedic manual physical therapists use six characteristics when describing a manipulative technique. These included:

1. Rate of force application – a description of the rate at which the force should be applied
2. Location in range of the available movement – a description of the point in the range at which the motion is intended to occur, e.g. at the beginning, towards the middle or at the end point of the available range of movement
3. Direction of the force – a description of the direction in which the therapist imparts the force
4. Target of the force – a description of the location at which the therapist intends to apply the force; this may be a specific spinal level, or more generally across a particular region of the spine, e.g. lower lumbar
5. Relative structural movement – a description of which structure (or region) is intended to remain stable and which structure (or region) is intended to move; the moving structure (or region) is described first and the stable segment second, separated by the word 'on', e.g. lower cervical spine on the upper thoracic spine
6. Patient position – a description of the position of the patient, e.g. supine, left side-lying, or prone.

Although the model proposed by the AAOMPT task force provided a step in the right direction towards improving accuracy and consistency in describing these interventions within the physical therapy profession, it remains to be seen whether it will serve as a bridge for improving descriptions of these interventions between the various professions.

Most clinicians would agree that there is a difference between spinal manipulation and spinal mobilization. Manipulation of the spine is said to differ from mobilization because, theoretically, during a manipulation the rate of vertebral joint displacement does not allow the patient to prevent joint movement (Maitland 1986). Mobilization of the spine involves cyclic, rhythmic, low-velocity (non-thrust) passive motion that can be stopped by the patient (Maitland 1986). Therefore, the speed of the technique (not necessarily the amount of force) is what should differentiate a manipulative technique from a mobilization technique.

Evidence for Spinal Manipulative Therapy

Despite a recent upsurge in clinical research into the efficacy of SMT for mechanical low back pain (LBP), results remain equivocal at best. It is sad to note that there is still a persistent myth within the medical community that 'most people with LBP will get better no matter what you do'. This has been based upon clinical experience, where family physicians would note that 9 out of 10 patients with an acute episode of non-specific LBP would recover (no matter what treatment was administered) within a month or two. However, a British study involving 490 individuals consulting their general practitioner (family physician) with LBP found that, whereas 92% of the individuals discontinued consultation within 3 months, only 20% had fully recovered within 12 months (Croft et al 1998). Another similar study followed 323 patients with LBP receiving physical therapy or chiropractic treatment. The study found that only 18% of patients reported no recurrence of symptoms over 1 year, and 58% sought additional healthcare (Skargren et al 1998). These, and similar studies, should effectively dispel the myth that LBP is a self-limiting condition and indicate that it deserves early attention in order to avoid longer-term disability. There is now a common consensus among healthcare providers that: (a) we can diagnose definite pathology in only about 15% of patients with LBP, (b) there is very little relationship between physical pathology and associated pain and disability, (c) we continue to regard LBP as an injury – however, most episodes occur spontaneously with normal everyday activities, (d) high-tech imaging such as magnetic resonance imaging (MRI) tells us very little about simple LBP, and indeed it appears to contribute to the problem of unwanted and unnecessary surgical procedures, and (e) the exact pathoanatomical lesion remains resistant to traditional clinical triage in the majority of patients with LBP. (Readers are referred to Chs 16 and 21 for further information on mechanical LBP and chronic LBP advances.)

Around the turn of this century, there was growing evidence for SMT but the conclusions were often conflicting. There were just as many randomized controlled trials in support of manipulation as there were against, and systematic reviews were evenly split on the evidence. Adding to the confusion, there were a variety of conclusions being drawn in national practice guidelines for the management of LBP (Koes et al 2001). A review of the research into SMT for LBP around the time finds that most studies had significant flaws in design methodology in that an incorrect assumption was being made that subjects with LBP were a homogeneous sample group. One example of such studies is the United Kingdom back pain exercise and manipulation (UK BEAM) randomized trial on the effectiveness of physical treatments for LBP in primary care (UK BEAM Trial Team 2004). In that study, 1334 patients with LBP were randomized into four groups and received 'best care' in general practice, 'best care' plus exercise classes, 'best care' plus spinal manipulation, or 'best care' plus spinal manipulation followed by exercise classes. The outcome measure used in the study was the Roland Morris disability questionnaire at 3 and 12 months, compared with baseline. The results demonstrated that all groups improved over time and that the addition of manipulation and / or exercise provided only small to moderate benefits over 'best care' at 3 months and only a small benefit over 'best care' at 12 months. The significant flaw with this study (and many others at the time) was that its use of broad inclusion criteria (i.e. LBP) resulted in a heterogeneous sample that may have included many patients for whom no benefit with manipulation would have been expected, thus masking the intervention's true value (Childs & Flynn 2004). The take-home message was that not all patients with LBP are the same, and this was something that certainly resonated with clinicians, who were well aware that certain patients with LBP were more likely to benefit from a manipulative technique, whereas other patients would not.

A classification-based approach was therefore proposed so that patients with LBP could be classified into more homogeneous subgroups. Classification systems for patients with LBP have been reported in the literature since the mid 1980s, with some systems designed to aid in prognosis, some designed to identify pathology and others designed to determine the most appropriate treatment (Riddle 1998). A treatment-based classification approach was proposed by physical therapy researchers in 1995, with one subgroup defined as those with LBP more likely to respond to manipulation (Delitto et al 1995); however, the criteria for membership of that LBP subgroup had not been determined through research. This became the 1997 agenda for primary care research on LBP: identifying the different varieties and subgroups of LBP within the treatment-based classification system and determining the criteria for membership. In other words, the treatment-based classification approach would be a way of knowing ahead of time which patients would be helped by which treatment interventions. As well as a classification system for patients with LBP, significant strides have also been made towards developing a similar classification system for patients with neck pain (Childs et al 2004a). (Ch 16 details the treatment-based classification approach for mechanical LBP.)

Clinical Prediction Rules

Clinical prediction rules (CPR) have been utilized within the healthcare community for many years. They are simply tools to assist in the clinical decision-making process. They can be designed to improve diagnostic accuracy or to predict a particular outcome, and examples of CPR in the medical literature include: accuracy of diagnosing ankle fractures (Ottawa ankle rule) (Stiell et al 1992), when to order cervical spine radiographs (Canadian C-spine rule) (Stiell et al 2001) and how to diagnose cervical radiculopathy (Wainner et al 2003). A CPR for classifying patients with LBP who demonstrate short-term improvement with SMT was developed in 2002 (Flynn et al 2002). This was a prospective, cohort study of patients with non-radicular LBP referred to physical therapy. In simple terms, the researchers admitted 71 consecutive patients with LBP who did not present with any exclusion criteria (factors that would present precautions or contraindications for manipulation), and conducted a standardized battery of subjective and objective (physical) tests. Upon completion of the testing, and regardless of the findings or the testing, all patients underwent a standardized SMT treatment programme. Using the model for standardized manipulation terminology discussed earlier in this chapter, clinicians gave all participants a 'high-velocity, end-range rotational manipulation to the lumbar spine on the lower thoracic spine with the patient in supine with contralateral lateral flexion'.

Subjects were then asked to return after 48 hours and complete a post-treatment Oswestry Disability Index (ODI); if there was an improvement of at least 50% compared with the pre-treatment ODI score, patients were classified as having experienced success with the manipulation. If they did not report an improvement of at least 50% in their ODI, they were given a second manipulation treatment session and asked to return after another 48 hours, whereupon they completed a third ODI and were finally classified as having experienced success or not. The researchers discovered that 32 (45%) of the subjects had experienced success with the manipulation intervention (Flynn et al 2002). Their next task was to determine the different characteristics (examination variables) existing between the groups. Each of the examination variables collected was analysed for univariate accuracy in predicting success, and these were then combined into a multivariate CPR. A CPR with five variables (symptom duration, fear-avoidance beliefs score, lumbar hypomobility, hip internal rotation range of motion, and no symptoms distal to the knee) was identified. When four or more of these variables were present in a subject with LBP, the positive likelihood ratio was 24.38, which raised the pre-test probability of experiencing success from 45% to a post-test probability of success of 95% (Flynn et al 2002). This was a significant finding that would greatly change the landscape of SMT for LBP. The next step required was to conduct a randomized controlled clinical trial to validate the rule.

That validation study was published in 2004 (Childs et al 2004b). In that study, 131 consecutive patients with LBP, aged 18 to 60 years, were randomly assigned to receive either manipulation plus exercise or exercise alone by a physical therapist for 4 weeks. Once allocated to the treatment groups, all subjects were examined according to the CPR criteria (symptom duration, symptom location, fear-avoidance beliefs, lumbar mobility and hip rotation range of motion) and classified as being either positive (at least 4 out of 5) or negative according to the rule (less than 4 out of 5). Outcome measures were disability (ODI) and pain at 1 week, 4 weeks and 6 months compared with baseline. There was a significant difference in outcomes between patients who were positive on the rule and received manipulation compared with patients who were either negative on the rule and received manipulation, positive on the rule and received exercise only, or negative on the rule and received exercise only. A patient who was positive on the rule and received manipulation was found to have a 92% chance of a successful outcome, with an associated number needed to treat (NNT) for benefit at 4 weeks of 1.9 (95% CI 1.4–3.5) (Childs et al 2004b). This meant that only two patients with LBP who are positive on the rule need be treated with manipulation in order to prevent one patient from failing to achieve a successful outcome. It is widely accepted that patients with persistent disability are at increased risk of chronic, disabling episodes of LBP, and this study demonstrated that decision making based on the CPR could help prevent progression to chronic disability. In a follow-up analysis of the study, it was found that patients with LBP who were positive on the rule and completed the exercise intervention without manipulation were eight (95% CI 1.1, 63.5) times more likely to experience a worsening in disability at 1 week than patients who actually received manipulation (Childs et al 2006). The authors noted that the risks associated with harm due to lumbopelvic manipulation were almost negligible and concluded that the risk of not offering manipulation was real, and a more proactive approach seemed to be warranted (Childs et al 2006).

Some researchers immediately questioned the validity of the newly validated CPR for LBP. Hancock et al (2008) performed a secondary analysis of a randomized controlled trial investigating the efficacy of SMT in 239 patients with non-specific LBP. Patients received SMT or placebo two to three times per week for up to 4 weeks, and outcomes were pain and disability measured at 1, 2, 4 and 12 weeks. These researchers reported that the CPR did no better than chance in identifying patients with LBP most likely to benefit from SMT, and they concluded (incorrectly, as we shall see) that the CPR proposed by Childs et al (2004b) did not generalize to patients presenting to primary care with acute LBP who received a course of SMT. However, it is important to recognize that these authors defined SMT as *either* thrust manipulation *or* non-thrust mobilization. Furthermore, they reported that the majority of the patients in their study (97%) received a variety of non-thrust mobilization and only a small proportion (3%) actually received thrust manipulation techniques. In a follow-up letter to the editor, Hebert and Perle (2008) pointed out the problem with the authors' definition of SMT and made the argument that the findings in the above study did not actually test the validity of the CPR; instead they made the case for the implementation of the rule in the same manner as it was developed, validated and examined in other clinical settings.

The issue of differences in outcome between thrust manipulation and non-thrust mobilizations was brought to further light by a more recent study. Cook et al (2013) found no significant difference in outcomes (i.e. pain, disability, reported rate of recovery, total visits, or days of care) between early use of manipulation (thrust) and mobilization (non-thrust) in 149 subjects with LBP. However, to qualify for the study, patients with LBP had to demonstrate a within-session change (improvement in pain and / or range of motion) during the assessment phase of the clinical examination – specifically during the passive accessory examination. The examination required the therapist to localize the most comparable response (reproduction of the chief complaint of the symptoms identified by the patient) during a passive accessory mobilization (either unilateral or central) to a specific level of the lumbar spine. Only patients with an identifiable comparable level *and* a within-session change were able to continue in the study. This may well have biased the results of the study in favour of non-thrust mobilization as only those patients who demonstrated improvement (albeit within-session) with mobilization (non-thrust) were allowed to continue in the study. The authors admitted that 'this process may have self-selected subjects for non-thrust mobilization since the procedure used to define a within-session change is also similar to the non-thrust mobilization used during treatment' (Cook et al 2013, p 197).

It would appear therefore that, for the time being, the decision to use either thrust manipulation or non-thrust mobilization might well be left to therapists (who may be more skilled / comfortable with one over the other) and patients with LBP (who may have a preference or belief that one will be more effective than the other).

The Audible Pop

For most practitioners of SMT, the aim of the technique is to achieve joint cavitation, which is accompanied by a 'popping' or 'cracking' sound (Gibbons & Tehan 2004). Despite the many theories, there is currently no evidence about what causes the characteristic 'cracking' sound or 'audible release'. Brodeur (1995) completed a review of the literature on the audible release associated with manipulation and reported that it is theorized that the audible release is caused by a cavitation process whereby a sudden decrease in intracapsular pressure causes dissolved gasses within the synovial fluid to be released into the joint cavity. However, a clinical trial investigating the effect of manipulation on the size and density of cervical zygapophyseal joint spaces in 22 asymptomatic subjects using CT and plain film radiography found no evidence of gas in the joint space, or of an obvious increase in zygapophyseal joint space width immediately after the manipulation (Cascioli et al 2003). Similar studies have failed to support such a theory of gas in the joint (Cramer et al 2011).

Another review of the literature (Evans 2002) to 'critically discuss previous theories and research of spinal HVLA thrust manipulation, highlighting reported neurophysiological effects that seem to be uniquely associated with cavitation of synovial fluid' found that there appeared to be two separate modes of action from zygapophyseal HVLA thrust manipulation: 'mechanical' effects and 'neurophysiological' effects. Evans (2002) also reported that the intra-articular 'mechanical' effects of zygapophyseal HVLA thrust manipulation seemed to be absolutely separate from, and irrelevant to, the occurrence of reported 'neurophysiological' effects (Evans 2002). It is safe to say that, currently, we do not know how or why manipulation might work in patients with LBP. What we do know, however, is that there are some patients with LBP who do benefit from manipulation, and the development and validation of CPRs is helping us to determine in advance who those patients are.

Most clinicians who utilize SMT consider that their manipulative technique has been correctly performed when there is an audible release or pop in the targeted joint. However, scientific research has suggested that this audible release may not matter. Flynn et al (2006) conducted a secondary analysis of their CPR studies to determine the relationship between an audible pop with spinal manipulation and the improvement in pain and function noted in patients with LBP. Therapists recorded whether an audible pop was heard by either the patient or the therapist during the treatment interventions, and an audible pop was perceived in 59 (84%) of the patients. However, no differences were detected at baseline, or at any follow-up period, in the level of pain, the Oswestry score, or lumbopelvic range of motion based on whether a pop was achieved. The results suggested that a perceived audible pop may not relate to improved outcomes from high-velocity thrust manipulation for patients with non-radicular LBP at either an immediate or a longer term follow-up.

Clinicians also seek to localize their manipulative techniques to specific joint(s) that require them and avoid unwanted stress on adjacent joints. Spinal manipulative techniques are taught and then performed with a specific (sometimes biomechanical) intent. However, an evaluation study (Ross et al 2004) using accelerometers to locate the joints that produced an audible sound in response to manipulation (cavitation) during spinal manipulative techniques found that both the accuracy and the specificity of the manipulation were poor. In this particular study, 64 asymptomatic subjects received thoracic and lumbar spinal manipulative procedures from 28 clinicians (all were Canadian chiropractors with a range of clinical experience from 1 to 43 years); its findings were that, for the lumbar spine, SMT was accurate 'about half the time' (57 / 124) and, for the thoracic spine, SMT appeared to be more accurate (29 / 54) (Ross et al 2004). However, most of the procedures were associated with multiple cavitations, and, in most cases, at least one cavitation emanated from the target joint. This may have skewed results towards greater accuracy.

Some authors have questioned whether SMT need be specific in terms of localization of motion (Cleland & Childs 2005; Flynn 2006). Several studies using posterior-to-anterior (PA) non-thrust mobilization techniques reported that there was no difference in outcomes for pain based on whether the most painful segment was treated, or whether a randomly selected segment was treated (Beneck et al 2005; Landel et al 2008; Aquino et al 2009). However, caution should be used when generalizing the results of such studies to all SMT techniques. If clinicians were to accept that it is neither necessary nor possible to be specific with SMT techniques, then one possible consequence might be unwanted adverse responses. As noted previously, poorly localized and excessively forceful manipulative techniques may provoke adverse responses. Therefore, to minimize risks associated with SMT, the clinician should either carefully select patients when deciding to use less specific manipulative techniques or use techniques that attempt to be more specific and localized.

Spinal Positioning and Locking

In both physical therapy and osteopathic manipulative techniques, spinal locking can be used in order to localize forces and achieve cavitation at a specific vertebral segment (Stoddard 1972; Downing 1985; Beal 1989; Kappler 1989; Nyberg 1993; Greenman 1996; Hartman 1997a). This locking can be achieved by facet apposition, ligamentous myofascial tension, or a combination of the two (Stoddard 1972; Downing 1985; Beal 1989; Nyberg 1993; Greenman 1996; Hartman 1997a). This principle is used to position the spine in such a way as to localize the leverage or force moment to one joint without placing undue strain on adjacent segments. The osteopathic profession uses the following nomenclature to classify spinal motion based upon the coupling of side-bending and rotation movements (Gibbons & Tehan 2004): in *type 1 movement*, side-bending and rotation occur in opposite directions; in *type 2 movement*, side-bending and rotation occur in the same direction. It is proposed that locking by facet apposition can be achieved when the spine is placed in a position opposite to that of normal coupling behaviour.

A systematic review of the literature on coupling behaviour of the cervical spine found that there was 100% agreement in coupling direction in the lower cervical vertebral segments (C2–C3 and below) (Cook et al 2006). Normal coupling behaviour is type 2 (i.e. left side-bending coupled with left rotation, and vice versa) and therefore facet locking can be achieved by producing type 1 movement (i.e. left side-bending coupled with right rotation and vice versa) (Cook et al 2006).

The available research relating to coupled movements of side-bending and rotation in the thoracic and lumbar spine is inconsistent (Panjabi et al 1989; Oxland et al 1992; Steffen et al 1997; Harrison et al 1999; Plaugher & Burrow 1999; Feipel et al 2001; Keller et al 2003; Legaspi & Edmond 2007). There is some evidence that spinal posture and positioning alter coupling behaviour in the thoracic and lumbar spine (Panjabi et al 1989; Steffen et al 1997; Harrison et al 1999). Specifically in the flexed position, the coupling of side-bending and rotation is to the same side, and in the neutral / extended position the coupling of side-bending and rotation occurs to the opposite sides. Although the research doesn't validate any single model for spinal positioning and locking in the thoracic and lumbar spine, many educators continue to find this model useful for learning and motor skill acquisition with manipulative therapy techniques.

For neutral / extension positioning, normal coupling behaviour of side-bending and rotation are to the opposite side (type 1). Therefore, facet apposition locking can be achieved through side-bending and rotation to the same side. For flexion positioning, normal coupling behaviour of side-bending and rotation are to the same side (type 2); therefore, facet apposition locking can be achieved through side-bending and rotation to the opposite side.

Safety and Manipulative Techniques

Studies show that, when it comes to manipulation in the lumbar spine, serious risks are very minimal. Haldeman and Rubinstein (1992) completed a review of the literature and, over a period of 77 years, found just 10 episodes of cauda equina syndrome following lumbar spinal manipulation. This equates to an estimated risk of less than 1 per 10 million manipulations. Shekelle et al (1992) estimated the rate of occurrence of cauda equina syndrome as a complication of lumbar spinal manipulation to be in the order of less than 1 case per 100 million manipulations. Finally, Bronfort (1999) reported that overall serious complications of lumbar spinal manipulation seemed to be rare.

Possible causes of complications from spinal manipulative techniques to the lumbar spine primarily involve one of two factors: (1) incorrect patient selection, and (2) poor manipulative technique. The clinician providing spinal manipulation for a patient with LBP should have:

- a mechanical or clinical-reasoning diagnosis for the use of manipulation
- an awareness of the possible complications
- conducted an adequate palpation assessment
- appropriately and adequately progressed through mobilization grades before coming to manipulation
- patient consent.

To avoid complications associated with poor manipulative technique, the clinician should:

- avoid excessive force
- avoid excessive amplitude of movement
- avoid excessive leverage of forces
- avoid inappropriate combination of leverages
- use the correct plane of thrust
- use correct patient positioning
- use correct therapist positioning
- obtain patient feedback in the pre-thrust positioning.

Spinal manipulative techniques require a level of skill and care that can be obtained only through appropriate and adequate clinical practice.

Contraindications and precautions

As with any therapeutic intervention, due consideration must be given to the risk–benefit ratio; that is, the benefit to the patient of providing the therapeutic intervention must outweigh any potential risk associated with the intervention. Clinicians should always be aware of any contraindications and precautions for SMT. Is there a difference between a contraindication and a precaution? A contraindication means that a manipulative technique should not be used under any circumstances, whereas a precaution means that, depending upon the skill, experience and training of the practitioner, the type of technique selected, the amount of leverage and force used, and the age, general health and physical condition of the patient, it may not be the wisest choice to use a manipulative technique. Boxes 22.1 and 22.2 provide some of the better-known and commonly accepted contraindications and

Box 22.1 Contraindications for spinal manipulative therapy

Bony issues

Any pathology that may have led to bony compromise:

- Tumour, e.g. metastases
- Infection, e.g. tuberculosis, osteomyelitis
- Metabolic, e.g. osteomalacia, osteoporosis
- Congenital, e.g. dysplasia
- Iatrogenic, e.g. long-term corticosteroid medication
- Inflammatory, e.g. severe rheumatoid arthritis
- Traumatic, e.g. fracture

Neurological issues

- Cervical myelopathy
- Cord compression
- Cauda equina syndrome
- Nerve root compression with increasing neurological deficit

Vascular issues

- Diagnosed vertebrobasilar insufficiency
- Aortic aneurysm
- Bleeding diatheses, e.g. severe haemophilia
- Lack of mechanical or clinical-reasoning diagnosis
- Lack of patient consent

Box 22.2 Precautions for spinal manipulative therapy

- Adverse reaction to previous manual therapy
- Disc herniation or prolapse
- Pregnancy
- Spondylolisthesis
- Psychological dependence upon manipulative techniques
- Ligamentous laxity

As a general rule, safety in manipulation is best provided by gradual progression of the strength of the technique (grades of mobilization) coupled with continual assessment and reassessment (Maitland, 1986).

How can we make manipulative techniques safer?

- Appropriate clinician training
- Take a thorough patient history
- Perform a thorough physical examination
- Use astute clinical reasoning skills
- Using graded mobilizations prior to the application of any manipulative procedure

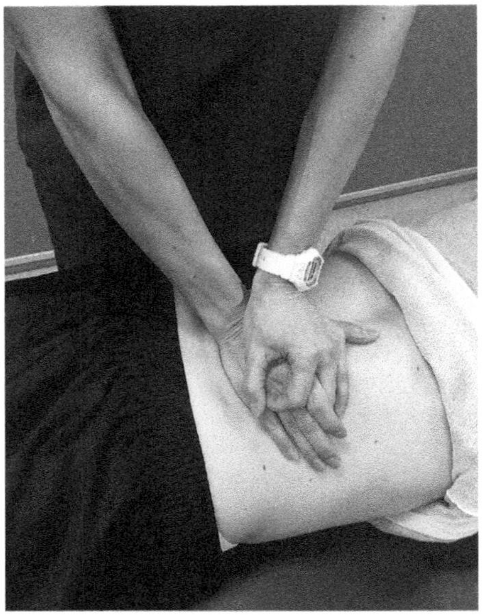

Figure 22.1 Central posterior-to-anterior mobilization.

precautions for manipulative techniques and offer some advice on making manipulation safer.

Spinal Mobilization and Manipulation Techniques

The techniques presented within this chapter are developed from Geoff Maitland, PT (Maitland 1986) and also from techniques taught by Laurie Hartman, DO, PhD (Hartman 1997b). The emphasis with any manual therapy technique should be to minimize the occurrence of moderate to severe adverse response as presented by Carnes et al (2010) and maximize outcomes in terms of decreased pain and increased function. These interventions can be subdivided into passive accessory intervertebral motions and passive physiological intervertebral motions.

Central posterior-to-anterior mobilization

The patient is prone in a position of greatest comfort where signs and symptoms are minimized. The therapist should assume a comfortable stance and adjust the treatment table to a comfortable height and then assume a pisiform contact on the desired spinous process (Fig. 22.1). The mobilization technique may be graded through forces as described by Maitland (1986). The force is directed towards the treatment table by the therapist shifting his / her weight forwards through the arms and hands, and the motion imparted should be slow, rhythmic and through a relatively short range. Most clinicians will use either a larger amplitude grade III oscillation or a smaller amplitude grade IV oscillation, and perform the mobilization for repeated bouts of 45 to 60 seconds, then reassess the patient for within-session changes to symptoms and range of motion.

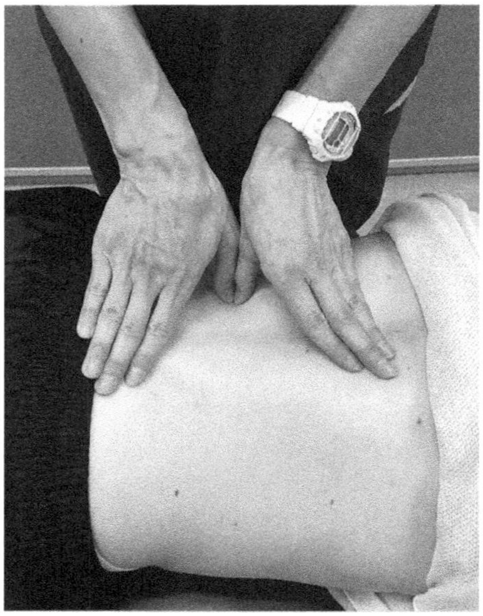

Figure 22.2 Unilateral posterior-to-anterior mobilization.

Unilateral posterior-to-anterior mobilization

The patient is prone in as comfortable a position as possible to minimize signs and symptoms. The therapist assumes a comfortable stance with the treatment table correctly adjusted, and makes contact with both thumb pads directly over the multifidus muscle and underlying zygapophyseal joint (Fig. 22.2). The mobilization technique is similarly graded through forces, as described by Maitland (1986). The force is usually directed downwards towards the treatment table, but can also be applied in a medial / lateral or cephalad / caudad direction based on patient feedback and response. As with the central PA mobilizations, they are generally applied as a larger amplitude grade III oscillation or a smaller amplitude grade

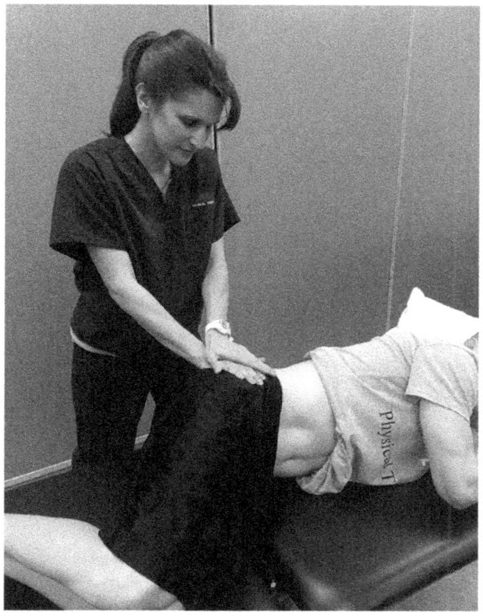

Figure 22.3 Lumbar rotation mobilization grade I.

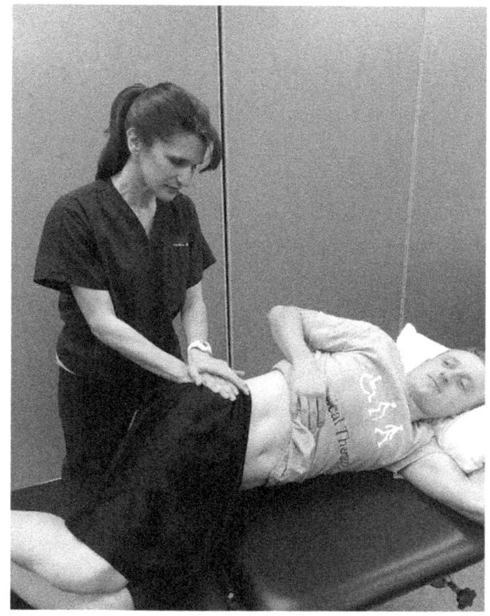

Figure 22.4 Lumbar rotation mobilization grade II.

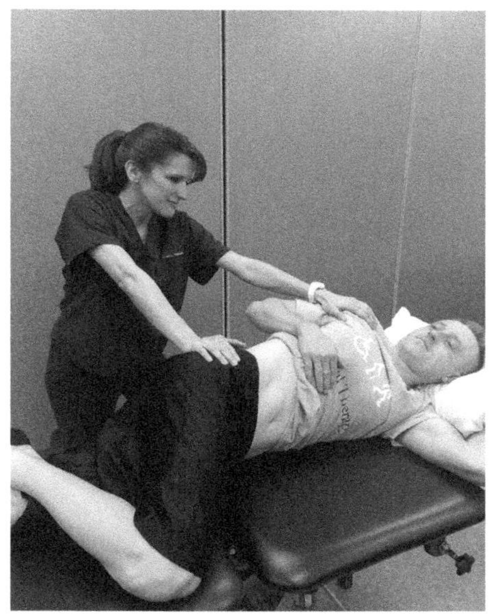

Figure 22.5 Lumbar rotation mobilization grade III.

IV oscillation for repeated bouts of 45 to 60 seconds, then the patient should be reassessed for within-session changes to symptoms and range of motion.

Lumbar rotation mobilization: grades I–IV

The patient is in side-lying with hips and knees flexed to maximum comfort. This technique is also graded through forces as described by Maitland (1986), so that grade I mobilization is performed with the lumbar spine in neutral rotation (Fig. 22.3). The therapist assumes a comfortable stride stance and places both hands above the patient's greater trochanter and immediately posterior to the anterior superior iliac spine (ASIS). Very few clinicians would use a grade I mobilization; however, it may be appropriate for a patient in severe discomfort as a gentle non-threatening mobilization that can then be progressed through a larger range of motion.

The grade II mobilization requires a larger amplitude motion and can be assisted by the patient placing the elbow behind the trunk (Fig. 22.4). During oscillations, the pelvis and shoulder girdles can be rhythmically moved in a comforting and hopefully pain-free range. To progress to a grade III rotation mobilization, the therapist can now apply forces through the hip and same-side shoulder (Fig. 22.5). This is typically performed through larger amplitude and kept short of end-range lumbar (trunk) rotation.

Grade IV mobilization is best performed facing the patient. The patient is placed in side-lying and rotation of the lumbar spine (trunk) is introduced (Fig. 22.6). The therapist takes up an axillary hold with the left forearm and uses the left hand to palpate and provide some 'fixation' at the desired level. He or she can then use the right forearm and hand to apply the rotation force up to the 'fixated' level. The rotation oscillations are generated through the therapist's body rather than the arms through trunk rotation while in a comfortable stride stance.

As with all other non-thrust mobilizations, oscillations are provided in two or three bouts of 45 to 60 seconds, then the patient should be reassessed for within-session changes to symptoms and range of motion.

Lumbopelvic regional manipulation

Using the terminology as recommended by Mintken et al (2008), this can be described as a high-velocity end-range rotation thrust to the lumbopelvic region, pelvis on lumbar spine with patient supine. It has traditionally been described as the anterior innominate technique (Fig. 22.7). The patient lies supine and the therapist moves the patient's pelvis towards him / her, then moves the feet and shoulders in the opposite direction to introduce left side-bending of the trunk. The therapist then places the patient's left foot and ankle on top

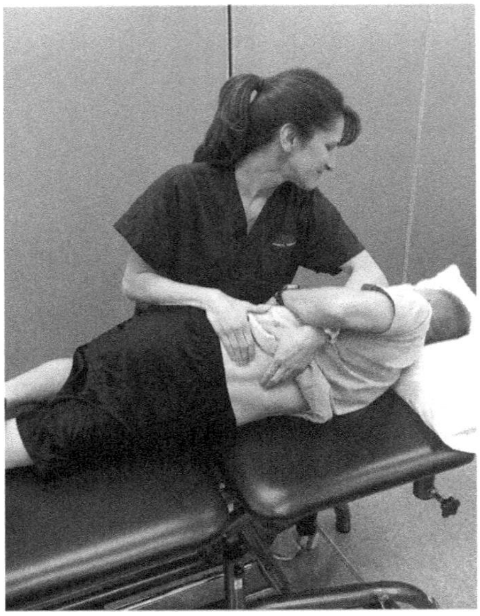

Figure 22.6 Lumbar rotation mobilization grade IV.

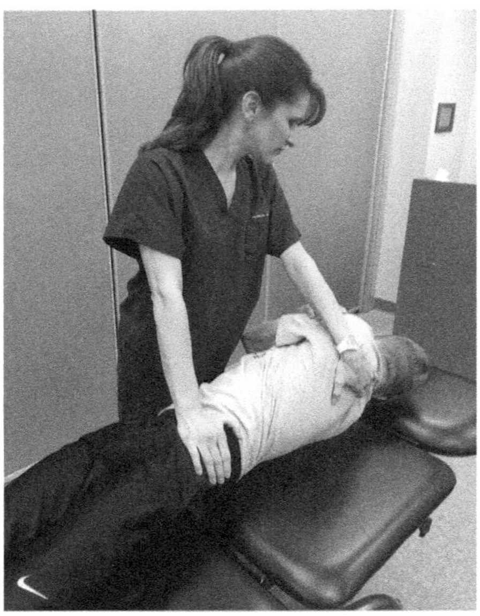

Figure 22.7 Lumbopelvic regional manipulation.

of the right ankle and asks the patient to clasp the fingers behind the neck, or asks patient to fold the arms across the chest (based on comfort for patient). The therapist then rotates the patient's trunk to the right while maintaining left trunk side-bending (it is important not to lose this side-bending). The therapist then grasps the patient's left scapular and thorax with the left hand and places the palm of the right hand directly over the ASIS. At this point, any necessary adjustments to achieve pre-thrust tension can be made.

The thrust is applied through the ASIS in a curved plane towards the couch. The therapist's left forearm, wrist and hand over the patient's scapula and thorax do not apply a thrust, but rather act as stabilizers only.

Lumbar rotation in neutral or extension manipulation

Using the terminology as recommended by Mintken et al (2008), this can be described as a high-velocity end-range rotation thrust to upper lumbar spine on lower lumbar spine with patient side-lying and lumbar spine in neutral or slightly extended. It has traditionally been described as the side-lying rotation technique or rotation gliding thrust in neutral positioning (Fig. 22.8A). The patient is in right side-lying, and the therapist places the patient's right leg and spine in a straight line to achieve neutral / extension positioning. The left hip is flexed to approximately 90° so that the left knee is also flexed and the dorsum of left foot can be placed just behind the right calf / knee. The therapist begins by introducing left rotation of the upper body down to desired level while avoiding the introduction of any spine flexion, and then takes up axillary hold with the left forearm and hand (Fig. 22.8B). Standing close to the couch, feet spread and with one leg behind the other, the therapist maintains an upright posture facing the patient's upper body then places the right forearm in the region between the gluteus medius and maximus to rotate the patient's pelvis and lumbar spine towards him / her until motion is palpated at the desired segment (pre-tension). The therapist then rotates the patient's upper body away until tension is sensed at the desired segment, and then rolls the patient about 10–15° towards him / her and can make any necessary adjustments to achieve pre-thrust tension.

The thrust is applied with the right forearm against the pelvis and the direction is down towards the couch by applying exaggerated pelvic rotation towards him / her. The left arm against the patient's axillary region does not apply a thrust, but rather acts as stabilizer only.

Lumbar rotation in flexion manipulation

Using the terminology as recommended by Mintken et al (2008), this can be described as a high-velocity end-range rotation thrust to upper lumbar spine on lower lumbar spine with patient side-lying and lumbar spine in slight flexion (Fig. 22.9). This uses the osteopathic principles where the lumbar spine, in flexion, has ipsilateral coupling motions and, therefore, facet apposition locking can be achieved by combining lateral flexion with contralateral rotation. The patient is in right side-lying and a rolled towel is placed under the lumbar spine to introduce lateral flexion to the right. The lumbar rotation will be to the left, thereby providing contralateral motions to counter the normal ipsilateral coupling behaviour. The therapist places the patient's right leg and hip in slight flexion to achieve lumbar flexion positioning. The left hip is flexed to approximately 90° so that the left knee is also flexed and the dorsum of the left foot can be placed just behind the right calf / knee. The therapist begins by introducing left rotation of the upper body down to desired level while avoiding the introduction of any spine flexion, and then takes up axillary hold with the left forearm and hand. Standing close to the couch, feet spread and with one leg behind the other, the therapist maintains an upright posture facing the patient's upper body, then places the right forearm in the region

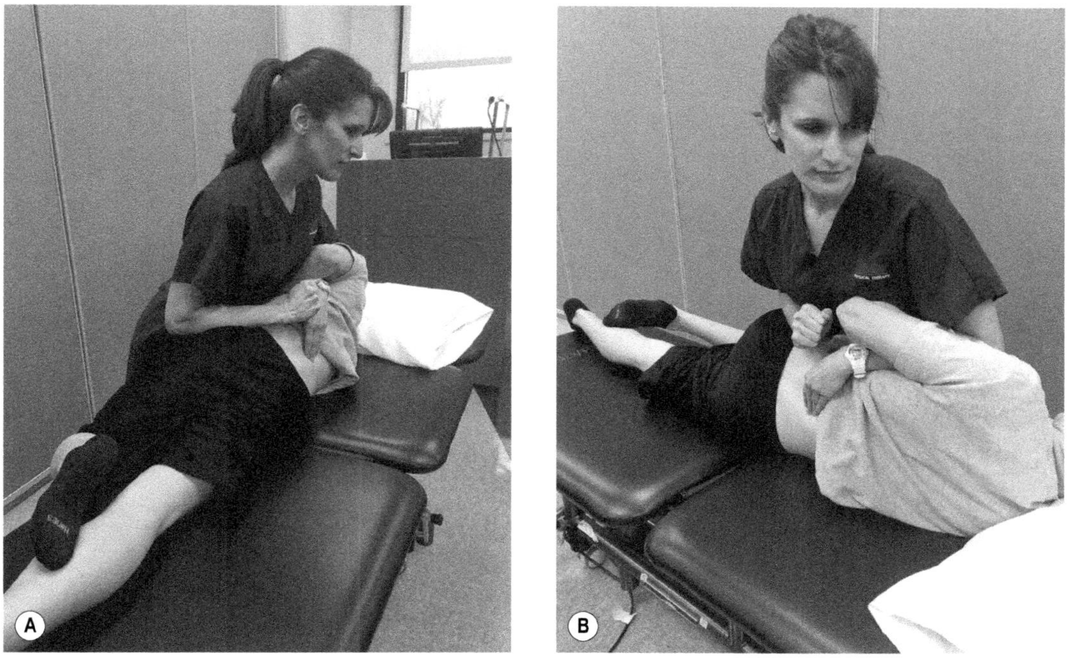

Figure 22.8 Lumbar rotation in neutral or extension manipulation: (**A**) caudal view, (**B**) cranial view.

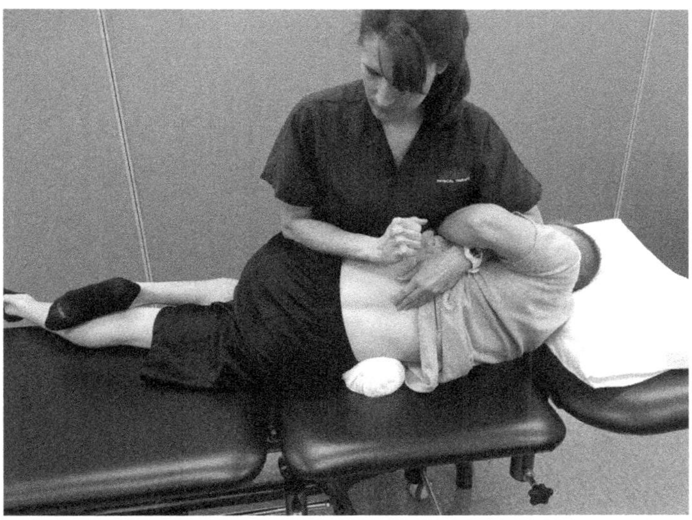

Figure 22.9 Lumbar rotation in flexion manipulation.

between gluteus medius and maximus to rotate the patient's pelvis and lumbar spine towards him / her until motion is palpated at the desired segment (pre-tension). The therapist then rotates the patient's upper body away until tension is sensed at the desired segment, and finally rolls the patient about 10–15° towards him / her and can make any necessary adjustments to achieve pre-thrust tension.

The thrust is applied with the right forearm against the pelvis and the direction is down towards the couch by applying exaggerated pelvic rotation towards him / her. The left arm against the patient's axillary region does not apply a thrust, but rather acts as stabilizer only.

Conclusion

Great strides have been made in recent years in our understanding of the various factors that are associated with successful management of LBP through the use of manipulation and non-thrust mobilization. A significant advancement has been the acknowledgement that not all patients with LBP are the same and, accordingly, not all will respond favourably to one specific treatment intervention. Use of the classification-based approach when evaluating an individual with LBP can help the clinician in determining the most beneficial treatment approach, and clinical prediction rules may also be useful. Ultimately, sound clinical reasoning will be required so that the therapist can provide the most appropriate intervention for the specific patient with LBP in the clinic.

References

Aquino RL, Caires PM, Furtado FC, et al. 2009. Applying joint mobilization at different cervical vertebral levels does not influence immediate pain reduction in patients with chronic neck pain: a randomized clinical trial. J Man Manip Ther 17: 95–100.

Beal M. 1989. Teaching the basic principles of osteopathic manipulative techniques. In: Beal M (ed) The principles of palpatory diagnosis and manipulative technique. Newark: American Academy of Osteopathy, pp 162–164.

Beneck GJ, Kulig K, Landel RF, et al. 2005. The relationship between lumbar segmental motion and pain response produced by a posterior-to-anterior force in persons with nonspecific low back pain. J Orthop Sports Phys Ther 35: 203–209.

Brodeur R. 1995. The audible release associated with joint manipulation. J Manipulative Physiol Ther 18: 155–164.

Bronfort G. 1999. Spinal manipulation: current state of research and its indications. Neurol Clin 17: 91–111.

Carnes D, Mullinger B, Underwood M. 2010. Defining adverse events in manual therapies: a modified Delphi consensus study. Man Ther 15: 2–6.

Cascioli V, Corr P, Till Ag AG. 2003. An investigation into the production of intra-articular gas bubbles and increase in joint space in the zygapophyseal joints of the cervical spine in asymptomatic subjects after spinal manipulation. J Manipulative Physiol Ther 26: 356–364.
Childs JD, Flynn TW. 2004. Spinal manipulation for low back pain. Ann Intern Med 140: 665; author reply 665–666.
Childs JD, Flynn TW, Fritz JM. 2006. A perspective for considering the risks and benefits of spinal manipulation in patients with low back pain. Man Ther 11: 316–320.
Childs JD, Fritz JM, Piva SR, et al. 2004a. Proposal of a classification system for patients with neck pain. J Orthop Sports Phys Ther 34: 686–696.
Childs JD, Fritz JM, Flynn TW, et al. 2004b. A clinical prediction rule to identify patients with low back pain most likely to benefit from spinal manipulation: a validation study. Ann Intern Med 141: 920–928.
Cleland JA, Childs JD. 2005. Does manual therapy technique matter? Orthop Division Rev 27–28.
Cook C, Hegedus E, Showalter C, et al. 2006. Coupling behavior of the cervical spine: a systematic review of the literature. J Manipulative Physiol Ther 29: 570–575.
Cook C, Learman K, Showalter C, et al. 2013. Early use of thrust manipulation versus non-thrust manipulation: a randomized clinical trial. Man Ther 18: 191–198.
Cramer GD, Ross K, Pocius J, et al. 2011. Evaluating the relationship among cavitation, zygapophyseal joint gapping, and spinal manipulation: an exploratory case series. J Manipulative Physiol Ther 34: 2–14.
Croft PR, Macfarlane GJ, Papageorgiou AC, et al. 1998. Outcome of low back pain in general practice: a prospective study. BMJ 316: 1356–1359.
Delitto A, Erhard RE, Bowling RW. 1995. A treatment-based classification approach to low back syndrome: identifying and staging patients for conservative treatment. Phys Ther 75: 470–485
Downing C. 1985. Principles and practice of osteopathy. London: Tamor Pierston.
Evans DW. 2002. Mechanisms and effects of spinal high-velocity, low-amplitude thrust manipulation: previous theories. J Manipulative Physiol Ther 25: 251–262.
Feipel V, De Mesmaeker T, Klein P, et al. 2001. Three-dimensional kinematics of the lumbar spine during treadmill walking at different speeds. Eur Spine J 10: 16–22.
Flynn TW. 2006. There's more than one way to manipulate a spine. J Orthop Sports Phys Ther 36: 198–199.
Flynn T, Fritz J, Whitman J, et al. 2002. A clinical prediction rule for classifying patients with low back pain who demonstrate short-term improvement with spinal manipulation. Spine 27: 2835–2843.
Flynn TW, Childs JD, Fritz JM. 2006. The audible pop from high-velocity thrust manipulation and outcome in individuals with low back pain. J Manipulative Physiol Ther 29: 40–45.
Gibbons PF, Tehan P. 2004. Manipulation of the spine, thorax and pelvis. An osteopathic perspective. London: Churchill Livingstone.
Greenman PE. 1996. Principles of manual medicine, 2nd edn. Baltimore: Lippincott Williams & Wilkins.
Haldeman S, Rubinstein SM. 1992. Cauda equina syndrome in patients undergoing manipulation of the lumbar spine. Spine 17: 1469–1473.
Hancock MJ, Maher CG, Latimer J, et al. 2008. Independent evaluation of a clinical prediction rule for spinal manipulative therapy: a randomised controlled trial. Eur Spine J 17: 936–943.
Harrison DE, Cailliet R, Harrison DD, et al. 1999. Lumbar coupling during lateral translations of the thoracic cage relative to a fixed pelvis. Clin Biomech 14: 704–709.
Hartman L. 1997a. Handbook of osteopathic technique, 3rd edn. London: Chapman & Hall.
Hartman L. 1997b. Handbook of osteopathic technique. Cheltenham, UK: Nelson Thornes.
Hebert JJ, Perle SM. 2008. Letter to the editor concerning 'Independent evaluation of a clinical prediction rule for spinal manipulative therapy: a randomised controlled trial' (M. Hancock et al.). Eur Spine J 17: 1401–1402; author reply 1403–1404.
Kappler RE. 1989. Direct application techniques. In: Beal M (ed) The principles of palpatory diagnosis and manipulative technique. Newark: American Academy of Osteopathy, pp 165–168.
Keller TS, Colloca CJ, Gunzburg R. 2003. Neuromechanical characterization of in vivo lumbar spinal manipulation. Part I. Vertebral motion. J Manipulative Physiol Ther 26: 567–578.
Koes BW, van Tulder MW, Ostelo R, et al. 2001. Clinical guidelines for the management of low back pain in primary care: an international comparison. Spine 26: 2504–2513.
Landel R, Kulig K, Fredericson M, et al. 2008. Intertester reliability and validity of motion assessments during lumbar spine accessory motion testing. Phys Ther 88: 43–49.
Legaspi O, Edmond SL. 2007. Does the evidence support the existence of lumbar spine coupled motion? A critical review of the literature. J Orthop Sports Phys Ther 37: 169–178.
Maitland GD. 1986. Vertebral manipulation, 5th edn. Ontario: Butterworths.
Mintken PE, DeRosa C, Little T, et al. 2008. AAOMPT clinical guidelines: a model for standardizing manipulation terminology in physical therapy practice. J Orthop Sports Phys Ther 38: A1–A6.
Nyberg R. 1993. Manipulation: definition, types, application. In: Basmajian J, Nyberg R, eds. Rational manual therapies. Baltimore: Lippincott Williams & Wilkins, pp 21–47.
Oxland TR, Crisco JJ 3rd, Panjabi MM, et al. 1992. The effect of injury on rotational coupling at the lumbosacral joint. A biomechanical investigation. Spine 17: 74–80.
Panjabi M, Yamamoto I, Oxland T, et al. 1989. How does posture affect coupling in the lumbar spine? Spine 14: 1002–1011.
Plaugher G, Burrow MN. 1999. Three-dimensional spinal coupling mechanics: Part I. A review of the literature. J Manipulative Physiol Ther 22: 350–352.
Riddle DL. 1998. Classification and low back pain: a review of the literature and critical analysis of selected systems. Phys Ther 78: 708–737.
Ross JK, Bereznick DE, McGill SM. 2004. Determining cavitation location during lumbar and thoracic spinal manipulation: is spinal manipulation accurate and specific? Spine 29: 1452–1457.
Shekelle PG, Adams AH, Chassin MR, et al. 1992. Spinal manipulation for low-back pain. Ann Intern Med 117: 590–598.
Skargren EI, Carlsson PG, Oberg BE. 1998. One-year follow-up comparison of the cost and effectiveness of chiropractic and physiotherapy as primary management for back pain. Subgroup analysis, recurrence, and additional health care utilization. Spine 23: 1875–1883.
Steffen T, Rubin RK, Baramki HG, et al. 1997. A new technique for measuring lumbar segmental motion in vivo. Method, accuracy, and preliminary results. Spine 22: 156–166.
Stiell IG, Greenberg GH, McKnight RD, et al. 1992. A study to develop clinical decision rules for the use of radiography in acute ankle injuries. Ann Emerg Med 21: 384–390.
Stiell IG, Wells GA, Vandemheen KL, et al. 2001. The Canadian C-spine rule for radiography in alert and stable trauma patients. JAMA 286: 1841–1848.
Stoddard A. 1972. Manual of osteopathic technique, 2nd edn. London: Hutchinson.
UK BEAM Trial Team. 2004. United Kingdom back pain exercise and manipulation (UK BEAM) randomised trial: effectiveness of physical treatments for back pain in primary care. BMJ 329: 1377.
Wainner RS, Fritz JM, Irrgang JJ, et al. 2003. Reliability and diagnostic accuracy of the clinical examination and patient self-report measures for cervical radiculopathy. Spine 28: 52–62.

Chapter 23

Therapeutic Exercise for Mechanical Low Back Pain

Carol Kennedy, Lenerdene Levesque

CHAPTER CONTENTS

Evidence for exercise in low back pain	255
Mobility exercises	256
Motor control: stabilization, motor pattern retraining, strength	259
Exercises	259
Abdominal draw-in manoeuvre	259
Adding lower limb challenges	260
Abdominal curl-up	260
Multifidus activation exercises	261
Bridge exercises in supine	262
Quadruped	262
Side plank/horizontal side support	263
Front plank/prone bridge	264
Exercises on unstable surfaces	264
Motor pattern retraining/functional integration	266
Pilates/yoga	267
Balance/proprioception	268
Higher level strengthening exercises	269
Exercise parameters	270
Conclusion	271

Evidence for Exercise in Low Back Pain

Exercise therapy is a commonly used intervention in the conservative management of mechanical low back pain (LBP). A Cochrane review conducted by Hayden et al (2005) found that exercise therapy significantly reduced pain and improved function in adults with chronic LBP. A more recent systematic review also found evidence for the effectiveness of exercise therapy compared with 'usual care' for reducing chronic pain intensity and disability at short-term follow-up (van Middelkoop et al 2010). Systematic reviews and clinical practice guidelines on the management of acute LBP do not, however, recommend exercise therapy and they have found strong evidence that exercise therapy is no more effective than no treatment or other conservative treatment for acute LBP (van Middelkoop et al 2010; Delitto et al 2012).

Various types of low back exercises have been described in the literature including mobility, stretching, stabilization, muscle strengthening from low load to high load, motor control, balance / coordination, graded activity and aerobic. Van Middelkoop et al (2010) found no evidence that one particular type of exercise is more effective than any other. In an earlier systematic review of 14 randomized controlled trials, however, Macedo et al (2009) found motor control exercises to be more effective than minimal intervention and beneficial when added to another intervention in reducing pain and disability for people with persistent LBP. A more recent meta-analysis concluded that, in patients with chronic or recurring LBP, motor control exercises were superior to general exercise, manual therapy and minimal intervention with regard to disability and pain (Bystrom et al 2013). Haladay et al (2013) evaluated the quality of systematic reviews on specific stabilization exercises for chronic LBP and found several high-quality reviews indicating that they are beneficial and should be considered as part of the treatment plan for this population.

Classification systems have been proposed, throughout the literature, suggesting that subgroups of patients may respond differently to various types of exercise programmes; however, it remains unclear as to which patients benefit most from which type of exercise (van Middelkoop et al 2010). Hicks et al (2005) derived a clinical prediction rule (CPR) to assist in identifying those patients who may respond to a stabilization-focused exercise programme. The four clinical variables included: (1) age <40 years, (2) positive prone instability test, (3) straight leg raise >91° and (4) presence of aberrant trunk movements with lumbar flexion. Rabin et al (2014) were unable to validate the rule in a recent randomized controlled trial, but did find that a modified version of the CPR containing only two of the original four items (presence of aberrant movement and a positive prone instability test) demonstrated better predictive validity in identifying those most likely to succeed with a stabilization programme.

Choi et al (2010) conducted a Cochrane review evaluating the effectiveness of exercises on the prevention of recurrence of LBP and reported moderate-quality evidence that post-discharge exercise programmes can prevent the number of recurrences of LBP. The American Physical Therapy Association (APTA) Low Back Pain Clinical Practice Guidelines recommend 'that clinicians should consider using trunk coordination, strengthening and endurance exercises to reduce LBP and disability in patients with subacute and chronic LBP with movement impairments' (Delitto et al 2012, p A2).

The effectiveness of stretching in the management of LBP has received little attention. Many of the studies that have investigated the use of stretching exercises for LBP also include other forms of exercise, most often stabilization. Although this is consistent with current practice, it does make it difficult to determine the effectiveness of stretching as an isolated intervention. Purepong et al (2012) found a significant improvement in pain and disability along with increased lumbar mobility following 2 weeks of flexibility exercises including flexion, extension and rotation. Franca et al (2012) compared two types of exercise in the treatment of LBP – stretching and segmental stabilization – and found that, although both resulted in pain relief and improved disability, the segmental stabilization group exhibited significantly higher gains in the variables associated with LBP than the stretching group. In a study investigating stretching in the management of LBP in nurses, 81% of the experimental group experienced a moderate to high level of back pain relief (Chen et al 2012). In the systematic review by Hayden et al (2005), both stretching and strengthening exercise programmes demonstrated the largest improvement over other comparisons.

Clinical Practice Guidelines recommend that patient preferences should be considered and that exercises should be individualized and supervised (Delitto et al 2012). In a recent systematic review of 15 qualitative studies, Slade et al (2014) found that the participants considered supervision of exercise programmes to be important, and that therapists should demonstrate exercises and observe and provide feedback and corrections rather than simply provide a printed list of exercises. The patient's feelings of self-efficacy with respect to exercising and fear-avoidance beliefs were associated with decisions whether to exercise or not, and patients felt that the ongoing support of the healthcare professional encouraged them to adhere to exercises. In a recent prospective study, Cecchi et al (2014) attempted to identify predictors of response to exercise therapy for chronic LBP. They concluded that individually designed exercise programmes were associated with clinically significant functional improvement both on discharge and at 1 year. Severe baseline pain intensity was associated with an unfavourable outcome and was considered a poor prognostic indicator. At 1 year after discharge, younger age and better mental health predicted improved outcome, whereas the use of medications and previous LBP treatments were associated with a poor response. Most importantly, these authors noted that adherence to an individually designed exercise programme improved long-term functional outcome (Cecchi et al 2014).

Nevertheless, the parameters for exercise prescription – intensity, duration and frequency – have not been well established in the literature, although some guidelines will be discussed later in this chapter.

Mobility Exercises

A decrease in spinal mobility is a common feature in the presentation of LBP. There are several ways to approach an exercise prescription that is meant to address an impairment of lumbar mobility. Mobility exercises can include repeated movements in a particular direction, specific articular mobility exercises and / or muscle stretching. Adverse tension in the neuromeningeal system can also reduce mobility in the lumbar spine. This topic is addressed in Chapter 65, and the reader is directed to that chapter for further information. Full mobility of the sacroiliac and hip joints as well as the thorax is also essential for optimal function, but exercises for these regions are beyond the scope of this chapter (see Chs 24 and 38 respectively).

McKenzie popularized the use of repeated movements to evaluate the response of symptoms to mechanical loading (McKenzie & May 2003). A centralization phenomenon occurs when repeated movements cause the pain either to move proximally towards the midline of the spine or to decrease peripherally. Directional preference is the direction that results in either centralization or a reduction in symptoms. The most common directional preference is extension, with 80% of subjects falling into that category (Long et al 2004). A recent systematic review reported mixed results for the efficacy of the McKenzie approach for treatment of LBP, but concluded that there was some evidence in the short and intermediate term for those presenting with a directional preference (Surkitt et al 2012). For patients with acute or subacute LBP, if there is a clear directional preference, and especially when a centralization phenomenon also occurs, the use of specific mobility exercises in that preferred direction appears to be more effective, at least in the short term (Aina et al 2004; Clare et al 2004; Long et al 2004). Delitto et al (2012, p A2), in their Clinical Practice Guidelines for Low Back Pain, concluded that there was strong evidence that 'Clinicians should consider using repeated exercises in a specific direction determined by treatment response to improve mobility and reduce symptoms in patients with acute, subacute, or chronic low back pain with mobility deficits'. (Readers are referred to Ch 7 for further discussion on McKenzie method.)

Extension exercises are suggested for those who present with back pain with or without leg pain that is reduced with repeated extension or worsened with flexion, or those who have a limitation of the extension motion (Fig. 23.1). Usually this patient group prefers standing and walking over sitting. Flexion exercises are indicated for those with a restriction of this motion, particularly if the flexed position or repeated movements improve the pain (Fig. 23.2). Patients with lumbar stenosis or spondylolisthesis commonly fall into this category. They prefer to sit or pelvic tilt and tend to respond better if manual therapy is included as a component of treatment (Whitman et al 2006). Lateral shift, side-flexion or rotation exercises are used when there is a visible lateral shift present or to restore a loss of those specific movements (Figs 23.3, 23.4). Box 23.1 illustrates various options for restoring lumbar spinal mobility.

A multimodal approach to the treatment of LBP would include the use of various mobilization and manipulation techniques along with exercise programmes. Mobility exercises can be general or localized, and tailored to maintain or to further increase the spinal mobility gained with the manual therapy component of the treatment. Self-mobilization techniques as popularized by Mulligan can be used to reinforce the segmental spinal mobility gained during treatment (Mulligan 2004; Vicenzino et al 2011). A self-mobilization exercise requires the use of a belt, strap or hand; the purpose of this is to localize to the involved segment by the patient pulling up on the strap in a vertical direction along the plane of the facet joints. Self-mobilizations can be performed in

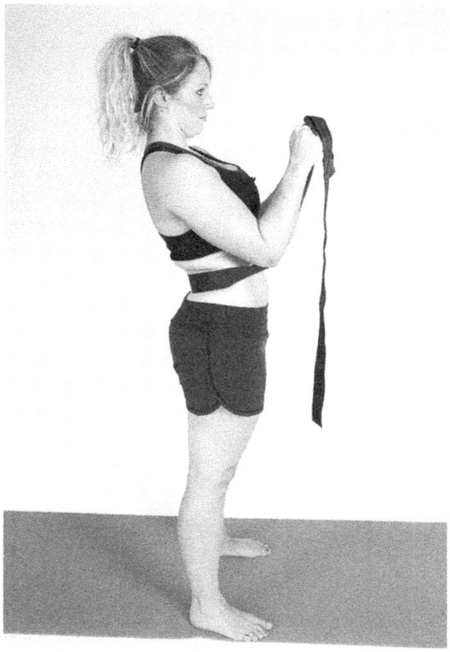

Figure 23.1 Extension self-mobilization. A belt is used to lift up to unload the affected level and the patient extends back over that support. The movement should be pain free.

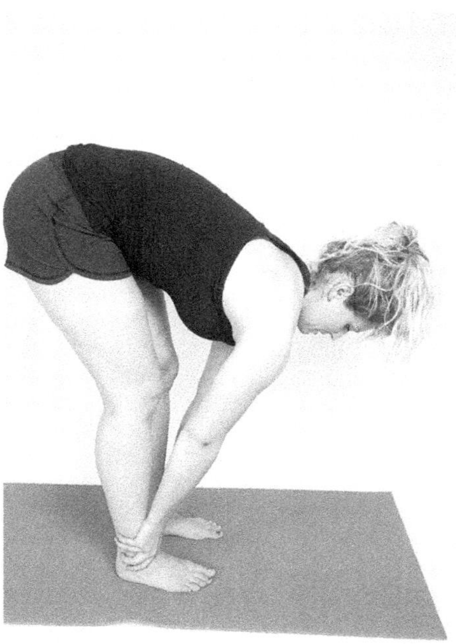

Figure 23.2 Jackknife. The patient bends over, flexing at the hips and knees, grasps the ankles and then extends the knees until they feel a stretch in either the lumber spine or posterior leg. This exercise can be used as a lumbar flexion flexibility exercise, erector spinae or hamstring muscle stretch.

various positions and directions (see Fig. 23.1). The exercise is usually repeated 10 times up to 10 times per day once it has been determined to be of benefit.

Janda (1987) suggested that the following muscles tend to tighten in subjects with LBP: the lumbar extensors, quadratus lumborum (QL), hip flexors, hip adductors, hamstrings, deep

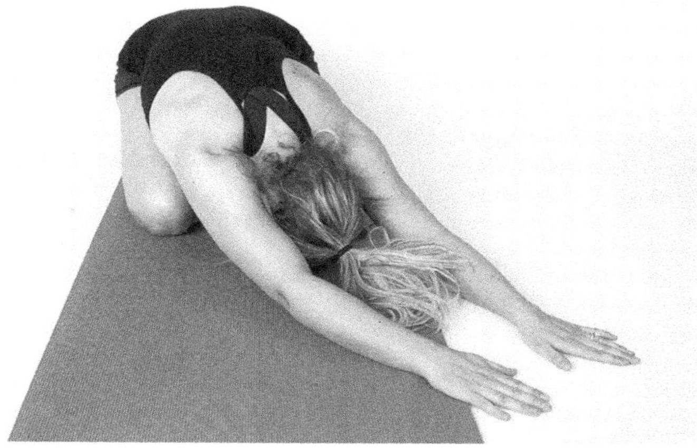

Figure 23.3 Child's pose with side-flexion. The patient sits back on the heels from the quadruped position with the arms forward and then moves the arms to one side to add a side-flexion component. This exercise can be used to regain lumbar side-flexion mobility and to obtain an erector spinae stretch, as well as stretching the quadratus lumborum, preferentially on the convex side.

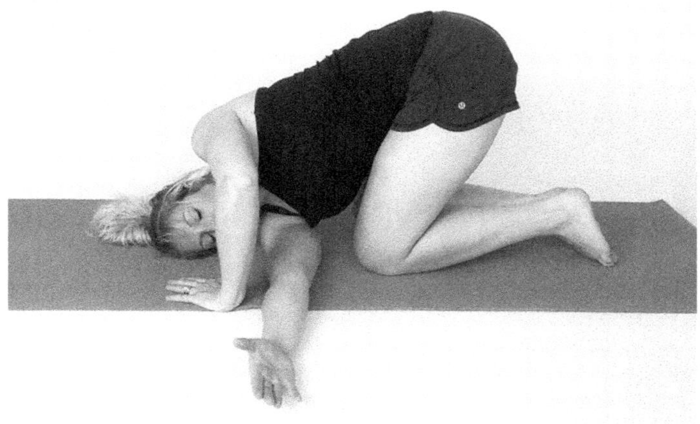

Figure 23.4 Thread the needle. From the quadruped position, the arm is threaded under the body to reach through to the opposite side. This creates a rotational stretch of the spine and can also be used to stretch the latissimus dorsi.

hip external rotators and tensor fasciae latae (TFL) / iliotibial band (ITB). In the literature, there is a lack of studies investigating the presence of muscle tightness specifically in subjects with LBP. Kujala et al (1992) investigated the association between various characteristics such as spinal mobility, general mobility, muscle length and strength and LBP in 12-year-olds and found an association only between LBP and tightness of the hip flexors. Bach et al (1985) found that, although runners had tighter hamstrings than non-runners, there was no correlation between hip muscle tightness and LBP in the runners.

With any stretching exercise it is important to monitor the postural control of other adjacent regions. It is common that, if one region is tight, an adjacent region may become relatively more mobile to compensate for that lack of motion; Sahrmann (2002) uses the phrase 'relative flexibility' to describe this phenomenon. Lengthening of a muscle becomes more focused if the relatively mobile section is controlled through either active muscular effort or specific

Box 23.1 Mobility exercise options

A. Extension

- Prone press-up
  - elbows→full press-up (sloppy push-up)
  - symmetrical→asymmetrical (unilateral/diagonal)
- Prone unilateral leg lift
- Supine anterior pelvic tilt
- Quadruped extension
- Standing back arch
  - from above/from below
- Forward lean at wall – extend from below
  - +side-flexion for unilateral
- Self-mobilization
  - use of hand/strap to localize

B. Flexion

- Supine knee to chest
  - double/single
- Pelvic tilt
  - supine→to full curl-up bridge
  - standing
- Forward curl
  - sitting (use therapy ball as roll-out)
  - standing (one leg up for unilateral)
- Jackknife
- Quadruped – flexion cat curl
- Quadruped sit-back (prayer stretch/child's pose)
  - use ball roll-out
  - add side-flexion for unilateral
- Flexion over end of bed
  - utilize contract–relax
- Self-mobilization
  - use of hand/strap to localize

C. Side-flexion/lateral glide

- Standing lateral glide automobilization/stretch
- Side-lean into wall
- Side-flexion back to wall (more extension)
  - reach rather than collapse
- Side-flexion in child's pose (more flexion)
- Pole side-flexion
- Lateral pelvic tilt/hip hike-drop
  - supine/standing
- Side-lying
  - legs drop over the edge of bed
  - over a roll/bolster
  - with arms overhead
- Yoga triangle pose

D. Rotation

- Quadruped – thread the needle (more flexion)
- Pole rotation
- Spinal twist
  - supine
  - side-lying
  - rotation with chair/wall assist
  - diagonal rotation in standing
  - into flexion (towards floor)
  - into extension (overhead)
- Yoga pose – warrior 2

positioning while the muscle is being stretched. Patients must be taught how to identify and control any unwanted movement to ensure an optimal stretch.

Specific myofascial extensibility exercises for the erector spinae (ES) muscle could include any of the flexion exercises listed in Box 23.1B. Using clinical reasoning, the choice of the optimal exercise would be dependent on the features of the patient's LBP. The jackknife stretch (see Fig. 23.2) for example, could address both the ES and the hamstrings length, but is performed in a position that would create substantial load on the lumbar spine as well as increase neuromeningeal tension. If spinal compression intolerance was a concern, a supine knee-to-chest stretch for the ES muscle and stretch of the hamstrings in supine would lessen the loading and therefore be more appropriate. Child's pose (see Fig 23.3) could be another option for stretching the ES muscle and adding side-flexion provides a unilateral focus in cases of asymmetrical tightness and would also lengthen a tight QL. During lengthening procedures for muscles attaching to the lumbar spine and pelvis, lumbopelvic stability must be monitored and maintained. Shortening of the latissimus dorsi muscle tends to pull the lumbar spine into a lordotic posture, and this lordosis must be controlled during any lengthening exercise for this muscle. Again the side-flexed child's pose position will prevent that tendency to lordose and having the arms overhead in a position of external rotation would further stretch the latissimus dorsi.

Although there are several studies that have compared different types of hamstring-stretching exercises (i.e. passive, active, static, dynamic, proprioceptive neuromuscular facilitation (PNF)), there is no clear indication as to which type is superior (Fasen et al 2009; Puentedura et al 2011; Ayala et al 2013). PNF stretching may result in earlier increases in length, but a passive stretch may be more effective over time. Borman et al (2011) determined that, despite significant increases in hamstring muscle length following stretching regimens, there was no change in lumbar mobility or curvature. Kang et al (2013) observed an immediate increase in hip flexion and decrease in lumbar flexion in the preparation phase of stooped lifting in subjects following therapist-assisted hamstring stretching. Sairyo et al (2013), in a pilot study, found the jackknife hamstring stretch exercise (see Fig. 23.2) to be effective for increasing hamstring length in both healthy adults and young athletes with LBP.

Winters et al (2004) reported that a passive stretch exercise (lunge and propped prone hip extension) was equal to an active exercise (prone active hip extension with knee flexed and knee extended) in lengthening tight hip flexors in subjects with LBP or lower extremity injuries.

Stretching of the TFL can be achieved using either the flexed or bent knee Ober's position, with conflicting reports as to which position is more effective (Gajdosik et al 2003; Wang et al 2006). Adding an overhead arm stretch to the opposite side seems to add further stretch when the traditional standing cross-leg stretch is used (Fredericson et al 2002). (See Ch 38 for further details on stretching the muscles of the hip.)

Motor Control: Stabilization, Motor Pattern Retraining, Strength

Specific stabilization or recruitment exercises are based on Panjabi's theoretical model that spinal stability depends on three systems: the passive osseoligamentous system, an active muscular system and a neural control system (Panjabi 1992). Bergmark (1989) divided the muscular system into a local (deep) system, controlling intervertebral motion, and a global (superficial) system, responsible for generating spinal motion. For the lumbosacral spine, the local muscles that have been identified as having a major role in spinal stability include the transversus abdominis (TrA), multifidus, pelvic floor and diaphragm. The evidence suggests that the function and structure of these muscles are altered in patients with LBP. The anticipatory contraction of the TrA and lumbar multifidus has been observed to be delayed, and morphological changes such as fatty infiltration and type I and II muscle fibre atrophy have been reported in the multifidus muscle, in individuals with LBP (Hides et al 1994; Hodges 2001; MacDonald et al 2009).

Motor control exercises have been developed to retrain optimal movement patterns and control of spinal motion. However, it has yet to be established which subgroup of patients would be most likely to benefit from this type of exercise. Debate remains over whether motor control exercises should focus on isolated contraction of the local muscles or whether exercises should aim at engaging all abdominal and back extensor muscles to ensure spinal stability (Bystrom et al 2013). Hodges (2011) postulated that isolated activation of the local musculature appears to be necessary to restore optimal control of movement and posture. The work by Tsao et al (2010) reported improved recruitment of the lumbar multifidus musculature with reduced coactivation of the superficial trunk muscles after skilled motor control training. The intervention involved cognitive attention to the activation of the multifidus and also included techniques such as motor imagery, anatomical description, palpation and coactivation with the pelvic floor musculature. An important observation made by these authors was that motor control exercises appear to be dependent on conscious and precise correction of movement (Tsao et al 2010).

Motor control exercise programmes have often been described in two stages (Costa et al 2009; Macedo et al 2012). The first stage involves training the coordinated activity of the trunk muscles including isolated activation of the deeper muscles (TrA and multifidus) while reducing the overactivity of the superficial muscles. Stage two focuses on the progression of the exercises through a range of functional activities using static and dynamic tasks: coordination / dissociation of trunk and limb movement, maintenance of optimal truck stability, postural correction and improvement of movement patterns. Hides et al (1996) found that local activation strategies could reverse the atrophy of multifidus in patients with acute LBP. Danneels et al (2001) suggested that, in chronic LBP patients, progressive strengthening involving high-load exercise was necessary to cause hypertrophy of multifidus, which was then associated with a decrease in pain.

Exercises

The following section is an evidence-informed description of commonly prescribed stabilization and motor control exercises for mechanical LBP. Many of the electromyographic (EMG) and real-time ultrasound studies reported here have been performed on normal subjects and this should be considered when generalizing these observations to clinical practice. Further studies on muscle activation during these various exercises in subjects with LBP would give more guidance for exercise choices in this patient population.

Abdominal draw-in manoeuvre

The abdominal draw-in manoeuvre is one of the essential exercises used to isolate / activate the TrA muscle (Fig. 23.5). Teyhen et al (2008), using ultrasound imaging in a group of healthy subjects, found that the abdominal draw-in manoeuvre preferentially activated the TrA with minimal changes in the internal oblique (IO). Individuals with unilateral lumbopelvic pain demonstrated a 20.9% smaller increase in the

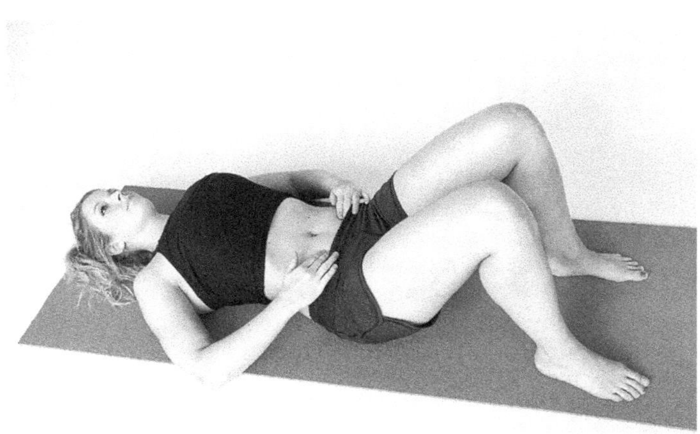

Figure 23.5 Abdominal draw-in manoeuvre. In supine the patient palpates the abdominal muscle activity and monitors for any substitution errors. On expiration, the patient is instructed to 'hollow' the abdomen; a pelvic floor activation cue may also be used to facilitate the isolated activation of the deep stability muscles.

thickness of the TrA muscle during the abdominal draw-in manoeuvre, compared with controls (Teyhen et al 2009). Other investigators have found that those who met the criteria for the stabilization classification of LBP (Fritz et al 2007) demonstrated a 50% increase in thickness during the contraction (Kiesel et al 2007). Various strategies have been suggested to facilitate the activation of TrA during this exercise, including palpation, contraction on expiration along with the instruction to 'hollow', and identification and correction of substitution strategies such as exaggeration of a posterior pelvic tilt. Co-contraction of the pelvic floor muscles, an integral component of the deep stabilization muscle system, can also be used to facilitate contraction of the TrA (Sapsford et al 2001). After a brief period of hollowing instruction, Bjerkefors et al (2010), using EMG recordings, found that a group of healthy subjects were able to activate the TrA independently of the rectus abdominis (RA). They were also able to integrate the TrA activation into basic exercises performed in supine, bridging and quadruped positions. This exercise can be performed in various positions and Mew (2009) found significantly greater thickness of the TrA with greater specificity in relation to IO and external oblique (EO) when the abdominal draw-in manoeuvre was performed in standing.

Chon et al (2010) examined the effect of an irradiation technique, a form of proprioceptive neuromuscular facilitation used to increase selectively the number of active motor unit recruitments. They applied resistance to strong ankle dorsiflexion in combination with the abdominal draw-in manoeuvre, proposing that the irradiation technique may stimulate the deep target muscle TrA. Using EMG and ultrasound imaging, they found that the addition of resisted ankle dorsiflexion enhanced TrA muscle activity, with associated increased thickness. Although this study provides empirical evidence, perhaps in those individuals who have difficulty in recruiting the TrA this could have important clinical implications.

The pressure biofeedback unit (PBU) has been used as a clinical tool to provide feedback for a successful abdominal draw-in manoeuvre in the prone or supine positions. In the prone position, the pressure sensor is placed under the lower abdomen, the lower edge in line with the anterior superior iliac spine, and is inflated to 70 mmHg. The patient is instructed to draw the lower abdomen gently off the PBU and hold the position. When the correct isolated contraction is performed, the pressure should decrease by approximately 6–8 mmHg up to a maximum of 10 mmHg in the holding position (Richardson et al 1999). In supine crook lying, the pressure biofeedback unit is placed in the lumbar lordosis and inflated to a base pressure of 40 mmHg where an isolated contraction can be performed and the pressure changes monitored. As a progression, the patient can be asked to perform a lower limb challenge while maintaining the pressure, for example a bent knee fall-out. A pressure increase of more than 10 mmHg indicates posterior tilt and uncontrolled flexion.

Adding lower limb challenges

According to Sahrmann (2002), the most important aspect of abdominal muscle performance is achieving the control that is necessary to: (1) appropriately stabilize the spine, (2)

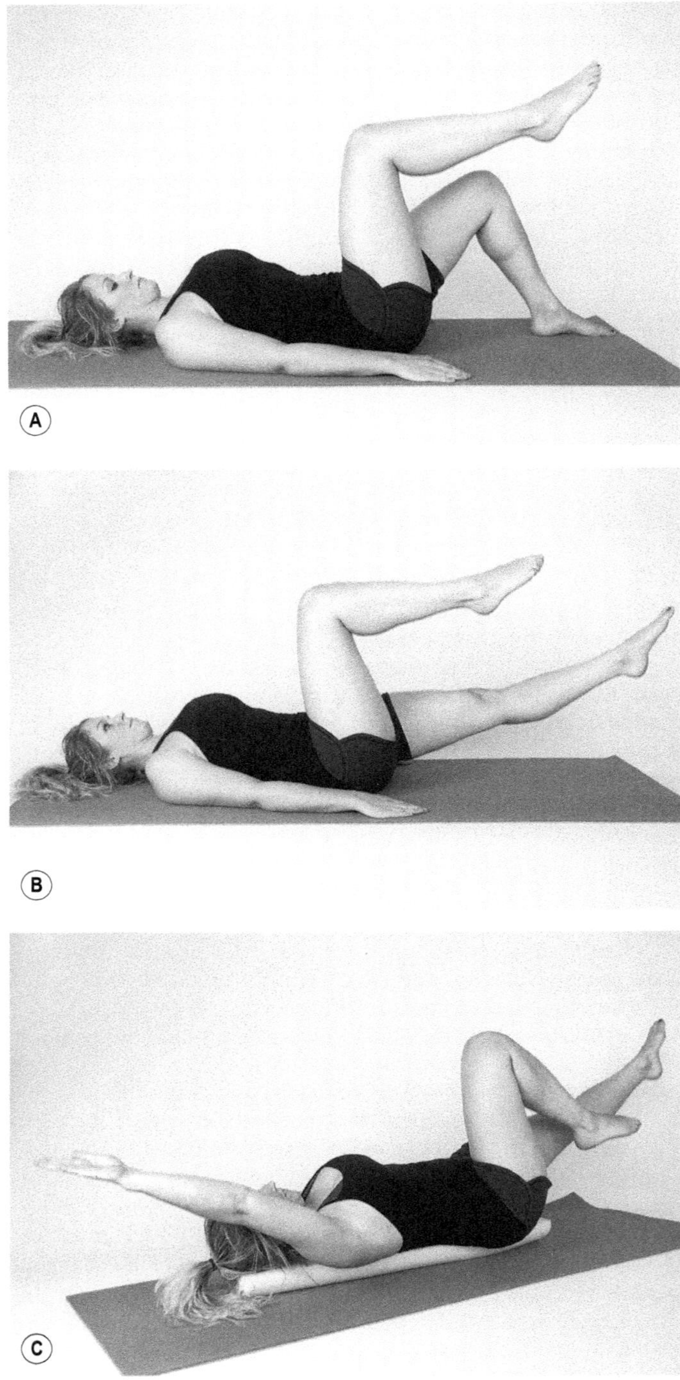

Figure 23.6 Limb load progressions. Various lower and upper limb movements can be added to challenge the ability of the deep muscles to maintain the lumbar neutral posture. All limb movements are preceded by the abdominal draw-in manoeuvre and this is maintained throughout the exercise.(**A**) In crook-lying, one leg is lifted to 90° hip flexion and then returned to the start position, alternating between legs. (**B**) Starting in crook-lying, one leg is lifted to 90° hip flexion and held there. The second leg is also lifted to 90° and then extended and returned without touching the supporting surface. Legs are alternated for the number of repetitions that can be performed without losing control of spinal neutral. (**C**) A modified 'dead bug' exercise can be performed on a foam roller to increase the abdominal muscle activation and stability challenge.

maintain optimal alignment and movement relationships between the pelvis and spine, and (3) prevent excessive stress and compensatory motions of the pelvis during movements of the extremities.

Various exercises have been described by Sahrmann (2002) based on the concept of leg loading to challenge lumbopelvic control. These exercises require the deep and superficial muscles to work synergistically in a static supporting role (Richardson et al 1999). The patient begins in a position of hip and knee flexion in supine-lying and prior to each exercise performs the abdominal draw-in manoeuvre. Initially low-load challenges such as a bent knee fall-out, lifting one foot with the other foot on the floor (Fig. 23.6A) or holding one knee to the chest and lifting the other foot can be introduced. The exercises then become progressively more difficult involving higher loads, such as unsupported extension of one leg (Fig. 23.6B) or adding arm and leg movements on an unstable surface (Fig. 23.6C). The patient should aim to perform 10 repetitions correctly before moving on to the next level. A neutral spine position should be maintained throughout the exercise and the patient should breathe normally. As described earlier, a PBU could be utilized to assist the patient in monitoring this while practising in the clinic. In cases where patients are having difficulty with the patterning, they can be instructed to place their hands such that their palms rest over the anterior superior iliac spine (ASIS) and fingers rest on the lower abdominal wall. This allows them to monitor both the deep abdominal muscle contraction and any pelvic motion that could indicate loss of spinal neutral.

Abdominal curl-up

The abdominal curl-up has been found to have the highest abdominal muscular challenge with the least amount of spinal compression (Axler & McGill 1997). In the supine position, with hands placed under the lumbar spine to maintain a neutral position and one knee flexed, the patient is instructed to pivot about the sternum and lift the shoulder blades off of the mat while maintaining a neutral neck position and to hold for 5 seconds (Fig. 23.7A) (McGill & Karpowicz 2009). This exercise is progressed by elevating the elbows from the table, placing the hands on the forehead (Fig. 23.7B) or forward reaching, pre-bracing the abdominal wall and breathing deeply during the exercise (McGill & Karpowicz 2009). Teyhen et al (2008) investigated six common abdominal strengthening exercises using ultrasound imaging and found the greatest changes in muscle thickness of the TrA during the side bridge and the abdominal curl-up.

The traditional bent knee sit-up (Fig. 23.8) requiring more than 30° of lumbar flexion has been shown to increase the compressive load through the lumbar spine, with potential risk of injury, and may not be appropriate for individuals who need to minimize the amount of lumbar flexion or compressive forces. Several studies have shown higher EO muscle activity during the bent knee sit-up compared with the curl-up, which may be indicated for higher intensity strength training, but there was also greater activity of the rectus femoris (Escamilla et al 2006a, 2006b, 2010). Escamilla et al (2010) reported that the curl-up generated relatively low rectus femoris and lumbar paraspinal activity and relatively high RA, EO and IO activity, perhaps making it a better choice for some individuals.

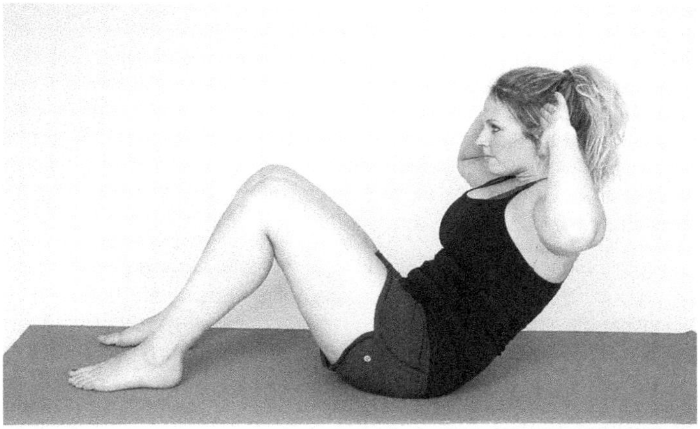

Figure 23.8 Bent knee sit-up. The traditional abdominal-strengthening exercise can be performed with hands by the head, reaching forward or across the chest to modify the difficulty.

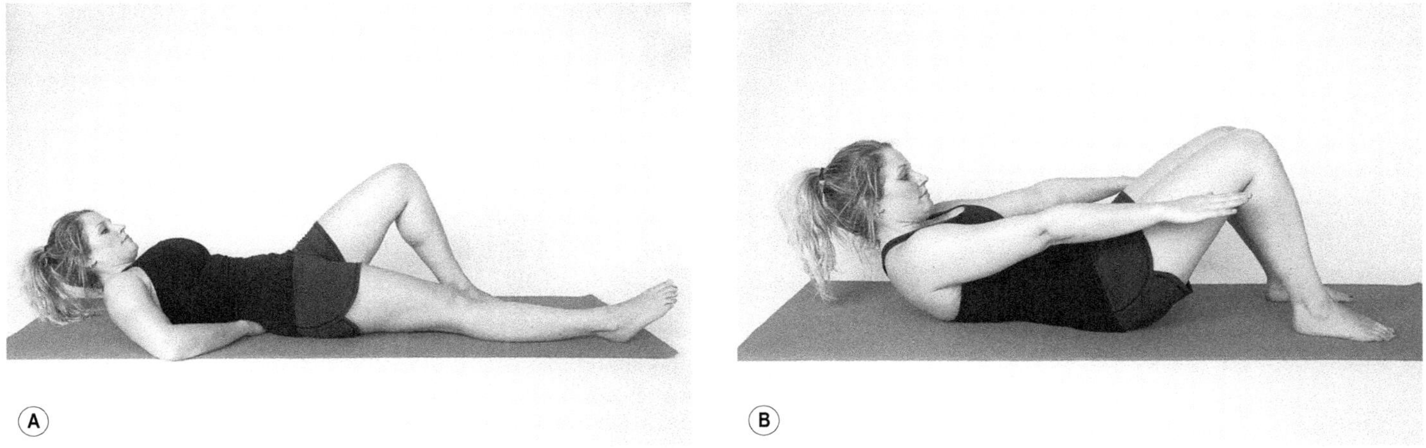

Figure 23.7 Abdominal curl-up progressions. (**A**) The initial curl-up position is shown ensuring the patient pivots about the sternum as the shoulder blades are lifted off of the mat. (**B**) The exercise can be progressed by reaching with the arms, or putting hands on the forehead.

Multifidus activation exercises

Researchers using real-time ultrasound and magnetic resonance imaging (MRI) demonstrated decreased cross-sectional area of the multifidus muscle in patients with chronic LBP (Danneels et al 2000; Barker et al 2004; Hides et al 2008b). In individuals with unilateral chronic LBP, Hides et al (2008a) documented asymmetry, with the smaller multifidus muscle being found ipsilateral to the symptoms. This atrophy appeared to be localized, suggesting that exercises should address this specific localized muscle impairment. Exercises to activate the multifidus selectively continue to be a challenging task for both clinicians and patients. Using ultrasound imaging in individuals with chronic LBP, Hides et al (2011) demonstrated that the ability to contract the multifidus was related to the ability to contract the TrA, with the odds of a good multifidus contraction being 4.5 times higher for patients who had a good contraction of the TrA. Palpation can be used as a facilitation technique and during a contraction of the multifidus a symmetrical deep tensioning should be palpated close to the midline (Richardson et al 2004). As illustrated in Figure 23.9A–C, various positions can be utilized in an attempt to target activation of the multifidus muscle. The multifidus has also been shown to contribute to proprioception and repositioning accuracy (Brumagne et al 2000). Visual / motor imagery, a process in which the individual imagines performing a motor task without any apparent motion of the body segments, may be a useful tool in retraining activation of the multifidus (Hodges et al 2013). Diane Lee (Lee & Lee 2011) suggests using the following cues:

Imagine a line connecting your groin (or back of your pubic bone) to the part of multifidus in your low back you are trying to train (wake up). Connect along this line and then gently think about suspending (lifting) the lumbar vertebra 1 mm above the one below.

According to Lee, the therapist should observe and correct compensation strategies such as rotation of the pelvis, anterior tilting, hiking of the hip or gripping with the buttock muscles. Various facilitation and correction techniques are outlined in Box 23.2 and can be applied to all of the exercises.

Box 23.2 Motor control facilitation techniques

- Palpation / observation / identification of compensation strategies
- Maintain neutral spine position – control lumbopelvic-trunk rotation
- Co-contract with other muscles – TrA with pelvic floor and multifidus with TrA
- Incorporate relaxed breathing
- Reduce activity of overactive or dominant muscles
- Manual facilitation / taping
- Feedback – ultrasound, pressure biofeedback unit
- Visual / motor imagery
- Correct faulty movement patterns
- Incorporate muscle activation into functional movements and postures

Bridge exercises in supine

Bridging exercises are commonly used in stabilization programmes to improve motor control and to enhance trunk stability and gluteal muscle activity. The patient is instructed to perform the abdominal draw-in manoeuvre initially and to squeeze the gluteal muscles prior to lifting the pelvis. It is important to eliminate hamstring dominance; McGill (2010) suggests palpating the hamstrings and, if active, the patient can be cued to use knee extension to push the feet into the surface to decrease hamstrings activation and use slight hip external rotation to ensure gluteal activation. It has been documented that multifidus activity measured by surface EMG is high during a back-bridge exercise (Ekstrom et al 2007; Okubo et al 2010). Okubo et al (2010) reported relatively high bilateral activation of the ES during the basic bridge exercise and the bridge with one leg extended (Fig. 23.10). These authors proposed that the need to extend the spine against gravity during the bridging exercise might account for this higher activity. In a recent EMG study, Kim et al (2013) investigated whether incorporating arm movements into bridge exercises on the floor or on a therapeutic ball changed the EMG activity of selected trunk muscles (Fig. 23.11). They found increased IO activity during bridging on a therapeutic ball and when arm movements were integrated into the exercise. Elevation of one leg during the traditional back bridge elicited the largest increase in IO activity on the side of the raised leg to control the tendency of the pelvis to rotate downwards (Garcia-Vaquero et al 2012). Progression of the bridge exercise to can include the addition of unstable surfaces such as lying on a foam roll, and limb challenges with or without resistance, such as elastic resistance around the knees (Fig. 23.12) (Jeon et al 2013).

Quadruped

Patients are taught to activate the stability muscles to maintain a neutral spine posture while performing various limb load challenges in the quadruped position. Teyhen et al (2009) found that the quadruped opposite arm and leg lift exercise generated preferential changes in TrA with minimal changes in IO thickness. Stevens et al (2007) using EMG measurements during single-leg extension and opposite arm and leg extension in the quadruped position found the highest muscle activity (>20% maximal voluntary contraction MVC) in the ipsilateral multifidus and gluteus maximus. Garcia-Vaquero et al (2012) found that, in this position, the IO on the side of the raised arm paired with the contralateral EO to stabilize, whereas ES activity was higher on the side corresponding to the elevated leg; they concluded that this was likely to be due to the increased torque produced with elevation of the leg. During the performance of this exercise, it is important that the patient maintains a neutral spine position and that the motion takes place about the shoulder and the hip, avoiding trunk rotation. Progressions could include opposite arm and leg elevation, quick short arc movements of the limbs, drawing imaginary patterns with the hand or foot (McGill & Karpowicz 2009), adding resistance (free weights / elastic) (Fig. 23.13A) and the use of an unstable surface (e.g. foam roll, sizzle, BOSU®, Swiss ball; Fig. 23.13B).

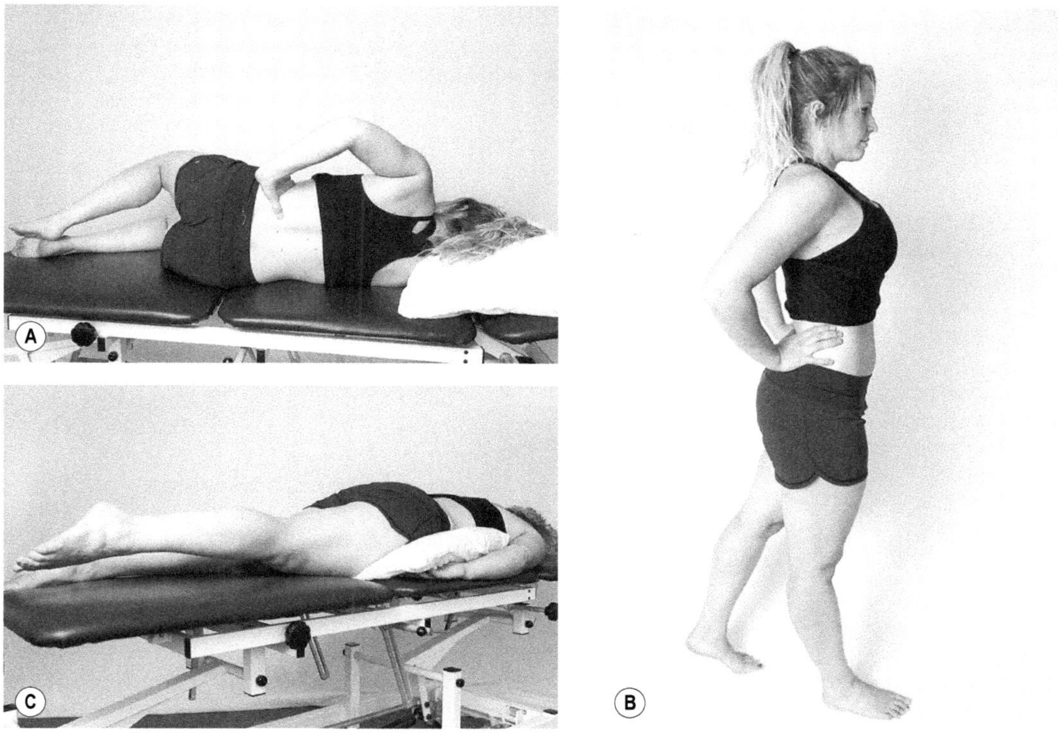

Figure 23.9 Multifidus activation exercises. Isolation of the multifidus can be performed in various positions and facilitated through palpation of muscle tension developing at the desired spinal segment. (**A**) Side-lying: the patient palpates for a tensioning of the muscle while performing a clam shell (lifting the top knee). (**B**) Standing: the patient palpates and accentuates the muscle tensioning while transferring load by pushing off to the forward leg in step stance. (**C**) Prone: a single-leg lift is performed to activate a multifidus contraction.

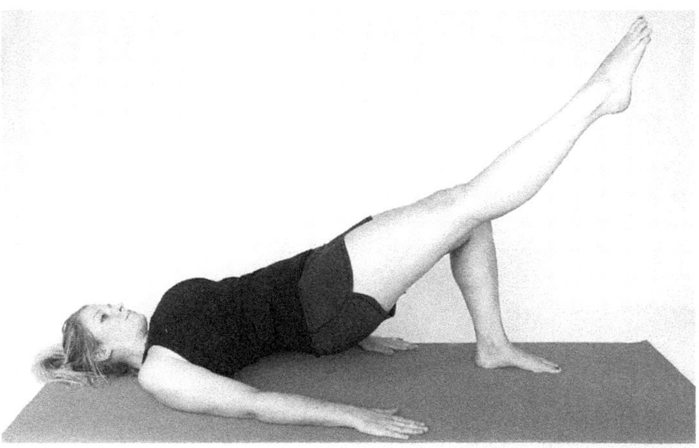

Figure 23.10 Supine bridge with leg lift. Maintaining a neutral lumbopelvic posture, one leg is lifted off the supporting surface in the bridge position. The exercise would be made more difficult by bringing the arms off the floor; the hands can be placed on the pelvis to monitor that position.

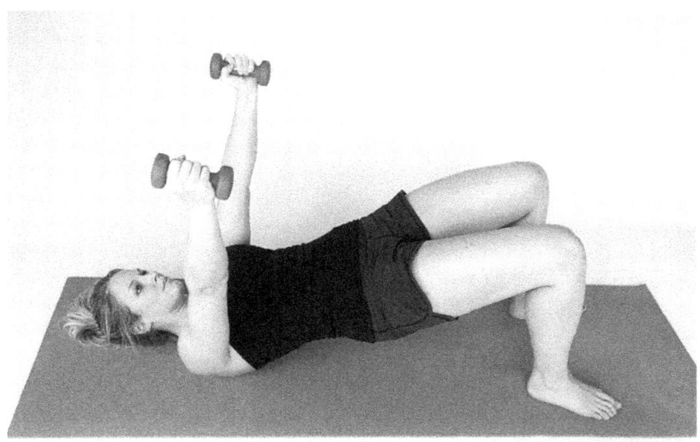

Figure 23.11 Supine bridge with arm load. Incorporating arm movements with or without resistance during a supine-bridge exercise increases activation of the abdominal muscles.

Side plank/horizontal side support

The side-plank exercise has been found to activate the IO, the EO and the QL with low lumbar loading (McGill et al 1996; McGill 1997). As illustrated in Figure 23.14, there are various progressions to this exercise: (1) side bridge with the knees on the ground and the hand on the deltoid to stabilize the shoulder (Fig. 23.14A); (2) knees on the ground and the hand on the waist / pelvis; (3) full side plank, knees extended (Fig. 23.14B); (4) single leg support – adding hip flexion, extension or abduction of the uppermost leg (Fig. 23.14C); (5) rolling from the side bridge into the front plank and then back into the opposite side bridge, ensuring minimal rotation between the pelvis and the rib cage (McGill & Karpowicz 2009). McGill emphasizes that this exercise should be initiated with a 'hip-hinge' movement in which the hips are extended in a squat-like manner to neutral and the trunk should maintain a neutral alignment.

A number of investigators have demonstrated the highest activation of the oblique abdominals (42–57% MVC) during this exercise (Kavcic et al 2004; Lehman et al 2005). Garcia-Vaquero et al (2012) demonstrated similar results, but also found the highest activation levels (14–30% MVC) on the lower side compared with the uppermost side (3–10% MVC). These authors postulated that the lateral orientation of the oblique muscles offers the greatest support to the trunk during a side-bridge exercise. They did, however, find that RA and ES on the lower side were also active (16% MVC), suggesting coactivation of muscles on the lower side so as to stabilize. Elevation of the leg during the side bridge with the hip flexed / extended resulted in the highest muscle activation, with IO on the support side increasing as much as 20% MVC compared with the conventional side bridge. Himes et al (2012) compared the activation of TrA during the side-bridge exercise progressions in healthy controls and in individuals with recurrent LBP, and found that TrA contracted similarly during the exercise in both groups. These authors recommended that this exercise could be used in patients with LBP as long as the progressions remained pain free and adequate time was spent on instruction and cueing proper technique.

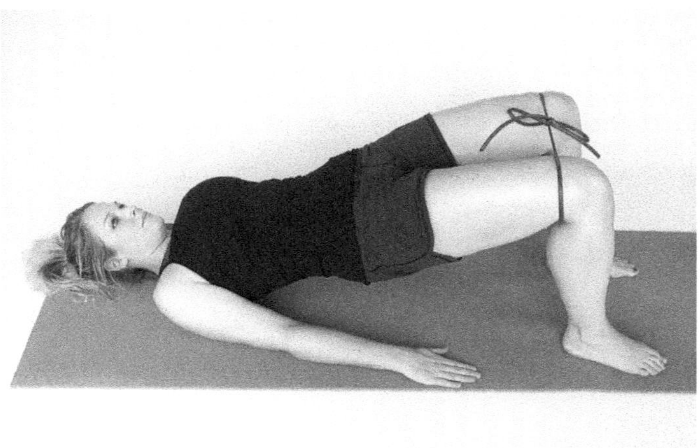

Figure 23.12 Supine bridge with leg load. Elastic resistance around the legs for hip external rotation will encourage increased gluteal muscle activity.

Front plank/prone bridge

The front plank or prone bridge is used to activate and strengthen both the deep and the superficial abdominal wall muscles. The easiest form of this exercise would have the patient performing it with the knees bent and the shoulder supported, as illustrated in Figure 23.15. The main muscle maintaining posture and stability during the prone bridge exercise is the RA (25–47% MVC) along with activation of the EO, which varies anywhere between 16% and 50% MVC (Lehman et al 2005; Ekstrom et al 2007; Imai et al 2010; Garcia-Vaquero et al 2012). Garcia-Vaquero et al (2012) described changes in the muscle recruitment patterns when single-leg support was added to conventional bridging exercises. Elevation of the leg during the front bridge (Fig. 23.16) resulted in slight lowering of RA activation, whereas the IO on the opposite side of the raised leg and the EO on the side of the raised leg increased slightly (3–4% MVC) to control the rotational torque (Garcia-Vaquero et al 2012). Although creating a higher challenge, the combination of the increased rotational torque and high trunk muscle activation may generate increased compressive loads on the spine and so this should be considered when prescribing this exercise with individuals with LBP.

Exercises on unstable surfaces

Additions of unstable surfaces, such as a Swiss ball or a BOSU®, are commonly used to increase the muscular demand required to maintain trunk stability (Imai et al 2010). The Swiss ball should be appropriately sized for the patient and inflated according to the patient's weight so that when he / she is sitting erect and centred on the ball with feet together and flat on the floor, the hips and knees should be flexed approximately 90° and thighs parallel to the floor. Some authors have shown enhanced activity of the global trunk musculature such as the EO and RA, compared with the local stabilizers

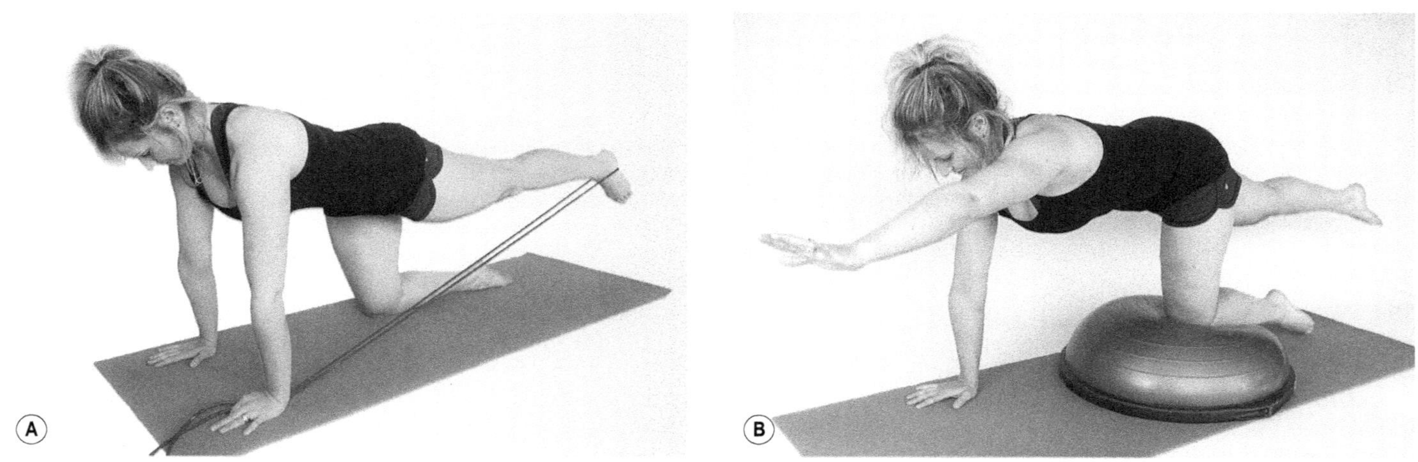

Figure 23.13 Quadruped exercises. (**A**) Resisted leg lift: elastic resistance can be added to a leg-lift challenge in the quadruped position. (**B**) The BOSU® provides an unstable base to increase further the challenge of an opposite arm and leg lift exercise.

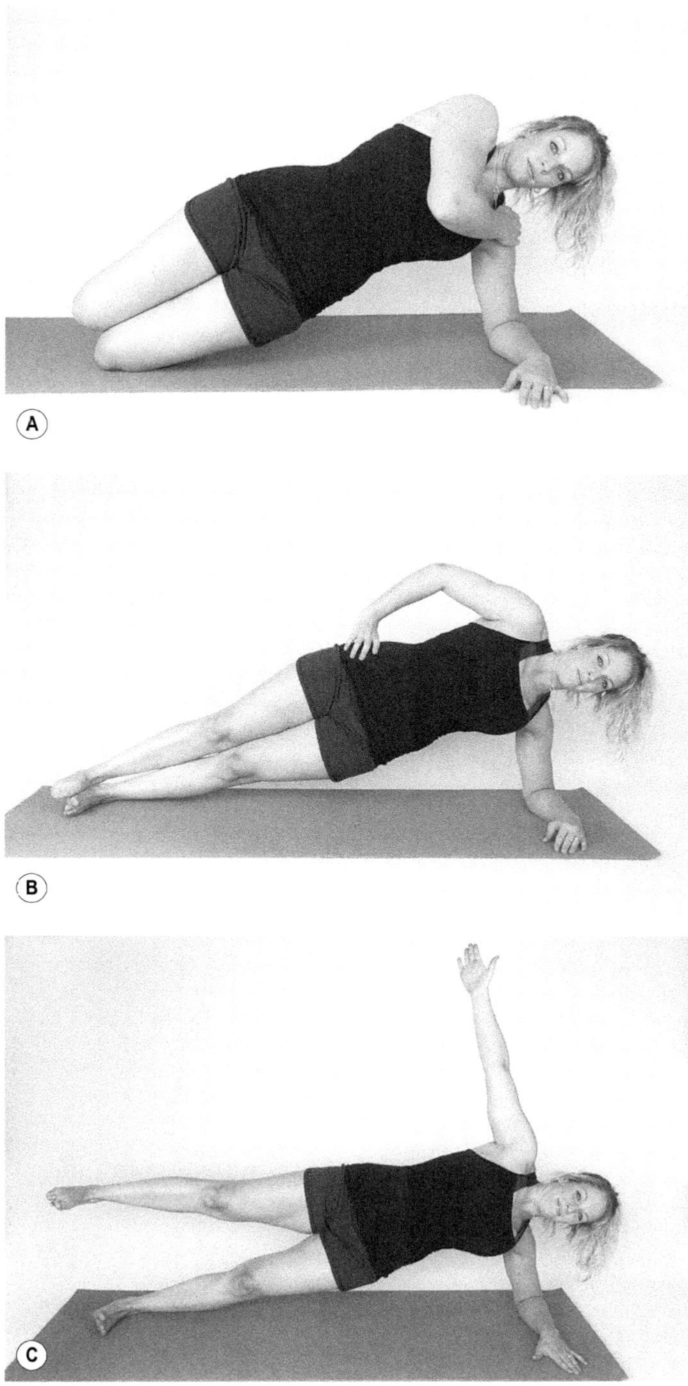

Figure 23.14 **Side plank.** (**A**) The easiest form of side plank is with bent knees and the arm supporting the opposite shoulder. (**B**) The side plank is progressed on to extended legs. (**C**) Adding a leg and arm lift in the full side-plank position further challenges stability and increases activation of the abdominal muscles.

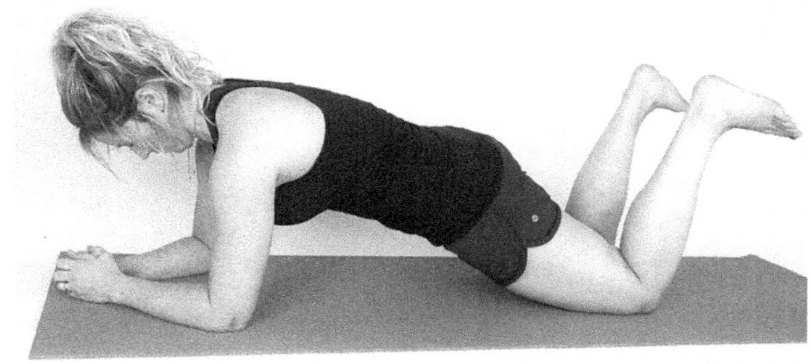

Figure 23.15 **Front plank.** The easiest form of the front plank is performed by lifting the hips off the supporting surface with the knees on the ground.

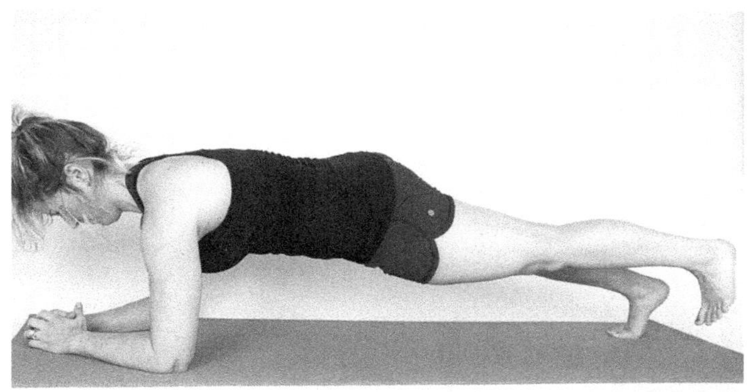

Figure 23.16 **Front plank with leg lift.** Adding a hip extension leg lift to the full front plank will challenge stability control and increase activity in the oblique abdominals.

(Imai et al 2010). The prone bridge exercise on a Swiss ball (Fig. 23.17A) produces the highest RA and EO activity (Lehman et al 2005; Imai et al 2010; Czaprowski et al 2014). The introduction of a BOSU® (Fig. 23.17B) or Swiss ball to the side-bridge exercise has been found to lead to a significant increase in TrA and EO activity (Imai et al 2010; Czaprowski et al 2014). Imai et al (2010) propose that the unstable surface requires greater muscle activity to control the rotation and lateral flexion torque generated through the trunk with this exercise. In contrast, for the back-bridge exercise, several authors have found that trunk muscle activity is not influenced by surface stability (Stevens et al 2006; Ekstrom et al 2008; Imai et al 2010). Czaprowski et al (2014) analysed EMG activity levels as well as relative activation of the deep to superficial abdominal muscles during prone, supine and side bridges on a stable surface, BOSU® or Swiss ball. There are several clinical implications arising from their research findings. If the goal is to use a low-load exercise generating low muscle activity, the supine bridge on a stable or unstable surface is appropriate, whereas if the aim is to strengthen the entire abdominal wall then the prone-bridge exercise on a Swiss ball is a good choice. Abdominal muscle activity during the side bridge is significantly higher than the activity during any of the supine-bridge exercises. Alternatively, if the goal is to maximize the activity of the deep abdominal muscles relative to the RA, then the prone and side bridge on the BOSU® or a stable surface would be the best choice.

There are several higher level Swiss ball exercises that may be used for athletic individuals or in the later stages of motor control training (Fig. 23.18A–B). Escamilla et al (2010)

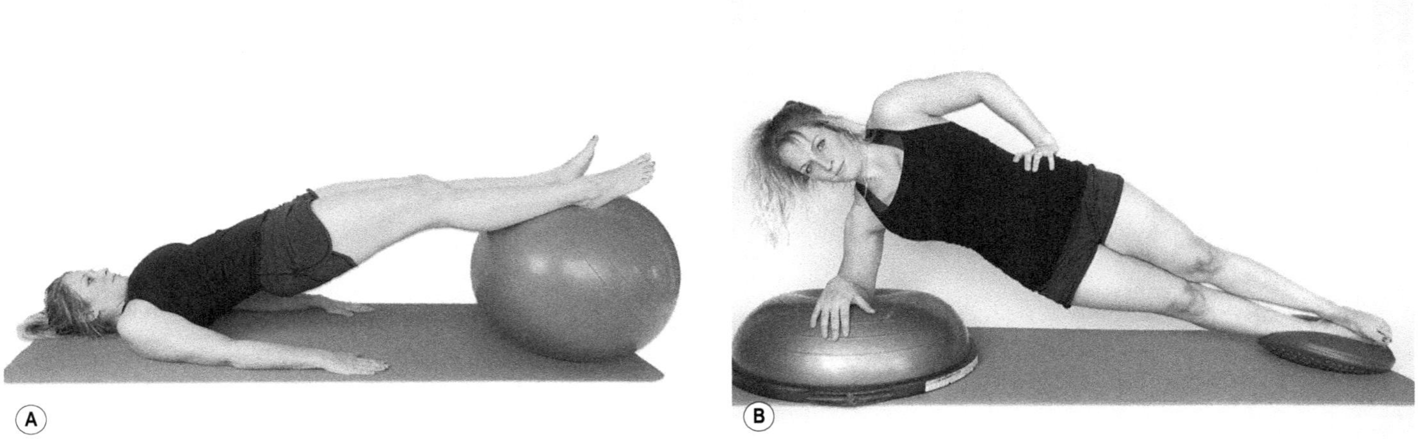

Figure 23.17 Adding unstable surfaces. The additional of unstable surfaces increases the muscular demand required for trunk stability. (**A**) A supine bridge performed with both legs on a Swiss ball. (**B**) Side bridge on a BOSU® and a sizzle.

investigated the effect of eight advanced Swiss ball exercises (roll-out, pike, skier, hip extension, decline push-up and sitting march) and two traditional abdominal exercises (crunch and bent knee sit-up) on activation of the lumbopelvic–hip musculature. These authors found that the pike and the roll-out were the most effective in recruiting the core muscles but that they also required the greatest effort and were the most difficult (Escamilla et al 2010). Exercises that generated more than 60% MVC (roll-out and pike) were suggested to be more conducive to developing muscle strength, whereas those that generated less than 20% MVC (sitting march, crunch) would be more appropriate for endurance training.

Motor Pattern Retraining/Functional Integration

Motor pattern retraining involves identifying faulty movement patterns, isolating the component of the movement and then practising the corrected pattern. Retraining into functional tasks specific to the patient's individual needs is then incorporated (O'Sullivan 2000). Motor learning strategies have been applied to the management of chronic LBP and involve the transition through three phases proposed by Fitts and Posner (1967): (1) cognitive, (2) associative, and (3) autonomous (O'Sullivan 2000; Hodges et al 2013).

The **cognitive phase** requires a high level of awareness in order to isolate the co-contraction of the deep local system without superficial global muscle activation (O'Sullivan 2000). During this time, the patient is improving the perception of the skill with conscious attention to detail and correction of errors (Hodges et al 2013). Various facilitation techniques can be used such as instructions, feedback, visual cues, mental imagery and optimal postures (Hodges et al 2013).

In the **associative phase**, the focus is on refining a particular movement pattern (O'Sullivan 2000). Two or three faulty and pain-provocative movement patterns are identified and broken down into component movements (O'Sullivan 2000). In this phase, repeated practice of the skill for thousands of repetitions is required to develop and solidify a motor pattern. Initially simple tasks are performed in unloaded positions,

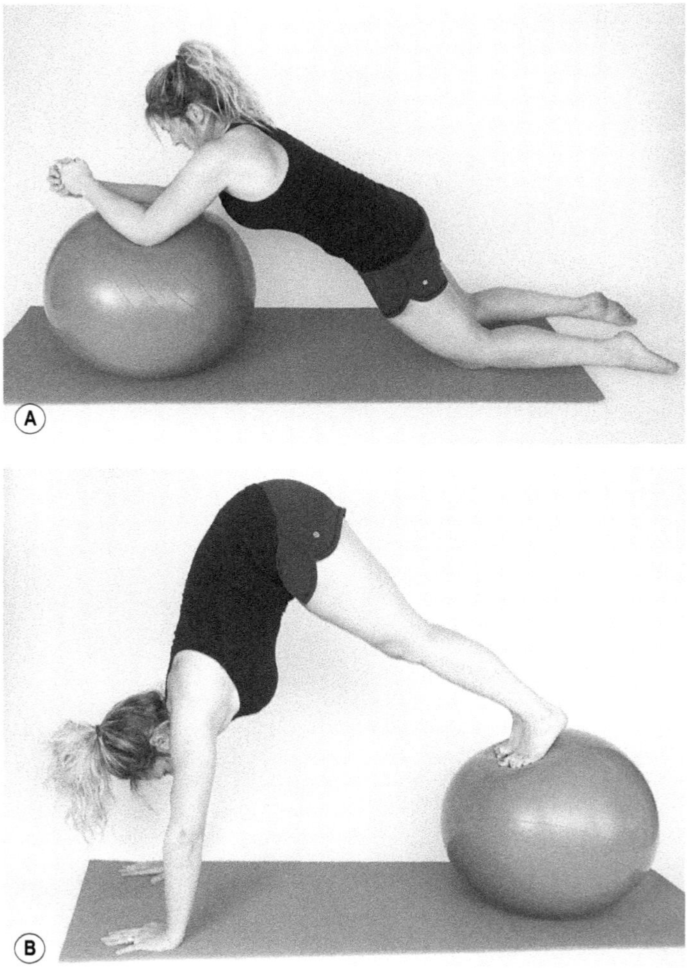

Figure 23.18 High-level Swiss ball exercises. (**A**) Roll-out: in a front-plank position the patient rolls the ball forwards and backwards while maintaining trunk control. (**B**) Pike: performing a pike motion with feet on the ball is a high-end challenge for the stability musculature, movement pattern control and balance.

with gradual progression to more-demanding complex functional tasks adding load and speed. Patients are encouraged to focus on consistency of performance (Hodges et al 2013).

The final phase is the **autonomous phase,** in which the objective of the exercises is to facilitate automatic correction of movement / postural faults with minimal conscious effort. This would promote dynamic stabilization of the spine in an automatic manner during functional activities (O'Sullivan 2000; Hodges et al 2013).

Evaluation and correction / training of posture is an integral component of the rehabilitation of mechanical LBP and could be considered the first step in developing movement pattern exercises. Prolonged sitting may produce increased mechanical stress and has been reported as a potential factor related to the development of LBP. Dankaerts et al (2006) investigated the sitting postures of asymptomatic individuals and chronic LBP patients and found that patients with LBP have a tendency to adopt postures near the end range of spinal motion away from the neutral position with less ability to change their posture. O'Sullivan (2000) classified two different subgroups: those who sit with a more kyphotic lumbar spine assuming an end-range flexion posture and those with a hyperlordotic sitting strategy. He also reported that LBP patients demonstrate a reduced ability to adopt and maintain a neutral (mid-range) position. LBP patients demonstrate greater neutral-spine-repositioning deficits and higher abdominal activity compared with healthy subjects (O'Sullivan et al 2006; Sheeran et al 2012).

There is little consensus in the literature as to the best sitting posture. It has been proposed that an optimal sitting posture for subjects with LBP is a neutral spine position involving slight lumbar lordosis and a relaxed thorax (O'Sullivan et al 2006). This 'ideal posture' is associated with less overactivation of the superficial muscles and encourages greater activity of the deeper trunk muscles along with a more relaxed breathing pattern (Claus et al 2009; Lee et al 2010; O'Sullivan et al 2012, Hodges et al 2013). This will obviously vary between individuals and so, when determining the best sitting posture for an individual with LBP, the clinician needs to consider a number of factors such as the underlying pathology, spinal mobility, pain and provocative postures. Verbal instructions such as 'grow tall' or 'roll forwards on your sit bones' to increase lumbar lordosis, or 'imagine lengthening your spine' to reduce thoracic kyphosis can be used to facilitate postural correction (Lee & Lee 2011). As an exercise, the patient may be asked to use their optimal cues to achieve a neutral spine, to hold that posture for the count of 10 and repeat 10 times, and to perform this every hour throughout the day to assist in habituation.

In a recent EMG study, Park et al (2013) found altered distribution of EMG activity between the ES, QL and psoas major (PM) in patients with LBP. Those subjects presenting with high ES EMG activity in a slight lordotic sitting posture had lower PM and QL activity, whereas those with lower ES activity in this posture had greater PM and QL activity. This preliminary information would suggest that, in some patients with LBP, the PM and QL muscles may need to be down-trained or stretched, whereas in others PM and QL recruitment exercises would be more appropriate.

Patients with LBP often move their whole spine as a block, being unable to isolate and dissociate movement between regions. Once the neutral spine posture has been achieved, dissociation tasks can be added. The sitting-forward lean can be used to train dissociation of spinal and hip flexion. After finding the neutral spine position, the patient is instructed to hinge at the hips to bring the trunk forwards while maintaining the neutral spine posture (Lee & Lee 2011). The 'waiter's bow' exercise (Fig. 23.19), executed in a similar manner in standing, could be used as a progression (Sahrmann 2002).

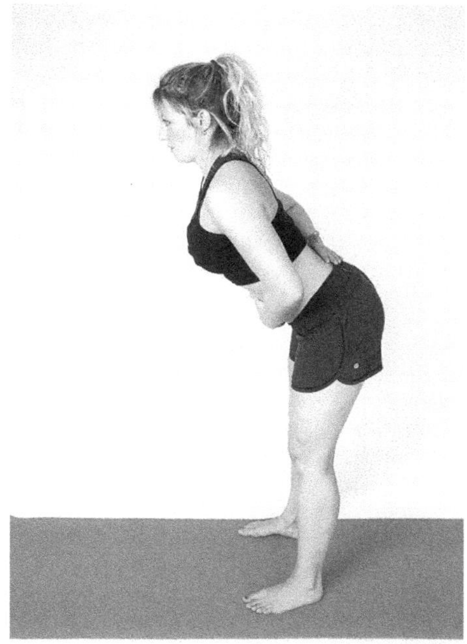

Figure 23.19 Waiter's bow. To practise hip–trunk dissociation patterning, the patient finds and maintains the neutral spine position and then hinges at the hips to bring the trunk forward without losing control of the neutral spine position.

In the quadruped position, patients can be taught to maintain a neutral lumbopelvic region while flexing and extending the thoracic spine in a slow and controlled manner. The opposite dissociation pattern can also be practised: maintaining thoracic neutral while flexing and extending the lumbopelvic region, initiating through anterior and posterior pelvic rotation. This lumbar / thoracic dissociation pattern can also be practised in the sitting position, initially on the stable surface of a chair, then progressing to a Swiss ball. Further progressions may include postural control in more difficult positions or increased loading, as well as integrating the postural control into more complicated movement patterns, some of which have already been discussed (quadruped opposite arm and leg, planks, various bridging exercises). From here, further specific functional integration exercises should relate directly to the patient's needs regarding occupation, hobby and sport activities.

Pilates / Yoga

Both pilates and yoga can be used to incorporate full-body activity integrating motor patterning into functional movements. Pilates-based therapeutic exercise, often referred to as clinical pilates, is becoming more common as an intervention for patients with LBP. Wells et al (2012), through a systematic review of the literature, developed a definition for pilates as a 'mind–body exercise that focuses on strength, core stability, flexibility, muscle control, posture and breathing'. To date, the research findings for the benefit of clinical pilates in the treatment of LBP are inconsistent in their results and conclusions (Lim et al 2011; Pereira et al 2011; Posadzki et al 2011; Wajswelner et al 2012; Aladro-Gonzalvo et al 2013; Wells et al 2013). A recent meta-analysis concluded that, in subjects with chronic LBP, pilates was moderately superior to other physiotherapeutic interventions in reducing disability but not pain, and also provided moderate to superior pain relief compared with minimal intervention (Aladro-Gonzalvo et al 2013). However, due to the small volume, poor quality and presence of co-interventions in many studies, the evidence supporting the use of pilates to reduce pain and disability in chronic LBP is inconclusive and the authors warn that any conclusions should be met with caution (Aladro-Gonzalvo et al 2013; Wells et al 2013).

One randomized clinical trial found that the use of a pilates-based exercise programme in patients with non-structural scoliosis reduced the degree of curvature, increased flexibility and decreased pain, compared with controls (Alves de Araujo et al 2012). Stolze et al (2012) developed a preliminary CPR to identify those patients most likely to benefit from a pilates-based exercise programme for LBP. Five variables were identified: total trunk flexion of 70° or less, current symptom duration of 6 months or less, no leg symptoms in the past week, body mass index of 25 kg / m^2 or more, and left or right average hip rotation of 25° or greater. If three or more of the five variables were present, the probability of a successful outcome increased from 54% to 93%. This rule has yet to be validated.

Yoga includes a number of components that theoretically could benefit the patient with LBP. Strengthening, stretching, balance, breathing and relaxation, as well as attention to alignment and postural control, could all contribute to the positive response that some patients receive from participating in this exercise approach. Sherman et al (2013) explored the factors that mediated the response to either yoga or an intensive stretching programme in LBP. Participation in exercise and self-efficacy were the strongest mediators for both types of exercise. Relaxation, awareness and the benefits of breathing were also important mediators for the yoga group. Tekur et al (2012) found greater reduction in pain, anxiety and depression and larger improvement of spinal mobility following a 7-day intensive residential yoga programme compared with physiotherapeutic exercises. Posadzki and Ernst (2011), in their systematic review, found that the majority of the studies were positive for the use of yoga in the treatment of LBP, but felt that definitive claims needed to be treated with caution because of the small number of studies and the inconsistency of results, as well as the many different types of yoga.

Balance / Proprioception

Balance deficits and poor position sense have been reported to be present in individuals with chronic LBP (Brumagne et al 2000; Newcomer et al 2000; Hodges et al 2013). Balance may be compromised as a result of sensory or motor impairments such as visual, vestibular or somatosensory deficits, poor coordination and an inability to move or involve the trunk in postural adjustments (Hodges et al 2013). A recent systematic review by Mazaheri et al (2013) examined LBP and postural sway and concluded that increased sway is present in some, but not all, LBP patients. Incorporation of trunk balance and proprioceptive retraining may be required to restore optimal function in patients with chronic LBP. Gatti et al (2011), in a randomized controlled trial, investigated the efficacy of trunk balance training in patients with chronic LBP. The balance exercises were performed in sitting, kneeling, quadruped and supine positions. The participants were asked to maintain the position for a period ranging from 30 seconds to 2 minutes. Once achieved the exercise was progressed in difficulty by changing the base of support, closing the eyes or by adding head or upper limb movement (Fig. 23.20A). The authors concluded that trunk balance exercises combined with

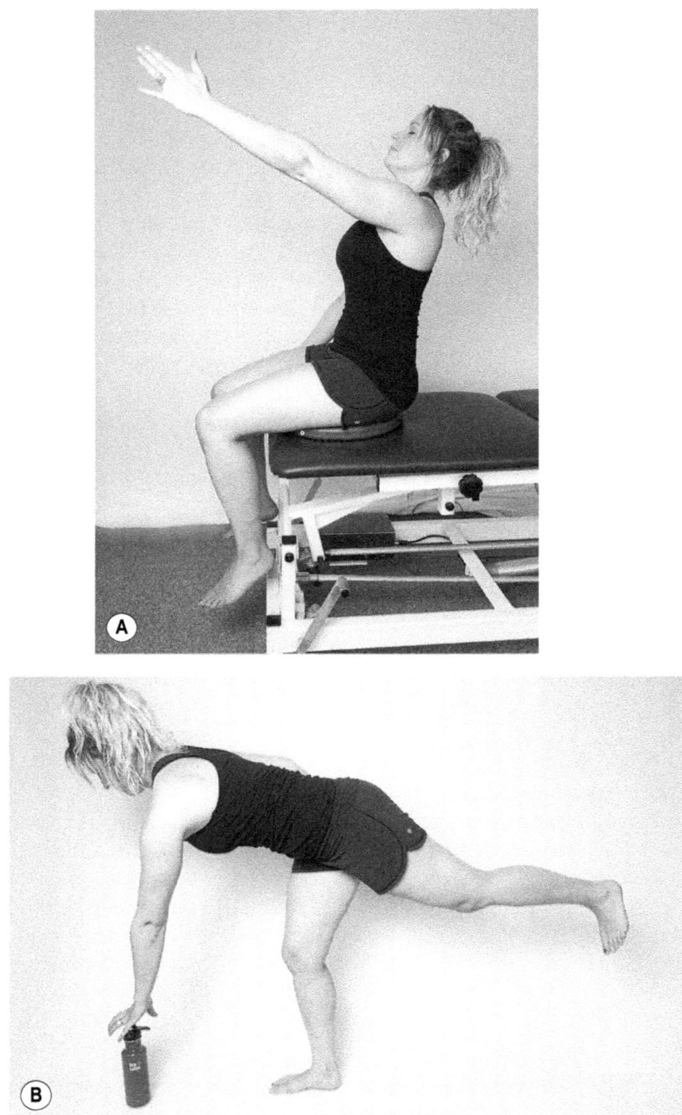

Figure 23.20 Balance exercises. (**A**) Sizzel sitting balance: a sizzle can provide an unstable sitting base; the patient can provide further challenge by closing the eyes, lifting the arm and extending the head backwards. (**B**) Single leg balance-reach: standing on one leg, the patient maintains lumbopelvic neutral and good alignment of the lower extremity while flexing forward at the hip to reach and pick up an object, challenging balance and motor control..

flexibility exercises were more effective than a combination of strength and flexibility exercises in reducing pain and improving the physical component of the quality of life in patients with chronic LBP (Gatti et al 2011). Other choices of balance exercises should take into consideration the specific requirements of the particular patient and could include functional patterns (Fig. 23.20B).

Higher Level Strengthening Exercises

For those patients with LBP who are returning to high-level sport or physically demanding work situations, higher load strengthening exercise progressions for both the anterior and posterior muscle groups should be included when building a comprehensive rehabilitation exercise programme. Although impairment of the deeper muscle system with inhibition and altered recruitment strategies has been identified in response to LBP, the superficial system can also become weak and, as such, targeted strength training may be required to regain optimal function. Strength training requires muscle overload and resistance and, other than the weight of the body against gravity, this can be achieved by using free weights or elastic tubing. Specialized equipment such as isokinetic machines and Roman chairs can also be used, although the lack of evidence of superiority makes it difficult to justify the cost of some of this equipment (Mayer et al 2008). This stage of the rehabilitation programme should be reserved for the period after pain has subsided and faulty patterning has been addressed. Strength can be trained by utilizing functional activities such as pushing, pulling, lifting, carrying and twisting.

McGill (2010) suggests that asymmetric kettlebell or suitcase carrying challenges the lateral musculature (QL and oblique muscles) as well as the opposite gluteal muscles. Although McGill and Marshall (2012) found unique muscle recruitment patterns during kettlebell swing exercises, he did recommend caution in using these exercises with patients because of the high shear forces generated.

Chop and lift exercises (Fig. 23.21) utilize functional PNF patterns and can be adapted to half kneeling, tall kneeling and standing with progressive increases in resistance, and can also be modified to correspond to patterns required for a specific sport or occupation. The movement patterns, both up and across into extension and down and across into flexion, encourage core and trunk stabilization with a triplanar rotational control and strengthening component.

Squats and lunges can be loaded with a weighted barbell to provide a symmetrical load, or with a single-sided kettlebell (Fig. 23.22) to increase the side-flexion and rotational control challenge. The use of straps while performing inverted rows or push-ups also creates a higher level of stability challenge during the strengthening exercise. A weight held while performing spinal rotation from a supine on ball bridge position (Fig. 23.23) increases the strength and stability challenge. Pull-ups, chin-ups and deadlifts are options for strengthening, but it is important to use clinical reasoning to determine which exercises are appropriate choices for a certain patient, taking into account the pathology, stage of healing, irritability and level of motor patterning control.

Many exercises may appear quite strenuous and yet create only moderate-intensity muscle contraction – as demonstrated for the floor walk-out, side walk-out and bowler's squat exercises (McGill et al 2009). Much of the difficulty is in the coordination and control and, although this could still be quite useful in the management of LBP, it will not necessarily provide the muscle overload stimulus required for strengthening.

Although Mayer et al (2008) found in their systematic review that, in the short term, lumbar extensor strengthening exercises were more effective than no treatment in improving pain and disability, there was no clear benefit of lumbar extensor strengthening exercises compared with other exercise programmes. High-intensity lumbar strengthening appears to be superior to low intensity in improving muscular strength and endurance. Slade and Keating (2006) in their systematic

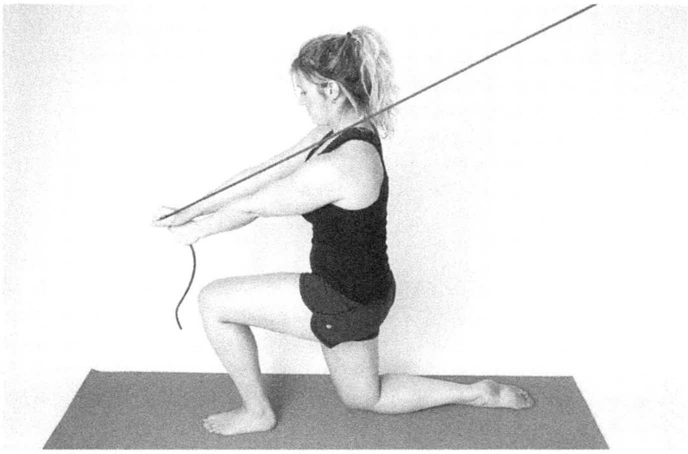

Figure 23.21 Chop exercises. A chop exercise against elastic resistance can be performed in a lunge position to challenge stability and balance further.

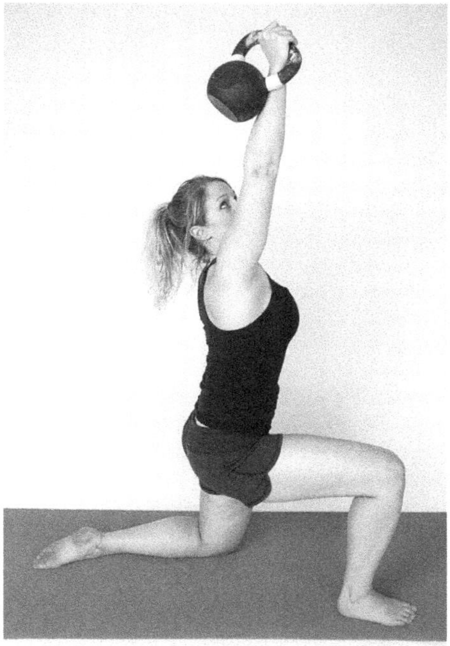

Figure 23.22 Kettlebell lift exercise. An overhead lift exercise can be performed in a lunge position using a kettlebell to provide resistance. Attention is given to proper form throughout the movement pattern.

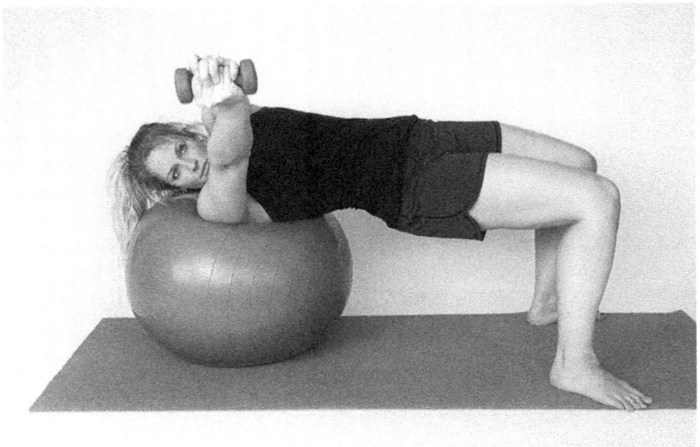

Figure 23.23 Trunk rotation control. In a supine bridge with shoulders supported on a Swiss ball and extended arms holding a weight, the patient rotates the trunk in a controlled pattern, maintaining optimal spinal alignment.

review reported similar results, but also stated that higher intensity programmes and those that included motivational strategies appeared to be of greater benefit than did less-intensive programmes. De Ridder et al (2013) found higher levels of lumbar extensor EMG activity during trunk extension exercises compared with leg extension exercises. There was no difference in the level of recruitment between deep and superficial muscles and also no difference in recruitment patterns with different types of contraction (i.e. isometric, concentric, eccentric). Strengthening through the full range beyond neutral into hyperextension does not seem to give any added benefit for strength or pain and disability, and so it may be safer to limit the range of lumbar extension when performing these exercises (Mayer et al 2008; Steele et al 2013). Danneels et al (2001) found that the lumbar extensor cross-sectional area significantly increased in the lumbar strengthening groups (prone back extension exercises) but not in the stabilization group. When progressing to higher intensity strength exercises, the magnitude of loading on the spine must also be considered relative to the current status of the patient's condition. In quadruped position, a single leg lift creates around 2000 Newton (N) of compression, an opposite arm and leg lift creates 3000 N, while a prone simultaneous bilateral arm and leg lift imposes over 4000 N of compressive force on the spine (Callagan et al 1998).

Exercise Parameters

The parameters for exercise prescription–intensity, duration, frequency, etc–have not been well established in the literature. The dosage of a specific exercise depends on several factors including the aim of the exercise (recruitment / patterning, strength, endurance, mobility, stretching), the ability to perform the exercise properly, the patient's tolerance (age), and the presence of pain and irritability of the condition.

In 2011 the American College of Sport Medicine (ACSM) updated their guidelines for exercise prescription (Garber et al 2011). Based on the available research, they grade the strength of evidence guiding the choice of doses for different types of exercise. They suggest that 2–4 sets of 8–12 repetitions (reps) at 60–70% of 1repetition maximum (RM), performed 2–3 times per week with 2–3 minutes rest between sets, is optimal for developing muscle strength. The intensity should be increased for more experienced strength trainers and decreased for sedentary or older adults. Two sets of 15–20 reps at 50% 1 RM, 2–3 times per week is considered to be more appropriate for improving endurance. McGill (2007) suggests building up to a 10-second hold and then increasing repetitions rather than the duration of the hold to improve endurance. McGill also advocates using the 'Russian descending pyramid' to design sets and repetitions, proposing that the pyramid provides a way for the patient to build endurance without becoming fatigued, which could then result in poor motor patterning. Postures are held for 8–10 seconds. If X repetitions are performed in set 1, $X-1$ reps are performed in set 2, $X-2$ reps are performed in set 3, and so on.

For flexibility, daily stretching (with a minimum of 3–4 days / week) to the point of slight discomfort, performing 2–4 reps held for 10–30 seconds (30–60 for older adults) for a total stretching time of 60 seconds is proposed, although there is not as much evidence available to guide these suggestions as there is for strength training (Garber et al 2011). Stretching will be more effective if performed following a light- to moderate-intensity warm-up. Flexibility exercises including static (active or passive), dynamic, ballistic or PNF stretching (contract–relax, hold–relax, reciprocal inhibition) have all been shown to be effective. For PNF stretching, the ACSM suggest a 20–75% maximum voluntary contraction held for 3–6 seconds, followed by a 10–30-second passive stretch. A review article by Sharman et al (2006) concluded that PNF was superior to other stretching methods. They suggested that the evidence supports a sequence of a 3–15-second low-intensity (<20% MVC) static contraction of the target muscle, followed by an active stretch produced by the antagonist until the stretch sensation abates. They state that a minimum of one repetition performed twice a week is required to gain range. Regardless of the type of stretching used, any gains in range are quickly lost when stretching is stopped. Although it has been suggested in the scientific literature that stretching performed just prior to activity results in decreased performance, Kay and Blazevich (2011), in a systematic review of 106 studies, determined that the detrimental effects of stretching were mainly limited to longer duration stretches of greater than 60 seconds.

There is no specific research to guide the dosage for articular mobility exercises. Clinically, 10–15 repetitions held from 2 to 10 seconds are commonly used. If the aim is for a capsular stretch, the hold time could be increased towards 30 seconds. A rocking motion could be used at end of range to mimic a joint mobilization technique, if that was found to be more effective. For self-mobilization exercises, the Mulligan approach suggests using 3 sets of 10 repetitions daily to gain mobility at a specific spinal segment (Hing et al 2008). The McKenzie programme suggests 1–2 sets of 8–15 repetitions performed rhythmically without a sustained hold, to the point of pain onset, and attempting to increase that range with each repetition. This is done every 1–2 hours for a minimum of 6 times per day (Ford et al 2011).

The ACSM found minimal evidence to guide the prescription of neuromotor exercises. Quality and precision in the performance of these exercises is considered more important than the quantity in a single session. Initially patients are

Table 23.1 **Exercise parameters**

Mode of exercise	Intensity	Sets	Reps	Duration	Rest	Frequency
Recruitment/isolation motor patterning	Low load	1–3	10	10 s hold	2 min	multiple ×/day
Strength	60–70% MVC	2–4	8–12		2–3 min	2–3 ×/week
Endurance	50% MVC	2	15–20	10 s hold	2–3 min	2–3 ×/week
Stretch	Slight discomfort	1	2–4	10–30 s hold *or* total stretch time = 60 s 30–60 s hold for older adults		minimum 3–4 ×/week
PNF stretch	20–75% MVC for resistance		1	3–15 s contraction 10–30 s passive stretch		2 ×/week
Mobility exercises: articular	Stretch sensation	1	10–15	2–10 (up to 30) s hold		>1×/day
Mulligan	Pain-free	3	10	Overpressure		Daily
McKenzie	To point of pain onset	1–2	8–15	Rhythmically		Every 2 hours – minimum 6×/day

instructed to perform only the number of exercises they can complete correctly and this could be as few as 3–5 repetitions. Cues should therefore be given to ensure that they are accurately monitoring their movement patterns. Motor learning principles suggest that multiple repetitions are needed to retrain and solidify new motor patterns. Identifying recurring activities in the day that could provide a cue to remind patients to perform at least a couple of repetitions of an exercise may assist in accomplishing this. Experts in this field recommend gradually building up to 1–3 sets of 10 repetitions held for 10-second holds with 2-minute rests between sets, performed multiple times a day (Tsao & Hodges 2007; Lee & Lee 2011). Table 23.1 provides a summary of suggested parameters for exercise prescription.

Conclusion

Exercise therapy is beneficial for patients with chronic LBP. However, further research is required to determine which subgroups will benefit from which type of exercise. Exercise dosage, intensity and frequency have yet to be fully determined in the literature. A sound clinical reasoning framework within a bio-psychosocial model should be applied and exercise prescription should consider the individual needs and clinical features of the LBP patient. In this chapter, we have provided an evidence-informed overview of current exercise approaches with various examples for clinicians to consider.

References

Aina A, May S, Clare H. 2004. The centralization phenomenon of spinal symptoms: a systematic review. Man Ther 9: 134–143.

Aladro-Gonzalvo A, Araya-Vargas G, Machado-Díaz M, et al. 2013. Pilates-based exercise for persistent, non-specific low back pain and associated functional disability: a meta-analysis with meta-regression. J Bodyw Mov Ther 17: 125–136.

Alves de Araujo M, Bezerra da Silva E, Mello D, et al. 2012. The effectiveness of the Pilates method: reducing the degree of non-structural scoliosis, and improving flexibility and pain in female college students. J Bodyw Mov Ther 16: 191–198.

Axler CT, McGill SM. 1997. Low back loads over a variety of abdominal exercises: searching for the safest abdominal challenge. Med Sci Sports Exer 29: 804–811.

Ayala F, Sainz de Baranda P, De Ste Croix M. 2013. Comparison of active stretching technique in males with normal and limited hamstring flexibility. Phys Ther Sport 14: 98–104.

Bach K, Green D, Jensen G, et al. 1985. A comparison of muscular tightness in runners and non-runners and the relation of muscular tightness to low back pain in runners. J Orthop Sports Phys Ther 6: 315–323.

Barker K, Shamley D, Jackson D. 2004. Changes in the cross-sectional area of multifidus and psoas in patients with unilateral back pain. Spine 29: E515–E519.

Bergmark A. 1989. Stability of the lumbar spine: a study in mechanical engineering. Acta Orthop Scand Suppl 230: 1–54.

Bjerkefors A, Ekblom MM, Josefsson K, et al. 2010. Deep and superficial abdominal muscle activation during trunk stabilization exercises with and without instruction to hollow. Man Ther 15: 502–507.

Borman N, Trudelle-Jackson E, Smith S. 2011. Effect of stretch positions on hamstring muscle length, lumbar flexion range of motion, and lumbar curvature in healthy adults. Physiother Theor Pract 27: 146–154.

Brumagne S, Cordo P, Lysens R, et al. 2000. The role of paraspinal muscle spindles in lumbosacral position sense in individuals with and without low back pain. Spine 25: 989–994.

Bystrom MG, Rasmussen E, Grooten WJA. 2013. Motor control exercises reduces pain and disability in chronic and recurrent low back pain. Spine 38: E350–E358.

Callaghan J, Gunning J, McGill S. 1998. The relationship between lumbar spine load and muscle activity during extensor exercises. Phys Ther 78: 8–18.

Cecchi F, Pasquini G, Paperini A, et al. 2014. Predictors of response to exercise therapy for chronic low back pain: result of a perspective study with one year follow-up. Eur J Phys Rehabil Med 50(2): 143–151.

Chen HM, Wang HH, Chen CH, et al. 2012. Effectiveness of a stretching exercise program on low back pain and exercise self-efficacy among nurses in Taiwan: a randomized clinical trial. Pain Manag Nurs 15(1): 283–291. doi: 10.1016/j.pmn.2012.10.003.

Choi BK, Verbeek JH, Tam WW, et al. 2010. Exercises for prevention of recurrences of low-back pain. Cochrane Database Syst Rev 1: CD006555.

Chon SC, Chang KY, You JH. 2010. Effect of the abdominal draw-in maneuver in combination with ankle dorsiflexion in strengthening the transverse abdominal muscle in healthy young adults: A preliminary, randomized, controlled study. Physiotherapy 96: 130–136.

Clare H, Adams R, Maher C. 2004. A systematic review of efficacy of McKenzie therapy for spinal pain. Austr J Physiother 50: 209–216.

Claus A, Hides J, Moseley GL, et al. 2009. Is 'ideal' sitting real? Measurement of spinal curves in four sitting postures. Man Ther 14: 404–408.

Costa LO, Maher CG, Latimer J, et al. 2009. Motor control exercise for chronic low back pain: a randomized placebo-controlled trial. Phys Ther 89: 1275–1286.

Czaprowski D, Afeltowicz A, Gebicka A, et al. 2014. Abdominal muscle EMG-activity during bridge exercises on stable and unstable surfaces. Phys Ther Sport 15(3): 162–168. doi: 10.1016/j.ptsp.2013.09.003.

Dankaerts W, O'Sullivan P, Burnett A, et al. 2006. Altered patterns of superficial trunk muscle activation during sitting in nonspecific chronic low back patients: importance of sub-classification. Spine 31: 2017–2023.

Danneels L, Vanderstraeten G, Cambier D, et al. 2000. CT imaging of trunk muscles in chronic low back pain patients and healthy control subjects. Eur Spine J 9: 266–272.

Danneels L, Vanderstraeten G, Cambier D, et al. 2001. Effects of three different training modalities on the cross sectional area of the lumbar multifidus muscle in patients with chronic low back pain Br J Sports Med 35: 186–191.

De Ridder E, Van Oosterwijck J, Vleeming A, et al. 2013. Posterior muscle chain activity during various extension exercises: an observational study. BMC Musculoskel Dis 14: 204.

Delitto A, George SZ, van Dillen L, et al. 2012. Low back pain Clinical Practice Guidelines linked to the International Classification of Functioning, Disability, and Health from the Orthopaedic Section of the American Physical Therapy Association. J Orthop Sports Phys Ther 42: A1–A57.

Ekstrom RA, Donatelli RA, Carp KC. 2007. Electromyographic analysis of core trunk, hip, and thigh muscles during 9 rehabilitation exercises. J Orthop Sports Phys Ther 37: 754–762

Ekstrom RA, Osborn RW, Hauer PL. 2008. Surface electromyographic analysis of the low back muscles during rehabilitation exercises. J Orthop Sports Phys Ther 38: 736–745.

Escamilla RF, Babb E, DeWitt R, et al. 2006a. Electromyographic analysis of traditional and nontraditional abdominal exercises: implications for rehabilitation and training. Phys Ther 86: 656–671.

Escamilla RF, McTaggart MS, Fricklas EJ, et al. 2006b. An electromyographic analysis of commercial and common abdominal exercises: implications for rehabilitation and training. J Orthop Sports Phys Ther 36: 45–57.

Escamilla RF, Lewis C, Bell D, et al. 2010. Core muscle activation during Swiss ball and traditional abdominal exercises. J Orthop Sports Phys Ther 40: 265–276.

Fasen J, O'Connor A, Schwartz S, et al. 2009. A randomized controlled trial of hamstring stretching: comparison of four techniques. J Strength Conditioning Res 23: 660–667.

Fitts PM, Posner MI. 1967. Human performance. Belmomt CA: Brooks / Cole Garber.

Ford J, Surkitt L, Hahne A. 2011. A classification and treatment protocol for low back disorders Part 2 – Directional preference management for reducible discogenic pain. Phys Ther Rev 16: 423–437.

Franca F, Burke T, Caffaro R, et al. 2012. Effects of muscular stretching and segmental stabilization on functional disability and pain in patients with chronic low back pain: a randomized control trial. J Manipulative Physiol Ther 36: 279–285.

Fredericson M, White J, MacMahon J, et al. 2002. Quantitative analysis of the relative effectiveness of 3 iliotibial band stretches. Arch Phys Med Rehabil 83: 589–592.

Fritz J, Cleland JA, Childs JD. 2007. Subgrouping patients with low back pain: evolution of a classification approach to physical therapy. J Orthop Sports Phys Ther 37(6): 290–302.

Gajdosik R, Sandler M, Marr H. 2003. Influence of knee positions and gender on the Ober test for length of the iliotibial band. Clin Biomech 18: 77–79.

Garber C, Blissmer B, Deschenes M, et al. 2011. Quantity and quality of exercise for developing and maintaining cardiorespiratory, musculoskeletal, and neuromotor fitness in apparently healthy adults: guidance for prescribing exercise. Med Sci Sports Exerc 43: 1334–1359.

García-Vaquero MP, Moreside JM, Brontons-Gil E, et al. 2012. Trunk muscle activation during stabilization exercises with single and double leg support. J Electromyogr Kinesiol 22: 398–406.

Gatti R, Faccendini S, Tettamanti A, et al. 2011. Efficacy of trunk balance exercises for individuals with chronic low back pain: a randomized clinical trial. J Orthop Sports Phys Ther 41: 542–552.

Haladay DE, Miller SJ, Challis J, et al. 2013. Quality of systematic reviews on specific spinal stabilization exercise for chronic low back pain. J Orthop Sports Phys Ther 43: 242–250.

Hayden JA, van Tulder MW, Malmivaara A, et al. 2005. Exercise therapy for treatment of non-specific low back pain. Cochrane Database Syst Rev 3: CD000335.

Hicks GE, Fritz JM, Delitto A, et al. 2005. Preliminary development of a clinical prediction rule for determining which patients with low back pain will respond to a stabilization exercise program. Arch Phys Med Rehabil 86: 1753–1762.

Hides JA, Stokes MJ, Saide M, et al. 1994. Evidence of lumbar multifidus muscle wasting ipsilateral to symptoms in patients with acute / sub-acute low back pain. Spine 19: 165–172.

Hides JA, Richardson CA, Jull GA. 1996. Multifidus muscle recovery is not automatic after resolution of acute, first-episode low back pain. Spine 21: 2763–2769.

Hides J, Gilmore C, Stanton W, et al. 2008a. Multifidus size and symmetry among chronic LBP and asymptomatic subjects. Man Ther 13: 43–49.

Hides J, Stanton W, McMahon S, et al. 2008b. Effect of stabilization training on multifidus muscle cross-sectional area among young elite-cricketers with low back pain. J Orthop Sports Phys Ther 38: 101–108.

Hides J, Stanton W, Mendis MD, et al. 2011. The relationship of transversus abdominis and lumbar multifidus clinical muscle tests in patients with chronic low back pain. Man Ther 16: 573–577.

Himes ME, Selkow NM, Gore MA, et al. 2012. Transversus abdominis activation during a side-bridge exercise progression is similar in people with recurrent low back pain and healthy controls. J Strength Condit Res 26: 3106–3112.

Hing W, Bigelow R, Bremner T. 2008. Mulligan's mobilisation with movement: a review of the tenets and prescription of MWMs. N Z J Physiother 36: 144–164.

Hodges PW. 2001. Changes in motor planning of feedforward postural responses of trunk muscles in low back pain. Exp Brain Res 141: 261–266.

Hodges PW 2011. Pain and motor control: from the laboratory to rehabilitation. J Electromyogr Kinesiol 21: 220–228.

Hodges PW, Van Dillen LR, McGill S, et al. 2013. Integrated clinical approach to motor control interventions in low back and pelvic pain. In: Hodges P (ed) Spinal control: the rehabilitation of back pain. Edinburgh: Churchill Livingstone, Ch 21.

Imai A, Kaneoka K, Okubo Y, et al. 2010. Trunk muscle activity during lumbar stabilization exercises on both a stable and unstable surface J Orthop Sports Phys Ther 40: 369–375.

Janda V 1987. Muscles and motor control in low back pain: assessment and management. In: Twomey LT (ed) Physical therapy of the low back. New York: Churchill Livingstone, pp 238–278.

Jeon JK, Lim HS, Shin SR, et al. 2013. Effects of three bridging exercises on local and global muscles of middle aged women. J Phys Ther Sci 25: 853–856.

Kang MH, Jung DH, An DH, et al. 2013. Acute effects of hamstring-stretching exercises on the kinematics of the lumbar spine and hip during stoop lifting. J Back Musculoskelet Rehabil 26: 329–336.

Kavcic N, Grenier S, McGill SM. 2004. Quantifying tissue loads and spine stability while performing commonly prescribed low back stabilization exercises. Spine 29: 2319–2329.

Kay A, Blazevich A. 2011. Effect of acute static stretch on maximal muscle performance: a systematic review. Med Sci Sports Exerc 44: 154–164.

Kiesel KB, Underwood FB, Mattacola CG, et al. 2007. A comparison of select trunk muscle thickness change between subjects with low back pain classified in the treatment-based classification system and asymptomatic controls J Orthop Sports Phys Ther 37: 596–607.

Kim MJ, OH DW, Park HJ. 2013. Integrating arm movement into bridge exercise: effect on EMG activity of selected trunk muscles. J Electromyogr Kinesiol 23: 1119–1123.

Kujala U, Salmenin J, Taimela S, et al. 1992. Subject characteristics and low back pain in young athletes and non-athletes. Med Sci Sports Exerc 24: 627–632.

Lee D, Lee LJ. 2011. The pelvic girdle: an integration of clinical expertise and research. Edinburgh: Churchill Livingstone.

Lee LJ, Chang AT, Coppieters MW, et al. 2010. Changes in sitting posture induce multiplanar changes in chest wall shape and motion with breathing. Resp Physiol Neurobiol 170: 236–245.

Lehman GJ, Hoda W, Oliver S. 2005. Trunk muscle activity during bridging exercises on and off a Swiss ball. Chir Osteopathy 13: 14.

Lim E, Poh R, Low A, et al. 2011. Effects of Pilates-based exercises on pain and disability in individuals with persistent nonspecific low back pain: a systematic review with meta-analysis J Orthop Sports Phys Ther 41: 70–80.

Long A, Donelson R, Fung F. 2004. Does it matter which exercise? A randomized control trial of exercise for low back pain. Spine 29: 2593–2602.

MacDonald D, Moseley L, Hodges PW. 2009. Why do some patients keep hurting their back? Evidence of ongoing back muscle dysfunction during remission from recurrent back pain. Pain 142: 183–188.

Macedo LG, Maher CG, Latimer J, et al. 2009. Motor control exercise for persistent, nonspecific low back pain: a systematic review. Phys Ther 89: 9–25.

Macedo LG, Latimer J, Maher CG, et al. 2012. Back pain: a randomized controlled trial activity in patients with chronic nonspecific low back pain. Phys Ther 92: 363–377.

Mayer J, Mooney V, Dagenais S. 2008. Evidence-informed management of chronic low back pain with lumbar extensor strengthening exercises. Spine J 8: 96–113.

Mazaheri M, Coenen P, Parnianpour M, et al. 2013. Low back pain and postural sway during quiet standing with and without sensory manipulation: a systematic review. Gait Posture 37: 12–22.
McGill SM. 1997. Distribution of tissue loads in the low back during a variety of daily and rehabilitation tasks. J Rehabil Res Develop 34: 448–458.
McGill SM. 2007. Low back disorders: evidence-based prevention and rehabilitation, 2nd edn. Windsor, ON: Human Kinetics.
McGill SM. 2010. Core training: evidence translating to better performance and injury prevention. J Strength Condit 32: 33–45.
McGill SM, Karpowicz A. 2009. Exercises for spine stabilization: motion / motor patterns, stability progressions and clinical technique Arch Phys Med Rehabil 90: 118–126.
McGill SM, Marshall L. 2012. Kettlebell swing, snatch and bottoms-up carry: back and hip muscle activation, motion, and low back loads. J Strength Condition Res 26: 16–27.
McGill SM, Juker D, Kropf P. 1996. Quantitative intramuscular myoelectric activity of quadratus lumborum during a wide variety of tasks. Clin Biomech 11: 170–172.
McGill SM, Karpowicz A, Fenwick C, et al. 2009. Exercises for the torso performed in a standing posture: spine and hip motion patterns and spine load. J Strength Condition Res 23: 455–464.
McKenzie R, May S. 2003. The lumbar spine mechanical diagnosis and therapy. Waikanae, NZ: Spinal Publications.
Mew R. 2009. Comparison of changes in abdominal muscle thickness between standing and crook lying during active abdominal hollowing using ultrasound imaging. Man Ther 14: 690–695.
Mulligan B. 2004. Manual therapy nags, snags, MWMs etc., 5th edn. Wellington, NZ: Plane View Services.
Newcomer KL, Laskowski ER, Yu B, et al. 2000. Differences in repositioning error among patients with low back pain compared with control subject. Spine 25: 2488–2493.
Okubo Y, Kaneoka K, Imai A, et al. 2010. Electromyographic analysis of transversus abdominis and lumbar multifidus using wire electrodes during lumbar stabilization exercises. J Orthop Sports Phys Ther 40: 743–750.
O'Sullivan PB. 2000. Lumbar segmental 'instability': clinical presentation and specific stabilizing exercise management Man Ther 5: 2–12.
O'Sullivan P, Dankaerts W, Burnett A, et al. 2006. Effect of different upright sitting postures on spinal–pelvic curvature and trunk muscle activation in a pain-free population. Spine 31: E707–E712.
O'Sullivan K, O-Sullivan P, O-Sullivan L, et al. 2012. What do physiotherapists consider to be the best sitting spinal posture? Man Ther 17: 432–437.
Panjabi MM. 1992. The stabilizing system of the spine: Part 2. Neutral zone and instability hypothesis. J Spinal Dis 5: 390–396.
Park R, Tsao H, Claus A, et al. 2013. Recruitment of discrete regions of the psoas major and quadratus lumborum muscles is changed in specific sitting postures in individuals with recurrent low back pain. J Orthop Sports Phys Ther 43: 833–840.
Pereira L, Obara K, Dias J, et al. 2011. Comparing the Pilates method with no exercise or lumbar stabilization for pain and functionality in patients with chronic low back pain: systematic review and meta-analysis. Clin Rehabil 26: 10–20.
Posadzki P, Ernst E. 2011. Yoga for low back pain: a systematic review of randomized clinical trials. Clin Rheumatol 30: 1257–1262.
Posadzki P, Lizis P, Hagner-Derengowska M. 2011. Pilates for low back pain: a systematic review. Compl Ther Clinical Pract 17: 85–89.
Puentedura E, Huijbregts P, Celeste S, et al. 2011. Immediate effects of quantified hamstring stretching: hold–relax proprioceptive neuromuscular facilitation versus static stretching. Phys Ther Sport 12: 122–126.
Purepong N, Jitvimonrat A, Boonyong S, et al. 2012. Effect of flexibility exercise on lumbar angle: A study among non-specific low back pain patients. J Bodywork Mov Ther 16: 236–243.
Rabin A, Shashua A, Pizem K, et al. 2014. A clinical prediction rule to identify patients with low back pain who are likely to experience short-term success following lumbar stabilization exercises: a randomized controlled validation study. J Orthop Sports Phys Ther 44(1): 6–18.
Richardson CA, Hodges PW, Hides J. 1999. Therapeutic exercise for spinal segmental stabilization in low back pain. Edinburgh: Churchill Livingstone.
Richardson CA, Hodges PW, Hides JA. 2004. Therapeutic exercise for lumbopelvic stabilisation: a motor control approach for the treatment and prevention of low back pain. Edinburgh: Churchill Livingstone.
Sahrmann S. 2002. Diagnosis and treatment of movement impairment syndromes. St Louis, MO: CV Mosby.
Sairyo K, Kawamura T, Mase Y, et al. 2013. Jack-knife stretching promotes flexibility of tight hamstrings after 4 weeks: a pilot study. Eur J Orthop Surg Traumatol 23: 657–663.
Sapsford RR, Hodges PW, Richardson CA, et al. 2001. Co-activation of the abdominal and pelvic floor muscles during voluntary exercises. Neurourol Urodyn 20: 31–42.
Sharman M, Cresswell A, Riek S. 2006. Proprioceptive neuromuscular facilitation stretching: Mechanisms and clinical implications. Sports Med 36: 929–939.
Sheeran L, Sparkes V, Caterson B, et al. 2012. Spinal position sense and trunk muscle activity during sitting and standing in non specific chronic low back pain. Spine 37: E486–E495.
Sherman K, Wellman R, Cook A, et al. 2013. Mediators of yoga and stretching for chronic low back pain. Evid Based Complement Alternat Med 2013: 130818.
Slade S, Keating J. 2006. Trunk-strengthening exercises for chronic low back pain: a systematic review. J Manipulative Physiol Ther 29: 163–173.
Slade SC, Patel S, Underwood M, et al. 2014. What are patient beliefs and perceptions about exercise fro non-specific chronic low back pain? A systematic review of qualitative studies. Clin J Pain 30(11):995–1005. doi: 10.1097/AJP.0000000000000044.
Steele J, Bruce-Low S, Smith D, et al. 2013. A randomized controlled trial of limited range of motion lumbar extension exercise in chronic low back pain. Spine 38: 1245–1252.
Stevens VK, Bouche KG, Mahieu NN, et al. 2006. Trunk muscle activity in healthy subjects during bridging stabilization exercises. BMC Musculoskel Dis 7: 75.
Stevens VK, Vleeming A, Bouche KG, et al. 2007. Electromyographic activity of trunk and hip muscles during stabilization exercises in four-point kneeling in healthy volunteers. Eur Spine J 16: 711–718.
Stolze L, Allison S, Childs J. 2012. Derivation of a preliminary clinical prediction rule for identifying a subgroup of patients with low back pain likely to benefit from Pilates-based exercise. J Orthop Sports Phys Ther 42: 425–436.
Surkitt L, Ford J, Hahne A, et al. 2012. Efficacy of directional preference management for low back pain: a systematic review. Phys Ther 92: 652–665.
Tekur P, Nagarathna R, Chametcha S, et al. 2012. A comprehensive yoga program improves pain, anxiety and depression in chronic low back pain patients more than exercise: an RCT. Complementary Ther Med 20: 107–118.
Teyhen DS, Rieger JL, Westrick RB, et al. 2008. Changes in deep abdominal muscle thickness during common trunk-strengthening exercises using ultrasound imaging. J Orthop Sports Phys Ther 38: 596–605.
Teyhen DS, Bluemle LN, Dolbeer JA, et al. 2009. Changes in lateral abdominal wall thickness during the abdominal drawing-in maneuver in patients with lumbopelvic pain J Orthop Sports Phys Ther 39: 791–798.
Tsao H, Hodges PW. 2007. Immediate changes in feed-forward postural adjustments following voluntary motor training. Exp Brain Res 181: 537–546.
Tsao H, Druiee TR, Schollum TM, et al. 2010. Motor training of the lumbar paraspinal muscles induces immediate changes in motor coordination in patients with recurrent low back pain. J Pain 11: 1120–1128.
van Middelkoop M, Rubinstein SM, Verhagen AP, et al. 2010. Exercise therapy for chronic nonspecific low-back pain. Best Practice Res Clin Rheumatol 24: 193–204. doi: 10.1016/j.berh.2010.01.002.
Vicenzino B, Hing W, Rivett D, et al. 2011. Mobilization with movement: the art and science. Edinburgh: Churchill Livingstone.
Wajswelner H, Metcalf B, Bennell K. 2012. Clinical Pilates versus general exercise for chronic low back pain: randomized trial. Med Sci Sports Exer 44: 1197–1205.
Wang T, Jan M, Lin K, et al. 2006. Assessment of stretching of the iliotibial tract with Ober and modified Ober tests: an ultrasonographic study. Arch Phys Med Rehabil 87: 1407–1411.
Wells C, Kolt G, Bialocerkowski A. 2012. Defining Pilates exercise: a systematic review. Complem Ther Med 20: 253–262.
Wells C, Kolt G, Marshall P, et al. 2013. Effectiveness of Pilates exercise in treating people with chronic low back pain: a systematic review of systematic reviews. BMC Med Res Methodol 13: 1–12.
Whitman J, Flynn T, Childs J, et al. 2006. A comparison between two physical therapy treatment programs for patients with lumbar spinal stenosis: a randomized clinical trial. Spine 31: 2541–2549.
Winters M, Blake C, Trost J, et al. 2004. Passive versus active stretching of hip flexor muscles in subjects with limited hip extension: A randomized clinical trial. Phys Ther 84: 800–807.

24 Chapter

Sacroiliac Joint as a Source of Pain: Diagnosis and Management

Kenneth E. Learman

CHAPTER CONTENTS

Introduction	274
Prevalence	274
Economic impact	275
Anatomy and biomechanics	275
Pathology and pathomechanics	277
Diagnosis	277
Medical diagnosis	277
Clinical diagnosis: subjective examination	278
Clinical diagnosis: physical examination	278
Clinical examination summary	283
Prognosis	283
Treatment	284
Exercise therapy	284
Manual therapy	286
Sacroiliac belts	288
Conclusion	288

Introduction

The sacroiliac joint (SIJ) as a source of low back pain has been enigmatic, although the capacity of the SIJ to be a pain generator has been known for more than 100 years. The controversy surrounds the types of pathomechanical problems related to the SIJ, the methods to treat those problems and the prevalence rates of SIJ pathology. The SIJ meets the requirements for pain generation as the joint is innervated. However, the exact nature and extent of that innervation is not conclusively known currently (Bogduk 2005), due in part to the lack of extensive study, the potential variability and the multisegmental contributions. It is believed that unencapsulated and encapsulated fibres innervate the joint itself and the surrounding structures in a multisegmental fashion, and it has been proposed that these are fibres originating from lower lumbar (Ikeda 1991) and sacral nerve roots (Grob et al 1995) , with possible contribution from more proximal root levels (Zelle et al 2005). Moreover, the complexity of the innervation makes the use of nerve blocks for further exploration of SIJ pathology exceedingly difficult. More conclusively, however, injections of the SIJ can produce pain with contrast medium and eliminate pain with lidocaine (Xylocaine) (Fortin et al 1994a). Early work by Goldtwait and Osgood (1905) suggested that the SIJ could contribute to pain in the low back and legs. Furthermore, as early as 1920, a radiographic study was published identifying movement and pain during pregnancy as the result of pelvic ring pathology (Lynch 1920).

Low back and lower extremity pain that is associated with pathology of the SIJs can be divided into two main classifications: those of non-mechanical and those of mechanical origin (Cook 2012). The former pathology can be further broken down into many subgroups, such as infectious conditions (bacterial or fungal), inflammatory pathologies of many subtypes, tumours, metabolic disorders and fractures (Huijbregts 2004). The examination and treatment of inflammatory and infectious pathologies related to medical diagnoses are beyond the scope of this text. The primary goal for the orthopaedic manual clinician is to be able to identify those patients who may have non-mechanical pathology so as to refer them for appropriate diagnostic testing. As will be discussed further, this can be a difficult task.

Mechanical disorders of the SIJ can also be further categorized into sacroiliac joint pain (SIJP) syndromes and sacroiliac joint dysfunctions (SIJD). Several authors have proposed a working definition of SIJD as a state where aberrant mobility within the joint's range of motion results in positional faults between the sacrum and the ilium (Dreyfuss et al 1994; van der Wurff et al 2000a; Laslett 2008). SIJP can be defined as any pain condition arising from the SIJ itself or surrounding structures. In addition, pelvic girdle pain (PGP) expands our working definition of SIJP to include pathology associated with the pubic symphysis anteriorly or combinations of the SIJ and pubic symphysis.

Prevalence

The reported prevalence estimates of SIJ pathology have proven to be an epidemiological challenge. Two major methodological problems with prevalence studies for SIJ pathology are a lack of a universally accepted diagnostic standard and subject sampling strategies. Current diagnostic standards include a predetermined response to a fluoroscopic-guided intra-articular injection (IAI). Using this diagnostic standard, studies might suggest that SIJ pathology occurs in 13–30% of chronic low back pain. A study of 54 patients with clinical presentation considered to be consistent with SIJ found that 18.5% (with a 95% CI of 9–26%) responded to an SIJ double IAI (Maigne et al 1996). Schwarzer et al (1995) found that up to 30% of low back pain may be the result of the SIJ, with a more conservative estimate of at least 13%. Young et al (2003) found that 22 of 81 patients with chronic low back pain responded to an SIJ IAI, yielding a prevalence rate of 27%. Irwin et al (2007) examined 158 patients with chronic low back pain and found that 26.6% responded to a dual IAI. A recent study found that 41% of all patients with low back and leg pain had mechanical pain of the SIJ (Visser et al 2013). Dreyfuss et al (1996) used a single-IAI technique on 85 subjects with possible SIJP and found a 53% response rate. In contrast, one study with more broadly applied inclusion criteria determined through IAIs that SIJ prevalence rates were as low as 2% (Manchikanti et al 2001).

Several studies have used clinically derived diagnostic criteria for determining the presence of SIJ pathology. Schmid (1985) found a prevalence rate of 35% when 467 of 1344 patient cases demonstrated positive clinical criteria for SIJ pathology. This study benchmarked 7 out of 14 clinical predictors to determine SIJ pathology. Cibulka and Koldehoff (1999) studied the diagnostic accuracy of a cluster of tests used for diagnosing SIJD and found that 86 of 105 patients (81.9%) with acute to subacute low back pain tested positive. A recent cross-sectional study revealed that 72.3% of subjects with imaging-confirmed herniated disc pathology also displayed clinical signs and symptoms consistent with SIJ pathology (Madani et al 2013). This study used a standard of at least four anatomical and two pain provocation tests as a diagnostic threshold (Madani et al 2013).

The clinical prevalence rates might be dependent upon the types of patients we examine. A study of 1460 pregnant Danish women found that 20.1% had pregnancy-related PGP. The 293 women with pelvic pain could be further broken down into four distinct categories: single-sided SIJP (5.5%), bilateral SIJP (6.3%), symphysiolysis (2.3%), and pelvic girdle syndrome (pain in all three pelvic joints 6.0%) and a miscellaneous category of mixed presentation (Albert et al 2002). This study attempted to categorize PGP into homogeneous groups from a heterogeneous population. Furthermore, a recent cross-sectional study suggests that the prevalence of PGP related to pregnancy could be much higher, at 60.4%, with 20% of the subjects reporting severe pain of >5 on the Numeric Pain Rating Scale (Mens et al 2012).

As previously stated, there have been significant methodological differences within epidemiological research, including the diagnostic benchmark used. Even within the use of diagnostic blocks there have been methodological differences, including variable thresholds of pain relief used to determine results; these differences will be further defined later in this chapter under diagnostic procedures. There have also been variations in subject selection between diagnostic studies (Manchikanti et al 2001). A common selection bias is to identify and study patients who are already suspected to have SIJ pathology, which may artificially inflate the prevalence rate. Manchikanti et al (2001) report selecting individuals with clinical presentation typical of SIJ pathology as appropriate candidates for the SIJ diagnostic block and bypassing this diagnostic test in those who did not satisfy those criteria. Many studies using diagnostic blocks for determining causation of low back pain have employed a strategy that assumes low back pain could be caused by only a single pathology (Manchikanti et al 2001). Nevertheless, multifactorial pain generation is theoretically possible when less than complete resolution of symptoms is the diagnostic standard, even though studies suggest that it may be a rare occurrence (Schwarzer et al 1994; Laslett et al 2005b). Finally, most studies that have attempted to identify the source of low back pain have focused on subjects with chronic or persistent pain as one would not wish to subject patients with acute, potentially benign pain to invasive interventional radiological procedures. Therefore, little is known about the prevalence of SIJ in acute low back and leg pain and there are still gaps in our knowledge about chronic low back pain.

Economic impact

The economic and societal costs of SIJP are also difficult to estimate. With great variation in the estimates of the contribution of SIJP to overall low back pain, the economic burden to society is essentially unknown, even though the economic burden of low back pain in general is well known. If we can conservatively estimate, however, that between 5% and 10% of chronic low back pain is SIJP in origin, it becomes evident that, based on a recent systematic review of the literature on healthcare costs related to low back pain (Dagenais et al 2008), SIJP may cost Western nations more than $10 billion annually.

Anatomy and Biomechanics

The pelvic ring is composed of the two innominates and the sacrum. Each innominate is composed of the ilium, ischium and pubis bones, which begin fusing during puberty with completion of this process by an individual's mid twenties. The sacrum comprises five vertebrae, which also begin fusing in puberty, but this completes only in the fourth decade of life. The innominates are held together anteriorly through a strong joint, the pubic symphysis – a cartilaginous joint with a fibrocartilaginous disc interfacing the joint surfaces. The superior, inferior and posterior pubic ligaments stabilize the joint through their connections across the joint line. Anteriorly, the pubic symphysis is supported by expansions from the rectus abdominis, the internal obliques, the transversus abdominis superiorly and the adductor longus inferiorly.

Posteriorly, the ring is formed by the wedge-shaped sacrum acting as a keystone between the innominates through the SIJ. The SIJ is a hybrid joint with synovial and syndesmotic portions. The anterior, synovial component of the SIJ is an irregular, L-shaped joint with furrows and ridges within the articular surfaces themselves that serve to encourage stability further (Snijders et al 1993a, 1993b). The pattern of ridges within the joint and the general shape of the joint itself can be highly variable between individuals, but there are consistently irregularities that serve to limit the mobility of these synovial joints. In youth, the articular surfaces are generally smooth, but with irregularity to the pattern of furrows and ridges beginning in the second to third decade and continuing to develop throughout life. Furthermore, it has been identified that anterior bony bridges may develop with age, further reducing SIJ movement from spontaneous fusion (Dar et al 2008). Posteriorly, the SIJ is a syndesmotic joint where strong ligaments extend from the sacral to the iliac tuberosities.

There are numerous ligaments that assist in providing stability to the SIJ. Anteriorly, the broad anterior sacroiliac ligament assists in preventing joint surface separation of the SIJ. Posteriorly, the interosseous sacroiliac ligament (ISL) runs between the ventromedial surface of the posterior superior iliac spine (PSIS) and the dorsolateral surface of the sacrum, creating the syndesmosis. The ligament itself is very dense and thick and lies dorsal to the SIJ. The size and position of the ligament allow it to support congruency of the joint surfaces, thereby resisting movement of the SIJ in all planes of motion.

Superficial to the interosseous ligament runs the posterior sacroiliac ligament (PSL). This has three distinct bands that differ in length. The longer band, also known as the long dorsal ligament, runs from the inferior tip of PSIS to the third and fourth segments of the sacrum (Vleeming et al 1996). Its fibres become taut during anterior rotation of the innominate (sacral counternutation). The short band of the PSL assists the ISL in supporting bony congruency of the SIJ.

The sacrospinous ligament runs from the lateral margin of the sacrum to the iliac spine. The sacrotuberous ligament runs from the lower sacral tubercles, the PSIS and the lateral margin of the sacrum to the medial portion of the ischial tuberosity. The sacrospinous and sacrotuberous ligaments become taut during posterior rotation of the innominate (sacral nutation). The sacrotuberous ligament's superior attachment is consistent with the long dorsal ligament, and its deep portion is consistent with the sacrospinous ligament. These interconnections create an interdependence of function: when one ligament becomes taut, it increases tension in the other ligament (Vleeming et al 1996). This tension modulation system prevents one ligament from becoming lax during SIJ loading, which would compromise stability (Pool-Goudzwaard et al 1998).

The superficial fibres of the sacrotuberous ligament attach at the ischial tuberosity and are consistent with the long head of biceps femoris muscle. In addition to the biceps femoris, the gluteus, latissimus dorsi and multifidus muscles have attachments with the ligamentous complex around the SIJ and lumbosacral junction through the thoracolumbar fascia; this provides dynamic stability during functional movement (Mens et al 2000). Anteriorly, the transversus abdominis and internal obliques pull medially on the ASIS and increase tension through the thoracodorsal fascia to increase tension throughout the pelvic system (Vleeming et al 1995).

There is variability in SIJ anatomy, which has been demonstrated by CT scan (Prassopoulos et al 1999). Pelvic morphology itself has been repeatedly demonstrated to be variable; asymmetries in the pelvis have been reported using CT scan (Badii et al 2003), cadaveric assessment of bony landmark angles (Preece et al 2008) and via instrumented palpation (Petrone et al 2003). The angle created by a straight line taken from ASIS through the PSIS with a straight line from the anterior pubis through the ASIS has been noted to vary between pelvises by as much as 23° (Preece et al 2008). When these angles are compared bilaterally within a pelvis, variability of up to 11° has been observed, with up to 16 mm difference in innominate height (Preece et al 2008).

Biomechanically, the SIJ rotates and translates in three planes, each around an instantaneous axis of rotation that lies midway between the posterior superior iliac spines (Smidt et al 1995). Because the SIJ both rotates and translates in each of three distinct planes, it is said to have six degrees of freedom for movement. The x-axis is transverse and runs mediolaterally through the bilateral PSIS and is the axis for nutation and counternutation of the sacrum. The y-axis is vertical and is the axis for the sacrum to rotate in the transverse plane, and would account for anterior translation of one SIJ with concomitant posterior translation for the contralateral SIJ. The z-axis runs anterior to posterior through the mid-sacrum and serves as the axis of sacral rotation in the frontal plane. Combination axes such as the right and left oblique axes have also been proposed (Mitchell 1958) and serve as the theoretical basis for a number of the proposed SIJD categories such as sacral torsions. To date, however, this author is unaware of any imaging data that validate these theories, and DeStefano (2011) acknowledges that their biomechanics are unknown and their existence is largely hypothetical. Axes of motion are complicated, and that which is taught is oversimplified, making it difficult to apply the proposed mechanics to the clinical assessment and treatment of SIJ pathology (Harrison et al 1997).

The SIJ has minimal movement exhibited by a systematic review reporting that seven manuscripts confirmed that rotational movements were –1.1° / 2.2° of movement along the x-axis, –0.8° / 4.0° along the y-axis and –0.5° / 8.0° along the z-axis (Goode et al 2008). In terms of translation, the movements averaged –0.3 / 8.0 mm in the x-axis, –0.2 / 7.0mm in the y-axis and –0.3 / 6.0 mm in the z-axis (Goode et al 2008). Data derived from roentgen stereophotogrammetric analysis (RSA), the most reliable and valid technique, tend to favour the lower end of the reported range. Movement is more restricted in weight-bearing (Sturesson et al 2000) than in non-weight-bearing, which is likely to be a result of the additional compressive forces placed upon the SIJ through trunk-loading in form and force closure (Pool-Goudzwaard et al 1998). During function, movement of the pubic symphysis occurs and is accompanied by deformation of the innominates (Pool-Goudzwaard et al 2012). This, in fact, probably complicates all attempts to identify mechanical and positional abnormalities in the low back pain population if they are indeed present.

Functionally, the SIJ has no muscular attachments that could result in active movement at the joint. Nevertheless, movement at the SIJ does occur passively. The SIJ and pubic symphysis are primarily joints that provide an avenue for force translation and dissipation (Snijders et al 1993a) between the lower body and trunk. The small amounts of movement outlined above would suggest that movement of these joints is not important for body positioning but rather forces attenuation. It has been hypothesized that the SIJ is necessary to dissipate forces transferring through the ring and hence prevent fractures. Sacral insufficiency fractures have been noted in populations that either have reduced natural movement through age and/or weakened bony structures of the sacrum (Grasland et al 1996). Elderly women, and those that repetitively load the pelvic ring at high levels with a weakened sacrum (Myburgh et al 1990), such as high-mileage running females (Wentz et al 2011) are examples.

There would appear to be two types of stabilization in the pelvic ring: form closure and force closure (Vleeming et al 1990a, 1990b; Snijders et al 1993a, 1993b). Form closure is the component of stabilization that is provided by the passive structures of the stabilization system. The wedge-shaped sacrum forces down into the ilia structurally as a keystone, evidenced by a reduction in SIJ movement during weight-bearing activities (Sturesson et al 2000). The posteriorly facing facets that articulate with the fifth lumbar vertebra assist in preventing anterior shearing of the lumbar spine on the nutated sacrum. The strong ligamentous system resists the separation of the ilia as the sacrum wedges in between them. The ground reaction forces translate proximally through the femurs, forcing the ilia together and stabilizing the pubic symphysis. It would seem that the greatest amount of stability would occur during equal weight-bearing. Alternatively, some of the highest SIJ loads occur during unilateral jumping and landing, making additional systems of stabilization necessary.

Force closure is the external stabilization being produced on the SIJ by muscles that can increase tension in the stabilizing system. Any muscle that can directly impact tension through the thoracolumbar fascia or the stabilizing ligaments of the SIJ or pubic symphysis can produce greater stability in the SIJ. There have been reported to be two slings that assist with force closure: a posterior sling and an anterior sling (Vleeming et al 1995). The posterior sling is made up of the hamstring muscle, the ipsilateral gluteus maximus and the contralateral multifidi and latissimus dorsi muscles. Anteriorly, the sling comprises the internal oblique and transversus abdominis and the contralateral adductor muscle group. These two slings work in concert to create additional tension in the SIJ as needed. More recent evidence suggests that a simple co-contraction of the multifidi and the transversus abdominis will stiffen the SIJ to a greater extent than targeting the diagonal pattern muscle of the pelvic slings (Richardson et al 2002). Nevertheless, an additional force for stabilization has been identified and is available and provided through the anterior (Richardson et al 2002) and posterior slings (van Wingerden et al 2004). Because of the anatomical interdependence of attachments outlined above, it becomes apparent that form and force closure are not mutually exclusive systems. As the sacrum rocks forwards into nutation tightening, the majority of the ligaments around the SIJ and the muscular components of the lumbopelvic system provide greater stabilizing force closure by pulling the structures together and increasing form closure by increasing tension through the ligaments.

Pathology and Pathomechanics

It has long been proposed that large external forces placed upon the SIJ can cause the joint to move internally and perhaps become stuck in a faulty position. The clinician would carefully examine the patient's posture and feel for abnormalities in position or movement – often a position that would presumably alter the stress placed on the SIJ, thereby causing a change in segmental positioning based on changing stress. It was believed that the furrows and ridges within the joint would provide a mechanism for the joint to get 'stuck' in an altered position, thereby creating pain. This philosophy has been taught and practised by numerous manual therapy professions. However, even though this hypothesis seems reasonable and is theoretically possible, there has not been a single biomechanical study published to this author's knowledge that has identified positional faults of the SIJ, nor has a single article been published to suggest that SIJ manipulation can and will change the position of the joint surfaces. On the contrary, more evidence has been produced to suggest that this is highly unlikely (Laslett 2008), and one study has provided evidence to refute this theory by identifying that SIJ manipulation does not alter the joint position (Tullberg et al 1998).

More recently, it has been surmised that most mechanical pain is related to some asymmetry of stabilization of the SIJ and / or pubic symphysis. This theory might suggest that, with altered stability, there would be pathological movement in the SIJ. This has not been shown to be the case, however. Sturesson (1999) identified that there was no measurable difference in movement between the symptomatic and asymptomatic sides. PGP is more associated with asymmetrical laxity of the pelvis, not generalized laxity of the SIJs (Vleeming et al 1996, 2008; Pool-Goudzwaard et al 1998; Damen et al 2001, 2002; Richardson et al 2002). When excessive asymmetric laxity is found in an SIJ through the active straight leg raise test (ASLR) or Doppler ultrasound (Damen et al 2001), excess movement is noted anteriorly at the pubic symphysis and not posteriorly in the ipsilateral SIJ (Mens et al 1999). Asymmetrical stability may be the result of altered muscle recruitment of the stabilizers on the side of pathology as evidenced by electromyographic study (Hungerford et al 2003).

Diagnosis

Medical diagnosis

As with any presumed neuro-musculoskeletal pathology, the first diagnostic question to answer is whether or not there is a serious or sinister medical problem that may be the source of the patient's pain (Murphy & Hurwitz 2007). Appropriate screening for medical, non-mechanical pathology must be performed (Huijbregts 2004; Sizer et al 2007).

As previously stated, the best external evidence for diagnosis of SIJP is a fluoroscopically guided IAI that results in at least an 80% reduction in pain as the gold standard (Chou et al 2004). This test is simply not routinely done in clinical practice, but is reserved for individuals with recalcitrant back pain referred for interventional radiology; therefore, only a select few will have the advantage of these test results. This procedure is not without its limitations, however. Intra-articular injections should only diagnose intra-articular problems, and not pain coming from periarticular structures such as the long dorsal ligament (Murakami et al 2007). There is also evidence that the reliability of the anaesthetic infiltrating the joint may be limited and that some may leak out into the surrounding tissues, confounding the diagnosis of a specific structure (Berthelot et al 2006). Conversely, periarticular structures may not be impacted by the injection if the anaesthetic doesn't leak out. Bearing these limitations mind, it is clear that false positives and false negatives exist with the IAI. Additionally, different thresholds of pain relief to dichotomize test results have ranged from 50% pain relief (van der Wurff et al 2006) to ≥90% (Dreyfuss et al 1996; Broadhurst & Bond 1998). Other frequently used thresholds include 70% (Broadhurst & Bond, 1998), 75% (Schwarzer et al 1995; Maigne et al 1996) and 80% (Slipman et al 2000; Fukui & Nosaka 2002; Laslett et al 2003, 2005a). Nevertheless, considering the limitations of imaging and other forms of diagnostic tests, although the injection may not be ideal it is better than any of the other available options for diagnosing pain arising from the SIJ region.

Imaging can be used to diagnose sacroiliitis; however, there are limitations to this technique. A recent MRI study examined 691 patients with suspected sacroiliitis and found that 41% showed no abnormal findings. Sacroiliitis appeared in 36%, but other pathologies of the lumbar spine and hip, SIJ degeneration and more problematic diagnoses such as tumours (1.6%), fractures (1.2%) and infections (0.6%) were also present (Jans et al 2013). An important point to note is that the belief of clinical sacroiliitis was not particularly discriminative, which may be considered as consistent with other studies that have attempted to isolate historical and clinical features of SIJ pathology.

Clinical diagnosis: subjective examination

A careful history assists the clinician in identifying potential conditions of the SIJ that are non-mechanical in nature. Unfortunately, many of the symptoms associated with inflammatory and infectious pathologies present with complaints similar to those associated with mechanical pathologies (Peloso & Braun 2004). There are no particular symptoms associated with the mechanical pain patterns in the SIJ, and this may be due in part to the basic problem of identifying mechanical pathologies as either SIJP or SIJD (Laslett 2008). The low back pain literature frequently uses the terms SIJP and dysfunction interchangeably, although we have little evidence to suggest that it is conceptually valid (Laslett 2008). The inability to differentiate the SIJP accurately as being of either mechanical origin or from an inflammatory process makes the clinical examination challenging. SIJP associated with mechanical causes may respond to conservative care. A failure to do so may be an indication for medical physician referral (Cook 2012).

Researchers have explored the use of pain maps to identify particular patterns associated with SIJ pathology. A rectangular area of approximately 3 cm wide × 10 cm long just distal to the PSIS has been proposed to be a primary area of pain for SIJ (Fortin et al 1994a, 1994b). This pain map was identified by injecting the joint of healthy subjects with contrast media to stimulate discomfort, followed by Xylocaine, and identifying the local region demonstrating hyperaesthesia to light touch. This same region has also been identified by other investigators (Broadhurst et al 2004). Contradictory findings have also been reported, however. Slipman et al (2000) found that there was no specific pain patterning for SIJ. Additionally, van der Wurff et al (2006) found that pain areas were not selective for SIJ pathology but that intensity of pain may be more selective; subjects who responded to a local anaesthetic block reported the greatest pain intensity in Fortin's region just inferior to the PSIS whereas non-responders had most pain over the region of the ischial tuberosity. In addition, pain reduction responses to anaesthetic injections, although usually localized to Fortin's area (94%), have also demonstrated referral to other regions of the lower quarter extending from the upper lumbar area (6%) and abdomen (2%) to the foot (12%) (Slipman et al 2000). This variability in somatic pain referral, with significant overlap in lumbar pathologies, is likely due to the complex and variable innervation noted earlier, with a proposed contribution of both lumbar and sacral roots (Vleeming et al 2012). The long dorsal ligament, which courses through Fortin's area, is frequently painful in patients with low back pain. Vleeming et al (1996) found that 44% of women and 47% of men with non-specific low back pain reported this area to be very tender to palpation; however, it is not diagnostically specific to SIJP.

Young et al (2003) found that pain that is felt on rising from sitting was significantly associated with SIJP, as was an absence of midline pain and unilateral pain below the L5 spinous process. Patients were 28 times more likely to have SIJP when they had concurrent pain upon rising and a positive cluster of three of out of five pain provocation tests. When examined specifically for diagnostic accuracy, pain on rising from sitting was found to be poor (Cook et al 2007). Therefore, historical factors associated with SIJ pathology are currently lacking in diagnostic accuracy. Historical features, as part of a comprehensive examination, may be helpful in identifying SIJ pathology but are not conclusive in and of themselves (Huijbregts 2004).

Clinical diagnosis: physical examination

There are a number of categories of tests used to classify different musculoskeletal pathologies. Active and passive ranges of motion are often used, as well as special tests. The latter can be further subclassified into three distinct forms of tests: positional palpation tests, tests for symmetry or predictable motion, and symptom provocation tests (Huijbregts 2004). Each of these classes of examination will be discussed.

Active physiological movements are frequently used in the examination of axial skeletal disorders. Active movements such as walking have been reportedly associated with pelvic pain associated with pregnancy (Rost et al 2004). However, other authors have suggested that active movements are not associated with SIJ pathology (Schwarzer et al 1995; Maigne et al 1996). Repeated active movements should be performed in an effort to identify the presence of the centralization phenomenon. When centralization is present a discogenic problem is indicated, lessening the likelihood that SIJP is the problem even though symptom provocation tests for SIJP are positive (Laslett et al 2005c).

Passive physiological tests are also frequently used in the examination of proposed SIJ pathology. Passive innominate rotations into end range have the capacity to stretch intra- and periarticular structures into end range. Pain provocation with these tests may indicate SIJ pathology. Exact identification of the structure involved is highly unlikely, but the behaviour of the symptoms with single and repeated passive rotations may indicate a possible method of treatment.

One study suggested that the presence of asymmetry of hip rotation was associated with SIJD (Cibulka et al 1998). An additional study demonstrated that hip range of motion could be enhanced following an SIJ manipulation (Pollard & Ward 1998). Interestingly, hip internal rotation (IR) of at least 35° in at least one hip was one of the predictor variables of who would do well with an SIJ manipulation (Flynn et al 2002). Nevertheless, in that study no specific SIJ test predicted success, reducing the likelihood that SIJP was the problem.

Passive accessory techniques are also frequently used in the diagnosis of low back pain and SIJP. Currently, there are no studies examining the benefit of passive accessory techniques for SIJ pathology (Cook 2012). A proposed diagnostic feature of passive accessory techniques may be to help rule in / out lumbar pathology. If the patient has the primary pain around the L5 spinous process or higher and the primary pain can be provoked by either a central or unilateral posterior–anterior (PA) glide, it is less likely to be SIJ in origin. If the patient's symptoms can be centralized with repeated PA pressures in the lumbar spine, lumbar pathology is likely. If PA glides on the sacrum are applied and result in alteration of symptoms, SIJ pathology may be ruled in and a potential treatment option is identified (Cook 2012).

Positional palpation tests are clinical tests used to diagnose SIJD that rely heavily upon the perception of asymmetrical bony alignment, whereas tests for symmetrical or predictable motion are special tests that attempt to assess SIJ movement qualitatively. Palpatory examination of the pelvis is the foundation of the osteopathic approach to treatment of pelvic pain (DeStefano 2011). In addition, many clinicians from various healthcare professions have adopted this methodology for assessment and treatment of pelvic and SIJ disorders. A fundamental limitation of this methodology, however, is the low degree of both reliability and diagnostic accuracy. The diagnosis of SIJ pathology based on palpation and movement tests and their symmetry fundamentally depends on the philosophy that there is easily palpable or measureable movement in the SIJ and that bony landmarks within the pelvic ring are directly palpable and symmetrical. As stated previously, however, this clinical premise appears to be inaccurate; as the movement of the SIJ is no more than a few degrees of rotation or a couple of millimetres of translation, it would appear that the SIJ is not a typical joint. Recognition of this philosophical limitation makes it easy to see why the diagnostic accuracy of clinical diagnostic tests for movement and symmetry is poor. Numerous studies have examined the intra-rater and inter-rater reliability of tests performed to establish symmetry of bony landmarks and SIJ movement, and have found the results to range from 'only slightly better than chance' to 'fair' (van der Wurff et al 2000b; Huijbregts 2004). Furthermore, although it would seem reasonable that greater training would improve reliability, this hypothesis has been refuted by two studies that found better reliability among novice clinicians (Herzog et al 1989; Mior et al 1990). There are other more-comprehensive reviews of the literature that provide more detailed data regarding these facts and the reader is referred to these (Huijbregts 2004; Stovall & Kumar 2010; Cook 2013). A recent study reported that the assessment of pelvic motion reliability can be enhanced to ≥0.97 with the use of an electromagnetic tracking device, but this type of instrumentation is not readily available to the clinician (Adhia et al 2012).

The validity of a clinical test can be defined as the extent to which the test measures the intended construct. Tests for SIJ symmetry of motion and palpation fail to achieve meaningful reliability – an underlying principle of validity; therefore, they cannot be considered as clinically valid (Huijbregts 2004; Laslett 2008). In addition, numerous studies have examined the validity of palpatory and motion symmetry tests and have consistently found it to be limited (Huijbregts 2004). Tullberg et al (1998) examined concurrent validity by having three investigators examine 10 individuals before and after an SIJ manipulation for symmetry of iliac crest, ASIS and PSIS in standing, supine and prone. There was substantial agreement that most individuals experienced correction of asymmetry following the SIJ manipulation; however, the RSA determined that no observable change in SIJ position occurred. Another study using RSA that examined SIJ movement during the standing flexion test in 22 patients with single-sided SIJD found that the motions of the SIJ were too small to be detected manually – causing the authors to conclude that the test was not clinically useful (Sturesson et al 2000). This suggests that the asymmetrical positions often associated with SIJD are likely to be the product of local muscular forces producing strain on the pelvis, which gives the illusion of SIJ positional faults (Tullberg et al 1998).

Anatomical asymmetry in form (Preece et al 2008) and fusion (Dar et al 2008) further challenge the validity of position- and movement-based tests. Bony asymmetry will produce false positives, which has been shown clinically by asymptomatic individuals demonstrating positive clinical tests (Dreyfuss et al 1994). Furthermore, the establishment of diagnostic accuracy in these tests is a challenge. Currently, there is no established benchmark standard for diagnosing SIJD. Diagnostic blocks can establish SIJP, but pain may be due to factors other than dysfunction, thus contributing to poor diagnostic accuracy (Laslett 2008). Because of these diagnostic limitations, McGrath (2006) questioned their clinical use and suggested the need to teach tests for symmetry of position and movement within the osteopathic educational system.

Clinicians often cluster tests in an attempt to enhance the clinical meaning of the results. Most tests when considered independently lack sufficient diagnostic accuracy to determine the appropriate clinical course of action. Clinical reasoning suggests that interpretation of the meaning of all available clinical data in an interdependent manner enhances the process. One test item cluster of symmetry tests – the standing flexion test, sitting PSIS symmetry test, supine to sit test for medial malleoli symmetry and prone knee flexion test – has shown moderately strong diagnostic power (LR+ 6.83), but the study failed to use a benchmark standard in confirming the SIJ diagnosis (Cibulka & Koldehoff 1999). The diagnostic accuracy in this study was based on the presence or absence of low back pain, which cannot be discriminatively defined as SIJD.

Symptom provocation tests require an alteration of the patient's perceived pain. Provocation tests have also demonstrated variability in both intra-rater and inter-rater reliability, which ranged from poor to substantial (Huijbregts 2004). The reliability of provocational tests is nevertheless greater than that of tests of symmetry, providing a stronger foundation for diagnostic accuracy (Laslett & Williams 1994). A recent systematic review suggested that the diagnostic accuracy of

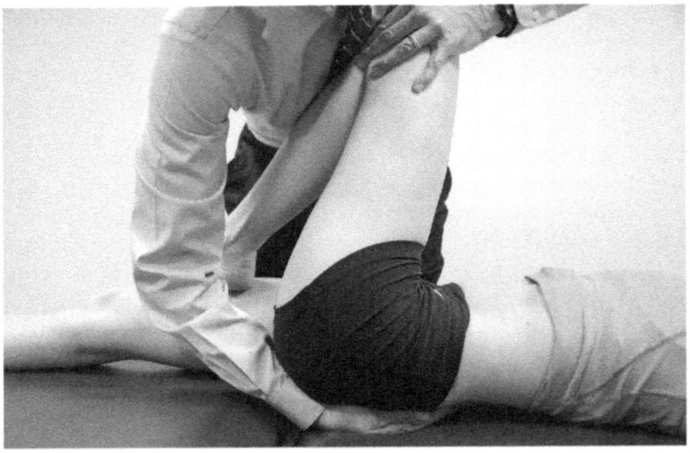

Figure 24.1 Thigh thrust test.

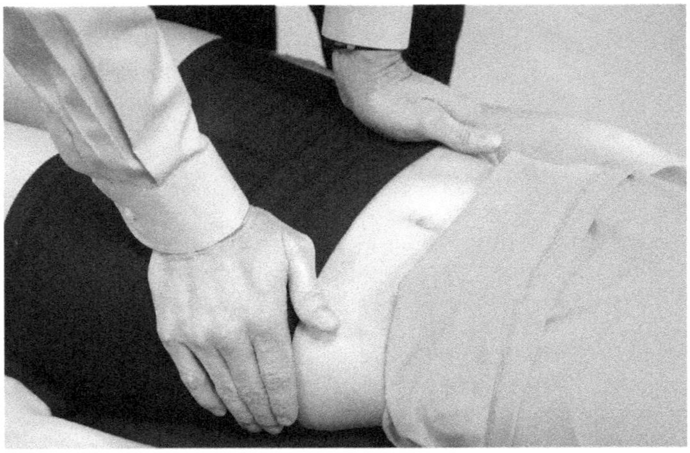

Figure 24.2 Sacroiliac distraction test.

provocation testing for SIJ dysfunction is fair (Simopoulos et al 2012). No single provocation test is very diagnostic though; therefore, clusters of tests have been proposed to enhance the likelihood of coming to a reliable conclusion. In addition, an earlier systematic review of the criteria for SIJP as determined by the International Association Society for the Study of Pain (IASP) suggested that clustering provocational tests yields satisfactory diagnostic accuracy (Szadek et al 2009).

Laslett et al (2003) first proposed a five-test-item cluster in which three of the five tests should be found positive in order to provide a positive likelihood ration of 4.16; the five tests in question included the thigh thrust test, the compression test, the distraction test, the torsional stress test (Gaenslen's test) and the sacral stress test. The reliability of this five-test-item cluster has been found to be satisfactory, at kappa=0.70 (Laslett & Williams 1994; Kokmeyer et al 2002). Subsequent research identified that similar diagnostic accuracy could be obtained with only four tests (i.e. when the Gaenslen's test was removed from the original test-item cluster) with at least two being positive (Laslett et al 2005a). The detailed descriptions of these tests are as follows:

- **Thigh thrust test:** The patient lies in supine with the hip flexed to 90° and adducted sufficiently to control hip rotation. The examiner places one hand under the sacrum, avoiding the PSIS of the testing side, and places a force posteriorly through the thigh to stress the SIJ (Fig. 24.1).
- **Distraction test:** The patient lies supine while the examiner applies an equal force posteriorly through both ASISs (Fig. 24.2).
- **Compression test:** The patient lies in side-lying with hips and knees comfortably flexed for positioning. The examiner applies a force towards the table through the uppermost iliac crest (Fig. 24.3).
- **Sacral thrust:** The patient lies in prone while the examiner performs a posterior-to-anterior force towards the table through the centre of the sacrum (Fig. 24.4).
- **Gaenslen's test:** The patient lies supine with one leg in maximum hip and knee flexion and the other hip in extension. Pelvic torsion is created with overpressure through both legs. This test is repeated on the contralateral side (Fig. 24.5).

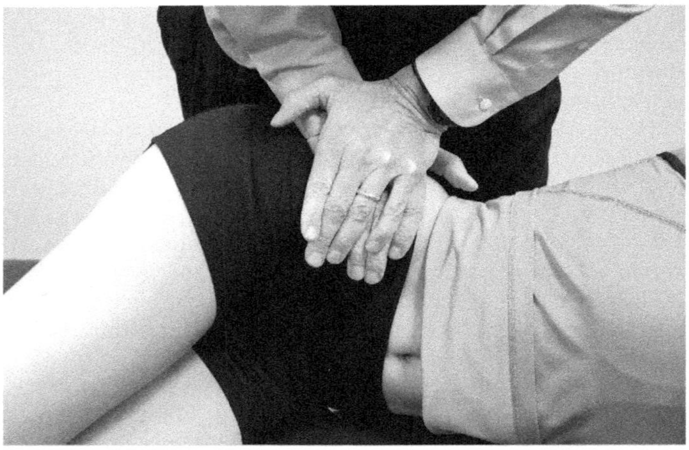

Figure 24.3 Sacroiliac compression test.

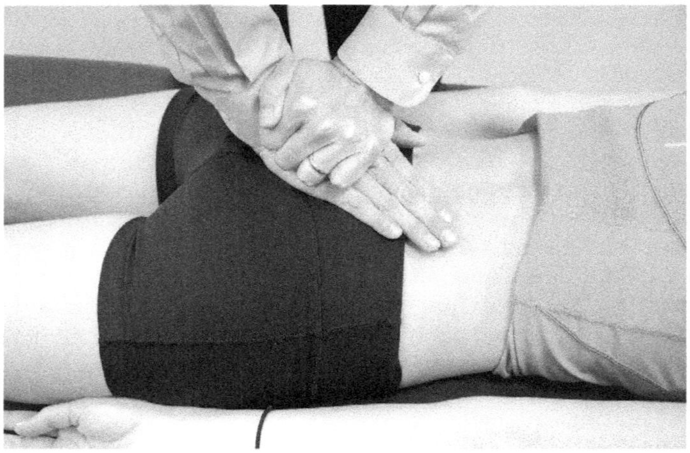

Figure 24.4 Sacral thrust test.

Any of these tests are positive if they reproduce the patient's comparable, familiar symptoms. The patient is instructed to ignore discomfort related to the examiner's hand placement

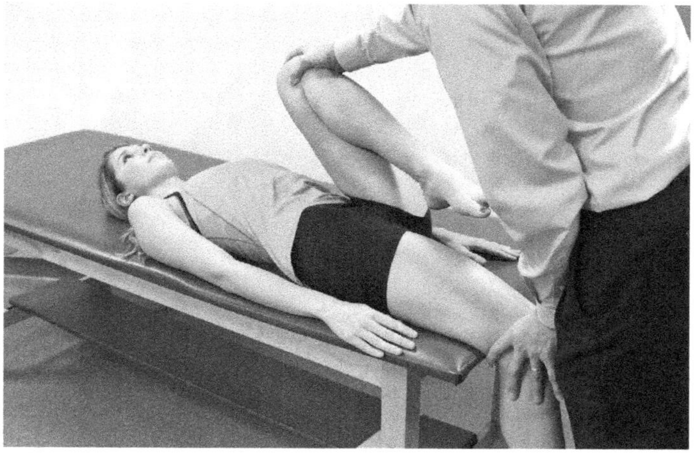

Figure 24.5 **Gaenslen's test.**

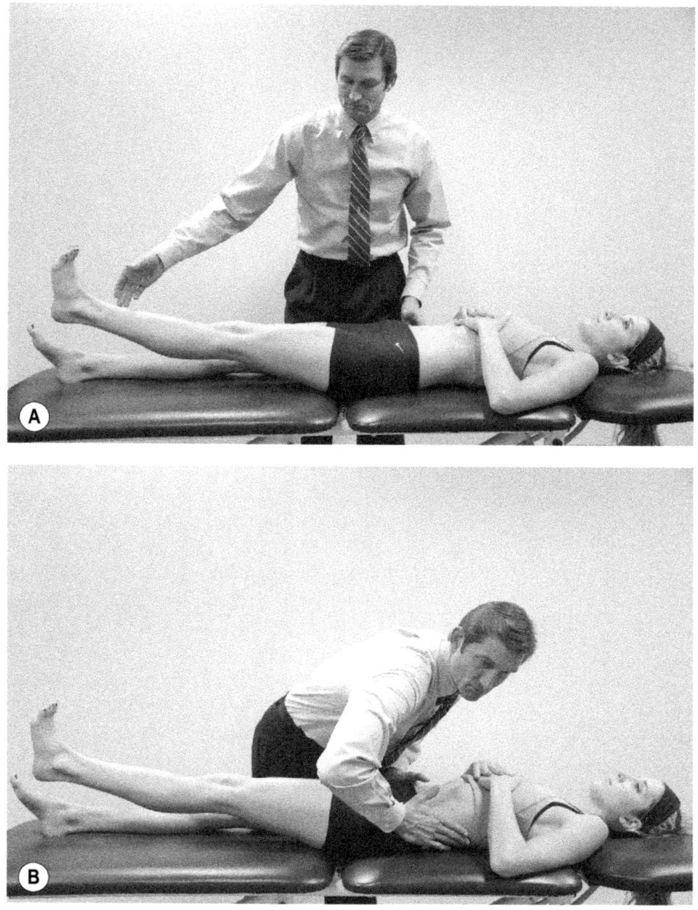

Figure 24.6 **Active straight leg raise test:** (**A**) without and (**B**) with compression by the therapist.

during the test. A potential source of variability has been reported when forces are applied asymmetrically so care should be taken to maintain equal forces side to side for tests that require bilateral contact (Levin et al 2001). A second potential source of error may occur if the force applied is not maintained for a sufficient period of time to create irritation in the SIJ. Levin and Stenstrom (2003) found that it took up to 20 seconds to provoke pain in individuals with SIJP, which may be explained by the large size, relative stability and general functional requirement of the SIJ to transfer large loads during weight-bearing activities.

As stated earlier, PGP can be subgrouped into four distinct categories with a fifth category of mixed presentation (Albert et al 2002). This classification system has been found to be reliable, with a kappa coefficient of 0.78 (Cook et al 2007). PGP is also best classified with the use of clusters of provocational tests. Albert et al (2000) found that SIJP was best classified with the use of the thigh thrust, Patrick's test and Menell's test, whereas the pubic symphysis classes were best identified using palpation of the pubic symphysis and Trendelenburg's test. A small study examining the diagnostic accuracy of specific examination procedures found the best single test to be the active straight leg raise, with a LR+ of 3.2 (Cook et al 2007); however, when the researchers clustered the ASLR with Gaenslen's test and the thigh thrust, with the requirement that at least two of the tests be positive, they found this raised the LR+ only slightly, to 3.5. From this study, the best clustering of examination findings was found to be a single positive provocative test from a lunge, hip manual muscle test, or hip range of motion, which produced an LR+ of 4.2 (Cook et al 2007); this study sample was too small, however, to subclassify diagnostic accuracy based on PGP class and doing so might improve the diagnostic accuracy of the examination findings.

Kristiansson et al (1996) found that provocational tests for the pelvic girdle produced adequate diagnostic accuracy for pregnancy-related PGP in a sample of 200 women. The Patrick's test and palpation of the long dorsal ligament were included in this study. Additionally, symptom provocation with resisted hip abduction has been associated with aberrant movement of the SIJ and symphysis pubis (Rost et al 2004). The following are descriptions of the additional provocational tests for PGP:

- **Active straight leg raise**: The patient lies supine and attempts to raise the heel of the involved leg 6 inches off the mat (Fig. 24.6A). The examiner then compresses the pelvis and the test is repeated (Fig. 24.6B). The test is positive if the patient reports primary pain while raising the heel on the first attempt, then reduced or eliminated pain on the second attempt.
- **Lunge test**: The standing patient steps forward with the involved leg, then lunges until the trailing knee reaches the floor. The test is repeated on the other side. A positive test is reproduction of the primary complaint of pain (Fig. 24.7).
- **Patrick's test**: The patient lies supine and the involved leg is flexed and externally rotated. The examiner then stabilizes the opposite ASIS and applies a downward force through the flexed knee (Fig. 24.8).
- **Trendelenburg's test**: The patient stands on the involved leg and the examiner observes for a drop of the non-weight-bearing hip. The test is positive if the primary pain is also provoked (Fig. 24.9).
- **Resisted hip abduction provocation test**: This test is carried out as the standard manual muscle test for hip abduction. The test is positive if it reproduces the patient's primary complaint of pain (Fig. 24.10).
- **Pubic symphysis compression test**: The patient lies supine and direct AP pressure is applied over the

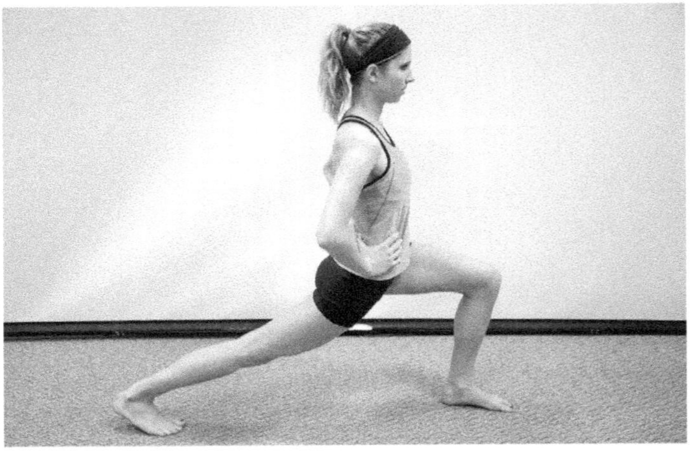

Figure 24.7 Lunge test.

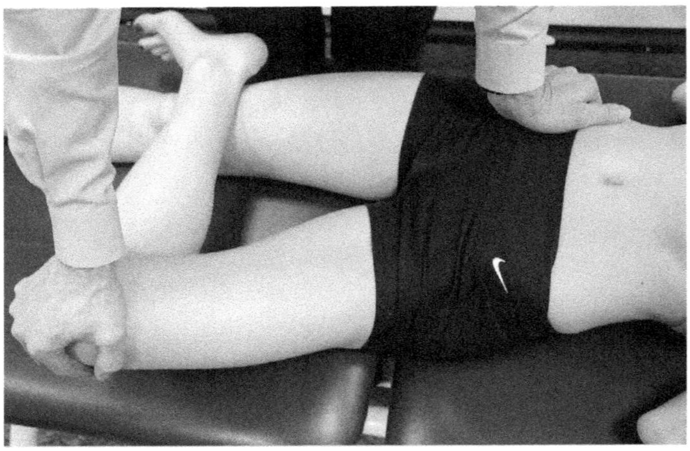

Figure 24.8 Patrick's test.

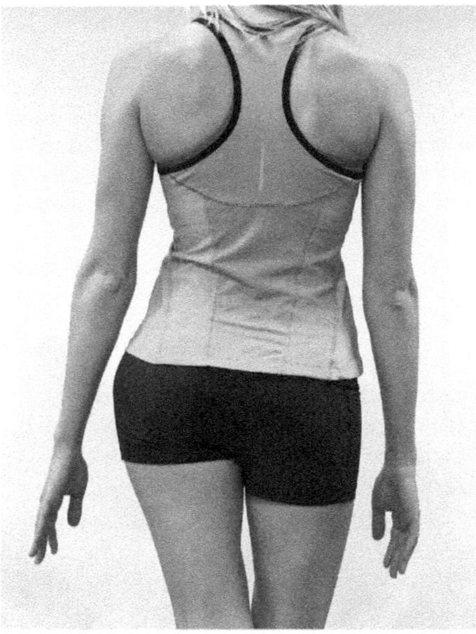

Figure 24.9 Modified Trendelenburg's test.

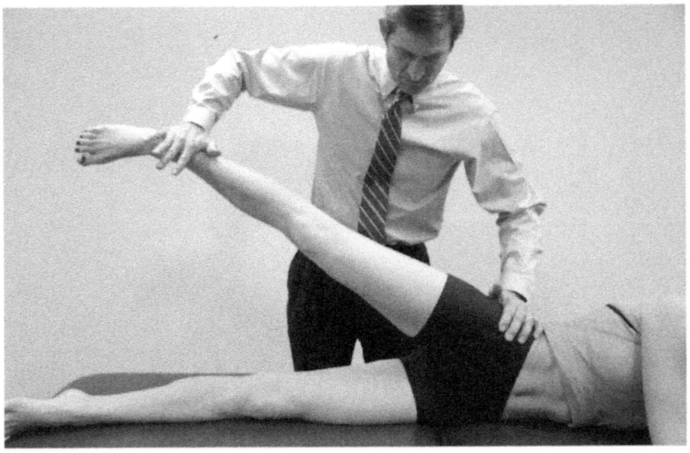

Figure 24.10 Hip abduction manual muscle test.

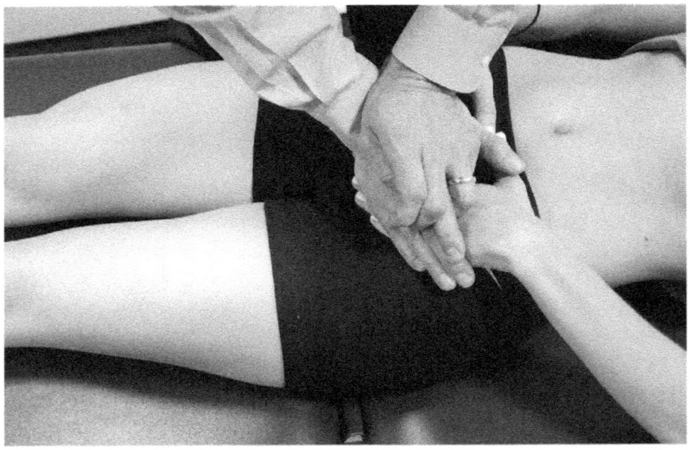

Figure 24.11 Pubic compression test.

symphysis. A positive test is provocation of symptoms comparable to the patient's primary complaint (Fig. 24.11).

- **Palpation of the long dorsal ligament**: The patient lies in prone and the examiner palpates just distally and slightly medially to the PSIS and uses medial-to-lateral strumming across the ligament, looking for tenderness and reproduction of the patient's primary complaint of pain (Fig. 24.12).
- **Palpation of the sacrotuberous ligament**: The patient lies in prone and the inferior lateral angles (ILAs) of the sacrum are palpated. The examiner drops slightly inferiorly and laterally to the ILAs and palpates deeply into the soft tissue to determine whether it reproduces the comparable pain (Fig. 24.13).

Bearing these issues in mind, it seems reasonable for the clinician to attempt to identify individuals who are experiencing SIJP, rather than patients who might have SIJD (van der Wurff et al 2000b; Laslett 2006). To identify patients with SIJP, a strategy of pain provocation tests is advocated. Once it has been determined that the low back pain is arising from the SIJ, the therapist should then adopt a strategy to identify

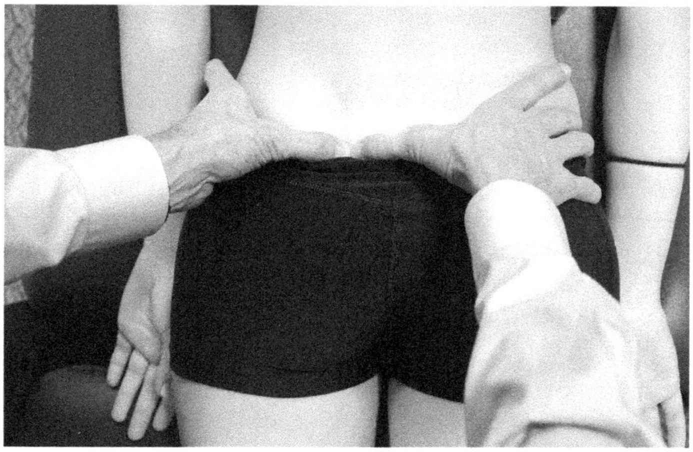

Figure 24.12 Long dorsal ligament palpation.

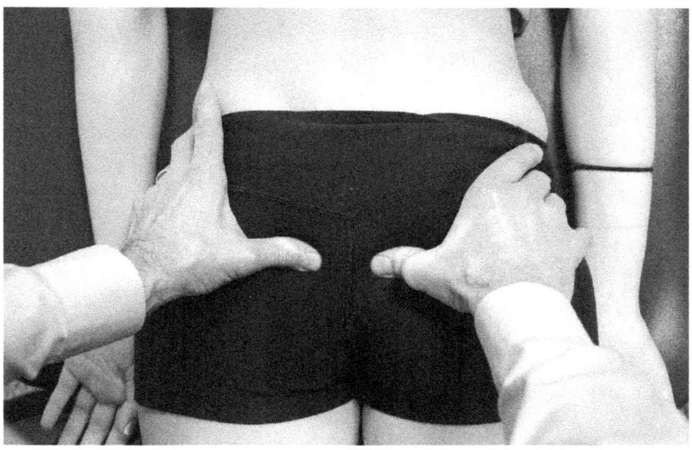

Figure 24.13 Sacrotuberous ligament palpation.

which directional movement might be the source of irritation, thereby elucidating a potential intervention approach to the condition (Laslett 2006). In addition, a precursor to provoking the SIJ may be to rule out lumbar spine pathology as more low back pain can be attributed to the lumbar spine than to the SIJ and SIJ provocational tests may be positive in individuals who have low back pain demonstrating the centralization phenomenon. Several studies have suggested that the centralization phenomenon is peculiar and highly specific to discogenic pathology (Young et al 2003; Laslett et al 2005c; Laslett 2006), so it can be assumed that positive SIJ provocational tests in the presence of centralization can be classified as false positives. If mechanical provocation of the lumbar spine reproduces the patient's pain, it would seem more likely that the lumbar spine is the region of choice for directing the intervention. Only after ruling out the lumbar spine, and specifically the centralization phenomenon, does it make sense to attempt to rule in the SIJ (Laslett et al 2005c; Cook 2012). In a systematic review to evaluate the clinical usefulness of spine special tests, Hancock et al (2007) found the only test that was useful for identifying discogenic pathology was centralization. In addition, clusters of provocation tests were the only method of identifying SIJ pathology. Therefore, the decision process presented here is consistent with these findings.

Clinical examination summary

During history taking, the individual with SIJ-related pain often reports primary symptoms distal to the L5 spinous process that are both unilateral and often focused in the region just distal to the PSIS. These symptoms frequently refer to the leg and may be present all the way down to the foot or even on occasion refer into the groin, lumbar spine or abdomen (Slipman et al 2000). Older patients with a history of symptoms below the knee are far less likely to have SIJP. The history may include a unilateral trauma, including a fall on the buttock or a mis-step on the side of pain. Further, the patient may report that symptoms increase when they rise from sitting. These historical features enhance the likelihood of SIJ pathology, but certainly are far from diagnostic.

The objective examination should thoroughly rule out the presence of lumbar pathology, specifically targeting centralization because, as mentioned above, subjects with discogenic back pain are known to demonstrate a positive response to the pain provocation manoeuvres recommended for ruling in SIJ pathology. Aside from assessing for the centralization phenomenon, active range of motion testing adds little diagnostic value to the objective examination (Huijbregts 2004). Passive physiological and passive accessory motions of the lumbar spine can be used to rule in / out lumbar involvement. Positional palpatory tests and tests for motion symmetry are not currently recommended for diagnosing SIJD since they have limited reliability, validity or diagnostic accuracy. Once lumbar pathology has been ruled out, however, a cluster of symptom provocation tests is recommended to assist the clinician in potentially ruling in SIJP.

Once SIJP has been found to be likely, passive physiological motions of the innominates and passive accessories around the sacrum can be used to identify potential manual therapy treatment options. If these tests are equivocal, stabilization asymmetry may be an issue. The PGP provocational tests then could be performed to rule in pelvic instability.

The recommendations above are consistent with the three criteria the IASP described to diagnose SIJ pathology – that is, the pain needs to be near the SIJ, provocational tests for pain in the SIJ are positive and the pain can be relieved through the use of intra-articular injections (Merskey & Bogduk 1994).

Prognosis

Few studies have focused on prognosis for SIJP. Studies that have addressed the prognosis of low back pain in general report that most low back pain resolves satisfactorily within a relatively short period of time. Bearing this in mind, it would seem that acute SIJP would be included in these statistics if it had not been differentiated in the diagnosis. However, most studies that have addressed SIJ pathology include patients with chronic low back pain, indicating a poorer prognosis since the condition has already become persistent in nature.

Pregnancy-related pelvic pain has been examined in a large trial which found that 62.5% of women had no pain within a month after delivery and 91.4% were pain free at 2 years (Albert et al 2001). However, the longitudinal follow-up of 341 patients revealed that differences between classification groups existed, as no subjects from the group with symphysiolysis pain still had pain after 6 months post delivery, yet 21% of subjects in the pelvic girdle syndrome group (with daily pain in all three pelvic joints) still had symptoms after 2 years. The study's conclusion was that post-partum PGP had an excellent prognosis for recovery in every group except the pelvic girdle syndrome group, which had a much poorer prognosis since over three times more subjects had pain in that group than in the other four groups combined (Albert et al 2001).

If all conservative care fails to provide adequate pain relief, surgical fusion of the SIJ is an available option. Numerous studies have demonstrated that surgical correction of recalcitrant SIJP is effective in providing adequate relief allowing return to normal function (Belanger & Dall 2001; Rudolf 2012; Cummings & Capobianco 2013; Sachs & Capobianco 2013; Smith et al 2013); however, the procedure is not without its critics, who cite high complication and residual pain rates in patients receiving SIJ fusions (Shaffrey & Smith 2013). Sachs and Capobianco (2013), in contrast, reported few postoperative complications in 40 patients having a minimally invasive SIJ fusion, and a 7.8-point improvement in the mean low back pain score, which decreased from 8.7 pre-surgery to 0.9 at 1-year follow-up. The minimally invasive surgical approach requires less recovery time and results in better pain and disability relief following surgery than the open approach – as identified by a retrospective examination of 263 patients treated by seven surgeons (Smith et al 2013). A recent study reported that the cost of minimally invasive SIJ fusions compares favourably with the lifetime cost of non-operative conservative care (Ackerman et al 2013).

Treatment

Intra-articular injections are the diagnostic reference standard for SIJ pathology, but are also a treatment technique. The use of IAI for the treatment of SIJ pathology is technically demanding so it is guided by an imaging technique to ensure proper placement of the medication into the SIJ. One study found that, despite a low rate of actual SIJ joint infiltration, there were similar outcomes for pain relief between those patients in whom the injection penetrated the joint and those in whom the injection was noted to have missed the joint (Hartung et al 2010).

Exercise therapy

There are two main types of active exercise prescribed for SIJ pathology: stabilization exercises and exercise for movement enhancement. Stabilization exercises are used to create tension within the thoracolumbar fascia and the other ligaments that stabilize the SIJ. This enhances the band-like tension in the posterior aspect of the sacral region, increasing force tension in the pelvic ring. Movement-based exercises are used to stretch the innominate in one direction or another so as to improve mobility and energy load transfer.

Multiple studies have questioned the benefit of a stabilization exercise programme for the treatment of SIJP or pelvic ring instability (Mens et al 2000; Nilsson-Wikmar et al 2005). One study found no between-group differences for an exercise programme that emphasized the diagonal muscle patterns of the anterior sling (Mens et al 2000). Conversely, there is evidence that stabilization may be effective in treating pelvic pain. Elden et al (2005) found that a stabilization approach incorporating modified multifidi and transversus abdominis muscles was clinically more effective than standard, non-exercising conservative care alone – although this study also found that acupuncture was also clinically more effective than standard care alone and was slightly more effective than the stabilization exercises. Stuge et al (2004a) examined the effects of a stabilization exercise programme in a sample of 81 subjects with PGP that focused on a combination of local muscle stabilizers, the multifidi (Fig. 24.14) and transversus abdominis (Fig. 24.15) muscles, and progressed to include global prime movers. Figs 24.16–24.22 provide some examples of global stabilization exercises. This study compared stabilization exercises with a control group over a 20-week programme and found that the stabilization group experienced improved pain and functional outcomes, which were maintained at both 1-year (Stuge et al 2004a) and 2-year follow-ups (Stuge et al 2004b). A comparison of the contradictory results obtained between this and an earlier randomized

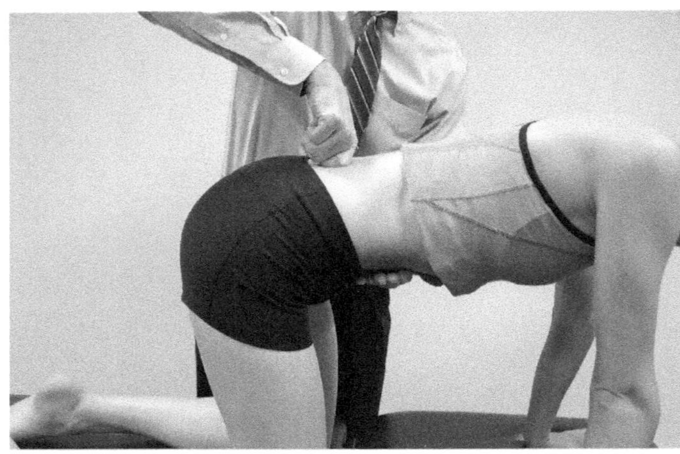

Figure 24.14 Multifidus muscle isolation contraction exercise.

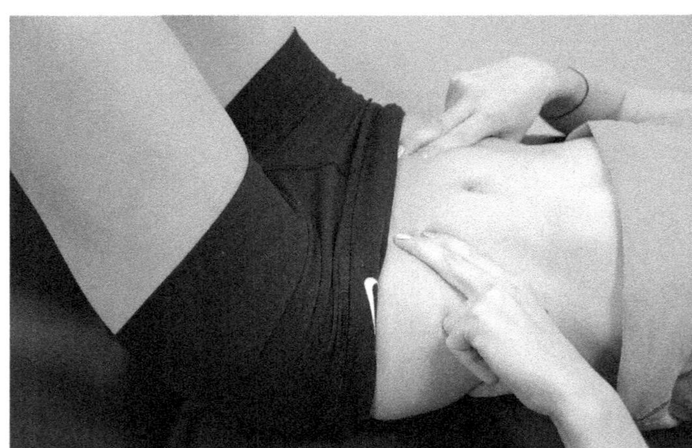

Figure 24.15 Transversus abdominis muscle isolation contraction exercise.

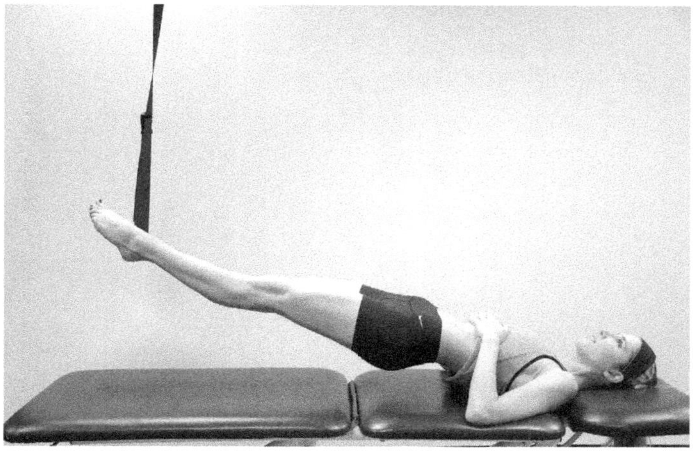

Figure 24.16 Single-leg, sling-supported bridge exercise.

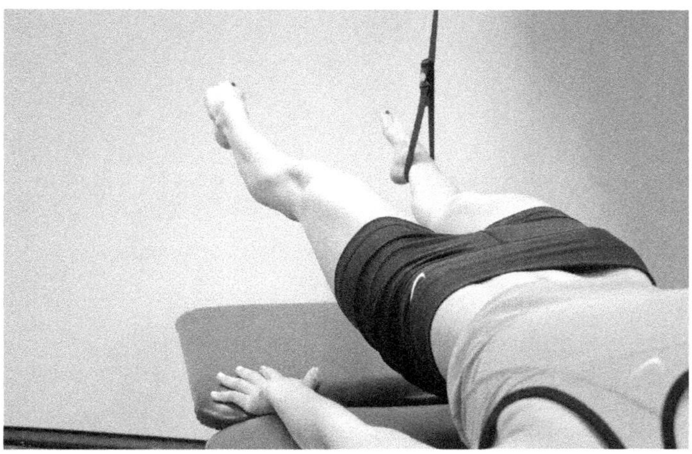

Figure 24.17 Single-leg, sling-supported bridge with active hip abduction exercise.

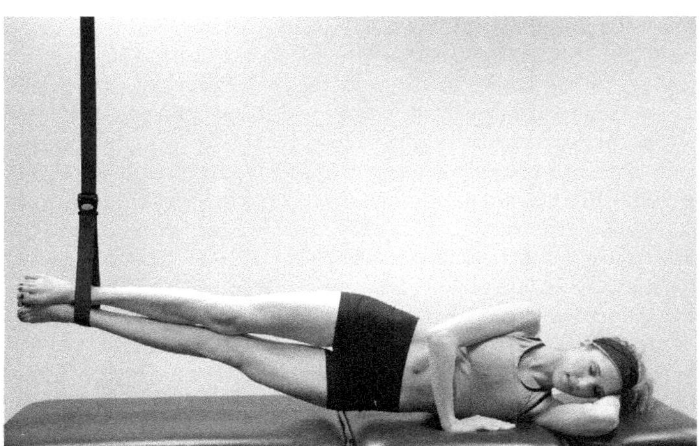

Figure 24.18 Sling-supported side-plank exercise.

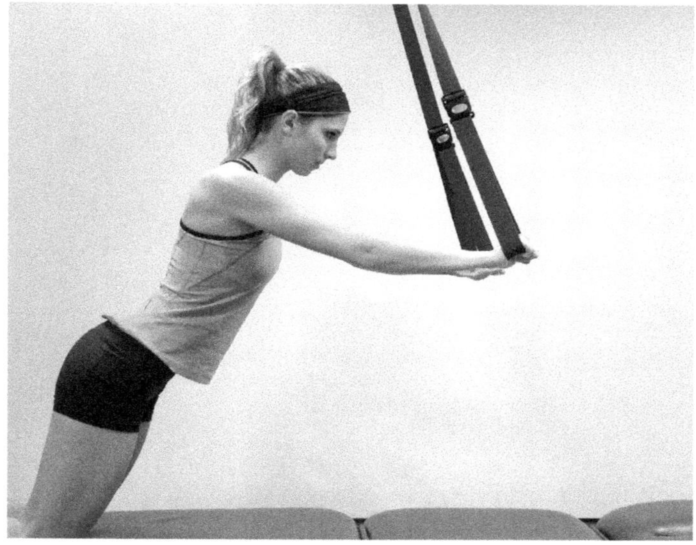

Figure 24.19 Sling-supported forward trunk lean exercise.

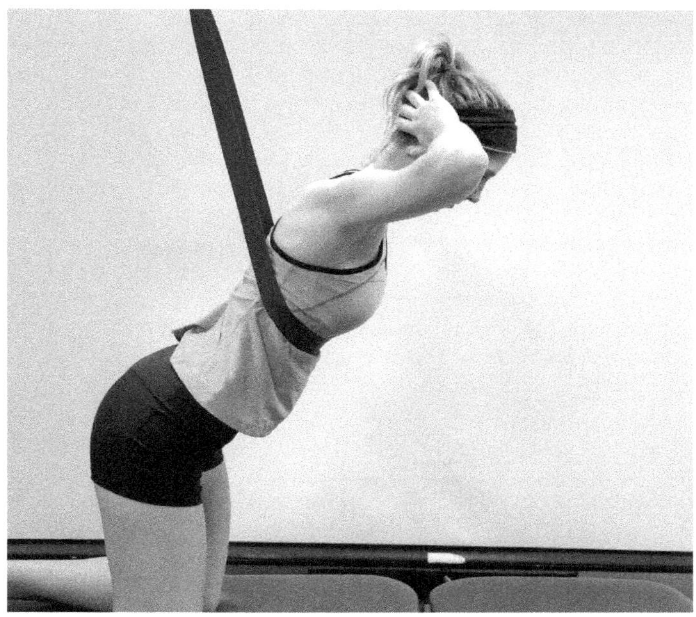

Figure 24.20 Sling-supported trunk extension exercise.

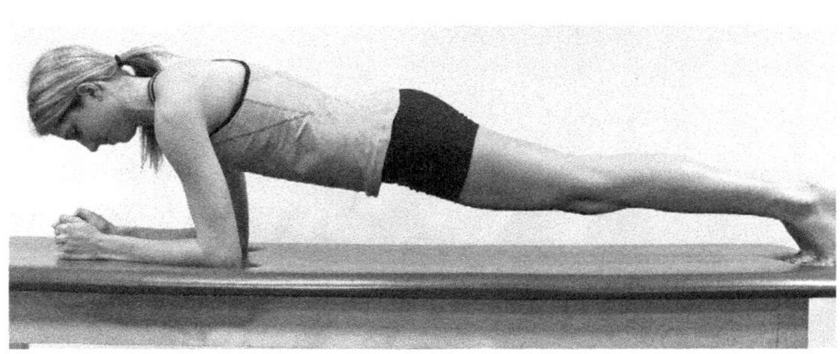

Figure 24.21 Standard plank exercise.

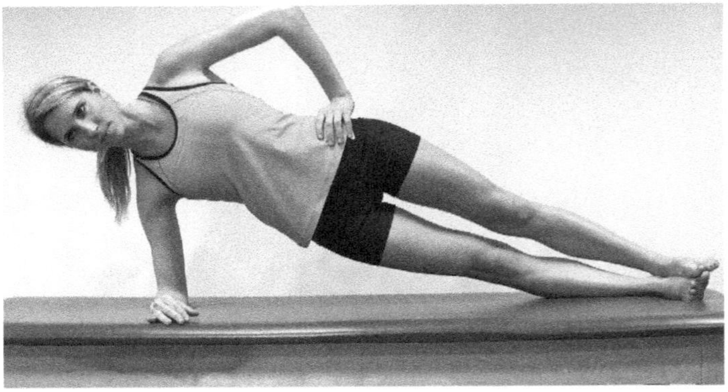

Figure 24.22 Standard side-plank exercise.

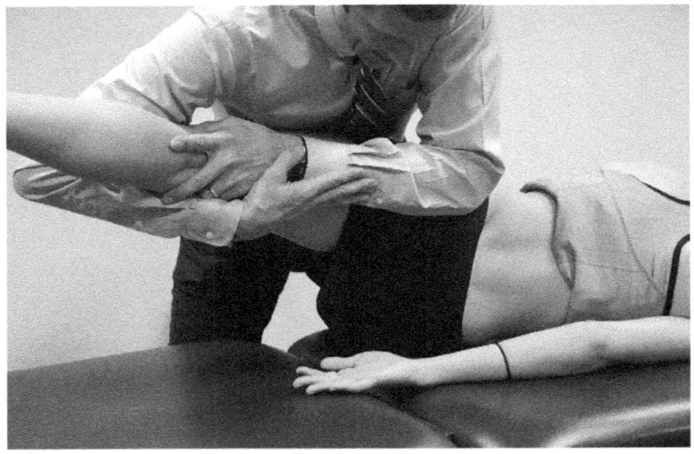

Figure 24.23 Non-thrust or thrust manipulation to rotate the innominate anteriorly.

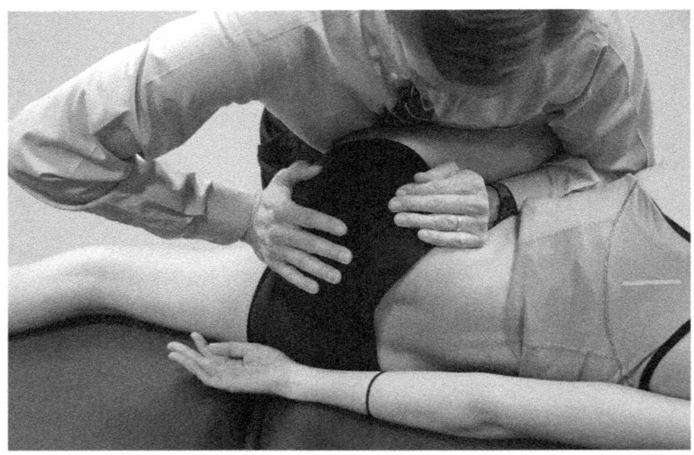

Figure 24.24 Non-thrust or thrust manipulation to rotate the innominate posteriorly.

controlled trial reporting no effect (Mens et al 2000) identified several key differences in the methods used, including the training and the supervision of the exercises provided (Stuge et al 2006a). Another potential key difference involved the theoretical implication of the exercises chosen. As previously stated, a study by Richardson et al (2002) identified that an isolated contraction of transversus abdominis and the multifidi produced greater stiffening of the SIJ than the other identified stabilizers of both the anterior and posterior pelvic slings. The studies by Elden et al (2005) and Stuge et al (2004a) emphasized the isolated muscle groups, whereas Mens et al (2000) had focused on the anterior sling muscles only. The importance of the deeper stabilizers has been identified in an observational study by Stuge et al (2006b). This sstudy identified key differences in the deep stabilizer muscles between women who had recovered from PGP and women currently experiencing PGP, including the ability to contract the pelvic floor muscles and the thickness of the transversus abdominis and internal obliques during a contraction.

Manual therapy

Manual therapy can be broadly divided into two subcategories of treatment: thrust manipulation and non-thrust manipulation. Thrust manipulation involves placing the joint in end-range position and applying high-velocity low-amplitude thrusts in the desired direction so as to increase available movement. Non-thrust manipulation involves placing the segment in the desired position and applying either an oscillatory force or a sustained force in the desired direction for a specified period of time. Marshall and Murphy (2006) found that an SIJ manipulation produced an immediate and significant increase in feed-forward activity of the deep trunk stabilizers in those with impaired feed-forward response times. The exact impact of this alteration in feed-forward mechanisms in terms of improvement in pain and disability remain unknown, however. Multiple case reports have nevertheless suggested that manual therapy for probable SIJP may be effective.

Bashir (2011) found that multiple sessions of rotational manipulation of the SIJ reduced pain and disability in a 38-year-old patient with probable SIJP. In this particular study, the investigator appropriately applied clinical tests of provocation and performed multiple movement tests to rule out lumbar pathology before testing for SIJP. Similarly, Horton and Franz (2007) found that exercise therapy involving rotational mobilization of the innominate in the direction of preference (anteriorly in this case) reduced pain and disability in a patient who had first been identified as having SIJP by ruling out centralization through a mechanical diagnosis therapy examination and ruling in SIJP through a test-item cluster. Figures 24.23–24.24 summarize potential rotational non-thrust / thrust manipulation techniques used in the clinic, and Figure 24.25 shows a home exercise programme usually used in combination with SIJ manipulation. Although in neither of the above case reports was SIJP diagnosed by IAI, the clinical examinations certainly met the standards set out by many investigators.

A small randomized clinical trial has examined the effect of two different thrust manipulation techniques on a sample of subjects diagnosed with SIJ using a test-item cluster of provocational tests (Kamali & Shokri 2012). The manipulation techniques included the SIJ thrust (Fig. 24.26) (Flynn et al 2002) and a neutral-gapping (Fig. 24.27) technique (Cook et al 2013). The outcomes would suggest that a combination of the two techniques results in improved outcomes over an intervention using the SIJ manipulation technique alone. The results also suggest that both procedures produced significant

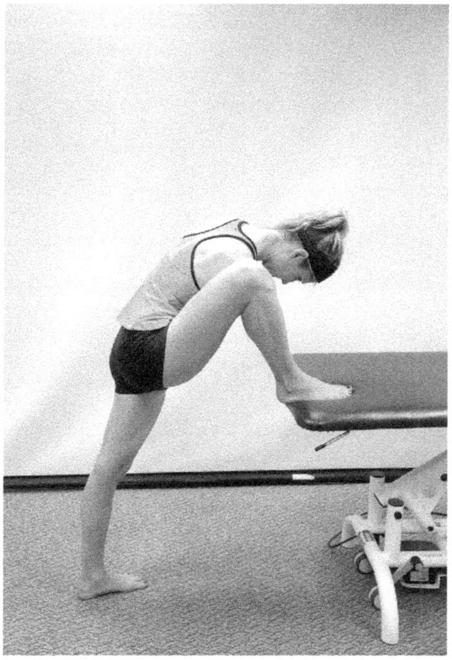

Figure 24.25 **Self-correction exercise to achieve posterior rotation of the innominate.**

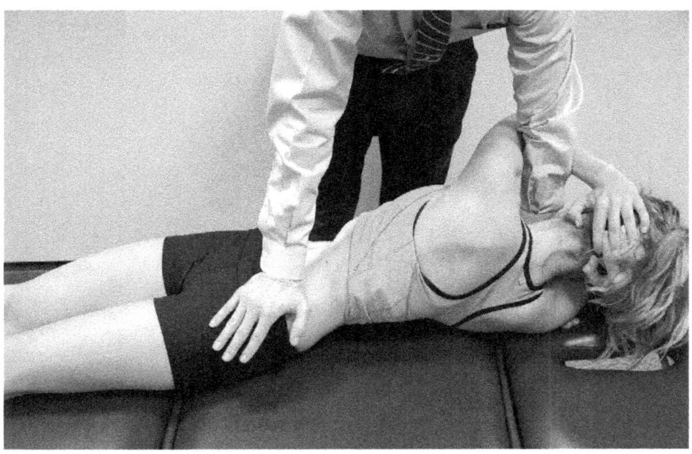

Figure 24.26 **Sacroiliac thrust manipulation.**

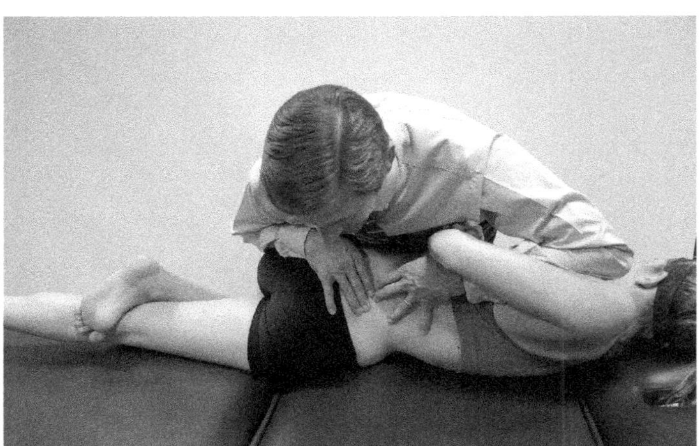

Figure 24.27 **Rotational neutral-gapping manipulation.**

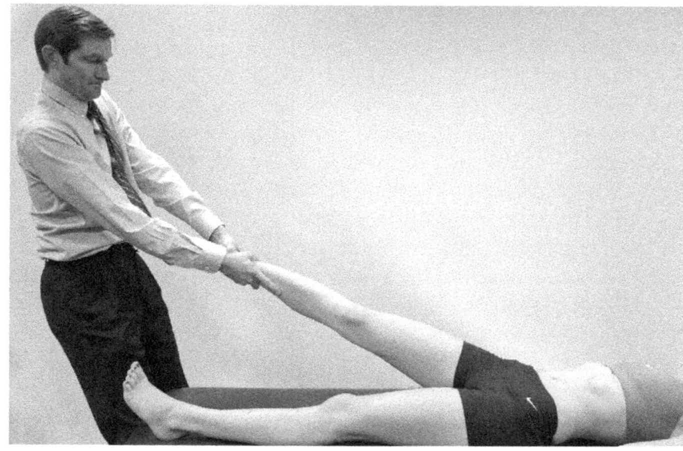

Figure 24.28 **Long-leg distraction manipulation for the sacroiliac joint.**

and clinically meaningful changes in both pain and disability following a single session of manipulative therapy for subjects with clinically diagnosed SIJP (Kamali & Shokri 2012). An additional thrust manipulation technique that has been purported to impact the SIJ is a long-leg distraction with the hip in end-range internal rotation to reduce passive hip movement (Fig. 24.28).

A small randomized clinical trial comparing orthopaedic manual therapy, exercise therapy and neuroemotional training for the treatment of pregnancy-related pelvic pain demonstrated a trend towards greater improvement in both manual therapy and exercise therapy than in neuroemotional training, but the between-group differences were not significant (Peterson et al 2012). The authors concluded that a larger trial was warranted based on the encouraging results of the study as 50% of all the patients reported a clinically meaningful change in pain and disability.

Many professions have adopted the osteopathic approach to managing SIJ. Osteopathic treatment involves placing the segment in the desired position to emphasize isolation of the SIJ to available movement in a single or specific plane. A muscle energy technique or a direct technique with impulse is then applied to mobilize the segment in the direction of the lost motion. This form of treatment is guided by the palpatory examination used to identify the asymmetry in the lumbosacral region that the technique purports to correct. There are a number of named diagnostic categories of dysfunction and therefore positions for treatment identified using this system (see Ch 62 for details of muscle energy techniques). Since rotational motions for the innominates can frequently be provocative, a technique that emphasizes rotation may reduce pain; therefore, placing patients in Gaenslen's test position (see Fig. 24.5) and having them resist the overpressure may be an effective treatment. A potential problem with this system for treating SIJ pathology is the lack of specificity of the proposed treatment, as isolated treatments to the SIJ may be a fallacious assumption (Laslett 2008). A large, well-done derivation study for a clinical prediction rule to determine treatment success prescriptively with an SIJ manipulation determined that not one of the SIJ tests predicted clinical success (Flynn et al 2002). These results may suggest that either the tests don't identify SIJ pathology or the SIJ manipulation procedure impacts more than just the SIJ (Laslett 2008);

given the fact that lumbar hypomobility did predict treatment success (Flynn et al 2002), the latter seems more plausible. To date, this author is unaware of a single study that strongly supports the use of the examination and treatment techniques for the correction of SIJD as confirmed by IAI.

Nonetheless, this examination and treatment process is supported anecdotally by subjective reports of pain reduction after such treatment, the clinicians taking this as confirmation that the diagnostic system was indeed correct when the treatment has never been confirmed to impact the position of the SIJ and could just as easily be impacting the lumbar spine. The pain relief observed following SIJ manipulation, mobilization and muscle energy techniques is likely to be the result of the well-documented neurophysiological and reflexogenic changes that occur producing short-term pain relief (Bialosky et al 2009; Coronado et al 2010).

Sacroiliac belts

Sacroiliac belts have been found to reduce pregnancy-related pelvic pain significantly when applied just inferior to the ASIS rather than over the level of pubic symphysis (Mens et al 2006). A review article suggests that there is moderate evidence from 18 articles to support the use of external support for the pelvic ring for pain reduction, altered recruitment of stabilizers and altered kinematics of the lumbopelvic region (Arumugam et al 2012). One EMG study of 17 subjects found that application of the sacroiliac belt reduced muscle recruitment of the transversus abdominis and abdominal obliques during the active straight leg raise and treadmill walking tests (Hu et al 2010). A second study of 17 subjects using EMG during abdominal exercises on an unstable surface found that activity of the rectus abdominis, and both internal and external obliques, was reduced following the application of this belt (Kim et al 2013). These studies would suggest that the sacroiliac belt provided force closure to the system thus allowing the usual stabilizers to relax during the attempted exercise or functional activity.

Conclusion

SIJ pathology involves pain, instability or asymmetrical stability of the pelvic ring, or alteration / asymmetrical motion. Pain and / or stability issues are the far most likely and readily identifiable pathologies. Traditional examination and treatment based on notable pelvic asymmetries found during a palpatory and visual examination cannot be recommended for the following reasons. First, the pathology has not been verified by any benchmark gold standard such as radiographic evidence. Secondly, the tests used to identify the pathology clinically are generally unreliable, with a few tests having reliability coefficients no better than chance agreement. Nevertheless, we cannot conclude that the treatments purported to correct these faults are ineffective because it is entirely possible that they demonstrate a general neurophysiological effect that may reduce discomfort. Likewise, improvements in patients' complaints of pain cannot be used to determine that the examination principles are valid.

The best evidence for clinical diagnosis of SIJ pathology comes from tests that are classified as provocative in nature. Most of these tests lack sufficient diagnostic accuracy as stand-alone tests, but their clinical utility is greatly enhanced when performed in clusters following the exclusion of likely lumbar pathology through clinical screening. Use of a diagnostic and treatment algorithm proposed by Cook (2012) is consistent with current guidelines and is based on considerable research.

References

Ackerman SJ, Polly DW Jr, Knight T, et al. 2013. Comparison of the costs of nonoperative care to minimally invasive surgery for sacroiliac joint disruption and degenerative sacroiliitis in a United States Medicare population: potential economic implications of a new minimally-invasive technology. Clinicoecon Outcomes Res 5: 575–587.

Adhia DB, Bussey MD, Mani R, et al. 2012. Inter-tester reliability of non-invasive technique for measurement of innominate motion. Man Ther 17: 71–76.

Albert H, Godskesen M, Westergaard J. 2000. Evaluation of clinical tests used in classification procedures in pregnancy-related pelvic joint pain. Eur Spine J 9: 161–166.

Albert H, Godskesen M, Westergaard J. 2001. Prognosis in four syndromes of pregnancy-related pelvic pain. Acta Obstet Gynecol Scand 80: 505–510.

Albert HB, Godskesen M, Westergaard JG. 2002. Incidence of four syndromes of pregnancy-related pelvic joint pain. Spine 27: 2831–2834.

Arumugam A, Milosavljevic S, Woodley S, et al. 2012. Effects of external pelvic compression on form closure, force closure, and neuromotor control of the lumbopelvic spine: a systematic review. Man Ther 17: 275–284.

Badii M, Shin S, Torreggiani WC, et al. 2003. Pelvic bone asymmetry in 323 study participants receiving abdominal CT scans. Spine 28: 1335–1339.

Bashir F. 2011. Diagnosis and manipulative therapy of sacroiliac disorder. Int Musculoskeletal Med 33: 115–119.

Belanger TA, Dall BE. 2001. Sacroiliac arthrodesis using a posterior midline fascial splitting approach and pedicle screw instrumentation: a new technique. J Spinal Disord 14: 118–124.

Berthelot JM, Labat JJ, Le Goff B, et al. 2006. Provocative sacroiliac joint maneuvers and sacroiliac joint block are unreliable for diagnosing sacroiliac joint pain. Joint Bone Spine 73: 17–23.

Bialosky JE, Bishop MD, Price DD, et al. 2009. The mechanisms of manual therapy in the treatment of musculoskeletal pain: a comprehensive model. Man Ther 14: 531–538.

Bogduk N. 2005. Clinical anatomy of the lumbar spine and sacrum, 4th edn. Edinburgh, UK: Elsevier.

Broadhurst NA, Bond MJ. 1998. Pain provocation tests for the assessment of sacroiliac joint dysfunction. J Spinal Disord 11: 341–345.

Broadhurst NA, Simmons DN, Bond MJ. 2004. Piriformis syndrome: correlation of muscle morphology with symptoms and signs. Arch Phys Med Rehabil 85: 2036–2039.

Chou LH, Slipman CW, Bhagia SM, et al. 2004. Inciting events initiating injection-proven sacroiliac joint syndrome. Pain Med 5: 26–32.

Cibulka MT, Sinacore DR, Cromer GS, et al. 1998. Unilateral hip rotation range of motion asymmetry in patients with sacroiliac joint regional pain. Spine 23: 1009–1015.

Cibulka MT, Koldehoff R. 1999. Clinical usefulness of a cluster of sacroiliac joint tests in patients with and without low back pain. J Orthop Sports Phys Ther 29: 83–89.

Cook CE. 2012. Manual therapy of sacroiliac joint and pelvis. In: Cook CE (ed) Orthopedic manual therapy: an evidence-based approach, 2nd edn. Upper Saddle River, NJ: Pearson Prentice Hall, pp 301–336.

Cook CE. 2013. Physical examination tests for the sacroiliac joint and pelvis. In: Cook CE, Hegedus EJ (eds) Orthopedic physical examination tests: an evidence-based approach. Upper Saddle River, NJ: Pearson Prentice Hall, pp 325–372.

Cook C, Massa L, Harm-Ernandes I, et al. 2007. Interrater reliability and diagnostic accuracy of pelvic girdle pain classification. J Manipulative Physiol Ther 30: 252–258.

Cook C, Learman K, Showalter C, et al. 2013. Early use of thrust manipulation versus non-thrust manipulation: a randomized clinical trial. Man Ther 18: 191–198.

Coronado RA, Bialosky JE, Cook CE. 2010. The temporal effects of a single session of high-velocity, low-amplitude thrust manipulation on subjects with spinal pain. Phys Ther Rev 15: 29–35.

Cummings J Jr, Capobianco RA. 2013. Minimally invasive sacroiliac joint fusion: one-year outcomes in 18 patients. Ann Surg Innov Res 7: 12.
Dagenais S, Caro J, Haldeman S. 2008. A systematic review of low back pain cost of illness studies in the United States and internationally. Spine J 8: 8–20.
Damen L, Buyruk HM, Guler-Uysal F, et al. 2001. Pelvic pain during pregnancy is associated with asymmetric laxity of the sacroiliac joints. Acta Obstet Gynecol Scand 80: 1019–1024.
Damen L, Buyruk HM, Guler-Uysal F, et al. 2002. The prognostic value of asymmetric laxity of the sacroiliac joints in pregnancy-related pelvic pain. Spine 27: 2820–2824.
Dar G, Khamis S, Peleg S, et al. 2008. Sacroiliac joint fusion and the implications for manual therapy diagnosis and treatment. Man Ther 13: 155–158.
DeStefano LA. 2011. Pelvic girdle dysfunction. In: DeStefano LA (ed) Greenman's principles of manual medicine, 4th edn. Philadelphia, PA: Lippincott Williams & Wilkins, pp 327–389.
Dreyfuss P, Dryer S, Griffin J, et al. 1994. Positive sacroiliac screening tests in asymptomatic adults. Spine 19: 1138–1143.
Dreyfuss P, Michaelsen M, Pauza K, et al. 1996. The value of medical history and physical examination in diagnosing sacroiliac joint pain. Spine 21: 2594–2602.
Elden H, Ladfors L, Olsen MF, et al. 2005. Effects of acupuncture and stabilising exercises as adjunct to standard treatment in pregnant women with pelvic girdle pain: randomised single blind controlled trial. BMJ 330: 761.
Flynn T, Fritz J, Whitman J, et al. 2002. A clinical prediction rule for classifying patients with low back pain who demonstrate short-term improvement with spinal manipulation. Spine 27: 2835–2843.
Fortin JD, Aprill CN, Ponthieux B, Pier J. 1994a. Sacroiliac joint: pain referral maps upon applying a new injection / arthrography technique. Part II: Clinical evaluation. Spine 19: 1483–1489.
Fortin JD, Dwyer AP, West S, et al. 1994b. Sacroiliac joint: pain referral maps upon applying a new injection / arthrography technique. Part I: Asymptomatic volunteers. Spine 19: 1475–1482.
Fukui S, Nosaka S. 2002. Pain patterns originating from the sacroiliac joints. J Anesth 16: 245–247.
Goldtwait JE, Osgood RB. 1905. A consideration of the pelvic articulations from an anatomical, pathological and clinical standpoint. Boston Med Surg J 152: 593–601.
Goode A, Hegedus EJ, Sizer P, et al. 2008. Three-dimensional movements of the sacroiliac joint: a systematic review of the literature and assessment of clinical utility. J Man Manip Ther 16: 25–38.
Grasland A, Pouchot J, Mathieu A, et al. 1996. Sacral insufficiency fractures: an easily overlooked cause of back pain in elderly women. Arch Intern Med 156: 668–674.
Grob KR, Neuhuber WL, Kissling RO. 1995. [Innervation of the sacroiliac joint of the human]. Z Rheumatol 54: 117–122.
Hancock MJ, Maher CG, Latimer J, et al. 2007. Systematic review of tests to identify the disc, SIJ or facet joint as the source of low back pain. Eur Spine J 16: 1539–1550.
Harrison DE, Harrison DD, Troyanovich SJ. 1997. The sacroiliac joint: a review of anatomy and biomechanics with clinical implications. J Manipulative Physiol Ther 20: 607–617.
Hartung W, Ross CJ, Straub R, et al. 2010. Ultrasound-guided sacroiliac joint injection in patients with established sacroiliitis: precise IA injection verified by MRI scanning does not predict clinical outcome. Rheumatology 49: 1479–1482.
Herzog W, Read LJ, Conway PJ, et al. 1989. Reliability of motion palpation procedures to detect sacroiliac joint fixations. J Manipulative Physiol Ther 12: 86–92.
Horton SJ, Franz A. 2007. Mechanical diagnosis and therapy approach to assessment and treatment of derangement of the sacro-iliac joint. Man Ther 12: 126–132.
Hu H, Meijer OG, van Dieen JH, et al. 2010. Muscle activity during the active straight leg raise (ASLR), and the effects of a pelvic belt on the ASLR and on treadmill walking. J Biomech 43: 532–539.
Huijbregts P. 2004. Sacroiliac joint dysfunction: evidence-based diagnosis. Orthop Division Rev 8: 18–44.
Hungerford B, Gilleard W, Hodges P. 2003. Evidence of altered lumbopelvic muscle recruitment in the presence of sacroiliac joint pain. Spine 28: 1593–1600.
Ikeda R. 1991. [Innervation of the sacroiliac joint. Macroscopical and histological studies]. Nihon Ika Daigaku Zasshi 58(5): 587–596. [Article in Japanese.]
Irwin RW, Watson T, Minick RP, et al. 2007. Age, body mass index, and gender differences in sacroiliac joint pathology. Am J Phys Med Rehabil 86: 37–44.
Jans L, Van Praet L, Elewaut D, et al. 2013. MRI of the SI joints commonly shows non-inflammatory disease in patients clinically suspected of sacroiliitis. Eur J Radiol 3(1): 179–184. doi: 10.1016/j.ejrad.2013.10.001.
Kamali F, Shokri E. 2012. The effect of two manipulative therapy techniques and their outcome in patients with sacroiliac joint syndrome. J Bodyw Mov Ther 16: 29–35.
Kim YR, Kim JW, An DH, et al. 2013. Effects of a pelvic belt on the EMG activity of the abdominal muscles during a single-leg hold in the hook–lying position on a round foam roll. J Phys Ther Sci 25: 793–795.
Kokmeyer DJ, Van der Wurff P, Aufdemkampe G, et al. 2002. The reliability of multitest regimens with sacroiliac pain provocation tests. J Manipulative Physiol Ther 25: 42–48.
Kristiansson P, Svardsudd K, von Schoultz B. 1996. Back pain during pregnancy: a prospective study. Spine 21: 702–709.
Laslett M. 2006. Pain provocation tests for diagnosis of sacroiliac joint pain. Aust J Physiother 52: 229.
Laslett M. 2008. Evidence-based diagnosis and treatment of the painful sacroiliac joint. J Man Manip Ther 16: 142–152.
Laslett M, Williams M. 1994. The reliability of selected pain provocation tests for sacroiliac joint pathology. Spine 19: 1243–1249.
Laslett M, Young SB, Aprill CN, et al. 2003. Diagnosing painful sacroiliac joints: a validity study of a McKenzie evaluation and sacroiliac provocation tests. Aust J Physiother 49: 89–97.
Laslett M, Aprill CN, McDonald B, et al. 2005a. Diagnosis of sacroiliac joint pain: validity of individual provocation tests and composites of tests. Man Ther 10: 207–218.
Laslett M, McDonald B, Tropp H, et al. 2005b. Agreement between diagnoses reached by clinical examination and available reference standards: a prospective study of 216 patients with lumbopelvic pain. BMC Musculoskelet Disord 6: 28.
Laslett M, Oberg B, Aprill CN, et al. 2005c. Centralization as a predictor of provocation discography results in chronic low back pain, and the influence of disability and distress on diagnostic power. Spine J 5: 370–380.
Levin U, Nilsson-Wikmar L, Harms-Ringdahl K, et al. 2001. Variability of forces applied by experienced physiotherapists during provocation of the sacroiliac joint. Clin Biomech 16: 300–306.
Levin U, Stenstrom CH. 2003. Force and time recording for validating the sacroiliac distraction test. Clin Biomech 18: 821–826.
Lynch FW. 1920. The pelvic articulations during pregnancy, labor, and the puerperium: an x-ray study. Surg Gynecol Obstet 30: 575–580.
Madani SP, Dadian M, Firouznia K, et al. 2013. Sacroiliac joint dysfunction in patients with herniated lumbar disc: a cross-sectional study. J Back Musculoskelet Rehabil 26: 273–278.
Maigne JY, Aivaliklis A, Pfefer F. 1996. Results of sacroiliac joint double block and value of sacroiliac pain provocation tests in 54 patients with low back pain. Spine 21: 1889–1892.
Manchikanti L, Singh V, Pampati V, et al. 2001. Evaluation of the relative contributions of various structures in chronic low back pain. Pain Physician 4: 308–316.
Marshall P, Murphy B. 2006. The effect of sacroiliac joint manipulation on feed-forward activation times of the deep abdominal musculature. J Manipulative Physiol Ther 29: 196–202.
McGrath MC. 2006. Palpation of the sacroiliac joint: an anatomical and sensory challenge. Int J Osteopathic Med 9: 103–107.
Mens JM, Vleeming A, Snijders CJ, et al. 1999. The active straight leg raising test and mobility of the pelvic joints. Eur Spine J 8: 468–473.
Mens JM, Snijders CJ, Stam HJ. 2000. Diagonal trunk muscle exercises in peripartum pelvic pain: a randomized clinical trial. Phys Ther 80: 1164–1173.
Mens JM, Damen L, Snijders CJ, et al. 2006. The mechanical effect of a pelvic belt in patients with pregnancy-related pelvic pain. Clin Biomech 21: 122–127.
Mens JM, Huis in 't Veld YH, Pool-Goudzwaard A. 2012. Severity of signs and symptoms in lumbopelvic pain during pregnancy. Man Ther 17: 175–179.
Merskey H, Bogduk N. 1994. Classification of chronic pain: descriptions of chronic pain syndromes and definitions of pain terms, 2nd edn. Seattle, WA: IASP Press.
Mior SA, McGregor M, Schut B. 1990. The role of experience in clinical accuracy. J Manipulative Physiol Ther 13: 68–71.
Mitchell FL. 1958. Structural pelvic function. Carmel, CA: Yearbook of The American Academy of Osteopathy.
Murakami E, Tanaka Y, Aizawa T, et al. 2007. Effect of periarticular and intraarticular lidocaine injections for sacroiliac joint pain: prospective comparative study. J Orthop Sci 12: 274–280.
Murphy DR, Hurwitz EL. 2007. A theoretical model for the development of a diagnosis-based clinical decision rule for the management of patients with spinal pain. BMC Musculoskelet Disord 8: 75.

Myburgh KH, Hutchins J, Fataar AB, et al. 1990. Low bone density is an etiologic factor for stress fractures in athletes. Ann Intern Med 113: 754–759.

Nilsson-Wikmar L, Holm K, Oijerstedt R, et al. 2005. Effect of three different physical therapy treatments on pain and activity in pregnant women with pelvic girdle pain: a randomized clinical trial with 3, 6, and 12 months follow-up postpartum. Spine 30: 850–856.

Peloso PM, Braun J. 2004. Expanding the armamentarium for the spondyloarthropathies. Arthritis Res Ther 6: S36–S43.

Peterson CD, Haas M, Gregory WT. 2012. A pilot randomized controlled trial comparing the efficacy of exercise, spinal manipulation, and neuro emotional technique for the treatment of pregnancy-related low back pain. Chiropr Man Therap 20: 18.

Petrone MR, Guinn J, Reddin A, et al. 2003. The accuracy of the Palpation Meter (PALM) for measuring pelvic crest height difference and leg length discrepancy. J Orthop Sports Phys Ther 33: 319–325.

Pollard H, Ward G. 1998. The effect of upper cervical or sacroiliac manipulation on hip flexion range of motion. J Manipulative Physiol Ther 21: 611–616.

Pool-Goudzwaard AL, Vleeming A, Stoeckart R, et al. 1998. Insufficient lumbopelvic stability: a clinical, anatomical and biomechanical approach to 'a-specific' low back pain. Man Ther 3: 12–20.

Pool-Goudzwaard A, Gnat R, Spoor K. 2012. Deformation of the innominate bone and mobility of the pubic symphysis during asymmetric moment application to the pelvis. Man Ther 17: 66–70.

Prassopoulos PK, Faflia CP, Voloudaki AE, et al. 1999. Sacroiliac joints: anatomical variants on CT. J Comput Assist Tomogr 23: 323–327.

Preece SJ, Willan P, Nester CJ, et al. 2008. Variation in pelvic morphology may prevent the identification of anterior pelvic tilt. J Man Manip Ther 16: 113–117.

Richardson CA, Snijders CJ, Hides JA, et al. 2002. The relation between the transversus abdominis muscles, sacroiliac joint mechanics, and low back pain. Spine 27: 399–405.

Rost CC, Jacqueline J, Kaiser A, et al. 2004. Pelvic pain during pregnancy: a descriptive study of signs and symptoms of 870 patients in primary care. Spine 29: 2567–2572.

Rudolf L. 2012. Sacroiliac joint arthrodesis-MIS technique with titanium implants: report of the first 50 patients and outcomes. Open Orthop J 6: 495–502.

Sachs D, Capobianco R. 2013. Minimally invasive sacroiliac joint fusion: one-year outcomes in 40 patients. Adv Orthop 2013: 536128.

Schmid HJA. 1985. Iliosacrale diagnose und behandlung 1978–1982. Manuelle Medizin 23: 101–108. [Article in German.]

Schwarzer AC, Aprill CN, Derby R, et al. 1994. The relative contributions of the disc and zygapophyseal joint in chronic low back pain. Spine 19: 801–806.

Schwarzer AC, Aprill CN, Bogduk N. 1995. The sacroiliac joint in chronic low back pain. Spine 20: 31–37.

Shaffrey CI, Smith JS. 2013. Editorial: stabilization of the sacroiliac joint. Neurosurg Focus 35(2 Suppl): Editorial. doi: 10.3171/2013.V2.FOCUS13273.

Simopoulos TT, Manchikanti L, Singh V, et al. 2012. A systematic evaluation of prevalence and diagnostic accuracy of sacroiliac joint interventions. Pain Physician 15: E305–344.

Sizer PS Jr, Brismee JM, Cook C. 2007. Medical screening for red flags in the diagnosis and management of musculoskeletal spine pain. Pain Pract 7: 53–71

Slipman CW, Jackson HB, Lipetz JS, et al. 2000. Sacroiliac joint pain referral zones. Arch Phys Med Rehabil 81: 334–338.

Smidt GL, McQuade K, Wei SH, et al. 1995. Sacroiliac kinematics for reciprocal straddle positions. Spine 20: 1047–1054.

Smith AG, Capobianco R, Cher D, et al. 2013. Open versus minimally invasive sacroiliac joint fusion: a multi-center comparison of perioperative measures and clinical outcomes. Ann Surg Innov Res 7: 14.

Snijders CJ, Vleeming A, Stoeckart R. 1993a. Transfer of lumbosacral load to iliac bones and legs. Part 1: Biomechanics of self-bracing of the sacroiliac joints and its significance for treatment and exercise. Clin Biomech 8: 285–294.

Snijders CJ, Vleeming A, Stoeckart R. 1993b. Transfer of lumbosacral load to iliac bones and legs Part 2: Loading of the sacroiliac joints when lifting in a stooped posture. Clin Biomech 8: 295–301.

Stovall BA, Kumar S. 2010. Reliability of bony anatomic landmark asymmetry assessment in the lumbopelvic region: application to osteopathic medical education. J Am Osteopath Assoc 110: 667–674.

Stuge B, Laerum E, Kirkesola G, et al. 2004a. The efficacy of a treatment program focusing on specific stabilizing exercises for pelvic girdle pain after pregnancy: a randomized controlled trial. Spine 29: 351–359.

Stuge B, Veierod MB, Laerum E, et al. 2004b. The efficacy of a treatment program focusing on specific stabilizing exercises for pelvic girdle pain after pregnancy: a two-year follow-up of a randomized clinical trial. Spine 29: E197–E203.

Stuge B, Holm I, Vollestad N. 2006a. To treat or not to treat postpartum pelvic girdle pain with stabilizing exercises? Man Ther 11: 337–343.

Stuge B, Morkved S, Dahl HH, et al. 2006b. Abdominal and pelvic floor muscle function in women with and without long lasting pelvic girdle pain. Man Ther 11: 287–296.

Sturesson B. 1999. Load and movement of the sacroiliac joint. Malmo, Sweden: Lund University. [PhD thesis.]

Sturesson B, Uden A, Vleeming A. 2000. A radiostereometric analysis of movements of the sacroiliac joints during the standing hip flexion test. Spine 25: 364–368.

Szadek KM, van der Wurff P, van Tulder MW, et al. 2009. Diagnostic validity of criteria for sacroiliac joint pain: a systematic review. J Pain 10: 354–368.

Tullberg T, Blomberg S, Branth B, et al. 1998. Manipulation does not alter the position of the sacroiliac joint. A roentgen stereophotogrammetric analysis. Spine 23: 1124–1128.

van der Wurff P, Hagmeijer RH, Meyne W. 2000a. Clinical tests of the sacroiliac joint. A systematic methodological review. Part 1: Reliability. Man Ther 5: 30–36.

van der Wurff P, Meyne W, Hagmeijer RH. 2000b. Clinical tests of the sacroiliac joint. A systematic methodological review. Part 2: validity. Man Ther 5: 89–96.

van der Wurff P, Buijs EJ, Groen GJ. 2006. Intensity mapping of pain referral areas in sacroiliac joint pain patients. J Manipulative Physiol Ther 29: 190–195.

van Wingerden JP, Vleeming A, Buyruk HM, et al. 2004. Stabilization of the sacroiliac joint in vivo: verification of muscular contribution to force closure of the pelvis. Eur Spine J 13: 199–205.

Visser LH, Nijssen PG, Tijssen CC, et al. 2013. Sciatica-like symptoms and the sacroiliac joint: clinical features and differential diagnosis. Eur Spine J 22: 1657–1664.

Vleeming A, Stoeckart R, Volkers AC, et al. 1990a. Relation between form and function in the sacroiliac joint. Part I: Clinical anatomical aspects. Spine 15: 130–132.

Vleeming A, Volkers AC, Snijders CJ, et al. 1990b. Relation between form and function in the sacroiliac joint. Part II: Biomechanical aspects. Spine 15: 133–136.

Vleeming A, Pool-Goudzwaard AL, Stoeckart R, et al. 1995. The posterior layer of the thoracolumbar fascia. Its function in load transfer from spine to legs. Spine 20: 753–758.

Vleeming A, Pool-Goudzwaard AL, Hammudoghlu D, et al. 1996. The function of the long dorsal sacroiliac ligament: its implication for understanding low back pain. Spine 21: 556–562.

Vleeming A, Albert HB, Ostgaard HC, et al. 2008. European guidelines for the diagnosis and treatment of pelvic girdle pain. Eur Spine J 17: 794–819.

Vleeming A, Schuenke MD, Masi AT, et al. 2012. The sacroiliac joint: an overview of its anatomy, function and potential clinical implications. J Anat 221: 537–567.

Wentz L, Liu PY, Haymes E, et al. 2011. Females have a greater incidence of stress fractures than males in both military and athletic populations: a systemic review. Mil Med 176: 420–430.

Young S, Aprill C, Laslett M. 2003. Correlation of clinical examination characteristics with three sources of chronic low back pain. Spine J 3: 460–465.

Zelle BA, Gruen GS, Brown S, et al. 2005. Sacroiliac joint dysfunction: evaluation and management. Clin J Pain 21: 446–455.

PART 4

The Shoulder Region in Upper Extremity Pain Syndromes

25 Acromioclavicular Joint 293
Janette W. Powell, Ian Shrier and Peter A. Huijbregts

26 Sternoclavicular Joint 302
Erland Pettman

27 Rotator Cuff Lesions: Shoulder Impingement 309
Peter A. Huijbregts and Carel Bron

28 Glenohumeral Instability 321
Steven C. Allen, Russell S. VanderWilde and Peter A. Huijbregts

29 Superior Labrum Anterior-to-Posterior (SLAP) Lesions 333
Janette W. Powell and Peter A. Huijbregts

30 Frozen Shoulder 344
Carel Bron, Arthur de Gast and Jo L.M. Franssen

31 Joint Mobilization of the Shoulder 350
Wayne Hing, Jack Miller and César Fernández-de-las-Peñas

32 Motor Control of the Shoulder Region 358
Mary E. Magarey, Mark A. Jones and Samuel R. Baida

33 Therapeutic Exercises for the Shoulder Region 373
Johnson McEvoy, Kieran O'Sullivan and Carel Bron

Chapter 25

Acromioclavicular Joint

Janette W. Powell, Ian Shrier, Peter A. Huijbregts

CHAPTER CONTENTS

Introduction 293
Anatomy of the acromioclavicular joint 293
Biomechanics of the acromioclavicular joint 293
Pathology of the acromioclavicular joint 294
Diagnosis of the acromioclavicular joint 295
Management of the acromioclavicular joint 298
Conclusion 299

Introduction

Shoulder pain is the third most common cause for musculoskeletal consultation in primary care (Docimo et al 2008). Acromioclavicular joint (ACJ) pathology and dysfunction is a common component of shoulder pain (Hutchinson & Ahuja 1996; Magee & Reid 1996; Auge & Fischer 1998; Shaffer 1999; Debski et al 2001; Garretson & Williams 2003; Renfree & Wright 2003; Kiner 2004; Walton et al 2004; Powell & Huijbregts 2006; Codsi 2007; Docimo et al 2008; Simovitch et al 2009). The ACJ accounts for approximately 9–12% of shoulder injuries presenting for general medical care (Rudzki et al 2003; Docimo et al 2008; Fraser-Moodie et al 2008; Macdonald & Lapointe 2008; White et al 2008) and is one of the most frequently injured joints in certain sports – for example, in football, ice hockey, skiing, snowboarding, skating and rugby (Magee & Reid 1996; Renfree & Wright 2003; Powell & Huijbregts 2006; Petron & Hanson 2007; Fraser-Moodie et al 2008; White et al 2008). Overall, ACJ sprains / separations have been described as accounting for 40–50% of all athletic shoulder injuries (Debski et al 2001; Petron & Hanson 2007; Simovitch et al 2009) and are noted to be twice as common as complete ACJ disruptions (Petron & Hanson 2007; Fraser-Moodie et al 2008), which account for 12% of all dislocations affecting the shoulder girdle (Magee & Reid 1996). In addition to the ACJ, the clavicle is frequently injured with an incidence of 23 per 1000 athletic exposures for ice hockey and 17 per 1000 athletic exposures for lacrosse (Hutchinson & Ahuja 1996). The prevalence of atraumatic osteolysis of the distal clavicle has been reported to be as high as 27% in weightlifters (Auge & Fischer 1998). These numbers probably underestimate the true prevalence, as individuals with minor injuries or dysfunction might not seek medical care (Mehrberg et al 2004; Fraser-Moodie et al 2008). ACJ injuries are more common in males (Beim 2000; Mehrberg et al 2004; Petron & Hanson 2007; White et al 2008; Fraser-Moodie et al 2008) and over half occur in the under-30-years age group (Kiner 2004; Mehrberg et al 2004).

Anatomy of the Acromioclavicular Joint

Fraser-Moodie et al (2008) described the ACJ as the 'keystone' link between the scapula and the clavicle. It suspends the upper extremity from the axial skeleton (Shaffer 1999; Buss & Watts 2003; Nuber & Bowen 2003; Renfree & Wright 2003). A thin capsule surrounds the diarthrodial ACJ, which typically contains a fibrocartilaginous disc (Lemos 1998; Shaffer 1999; Beim 2000; Buss & Watts 2003; Garretson & Williams 2003; Renfree & Wright 2003; Docimo et al 2008; Fraser-Moodie et al 2008; Macdonald & Lapointe 2008; Rios & Mazzocca 2008; White et al 2008; Simovitch et al 2009). This intra-articular disc is variable in size and shape and may sometimes undergo rapid degeneration, beginning as early as the second decade of life (Beim 2000; Renfree & Wright 2003; Mehrberg et al 2004; Docimo et al 2008; White et al 2008; Simovitch et al 2009). The ACJ is reinforced by the acromioclavicular (AC) ligaments (superior, inferior, anterior and posterior), the robust coracoclavicular (CC) ligaments (conoid and trapezoid), the coracoacromial ligament, and the deltotrapezius aponeurosis (Fig. 25.1) (Lemos 1998; Shaffer 1999; Beim 2000; Buss & Watts 2003; Garretson & Williams 2003; Renfree & Wright 2003; Petron & Hanson 2007; Docimo et al 2008; Fraser-Moodie et al 2008; Macdonald & Lapointe 2008; Rios & Mazzocca 2008; White et al 2008; Simovitch et al 2009). Dynamic stabilization is provided by the deltoid and trapezius muscles (Lizaur et al 1994; Beim 2000; Buss & Watts 2003; Renfree & Wright 2003; Garretson & Williams 2003; Petron & Hanson 2007; Docimo et al 2008; Macdonald & Lapointe 2008; Rios & Mazzocca 2008; White et al 2008; Simovitch et al 2009).

Biomechanics of the Acromioclavicular Joint

Few studies have been published on ACJ kinematics (Teece et al 2008) but more recent three-dimensional imaging

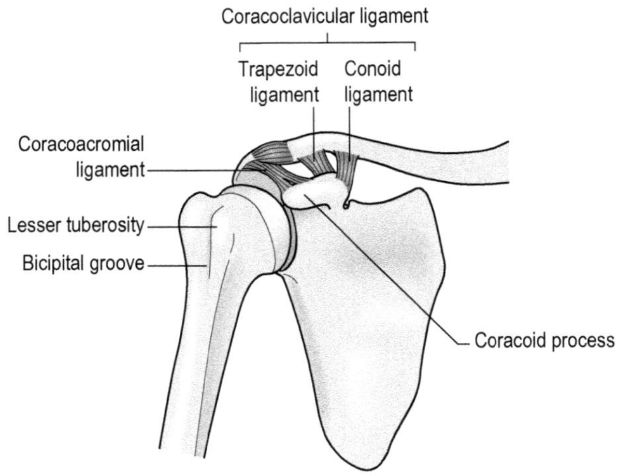

Figure 25.1 Normal anatomy of the acromioclavicular joint.

studies quantifying its motion suggest that the extent of movement has historically been underestimated (Sahara et al 2006, 2007; Fraser-Moodie et al 2008; Teece et al 2008). Sahara et al (2007) have noted that during abduction of the shoulder there is significant rotation of the clavicle and within the ACJ, with the clavicle acting as a screw axis (Sahara 2006). For example, in the anterior–posterior (AP) direction, the clavicle translated most posteriorly (1.9±1.3 mm) at 90° of abduction and most anteriorly (1.6±2.7 mm) at maximum abduction. When defining motion of the scapula with respect to the clavicle, this study noted that the scapula generally rotated about a specific screw axis passing through the insertions of both the AC and the CC ligaments on the coracoid process (Sahara et al 2006). Teece et al (2008) found that significant motion (internal rotation, upward rotation and posterior tilting) occurs at the ACJ during active humeral elevation, and discussed how abnormal motions at the ACJ will affect the position of the scapula on the thorax, and contribute to shoulder pathology and dysfunction. The same researchers observed, during active scapular plane abduction from rest to 90°, that average ACJ angular values demonstrated increased internal rotation (approximately 4.3°), increased upward rotation (approximately 14.6°) and increased posterior tilting (approximately 6.7°). That study did not analyse motion beyond 90° abduction, owing to technical limitations with clavicular tracking. These ACJ motions are of sufficient magnitude to warrant clinical attention with manual mobilization when these motions are abnormal or dysfunctional.

Pathology of the Acromioclavicular Joint

Box 25.1 summarizes the pathologies that may affect the ACJ (Hutchinson & Ahuja 1996; Magee & Reid 1996; Auge & Fischer 1998; Lemos 1998; Lehtinen et al 1999; Shaffer 1999; Debski et al 2001; Santis et al 2001; Garretson & Williams 2003; Renfree & Wright 2003; Kiner 2004; Walton et al 2004; Simovitch et al 2009). The ACJ can be acutely injured by direct blows to the shoulder or falls onto an upper extremity (ligament sprain / separations / dislocations). The ACJ is also vulnerable to repetitive overuse (osteolysis and degenerative joint disease) (Lemos 1998; Debski et al 2001; Nuber & Bowen 2003; Kiner 2004; Petron & Hanson 2007; Macdonald & Lapointe 2008; Rios & Mazzocca 2008; Simovitch et al 2009).

Acute injuries to the ACJ typically involve a direct fall onto the outer aspect of the shoulder, usually with the arm adducted (Beim 2000; Buss & Watts 2003; Garretson & Williams 2003; Rudzki et al 2003; Petron & Hanson 2007; Fraser-Moodie et al 2008; Simovitch 2009). This force drives the acromion inferiorly under the clavicle. The greater stability of the sternoclavicular joint (discussed in Ch 26) results in the majority of the impact dissipated in the ACJ structures, which leads to a systematic failure of stabilizing structures with progressive force (Beim 2000; Bradley & Elkousy 2003; Rudzki et al 2003; Petron & Hanson 2007; Fraser-Moodie et al 2008; Macdonald & Lapointe 2008; Rios & Mazzocca 2008; Simovitch et al 2009). The downward force with this injury initially stretches the AC ligaments; then, as the force continues, the AC ligaments tear and the CC ligaments are stressed (Tom et al 2009). As the downward force continues the CC ligaments tear, followed by the muscle attachments of the deltoid and trapezius muscles, resulting in a complete disruption to the ACJ (Tom et al 2009).

These sequential acute injuries have been defined and described by Tossy et al (1963). Rockwood et al (1996) modified and expanded these injury types to the system that is commonly used today (Fig. 25.2):

- **type I:** AC ligament sprain, CC ligament intact, deltoid and trapezius muscles intact
- **type II:** AC ligaments and ACJ disrupted, CC ligament sprain, deltoid and trapezius muscles intact
- **type III:** AC ligaments and ACJ disrupted and displaced, CC ligaments disrupted with CC interspace 25–100% larger than normal shoulder, deltoid and trapezius muscles usually detached
- **type IV:** AC ligaments disrupted and ACJ displaced, clavicle displaced posteriorly, CC ligaments disrupted

Box 25.1 Pathologies/dysfunctions affecting the acromioclavicular joint

Traumatic conditions
- Separation/dislocation (types I–VI)
- Fracture
- Subacromial bursitis
- Rotator cuff pathology

Infectious conditions
- Septic arthritis

Inflammatory conditions
- Rheumatoid arthritis
- Systemic lupus erythematosus
- Ankylosing spondylitis
- Gout

Degenerative joint disease
- Osteoarthritis
- Osteolysis

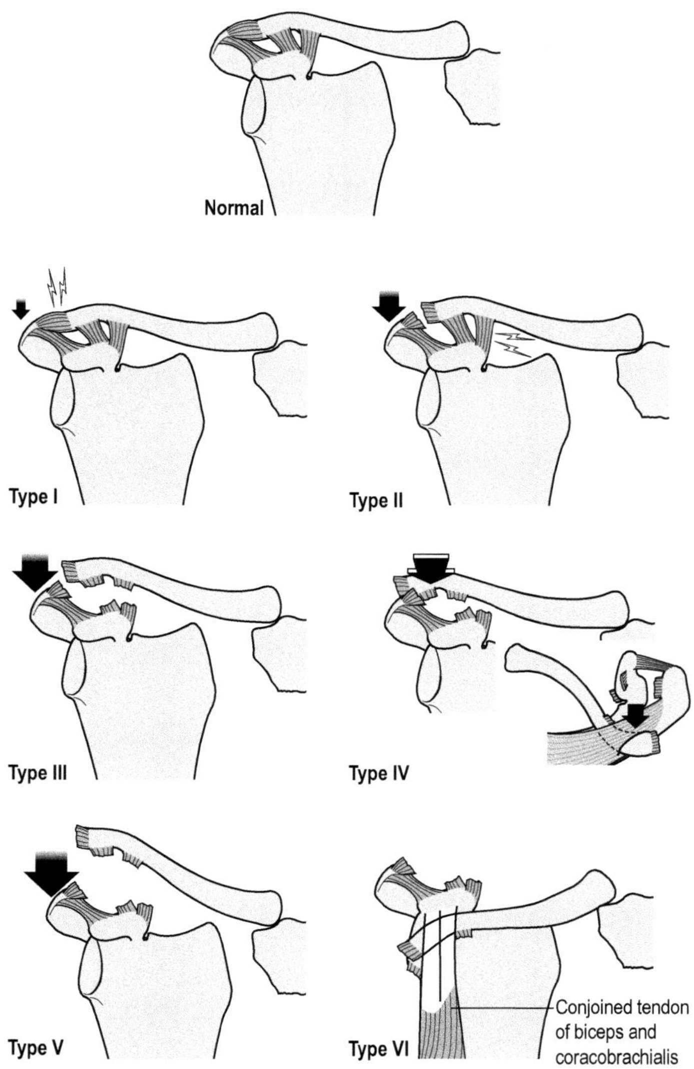

Figure 25.2 Types I–VI acromioclavicular joint sprain.

with wider CC interspace, deltoid and trapezius muscles detached

- **type V:** AC and CC ligaments disrupted, ACJ grossly displaced (100–300% more than normal shoulder), deltoid and trapezius muscles detached
- **type VI:** AC and CC ligaments disrupted and ACJ displaced, clavicle displaced inferiorly, deltoid and trapezius muscles detached (Tossy et al 1963; Simovitch et al 2009; Tom et al 2009).

A less common mechanism of acute injury to the ACJ would involve a fall onto an outstretched hand, or a direct blow to the elbow. These mechanisms drive the humeral head superiorly into the acromion (Beim 2000; Garretson & Williams 2003; Petron & Hanson 2007; White et al 2008). These indirect forces may result in the same injury patterns described above (Simovitch et al 2009), or may spare the CC ligaments when the scapula is driven superiorly and medially, injuring the AC ligaments in isolation (Mehrberg et al 2004; White et al 2008). Additionally the ACJ may be injured by a traction force applied to the upper extremity (Beim 2000; Garretson & Williams 2003).

Rios and Mazzocca (2008) describe an acute 'internal derangement' whereby the intra-articular disc is torn. Magee and Reid (1996) propose that intra-articular disc injuries are implicated in the 'clicking' that is sometimes heard and in some of the post-traumatic pain syndromes following ACJ injuries.

Although many ACJ injuries are due to a sudden force, repetitive loads may also cause injury to the region. Non-contact sports such as cycling, baseball and weightlifting have been associated with degenerative ACJ injuries (Bowen & Nuber 2003). For example, the compressive forces across the ACJ that are created during repeated forceful contraction by the deltoid, trapezius and pectoralis major muscles may contribute to osteolysis of the distal clavicle (Nuber & Bowen 2003; Renfree & Wright 2003). This repetitive stress to the subchondral bone can cause fatigue fractures and a hypervascular response leading to absorption of bone and an eventual clinically relevant osteolysis. The sequelae include demineralization, osteopenia, subchondral cyst formation and distal clavicle erosion (Nuber & Bowen 2003). It is often noted that the ACJ is required to transmit large loads across a very small surface area and this may contribute to failure with repetitive activity and overuse (Shaffer 1999; Beim 2000; Nuber & Bowen 2003; Renfree & Wright 2003; Docimo et al 2008).

In addition, degeneration of the ACJ intra-articular disc commences in the second decade of life and may be significant by the fourth decade (Garretson & Williams 2003). An incomplete fibrocartilaginous disc may play a significant role in the development of arthrosis (Beim 2000; Powell & Huijbregts 2006; Docimo et al 2008). Primary osteoarthritis and post-traumatic arthritis are noted to be prevalent in 50–60% of asymptomatic elderly individuals (Shaffer 1999; Docimo et al 2008; Rios & Mazzocca 2008). ACJ arthrosis, joint degradation, may be idiopathic, or result from injury and / or instability of this joint (Rios & Mazzocca 2008). The ACJ is also prone to inflammatory, septic and crystalline arthropathy (Garretson & Williams 2003; Renfree & Wright 2003).

Diagnosis of the Acromioclavicular Joint

The clinical presentation of an individual with acute ACJ injury typically involves a history of one of the mechanisms of injury described above: direct trauma to the shoulder with the arm adducted, fall onto an outstretched hand or elbow, or a traction injury to the upper extremity (Hutchinson & Ahuja 1996; Lemos 1998; Beim 2000; Buss & Watts 2003; Garretson & Williams 2003; Petron & Hanson 2007; Macdonald & Lapointe 2008; Rios & Mazzocca 2008; White et al 2008; Simovitch et al 2009). Individuals with isolated ACJ lesions typically note pain over the anterior and / or superior aspect of the shoulder. Although the pain is often localized to the region directly over the ACJ, it may radiate to the anterolateral neck, the trapezius–supraspinatus region and the anterolateral deltoid (Gerber et al 1998; Shaffer 1999; Petron & Hanson 2007; Fraser-Moodie et al 2008; Macdonald & Lapointe 2008; Rios & Mazzocca 2008).

Swelling, ecchymosis / erythema and deformity, if present, are easily observed as the ACJ is just under the skin (Hutchinson & Ahuja 1996; Shaffer 1999; Beim 2000; Mehrberg et al 2004; Petron & Hanson 2007; Fraser-Moodie et al 2008; Macdonald & Lapointe 2008; White et al 2008; Simovitch et al 2009; Tom et al 2009). Tenderness on palpation of the ACJ is reported as a common clinical finding associated with ACJ dysfunction (Hutchinson & Ahuja 1996; Magee & Reid 1996; Shaffer 1999; Beim 2000; Tallia & Cardone 2003; Buss & Watts 2003; Nuber & Bowen 2003; Mehrberg et al 2004; Walton et al 2004; Brukner & Khan 2006; Petron & Hanson 2007; White et al 2008; Docimo et al 2008; Fraser-Moodie et al 2008; Macdonald & Lapointe 2008; Rios & Mazzocca 2008; Park et al 2009; Simovitch et al 2009; Tom et al 2009). A number of physical examination tests have been proposed to stress the structures of the ACJ and assist in the clinical diagnosis of ACJ pathology. These include the active compression test (also known as O'Brien's sign) (Fig. 25.3) (O'Brien et al 1998; Maritz & Oosthuizen 2002; Chronopoulos et al 2004; Walton et al 2004), cross-body adduction test (also known as Scarf sign) (Fig. 25.4) (Maritz & Oosthuizen 2002; Chronopoulos et al 2004), acromioclavicular resisted extension test (Fig. 25.5) (Chronopoulos et al 2004), ACJ tenderness test (Maritz & Oosthuizen 2002; Walton et al 2004) and Paxinos sign (Fig. 25.6) (Walton et al 2004; Brukner & Khan 2006). Table 25.1 provides psychometric data on these clinical tests.

Powell and Huijbregts (2006) noted that research evidence supports the inclusion of the following tests, with the following interpretation, for the diagnosis of painful ACJ dysfunction:

- A negative finding on *any* of the following tests would *rule out* ACJ dysfunction: cross-body adduction test, tenderness on palpation of the ACJ, or Paxinos sign.
- A positive finding on *any* of the following tests would *rule in* ACJ dysfunction: active compression test, the cross-body adduction test, or acromioclavicular resisted extension test.
- A positive finding on *all* three tests used to rule in ACJ dysfunction (i.e. the cross-body adduction stress, active compression, and resisted acromioclavicular extension tests) *may be relevant* when considering a medical–surgical referral and associated higher risk interventions.

A number of authors note the value of ACJ local anaesthetic injections to assist and / or confirm the involvement of ACJ dysfunction in the clinical presentation when other associated shoulder injuries may be present (Parlington & Broome 1998; Shaffer 1999; Maritz & Oosthuizen 2002; Nuber & Bowen 2003; Tallia & Cardone 2003; Walton et al 2004; Chronopoulos et al 2004; Codsi 2007; Docimo et al 2008; Rios & Mazzocca 2008; Park et al 2009), and some consider it the criterion reference (gold standard) for the diagnosis of ACJ injury / pathology (Parlington & Broome 1998; Maritz & Oosthuizen 2002; Chronopoulos et al 2004; Walton et al 2004). If pain ceases with injection then only the ACJ is involved; if pain decreases with injection then other pathologies probably coexist; if pain is unaffected then the ACJ is probably not involved (Parlington & Broome 1998; Shaffer 1999; Maritz & Oosthuizen 2002; Tallia & Cardone 2003; Chronopoulos et al 2004; Walton et al 2004; Codsi 2007; Docimo et al 2008; Rios & Mazzocca 2008; Park et al 2009). However, injection into the ACJ is noted to have its challenges. It may be unsuccessful, particularly with regards injection targeting, due to the variability in ACJ anatomy, the obliquity of the joint, the small intra-articular region, and substantial joint space narrowing when diminished by osteophyte formation (Parlington & Broome 1998; Shaffer 1999; Bisbinas et al 2006; Codsi 2007; Rios & Mazzocca 2008). Parlington and Broome (1998) noted that non-image-guided intra-articular infiltrations were placed successfully in the ACJ in only 16 / 24 (67%) of cadaveric shoulders. Bisbinas et al (2006) found that only 40% of ACJ injections will be placed in the joint if performed without imaging guidance.

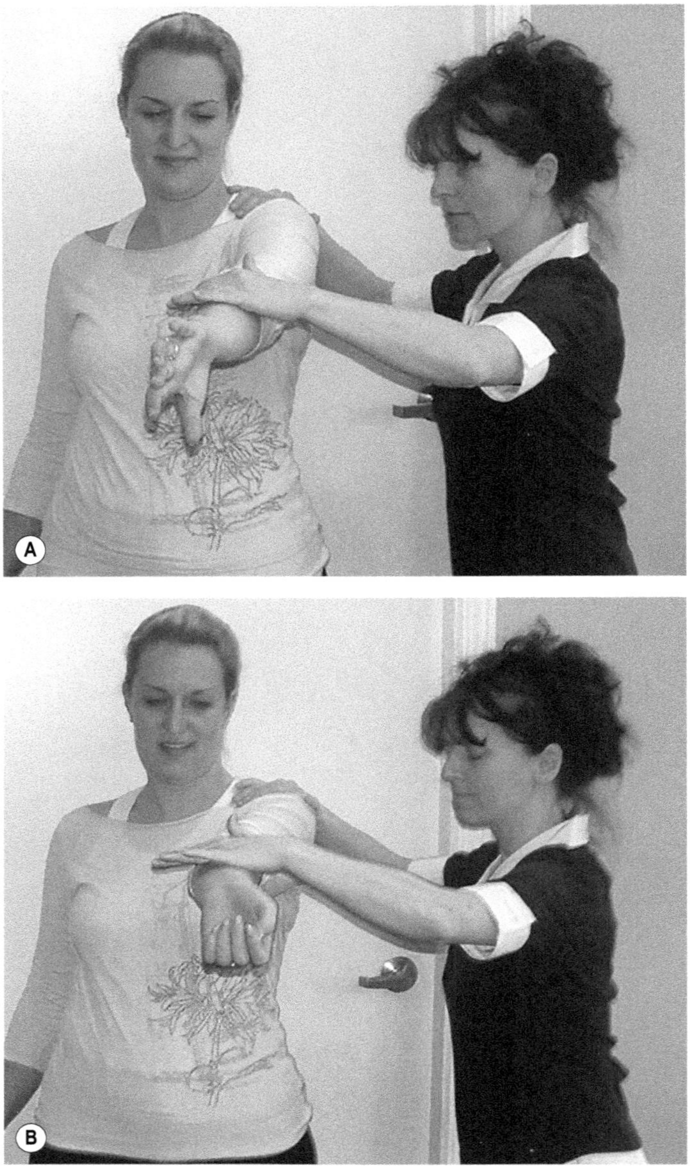

Figure 25.3 Active compression test: (**A**) Maximal internal rotation: the client stands with the involved arm straight and forward flexed to 90°. The arm is then horizontally adducted 10–15° and maximally internally rotated. The client then resists a downward force applied by the examiner to the distal arm. (**B**) Maximal external rotation: the test is then repeated in the same position with the arm maximally externally rotated; O'Brien et al (1998) did not quantify the amount of force used. This test is considered positive for ACJ dysfunction if the pain is localized to the ACJ on the first position and relieved or eliminated on the second position. Pain 'deep inside the shoulder', with or without a click, in the first position and eliminated or reduced in the second position is considered indicative of a glenoid labrum tear. (From Powell & Huijbregts 2006, with permission.)

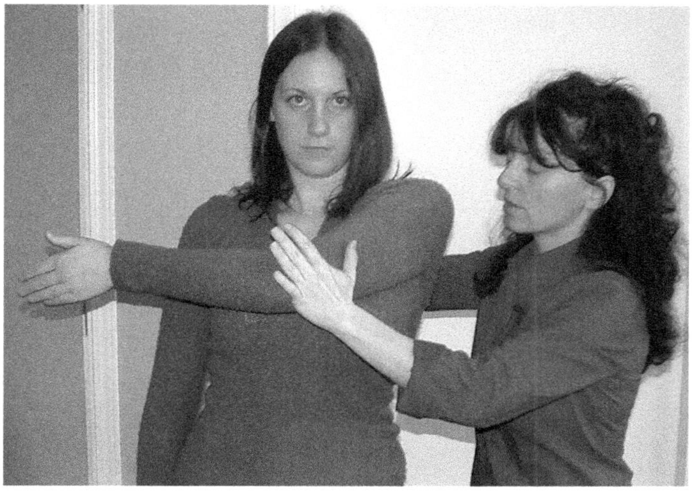

Figure 25.4 Cross-body adduction test. The client's arm is forward flexed to 90° and then horizontally adducted across the body. The literature is unclear on whether this test is active or passive. This test is considered positive if it causes pain localized to the ACJ. (From Powell & Huijbregts 2006, with permission.)

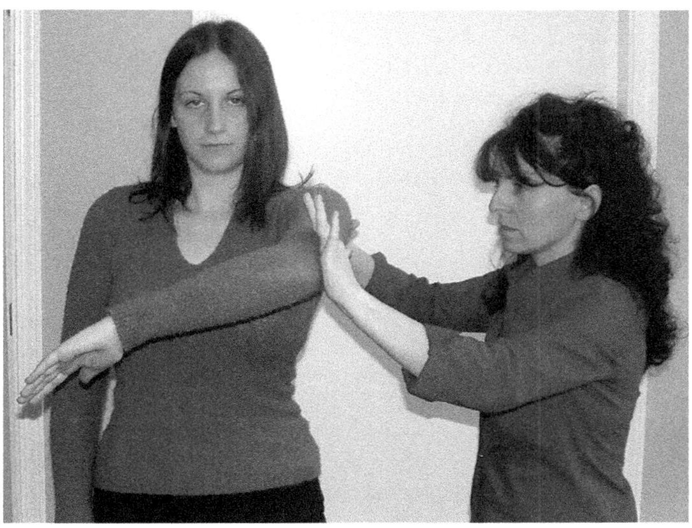

Figure 25.5 Acromioclavicular resisted extension test. The client's shoulder is flexed to 90°, then combined with maximal internal rotation and 90° of elbow flexion. The client is then asked to abduct the arm horizontally against resistance. This test is considered positive if it causes pain at the ACJ. (From Powell & Huijbregts 2006, with permission.)

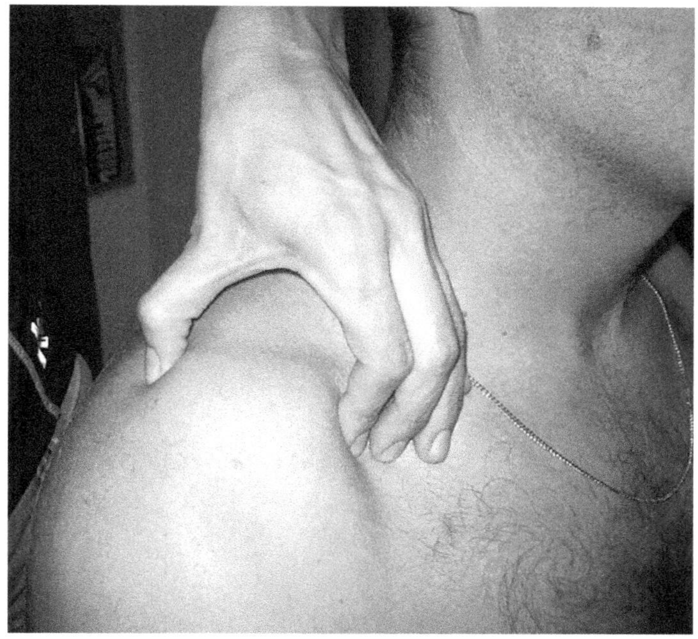

Figure 25.6 Paxinos sign. The patient sits with the arm relaxed by his/her side. The examiner's thumb is placed under the posterolateral aspect of the acromion; the index and long fingers (same or contralateral hand) are then placed superior to the mid-portion of the ipsilateral clavicle. The thumb applies an anterosuperior force concurrently while the fingers apply an inferior force. This test is considered positive if it causes or increases pain localized to the ACJ. (From Powell & Huijbregts, 2006 with permission.)

As a general principle, imaging is only necessary when it will change management. For acute injuries, history and clinical examination will usually rule out a fracture or an ACJ injury severe enough to require surgical intervention, and therefore imaging is often not recommended. If a fracture cannot be ruled out, or if the injury may benefit from surgery, standardized radiographs are essential to both the diagnosis and the classification (Shaffer 1999; Fraser-Moodie et al 2008; Nuber & Bowen 2003; Docimo et al 2008; White et al 2008; Simovitch et al 2009). These routine images include: true AP views, axillary views and the Zanca view (10–15° cephalic tilt) (Shaffer 1999; Beim 2000; Garretson & Williams 2003; Nuber & Bowen 2003; Mehrberg et al 2004; Docimo et al 2008; Fraser-Moodie et al 2008; Macdonald & Lapointe 2008; Rios & Mazzocca 2008; White et al 2008; Simovitch et al 2009). Views would ideally be taken of the uninvolved shoulder to provide normative comparison images (Shaffer 1999; Beim 2000; Garretson & Williams 2003; Simovitch et al 2009). Although stress views of the ACJ have been described to differentiate between type II and type III injuries, they are costly, uncomfortable, rarely add diagnostic information, do not affect management and are thus no longer recommended for routine use (Shaffer 1999; Beim 2000; Buss & Watts 2003; Garretson & Williams 2003; Petron & Hanson 2007; Rios & Mazzocca 2008; White et al 2008; Simovitch et al 2009). Rios and Mazzocca (2008) proposed the use of an AP radiograph of the involved shoulder with the arm adducted across the chest as a prognostic tool. Normal positioning, where the acromion does not overlap the clavicle, indicates a stable joint and directs the clinician to non-surgical management. Superimposition of the acromion and distal clavicle suggests instability and may indicate the need for surgical intervention (Rios & Mazzocca 2008).

In contrast to acute injuries, standardized radiographs are often essential to both the diagnosis and the classification of non-acute injuries (Shaffer 1999; Nuber & Bowen 2003; Docimo et al 2008; Fraser-Moodie et al 2008; White et al 2008; Simovitch et al 2009). Computed tomography (CT) can be utilized when investigating arthritic osseous changes (e.g. joint narrowing, erosions, subchondral cysts) (Docimo et al 2008; Macdonald & Lapointe 2008). Some authors recommend magnetic resonance imaging (MRI) and ultrasound when investigating capsular hypertrophy, effusions, subchondral oedema, subchondral fractures and ligamentous/

Table 25.1 Psychometric data for ACJ physical examination tests

	Active compression	Cross-body adduction	AC resisted extension	ACJ tenderness	Paxinos sign
Accuracy	0.53[1]; 0.92[2]; 0.97[3]	0.79[2]	0.84[2]	0.53[1]	0.65[1]
Sensitivity	0.16[1]; 0.41[2]; 0.68[4]; 1.0[3]	0.77[2];1.0[4]	0.72[2]	0.95[4]; 0.96[1]	0.7[1]
Specificity	0.90[1]; 0.93[3]; 0.95[2]	0.79[2]	0.85[2]	0.1[1]	0.5[1]
Positive predictive value	0.29[2]; 0.62[1]; 0.92[3]	0.2[2]	0.2[2]	0.52[1]	0.61[1]
Negative predictive value	0.52[1]; 0.97[2]; 1.0[3]	0.98[2]	0.98[2]	0.71[1]	0.7[1]
Positive likelihood ratio	1.6[1]; 8.2[2]; 13.3[3]	3.7[2]	4.8[2]	1.1[1]	1.6[1]
Negative likelihood ratio	0.0[3]; 0.6[2]; 0.9[1]	0.3[2]	0.3[2]	0.4[1]	0.4[1]

(Powell & Huijbregts 2006.)
1 Walton & Sadi (2008).
2 Chronopoulos et al (2004).
3 O'Brien et al (1998).
4 Maritz & Oosthuizen (2002).

aponeurosis injury (Shaffer 1999; Nuber & Bowen 2003; Petron & Hanson 2007; Docimo et al 2008; Fraser-Moodie et al 2008; Macdonald & Lapointe 2008). A recent study utilized ultrasound to identify abnormal movements in an injured ACJ that were not identified on standard imaging or stress radiographs (Peetrons & Bédard 2007; Rios & Mazzocca 2008). Isotope bone scanning may be useful in discriminating the source of symptoms (Shaffer 1999; Nuber & Bowen 2003; Fraser-Moodie et al 2008). Walton et al (2004) found that bone scans had relatively high sensitivity (82%) and specificity (70%) in the diagnosis of ACJ-related pain.

Management of the Acromioclavicular Joint

The goals of treatment for ACJ injuries are achieving painless range of motion of the shoulder, obtaining full strength and exhibiting no limitation in activity (Fraser-Moodie et al 2008; Macdonald & Lapointe 2008; White et al 2008). Conservative management is considered the standard of care for non-acute ACJ dysfunction and for types I and II ACJ injuries (Magee & Reid 1996; Bradley & Elkousy 2003; Buss & Watts 2003; Hootman 2004; Mehrberg et al 2004; Petron & Hanson 2007; Spencer 2007; Ceccarelli et al 2008; Docimo et al 2008; Fraser-Moodie et al 2008; Macdonald & Lapointe 2008; Rios & Mazzocca 2008; White et al 2008; Tom et al 2009). Although there is some controversy over the treatments of type III injuries, most authors now favour non-surgical intervention (Magee & Reid 1996; Bradley & Elkousy 2003; Buss & Watts 2003; Rudzki et al 2003; Hootman 2004; Mehrberg et al 2004; Brukner & Khan 2006; Petron & Hanson 2007; Spencer 2007; Ceccarelli et al 2008; Fraser-Moodie et al 2008; Macdonald & Lapointe 2008; Rios & Mazzocca 2008; White et al 2008; Murena et al 2009; Simovitch et al 2009; Tom et al 2009). Treatment of type III ACJ injuries is dependent on the injury severity and activity level of the patient. Surgical intervention is recommended for types IV, V and VI and for protracted pain / disability with ACJ dysfunction (Urist 1963; Bradley & Elkousy 2003; Hootman 2004; Mehrberg et al 2004; Petron & Hanson 2007; Rabalais & McCarty 2007; Macdonald & Lapointe 2008; Rios & Mazzocca 2008; White et al 2008; Simovitch et al 2009).

Conservative management can involve rest, splinting / bracing, physical therapy (including but not limited to manual therapy, active rehabilitation, taping, modalities including cold, heat, ultrasound, laser, electrical stimulation and iontophoresis), ACJ corticosteroid injections and anti-inflammatory and / or analgesic medication (Magee & Reid 1996; Shaffer 1999; Bradley & Elkousy 2003; Buss & Watts 2003; Lemos & Tolo 2003; Rudzki et al 2003; Buttaci et al 2004; Mehrberg et al 2004; Brukner & Khan 2006; Codsi 2007; Petron & Hanson 2007; Spencer 2007; Docimo et al 2008; Fraser-Moodie et al 2008; Macdonald & Lapointe 2008; Rios & Mazzocca 2008; White et al 2008; Simovitch et al 2009; Tom et al 2009). A structured active rehabilitation programme that involves the strengthening of the shoulder girdle muscles, including the deltoid, trapezius, sternocleidomastoid and subclavius as well as the rotator cuff and periscapular stabilizers, is recommended to prevent ongoing disability in individuals with AJC dysfunction / injury (Shaffer 1999; Bradley & Elkousy 2003; Buss & Watts 2003; Fraser-Moodie et al 2008; Simovitch et al 2009).

The literature suggests that 80–90% of conservatively managed individuals have good / satisfactory outcomes with regards to strength, motion and return to pre-injury levels of function (Rudzki et al 2003; Hootman 2004; Macdonald & Lapointe 2008; Rios & Mazzocca 2008; White et al 2008; Simovitch et al 2009). These studies used a variety of 'conservative treatments'. Simovitch et al (2009) proposed that non-surgical management often translates into benign neglect and suggested that inadequate rehabilitation explains some of the failures seen in non-surgical management. First, a good / satisfactory outcome in 80–90% of individuals does not necessarily mean that these subjects are free of pain or dysfunction (Bjerneld et al 1983; Rawes & Dias 1996; Schlegel et al 2001); up to one-third of those with type I and type II ACJ injuries had pain on activity at longer term follow-up (Galpiri et al 1985; Rawes & Dias 1996). Bergfeld et al (1978) found that 30% of individuals with type I ACJ injury and 42% of individuals with type II ACJ injury reported clicking and pain with push-ups and dips. An additional 9% and 23% of individuals with type I and II injuries respectively reported severe pain and limitation of activities. Mouhsine et al (2003) reported similar results, noting that 27% of individuals with type I and II ACJ injuries treated non-surgically developed chronic ACJ symptoms at a mean of 26 months post injury and required subsequent surgery. Unsatisfactory results have been reported in 10–50% of individuals undergoing conservative management, at times leading to a change of job and / or modification of recreational activities, even potentially requiring subsequent surgery (Fraser-Moodie et al 2008). These results underscore the need for investigators and clinicians to provide detailed information about 'conservative management' when reporting their results, just as a proper evaluation of studies on pharmaceuticals requires details on type, dose and frequency.

The importance of adequate rehabilitation was shown in a study of the non-surgical management of type III ACJ injuries (Simovitch et al 2009). Glick et al (1977) investigated 35 unreduced ACJ dislocations that were managed conservatively in a professional and competitive recreational athletic population and noted that all individuals who had a supervised rehabilitation programme were pain free. They concluded that the predominant reason for persistent pain and disability after a type III ACJ injury managed conservatively was inadequate rehabilitation. This proposition is supported by Gurd (1941) who noted that the shoulder can function normally despite an absent clavicle, as long as the shoulder girdle muscles are strengthened and maintained.

Despite the success of conservative treatment for the vast majority of injuries, there are indications for surgery. These include: ACJ tenderness with (1) evident abnormal signs on ACJ imaging results such as those seen in types IV, V and VI ACJ injuries, (2) a lack of response to conservative management and (3) an unwillingness or inability to modify, or refrain from, demanding physical activity (e.g. overhead sports, weight-training, manual labour) (Shaffer 1999; Schwarzkopf et al 2008; White et al 2008). When indicated, surgical outcomes are also successful but tend to have higher rates of complications, longer convalescence and longer periods away from work and sports (Petron & Hanson 2007; Spencer 2007). There are many surgical options for managing ACJ dysfunction and injury, including but not limited to open or arthroscopic procedures, distal clavicle resection, primary fixation of the ACJ, secondary stabilization of the ACJ via a linkage between the clavicle and coracoid process, dynamic stabilization of the ACJ via a musculotendinous (inferiorly directed force) transfer from distal clavicle to the coracoid process, ligament transfers and soft tissue reconstructions, and anatomical reconstruction (Magee & Reid 1996; Shaffer 1999; Bradley & Elkousy 2003; Buss & Watts 2003; Kwon & Iannotti 2003; Nuber & Bowen 2003; Buttaci et al 2004; Mehrberg et al 2004; Petron & Hanson 2007; Rabalais & McCarty 2007; Docimo et al 2008; Macdonald & Lapointe 2008; White et al 2008; Simovitch et al 2009; Murena et al 2009; Tom et al 2009).

A wide variety of surgical techniques have been described, but none has been shown to be significantly superior (Fraser-Moodie et al 2008). The later minimally invasive techniques are reported to show promise, but well-designed prospective studies need to be performed (Fraser-Moodie et al 2008; White et al 2008). Timing of surgery is controversial, with some authors advocating early reconstruction and others advocating that surgery be reserved for chronic symptomatic patients (Weinstein et al 1995; Bradley & Elkousy 2003; Buss & Watts 2003). Weinstein et al (1995) noted a trend to better outcomes when ligament reconstruction was done within the first 3 weeks after injury. Dumontier et al (1995) found no difference between early (<3 weeks) and late ligamentous reconstruction.

The evaluation of success or failure for a surgical intervention must include complications. Surgical complications include but are not limited to: hardware failure and migration, neurovascular injury, infection, fracture and osteolysis (Shaffer 1999; Bradley & Elkousy 2003; Kwon & Iannotti 2003; Lemos & Tolo 2003; Nuber & Bowen 2003; Rudzki 2003; Petron & Hanson 2007; Fraser-Moodie et al 2008; Rios & Mazzocca 2008; White et al 2008; Simovitch et al 2009). Many surgical options exist for the ACJ region and their goal is to minimize symptoms and maximize long-term function (Bradley & Elkousy 2003; Kwon & Iannotti 2003). Bradley and Elkousy (2003) reported that there is no correlation in the literature between anatomical reduction and improvements in pain, strength or motion. Fraser-Moodie et al (2008) note that, even though the many varied surgical techniques record a low rate of failure, the multiplicity of procedures, the lack of a generally accepted surgical method and the number of reports outlining the specific surgical complications infer that all ACJ surgical techniques carry a substantial risk of failure of the implant, leading to resubluxation of the joint. Partial resubluxation is not necessarily associated with poor outcomes and is often managed conservatively (Fraser-Moodie et al 2008). Complete resubluxation is associated with residual symptoms, and there are reports of successful revision operations (Fraser-Moodie et al 2008).

Conclusion

The vast majority of ACJ injuries are minor (grades I–II, with CC ligaments intact) and recover fully with adequate conservative management. Studies comparing adequate rehabilitation with surgery for grade III injuries (CC ligaments disrupted) also support the role of adequate rehabilitation as the primary treatment. The more severe injuries (e.g. posterior or inferior displacement of the clavicle) are rarer and there is some research suggesting these injuries should be treated surgically. Areas that are most likely to benefit from more research include:

- **long-term prognosis:** studying the sequelae of ACJ injury with validated relevant outcome measures (Hootman 2004)
- **diagnostic testing:** study of the validity of newer diagnostic manoeuvres such as Paxinos sign and cross-arm adduction AP radiographs (Rios & Mazzocca 2008) and understanding how best to combine the results of different tests for making management decisions
- **conservative treatment:** the comparison of different types of supervised rehabilitation in the management of types I, II and III ACJ injury and in chronic ACJ dysfunction (Hootman 2004; Spencer 2007; Ceccarelli et al 2008; Macdonald & Lapointe 2008; Simovitch et al 2009)

- **surgical treatment:** the timing of surgical interventions, including whether there are sometimes indications for early surgical intervention with type III ACJ injury (Rios & Mazzocca 2008).

References

Auge WK, Fischer RA. 1998. Arthroscopic distal clavicle resection for isolated atraumatic osteolysis in weight lifters. Am J Sports Med 26: 189–192.

Beim GM. 2000. Joint injuries. J Athl Train 35: 261–267.

Bergfeld JA, Andrish JT, Clancy WG. 1978. Evaluation of the acromio-clavicular joint following first- and second-degree sprains. Am J Sports Med 6: 153–159.

Bisbinas I, Belthur M, Said HG, et al. 2006. Accuracy of needle placement in ACJ injections. Knee Surg Sports Traumatol Arthrosc 14: 762–765.

Bjerneld H, Hovelius L, ThoHing J. 1983. Acromioclavicular separations treated conservatively: a 5-year follow-up study. Acta Orthop Scand 54: 743–745.

Bowen MK, Nuber GW. 2003. Acromioclavicular and sternoclavicular injuries. Clin Sports Med 22: xiii.

Bradley JP, Elkousy H. 2003. Decision making: operative versus nonoperative treatment of acromio-clavicular joint injuries. Clin Sports Med 22: 277–290.

Brukner P, Khan K. 2006. Clinical sports medicine. Sydney: McGraw-Hill Australia.

Buss DD, Watts JD. 2003. Acromioclavicular injuries in the throwing athlete. Clin Sports Med 22: 327–341.

Buttaci CJ, Stitik TP, Yonclas PP, et al. 2004. Osteoarthritis of the acromio-clavicular joint: a review of anatomy, biomechanics, diagnosis, and treatment. Am J Phys Med Rehabil 83: 791–797.

Ceccarelli E, Bondì R, Alviti F, et al. 2008. Treatment of acute grade III acromio-clavicular dislocation: a lack of evidence. J Orthoped Traumatol 9: 105–108.

Chronopoulos E, Kim TK, Park HB, et al. 2004. Diagnostic value of physical tests for isolated chronic acromioclavicular lesions. Am J Sports Med 32: 655–661.

Codsi MJ. 2007. The painful shoulder: when to inject and when to refer. Cleve Clin J Med 74: 473–488.

Debski RE, Parsons IM, Woo SLY, et al. 2001. Effect of capsular injury on acromio-clavicular joint mechanics. J Bone Joint Surg 83B: 1344–1351.

Docimo S, Kornitsky D, Futterman B, et al. 2008. Surgical treatment for acromio-clavicular joint osteoarthritis: patient selection, surgical options, complications, and outcome. Curr Rev Musculoskelet Med 1: 154–160.

Dumontier C, Sautet A, Man M, et al. 1995. Acromioclavicular dislocations: treatment by coracoacromial ligamentoplasty. J Shoulder Elbow Surg 4: 130–134.

Fraser-Moodie J, Shortt NL, Robinson CM. 2008. Injuries to the acromio-clavicular joint. J Bone Joint Surg 90B: 697–707.

Galpiri RD, Hawkins RJ, Grainger RW. 1985. A comparative analysis of operative versus nonoperative treatment of grade III acromioclavicular separations. Clin Orthop Relat Res 193: 150–155.

Garretson RB 3rd, Williams GR Jr. 2003. Clinical evaluation of injuries to the acromioclavicular and sternoclavicular joints. Clin Sports Med 22: 239–254.

Gerber C, Galantay RV, Hersche O. 1998. The pattern of pain produced by irritation of the acromio-clavicular joint and the subacromial space. J Shoulder Elbow Surg 7: 352–355.

Glick JM, Milburn LJ, Haggerty JF, et al. 1977. Dislocated acromio-clavicular joint: follow-up study of 35 unreduced acromioclavicular dislocations. Am J Sports Med 5: 264–270.

Gurd FB. 1941. The treatment of complete dislocation of the outer end of the clavicle: an hitherto undescribed operation. Ann Surg 113: 1094–1098.

Hootman JM. 2004. Acromioclavicular dislocation: conservative or surgical therapy. J Athl Train 39: 10–11.

Hutchinson MR, Ahuja GS. 1996. Diagnosing and treating clavicle injuries. Phys Sportsmed 24: 26–36.

Kiner A. 2004. Diagnosis and management of grade II acromio-clavicular joint separation. Clin Chiropract 7: 24–30.

Kwon YW, Iannotti JP. 2003. Operative treatment of acromio-clavicular joint injuries and results. Clin Sports Med 22: 291–300.

Lehtinen JT, Lehto MUK, Kaarela K, et al. 1999. Radiographic joint space in rheumatoid acromio-clavicular joints: a 15 year prospective follow-up study in 74 patients. Rheumatology 38: 1104–1107.

Lemos MJ. 1998. The evaluation and treatment of the injured acromio-clavicular joint in athletes. Am J Sports Med 26: 137–144.

Lemos MJ, Tolo ET. 2003. Complications of the treatment of the acromio-clavicular and sternoclavicular joint injuries, including instability. Clin Sports Med 22: 371–385.

Lizaur A, Marco L, Cebrian R. 1994. Acute dislocation of the acromio-clavicular joint. Traumatic anatomy and the importance of deltoid and trapezius. J Bone Joint Surg 76B: 602–606.

Macdonald PB, Lapointe P. 2008. Acromioclavicular and sternoclavicular joint injuries. Orthop Clin North Am 39: 535–545.

Magee DJ, Reid DC. 1996. Shoulder injuries. In: Zachazewski JE, Quillen WS (eds) Athletic injuries and rehabilitation. Philadelphia: WB Saunders, pp 509–542.

Maritz NGJ, Oosthuizen PJ. 2002. Diagnostic criteria for acromio-clavicular joint pathology. J Bone Joint Surg. 84A: 78.

Mehrberg RD, Lobel SM, Gibson WK. 2004. Disorders of the acromio-clavicular joint. Phys Med Rehabil Clin North Am 15: 537–555.

Mouhsine E, Garofalo R, Crevoisier X, et al. 2003. Grade I and II acromio-clavicular dislocations: results of conservative treatment. J Shoulder Elbow Surg 12: 599–602.

Murena L, Vulcano E, Ratti C, et al. 2009. Arthroscopic treatment of acute acromio-clavicular joint dislocation with double flip button. Knee Surg Sports Traumatol Arthrosc 17(12): 1511–1515.

Nuber GW, Bowen MK. 2003. Arthroscopic treatment of acromio-clavicular joint injuries and results. Clin Sports Med 22: 301–317.

O'Brien SJ, Pagnani MJ, Fealy S, et al. 1998. The active compression test: a new and effective test for diagnosing labral tears and acromio-clavicular joint abnormality. Am J Sports Med 26: 610–613.

Park GY, Park JH, Bae JH. 2009. Structural changes in the acromio-clavicular joint measured by ultrasonography during provocative tests. Clin Anat 22: 580–585.

Parlington PF, Broome GH. 1998. Diagnostic injection around the shoulder: hit and miss. A cadaveric study of injection accuracy. J Shoulder Elbow Surg 7: 147–150.

Peetrons P, Bédard JP. 2007. Acromio-clavicular joint injury: enhanced technique of examination with dynamic maneuver. J Clin Ultrasound 35: 262–267.

Petron DJ, Hanson RW Jr. 2007. Acromio-clavicular joint disorders. Curr Sports Med Rep 6: 300–306.

Powell JW, Huijbregts PA. 2006. Concurrent criterion-related validity of acromio-clavicular joint physical examination tests: a systematic review. J Man Manip Ther 14: E19–E29.

Rabalais RD, McCarty E. 2007. Surgical treatment of symptomatic acromio-clavicular joint problems: a systematic review. Clin Orthop Relat Res 455: 30–37.

Rawes ML, Dias J. 1996. Long-term results of conservative treatment for acromio-clavicular dislocation. J Bone Joint Surg 78B: 410–412.

Renfree KJ, Wright TW. 2003. Anatomy and biomechanics of the acromio-clavicular and sternoclavicular joints. Clin Sports Med 22: 219–237.

Rios CG, Mazzocca AD. 2008. Acromio-clavicular joint problems in athletes and new methods of management. Clin Sports Med 27: 763–788.

Rockwood CA Jr, Williams GR, Young DC. 1996. Injuries to the acromio-clavicular joint. In: Rockwood CA Jr, Bucholz RW, Green DP (eds) Fractures in adults. Philadelphia: Lippincott-Raven, pp 1341–1413.

Rudzki JR, Matava MJ, Paletta GA Jr. 2003. Complications of treatment of acromio-clavicular and sternoclavicular joint injuries. Clin Sports Med 22: 387–405.

Sahara W, Sugamoto K, Murai M, et al. 2006. 3D kinematic analysis of the acromio-clavicular joint during arm abduction using vertically open MRI. J Orthop Res 24: 1823–1831.

Sahara W, Sugamoto K, Murai M, et al. 2007. Three-dimensional clavicular and acromioclavicular rotations during arm abduction using vertically open MRI. J Orthop Res 25: 1243–1249.

Santis DD, Palazzi C, D'Amico E, et al. 2001. Acromioclavicular cyst and 'porcupine shoulder' in gout. Rheumatology 40: 1320–1321.

Schlegel TF, Burks RT, Marcus RI, et al. 2001. A prospective evaluation of untreated acute grade iii acromioclavicular separations. Am J Sports Med 29: 699–703.

Schwarzkopf R, Ishak C, Elman M, et al. 2008. Distal clavicular osteolysis: a review of the literature. Bull NYU Hosp Jt Dis 66: 94–101.

Shaffer BS. 1999. Painful conditions of the acromio-clavicular joint. J Am Acad Orthop Surg 7: 176–188.

Simovitch R, Sanders B, Ozbaydar M, et al. 2009. Acromio-clavicular joint injuries: diagnosis and management. J Am Acad Orthop Surg 17: 207–219.

Spencer EE Jr. 2007. Treatment of grade III acromio-clavicular joint injuries: a systematic review. Clin Orthop Relat Res 455: 38–44.

Tallia AF, Cardone DA. 2003. Diagnostic and therapeutic injection of the shoulder region. Am Fam Physician 67: 1271–1278.

Teece RM, Lunden JB, Lloyd AS, et al. 2008. Three-dimensional acromio-clavicular joint motions during elevation of the arm. J Orthop Sports Phys Ther 38: 181–190.

Tom A, Mazzocca AD, Pavlatos CJ. 2009. Acromio-clavicular joint injuries. In: Wilk KE, Reinold MM, Andrews J (eds) The athlete's shoulder. Philadelphia: Churchill Livingstone Elsevier, pp 303–313.

Tossy JD, Mead NC, Sigmond HM. 1963. Acromioclavicular separations: Useful and practical classification for treatment. Clin Orthop Relat Res 28: 111–119.

Urist MR. 1963. Complete dislocation of the acromio-clavicular joint. J Bone Joint Surg 45A: 1750–1753.

Walton DM, Sadi J. 2008. Identifying SLAP lesions: a meta-analysis of clinical tests and exercise in clinical reasoning. Phys Ther Sport 9: 167–176.

Walton J, Mahajan S, Paxinos A, et al. 2004. Diagnostic values of tests for acromio-clavicular joint pain. J Bone Joint Surg 86A: 807–812.

Weinstein DM, McCann PD, McIlveen SJ, et al. 1995. Surgical treatment of complete acromioclavicular dislocations. Am J Sports Med 23: 324–331.

White B, Epstein D, Sanders S, et al. 2008. Acute acromioclavicular injuries in adults. Orthopedics 31: 1219–1226.

26 Chapter

Sternoclavicular Joint

Erland Pettman

CHAPTER CONTENTS

Introduction	302
Anatomy of the sternoclavicular joint	302
Biomechanics of the sternoclavicular joint	304
Pathology of the sternoclavicular joint	304
Patients requiring a medical/surgical consultation	304
Patients with indication for physical therapy intervention	305
Diagnosis of the sternoclavicular joint	305
Management of the sternoclavicular joint	306
Anterior disc/manubrial rotation mobilization (left shoulder)	306
Posterior disc/manubrial rotation mobilization (left shoulder)	306
Inferior clavicular/disc glide (right shoulder)	306
Posterior clavicular/disc glide (right shoulder)	306
Adjunct exercises	307
Conclusion	307

Introduction

A literature search on the sternoclavicular joint rapidly makes the reader aware that there are a very limited number of publications on this joint and these predominantly cover medical and surgical concerns. Anatomical and biomechanical references are designed, most often, to support medical or surgical interventions. From a physical therapy perspective, this joint would therefore appear to be the 'poor cousin' of the shoulder girdle in both interest and research. However, whilst bemoaning this fact, the reason almost certainly lies in the joint's inherent strength and stability. These factors will be covered in the sections on anatomy and biomechanics.

What is most interesting to the writer, however, is this joint's proposed ability to work in concert with the thoracic spine to facilitate the function of elevation through flexion/abduction without compromise to the neurovascular structures that supply the upper limb. With respect to our upper limbs, we must accept the fact that they enable us to be primate 'brachiates' (i.e. we are able to locomote with our upper limbs). Although as we get older and heavier this seems an unlikely premise, we need merely to view children at a playground or to study gymnasts to realize this is at least one of the functions of the human upper limb and something we have in common with all other primates.

All anatomy texts that the author has read describe the shoulder girdle as 'ending' at the manubrium. Emphasis is, therefore, placed on how the clavicle moves at the sternomanubrial articulation. The author's paper entitled 'The functional shoulder girdle' (Pettman 1984) inferred that, during functional movements of the shoulder girdle, there is indeed another biomechanical component to this joint that needs to be considered – *manubriosternal* motion (i.e. that dictated by the thoracic spine). Given the dearth of biomechanical research regarding this joint, this chapter must first present a proposed biomechanical model, based on observation and palpation, which might lead to further research. Within this proposal will be a clinically reasoned explanation of how thoracic and/or sternoclavicular dysfunction may directly affect glenohumeral joint function.

Anatomy of the Sternoclavicular Joint

Descriptive anatomy of this joint is well covered in texts such as *Gray's anatomy* (Standring 2008). Therefore, the emphasis here should be on functional and comparative anatomy. In embryological development the clavicle is present in almost all mammals. However, in quadrupeds the clavicle becomes a vestigial or rudimentary structure helping to provide muscle attachments that produce a muscular 'sling' to support the weight of the thorax, neck and head. A fully developed, osseous clavicle that connects the scapula to the manubrium only exists in primates. This bony strut enables primates to enjoy a very large range of upper limb motion, especially away from the midline of the body. Such motion gives primates the functional advantages of grasping, thrusting (throwing or punching) and brachiation (swinging).

Specialization of function within different primate groups appears to depend upon the position of the scapula bone (lateral or posterior to the thorax) (Chan 2007) and the curvature(s) of the clavicle (Voisin 2006). The distinctive 'S' shape of the human clavicle has been likened to a 'crank'. This enables our muscles to support a relatively heavy body weight during brachiation, but also to increase the power and velocity of upper limb movements such as throwing. However, that same 'S'-shaped clavicle does poorly with respect to compressive loading – its weak spot being the junction between the medial convexity and its lateral concavity. This fact is underscored by the finding that this mid-shaft region is the most prevalent site for clavicular fractures during compressive loading, such as a fall directly onto the shoulder or the outstretched hand (Denard et al 2005). Most fractures of this region are uncomplicated, but on rare occasion may lead to brachial plexus involvement, pulmonary dysfunction or even death (Kendall et al 2000).

The medial end of the clavicle bone presents a large, bulbous head. Its surface is concave horizontally and convex vertically, giving it a saddle-shaped appearance. Histological analysis of the clavicular head (Ellis & Carlson 1986), at least developmentally, shows plates of cartilage within the bone; this is a direct comparison with the head of the mandible (Wolford et al 1994) – as both are presumably designed to absorb extreme stresses and strains. The corresponding surface of the sternum has, reciprocally, an obvious concave surface vertically and a slight convexity horizontally. Since the articulating surface of the clavicular head is over twice that of the manubrial surface, this apparent incongruence, although enabling large amplitude of motion, makes the joint potentially very unstable. It is the role of the joint's ligamentous structures to maintain stability (Iannotti & Williams 1999). Ligaments of the sternoclavicular joint include the intra-articular ligament or disc, the interclavicular ligament, the capsular (superior) ligament and the costoclavicular ligament.

There is some disagreement over whether this intra-articular ligament serves primarily as a ligament or as an intra-articular disc, and this will be discussed later. The dense fibrous structure has a strong peripheral capsular attachment that completely divides the joint into separate cavities (DePalma 1959), which in itself hints at a discrete function for each of the joint's cavities. Occasionally, there may be some central connection between the two joint cavities, but this is believed to be secondary to wear and tear. Inferiorly, the disc arises from the synchondrosis of the first rib cartilage and the manubrium. Superiorly, it attaches to the superior and medial aspects of the medial clavicle at the lateral joint margin, but blends with the fibres of the capsular (superior) ligament.

The interclavicular ligament, as its name suggests, blends with the same ligament of the opposite side. Also, it is attached to the superior part of the manubrium and blends with the ipsilateral capsular (superior) ligament.

The capsular (superior) ligament, which is perhaps the strongest of the sternoclavicular joint ligaments, really represents anterosuperior and posterior reinforcement (or thickening) of the articular capsule, the anterosuperior being the thickest.

Working in concert, these above three ligaments afford both strength and static stability to the sternoclavicular joint with the shoulder girdles in a resting, weight-dependent position. This has been referred to as 'shoulder poise' where the distal end of the clavicle is passively supported slightly higher than its medial end. As a passive support mechanism, this represents a significant saving in muscular energy expenditure to help carry objects either on the shoulder girdles (e.g. a yoke, satchel and even a child) or by hand (e.g. hunted game, water containers and suitcases). Also, this passive shoulder poise is essential for efficiency during manual activities that require minimal shoulder girdle excursion (e.g. moulding clay, cooking and using the computer mouse). With regard to stability, the most important of the above three ligaments appears to be the capsular (superior) ligament. Cadaveric experiments (Bearn 1967) have clearly demonstrated that static 'clavicular poise' is independent of myofascial support, or even support from the interclavicular and intra-articular disc ligaments. Once the capsular ligament is torn, minimal force is needed to tear the intra-articular ligament, leading to superior dislocation and disruption of the sternoclavicular joint. If the posterior part of the capsular ligament also fails then posterior dislocation is possible, which may lead to more serious health or even life-threatening complications due to compression of mediastinal structures.

The costoclavicular ligament is also called the rhomboid ligament because of the orientation of its fibres. For this ligament, there appears to be some disagreement as to its actual morphology (Tubbs et al 2009). Traditionally the ligament has been described as a 'flattened' cone. The best way to visualize this is to take a polystyrene paper cup and draw oblique parallel lines around its perimeter. If it were then squashed flat, the drawn lines would resemble a rhomboid if viewed from anterior and posterior; however, the lateral and medial margins of the cup would appear to continue the spiralling lines originally drawn. As such, the fibres of the ligament would indeed be capable of resisting clavicular motion in all directions and planes except for one: depression of the clavicle in neutral. The argument within the literature regarding its morphology is about whether there is an interposing bursa (or space) between the anterior and posterior sets of fibres or whether they form one solid mass. Regardless of the orientation, this ligament's fibres are clearly designed to resist any motion of the clavicle away from its neutral 'poise'. The anterior fibres appear particularly vulnerable to excessive elevation and protraction of the shoulder girdle, which this author believes, from cadaveric observation, is considered the close-packed position of the sternoclavicular joint.

During full elevation of the humerus (through flexion / abduction) the shoulder girdle (scapula and clavicle) moves into depression and retraction. The disagreement over whether the clavicle elevates or depresses (Ludewig et al 2004) is probably the result of different instructions given to the observed models. If the model is asked to elevate their hand as high as he / she can then elevation of the clavicle will result; however, this author believes that functional elevation requires a stable, depressed clavicle.

During full elevation, recruitment of the lower trapezius muscle coincides with activation of subclavius muscle (Konstant et al 1982). This would make sense as the motion probably coincides with the greatest stress placed on the sternoclavicular joint for either throwing or brachiation. The 'shunt' action of subclavius would now be most appropriate in terms of stability of the sternoclavicular joint. In this author's experience, most costoclavicular ligament injuries (treatable by physical therapy) occur when there is a forceful elevation thrust of the arm together with a corresponding elevation and protraction of the shoulder girdle. In this circumstance, the forced lateral displacement of the clavicle would not be resisted by the appropriate reflex shunt action of subclavius, rendering the anterior fibres susceptible to damage. Individuals who might perform such an action are limited to certain athletes (e.g. shot putters, javelin throwers, racquet players), but also those performing household tasks (e.g. cleaning a bathtub, painters).

Biomechanics of the Sternoclavicular Joint

At the sternoclavicular joint, the clavicle is clearly capable of moving through at least two cardinal planes – that is, the horizontal (35° of combined protraction and retraction) and vertical (30–35° degrees of elevation) planes (Iannotti & Williams 1999). The joint is therefore considered to possess two degrees of freedom, which are both pure swings. The largest displacement, however, is 45–50° of rotation (Iannotti & Williams 1999; Ludewig et al 2004) around the long axis of the clavicle (i.e. motion through a sagittal plane), but this author wonders whether this can truly be considered a degree of freedom?

As mentioned earlier, the joint is clearly divided into two separate anatomical compartments, suggesting two separate functions (similar to the temporomandibular joint). If the posterior edge of the lateral end of the clavicle is palpated during inspiration and expiration, rotation of the bone is clearly felt. This is because the clavicle is 'crank' shaped, and, as the manubrium rises with inspiration, elevation of the medial end of the clavicle produces a posterior rotation around its longitudinal axis. Since there is no other obvious displacement of the clavicle (shoulder girdle), it is assumed that the rotational motion at the sternoclavicular joint occurs within the medial component (disc / manubrium) of the joint. So it could well be argued that the sternoclavicular joint complex has, indeed, three degrees of freedom of motion.

The large, superficial head of the clavicle is easily palpated during motion of the shoulder girdle on a relatively stationary manubrium. From full retraction towards protraction, the most obvious motion initially appears as a posterior male (convex on concave) glide, but this glide occurs only through the first two-thirds of the range (from full retraction to neutral poise). After that point, as protraction continues an anterior rotation is apparent, representing a female (concave on convex) glide.

A similar change in glides is apparent when the joint is palpated from full depression to full elevation of the shoulder girdle – where there is an initial inferior male glide followed by a superior anterior female glide. Understanding that the male motion occurs at the disc / clavicle component and the female motion arises from the disc / manubrium component allows the clinician to use a very simple palpatory assessment technique to discern which component is in dysfunction, or indeed whether the whole complex might be deranged.

Considering the dearth of biomechanical research relevant to physical therapy, at this point the author sees fit to propose the following interaction between clavicular motion and manubrial motion during elevation of the arm through flexion and abduction, based on clinical experience and extrapolation of anatomical knowledge. As the arm is elevated through flexion / abduction, the initial motion appears to occur at the glenohumeral and acromioclavicular joints on a relatively fixed clavicle. The inferior angle of the scapula displaces laterally and anteriorly to produce an upward rotation of the scapula and its glenoid surface, the motion occurring at the acromioclavicular joint. At about 150° of elevation, the inferior angle stops moving. Presumably fixated by an isometric contraction of the lower serratus anterior muscle, the axis of shoulder girdle motion now shifts from the acromioclavicular joint to the sternoclavicular joint and the shoulder girdle is seen to depress and retract in the last 30–50° of arm elevation. It might be reasonably assumed that the clavicle should significantly rotate posteriorly. However, if the clavicle is palpated during this terminal range then minimal, if any, rotation is sensed. To solve this apparent conundrum, one must now study what is occurring at the manubrium.

As the arm is elevated beyond 150°, upper thoracic motion can be both seen and palpated. The upper thoracic spine extends, ipsilaterally rotates and side-bends towards the moving arm. The first thoracic vertebra, first rib and manubrium now all move in concert, dictated by thoracic spine motion. This is easily felt at the manubrium by palpating bilaterally just below the first rib cartilage. The manubrium also side-bends and rotates towards the elevating arm. So the manubrium is now moving under the clavicle, producing a relative anterior rotation of the sternoclavicular joint. This simultaneous motion of both the clavicle and the manubrium ensures that there is no resultant posterior rotation of the clavicle. The main question now is: why would this be necessary?

The deep cervical fascia blends with the posterior and superior periosteum of the clavicle. If the clavicle were to rotate posteriorly up to 45°, as has been suggested, the deep cervical fascia would undergo an extreme increase in tension, potentially compromising the neurovascular tissue passing through it – a distinct disadvantage for a brachiator.

Although not strictly a sternoclavicular joint disruption or injury, an inability of the thoracic spine to move appropriately during the final stages of arm elevation would prevent the disc / manubrium component of the sternoclavicular joint from derotating the clavicle. Clinically, individuals who perform habitual or sustained arm elevation in their recreational or work environment would potentially complain of signs or symptoms of abnormal neural tension within the arm and / or damage to distal shoulder girdle structures from mechanical compensation. For this reason, assessment of thoracic and manubrial motion should be a routine part of shoulder girdle assessment.

Pathology of the Sternoclavicular Joint

For the physical therapist, pathologies of the sternoclavicular joint are best divided into two main sections: those requiring a medical / surgical consultation and those with an indication for physical therapy intervention.

Patients requiring a medical / surgical consultation

The sternoclavicular joint is susceptible to any of the pathologies that affect synovial joints (Iannotti & Williams 1999; Higginbotham & Khun 2005). Whilst not attempting an exact medical diagnosis, the therapist needs nevertheless to be able to identify patients suffering from serious traumatic injuries and non-traumatic or degenerative arthritic conditions.

Dislocations, although uncommon, represent the greatest threat to articular function. They can occur in anterior, superior and posterior directions. Dislocations can be the result of direct trauma to the clavicle or manubrium, as may occur in motor vehicle accidents or sports. They can also result from indirect trauma, especially to the posterolateral shoulder (superior and posterior dislocations) and anterolateral shoulder (anterior dislocations) (Iannotti & Williams 1999).

The posterior dislocation is of greatest concern because of the threat to retrosternal structures such as the trachea and major blood vessels (Rodrigues 1843; Worman & Laegus 1967; Cooper et al 1992). If these structures are involved the patient may well be observed as having breathing problems and changes in skin colour due to vascular or airway compromise.

Dislocations tend not to be subtle. The therapist may suspect them from a history of extreme trauma, a gross loss of motion of the upper limb, and an obvious observable and palpable change in the natural contours of the sternoclavicular joint. During palpation of motion (described later) the therapist may detect gross disruption of the anticipated (male-to-female) motion sequence.

Although the clavicle is the first long bone to begin ossification, it is the last to complete it. The epiphysis of the medial end of the clavicle ossifies in the 18th–20th year and fuses with the shaft between the 23rd and 25th years. Direct and indirect trauma to the medial end of the clavicle may result in epiphyseal disruption, even fracture; these closely resemble the presentation of a dislocation, and only medical examination can provide an accurate differential diagnosis (Iannotti & Williams 1999).

Hyperostosis at the sternoclavicular joint (Dihlmann et al 1993; Noble 2003), felt initially by the therapist as an apparent bony hypertrophy of either the clavicular head or the manubrium, could signify serious pathology and a medical consult is certainly warranted (Fritz et al 1992). However, the author has seen two cases of physeal trauma where fracture or disruption were ruled out but the trauma resulted in benign hyperostosis of the head of the clavicle. Apart from the distressing cosmetic appearance, joint function and stability in these two cases appeared normal.

The sternoclavicular joint has been shown to suffer from almost all potential causes of non-traumatic arthritis, the more common of these including septic arthritis, rheumatoid arthritis, tuberculosis and ankylosing spondylitis. The author has rarely seen gouty arthritis as is mentioned in the literature (Kearn et al 1999), but clearly it cannot be ruled out. However, the presentation of a painful, hot and swollen joint with no history of injury should immediately raise enough concern for the therapist to request a medical consultation.

Patients with indication for physical therapy intervention

These patients will include those with sprains and strains of the sternoclavicular joint. Acute traumatic arthritis may present with enough pain, swelling and dysfunction that a medical consult should be sought. They are most effectively treated with a resting sling and subsequent referral to physical therapy.

The location of pain from sternoclavicular joint injury is most commonly within the joint itself, but distal referral (e.g. to the neck, shoulder and arm) is also possible (Hassett & Barnsley 2001). With subacute and chronic (traumatic) arthritis, the therapist's main concern is whether joint motion has been lost, and if so assess which component of the joint is responsible.

Another concern would be the possibility of a ligamentous sprain. The author is unaware of any confirmed discrete tests for the intra-articular disc ligament, capsular ligament or interclavicular ligament. However, if articular motion is normal but localized pain is reproduced by overpressure of shoulder girdle movements, a ligamentous injury must be suspected. Accurate palpation followed by deep transverse friction massage (DTFM) and ultrasound would appear to be the treatment of choice.

Unlike the other ligaments, the costoclavicular ligament can be stressed discretely. With the patient in contralateral side-lying, the therapist moves the (affected side) glenohumeral joint into extension and adduction. Applying pressure through the elbow, the therapist then pushes the shoulder girdle into full elevation and protraction. Continued pressure through the patient's elbow now provides a lateral distractive force to the sternoclavicular joint, maximally stressing the costoclavicular ligament. In this author's opinion and experience, the anterior fibres are those most likely to be injured. They are accessible to DTFM if the shoulder girdle is positioned into depression and retraction (posterior rotation of the clavicle).

Osteoarthrosis is suspected when crepitation or even 'clunking' is detected during motion palpation. One paper on cadaveric dissection of the sternoclavicular joints (Hagemann & Ruttner 1979) suggested that 80% of people over 50 may have osteoarthrosis of this joint. However, as cadaveric dissection can rarely be correlated with symptoms, it is unclear for how much symptomatology this condition is responsible. In the author's experience, minor, asymptomatic joint crepitation is common in the presence of normal joint function and should probably be ignored. However, if the crepitation or clunking is significant, or corresponds to the reproduction of the patient's symptoms, then a medical consult should be sought. The degenerative state of the joint may help in an eventual prognosis, but also in determining the appropriate magnitude of force used in physical therapy procedures (Frosi et al 2004). It is worth remembering that all resisted forces on the upper limb must ultimately be transferred to the sternoclavicular joint.

Diagnosis of the Sternoclavicular Joint

As was inferred earlier, the size of the clavicular head, coupled with the fact it is located so superficially, enables the therapist to palpate sternoclavicular joint motion easily. Following the taking of a history and observation, the therapist palpates the anterior surface of the head of the clavicle.

From a position of full retraction, the patient is instructed to pull the shoulder girdles into protraction. In normal motion, the therapist should be able to feel the head of the clavicle move initially posteriorly (male clavicular / disc

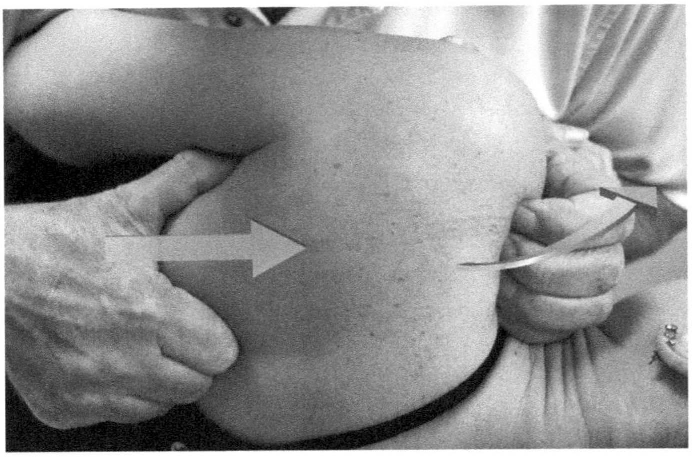

Figure 26.1 Mobilization for anterior rotation of the female component (elevation and protraction).

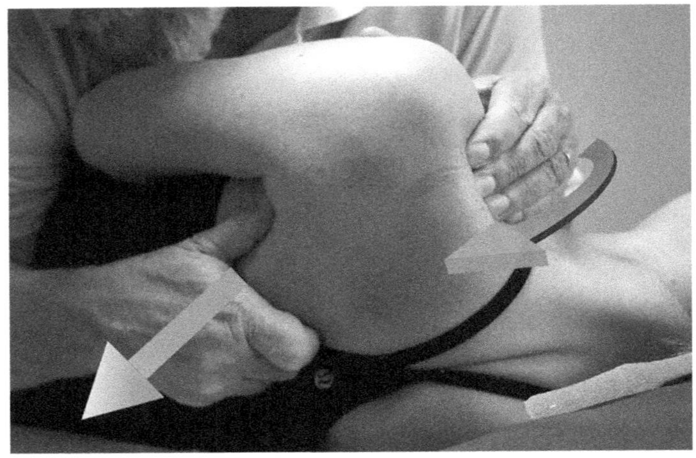

Figure 26.2 Mobilization of posterior rotation of the female component (depression and retraction).

motion). At the position of neutral 'poise' the motion should be felt to change to a female (disc / manubrial motion) anterior glide (roll). From a position of full depression, the patient is instructed to lift the shoulder girdles into elevation. In normal motion, the therapist should be able to feel the head of the clavicle move initially inferiorly (male clavicular / disc motion). At mid-range this motion is felt to change to a female superior / anterior roll. This simple test enables the therapist to decide which articular component is lacking.

Management of the Sternoclavicular Joint

Options for physical therapy management have been provided above in the section on pathology. The emphasis in this section will be on manual therapy intervention and adjunct exercises for patients with mechanical sternoclavicular joint dysfunction. Techniques address either disc / manubrial restrictions (anterior and posterior rotation) or clavicular / disc restrictions (inferior glide and posterior glide).

Anterior disc/manubrial rotation mobilization (left shoulder)

The patient is placed on the right side lying facing the therapist. The therapist stands facing the patient. The therapist's left middle and ring finger tips are tucked posterior and inferior to the lateral edge of the patient's left clavicle. The therapist's right hand grasps the inferior angle of the scapula; the left hand passively draws the patient's left shoulder girdle into elevation and protraction until anterior rotation is sensed to cease (Fig. 26.1).

The therapist instructs the patient to take a short in-breath, followed by a long out-breath. As the patient breathes out, increased anterior rotation of the clavicle is taken up by passively increasing elevation and protraction, and also by the therapist's left hand pulling the posterior edge of the clavicle upward and forward. The procedure is repeated until no further motion can be elicited.

Posterior disc/manubrial rotation mobilization (left shoulder)

The patient's starting position is the same as described above. In this technique, and in contrast to the above technique for anterior rotation, the therapist's middle and ring fingers are over the superior aspect of the posterior edge of the lateral clavicle. The therapist moves the shoulder girdle into depression and retraction until posterior rotation of the clavicle ceases (Fig. 26.2).

The patient is instructed to take a short out-breath followed by a long in-breath. As increased posterior rotation of the clavicle is detected, the therapist pushes the patient's shoulder girdle into further depression and retraction with an accompanying push on the posterior edge of the clavicle inferiorly by the therapist's left fingers. This procedure is repeated until no further motion can be elicited.

Inferior clavicular/disc glide (right shoulder)

The patient is supine. The therapist is standing adjacent to the patient's opposite shoulder girdle. The therapist's left thumb pad or thenar eminence is placed over the superior aspect of the head of the patient's right clavicle. The therapist's right hand draws the patient's right shoulder girdle into elevation until the inferior glide of the clavicular head ceases (Fig. 26.3).

The therapist then instructs the patient to resist an attempt to push the right shoulder girdle into depression. An inferior glide of the right clavicular head will be detected and this motion slack is taken up by pressure from the therapist's left thumb. Any slack in right girdle elevation is now taken up by the therapist's right hand. This procedure is repeated until no further motion is perceived.

Posterior clavicular/disc glide (right shoulder)

The patient is supine. The therapist stands on the opposite side to the joint being treated, then grasps the patient's right shoulder with the left hand and instructs the patient to place

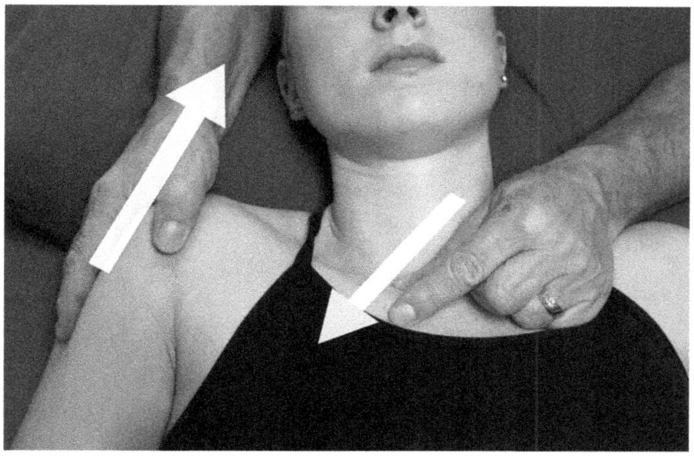

Figure 26.3 **Mobilization of the inferior male glide (elevation).**

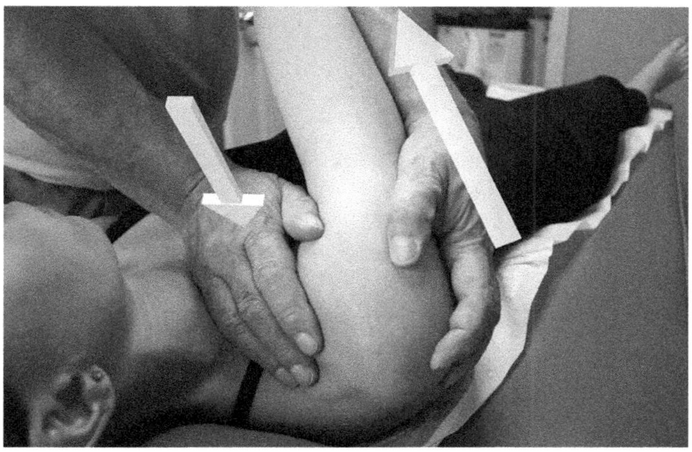

Figure 26.4 **Mobilization of the posterior male glide (protraction).**

his / her right hand on the therapist's left arm. The therapist's right thumb or thenar eminence is placed over the anterior surface of the head of the patient's right clavicle (Fig. 26.4).

The patient is instructed to resist the therapist's attempt to push the patient's right shoulder girdle into retraction. A posterior motion of the clavicular head will be noted and the therapist's right thumb takes up the slack. Any increased protraction is taken up by therapist's left hand. This procedure is repeated until no further motion is perceived.

Adjunct exercises

Active exercises to maintain the range of motion of the sternoclavicular joint gained by passive mobilizations should simply be instructed in functional sets – that is, they should have an emphasis either on a combination of elevation and protraction or on a combination of depression and retraction. With regard to normal sternoclavicular joint function, however, the author cannot overemphasize the need for normal thoracic joint motion. Manual mobilization and manipulation techniques to restore mobility in this region have been described in Chapter 13 and should be reviewed and included for optimal management of patients with sternoclavicular joint dysfunction as indicated by the examination findings. Addressing this component of sternoclavicular joint dysfunction may also necessitate the patient to perform additional thoracic spine exercises to facilitate shoulder girdle depression and retraction (extension and ipsilateral side-bending / rotation of the thoracic spine) or girdle elevation and protraction (flexion and contralateral side-bending / rotation of the thoracic spine).

Conclusion

The sternoclavicular joint seems to be poorly understood and more poorly researched, but it is accepted that this is, in part, due to the rarity of significant injury to the joint. However, as physical therapists continue to gain the privilege of direct access to patients, it is essential they become aware of how to differentiate between pathological conditions of this joint that may be either health or life threatening demanding a medical consult and those that require a physical therapy intervention. Also, much more work is required by all interested parties to investigate the biomechanical role of the thorax in sternoclavicular joint function and its potential patho-biomechanical interaction with upper limb function.

References

Bearn JG. 1967. Direct observations on the function of the capsule of the sterno-clavicular joint in the clavicular support. Anatomy 101: 159–170.

Chan LK. 2007. Scapular position in primates. Folia Primatol 7: 19–35.

Cooper GJ, Stubbs D, Walker DA, et al. 1992. Posterior sterno-clavicular joint dislocation: a novel method of external fixation. Injury 23: 565–567.

Denard PJ, Koval KJ, Cantu RV, et al. 2005. Management of midshaft clavicle fractures in adults. Am J Orthop 34 (11): 527–536.

DePalma AF. 1959. The role of the disks of the sterno-clavicular and the acromioclavicular joints. Clin Orthop Relat Res 13: 222–233.

Dihlmann W, Schnabel A, Gross WL. 1993. The acquired hyperostosis syndrome: a little known skeletal disorder with distinctive radiological and clinical features. J Clin Invest 72: 4–11.

Ellis E, Carlson DS. 1986. Histological comparison of the costochondral, sterno-clavicular and temporomandibular joints during growth in *Macaca mulatta*. J Oral Maxillofac Surg 44: 312–321.

Fritz P, Baldauf G, Whilke HJ, et al. 1992. Hyperostosis: its progression and radiological features. Ann Rheum Dis 51: 658–664.

Frosi G, Sulli A, Testa M, et al. 2004. The sterno-clavicular joint: anatomy, biomechanics, clinical features and aspects of manual therapy. Reumatismo 56: 82–88. [Article in Italian.]

Hagemann R, Ruttner JR. 1979. Arthrosis of the sterno-clavicular joint. Z Rheumatol 38: 27–28.

Hassett G, Barnsley L. 2001. Pain referral from the sterno-clavicular joint: a study in normal volunteers. Rheumatology 40: 859–862.

Higginbotham TO, Khun JE. 2005. Atraumatic disorders of the sternoclavicular joint. J Am Acad Orthop Surg 13: 138–145.

Iannotti JP, Williams GR. 1999. Disorders of the shoulder. Philadelphia: Lippincott Williams & Wilkins.

Kearn A, Schunk A, Thelan M. 1999. Gout in the area of the cervical area and sterno-clavicular joint. Rofo 170: 515–517.

Kendall KM, Burton JH, Cushing B. 2000. Fatal subclavian artery transection from isolated clavicle fracture. Trauma 42: 316–318.

Konstant W, Stern J, Fleagle J, et al. 1982. Function of the subclavius muscle in a non-human primate, the spider monkey. Folia Primatol 38: 170–182.

Ludewig P, Bahrens S, Spoden S, et al. 2004. Three-dimensional clavicular motion during arm elevation: reliability and descriptive data. J Orthop Sports Phys Ther 34: 140–149.

Noble JS. 2003. Degenerative sterno-clavicular arthritis and hyperostosis. Clin Sports Med 22: 407–422.

Pettman E. 1984. The functional shoulder girdle. Vancouver: International Federation of Orthopaedic Manipulative Therapists (IFOMT).

Rodrigues H. 1843. Case of dislocation, inwards, of the internal extremity of the clavicle. Lancet 1: 309–310.
Standring S (ed). 2008. Gray's anatomy: the anatomical basis of clinical practice, 40th edn. Edinburgh: Churchill Livingstone, pp 777–822.
Tubbs SR, Shah NA, Sullivan BP, et al. 2009. The costoclavicular ligament revisited: a functional and anatomical study. J Morphol Embryol 50: 475–479.
Voisin JL. 2006. Clavicle, a neglected bone: morphology and relation to arm movements and shoulder architecture in primates. Anat Rec A 288A: 944–953.
Wolford LM, Cottrell DA, Henry C. 1994. Sterno-clavicular grafts for temporomandibular reconstruction. J Oral Maxillofac Surg 52: 119–128.
Worman LM, Laegus C. 1967. Intrathoracic injury following retrosternal dislocation of the clavicle. J Trauma 7: 416–423.

Chapter 27

Rotator Cuff Lesions: Shoulder Impingement

Peter A. Huijbregts, Carel Bron

CHAPTER CONTENTS

Introduction	309
Anatomy	309
Biomechanics	310
Pathology of the rotator cuff	311
Diagnosis of shoulder impingement	313
Prognosis	315
Management	315
Conclusion	318

Introduction

Shoulder complaints are common. A Dutch study indicated a point-prevalence of 20.9% in the general population (Picavet et al 2000). Another Dutch study indicated a yearly incidence of 11.2 per 1000 patients in general medical practice, with 41% of the patients seeking care for shoulder complaints diagnosed with impingement (van der Windt et al 1995). A UK study found that, at 16%, shoulder problems were the third most common cause of musculoskeletal disease in primary care (Urwin et al 1998). Shoulder complaints are also a common reason for patients to seek therapy. In a survey of US outpatient physical therapy services (Boissonnault 1999), 11% of 1258 patients indicated the shoulder as their chief area of complaints.

Although descriptions of rotator cuff tears can be found in the medical literature as early as the 18th century (Limb & Collier 2000), and Codman (1906, 1934) and Goldthwait (1909) in the early 20th century had made significant contributions to our understanding of anatomy and pathology of the subacromial region, it was the description and classification by Neer (1972) into stage I (oedema and haemorrhage), stage II (tendonitis with fibrosis) and stage III (partial- to full-thickness rotator cuff tears) impingement that truly brought subacromial impingement to the diagnostic forefront. However, the development in our understanding of impingement has not stopped there and today, in addition to primary or subacromial impingement, we recognize secondary, internal and coracoid impingement as distinct and relevant clinical presentations. Similarly, an understanding of relevant intrinsic pathological mechanisms has complemented the sole emphasis on extrinsic aetiology by Neer (1972). Together with this increased knowledge has come an increasing role for conservative management of patients with these conditions.

Anatomy

Anatomical structures relevant to the various types of impingement are the rotator cuff tendons, the tendon of the long head of the biceps, the subacromial / subdeltoid bursa, the coracoacromial arch, the glenohumeral capsuloligamentous structures (Ch 28) and the glenoid labrum (Ch 29). (As the movement of the shoulder is dependent on the other components of the shoulder girdle as well as the cervical and thoracic spine, the reader is also referred to the other relevant chapters of this text for more details on anatomy.)

The rotator cuff consists of the supraspinatus, infraspinatus, teres minor and subscapularis muscles. Even macroscopically, the tendons of these muscles can be seen to fuse into a single structure. The supraspinatus and infraspinatus muscles join some 1.5 cm proximal to their insertion, whereas the infraspinatus in turn merges with the teres minor proximal to their musculotendinous junction (Clark & Harryman 1992). Even though the anterior portion of the supraspinatus and the superior portion of the subscapularis are separated by the rotator interval, through which the coracoid process projects medially, the fibres from the supraspinatus and subscapularis also merge and interweave to form a sheath around the biceps tendon (Clark & Harryman 1992; Carr & Harvie 2005). These interconnected fibres from the subscapularis and supraspinatus tendons, together with the superior glenohumeral and coracohumeral ligament, form a tenoligamentous sling, called the biceps pulley, that keeps the long head of the biceps tendon stabilized as it courses across the glenohumeral joint to the bicipital sulcus (Choi et al 2004; Habermeyer et al 2004).

Microscopically, an even greater anatomical interdependence becomes apparent. At the level of the supraspinatus, infraspinatus and subjacent capsuloligamentous structures, there are five distinct layers to the cuff–capsule complex (Clark & Harryman 1992):

1. The most superficial layer is 1 mm thick and consists of fibres of the coracohumeral ligament, coursing through

the rotator interval and oriented obliquely to the axis of each muscle.

2. The second layer is 3–5 mm thick and consists of closely packed parallel tendon fibres grouped in large bundles that also form the roof of the biceps tendon sheath.
3. The third layer is 3 mm thick and consists of smaller tendon fascicles with a less uniform orientation, where fibre bundles intersect at a 45° angle and extensive interdigitations occur between the supraspinatus and infraspinatus tendons.
4. The fourth layer consists of loose connective tissue with some thick collagen fibre bands located mostly on the extra-articular side of this layer.
5. The deepest layer is only 1.5–2 mm thick and is made up of interwoven collagen fibrils that make up the 'true' glenohumeral capsule.

The subscapularis tendon consists of 4–6 thick collagen fibre bundles. The most proximal of these bundles passes under the biceps tendon to form the floor of its sheath interwoven with some fibres from the supraspinatus. In this groove, these interwoven tendons become fibrocartilaginous. The superior and middle glenohumeral ligaments run under the subscapularis tendon and separate the tendon from the capsule with a structure similar to that described for the fourth layer of the supraspinatus region above (Clark & Harryman 1992).

Although extensively interwoven with the other local structures, as described above, the tendinous segments of the rotator cuff are thickened along the axes of the four muscles (Clark & Harryman 1992). Clinically most relevant is that the strong central tendon of the bipennate supraspinatus muscle along its course migrates anteriorly, leaving a stress riser at the junction between its thick leading edge and the weaker posterior two-thirds, which is where 96% of all rotator cuff tears initiate (Bunker 2002).

The vascular anatomy of the rotator cuff has been a contentious issue. Rathbun and Macnab (1970) reported an avascular area near the supraspinatus insertion, especially with adduction, that corresponds with the area where tears first occur. Biberthaler et al (2003) also noted a significant reduction in capillary density at the edge of degenerative rotator cuff lesions. Other sources have reported no such hypovascularity (Moseley & Goldie 1963; Bunker 2002; Carr & Harvie 2005), or have even shown hypervascularity in patients with symptomatic impingement (Chansky & Iannotti 1991). An impaired, but also increased, blood supply may be a secondary event rather than a factor in the aetiology of rotator cuff lesions (Carr & Harvie 2005).

The coracoacromial arch defines the subacromial space and consists of the acromion and coracoid processes with, spanned between them, the coracoacromial ligament. Between the head of the humerus and the coracoacromial arch, in a space measuring 1–1.5 cm on radiographs taken in the anatomical position, are located the subacromial bursa, the rotator cuff tendons and the tendon of the long head of the biceps (Limb & Collier 2000). Apart from having a mechanical role, variations in the anatomy of the long head of the biceps have been associated with the aetiology of rotator cuff lesions. Dierickx et al (2009) noted the role of the double-origin biceps variant in causing impingement and tears in young patients. Variations in the shape of the acromion have been suggested as playing a role in impingement; Bigliani et al (1986) described a flat (type I), a curved (type II), and a hooked (type III) acromion and related these types with increasing occurrence of impingement.

Biomechanics

Although a simplification, within the context of impingement we can divide the muscles of the glenohumeral joint into prime movers and stabilizers. Normal glenohumeral motion consists of a roll–gliding combination that keeps the humeral head centred on the glenoid. Due to their orientation, the large prime mover muscles impart not only rolling but also significant translational forces on the head of the humerus. The latissimus dorsi and the teres major, for example, can impart an inferior glide (Halder et al 2001), whereas the deltoid will cause a superior glide (Limb & Collier 2000). Although a superior translation of the humeral head can be easily seen to cause narrowing of the subacromial space and subsequent impingement, decentring of the humeral head on the glenoid in any direction will cause excessive tensile, compressive and shear forces in active and passive structures that predispose the patient to eventual pathology.

Described in more detail in Chapter 28, the glenohumeral capsuloligamentous structures serve as stabilizers mainly near or at the end range of motions. Negative intra-articular pressure, which is lost in the case of a full-thickness rotator cuff tear, further contributes to glenohumeral stability (Hurschler et al 2000). However, the main stabilizers of the glenohumeral joint are the rotator cuff muscles. In the context of this muscular stabilization, two force couples are relevant (Parsons et al 2002). In the coronal plane both the deltoid and supraspinatus muscles contribute to abduction. Whereas the supraspinatus throughout abduction has a predominant vector compressing the humeral head into the glenoid, this component increases for the deltoid as abduction progresses (Fig. 27.1). However, during early abduction the predominant vector for the deltoid muscle is directed cranially, thus compressing the humeral head against the subacromial structures and the coracoacromial arch. Most relevant to keeping the humeral head centred throughout motion – and likely explaining the noted prevalence of asymptomatic rotator cuff tears involving solely the supraspinatus (Sher et al 1995) – is the transverse plane force couple formed by the subscapularis, infraspinatus and teres minor muscles (Fig. 27.2). The frontal

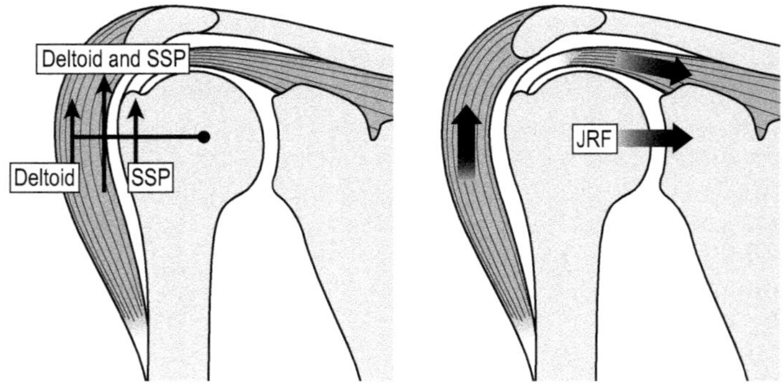

Figure 27.1 Frontal plane force couple. SSP = supraspinatus; JRF = joint reaction force.

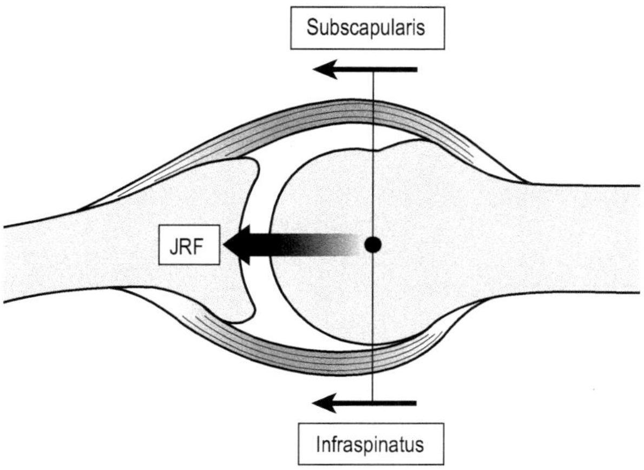

Figure 27.2 Transverse plane force couple. JRF = joint reaction force.

and coronal plane force couples together counteract the cranially directed force imposed by the deltoid muscle (Lo & Burkhart 2002).

Traditionally, the rotator cuff muscles were thought of as humeral head depressors maintaining a physiological subacromial space against mainly the deltoid imparting superior translation. However, the rotator cuff muscles are poorly positioned to produce effective depression of the humeral head (Halder et al 2001). More likely, their true or main role is in producing the compressive forces required for concavity compression. Concavity compression is a mechanism in which compression of the convex humeral head into the concave glenoid fossa stabilizes it against translating forces. Glenohumeral stability is thereby related to the depth of the concavity as well as the magnitude of the compressive force. This clarifies the important role in stability not only of the rotator cuff but also of glenoid morphology and an intact glenoid rim, labrum and closely associated capsuloligamentous structures responsible for the glenoid concavity (Lippitt et al 1993).

Although the tendon of the long head of the biceps is often functionally considered part of the rotator cuff, research evidence with regard to its biomechanical role is equivocal, ranging from it having no role at the shoulder to it being a major depressor of the humeral head (Krupp et al 2009). The most likely role of the biceps tendon (as well as the coracoacromial arch) is that of a static restraint to superior translation of the humeral head. In normal shoulders the active role in stability for the biceps tendon seems limited to a position of abduction and maximal external rotation – as occurs in the late cocking phase of an overhead-throwing motion where contraction of the biceps adds to torsional stiffness of the glenohumeral joint and reduces anterior translation (Itoi et al 1993; Rodosky et al 1994). However, confirming both authors' clinical observations, the biceps tendon may have a greater role in shoulders with rotator cuff deficiency: Kido et al (2000) showed that it acted as a humeral head depressor limiting upward translation not just at 90° but also at 0° and 45° of abduction in patients with a rotator cuff tear.

Clinically, function and biomechanics of the glenohumeral joint cannot be discussed in isolation. The glenohumeral joint assumes the required positions in space by the grace of scapular movement. Scapulothoracic movement in turn is made possible by adequate mobility and neuromuscular function in the acromioclavicular, sternoclavicular and upper thoracic joints, discussed in greater detail in Chapters 25 and 26. Adequate neuromuscular function of the scapulothoracic joint, thoracic posture and the degree of thoracic kyphosis also determine scapular movement (Ludewig & Reynolds 2009).

In the context of scapulothoracic contribution to shoulder motion, clinicians often refer to the scapulothoracic rhythm. At its least complex, a normal scapulothoracic rhythm has been defined as a scapula that remains stable during the initial 30° of shoulder abduction or 60° of flexion and then smoothly and continuously rotates upwards during elevation, followed by a smooth and continuous downward rotation when the arm moves back to neutral without evidence of scapular winging (Kelley 1995; McClure et al 2009). Normal relative contribution of glenohumeral and scapulothoracic motion to elevation motions of the shoulder are suggested to be 2:1, meaning that 120° occurs in the glenohumeral joint versus 60° in the scapulothoracic joint (Kelley 1995). However, research has shown that the exact contribution throughout motion has high inter-individual variability, is affected by adding resistance to motion and differs between active and passive motions (Kelley 1995; Ludewig & Reynolds 2009). This makes a reliable and valid clinical diagnosis of relevant scapulothoracic dyskinesis problematic. Using a more three-dimensional orthogonal biomechanical rather than a clinical perspective to describe motion, one can describe normal shoulder function as depending on the ability of the scapula to produce sufficient frontal plane upward rotation and sagittal plane posterior tilt during elevation motions (Fig. 27.3); in a transverse plane initially the scapula may internally rotate to some extent but in end range it is externally rotated (Ludewig & Reynolds 2009).

Pathology of the Rotator Cuff

When Neer (1972) classified impingement into stages I–III he described what is now known as primary impingement. In primary impingement the combination of repetitive overhead activity and external narrowing of the subacromial space is thought to be responsible for tendon injury. Mechanical compression occurs between the tendons and the coracoacromial arch. Causes of subacromial narrowing include acromial variants such as an unfused anterior acromial epiphysis or os acromiale, malunion or non-union after acromial fracture, and acromioclavicular separation or degeneration with inferior osteophytic spurring (Pyne 2004). Although acromial morphology, especially a type II or III acromion, has been suggested as a cause of primary impingement, prevalence of these variants increases with age and it has been suggested that they are traction spurs due to tension in the coracoacromial ligament resulting from rather than causing impingement (Shah et al 2001; Bunker 2002).

Secondary impingement is associated with glenohumeral instability. This primary instability has to be thought of as a continuum that ranges from minor or functional instability often indicated only by history findings to more pronounced instability that presents with physical examination and at times even imaging findings (Belling Sørensen & Jørgensen 2000). Congenital laxity, labral and rotator cuff tears, and

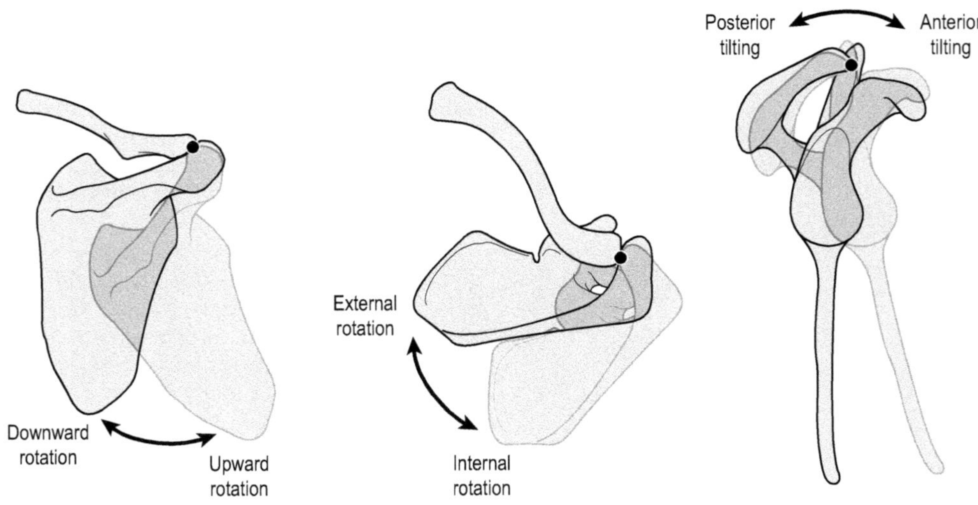

Figure 27.3 Scapular motions.

posterior glenohumeral capsular tightness have all been implicated in secondary impingement (Pyne 2004). Neuromuscular insufficiency (initially without musculotendinous lesions) can lead to decreased efficiency of the concavity compression mechanism. Probably indicative of insufficient active stabilization, glenohumeral proprioceptive acuity is decreased in patients with impingement (Machner et al 2003) but also with muscle fatigue in asymptomatic subjects, especially in the injury-prone late cocking position (Carpenter et al 1998; Tripp et al 2004). Neuromuscular insufficiency may go beyond decreased proprioception, coordination and endurance. Ganssen and Irlenbusch (2002) showed selective fast-twitch muscle fibre atrophy in the supraspinatus more than in the deltoid muscle with progressively worse rotator cuff lesions. Especially relevant for the active older population is that with age there seems to be an increase in muscle activity in the rotator cuff (infraspinatus and supraspinatus) and deltoid muscles required for shoulder motions (Gaur et al 2007). Higher demand may lead to earlier fatigue and impaired active stabilization in the elderly compared with younger subjects.

Reflecting the role of the glenohumeral joint as part of the multijoint shoulder girdle, scapular dyskinesis has been suggested as a cause for secondary but also internal impingement (Ludewig & Reynolds 2009). We have discussed above the role of the acromioclavicular, sternoclavicular and upper thoracic joints and the influence of increased thoracic kyphosis and thoracic flexion postures. Soft tissue tightness – as often found in, for example, the pectoralis minor muscle and the levator scapulae muscle – might result in inadequate posterior scapular tilt. We also need to consider the role of scapulothoracic neuromuscular fatigue and dyscoordination. Ludewig and Reynolds (2009) described decreased serratus anterior and increased upper trapezius muscle activity. External rotator fatigue significantly reduced scapular upward rotation, posterior tilt and external rotation during shoulder elevation, thereby decreasing the amount of subacromial space (Tsai et al 2003). Cools et al (2003) showed significant delays in muscle activation of the middle and lower trapezius muscle in subjects with impingement compared with asymptomatic controls. Indicating the possible role of pain-related inhibition in scapular dyskinesis, Falla et al (2007) demonstrated that an acute bout of upper trapezius pain was sufficient to result in altered motor control of this muscle, not only locally at the site of pain but also in non-painful regions within the muscle and on the contralateral side. A modification of motor strategy that results in compensatory muscle activity is likely to lead to muscle overload and perpetuate pain and dyskinesis.

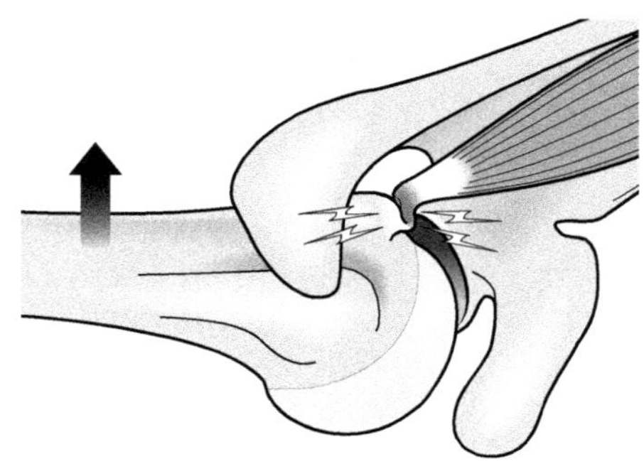

Figure 27.4 Posterosuperior glenoid impingement.

The most common type of internal impingement is posterosuperior internal impingement whereby the articular side of the supraspinatus tendon is impinged between the posterosuperior labrum and glenoid and the greater tuberosity (Fig. 27.4) (Belling Sørensen & Jørgensen 2000). This contact between the supraspinatus and the posterosuperior structures is actually a normal and physiological occurrence during abduction–external rotation, but it is likely that in higher level throwing athletes – perhaps secondary to concurrent minor instability or scapular dyskinesis – it may lead to fraying of the tendon and labrum, and symptoms are especially located in the posterior shoulder during the late cocking phase of throwing (Pyne 2004). It is of differential diagnostic relevance that shoulder pain in the late cocking phase may also be due to the overstretching of the subscapularis muscle. Myofascial trigger points in the subscapularis may produce referred pain in the posterior shoulder. Trigger points in the posterior deltoid and the teres minor muscle may also produce posterior shoulder pain owing to their concentric contraction in a shortened position during late cocking (Simons et al 1999).

Although very infrequently encountered in both authors' clinical practice, with anterosuperior internal impingement there is contact occurring between the biceps pulley and the anterosuperior labrum when the shoulder is flexed and internally rotated. This causes damage to the anterosuperior labrum, the tendon of the long head of the biceps, the biceps pulley, the superior part of the insertion of the subscapularis and sometimes the anterior fibres of the insertion of supraspinatus that are normally unaffected in degenerative or tensile rotator cuff lesions. Anterosuperior internal impingement may be responsible for the infrequent (4%) anterosuperior rotator cuff tear (Bunker 2002; Habermeyer et al 2004).

With coracoid impingement, the tendon of the subscapularis (and occasionally the long head of the biceps tendon) is impinged between the lesser tuberosity and the coracoid process. This impingement occurs especially during flexion, internal rotation and cross-body adduction of the shoulder. Coracoid impingement may occur after arthroscopy, glenoplasty, tenodesis of the long head of the biceps, acromioplasty, coracoid or glenoid fracture with malunion, but can also be related to congenital or acquired deformities of the humeral head or coracoid apophysis, anterior glenohumeral instability, and chronic overuse in a flexion–adduction–internal rotation position (Ferrick 2000; Radas & Pieper 2004).

Impingement can produce or contribute to lesions that vary across a spectrum ranging from inflammatory tendonitis, bursitis and degenerative tendinosis to partial- or full-thickness rotator cuff tears. We discussed earlier the stress riser at the junction of the thick leading edge and the weaker posterior two-thirds of the supraspinatus tendon, where most tears due to primary impingement initiate. Located some 7 mm behind the biceps pulley, an articular side rim-rent tear starts at this weak point and gradually peels back further off its insertion into the superior facet of the greater tuberosity until it emerges on the bursal side – and has thus evolved from a partial-thickness to a full-thickness tear. Decreased concavity compression allows for superior subluxation of the humeral head and secondary impingement. The cuff tear can either extend slowly over time or give way more suddenly with trauma, progressing from a small (<1 cm) to a moderate tear (1–3 cm). The superior capsule loosened from its humeral insertion contracts and pulls the cuff to which it is merged back towards the glenoid. As the coracohumeral ligament, which reinforces the superior capsule, retracts towards the coracoid it pulls the strong leading edge of the supraspinatus tendon with it. As the tear thus evolves into a large (3–5 cm) tear, the humeral head 'pops' up through the hole and causes an inferior subluxation of the leading edge of the supraspinatus tendon anteriorly and the infraspinatus tendon posteriorly.

Although the infraspinatus tendon rarely tears, it is hard to retrieve, even surgically, from behind the acromion and therefore many surgeons often assume it to be torn. Either way, in its new mechanically disadvantageous position and due to atrophy it becomes non-functional – making the question of whether or not it really tears a moot point. The tendon of the long head of the biceps starts to hypertrophy and fray. As the lesion extends into a massive tear (>5 cm), in some 16% of patients with cuff tearing the biceps pulley and the superior margin of the subscapularis also give way, which can lead to biceps tendon subluxation or even tearing, which thus removes one more stabilizing force in the rotator-cuff-deficient shoulder. As the humeral head subluxes anteriorly and superiorly through the now massive tear, arthritic changes between the humeral head and acromion may ensue. This leads to the end stage of cuff tear arthropathy, or Milwaukee shoulder, which is identified on a radiograph by massive rotator cuff calcifications (Bunker 2002; Hughes & Bolton-Maggs 2002). Isolated subscapularis tendon tears are very rare and may be solely associated with anterosuperior internal impingement (Bunker 2002) – although one might, with its impingement of the subscapularis, implicate coracoid impingement as well.

Although all above types of impingement would seem to strongly favour an extrinsic mechanical aetiology for rotator cuff lesions, intrinsic mechanisms are likely to also play a role, especially in the more chronic degenerative tendinopathies. As we have discussed, evidence for the role of hypovascularity as an intrinsic factor is equivocal. However, immobilization, age-related changes, genetic disorders, endocrine and metabolic influences, rheumatic diseases, nutritional deficiencies and tensile overload all need to be considered as relevant intrinsic factors in the aetiology of rotator cuff injuries. As these factors impact on prognosis they will be discussed in more detail in that section.

Diagnosis of Shoulder Impingement

Shoulder impingement often presents with a poorly localized pain in the anterior to lateral shoulder. The pain may be present at rest or at night, but is most pronounced with movement, especially overhead. Associated symptoms may include weakness, crepitus and stiffness. A history of repetitive overhead use in sports or work (e.g. throwing, painting, carpentry) may be elicited (Pyne 2004; Boyles et al 2009). Secondary and posterosuperior internal impingements occur mostly in athletes under 35 years of age engaging in overhead activity, such as throwing or racket sports, gymnastics and swimming (Belling Sørensen & Jørgensen 2000). Anterosuperior internal impingement is more prevalent in middle-aged men who are still active in sports, with pain especially on flexion and internal rotation movements (Bunker 2002). Chronic overuse in a flexion–adduction–internal rotation position, pain more consistently in midrange than in end range of shoulder flexion and tenderness indicated over the coracoid may all suggest coracoid impingement (Ferrick 2000).

Northover et al (2007) studied risk factors for primary impingement. Activities that increased the risk of primary impingement included occupations with heavy manual labour (OR 3.81; 95% CI 1.93–7.51) and / or overhead work (OR 3.83; 95% CI 2.15–6.84), weight-training (OR 2.39; 95% CI 1.07–5.05) and swimming (OR 1.98; 95% CI 1.11–3.53). Work involving hammering (OR 2.47; 95% CI 1.12–5.44) and using vibrating tools (OR 1.95; 95% CI 0.973–3.93) also increased the likelihood of impingement, but these risk factors may have not been independent risk factors but rather associated with heavy labour. A medical history that included diabetes (OR 3.34; 95% CI 1.26–8.85) and generalized osteoarthritis (OR 2.39; 95% CI 1.41–4.07) also served as a risk factor.

Generally, pain levels in patients with impingement are at best moderate and severe pain may indicate pathology requiring referral for medical diagnosis and (co)management, if for no other reason than adequate pain control. A build-up of calcium hydroxyapatite crystals within the tendon is characteristic of calcifying tendinopathy. In the shoulder, the supraspinatus tendon is most commonly affected, with deposits located 1–1.5 cm proximal to its humeral insertion. Although calcific deposits in the rotator cuff tendons are often asymptomatic, in cases of sudden-onset severe pain where the patient is reluctant to move the shoulder actively or passively and where increased temperature is noted on palpation the clinician needs to consider calcifying tendinopathy during its resorption phase. Symptoms are due to exudation of cells, rupture of the calcific deposit into the bursa, and vascular proliferation. This acute episode can last up to 2 weeks, whereas the subsequent subacute episode with pain and restricted movement lasts 3–8 weeks (Hughes & Bolton-Maggs 2002).

As data on diagnostic accuracy of history items are not available and the above-mentioned history items are obviously not very specific, the clinician needs to depend to a greater extent on physical examination. Patients with pathology ranging from impingement to massive tears have noted decreases in shoulder flexion and external rotation (at 0° and 90°) range of motion compared with the contralateral shoulder (McCabe et al 2005). Clinically both authors have also noted painfully decreased mobility in the hand-behind-the back test for the full spectrum of impingement.

A painful arc sign is defined as pain on active frontal or scapular plane elevation that is most pronounced during mid-range (60–120°). Sensitivity of the painful arc sign in the diagnosis of rotator cuff tears was 0.45–0.98 and for impingement the sensitivity was 0.33–0.71. Specificity for rotator cuff tears was 0.10–0.79 and for impingement it was 0.47–0.81 (Çalis et al 2000; Litaker et al 2000; Park et al 2005). Considering the wide range of diagnostic accuracy statistics, this sign can hardly be considered (as it often is) pathognomonic for rotator cuff lesions.

Rotator cuff lesions can affect findings on strength tests due to pain and / or tearing. Patients with the full spectrum of impingement have significant decreases in shoulder strength in abduction (at 10° and 90°), external rotation (at 90°) and on the empty can test (resisted scapular plane elevation with internal rotation) when compared with the contralateral shoulder. Note that weakness of greater than 50% compared with the other arm for abduction at 10° is indicative of a large or massive rotator cuff tear (McCabe et al 2005). Weakness on the empty can test, weakness on external rotation and a positive impingement sign provide a 98% (95% CI 89–100%) probability that a (partial- or full-thickness) rotator cuff tear is present. Any two of three positive tests in a patient aged over 60 also provide the exact same post-test probability of a rotator cuff tear (Murrell & Walton 2001).

Although Neer impingement test was originally described (Neer 1972) with a retest after subacromial anaesthetic infiltration (Northover et al 2007), in physical therapy literature this test is generally described as the clinician preventing scapular rotation with one hand while passively elevating the patient's arm in the scapular of sagittal plane. Pain at end range is considered to be a positive finding. The Hawkins–Kennedy impingement test involves the clinician facing the patient and raising the arm to 90° flexion, followed by internal rotation, with pain again considered a positive finding. Hegedus et al (2008) performed a meta-analysis of these tests and provided a pooled sensitivity of 0.79 (95% CI 0.75–0.82) and a pooled specificity of 0.53 (95% CI 0.48–0.58) for the Neer test; for the Hawkins–Kennedy test the pooled sensitivity and specificity were 0.79 (95% CI 0.75–0.82) and 0.59 (95% CI 0.53–0.64) respectively. As Dinnes et al (2003) also have indicated, this means that these special tests can be helpful in ruling out a diagnosis of impingement when negative, but not in diagnosing it when positive.

After eliminating diagnostic accuracy studies of insufficient methodological quality, Hegedus et al (2008) noted the external rotation lag sign as a specific test for infraspinatus tears (98%) (although, as noted above, the infraspinatus probably does not truly tear but rather subluxes and atrophies) or any rotator cuff tear (98%). For the external rotation lag sign the patient is seated and the clinician stands behind the patient. The patient's elbow is passively flexed to 90° with the shoulder at 90° of scapular plane elevation. The shoulder is placed in maximal external rotation, less 5° (to avoid elastic recoil in the joint). The patient is asked to maintain this position actively as the clinician releases the wrist while maintaining support of the arm at the elbow. The test is positive when lag or angular drop occurs.

The Hornblower or Patte sign was noted as specific (92%) for absence or severe degeneration of the teres minor (Hegedus et al 2008). For this test, the clinician supports the patient's arm at 90° of scapular plane elevation with the elbow also flexed to 90°. The patient is asked to rotate the forearm externally against the resistance of the clinician's hand. If he / she is unable to do this, the test is considered to be positive.

Hegedus et al (2008) noted the bear hug (92%) and belly press test (98%) as specific for subscapularis tears. For the bear hug test, the patient places the palm of the involved side on the opposite shoulder, with the fingers extended so that he / she cannot resist by grabbing the shoulder. The patient is asked to keep the hand on the opposite shoulder as the clinician then attempts to pull the hand off the shoulder with an external rotation force applied perpendicular to the forearm. The test is positive if the patient cannot hold the hand against the shoulder; a 20% deficit with a 5-second static strength test compared with the opposite side measured with a tensiometer has also been described as a positive finding (Barth et al 2006). The belly press test has the patient press a flat hand on the abdomen while maintaining maximal internal rotation at the shoulder. If the patient is unable to maintain active internal rotation and the elbow drops back behind the frontal plane, the test is considered positive.

With bicipital injury defined as a tear, instability or intrasubstance tendinopathy, Kibler et al (2009) reported the bear hug (79%) and upper cut test (73%) as the most sensitive. The belly press test was noted as the most specific (85%). The upper cut test also produced the highest positive likelihood ratio (3.38). The upper cut test is performed with the involved shoulder in a neutral position, the elbow flexed 90°, the forearm supinated and the patient making a fist. The patient is then asked to rapidly bring the hand up and towards the chin, mimicking an upper cut punch, as the clinician resists this motion with his / her hand on the patient's fist. Pain or a painful pop over the anterior portion of the shoulder indicates a positive test.

In young athletes with shoulder pain, Meister et al (2004) validated the posterior impingement sign whereby the shoulder is brought into 90–110° of abduction, 10–15° of extension and maximal external rotation. Pain reproduced in the posterior shoulder constitutes a positive finding. In this study, sensitivity and specificity for the diagnosis of a posterior labral and / or articular side rotator cuff tear were 75.5% and 85%, respectively. When only athletes with a gradual onset of pain were considered, sensitivity increased to 95% and specificity to 100%, making this the only test described in the literature with established diagnostic accuracy relevant to internal impingement. Although admittedly not validated and solely based on biomechanical extrapolation and clinical experience, the first author attached further diagnostic relevance to relief of posterior shoulder symptoms on adding a posterior glide (relocation) to the test position.

Medical diagnostic options include diagnostic anaesthetic infiltration and imaging (Pyne 2004). Imaging relevant for patients with impingement includes plain radiography, ultrasonography, magnetic resonance imaging (MRI) and magnetic resonance arthrography (MRA). Plain radiography shows calcific deposits in the rotator cuff tendons in 2.7–20% of asymptomatic adults. Calcific deposits at the edge of some full-thickness rotator cuff tears indicate poor prognosis. Massive calcifications, as in Milwaukee shoulder or cuff arthropathy, indicate end-stage rotator cuff disease and severe glenohumeral osteoarthritis (Bunker 2002; Hughes & Bolton-Maggs 2002). Sclerosis of the underside of the acromion and upper greater tuberosity together with superior migration of the humeral head may indicate the presence of a large-to-massive rotator cuff tear. Lesions associated with frank instability such as a Hill–Sachs lesion, acromioclavicular abnormalities narrowing the subacromial space, acromial or coracoid abnormalities and acromial shape can all be identified with plain radiography (Limb & Collier 2000; Pyne 2004).

Ultrasonography is portable and offers high resolution, the option of dynamic imaging and the ability to correlate imaging directly with physical findings, all at a relatively low cost (Pyne 2004). Dinnes et al (2003) did a systematic review of the literature on diagnostic accuracy of tests for soft tissue disorders of the shoulder including the rotator cuff. If partial- and full-thickness cuff tears were combined, sensitivity for ultrasound was 0.33–1.00 and specificity was 0.43–1.00. For full-thickness tears, both sensitivity and specificity were higher than for diagnosis of all tears combined, but ranges were still wide with sensitivity at 0.58–1.00 and specificity at 0.78–1.00. For detection of partial-thickness tears, the pooled sensitivity of ultrasonography was low (0.67; 95% CI 0.61–0.73) but specificity remained high (0.94; 95% CI 0.92–0.96). Ultrasound, therefore, can be used with greater confidence for diagnosing than for ruling out partial- and full-thickness rotator cuff tears.

For any tear, pooled sensitivity of MRI was 0.83 (95% CI 0.79–0.86) and specificity was 0.86 (95% CI 0.83–0.88). For diagnosis of partial-thickness tears, the pooled sensitivity was low (0.44; 95% CI 0.36–0.51) but specificity remained high (0.90; 95% CI 0.87–0.92) (Dinnes et al 2003). MRI can be used with confidence for diagnosing partial- and full-thickness tears and for ruling out full- but not partial-thickness tears. However, it should be noted that MRI produces many false positives. For example, Sher et al (1995) found that in asymptomatic individuals under the age of 40 nobody had a tear, whereas 4% of those between the ages of 40 and 60 years had a tear, and 24% of those over the age of 60 years had a tear. Milgrom et al (1995) showed a similar correlation between age and the incidence of asymptomatic rotator cuff tears. Further questioning the diagnostic relevance of MRI, Krief and Huguet (2006) reported no correlation between pain or function and size or location of rotator cuff tears on MRI.

In the diagnosis of full-thickness tears, MRA had a pooled sensitivity of 0.95 (95% CI 0.82–0.98) and a specificity of 0.93 (95% CI 0.84–0.97) – making it a useful tool both to diagnose and to rule out full-thickness tears. Despite limited research evidence, Dinnes et al (2003) noted that, for partial tears, the diagnostic accuracy of MRA exceeded that of ultrasonography or MRI.

Prognosis

Research on prognostic indicators for patients with impingement syndrome is very limited. Brox and Brevik (1996) reported on indicators for success or failure with treatment in patients with stage II impingement. The best independent prognostic indicators for success were active treatment in the sense of arthroscopic surgery or supervised exercise (4.8; 95% CI 1.7–13.6), not being on sick leave (4.4; 95% CI 1.6–12.1) and not being on regular medication (OR 4.2; 95% CI 1.5–11.1). Reported shoulder-related work demands did not impact on sick leave. Taking regular medication was a prognostic factor for treatment failure that was particularly high in those patients who had no disease apart from the painful shoulder (OR 17.0), which indicates the need for careful pharmacological management.

Under pathology we briefly discussed intrinsic causes for rotator cuff tendon pathology. In addition to a role in aetiology, these causes predisposing the rotator cuff to degenerative tendon lesions will probably also affect prognosis and management choices, although specific quantitative study into their prognostic relevance has not been done. Box 27.1 lists diseases and conditions associated with tendon degeneration relevant not only to the rotator cuff tendons but also to all tendons (Leadbetter 1992; Archambault et al 1995; Buckwalter 1995; Jósza & Kannus 1997; Curwin 1998; Almekinders & Deol 1999; Dahners & Mullis 2004; Virchenko et al 2004; Broughton et al 2006; Hansen et al 2008).

Management

Physical therapy management options for patients with impingement syndrome include education, modalities, exercise, manual therapy and also taping interventions. Common medical management includes non-steroidal anti-inflammatory medication (NSAIDs), subacromial steroid infiltration and arthroscopic or open subacromial decompression surgery.

Given the role of thoracic flexion on scapulothoracic motion, education with regard to appropriate posture seems to be an obvious component of patient education. Bullock et al (2005) noted a significant increase in patients with impingement for shoulder flexion range, although not pain intensity, with erect compared with slouched sitting posture.

Box 27.1 Prognostic factors: diseases and conditions associated with tendon degeneration

- Genetic disorders
- Ehlers–Danlos syndrome
- Marfan syndrome
- Osteogenesis imperfecta
- Homocystinuria
- Hypercholesterolaemia
- Hypertriglyceridaemia
- Aspartylglycosaminuria
- Haemochromatosis
- Menke syndrome
- Larsen syndrome
- Congenital muscle dystrophies
- Endocrine and metabolic diseases/conditions
- Diabetes mellitus
- Stress
- Overtraining
- Premature menopause
- Diminished oestrogen levels
- Premenopausal hysterectomy
- Oral contraceptive use (increased estradiol)
- Hyperthyroidism
- Hyperparathyroidism
- Renal disease
- Dialysis
- Rheumatic diseases
- Rheumatoid arthritis
- Seronegative spondylarthropathies
- Nutritional deficiencies
- Decreased levels of vitamin A
- Decreased levels of vitamin C
- Decreased levels of copper
- Medications
- Corticosteroids
- Indometacin
- Naproxen
- Parecoxib used during early tendon healing
- Immobilization
- Ageing

Visual, manual and verbal feedback combined with education on faulty movement patterns provided significantly decreased electromyographic activity in the upper and middle trapezius, infraspinatus, serratus anterior, and anterior and middle deltoid muscles of patients with impingement both immediately after and 24 hours after movement training, whereas trunk, shoulder and clavicular kinematics improved during and immediately after training, especially in the subset of patients with elevated clavicular position; this supports the role of educating patients on correct movement patterns (Roy et al 2009).

Taping patients may support retraining of correct movement patterns. However, using asymptomatic subjects Cools et al (2002) showed that tape application intended to inhibit the upper and facilitate the lower trapezius had no effect on electromyographic activity in the serratus anterior, or all three portions of the trapezius, with resisted or unresisted flexion and abduction of the shoulder. The authors suggested altered timing as a possible explanation for the clinically observed effects of taping. In contrast, Selkowitz et al (2007) did show in patients with subacromial impingement that similar taping decreased upper trapezius and increased lower trapezius activity during a functional overhead-reaching task, and that it decreased upper trapezius activity during shoulder abduction in the scapular plane. Mechanisms suggested to be involved in taping include facilitation or augmentation of proprioceptive cutaneous input, tension when movement occurs outside of the movement pattern allowed by the taping application, and inhibition or facilitation by taping shortened overactive muscles in a lengthened position, whereas the tape might be used to hold lengthened underactive muscles in a shortened position. Various taping techniques appropriate for patients with impingement have been described in the literature (Morrissey 2000; Kneeshaw 2002) (Fig. 27.5). Morrissey (2000) suggested that, when the positive effect on the movement pattern or on symptoms was maintained, taping could be discontinued.

Laser therapy was not demonstrated to be superior to placebo for patients with rotator cuff tendinopathy (Green et al 2003). Ultrasound (RR 1.81; 95% CI 1.26–2.60) and pulsed electromagnetic field therapy (RR 19; 95% CI 1.16–12.43) resulted in improvement compared with placebo in alleviating pain in patients with calcific tendinopathy. There is no evidence of an effect for ultrasound in patients with other tendinopathies, however. Ultrasound also provided no additional benefit when used in combination with exercise interventions over that obtained with exercise alone (Green et al 2003). There also is strong evidence that extracorporeal shockwave therapy is no more effective than placebo in patients with impingement, with regard to functional limitations (Faber et al 2006).

Exercise therapy interventions for patients with impingement are intended to restore the frontal and transverse plane glenohumeral force couples and normalize scapular motion. Generally they consist of progressive resistive exercises for the rotator cuff and scapular muscles and stretching of tight structures, but they should also address the motor control deficits identified in patients with impingement. More detail on shoulder exercises is provided in Chapters 32 and 33. Exercise interventions have been supported in a number of recent randomized trials (Werner et al 2002; Walther et al 2004; Lombardi et al 2008) and systematic literature reviews for producing improvements in both pain and function (Green et al 2003; Faber et al 2006; Trampas & Kitsios 2006). In a Cochrane review (Green et al 2003), exercise was noted as effective in terms of short-term recovery in rotator cuff disease (RR 7.74; 95% CI 1.97–30.32) and of longer term benefit with regard to function (RR 2.45; 95% CI 1.24–4.86). It should be noted that in patients with Neer stage I–II impingement there are no significant between-group differences (at 6 and 12 weeks) with regard to pain and function for patients treated with a supervised exercise programme or a home programme in

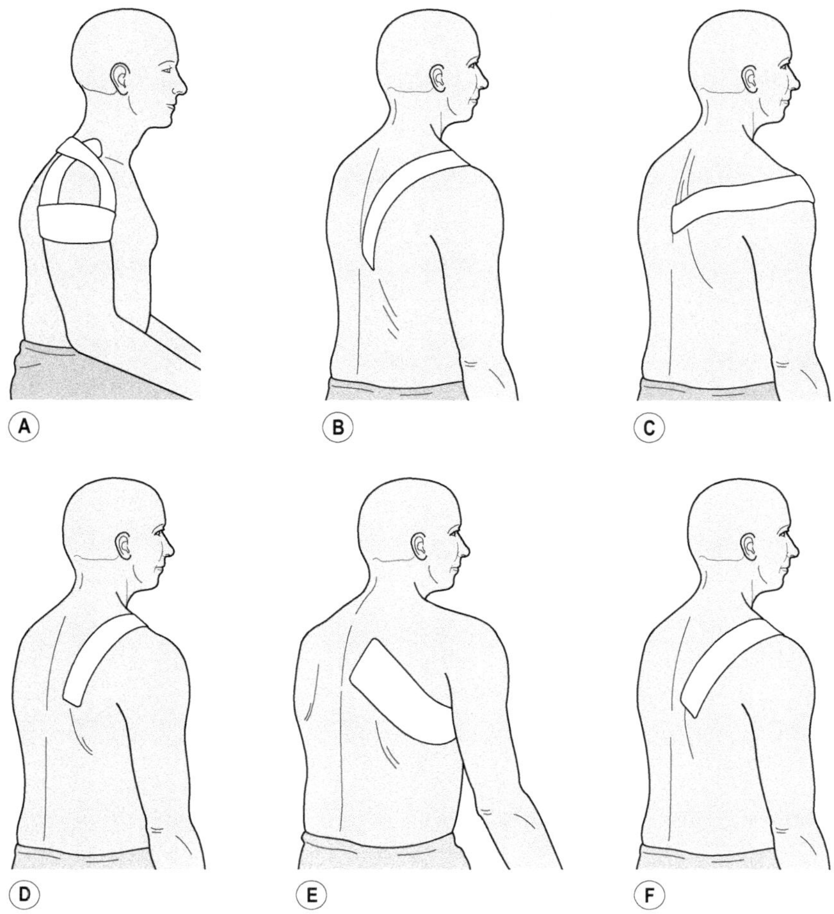

Figure 27.5 Taping techniques for the shoulder: (**A**) elevation of the shoulder girdle, (**B**) retraction/upward rotation, (**C**) retraction of the shoulder, (**D**) upper trapezius inhibition, (**E**) serratus anterior facilitation and inferior angle abduction, (**F**) acromioclavicular joint relocation.

which they are instructed by a physical therapist (Werner et al 2002; Walther et al 2004).

The presence and size of a full-thickness rotator cuff tear may limit potential for management with exercise and this underscores the importance of correct diagnosis. However, at least in a subset of patients with impingement, non-operative management is equally effective as open or arthroscopic decompression (Coghlan et al 2008). Haahr et al (2005) noted no between-group differences at 12 months for pain and function in patients treated with subacromial arthroscopic decompression or 19 sessions of rotator cuff and scapular strengthening augmented by thermotherapy and massage. Faber et al (2006) reported no significant difference between supervised exercise therapy and arthroscopic acromioplasty with regard to return to work status either at 6 months or at 2.5 years.

Some systematic reviews (Green et al 2003; Faber et al 2006) have supported a combination of manual therapy and exercise for patients with impingement in terms of improvements in pain and function. Manual therapy interventions may be appropriate for restrictions in the glenohumeral joint, shoulder girdle, cervical and thoracic spine, and ribs; these are discussed in more detail in Chapters 13, 14, 26 and 31.

Senbursa et al (2007) compared a home programme of rotator cuff and scapular strengthening exercises, active range of motion and stretching with 12 sessions of glenohumeral soft tissue and joint mobilization, ice application, stretching and strengthening exercises in patients with impingement. At 4 weeks there were significant between-group differences with regard to pain and function in favour of the manual therapy group. Kachingwe et al (2008) showed significant changes with regard to pain, pain-free range of motion, and function in patients with impingement treated with six sessions of supervised exercise only, supervised exercise with glenohumeral grade I–IV glide and traction mobilizations from midrange, supervised exercise with a Mulligan mobilization with movement (MWM) shoulder flexion technique, or a control group receiving only physician advice; there were no between-group differences. Although the statistical power in this pilot study was extremely limited, the three intervention groups had a greater improvement in function, and both manual therapy groups improved more with regard to pain measures. The active range of motion increased most for the MWM and least for the mobilization group.

Bergman et al (2004) compared medical care (consisting of oral analgesics or NSAIDs, education, advice, corticosteroid infiltrations and physical therapy referral for exercise, modalities, massage after 6 weeks) to medical care with up to six treatments of thrust and non-thrust manipulative interventions to the ribs and cervicothoracic spine over 12 weeks in patients with shoulder symptoms and dysfunction of cervicothoracic spine and adjacent ribs. At 12 weeks, 43% of the manipulation group and 21% of the medical care group reported full recovery. A 17-percentage point difference favouring manipulation still existed at 52 weeks. During intervention and at follow-up, consistent between-group differences in severity of the main complaint, shoulder pain and disability and general health favoured the manual therapy group.

Bang and Deyle (2000) showed significant between-group differences in function, pain and isometric strength of the shoulder in patients with impingement for a patient group that received thrust and non-thrust techniques to the glenohumeral joint, shoulder girdle, cervical and thoracic spine and ribs plus manual muscle stretching, massage and supervised exercise compared with a group receiving only the exercise intervention. Boyles et al (2009) showed significant within-group improvements at 48 hours for pain (measured with provocative shoulder and resisted tests and functional scores) in patients with impingement after receiving only mid-thoracic, cervicothoracic and rib thrust manipulation.

With regard to medical management, Green et al (2003) reported that, for rotator cuff disease, corticosteroid injections might at times be superior to physical therapy. Buchbinder et al (2003) noted that, for rotator cuff disease, subacromial steroid injection demonstrated a small benefit over placebo in some trials. The pooled results of three trials showed no benefit of subacromial steroid injection over NSAIDs. In the context of surgery, it should be noted that no significant differences have been reported in outcome between arthroscopic and open subacromial decompression, although four trials did report earlier recovery with arthroscopic decompression (Coghlan et al 2008).

Conclusion

Hegedus et al (2008) called impingement the final common pathway for all shoulder disorders, and we agree. It is not the diagnosis of impingement per se that is challenging, but rather elucidating the underlying aetiology. This requires a combination of clinical reasoning based on pathophysiological and patho-biomechanical extrapolation and a good command of relevant research knowledge, thereby epitomizing the evidence-informed paradigm. Future research is required with regard to clinical diagnosis of the various types of impingement discussed in this chapter, but also into implications of these various types on optimal patient management and on prognostic factors that can guide management decisions for patients at various points along the impingement spectrum.

References

Almekinders LC, Deol G. 1999. The effects of aging, anti-inflammatory drugs, and ultrasound on the in vitro response of tendon tissue. Am J Sports Med 27: 417–421.

Archambault DM, Wiley JP, Bray RC. 1995. Exercise loading of tendons and the development of overuse injuries, a review of current literature. Sports Med 20: 77–89.

Bang MD, Deyle GD. 2000. Comparison of supervised exercise with and without manual physical therapy for patients with shoulder impingement syndrome. J Orthop Sports Phys Ther 30: 126–137.

Barth JR, Burkhart SS, De Beer JF. 2006. The bear-hug test: a new and sensitive test for diagnosing a sub-scapularis tear. Arthroscopy 22: 1076–1084.

Belling Sørensen AK, Jørgensen U. 2000. Secondary impingement in the shoulder: an improved terminology in impingement. Scand J Med Sci Sports 10: 266–278.

Bergman GJD, Winters JC, Groenier KH, et al. 2004. Manipulative therapy in addition to usual medical care for patients with shoulder dysfunction and pain. Ann Intern Med 141: 432–439.

Biberthaler P, Wiedemann E, Nerlich A, et al. 2003. Microcirculation associated with degenerative rotator cuff lesions. J Bone Joint Surg 85A: 475–480.

Bigliani LU, Morrison DS, April EW. 1986. The morphology of the acromion and its relationship to rotator cuff tears. Orthop Trans 10: 228.

Boissonnault WG. 1999. Prevalence of comorbid conditions, surgeries, and medications in a physical therapy outpatient population: a multicentered study. J Orthop Sports Phys Ther 29: 506–525.

Boyles RE, Ritland BM, Miracle BM, et al. 2009. The short-term effects of thoracic spine thrust manipulation on patients with shoulder impingement syndrome. Man Ther 14: 375–380.

Broughton G, Janis JE, Attinger CE. 2006. Wound healing: an overview. Plast Reconstr Surg 117: 1eS–32eS.

Brox JI, Brevik JI. 1996. Prognostic factors in patients with rotator tendinosis (stage II impingement syndrome) of the shoulder. Scand J Prim Health Care 14: 100–105.

Buchbinder R, Green S, Youd JM. 2003. Corticosteroid injections for shoulder pain. Cochrane Database Syst Rev 1: CD004016. doi: 10.1002/14651858.CD004016.

Buckwalter JA. 1995. Pharmacological treatment of soft-tissue injuries. J Bone Joint Surg 77A: 1902–1914.

Bullock MP, Foster NE, Wright CC. 2005. Shoulder impingement: the effect of sitting posture on shoulder pain and range of motion. Man Ther 10: 28–37.

Bunker T. 2002. Rotator cuff disease. Curr Orthop 16: 223–233.

Çalis M, Akgün K, Birtane M, et al. 2000. Diagnostic values of clinical diagnostic tests in sub-acromial impingement syndrome. Ann Rheum Dis 59: 44–47.

Carpenter JE, Blasier RB, Pellizzon GG. 1998. The effect of muscle fatigue on shoulder joint position sense. Am J Sports Med 26: 262–265.

Carr A, Harvie P. 2005. Rotator cuff tendinopathy. In: Maffulli N, Renström P, Leadbetter WB (eds) Tendon injuries: basic science and clinical medicine. London: Springer, pp 101–118.

Chansky HA, Iannotti JP. 1991. The vascularity of the rotator cuff. Clin Sports Med 10: 807–822.

Choi CH, Kim SK, Jang WC, et al. 2004. Biceps pulley impingement. Arthroscopy 20: 80–83.

Clark JM, Harryman DT. 1992. Tendons, ligaments, and capsule of the rotator cuff: gross and microscopic anatomy. J Bone Joint Surg 74A: 713–725.

Codman EA. 1906. On stiff and painful shoulders: the anatomy of the sub-deltoid and sub-acromial bursa and its clinical importance. Sub-deltoid bursitis. Boston Med Surg J 154: 613–616.

Codman EA. 1934. The shoulder: rupture of the supraspinatus tendon and other lesions in or about the sub-acromial bursa. Boston: Thomas Todd.

Coghlan JA, Buchbinder R, Green S, et al. 2008. Surgery for rotator cuff disease. Cochrane Database Syst Rev 1: CD005619. doi: 10.1002/14651858.CD005619.

Cools AM, Witvrouw EE, Danneels LA, et al. 2002. Does taping influence electromyographic muscle activity in the scapular rotators in healthy shoulder? Man Ther 7: 154–162.

Cools AM, Witvrouw EE, Declerq GA, et al. 2003. Scapular muscle recruitment patterns: trapezius muscle latency with and without impingement symptoms. Am J Sports Med 31: 542–549.

Curwin SL. 1998. The aetiology and treatment of tendinitis. In: Harries M, Williams C, Stanish WD, et al. (eds) Oxford textbook of sports medicine. Oxford: Oxford University Press, pp 610–630.

Dahners LE, Mullis BH. 2004. Effects of non-steroidal anti-inflammatory drugs on bone formation and soft-tissue healing. J Am Acad Orthop Surg 12: 139–143.

Dierickx C, Ceccarelli E, Conti M, et al. 2009. Variations of the intra-articular portion of the long head of the biceps tendon: a classification of embryologically explained variations. J Shoulder Elbow Surg 18: 556–565.

Dinnes J, Loveman E, McIntyre L, et al. 2003. The effectiveness of diagnostic tests for the assessment of shoulder pain due to soft tissue disorders: a systematic review. Health Technol Assess 7(29): iii, 1–166.

Faber E, Kuiper JI, Burdorf A, et al. 2006. Treatment of impingement syndrome: a systematic review of the effects on functional limitations and return to work. J Occup Rehabil 16: 7–25.

Falla D, Farina D, Graven-Nielsen T. 2007. Experimental muscle pain results in reorganization of coordination among trapezius muscle subdivisions during repetitive shoulder flexion. Exp Brain Res 178: 385–393.

Ferrick MR. 2000. Coracoid impingement: a case report with review of the literature. Am J Sports Med 28: 117–119.

Ganssen HK, Irlenbusch U. 2002. Die neuromuskuläre Insuffizienz der Rotatorenmanschette ala Ursache des funktionellen Impingement: Muskelbioptische Untersuchungen am Schultergelenk. Z Orthop 140: 65–71.

Gaur DG, Shenoy S, Sandhu JS. 2007. Effect of aging on shoulder muscles during dynamic activities: an electromyographic analysis. Int J Shoulder Surg 1: 51–57.

Goldthwait JE. 1909. An anatomic and mechanical study of the shoulder joint, explaining many of the cases of painful shoulder, many of the recurrent dislocations and many of the cases of brachial neuralgia or neuritis. Am J Orthop Surg 6: 579–606.

Green S, Buchbinder R, Hetrick SE. 2003. Physiotherapy interventions for shoulder pain. Cochrane Database Syst Rev 2: CD004258. doi: 10.1002/14651858.CD004258.

Haahr JP, Østergaard S, Dalsgaard J, et al. 2005. Exercises versus arthroscopic decompression in patients with sub-acromial impingement: a randomized, controlled study in 90 cases with a one year follow up. Ann Rheum Dis 64: 760–764.

Habermeyer P, Magosch P, Pritsch M, et al. 2004. Anterosuperior impingement of the shoulder as a result of pulley lesions: a prospective arthroscopic study. J Shoulder Elbow Surg 13(1): 5–12.

Halder AM, Zhao KD, O'Driscoll SW, et al. 2001. Dynamic contributions to superior shoulder stability. J Orthop Res 19: 206–212.

Hansen M, Koskinen SO, Petersen SG, et al. 2008. Ethinyl oestradiol administration in women suppresses synthesis of collagen in tendon in response to exercise. J Physiol 586: 3005–3016.

Hegedus EJ, Goode A, Campbell S, et al. 2008. Physical examination tests of the shoulder: a systematic review with meta-analysis of individual tests. Br J Sports Med 42: 80–92.

Hughes PJ, Bolton-Maggs P. 2002. Calcifying tendonitis. Curr Orthop 16: 389–394.

Hurschler C, Wülker N, Mendila M. 2000. The effect of negative intra-articular pressure and rotator cuff force on gleno-humeral translation during simulated active elevation. Clin Biomech 15: 306–314.

Itoi E, Kuechle DK, Newman SR, et al. 1993. Stabilising function of the biceps in stable and unstable shoulders. J Bone Joint Surg 75B: 546–550.

Jósza L, Kannus P. 1997. Human tendons: anatomy, physiology, and pathology. Champaign, IL: Human Kinetics.

Kachingwe AF, Phillips B, Sletten E, et al. 2008. Comparison of manual therapy techniques with therapeutic exercise in the treatment of shoulder impingement: a randomized controlled pilot clinical trial. J Man Manip Ther 16: 238–247.

Kelley MJ. 1995. Biomechanics of the shoulder. In: Kelley MJ, Clark WA (eds) Orthopaedic therapy of the shoulder. Philadelphia: JB Lippincott.

Kibler WB, Sciascia AD, Hester P, et al. 2009. Clinical utility of traditional and new tests in the diagnosis of biceps tendon injuries and superior labrum anterior and posterior lesions in the shoulder. Am J Sports Med 37: 1840–1847.

Kido T, Etoi E, Konno N, et al. 2000. The depressor function of the biceps on the head of the humerus in shoulders with tears of the rotator cuff. J Bone Joint Surg 82B: 416–419.

Kneeshaw D. 2002. Shoulder taping in the clinical setting. J Bodyw Mov Ther 6: 2–8.

Krief OP, Huguet D. 2006. Shoulder pain and disability: comparison with MRI findings. Am J Radiol 186: 1234–1239.

Krupp RJ, Kevern MA, Gaines MD, et al. 2009. Long head of the biceps tendon pain: Differential diagnosis and treatment. J Orthop Sports Phys Ther 39: 55–70.

Leadbetter WB. 1992. Cell-matrix response in tendon injury. Clin Sports Med 11: 533–578.

Limb D, Collier A. 2000. Impingement syndrome. Curr Orthop 14: 161–166.

Lippitt S, Vanderhooft J, Harris S, et al. 1993. Gleno-humeral stability from concavity-compression: a quantitative analysis. J Shoulder Elbow Surg 2: 27–35.

Litaker D, Pioro M, Bilbeisi HE, et al. 2000. Returning to bedside: using the history and physical examination to identify rotator cuff tears. J Am Geriatr Soc 48: 1633–1637.

Lo IK, Burkhart SS. 2002. Sub-scapularis tears: arthroscopic repair of the forgotten rotator cuff tendon. Tech Shoulder Elbow Surg: 3: 282–291.

Lombardi I, Magri AG, Fleury AM, et al. 2008. Progressive resistance training in patients with shoulder impingement syndrome: a randomized controlled trial. Arthritis Rheum 59: 615–622.

Ludewig PM, Reynolds JF. 2009. The association of scapular kinematics and gleno-humeral joint pathologies. J Orthop Sports Phys Ther 39: 90–104.

Machner A, Merk H, Becker R, et al. 2003. Kinesthetic sense of the shoulder in patients with impingement syndrome. Acta Orthop Scand 74: 85–88.

McCabe RA, Nicholas SJ, Montgomery KD, et al. 2005. The effect of rotator cuff size on shoulder strength and range of motion. J Orthop Sports Phys Ther 35: 130–135.

McClure P, Tate AR, Kareha S, et al. 2009. A clinical method for identifying scapular dyskinesis. Part 1: Reliability. J Athl Train 44: 160–164.

Meister K, Buckley B, Batts J. 2004. The posterior impingement sign: diagnosis of rotator cuff and posterior labral tears secondary to internal impingement in overhand athletes. Am J Orthop 33: 412–415.

Milgrom C, Schaffler M, Gilbert S, et al. 1995. Rotator cuff changes in asymptomatic adults: the effect of age, hand dominance and gender. J Bone Joint Surg 77B: 296–298.

Morrissey D. 2000. Proprioceptive shoulder taping. J Bodyw Mov Ther 4: 189–194.

Moseley HF, Goldie I. 1963. The arterial pattern of the rotator cuff of the shoulder. J Bone Joint Surg 45B: 780–789.

Murrell GAC, Walton JR. 2001. Diagnosis of rotator cuff tears. Lancet 357: 769–770.

Neer CS. 1972. Anterior acromioplasty for the chronic impingement syndrome in the shoulder: a preliminary report. J Bone Joint Surg 54A: 41–50.

Northover JR, Lunn P, Clark DI, et al. 2007. Risk factors for development of rotator cuff disease. Int J Shoulder Surg 1: 82–86.

Park HB, Yokota A, Gill HS, et al. 2005. Diagnostic accuracy of clinical tests for the different degrees of sub-acromial impingement syndrome. J Bone Joint Surg 87A: 1446–1455.

Parsons IM, Apreleva M, Fu FH, et al. 2002. The effect of rotator cuff tears on reaction forces at the gleno-humeral joint. J Orthop Res 20: 439–446.

Picavet HSJ, Van Gils HWV, Schouten JSAG. 2000. Klachten van het bewegingsapparaat in de Nederlandse bevolking: prevalenties, consequenties en risicogroepen. Bilthoven: Centraal Bureau voor Statistiek.

Pyne SW. 2004. Diagnosis and current treatment options of shoulder impingement. Curr Sports Med Rep 3: 251–255.

Radas CB, Pieper HG. 2004. The coracoid impingement of the sub-scapularis tendon: a cadaver study. J Elbow Shoulder Surg 13: 154–159.

Rathbun JB, Macnab I. 1970. The microvascular patter of the rotator cuff. J Bone Joint Surg 52B: 540–553.

Rodosky MW, Harner CD, Fu FH. 1994. The role of the long head of the biceps muscle and superior glenoid labrum in anterior stability of the shoulder. Am J Sports Med 22: 121–130.

Roy JS, Moffett H, MacFadyen BJ, et al. 2009. Impact of movement training on upper limb motor strategies in persons with shoulder impingement syndrome. Sports Med Arthrosc Rehabil Ther Technol 1: 8.

Selkowitz DM, Chaney C, Stuckey SJ, et al. 2007. The effects of scapular taping on the surface electromyographic signal amplitude of shoulder girdle muscles during upper extremity elevation in individuals with suspected shoulder impingement syndrome. J Orthop Sports Phys Ther 37: 694–702.

Senbursa G, Baltasi G, Atay A. 2007. Comparison of conservative treatment with and without manual physical therapy for patients with shoulder impingement syndrome: a prospective, randomized clinical trial. Knee Surg Sports Traumatol Arthrosc 15: 915–921.

Shah NN, Bayliss NC, Malcolm A. 2001. Shape of the acromion: congenital or acquired. A macroscopic, radiographic, and microscopic study of acromion. J Shoulder Elbow Surg 10: 309–316.

Sher JS, Uribe JW, Posada A, et al. 1995. Abnormal findings on MRI of asymptomatic shoulders. J Bone Joint Surg 77B: 10–15.

Simons DG, Travell JG, Simons LS. 1999. Travell and Simons' myofascial pain and dysfunction: the trigger point manual. Vol. 1: Upper half of body, 2nd edn. Baltimore: Williams & Wilkins.

Trampas A, Kitsios A. 2006. Exercise and manual therapy for the treatment of impingement syndrome of the shoulder: a systematic review. Phys Ther Rev 11: 125–142.

Tripp BL, Boswell L, Gansneder BM, et al. 2004. Functional fatigue decreases 3-dimensional multi-joint position reproduction acuity in the overhead-throwing athlete. J Athl Train 39: 316–320.

Tsai NT, McClure PW, Karduna AR. 2003. Effects of muscle fatigue on 3-dimensional scapular kinematics. Arch Phys Med Rehabil 84: 1000–1005.

Urwin M, Symmons D, Allison T. 1998. Estimating the burden of musculoskeletal disease in the community. Ann Rheum Dis 57 649–655.

Van der Windt DA, Koes BW, De Jong BA, et al. 1995. Shoulder disorders in general practice: incidence, patient characteristics and management. Ann Rheum Dis 54: 959–964.

Virchenko O, Skoglund B, Aspenberg P. 2004. Parecoxib impairs early tendon repair but improves later remodeling. Am J Sports Med 32: 1743–1747.

Walther M, Werner A, Stahlschmidt T, et al. 2004. The sub-acromial impingement syndrome of the shoulder treated by conventional physiotherapy, self-training, and a shoulder brace: results of a prospective, randomized study. J Shoulder Elbow Surg 13: 417–423.

Werner A, Walther M, Ilg A, et al. 2002. Zentrierende Kräftigungstherapie beim einfachen subakromialen Schmerzsyndrom: Eigentrainung versus Krankengymnastik. Z Orthop 140: 375–380. [Article in German.]

Chapter 28

Glenohumeral Instability

Steven C. Allen, Russell S. VanderWilde, Peter A. Huijbregts

CHAPTER CONTENTS

Introduction	321
Anatomy	321
Biomechanics	322
Pathology	323
Diagnosis of glenohumeral instability	325
History	325
Examination	325
Stability tests	326
Laxity tests	326
Imaging	328
Prognosis	329
Clinical risk factors	329
Anatomical risk factors	330
Management of glenohumeral instability	330
Conclusion	331

Introduction

In Chapter 27, glenohumeral instability was discussed in the context of secondary impingement. In the authors' combined experience, patients presenting with shoulder pain often have underlying instability of the glenohumeral joint. However, glenohumeral instability presents a wide spectrum. At the one end of this spectrum is the minor instability (more appropriately classified as atraumatic, involuntary, recurrent, mostly anterior–inferior subluxation) with often only the history findings indicating its presence that responds well to conservative management. At the other end of the spectrum is the traumatic dislocation, at times with associated fractures and neurovascular or soft tissue damage, which often poses a surgical indication.

With regard to dislocation, Krøner et al (1989) reported an incidence of 0.17 per 1000 person-years in a general urban population. Owens et al (2009) reported an incidence in the general population of 0.08, versus 1.69 per 1000 person-years for military personnel. In about 98% of patients the shoulder dislocates anteriorly, whereas less than 2% of dislocations are posterior and only 0.5% are inferior (Walton et al 2002; Cicak 2004; Camarda et al 2009).

The glenohumeral joint can be unstable in anterior, posterior or multiple directions. Multidirectional instability (MDI) is symptomatic laxity in two or more directions, one of which is always inferior (Caplan et al 2007). It is important to distinguish instability from laxity, as the great majority of lax shoulders are not unstable (McFarland et al 2010). Objectively, laxity describes the extent to which the humeral head can be translated on the glenoid (Schenk & Brems 1998). In contrast, instability is an abnormal increase in glenohumeral translation that causes symptoms related to subluxation or dislocation. Shoulder instability becomes a clinically relevant pathology in the presence of: (a) abnormal and usually asymmetric laxity, (b) correlating symptoms, and (c) correlating pathological anatomy. When these three elements are present, an imbalance of the static and dynamic glenohumeral joint stabilizers occurs and the result is instability. Probably due to problems with definitive diagnosis, epidemiological data on shoulder instability are not available.

Many young athletic patients present to physical therapy with shoulder pain due to atraumatic, involuntary, recurrent, mostly anterior–inferior subluxation. However, therapists in a direct access role may also be confronted with patients with complaints at the other end of the spectrum and therefore need to be familiar also with the presentation of frank dislocations, so that they may recognize a patient in need of medical–surgical evaluation.

Anatomy

The anterior shoulder joint capsule has distinct bands, described as the superior (SGHL), middle (MGHL) and inferior (IGHL) glenohumeral ligaments. The humeral attachment of the SGLH lies just superior to the lesser tuberosity near the bicipital groove. The ligament courses anterior to the biceps tendon to attach to the anterosuperior labrum (Levine & Flatow 2000). The MGHL, the most variable (and at times absent) of the glenohumeral ligaments, arises from the humerus at the lesser tuberosity in association with the subscapularis tendon; its labral attachment lies just inferior to that of the SGHL. The humeral attachment of the inferior capsule or axillary pouch, which contains the anterior (AB-IGHL) and posterior (PB-IGHL) bands of the IGHL, runs from the 4 to the 8 o'clock position of the humeral head to attach

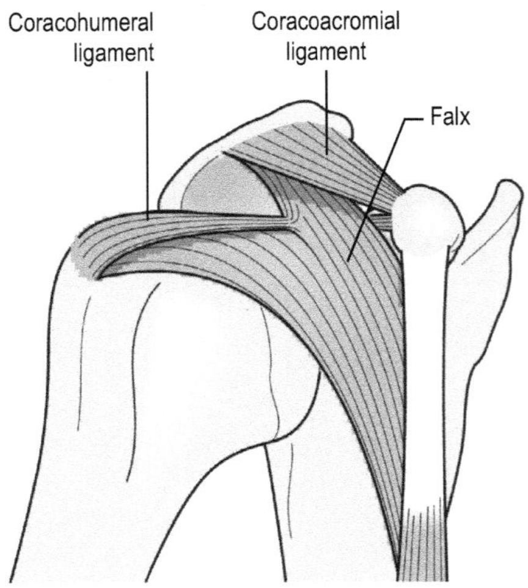

Figure 28.1 Falx attaching fibres of coracoacromial ligament directly to the conjoint tendon of the rotator cuff.

to the inferior labrum (Sugalski et al 2005). The posterior capsule extends from the PB-IGHL to the posterior band of the tendon of the long head of the biceps. It has been subdivided into the superior (SC), middle and posterior capsules. Although often assumed of minor biomechanical importance, it should be noted that the SC has a tissue thickness similar to that of the AB-IGHL (Bey et al 2005).

The coracohumeral ligament (CHL) arises from the lateral aspect of the coracoid process, and traverses horizontally beneath the coracoacromial ligament (CAL). It attaches to the greater and lesser tuberosities on each side of the bicipital groove. In the rotator interval between the inferior margin of the supraspinatus and the superior margin of the subscapularis, the CHL blends with the adjacent tendons and the underlying joint capsule. At the anterior joint capsule the anterior band of this ligament is superficial to and overlies the SGHL.

The CAL spans the superior aspect of the shoulder, running from the coracoid process to the anterior and inferior acromial processes. Lee et al (2001) described a falx or band of tissue that directly connects the fibres of the CAL to the conjoint tendon of the rotator cuff without attaching to the coracoid process (Fig. 28.1). In the rotator interval, the CHL is also connected via this falx to the CAL, and laxity or damage (also iatrogenic, as occurs during acromioplasty) to the CAL may compromise the tension in the CHL.

The intact labrum (discussed in detail in Ch 29) is fibrous throughout with a fibrocartilaginous transition zone at its attachment with the glenoid articular cartilage (Abboud & Soslowsky 2002). Firmly attached inferiorly and found to be looser superiorly and anteriorly, the labrum increases the depth of the glenohumeral socket by 50% (Cooper et al 1992). As noted above, it serves as the attachment sites for the glenohumeral ligaments and biceps tendon.

Biomechanics

All three bands of the glenohumeral joint capsule serve as the primary passive restraints to external rotation (Turkel et al 1981; O'Connell et al 1990). The SGHL contributes a primary restraint to external rotation in 0° of abduction. The CHL, intimate anatomically to the SGHL, also contributes a primary source of passive restraint to external rotation in this position (Neer et al 1992; Kuhn et al 2005). The MGHL is believed to be a more important contributor to anterior shoulder stability in 45° of abduction, possibly implicating it in midrange shoulder instability (O'Connell et al 1990; Kuhn et al 2005). Together the SGHL and CHL also limit inferior translation and posterior translation in the flexed, adducted and internally rotated shoulder (Levine & Flatow 2000).

The inferior portion of joint capsule acts as a 'hammock' that checks undue translation of the humeral head on the glenoid. In abduction, this entire complex moves beneath the humeral head and becomes taut. The AB-IGHL comes under the greatest tension in 90° of abduction, 10° of extension and end-range external rotation. The inferior complex moves anteriorly beneath the humeral head with external rotation limiting anterior translation (Levine & Flatow 2000). In cadaver tests of the AB-IGHL complex, the anterior drawer test at 60° abduction produced high strain at the insertion sites on both the humerus and glenoid. These two sites correspond to the most prevalent failure sites during tensile testing of the AB-IGHL; specifically the insertion site on the glenoid is a common site for an anterior labral tear (Bankart lesion). Kuhn et al (2005) reported that the entire IGHL, including the axillary pouch, was the most important restraint for external rotation in both positions of 15° and 60° abduction.

The PB-IGHL of the inferior recess comes under tension with abduction and internal rotation, as the complex moves posteriorly beneath the humeral head (Levine & Flatow 2000). The PB-IGHL has been implicated in the clinically observed stiff posterior shoulder. After the PB-IGHL, in the flexed and internally rotated shoulder the greatest tension is found in the posterior shoulder capsule, which indicates its role as another posterior stabilizer (Urayama 2001).

The CAL is a significant static stabilizer of the glenohumeral joint at lower elevations (Lee et al 2001). Previously it was thought to have no functional importance and surgically released during acromioplasty; however, compromise of the CAL allows for increased anterior and inferior translation of the internally and externally rotated shoulder in 0° and 30° of abduction, which indicates the potential for iatrogenic instability after acromioplasty.

The intact labrum contributes to the centring of the humeral head on the glenoid, and damage to the anteroinferior labrum allows migration of the humeral head towards the site of lesion. Fehringer et al (2003) concluded that precise centric position of the glenohumeral joint is well served by an intact labrum, especially in the midranges where the majority of ligaments are lax. The glenohumeral labrum elevates the glenoid edge, contributing to shoulder stability by effectively doubling the depth of the glenoid socket and serving as a 'chock block' to translation (Walton et al 2002), adding as much as 20% to the resistance to translation forces (Abboud & Soslowsky 2002). (In Chapter 27 the role of the labrum in the concavity compression mechanism contributing to glenohumeral stability was discussed.)

Stability, of course, is not solely provided by passive restraints. The transverse (subscapularis, infraspinatus and teres minor) and frontal plane (supraspinatus and deltoid) force couples of the concavity compression mechanism function as local stabilizers (Parsons et al 2002). Both the rotator cuff muscles and the prime movers of the shoulder provide muscle force vectors to the glenohumeral joint that have compressive and shear components (Lee et al 2000). The directions of these force vectors change substantially from 0° to 90° abduction, although the compressive component provided by the rotator cuff is consistently much larger than its shear component. The shear component can potentially stabilize or destabilize the joint, depending on its direction. The infraspinatus and teres minor generate a posterior shear in the late cocking phase of throwing, thereby contributing to anterior shoulder stabilization, whereas the supraspinatus generates a large anterior shear force in end range, thus destabilizing the joint in the anterior direction (Lee et al 2000). The pectoralis major similarly provides an anterior destabilizing force in the late cocking position (Labriola et al 2005). The latissimus dorsi and teres major produce more effective inferior shear forces than do infraspinatus and subscapularis; the role of the supraspinatus in this regard is only minimal (Halder et al 2001b). (In Chapter 27 the equivocal evidence on the role of the long head of the biceps tendon in stabilization was discussed.) The deltoid is a significant contributor to anterior stability in the position of apprehension, with all three heads contributing equally to stabilization (Kido et al 2003). The lateral deltoid is a key muscle restraint to inferior glenohumeral instability (Halder et al 2001a).

Pathology

Avulsion of the glenoid labrum in the anteroinferior quadrant, called a Bankart or Perthes lesion, is the most common pathology seen in anterior shoulder dislocation. It is disruption of the IGHL, and not solely the Bankart lesion, that is thought to allow for dislocation (Robinson & Dobson 2004). Bigliani et al (1992) showed that an intrasubstance ligament injury occurs before labral avulsion. An isolated IGHL injury renders the glenohumeral joint very unstable, even with intact dynamic stabilizers. The typical mechanism for anterior dislocation in the younger patient is indirect trauma to the abducted, extended and externally rotated arm, which occurs most commonly in overhead sports activities (Bohnsack & Wulker 2002). Primary anterior dislocation of the shoulder occurs commonly after low-energy falls in the elderly (Robinson & Dobson 2004). An impression fracture of the posterolateral humeral head, called a Hill–Sachs lesion, is also present in most patients with anterior instability (Cicak 2004; Robinson & Dobson 2004).

At less than 2% of all dislocations, dislocation in a posterior direction is uncommon. Posterior dislocation can be caused by a fall onto the outstretched arm, a weight 'getting away' from a weightlifter at terminal extension of a bench press, a football lineman unable to hold off an opponent with forces axially transmitted through the forward flexed arms, or a hockey player attempting to slow down velocity of a hit into the boards. It may also result from epileptic seizure or electric shock. Posterior dislocation may be associated with fractures of the surgical neck of the humerus or fractures of the tuberosities. Posterior shoulder dislocations with posterior labral detachment (reverse Bankart lesion) and a humeral anteromedial impression fracture (reverse Hill–Sachs lesion) need to be considered for surgery. Indications for surgical repair include recurrent subluxations or dislocations, or mechanical symptoms despite adequate rehabilitation (Seebauer & Keyl 1998; Cicak 2004; Kim et al 2005).

At 0.5% of all dislocations, inferior dislocations are even less common. Mechanisms of injury include direct axial loading through the humerus – as might occur when the patient tries to catch hold of something overhead when falling from a height. The other mechanism is violent forced abduction of an already-abducted shoulder. Impingement of the neck or proximal shaft of the humerus against the acromion levers the humeral head inferiorly out of the glenoid. The term 'luxatio erecta' refers to the presentation of patient with the arm abducted, elbow flexed, forearms pronated and hand above the head unable to lower the arm to the side. Associated injuries may include fractures of the acromion, clavicle, coracoid process, greater tuberosity and humeral head. Associated vascular injuries to the axillary vessels are often serious and require surgery, but are less common than axillary, radial or ulnar nerve, or brachial plexus injuries that mostly recover well, indicating their neuropraxic nature (Baba et al 2007; Camarda et al 2009). Mallon et al (1990) reviewed 80 cases and reported greater tuberosity fracture or rotator cuff injuries in 80%, neurological involvement in 60% and vascular compromise in 3.3% of cases.

Posterior subluxation is attributed to posterior compressive or tensile loading and forced hyperadduction (Robinson & Dobson 2004; Kim et al 2005) with pain attributed to excessive translation into the posterior recess. Recurrent posterior shoulder subluxation as a clinical entity has become increasingly recognized as a less common (2–5%) but important contributor to shoulder instability (Eckenrode et al 2009). A single traumatic event or repetitive cumulative trauma, as may occur in contact sports with high-energy forces directed to the posterior capsule, may lead to posterior glenohumeral instability. Glenoid retroversion and weakness of the external rotators have also been identified as potential contributors (Eckenrode et al 2009).

Excessive anterior translation of the humeral head during abduction–external rotation leads to plastic deformation of the AB-IGHL and anterior glenohumeral joint subluxation. This would also indicate that the degree of excessive laxity commonly found in the shoulder of throwing athletes might be on a progressive track of excessive motion and translation leading to symptoms that eventually manifest in labral injury and / or partial-thickness rotator cuff tears (Kuhn et al 2003). However, laxity and hypermobility are not instability and in fact are prerequisites for achieving higher degrees of speed and torque in the throwing shoulder (Huijbregts 1998). Considering its frequent association with anterior shoulder instability and subluxation, we believe it is important to review the various phases of overhead throwing and apply clinical reasoning to the kinetic chain to allow for the diagnosis of possible relevant patho-biomechanical faults.

The overhead throw (e.g. of a cricket ball) has five phases: wind-up, early cocking, late cocking phase, acceleration and follow-through (Fig. 28.2). The wind-up phase in the overhead baseball pitch is a preparatory phase, centred on flexion. A right-handed thrower has a flexion pattern of the left lower extremity with considerable hip and knee flexion. There also will be a flexion movement of the spine. Both hands are in contact with the ball and the shoulders are in

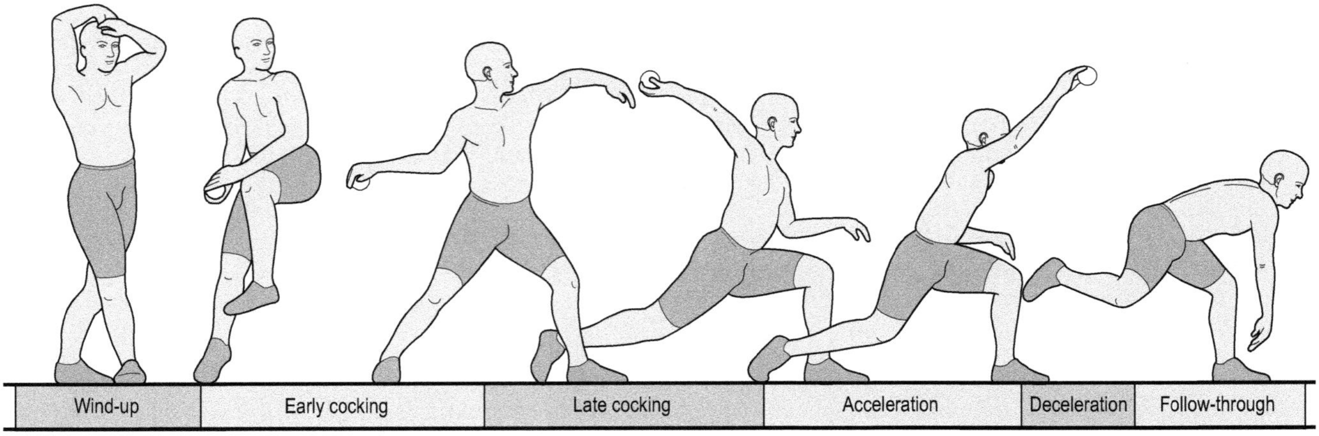

Figure 28.2 Five phases of the overhead-throwing motion.

an internal rotation–adduction position with bilateral elbow flexion. The pitcher is facing the batter with the left side of the body. Early cocking starts when the left hand loses contact with the ball. The right shoulder moves from adduction and internal rotation to abduction and external rotation. The pitcher steps with the previously flexed left leg in the direction of the batter, and the trunk moves into extension, right rotation and left side-bending. The late-cocking phase starts when the left foot of the pitcher hits the ground. This is the start of a derotation movement of the trunk and legs that will contribute to accelerating the ball. The right arm and ball still move in the same direction of horizontal abduction and external rotation.

Acceleration starts with the switch-over from shoulder external rotation to shoulder internal rotation. This rotation is the most important movement of the acceleration phase. In this phase, the shoulder also moves from horizontal abduction to horizontal adduction and back in the direction of horizontal abduction just prior to ball release. Ball release by the right hand marks the end of acceleration. The arm, which has been immensely accelerated for the throwing motion, now has to be decelerated. The left lower extremity moves into flexion and the trunk into flexion and left rotation. The right arm is moving into adduction and internal rotation. The first part (deceleration) of the follow-through phase is marked by high activity in the muscle complex of the right shoulder, with the second part of follow-through requiring adequate trunk and lower extremity movement to decrease the force requirements about the shoulder and reduce the potential for injury (Huijbregts 1998). The overhead throw is an extremely fast activity. Fleisig et al (1995) measured an average time of 0.139 ± 0.017 s from foot contact to ball release, a period that corresponds to the late cocking and acceleration phases combined.

Two critical instants are identified in the overhead throw that place unusually high demands on the shoulder complex. The first phase identified in late cocking reveals high torsional and compressive loads to the shoulder that may well exceed the plastic limit of the anteroinferior capsuloligamentous complex, resulting in pain and instability in this quadrant. The second critical instant occurs just after ball release in the early deceleration phase. Although torsional loading is significantly reduced and shear forces to the anterior restraints are low in this phase of throwing, the compressive loading to the shoulder joint is highest at 1100 N, constituting a more than 100% increase from compression during the first critical instant. Any unwanted translation of the humeral head in the presence of these compressive forces has the potential to produce damage to the capsule, the closely associated rotator cuff tendons and the labrum. Enormous demands are placed on both the active and passive restraints of the shoulder with – in addition to these high torques and forces – an external rotation range of motion of 140° at the end of late cocking, an internal rotation angular velocity of 7000° / s during acceleration and an angular deceleration of 500 000° / s^2 during deceleration (Huijbregts 1998).

In a throwing athlete with glenohumeral instability, the clinician should not limit the search for causative or contributory dysfunctions to the shoulder joint or even the shoulder girdle. As an example of relevant lower quadrant dysfunctions, a right sacral torsion present at left foot contact in the acceleration phase may lead to excessive compensation in the shoulder to attain the required arm velocity for competitive throwing. Also maximal lumbar extension and right-side bending are required in this phase of throwing, implying that an unresolved, chronic right posterolateral disc lesion may also place excessive demand on the shoulder girdle, as trunk motion in this quadrant may be limited. This same disc lesion in a more irritable back problem would compromise the derotation and deceleration of the throwing arm where flexion and left rotation of the trunk are required.

The overhead athlete may also be vulnerable in cases of lumbar instability or an increase in the neutral zone of a spinal motion segment (Panjabi 1992). If this instability is in a rotational plane to the right in the overhead thrower, the critical zone of acceleration may result in compensation higher up in the kinetic chain and subsequent injury to the glenohumeral joint. Unilateral weakness of the multifidus muscles of the lumbar spine may lead to subsequent atrophy in patients with unilateral back pain (Hides et al 1996). Asymmetrical contraction of this group of segmental muscles would result in torsional loading with excessive translation of the spinal motion segment and loss of form closure in the lumbosacral region (Lee 1989) – again exposing the glenohumeral joint higher up the kinetic chain to excessive shear or compression. A higher incidence of osteoarthrosis in the opposite hip from the throwing side in retired javelin throwers (Schmitt et al 2004) suggests the need to tolerate high torsional forces on the left hip in the right-handed overhead athlete. Weakness in the deep left hip rotators or gluteus medius in the deceleration phase of throwing or limited hip rotation mobility would be likely to compromise the safety margin for attenuating force requirements on the throwing shoulder that the contribution of the hip muscles in this phase would otherwise offer.

With regard to upper quadrant dysfunctions, scapular dynamics require adequate upward rotation, abduction and posterior tilting for optimal shoulder function in the throwing athlete (Magarey & Jones 1992). Muscle imbalances between the upper trapezius and serratus anterior may manifest in scapular winging owing to serratus anterior inhibition (Sahrmann 2002), thus compromising the well-coordinated movement of the scapula and humerus and the maintenance of centric position of the humeral head on the labrum. A hypertonic or stiff levator scapulae muscle, due to C4 facilitation from a cervical spine joint dysfunction, would tilt the scapula into downward rotation and inhibit the 'chock-block' mechanism offered by the labrum (Fowler & Pettman 1992; Walton et al 2002). This would increase strain in the structures, limiting inferior and anterior translation of the humeral head. The upper thoracic spine requires adequate rotation and side-bending to the right in a right-handed thrower. Hypomobility in this region of the thoracic spine is common and will directly impact the degree of stress placed on the anterior restraints to the glenohumeral joint.

Diagnosis of Glenohumeral Instability

Although it would be hard to imagine that a clinician would not recognize a luxatio erecta, the much more common patient with minor instability is much harder to diagnose, and even most posterior dislocations are missed on initial examination (Cicak 2004).

History

Patients with shoulder instability most often present with pain as their primary complaint. Somatic pain described as deep, aching and intermittent and located in the anterior or posterior shoulder joint is common. Trauma may suggest dislocation that may have spontaneously reduced, especially when in an anterior direction. In the section on pathology, we discussed mechanisms of injury that should make the clinician consider anterior, posterior and inferior dislocations. As noted above, posterior dislocations are often missed on initial examination, with the patient complaining only of subjective instability and pain with flexion, adduction and internal rotation (Cicak 2004).

In the introduction, we discussed how in physical therapy the commonly used diagnosis of minor instability would be more appropriately classified as atraumatic, involuntary, recurrent, mostly anterior–inferior subluxation. This type of instability is much more common, but hard to diagnose definitively. It is most often seen in young overhead-throwing athletes or gymnasts. Trauma may play a role, but is often more of a cumulative type with previous minor episodes of injury. Magarey and Jones (1992) have suggested the following (non-validated) history findings as indicative of minor shoulder instability: (1) apprehension with certain movements, (2) sensation of the joint slipping in and out, (3) pain worse with overhead activity, (4) painful catches through range, (5) painful intra-articular clicking or 'dead arm syndrome' during late cocking, (6) weakness in the late cocking position. Note, however, that at least some of these symptoms can hardly be considered specific; Schenk and Brems (1998) noted that patients with MDI might also present with pain in midrange positions.

Examination

As indicated above, the examination of a patient with shoulder instability should not be limited to the shoulder girdle but also include a search for causative or contributory dysfunctions throughout the kinetic chain in the upper and lower quadrants. Specific to the shoulder, though, a scanning examination must include assessment of three-dimensional posture. Winging of the scapula at rest and in 90° abduction can be appreciated with a posterior view and it indicates the need for specific muscle strength and flexibility tests. A side view may suggest muscle length restriction in the pectoralis minor, as evidenced by a shoulder held in protraction and elevation with scapular inferior border winging. A patient with an unreduced anterior or inferior dislocation may present with the humeral head visible and palpable on the chest wall out of the glenoid socket. Patients with unreduced posterior dislocation may present with the arm held and fixed in adduction and internal rotation.

Active range of motion in cardinal planes with overpressure and discrete resistance to muscles while on stretch (Cyriax 1978), as well as combined motions, are initial tests for provocation and assessing integrity. Easy to spot are patients with luxatio erecta, who are not able to lower their arms from the elevated position (Camarda et al 2009). Patients with posterior dislocation may have the humeral head caught on the posterior glenoid rim, thus locking the shoulder between 10° and 60° of internal rotation with no external rotation possible from this position (Cicak 2004). Should this initial screen not provoke the patient's symptoms, the clinician may suspect a remote source, including referred mechanical pain from the cervical spine or a non-mechanical aetiology. Note that, unless there has been recent trauma, there may well be a full or nearly full range of motion in the shoulder girdle. A neurovascular examination for compromise, especially in the patient with a possible dislocation, will complete the seated examination. Close inspection of the scapula from a posterior viewpoint during arm elevation will be helpful in the investigation of abnormal rhythm, lack of upward rotation and abduction, or medial border winging, as discussed in Chapter 32.

Magarey and Jones (1992) have suggested the following (non-validated) physical examination findings as indicative of minor instability: (1) excessive mobility or loss of normal end feel on instability tests with or without apprehension or intra-articular click, (2) full or excessive range of motion with end-range pain, (3) loose end feel with less of a ligamentous character, (4) external rotation at 90° abduction that is either limited by spasm or shows excessive range, (5) pain-free and strong rotator cuff contractions with the exception of an often-weak but pain-free infraspinatus. Again, though, note that many of these findings may not be very specific.

Stability tests

Special tests for clinical instability of the glenohumeral joint fall into two categories (Levy et al 1999; Ellenbecker et al 2002; Tibone et al 2002). Stability tests use provocation, apprehension and end feel to determine joint integrity towards end range, whereas laxity tests examine the mobility of a joint in functional and midranges of motion. Bahk et al (2007) concluded that special tests can add significantly to our assessment of the unstable shoulder but findings on clinical laxity examination and relevance to instability must be placed in perspective. If findings 'fit' they confirm and solidify the diagnosis. If findings on these tests do not fit with other history and examination findings, laxity alone means nothing except a 'loose shoulder', which is not a diagnosis but rather a physical exam finding. In the clinic of the second author, throwing-related MDI is often superimposed upon an already genetically loose shoulder capsule that subsequently becomes too loose and 'decompensates'. An important paradox is that it is partly the genetic laxity that initially allows these athletes to succeed at a high level in overhead athletic events such as throwing. Once they decompensate, however, the original advantage becomes a disadvantage.

Apprehension test

The patient is supine on the table, with the glenohumeral joint at the edge of the table but the scapula supported by the table. The patient's shoulder is at 90° of abduction, the elbow is flexed to 90° and the examiner's knee supports the elbow to prevent extension of the shoulder. The examiner then applies external rotation progressively until the patient can tolerate no further rotation, and the degree of rotation is recorded. In patients with anterior instability, a patient's report of apprehension and a feeling that the shoulder will come out of joint is considered to be a positive test. Some authors note that pain in this manoeuvre may be indicative of more subtle anterior instability. Sensitivity for this test for the diagnosis of traumatic anterior instability has been established at 52.78% and specificity at 98.91% (Lo et al 2004).

Relocation test

First described by Jobe et al (1989), the relocation test comprises the application of a posterior force to the humeral head in the position of apprehension as recorded in the above test; it is positive if it relieves the symptoms of apprehension. Although Lo et al (2004) proposed this test to differentiate a subtle instability in the overhead athlete from rotator cuff impingement, if pain was experienced in the apprehension test and improved with the relocation test the sensitivity and specificity with production and subsequent reduction of pain were both low – at 40% and 42.65% respectively. However, when considering solely diminished apprehension as a positive test finding, specificity was 100% for anterior shoulder instability – although sensitivity stayed low at 31.94%. Reduction of symptoms is usually associated with an increase in external rotation range.

Surprise (release) test

In this test, while holding the final position of the relocation test, the examiner's hand is quickly removed from the proximal humerus and the patient's response elicited. A positive test is indicated by a sudden return of the symptoms noted with the apprehension test. The surprise test was reported to have a sensitivity of 63.89% and specificity of 98.91% for the diagnosis of anterior instability (Lo et al 2004). Note, though, that the surprise test puts the shoulder into a more vulnerable position of greater external rotation than does the apprehension test. For this reason, to perform the surprise test safely and accurately we recommend that the apprehension and relocation tests be performed first. This will give the examiner an initial impression of where the patient feels vulnerable and thus allows careful placement of the posterior-directed force so as to apply and release it within the patient's comfort level. If the clinician performs a surprise test immediately this may not only startle the patient but also can acutely dislocate the shoulder.

Posterior shoulder instability has typically been examined with a load-and-shift test producing posterior translation, or by posterior joint line tenderness (Eckenrode et al 2009). Patients may also have a positive jerk test. This test is performed with the patient supine, and the arm to be tested in 90° abduction and internal rotation. An axial load is then applied as the arm is brought into horizontal adduction. The test is positive if the manoeuvre produces a palpable or audible clunk, as well as pain. Sensitivity and specificity were reported to be 73% and 98% respectively, in the diagnosis of a postero-inferior labral lesion (Kim et al 2005).

Laxity tests

Motion in any simple plane of the glenohumeral joint results in coupled motion in two additional planes. A strain-gauge analysis of the glenohumeral ligaments showed that, for each ligament tested, a tension-sharing relationship existed with transfer of tension among all ligaments (Terry 1991). Still, Fowler & Pettman et al (1992), in their teaching at the North American Institute of Orthopaedic Manual Therapy (NAIOMT), have proposed that the capsuloligamentous complex of the glenohumeral joint be tested in serial fashion to discriminate the predominant site of injury or loss of integrity. Using an electronic digital ruler, Sharp and Kisser (unpublished research 2009), in a physical therapy doctoral capstone research project at Andrews University in Berrien Springs, Michigan, provided preliminary validation for the selective tensioning suggested as the rationale for the following NAIOMT tests for the SGHL, MGHL and AB-IGHL.

NAIOMT SGHL / CHL test

With the patient supine, and the shoulder to be tested at the edge of the examination table with the scapula supported on the table, the shoulder is placed in 0° abduction and end-range external rotation is followed by an anterior glide of the proximal humerus (Fig. 28.3) so as to test the SGHL and the posterior or lateral band of the CHL. If the arm is now allowed to move into 10° extension, the anterior or medial band of the CHL comes more under tension (Fig. 28.4).

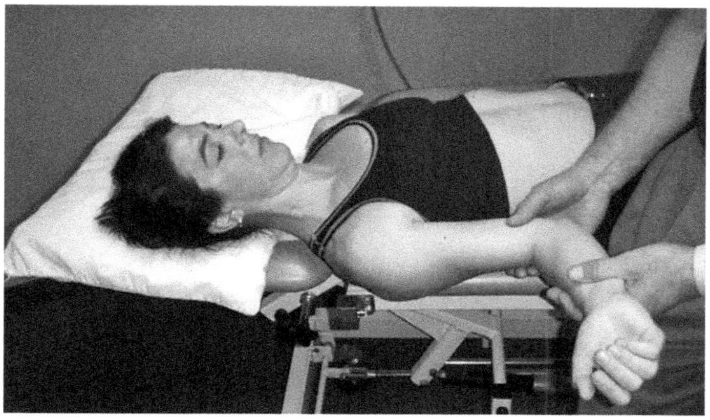

Figure 28.3 **NAIOMT SGHL / posterior CHL test.**

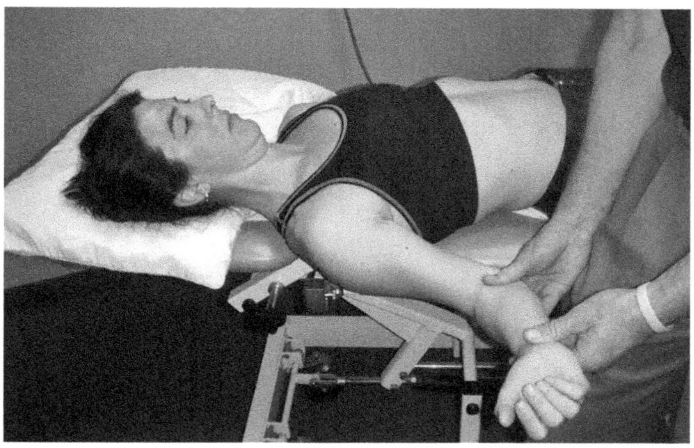

Figure 28.4 **NAIOMT SGHL / anterior CHL test.**

NAIOMT MGHL test

From the test position of 0° abduction, 10° extension and end-range external rotation, the examiner now moves the arm to 45° abduction and then applies an anterior medial glide in the plane of the glenohumeral joint surface (Fig. 28.5) to test the MGHL.

NAIOMT IGHL test

From the MGHL test position, the examiner now moves the arm to 90° abduction and applies an anterior medial glide to the proximal humerus to test the AB-IGHL (Fig. 28.6). The PB-IGHL is tested with the arm maintained in this position of 90° abduction and 10° extension, but now with full internal rotation, and a posterior lateral glide applied to the gleno-humeral joint (Fig. 28.7) (Fowler & Pettman 1992; Levine & Flatow 2000).

NAIOMT posterior capsule test

The examiner brings the arm to 90° flexion, followed by full internal rotation, then end-range horizontal adduction, and finally applies an axial stress to the proximal humerus in a postero- lateral direction to test the posterior capsule (Fig. 28.8) (Fowler & Pettman 1992; Urayama 2001).

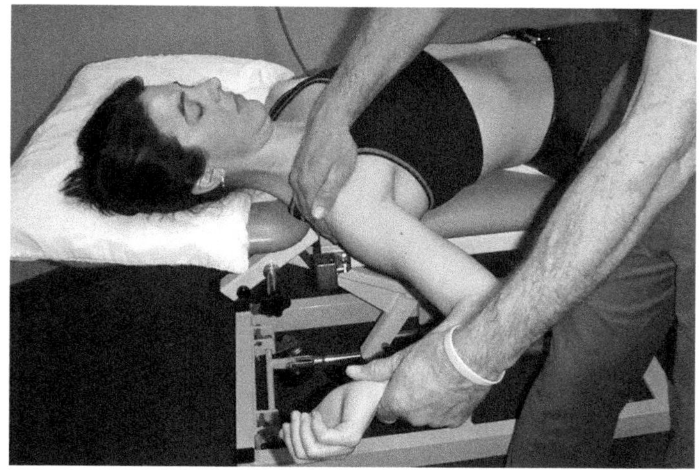

Figure 28.5 **NAIOMT MGHL test.**

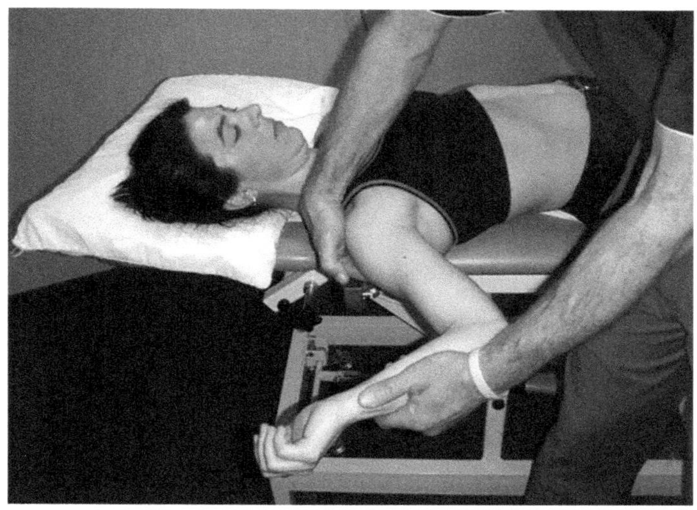

Figure 28.6 **NAIOMT AB-IGHL test.**

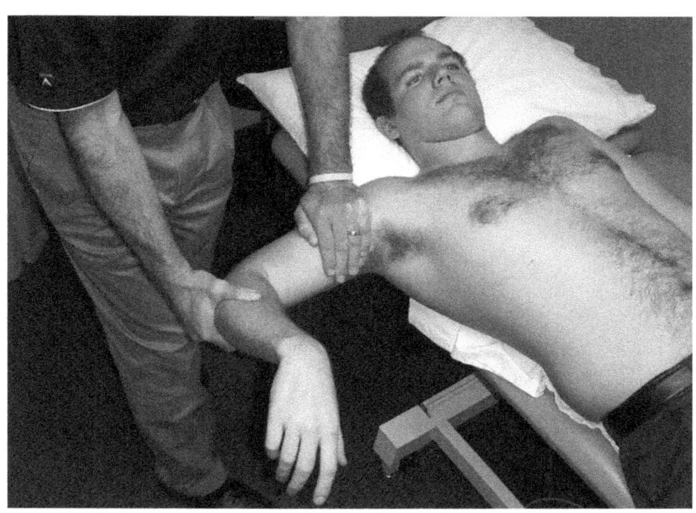

Figure 28.7 **NAIOMT PB-IGHL test.**

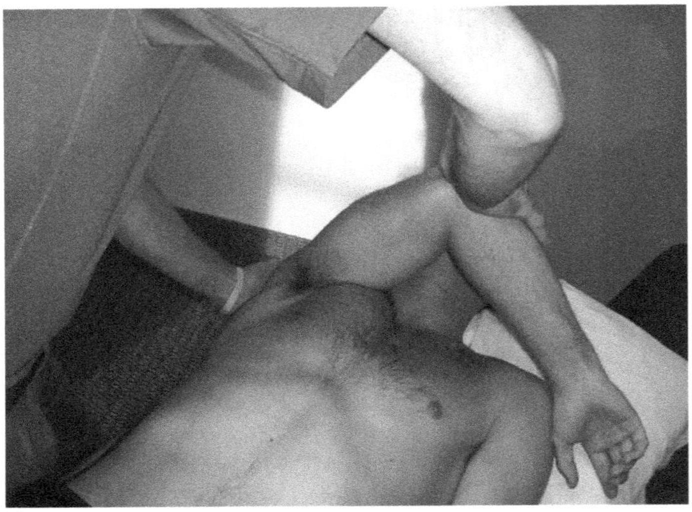

Figure 28.8 **NAIOMT posterior capsule test.**

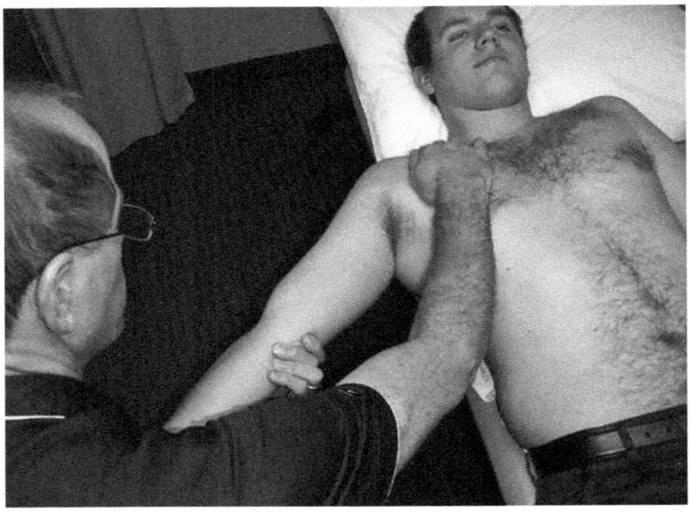

Figure 28.9 **NAIOMT sulcus sign in external rotation.**

NAIOMT sulcus stability test for AB- / PB-IGHL and inferior labrum

A sulcus sign or dimple created beneath the acromion when the subject's arm is axially tractioned inferiorly, usually in a seated position, was first described as the hallmark test for MDI if it also reproduces the patient's characteristic symptoms (Neer & Foster 1980). However, Bahk et al (2007) reported the test as provocative of a patient's symptoms in only a small number of symptomatic patients. The degree of laxity considered to be relevant has also been arbitrary, and McFarland et al (2003) suggested that the sulcus sign might lead to an overdiagnosis of MDI. Pettman (personal communication 2009) has suggested a modification of the sulcus sign. In this test, the examiner stabilizes the scapula by holding one hand in the axilla. With the other hand the examiner rotates the arm into external rotation and, while holding this position, applies an inferior force to assess for a sulcus sign, which is suggested as consistent with a possible labral lesion in the AB-IGHL complex (Fig. 28.9). If this sulcus sign is present in the same test with the arm in full internal rotation, a possible labral lesion in the PB-IGHL complex is suggested (Fig. 28.10).

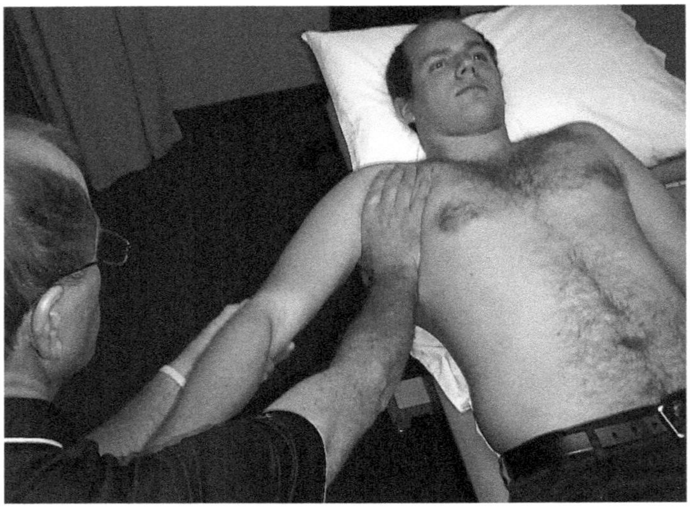

Figure 28.10 **NAIOMT sulcus sign in internal rotation.**

Imaging

From a medical–surgical perspective, in the vast majority of patients the diagnosis of instability is based on the history and physical examination in combination with plane radiographs. Plain radiographs are also important in ruling out fractures, which are often associated with dislocations. Whereas a standard anteroposterior view of the uncomplicated unstable shoulder may produce equivocal findings or may be hard to interpret, an axillary lateral view is helpful to visualize the presence and extent of a (reverse) Hill–Sachs lesion, but may be near impossible to obtain in a patient whose abduction is severely limited owing to the pain. The lateral scapular plane view is particularly helpful in determining the relationship of the humeral head to the glenoid. In anterior dislocations of the shoulder, the humeral head lies anterior to the glenoid; in posterior dislocations it is posterior (Workman et al 1992; Cicak 2004).

With a sensitivity of 97% and specificity of 91%, magnetic resonance imaging (MRI) has been show to have greater accuracy than plain radiography and arthroscopy in the diagnosis of Hill–Sachs lesions (Workman et al 1992). MRI is most useful for visualizing the rotator cuff in elderly patients who have sustained a dislocation and are at risk for a rotator cuff tear as a result of the dislocation. The second author considers magnetic resonance arthrography (MRA), with gadolinium contrast injected into the joint, to be the imaging study of choice for patients with mechanical symptoms where there is a clinical concern for labral or intra-articular pathology. MRA can be particularly valuable in the young athlete who is suspected of a dislocation, but who may clinically have suffered only a subluxation. In the opinion of the second author, in the young overhand athlete, a clear labral detachment (either an anterior or posterior Bankart tear) and a clear Hill–Sachs lesion on MRA (Fig. 28.11) would serve to confirm a dislocation and steer the treating physician towards a surgical

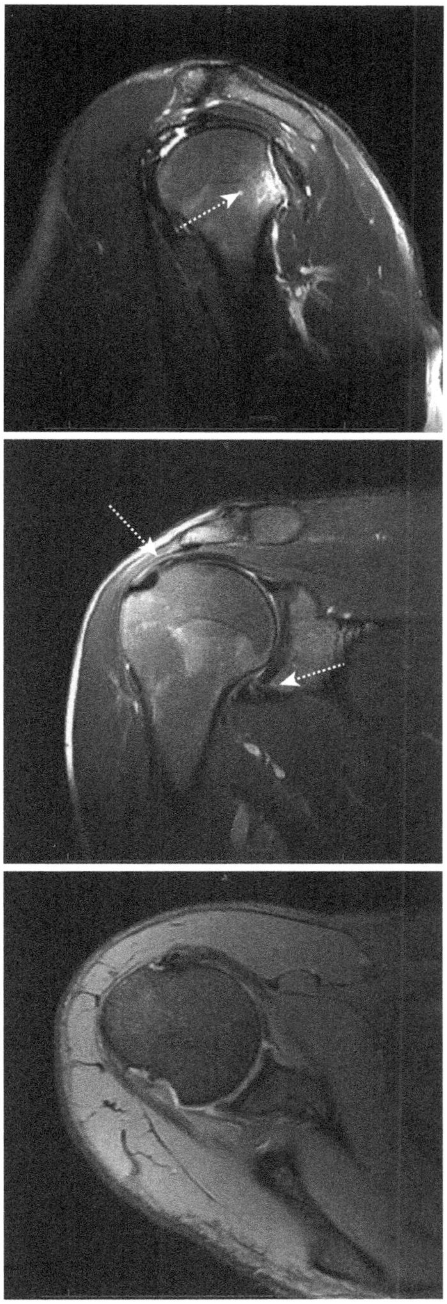

Figure 28.11 Hill–Sachs lesion on MRI.

repair – owing to the high risk of recurrent instability with non-operative management. Computed tomography (CT) can be a very useful tool for imaging bony defects such as a Hill–Sachs lesion or an anterior glenoid bone deficiency (Cicak 2004). This can be useful in surgical planning and for helping to determine the need for alternative procedures to address bony defects.

Prognosis

The challenge to the orthopaedic physical therapist is to determine which patients presenting with instability can be best managed on a conservative basis with a well-outlined and carefully managed programme, and which patients are best referred for further diagnostic testing and orthopaedic surgery consultation. Patients who may require surgical stabilization must not be delayed or missed as the long-term outlook for recurrence and morbidity associated with further insult to the articular cartilage is of primary concern. Although the authors did not study the possibly mitigating effect of conservative or surgical intervention, based on a case–control study Marx et al (2002) reported that the risk of developing severe arthrosis of the shoulder is between 10 and 20 times greater for patients who have had a previous dislocation.

In the clinical opinion of the second author, the young patient (less than 20 years of age) with a first-time traumatic anterior dislocation with a Bankart tear and Hill–Sachs lesion is the most obvious high-risk patient, and probably the only clear candidate for early surgery after a single instability episode (Arciero et al 1994). In addition, the elderly patient with a rotator cuff tear and weakness should be considered for surgery owing to the risk of pain and weakness, rather than risk of recurrent dislocation. All others should be considered for surgery when they fail non-operative management with persisting symptoms, or if they have recurrent dislocations or subluxation symptoms. Although the exact risk of recurrent instability is impossible to determine for any individual, risk factors have been identified that help us classify those individuals who are at increased risk of recurrent instability. Risks of recurrence can be broken down into the following clinical and anatomical risk factors.

Clinical risk factors

The age at which the first dislocation occurs is a very powerful prognosticator. In young patients aged less than 20 years, recurrence rates have ranged from 55% to 94%. Te Slaa et al (2004) reported 26% recurrence within 4 years; in this study, age was the most significant prognostic factor with recurrence in 64% of patients less than 20 years of age, versus only 6% of those older than 40 years. Kralinger et al (2002) also reported an age between 21 and 30 as the only factor associated with recurrence. Note that advancing age is, however, associated with an increased risk of falling leading to recurrent dislocation and an increasing incidence of rotator cuff tears.

Chronicity refers to the number of times that a patient has suffered a dislocation. Although rare, a truly chronically dislocated shoulder is one that has dislocated and remains dislocated. An acute dislocation is a shoulder that has just dislocated and is in need of reduction. More common clinically is the recurrent dislocation. The recurrent dislocator is the patient who reports both prior dislocations and subsequent reductions. The more often a patient has suffered with an instability episode, the more likely it is that a subsequent recurrence will take place. There is, however, no consensus on the number of instability episodes beyond which the risk becomes a certainty.

A traumatic aetiology is associated with a higher recurrence risk than either microtraumatic / overuse or atraumatic instability. Atraumatic instability, especially when associated with generalized ligamentous laxity, is in fact a risk factor for surgical failure. Volition is the patient's ability to reproduce the symptom or dislocation at will; some describe their 'trick shoulder' and can voluntarily demonstrate the ability to dislocate or subluxate their joint. These voluntary dislocators need careful screening for emotional and mental health issues, as although not an absolute surgical contraindication, surgery in this subset of patients needs to be very carefully considered only after failure of non-operative management and careful counselling of the patient and family.

Although perhaps considered by some as an indication of likely failure with conservative management, patients with MDI may benefit from conservative management. In addition, in a subset of patients with MDI, the natural history even without conservative intervention seems benign. Kuroda et al (2001) reported spontaneous recovery in 43 of 476 shoulders of patients followed for 3 years or longer. Although shoulder kinematics may not be restored with physical therapy in all patients with MDI, some of whom may rather require surgical intervention and postoperative physical therapy (Kiss et al 2010), conservative management has been shown to be effective in an as-yet not clearly identified subset of these patients and ultimately may be the key to a successful outcome. Glenohumeral instability can occur as a complete separation of the humerus from the glenoid socket, or as a partial separation or subluxation. Dislocations carry a higher risk of associated injury and recurrence.

Anatomical risk factors

Anatomical risk factors for recurrence include soft tissue and bony defects. Soft tissue defects include rotator cuff, labral and capsular tears. Bony defects include glenoid rim fractures and (reverse) Hill–Sachs lesions. A Hill–Sachs lesion is basically a dent in the humeral head caused by an impaction fracture that occurs as the head dislocates and impacts the anterior or posterior glenoid rim. An engaging Hill–Sachs lesion is a dent that hooks over the edge of the glenoid in a functional range of motion and, by levering, creates a high risk for recurrent anterior or posterior glenohumeral dislocation (Fig. 28.12). A large or engaging Hill–Sachs lesion constitutes a higher risk for recurrent dislocation.

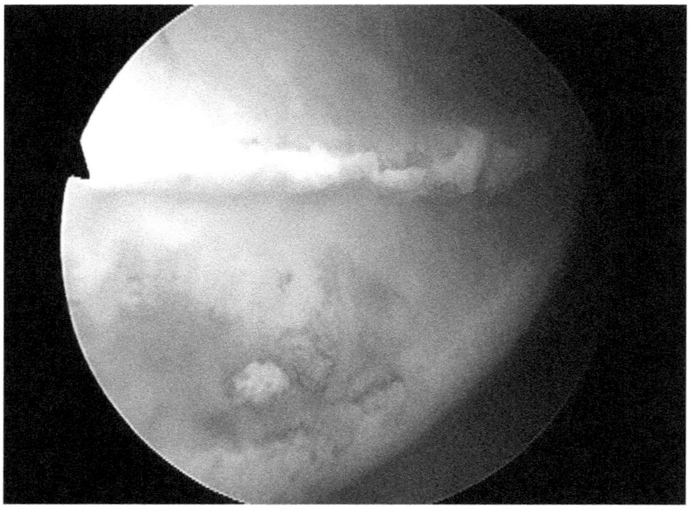

Figure 28.12 Hill–Sachs lesion.

Management of Glenohumeral Instability

Inferior and anterior dislocations are generally addressed with closed reduction, with the patient sedated (Baba et al 2007; Camarda et al 2009). Cicak (2004) suggested that closed reduction under general anaesthesia of a posterior dislocation is most likely to be successful in patients with a humeral head defect of less than 25% of the articular surface where the dislocation is present for less than 3 weeks. If closed reduction is unsuccessful the surgeon may have to progress to an open reduction. Although in some jurisdictions, such as most provinces in Canada, it is within the physical therapy scope of practice to reduce acute dislocations of extremity joints; nevertheless, the risk of associated fractures and neurovascular and other soft tissue damage, the lack of access to imaging and the inability to provide sedation clearly indicate the need for medical–surgical referral and management where possible. Surgical management may also include addressing the possibly present anatomical risk factors for recurrence addressed above.

In the past, patients post dislocation have often been temporarily immobilized with a sling that keeps the arm in adduction and internal rotation. Although bracing the limb in 15–20° of external rotation has been suggested as being anatomically more beneficial and leading to decreased recurrence (Itoi et al 2001, 2003; Funk & Smith 2005), more recent research has pointed out that the evidence is insufficient to support use of one immobilization method over the other, or even to support immobilization at all (Kralinger et al 2002; Handoll et al 2006; Smith 2006; Finestone et al 2009). It should also be noted that patient compliance with the required 3 weeks of full-time bracing is often limited, irrespective of the method used.

Although not providing sufficient operational definitions of specific interventions, Kralinger et al (2002) reported that participation of patients in physical therapy did not reduce risk of recurrence. In general, insufficient evidence is available to guide physical therapy management after closed reduction of traumatic anterior dislocation, which is perhaps reflective of insufficient methodological quality of studies in this area (Handoll et al 2006). A Cochrane review reported no differences, with regard to renewed injury or function, between open and arthroscopic stabilizing surgery for anterior shoulder instability in adults (Pulavarti et al 2009). Scheibel (2007) discussed the possibility of subscapularis dysfunction after open repairs and, considering the important role of this muscle in the transverse plane stabilizing force couple, this may present another reason to choose arthroscopic over open techniques. Limited evidence supports surgery in young, predominantly male adults with a first acute traumatic dislocation who are engaged in highly demanding physical activities for reducing recurrent dislocation or subluxation; however, no evidence is available to determine the best treatment for other patient groups (Handoll & Al-Maiyah 2004).

In the absence of research to guide conservative management of patients post dislocation, but also those patients with (minor) instability, therapists have had to depend on clinical reasoning and extrapolation from basic science research. Te Slaa et al (2004) did not report sports participation as a risk factor for dislocation, yet Kuroda et al (2001) reported an 8.7-fold increase in incidence of spontaneous recovery for those patients with atraumatic shoulder instability who discontinued playing overhead sports. Provision of education regarding adaptation in high-risk movements in sports seems a logical intervention. In athletes, this includes modification of the often ancillary weight-training activities. Fees et al (1998) suggested a grip width during the bench press of less than 1.5 times the biacromial distance in patients with anterior shoulder instability. Other suggested modifications included required assistance when lifting the bar from and onto the rack, decrease of the shoulder abduction angle during the bench press, alternation of flat and decline bench press to reduce the chance of microtraumatic injury, and elimination of the incline bench press and the behind-the-neck press and pull-down exercises, as well as the back-squat position, where the hands stabilize the bar on the shoulders. In patients with posterior shoulder instability, Fees et al (1998) suggested a grip width during the bench press of > 2 times the biacromial width, use of a shoulder abduction angle > 80°, horizontal abduction > 15° at the start and horizontal adduction < 20° at the finish of the bench press motion. They also proposed mandatory assists with (un)racking the bar and use of the flat bench press only, or preferably no bench press at all.

As discussed in Chapter 28, proprioceptive deficits have also been identified in patients with anterior glenohumeral joint instability as well as altered muscle activation (Myers et al 2004). Decreased rotator cuff coactivation and slower biceps brachii and pectoralis major activation were identified and restoration of their normal function, and thus should be part of any targeted rehabilitation programme for anterior instability. A defect in proprioception also may be a factor in the pathophysiology of MDI (Schenk & Brems 1998). Dynamic exercises incorporating proprioceptive neuromuscular facilitation (PNF) have been found to be effective in the early phases of shoulder rehabilitation (Padua et al 2004). Utilizing well-established principles of PNF to the upper quadrant such as rhythmic stabilization, eccentric-to-concentric loading and continuous movements associated with rotation (Knott & Voss 1968), therapists can easily implement and progress a programme even in the early stages. Closed kinetic chain exercises, initially on stable and later on unstable surfaces, can increase the accuracy of joint position sense and enhance stimulation of mechanoreceptors (Naughton et al 2005; Eckenrode et al 2009). Open-chain oscillatory exercises with the Bodyblade® can be used to provide more advanced open-chain dynamic stabilization (Buteau et al 2007). Exercises for muscular endurance and strength need to address both the local stabilizers in an attempt to restore at least the active (if not the passive) contribution to the concavity compression mechanism, as well as the prime movers required for functional movement and known to have an effect on glenohumeral stability. A careful progression needs to be both adapted to the patient's functional demands and rehabilitation goals and also based on a careful and educated impression of the therapist with regard to rehabilitation potential. Chapters 32 and 33 provide examples of exercises for motor control and other exercises relevant to the shoulder.

Conclusion

Shoulder instability can present a challenge to the orthopaedic physical therapist in differential diagnosis and management. Identification of patients at high risk for recurrence of shoulder dislocation indicates the need for referral to a shoulder specialist for likely surgical intervention. Further research on diagnostic and prognostic validity of our clinical tests, such as those outlined above, is necessary and would help drive outcome studies of conservative versus surgical management for possible subgroups of patients identified on the basis of our clinical tests. A clear indication of glenohumeral instability should not limit the therapists to management of the shoulder area alone. Patients with a history of shoulder instability should be examined for underlying biomechanical faults in both the upper and lower quadrants that may contribute to the instability in more dynamic activities.

References

Abboud AA, Soslowsky J. 2002. Interplay of the static and dynamic restraints in glenohumeral instability. Clin Orthop Relat Res 400: 48–57.

Arciero RA, Wheeler JH, Ryan JB, et al. 1994. Arthroscopic Bankart repair versus nonoperative treatment for acute, initial anterior shoulder dislocations. Am J Sports Med 22: 589–594.

Baba AN, Bhat JA, Paljor SD, et al. 2007. Luxatio erecta: inferior glenohumeral dislocation – a case report. Int J Shoulder Surg 1: 100–102.

Bahk M, Keyurapan E, Tasaki A. 2007. Laxity testing of the shoulder: a review. Am J Sports Med 35: 131–144.

Bey M, Hunter S, Kilambi N, et al. 2005. The structural and mechanical properties of the glenohumeral joint capsule. J Shoulder Elbow Surg 14: 201–206.

Bigliani LU, Pollockv RG, Soslowsky LJ, et al. 1992. Tensile properties of the inferior glenohumeral ligament. J Orthop Res 10: 187–197.

Bohnsack M, Wulker N. 2002. Arthroscopic anterior shoulder stabilization: combined multiple suture repair and laser-assisted capsular shrinkage. Injury 33: 795–799.

Buteau JL, Eriksrud O, Hasson SM. 2007. Rehabilitation of a glenohumeral instability utilizing the body blade. Physiother Theory Pract 23: 333–349.

Camarda R, Martorana U, D'Arienzo M. 2009. A case of bilateral luxatio erecta. J Orthop Traumatol 10: 97–99.

Caplan J, Julien TP, Michelson J, et al. 2007. Multidirectional instability of the shoulder in elite female gymnasts. Am J Orthop 36: 660–665.

Cicak N. 2004. Posterior dislocation of the shoulder. J. Bone Joint Surg 86B: 324–332.

Cooper DE, Arnoczky SP, O'Brien SJ, et al. 1992. Anatomy, histology and vascularity of the glenoid labrum: an anatomic study. J Bone Joint Surg 74A: 46–52.

Cyriax J. 1978. Textbook of orthopaedic medicine. Vol 1. London: Cassell.

Eckenrode BJ, Logerstedt DS, Sennett BJ. 2009. Rehabilitation and functional outcomes in collegiate wrestlers following a posterior shoulder stabilization procedure. J Orthop Sports Phys Ther 39: 550–559.

Ellenbecker T, Bailie D, Mattalino A, et al. 2002. Intrarater and interrater reliability of a manual technique to assess anterior humeral head translation of the glenohumeral joint. J Shoulder Elbow Surg 11: 470–475.

Fees M, Decker T, Snyder-Mackler L, et al. 1998. Upper extremity weight-training modifications for the injured athlete. Am J Sports Med 26: 732–742.

Fehringer EV, Schmidt GR, Boorman RS, et al. 2003 The anteroinferior labrum helps center the humeral head on the glenoid. J Shoulder Elbow Surg 12: 53–58.

Finestone A, Milgrom C, Radeva-Petrova DR, et al. 2009. Bracing in external rotation for traumatic anterior dislocation of the shoulder. J Bone Joint Surg 91: 918–921.

Fleisig G, Andrews J, Dillman C, et al. 1995. Kinetics of baseball pitching with implications about injury mechanisms. Am J Sports Med 23: 233–239.

Fowler C, Pettman E. 1992. North American Institute orthopaedic manual therapy (NAIOMT) upper quadrant course 600A. Portland, OR: NAIOMT.

Funk L, Smith M. 2005. Best evidence report. How to immobilize after shoulder dislocation? Emerg Med J 22: 814–815.

Halder AM, Halder CG, Zhao KD, et al. 2001a. Dynamic inferior stabilizers of the shoulder joint. Clin Biomech 16: 138–143.

Halder AM, Zhao KD, O'Driscoll SW, et al. 2001b. Dynamic contributors to superior shoulder stability. J Orthop Res 19 (2): 206–212.

Handoll HHG, Al-Maiyah MA. 2004. Surgical versus non-surgical treatment for acute anterior shoulder dislocation. Cochrane Database Syst Rev 1: CD004325. doi: 10.1002/14651858.CD004325.pub2.

Handoll HHG, Hanchard NCA, Goodchild LM, et al. 2006. Conservative management following closed reduction of traumatic anterior dislocation of the shoulder. Cochrane Database Syst Rev 1: CD004962. doi: 10.1002/14651858.CD004962.pub2.

Hides JA, Richardson CA, Jull GA. 1996. Multifidus muscle recovery is not automatic after resolution of acute first episode low back pain. Spine 21: 2763–2769.

Huijbregts PA. 1998. Biomechanics and pathology of the overhead throwing motion: a literature review. J Man Manip Ther 6: 17–23.

Itoi E, Sashi R, Minagawa H, et al. 2001. Position of immobilization after dislocation of the glenohumeral joint: a study with use of magnetic resonance imaging. J Bone Joint Surg 83B: 661–667.

Itoi E, Hatakeyama Y, Kido T, et al. 2003. A new method of immobilization after traumatic anterior dislocation of the shoulder: a preliminary study. J Shoulder Elbow Surg 12: 413–415.

Jobe FW, Kvitne RS, Giangarra CE. 1989. Shoulder pain in the overhead or throwing athlete: the relationship of anterior instability and rotator cuff impingement. Orthop Rev 18: 963–975.

Kido T, Ito E, Lee SB, et al. 2003. Dynamic stabilizing function of the deltoid muscle in shoulders with anterior instability. Am J Sports Med 31: 399–403.

Kim SH, Park JS, Jeong WK, et al. 2005. The Kim test: a novel test for posteroinferior labral lesion of the shoulder: a comparison to the jerk test. Am J Sports Med 33: 1188–1192.

Kiss RM, Illyés A, Kiss J. 2010. Physiotherapy versus capsular shift and physiotherapy in multidirectional shoulder joint instability. J Electromyogr Kinesiol 20(3): 489–501. doi: 10.1016/j.jelekin.2009.09.001.

Knott M, Voss DE. 1968. Proprioceptive neuromuscular facilitation: patterns and techniques. London: Harper & Row.

Kralinger FS, Golser K, Wischatta R, et al. 2002. Predicting recurrence after primary anterior shoulder dislocation. Am J Sports Med 30: 116–120.

Krøner K, Lind T, Jensen J. 1989. The epidemiology of shoulder dislocations. Arch Orthop Trauma Surg 108: 288–290.

Kuhn JE, Lindholm SR, Huston LJ, et al. 2003. Failure of the biceps superior labral complex: A cadaveric biomechanical investigation comparing the late cocking and early deceleration positions of throwing. Arthroscopy 19: 373–379.

Kuhn JE, Huston LJ, Soslowsky LJ, et al. 2005. External rotation of the glenohumeral joint: Ligament restraints and muscle effects in the neutral and abducted positions. J Shoulder Elbow Surg 14 (Suppl): 39S–48S.

Kuroda S, Sumiyoshi T, Moriishi J, et al. 2001. The natural course of atraumatic shoulder instability. J Shoulder Elbow Surg 10: 100–104.

Labriola J, Lee T, Debski R, et al. 2005. Stability and instability of the glenohumeral joint: the role of shoulder muscles. J Shoulder Elbow Surg 14: 32S–38S.

Lee D. 1989. The pelvic girdle. Oxford: Churchill Livingstone.

Lee SB, Kyu-Jung K, O'Driscoll S, et al. 2000. Dynamic glenohumeral stability provided by the rotator cuff muscles in the mid-range and end-range of motion. J Bone Joint Surg 82A: 849–857.

Lee T, Black A, Tibone J, et al. 2001. Release of the coracoacromial ligament can lead to glenohumeral laxity: a biomechanical study. J Shoulder Elbow Surg 10: 68–72.

Levine WM, Flatow E. 2000. The pathophysiology of shoulder instability. Am J Sports Med 28: 910–917.

Levy A, Linter S, Kenter K, et al. 1999. Intra- and interobserver reproducibility of the shoulder laxity examination. Am J Sports Med 27: 460–463.

Lo IK, Nonweiler B, Woolfrey M, et al. 2004. An evaluation of the apprehension, relocation, and surprise tests for anterior shoulder instability. Am J Sports Med 32: 301–307.

Magarey M, Jones M. 1992. Clinical diagnosis and management of minor shoulder instability. Aust J Physiother 38: 269–279.

Mallon WJ, Bassett FH, Goldner RD. 1990. Luxatio erecta: the inferior glenohumeral dislocation. J Orthop Trauma 4: 19–24.

Marx RG, McCarthy EC, Montemurno TD, et al. 2002. Development of arthrosis following dislocation of the shoulder: a case–control study. J Shoulder Elbow Surg 11: 1–5.

McFarland TK, Kim EG, Park HB, et al. 2003. The effect of variation in definition on the diagnosis of multidirectional instability of the shoulder. J Bone Joint Surg 85A: 2145–2146.

McFarland EG, Garzon-Muvdi J, Jia X, et al. 2010. Clinical and diagnostic tests for shoulder disorders: a critical review. Br J Sports Med 44: 328–332.

Myers JB, Ju YY, Hwang JH, et al. 2004. Reflexive muscle activation alterations in shoulders with anterior glenohumeral instability. Am J Sports Med 32: 1013–1021.

Naughton J, Adams R, Maher C. 2005. Upper-body wobble board training effects on the post-dislocation shoulder. Phys Ther Sport 6: 31–37.

Neer CS, Foster CR. 1980. Inferior capsular shift for involuntary inferior and multidirectional instability of the shoulder: a preliminary report. J Bone Joint Surg 62A: 897–908.

Neer CS, Satterlee CC, Dalsey RM, et al. 1992. The anatomy and potential effects of contracture of the coracohumeral ligament. Clin Orthop Relat Res 280: 182–185.

O'Connell PW, Nuber GW, Mileski RA, et al. 1990. The contribution of the glenohumeral ligaments to anterior stability of the shoulder joint. Am J Sports Med 18: 579–584.

Owens BD, Dawson L, Burksv R, et al. 2009. Incidence of shoulder dislocation in the United States military: considerations from a high-risk population. J Bone Joint Surg 91A: 791–796.

Padua D, Guskiewicz K, Prentice W, et al. 2004. The effect of select shoulder exercises on strength, active angle reproduction, single-arm balance, and functional importance. J Sports Rehabil 13: 75–95.

Panjabi MM. 1992. The stabilizing system of the spine, part II: Neutral zone and instability hypothesis. J Spinal Disord 5: 390–396.

Parsons IM, Apreleva M, Fu FH, et al. 2002. The effect of rotator cuff tears on reaction forces at the glenohumeral joint. J Orthop Res 20: 439–446.

Pulavarti RS, Symes TH, Rangan A. 2009. Surgical interventions for anterior shoulder instability in adults. Cochrane Database Syst Rev 4: CD005077. doi: 10.1002/14651858.CD005077.pub2.

Robinson CM, Dobson R. 2004. Anterior instability of the shoulder after trauma. J Bone Joint Surg 86B: 469–479.

Sahrmann S. 2002. Diagnosis and treatment of movement impairment syndromes. St Louis: Mosby.

Scheibel M. 2007. Subscapularis dysfunction after open instability repair. Int J Shoulder Surg 1: 16–22.

Schenk TJ, Brems JJ. 1998. Multidirectional instability of the shoulder: pathophysiology, diagnosis, and management. J Am Acad Orthop Surg 6: 65–72.

Schmitt H, Brocal D, Lukoschek M. 2004. High prevalence of hip arthrosis in former elite javelin throwers and high jumpers: 41 athletes examined more than 10 years after retirement from competitive sports. Acta Orthop Scand 75: 34–39.

Seebauer L, Keyl W. 1998. Posterior shoulder joint instability. Classification, pathomechanism, diagnosis, conservative and surgical management. Orthopäde 27: 542–555.

Smith TO. 2006. Immobilization following traumatic anterior glenohumeral joint dislocation: a literature review. Injury 37: 228–237.

Sugalski M, Wiater JM, Levine W, et al. 2005. An anatomic study of the humeral insertion of the inferior glenohumeral capsule. J Shoulder Elbow Surg 14: 91–95.

Te Slaa RL, Wijffels MP, Brand R, et al. 2004. The prognosis following acute primary glenohumeral dislocation. J Bone Joint Surg 86B: 58–64.

Terry GC. 1991. The stabilizing function of passive shoulder restraints. Am J Sports Med 19: 26–34.

Tibone J, Lee T, Csintalan R, et al. 2002. Quantitative assessment of glenohumeral translation. Clin Orthop Relat Res 400: 93–97.

Turkel SJ, Panio MW, Marshall J, et al. 1981. Stabilizing mechanisms preventing anterior dislocation of the glenohumeral joint. J Bone Joint Surg 63A: 1208–1217.

Urayama M. 2001. Function of the 3 portions of the inferior glenohumeral ligament: a cadaveric study. J Shoulder Elbow Surg 10: 589–594.

Walton J, Tzannes A, Callanan M, et al. 2002. The unstable shoulder in the adolescent athlete. Am J Sports Med 30: 758–767.

Workman TL, Burkhard TK, Resnick D, et al. 1992. Hill–Sachs lesion: comparison of detection with MR imaging, radiography, and arthroscopy. Radiology 185: 847–852.

Chapter 29

Superior Labrum Anterior-to-Posterior (SLAP) Lesions

Janette W. Powell, Peter A. Huijbregts

CHAPTER CONTENTS

Introduction	333
Anatomy	334
Biomechanics	335
Pathology	336
Diagnosis	337
Management	340
Prognosis	341
Conclusion	341

Introduction

Superior labrum anterior-to-posterior (SLAP) lesions have been discussed and investigated since Andrews et al first described this pathology in 1985. SLAP lesions involve the superior glenoid labrum extending anteriorly and posteriorly (Andrews et al 1985; Snyder et al 1990; D'Alessandro et al 2000; Kim et al 2003; Bedi & Allen 2008; Dodson & Altchek 2009). SLAP lesions not only involve the superior glenoid labrum, but can also affect the biceps tendon and glenohumeral ligament attachments (D'Alessandro et al 2000; Dessaur & Magarey 2008). SLAP lesions are often complex injuries with a spectrum of locations and varied types of tissue defects in the glenoid labrum and its associated structures (D'Alessandro et al 2000; Lebolt et al 2006; Bedi & Allen 2008).

These variants, in addition to age-related changes in the superior labrum, have thwarted an understanding of the precise epidemiology of SLAP lesions (Bedi & Allen 2008). Their prevalence has been reported in the literature to range between 6% and 76% of all shoulder injuries evaluated arthroscopically, but even independent of their large range the relevance of this reported prevalence to primary care settings is unclear (Snyder et al 1990; Liu et al 1996a; Mileski & Snyder 1998; D'Alessandro et al 2000; Higgins & Warner 2001; Huijbregts 2001; Musgrave & Rodosky 2001; Kim et al 2002, 2003; Guanche & Jones 2003; Wilk et al 2005; Lebolt et al 2006; Barber et al 2007; Funk & Snow 2007; Bedi & Allen 2008; Walsworth et al 2008; Dodson & Altchek 2009). Without supplying specific quantitative data, these lesions have been described as common occurrences in the athletic population, particularly in overhead / throwing athletes (Lebolt et al 2006; Funk & Snow 2007; Bedi & Allen 2008; Dodson & Altchek 2009). However, a number of authors note the challenge of determining the clinical relevance of a SLAP lesion when there are coexisting lesions in the shoulder (Musgrave & Rodosky 2001; Stetson & Templin 2002; McFarland et al 2002; Kim et al 2003, 2007; Dodson & Altchek 2009). Difficulties associated with investigations of SLAP lesions include the variability of pathological findings, clinical features and the prevalence – all of which can vary depending on the population studied (Kim et al 2003).

SLAP lesions have been classified into types on the basis of their morphological pattern. Snyder et al (1990) classified these pathological variations into four types (Fig. 29.1):

- **type I:** degenerative fraying with no detachment of the biceps insertion
- **type II:** detachment of the biceps insertion
- **type III:** a bucket-handle tear of the superior aspect of the labrum with an intact biceps tendon insertion to bone
- **type IV:** an intrasubstance tear of the biceps tendon with a bucket-handle tear of the superior aspect of the labrum.

The type II SLAP lesions have been further divided into three subtypes (Fig. 29.2) depending on whether the detachment of the labrum involves solely the anterior aspect of the labrum, solely the posterior aspect, or both aspects. The above classification system has been expanded to include an additional three types (D'Alessandro et al 2000; Higgins & Warner 2001; Huijbregts 2001; Musgrave & Rodosky 2001; Parentis et al 2002; Kim et al 2003; Nam & Snyder 2003; Wilk et al 2005), as follows:

- **type V:** a Bankart lesion that extends superiorly to include a type II SLAP lesion
- **type VI:** an unstable flap tear of the labrum in conjunction with a biceps tendon separation
- **type VII:** a superior labrum and biceps tendon separation that extends anteriorly, inferior to the middle glenohumeral ligament.

The prevalence of the various types of SLAP lesions as reported in the literature again shows wide ranges: type I 20–74%, type II 21–70%, type III 1–9%, and type IV 4–10% (Snyder et al 1995; Kim et al 2003; Kampa & Clasper 2005). The prevalence of associated pathology, with other intra-articular lesions, has been reported to range from 62% to 88% (Snyder et al 1995; Mileski & Snyder 1998; Kim et al 2003).

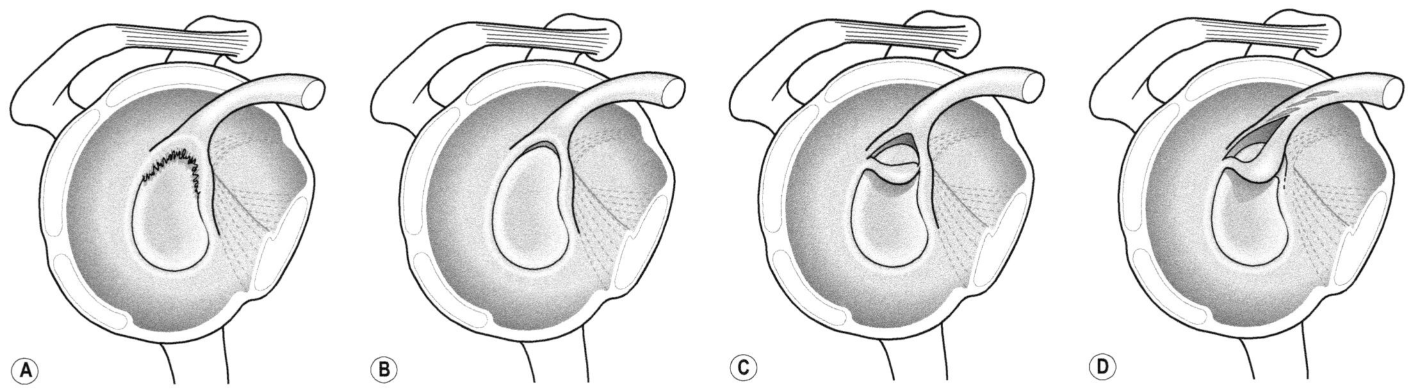

Figure 29.1 Classification of superior glenoid or superior labrum and biceps anchor (SLAP) lesions: (**A**) type I, degenerative fraying of the superior labrum with the edge still firmly attached to the glenoid; (**B**) type II, detachment of the superior labrum and biceps tendon from the glenoid with resultant destabilization of the biceps anchor; (**C**) type III, bucket-handle tear of superior labrum. The remaining labrum and biceps anchor are stable; (**D**) type IV, bucket-handle tear of superior labrum with extension into the biceps tendon.

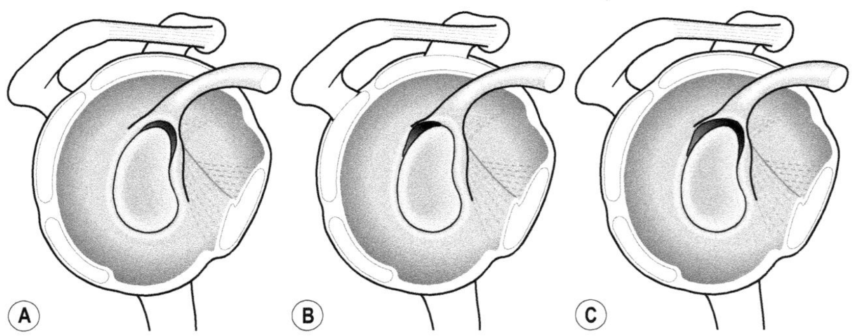

Figure 29.2 Subtypes of type II SLAP lesions: (**A**) anterior, (**B**) posterior, (**C**) combined anterior–posterior.

Anatomy

The glenoid labrum is a triangular fibrocartilaginous structure that sits on the periphery of the glenoid rim. It is a transitional connective tissue, typically an ovoid circumferential rim, that lies between the articular surface of the glenoid fossa and the fibrous capsule of the glenohumeral joint (D'Alessandro et al 2000; Higgins & Warner 2001; Musgrave & Rodosky 2001; Wilk et al 2005). Musgrave and Rodosky (2001) describe this labral rim as being approximately 3 mm high and 4 mm wide. The depth of the glenoid fossa is doubled with the labrum and the surface contact area between the humeral head, and the glenoid is greatly enhanced by the labrum (Higgins & Warner 2001; Huijbregts 2001; Musgrave & Rodosky 2001, Wilk et al 2005). The superior labrum is triangular in cross-section, is 'loosely' attached to the glenoid with a free edge and is commonly described as 'meniscal' in its morphology (Huijbregts 2001; Musgrave & Rodosky 2001; Nam & Snyder 2003; Wilk et al 2005; Dessaur & Magarey 2008). The inferior labrum, in contrast, is rounded and firmly attached (Huijbregts 2001; Musgrave & Rodosky 2001; Nam & Snyder 2003; Wilk et al 2005).

The blood supply to the labrum arises mostly from its peripheral attachment to the capsule and is from a combination of the suprascapular artery, the circumflex scapular branch of the subscapular artery and the posterior circumflex humeral arteries (Huijbregts 2001; Nam & Snyder 2003; Wilk et al 2005). The literature on the extent and localization of vascularization of the glenoid labrum is contradictory, with some authors describing only vascularization of the peripheral labrum, which in addition is more extensive posteriorly and inferiorly than (antero)superiorly (Cooper et al 1992; Huijbregts 2001; Nam & Snyder 2003; Wilk et al 2005, Dessaur & Magarey 2008), whereas other authors have described more global vascularization (Prodromos et al 1990). The question of whether the superior labrum is indeed a vascular structure has important implications in terms of the healing potential of a SLAP lesion (D'Alessandro et al 2000; Dessaur & Magarey 2008); vascularity of the labrum appears to decrease with increasing age (Huijbregts 2001; Nam & Snyder 2003; Wilk et al 2005).

Other glenohumeral structures, including the superior and middle glenohumeral ligaments and the biceps tendon, are noted to be continuous and intimately related with the superior labrum (D'Alessandro et al 2000; Huijbregts 2001; Musgrave & Rodosky 2001; Parentis et al 2002; Wilk et al 2005; Dessaur & Magarey 2008). The anterosuperior labrum is one of the most variable areas of glenohumeral anatomy (Fig. 29.3). It is important that normal variants of this anatomy are recognized as non-pathological (D'Alessandro et al 2000; Higgins & Warner 2001; Huijbregts 2001; Musgrave & Rodosky 2001; Kim et al 2003; Wilk et al 2005). A sublabral recess or foramen has been reported in up to 73% of normal shoulders and consists of an opening or hole between the labrum and glenoid rim (Musgrave & Rodosky 2001). Its size can vary from only a few millimetres to spanning the entire anterosuperior quadrant (Fig. 29.4A) (D'Alessandro et al

2000; Huijbregts 2001; Musgrave & Rodosky 2001; Nam & Snyder 2003; Wilk et al 2005). The Buford complex represents another anatomical variant and is described as a cord-like thickening of the middle glenohumeral ligament and absence of the anterosuperior labrum (Fig. 29.4C). This complex is reported to be less common, with prevalence ranging between 1.5% and 5% (Musgrave & Rodosky 2001; Bents & Skeete 2005; Wilk et al 2005). Relevant to accurate diagnosis is the finding that, in normal variants, the edges of both the labrum and glenoid can be expected to be smooth without the fraying or haemorrhage that when noted on arthroscopy would be more suggestive of a pathological detachment (D'Alessandro et al 2000; Higgins & Warner 2001; Huijbregts 2001; Musgrave & Rodosky 2001; Wilk et al 2005).

The anatomy of the origin of the tendon of the long head of biceps (LHB) is noted to be highly variable (Barber et al 2007; Ghalayini et al 2007; Dierickx et al 2009). Studies have reported that between 25% and 60% of LHB tendons originate from the supraglenoid tubercle, with the remainder originating from the superior glenoid labrum (Pal et al 1991; Vangsness et al 1994; Ghalayini et al 2007; Krupp et al 2009). Other variations that have been described include a split tendon from a single origin, a double tendon origin from the capsule, labrum or tuberosity, medial and / or lateral tendon–capsular adhesions, medial and / or lateral tendon–rotator cuff adhesions, and even a complete absence of the LHB tendon (Dierickx et al 2009). It is additionally noted that a greater portion of the LHB attachment to the labrum is to the posterior labrum (Vangsness et al 1994; Dierickx et al 2009). The variable attachment of this biceps anchor may make it difficult to differentiate pathological detachment of the biceps anchor from a normal meniscoid labrum with a sublabral recess or a Buford complex (D'Alessandro et al 2000; Higgins & Warner 2001; Huijbregts 2001; Musgrave & Rodosky 2001; Kim et al 2003; Nam & Snyder 2003; Wilk et al 2005; Barber et al 2007).

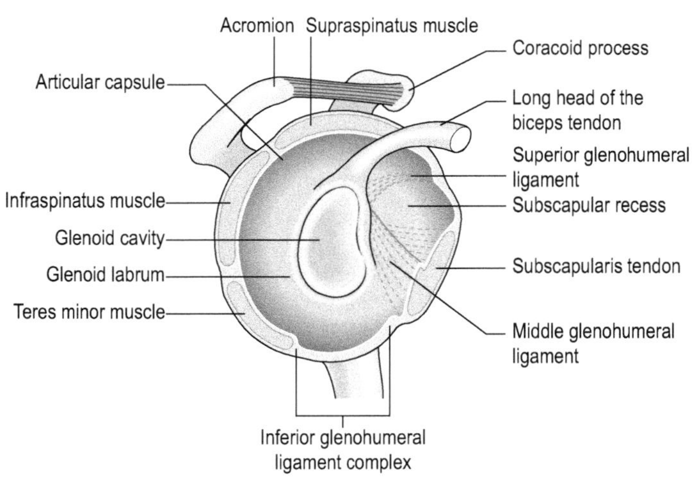

Figure 29.3 Arthroscopic anatomy of the glenohumeral joint.

Biomechanics

The labrum appears to serve as a buttress assisting in controlling glenohumeral translation, similar to a 'chock-block' (Wilk et al 1997, 2005; Huijbregts 2001). Labral damage disrupts the circular configuration and the hoop stresses, rendering this 'chock-block' mechanism less effective (Howell & Galinat 1989; Huijbregts 2001). Resection of the labrum has been shown to reduce the concavity-compression stabilization of the glenohumeral joint by 10–20% (Lippitt et al 1993; Wilk et al 1997; Halder et al 2001). The labrum has also been described as functioning like a seal, whereby labral injury results in a loss of negative intra-articular pressure thereby diminishing glenohumeral joint stability (Huijbregts 2001).

The biceps–labrum complex has been shown to be an important stabilizer of the glenohumeral joint (Bedi & Allen 2008). Andrews et al (1985) noted that electrical stimulation of the biceps during arthroscopy led to humeral head compression within the glenoid. Increased glenohumeral translation has been demonstrated when the long head of the biceps tendon has been destabilized (Pagnani et al 1995; Warner & McMahon 1995; Pradhan et al 2001). Warner and McMahon (1995) observed up to 6 mm of superior humeral migration during active abduction in individuals with isolated LHB tendon tears compared with their intact contralateral shoulders. Kim et al (2001) reported that maximal biceps activity occurred when the shoulder was in the abducted and externally rotated position in patients with anterior instability. SLAP lesions result in significant increases in strain of the anterior band of the glenohumeral ligament with shoulder abduction and external rotation, suggesting a key role of the superior labrum in glenohumeral stability (Rodosky et al 1994). Pagnani et al (1995) found that a complete lesion of the superior portion of the labrum was associated with significant increases in glenohumeral translation and that a simulated SLAP lesion resulted in a 6 mm increase in anterior glenohumeral translation. Rodosky et al (1994) observed that a SLAP lesion contributed to anterior shoulder instability by

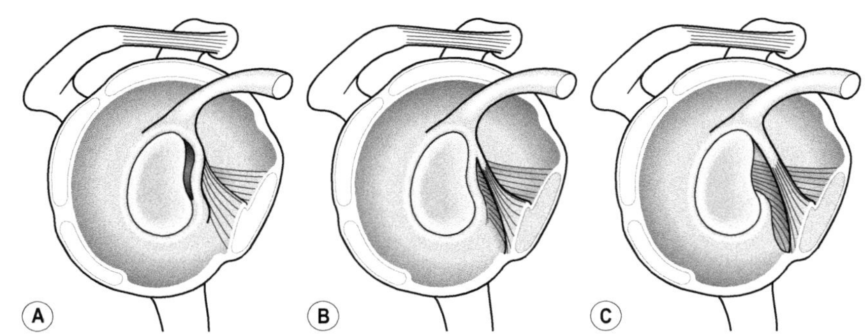

Figure 29.4 Normal anatomical variants of the anterosuperior glenoid labrum and glenohumeral ligaments: (**A**) sublabral foramen, (**B**) cord-like middle glenohumeral ligament, (**C**) Buford complex (cord-like middle glenohumeral ligament with absence of anterosuperior labral tissue).

decreasing the shoulder's resistance to torsion and placing a greater strain on the inferior glenohumeral ligament. Panossian et al (2005) demonstrated how a type II SLAP lesion increased total glenohumeral range of motion, in addition to anteroposterior and inferior translation.

Pathology

Associated pathology is commonly encountered with SLAP lesions, most notably concomitant rotator cuff tears and other labral pathology (Dodson & Altchek 2009). Andrews and Carson (1984) noted that 45% of individuals (and 73% of baseball pitchers) with SLAP lesions also had partial-thickness tears of the supraspinatus. Mileski and Snyder (1998) reported that 29% of their individuals with SLAP lesions had partial-thickness rotator cuff tears, 11% complete rotator cuff tears, and 22% Bankart lesions. They also noted that type I lesions were typically associated with rotator cuff pathology, while types III and IV were associated with traumatic instability. Additionally they observed that, in patients with type II lesions, older individuals tended to have associated rotator cuff pathology while younger individuals had associated anterior instability.

Dodson and Altcheck (2009) explained how recognition of these associated lesions facilitates insight into the biomechanical aetiology of SLAP lesions. There are several proposed mechanisms for SLAP lesions. These mechanisms can be divided into acute traumatic events and chronic repetitive injuries that lead to failure (Dodson & Altchek 2009). Acute traumatic events, such as falling onto an outstretched arm or a direct lateral blow to the shoulder, may result in a SLAP lesion from impaction of the humeral head against the superior labrum and the biceps anchor (D'Alessandro et al 2000; Funk & Snow 2007; Bedi & Allen 2008; Dodson & Altchek 2009). Sudden inferior pulls on the arm, such as when losing control of a heavy object, anterior traction while water skiing, or superior traction when grasping overhead to stop a fall, are traumatic mechanisms of injury described in the literature (Maffet et al 1995; D'Alessandro et al 2000; Barber et al 2007; Bedi & Allen 2008). SLAP lesions in the throwing athlete have also been postulated to be traction injuries of the biceps–labrum complex (Higgins & Warner 2001; Funk & Snow 2007). Andrews and Carson (1984) theorized that SLAP lesions in overhead-throwing athletes were the result of the high eccentric activity of the biceps muscle, creating tension on the long head of the biceps tendon during the arm deceleration and follow-through phases of throwing. The sudden tensile load on the biceps was suggested to avulse the biceps–labrum complex (Andrews & Carson 1984; Higgins & Warner 2001). Subsequent research with electrical stimulation applied to the biceps during arthroscopy have, indeed, noted that biceps activation caused the biceps anchor to separate from the glenoid (Andrews et al 1985). Electromyographic studies showing increased biceps activity after ball release support this theory (Jobe et al 1984; Glousman et al 1988; D'Alessandro et al 2000).

Repetitive overhead activity has been hypothesized as a common mechanism for producing SLAP lesions (Funk & Snow 2007; Dodson & Altchek 2009). The traction injury mechanism described above has also been postulated to result in repetitive micro- rather than macrotrauma (avulsion), progressively leading to structural failure of the biceps–labrum complex (D'Alessandro et al 2000). Burkhart and Morgan (1998) hypothesized that a 'peel-back' mechanism may produce a SLAP lesion in the overhead athlete. They theorized that, when the shoulder is placed in abduction and maximal external rotation, the rotation causes a torsional force at the base of the biceps. Pradhan et al (2001) measured superior labral strain during each phase of the throwing motion and reported increased superior labral strain during the late cocking phase of throwing, which supports the concept of the 'peel-back' mechanism.

Additional authors (Walch et al 1992; Jobe 1995) have demonstrated contact between the posterior–superior labrum and the rotator cuff when the arm is in an abducted and externally rotated position, which simulates the late cocking phase of throwing. Shepard et al (2004) simulated each of the aforementioned mechanisms in nine pairs of cadaveric shoulders that were loaded to biceps anchor failure in either a position of inline loading (similar to the deceleration phase of throwing) or in a simulated peel-back mechanism (similar to the late cocking phase of throwing). Their results showed that all of the simulated peel-back group failures resulted in a type II SLAP lesion, whereas the majority of the simulated inline-loading group failures occurred in the mid-substance of the biceps tendon. Additionally, the biceps anchor demonstrated a significantly higher strength with inline loading as opposed to the ultimate strength during the 'peel-back' mechanism. These results support the theory of peel-back as the predominant mechanism, but does not exclude a combination of mechanisms in the aetiology of SLAP lesions (Dodson & Altchek 2009).

A number of authors have reported an association between SLAP lesions and glenohumeral instability (Cordasco et al 1993; Rodosky et al 1994; Pagnani et al 1995; D'Alessandro et al 2000; Higgins & Warner 2001; Kim et al 2001; Pradhan et al 2001; Parentis et al 2002; Panossian et al 2005; Bedi & Allen 2008; Dodson & Altchek 2009). However, the exact cause-and-effect relationship of instability and SLAP lesions is still unclear (Liu et al 1996b; Higgins & Warner 2001; Parentis et al 2002). It may be that instability allows for a pathological range of motion that facilitates the peel-back mechanism, or conversely that SLAP lesions allow for excessive glenohumeral translation, which then leads to instability (Huijbregts 2001; Parentis et al 2002; Dodson & Altchek 2009).

Internal impingement is another proposed mechanism whereby the superior labrum is subjected to shear and direct contact, in the position of maximal shoulder abduction and external rotation, between the greater tubercle of the humerus and the posterosuperior rim of the glenoid (Bedi & Allen 2008; Cools et al 2008; Heyworth & Williams 2009). Recurrent abutment, between the articular side of the rotator cuff, the posterosuperior labrum and the glenoid rim, ultimately precipitates articular-sided rotator cuff tears and posterosuperior labral lesions (Higgins & Warner 2001; D'Alessandro et al 2000; Bedi & Allen 2008; Heyworth & Williams 2009). A range of theories has been proposed regarding internal impingement and the role that this plays in shoulder dysfunction and SLAP lesions (Wilk et al 2005; Heyworth & Williams 2009). Also a number of clinical findings have been associated with internal impingement including glenohumeral internal rotation deficit, SICK scapula syndrome, posterior humeral head lesions, posterior glenoid bony injury and Bankart and inferior glenohumeral ligament lesions (Heyworth & Williams 2009).

A variety of aetiological mechanisms have been implicated for SLAP lesions (D'Alessandro et al 2000; Higgins & Warner 2001; Huijbregts 2001; Musgrave & Rodosky 2001; Parentis et al 2002; Burkhart et al 2003; Nam & Snyder 2003; Wilk et al 2005; Bedi & Allen 2008; Heyworth & Williams 2009). Musgrave and Rodosky (2001) suggested that different mechanisms of injury were likely to be operational in the various SLAP-lesion types. It is probable that the varied pathoanatomy and / or pathomechanics of these different types of SLAP lesions significantly alter the clinical presentation (Kim et al 2003; Wilk et al 2005). Kim et al (2003) noted how the rarity of some of the types of SLAP lesions limits the statistical evaluation of some factors that might be important in understanding the pathophysiology of such lesions. Kim et al (2003) and Rao et al (2003) reported a positive association between anterosuperior labral anatomical variants and anterosuperior labral fraying. These authors postulated that anatomical variants influenced glenohumeral biomechanics and predisposed the shoulder to SLAP lesions (Kim et al 2003; Rao et al 2003; Bedi & Allen 2008). A retrospective review by Bents and Skeete (2005) supported this postulation: they found the presence of a Buford complex correlated with the presence of a SLAP lesion in patients. Additionally, a split biceps tendon has been associated with a displaced superior labrum in a type IV lesion (Parentis et al 2002, Nam & Snyder 2003).

Diagnosis

Clinical diagnosis of the SLAP lesion is difficult (Musgrave & Rodosky 2001; Dodson & Altchek 2009). The clinical presentation and correct diagnosis, even when using arthroscopy findings as a gold standard, are complicated by the variability of 'normal' anatomy of the superior labrum (D'Alessandro et al 2000; Higgins & Warner 2001; Huijbregts 2001; Musgrave & Rodosky 2001; Kim et al 2003; Nam & Snyder 2003; Wilk et al 2005). Adding to these intrinsic complexities, these lesions are often associated with additional concomitant shoulder pathology that influences patient presentation (Mileski & Snyder 1998; Musgrave & Rodosky 2001; Huijbregts 2001; Parentis et al 2002; Kim et al 2003; Wilk et al 2005). A number of authors note the difficulty in clinically differentiating, via examination, a SLAP lesion from concomitant pathology; they report that, despite efforts seen in literature to find clinical tests for the identification of SLAP lesions, a significant number of patients with such lesions are discovered only at arthroscopy (D'Alessandro et al 2000; Kim et al 2003; Wilk et al 2005). Thus, extra- and intra-articular shoulder pathologies confuse the clinical diagnostic process (Musgrave & Rodosky 2001).

Funk and Snow (2007) noted that the most common presenting clinical symptoms with SLAP injuries were mechanical symptoms such as 'locking, catching, popping, or snapping' in the shoulder. Walsworth et al (2008) investigated the diagnostic yield of history findings for glenoid labral tears (including SLAP lesions); a combined patient report of popping or catching and a positive crank (specificity 91%, +LR3.0) or anterior slide test (specificity 100%, +LR∞) suggested the presence of a labral tear. In the absence of a patient report of popping or clicking, having a negative anterior slide test or a negative crank test suggested absence of a labral tear (–LR0.31 and 0.33, respectively). Age as a predictor for such lesions has been investigated by Liu et al (1996a) and Walsworth et al (2008) but has not been noted to be of diagnostic utility, although Liu et al (1996a) noted a tendency for younger individuals (<35 years) to have such lesions.

From a retrospective study, Kampa and Clasper (2005) reported that individuals with a history of trauma or symptoms of instability were more likely to have a SLAP lesion than those presenting with atraumatic aetiologies ($p<0.0001$). Without providing research data, Barber et al (2007) suggested that clinically relevant SLAP injuries were most often found in the dominant arm of men <40 years of age who had participated in high-performance overhead activities for many years, patients with a specific history of shoulder trauma, or patients with shoulder instability. Barber et al (2007) additionally noted that a fall onto an outstretched hand or a prior motor vehicle accident in which the patient was wearing a seat-belt was suggestive of a SLAP injury.

As many as 21 different clinical tests have been described and investigated for their value in the diagnosis of SLAP lesions. There exists a large variation in the positions and movements used to reproduce symptoms and many authors report that no clinical test is sensitive and specific enough for the accurate diagnosis of SLAP lesions, noting the need for arthroscopic visualization for diagnosis (Mirkovic et al 2005; Bedi & Allen 2008; Dessaur & Magarey 2008; Powell et al 2008; McCaughey et al 2009). In addition, methodological inadequacies have been prevalent in research of SLAP lesion clinical tests (Dessaur & Magarey 2008; Meserve et al 2008; Powell et al 2008; Walsworth et al 2008; Walton & Sadi 2008; Munro & Healy 2009).

It is possible, and maybe even probable, that the varied pathoanatomy and / or pathomechanics of the differing types of SLAP lesions significantly alter the clinical presentation and clinical findings (D'Alessandro et al 2000; Huijbregts 2001; Musgrave & Rodosky 2001; Parentis et al 2002; Nam & Snyder 2003; Wilk et al 2005; Dessaur & Magarey 2008; Ebinger et al 2008; Dodson & Altchek 2009; Kibler et al 2009). Ebinger et al (2008) proposed that the flexion resistance test has high specificity for type II SLAP lesions. The speed test and O'Brien test have been reported to be highly specific for anterior type II SLAP lesions, whereas the modified Jobe relocation test has been reported as highly sensitive and highly specific for posterior SLAP lesions (D'Alessandro et al 2000; Burkhart & Morgan 2001; Burkhart et al 2003; Wilk et al 2005). The anterior scapular slide test has been reported to be useful for detecting anterior SLAP lesions (Burkhart & Morgan 2001; Burkhart et al 2003). Huijbregts (2001) reported that the SLAP-prehension test showed greater sensitivity for identifying types II–IV SLAP lesions and that the active compression (O'Brien) test, the provocation test and the biceps load test were useful for distinguishing between stable and unstable SLAP lesions. However, type-specific diagnostic utility statistics have yet to be reported (Powell et al 2008).

The clinical recommendations for the utilization of clinical SLAP lesion tests are varied. There are inconsistencies in the recommendations based on the various reviews available on this topic. Hegedus et al (2008) proposed, with caution, that the biceps load II test appeared diagnostic for SLAP lesions.

Cools et al (2008) proposed the inclusion of the speed test, the active compression test and the biceps load II test when investigating SLAP lesions. Meserve et al (2008) proposed that the active compression test should be utilized to rule out a SLAP lesion and that the speed test should be used to rule in a SLAP lesion when the active compression test or crank test have positive findings. Meserve et al (2008) reported that a positive sign on all three tests (active compression test, crank test, speed test) increases the probability that a SLAP lesion is present. Meserve et al (2008) and Pandya et al (2008) claimed the active compression test to be one of the best tests for diagnosing SLAP lesions. Oh et al (2008) concluded from a study of multitest regimens that combinations of two relatively sensitive clinical tests and one relatively specific clinical test increase the diagnostic efficacy of superior labrum anterior and posterior lesions.

Based on their systematic review of the diagnostic accuracy research, the current authors recently recommended the inclusion of the following clinical tests with the following interpretation for the diagnosis of SLAP lesion (with diagnostic accuracy data in Table 29.1):

- a negative finding on the passive compression test (Fig. 29.5) to *rule out* a SLAP lesion;
- a positive finding on the anterior apprehension manoeuvre (Fig. 29.6) (Guanche & Jones 2003), the anterior slide test (Fig. 29.7) (Kibler 1995; Powell et al 2008), the Jobe relocation test (Fig. 29.8) (Cook & Hegedus 2007), the passive compression test, the speed test and the Yergason test, or on a combination of positive findings on the Jobe relocation test and the active compression test or the Jobe relocation test and the anterior apprehension manoeuvre, to *rule in* a SLAP lesion.

The active compression test has been described in Chapter 28. In contrast to pain localized to the top of the shoulder in the

Table 29.1 **Psychometric data for SLAP-lesion clinical examination tests**

	Passive compression	Anterior apprehension	Anterior slide	Jobe relocation	Speed	Yergason	Active compression
Accuracy	0.84	0.59	0.54–0.86	0.56	0.56–0.57	0.61–0.63	0.54–0.98
Sensitivity	0.82	0.4–0.83	0.05–0.78	0.44–1.0	0.04–0.48	0.09–0.43	0.47–1.0
Specificity	0.86	0.4–0.87	0.81–0.93	0.4–0.87	0.67–1.0	0.79–1.0	0.1–0.98
Positive predictive value	0.87	0.53–0.9	0.05–0.64	0.32–0.91	0.35–1.0	0.46–1.0	0.1–0.94
Negative predictive value	0.8	0.33–0.75	0.56–0.90	0.34–0.71	0.26–0.72	0.25–0.71	0.1–1.0
Positive likelihood ratio	5.72	1.38–3.07	0.50–9.22	1.07–3.39	0.0–1.47	0.0–2.05	0.78–66
Negative likelihood ratio	0.21	0.43–0.72	0.24–1.10	0.63–0.94	0.6–0.94	0.72–1.29	0.0–2.0

(From: Kibler 1995; O'Brien et al 1998; Hamner et al 2000; McFarland et al 2002; Stetson & Templin 2002; Guanche & Jones 2003; Holtby & Razmjou 2004; Myers et al 2005; Nakagawa et al 2005; Parentis et al 2006; Kim et al 2007; Powell et al 2008.)

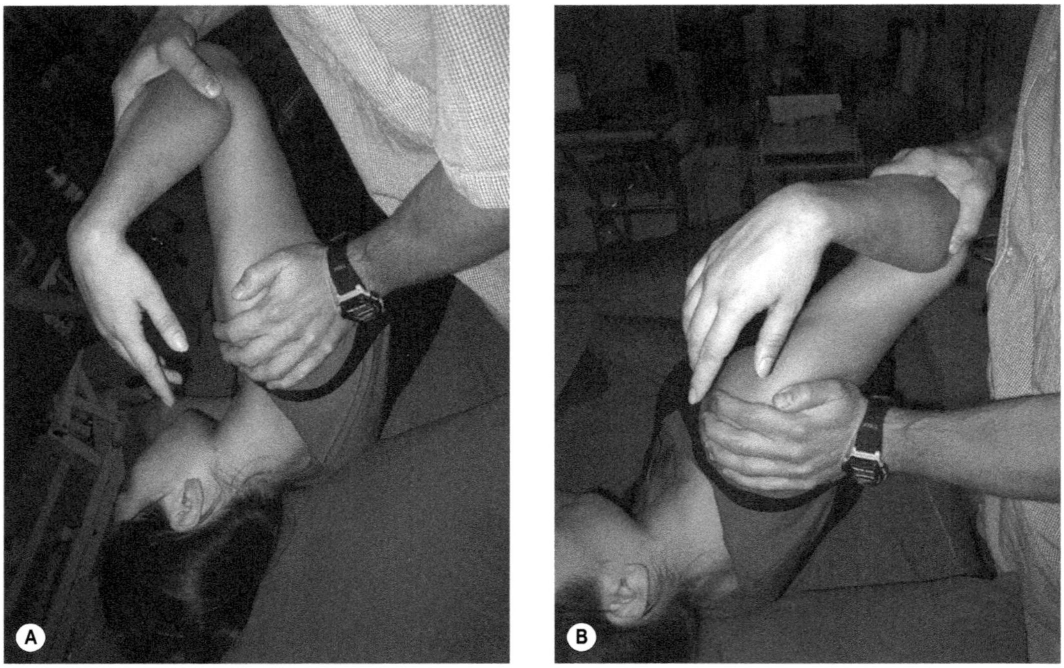

Figure 29.5 Passive compression test: (**A**) start position: the clinician rotates the patient's involved arm externally with 30° of abduction and pushes the arm proximally while extending the shoulder, which results in the passive compression of the superior labrum onto the glenoid; (**B**) end position. (From Powell et al 2008, with permission.)

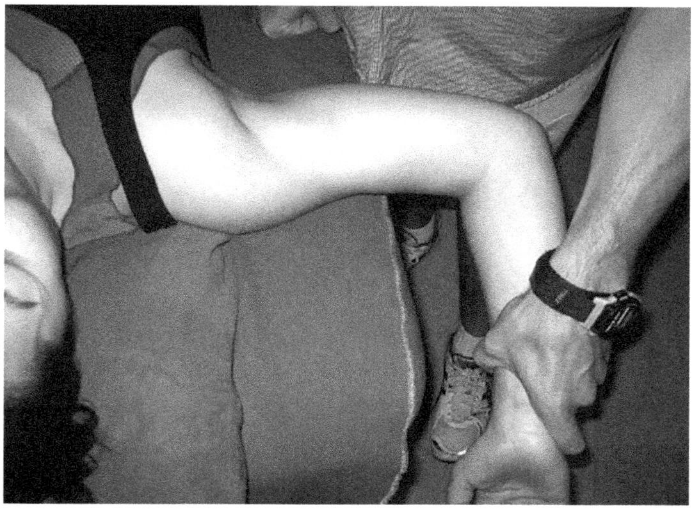

Figure 29.6 Anterior apprehension manoeuvre. The patient is supine and the examiner abducts the arm to 90° with the elbow in 90° of flexion and then progressively externally rotates the involved shoulder. A positive test is indicated by a look or feeling of apprehension or alarm on the patient's face and the patient's resistance to further motion. The patient might also state that the feeling experienced is what it felt like when the shoulder was previously dislocated. (From Powell et al 2008, with permission.)

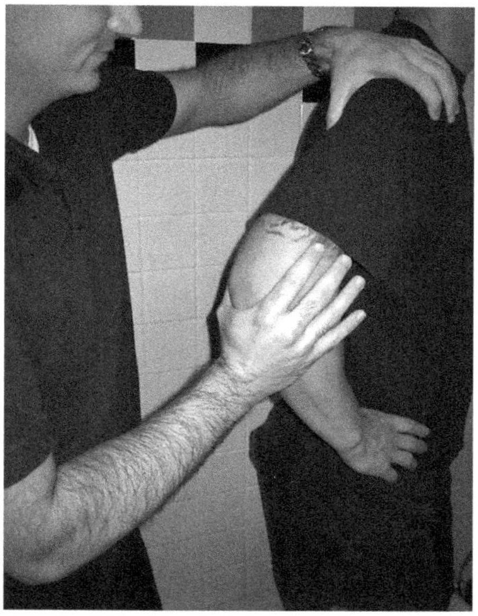

Figure 29.7 Anterior slide test. The patient is examined standing or sitting with hands on hips and the thumbs pointing posteriorly. One of the examiner's hands is positioned at the top of the shoulder from the posterior direction, with the last segment of the index finger extending over the anterior aspect of the acromion at the glenohumeral joint. The examiner's other hand is placed behind the elbow and a forward and a slightly superiorly directed force is applied to the elbow and upper arm. The patient is asked to push back against the clinician's force. Pain localized to the front of the shoulder under the examiner's hand and/or a pop or click in the same area is considered a positive result. This test is also considered positive if the patient reported this testing manoeuvre reproduces their presenting symptoms as associated with overhead activity. (From Powell et al 2008, with permission.)

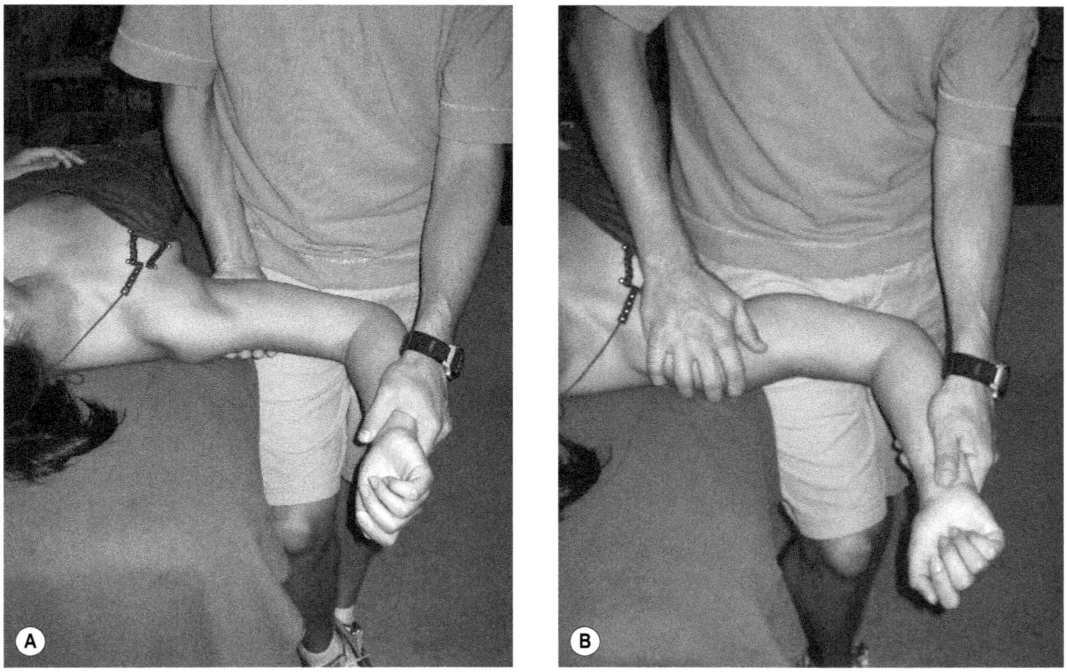

Figure 29.8 Jobe relocation test: (**A**) The patient is supine and the test performed at 90° of shoulder abduction with the involved shoulder in maximal external rotation. Initially an anterior force is applied to the proximal humerus. (**B**) A posterior force is applied to the proximal humerus. Pain that occurs with the anterior force and is relieved or diminished pain with the posterior force is considered a positive test finding. (From Powell et al 2008, with permission.)

internally rotated position that is relieved in the externally rotated position, which is considered indicative of acromioclavicular dysfunction, pain 'deep inside the shoulder,' with or without a click in the first position and eliminated or reduced in the second position, is considered indicative of a glenoid labrum tear (O'Brien et al 1998; Powell & Huijbregts 2006). In the context of diagnosis, the greatest value should be placed on a positive finding on the passive compression test owing to the strength of its positive likelihood ratio (Powell et al 2008).

Different imaging tests (magnetic resonance imaging (MRI), ultrasonography or computed tomography) may be useful in confirming the presence of a SLAP lesion, but they are reported to have a sensitivity of only 60–90%. The value of imaging studies has been questioned in the orthopaedic literature (Luime et al 2004). Approximately 10–20% of patients with a normal reading on shoulder MRI or ultrasonography may still have a SLAP lesion (Mileski & Snyder 1998; Mimori et al 1999; D'Alessandro et al 2000; Burkhart & Morgan 2001; Parentis et al 2002; Stetson & Templin 2002; Burkhart et al 2003; Nam & Snyder 2003; Holtby & Razmjou 2004; Luime et al 2004; Mirkovic et al 2005; Nakagawa et al 2005; Wilk et al 2005; Parentis et al 2006; Swearingen et al 2006; Jones & Galluch 2007; Dessaur & Magarey 2008; Calvert et al 2009). Therefore, definitive diagnosis requires arthroscopy (D'Alessandro et al 2000; Burkhart & Morgan 2001; Nam & Snyder 2003; Bedi & Allen 2008).

Standard multiplanar T1- and T2-weighted MRI images can detect supraglenoid cysts, which have been associated with type II SLAP lesions. These cysts can arise as a result of labral injury with a communication through the capsule (Nam & Snyder 2003). MR arthrography with gadolinium may offer improved visualization (Nam & Snyder 2003; Clifford 2007; Bedi & Allen 2008; Magee 2009). Bencardino et al (2000) reported 89% sensitivity, 91% specificity and 90% accuracy for the diagnosis of SLAP lesions with gadolinium-enhanced MR arthrography compared with a gold standard of arthroscopic findings. However, false-positive and false-negative results do occur (Burkhart & Morgan 2001; Parentis et al 2002; Nam & Snyder 2003; Clifford 2007).

SLAP lesions may be visualized on the coronal oblique sequence as a deep cleft between the superior labrum and the glenoid that extends well around and below the biceps anchor (Fig. 29.9). Often the contrast medium will dissipate into the labral fragment, causing it to appear ragged / frayed or indistinct. The axial view is sometimes helpful to view the displaced superior labral fragment. Normal labral variants must be kept in mind when viewing these labral images, as these congenital variations of the anterosuperior labrum can be misleading and can complicate results (Parentis et al 2002; Clifford 2007). If there is an associated labral split or biceps tear, as seen in a type III or IV lesion, the displaced fragment may be difficult to visualize unless the superior labral area is carefully examined.

Standard radiographs (AP, axillary and outlet views) cannot identify a SLAP lesion, but assessment of the acromial morphology and the acromioclavicular joint are useful when the clinician is considering associated disorders (D'Alessandro et al 2000; Bedi & Allen 2008; Dodson & Altchek 2009). Although radiographs are usually normal in isolated SLAP lesions, other potential sources of abnormalities can be evaluated (Wilk et al 2005). As the clinical presentation of SLAP

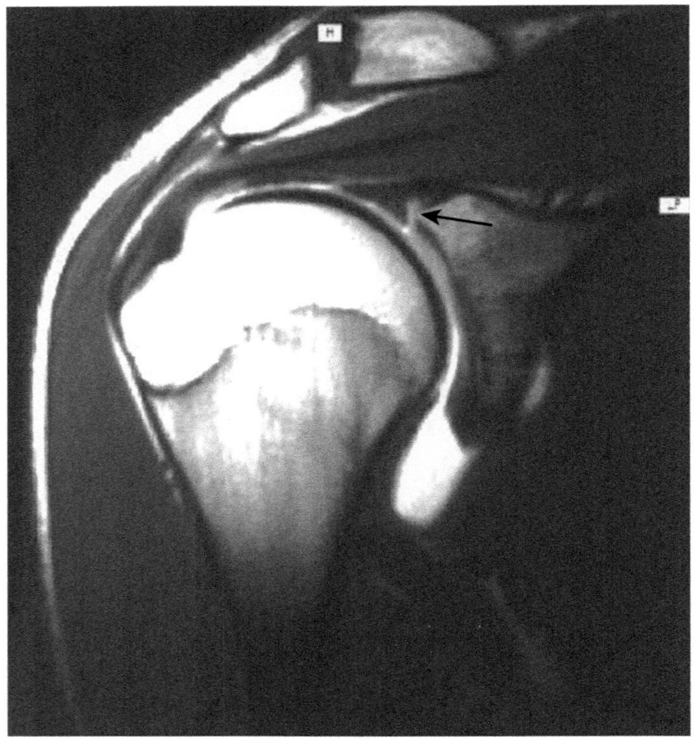

Figure 29.9 Coronal T1-weighted image of a SLAP lesion from an MR arthrogram. Contrast material is interposed between the superior labrum and the glenoid (arrow). The labrum is displaced (arrowhead). (From Powell et al 2008, with permission.)

lesions is often unclear, radiographic and imaging studies are frequently used to aid in the diagnosis. Imaging options enhance the diagnostic 'picture' by enabling the clinician to determine the presence or absence of common concomitant pathology for SLAP lesions. The clinical value of these diagnostic tools should not be underestimated in the clinically complex SLAP lesions.

Management

Different types of SLAP lesions seem to respond to different types of interventions (D'Alessandro et al 2000; Huijbregts 2001; Parentis et al 2002, 2006; Nam & Snyder 2003; Wilk et al 2005). Some authors (D'Alessandro et al 2000; Bedi & Allen 2008) propose an initial trial of conservative management for SLAP lesions, whereas others (Mileski & Snyder 1998; Wilk et al 2005; Dodson & Altchek 2009) propose that conservative management will be unsuccessful. However, the natural history of SLAP lesions is unknown and data regarding the efficacy of conservative treatments for SLAP lesions are not available (D'Alessandro et al 2000). Vascularization, and thereby healing potential, is a prerequisite for optimal conservative management (Powell et al 2008; Huijbregts 2001).

Treatment goals for conservative management would include the reduction of pain and mechanical symptoms, and the restoring and optimizing of glenohumeral and also scapulothoracic, acromioclavicular, sternoclavicular and thoracic motion, strength and function. Dodson and Altcheck (2009) describe conservative management as including relative rest from aggravating activities; anti-inflammatory medication; restoration of normal shoulder motion – including addressing glenohumeral internal rotation deficit, if present; strengthening of the shoulder girdle musculature to restore normal scapulothoracic motion; and progression to advanced conditioning activities that include trunk, core, rotator cuff and scapulothoracic musculature and sport / acrobatic / functional skills.

Cordasco et al (1993) stated that SLAP lesions are the result of instability and should not be considered isolated lesions. Shear forces at the glenohumeral joint have been hypothesized to play a role in producing the labral lesion (Snyder et al 1990; Bey et al 1998). Muscle force has been hypothesized to compress the humeral head into the labrum, which normally prevents it from rolling up and over the labrum (Howell & Galinat 1989) but in the case of instability imparts excessive shear and compressive forces to the labrum. Addressing glenohumeral instability would therefore be a treatment priority (Huijbregts 2001). Liu et al (1996a) suggested an intensive 3-month programme of activity modification, non-steroidal anti-inflammatory medications and physical therapy for patients with mild instability and labral tears. The physical therapy programme they described involves passive range of motion followed by active range of motion of the shoulder, strengthening of the rotator cuff and scapular stabilizers, and finally functional and sport-specific activities. Patients who experience relief are thought to have had pain as a result of the instability. It has been questioned whether the pain that individuals with a SLAP lesion complain of is the result of the labral tear itself or the instability (Liu et al 1996b; Huijbregts 2001).

Musgrave and Rodosky (2001) reported that SLAP lesions should be treated based on the type with which an individual presents. They proposed debridement of type I lesions with preservation of the biceps anchor, whereas Wilk et al (2005) suggested conservative management for type I lesions. Type II lesions, due to the disruption of the biceps attachment and consequent glenohumeral instability, commonly require surgical repair for optimal stabilization and restoration of function (D'Alessandro et al 2000; Musgrave & Rodosky 2001; Parentis et al 2002, 2006; Nam & Snyder 2003; Panossian et al 2005; Wilk et al 2005; Bedi & Allen 2008; Dodson & Altchek 2009). The bucket-handle tear of a type III lesion is typically excised, with care taken to avoid destabilization of the middle glenohumeral ligament, particularly if a cord-like middle glenohumeral ligament is present (D'Alessandro et al 2000; Higgins & Warner 2001; Musgrave & Rodosky 2001; Bedi & Allen 2008; Dodson & Altchek 2009). Management of type IV lesions is somewhat dependent on the extent of injury to the biceps tendon. When the biceps involvement is less than 30% then the torn tissue is excised and the superior labrum repaired; if the biceps involvement is more extensive then either it is repaired or a tenodesis is performed (Mileski & Snyder 1998; D'Alessandro et al 2000; Higgins & Warner 2001; Musgrave & Rodosky 2001; Parentis et al 2002; Wilk et al 2005; Bedi & Allen 2008; Dodson & Altchek 2009). SLAP lesion types V, VI and VII are treated similarly to types I to IV, but there is additional treatment for the associated pathology (type V – Bankart repair and biceps anchor stabilization, type VI – flap debridement and biceps anchor stabilization, type VII – repair of middle glenohumeral ligament and biceps anchor stabilization) (Musgrave & Rodosky 2001; Parentis et al 2002; Wilk et al 2005; Bedi & Allen 2008). Suture anchor repair is preferred over biodegradable sutureless implants, which have been associated with complications such as synovitis, chondral injury and mechanical failure (Bedi & Allen 2008).

SLAP lesions that are complex, such as those involving rotator cuff tears, those associated with glenohumeral joint instability, or those with concomitant biceps tendon pathology, are likely to respond to different management strategies from isolated SLAP lesions (D'Alessandro et al 2000; Kim et al 2003; Nam & Snyder 2003; Panossian et al 2005, Wilk et al 2005). Concomitant shoulder disorders should be addressed and their management may even be critical to ensure a successful outcome (Mileski & Snyder 1998; Higgins & Warner 2001, Dodson & Altchek 2009). SLAP lesions identified at arthroscopy may not be pathological or clinically significant, but rather are part of a constellation of generalized degenerative changes (Lebolt et al 2006; Bedi & Allen 2008).

Prognosis

Information on the natural history of SLAP lesions is lacking. Outcome data, and therefore prognosis, for conservatively managed SLAP lesions are also unknown. Conservative management of SLAP lesions (regardless of type) is often reported to be unsuccessful, but outcome data are not provided (Mileski & Snyder 1998; Wilk et al 2005; Dodson & Altchek 2009). Further, long-term results with simple debridement of lesions are often reported to be poor, but again outcome data are rarely provided (Mileski & Snyder 1998; Wilk et al 2005).

Cordasco et al (1993) reported deterioration of clinical outcomes with longer follow-up (78% pain relief at 1 year, 63% at 2 years) after SLAP lesion debridement, with only 45% of individuals returning to their preoperative level of function. Abbot et al (2009) reported that, in older patients (>45 years) who presented for management of rotator cuff injury and type II SLAP lesion, those who had debridement rather than SLAP repair with concomitant rotator cuff repair had significantly better function, pain relief and range of motion.

The majority of the SLAP lesion surgical outcomes published report that 80–90% of individuals have good or excellent results, at short-term or intermediate follow-up after surgical repair of type II SLAP lesions (D'Alessandro et al 2000; Bedi & Allen 2008; Dodson & Altchek 2009). Dodson and Alcheck (2009) noted a lack of long-term follow-up studies following type II SLAP lesion repairs and suggested that surgical repair of type II SLAP lesions in overhead athletes with a non-traumatic incident may be less successful than in other individuals. Bedi and Allen (2008) reported that individuals with traumatic-onset, isolated type II SLAP lesions who then had surgical repair reported greater subjective satisfaction than did individuals with insidious SLAP injury.

Conclusion

In summary, individuals who present with pain or dysfunction of the shoulder may have sustained an injury to the superior labrum. If present, the severity of a SLAP lesion is widely variable and may, or may not, be clinically significant.

SLAP lesions are often associated with other intra-articular shoulder injuries, and the examining clinician should have a high index of suspicion for coexisting pathology. SLAP lesions are difficult to identify clinically. There is a paucity of evidence-based guidance for the clinical examination and the optimal management strategy to employ. There is widespread agreement that a traumatic labral injury where the biceps origin is disrupted (types II, IV, V, VI and VII) needs surgical management, yet long-term outcome studies have not been published to support this. Further studies are needed to gain a better understanding of the causes of SLAP lesions, to improve clinical diagnoses and to determine the optimal management strategy for such lesions. Areas that are most likely to benefit from more research include:

- **long-term prognosis:** studying the sequelae of SLAP injury with validated relevant outcome measures
- **diagnostic testing:** (a) study of the diagnostic utility for type-specific clinical tests would allow the clinician to differentiate within SLAP lesions those best managed conservatively from those best managed surgically (Huijbregts 2001; Powell et al 2008); (b) further diagnostic accuracy investigation into more recently proposed clinical tests for SLAP lesions including the biceps load II, passive compression and resisted supination external rotation tests (Dessaur & Magarey 2008; Meserve et al 2008); (c) study of the combination(s) or clustering of history components and clinical tests for determining the presence or absence of type-specific SLAP lesions (Dessaur & Magarey 2008; Meserve et al 2008; Walsworth et al 2008)
- **conservative treatment:** the comparison of different types of supervised rehabilitation in the management of the varied types of SLAP lesions (Huijbregts 2001)
- **surgical treatment:** study of the long-term outcomes of surgically managed SLAP lesions.

References

Abbot AE, Li X, Busconi BD. 2009. Arthroscopic treatment of concomitant superior labral anterior posterior (SLAP) lesions and rotator cuff tears in patients over the age of 45 years. Am J Sports Med 37: 1358–1362.

Andrews JR, Carson WG. 1984. The arthroscopic treatment of glenoid labrum tears in the throwing athlete. Orthop Trans 8: 44.

Andrews JR, Carson WG, McLeod WD. 1985. Glenoid labrum tears related to the long head of the biceps. Am J Sports Med 13: 337–341.

Barber A, Field LD, Ryu R. 2007. Biceps tendon and superior labrum injuries: decision-marking. J Bone Joint Surg 89A: 1844–1855.

Bedi A, Allen AA. 2008. Superior labral lesions anterior to posterior–evaluation and arthroscopic management. Clin Sports Med 27: 607–630

Bencardino JT, Beltran J, Rosenberg ZS, et al. 2000. Superior labrum anterior–posterior lesions: diagnosis with MR arthrography of the shoulder. Radiology 214: 267–271.

Bents RT, Skeete KD. 2005. The correlation of the Buford complex and SLAP lesions. J Shoulder Elbow Surg 14: 565–569.

Bey MJ, Elders GJ, Huston LJ, et al. 1998. The mechanism of creation of superior labrum, anterior and posterior lesions in a dynamic biomechanical model of the shoulder: the role of inferior subluxation. J Shoulder Elbow Surg 7: 397–401.

Burkhart SS, Morgan CD. 1998. The peel-back mechanism: its role in producing and extending posterior type II SLAP lesions and its effect on SLAP repair rehabilitation. Arthroscopy 14: 637–640.

Burkhart SS, Morgan C. 2001. SLAP lesions in the overhead athlete. Orthop Clin North Am 32: 431–441.

Burkhart SS, Morgan CD, Kibler WB. 2003. The disabled throwing shoulder: spectrum of pathology. Part II: Evaluation and treatment of SLAP lesions in throwers. Arthroscopy 19: 531–539.

Calvert E, Chambers GK, Regan W, et al. 2009. Special physical examination tests for superior labrum anterior posterior shoulder tears are clinically limited and invalid: a diagnostic systematic review. J Clin Epidemiol 62: 558–563.

Clifford PD. 2007. Superior labral anterior to posterior (SLAP) tears. Am J Orthop 36: 685–686.

Cook C, Hegedus E. 2007. Orthopedic physical examination tests: an evidence-based approach. Upper Saddle River, NJ: Prentice Hall.

Cools AM, Cambier D, Witvrouw EE. 2008. Screening the athlete's shoulder for impingement symptoms: a clinical reasoning algorithm for early detection of shoulder pathology. Br J Sports Med 42: 628–635.

Cooper DE, Arnoczky SP, O'Brien SJ, et al. 1992. Anatomy, histology, and vascularity of the glenoid labrum. J Bone Joint Surg 74A: 46–52.

Cordasco FA, Steinmann S, Flatow EL, et al. 1993. Arthroscopic treatment of glenoid labral tears. Am J Sports Med 21: 425–430.

D'Alessandro, DR Fleischli JE, Connor PM. 2000. Superior labral lesions: diagnosis and management. J Athl Train 35: 286–292.

Dessaur WA, Magarey ME. 2008. Diagnostic accuracy of clinical tests for superior labral anterior posterior lesions: a systematic review. J Orthop Sports Phys Ther 38: 341–352.

Dierickx C, Ceccarelli E, Conti M, et al. 2009. Variations of the intra-articular portion of the long head of the biceps tendon: a classification of embryologically explained variations. J Shoulder Elbow Surg 18: 556–565.

Dodson CC, Altchek DW. 2009. SLAP lesions: an update on recognition and treatment. J Orthop Sports Phys Ther 39: 71–80.

Ebinger N, Magosch P, Lichtenberg S, et al. 2008. A new SLAP test: the supine flexion resistance test. Arthroscopy 24: 500–505.

Funk L, Snow M. 2007. SLAP tears of the glenoid labrum in contact athletes. Clin J Sport Med 171–174.

Ghalayini SR, Board TN, Srinivasan MS. 2007. Anatomic variations in the long head of biceps: contribution to shoulder dysfunction. Arthroscopy 23: 1012–1018.

Glousman R, Jobe F, Tibone J, et al. 1988. Dynamic electromyographic analysis of the throwing shoulder with gleno-humeral instability. J Bone Joint Surg 70A: 220–226.

Guanche CA, Jones C. 2003. Clinical testing for tears of the glenoid labrum. Arthroscopy 19: 517–523.

Halder AM, Kuhl SG, Zobitz ME, et al. 2001. Effects of the glenoid labrum and gleno-humeral abduction on stability of the shoulder joint through concavity-compression: an in vitro study. J Bone Joint Surg 83A: 1062–1069.

Hamner DL, Pink MM, Jobe FW. 2000. A modification of the relocation test: Arthroscopic findings associated with a positive test. J Shoulder Elbow Surg 9: 263–267.

Hegedus EJ, Goode A, Campbell S, et al. 2008. Physical examination tests of the shoulder: a systematic review with meta-analysis of individual tests. Br J Sports Med 4: 280–292.

Heyworth BE, Williams RJ. 2009. Internal impingement of the shoulder. Am J Sports Med 37: 1024–1037.

Higgins LD, Warner JP. 2001. Superior labral lesions: anatomy, pathology, and treatment. Clin Orthop 390: 73–82.

Holtby R, Razmjou H. 2004. Accuracy of the Speed's and Yergason's tests in detecting biceps pathology and SLAP lesions: comparison with arthroscopic findings. Arthroscopy 20: 231–236.

Howell SM, Galinat BJ. 1989. The glenoid-labral socket. Clin Orthop 243: 122–125.

Huijbregts PA. 2001. SLAP lesions: structure, function, and physical therapy diagnosis and treatment. J Man Manip Ther 9: 71–83.

Jobe CM. 1995. Posterior superior glenoid impingement: expanded spectrum. Arthroscopy 11: 530–536.

Jobe FW, Moynes DR, Tibone JE, et al. 1984. An EMG analysis of the shoulder in pitching. A second report. Am J Sports Med 12: 218–220.

Jones GL, Galluch DB. 2007. Clinical assessment of superior glenoid labral lesions. Clin Orthop Relat Res 455: 45–51.

Kampa RJ, Clasper J. 2005. Incidence of SLAP lesions in a military population. J R Army Med Corps 151: 171–175.

Kibler WB. 1995. Specificity and sensitivity of the anterior slide test in throwing athletes with superior glenoid labral tears. Arthroscopy 11: 296–300.

Kibler WB, Sciascia AD, Hester P, et al. 2009. Clinical utility of traditional and new tests in the diagnosis of biceps tendon injuries and superior labrum anterior and posterior lesions in the shoulder. Am J Sports Med 37(9): 1840–1847.

Kim SH, Ha KI, Ahn JH, et al. 2001. Biceps load test II: a clinical test for SLAP lesions of the shoulder. Arthroscopy 17: 160–164.

Kim SH, Ha KI, Kim SH, et al. 2002. Results of arthroscopic treatment of superior labral lesions. J Bone Joint Surg 84A: 981–985.

Kim TK, Queale WE, Cosgarea AJ, et al. 2003. Clinical features of the different types of SLAP lesions: an analysis of one hundred and thirty-nine cases. J Bone Joint Surg 85A: 66–71.

Kim YS, Kim JM, Ha KY, et al. 2007. The passive compression test: a new clinical test for superior labral tears of the shoulder. Am J Sports Med 35: 1489–1494.

Krupp RJ, Kevern MA, Gaines MD, et al. 2009. Long head of the biceps tendon pain: differential diagnosis and treatment. J Orthop Sports Phys Ther 39: 55–70.

Lebolt JR, Cain EL, Andrews JR. 2006. SLAP lesions, 2007. Am J Orthop 35: 554–557.

Lippitt SB, Vanderhooft JE, Harris SL, et al. 1993. Gleno-humeral stability from concavity-compression: a quantitative analysis. J Shoulder Elbow Surg 2: 27–35.

Liu SH, Henry MH, Nuccion SL. 1996a. A prospective evaluation of a new physical examination in predicting glenoid labral tears. Am J Sports Med 24: 721–725.

Liu SH, Henry MH, Nuccion S, et al. 1996b. Diagnosis of glenoid labral tears. A comparison between magnetic resonance imaging and clinical examinations. Am J Sports Med 24: 149–154.

Luime JJ, Verhagen AP, Miedema HS, et al. 2004. Does this patient have an instability of the shoulder or a labrum lesion? JAMA 292: 1989–1999.

Maffet MW, Gartsman GM, Moseley B. 1995. Superior labrum–biceps tendon complex lesions of the shoulder. Am J Sports Med 23: 93–98.

Magee T. 2009. 3-T MRI of the shoulder: is MR arthrography necessary? AJR Am J Roentgenol 192: 86–92.

McCaughey R, Green RA, Taylor NF. 2009. The anatomical basis of the resisted supination external rotation test for superior labral anterior to posterior lesions. Clin Anat 22: 665–670.

McFarland EG, Kim TK, Savino RM. 2002. Clinical assessment of three common tests for superior labral anterior–posterior lesions. Am J Sports Med 30: 810–815.

Meserve BB, Cleland JA, Boucher TR. 2008. The anatomical basis of the resisted supination external rotation test for superior labral anterior to posterior lesions. Am J Sports Med 37: 2252–2258.

Mileski RA, Snyder SJ. 1998. Superior labral lesions in the shoulder: pathoanatomy and surgical management. J Am Acad Orthop Surg 6: 121–131.

Mimori K, Muneta T, Nakagawa T, et al. 1999. A new pain provocation test for superior labral tears of the shoulder. Am J Sports Med 27: 137–142.

Mirkovic M, Green R, Taylor N, et al. 2005. Accuracy of clinical tests to diagnose superior labral anterior and posterior (SLAP) lesions. Phys Ther Rev 10: 5–14.

Munro W, Healy R. 2009. The validity and accuracy of clinical tests used to detect labral pathology of the shoulder – a systematic review. Man Ther 14: 119–130.

Musgrave DS, Rodosky MW. 2001. SLAP lesions: current concepts. Am J Orthop 30: 29–38.

Myers TH, Zemanovic JR, Andrews JR. 2005. The resisted supination external rotation test: a new test for the diagnosis of superior labral anterior posterior lesions. Am J Sports Med 33: 1315–1320.

Nakagawa S, Yoneda M, Hayashida K, et al. 2005. Forced shoulder abduction and elbow flexion test: a new simple clinical test to detect superior labral injury in the throwing shoulder. Arthroscopy 21: 1290–1295.

Nam EK, Snyder SJ. 2003. The diagnosis and treatment of superior labrum, anterior and posterior (SLAP) lesions. Am J Sports Med 31: 798–810.

O'Brien SJ, Pagnani MJ, Fealy S, et al. 1998. The active compression test: a new and effective test for diagnosing labral tears and acromioclavicular joint abnormality. Am J Sports Med 26: 610–613.

Oh JH, Kim JY, Kim WS, et al. 2008. The evaluation of various physical examinations for the diagnosis of type II superior labrum anterior and posterior lesion. Am J Sports Med 36: 353–359.

Pagnani MJ, Deng XH, Warren RF, et al. 1995. Effect of lesions of the superior portion of the glenoid labrum on gleno-humeral translation. J Bone Joint Surg 77A: 1003–1010.

Pal GP, Bhatt RH, Patel VS, 1991. Relationship between the tendon of the long head of biceps brachii and the glenoidal labrum in humans. Anat Rec 229: 278–280.

Pandya NK, Colton A, Webner D, et al. 2008. Physical examination and magnetic resonance imaging in the diagnosis of superior labrum anterior–posterior lesions of the shoulder: a sensitivity analysis. Arthroscopy 24(3): 311–317.

Panossian VR, Mihata T, Tibone JE, et al. 2005. Biomechanical analysis of isolated type II SLAP lesions and repair. J Shoulder Elbow Surg 14: 529–534.

Parentis MA, Mohr KJ, ElAttrache NS. 2002. Disorders of the superior labrum: review and treatment guidelines. Clin Orthop 400: 77–87.

Parentis MA, Mohr KJ, Yocum LA. 2006. An evaluation of the provocative tests for superior labral anterior posterior lesions. Am J Sports Med 34: 265–268.

Powell JW, Huijbregts PA. 2006. Concurrent criterion-related validity of acromio-clavicular joint physical examination tests: a systematic review. J Man Manip Ther 14: E19–E29.

Powell JW, Huijbregts PA, Jensen R. 2008. Diagnostic utility of clinical tests for SLAP lesions: a systematic literature review. J Man Manip Ther 16: E58–E79.

Pradhan RL, Itoi E, Hatakeyama Y, et al. 2001. Superior labral strain during the throwing motion. A cadaveric study. Am J Sports Med 29: 488–492.

Prodromos CC, Ferry JA, Schiller AL, et al. 1990. Histological studies of the glenoid labrum from fetal life to old age. J Bone Joint Surg 72A: 1344–1348.

Rao AG, Kim TK, Chronopoulos E, et al. 2003. Anatomical variants in the anterosuperior aspect of the glenoid labrum: a statistical analysis of seventy-three cases. J Bone Joint Surg 85A: 653–659.

Rodosky MW, Harner CD, Fu FH. 1994. The role of the long head of the biceps muscle and superior glenoid labrum in anterior stability of the shoulder. Am J Sports Med 11: 121–130.

Shepard MF, Dugas JR, Zeng N, et al. 2004. Differences in the ultimate strength of the biceps anchor and the generation of type II superior labral anterior posterior lesions in a cadaveric model. Am J Sports Med 32: 1197–1201.

Snyder SJ, Karzel RP, Del Pizzo W, et al. 1990. SLAP lesions of the shoulder. Arthroscopy 6: 274–279.

Snyder SJ, Banas MP, Karzel RP. 1995. An analysis of 140 injuries to the superior glenoid labrum. J Shoulder Elbow Surg 4: 243–248.

Stetson WB, Templin K. 2002. The crank test, the O'Brien test, and routine magnetic resonance imaging scans in the diagnosis of labral tears. Am J Sports Med 30: 806–809.

Swearingen JC, Mell AG, Langenderfer J, et al. 2006. Electromyographic analysis of physical examination tests for types II superior labrum anterior–posterior lesions. J Shoulder Elbow Surg 15: 576–579.

Vangsness CT, Jorgenson SS, Watson T, et al. 1994. The origin of the long head of the biceps from the scapula and glenoid labrum. An anatomical study of 100 shoulders. J Bone Joint Surg 76B: 951–954.

Walch G, Boileau P, Noel E, et al. 1992. Impingement of the deep surface of the infraspinatus tendon on the posterior glenoid rim. J Shoulder Elbow Surg 1: 238–245.

Walsworth MK, Doukas WC, Murphy KP, et al. 2008. Reliability and diagnostic accuracy of history and physical examination for diagnosing glenoid labral tears. Am J Sports Med 36: 162–168.

Walton DM, Sadi J. 2008. Identifying SLAP lesions: a meta-analysis of clinical tests and exercise in clinical reasoning. Phys Ther Sport 9: 167–176.

Warner JJ, McMahon PJ. 1995. The role of the long head of the biceps brachii in superior stability of the gleno-humeral joint. J Bone Joint Surg 77A: 366–372.

Wilk KE, Arrigo CA, Andrews JR. 1997. Current concepts: the stabilizing structures of the gleno-humeral joint. J Orthop Sports Phys Ther 25: 364–379.

Wilk KE, Reinold MM, Dugas JR, et al. 2005. Current concepts in the recognition and treatment of superior labral (SLAP) lesions. J Orthop Sports Phys Ther 35: 273–291.

30 Chapter

Frozen Shoulder

Carel Bron, Arthur de Gast, Jo L.M. Franssen

CHAPTER CONTENTS

Introduction 344
Incidence 344
Pathology 344
Natural history and prognosis 345
Diagnosis 346
  History 346
  Physical examination 347
Treatment 347
  Recalcitrant frozen shoulders 348
  Prevention of frozen shoulder 348
Conclusion 348

Introduction

Frozen shoulder (FS) or adhesive capsulitis is, although known for more than a century, still an enigmatic and poorly defined shoulder disorder. The earliest case report was published in 1872 by the French surgeon Duplay (1872), who used the term 'peri-arthrite scapulo-humerale' when he described a disorder similar to the condition we know nowadays as frozen shoulder. This latter term was introduced several decades later by Codman (1934). Finally, Neviaser (1945), an orthopaedic surgeon also used the term 'adhesive capsulitis' based on his arthrographic and intra-articular findings.

Codman (1934) stated that the frozen shoulder was 'difficult to define, difficult to treat, and difficult to explain from the point of view of pathology'. Obviously, not much has changed as the years have passed. The three terms 'frozen shoulder', 'adhesive capsulitis' and 'peri-arthrite scapulo-humerale' (although the last one from Duplay is now somewhat outdated) are all used to describe a clinical condition of pain and severe (more than 50%) restricted passive range of motion (PROM) of the glenohumeral joint in all directions (flexion, extension, abduction, adduction and internal–external rotations). The aetiology of FS is usually unknown. Patients occasionally mention a variety of activities or circumstances that they associate with the start of their complaints. Still, the exact cause of FS remains to be established.

It is common usage to differentiate between a primary and a secondary frozen shoulder (Lundberg 1969). Primary FS is idiopathic and not related to other diseases, whereas secondary FS is defined as being related to known systemic pathology, such as diabetes mellitus, thyroid disease or Parkinson's disease, or occurring post surgery, post trauma or after a period of immobilization. It is difficult to differentiate, but one might suffer from post-surgical shoulder stiffness, which is not the same as secondary post-surgical FS.

In this chapter we will focus on primary FS, which encompasses the following clinical criteria: (1) restriction of shoulder motion without major shoulder injury; (2) global stiffness of the shoulder joint in all directions, without the loss of strength, joint stability, or joint surface integrity; and (3) plain shoulder radiographs demonstrating a normal glenohumeral joint space and no periarticular abnormalities, although some osteopenia of the proximal humerus and glenoid may be seen.

Incidence

FS has an incidence of 3–5% in the general population, and is a common shoulder disorder in orthopaedic practice. In the Netherlands it is calculated that 1 in 105 shoulder patients who consult a general practitioner is diagnosed with primary FS. FS is more common among patients with diabetes, affecting 20% or more of such patients (Balci et al 1999; Kordella 2002; Tighe & Oakley 2008).

Pathology

Normal functional limits of the glenohumeral joint are determined by skeletal morphology, articular surface area and the flexibility of the connection joint capsule, ligaments, musculotendinous units and integument. In a glenohumeral joint with smooth articular surfaces, shoulder stiffness occurs as a result of (1) stiffening of the joint capsule, ligaments or muscle–tendon units, (2) adhesions along the gliding surfaces between the rotator cuff and its surroundings, adhesions in the biceps tendon mechanism and (3) extra-articular adhesions. These restrictions can occur independently or in combination. In primary FS the glenohumeral functional restriction most probably starts in the glenohumeral joint capsule, and during the course of the disease the stiffness may encompass soft tissue structures outside the joint.

The pathological process in primary FS is not clear, although several authors have tried to elucidate it (Hannafin & Chiaia 2000; Cleland & Durall 2002; Uhthoff & Boileau 2007; Schultheis et al 2008). It is generally accepted that underlying FS is an inflammatory process of the synovial membrane, which is subsequently followed by a fibrotic reaction of the fibrous layer. There is still disagreement over whether or not the underlying pathology is an inflammatory process, but arthroscopy shows a hyperaemic and swollen synovial membrane. The recent discovery of several cytokines in the joint capsule in patients with FS supports the inflammation theory. The synovial reaction (or inflammation) eventually leads to fibrosis of the underlying layer of the glenohumeral capsule (fibrous membrane). Especially in the area of the coracohumeral ligament (CHL) and the rotator cuff interval, scar formation and contracture formation are initiated by the expression of vimentin (a cytocontractile protein that is usually seen in fibromyocytes), while in the entire joint capsule there is fibroplasia (thickening of the joint capsule) but without contraction.

Another important outcome is the need for a distinction between fibroplasia and contracture. Uhthoff and Boileau (2007) found that, although fibroplasia involves the entire capsule, the presence of cytocontractile proteins is limited to the anterior capsular part. Further, fibroplasia involves the entire joint capsule to an almost identical degree, with no preferential involvement of the anterior capsule. From this, it follows that the reduced range of motion of the primary FS is primarily attributable to the contracture of anterior capsular structures, particularly the CHL and the capsule at the rotator interval as seen by the selective expression of the cytocontractile protein vimentin. The above finding also confirms the clinical experience that surgical division of these structures is usually sufficient to restore the lost range of motion. Yang et al (2009) studied the anatomical relationship of the CHL in 14 normal cadaveric shoulders. In most of the cases (11 of 14) the CHL (Fig. 30.1) inserted into the rotator cuff interval and the supraspinatus tendon, while in four the tendon of the subscapularis was also involved. The dissimilarity in the insertion of the CHL may be one of the reasons for different clinical pictures seen with, for example, more or less limitation of external rotation.

Although it is still controversial whether the CHL is a separate entity or just a thickening of the glenohumeral capsule, Yang et al (2009) concluded, based upon their findings, that the CHL position, morphology and origin are relatively unchanged, but that its insertion varies greatly and that the CHL is a more capsular than a ligamentous structure based on its histological features. Finally, although Neviaser (1945) was convinced of the formation of intra-articular adhesion between parts of the joint capsule (especially in the axillary recess) and the articular cartilage, there is nevertheless no scientific evidence that this really exists.

Despite all the scientific work that has been done on primary FS, the question still remains as to what is the trigger for the cascade of inflammatory and fibrogenetic processes. There is, however, some knowledge about factors that predispose to shoulder stiffness, including: (1) age, (2) minor injuries with no detectable structural damage to the glenohumeral joint, (3) non-shoulder surgery (e.g. cervical neck dissection, thoracotomy, sternotomy and intervention cardiology), (4) immobility, (5) cervical disease such as intervertebral disc degeneration in the lower regions of the cervical spine, (6) thyroid disorders, (7) diabetes mellitus and (8) cardiac and pulmonary disease.

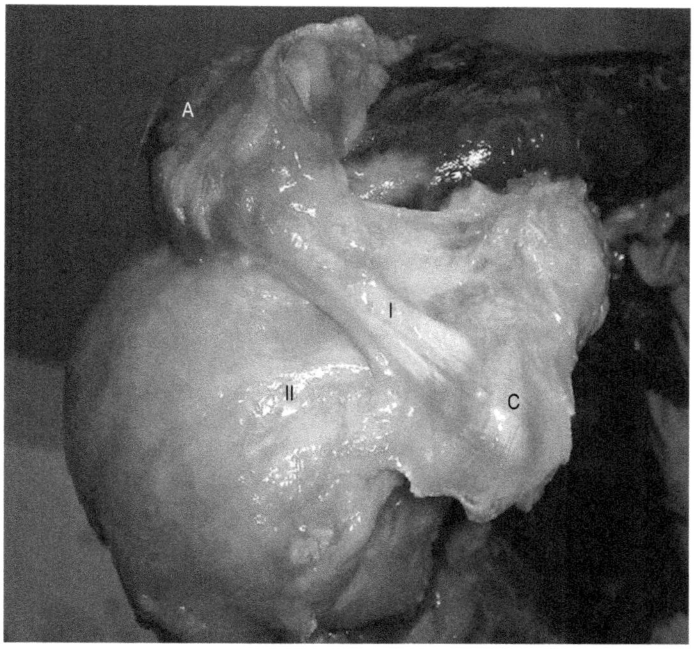

Figure 30.1 The coracohumeral ligament (II) shown in a normal cadaveric right shoulder. Other visible structures are the coracoacromial ligament (I), the acromion (A) and the coracoid process (C). (From Yang et al 2009, with permission.)

Primary FS seems to be strongly associated with Dupuytren's disease (Bunker & Anthony 1995; Smith et al 2001). Smith et al (2001) confirmed that Dupuytren's disease was commonly seen in patients with frozen shoulder (52%), and this finding suggests that the two conditions may share a common biochemical pathway that leads to contracture. Bunker and Anthony (1995) found that the histological appearances of the tissues excised from primary FS patients and those from patients with Dupuytren's contractures of the hand were similar.

Some authors also recognize similarities with reflex dystrophy (Sudeck's dystrophy, or complex regional pain syndrome type I, as it is referred to nowadays) (Hertel 2000; Muller et al 2000).

Natural History and Prognosis

Knowledge of the natural history of primary FS is crucial for making treatment decisions. The natural history of FS is not fully understood and remains controversial, as many reports of long-term follow-up concern the evaluation of patient groups who have received particular treatment regimens.

Some authors have described FS as a self-limiting disease with an average duration of 1–3 years, but a substantial part of the population presents with substantial limitations in glenohumeral passive range of motion for up to 10 years after the onset of their FS (Miller et al 1996). Nevertheless, some discrepancy may exist between the patient's recognition of

Box 30.1 Stages of frozen shoulder

Stage 1: Freezing, synovitis (duration 3–9 months)

There is increasing pain during rest and movement. As the patient is often not able to lie down on the affected side, sleep may be disturbed. When the patient makes a sudden movement (this may often be called a 'wrong movement') it can take several minutes (up to 15) before the pain subsides. The pain is very severe and is often scored on a visual analogue scale as reaching 9 or 10.

In this phase it might be quite difficult to diagnose the primary FS, because of the absence of PROM limitation. Therefore in this stage patients are often diagnosed with subacromial tendinitis or bursitis. At the end of the freezing phase, the limitation of PROM becomes progressively worse.

Stage 2: Frozen (duration 4–12 months)

There is hypertrophy of the glenohumeral joint capsule and contracture of the coracohumeral ligament and the rotator cuff interval (Omari & Bunker 2001; Uhthoff & Boileau 2007).

In this phase, pain will diminish gradually, owing to the recovery of the inflammatory process. Pain may be completely absent during rest but pain felt at the end of the (significantly limited) range of motion is still present. Sleeping is still disturbed because lying on either side is still not possible owing to the severe restriction of PROM (Cleland & Durall 2002). Although there is some muscular atrophy due to inactivity of the shoulder, severe loss of strength will not occur during the course of FS. The PROM is limited by about 50% or even more in all directions.

Stage 3: Thawing (between 12 and 42 months)

This stage is characterized by gradually improving PROM.

functional limitation and the clinically measured objective restrictions of the PROM. This can be explained by the fact that shoulder pain is usually more incapacitating than is restriction of glenohumeral PROM as such.

To our knowledge, recurrence of primary FS in the same shoulder joint does not occur, although one case report has been published (Cameron et al 2000). In this case the patient fully recovered within 6 weeks, which is very unusual for a FS. Therefore we doubt that this is indeed the first case report of a recurrent FS; most probably, it is an example of mistaking a shoulder complaint for FS, which often happens. In a large (269 shoulders) retrospective study on the long-term (5 years) outcome in primary FS, Hand et al (2008) reported no recurrences. Simultaneous bilateral presentation of FS is rare, but an FS developing over time in the opposite shoulder may be seen in up to approximately 35% of cases.

FS is classically characterized by three clinical phases: (1) freezing phase, (2) frozen phase, and (3) thawing phase (Neviaser 1945) (Box 30.1). However, some authors use a classification of four stages, where the first stage is divided into a painful pre-freezing stage and a freezing stage where the PROM gradually decreases (Neviaser & Neviaser 1987; Hannafin & Chiaia 2000; Sheridan & Hannafin 2006; Schultheis et al 2008).

Patient education is one of the important aspects of the treatment. The clinician explaining the benign nature of the

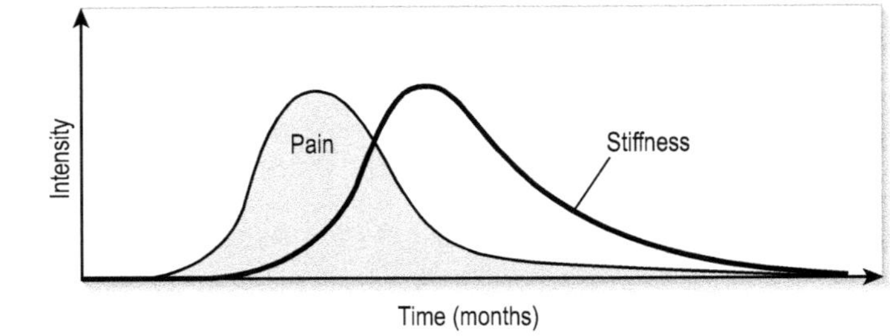

Figure 30.2 The natural history of the self-limiting form of primary frozen shoulder according to Hertel. (From Hertel R, 2000. Orthopäde 29: 845–851, with permission.)

primary FS helps to reassure the patient. Although primary FS is seen as a self-limiting disease, this is probably especially true for the inflammatory processes during the first stages. However, the PROM restriction occasionally persists for several years and might result in major limitations in daily activities. Therefore it might be useful for therapist to instruct patients to perform gentle stretching exercises in the thawing phase. Very few cases will result in a refractory primary frozen shoulder in which more rigorous interventions are needed. According to Tasto and Elias (2007), about 10–15% of patients continue to suffer from continuous pain and limited motion, needing up to 10 years to recover fully. Figure 30.2 shows the natural history of the self-limiting form of primary FS.

Diagnosis

The diagnosis of a primary FS should be easy. The history is generally clear, physical examination only requires few diagnostic shoulder tests, and even fewer additional diagnostic tools are necessary. Still, FS is chosen as the most frequently misdiagnosed shoulder complaint in patients referred for a second opinion. FS is characterized by three phases, and the practitioner's clinical challenge consists of discriminating the exact phase and appropriate duration of symptoms or signs. (For details of these phases see Box 30.1.)

History

Patients who present at the clinic are usually aged between 40 and 70 years, and women are more frequently affected than men (Hannafin & Chiaia 2000). The right and left shoulders are involved with equal frequency. Even when patients within the typical age group present themselves with a painful and stiff shoulder, and the diagnosis of FS seems obvious, nevertheless other diagnoses, such as neoplasias (Quan et al 2005; Sano et al 2010), glenohumeral infection, calcific bursitis or tendinitis, rotator cuff lesions and glenohumeral osteoarthritis, have to be considered.

The pain is usually experienced in the shoulder region, the deltoid insertion and upper arm, but it often radiates to the neck and to more distal regions of the upper extremity. In the freezing phase the pain is felt during rest and intensified during both movement and sleep. The amount of pain strongly depends on the clinical phase of the disease.

Physical examination

Examination starts with both shoulders exposed. The alignment and symmetry of both shoulder girdles and the cervical spine are assessed. The cervical spine is assessed for muscle spasm and local tenderness. Both shoulders are checked for signs of muscle atrophy, former trauma and pathological swelling. Next, the affected shoulder is palpated. Patients with FS typically demonstrate tenderness in the region of the rotator cuff and subacromial bursa, deltoid insertion and along the course of the biceps tendon. A painful biceps tendon is often confounded with a taut band in the anterior deltoid, which is much more accessible to palpation than the biceps tendon, which lies deep in the biceps groove underneath a tight transverse ligament. Myofascial trigger points (TrPs) may be found in almost all shoulder muscles, but most often in the subscapularis, infraspinatus, teres minor, teres major, deltoid and trapezius muscles. According to Simons et al (1999), the shoulder becomes more restricted in external rotation (up to 45% or more) when TrPs in the subscapularis muscle become progressively active, whereas TrPs in the teres major muscle may be responsible for a restriction in abduction. It is unclear whether TrPs in the subscapularis mimic a primary FS, or whether they initiate it. Simons et al (1999) propose to make a distinction between severely restricted motion due to active TrPs in the shoulder musculature and adhesive capsulitis as a result of true fibrosis (see Ch 59 for muscle TrPs).

During assessment of the mobility of the shoulder, particular attention should be paid to the contribution of the glenohumeral joint to the total active and passive range of motion (Fig. 30.3). Only then can FS be clinically distinguished from other diseases that limit shoulder mobility.

In the pre-freezing and freezing phases, pain is the most limiting factor and the characteristic global restriction of the glenohumeral joint may be less clear. In the frozen phase, the characteristic global limitation of PROM of the glenohumeral joint is present. In the thawing phase, the global limitation fades out and usually the contracture of the rotator interval causes a marked limitation of external rotation.

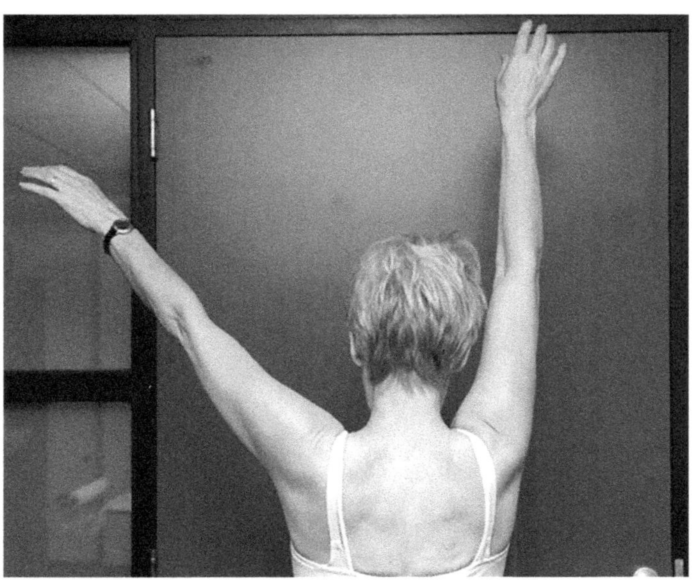

Figure 30.3 Patient with frozen left shoulder during shoulder abduction.

Isometric strength testing of the shoulder muscles in a pain-free shoulder position with the arm at the side of the body is usually non-provocative and reveals nearly normal strength.

Treatment

Treatment regimens depend on the stage of the FS. In the pre-freezing (first phase) or freezing phase (second phase), the chief complaint of the patient is the extreme pain. Treatment therefore has to be aimed at pain relief using intra-articular injections of corticosteroids (Buchbinder et al 2003), oral non-steroidal anti-inflammatory drugs (NSAIDs) or suprascapular nerve block (Harmon & Hearty, 2007), or treating the TrPs in the surrounding shoulder muscles (Simons et al 1999; Jankovic & van Zundert 2006).

In one study (Brue et al 2007), the use of corticosteroids did not make any difference in long-term outcome compared with physiotherapy, although it could provide some pain relief in the early stages. Myofascial TrPs may occur in rotator cuff muscles, especially in the subscapularis muscle and in the thoracoscapular muscles; however, manual treatment of the subscapularis muscle may be difficult because the muscle is poorly accessible in severely restricted shoulder joints. Therefore TrP dry needling using a Japanese needle plunger to position the needle deep into the muscle is a good option (Fig. 30.4). The other shoulder muscles can be treated either manually or by TrP dry needling (see Ch 61 for TrP dry needling). In some cases, the application of cold-packs or hot-packs (or hot shower) may be beneficial. The patient can apply this several times a day, as often as necessary.

In the freezing phase, it is not useful to perform glenohumeral joint mobilization – either because of the lack of PROM restriction (in the pre-freezing phase) or because the patient will respond with increasing pain during mobilization

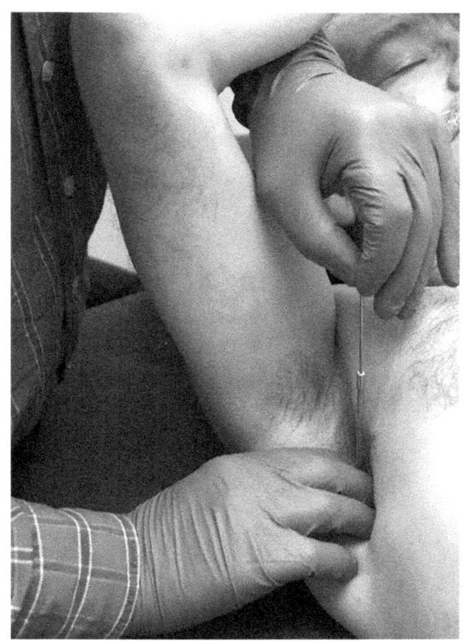

Figure 30.4 Dry needling of subscapularis muscle using a Japanese needle plunger.

and subsequently with increasing joint limitation. It is essential to explain to patients the nature of the disease and advise them to stop exercising. They have to be encouraged to do everything that diminishes the pain, as less pain may lead to diminishing of the inflammation process and hence probably to less fibrosis (Hannafin et al 1994; Marx et al 2007).

In the frozen phase, the pain will rapidly decrease as the inflammatory process recedes and anti-inflammatory drugs are no longer indicated. Over-the-counter painkillers may be taken on an irregular basis. However, there is great variety in the treatment options that have been advised for improving the PROM, which reflects the poor consensus of opinions over the best-available treatment. Due to the benign natural course, the authors consider that the best choice is to start with a conservative, non-surgical intervention. A supervised physical therapy treatment or a gentle home stretching programme may be sufficient. End-range mobilization has been shown to be more effective, but the benefits are small (Vermeulen et al 2006), and rigorous mobilization or stretching is not more beneficial per se than gentle mobilization. In the frozen phase one might prefer a milder mobilization technique as this produces less pain during and after the treatment sessions. Occasionally new treatment options are invented. Ruiz (2009) presented a single case report in which he described positional stretching of the CHL; the patient regained considerable glenohumeral range of motion within 4 weeks, which could not be due to natural recovery alone. Gaspar and Willis (2009) presented in a controlled, cohort study a new intervention, called dynamic splinting; due to methodological flaws, however, firm conclusions cannot be made.

In the thawing phase, gentle mobilization may be applied (Diercks & Stevens 2004; Vermeulen et al 2006). In this phase the recovery is mostly due to the natural course of recovery and it is the opinion of the authors that mobilization does not add much benefit (Miller et al 1996; Diercks & Stevens 2004). Recently, Kelley et al (2009) proposed a model for guiding rehabilitation. Because of the lack of evidence to determine which patients may need formal supervised therapy rather than simply a home programme, the researchers propose a patient-centred approach in which the decision is made based on the physician's and patient's preference, with input from the therapist after initial evaluation (Yang et al 2008).

As range of motion is gradually regained, the patient will carefully start to use the affected arm in daily activities. This in itself will help to exercise the shoulder and arm muscles and hence additional exercises are rarely needed.

Recalcitrant frozen shoulders

Although most cases of primary FS recover within months, it might be necessary in a very few cases (especially when the patient or his / her physician or physical therapist is impatient) to use more rigorous treatment options. These interventions include manipulation under anaesthesia, glenohumeral joint distension and arthroscopic capsular release.

Closed manipulation under anaesthesia may be effective in terms of joint mobilization; however, the method can cause iatrogenic damage, which includes haemarthrosis, rupture of the glenohumeral capsule, superior labrum anterior–posterior (SLAP) lesions, Bankart lesions, tendinous or ligamentous ruptures, fractures of the humerus and axillary nerve lesions (Loew et al 2005). Also closed manipulation under anaesthesia is contraindicated in patients with significant osteopenia, recent surgical repair of soft tissue about the shoulder, fractures, neurological injury or instability (Hannafin & Chiaia 2000).

Glenohumeral joint distension using saline either in combination with or without corticosteroids seems to be beneficial only in the short term. The technique is also often poorly tolerated because of the pain that is experienced during the procedure (Manske & Prohaska 2008).

More recently, arthroscopy has been advocated for confirmation of diagnosis as well as for selective release of the contracted parts of the capsule (Brue et al 2007). Release of the CHL and the rotator cuff interval is particularly effective in increasing the range of motion in external rotation, abduction and elevation. In cases with a decreased internal rotation and adduction (cross-body adduction), release of the posterior capsule is performed. Arthroscopic release prior to or following a closed manipulation is considered to be an effective and relatively safe procedure, with less iatrogenic damage than that seen after closed manipulation under anaesthesia.

Prevention of frozen shoulder

Patients with severe shoulder complaints are often advised to perform mobilizing or stretching exercises to prevent the development of FS. However, the authors strongly believe that it is impossible for the patient to succeed in this, or even to slow down the development of FS, by performing exercises. If doctors or therapists insist on an exercise regimen, patients will then feel a responsibility for their FS that they should not.

Conclusion

The frozen shoulder is still a challenge for physicians, therapists and researchers as there is still controversy over the aetiology, the pathophysiology, the diagnosis and the optimal treatment strategy. Most important, though, is that the prognosis in most cases is good. About 80–90% of all patients will eventually fully recover, although improvement may take up to 10 years. Recurrence of the primary frozen shoulder in the same shoulder does not occur. Patient education about the natural history and good prognosis is an important aspect of the treatment. The treatment is mainly conservative and depends largely on the stage of the frozen shoulder. In the freezing stage the treatment is aimed at inhibiting the pain and diminishing the inflammation, whereas in the frozen stage it is aimed at regaining the range of motion. It is the authors' preferred treatment to search for the least painful approach. Recalcitrant frozen shoulders are very rare and patience has to be exercised before surgery is considered. If necessary, arthroscopic release of carefully selected structures seems to be beneficial in restoring the range of motion in refractory frozen shoulder. Recently, new stretching techniques and devices have been published, but further research is needed to see whether these can be of additional value. The bottom-line message for therapists, physicians and patients should be to remain patient during the natural course of the primary frozen shoulder.

References

Balci N, Balci MK, Tuzuner S. 1999. Shoulder adhesive capsulitis and shoulder range of motion in type II diabetes mellitus: association with diabetic complications. J Diabetes Complications 13: 135–140.

Brue S, Valentin A, Forssblad M, et al. 2007. Idiopathic adhesive capsulitis of the shoulder: a review. Knee Surg Sports Traumatol Arthrosc 15: 1048–1054.

Buchbinder R, Green S, Youd JM. 2003. Corticosteroid injections for shoulder pain. Cochrane Database Syst Rev 1: CD004016.

Bunker TD, Anthony PP. 1995. The pathology of frozen shoulder: a Dupuytren-like disease. J Bone Joint Surg Br 77: 677–683.

Cameron RI, McMillan J, Kelly IG. 2000. Recurrence of a 'primary frozen shoulder': a case report. J Shoulder Elbow Surg 9: 65–67.

Cleland J, Durall C. 2002. Physical therapy for adhesive capsulitis: systematic review. Physiotherapy 88: 450–457.

Codman EA. 1934. The shoulder. Boston: Thomas Odd.

Diercks RL, Stevens M. 2004. Gentle thawing of the frozen shoulder: a prospective study of supervised neglect versus intensive physical therapy in seventy-seven patients with frozen shoulder syndrome followed up for two years. J Shoulder Elbow Surg 13: 499–502.

Duplay S. 1872. De la periarthrite scapulo-humerale et des raideurs de l'épaule qui en sont la consequence. Arch Gen Med 20: 513–542.

Gaspar PD, Willis FB. 2009. Adhesive capsulitis and dynamic splinting: a controlled, cohort study. BMC Musculoskelet Disord 10: 111.

Hand C, Clipsham K, Rees JL, et al. 2008. Long-term outcome of frozen shoulder. J Shoulder Elbow Surg 17: 231–236.

Hannafin JA, Chiaia TA. 2000. Adhesive capsulitis. A treatment approach. Clin Orthop Relat Res 1: 95–109.

Hannafin JA, DiCarlo EF, Wickiewicz TL, et al. 1994. Adhesive capsulitis: capsular fibroplasia of the glenohumeral joint. J Shoulder Elbow Surg 3 (Suppl): 5.

Harmon D, Hearty C. 2007. Ultrasound-guided suprascapular nerve block technique. Pain Physician 10: 743–746.

Hertel R. 2000. The frozen shoulder. Orthopade 29: 845–851.

Jankovic D, van Zundert A. 2006. The frozen shoulder syndrome. Description of a new technique and five case reports using the subscapular nerve block and subscapularis trigger point infiltration. Acta Anaesthesiol Belg 57: 137–143.

Kelley MJ, McClure PW, Leggin BG. 2009. Frozen shoulder: evidence and a proposed model guiding rehabilitation. J Orthop Sports Phys Ther 39: 135–148.

Kordella T. 2002. Frozen shoulder and diabetes. Frozen shoulder affects 20 percent of people with diabetes. Proper treatment can help you work through it. Diabetes Forecast 55: 60–64.

Loew M, Heichel TO, Lehner B. 2005. Intraarticular lesions in primary frozen shoulder after manipulation under general anesthesia. J Shoulder Elbow Surg 14: 16–21.

Lundberg BJ. 1969. The frozen shoulder. Clinical and radiographical observations. The effect of manipulation under general anesthesia. Structure and glycosaminoglycan content of the joint capsule. Local bone metabolism. Acta Orthop Scand 119: 1–59.

Manske RC, Prohaska D. 2008. Diagnosis and management of adhesive capsulitis. Curr Rev Musculoskelet Med 1: 180–189.

Marx RG, Malizia RW, Kenter K, et al. 2007. Intra-articular corticosteroid injection for the treatment of idiopathic adhesive capsulitis of the shoulder. HSS J 3(2): 202–207. doi: 10.1007/s11420-007-9044-5.

Miller MD, Wirth MA, Rockwood CA. 1996. Thawing the frozen shoulder: the 'patient' patient. Orthopedics 19: 849–853.

Muller LP, Muller LA, Happ J, et al. 2000. Frozen shoulder: a sympathetic dystrophy? Arch Orthop Trauma Surg 120: 84–87.

Neviaser JS. 1945. Adhesive capsulitis of the shoulder: a study of the pathological findings in periarthritis of the shoulder. J Bone Joint Surg Am 27: 211–222.

Neviaser RJ, Neviaser TJ. 1987. The frozen shoulder. Diagnosis and management. Clin Orthop Relat Res 223: 59–64.

Omari A, Bunker TD. 2001. Open surgical release for frozen shoulder: surgical findings and results of the release. J Shoulder Elbow Surg 10: 353–357.

Quan GM, Carr D, Schlicht S, et al. 2005. Lessons learnt from the painful shoulder; a case series of malignant shoulder girdle tumours misdiagnosed as frozen shoulder. Int Semin Surg Oncol 2: 2.

Ruiz JO. 2009. Positional stretching of the coracohumeral ligament on a patient with adhesive capsulitis: a case report. J Man Manip Ther 17: 58–63.

Sano H, Hatori M, Mineta M, et al. 2010. Tumors masked as frozen shoulders: a retrospective analysis. J Shoulder Elbow Surg 19(2): 262–266. doi: 10.1016/j.jse.2009.05.010.

Schultheis A, Reichwein F, Nebelung W. 2008. Frozen shoulder: diagnosis and therapy. Orthopade 37: 1065–1072.

Sheridan MA, Hannafin JA. 2006. Upper extremity: emphasis on frozen shoulder. Orthop Clin North Am 37: 531–539.

Simons DG, Travell JG, Simons LS. 1999. Myofascial pain and dysfunction. The trigger point manual. Vol I. Upper half of body, 2nd edn. Baltimore, MD: Lippincott Williams & Wilkins.

Smith SP, Devaraj VS, Bunker TD. 2001. The association between frozen shoulder and Dupuytren's disease. J Shoulder Elbow Surg 10: 149–151.

Tasto JP, Elias D. 2007. Adhesive capsulitis. Sports Med Arthrosc 15: 216–221.

Tighe CB, Oakley WS. 2008. The prevalence of a diabetic condition and adhesive capsulitis of the shoulder. South Med J 101: 591–595.

Uhthoff HK, Boileau P. 2007. Primary frozen shoulder: global capsular stiffness versus localized contracture. Clin Orthop Relat Res 456: 79–84.

Vermeulen HM, Rozing PM, Obermann WR, et al. 2006. Comparison of high-grade and low-grade mobilization techniques in the management of adhesive capsulitis of the shoulder: randomized controlled trial. Phys Ther 86: 355–368.

Yang JL, Chang CW, Chen SY, et al. 2008. Shoulder kinematic features using arm elevation and rotation tests for classifying patients with frozen shoulder syndrome who respond to physical therapy. Man Ther 13: 544–551.

Yang HF, Tang KL, Chen W, et al. 2009. An anatomic and histologic study of the coracohumeral ligament. J Shoulder Elbow Surg 18: 305–310.

31 Chapter

Joint Mobilization of the Shoulder

Wayne Hing, Jack Miller, César Fernández-de-las-Peñas

CHAPTER CONTENTS

Introduction	350
Passive mobilization interventions of the glenohumeral joint	350
Inferior glide	351
Posterior glide	351
Posterior glide in flexion	352
Inferior and anterior glide	352
Anteroposterior or lateral–medial glide at end-of-range elevation	352
Mobilization with movement of the shoulder complex	352
Overhead elevation mobilizations with movement	353
Overhead elevation: progression of range of motion	354
Hand behind back	355
Horizontal adduction motion	356
Conclusion	357

Introduction

A fully functional upper limb is dependent on the optimal pain-free mobility of the shoulder girdle. Shoulder pain and dysfunction limit our ability to utilize the upper extremity in activities of daily living, resulting in recreational, occupational and societal disabilities. This chapter has been organized to highlight the concept of the restoration of upper limb functional tasks through a continuum of manual therapy interventions to the shoulder joint and shoulder girdle complex. The techniques demonstrated in this chapter are focused on achieving the optimization of upper limb functional activities including passive mobilizations, and mobilization with movement (MWM) focusing on overhead elevation, cross-body motion and placing the hand behind the back. The progression of the techniques, by involving active participation of the patient, will be determined by key subjective and objective parameters such as patient irritability, severity of pain, stage of pathology and recovery, the available range of motion and the effect of upper limb load-bearing forces (Hing et al 2003).

Manual therapy procedures used to restore mobility and function of the shoulder girdle have been developed and described by a variety of authors (Kaltenborn et al 2002; Mulligan 2003; Hengeveld et al 2005). A dispassionate perspective on these apparently diverse approaches reveals that, although each may have highly original components, they are invariably progressions of previously established work and form an evolutionary continuum (Miller 1999). This chapter will highlight different mobilizations of the shoulder joint that have been demonstrated clinically to be safe and effective and are, at least partially, evidence based.

Passive Mobilization Interventions of the Glenohumeral Joint

Translatoric accessory joint mobilization techniques are well established and form the basis of much of the curriculum of both entry level and postgraduate manual therapy training programmes. Originally developed by physical therapists such as Kaltenborn and Evjenth from Norway (Kaltenborn et al 2002), orthopaedic manual therapy (OMT) utilizes a clinical-reasoning paradigm based on the manual therapist's perception of joint restriction as revealed by passive movement examination and the application of the concave–convex rule. According to the concave–convex rule, the direction of the glide is determined by considering the geometry of the moving articular surfaces. In such a manner, when the convex surface moves, it glides in the opposite direction to the concave surface. In the glenohumeral joint, the glenoid fossa (concave surface) is considered to be stable while the humeral head (convex surface) is usually mobilized during a physiological shoulder movement. Nevertheless, the validity of this rule has been questioned (Brandt et al 2007).

In addition, passive translatoric accessory mobilizations can be performed parallel to or perpendicular to the treatment plane as determined by the specific orientation of the joint surfaces. Mobilizations are graded in their range and sustained for specific durations according to their intended therapeutic goal(s), including pain relief and improvement of joint mobility. In fact, a cadaveric study found that greater gain in mobility is obtained at the end-range position during axial distraction mobilization of the glenohumeral joint (Hsu et al 2009). This would be important for clinical practice if the aim of the treatment were to increase available range of motion.

The conceptual model is that joint capsule contracture must be passively elongated through tissue creep, effected by sustained passive mobilization techniques into the tissue barrier. This hypothesis is supported by an animal study where immobilization of the rat shoulder induced synovial hyperplasia of the joint capsule, adhesion of subscapular bursa and an increase of the capsular content of types I and III collagen (Liu et al 2011). Therefore, technique repetition and an appropriate self-treatment regimen along with consideration of associated soft tissue dysfunction, neurophysiological and motor control factors are proposed to provide short- and long-term positive outcomes. There is little evidence demonstrating the efficacy of passive mobilization interventions in the shoulder region. Vermeulen et al (2006) found that application of shoulder joint mobilization techniques was effective for improving glenohumeral joint mobility and reducing disability in subjects with adhesive capsulitis of the shoulder.

Maricar et al (2009) demonstrated that the inclusion of Maitland accessory glenohumeral mobilizations including anterior–posterior mobilization in shoulder flexion and longitudinal caudal mobilization in shoulder abduction induced better outcomes when added to an exercise programme. Surenkok et al (2009) reported that manual mobilization of the shoulder complex increased the range of motion and decreased pain intensity in patients with shoulder pain.

Passive mobilization procedures directed at the shoulder region are designed to increase the accessory and physiological ranges of joint mobility, with the therapeutic goals of improving the patient's range of motion and function. The shoulder joint generally responds well to OMT procedures; however, it may also react poorly in cases of high irritability. The inability to sleep on the affected shoulder, continual pain at rest and pain of shoulder origin radiating below the elbow are generally accepted indicators of high levels of irritability and may indicate the need to approach the patient with caution.

In the following sections we describe some of the passive mobilization interventions targeted to the glenohumeral joint that are most commonly used in clinical practice.

Inferior glide (Fig. 31.1)

This glenohumeral mobilization is indicated to increase the range of passive caudal glide of the head of the humerus on the glenoid fossa and to decrease pain related to a superiorly positioned humeral head. Subacromial impingement syndromes that are improved by a caudal glide of the humerus during overhead lifting (Flatow et al 1994) may respond well to this mobilization. For this purpose, the patient is supine lying close to the edge of the bed. The humerus is maintained in neutral internal / external rotation. The therapist grasps the arm close to the joint line with the web space of one hand cupping the superior aspect of the humeral head, while the other hand supports the weight of the extremity. A caudal / inferior glide is imparted to the humerus along joint plane of glenoid fossa. The glenoid can be stabilized by a towel under the scapula and / or a harness. In irritable cases the therapist may want to begin with the patient's arm by the side in minimal abduction. Progression to increasing ranges of abduction may be attempted in non-irritable cases. As reported by Hsu et al (2009), the mobilization should be conducted at the pain-free end-range position.

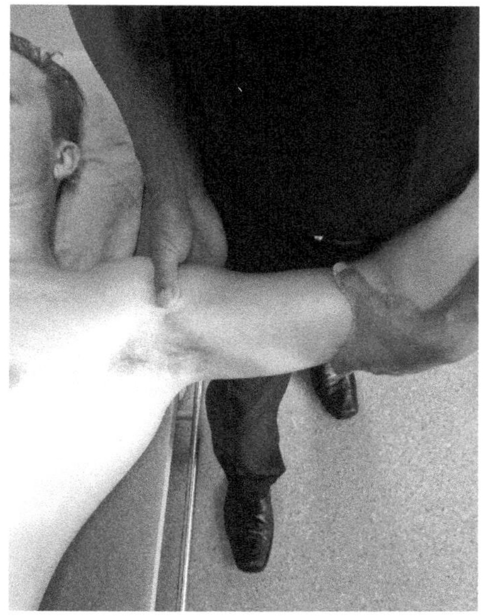

Figure 31.1 Inferior glide of the glenohumeral joint (humeral head).

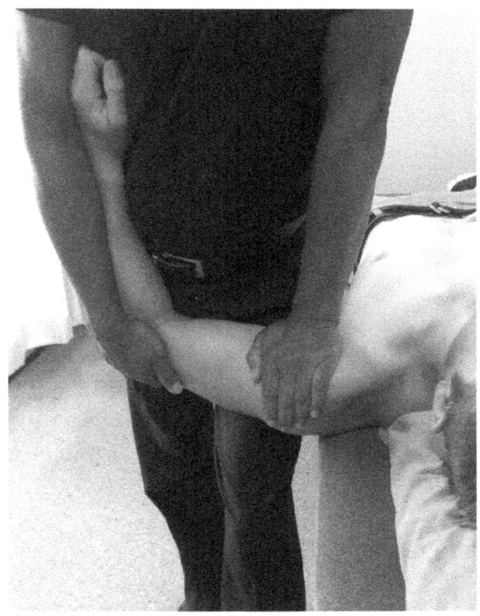

Figure 31.2 Posterior glide of the glenohumeral joint (humeral head).

Posterior glide (Fig. 31.2)

This mobilization is indicated to increase the available range of passive posterior glide of the head of the humerus and to decrease pain related to an anteriorly positioned humeral head (Dashottar & Borstad 2012). For this technique, the patient is supine with the arm in neutral internal / external rotation and the cervical spine neutral. The therapist is standing at the side of the bed. The cephalic hand cups the humeral head with the palm, and the caudal hand supports the upper arm / forearm in a slightly flexed and abducted position. The therapist applies a posterior–lateral glide of the humerus head along the joint plane of glenoid fossa. Clinicians should ensure the glide is translatoric by moving both hands equally in a posterior–lateral direction, avoiding contact with the coracoid process.

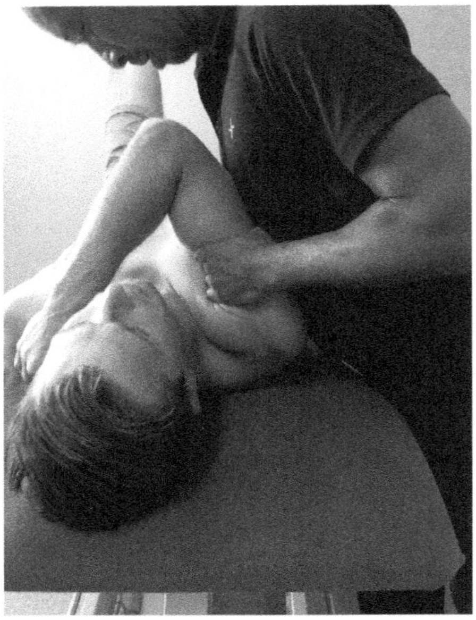

Figure 31.3 Posterior glide of the glenohumeral joint in flexion (humeral head).

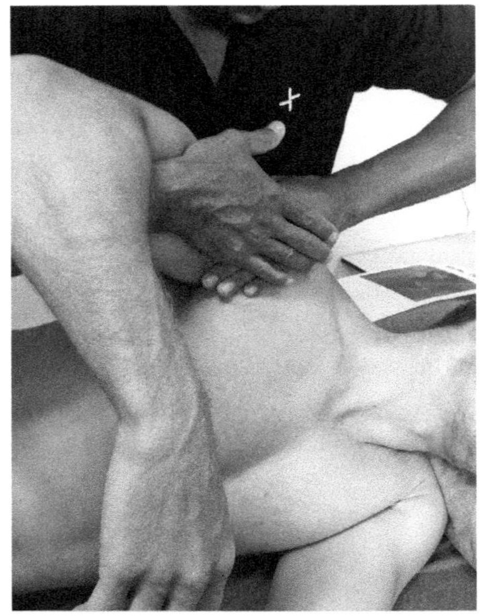

Figure 31.4 Inferior and anterior glide of the glenohumeral joint (humeral head).

Posterior glide in flexion (Fig. 31.3)

This mobilization is indicated for non-irritable patients with internal impingement syndrome and loss of cross-body movement. It can be also effective for patients with posterior capsule tightening. For this purpose, the patient is supine close to the edge of the bed; the scapula may be stabilized by a folded towel placed on the bed. The arm is flexed to 90° and internally rotated such that the therapist's hand rests on the patient's sternum. The therapist then grasps the patient's arm close to the humeral head and stabilizes the elbow with his / her sternum. A posterior glide of the humerus may now be performed with both hands. Additional ranges of arm adduction may be used as the patient's range of cross-body movement improves.

Inferior and anterior glide (Fig. 31.4)

This mobilization is indicated in cases where restoration of internal rotation is the desired rehabilitation goal. The patient is side-lying with the arm in 45° of abduction and 80° of internal rotation (when possible) with the hand resting on the abdomen. The therapist stands behind the patient clasping the humerus proximally and using the abdomen to stabilize the distal end. The therapist may next induce an inferior and anterior translatoric glide to the humeral head while monitoring and varying the amount of abduction / adduction of the arm, according to patient irritability.

Anteroposterior or lateral–medial glide at end-of-range elevation (Fig. 31.5)

This mobilization is indicated for recovery of end-range elevation in non-irritable cases. The patient lies prone with the arm resting on the bed in maximum pain-free overhead elevation. The amount of internal / external rotation may be varied depending on the goals of treatment. The therapist stands by the side of the bed stabilizing the scapula and controlling the position of the humerus with the palms of the hands. The thumb pads are placed over the posterior aspect of the humeral head and an anterior–posterior or lateral–medial mobilization force can be applied. The beginning range of arm elevation may be progressed as determined by patient irritability. Yang et al (2012) reported that end-range mobilizations were more effective than a standardized physical therapy programme in a subgroup of subjects with frozen shoulder.

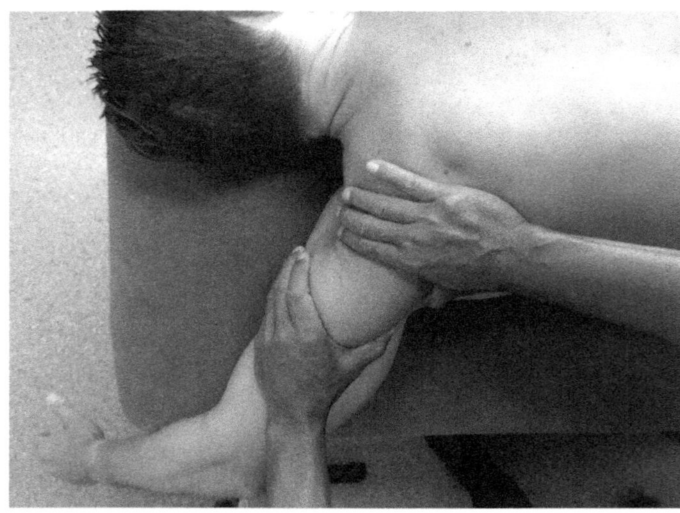

Figure 31.5 Anteroposterior or lateral–medial glide of the glenohumeral joint (humeral head) at end-of-range elevation.

Mobilization with Movement of the Shoulder Complex

A growing body of evidence has demonstrated the value of combining traditional OMT therapy mobilizations concurrently with patients' pain-limited physiological movements.

Termed 'mobilizations with movement' (MWMs), this concept was developed by Brian Mulligan of New Zealand (Mulligan 2003) and built on the foundations of OMT. Within the Mulligan concept, the management of the patient requires the identification of a comparable sign or client-specific impairment measure (CSIM) as a baseline measure to evaluate treatment effectiveness, often measured as a functionally limited motor activity. This clinically measurable functional deficit becomes the benchmark against which the effectiveness of the intervention(s) is continually reassessed (Vicenzino et al 2011).

The clinical-reasoning paradigm of selection and progression of MWMs rests on the patient's individual response to selected trial mobilizations as measured by pain-free improvement in the identified CSIM. The therapist must continuously monitor the patient's reaction to ensure that minimal to no pain is recreated. Utilizing their knowledge of joint arthrology, a well-developed sense of tissue tension and active clinical reasoning, the therapist investigates various combinations of mobilization directions to find the ideal treatment plane and grade of movement. While sustaining the pain-free accessory mobilization, the patient is requested to perform the previously identified pain-restricted CSIM. The CSIM may now be significantly improved – that is, increased range of motion, and a significant decrease in, or ideally absence of, the original pain. Failure to improve the CSIM would indicate that the therapist has not found the correct contact point, treatment plane, grade or direction of mobilization, or spinal segment, or that the technique is not indicated. The previously restricted and / or painful CSIM is repeated by the patient, initially as a trial treatment progressing up to sets of 10, while the therapist continues to maintain the appropriate accessory glide. Further gains are expected with repetition during a treatment session, which typically involves three to four sets of 10 repetitions. Repetition of the CSIM and pain-free end-range loading in the form of passive overpressure appears to be critical to achieve durable results (Miller 1999; Mulligan 2003; Hing et al 2008). As with all manual therapy concepts, a properly structured subjective and objective assessment of the patient and continuous reflective clinical reasoning (Jones & Rivett 2004) are mandatory both within the patient's assessment and during treatment sessions.

The theoretical model of the effect of MWMs is that either a positional fault of bony positional malalignment or a neuromechanical dysfunction is corrected or affected by the mobilization component of the procedures. Nevertheless, the biomechanical hypothesis that MWM reverses positional faults requires further investigation (Vicenzino et al 2007). In place of the therapist's perception of passive accessory movement restriction and the concave–convex rule, the specific direction and grade of mobilization are determined by the patient's reports of an accessory direction of preference of pain abolition and objective improvements in CSIM function (Miller 2006; Hing et al 2009). Self-treatment procedures along with the application of sports adhesive tape are often used to maintain gains achieved in the clinical setting.

Some case reports have demonstrated that the application of MWM over the shoulder complex was effective for reducing shoulder pain and disability in subjects with shoulder pain (Scaringe et al 2002) or subacromial impingement (DeSantis & Hasson 2006). Other randomized controlled trials reported immediate positive effects in range of motion and pressure pain sensitivity in subjects with shoulder pain (Kachingwe 2008; Teys et al 2008) or frozen shoulder (Yang et al 2007) after the application of MWM over the shoulder complex. Doner et al (2013) demonstrated that MWM leads to better improvements in terms of pain, range of motion, shoulder scores, and patient and physiotherapist satisfaction than passive stretching for adhesive capsulitis. A systematic review concluded that the efficacy of MWM at peripheral joints is well established for various joints and pathologies, demonstrating positive effects (Hing et al 2009).

Overhead elevation mobilizations with movement

Individuals with shoulder dysfunction usually report that regaining a functional range of overhead elevation is often of prime importance. In highly irritable and restricted cases the patient may initially need to be treated in a non-gravity-dependent, recumbent position with a graduated progression to upright gravity-dependent postures and resisted load-bearing environments. The clinical selection of the appropriate initial procedure and the appropriate progression of loads will always be dependent on the findings at assessment, ongoing re-evaluation and active clinical reasoning.

Mobilization with movement – elevation (Fig. 31.6)

This mobilization is indicated to reposition the humeral head in the glenoid fossa while restoring functional range of overhead elevation, and to increase active range of pain-free elevation during a trial treatment. The patient is sitting or standing, depending on the height of the therapist and patient with the cervical spine neutral. The therapist stands on the contralateral side of the patient, then with one hand makes manual contact with the anterior humeral head with the cup of the hand, while the other hand stabilizes the scapula posteriorly. The technique consists of the application of a posterior–lateral glide along the joint plane of the glenoid fossa while the patient is asked to perform a simultaneous active shoulder elevation through the scaption plane (30° from frontal plane). It is important to allow normal scapulothoracic movement throughout the technique to ensure that the patient elevates the arm fully to achieve end-range loading, and progressing to resistance loading with the use of soft weights or elastic tubing as tissue irritability decreases. Hsu et al (2000), in a cadaveric study, found that the application of an

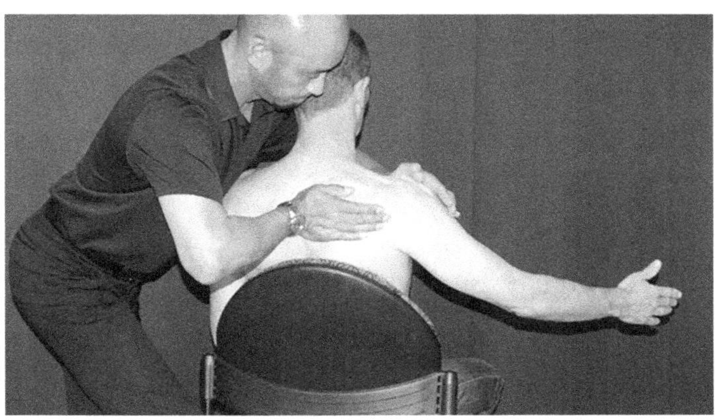

Figure 31.6 Mobilization with movement – elevation.

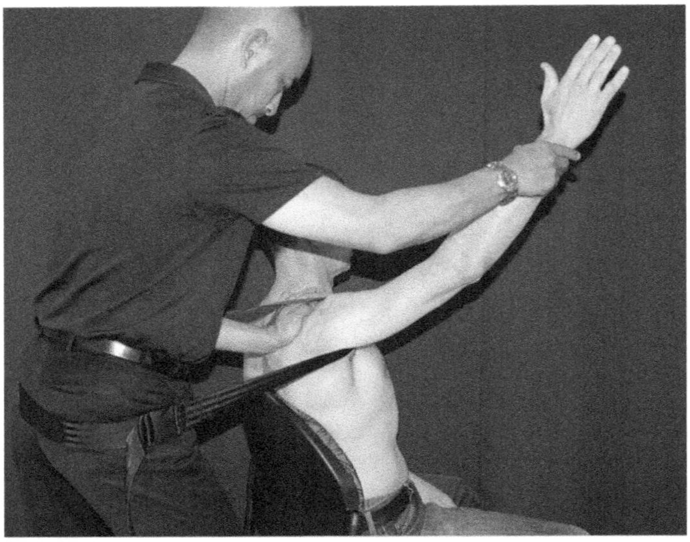

Figure 31.7 Mobilization with movement – elevation, belt assisted.

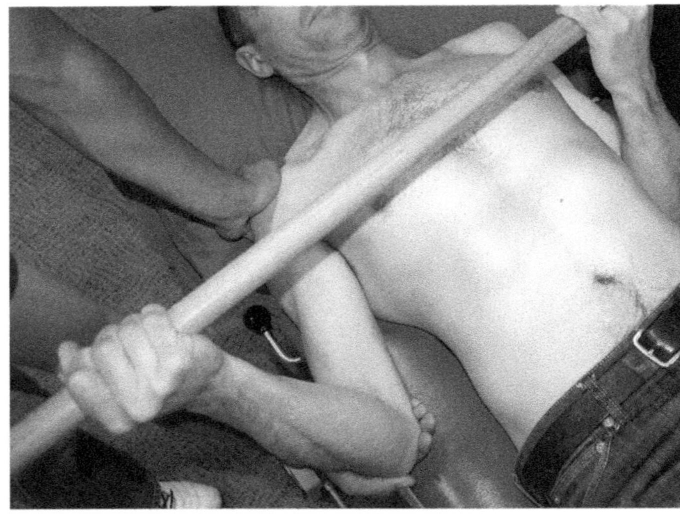

Figure 31.8 Mobilization with movement – end-range elevation (external rotation).

anterior–posterior glide towards the end of range of abduction was effective in improving the range of glenohumeral abduction. In a posterior cadaveric study, the same authors reported that this MWM technique is effective in changing the joint kinematic characteristics during glenohumeral abduction (Ho & Hsu 2009).

Mobilization with movement – elevation, belt assisted (Fig. 31.7)

This mobilization is indicated in larger patients who require a greater mobilization force than is available through a manual mobilization technique. The aim of the mobilization is to reposition the humeral head in the glenoid fossa while restoring the functional range of overhead elevation and to increase the active range of pain-free elevation. The patient is sitting on the chair with the spine fully supported but the scapula exposed and the cervical spine in neutral. The therapist stands posterior to the patient. The mobilization belt is looped around the therapist's buttocks and over the humeral head of the patient. One hand is placed over the scapula, thus stabilizing the scapula to the chest wall but allowing normal scapulothoracic movement. The technique consists of the application of a posterior–lateral glide along the joint plane of the glenoid fossa, while the patient is asked to perform a simultaneous active shoulder elevation through the scaption plane (30° from frontal plane). Note: the clinician should ensure the belt is on the humeral head and does not impede elevation of the arm, and also ensure the patient elevates the arm fully to achieve end-range loading. The mobilization progresses to resistance loading with the use of soft weights or elastic tubing as tissue irritability decreases.

Overhead elevation: progression of range of motion

During normal arm elevation the humerus undergoes a conjunct external rotation, which is often referred to as Codman's paradox (Cheng 2006). In order to accomplish full overhead elevation it may be necessary to ensure the recovery of external rotation of the glenohumeral joint, first in neutral, then in increasing degrees of elevation and culminating in the position originally described by Maitland (Hengeveld et al 2005) as 'the upper quadrant'. Additionally, in order to achieve full elevation, the therapist may need to progress into an inferior glide of the humerus (see Fig. 31.1) and consider the significant involvement of the full shoulder girdle complex.

Mobilization with movement – end-range elevation (external rotation) (Fig. 31.8)

This mobilization is indicated where the patient presents with a loss of functional range of external rotation or restriction of elevation due to loss of conjunct external rotation at or above 90° elevation. The patient is lying supine with the shoulder slightly abducted to the comfortable range, with the elbow flexed to 90° and the cervical spine neutral. The therapist stands at the side of the patient, and with the cephalic hand cups the head of the humerus with the palm, while the caudal hand supports the upper arm. The mobilization consists of the application of a posterior–lateral glide in the treatment plane of the scapula by the cephalic hand. Additional inferior glide can be applied with the caudal hand of the therapist, allowing the humerus to translate posteriorly. The patient performs passive external rotation using the unaffected hand to passively push the hand of the affected arm laterally with a short stick while the therapist maintains the patient's elbow at their side, creating a 'spin' of the humerus into external rotation. Clinicians should ensure that the posterior mobilization force is maintained until the patient returns to a neutral position. The technique can progress into greater ranges of abduction / elevation (the quadrant position).

Mobilization with movement – end-range elevation (inferior glide) (Fig. 31.9)

This mobilization is indicated for patients with end-range loss of elevation. The patient is lying supine with the scapula

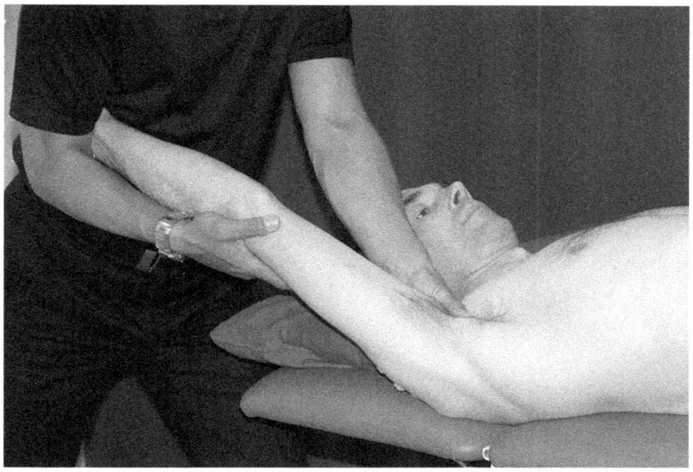

Figure 31.9 **Mobilization with movement – end-range elevation (inferior glide).**

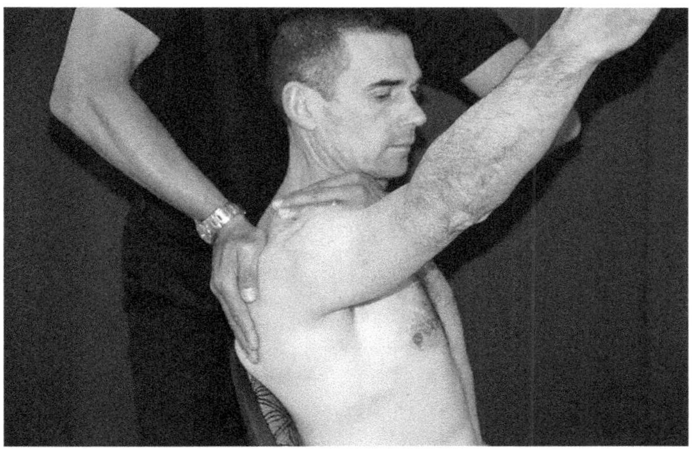

Figure 31.10 **Mobilization with movement – elevation (shoulder girdle).**

supported by the bed surface or a small folded towel. The therapist is standing at the head of the bed. The therapist grips the anterior forearm and posterior humerus in order to control elbow flexion. The technique consists of applying a posterior–caudal glide at the end-of-range elevation. The patient is asked to perform active arm elevation through scaption. The clinician should ensure that the humerus is in external rotation, and does not allow the elbow to bend / flex.

Mobilization with movement – elevation (shoulder girdle) (Fig. 31.10)

This mobilization is indicated in patients with observable winging or dyskinesis of scapulohumeral rhythm, or those with persistent shoulder pain with active elevation not responding to treatment of the glenohumeral joint. The patient is sitting on a chair with a low back and the cervical spine in neutral. The therapist is standing on the contralateral side of the patient. The posterior hand contacts the superior edge of the lateral one-third of the spine of the scapula while the anterior hand provides stability to the medial half of the clavicle. The technique consists of gliding the scapula inferomedially, rotating the scapula externally and controlling any winging of the scapula bone. The patient is asked to perform a simultaneous active arm elevation through scaption. Finally, an assistant may also provide an additional posterior–caudal glide of the humerus during elevation. Lewis (2015) reported that this particular procedure exerts a significant benefit in the recovery of motion in patients with frozen shoulder. Some important points are: (a) progression into a closed chain position may be accomplished by having the patient adopt a four-point kneeling stance, and (b) having the patient sit back on the heels will recreate controlled weight-bearing forces on the shoulder girdle during the application of a mobilization with movement, which should now render the activity pain free.

Hand behind back

This movement is a multiplane movement requiring a combination of shoulder extension, internal rotation and adduction components. Occasionally limited by significant pain, this motion is often avoided by patients with impairments of the shoulder with a resulting loss of function including the ability to effectively dress, reach for a wallet and undertake personal hygiene.

Mobilization with movement – hand behind back (Fig. 31.11)

This mobilization is indicated in patients with pain or with a loss of the hand-behind-back movement. The patient is standing with the contralateral hip supported by a treatment plinth to counteract the adductory forces. A mobilization belt is draped over the contralateral shoulder, and is held anteriorly by the free hand and posteriorly by the involved arm hand. The therapist stands at the side of the patient, placing the posterior hand high in the axilla with the palm facing away from the patient, while the anterior hand is supinated fully to grip the distal humerus with the thumb hooked into the cubital fossa of the patient. For this technique, the therapist stabilizes the scapula with the cephalic hand and medially directed force from the posterior hand. The mobilization consists of an inferior glide of the humerus with the thumb of the anterior hand in the cubital fossa. The patient simultaneously moves the hand behind the back by pulling on the belt. Clinicians should ensure the patient does not attempt to lift the hand away from the back and ensure that the posterior hand force in the axilla is adductory and cephalic so as to stabilize the scapula.

Mobilization with movement – hand behind back, belt assisted (Fig. 31.12)

This technique is indicated in larger patients, or with smaller therapists, and in those patients with pain or loss of hand-behind-back movement. The patient is standing with the contralateral hip supported by a treatment plinth to counteract adductory forces. The mobilization belt is draped over the contralateral shoulder and held anteriorly by the free hand and posteriorly by the involved-side hand. One of the therapist's hands is placed high in the axilla with the palms facing away from patient. The mobilization belt is folded in half and hooked into the cubital fossa of the patient, and the heel of one of the therapist's feet in the belt loop with the toe on the floor so as to control the belt force. For this technique, the therapist stabilizes the scapula with the cephalic hand and a

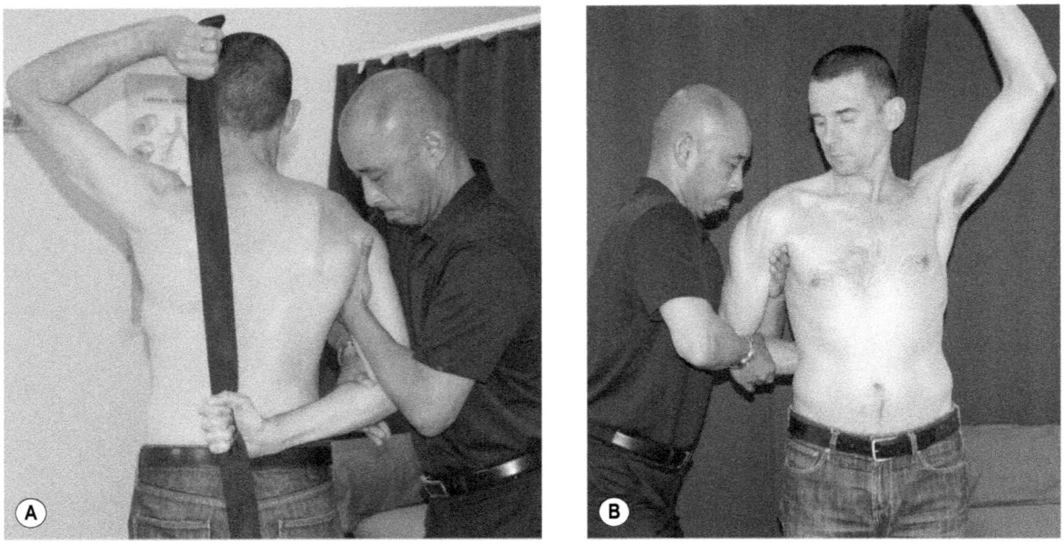

Figure 31.11 Mobilization with movement – hand behind back: (**A**) posterior view, (**B**) anterior view.

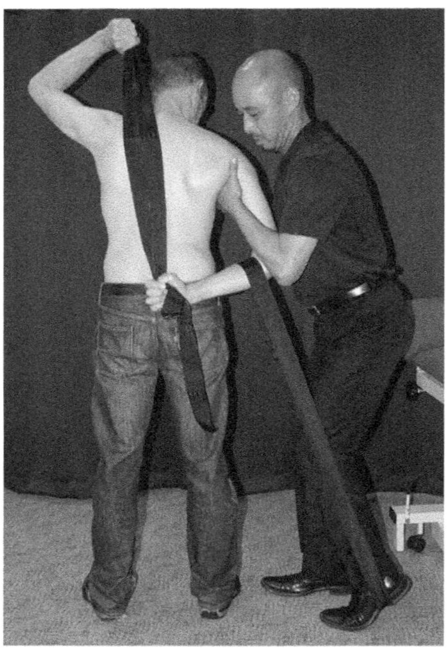

Figure 31.12 Mobilization with movement – hand behind back, belt assisted.

medially directed force from the posterior hand. The mobilization consists of an inferior glide of the humerus, done by pulling on the belt by dorsal flexing the foot. The patient simultaneously moves the hand behind the back by pulling on the belt. The clinician should ensure that the patient does not attempt to lift the hand away from the back. Some important points are: (a) to ensure that the hand force in the axilla is adductory and cephalic to stabilize the scapula, and (b) to use gentle pressure from the belt with the heel on the floor for control.

Horizontal adduction motion

Reaching across the body to the opposite shoulder is an activity involving multiple articulations in addition to the glenohumeral joint. Optimal functioning of the acromioclavicular (AC) and the sternoclavicular (SC) joints is intimately associated with normal pain-free performance of cross-body motion. Spinal mobilizations with upper extremity movement may render shoulder movements pain free and restore functional mobility when the neck is involved in dysfunction of the upper quadrant.

Mobilization with movement – horizontal adduction (AC/SC joints) (Fig. 31.13)

This technique is indicated when there is pain reaching across the body towards the contralateral shoulder in the transverse plane. The patient is seated on a low-back chair with the cervical spine neutral. The therapist stands behind the patient with the hypothenar portion of the hand on the superior surface of the patient's distal clavicle bone. The technique consists of an inferior glide of the clavicle, while the patient is asked to perform a simultaneous cross-body movement towards the contralateral shoulder or rib cage. Some important points are: (a) the presence of moderate pain-free crepitus is normal, and (b) the therapist should begin with gentle active movement, progressing to more vigorous motion as irritability decreases.

Spinal mobilization with upper extremity movement – horizontal adduction (Fig. 31.14)

This technique is indicated when there is pain with cross-body movement related to cervical dysfunction. The patient is seated with cervical spine in neutral. The therapist stands behind the patient, with the side of one thumb contacting the lateral slope of the involved cervical vertebrae spinous process. This thumb may be reinforced by the contralateral thumb or index fingertip. The mobilization intervention consists of applying a medial translation / rotation of the targeted cervical vertebrae, while the patient is asked to perform a simultaneous cross-body movement towards the contralateral shoulder or rib cage. Some important points are: (a) that the mobilization force controls, but does not block, the normal ipsilateral rotation of the cervical vertebrae and spinous process, and (b) the therapist should begin with gentle active

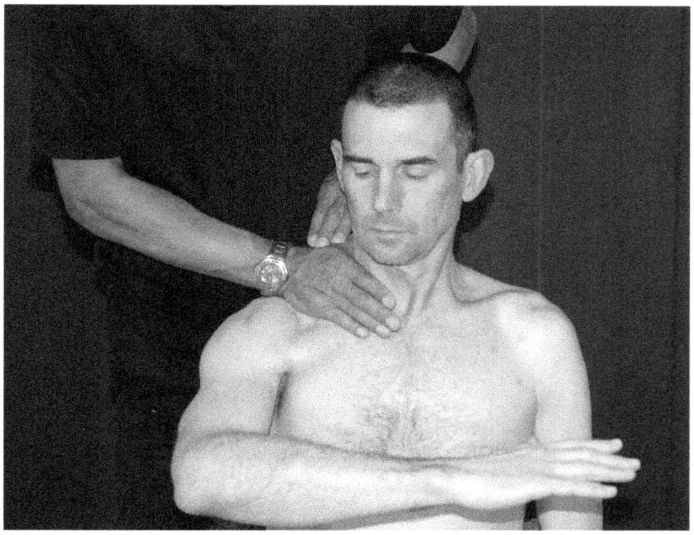

Figure 31.13 **Mobilization with movement – horizontal adduction (AC/SC joints).**

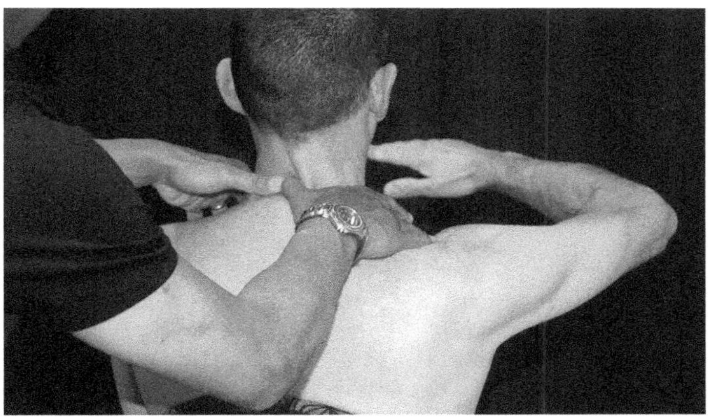

Figure 31.14 **Spinal mobilization with upper extremity movement – horizontal adduction.**

movement, progressing to more vigorous motion as irritability decreases.

Conclusion

The inclusion of passive intra-articular mobilizations and mobilization with movement interventions of the shoulder region into a multimodal approach in patients with neck and arm pain syndromes should be considered in order to improve the function and decrease the disability of the patient. The intensity and progression of the mobilizations should be adapted to the irritability of the tissue of the patient.

References

Brandt C, Sole G, Krause MW, et al. 2007. An evidence-based review on the validity of the Kaltenborn rule as applied to the glenohumeral joint. Man Ther 12: 3–11.

Cheng PL. 2006. Simulation of Codman's paradox reveals a general law of motion. J Biomech 39: 1201–1207.

Dashottar A, Borstad J. 2012. Posterior glenohumeral joint capsule contracture. Shoulder Elbow 1: 4.

DeSantis L, Hasson SM. 2006. Use of mobilization with movement in the treatment of a patient with sub-acromial impingement: a case report. J Manual Manipul Ther 14: 77–87.

Doner G, Guven Z, Atalay A, et al. 2013. Evalution of Mulligan's technique for adhesive capsulitis of the shoulder. J Rehab Med 45: 87–91.

Flatow E, Soslowsky J, Ticker J, et al. 1994. Excursion of the rotator cuff under the acromion. Patterns of subacromial contact. Am J Sports Med 22: 7779–7788.

Hengeveld E, Banks K, Maitland GD (eds). 2005. Maitland's peripheral manipulation, 4th edn. Edinburgh: Elsevier / Butterworth Heinemann.

Hing WA, Reid DA, Monaghan M. 2003. Manipulation of the cervical spine. Man Ther 8: 2–9.

Hing WA, Bigalow R, Bremner T. 2008. Mulligan's mobilisation with movement: a review of the tenets and prescription of MWMs. N Z J Physiother 36: 34–54.

Hing WA, Bigalow R, Bremner T. 2009. Mulligans mobilisation with movement: a systematic review. J Manual Manipul Ther 17:E39–E66.

Ho KY, Hsu AT. 2009. Displacement of the head of humerus while performing 'mobilization with movements' in glenohumeral joint: a cadaver study. Man Ther 14: 160–166.

Hsu AT, Ho L, Ho S, et al. 2000. Joint position during anterior–posterior glide mobilization: its effect on glenohumeral abduction range of motion. Arch Phys Med Rehabil 81: 210–214.

Hsu AT, Chiu JF, Chang JH. 2009. Biomechanical analysis of axial distraction mobilization of the glenohumeral joint: a cadaver study. Man Ther 14: 381–386. doi: 10.1016/j.math.2008.06.003.

Jones MA, Rivett DA (eds). 2004. Clinical reasoning for manual therapists, 1st edn. Edinburgh: Butterworth Heinemann.

Kachingwe A, Phillips B, Plunkett S. 2008. Comparison of manual therapy techniques with therapeutic exercise in the treatment of shoulder impingement: a randomized controlled clinical trial. J Man Manip Ther 16: 238–247.

Kaltenborn FM, Evjenth O, Kaltenborn TB, et al. 2002. Manual mobilization of the joints: the Kaltenborn method of joint examination and treatment: the extremities, 6th edn. Oslo: Olaf Norlis Bokhandel.

Lewis J. 2015. Frozen shoulder contracture syndrome – aetiology, diagnosis and management. Man Ther 20: 2–9.

Liu YL, Ao YF, Cui GQ, et al. 2011. Changes of histology and capsular collagen in a rat shoulder immobilization model. Chin Med J 124: 3939–3944.

Maricar N, Shacklady C, McLoughlin L. 2009. Effect of Maitland mobilization and exercises for the treatment of shoulder adhesive capsulitis: a single-case design. Physiother Theory Pract 25: 203–217.

Miller J. 1999. The Mulligan concept: the next step in the evolution of manual therapy. Can Physiother Assoc Orthop Division Rev March / April: 9–13.

Miller J. 2006. The Mulligan concept: how: clinical application, when: clinical reasoning, why: clinical research. Can Physiother Assoc Orthop Division Rev May / June: 22–28.

Mulligan BR. 2003. Manual therapy: NAGS, SNAGS, MWMS, etc., 3rd edn. Wellington, NZ: Plane View Services.

Scaringe J, Kawaoka C, Studt T. 2002. Improved shoulder function after using spinal mobilisation with arm movement in a 50 year old golfer with shoulder, arm and neck pain. Topics Clin Chiropr 9: 4453.

Surenkok O, Aytar A, Baltaci G. 2009. Acute effects of scapular mobilization in shoulder dysfunction: a double-blind randomized placebo-controlled trial. J Sport Rehabil 18: 493–501.

Teys P, Bisset L, Vicenzino B. 2008. The initial effects of a Mulligan's mobilization with movement technique on range of movement and pressure pain threshold in pain-limited shoulders. Man Ther 13: 37–42.

Vermeulen HM, Rozing PM, Obermann WR, et al. 2006. Comparison of high-grade and low-grade mobilization techniques in the management of adhesive capsulitis of the shoulder: randomized controlled trial. Phys Ther 86: 355–368.

Vicenzino B, Paungmali A, Teys P. 2007. Mulligan's mobilization-with-movement, positional faults and pain relief: current concepts from a critical review of literature. Man Ther 12: 98–108.

Vicenzino B, Hing WA, Rivett D, et al. 2011. Mobilisation with movement: the art and the science. London: Elsevier.

Yang JL, Chang CW, Chen SY, et al. 2007. Mobilization techniques in subjects with frozen shoulder syndrome: randomized multiple-treatment trial. Phys Ther 87: 1307–1315.

Yang JL, Jan MH, Chang CW, et al. 2012. Effectiveness of the end-range mobilization and scapular mobilization approach in a subgroup of subjects with frozen shoulder syndrome: a randomized control trial. Man Ther 17: 47–52.

32 Chapter

Motor Control of the Shoulder Region

Mary E. Magarey, Mark A. Jones, Samuel R. Baida

CHAPTER CONTENTS

Introduction 358
Motor control 358
Motor control and joint stability 358
Evidence of altered motor control around the scapula 359
Evidence of altered motor control around the glenohumeral joint 360
Evaluation of motor control around the shoulder girdle 360
Postural assessment 360
Evaluation of isolated motor control around the shoulder 366
Management of motor control impairments around the shoulder girdle 367
Management of shoulder motor control through patient examples 368
Conclusion 371

Introduction

Motor control around the shoulder, its examination and management, are vast and complex topics. In this chapter we provide a brief background of motor control theory and the evidence in support of impairments in motor control around the shoulder, together with a summary of the principles of motor learning in the context of shoulder rehabilitation. The focus is on control aspects of the scapulothoracic and glenohumeral joints as directly relevant to shoulder function. Although the focus is on evaluation and management associated with motor control abilities and impairments, evaluation for and management of impairments in pain, range of movement, strength, endurance, power and technique must also be addressed in a holistic context, with appropriate diagnostic considerations and a thorough bio-psychosocial approach. The influence of the remainder of the kinetic chain on shoulder function and of shoulder girdle influence on arm function should also be acknowledged and considered in both examination and management.

Motor Control

Motor control theories explain the central nervous system's ability to organize mechanisms and systems essential for regulating movement, posture and stability. These address both sensory (particularly, vision, audition and proprioception) and motor systems with consideration of the complex interaction between the individual, the task and the environment (Schmidt & Lee 2005; Shumway-Cook & Woollacott 2012). Motor behaviour is considered to be pre-structured generalized neuronal coding about the order of events, their relative timing and the relative force required across different tasks. For example, the sequencing of muscle activity and joint motion for shoulder elevation is included in a motor programme of elevation, which is supplemented by rules that specify the parameters related to the particular way the programme is executed according to the task, such as speed (Schmidt & Lee 2005). Targeted motor training can be used to strengthen, modify or reacquire such motor patterns. In order for the brain to encode new or modified movement it must continually remodel its neural circuitry for behavioural changes to take place (Kleim & Jones 2008). Pain and / or perceived threat can also drive motor behavioural changes. Adaptation involves a protective process that helps prevent injury by generating a withdrawal reflex from the noxious stimulus and / or an unpleasant sensation that results in complex behavioural strategies used to avoid replication of that sensation (Latremoliere & Woolf 2009). With regards to rehabilitation programmes, approaches to motor control and learning must recognize the breadth of potential neural changes, both short and long term and in different tasks and environments (Hodges 2011; Shumway-Cook & Woollacott 2012). A primary goal of rehabilitation is to promote neuroplasticity, such that long-lasting and advantageous modifications in motor control strategies can be achieved (Boudreau et al 2010a). This must be balanced with treatment interventions to address potential psychosocial factors contributing to a pain and / or disability experience.

Motor control and joint stability

Motor control and joint stability are closely linked and should be considered as a dynamic process of controlling static position while allowing movement with control (Hodges 2004). Panjabi's now-familiar model of three inter-related systems responsible for control of the neutral zone (Panjabi 1992a, 1992b, 1996) forms the basis for much recent work in relation to function and differences in behaviour of different types of muscles. As a result, two groups of muscles have been identified that fulfil different roles – 'stabilizers' or 'local system' and 'mobilizers' or 'global system' (Hodges 2004; Magee & Zachazewski 2007). Although this categorization is debated (McGill 2007) and further research is needed to clarify this distinction and its clinical efficacy, we find this construct helpful in focusing assessment and treatment procedures, with excellent results.

It has been established that motor coordination can be altered with musculoskeletal pain syndromes (Kofler et al 1998; Tsao et al 2010). Hodges (2011) has put forward a model comprising five key principles, which helps better understand the relationship between motor control, pain and neural plasticity. This model provides explanation of the multiple mechanical adaptation strategies that may be implemented by the brain depending on the individual (experience, anthropometrics, posture) and the task (Hodges & Tucker 2011). The majority of changes are driven from reorganization of movement representations in the primary motor cortex (Hodges 2011). Examination is recommended of all components of the neuromuscular system including dysfunction of synergistic control, timing of muscle activation, patterns of co-contraction and proprioceptive control in patients with musculoskeletal pain, especially pain of long duration and / or intensity. This recommendation, built on the hypothesis related to the relationship between afferent nociceptive input and motor control and the principles of motor learning, forms the foundation of our approach to evaluation and management of patients with shoulder dysfunction.

Evidence of altered motor control around the scapula

Alterations to muscle function around the scapula have been demonstrated in the presence of cervical pain or headaches (Nederhand et al 2000; Falla 2004; Szeto et al 2005, 2009; Falla et al 2007; Jull et al 2008). With respect to the shoulder, a consistent recruitment pattern has been demonstrated in asymptomatic shoulders that is related to active abduction in the scapular plane (Wadsworth & Bullock-Saxton 1997; Moraes et al 2008) or response to sudden release from an abducted position (Cools et al 2002, 2003) and reaching tasks (Roy et al 2008). The upper trapezius muscle is activated first, followed by the serratus anterior, the middle trapezius and finally the lower trapezius muscles. The temporal characteristics are delayed but not changed by fatigue in asymptomatic subjects (Moraes et al 2008).

A reasonably consistent pattern of decreased activity has been demonstrated in both the lower trapezius and the serratus anterior, and increased activity in the upper trapezius in patients experiencing shoulder pain or pathology during different tasks (Glousman et al 1988; Scovazzo et al 1991; Pink et al 1993; Ludewig & Cook 2000; Cools et al 2003, 2004, 2005; McClure et al 2006; Cools et al 2007a; Roy et al 2008). Kibler (1998) and Kibler et al (2013) observed that inhibition of the lower trapezius and serratus anterior muscles appears to be a non-specific response to shoulder pain irrespective of the pathology. The lower trapezius has a predominance of type I fibres, whereas the upper trapezius has predominantly type II (Simons et al 1999); this implies that the lower trapezius is best suited for postural and stabilizing roles and the upper trapezius for phasic activity. Findings of delayed and / or reduced activity in the lower trapezius and serratus anterior in response to shoulder pain coupled with increased activity in the upper trapezius, although not universally reported, lend support to this hypothesis. These results support findings from other body regions of a neuromuscular impairment associated with pain in an adjacent joint (Cowan et al 2001, 2002, 2003; Hodges 2004; Colné & Thoumie 2006; Hertel & Olmsted-Kramer 2007; Jull et al 2008).

Altered scapular position is common in association with shoulder pain, with typical patterns identified and given various names. A very common pattern is the 'scapular downwardly rotated syndrome' (Sahrmann 2002), also termed 'type 1 scapular dyskinesis' (Kibler et al 2002, 2003) – one of the impairment patterns identified under the acronym of 'SICK' scapula (**S**capular malposition, **I**nferior medial border prominence, **C**oracoid pain and malposition and dys**K**inesis of scapular movement) (Burkhart et al 2003). This pattern appears to be associated with insufficiency of the upward rotation force couple and overactivity or increased tone in the antagonist muscles, in particular levator scapulae, rhomboids and pectoralis minor (Kibler & McMullen 2003). Kibler et al (2013), summarizing the findings of a recent 'scapular summit', observed that contemporary thinking is that scapular static position is of less significance than impaired scapular movement patterns during arm movement, such that the focus on naming different static positions and taking objective measures is down-played.

The serratus anterior and lower trapezius muscles are important components of the scapular upward rotation force couple, particularly above 60° of arm elevation (Bagg & Forrest 1986, 1988). Decreased activity in the lower trapezius and serratus anterior associated with arm elevation (Ludewig & Cook 2000; Cools et al 2007a) in patients with subacromial pain supports the observation of delayed or reduced upward rotation in the clinical setting. Increased upper trapezius activity under a heavier load (Ludewig & Cook 2000) and in the upper ranges of elevation (Cools et al 2007a) possibly reflects a compensation for decreased activity in the lower trapezius and serratus anterior and / or an attempt to overcome the increased tone in the antagonists.

A second altered scapular posture, an elevated scapula, is described as type III scapular dyskinesis (Kibler et al 2002, 2003). This pattern appears to present in association with either shoulder stiffness into elevation or major rotator cuff dysfunction, such that the deltoid / rotator cuff force couple is disrupted and the humeral head translates superiorly to abut against the undersurface of the acromion. Increased activity in the upper trapezius and levator scapulae is dominant.

Not all responses to shoulder pain are consistent (Cools et al 2003, 2004, 2005, 2007a), which possibly reflects the different patterns demonstrated in subgroups within sample populations with the same diagnosis (Graichen et al 2001; Hébert et al 2002; Roy et al 2008). The observation of variations in patterns of muscle activity supports the need to address each patient's impairment individually during assessment and management.

Altered scapular positioning and scapular plane elevation are frequently associated with increased thoracic kyphosis, cervical flexion or forward head posture (Crawford & Jull 1993; Greenfield et al 1995; Ludewig & Cook 1996; Bullock et al 2005), which supports the kinematic relationship of spinal posture, scapular posture and shoulder elevation. Although spinal posture may not be correlated with specific shoulder pathology (Lewis et al 2005a, 2005b), its relationship to shoulder elevation impairment warrants attention in rehabilitation.

Clearly, when considering rehabilitation of the shoulder, attention to the scapular muscle impairments, particularly those related to motor control, is imperative (Ebaugh et al 2005; Kibler et al 2013). Equally the shoulder should not be considered in isolation from the cervical and thoracic spine (Jull et al 2008) and the control and movement patterns of the lumbar spine, pelvis and lower limbs (Kibler 1998, 2013). Although the focus in this chapter is on motor control of the shoulder, the important contributions of these other areas must not be forgotten.

Evidence of altered motor control around the glenohumeral joint

Evidence related to local stabilizing muscle function around the glenohumeral joint is less robust, with only two studies reporting on specific rotator cuff control. David et al (2000) demonstrated that, during isokinetic glenohumeral rotation, the rotator cuff and biceps brachii when considered as a group were always activated prior to the superficial muscles, deltoid and pectoralis major in asymptomatic shoulders and there was always an element of co-contraction, regardless of direction or speed of rotation. The rotator cuff group was also always activated before movement of the isokinetic device's lever arm. This finding supports the hypothesis that the rotator cuff functions in a joint-stabilizing role. Delayed activation of the rotator cuff / biceps in individuals with unstable shoulders was also demonstrated in a clinical but not a research setting.

Hess et al (2005) demonstrated delayed activation of the subscapularis during a reaction time test into external rotation in throwers with painful shoulders compared with a matched group of asymptomatic volunteers, hypothesizing that subscapularis fulfilled a joint stabilization role. However, their testing protocol required use of the infraspinatus as a prime mover. Lumbar spine research demonstrates that competing demands on the central nervous system lead to an alteration in muscle use (Hodges 2004) so that, when required to function in its primary role, a muscle's secondary stabilizing role is compromised.

Ginn et al (2009) demonstrated from EMG research that the rotator cuff does not function at equal loads through all activities; rather, the majority of activation is direction specific. The antagonist cuff muscle was activated at approximately 6% maximal voluntary contraction (MVC) during each of the movements. However, given that only 1–3% MVC is required to stiffen a joint (Cholewicki & McGill 1996), their findings do not disprove the stabilization role. There is also a wealth of biomechanical literature that supports a stabilization role for the rotator cuff (Clark & Harryman 1992; Wuelker et al 1995; Burkhart 1996; Kibler 1998; Lee et al 2000), particularly the subscapularis and infraspinatus / teres minor muscles (Burkhart 1996). Given that the lower fibres of the subscapularis attach directly to the medial lip of the bicipital groove (Morag et al 2011) and those of the teres minor muscle attach to the lateral lip (Drake et al 2009), these two muscles are ideally placed biomechanically to fulfil a stabilization role. Independent innervation for these muscles (the lower subscapularis nerve for the lower subscapularis and the axillary nerve for the teres minor, the most common derivation of the lower subscapular being the axillary nerve) also indicates the potential for their function to differ from that of the infraspinatus (suprascapular nerve) and upper subscapularis (upper subscapularis nerve) (Kasper et al 2008; Morag et al 2011).

Evaluation of Motor Control around the Shoulder Girdle

The assessments described below are used to guide motor control retraining. Impairments in motor control exist within a continuum and manifest as poor postural awareness combined with an inability to produce smooth, kinematically correct movements through a full range without compensation under varying demands of posture, load and speed. Whereas severe impairments will be apparent even in gravity-eliminated positions, lesser impairments will often be evident only in certain ranges of movement, loads (Ludewig & Cook 2000; McClure et al 2001, 2006) and speeds (Roy et al 2008) and during distracting tasks (Hodges 2004). Equally, side-to-side comparison provides evidence of bilateral movement dysfunction, possibly indicating a predisposition to impairment (Hébert et al 2002; McClure et al 2006), and / or physiological processes occurring throughout higher processing centres in the central nervous system (Sterling et al 2001; Kleim & Jones 2008; Shumway-Cook & Woollacott 2012), and a poorer prognosis with respect to change. With the aim of converting identified motor control impairments into retraining exercises, each assessment evaluates where (range, posture, load, speed) the patient has control and where that control is lost, and attends to all components in the kinetic chain (upper and lower trunk, scapula, glenohumeral). The assessment is varied with respect to position (against gravity versus gravity eliminated or assisted) to identify the position / function in which control is sufficient to initiate retraining.

Postural assessment

Detailed evaluation of posture allows formation of initial hypotheses in relation to potential impairments in motor control. Postural abnormalities may be associated with movement and control impairments, although an association must not be assumed. Such hypotheses must be tested with movement, resistive and palpatory assessment and specific postural impairment correction during provocative active movements to ascertain the effect (Lewis et al 2005a). Static posture should be assessed in positions relevant to the patient's function and symptom production, not just in a standardized starting position. In addition to visual assessment, the scapular slide test (Kibler 1998, 2003) is a validated measure of scapular resting position – although resting position is not necessarily correlated with function and more objective measures of spinal posture are available (Jull et al 2008).

If an apparent postural impairment is identified, its association with the patient's presenting condition should be tested to determine its direct or indirect relevance by assessing whether alteration of the impairment, either passively or actively, influences the patient's symptoms or sense of 'normalcy'. Although not confirmatory, alteration in response to postural correction and the ability to achieve a corrected position provide an indication of the significance of the positional fault to their symptom presentation, level of awareness or control impairment.

Evaluation of movement impairments and awareness

The focus of this movement assessment is not 'diagnostic' of structural symptom sources, but rather on impairments of awareness, movement and control; however, this should always be undertaken with appropriate caution and monitoring of symptom provocation.

All active movements of the shoulder girdle provide an indication of motor control, in addition to movement awareness, dissociation, relative activity within and between force couples, more so than specific strength or endurance. Therefore, all active shoulder movements should be examined as part of an evaluation of motor control. Any movement impairments are evaluated for their relevance to provocation of symptoms. Assistance with active movement, such as the scapular assistance test (SAT) (Kibler et al 2002, 2006; Kibler 2003; Cools et al 2008) (Fig. 32.1, Box 32.1) to facilitate scapular upward rotation or passive posterior translation for an anteriorly placed humeral head will, for example, often improve movement and lessen symptoms.

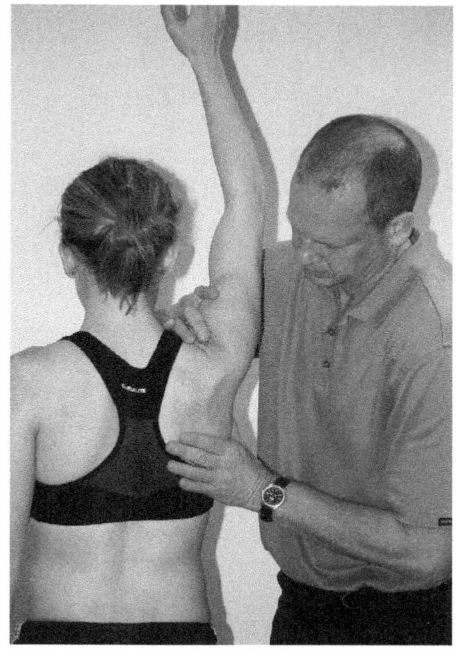

Figure 32.1 Scapular assistance test. (From Kibler 2003; Kibler et al 2002, 2006, with permission.)

Box 32.1 Description/discussion of tests

Figure 32.1

The scapular assistance test involves the therapist providing manual assistance to upward rotation of the scapula during glenohumeral elevation through flexion, abduction or scapular plane abduction.

Figure 32.2

Strength of the rotator cuff muscles is more accurately evaluated when the scapula is supported in a retracted position, such that it provides a stable base from which the rotator cuff can work. The therapist maintains the scapula in a retracted position with manual pressure while providing manual resistance to the arm for the relevant rotator cuff test.

Figure 32.3

A shoulder shrug in standing with the arms by the side demonstrates the patient's ability to elevate the shoulder girdles to full passive range, the pattern of activation associated with the movement and symmetry between sides. Shoulder shrug is frequently accompanied by significant low cervical flexion and upper cervical extension, scapular elevation combined with protraction and apparent glenohumeral internal rotation, possibly representing a dominance of the levator scapulae over the upper trapezius, as the forward-poking head lengthens the upper component of the muscle, thus allowing it more leverage to complete the movement at its distal end. The accompanying scapular movement is reflective of the dominance of the levator scapulae and pectoralis minor. Correction of this movement pattern leads to an inability to raise the scapulae to their full passive range. A tape or ruler can be used to measure vertical distance between the ear lobe and the shoulder girdle to provide an objective outcome measure.

The hypothesized basis for this test is that, in the elevated arm position, the upper trapezius is in its maximally shortened position, so if lengthened in its resting posture, as with a downwardly rotated scapula, attaining the same level of shoulder shrug as with the arms by the side will be difficult. Lack of passive flexibility or overactivity in the levator scapulae, rhomboids or latissimus dorsi will limit the passive range of shoulder shrug in this position. An equivalent measure may be taken to compare the range in the two positions.

Figure 32.4

Glenohumeral rotations, particularly in 90° of abduction/flexion, demonstrate the ability to move the glenohumeral joint on a stable scapula and an awareness of dissociation of the arm from the scapula. Differences in the ability to dissociate in standing and in prone/supine provide indication of the effect of load on the scapular stabilizers and rotator cuff during this task.

This analysis can be made more objective by measuring the distance moved by the acromion from its neutral start position during the arm movement. Ideally, movement should be minimal. Excessive scapular movement leads to greater acromial movement from its resting position.

Continued

Box 32.1 Description/discussion of tests—cont'd

Figure 32.5

Evaluation of awareness of scapular movement can be undertaken using scapular proprioceptive neuromuscular facilitation (PNF) patterns. Given that the movements involved are unfamiliar to the patient, several steps are taken in this evaluation:

- Explain the direction of movement required, using cues such as 'Take the point of your shoulder towards the corner of your eye', while at the same time touching the corresponding acromial angle and outer corner of the eye and doing the movement with the patient passively, using traditional PNF hand-holds and principles. For the opposite direction, cue 'Take the point of your shoulder blade (while touching it with your fingers) down towards the opposite hip/back pocket' and again guide the patient in the appropriate movement direction.
- Talk the patient through the movement while performing it passively, ensuring availability of full passive range.
- Ask the patient to assist with the movement, following which unassisted performance determines the patient's ability to replicate it.
- If the patient has difficulty grasping the feel of the movement, further facilitation can be given by means of verbal encouragement, resistance to the movement through range, holds at end of range with slow eccentric contraction and reversals, etc. (Fig. 32.5A).
- In patients with poor awareness or control, the scapula tends to follow a curvilinear path rather than a diagonal one, with jerky uncoordinated movement. Frequently, the scapula moves into excessive protraction and anterior tilt when attempting the 'up-and-forward' direction in particular, as demonstrated in Figure 32.5B. Such an inability to control the movement in a direct diagonal and to the desired end point is an indication that use of PNF as a hands-on facilitation may be indicated in the early stages of rehabilitation.

Figure 32.6

The test is performed in side-lying, with tested arm uppermost and supported on the therapist's arm in approximately 120° elevation, such that the therapist can apply progressively increased resistance into scapular protraction, glenohumeral elevation and external rotation, with the heel of the other hand against the lateral border of the scapula used to assess and resist scapular upward rotation. The activation can be tested isometrically, isotonically both concentrically and, at higher levels, eccentrically. Poor activation is felt as a sluggish response of the scapula to resistance and/or more 'give' to the movement. The test may be progressed from simply holding the arm while applying resistance to the scapula to resisting protraction and elevation/external rotation on the arm concurrent with upward rotation on the scapula.

Figure 32.7

Evaluation in four-point kneeling:

- Initially, spontaneous posture is noted with respect to spinal, scapular, shoulder and hip alignments and the position maintained for an arbitrary period (e.g. 2 minutes) while observing for fatigue. Typical compensation strategies include locking the elbows into full extension; arms into end-range rotation; dropping the trunk forward, leading to a passive scapular retraction and thoracic extension, increased lumbar lordosis, forward head posture and cervical flexion; elevation of the shoulder girdle towards the ears; scapular winging or tremor of the arm and/or shoulder girdle muscles. Asymmetries from neutral are highlighted to the patient and correction is facilitated by passive guidance if necessary. In this context, neutral refers to normal spinal curves and scapular posture, taking account of the patient's individual spinal mobility. The patient's abilities and impairments are then recorded.
- The patient is instructed to shift the weight onto one hand, initially without lifting the other arm and then in conjunction with arm elevation so that the pattern of head on neck, trunk, scapular and arm control can be further evaluated. Again, impairments are recorded. This assessment may be taken through further steps to increase the challenge to match relevant sporting requirements. Raising the diagonally opposite arm and leg, in a full push-up position, undertaking the assessment with the legs and trunk on an unstable surface, such as a gym ball, or the hand balancing on an unstable surface, such as a slide mat, spin disk or ball, all provide additional challenge to the system and may highlight impairments. These steps also integrate the whole kinetic chain so impairments more distant to the shoulder may be identified.

Figure 32.8

Evaluation in four-point kneeling:

- During evaluation of spinal dissociation, a frequent finding is an inability to position the head in neutral without concomitant thoracic and lumbar extension. An instruction to extend the neck frequently leads to a whole-spine extension pattern. A request for pelvic neutral may have a similar effect, with the patient unable to isolate the lumbar spine movement.
- With pro/retraction of the scapula, the chest 'drops through' the scapulae on retraction and is elevated between them on protraction. Typically, a patient with shoulder pain is unable to perform this movement independently of thoracic flexion/extension. An inability to protract (i.e. push-up plus position) is also often observed. Education about the impairment and facilitation of an improved movement is undertaken to determine how 'fixed' the impairment is in the patient's motor patterning and, therefore, how significant it might be in the context of the presenting problem.

Figure 32.9

The therapist palpates the humeral head with one hand, ensuring no restraint of humeral head movement. This hand feels for humeral head translation or altered quality of movement through each stage of the test. The therapist also observes scapular and spinal control and movement, and enquires about provocation of symptoms.

- With the patient's arm by the side, elbow flexed to 90° and neutral forearm rotation, manual resistance is applied slowly through the wrist to an isometric contraction. This contraction is repeated in as many positions as appropriate for the

Box 32.1 Description/discussion of tests—cont'd

particular patient's presentation. Do not stop in the sequence of positions when an impairment is noted, as activity regularly performed at higher range, such as throwing, may lead to better function in this range. The movement is repeated from the neutral start position into the opposite rotation.

- In most instances, at least three elevation positions are tested: neutral, 45–60° elevation and an end position relevant to function (e.g. 110° elevation in the scapular plane for a thrower or full elevation for a swimmer, mimicking the 'catch' position).
- The test procedures are repeated using an isotonic contraction through the full available range, first in one rotation and then the other, ensuring that the movement is one of pure rotation.
- If no impairment is detected through any part of the test, it is repeated at higher speed, with an eccentric component, quick reversals or with increased load. Occasionally, the resistance of the therapist's hand is sufficient to facilitate co-contraction. Asking the patient to repeat the test movements with a small weight in the hand may lead to altered humeral head control, or the patient may be able to feel when control is lost even if the therapist cannot.
- Once a position of impairment is detected, whether isometrically or dynamically, small variations of positions are evaluated until a position of control is found as close to where control is lost as possible. If impairment on the dynamic rotary stability test (DRST) is prioritized for inclusion in a management plan, this would be the position where training is commenced.

Figure 32.10

- The start position is usually sitting with the arm supported in 60–90° scapular plane elevation, neutral rotation. The start position must be pain free, with a relaxed scapula and relatively neutral spinal position. The therapist palpates the axillary aspect of subscapularis with the tips of the middle two fingers, usually from a posterior direction, with the pads adjacent to the latissimus dorsi on the posterior axillary wall. Concurrently, the therapist places the pad of the thumb vertically along the tendon of the infraspinatus/teres minor so that activation of both components of the force couple can be palpated simultaneously. Finding the subscapularis tendon may be difficult on some people, especially those with a superiorly translated humeral head or hypertrophy of either the latissimus dorsi or pectoralis major. Confirmation of correct positioning is made by gentle resistance into first one rotation and then the other while the therapist feels for increased tone in the relevant tendon.
- Very gentle traction is applied to the humerus and the patient asked to 'draw the arm into the socket'. The therapist palpates both tendons to evaluate levels of contraction while monitoring unwanted activation in other muscles. Manual facilitation by pressure on the tendons may be useful, reinforced by verbal encouragement and visual imagery. This is an unfamiliar task, so initial assessment should be on the non-affected side.
- If co-contraction can be felt but only in association with superficial muscle activity, training is undertaken to reduce the extraneous activity. If no co-contraction can be facilitated, further tactile stimulation and/or imagery may help. For example, the anteriorly unstable shoulder may respond to instruction to 'draw the arm up and back' in association with a traction force combined with gentle internal rotation, thus biasing the facilitation to the external rotators. The superiorly placed humeral head may respond better to a suggestion to 'draw in and gently push down on my finger in your armpit' in conjunction with pressure on the subscapularis, although excessive activation of latissimus dorsi and pectoralis major may be the result of this suggestion. Persistence with facilitation and multiple trials may be needed to achieve success. In the future, biofeedback with real-time ultrasound is planned to facilitate training.
- Once the co-contraction can be achieved, a benchmark is established to form the basis for a home programme and further training, during which the patient must be able to find the subscapularis tendon and co-contract without the traction facilitation. An arbitrary 10 repeats of 10-second holds with slow, smooth build-up and release of contraction is used as a goal before progression. Once this can be achieved, the direction of progression depends on the presentation of the patient. If an athlete whose primary range of poor control is in elevation, progression is quickly made into positions within the DRST where control was lost, whereas the patient with pathology of the rotator cuff or subacromial bursa may need much slower and more deliberate co-contraction training before any load is applied to the arm.

Figure 32.11

The patient drives the hands forwards and upwards in a position of elevation, external rotation and elbow extension, thus facilitating the upward rotation component of the movement. Slight tension maintained on a lighter weight Theraband® into glenohumeral external rotation ensures that the patient does not drift into internal rotation and scapular position of downward rotation/anterior tilt. The lumbar and cervical spines must be maintained in a neutral position.

Figure 32.12

The Theraband® is looped over the shoulder and under the opposite foot. The patient catches hold of the Theraband® and steps through the loop. Placing the foot behind in a walk–stand position provides a downward-and-backward force on the shoulder, which facilitates correct movement of the acromion towards the corner of the eye. Maintenance of a chin tuck, arm external rotation and a neutral lumbar spine will all assist correct movement of the scapula.

The reverse 'downward-and-backward' pattern can also be trained by placing the Theraband® over a door and shutting the door while looping the Theraband® under the axilla. A small towel placed in the axilla makes this more comfortable. The patient stands facing the door so that the Theraband® pulls the shoulder girdle up and forwards and works the scapula down and back towards the opposite hip.

Active physiological glenohumeral movements that are most useful from a motor control perspective include:

- **flexion, abduction, scapular plane abduction:** all provide an indication of relative scapular to glenohumeral contribution, timing of movement of each component and a visual impression of activation of the key muscle groups
- **glenohumeral rotations, particularly in 90° abduction/flexion:** these demonstrate the ability to move the glenohumeral joint on a stable scapula and an awareness of dissociation of the arm from the scapula.

Traditional manual muscle tests provide an indication of the strength of specific movement directions, but not individual muscles, as both stabilizer and mobilizer muscles contribute to the generation of force. Observation of relative control of the scapula and glenohumeral joint during maximal strength tests is useful, but it does not identify specific individual muscle dysfunction, only a faulty movement pattern under load. Evaluation and possible correction of scapular position, for example with the scapular retraction test (Kibler et al 2006), during manual muscle testing is essential to determine whether the scapula is fulfilling its stabilizing role (Fig. 32.2).

Evaluation of specific motor control impairments around the scapula

On the basis of the evidence and clinical experience, we use the following key movement impairment tests to gain a broad picture of the ability and level of impairment of the axioscapular muscles. If movement impairment is noted, its significance is evaluated using the principles as outlined above. These assessments are by no means exhaustive, but representative of those commonly found useful.

Shoulder shrug (Roberts 2009)

A shoulder shrug in standing position with the arms both by the side and overhead demonstrates the patient's ability to elevate the shoulder girdles to the full passive range, the pattern of activation and movement symmetry and the effect of the altered muscle balance in different arm positions. A tape or ruler can be used to measure the vertical distance between the ear lobe and the shoulder girdle to provide an objective outcome measure (Fig. 32.3A,B).

Scapular control through glenohumeral rotations in prone and supine (Sahrmann 2002)

Glenohumeral rotations in 90° abduction or flexion demonstrate the ability to move the glenohumeral joint on a stable scapula and an awareness of dissociation between arm and scapular movement (Fig. 32.4). Poor awareness leads to excessive scapular elevation, anterior tilt and protraction during

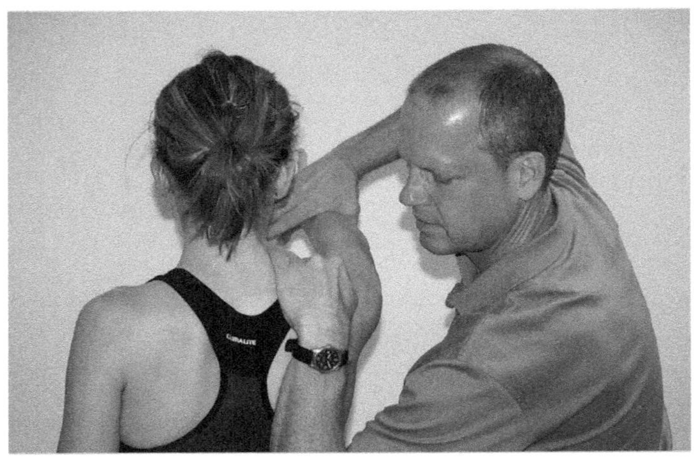

Figure 32.2 Scapular retraction test.

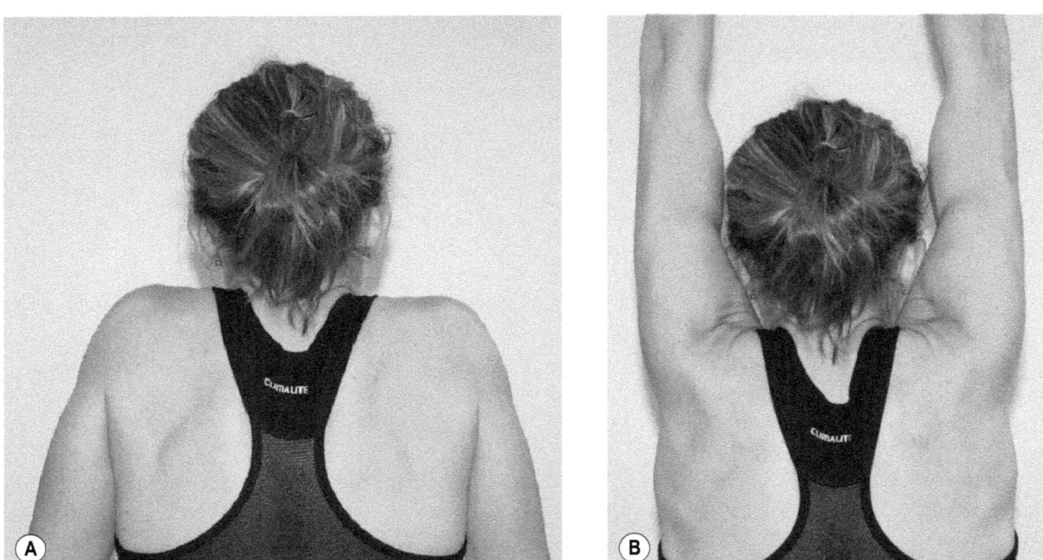

Figure 32.3 Shoulder shrug: (**A**) with arms by the side, (**B**) with arms in full elevation.

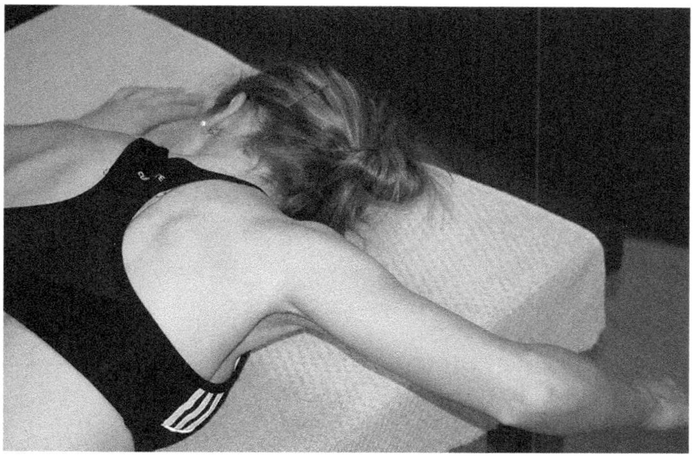

Figure 32.4 Glenohumeral rotation on a stable scapula.

internal rotation and the reverse on external rotation, or simply an inability to maintain a stable position. Measurement of acromial movement from neutral start position during the arm movement makes the test more objective. Such testing should be initiated from the least-challenging position (upper arm supported) and progressed through more challenging positions to identify where control exists and where it is lost. If later chosen as part of a retraining programme, the task must be controlled while still having sufficient challenge and variability to optimize motor learning.

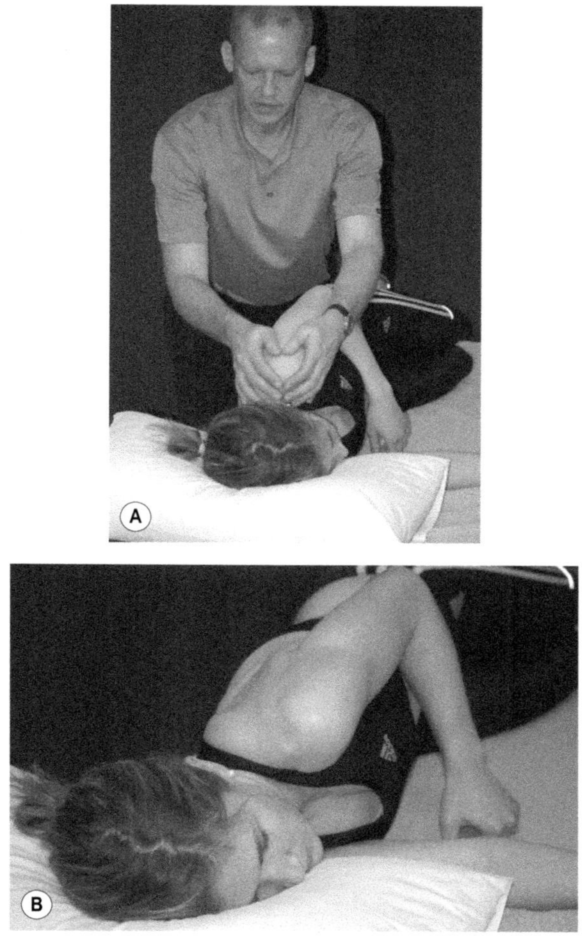

Figure 32.5 Evaluation of scapular movement awareness using scapular PNF patterns: (**A**) manual correction and guidance into a more normal movement pattern, (**B**) poor movement pattern during scapular movement in an up-and-forward direction.

Scapular PNF patterns (Voss et al 1985)

Awareness of movement of the scapula in isolation from the arm is difficult. Use of the scapular component of the traditional PNF diagonal arm patterns provides useful information on the kinaesthetic awareness of the scapula (Fig. 32.5). Given that this is an unfamiliar movement, it is unreasonable to expect a patient to perform it without some facilitation and education. More detailed description of these tests can be found in Magarey and Jones (2003a).

Evaluation of range and control of scapular upward rotation

Scapular upward rotation occurs actively in conjunction with elevation of the arm. Therefore, the optimal position in which to evaluate activity in the upward rotation force couples is with the arm in elevation greater than 90°, with resistance applied through the arm to glenohumeral elevation and external rotation and through the lateral border and inferior angle of the scapula against upward rotation (Fig. 32.6). The stage of the assessment, the quality of contraction of this important force couple, the load applied through the arm and the number of repetitions are all useful clinical outcome measures.

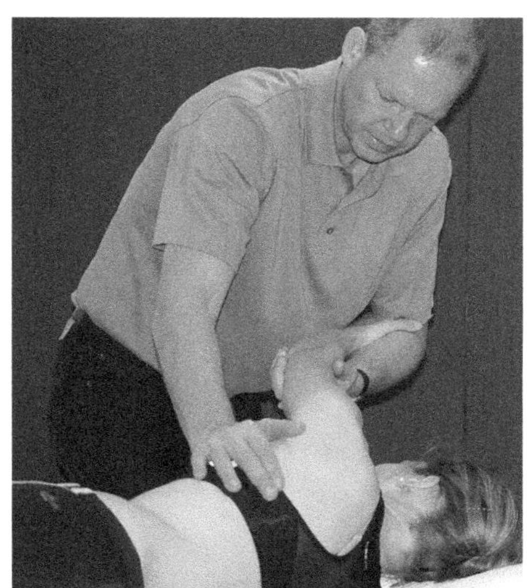

Figure 32.6 Evaluation of scapular upward rotation in glenohumeral elevation.

Evaluation in four-point kneeling

Four-point kneeling, although not particularly functional in itself, is useful for assessing patients' dissociation and control capabilities. The evaluation steps can also be applied in prone position on the elbows, or modified plantigrade (i.e. standing with hands supported on table or wall) with the aim of identifying where the patient has control and where that control is lost, thereby providing an effective starting position for retraining. Positional and movement impairments of the scapula and humerus are observed and loss of control / position from either identified as the limiting factor.

Steps in the evaluation include:

- observation of spontaneous posture and muscular endurance with a sustained hold
- scapular and glenohumeral control during weight shift from one arm to the other (Fig. 32.7)
- dissociation (the ability to isolate movement of one body part from another) of different regions of the spine and between spine and scapula (Fig. 32.8)
- control of scapular and cervical movements
- endurance of pro / retraction while weight-bearing on one or both hands and with trunk movement on a fixed hand.

All components can be progressed to more challenging situations, such as with the trunk on a gym ball or hand on an unstable surface, as appropriate for the patient. More detailed description of these tests can be found in Magarey and Jones (2003a). In addition, Ellenbecker and Cools (2010) have provided an excellent summary of recent research related to evaluation of scapular muscle function, which is further discussed in the report of the recent scapular summit (Kibler et al 2013). Readers are encouraged to review these papers for further suggestions.

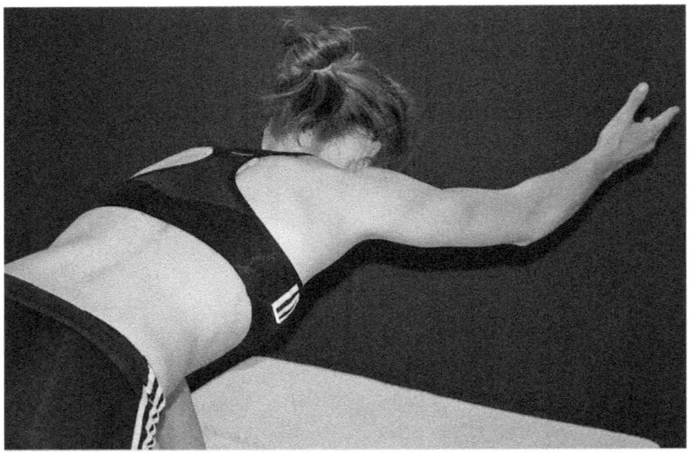

Figure 32.7 Evaluation in four point kneeling. Scapular and glenohumeral control in a single arm loaded position.

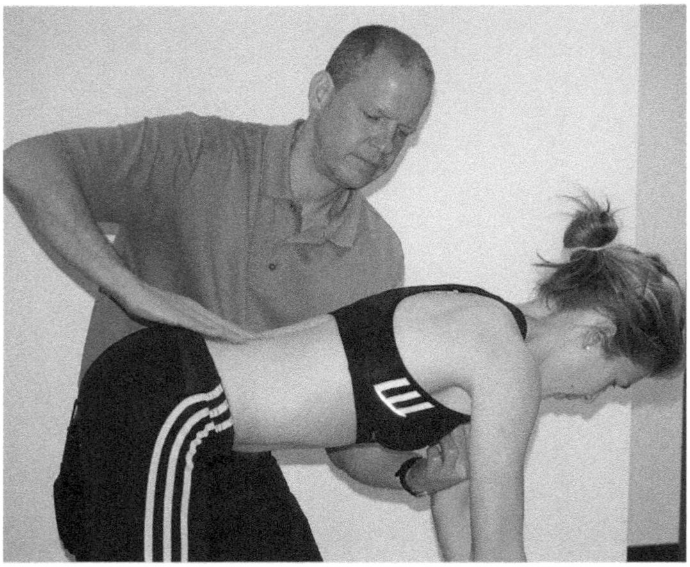

Figure 32.8 Dissociation evaluation in four-point kneeling. Scapular protraction in a spinal neutral position.

Evaluation of thoracic extension and control of scapular retraction

The patient's ability to perform thoracic extension in a relatively segmental fashion provides an indication of the priority for its retraining during rehabilitation. One effective evaluation is facilitated intersegmental extension from C7 to T7 / T8 over a gym ball, the patient's trunk remaining in contact with the ball to reduce the lumbar spine contribution. Once relative segmental thoracic extension is achieved, assessment is progressed by addition of scapular retraction and arm movements.

Evaluation of isolated motor control around the shoulder

Dynamic rotary stability test (Magarey & Jones 2003a, 2003b)

The DRST is used to evaluate the rotator cuff's ability to maintain the humeral head centred in the glenoid when loaded through rotation. The DRST is predicated on the knowledge that the humeral head should remain centred in the glenoid throughout the range of rotation in any position of elevation, except at end range, where coupled translation forces the humeral head to translate (Harryman et al 1990; Terry et al 1991). When dynamic control is lacking, the humeral head is felt to translate anteriorly, posteriorly or superiorly when the rotator cuff is loaded. In more subtle situations, any symptom provocation, alteration in the contraction quality or compensation elsewhere alerts the examiner to dysfunction without the sensation of humeral head translation. The patient's subjective sensation of 'stability' during testing is also informative.

The DRST is undertaken in different parts of the elevation range starting from neutral and progressing towards the patient's symptomatic functional position(s) (Fig. 32.9A–B). The number of positions in which the test is performed depends on the irritability of the condition, the general physical status of the patient, the clarity with which the patient can identify the symptomatic position(s) and the demands placed on the shoulder by the patient. The aim is to find the position(s) in range where the patient has humeral head control as close as possible to the position at which control is lost when an isometric and progressively challenging dynamic load is applied to the arm. The amount of resistance added is light / moderate, as the assessment is of the ability to stabilize, rather than of rotation strength. All movements are performed in one direction first rather than alternately, as patients find this easier. If lack of control is identified, rehabilitation can be undertaken starting from positions of control to facilitate activation of the rotator cuff and then progressing to more

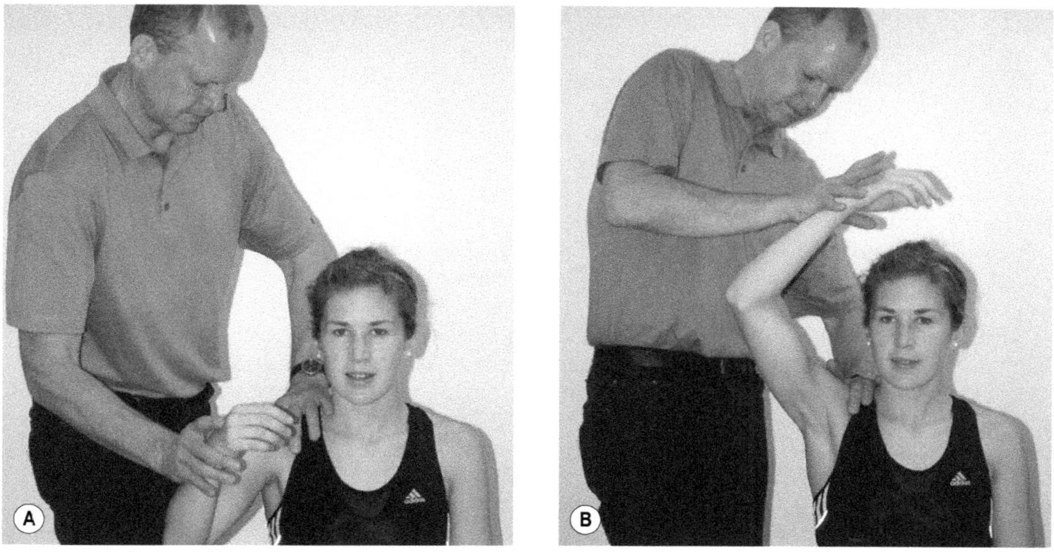

Figure 32.9 **Dynamic rotary stability test:** (**A**) evaluation of humeral head movement during isometric rotation in low range of elevation, (**B**) evaluation of humeral head movement during isometric rotation in high range of elevation. (From Magarey & Jones 2003a, 2003b.)

challenging positions. More detailed description of this test may be found in Magarey and Jones (2003b).

Dynamic relocation test (Magarey & Jones 2003a, 2003b)

The DRT is a test of the ability of the rotator cuff, particularly the lower elements, to stabilize the humeral head in the glenoid by means of co-contraction against a destabilizing load. Once the ability to isolate the co-contraction has been determined in an optimal position, it can be evaluated in different positions and during different tasks. If a patient is unable to achieve more than the very basic levels of the DRST, assessment should start with the DRT. The principles of testing are similar to those for the craniocervical flexion test (Jull et al 2008) and transversus abdominis activation (Hodges 2004).

Patient education about test performance is important as it is an unfamiliar task. Use of diagrams and / or anatomical models / apps is helpful so that the patient understands that the movement required is one of a subtle 'drawing in' of the humeral head to the glenoid via co-contraction of the infraspinatus / teres minor and lower subscapularis with minimal involvement of the superficial muscles, in response to a gentle longitudinal movement applied to the arm (Fig. 32.10). Occasionally, a patient's ability to co-contract is enhanced in a loaded, closed kinetic chain position. More detailed description of this test may be found in Magarey and Jones (2003b).

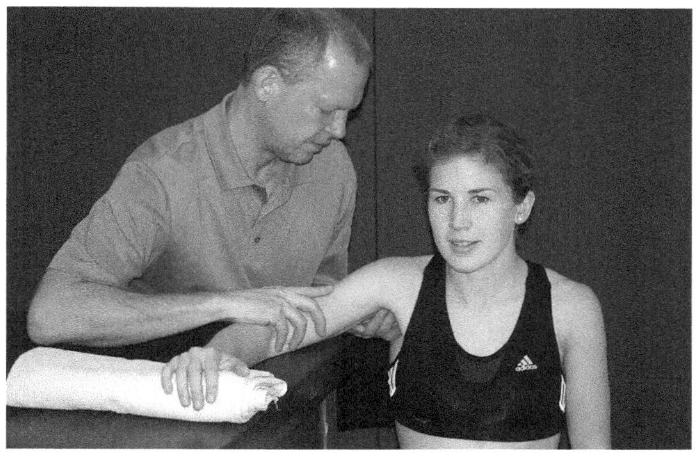

Figure 32.10 **Dynamic relocation test.** (From Magarey & Jones 2003a, 2003b.)

Management of Motor Control Impairments around the Shoulder Girdle

Motor learning refers to the acquisition or modification of movement (Shumway-Cook & Woollcott 2012). This process has been demonstrated in both sensory and motor areas of the human cortex as a result of manipulation of practice or experience (Boniface & Ziemann 2003). The physiological processes of motor learning are distributed throughout many different brain structures involving multiple processing levels. The neural modifiability can be seen as a continuum from short-term to long-term changes that lead to the (re) acquisition of relatively permanent movement capability (Schmidt & Lee 2005; Shumway-Cook & Woollcott 2012). Rehabilitation strategies should be tailored to the individual's specific neuromuscular impairments and motor control capabilities, which may vary in different body segments and over different tasks, together with consideration of their goals and any potential psychosocial issues that may increase the brain's threat appraisal (Latremoliere & Woolf 2009; Hodges 2011).

Although the Fitts and Posner (1967) (cognitive, associative, autonomous) model of motor learning is perhaps more familiar, Vereijken et al (1992) described another three-stage (novice, advanced, expert) theory of motor learning that accounts for reductions in body degrees of freedom seen in child development and new skill acquisition in general. Given that much research around disruptions to motor control relates to freezing of degrees of freedom (Cowan et al 2001, 2002, 2003; Hodges 2004; Colné & Thoumie 2006; Hertel &

Olmsted-Kramer 2007; Jull et al 2008; Hodges et al 2009), we feel that this model complements and adds to the useful model of Fitts and Posner (1967). The novice stage involves the learner freezing degrees of freedom by co-contracting agonists and antagonists to constrain a joint so as to simplify the movement, as with the rigid bracing of the wrist when first learning to use a hammer. Degrees of freedom are progressively released through the advanced and expert stages, thus enabling movement at more joints and more sophisticated muscle synergies across multiple joints until smooth, coordinated movements are performed. This theory offers a rationale for the clinical effectiveness of strategic posturing and external support that is commonly used in early stages of rehabilitation, such as retraining the co-contraction of the lower subscapularis and infraspinatus / teres minor with the arm initially supported in a stabilized scapular and glenohumeral neutral position. Decreasing the degrees of freedom required at the scapula through external support of the table and neutral positioning simplifies the task, allowing the patient to focus on the correct activation.

Shoulder complex rehabilitation exercises should be individualized to specific impairments identified from the examination as potentially contributing to the patient's activity (e.g. shoulder elevation or throwing) (as described in Case Report 1) and participation limitations (e.g. in activities of daily living or sport) (as described in Case Report 2) (Graichen et al 2001; Hébert et al 2002; Roy et al 2008). The focus in relation to motor learning theory and research in this chapter is limited to retraining of skills with which patients are already familiar, rather than learning new skills. Although this focus implies commencing with the associative / advanced stage of motor skill development, pre-existing impairments in posture and movement patterns commonly require that attention be given to the cognitive / novice stage to ensure understanding and correct performance (e.g. retraining shoulder elevation with less scapular protraction). Such impairments are commonly the result of short-term motor adaptations that can occur post injury and, if maintained, may compromise the quality of movement, decrease the variability of movement and increase the load on specific structures / tissues (Hodges 2011). Awareness training is generally started in neutral positions, whereas control training is commenced from neutral or a position close to the position of impairment where the action / hold can be performed correctly.

Patients' understanding and motivation, goal setting, quality practice, repetition and feedback (Monfils et al 2005; Schmidt & Lee 2005; Sousa 2006; Kleim & Jones 2008; Shumway-Cook & Woollacott 2012) all facilitate motor learning. Understanding, where explanations are meaningful to the individual, enhances patient motivation, attention and learning. The more thoroughly the information is processed, the deeper is the learning and more likely the transfer to new situations outside the therapeutic setting (Sousa 2006). Explanations of assessment findings and management recommendations, linked to research and successful clinical outcomes, use of anatomical pictures, models and apps, and opportunities to ask questions and summarize main points all promote deeper learning.

Goal setting also facilitates motivation and learning. Specific, absolute goals of moderate difficulty produce better performance than either vague (e.g. 'do your best') (Kyllo & Landers 1995; Schmidt & Lee 2005) or no goals. Specific goals, both short and long term, assist patient focus and facilitate performance while providing a reference for monitoring progress (Kyllo & Landers 1995).

Practice is recognized as the single most important variable influencing learning, with changes occurring rapidly (within 15 minutes) and continuing to evolve with extended training (Schmidt & Lee 2005; Boudreau et al 2010b; Shumway-Cook & Woollacott 2012). Whereas synaptic connections are strengthened through experience, complexity of task, variability, level of attention and repetition (Spitzer 1999; Perez et al 2004; Boudreau et al 2010b), success during exercise enhances learning; this necessitates the choosing of exercises that can be successfully achieved with good kinematic control and no symptom aggravation (Hodges 2011). Motor adaptations need to continue beyond the resolution of pain and therefore, to restore optimal control, interventions must continue to incorporate the above strategies that target higher levels of processing (Hodges & Tucker 2011).

Augmented feedback regarding performance of a movement or exercise is considered to be critical to motor learning, second only to practice itself (Schmidt & Lee 2005; Hodges & Tucker 2011). Performance feedback can be provided visually, as with video, real-time ultrasound, through EMG-based biofeedback, through tactile reinforcement or verbally, typically highlighting some aspect of the movement pattern that is difficult to perceive (e.g. recognition of spinal posture / movement during shoulder elevation). Inherent feedback refers to sensory information directly available to the individual during or resulting from the execution of a movement. Understanding when control is lost is essential for home motor control exercises to ensure that exercises are not continued past this point, which would potentially reinforce incorrect movement patterns. For example, although patients cannot see the loss of scapular control, by drawing their attention to their scapula the therapist can teach them to recognize the local sensation associated with control and loss of control; they thereby learn to continue the exercise only to the point where that sensation occurs. Use of facilitatory taping with a product such as Dynamic Tape® (www.dynamictape.com) can enhance learning of new scapular motor patterns.

Management of shoulder motor control through patient examples

Two patient case studies are presented below as examples of implementation of the suggestions above and to highlight clinical reasoning and implementation of motor learning principles.

Case Report 1

Tom – baseball player with shoulder pain

Tom was a 19-year-old left-hand-dominant elite baseball player with painful shoulder with throwing. He presented with deep, moderately severe superior shoulder pain associated primarily with the late cocking phase of a throw. The onset was gradual through the previous baseball season and he was keen to address it in the off-season. There were no red flag issues to consider, no apparent frank rotator cuff or labral pathology, cervical or neurodynamic involvement.

Tom had a good range of movement but poor awareness of dissociation of different regions of his spine and between the spine and scapula, leading to poor ability to stabilize the scapula or arm. He stood with poor spinal posture, particularly thoracic kyphosis and a forward head posture. Active assisted correction was possible but could not be maintained. His scapula was downwardly rotated and anteriorly tilted (type I / III dyskinesis combined) (Kibler et al 2002) so that his arm hung in medial rotation. His ability to dissociate in four-point kneeling was inadequate as he was unable to sustain good scapular position without fatigue-related compensations. Increased 'give' to resistance on the lateral scapular border was evident on upward rotation to his unaffected side. A DRST demonstrated poor isometric control of his humeral head in 110° scapular elevation with both rotations, the position relevant to his throwing, and at 90° with slow isotonic rotations. With facilitation, Tom was able to achieve good contraction and control in neutral with the DRT.

Tom's management consisted of education about the relevance of his postural and movement impairments to his throwing pain, followed by spinal and scapular postural correction and dissociation training in both sitting and four-point kneeling, which was later progressed to standing and positions relevant for throwing. Retraining of the upward rotation of his scapula, with hands-on facilitation / feedback, was followed by a home programme ensuring the maintenance of a neutral spine, glenohumeral external rotation and elbow extension as he drove forwards through his hands (Fig. 32.11). As Tom improved, the training was progressed to closed kinetic chain activities such as a slide board in four-point kneeling and push-up position, concentric and eccentric load, always focusing on good positioning.

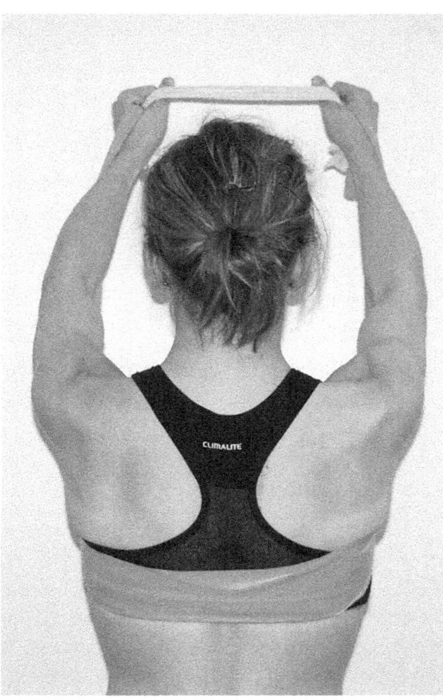

Figure 32.11 Home exercise for retraining scapular upward rotation.

Isolation training for glenohumeral stabilization was not warranted as Tom was able to learn the technique quickly and integrate it into the DRST, to which training was directed immediately close to positions of lost control, both isometrically and isotonically, and stopping when he felt humeral head translation or lost control of his scapular position – both of which required explicit sensory recognition training for him to recognize. Over time, he increased the speed and range of movement, as required for throwing, and later increased the load.

Attention to Tom's throwing technique and the rest of his kinetic chain was an integral part of his management, with strengthening and skill training built around dynamic control. If any given strengthening exercise resulted in loss of control, the task was judged too challenging and modified in position or load. For each task, frequent practice in as many different environments as practical was encouraged to facilitate motor learning (Schmidt & Lee 2005). Based on research by Boudreau et al (2010b), changes in cortical plasticity have been shown to occur over short intervals (60 within-session task repetitions over a period of 10–15 minutes). If Tom was not able to maintain control over any parameters of a specific task, the achievement of these was set as a short-term goal. Once achieved, these parameters were then progressively made more challenging with lengths of hold, sequence of movements, complexity of tasks, load, repetitions and other cognitively distracting tasks added to challenge the neuromuscular system further.

Tom was provided with thoracic extension facilitation training over the gym ball, learning intersegmental thoracic extension and then loaded endurance exercises into extension. As a result of the postural training and maintenance of good cervical posture throughout these exercises, inclusion of formal craniocervical flexor training was not necessary. Later progressions were added to challenge his spinal control and endurance further in conjunction with arm movements.

The need to lose co-contraction is part of the autonomous / expert stage of learning associated with skilled activity (Shumway-Cook & Woollacott 2012) such that the task becomes a feed-forward mechanism not a feedback one. As Tom's control of the DRST position improved and he returned to throwing, it is likely that he lost the majority of the co-contraction included while refining his technique. Loss of co-contraction in skilled pitchers (Glousman et al 1988) and elite swimmers (Carr et al 1998) compared with untrained controls supports the need to increase degrees of freedom with development of skill (Vereijken et al 1992). However, intermittent but regular co-contraction training is recommended, as clinical experience demonstrates a tendency to lose this ability with the potential to lead to higher risk of injury. Such control is still required for activities requiring high degrees of accuracy (Gribble et al 2003).

Case Report 2

Joan – office worker with full-thickness rotator cuff tear

Joan was a 59-year-old right-hand-dominant office worker with MRI-confirmed full-thickness rotator cuff tear involving the supraspinatus and a small portion of the infraspinatus, coupled with a thickened swollen subacromial bursa. She presented with sharp severe left subacromial pain on quick movements, an inability to raise her arm above 90° elevation because 'it won't go' and difficulty in sleeping because of pain. Three weeks previously, her dog had pulled suddenly on the leash and she felt something 'give' in her shoulder. Joan had a history of 'nuisance value' discomfort in her shoulder and neck pain with prolonged computer use. She had difficulty with hand-behind-back activities, brushing her hair and reaching to the top cupboard because of painful limitation of movement. However, the pain settled quickly. There were no neurological symptoms, vertebrobasilar insufficiency issues or red flags. As a result of painful restricted range, Joan's motor control assessment was limited.

Joan's key postural impairments included increased thoracic kyphosis, a forward head posture, elevation of her left acromion compared with the right, apparent increased tone in both the levator scapulae and upper trapezius, and wasting of the supraspinatus. Correction of spinal posture was impossible owing to low cervical / upper thoracic stiffness on extension. Active shoulder elevation of 80° led to immediate humeral superior translation and scapular elevation, while assistance to scapular upward rotation gained a further 30° before pain increased. Pain and weakness prevented Joan from holding this position.

Joan's movement awareness on scapular PNF patterns was poor, even with facilitation. DRT was taught initially on her right shoulder where she could activate the rotator cuff well; however, she had great difficulty in the left shoulder, and was eventually able to create only a weak pain-free co-contraction, sustained for 3–4 seconds.

Joan's rotator cuff tear was not large but extended into the infraspinatus, such that it disrupted the biomechanics of the shoulder (Burkhart 1996). Therefore, the lower rotator cuff force couple was unable to control superior humeral migration during active elevation. The motor control approach required focusing on the scapula and rotator cuff concurrently as the movement impairment was so closely linked. Joan's accessory movement of the lower cervical and upper thoracic spine revealed significant stiffness, which also contributed to her loss of shoulder elevation.

The priorities for Joan's treatment were very different to those for Tom. Isolated rotator cuff training with the dynamic relocation manoeuvre was appropriate in conjunction with retraining scapular movement patterns. Passive mobilization and mobility exercises improved her spinal range, following which awareness and intersegmental control were facilitated with training. Joan's poor cervical posture and previous cervical pain meant that craniocervical flexor evaluation and training were appropriate and integrated (Jull et al 2008).

Scapular PNF patterns were used to facilitate improved scapular awareness and movement. Tactile and verbal stimulation of correct movement was complemented with a home programme (Fig. 32.12).

Dynamic relocation training was initiated in a pain-free neutral position, and she gradually built up her capacity to 10 sets of 10-second holds of good-quality contraction.

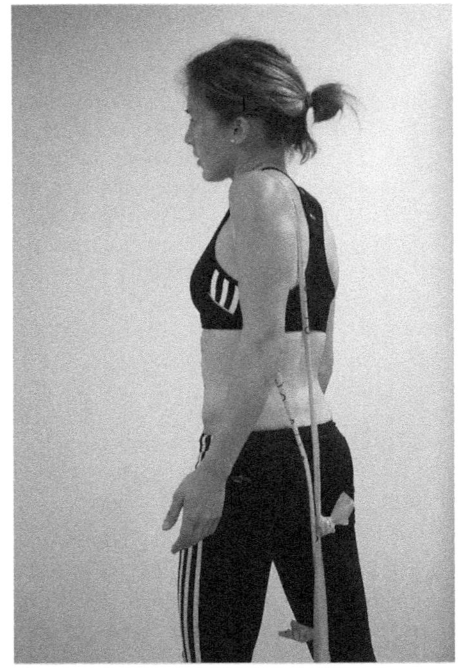

Figure 32.12 Home exercise for retraining scapular movement awareness in the PNF pattern of 'up & forward'.

Training was then progressed into increased ranges of elevation, always with the arm supported and pain free. Only when Joan could perform 10 sets of 10 holds in each position was she progressed to taking the weight of her arm. Gradually, she was able to support her arm in each training position and could start to work into functional positions through elevation with controlled scapulohumeral and glenohumeral movement. To optimize improvements in performance, it is vital that control is trained with skilled, precise tasks prior to re-integration of higher load exercises (Remple et al 2001; Boudreau et al 2010b).

Once Joan could perform the PNF patterns well, side-lying scapular upward rotation training was instigated in the increased range available, initially with no load through the arm, then later adding a protraction load but upward rotation stimulus only to the lateral scapular border, with progression focused on increased elevation range rather than load, again with an associated home programme.

Concurrently, Joan worked with a series of scapular retraining exercises focused on facilitating lower trapezius / lower serratus anterior activity while reducing activation of the upper trapezius muscle (Kibler et al 2008). 'Low row' and 'lawn mower' exercises could be performed pain free without loss of scapular or humeral head control quite early in the programme.

Tom's problems were largely a result of poor movement awareness and technique combined with inadequate postural awareness, endurance and explosive power for throwing. Joan's poor movement patterns, however, were much more entrenched and associated with spinal stiffness, pathology within the tissues and provocation of pain. Reduction in pain and increase in range probably resulted at least in part from improved spinal and shoulder girdle movement patterns plus reduced superior humeral translation, reducing the compressive force through the irritated subacromial bursa. As a result of her initial poor ability to control the humeral head position, isolation training of the rotator cuff was warranted, combined with progressive scapular training. Progression was slow for Joan, whereas for Tom it was quick.

The training programmes chosen incorporated exercises from or were similar to those recommended by Cools et al (2007b) and Kibler et al (2006, 2008). While not exhaustive, this approach to management of poor motor control is effective and applicable across a range of presentations of patients with shoulder pain.

Conclusion

Our approach to motor control evaluation and management has not been validated in formal research but is based on strong evidence, sound clinical reasoning and experience. Although we readily acknowledge that motor control retraining extends beyond regaining control of the neutral zone, for the purposes of this chapter the main focus has been on the early stages as progressive loading is covered in Chapter 33. Building more functional retraining on the basis of sound motor control enhances the benefits of more advanced training and improves chances of successful management.

References

Bagg SD, Forrest WJ. 1986. Electromyographic study of the scapular rotators during arm abduction in the scapular plane. Am J Phys Med Rehabil 65: 111–124.

Bagg SD, Forrest WJ. 1988. A biomechanical analysis of scapular rotation during arm abduction in the scapular plane. Am J Phys Med Rehabil 67: 238–245.

Boniface SJ, Ziemann U. 2003. Plasticity in the human nervous system: investigations with transcranial magnetic stimulation. New York: Cambridge University Press.

Boudreau SA, Farina D, Falla D. 2010a. The role of motor learning and neuroplasticity in designing rehabilitation approaches for musculoskeletal pain disorders. Man Ther 15: 410–414.

Boudreau SA, Hennings K, Svensson P, et al. 2010b. The effects of training time, sensory loss and pain on human motor learning. J Oral Rehabil 37: 704–718.

Bullock MP, Foster NE, Wright CC. 2005. Shoulder impingement: the effect of sitting posture on shoulder pain and range of motion. Man Ther 10: 28–37.

Burkhart SS. 1996. A unified biomechanical rationale for the treatment of rotator cuff tears: debridement versus repair. In: Burkhead WZ (ed) Rotator cuff disorders. Baltimore: Williams & Wilkins, pp 293–312.

Burkhart SS, Morgan C, Kibler WB. 2003. The disabled throwing shoulder: spectrum of pathology. Part III: The SICK scapula, scapular dyskinesis, the kinetic chain, and rehabilitation. Arthroscopy 19: 641–661.

Carr A, David G, Magarey ME, et al. 1998. Rotator cuff muscle performances during glenohumeral joint rotations: an isokinetic and electromyographic study of freestyle swimmers. Proceedings, Australian Conference of Science & Medicine in Sport, 13–16 October, Adelaide. Online. Abstract available: http://fulltext.ausport.gov.au/fulltext/1998/acsm/smabs084.htm.

Cholewicki J, McGill SM. 1996. Mechanical stability of the in vivo lumbar spine: implications for injury and chronic low back pain. Clin Biomech 11: 1–15.

Clark JC, Harryman DT. 1992. Tendons, ligaments and capsule of the rotator cuff. J Bone Joint Surg 74A: 5713–5725.

Colné P, Thoumie P. 2006. Muscular compensation and lesion of the anterior cruciate ligament: contribution of the soleus muscle during recovery from a forward fall. Clin Biomech 21: 849–859.

Cools AM, Witvrouw EE, Declercq GA, et al. 2002. Scapular muscle recruitment pattern: electromyographic response of the trapezius muscle to sudden shoulder movement before and after a fatiguing exercise. J Orthop Sports Phys Ther 32: 222–229.

Cools AM, Witvrouw EE, Declercq GA, et al. 2003. Scapular muscle recruitment patterns: trapezius muscle latency with and without impingement symptoms. Am J Sports Med 31: 542.

Cools AM, Witvrouw EE, Declercq GA, et al. 2004. Evaluation of isokinetic force production and associated muscular activity in the scapular rotators during a protraction–retraction movement in overhead athletes with impingement symptoms. Br J Sports Med 38: 64–68.

Cools AM, Witvrouw EE, Maheu NN, et al. 2005. Isokinetic scapular muscle performance in overhead athletes with and without impingement symptoms. J Athletic Train 40: 104–110.

Cools AM, Declearcq GA, Cambier DC, et al. 2007a. Trapezius activity and intramuscular balance during isokinetic exercise in overhead athletes with impingement symptoms. Scand J Med Sci Sports 17: 25–33.

Cools AM, Dewitte V, Lanszweert F, et al. 2007b. Rehabilitation of scapular muscle balance: which exercises to prescribe? Am J Sports Med 35: 1744–1751.

Cools AM, Cambier D, Witvrouw EE. 2008. Screening the athlete's shoulder for impingement symptoms: a clinical reasoning algorithm for early detection of shoulder pathology. Br J Sports Med 42: 628–635.

Cowan SM, Bennell KL, Hodges PW, et al. 2001. Delayed onset of electromyographic activity of vastus medialis obliquus relative to vastus lateralis in subjects with patellofemoral pain syndrome. Arch Phys Med Rehabil 82: 183–189.

Cowan SM, Hodges PW, Bennell KL, et al. 2002. Altered vastii recruitment when people with patelloremoral pain syndrome complete a postural task. Arch Phys Med Rehabil 83: 989–995.

Cowan SM, Bennell KL, Hodges PW, et al. 2003. Simultaneous feedforward recruitment of the vasti in untrained postural tasks can be restored by physical therapy. J Orthop Res 21: 553–558.

Crawford HJ, Jull GA. 1993. The influence of thoracic range and posture on range of arm elevation. Physiother Theor Pract 9: 143–148.

David G, Magarey M, Jones M, et al. 2000. EMG and strength correlates of selected shoulder muscles during rotations of the glenohumeral joint. Clin Biomech 15: 95–102.

Drake R, Vogl AW, Mitchell AWM. 2009. Gray's anatomy for students, 2nd edn. Philadelphia: Churchill Livingstone.

Ebaugh DD, McClure PW, Karduna A. 2005. Three dimensional scapulothoracic motion during active and passive arm elevation. Clin Biomech 20: 700–709.

Ellenbecker TS, Cools A. 2010. Rehabilitation of shoulder impingement syndrome and rotator cuff injuries: an evidence-based review. Br J Sports Med 44: 319–327.

Falla D. 2004. Unravelling the complexity of muscle impairment in chronic neck pain. Man Ther 9: 125–133.

Falla D, Farina D, Graven-Neilsen T. 2007. Experimental muscle pain results in reorganization of coordination among trapezius muscle subdivisions during repetitive shoulder flexion. Exp Brain Res 178: 385–393.

Fitts PM, Posner MI. 1967. Human performance. Belmont CA: Brooks/Cole.

Ginn K, Boetcher C, Cathers I. 2009. Are rotator cuff muscles functioning to stabilise the shoulder joint during isometric flexion, extension and rotation contractions. Proceedings, Sports Physiotherapy Australia Conference, Sydney Australia.

Glousman R, Jobe F, Tibone J, et al. 1988. Dynamic electromyographic analysis of the throwing shoulder with glenohumeral instability. J Bone Joint Surg 70A: 220–226.

Graichen H, Stammberger T, Bonkl H, et al. 2001. Three-dimensional analysis of shoulder girdle and supraspinatus motion patterns in patients with impingement syndrome. J Orthop Res 19: 1192–1198.

Greenfield B, Catlin PA, Coats PW, et al. 1995. Posture in patients with shoulder overuse injuries and healthy individuals. J Orthop Sports Phys Ther 21: 287–295.

Gribble PL, Mullin LI, Cothros N, et al. 2003. Role of co-contraction in arm movement accuracy. J Neurophysiol 89: 2396–2405.

Harryman DT, Sidles JA, Matsen FA. 1990. The humeral head translates on the glenoid with passive motion. In: Post M, Morrey BF, Hawkins RJ (eds) Surgery of the shoulder. St Louis, MO: Mosby Year Book, p 186.

Hébert LJ, Moffet H, McFadyen BJ, et al. 2002. Scapular behaviour in shoulder impingement syndrome. Arch Phys Med Rehabil 83: 60–69.

Hertel J, Olmsted-Kramer LC. 2007. Deficits of time-to-boundary measures of postural control with chronic ankle instability. Gait Posture 25: 33–39s.

Hess SA, Richardson C, Darnell R, et al. 2005. Timing of rotator cuff activity during shoulder external rotation in throwers with and without shoulder pain. J Orthop Sports Phys Ther 35: 812–820.

Hodges PW. 2004. Lumbopelvic stability: a functional model of the biomechanics and motor control. In: Richardson C, Hodges PW, Hides J (eds) Therapeutic exercise for lumbo-pelvic stabilization. A motor control approach for the treatment and prevention of low back pain. Edinburgh: Churchill Livingstone, pp 13–28.

Hodges PW. 2011. Pain and motor control: from the laboratory to rehabilitation. J Electromyogr Kinesiol 21: 220–228.

Hodges PW, Tucker K. 2011. Moving differently in pain: a new theory to explain the adaptation to pain. Pain 152: S90–S98.

Hodges P, Van HW, Dawson A, et al. 2009. Changes in the mechanical properties of the trunk in low back pain may be associated with recurrence. J Biomech 42: 61–66.

Jull GA, Sterling M, Falla D, et al. 2008. Whiplash, headache and neck pain. Edinburgh: Churchill Livingstone, Elsevier.

Kasper JC, Itamura JM, Tibone JE, et al. 2008. Human cadaveric study of subscapularis muscle innervation and guidelines to prevent denervation. J Shoulder Elbow Surg 17: 659–662.

Kibler WB. 1998. The role of the scapula in athletic shoulder function. Am J Sports Med 26: 325–337.

Kibler WB. 2003. Management of the scapula in glenohumeral instability. Techniques Shoulder Elbow Surg 4(3): 89–98.

Kibler WB, McMullen J. 2003. Scapular dyskinesis and its relation to shoulder pain. J Am Acad Orthop Surg 11: 142–151.

Kibler WB, Uhl TL, Maddux JW, et al. 2002. Qualitative clinical evaluation of scapular dysfunction: a reliability study. J Shoulder Elbow Surg 11: 550–556.

Kibler WB, Sciascia A, Dome D. 2006. Evaluation of apparent and absolute supraspinatus strength in patients with shoulder injury using the scapular retraction test. Am J Sports Med 34: 1643–1647.

Kibler WB, Sciascia AD, Uhl TL, et al. 2008. Electromyographic analysis of specific exercises for scapular control in early phases of shoulder rehabilitation. Am J Sports Med 36: 1789–1798.

Kibler WB, Ludewig PM, McClure PW, et al. 2013. Clinical implications of scapular dyskinesis in shoulder injury: the 2013 consensus statement from the scapular summit. Br J Sports Med 47: 877–885.

Kleim JA, Jones TA. 2008. Principles of experience-dependent neural plasticity: implications for rehabilitation after brain damage. J Speech Lang Hear Res 51: S225–S239.

Kofler M, Glocker FX, Leis AA, et al. 1998. Modulation of upper extremity motoneurone excitability following noxious finger tip stimulation in man: a study with transcranial magnetic stimulation. Neurosci Lett 246: 97–100.

Kyllo LB, Landers DM. 1995. Goal setting in sport and exercise: a research synthesis to resolve the controversy. J Sport Exercise Psychol 17: 117–177.

Latremoliere A, Woolf CJ. 2009. Central sensitization: a generator of pain hypersensitivity by central neural plasticity. J Pain 10: 895–926.

Lee BS-B, Kim K-J, O'Driscoll SW, et al. 2000. Dynamic glenohumeral stability provided by the rotator cuff muscles in the mid-range and end-range of motion. J Bone Joint Surg 82A: 849–857.

Lewis JS, Green A, Wright C. 2005a. Sub-acromial impingement syndrome: the role of posture and muscle balance. J Shoulder Elbow Surg 14: 385–392.

Lewis JS, Wright C, Green A. 2005b. Sub-acromial impingement syndrome: the effect of changing posture on shoulder range of movement. J Orthop Sports Phys Ther 35: 72–87.

Ludewig PM, Cook TM. 1996. The effect of head position on scapular orientation and muscle activity during shoulder elevation. J Occup Rehabil 6: 147–158.

Ludewig PM, Cook TM. 2000. Alterations in shoulder kinematics and associated muscle activity in people with symptoms of shoulder impingement. Phys Ther 80: 276–291.

Magarey ME, Jones MA. 2003a. Dynamic evaluation and early management of altered motor control around the shoulder complex. Man Ther 8: 195–206.

Magarey ME, Jones MA. 2003b. Specific evaluation of the function of force couples relevant for the stabilization of the glenohumeral joint. Man Ther 8: 247–253.

Magee DJ, Zachazewski JE. 2007. Principles of stabilization training. In: Magee DJ, Zachazewski JE, Quillen WS (eds) Scientific foundations and principles of practice in musculoskeletal rehabilitation. St Louis, MO: Saunders, Elsevier, pp 388–431.

McClure PW, Michener LA, Sennett BJ, et al. 2001. Direct 3-dimensional measurement of scapular kinematics during dynamic movements in vivo. J Shoulder Elbow Surg 10: 269–277.

McClure PW, Michener LA, Karduna AR. 2006. Shoulder function and 3-dimensional scapular kinematics in people with and without shoulder impingement syndrome. Phys Ther 86: 1075–1090.

McGill S, 2007. Low back disorders. Evidence-based prevention and rehabilitation. Champaign, IL: Human Kinetics.

Monfils M-H, Plautz EJ, Kleim JA. 2005. In search of the motor engram: motor map plasticity as a mechanism for encoding motor experience. Neuroscientist 11: 471–483.

Moraes GFS, Faria CDCM, Teixeira-Salmela LF. 2008. Scapular muscle recruitment patterns and isokinetic strength ratios of the shoulder rotator muscles in individuals with and without impingement syndrome. J Shoulder Elbow Surgery 17: 48S–53S.

Morag Y, Jamadar DA, Miller B, et al. 2011. The subscapularis: anatomy, injury and imaging. Skeletal Radiol 40: 255–269.

Nederhand NJ, Hermens HJ, Ijzman MJ, et al. 2000. Cervical muscle dysfunction in chronic whiplash-associated disorder grade 2: the relevance of the trauma. Spine 27: 1056–1061.

Panjabi MM. 1992a. The stabilizing system of the spine. Part I: function, dysfunction, adaptation and enhancement. J Spinal Dis 5: 383–389.

Panjabi MM. 1992b. The stabilizing system of the spine. Part II: neutral zone and instability hypothesis. J Spinal Dis 5: 390–396.

Panjabi MM. 1996. Low back pain and spinal instability. In: Weinstein JN, Gordon SL (eds) Low back pain: a scientific and clinical overview. Rosemont, IL: American Academy of Orthopaedic Surgeons, pp 367–384.

Perez MA, Lungholt KS, Nyborg K, et al. 2004. Motor skill training induces changes in the excitability of the leg cortical area in healthy humans. Exp Brain Res 159: 197–205.

Pink M, Jobe FW, Perry J, et al. 1993. The painful shoulder during butterfly swimming. An electromyographic and cinematico-graphic analysis of 12 muscles. Clin Orthop Relat Res 288: 60–72.

Remple MS, Bruneau RM, Vandenberg PM, et al. 2001. Sensitivity of cortical movement representations to motor experience: evidence that skill learning but not strength training induces cortical reorganization. Behavioural Brain Res 123: 133–141.

Roberts PD. 2009. Movement analysis and training. [Educational lecture notes, MA Musculoskeletal and Sports Physiotherapy, University of South Australia.]

Roy JS, Moffet H, McFadyen BJ. 2008. Upper limb motor strategies in persons with and without shoulder impingement syndrome across different speeds of movement. Clin Biomech 23: 1227–1236.

Sahrmann S. 2002. Diagnosis and treatment of movement impairment disorders. St Louis, MO: Mosby.

Schmidt RAS, Lee TD. 2005. Motor control and learning: a behavioral emphasis. Champaign, IL: Human Kinetics.

Scovazzo ML, Browne A, Pink M, et al. 1991. The painful shoulder during freestyle swimming: an electromyographic and cinematographic analysis of 12 muscles. Am J Sports Med 6: 577–582.

Shumway-Cook A, Woollcott MH. 2012. Motor control: translating research into clinical practice. Philadelphia: Wolters Kluwer Health / Lippincott Willams & Wilkins.

Simons DG, Travell JG, Simons LS. 1999. Travell and Simon's myofascial pain and dysfunction: the trigger point manual, 2nd edn. Vol 2. Baltimore, MD: Williams & Wilkins

Sousa D. 2006. How the brain learns. Thousand Oaks, CA: Corwin Press, chs 2–4.

Spitzer M. 1999. Learning. In: Spitzer M. The mind within the net: models of learning, thinking and acting. Cambridge, MA: MIT Press, Ch 3, pp 39–63.

Sterling M, Jull G, Wright A. 2001. The effect of musculoskeletal pain on motor activity and control. J Pain 2: 135–145.

Szeto GPR, Straker L, O'Sullivan PB. 2005. A comparison of symptomatic and asymptomatic office workers performing monotonous keyboard work 2: neck and shoulder kinematics. Man Ther 10: 281–291.

Szeto GPR, Straker LM, O'Sullivan PB. 2009. Neck–shoulder muscle activity in general and task-specific resting postures of symptomatic computer users with chronic neck pain. Man Ther 14: 338–345.

Terry GC, Hammon D, France P, et al. 1991. The stabilizing function of passive shoulder restraints. Am J Sports Med 19: 26–34.

Tsao H, Galea MP, Hodges PW. 2010. Driving plasticity in the motor cortex in recurrent low back pain. Eur J Pain 14: 832–839.

Vereijken B, van Emmerik REA, Whiting HTA, et al. 1992. Free(z)ing degrees of freedom in skill acquisition. J Motor Behavior 24: 739–749.

Voss DE, Ionta MK, Myers BJ. 1985. Proprioceptive neuromuscular facilitation. Patterns and techniques, 3rd edn. Philadelphia: Harper & Row.

Wadsworth DJ, Bullock-Saxton JE. 1997. Recruitment patterns of the scapular–rotator muscle in freestyle swimmers with sub-acromial impingement. Int J Sports Med 18: 618–624.

Wuelker N, Roetman B, Roessig S. 1995. Coracoacromial pressure recordings in a cadaveric model. J Shoulder Elbow Surgery 4: 462–467.

Chapter 33

Therapeutic Exercises for the Shoulder Region

Johnson McEvoy, Kieran O'Sullivan, Carel Bron

CHAPTER CONTENTS

Introduction	373
Clinical background	373
Shoulder exercise: evidence	374
Principles of exercise	374
Posture	376
Stretching	376
Isometric exercise of the shoulder	378
Isotonic exercises of the shoulder	378
Supraspinatus muscle	379
Infraspinatus and teres minor muscles	379
Subscapularis muscle	380
Trapezius muscle	380
Serratus anterior muscle	381
Functional exercises	381
Conclusion	383

Introduction

Therapeutic exercise is a cornerstone of physiotherapy practice and was initially referred to as **medical gymnastics**. The development of medical gymnastics in physical therapy has had many diverse influences including Dr Francis Fuller, author of *Medicina gymnasticia* (1740), Swedish gymnast Per Henrik Ling (1776–1839) and the Dutch physical education teacher and physician Dr Johann Georg Mezger (1838–1909) (Barclay 1994; Terlouw 2007). More recently Kendall (2002) summed up the role of therapeutic exercise in physical therapy: 'Central to the practice of physical therapy is the prevention of movement dysfunction and the rehabilitation through restoration and maintenance of active movement – in other words, therapeutic exercise in its broadest sense'. The focus of this chapter is to introduce general principles of therapeutic exercise for the shoulder, and to stimulate clinical reasoning and rational rehabilitation. The chapter will briefly discuss posture, stretching and strengthening of a selection of muscles, without focusing on one specific clinical population.

Clinical Background

Essential to an understanding of therapeutic exercise is an in-depth knowledge of anatomy, physiology and function, specifically related to the neuromuscular and musculoskeletal systems (Kendall 2002). The shoulder is a complex functional system producing movement of the arm on the trunk and allowing the upper limb and hand to be dynamically moved and positioned for function. The shoulder consists of the scapula, clavicle and humerus, giving rise to the sternoclavicular, clavicular, humeral and scapulothoracic joints, and has a close relationship to the neck, thorax and ribs. The shoulder is supported by capsular, ligamentous and muscular systems with complex neuromuscular processing that offer a wide range of motion, but with a subsequent compromise in joint stability. This trade-off in stability makes the shoulder potentially vulnerable to dysfunction and injury, and stability is often the main focus of therapeutic exercise for the shoulder complex. Readers should refer to the appropriate chapters of this book and other texts for a comprehensive review of shoulder anatomy, biomechanics, kinesiology and pathomechanics (Donatelli 2004a; Oatis 2004). Further, knowledge of connective tissue properties, force applications, tissue injury (bone, ligament, tendon, muscle, fascia, nerve, etc.) and tissue-healing concepts and timelines (inflammation, proliferation, maturation) is an important precursor to the development of a suitable and safe therapeutic exercise programme (Tippet & Voight 1995; Paris & Loubert 1999; Houglum 2005).

Prior to the development of a rehabilitation programme for the shoulder complex a comprehensive assessment and physical examination should be performed with reference to the principles of physical therapy practice so as to ascertain pertinent information and physical characteristics of the individual patient. Indications for therapeutic exercise of the shoulder are listed in Box 33.1 and are diverse; they include specific and non-specific musculoskeletal, orthopaedic, surgical and neurological conditions and dysfunctions, and also postural and performance enhancement and injury prevention strategy.

Box 33.1 Indications for therapeutic shoulder exercises

- Glenohumeral joint lesions, dysfunctions and instability
- Rotator cuff lesions and dysfunctions
- Subacromial impingement syndrome
- Acromioclavicular joint lesions and dysfunctions
- Sternoclavicular joint lesions and dysfunctions
- Superior labrum anterior-to-posterior (SLAP) lesions
- Adhesive capsulitis (frozen shoulder)
- Arthropathies: arthrosis, arthritis, rheumatoid arthritis
- Post fracture and trauma
- Soft tissue injuries and syndromes
- Sports injuries
- Myofascial pain and dysfunction from trigger points
- Hypermobility syndromes
- Postural dysfunction
- Movement disorders
- Performance enhancement and performance optimization
- Injury prevention
- Post shoulder surgery and arthroscopy
- Shoulder replacement
- Thoracic surgery with shoulder involvement (e.g. mastectomy)
- Spinal cord injuries and nerve root syndromes
- Peripheral nerve injuries
- Central nervous system disorders (e.g. hemiplegia)

Shoulder Exercise: Evidence

A wide variety of shoulder disorders have demonstrated alterations in shoulder range of motion (Hall & Elvey 1999; Vermeulen et al 2002; McClure et al 2006), scapular kinematics (Lukasiewicz et al 1999; Ludewig & Cook 2000; McClure et al 2006; Roy et al 2009; Tate et al 2009), scapular and rotator cuff muscle activation (Ludewig & Cook 2000; Cools et al 2007; Moraes et al 2008; Myers et al 2009), humeral translation (Chen et al 1999; Ludewig & Cook 2002), repositioning sense (Naughton et al 2005) and shoulder strength (McClure et al 2006; Lombardi et al 2008; Baydar et al 2009; Bigoni et al 2009). Therefore, therapeutic exercises are commonly advocated to address these dysfunctions in mobility, posture, muscle activation, proprioception and strength.

Overall, the evidence that therapeutic exercise is effective for non-specific shoulder pain is mixed (Smidt et al 2005), similar to other approaches including manual therapy (Ho et al 2009) and acupuncture (Green et al 2005). However, exercise appears to be as effective for non-specific shoulder pain as more expensive treatments such as multidisciplinary bio-psychosocial rehabilitation (Karjalainen et al 2001). Furthermore, when specific shoulder disorders are considered there is little evidence that alternative approaches are superior to therapeutic exercise. For example medium- and long-term outcomes after therapeutic exercise in adhesive capsulitis are similar to those after other treatments including arthrographic distension (Buchbinder et al 2008) and corticosteroid injection (Winters et al 1997, 1999; Buchbinder et al 2003). There is also evidence that combining corticosteroid injection with physiotherapy including therapeutic exercise results in greater improvement than either treatment in isolation (Carette et al 2003).

The use of therapeutic exercise in the management of specific disorders including subacromial impingement syndrome (SAIS) and rotator cuff lesions is supported by much research (Bang & Deyle 2000; Desmeules et al 2003; Green et al 2003; Michener et al 2004; Dickens et al 2005; Jonsson et al 2006; Trampas & Kitsios 2006; Senbursa et al 2007; Lombardi et al 2008; Baydar et al 2009; Chen et al 2009; Kuhn 2009; Roy et al 2009). Furthermore, outcomes following conservative treatment (incorporating therapeutic exercise) appear to be similar to those after surgical intervention in SAIS and rotator cuff lesions (Haahr & Andersen 2006; Dorrestijn et al 2009). This key role of therapeutic exercise in shoulder rehabilitation is emphasized by the fact that good clinical outcomes have been associated with normalization of scapular kinematics (Roy et al 2009) and recovery of strength (Nho et al 2009).

Principles of Exercise

A clinical assessment should be completed prior to exercise prescription and clinicians should remain cognisant of the various facets of an exercise programme and suit the needs to the individual patient: posture, flexibility and stretching, stability, strengthening, proprioception and functional progression (Tippet & Voight 1995; Lephart & Fu 2000; Alter 2004; Donatelli 2004b, 2006; Kraemer & Ratamess 2004; Weerapong et al 2004; Houglum 2005; Kendall et al 2005; MacIntosh et al 2006). It is important for the clinician to gather information including the subjective history, objective examination, special tests, functional ability, impairment, dysfunctions, diagnosis and any other pertinent information. Two-way communication with other team members (e.g. medical, surgical, psychological, coach, strength and conditioning, etc.) is essential in order to enhance the overall physical therapy plan of care, and set appropriate and safe goals. Clinicians should employ evidence-based practice and clinical reasoning with respect to current research, and patient-orientated goals as the basis for rational rehabilitation (Cicerone 2005). Safety is of paramount importance and clinicians should ensure that exercises are suitable and safe for individual patients. Furthermore, since painful sensory input may alter motor output during exercise, reduction of the pain where possible with appropriate physical, pharmacological and / or psychological strategies is an important part of the rehabilitation process.

There are three phases of a therapeutic exercise programme, which are worked through progressively based on the requirements of the individual patient; these include: (1) posture, joint range of motion and flexibility, (2) muscle strength and endurance, and (3) functional aspects including proprioception, coordination and agility (Houglum 2005). For example, the exercise prescription and goals of a patient with adhesive capsulitis will differ significantly from those of a patient with humeral instability. Principles for guiding rehabilitation include avoidance of aggravation, timing of

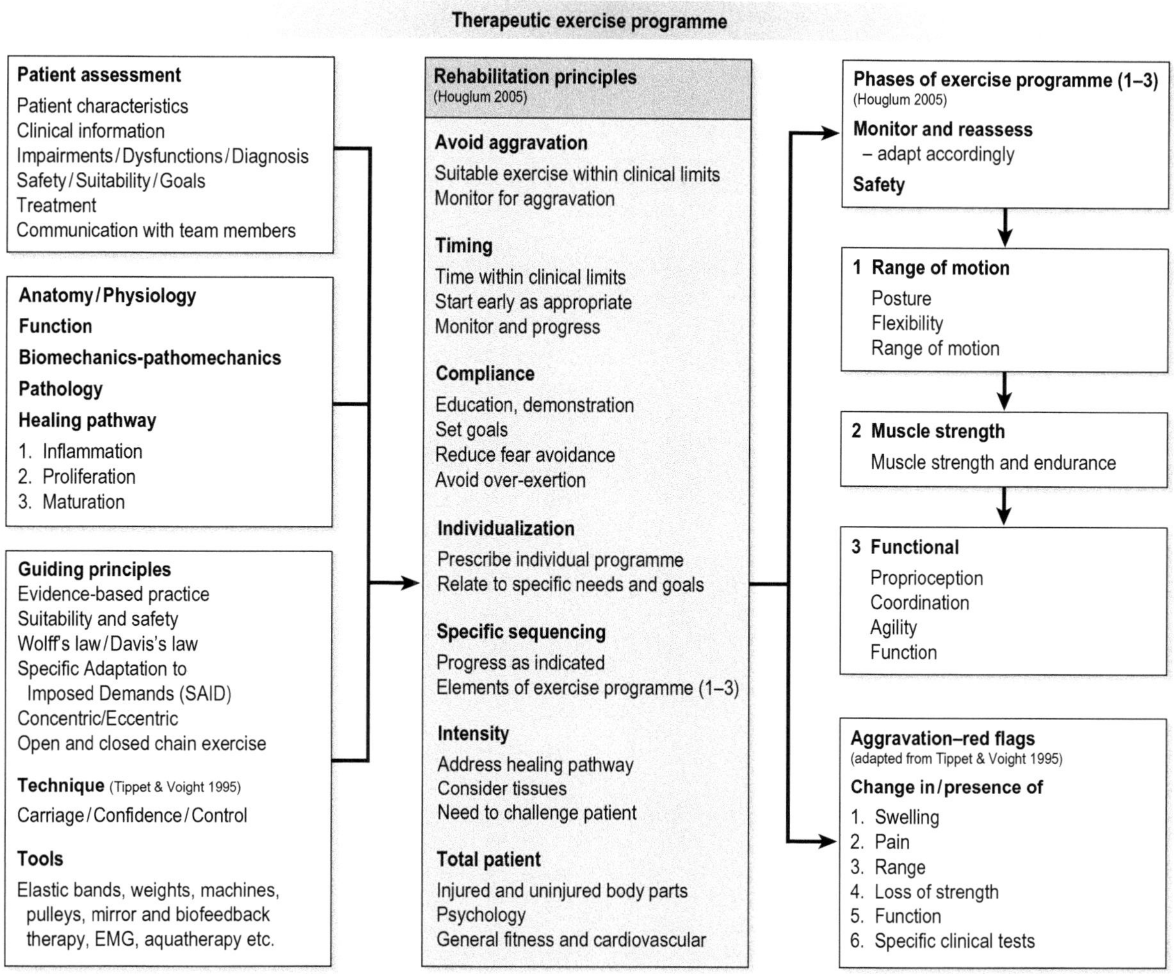

Figure 33.1 Principles of therapeutic exercise.

exercise, compliance, individualization, specific sequencing, intensity and total patient approach (Houglum 2005); these principles are presented in Figure 33.1.

Exercise programmes should be progressive and graded according to the stage of healing and should not aggravate pain, swelling or result in deterioration in other clinical signs such as range of motion, strength and function (see Fig. 33.1) (Tippet & Voight 1995). The ability to perform exercises with appropriate skill should be monitored closely (Tippet & Voight 1995). These authors referred to the three 'C's: (1) carriage – appropriate weight shift, weight acceptance and symmetry of movement, (2) confidence – verbal and non-verbal communication, speed and deliberateness of exercise performed, and (3) control – smooth unrestricted automatic movements with skilled task performance (Tippet & Voight 1995).

Bone and soft tissues adapt according to the stresses placed upon them, which highlights the importance of appropriate loading of tissue in a graded progressive manner to enhance healing, and has been described by Wolff's law and Davis's law respectively (Wolff 1986; Tippet & Voight 1995). These principles also apply to the hypertrophy of uninjured tissues; for example, it has been demonstrated that baseball athletes have thicker biceps and supraspinatus tendons compared with non-athletes (Wang et al 2005). On the other hand, overloading of bone and soft tissue can result in injury such as bone stress fracture or tendon failure.

The principle of specific adaptations to imposed demands (SAID) refers to the body's ability to change according to specific demands placed upon it and therefore has implications for rehabilitation design in that exercises should mimic the expected functional stressors of the individual patient as much as possible (Houglum 2005). Implementing variance of activities and rest phases is important so as to allow adaptation. An example of the relevance of these principles is when considering the introduction of eccentric strength training into the rehabilitation programme. Eccentric strength training programmes appear to be effective in the management of knee and ankle tendon pathology (Alfredson et al 1998; Young et al 2005). There has been less research on eccentric programmes for rotator cuff tendon pathology; however, initial results are encouraging (Jonsson et al 2006). Eccentric programmes are, however, associated with muscle damage (Clarkson & Hubal 2002). Before placing such high stresses on previously injured tissues, basic isometric and isotonic strength programmes should be already in place. Further, the introduction of such eccentric training programmes should be progressed.

Shoulder muscle balance ratios have been reported, including ratios between the external and internal rotators of 1.5:1 (66%) for both fast and slow isokinetic torque arm speed in normal subjects (Ivey et al 1985). Ratios have also been presented for professional baseball pitchers (Ellenbecker & Mattalino 1997). Clinicians should consider these ratios in exercise programme design. A discussion of isokinetics is beyond the scope of this chapter, but has been reviewed by Ellenbecker and Davies (2000).

The following sections will discuss, posture, stretching and strengthening (isometric and isotonic) and briefly mention functional exercise. Specific parameters for timing and repetitions of stretching and strengthening will be covered under each appropriate section.

Posture

Postural assessment is an important part of the objective evaluation and ideal static postural alignments have been suggested (Kendall et al 2005). However, it is important to assess both static and dynamic postures to ascertain the patient's functional movement and ability to self-correct a static habitus. An example of this is a boxer, who enhances a hyperkyphotic and rounded shoulder posture to reduce his target size for strategic advantage, but when dynamically tested may be able to self-correct the seemingly poor posture.

It is important to assess for muscle length, joint mobility and muscle control. Altered posture may be related to muscle imbalances and altered joint position, which ultimately could result in movement dysfunction and pain. Deviations in normal upright positions may include a forward head position, an exaggerated curve in the thoracic kyphosis, and rounded shoulders. Deviations in scapular kinematics may present in multiple planes, including changes in scapular elevation, protraction, tilt and rotation, affecting the size of the subacromial space (Solem-Bertoft et al 1993), as well as both activation (Roy et al 2009) and mechanical advantage (Kibler et al 2006) of muscular structures. It has been demonstrated that the size of the subacromial space is reduced in the presence of thoracic hyperkyphosis (Raine & Twomey 1997; Gumina et al 2008) and shoulder protraction (Solem-Bertoft et al 1993). It is, however, uncertain whether a strong correlation exists between narrowing of the subacromial space and shoulder symptoms (Graichen et al 2001; Roberts et al 2002; Hinterwimmer et al 2003; Lewis et al 2005; Mayerhoefer et al 2009). In fact, although it has been assumed that there is a definitive association between these postural deviations, a study of 160 asymptomatic subjects found no such correlation (Raine & Twomey 1997). Therefore, although there may be a relationship between posture and subacromial space, this is not yet fully understood.

Thoracic kyphosis and forward shoulder position influence the length of the upper back and scapular muscles and place the intervertebral joints in an end-range position (Griegel-Morris et al 1992). The sustained strain on these soft tissues may lead to upper back pain or shoulder pain. In the front of the body the pectoral muscles may shorten (Borstad & Ludewig 2006; Muraki et al 2009). Sustained muscle shortening may lead to the development or activation of myofascial trigger points (Simons et al 1999). Referred pain from the pectorals may be felt in the front of the shoulder and arm (Simons et al 1999) and sometimes even in the upper back region (Dejung et al 2003). (See Ch 59 for a review of these mechanisms and muscle referral patterns.)

Sustained contractions impair normal blood flow in skeletal muscles. Optimal posture allows muscles the opportunity to relax in between contractions, which permits and facilitates recovery of circulation (Otten 1988; Sjogaard & Sogaard 1998; Palmerud et al 2000). Combining postural exercises with myofeedback / EMG is helpful when teaching patients how to use their muscles in an economic and healthy manner (Peper et al 2003; Voerman et al 2006). Though there is a wide range of postures, clinicians should consider the optimal posture for each patient and individualize exercise programmes, rather than focusing on an idealized posture suitable for all. Assumption of an appropriate upright trunk posture can change muscle activation and modify range of motion and symptoms (Bullock et al 2005). Scapular taping can be used as a temporary means of altering scapular muscle activation (Selkowitz et al 2007). Furthermore, Lucas et al (2004) demonstrated that latent trigger points can alter muscle activation patterns of the shoulder as assessed by EMG and subsequently reported that dry needling and stretch, when compared with placebo ultrasound, was found to improve the muscle activation patterns significantly and similar to controls.

Treatment for postural dysfunctions may include manual therapies, including: joint mobilization and manipulation, massage and myofascial trigger point release, myofascial release techniques, trigger point dry needling, biofeedback and EMG, stretching, stability and strengthening and cognitive and behavioural strategies.

Stretching

Flexibility and stretching is a broad topic with conflicting opinions in the literature, and a full discussion of this topic is beyond the scope of this chapter. Readers are referred elsewhere for a comprehensive review of stretching (Alter 1996; Weerapong et al 2004). A rehabilitation programme of the shoulder may incorporate a muscle-stretching programme, which is usually employed for muscle lengthening and associated clinical implications, pain inhibition and potential injury prevention.

It has been reported that alterations in scapular movement are related to changes in myofascial length (Borstad & Ludewig 2005; Borstad 2006). The addition of appropriate manual therapy techniques may increase the effectiveness of therapeutic exercise (Winters et al 1997; Conroy & Hayes 1998; Bang & Deyle 2000; Desmeules et al 2003; Bergman et al 2004; Michener et al 2004; Senbursa et al 2007; Boyles et al 2009). These techniques may include soft tissue techniques, passive stretching and joint mobilization, and may increase range of motion in subjects with shoulder pain (Vermeulen et al 2006; Johnson et al 2007). Therapeutic exercise alone, however, may be as effective as adding passive joint mobilizations to therapeutic exercise (Trampas & Kitsios 2006; Chen et al 2009). (Different joint mobilization techniques are described in detail in Ch 31.)

A muscle-stretching programme should be based on assessment of muscle length and end feel. Muscles and fascia may

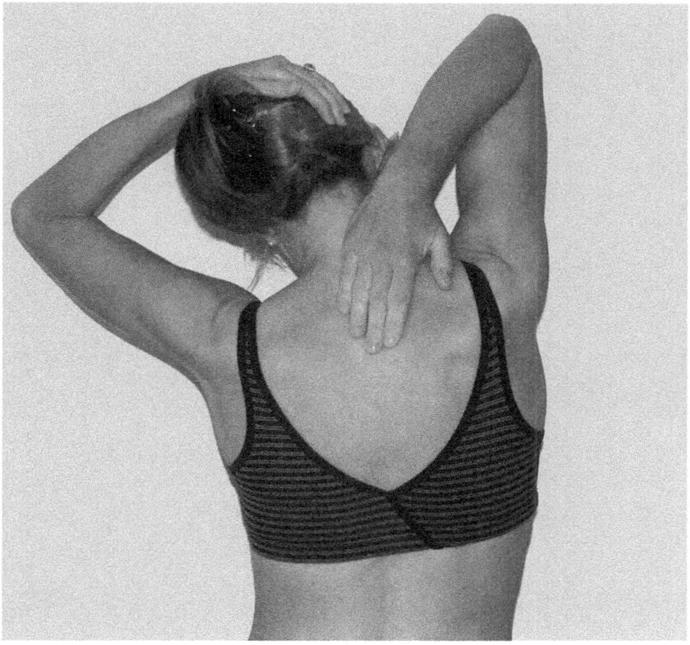

Figure 33.2 **Levator scapula stretch.** Ipsilateral arm-elevated position is proposed to assist in isolating the levator scapula from the upper trapezius.

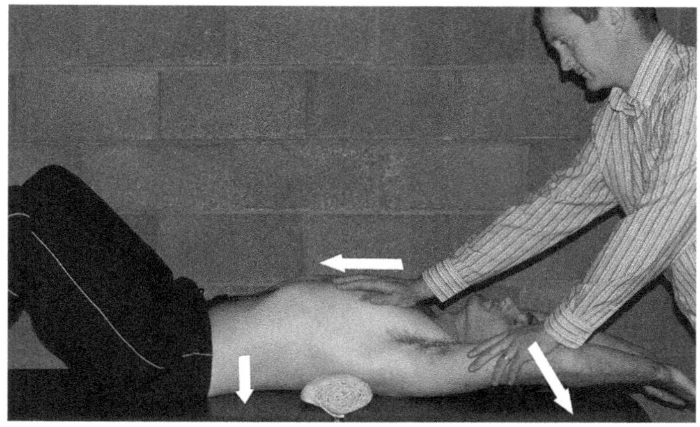

Figure 33.3 **Pectoral and latissimus dorsi, clinician-assisted stretch.** The patient maintains a neutral lumbar spine and a towel can be used to reduce thoracic kyphosis. The clinician applies a low-grade smooth stretch against soft tissue barrier. For appropriate modesty, the patient's opposite hand can be placed across the chest and the clinician's hand can be placed on top. Contract relax application can also be added to augment stretch.

present with neuromuscular, viscoelastic or connective tissue alterations (Chaitow & Liebenson 2001). It is important to evaluate muscle length, and its influence on the length–tension relationship should not be overlooked (Janda 1993; Sahrmann 2002; Ekstrom & Osborn 2004; Kendall et al 2005). Though individual patients will present with varying degrees of muscle length, the following patterns, as outlined by Janda and others, are often seen in clinic practice (Chaitow & Liebenson 2001):

- **short muscles and often facilitated:** pectoralis major and minor, latissimus dorsi, levator scapula, upper trapezius (at times)
- **long muscles and often inhibited:** serratus anterior, lower and middle trapezius.

A stretch for the levator scapula and a clinician-assisted stretch for the pectorals and latissimus dorsi muscles are presented in Figures 33.2 and 33.3 respectively. Other self-stretch exercises for the pectorals and latissimus dorsi may include the doorway stretch and one-sided unilateral self-stretch of the pectoralis minor, which has been shown to be superior to a supine manual stretch and a sitting manual stretch (Borstad & Ludewig 2006).

Muscle-stretching techniques include static, ballistic, dynamic and proprioceptive neuromuscular facilitation (Weerapong et al 2004; Houglum 2005). Other techniques have been described including post-isometric relaxation (Lewit & Simons 1984; Lewit 1986, 1999), muscle energy technique (Greenman 1989; Chaitow & Crenshaw 2006), activated isolated stretching (Mattes 1995) and spray and stretch (Travell & Simons 1983; Simons et al 1999; Kostopoulos & Rizopoulos 2008). Stretching has been employed for the treatment of pain, especially in relation to the treatment of myofascial trigger points (Simons et al 1999).

The recommended duration of static stretching varies, but it is reasonable to recommend a 15–30-second hold with 3–5 repetitions (Taylor et al 1990; Houglum 2005) repeated daily or several times / day. Good form should be maintained during stretching technique, which should be smooth and within the clinical limits of the presenting problem. Longer hold times up to and beyond 5 minutes have been recommended for fascial tissue release (Barnes 1999).

Patients with a history of subluxation, dislocation, hypermobility of the shoulder or general hypermobility syndrome need to be identified, as a stretching programme may be inappropriate and potentially detrimental in these individuals. The patient history, muscle length tests, joint end feel, passive joint tests and the Beigthon score (Alter 1996) may assist the clinician in identifying hypermobility and instability. Up to 11.7% of people have some form of joint hypermobility, and this has been reported to be up to three times more prevalent in females than in males (Hakim & Grahame 2003; Seckin et al 2005).

The majority of current research does not support the hypothesis that stretching prevents injury (Shrier 1999; Weerapong et al 2004). However, there is some evidence to suggest that lower limb stretching can reduce the risk of injury (Hartig & Henderson 1999; Amako et al 2003; Jamtvedt et al 2009), or the rate of return from injury (Malliaropoulos et al 2004). Interestingly, though, reviewed research on stretching has demonstrated a negative effect on muscle strength and functional performance (Weerapong et al 2004). Further, the fact that most research has focused on the lower extremities raises validity issues about the validity of extrapolating the findings to the upper extremity. However, clinicians should consider these issues when prescribing flexibility programmes, especially in relation to performance athletes and players. More research is required to assist in a better understanding of the role of stretching in injury management and prevention.

External rotation is fundamental for elevation and shoulder function and it is important to restore passive and active external rotation (Donatelli 2004a). External rotation is

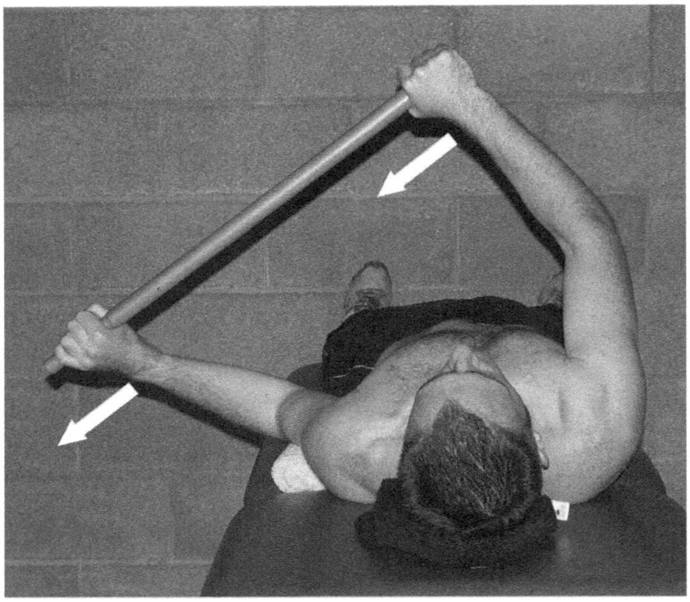

Figure 33.4 Subscapularis stretch, self-assisted stretch with cane. The supine position offers stability of the scapula while external rotation of the glenohumeral joint is assisted with self-control using the cane. A towel is placed under the elbow to maintain alignment of the humerus.

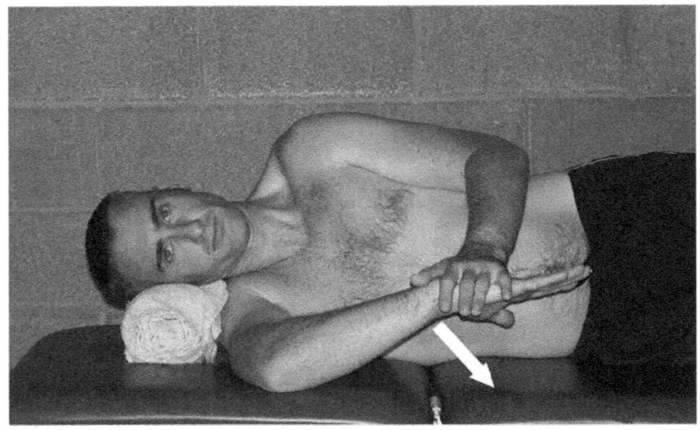

Figure 33.5 Sleeper stretch. The 90° position stabilizes the scapula and downward pressure is applied with a self-stretch to the opposite hand into internal rotation.

primarily limited at 0° by the subscapularis, at 45° of abduction by the subscapularis, middle and inferior humeral ligament and at 90° of abduction by the inferior humeral ligament (Turkel et al 1981). Muscle length testing of the subscapularis is carried out with the arm in neutral and testing into external rotation (Donatelli 2004b). An auto-assisted stretch for the subscapularis, using a cane, is presented in Figure 33.4. The stretching position, for example at 0°, 45°, 90° abduction, etc., should be based on any restrictions of the subscapularis and humeral capsule and ligaments identified from the physical assessment. The contribution of the humeral joint capsule (and other posterior soft tissue structures including the infraspinatus, teres minor and deltoid) to shoulder movement should not be overlooked and has been proposed to be particularly important in certain shoulder disorders, including SAIS (Donatelli 2004a). Reduced cross-body adduction has been linked to tightness of the posterior capsule, and associated with abnormal humeral translation (Ludewig & Cook 2002). Cross-body adduction and the 'sleeper stretch' (internal rotation of the shoulder in 90° of shoulder flexion) have been recommended as stretches for posterior shoulder capsular tightness (Cooper et al 2004; McClure et al 2007; Laudner et al 2008). The 'sleeper stretch' is presented in Figure 33.5. However, modification into less shoulder flexion may be necessary if symptoms are aggravated in this position.

Isometric Exercise of the Shoulder

Isometric exercise is usually utilized in the early phase of rehabilitation to minimize muscle atrophy when movement of the shoulder is limited. Studies have demonstrated up to a 41% decrease in isometric strength after immobilization of the upper extremity for 5–6 weeks, with significant decreases in muscle fibre area by 33% and 25% for fast- and slow-twitch fibres respectively (MacDougall et al 1980). During immobilization of the upper limb, strength training with maximal isometric exercise 5 days / week of the free limb may prevent atrophy of the immobilized limb (Farthing et al 2009). Further research has suggested that adding a 0.5 kg weight to the ipsilateral hand during isometric and dynamic shoulder exertions increases shoulder muscle activity by 4% maximum voluntary excitation (Antony & Keir 2010). Static exercises for the shoulder are presented in Figure 33.6. A belt is employed to allow multidirectional static exercises; however, other options include resistance against a wall. A hand-held weight of 0.5 kg is used to assist in increasing shoulder muscle activity (Antony & Keir 2010). Suggested parameters for isometric exercises include pain-free 5- to 10-second holds with 10 repetitions, graded to maximal contraction and repeated several times per day with progression as indicated (Houglum 2005).

Isotonic Exercises of the Shoulder

There is a plethora of exercises for the shoulder girdle, and research employing EMG has aimed at identifying exercises that target specific shoulder muscles; here we briefly review a selection of exercises that target the rotator cuff, trapezius and serratus anterior muscles. For a further expansion of this, readers are recommended to review other publications (Ekstrom & Osborn 2004; Houglum 2005; Reinold et al 2009). When designing a strengthening programme, the clinician should target muscles identified as weak during the evaluation and, on the basis of this, prescribe suitable exercises. The clinician should prescribe the specific exercise, resistance (or none), repetitions, sets and frequency of the programme. This programme should be monitored, adjusted and advanced progressively. A programme can be initiated with or without weight, as appropriate. Recommendations have been made in relation to exercise repetitions (reps) and include 1–6 reps for strength, 6–12 for hypertrophy and 12–15 for endurance (Kraemer & Ratamess 2004). The weight used is appropriate to cause fatigue towards the end of the stated number of repetitions. It has been found that two

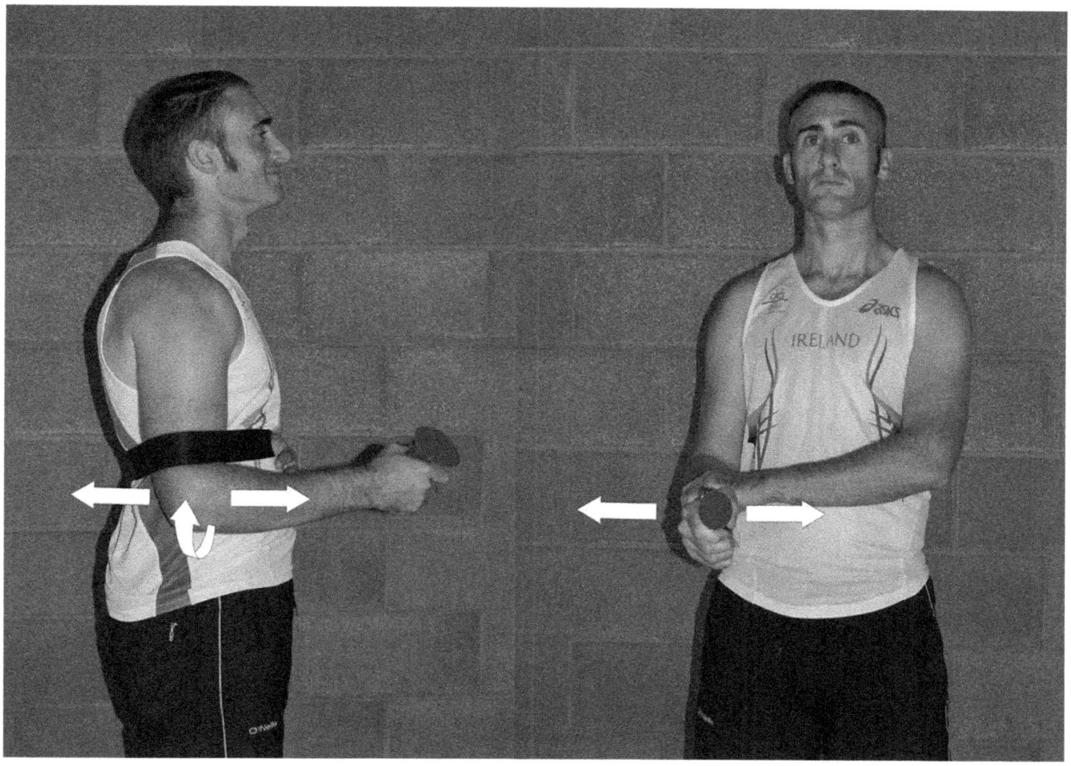

Figure 33.6 Isometric exercises for the shoulder. The use of a belt allows the patient to perform isometric exercise in multiple directions. This can be also done against a wall. Internal and external rotation is performed with self-assisted resistance. The use of a hand-held weight of 0.5 kg has been shown to assist in increasing shoulder muscle EMG by 4%. The arrows indicate direction of force, but as an isometric exercise there is no movement.

to six sets per exercise produced significant increases in muscular strength in both trained and untrained individuals (Kraemer & Ratamess 2004).

Other recommendations include 6–15 repetitions of two sets where the patient can control the weight, progressing to 20–25 repetitions of three sets (Houglum 2005). When this is reached, the weight then is progressed accordingly and the process started again with 6–15 repetitions of two sets, etc. (Houglum 2005). There are various exercise progressions that can be considered including that of Delorme and Watkins (1948), Oxford technique (Zinovieff 1951) and daily adjusted progressive resistive exercise (Knight 1985; Houglum 2005). The clinician should consider the principles of exercise as outlined in Figure 33.1 when prescribing strength programmes. The rotator cuff muscles are important stabilizers of the humeral joint and assist in stabilizing the humerus in the glenoid by compression and preventing shear and upward movement of the humeral head during arm movements (Oatis 2004). Other muscles assist in stabilizing the scapulothoracic complex and in dynamic stability (Oatis 2004) and these muscle-specific exercises are covered below. For muscles such as the deltoid, levator scapulae and rhomboids, and indications for strengthening, readers are recommended to review the article by Reinold et al (2009).

Supraspinatus muscle

The supraspinatus is the most superior of the rotator cuff muscles and lies deep to the subacromial bursa and the coracoacromial ligament within the subacromial space (Oatis 2004). The reported actions of this muscle include abduction, external rotation and stabilization of the shoulder (Oatis 2004). Activity of the supraspinatus increases with increased loading during abduction and scaption movements, peaking at 30–60° of elevation (Reinold et al 2009). Reinold et al (2007) demonstrated that EMG activity was similar across three exercises: full can, empty can and prone full can. The full-can exercise results in significantly less activity of the middle and posterior deltoid, which may reduce harmful shear force on the humeral joint from deltoid activity (Reinold et al 2007, 2009). In addition, it reduces the potential for subacromial impingement because of the external rotation component (Ekstrom & Osborn 2004). Moreover, this exercise has been recommended by previous research (Kelly et al 1996). The full-can exercise in the plane of the scapula with external rotation of the shoulder is presented in Figure 33.7.

Infraspinatus and teres minor muscles

The actions of the infraspinatus and teres minor are primarily external rotation and functionally assisting the stability of the humeral joint during elevation movements (Reinold et al 2009). Stabilization of the shoulder by these muscles is also achieved by opposing superior and anterior humeral head translation (Reinold et al 2009). The infraspinatus has potentially a role in abduction and horizontal abduction, with the teres minor involved in adduction, the difference apparently being due to different moment arms (Oatis 2004). EMG analysis demonstrated the best isolation of the infraspinatus in 0° abduction with 45° of medial rotation from neutral (Kelly et al 1996), and Reinold et al (2009) suggested incorporating this position as an exercise to any rehabilitation programme when focusing on increasing external rotation strength. Addition of a roll support between the arm and the trunk (Fig. 33.8) has been shown to increase EMG activity in the infraspinatus and teres minor muscles by up to 25% (Reinold et al 2004, 2009).

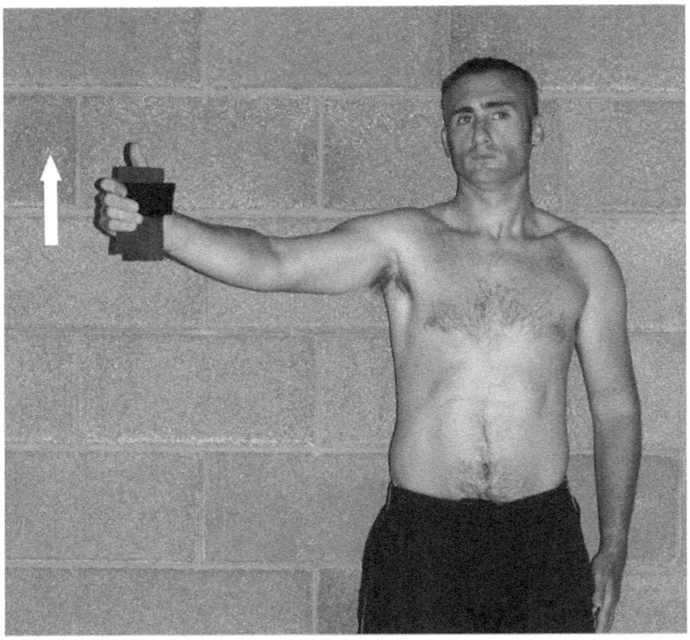

Figure 33.7 Supraspinatus full-can strengthening. This is carried out in the plane of the scapula, slowly and controlled with the thumb up to ensure a degree of external rotation.

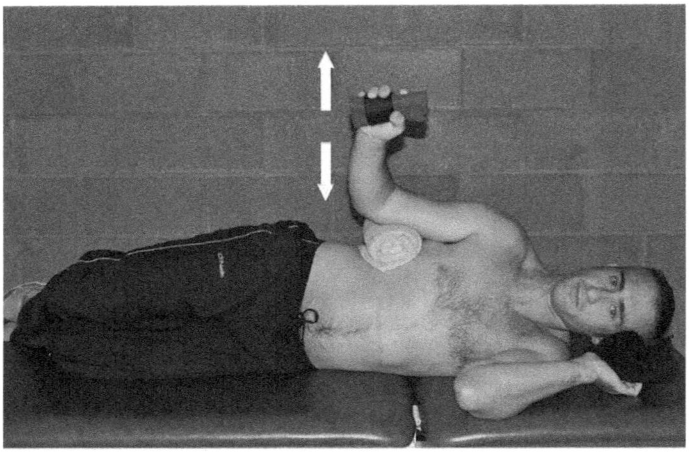

Figure 33.8 Infraspinatus and teres minor muscles strengthening. In side-lying, the arm is brought from internal into external rotation. A towel positioned between the arm and trunk has been shown to increase EMG of the muscles by 25%.

A second exercise worth considering is standing external rotation in the scapular plane (45° of abduction) (Fig. 33.9) as this has demonstrated good EMG activation of the infraspinatus and teres minor (Reinold et al 2004), and isokinetic external rotational strength values in the plane of the scapula have been reported to be significantly higher than in the frontal plane (Greenfield et al 1990).

Other exercises for external rotation have been recommended that place the shoulder in a more compromised position (e.g. external rotation in 90° abduction) and clinicians should carefully consider the appropriateness of these exercises in the presence of capsulolabral dysfunction and pathology (Reinold et al 2009).

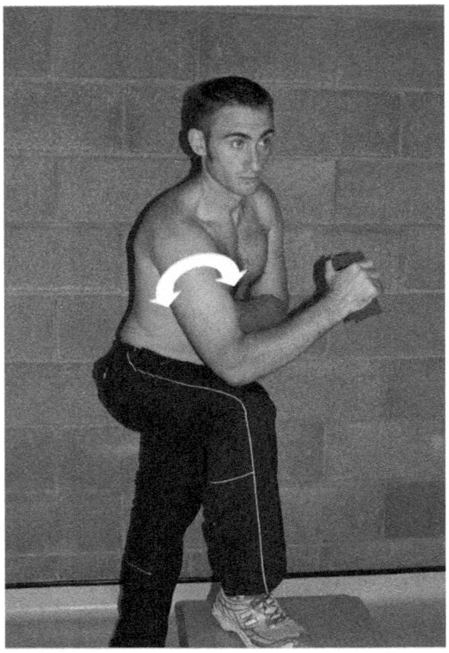

Figure 33.9 External rotation in the plane of the scapula. The shoulder is rotated from internal to external rotation.

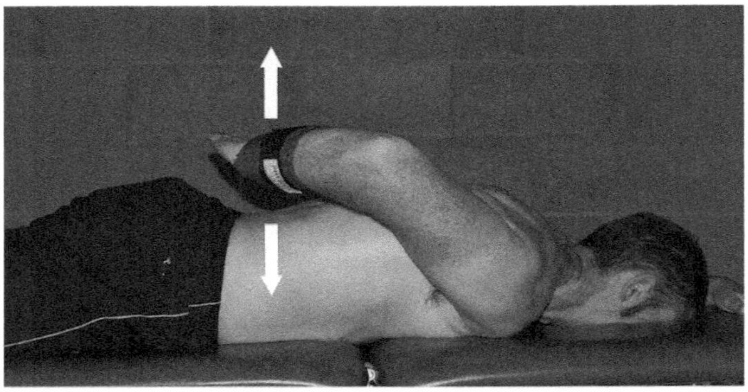

Figure 33.10 Subscapularis strengthening (Gerber's lift-off test). The hand is raised upwards from the trunk.

Subscapularis muscle

The subscapularis is the largest of the rotator cuff muscles and acts to rotate internally, flex, extend, abduct, adduct, adduct horizontally and stabilize the shoulder, with broad agreement that internal rotation and stabilization are the primary roles (Oatis 2004). Subscapularis weakness leads to significant decrease in internal rotation strength and may contribute to anterior instability of the shoulder (Oatis 2004). The lift-off test as described by Gerber and Krushell (1991) has been demonstrated to isolate the subscapularis (Greis et al 1996; Kelly et al 1996). The lift-off exercise for the subscapularis muscle is presented in Figure 33.10.

Trapezius muscle

The trapezius is an expansive muscle that has three distinct muscle sections: upper, middle and lower, with each having

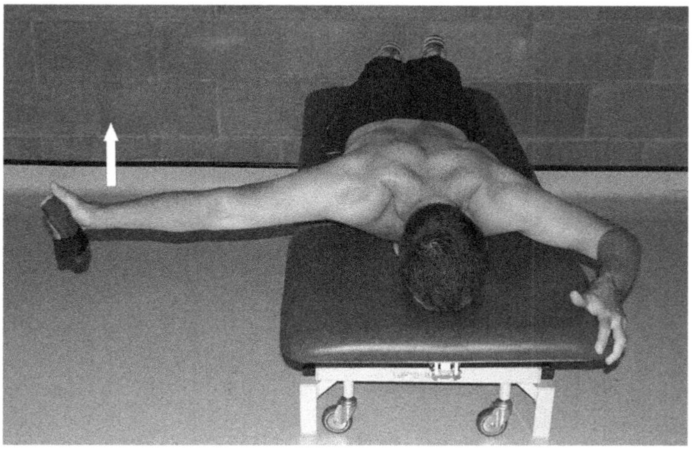

Figure 33.11 Trapezius strengthening. This targets the upper, middle and lower sections of the trapezius muscle. The thumb is maintained in an upright position.

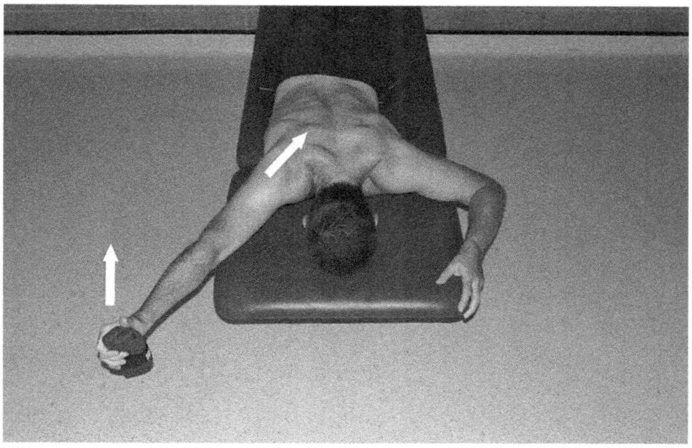

Figure 33.12 Trapezius strengthening. This targets mainly the lower fibres of trapezius performed at approximately 120–135° of abduction or with the arm positioned in line with the lower fibres of the trapezius.

a distinct function and combining to assist in the overall function of the trapezius (Oatis 2004). The actions of the three sections have been reported as follows (Oatis 2004): upper trapezius – elevation of the scapula, adduction and upward rotation of the scapula; middle trapezius – adduction of the scapula; and lower trapezius – depression, adduction and upward rotation of the scapula. In particular, the upper and lower trapezius form an anatomical force couple that assists in stabilizing the scapula, and maintaining a balance between these muscle segments is important for optimal function (Oatis 2004). Furthermore, the lower fibres have been reported to play an important role in posterior tilt and upward rotation of the scapula during shoulder elevation (Ludewig et al 1996). Therefore, the lower trapezius and serratus anterior comprise an important target for rehabilitation and prevention of shoulder dysfunction and impingement syndromes (Ludewig & Cook 2000). With regard to exercises for the upper trapezius, the shoulder shrug has been reported to produce the greatest EMG activity (Ekstrom et al 2003). However, it has been further reported that the shrug exercise also highly activates the levator scapula and so if this needs to be avoided, owing to the levator scapulae action of scapular downward rotation, the military press may be more appropriate (Ekstrom & Osborn 2004).

For the middle trapezius, abduction and external rotation of the shoulder at 90° in prone (Fig. 33.11) has been shown to induce good EMG activity and is considered a suitable exercise (Moseley et al 1992; Ekstrom & Osborn 2004; Reinold et al 2009). This exercise has also been recommended for strengthening the trapezius as a whole, owing to high EMG activity in the upper, middle and lower muscle segments (Ekstrom et al 2003; Ekstrom & Osborn 2004).

The lower trapezius has been shown to be best activated with the arm raise overhead exercise in the prone position, performed at approximately 120° (Reinold et al 2009) to 135° of abduction or with the arm positioned in line with the lower fibres of trapezius (Fig. 33.12) (Ekstrom et al 2003; Ekstrom & Osborn 2004).

Serratus anterior muscle

The serratus anterior muscle action has been reported as protraction, abduction, upward rotation and elevation of the scapula; the muscle functions in actions such as pushing a revolving door and weakness may lead to winging of the scapula and difficulty with overhead activities (Oatis 2004). Shoulder abduction in the plane of the scapula above 120° (to avoid painful arc) in the standing position has demonstrated more EMG activity in the serratus anterior than does straight scapular protraction (Fig. 33.13). The increased serratus anterior activation should, however, be balanced against the increased risk of impingement when exercises are performed in elevation (Roberts et al 2002). Other recommended exercises for the serratus anterior include the dynamic hug, push-up with a plus and punch exercises (Decker et al 1999; Reinold et al 2009).

Functional Exercises

The daily tasks and movements performed by the individual should be considered when prescribing therapeutic exercise, so that the exercises take into account the specific functional demands of that person. Functional progression may include movement from isolated plane to multiplane strengthening (Fig. 33.14) and eventually plyometric exercise (Houglum 2005). Upper limb tasks are commonly open kinetic chain movements. In athlete subjects with recurrent anterior shoulder dislocation, rehabilitation near / in the zone of instability is indicated in late-stage rehabilitation and therefore tasks that load the rotator cuff in semi-compromised positions may help replicate the stability action required on return to sport. Closed chain and stability exercises (Figs 33.15 and 33.16) for the shoulder girdle are important to assist in motor control and re-education (Houglum 2005) and are discussed in Chapter 32. The shoulder girdle relationship to the kinetic

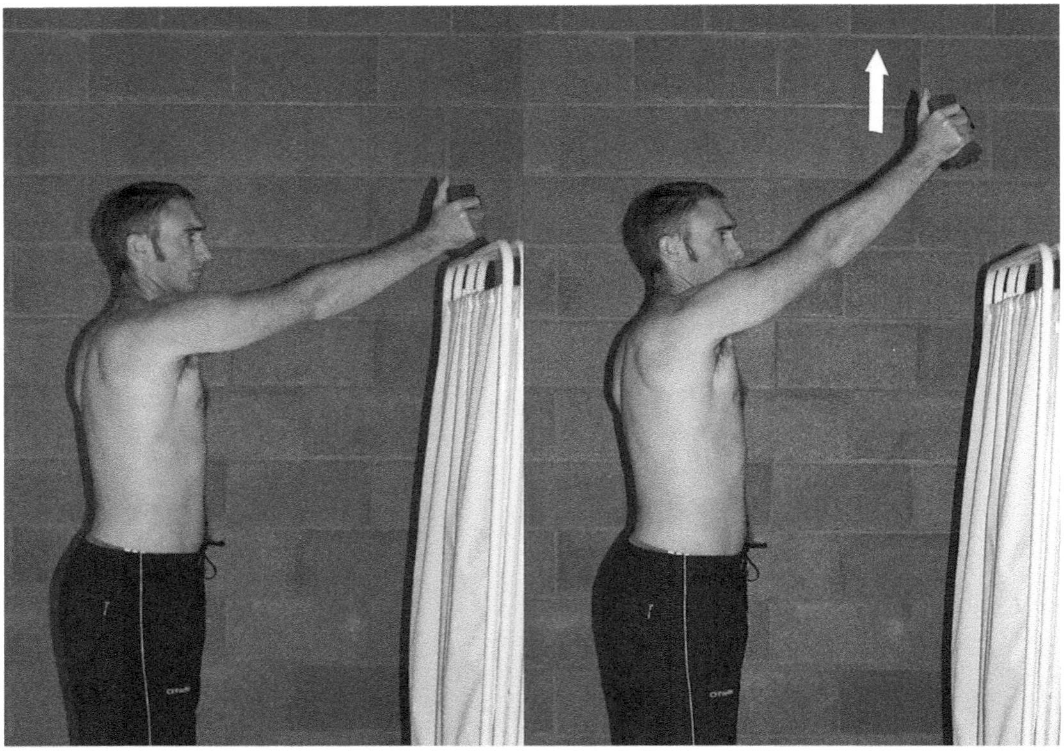

Figure 33.13 Serratus anterior strengthening. Shoulder abduction is performed in the plane of the scapula above 120° (to avoid painful arc) in the standing position.

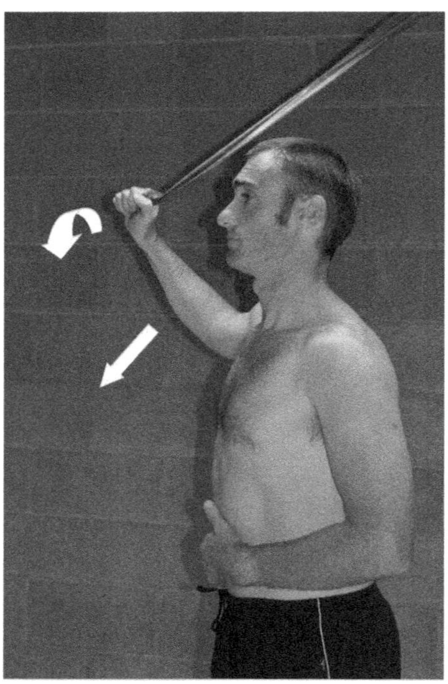

Figure 33.14 Proprioceptive neuromuscular facilitation with elastic band. Elastic bands can assist with creating open chain coordinated movements that mimic functional patterns.

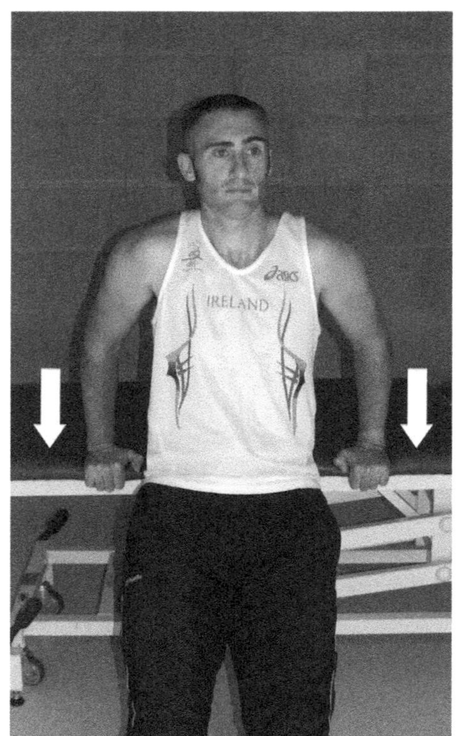

Figure 33.15 Shoulder dip. This is a closed chain kinetic loading and proprioceptive exercise.

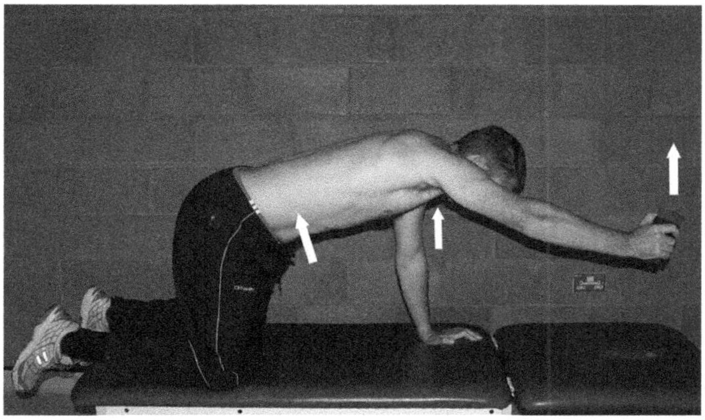

Figure 33.16 **Prone knee, single-arm raise.** The abdominals are primed prior to the lift. This offers a closed chain exercise for weight-bearing shoulder and a dynamic open chain exercise for the opposite arm. This exercise can be advanced to alternative arm and leg lift for stability.

chain should be considered in the overall management of the patient and exercise programmes may incorporate standing balance and eye–hand coordination tasks, etc. (Donatelli 2006). A common barrier to shoulder rehabilitation is difficulty in replicating the therapeutic exercise correctly at home, possibly owing to reduced positional sense (Naughton et al 2005). Tasks that challenge the proprioceptive acuity and load-bearing ability of the shoulder region may help to restore positional sense awareness (see Figs 33.14–33.16). Clinicians can also incorporate the use of exercise equipment to assist in functional progression, including elastic bands, pulleys, Theraballs, wobble boards, proprioceptive exercise devices and feedback devices such as mirrors, etc.

Conclusion

Therapeutic exercises can play an important role in the management of shoulder pain. This chapter has outlined some basic principles on the type of exercise that may be indicated in the clinical setting, especially in relation to strength of the rotator cuff and stabilizers of the scapula. Clinicians should remain cognisant of the need for a comprehensive assessment and ensure safe and suitable exercise prescription and progression. The nature, intensity and volume of exercise prescribed must be matched to the clinical presentation. Individual therapists may use the principles outlined in this chapter as a guide when prescribing a therapeutic exercise programme that is suitable for the needs of each individual patient or athlete. Further research is required and should focus on identifying exercises to suit the specific patient presentation.

Acknowledgements

Thank you to the photographic volunteers: Derek Malone, Irish Paralympic athlete and S.M.

References

Alfredson H, Pietilä T, Jonshon P, et al. 1998. Heavy-load eccentric calf muscle training for the treatment of chronic Achilles tendinosis. Am J Sports Med 26: 360–366.

Alter MJ. 1996. Science of flexibility, 2nd edn. Champaign, IL: Human Kinetics.

Alter MJ. 2004. Science of flexibility, 3rd edn. Champaign, IL: Human Kinetics.

Amako M, Oda T, Masuoka K, et al. 2003. Effect of static stretching on prevention of injuries for military recruits. Mil Med 168: 442–446.

Antony NT, Keir PJ. 2010. Effects of posture, movement and hand load on shoulder muscle activity. J Electromyogr Kinesiol 20: 191–198.

Bang M, Deyle G. 2000. Comparison of supervised exercise with and without manual physical therapy for patients with shoulder impingement syndrome. J Orthop Sports Phys Ther 30: 126–137.

Barclay J. 1994. In good hands: the history of the Chartered Society of Physiotherapy 1894–1994. Oxford: Butterworth Heinemann.

Barnes J. 1999. Myofascial release. In: Hammer WI (ed) Functional soft tissue examination and treatment by manual methods: new perspectives, 2nd edn. Gaithersburg, MD: Aspen Publishers, x, p 625.

Baydar M, Akalin E, El O, et al. 2009. The efficacy of conservative treatment in patients with full-thickness rotator cuff tears. Rheumatol Int 29: 623–628.

Bergman G, Winters J, Groenier K, et al. 2004. Manipulative therapy in addition to usual medical care for patients with shoulder dysfunction and pain: a randomized, controlled trial. Ann Intern Med 141: 432–439.

Bigoni M, Gorla M, Guerraio S, et al. 2009. Shoulder evaluation with isokinetic strength testing after arthroscopic rotator cuff repairs. J Shoulder Elbow Surg 18: 178–183.

Borstad J. 2006. Resting posture variables at the shoulder: evidence to support a posture-impairment association. Phys Ther 86: 549–557.

Borstad J, Ludewig P. 2005. The effect of long versus short pectoralis minor resting length on scapular kinematics in healthy individuals. J Orthop Sports Phys Ther 35: 227–238.

Borstad JD, Ludewig PM. 2006. Comparison of three stretches for the pectoralis minor muscle. J Shoulder Elbow Surg 15: 324–330.

Boyles RE, Ritland BM, Miracle BM, et al. 2009. The short-term effects of thoracic spine thrust manipulation on patients with shoulder impingement syndrome. Man Ther 14: 375–380.

Buchbinder R, Green S, Youd JM, et al. 2003. Corticosteroid injections for shoulder pain. Cochrane Database Syst Rev 1: CD004016.

Buchbinder R, Green S, Youd JM, et al. 2008. Arthrographic distension for adhesive capsulitis. Cochrane Database Syst Rev 23(1): CD007005. doi: 10.1002/14651858.CD007005.

Bullock M, Foster N, Wright C. 2005. Shoulder impingement: the effect of sitting posture on shoulder pain and range of motion. Man Ther 10: 28–37.

Carette S, Moffet H, Tardif J, et al. 2003. Intra-articular corticosteroids, supervised physiotherapy, or a combination of the two in the treatment of adhesive capsulitis of the shoulder: a placebo-controlled trial. Arthritis Rheum 48: 829–838.

Chaitow L, Crenshaw K. 2006. Muscle energy techniques: with accompanying DVD. Edinburgh: Churchill Livingstone Elsevier.

Chaitow L, Liebenson C. 2001. Muscle energy techniques. Edinburgh: Churchill Livingstone Elsevier.

Chen S, Simonian P, Wickiewicz T, et al. 1999. Radiographic evaluation of gleno-humeral kinematics: a muscle fatigue model. J Shoulder Elbow Surg 8: 49–52.

Chen J, Ginn KA, Herbert R, et al. 2009. Passive mobilisation of shoulder region joints plus advice and exercise does not reduce pain and disability more than advice and exercise alone: a randomised trial. Aust J Physiother 55: 17–23.

Cicerone KD. 2005. Evidence-based practice and the limits of rational rehabilitation. Arch Phys Med Rehabil 86: 1073–1074.

Clarkson PM, Hubal MJ. 2002. Exercise-induced muscle damage in humans. Am J Phys Med Rehabil 81: S52S69.

Conroy D, Hayes K. 1998. The effect of joint mobilisation as a component of comprehensive treatment for primary shoulder impingement syndrome. J Orthop Sports Phys Ther 28: 3–14.

Cools A, Witvrouw E, Declercq G, et al. 2007. Scapular muscle recruitment patterns: trapezius muscle latency with and without impingement symptoms. Am J Sports Med 31: 542–549.

Cooper J, Donley P, Morgan C, et al. 2004. Throwing injuries. In: Donatelli R (ed) Physical therapy of the shoulder. St Louis, MO: Churchill Livingstone, pp 29–78.
Decker MJ, Hintermeister RA, Faber KJ, et al. 1999. Serratus anterior muscle activity during selected rehabilitation exercises. Am J Sports Med 27: 784–791.
Dejung B, Gröbli C, Colla F, et al. 2003. Triggerpunkttherapie. Bern: Hans Huber.
Delorme TL, Watkins AL. 1948. Technics of progressive resistance exercise. Arch Phys Med Rehabil 1(29): 263–273.
Desmeules F, Côté CH, Fremont P, et al. 2003. Therapeutic exercise and orthopedic manual therapy for impingement syndrome: a systematic review. Clin J Sport Med 13: 176–182.
Dickens V, Willimas J, Bhamra M. 2005. Role of physiotherapy in the treatment of sub-acromial impingement syndrome: a prospective study. Physiotherapy 91: 159–164.
Donatelli R. 2004a. Functional anatomy and mechanics. In: Donatelli R (ed) Physical therapy of the shoulder. St Louis, MO: Churchill Livingstone, pp 11–28.
Donatelli R. 2004b. Physical therapy of the shoulder. St Louis, MO: Churchill Livingstone.
Donatelli R. 2006. Sports-specific rehabilitation. St Louis, MO: Churchill Livingstone Elsevier.
Dorrestijn O, Stevens M, Winers J, et al. 2009. Conservative or surgical treatment for sub-acromial impingement syndrome? A systematic review. J Shoulder Elbow Surg 18: 652–660.
Ekstrom R, Osborn R. 2004. Muscle length testing and electromyographic data for manual strength testing and exercises for the shoulder. In: Donatelli R (ed) Physical therapy of the thoulder. St Louis, MO: Churchill Livingstone, pp 435–463.
Ekstrom RA, Donatelli RA, Soderberg GL. 2003. Surface electromyographic analysis of exercises for the trapezius and serratus anterior muscles. J Orthop Sports Phys Ther 33: 247–258.
Ellenbecker TS, Davies GJ. 2000. The application of isokinetics in testing and rehabilitation of the shoulder complex. J Athl Train 35: 338–350.
Ellenbecker TS, Mattalino AJ. 1997. Concentric isokinetic shoulder internal and external rotation strength in professional baseball pitchers. J Orthop Sports Phys Ther 25: 323–328.
Farthing JP, Krentz JR, Magnus CR. 2009. Strength training the free limb attenuates strength loss during unilateral immobilization. J Appl Physiol 106: 830–836.
Gerber C, Krushell RJ. 1991. Isolated rupture of the tendon of the subscapularis muscle. Clinical features in 16 cases. J Bone Joint Surg Br 73: 389–394.
Graichen H, Bonel H, Stammberger T, et al. 2001. Sex-specific differences of subacromial space width during abduction, with and without muscular activity, and correlation with anthropometric variables. J Bone Joint Surg 10: 129–135.
Green S, Buchbinder R, Hetrick S. 2003. Physiotherapy interventions for shoulder pain. Cochrane Database Syst Rev 2: CD004258.
Green S, Buchbinder R, Hetrick S. 2005. Acupuncture for shoulder pain. Cochrane Database Syst Rev 2: CD005319.
Greenfield BH, Donatelli R, Wooden MJ, et al. 1990. Isokinetic evaluation of shoulder rotational strength between the plane of scapula and the frontal plane. Am J Sports Med 18: 124–128.
Greenman PE. 1989. Principles of manual medicine. Baltimore, MD: Williams & Wilkins.
Greis PE, Kuhn JE, Schultheis J, et al. 1996. Validation of the lift-off test and analysis of sub-scapularis activity during maximal internal rotation. Am J Sports Med 24: 589–593.
Griegel-Morris P, Larson K, Mueller-Klaus K, et al. 1992. Incidence of common postural abnormalities in the cervical, shoulder, and thoracic regions and their association with pain in two age groups of healthy subjects. Phys Ther 72: 425–431.
Gumina S, Di Giorgio G, Postacchini F, et al. 2008. Sub-acromial space in adult patients with thoracic hyperkyphosis and in healthy volunteers. Chir Organi Mov 91: 93–96.
Haahr JP, Andersen JH. 2006. Exercises may be as efficient as subacromial decompression in patients with subacromial stage II impingement: 4–8-years' follow-up in a prospective, randomized study. Scand J Rheumatol 35: 224–228.
Hakim A, Grahame R. 2003. Joint hypermobility. Best Pract Res Clin Rheumatol 17: 989–1004.
Hall T, Elvey R. 1999. Nerve trunk pain: physical diagnosis and treatment. Man Ther 4: 63–73.
Hartig DE, Henderson JM. 1999. Increasing hamstring flexibility decreases lower extremity overuse injuries in military basic trainees. Am J Sports Med 27: 173–176.
Hinterwimmer S, Von Eisenhart-Rothe R, Siebert M, et al. 2003. Influence of adducting and abducting muscle forces on the sub-acromial space width. Med Sci Sports Exerc 35: 2055–2059.
Ho C, Sole G, Munn J. 2009. The effectiveness of manual therapy in the management of musculoskeletal disorders of the shoulder: a systematic review. Man Ther 14: 463–474.
Houglum PA. 2005. Therapeutic exercise for musculoskeletal injuries. Champaign, IL: Human Kinetics.
Ivey FM, Calhoun JH, Rusche K, et al. 1985. Isokinetic testing of shoulder strength: normal values. Arch Phys Med Rehabil 66: 384–386.
Jamtvedt G, Herbert RD, Flottorp S, et al. 2009. A pragmatic randomised trial of stretching before and after physical activity to prevent injury and soreness. Br J Sports Med 44(14): 1002–1009.
Janda V. 1993. Muscle strength in relation to muscle length, pain, and muscle imbalance. In: Harms-Ringdahl K (ed) Muscle strength. Edinburgh: Churchill Livingstone, pp 83–91.
Johnson A, Godges J, Zimmerman G, et al. 2007. The effect of anterior versus posterior glide joint mobilization on external rotation range of motion in patients with shoulder adhesive capsulitis. J Orthop Sports Phys Ther 37: 88–99.
Jonsson P, Wahlstrom P, Ohberg L, et al. 2006. Eccentric training in chronic painful impingement syndrome of the shoulder: results of a pilot study. Knee Surg Sports Traumatol Arthrosc 14: 76–81.
Karjalainen K, Malmivaara A, Van Tulder M, et al. 2001. Multidisciplinary biopsychosocial rehabilitation for neck and shoulder pain among working age adults: a systematic review within the framework of the Cochrane Collaboration Back Review Group. Spine 26: 174–181.
Kelly BT, Kadrmas WR, Speer KP. 1996. The manual muscle examination for rotator cuff strength. An electromyographic investigation. Am J Sports Med 24: 581–588.
Kendall FP. 2002. Kendall urges a return to basics. PT Bulletin Online 3.
Kendall F, Kendall McCreary E, Provance P, et al. 2005. Muscles: testing and function with posture and pain. Baltimore, MD: Lippincott Williams & Wilkins.
Kibler W, Sciascia A, Dome D. 2006. Evaluation of apparent and absolute supraspinatus strength in patients with shoulder injury using the scapular retraction test. Am J Sports Med 34 1643–1647.
Knight KL. 1985. Guidelines for rehabilitation of sports injuries. Clin Sports Med 4: 405–416.
Kostopoulos D, Rizopoulos K. 2008. Effect of topical aerosol skin refrigerant (spray and stretch technique) on passive and active stretching. J Bodyw Mov Ther 12: 96–104.
Kraemer WJ, Ratamess NA. 2004. Fundamentals of resistance training: progression and exercise prescription. Med Sci Sports Exerc 36: 674–688.
Kuhn JE. 2009. Exercise in the treatment of rotator cuff impingement: a systematic review and a synthesized evidence-based rehabilitation protocol. J Shoulder Elbow Surg 18: 138–160.
Laudner KG, Sipes RC, Wilson JT. 2008. The acute effects of sleeper stretches on shoulder range of motion. J Athl Train 43: 359–363.
Lephart SM, Fu FH. 2000. Proprioception and neuromuscular control in joint stability. Champaign, IL: Human Kinetics.
Lewis JS, Green A, Wright C. 2005. Subacromial impingement syndrome: the role of posture and muscle imbalance. J Shoulder Elbow Surg 14: 385–392.
Lewit K. 1986. Postisometric relaxation in combination with other methods of muscular facilitation and inhibition. Manual Med 2: 101–104.
Lewit K. 1999. Manipulative therapy in rehabilitation of the locomotor system. Oxford: Butterworth-Heinemann.
Lewit K, Simons DG. 1984. Myofascial pain: relief by post-isometric relaxation. Arch Phys Med Rehabil 65: 452–456.
Lombardi IJ, Magri A, Fleury A, et al. 2008. Progressive resistance training in patients with shoulder impingement syndrome: a randomized controlled trial. Arthritis Rheum 59: 615–622.
Lucas KR, Polus BI, Rich PS. 2004. Latent myofascial trigger points: their effect on muscle activation and movement efficiency. J Bodyw Mov Ther 8: 160–166.
Ludewig PM, Cook T. 2000. Alterations in shoulder kinematics and associated muscle activity in people with symptoms of shoulder impingement. Phys Ther 80: 276–291.
Ludewig PM, Cook T. 2002. Translations of the humerus in persons with shoulder impingement symptoms. J Orthop Sports Phys Ther 32: 248–259.

Ludewig PM, Cook TM, Nawoczenski DA. 1996. Three-dimensional scapular orientation and muscle activity at selected positions of humeral elevation. J Orthop Sports Phys Ther 24: 57–65.

Lukasiewicz A, McClure P, Michener L, et al. 1999. Comparison of 3-dimensional scapular position and orientation between subjects with and without shoulder impingement. J Orthop Sports Phys Ther 29: 574–583.

MacDougall JD, Elder GC, Sal DG, et al. 1980. Effects of strength training and immobilization on human muscle fibres. Eur J Appl Physiol Occup Physiol 43: 25–34.

MacIntosh BR, Gardiner PF, McComas AJ. 2006. Skeletal muscle: form and function. Leeds, Champaign, IL: Human Kinetics.

Malliaropoulos N, Papalexandris S, Papalada A, et al. 2004. The role of stretching in rehabilitation of hamstring injuries: 80 athletes follow-up. Med Sci Sports Exerc 36: 756–759.

Mattes AL (ed). 1995. Active isolated stretching. Sarasota, FL: Aaron Mattes Therapy.

Mayerhoefer ME, Breitenseher MJ, Wurnig C, et al. 2009. Shoulder impingement: relationship of clinical symptoms and imaging criteria. Clin J Sport Med 19: 83–89.

McClure PW, Michener LA, Karduna AR. 2006. Shoulder function and 3-dimensional scapular kinematics in people with and without shoulder impingement syndrome. Phys Ther 86: 1075–1090.

McClure P, Balaicuis J, Heiland D, et al. 2007. A randomized controlled comparison of stretching procedures for posterior shoulder tightness. J Orthop Sports Phys Ther 37: 108–114.

Michener L, Walsworth M, Burnet E. 2004. Effectiveness of rehabilitation for patients with sub-acromial impingement syndrome: a systematic review. J Hand Ther 17: 152–164.

Moraes G, Faria C, Teixeira-Salmela L. 2008. Scapular muscle recruitment patterns and isokinetic strength ratios of the shoulder rotator muscles in individuals with and without impingement syndrome. J Shoulder Elbow Surg 17: 48S–53S.

Moseley JB, Jobe FW, Pink M, et al. 1992. EMG analysis of the scapular muscles during a shoulder rehabilitation program. Am J Sports Med 20: 128–134.

Muraki T, Aoki M, Izumi T, et al. 2009. Lengthening of the pectoralis minor muscle during passive shoulder motions and stretching techniques: a cadaveric biomechanical study. Phys Ther 89: 333–341.

Myers JB, Hwang JH, Pasquale MR, et al. 2009. Rotator cuff coactivation ratios in participants with subacromial impingement syndrome. J Sci Med Sport 12: 603–608.

Naughton J, Adams R, Maher C. 2005. Upper-body wobbleboard training effects on the post-dislocation shoulder. Phys Ther Sport 6: 31–37.

Nho SJ, Brown BS, Lyman S et al. 2009. Prospective analysis of arthroscopic rotator cuff repair: prognostic factors affecting clinical and ultrasound outcome. J Shoulder Elbow Surg 18: 13–20.

Oatis CA. 2004. Kinesiology: the mechanics and pathomechanics of human movement. Baltimore, MD: Lippincott Williams & Wilkins.

Otten E. 1988. Concepts and models of functional architecture in skeletal muscle. Exerc Sport Sci Rev 16: 89–137.

Palmerud G, Forsman M, Sporrong H, et al. 2000. Intramuscular pressure of the infra- and supraspinatus muscles in relation to hand load and arm posture. Eur J Appl Physiol 83: 223–230.

Paris S, Loubert P. 1999. Foundations of clinical orthopaedics. St Augustine, FL: Institute of Physical Therapy, University of St Augustine.

Peper E, Wilson VS, Gibney KH, et al. 2003. The integration of electromyography (SEMG) at the workstation: assessment, treatment, and prevention of repetitive strain injury (RSI). Appl Psychophysiol Biofeedback 28: 167–182.

Raine S, Twomey LT. 1997. Head and shoulder posture variations in 160 asymptomatic women and men. Arch Phys Med Rehabil 78: 1215–1223.

Reinold MM, Wilk KE, Fleisig GS, et al. 2004. Electromyographic analysis of the rotator cuff and deltoid musculature during common shoulder external rotation exercises. J Orthop Sports Phys Ther 34: 385–394.

Reinold MM, Macrina LC, Wilk KE, et al. 2007. Electromyographic analysis of the supraspinatus and deltoid muscles during 3 common rehabilitation exercises. J Athl Train 42: 464–469.

Reinold MM, Escamilla RF, Wilk KE. 2009. Current concepts in the scientific and clinical rationale behind exercises for glenohumeral and scapulothoracic musculature. J Orthop Sports Phys Ther 39: 105–117.

Roberts C, Davila J, Hushek S, et al. 2002. Magnetic resonance imaging analysis of the subacromial space in the impingement sign positions. J Shoulder Elbow Surg 11: 595–599.

Roy JS, Moffet H, Hébert LJ, et al. 2009. Effect of motor control and strengthening exercises on shoulder function in persons with impingement syndrome: a single-subject study design. Man Ther 14: 180–188.

Sahrmann S. 2002. Diagnosis and treatment of movement impairment syndromes. St Louis, MO: Mosby.

Seckin U, Tur BS, Yilmaz O, et al. 2005. The prevalence of joint hypermobility among high school students. Rheumatol Int 25: 260–263.

Selkowitz D, Chaney C, Stuckey S, et al. 2007. The effects of scapular taping on the surface electromyographic signal amplitude of shoulder girdle muscles during upper extremity elevation in individuals with suspected shoulder impingement syndrome. J Orthop Sports Phys Ther 37: 694–702.

Senbursa G, Baltacı G, Atay A. 2007. Comparison of conservative treatment with and without manual physical therapy for patients with shoulder impingement syndrome: a prospective, randomized clinical trial. Knee Surg Sports Traumatol Arthrosc 15: 915–921.

Shrier I. 1999. Stretching before exercise does not reduce the risk of local muscle injury: a critical review of the clinical and basic science literature. Clin J Sport Med 9: 221–227.

Simons DG, Travell JG, Simons L. 1999. Travell and Simons' myofascial pain and dysfunction: the trigger point manual. Baltimore, MD: Williams & Wilkins.

Sjogaard G, Sogaard K. 1998. Muscle injury in repetitive motion disorders. Clin Orthop Relat Res 351: 21–31.

Smidt N, De Vet H, Bouter L, et al. 2005. Effectiveness of exercise therapy: a best-evidence summary of systematic reviews. Aust J Physiother 51: 71–85.

Solem-Bertoft E, Thuomas KA, Westerberg CE. 1993. The influence of scapular retraction and protraction on the width of the subacromial space. An MRI study. Clin Orthop Relat Res 296: 99–103.

Tate A, McClure P, Kareha S, et al. 2009. A clinical method for identifying scapular dyskinesis. Part 2: Validity. J Athl Train 44: 165–173.

Taylor DC, Dalton JD, Seaber AV, et al. 1990. Viscoelastic properties of muscle-tendon units. The biomechanical effects of stretching. Am J Sports Med 18: 300–309.

Terlouw TJ. 2007. Roots of physical medicine, physical therapy, and mechanotherapy in the Netherlands in the 19th century: a disputed area within the healthcare domain. J Man Manip Ther 15: E23–E41.

Tippet SR, Voight ML. 1995. Functional progression for sports rehabilitation. Champaign, IL: Human Kinetics.

Trampas A, Kitsios A. 2006. Exercise and manual therapy for the treatment of impingement syndrome of the shoulder: a systematic review. Phys Ther Rev 11: 125–142.

Travell JG, Simons DG. 1983. Myofascial pain and dysfunction: the trigger point manual. Baltimore, MD: Williams & Wilkins.

Turkel SJ, Panio MW, Marshall JL, et al. 1981. Stabilizing mechanisms preventing anterior dislocation of the glenohumeral joint. J Bone Joint Surg Am 63: 1208–1217.

Vermeulen HM, Stokdijk M, Eilers PH, et al. 2002. Measurement of three dimensional shoulder movement patterns with an electromagnetic tracking device in patients with a frozen shoulder. Ann Rheum Dis 61: 115–120.

Vermeulen HM, Rozing PM, Obermann WR, et al. 2006. Comparison of high-grade and low-grade mobilization techniques in the management of adhesive capsulitis of the shoulder: randomized controlled trial. Phys Ther 86: 355–368.

Voerman GE, Vollenbroek-Hutten MM, Hermens HJ. 2006. Changes in pain, disability, and muscle activation patterns in chronic whiplash patients after ambulant myofeedback training. Clin J Pain 22: 656–663.

Wang HK, Lin JJ, Pan SL, et al. 2005. Sonographic evaluations in elite college baseball athletes. Scand J Med Sci Sports 15: 29–35.

Weerapong P, Hume PA, Kolt GS. 2004. Stretching: mechanisms and benefits for sport performance and injury prevention. Phys Ther Rev 9: 189–206.

Winters J, Sobel J, Groenier K, et al. 1997. Comparison of physiotherapy, manipulation and corticosteroid injection for treating shoulder complaints in general practice: randomised, single blind study. BMJ 314: 1320–1325.

Winters J, Jorritsma W, Groenier K, et al. 1999. Treatment of shoulder complaints in general practice: long-term results of a randomised, single blind study comparing physiotherapy, manipulation, and corticosteroid injection. BMJ 318: 1395–1396.

Wolff J. 1986. The law of bone remodelling. Berlin, New York: Springer–Verlag.

Young M, Cook J, Purdam C, et al. 2005. Eccentric decline squat protocol offers superior results at 12 months compared with traditional eccentric protocol for patellar tendinopathy in volleyball players. Br J Sports Med 39: 102–105.

Zinovieff AN. 1951. Heavy-resistance exercises: the 'Oxford technique'. Br J Phys Med 14: 129–132.

PART 5

The Hip Region in Lower Extremity Pain Syndromes

34 Hip Osteoarthritis 389
Alexis A. Wright

35 Other Hip Disorders: Muscle, Labrum and Bursa 397
John Dewitt and David Kohlrieser

36 Postoperative Management of Hip Disorders 413
Robert C. Manske and Erik Meira

37 Joint Mobilization and Manipulation of the Hip 421
Jack Miller and Wayne Hing

38 Therapeutic Exercises for the Lower Quadrant 426
Carol Kennedy and Lenerdene Levesque

Chapter 34

Hip Osteoarthritis

Alexis A. Wright

CHAPTER CONTENTS

Introduction 389
Prevalence 389
Economic impact 390
Anatomy 390
Pathomechanics 390
Diagnosis 390
Risk factors 391
Clinical presentation 392
Prognosis 392
Treatment 392
Non-pharmacological treatment 392

Introduction

Osteoarthritis (OA), or degenerative joint disease, is the most common form of arthritis, and remains one of the few chronic diseases of ageing for which there is little effective treatment (Lane 2007; Felson 2009). OA accounts for more mobility disability in the elderly than any other disease, and ranks as one of the leading sources of disability as measured by disability adjusted life years (DALYs) and years lived with disability (YLDs) in people from the United States (Michaud et al 2006; Felson 2009).

OA is characterized by joint pain and dysfunction and, in its advanced stages, joint contractures, muscle atrophy and limb deformity (Buckwalter & Martin 2006). Although pain, reduced function and participation restriction can be important consequences of OA, structural changes commonly occur without accompanying symptoms (National Institute for Health and Clinical Excellence (NICE) 2008).

Any synovial joint can develop osteoarthritis, but the knees, hips and small hand joints are the peripheral sites most commonly affected (NICE 2008). OA develops most commonly in the absence of a known cause of joint degeneration – a condition referred to as primary or idiopathic OA. Less frequently, it develops as a result of joint degeneration caused by injury or a variety of hereditary, congenital, metabolic, neuropathic, inflammatory or other medical causes – referred to as secondary OA (Buckwalter et al 2004).

Although there is no currently known cure for OA, disease-related factors such as impaired muscle strength and decreased function are potentially amenable to intervention (Fransen et al 2003). However, the frequency and chronicity of OA, coupled with the lack of effective preventive measures or cures, make this disease a substantial economic burden for patients, healthcare systems, businesses and nations (Buckwalter & Martin 2006).

Prevalence

Epidemiological research in OA faces some specific problems relative to prevalence estimates, which are primarily due to the difficulty of making a correct diagnosis given the range of signs and symptoms associated with OA. In fact, multiple definitions of OA are in existence, including radiographic OA, symptomatic OA and self-reported OA. Based on a recent systematic review (Pereira et al 2011), the overall prevalence of hip OA has been reported as 10.9%. Using only radiographic criteria, prevalence estimates ranged from 1% in China and Japan to 45% in Tasmania. Using symptomatic criteria, prevalence estimates ranged from 0.9% in Greece to 7.4% in Spain. In the United States of America (USA) alone, crude prevalence of symptomatic radiographic hip OA has been reported as in the range of 4–18% depending on age and gender (Jordan et al 2009).

The prevalence of OA increases with age and recent estimates suggest that, if the prevalence of OA remains stable, the number of older adults with arthritis or other chronic musculoskeletal joint symptoms is projected to reach 41.1 million by 2030 (Nho et al 2013). Gender prevalence rates are contradictory in the literature, however, with some studies reporting higher rates in women and others higher rates in men (Lawrence et al 2008; Dagenais et al 2009). It has recently been suggested that men have a higher prevalence of hip OA before the age of 50 years, after which women have a higher prevalence (Dagenais et al 2009). It has also been suggested that the higher incidence of hip OA in older women may be a result of hormonal changes after menopause (Dagenais et al 2009).

Economic Impact

Available approximations rank OA as a major worldwide cause of economic loss (Buckwalter et al 2004). It has been estimated that the ageing population will give rise to a higher prevalence of disabling OA, as the number of people aged over 65 years is expected to nearly double from 12.9% to 20.0% by 2030 (Croft 2005; Nho et al 2013). An ageing population, along with escalations in obesity and physical inactivity (Felson 2000; Yelin et al 2007), would increase the economic burden to society of disablement due to OA.

In the USA, the annual cost to society in medical care and lost wages attributable to arthritis and other rheumatic conditions is currently estimated at US $128 billion ($80.8 billion in direct costs and $47.0 billion in indirect costs), which is equivalent to 1.2% of the 2003 US gross domestic product (Centers for Disease Control and Prevention 2007). OA is suggested to be responsible for greater than US $65 billion of the total costs indicated (Elders 2000). Direct costs include diagnostic services, pharmacological and non-pharmacological therapies, visits to healthcare professionals, surgical interventions and the purchase of adaptive equipment (Maetzel et al 2004; Yelin et al 2007; Loza et al 2009). Indirect medical costs include compensation payments for lost labour / productivity, care seeking and care by non-professionals and family members (Loza et al 2009; Nho et al 2013). Estimated total annual disease costs are approximately $5700 per patient (US dollars fiscal year 2000) (Maetzel et al 2004). Medical costs were 30% higher among OA patients than non-arthritic controls, which highlights the increasing economic burden of OA in society (Maetzel et al 2004). Estimated costs of job-related OA are $3.4 to $13.2 billion per year (Buckwalter & Martin 2006).

Direct costs appear to account for the majority of the total cost associated with OA (Loza et al 2009). It also appears that higher total costs were associated with increasing age, increasing numbers of comorbidities, poor health-related quality of life and worsening global health status (Maetzel et al 2004; Gupta et al 2005; Yelin et al 2007; Loza et al 2009).

The ability to prevent the onset of various types of arthritis is quite limited, therefore the blunting of this growing economic impact will require cost-effective efforts to decrease mean medical expenditures and to reduce the proportion of adults who are limited in their ability to work for pay. The latter may be achieved with greater use of currently underutilized interventions, such as physiotherapy, which have been shown to reduce the disability associated with arthritis (Yelin et al 2007).

Anatomy

Osteoarthritis can be defined as a pathological disease process affecting the synovial joints that is characterized by focal areas of articular cartilage degradation followed by subsequent thickening of the subchondral bone, new bony outgrowths at joint margins (osteophytes), mild to moderate synovial inflammation and thickening of the capsule (Lane 2007; Felson 2009). Contrary to popular belief, OA is not caused by ageing and does not necessarily progress (Felson 2009). Rather, it is a metabolically active, dynamic process that involves all joint tissues (cartilage, bone, synovium / capsule, ligaments and muscles) and function. Fibrocartilage degeneration including the labrum is integral to the disease, and changes in the load-distributing function of this fibrocartilage may induce injury to adjacent hyaline cartilage (Felson 2009). This combination of tissue loss and new tissue synthesis supports the view of OA as a repair process of synovial joints (NICE 2008). A variety of joint traumas may trigger the need to repair. OA has a slow but efficient repair process that often compensates for the initial trauma, resulting in a structurally altered but symptom-free joint (NICE 2008; Felson 2009). In some people, either because of overwhelming trauma or compromised repair potential, the process cannot compensate, resulting in continuing tissue damage and eventual presentation with symptomatic OA. This explains the extreme variability in clinical presentation and outcome that can be observed between individuals (NICE 2008).

Pathomechanics

It has been proposed that OA is almost always caused by increased forces across a local area of a joint from: (1) abnormal anatomy (congenital or acquired) leading to increased focal stress, (2) excess overall load from either an acute injury or a chronic obesity, or (3) a combination of both anatomy and excess load (Felson 2013). Two examples of anatomical abnormalities associated with development of hip OA include congenital dysplasia and femoroacetabular impingement (FAI). Congenital dysplasia increases the risk of hip OA by placing increased focal stress on a small area of the acetabulum, which provides insufficient coverage of the femur. The anatomical abnormalities associated with FAI (which include cam and pincer deformities) are major risk factors predisposing to later life hip OA, suggesting mechanical abnormalities as causes of this disease.

Generally, once joint injury has occurred, a vicious cycle of joint damage follows. Typically, the area of focal stress is subjected to increased loads leading to increased cartilage damage, releasing debris into the joint space, which is ingested by the synovium causing secondary inflammation and excess fluid release (Felson 2013). This is followed by underlying bone remodelling and damage, which may create additional and more severe areas of increased stress that place the joint at risk of more damage (Felson 2013).

Diagnosis

Physicians frequently diagnose OA based on the patient's history and physical findings, which is then confirmed by radiography, as radiographs represent the current gold standard for diagnosing hip OA (Reijman et al 2004). The fundamental radiological and pathological characteristic of OA of the hip is joint space narrowing; consequently, the best radiological criterion used to detect OA of the hip is the measurement of joint space width (Reijman et al 2004).

Radiographs, though usually helpful in the diagnosis of severe hip OA, are not always beneficial in the diagnosis of mild or moderate hip OA. In patients with severe hip OA, radiographs typically show joint space narrowing, sclerosis or osteophytes; however, patients with early OA often do not show these kinds of radiographic changes (Cibulka & Threlkeld 2004). The correlation between radiographic changes and the clinical presentation of the disease varies considerably among patients (Buckwalter & Martin 2006). Some people with minimal radiographic changes have severe symptoms, whereas other people with radiographic evidence of advanced joint degeneration have minimal symptoms (Birrell et al 2005; Buckwalter & Martin 2006; Dieppe et al 2009). Changes in pain and function appear to have little relation to the trajectory of structural progression as evidenced by radiology (Felson 2009). Thus, sole reliance on radiographs to determine OA of the hip, especially in patients with early or mild hip OA, can result in false-negative diagnosis (Cibulka & Threlkeld 2004).

In addition to changes in the synovial joint, which are usually observed by plain radiographs, diagnosis of the clinical syndrome of OA requires the presence of chronic joint pain (Buckwalter & Martin 2006). Clinical criteria for the classification of patients with hip pain associated with OA were developed by the American College of Rheumatology (Altman et al 1991). Clinical diagnosis of hip OA is confirmed when patients present with either one of the following cluster of clinical findings: (1) hip pain, hip flexion less than 115° degrees, and hip internal rotation less than 15° degrees, or (2) hip pain with internal rotation of the hip, duration of morning stiffness of the hip less than or equal to 60 minutes, and age greater than 50 years (sensitivity 86%, specificity 75%) (Altman et al 1991; Cibulka & Threlkeld 2004). Cibulka et al (2009) suggested that the following clinical criteria are typically present in individuals who have radiographic findings consistent with hip OA: reports of moderate pain in the lateral or anterior hip with weight-bearing, age greater than 50 years, limited passive hip joint range of motion in at least two of six directions (flexion, extension, abduction, adduction, internal rotation and external rotation) and morning stiffness that improves in less than 1 hour.

Although clinical examination findings are often used to determine the location and irritability of a patient's symptoms, the diagnostic accuracy of several commonly used examination procedures has not been thoroughly studied for diagnosing OA of the hip in patients with hip pain (Sutlive et al 2008). The importance of identifying key clinical examination findings that are diagnostic of hip OA assists healthcare providers in initiating early management, and making referrals to appropriate providers when needed (Sutlive et al 2008). A recent study of patients with hip symptoms identified five possible clinical predictors for a diagnosis of hip OA as defined by a Kellgren and Lawrence score of ≥2: pain with squatting, a positive scour test, pain with active hip flexion, pain with active hip extension and passive range of hip internal rotation less than 25° (Sutlive et al 2008). The Kellgren and Lawrence scale is used to grade the severity of radiography-confirmed OA. A score of ≥2 would indicate at least definitive narrowing of joint space with associated osteophytes. The higher the grade (up to grade 4), the more severe is the joint space narrowing and presence of osteophytes The positive likelihood ratio (LR+) when at least three out of the five symptoms were present was found to be 5.2 (Sutlive et al 2008), which increases the probability of having hip OA from a pre-test probability of 29% (21 / 72) to a post-test probability of 68% – suggesting that clinical examination findings are capable of identifying patients with hip pain who are likely to have hip OA. Pre-test probability in this study was based on the number of patients presenting with a chief complaint of unilateral pain in the buttock, groin or anterior thigh, with corresponding radiographic confirmation of hip OA, defined as a Kellgren and Lawrence score of 2 of higher (Sutlive et al 2008).

A clinical method for detecting early OA of the hip gives the clinician an opportunity for early intervention, thus improving the chances of clinical success and potentially limiting or delaying progression. Improvement in the clinical diagnosis of hip OA may also minimize the costs associated with unnecessary radiographic procedures and, importantly, avoid the risks of radiation exposure (Sutlive et al 2008). Currently, radiographs are still considered the gold standard for proper diagnosis of hip OA. However, additional validation studies of the current clinical prediction rule for diagnosing hip OA could eventually lead to reduced costs associated with radiography if it is determined that clinical diagnosis of hip OA is sufficient for referral for early treatment management strategies, such as physiotherapy. Perhaps radiography could be spared until conservative treatment management strategies have failed, deeming surgery a viable option.

Risk factors

Osteoarthritis can be defined as a complex disorder with multiple risk factors. Such risk factors are divisible into genetic factors (genetic predisposition), constitutional factors (ageing, gender, greater bone density) and biomechanical factors (joint laxity, muscle weakness, joint malalignment, joint injury, occupational / recreational usage) (Felson 2000; NICE 2008). Age, hip developmental disorders and previous hip joint injury show the strongest evidence as risk factors for hip OA. A number of studies have demonstrated an association between developmental disorders, including Legg–Calve–Perthes disease, congenital hip dislocation, or slipped capital femoral epiphysis, and premature OA of the hip (Felson 2000; Jacobsen & Sonne-Holm 2005; Cibulka et al 2009; Novais & Millis 2012; Kim 2012). There is limited evidence suggesting that acetabular dysplasia and femoroacetabular impingement are associated with hip OA (Harris-Hayes & Royer 2011). Participation in weight-bearing sports, occupations that require prolonged standing, lifting or moving of heavy objects, major musculoskeletal injuries and vitamin D deficiency have also been identified as potential risk factors (Cooper et al 1998; Tanzer & Noiseux 2004; Lane 2007; Das & Farooqi 2008; Juhakoski et al 2009; Sulsky et al 2012). A recent systematic review with meta-analysis reported a small but significant association (relative risk (RR) 1.11; 95% CI 1.07, 1.16; $p<0.01$) between body mass index (BMI) and the development of hip OA (Jiang et al 2011). The authors found that a 5-unit increase (5 kg / m^2) in BMI was significantly associated with an 11% increased risk of hip OA (Jiang et al 2011). However, the most important and over-riding risk factor for hip OA in all populations is age (Buckwalter & Martin 2006; Cibulka et al 2009). OA of the hip primarily affects middle-aged and elderly people, most often those over 60 years (Tepper & Hochberg 1993; Buckwalter & Martin 2006; Quintana et al 2008).

Importantly, many environmental / lifestyle risk factors are modifiable (muscle weakness) or avoidable (recreational joint trauma), which has important implications for secondary and primary prevention (NICE 2008).

Clinical presentation

Clinical presentation of OA of the hip is characterized by pain, stiffness, reduced movement or function, and variable degrees of local inflammation (Hunter & Felson 2006; Juhakoski et al 2008). Most people with OA seek medical attention because of joint pain (Buckwalter & Martin 2006); the pain is often described as a deep, aching, poorly localized discomfort that has been present for years (Buckwalter & Martin 2006). Early on in disease, patients typically report a gradual onset of hip pain that is episodic, with known precipitants and self-limiting pain episodes (Lane 2007). As OA progresses, pain becomes more constant, with unanticipated episodes of sharp pain. Consistent pain tends to occur when structural disease is advanced. Progressive OA is also associated with morning stiffness, pain at rest or at night, decreased active joint movement, lower limb weakness, slower gait, reduced aerobic capacity and decreased mobility (Vogels et al 2003; Buckwalter & Martin 2006; Lane 2007; Arnold & Faulkner 2009). Existing literature has identified consistent evidence of generalized muscle strength deficit of 20% of the affected lower extremity in individuals with unilateral hip OA relative to the contralateral leg and healthy controls (Loureiro et al 2013). These various impairments can lead to diverse disabilities associated with walking, climbing stairs, getting in and out of a car, cycling, putting on shoes, and social participation (Vogels et al 2003).

Further, disability is associated with the ability to cope with pain and psychological well-being (van Baar et al 1998a). Patients suffering from painful OA are subject to psychological distress, depression, sleep disorders and possible neuropathic elements, all of which have implications for treatment. Depressive symptoms are far more common in patients with painful hip OA than was previously recognized (Felson 2009). Negative affect is hypothesized to enhance a vicious circle consisting of avoidance of pain-related activities, muscle weakness, instability of joints, pain and disability (Dekker et al 1993). Patients may feel withdrawn and express general disinterest in social activities (Dosanjh et al 2009). This is exacerbated as older patients are more likely to believe that arthritis is a natural part of growing old, that people should expect that when they get older they will not be able to walk as well, and that people should expect to live with pain as they grow older (Appelt et al 2007). These beliefs that medical conditions are a natural part of ageing are associated with decreased utilization of preventative healthcare services, which in turn impacts on functional health and longevity (Goodwin et al 1999).

Prognosis

Although physicians and patients commonly regard OA as relentlessly progressive, the disease does not necessarily follow this course (Buckwalter & Martin 2006). Some patients with hip OA experience little change in pain or function and little structural progression, whereas others note a rapid downhill course to the point where the patient is disabled within a few years of the onset of the disease (Buckwalter & Martin 2006). In contrast, some hips heal spontaneously with restoration of radiographic cartilage space and decreased pain (Guyton & Brand 2002; NICE 2008). There is limited evidence that functional status and pain in hip OA do not change during the first 3 years of follow-up (van Dijk et al 2006). However, at the individual level, considerable variation occurs. Prognostic factors for worsening of limitations in activities in patients with hip OA include avoidance of activity, reduced range of motion at 1 year, increased pain, higher comorbidity count, higher age, higher educational level, reduced range of motion at baseline, the presence of moderate to severe cardiac disease, and poor cognitive functioning (Dekker et al 2009; van Dijk et al 2010; Pisters et al 2012). A recent trial identified that higher educational level, absence of knee OA and comorbidities, supervised exercise training and habitual conditioning physical activity predicted a lower presence of pain and better functional status in patients with hip OA (Juhakoski et al 2013).

Progression of hip OA is commonly associated with migration of the femoral head in a superior–lateral direction, smaller joint space width at entry and atrophic bone response (Lievense et al 2002; Cheng et al 2010). Conflicting evidence exists for the association between progression of hip OA and older age at entry, female gender, BMI and progression of yearly mean narrowing (Lievense et al 2002; Cheng et al 2010). There is strong evidence for no relationship between BMI or weight and progression, and limited evidence for no relationship between hip dysplasia and progression of hip OA (Lievense et al 2002).

A few studies have attempted to identify variables associated with response to physical therapy interventions. Although the results are mixed, the variables of female gender, absence of depressive symptoms, history of complementary medicine use, low comorbidity count, unilateral hip pain, age ≤58 years, pain severity ≥6 / 10, 40-metre self-paced walk test ≤25.9 seconds and duration of symptoms ≤1 year have been identified as positive predictors of outcome (Weigl et al 2006; Wright et al 2011).

Treatment

Pain relief and preservation of function remain the primary treatment objectives for patients with OA of the hip. Management of OA should be administered on an individual basis and modified according to the response obtained (Hunter & Felson 2006; Bennell et al 2011; Fernandes et al 2013). A number of international clinical guidelines advocate non-pharmacological treatments as the first line of management, followed by pharmacological treatment and finally surgery (American College of Rheumatology Subcommittee on Osteoarthritis Guidelines 2000; Ottowa Panel 2005; Zhang et al 2005, 2008; NICE 2008).

Non-pharmacological treatment

A variety of interventions have been described for the treatment of hip OA with fair evidence to support the benefits of physiotherapy intervention in these patients. Recently, the European League of Associations for Rheumatology (EULAR) convened a group of experts producing an evidence-based clinical guideline for non-pharmacological management of people with hip or knee OA (Fernandes et al 2013). A combined treatment approach including the following core non-pharmacological interventions for managing patients with hip and knee OA has been recommended (Fernandes et al 2013): (1) information and education regarding OA, (2) addressing a regular individualized exercise regimen and (3) addressing weight loss if the patient is overweight or obese. Further, the UK clinical guidelines for management of hip OA recommend inclusion of manual therapy in conservative treatment programmes, which are described below (NICE 2008).

Patient education

Studies have shown the benefit of patient education in the self-management of patients with arthritis in decreasing pain, improving function, and reducing stiffness, fatigue and medication usage (Hughes et al 2004, 2006; Walsh et al 2006; Fernandes et al 2010, 2013). Education may come in the form of Hip School (Klassbo et al 2003), which highlights the need for educating patients with hip OA, especially their understanding about the importance of preserving hip range of motion and muscle function, what therapy is effective and what is not, and when surgery is likely to be indicated (Cibulka et al 2009; Bennell et al 2011). Additional educational advice should focus on activity and lifestyle changes, including both exercise and weight loss. Clinicians may want to consider behavioural change strategies such as goal setting for physical activity, weight changes and regular exercise (Fernandes et al 2010). Intervention strategies regarding education on weight loss may include strategies on reducing caloric intake through use of meal plans, reduction of fats and sugars, reduced portion sizes, and self-monitoring strategies (Fernandes et al 2010).

Exercise therapy

Typically, exercise therapy consists of a combination of range of motion / flexibility exercises, muscle strengthening exercises and aerobic conditioning / endurance exercises (Cibulka et al 2009). The goals of prescribed exercise should be individualized and agreed between the patient and the healthcare professional. In general, the goal here is to increase hip range of motion and strengthen both the hip and knee musculature so as to decrease the excess load absorbed by the joint when hip / knee musculature is weak. Treatment typically involves one to three sessions per week, for 30 minutes duration for up to 12 weeks (van Baar et al 1998b; Bennell et al 2011). One important aspect of therapy in patients with OA of the hip or knee lies in encouraging the continuation of exercise both during and after treatment (Vogels et al 2003; NICE 2008).

Many of the published articles reporting on the benefits of exercise therapy in lower extremity OA include both studies where participants have either hip or knee OA and those presenting results of joint-specific exercise specific to patients with hip OA alone. A recent systematic review with meta-analysis identified 60 trials (44 knee, 2 hip, 14 mixed) studying the effectiveness of exercise in lower limb OA (Uthman et al 2013). Based on their findings, the authors reported that there is firm evidence for a beneficial effect of exercise intervention over no exercise for both pain and function in people with lower limb OA, although a majority of the evidence was from trials in patients with knee OA. The authors also found interventions combining strengthening with flexibility and aerobic exercise to be the most effective in terms of improving both pain and function (Uthman et al 2013).

There is conflicting evidence, however, with regards the effectiveness of exercise in reducing pain and improving function and overall quality of life in people with hip OA (Hernandez-Molina et al 2008; Fransen et al 2009, 2014; McNair et al 2009). A Cochrane systematic review (Fransen et al 2009) found that, in people with hip OA, land-based exercise may reduce pain slightly but may not improve physical function. An additional systematic review (McNair et al 2009) was in agreement with these findings, suggesting there is insufficient evidence to support the use of land-based exercise therapy as a treatment for decreasing pain, improving function or enhancing quality of life in patients with OA of the hip. However, a meta-analysis by Hernandez-Molina et al (2008) reported the effectiveness of range of motion and strengthening exercises (including hydrotherapy) in patients with OA of the hip, following data extraction on patients with hip OA from trials where hip and knee OA were originally combined (Hernandez-Molina et al 2008). These authors found hip-strengthening exercises to have a beneficial effect (effect size –0.46; 95% CI –0.64, –0.28; $p<0.001$) in reducing pain and improving function in patients with hip OA (Pisters et al 2007; Hernandez-Molina et al 2008). Pisters et al (2010) further suggested that a behavioural graded activity programme consisting of gradual reintegration of activity, individualized treatments and additional booster sessions following cessation of treatment may reduce the risk for joint replacement surgery in the long term in patients with hip OA. Two additional randomized controlled trials (Abbott et al 2013; French et al 2013) further support the use of exercise therapy in improving pain, function and patient-perceived improvement amongst patients with hip OA.

Manual therapy

Manual therapy techniques are designed to improve the mobility of restricted joints, connective tissue or skeletal muscles, and are directed at influencing joint function and pain. They include mobilization, manipulation, soft tissue techniques and sustained stretches (NICE 2008; Bennell et al 2011). There is fair evidence for manual therapy for short-term and long-term treatment of hip OA to increase hip joint range of motion, improve function and reduce pain in patients with mild hip OA (Hoeksma et al 2004; MacDonald et al 2006; Cibulka et al 2009; Brantingham et al 2009; Abbott et al 2013; French et al 2013). One study reported on the benefits of manual therapy over exercise therapy in terms of general improvement, hip function and pain in some patients with mild hip OA (Hoeksma et al 2004). Specifically, following treatment the success rate of manual therapy was 81%, versus 50% for exercise therapy. Two recent randomized controlled trials reported on the benefits of manual therapy, either alone or in combination with exercise, with effects lasting up to 1 year (Abbott et al 2013; French et al 2013). In a recent

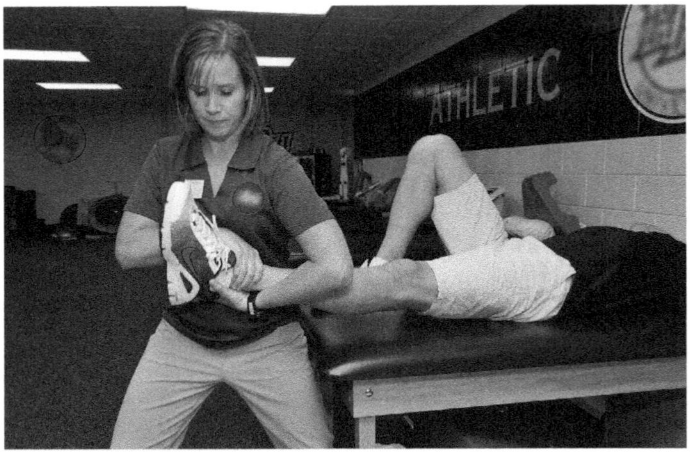

Figure 34.1 **Indirect distraction manipulation.**

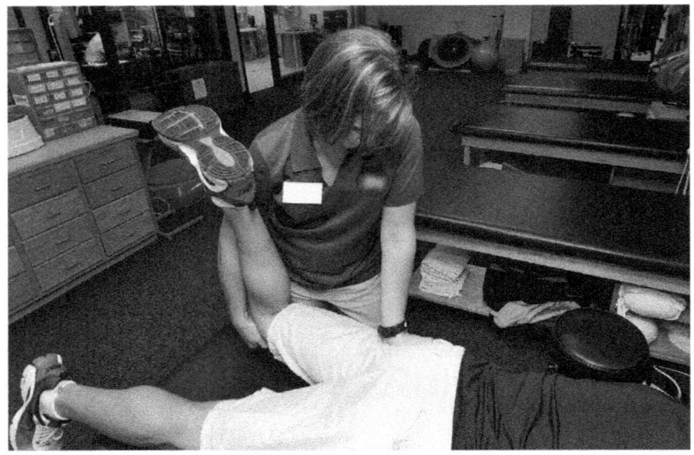

Figure 34.2 **Posterior-to-anterior mobilization of the hip.**

randomized controlled trial (Abbott et al 2013), manual therapy demonstrated the greatest benefit, compared with exercise therapy or a combination of exercise therapy and manual therapy, over usual care in terms of pain and function as reported by the Western Ontario and McMaster Osteoarthritis Index (WOMAC). Specifically, WOMAC scores improved by 22.9 points (170-point scale) in the manual therapy only group as compared with 12.4 points and 7.9 points for the exercise therapy and combined treatment group respectively (Abbott et al 2013). Benefits were seen at the 9-week follow-up and were maintained to 6 months and 1 year. In another recent randomized controlled trial (French et al 2013), improvements in hip function, hip range of motion and patient-perceived change were noted in both the exercise alone group and exercise plus manual therapy group, with higher patient satisfaction with outcome reported by the exercise plus manual therapy group. Given these results, manual therapy has been recommended to provide both short-term and long-term pain relief, and to improve hip mobility and function in patients with hip OA; however, the grade of recommendation remains moderate given that currently only a few high-quality randomized controlled trials (Hoeksma et al 2004; Abbott et al 2013; French et al 2013) support the recommendation. Here we describe some hip mobilization techniques commonly applied on patients with hip OA. (See Ch 37 for further manual therapies targeted to the hip joint.)

Indirect distraction manipulation (Fig. 34.1)

This technique is performed in supine. The clinician cradles the patient's ankle in both hands, and then takes up the slack to pre-position the patient's hip ready for the targeted motion – generally, the resting position of the hip includes a moderate degree of hip flexion and abduction with slight external rotation. The clinician then provides an inferior force while holding the ankle.

Posterior-to-anterior mobilization of the hip (Fig. 34.2)

The patient assumes a prone position. The clinician positions the hip in a neutral position. The clinician then passively glides the hip joint in a posterior–anterior direction using the heel of the hand.

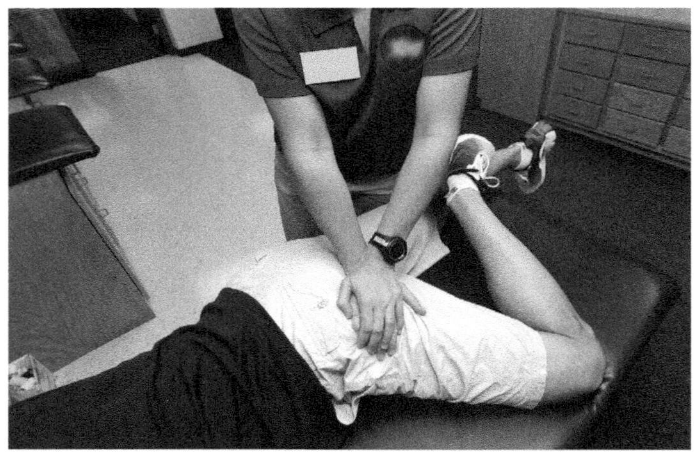

Figure 34.3 **Posterior-to-anterior mobilization in a 'figure 4' position.**

Posterior-to-anterior mobilization – 'figure 4' position (Fig. 34.3)

This technique is a modification of the posterior-to-anterior glide mobilization. The patient assumes a prone position with pre-positioning including flexion, abduction and external rotation of the hip. The clinician then applies a passive glide of the hip joint using the heel of the hand to apply the force in a posterior–anterior direction.

References

Abbott JH, Robertson MC, Chapple C, et al. 2013. Manual therapy, exercise therapy, or both, in addition to usual care, for osteoarthritis of the hip or knee: a randomized controlled trial. 1: clinical effectiveness. Osteoarthritis Cartilage 21: 525–534.

Altman R, Alarcon G, Appelrouth D, et al. 1991. The American College of Rheumatology criteria for the classification and reporting of osteoarthritis of the hip. Arthritis Rheum 34:505–514.

American College of Rheumatology Subcommittee on Osteoarthritis Guidelines. 2000. Recommendations for the medical management of osteoarthritis of the hip and knee. Arthritis Rheum 43: 1905–1915.

Appelt C, Burant CJ, Siminoff LA, et al. 2007. Arthritis-specific health beliefs related to aging among older male patients with knee and / or hip osteoarthritis. J Gerontol 62A: 184–190.

Arnold CM, Faulkner RA. 2009. Does falls-efficacy predict balance performance in older adults with hip osteoarthritis. J Gerontol Nurs 35: 45–52.

Bennell KL, Egerton T, Pua YH, et al. 2011. Building the rationale and structure for a complex physical therapy intervention within the context of a clinical trial: a multimodal individualized treatment for patients with hip osteoarthritis. Phys Ther 91: 1525–1541

Birrell F, Lunt M, Macfarlane G, et al. 2005. Association between pain in the hip region and radiographic changes of osteoarthritis: results from a population-based study. Rheumatology 44: 337–341

Brantingham JW, Globe G, Pollard H, et al. 2009. Manipulative therapy for lower extremity conditions: expansion of literature review. J Manipulative Physiol Ther 32: 53–71.

Buckwalter JA, Martin JA. 2006. Osteoarthritis. Adv Drug Deliv Rev 58(2): 150–167.

Buckwalter JA, Saltzman C, Brown T. 2004. The impact of osteoarthritis. Clin Orthop Relat Res 427S:S6–S15.

Centers for Disease Control and Prevention. 2007. National and state medical expenditures and lost earnings attributable to arthritis and other rheumatic conditions – United States, 2003. MMWR 56: 4–7.

Cheng PP, Gossec L, Dougados M. 2010. What are the best markers for disease progression in osteoarthritis (OA)? Best Pract Res Clin Rheumatol 24: 81–92.

Cibulka MT, Threlkeld J. 2004. The early clinical diagnosis of osteoarthritis of the hip. J Orthop Sports Phys Ther 34: 461–467.

Cibulka MT, White D M, Woehrle J, et al. 2009 Hip pain and mobility deficits – hip osteoarthritis. Clinical practice guidelines linked to the international classification of functioning, disability, and health from the othopaedic section of the American Physical Therapy Association. J Orthop Sports Phys Ther 39: A1–A25.

Cooper C. Inskip H, Croft P, et al. 1998. Individual risk factors for hip osteoarthritis: obesity, hip injury, and physical activity. Am J Epidemiol 147: 516–522.

Croft P. 2005. The epidemiology of osteoarthritis: Manchester and beyond. Rheumatology 44S: iv27–iv32.

Dagenais S, Garbedian S, Wai EK. 2009. Systematic review of the prevalence of radiographic primary hip osteoarthritis. Clin Orthop Relat Res 467: 623–637.

Das SK, Farooqi A. 2008. Osteoarthritis. Best Pract Res Clin Rheumatol 22: 657–675.

Dekker J, Tola P, Aufdemkampe G, et al. 1993. Negative affect, pain and disability in osteoarthritis patients: the mediating role of muscle weakness. Behav Res Ther 31: 203–206.

Dekker J, Van Dijk GM, Veenhof C. 2009. Risk factors for functional decline in osteoarthritis of the hip or knee. Curr Opin Rheumatol 21: 520–524.

Dieppe P, Judge A, William S, et al. 2009. Variations in the pre-operative status of patients coming to primary hip replacement for osteoarthritis in European orthopaedic centres. BMC Musculoskelet Disord 10:19. doi: 10.1186/1471-2474-10-19.

Dosanjh S, Matta JM, Bhandari M, for the Anterior Tha Research Collaborative (Athac). 2009. The final straw: a qualitative study to explore patient decisions to undergo total hip arthroplasty. Arch Orthop Trauma Surg 129: 719–727.

Elders MJ. 2000. The increasing impact of arthritis on public health. J Rheumatol Suppl 60: 6–8.

Felson DT. 2000. Osteoarthritis: new insights. Ann Intern Med 133: 635–646.

Felson DT. 2009. Developments in the clinical understanding of osteoarthritis. Arthritis Res Ther 11: 203.

Felson DT. 2013. Osteoarthritis as a disease of mechanics. Osteoarthritis Cartilage 21: 10–15.

Fernandes L, Storheim K, Sandvik L, et al. 2010. Efficacy of patient education and supervised exercise vs patient education alone in patients with hip osteoarthritis: a single blind randomized clinical trial. Osteoarthritis Cartilage 18: 1237–1243.

Fernandes L, Hagen KB, Bijlsma J, et al. 2013. EULAR recommendations for the non-pharmacological core management of hip and knee osteoarthritis. Ann Rheum Dis 72: 1125–1135.

Fransen M, Mcconnell S, Bell M. 2003. Exercise for osteoarthritis of the hip or knee. Cochrane Database Syst Rev 3: CD004286.

Fransen M, Mcconnell S, Hernandez-Molina G, et al. 2009. Exercise for osteoarthritis of the hip. Cochrane Database Syst Rev 3: CD007912. doi: 10.1002/14651858.CD007912.

Fransen M, Mcconnell S, Hernandez-Molina G, et al. 2014. Exercise for osteoarthritis of the hip. Cochrane Database Syst Rev 4: CD007912. doi: 10.1002/14651858.CD007912.pub2.

French HP, Cusack T, Brennan A, et al. 2013. Exercise and manual physiotherapy arthritis research trial (EMPART) for osteoarthritis of the hip: a multicenter randomized controlled trial. Arch Phys Med Rehabil 94: 302–314.

Goodwin JS, Black SA, Satish S. 1999. Aging versus disease: the opinions of older black, Hispanic, and non-Hispanic white Americans about the causes and treatment of common medical conditions. J Am Geriatr Soc 47: 973–979.

Gupta S, Hawker GA, Laporte A, et al. 2005. The economic burden of disabling hip and knee osteoarthritis (OA) from the perspective of individuals living with this condition. Rheumatology 44: 1531–1537.

Guyton GP, Brand RA. 2002. Apparent spontaneous joint restoration in hip osteoarthritis. Clin Orthop Relat Res 44: 302–307.

Harris-Hayes M, Royer NK. 2011. Relationship of acetabular dysplasia and femoroacetabular impingement to hip osteoarthritis: a focused review. PM R 3: 1055–1067.

Hernandez-Molina G, Reichenback S, Zhang B, et al. 2008. Effect of therapeutic exercise for hip osteoarthritis pain: results of a meta-analysis. Arthritis Rheum 59: 1221–1228.

Hoeksma HL, Dekker J, Ronday HK, et al. 2004. Comparison of manual therapy and exercise therapy in osteoarthritis of the hip: a randomized clinical trial. Arthritis Rheum 51: 722–729.

Hughes SL, Seymour RB, Campbell R, et al. 2004. Impact of the fit and strong intervention on older adults with osteoarthritis. Gerontologist 44: 217–228.

Hughes SL, Seymour RB, Campbell RT, et al. 2006. Long-term impact of Fit and Strong! on older adults with osteoarthritis. Gerontologist 46: 801–814.

Hunter DJ, Felson D. 2006. Osteoarthritis. BMJ 332: 639–642.

Jacobsen S, Sonne-Holm S. 2005. Hip dysplasia: a significant risk factor for the development of hip osteoarthritis. A cross-sectional survey. Rheumatology (Oxford) 44: 211–218.

Jiang L, Rong J, Wang Y, et al. 2011. The relationship between body mass index and hip osteoarthritis: a systematic review and meta-analysis. Joint Bone Spine 78: 150–155.

Jordan JM, Helmick CG, Renner JB, et al. 2009. Prevalence of hip symptoms and radiographic and symptomatic hip osteoarthritis in African Americans and Caucasians: the Johnston County Osteoarthritis Project. J Rheumatol 36: 809–815.

Juhakoski R, Tenhonen S, Anttonen T, et al. 2008. Factors affecting self reported pain and physical function in patients with hip osteoarthritis. Arch Phys Med Rehabil 89: 1066–1073.

Juhakoski R, Heliovaara M, Impivaara O, et al. 2009. Risk factors for the development of hip osteoarthritis: a population-based prospective study. Rheumatology 48: 83–87.

Juhakoski R, Malmivaara A, Lakka TA, et al. 2013. Determinants of pain and functioning in hip osteoarthritis – a two-year prospective study. Clin Rehabil 27: 281–287.

Kim, HK. 2012. Pathophysiology and new strategies for the treatment of Legg–Calve–Perthes disease. J Bone Joint Surg Am 94: 659–669.

Klassbo M, Larsson G, Harms-Ringdahl K. 2003. Promising outcome of a hip school for patients with hip dysfunction. Arthritis Rheum 49: 321–327.

Lane NE. 2007. Osteoarthritis of the hip. N Engl J Med 357: 1413–1421.

Lawrence RC, Felson DT, Helmick CG, et al. 2008. Estimates of the prevalance of arthritis and other rheumatic conditions in the United States. Part II. Arthritis Rheum 58: 26–35.

Lievense AM, Bierma-Zeinstra SM, Verhagen AP, et al. 2002. Prognostic factors of progress of hip osteoarthritis: a systematic review. Arthritis Rheum 47: 556–562.

Loureiro A, Mills PM, Barrett RS. 2013. Muscle weakness in hip osteoarthritis: a systematic review. Arthritis Care Res 65: 340–352.

Loza E, Lopez-Gomez JM, Abasolo L, et al.; the Artrocad Study Group. 2009. Economic burden of knee and hip osteoarthritis in Spain. Arthritis Rheum 61: 158–165.

MacDonald CW, Whitman JM, Cleland JA, et al. 2006. Clinical outcomes following manual physical therapy and exercise for hip osteoarthritis: a case series. J Orthop Sports Phys Ther 36: 588–599.

Maetzel A, Li LC, Pencharz J, et al; Community Hypertension and Arthritis Project Study Team. 2004. The economic burden associated with osteoarthritis, rheumatoid arthritis, and hypertension: a comparative study. Ann Rheum Dis 63: 395–401.

McNair PJ, Simmonds MA, Boocock MG, et al. 2009. Exercise therapy for the management of osteoarthritis of the hip joint: a systematic review. Arthritis Res Ther 11: R98.

Michaud CM, Mckenna MT, Begg SJ, et al. 2006. The burden of disease and injury in the United States 1996. Popul Health Metr 4: 11.

National Institute for Health and Clinical Excellence (NICE). 2008. Osteoarthritis: the care and management of osteoarthritis in adults. London: NICE. Online. Available: http://www.nice.org.uk/guidance/CG59. Accessed 20 Nov 2014.

Nho SJ, Kymes SM, Callaghan JJ, et al. 2013. The burden of hip osteoarthritis in the United States: epidemiologic and economic considerations. J Am Acad Orthop Surg 21: S1–S6.

Novais EN, Millis MB. 2012. Slipped capital femoral epiphysis: prevalence, pathogenesis, and natural history. Clin Orthop Relat Res 470: 3432–3438.

Ottowa Panel. 2005. Ottawa Panel evidence-based clinical practice guidelines for therapeutic exercises and manual therapy in the management of osteoarthritis. Phys Ther 85: 907–971.

Pereira D, Peleteiro B, Araujo J, et al. 2011. The effect of osteoarthritis definition on prevalence and incidence estimates: a systematic review. Osteoarthritis Cartilage 19: 1270–1285.

Pisters MF, Veenhof C, Van Meeteren NLU, et al. 2007. Long-term effectiveness of exercise therapy in patients with osteoarthritis of the hip or knee: a systematic review. Arthritis Rheum 57: 1245–1253.

Pisters MF, Veenhof C, Schellevis FG, et al. 2010. Long-term effectiveness of exercise therapy in patients with osteoarthritis of the hip or knee: a randomized controlled trial comparing two different physical therapy interventions. Osteoarthritis Cartilage 18: 1019–1026.

Pisters MF, Veenhof C, Van Dijk GM, et al. 2012. The course of limitations in activities over 5 years in patients with knee and hip osteoarthritis with moderate functional limitations: risk factors for future functional decline. Osteoarthritis Cartilage 20: 503–510.

Quintana JM, Arostegui I, Escobar A, et al. 2008. Prevalence of knee and hip osteoarthritis and the appropriateness of joint replacement in an older population. Arch Intern Med 168: 1576–1584.

Reijman M, Hazes JM, Koes BW, et al. 2004. Validity, reliability, and applicability of seven definitions of hip osteoarthritis used in epidemiological studies: a systematic appraisal. J Orthop Sports Phys Ther 63: 226–232.

Sulsky SI, Carlton L, Bochmann F, et al. 2012. Epidemiological evidence for work load as a risk factor for osteoarthritis of the hip: a systematic review. PLoS ONE 7: e31521.

Sutlive TG, Lopez HP, Schnitker DE, et al. 2008. Development of a clinical prediction rule for diagnosing hip osteoarthritis in individuals with unilateral hip pain. J Orthop Sports Phys Ther 38: 542–550.

Tanzer M, Noiseux N. 2004. Osseous abnormalities and early osteoarthritis: the role of hip impingement. Clin Orthop Relat Res (429): 170–177.

Tepper S, Hochberg M. 1993. Factors associated with hip osteoarthritis: data from the first national health and nutrition examination survey (NHANES-I). Am J Epidemiol 137: 1087–1088.

Uthman OA, Van Der Windt DA, Jordan JL, et al. 2013. Exericse for lower limb osteoarthritis: systematic review incorporating trial sequential analysis and network meta-analysis. BMJ 347: f5555.

Van Baar ME, Dekker J, Lemmens JA, et al. 1998a. Pain and disability in patients with osteoarthritis of hip or knee: the relationship with articular, kinesiological, and psychological characteristics. J Rheumatol 25: 125–133.

Van Baar ME, Dekker J, Oostendorp RA, et al. 1998b. The effectiveness of exercise therapy in patients with osteoarthritis of the hip or knee: a randomized clinical trial. J Rheumatol 25: 2432–2439.

Van Dijk GM, Dekker J, Veenhof C, et al. 2006. Course of functional status and pain in osteoarthritis of the hip or knee: a systematic review of the literature. Arthritis Rheum 55: 779–785.

Van Dijk GM, Veenhof C, Spreeuwenberg MA, et al. 2010. Prognosis of limitations in activities in osteoarthritis of the hip or knee: a 3 year cohort study. Arch Phys Med Rehabil 91: 58–66.

Vogels EM, Hendriks HJ, Van Baar ME, et al. 2003. KNGF–clinical practice guidelines for physical therapy in patients with osteoarthritis of the hip or knee. Royal Dutch Society for Physical Therapy V-06. Online. Available: http://www.ifompt.com/site/ifompt/files/pdf/Osteoarthr.H-K.Gln.pdf. Accessed 20 Nov 2014.

Walsh NE, Mitchell HL, Reeves BC, et al. 2006. Integrated exercise and self management programmes in osteoarthritis of the hip and knee: a systematic review of effectiveness. Phys Ther Rev 11: 289–297.

Weigl M, Angst F, Aeschlimann A, et al. 2006. Predictors for response to rehabilitation in patients with hip or knee osteoarthritis: a comparison of logistic regression models with three different definitions of responder. Osteoarthritis Cartilage 14: 641–651.

Wright AA, Cook CE, Flynn TW, et al. 2011. Predictors of response to physical therapy intervention in patients with primary hip osteoarthritis. Phys Ther 91: 510–524.

Yelin E, Murphy L, Cisternas MG, et al. 2007. Medical care expenditures and earnings losses among persons with arthritis and other rheumatic conditions in 2003, and comparisons with 1997. Arthritis Rheum 56: 1397–1407.

Zhang W, Doherty M, Arden N, et al. 2005. EULAR evidence based recommendations for the management of hip osteoarthritis: report of task force of the EULAR standing committee for international clinical studies including therapeutics (ESCISIT). Ann Rheum Dis 64: 669–681.

Zhang W, Moskowitz RW, Nuki G, et al. 2008. OARSI recommendations for the management of hip and knee osteoarthritis. Part II: OARSI evidence-based, expert consensus guidelines. Osteoarthritis Cartilage 16: 137–162.

Chapter 35

Other Hip Disorders: Muscle, Labrum and Bursa

John Dewitt, David Kohlrieser

CHAPTER CONTENTS

Introduction 397
Iliotibial band syndrome 397
- Epidemiology 397
- Pathomechanics 397
- Diagnosis and clinical examination 398
- Manual therapy treatment 398
- Prognosis 399
- Summary 399

Hip flexor tendinopathy (internal snapping hip syndrome) 400
- Epidemiology 400
- Pathomechanics 400
- Diagnosis and clinical examination 400
- Treatment 400
- Prognosis 401
- Summary 401

Gluteus medius tendinopathy 401
- Epidemiology 401
- Pathomechanics 401
- Patient history 402
- Diagnosis and clinical examination 402
- Treatment 403
- Prognosis 404
- Summary 405

Adductor tendinopathy 405
- Epidemiology 405
- Pathomechanics 405
- Patient history 405
- Diagnosis 406
- Treatment 406
- Summary 407

Sports hernia 407
- Epidemiology 407
- Pathomechanics 408
- Diagnosis and clinical examination 408
- Treatment 409
- Prognosis 409
- Summary 409

Conclusion 409

Introduction

Pain and discomfort experienced around the hip joint can be referred from many extra-articular structures. The anatomical and biomechanical complexity of this region can pose a significant challenge to professionals in diagnosing and treating these pathologies effectively owing to overlapping symptoms or coexisting conditions. Extra-articular disorders can produce significant pain and disability, making a prompt and accurate diagnosis imperative. Knowledge of best practice improves treatment efficiency and patient quality of life.

Iliotibial Band Syndrome

Epidemiology

Iliotibial band syndrome (ITBS) is a common knee injury in athletes. The most commonly reported symptom is lateral knee pain due to inflammation of the distal aspect of the iliotibial band (ITB). The ITB is a thick fascia band that crosses both the hip and knee joints. In some athletes, the repetitive movement of the knee produces inflammation resulting in pain (Khaund & Flynn 2005). ITBS is more common in endurance athletes and is the most common running injury occurring at the lateral knee, with reported incidence rates between 1.6% and 12% (Lavine 2010). In cyclists, ITBS has been reported as accounting for 15% of all overuse injuries at the knee (Holmes et al 1993; Lavine 2010). It therefore is important for medical professionals treating these individuals to understand the risk factors, pathomechanics and most effective / efficient treatment practices related to this condition.

Pathomechanics

Injury is thought to occur from excessive friction between the ITB and lateral femoral condyle as the knee is flexed beyond 30° (Fredericson & Wolf 2005). There is some debate over whether the symptoms are from friction or compression of structures around the lateral femoral condyle. Anatomical studies support the idea that the ITB is not a separate band, but rather a thickening of the lateral fascia firmly connected to the linea aspera (Fairclough et al 2007), and it has been proposed that the perception of ITB movement is due to repetitive cycles of tightening, which causes repetitive compression on the tissues deep to the ITB (Lavine 2010).

Both intrinsic and extrinsic factors have been identified that may be associated with development of ITBS. Anatomical factors, including tightness of the ITB–TFL (tensor fascia lata) complex, hip abductor weakness, increased Q-angle, leg length differences, and altered knee, hindfoot and forefoot alignment have been associated with increased risk of ITBS. These factors are theorized to increase strain or friction at the distal ITB and femoral condyle during repetitive activities (Fredericson & Wolf 2005; Baker et al 2011; Saikia & Tepe 2012).

Strength deficits throughout the hip abductor complex can also have a role in development of this condition. Weakness of this muscle group results in contralateral pelvic drop, increased ipsilateral hip adduction and internal rotation, which potentially increase the strain on the ITB. Fredericson et al (2000a, 2000b) found that individuals who completed a gluteal-strengthening programme not only increased their hip abduction strength, but also reported decreased pain and improved ability to return to activity. Runners with ITBS had decreased hip abductor strength in their affected lower extremity compared with their uninvolved lower extremity and with a control group (Fredericson et al 2000a). In another study (Fredericson & Weir 2006), 50 marathon runners were evaluated at the beginning of their training programme and it was found that those 7 runners who developed ITBS had increased peak hip adduction compared with the uninjured runners; the increased hip adduction range of motion during stance phase was theorized to occur from decreased hip abductor strength and the decreased eccentric control of this motion.

The alignment of the lower extremity and / or weakness of the abductor complex may predispose the individual to developing ITBS. A Trendelenburg gait pattern may lead to excessive tension through the lateral hip and ITB, due to increased varus torque at the knee region (Baker et al 2011). A second observable movement pattern that may increase stress through the ITB is a contralateral pelvic drop with increased femoral adduction and valgus positioning at the knee of the stance leg (Baker et al 2011).

Patients affected by ITBS report sharp and occasionally burning pain localized to the lateral aspect of the knee. The majority of these patients are active and involved in endurance sports such as running and / or cycling (Barber & Sutker 1992; Fredericson & Wolf 2005). Several training factors associated with ITBS include always running in one direction on a track, increased weekly mileage, and routes that include downhill running. Downhill running places an individual at risk for developing ITBS due to decreased knee flexion at foot strike, which increases friction between the distal iliotibial band and lateral femoral condyle (Linderburg et al 1984; Barber & Sutker 1992; Fredericson & Wolf 2005).

Diagnosis and clinical examination

Patients may exhibit occasional swelling and localized tenderness along the distal ITB. Palpable tenderness is localized to an area 2–3 cm proximal to lateral joint line. This is the region where the ITB moves directly over, or produces compression at, the lateral femoral condyle with flexion and extension of the knee joint. If present, pitting oedema and complaints of snapping are localized to this area (Fredericson & Wolf 2005). Pain and / or paraesthesia is also localized in this area, but less commonly can extend along the length of the ITB (Fredericson & Wolf 2005).

The clinician should assess the presence of any myofascial restrictions and / or trigger points. Trigger points may be the cause or the result of the ITBS and are typically found in the vastus lateralis, gluteus minimus, piriformis and distal biceps femoris muscles (Fredricson et al 2000a; Fredericson & Wolf 2005).

Pes planus deformity can contribute to the development of ITBS from increasing strain on ITBS due to increased internal rotation of the lower leg and thigh. This fault may exaggerate the effects of gluteal muscle weakness, leading to excessive adduction and internal rotation of the lower extremity during single-leg activities (Fredericson & Wolf 2005; Bauer & Duke 2012). If any asymmetries are identified between anatomical landmarks at the pelvis or lower extremities, the examiner must rule out a leg length discrepancy.

Extensibility of the gastrocnemius / soleus complex must be assessed, as tightness throughout this complex can cause decreased ankle dorsiflexion, which produces increased knee flexion and ankle pronation during running or closed kinetic chain activities (Baker et al 2011). The modified Thomas test and Ober test are included to determine tightness of the anterior and lateral hip muscles.

Further special testing should include the Noble compression test, which is used determine whether the pain associated with ITBS can be reproduced proximal to the lateral femoral condyle (Magee 2002; Fredericson & Weir 2006). Unfortunately none of these tests have been examined for their diagnostic utility in identifying ITBS. Strength testing of the hip musculature should also be performed.

The Trendelenburg test is performed by having the patient stand on one leg while the opposite foot is lifted off the ground. Once the patient is balanced he / she is asked to hike the non-stance pelvis as high as possible. This position is then maintained for 30 seconds. A test is considered positive if the patient is unable to assume the start position or the pelvis begins to drop; this indicates weakness of the hip abductors on the stance limb (Hardcastle & Nade 1985; Youdas et al 2007). Any increased lateral trunk flexion, contralateral pelvic drop, or increased knee valgus or ankle / foot pronation could indicate decreased functional hip and core strength and so predispose the athlete to injury (Youdas et al 2007; Hollman et al 2009; Baker et al 2011).

It is recommended that further functional testing (e.g. a step-down test, an anterior ipsilateral reach test and a frontal plane overhead reach test) be included in the evaluation of an individual with symptoms consistent with ITBS. Functional tests such as the forward step-down test may identify weakness or compensatory patterns that the patient is able to see and understand (Baker et al 2011).

Manual therapy treatment

Fredericson and Wolf (2005) recommended dividing the rehabilitation programme into phases, consisting of acute, subacute, recovery and strengthening, and finally return to running phases. The goal of the acute phase is to reduce the inflammation that is creating pain and symptoms at the distal ITB (Fredericson & Wolf 2005). The use of oral non-steroidal anti-inflammatory drugs (NSAIDs), soft tissue mobilization, and stretching is recommended in the acute phase of injury and treatment (Fredericson & Wolf 2005; Baker et al 2011). The use of ice massage has also been found to be beneficial in this early period of injury and recovery (Fredericson & Wolf 2005). The most important aspect of the acute phase of management is patient education and activity modification. Without avoidance or significant reduction in the volume of aggravating activities, measures to decrease pain and inflammation will be ineffective. The patient should be recommended to exercise below the repeatable time that provokes symptoms. In more severe cases, it is recommended that the only exercise an athlete may perform is swimming. A local corticosteroid injection is recommended if visible swelling remains after 3 days and is not responding to physical therapy, other modalities and NSAIDs (Fredericson & Wolf 2005; Baker et al 2011). However, no studies to date have examined the effectiveness of this approach in a population of patients with ITBS.

As the acute inflammation and pain resolve, the athlete should be progressed into the subacute phase. The goals of this phase are to improve flexibility throughout the ITB–TFL complex, allowing athletes to perform strengthening exercises without exacerbation of symptoms (Fredericson & Wolf 2005; Baker et al 2011). Various studies recommend using standing ITB stretches (Fredericson et al 2002; Fredericson & Wolf 2005). The clinician should also address any myofascial restrictions and / or trigger points at the lateral hip or thigh. Contractures, adhesions or trigger points should be addressed before initiating strengthening exercises. There are a variety of treatment techniques that can be used to target restrictions (see Chs 59–63). In fact, a combination of soft tissue techniques with isolated stretching and a foam roll has been recommended (Fredericson & Weir 2006).

The recovery or strengthening phase should be initiated once myofascial restrictions have been addressed and normal flexibility has been established (Fredericson & Weir 2006; Baker et al 2011). The goal of the strengthening phase is to improve the gluteus medius and maximus strength in order to increase dynamic control of the lower extremity during functional activities (Baker et al 2011). All strengthening exercises should be pain free and the volume of progressive resistance exercises should be progressed from 5–8 repetitions of each up to 2–3 sets of 8–15 repetitions. Exercises should be performed bilaterally, even if the patient is symptomatic only on one leg (Fredericson & Wolf 2005; Fredericson & Weir 2006). A hip abductor strengthening programme, progressing from open chain side-lying leg lifts to closed chain single-leg forward step-downs and lateral pelvic drop exercises, allowed 22 of 24 runners with ITBS to return to their previous activity levels after 6 months (Fredericson et al 2000a). Beneficial results have been reported from the inclusion of triplanar and functional movements into the rehabilitation programmes so as to place greater eccentric demands on the gluteal musculature (Fredericson & Weir 2006). A recent EMG study (Selkowitz et al 2013) has provided direction to gluteal strengthening programmes; 11 exercises were compared and the results supported the inclusion of unilateral and bilateral bridges, quadruped hip extension with knee flexed and extended, clamshells, side-stepping with band, and squats in a gluteal strengthening exercise programme. (See Ch 38 for further detail on muscle strengthening of the lower extremity musculature.)

The return to sport participation is initiated once the athlete can perform all the above exercises without pain and with proper technique and form. The clinician should ensure that the athlete has full range of motion, normalized and symmetrical gluteal muscle strength, and normalized flexibility. It is recommended that there is a negative Noble compression test prior to attempting any return to sport activities. Runners and cyclists should be educated to return to training every other day and only on level ground. They should increase the distance and frequency of training incrementally while monitoring for any signs or symptoms of ITBS (Fredericson & Wolf 2005; Baker et al 2011). Athletes should run no more than every other day during the first week of their return to running progression, and should be instructed to begin with easy sprints on level ground while avoiding any downhill running during the first couple of weeks. Faster paced running has been shown to increase the knee flexion angle beyond the zone of impingement at foot strike, which decreases the chance of re-injury. The athlete is then counselled to increase the distance and frequency of running gradually over the next 3–4 weeks. It has been reported that the majority of patients are able to return to their previous level of activity at 6 weeks (Fredericson & Weir 2006).

Prognosis

If an athlete is willing to modify the training routine and has addressed the factors associated with ITBS, a full return to sport participation is likely. The majority of athletes with ITBS are able to return to running or playing sports after following a structured rehabilitation plan (Fredericson & Weir 2006). Fredericson et al (2000a) provided evidence to support an athlete's ability to return to previous level of activity within 6 months after completing a gluteal-muscle-strengthening programme.

Summary

The diagnosis of ITBS is usually based on the history and clinical exam. A thorough musculoskeletal exam is included to identify any impairment that may be contributing to symptoms (Fredericson & Weir 2006). Overall, the literature supports conservative management of ITBS in runners, including anti-inflammatory medication, corticosteroid injection, stretching, gluteal-muscle-strengthening exercises and patient education about training parameters (Van der Worp et al 2012). Many factors associated with training programmes, such as downhill running, running on a track and rapid increase in mileage, may predispose an athlete to injury and should be addressed. A structured rehabilitation programme broken up into phases is recommended. The majority of patients are able to return to previous level of activity with conservative management alone. In rare, unresponsive or recurring cases surgery may be considered (Fredericson & Weir 2006).

Hip Flexor Tendinopathy (Internal Snapping Hip Syndrome)

Epidemiology

The iliopsoas muscle will often create mechanical snapping sensations, which are referred to as 'internal' snapping hip syndrome. Symptoms may range from a non-painful annoyance to pain and snapping. Non-painful snapping hip syndrome occurs in approximately 5–10% of the population; however, this proportion may increase in populations of athletes who must make excessive hip motions (Teitz et al 1997; Byrd 2005). Snapping hip syndrome has been reported in athletic populations including soccer players, weightlifters and runners (Keskula et al 1999; Gruen et al 2002; Konczak & Ames 2005). Females tend to be at higher risk for snapping hip syndrome, with reports ranging from 62% to 86%, which may be attributed to the greater frequency of associated labral pathology (Pelsser et al 2001; Hoskins et al 2004; Lewis 2010). Snapping hip syndrome seems to have the greatest frequency within the elite ballet community; a study by Winston et al (2007) reported a prevalence of as high as 90% in professional ballet dancers, with most complaining of bilateral symptoms. Voluntary reproduction of snapping was found in 60% of confirmed cases, with the majority stemming from the iliopsoas tendon (Winston et al 2007).

Pathomechanics

Internal snapping hip syndrome is attributed to the iliopsoas tendon subluxing over two common bony landmarks as it crosses the anterior hip: the femoral head / joint capsule and the iliopectineal eminence (Byrd 2005). Snapping typically occurs with hip motion from a flexed, abducted and externally rotation position into extension, adduction and internal rotation. The snapping is often audible and can be reproducible voluntarily (Winston et al 2007). An alternative soft tissue theory has been described, which suggests that the iliopsoas tendon actually flips around the iliacus muscle as the hip is moved from an abducted, flexed and externally rotated position to neutral (Fig. 35.1) (Deslandes et al 2008). An imaging study by Deslandes et al (2008) identified this 'flipping' phenomenon in 14 of 18 snapping hip syndrome cases, while the remaining four were due to a bifid iliopsoas. Other less common causes include one part of a bifid iliopsoas tendon head flipping over the other, as far as well over a paralabral cyst (Deslandes et al 2008), stenosing tenosynovitis of the iliopsoas insertion (Micheli 1983) and a bony ridge at the lesser tubercle (Schaberg et al 1984).

Acute inflammation and chronic degeneration associated with tendinopathy will often cause pain during resisted hip flexion; however, this is not a consistent finding (Winston et al 2007; Tibor & Sekiya 2008). Patients typically report difficulty in standing from a seated position, running, cycling or getting into and out of a car (Taylor & Clarke 1995; Keskula et al 1999; Gruen et al 2002; Little & Mansoor 2008).

Diagnosis and clinical examination

Reproduction of iliopsoas snapping is commonly performed when the leg is brought into extension from a flexed, abducted and externally rotated position (FABER) (Gruen et al 2002; Hoskins et al 2004; Wahl et al 2004). Subluxation of the iliopsoas at the iliopectineal eminence can often be felt and reduced with manual pressure applied during the movement so as to prevent the lateral to medial movement (Gruen et al 2002). Although the diagnostic accuracy of special tests has not been reported, Winston et al (2007) reported snapping in 24% of ballet dancers moving in extension from a FABER position; interestingly, these patients were able to sublux the iliopsoas voluntarily more than 90% of the time.

Treatment

Management for internal snapping hip syndrome initially includes rest, activity modification and oral NSAIDs. Peritendon and intrabursal injections followed by physical therapy may be warranted if symptoms persist (Wahl et al 2004). Favourable outcomes have been reported with iliopsoas stretching (Jacobson & Allen 1990; Taylor & Clarke 1995; Gruen et al 2002), ultrasound (Taylor & Clarke 1995) and strengthening of hip muscles (Gruen et al 2002). Gruen et al (2002) reported a 63% success rate by utilizing concentric hip rotator strengthening and eccentric training of the hip flexors and extensors. Neuromuscular activation and myofascial

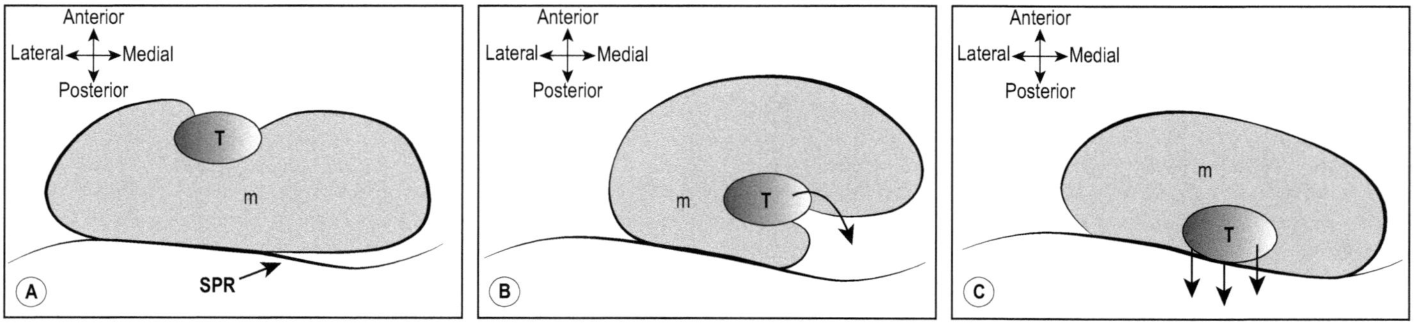

Figure 35.1 Causation of snapping iliopsoas tendon, transverse oblique view above the level of the hip joint: (**A**) As the hip is flexed, abducted, and externally rotated, the iliopsoas tendon (T) rolls laterally over part of the iliac muscle (m) that becomes interposed between the tendon and superior pubic ramus (SPR). (**B**) As the hip joint is brought back to neutral position, the tendon (T) follows a reverse path (medially and posteriorly) and part of its muscle (m) becomes trapped between its tendon and the superior pubic ramus. (**C**) At one point, the muscle (m) is suddenly released laterally, allowing abrupt return of the tendon (T) against the pubic bone, producing an audible snap.

release techniques to impaired tissue can help resolve symptoms and enhance return to pre-injury activity (Konczak & Ames 2005). Although good results have been reported, few randomized clinical trials exist.

If conservative management fails then surgical intervention may be warranted. Arthroscopic release or lengthening of the iliopsoas is often used to correct symptomatic snapping (Ilizaliturri et al 2005). A complete release of the iliopsoas tendon may be performed at the pelvic brim, femoral head (transcapsular) or lesser trochanter, with exception of the iliacus muscle fibres that directly insert into the lesser trochanter (Ilizaliturri et al 2009). No differences have been reported between locations, and good functional results are obtained at follow-up regardless of the release site (Ilizaliturri et al 2009). Fractional lengthening of the iliopsoas tendon has also been reported with good outcomes (Gruen et al 2002). Active hip flexion is restricted for the first 4 weeks following surgery. Isometric hip flexion strengthening can begin at 6 weeks following release, with gradual progression and restoration of hip strength and neuromuscular stability.

Complications following surgical correction may include recurrent snapping, heterotrophic ossification, femoral nerve palsy, persistent anterior hip pain, hip flexor weakness and wound infection (Gruen et al 2002; Ilizaliturri et al 2005, 2009; McCulloch & Bush-Joseph 2006; Flanum et al 2007). Of these, long-term hip flexor weakness is the most commonly reported impairment. Because labral pathology may be present with internal snapping hip syndrome, an intra-articular evaluation should be performed to determine the need for surgical correction (Taylor & Clarke 1995; Gruen et al 2002; Ilizaliturri et al 2005; Flanum et al 2007).

Prognosis

Success rates between 36% and 63% have been reported for non-operative management using physical therapy (Taylor & Clarke 1995; Flanum et al 2007). A combination of a hip flexor stability programme and steroid injections in eight cases resulted in relief lasting between 2 and 8 months (Vaccaro et al 1995). Although optimal outcomes were reported, it should be noted that 50% of the cases eventually underwent surgical intervention (Vaccaro et al 1995). A case study by Wahl et al (2004) demonstrated high success rates with use of injections in professional athletes. Additionally, Hoskins et al (2004) reported an overall patient satisfaction of 89% at an average of 6 months post surgery in 92 patients. Although these outcomes appear positive, complications occurred in 40% of cases. Flanum et al (2007) also reported significant improvement following an endoscopic release, with improved hip scores as high as 90–96 points and no recurrence of snapping in a case series of six patients.

Summary

Internal snapping hip syndrome can be a common hip complication in young, active individuals, especially elite ballet dancers; however, most cases are asymptomatic and do not affect functional activity (Winston et al 2007). If pain is present and function is limited, non-operative management is usually effective, including hip flexor stretching, neuromuscular activation, rotational strengthening and activity modification (Lewis 2010). If symptoms continue to persist after 2–3 months of conservative management, surgical intervention is recommended. Imaging techniques, especially dynamic ultrasonography, are useful to identify the location and cause of subluxation. Careful inspection of the intra-articular anatomy should be performed to rule out labral pathology as the source of mechanical symptoms. Following endoscopic correction, good outcomes are expected; however, careful monitoring during rehabilitation should be utilized so as to avoid complications, especially chronic hip flexion weakness (Ilizaliturri et al 2009).

Gluteus Medius Tendinopathy

Epidemiology

Pain experienced at the greater trochanter is a common condition that may be referred from intra-articular or extra-articular structures. Previously diagnosed as trochanteric bursitis, the term 'greater trochanteric pain syndrome' better encompasses the array of problems in this region, which affects 10–25% of the population (Williams & Cohen 2009). The incidence peaks between the fourth and sixth decades of life, more females being affected than males (Bird et al 2001). Gluteal tendinopathies, including overuse of injury to gluteus medius and / or minimus tendons, are common causes of greater trochanteric pain (Klauser et al 2013). In the past, treatment consisted of physical therapy and local corticosteroid injection targeting the trochanteric bursa, which was believed to be the source of the reported pain and symptoms. However, the advancement and inclusion of magnetic resonance imaging (MRI) in diagnosis of greater trochanteric pain syndrome has identified gluteus medius injury to be present in a large proportion of these individuals, whereas bursitis is not present in isolation (Bird et al 2001). Lateral hip pain or greater trochanteric pain syndrome can be due to tendinitis and / or bursitis related to the gluteus medius and minimus tendons (Lequesne et al 2008).

Pathomechanics

The specific cause of gluteal muscle tendinopathy is not completely understood, but local micro-trauma and injury are often present (Connell et al 2003; Klauser et al 2013). Tendinopathy is often the result of overload; however, it is not just repetitive tensile loads that can lead to injury. Compressive loading can also lead to injury of tendons (Docking et al 2013). The gluteal tendons can be compressed beneath the iliotibial band when the hip is adducted; the amount of compression increases with a combination of flexion and internal or external rotation of the hip (Goom 2013). The combination of tensile and compressive loading of the tendon can lead to the pain and dysfunction associated with tendinopathy (Docking et al 2013). Muscle imbalances due to weakness or abnormal tightness throughout the hip region can predispose to injury; a commonly seen imbalance and / or abnormal movement pattern in such individuals is compensation with the TFL for hip abduction movements, which leads to weakness and atrophy of the posterior portion of gluteus medius (Bewyer & Bewyer 2003). Clinically this pattern presents as a weakened or lengthened posterior gluteus medius and a shortened strong TFL muscle.

Overuse injuries may occur from a low-magnitude stress over a long period of time – as in weight gain, postural habits and / or sleeping position (Bewyer & Bewyer 2003). Weight gain increases the demand on the gluteus medius during walking / running and standing. Postural habits, such as shifting the weight onto one leg with contralateral pelvic drop and / or prolonged side-lying positioning with the top leg adducted in front of other leg, can lead to adaptive lengthening of the posterior gluteus medius (Bewyer & Bewyer 2003). This pattern can result in bursal irritation and compression of gluteal tendons (Bewyer & Bewyer 2003). Other factors that have been linked to lateral hip pain in the athlete include a wide pelvis, leg-length discrepancy, excessive foot pronation and poor running surfaces (Robertson et al 2008). If excessive compression or tension continues without allowing a significant period for tissue repair and recovery, the tendon may begin to degenerate.

Patient history

Typically patients present with reports of non-specific hip and buttock pain that intensifies with prolonged standing, prolonged sitting, longer bouts of walking, stair negotiation and lying on the involved side (Bewyer & Bewyer 2003). Occasionally patients report early fatigue while walking, or walking with a limp (Lequesne et al 2008). The pain is described as an 'aching pain' at the lateral aspect of the hip (Bird et al 2001). Pain less commonly radiates into the groin and lateral thigh, and this referral pattern can potentially lead to patients being misdiagnosed with ipsilateral hip or lumbar spine pathology (Kingzett-Taylor et al 1999).

Diagnosis and clinical examination

Clinicians need to rely on the patient history and the clinical signs and symptoms in order to make an accurate diagnosis that will guide treatment (Woodley et al 2008). The clinical exam should include observation, functional movement tests, palpation, range of motion, resisted testing and special tests (Grumet et al 2010).

The clinician should identify whether any atrophy is present throughout the gluteal musculature, which could be due to compensatory patterns secondary to pain, injury, or entrapment of neural structures involving the sciatic, superior gluteal or inferior gluteal nerve. A retrospective evaluation of subjects with gluteus medius muscle atrophy indicated that four out of five subjects had gluteus medius tendon pathology as diagnosed with MRI (Woodley et al 2008).

Functional movement testing

Beyond the static postural assessment, the clinician should observe the patient completing a series of functional movements. These should include, but are not limited to, single-leg balance testing and gait. The patient's gait cycle is assessed in order to identify an antalgic or an abductor deficient pattern. A Trendelenburg gait pattern is characterized by a weak or dysfunctional abductor muscle complex. As the weakness progresses, a compensatory weight shift may occur towards the affected side in an attempt to unload the involved abductors (Poultsides et al 2012). If the single-leg stance can be held for 30 seconds, a reported sensitivity and specificity of 100% and 97.3% respectively have been identified (Lequesne et al 2008). The Trendelenburg test also provides value to the examination as it has been reported to have a sensitivity of 72.7% and a specificity of 76.9% in predicting a tendon tear (Bird et al 2001). There are many variations of single-leg balance testing recommended, but the intent of all of these tests is to evaluate the patient's proprioception and abductor muscle functioning (Poultsides et al 2012). Additionally, the single-leg stance test, single-leg squat test (Fig. 35.2) and star excursion balance test (Fig. 35.3) are recommended to assess hip abductor muscle functioning in a young athletic population with hip pain (Kivlan & Martin 2012).

Active and passive range of motion of the hip and trunk should be included to assist with the differential diagnosis by ruling in or out lumbar spine or intra-articular hip pathologies. The hip range of motion is typically normal in patients with abductor tendinopathy. Passive elongation of involved tendons will increase pain and should be kept in mind as the

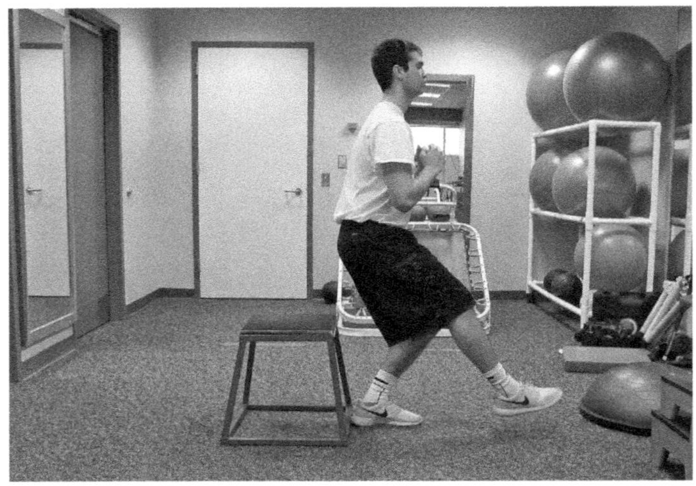

Figure 35.2 Single-leg squat test to assess hip abductor muscle functioning.

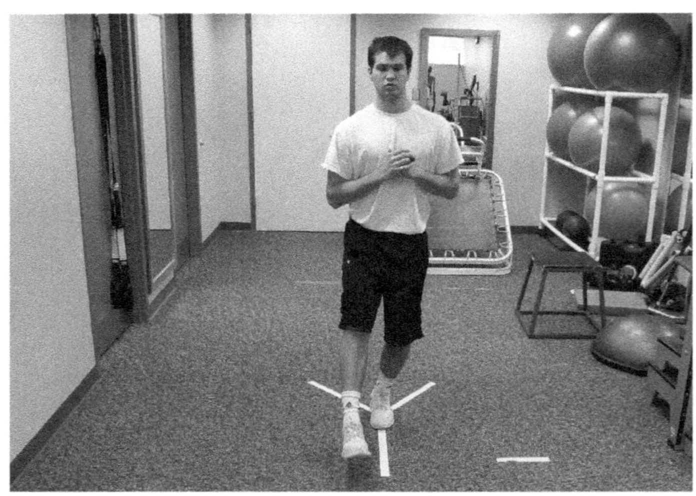

Figure 35.3 Star excursion balance test to assess hip abductor muscle functioning.

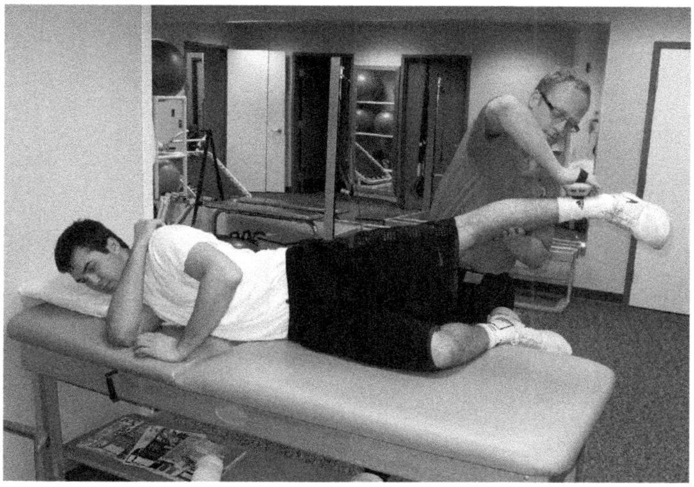

Figure 35.4 Hip abduction strength testing with a dynamometer.

range of motion is assessed. Passive external rotation with the hip in 90° of flexion is typically the only provocative movement during hip range of motion testing (Lequesne et al 2008). Occasionally, hip adduction beyond neutral increases symptoms owing to compression of the involved tendons.

Resisted hip abduction and resisted hip internal rotation are commonly recommended to assist in the diagnosis of greater trochanteric pain syndrome or gluteal tendinopathy. However, the sensitivity of resisted abduction test has been reported as 72.5%, and as 54.5% for resisted internal rotation (Bird et al 2001). The examiner should closely monitor the patient during hip abduction strength testing (Fig. 35.4) as many will compensate for gluteal musculature weakness with the TFL or the quadratus lumborum (Fredericson & Wolf 2005). The gluteus maximus strength is commonly assessed in the prone position with the knee positioned in 90° of flexion and neutral hip rotation (Baker et al 2011). General hip internal and external rotation strength can be measured in a variety of positions. The external derotation test is performed by having the patient lie in a supine position with the hip and knee flexed to 90°; the hip is then placed in external rotation. This position is typically painful in patients with gluteal tendinopathy, so the degree of external rotation should be reduced until the pain disappears. Patients are then instructed to internally rotate their leg against resistance; any reproduction of their pain is considered to be a positive test for gluteal tendinopathy or trochanteric bursitis. The sensitivity and specificity of this test have been reported to be 88% and 97.3% respectively (Lequesne et al 2008). The clinician should note any weakness, reproduction of pain and / or asymmetry between the lower extremities.

Beyond the balance and functional movement testing, several special tests provide information that can assist with differential diagnosis of lateral hip pain. The Patrick FABER test and the Ober test should be included in the exam. The FABER test is used to differentiate sacroiliac joint from hip joint pain in an abducted position (Grumet et al 2010; Poultsides et al 2012). The Ober test will allow the clinician to assess the tightness throughout the TFL / ITB complex that is potentially contributing to compression or irritation of the gluteal tendons with functional activities.

Palpation to the trochanter was reported to be the most provocative test included in clinical exam for lateral hip pain (Woodley et al 2008). Specifically, tenderness along the posterior aspect of the trochanter may be indicative of gluteus medius involvement, whereas tenderness anterior to the trochanter may be attributed to gluteus minimus pathology (Grumet et al 2010).

Treatment

Successful treatment of tendinopathy is dependent on accurate staging of the acuteness or chronicity of injury. In the early or reactive tendinopathy stage of injury, emphasis should be placed on reducing the physical demands placed on the involved tendon to allow healing and to prevent further progression of injury. Activity modification, including placing pillows between the knees while in a side-lying position, not crossing legs while sitting, and ensuring equal weight distribution while standing, have been recommended to reduce the amount of compression or tension placed through the involved tendons and musculature (Bewyer & Bewyer 2003). The use of a cane in the contralateral hand and carrying of external loads on the ipsilateral side are recommended in order to decrease demands on the gluteus medius during the stance phase of gait (Neumann & Cook 1985; Bewyer & Bewyer 2003). Although there is debate over whether or not tendinopathy is an inflammatory pathology, NSAIDs may nevertheless help to reduce tendon swelling (Cook & Purdam 2009).

Management of gluteus-medius-associated pain should include an initial period of 1–2 weeks of physical therapy. If symptoms do not improve after 2 weeks then an injection should be considered (Bewyer & Bewyer 2003), which has also been shown to be beneficial (Williams & Cohen 2009). If injection reduces symptoms then physical therapy should be continued. If no clear improvement is reported and no significant strength improvement is noted with continued physical therapy at 6 weeks, referral for further diagnostic imaging including MRI is recommended so as to determine the presence or severity of abductor tendon pathology (Bewyer & Bewyer 2003).

Strengthening exercises should be included in the initial management of this condition, but tailored to the stage of the injury, with loads that are appropriate to the strength as determined in the clinical exam. Strengthening exercises should be done with the muscle in shortened positions to facilitate normal muscle length in order to correct underlying imbalances and compensatory movement patterns (Bewyer & Bewyer 2003). Isometric exercises may be beneficial in the reactive stage of tendon pathology. The clinician needs to monitor performance of these exercises to ensure that the patient is not compensating with the TFL. Due to increased compression of the gluteal tendons with hip flexion combined with internal or external rotation, the clinician should consider avoiding certain common exercises, such as the clamshell, in the early phases (Goom 2013).

As pain and symptoms progress with early activity avoidance or / and reduced loading of the involved tendons, the strengthening component of the rehabilitation programme becomes more important. The performance of each prescribed exercise should be monitored to prevent any abnormal

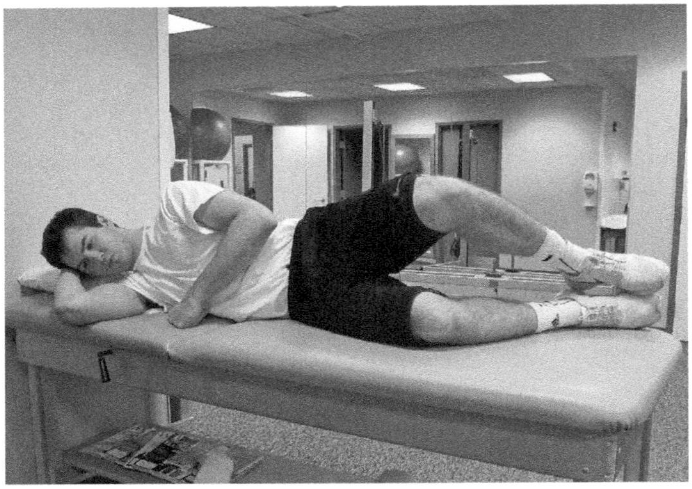

Figure 35.5 The clam exercise with knee flexed.

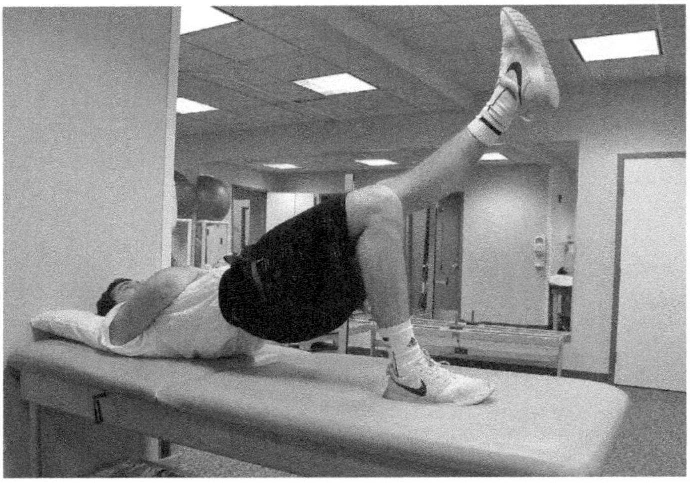

Figure 35.6 Unilateral bridge.

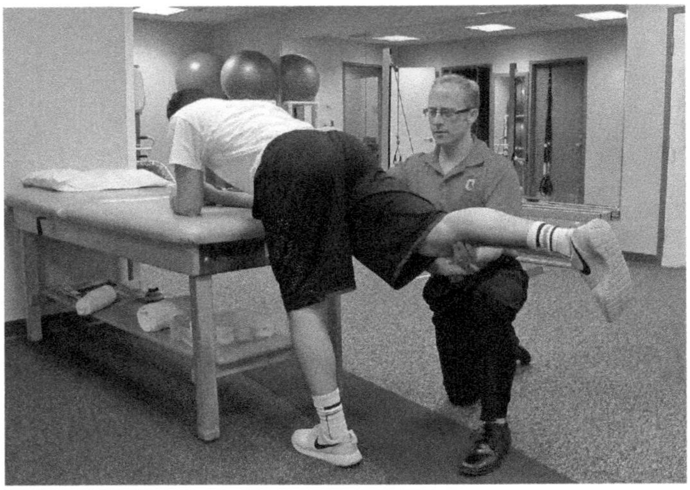

Figure 35.7 Quadruped hip extension with knee extended.

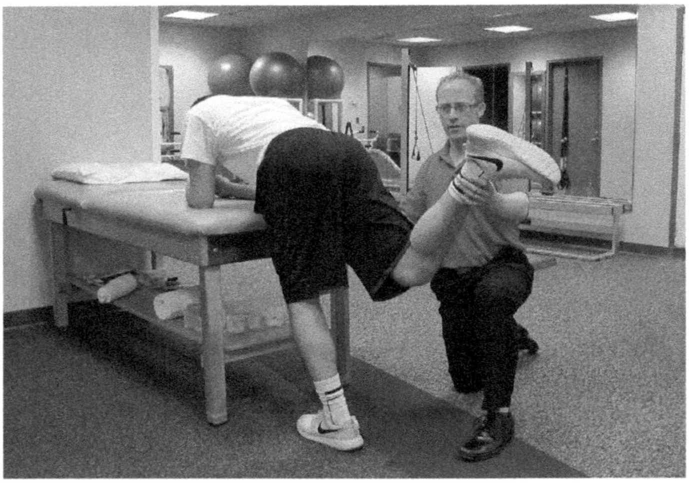

Figure 35.8 Quadruped hip extension with knee flexed.

movements or compensatory motions that could aggravate symptoms or limit strength gains in these individuals. Some studies have analysed common hip strengthening exercises in order to help guide the clinician in selecting the most appropriate or beneficial exercises in these patients. Bolgla and Uhl (2005) found that weight-bearing exercises required greater muscle activation; the results also indicated that side-lying hip abduction exercises generated greater muscle activation than standing non-weight-bearing hip abduction exercises. The authors concluded that, although the non-weight-bearing exercises produced less muscle activation, they may nevertheless benefit those patients who are unable to perform the weight-bearing or side-lying abduction exercises (Bolgla & Uhl 2005). A study completed by Selkowitz et al (2013) compared 11 common exercises in order to determine which exercises preferentially activated the gluteal musculature while minimizing TFL activity. The authors reported that the clam (Fig. 35.5), side-stepping, unilateral bridge (Fig. 35.6), quadruped hip extension with knee extended (Fig. 35.7) and quadruped hip extension with knee flexed (Fig. 35.8) were the most beneficial for maximizing gluteal activation with minimal TFL activity (Selkowitz et al 2013).

In the late tendon disrepair or degeneration stage, eccentric exercise should be used to load the tendon sufficiently. Eccentric exercise programmes have been shown to reduce pain levels, affecting tendon structure, and improve an individual's ability to return to former activity (Cook & Purdam 2009).

In patients who fail conservative treatment, surgical intervention is recommended (Williams & Cohen 2009). There are a variety of surgical interventions utilized to address recurring or lateral hip pain that is unresponsive to conservative measures; these include bursectomy, direct lengthening of the iliotibial band, trochanteric reduction osteotomy and gluteal tendon repairs.

Prognosis

The majority of greater trochanteric pain syndrome cases resolve with proper conservative treatment (Williams & Cohen 2009). However, it is difficult to determine prognosis or outcomes specific to gluteal tendinopathy owing to the challenging nature of clinical differential diagnosis in those presenting with lateral hip pain (Klauser et al 2013).

Conservative management including rest, physical therapy, a corticosteroid injection and various other modalities allowed 66% of those diagnosed with trochanteric bursitis to return to sport and 83% to return to manual labour after 3 months (Lustenberger et al 2011). In patients who fail conservative treatment, surgical intervention has been recommended (Williams & Cohen 2009). Comparisons between surgical interventions are difficult owing to the large number of pathologies that may refer pain to the lateral hip, limited amount of high-quality evidence available and large variability in outcome measures used (Lustenberger et al 2011).

Summary

Greater trochanteric pain syndrome is a commonly reported condition that was previously termed trochanteric bursitis. The pain and disability reported may be due to a variety of structures throughout the lateral hip. With advances in imaging techniques, gluteus medius and minimus tendinopathy has been identified as a primary cause of pain in these individuals. The examiner should take a thorough history and exam to help assist with this challenging clinical diagnosis and determine the functioning of the hip abductor complex. There is little evidence available to support best practice and guide physical therapy interventions. Generally treatment should focus on relative rest and avoidance of aggravating factors early on and then progress towards addressing lower extremity muscular imbalances contributing to the symptoms. Future research should be directed toward the development of prevention strategies and the effectiveness of specific rehabilitation programmes after accurate diagnosis of gluteal tendinopathy.

Adductor Tendinopathy

Epidemiology

Injury to the adductor muscle group is seen amongst sports that incorporate quick movements and changes of direction. Sports such as ice hockey, soccer and Australian-rules football appear to have some of the highest prevalences of adductor stains (Ekstrand & Gillquist 1983; Molsa et al 1997; Emery et al 1999; Tyler et al 2001; Kluin et al 2004; Crow et al 2010). Ten per cent of all injuries in Swedish hockey players involve an adductor muscle strain and a prevalence of 43% has been reported in Finnish ice hockey (Molsa et al 1997; Kluin et al 2004). Similarly, Tyler et al (2001) demonstrated an incidence of 3.2 strains per 1000 player-game exposures in the National Hockey League (NHL). Rates as high as 13–20 injuries per 1000 players per year have also been reported in the NHL, with an increased risk of groin and abdominal injuries during the pre-season period (Emery et al 1999). Within the soccer population, prevalences ranging as high as 31% have been reported (Ekstrand & Gillquist 1983). A recent study by Holmich et al (2013) reviewed groin-related injuries in sub-elite male soccer players and identified adductor-related groin pain as the most common cause of prolonged recovery, especially when combined with abdominal-related injuries.

Flexibility and strength have both been reported as risk factors for adductor injury. Studies in soccer players have shown a decrease in hip abduction motion to be a risk factor for groin strains (Ekstrand & Ringborg 2001; Arnason et al 2004). Despite this, other studies have found no relationship between hip abduction mobility and risk of groin injury (Tegner & Lorentzon 1991; Emery et al 1999; Emery & Meeuwisse 2001). Deficits in hip adduction strength have been demonstrated in athletes both before and after a groin-related injury. Tyler et al (2001) found that an 18% hip adductor strength deficit in NHL hockey players increased the risk of a future groin strain compared with uninjured players. In the same study, a decreased hip adduction to abduction strength ratio was also found in players suffering a groin-related injury. Adduction strength was 95% of abduction strength in uninjured players, but only 78% of abduction strength in injured players (Tyler et al 2001). Similarly, Crow et al (2010) showed decreased adductor strength immediately before and after the onset of groin pain in Australian football players. In contrast to these findings, a study of elite soccer players found no association with hip adductor strength and groin injury (Emery & Meeuwisse 2001). A previous history and / or presence of adductor injury are associated with recurrence of groin pain (Tyler et al 2001).

Pathomechanics

The cause of adductor strain or tendinopathy is often multifactorial, with two or more factors in 27% of cases (Ibrahim et al 2007). A thorough differential diagnosis is essential to determine the pain generator and rule out pathology of the hip, lumbosacral spine and abdominal region, as presence of groin pain is common with these conditions (Clohisy et al 2009). Quick movements in sports requiring eccentric activation of the adductor muscles may produce injury if strength or mobility deficits are present (Tyler et al 2001; Crow et al 2010). Imbalances in flexibility and strength have shown an association with muscle strains in the lower extremity. Deficits in general strength and flexibility have also been associated with injury in female collegiate athletes, although specific muscle groups were not identified (Knapik et al 1991). Conversely, Orchard et al (1997) demonstrated a relationship with strength deficits, but not flexibility, with hamstring injury. Specific to adductor injuries, Tyler et al (2001) demonstrated a relationship with injury and strength, noting a 17 times greater risk of injury if the adductor strength was less than 80% of the abductor strength. In professional hockey players, the incidence rates of adductor strains were reduced through an adductor-strengthening programme (Tyler et al 2002). Core musculature weakness and delayed onset of transversus abdominis muscle recruitment may also increase lower extremity and adductor injuries; however, debate still exists and additional research is needed to identify the causation (Maffey & Emery 2007; Hrysomallis 2009; Labella et al 2011; Herman et al 2012).

Patient history

Adductor strains are most commonly associated with ice hockey, rugby, soccer and Australian-rules football – sports that involve quick deceleration and changes of direction. Many of these athletes will report a chief complaint of groin pain after injury (Tyler et al 2001; Jansen et al 2008; Topol &

Reeves 2008) and can result from a single event or from repetitive micro-trauma (Avrahami & Choudur 2010). Soft tissue disruption may be present, depending on extent of the injury, and athletes will often complain of pain with sports-related activities that require adductor involvement (Lynch & Renstrom 1999).

Diagnosis

Diagnosis of an adductor strain is often formulated after a thorough history, clinical exam and imaging to ensure proper identification of the pathology. Clinical assessment of strength and flexibility of the adductors, iliopsoas and abdominal muscles should be highlighted, owing to alterations in anticipatory longstanding groin pain (Jansen et al 2010). Holmich et al (2004) demonstrated good (>0.60) intra- and inter-rater reliability of mobility and strength testing, with the exception of inter-rater reliability during iliopsoas strength testing, which was deemed unacceptable. One of the most valid and reliable clinical exams for identifying groin pain is the adductor squeeze test (Verrall et al 2007a). This is a reliable measure for adductor muscle strength and is the only measure to discriminate between athletes with and those without groin pain (Malliaras et al 2009). The test is reliable in the positions of 0°, 45° and 90° of hip flexion; however, Delahunt et al (2011) demonstrated the 45° position as optimal for eliciting adductor muscle activity.

MRI can be useful in identifying the location and degree of an adductor strain. This commonly occurs at the myotendinous junction; however, tendon avulsions may also be present (Lischuk et al 2010). Although not specific to the adductors, MRI results have been associated with functional outcomes, identifying longer recovery time based on cross-sectional involvement and fluid accumulation (Pomeranz & Heidt 1993). MRI may also be useful for identifying non-adductor-related causes of groin pain (Robinson et al 2004; Lischuk et al 2010). Conventional radiographs can be used to identify stress fractures, avulsion injuries and osseous abnormalities (Bencardino et al 2003).

Treatment

Initial management of adductor tendinopathy is focused on activity modification, rest, steroid injection, prolotherapy, lumbosacral strengthening and passive therapy modalities (Topol et al 2005; Tyler & Nicholas 2007; Topol & Reeves 2008). Holmich et al (1999) found significantly better outcomes utilizing a programme focused on active pelvic stabilization compared with one consisting of passive interventions including laser, cross-friction massage, stretching and transcutaneous electrical nerve stimulation. After a 7-month follow-up, 79% of patients completing the active stability programme were able to return to sports at the same or higher level, compared with only 14% in the passive treatment group (Holmich et al 1999). Verrall et al (2007b) demonstrated an 89% return to sport success rate after a programme using both passive modalities and exercise progression; however, almost half of patients were still symptomatic after their return. Inclusion of manual therapy may be beneficial as a component of a multimodal therapy programme; Weir et al (2010) reported short- and mid-term improvements using a combination of joint mobilizations and exercise, with a 77% success rate. They found that the inclusion of manual therapy may provide quicker results compared with a programme without this intervention; however, in this study the long-term outcomes and pain during sport were no different between groups. Tyler et al (2002) demonstrated an effective adductor strain prevention programme utilizing an adductor-strengthening programme. In this study, 33 out of 58 professional hockey players were determined to be at risk for adductor strain based on an adductor : abductor strength ratio of less than 80%. The prevention programme consisted of concentric, eccentric and functional strengthening exercise performed three times per week for 6 weeks (Box 35.1). Following the prevention programme, the incidence rate of adductor injuries decreased from 3.2 to 0.71 per 1000 player-game exposures.

Injection at the pubic cleft has been shown to improve outcomes in competitive and recreational athletes with adductor-related groin pain (Schilders et al 2007, 2009). Although all competitive athletes demonstrated immediate relief following the injection, only those with normal MRI findings had no recurrence of pain at 1-year follow-up (Schilders et al 2007). Almost the entire group with abnormal findings (16 of 17 cases) reported recurrence, on average at 5 weeks following the injection; however, when the same protocol was applied to recreational athletes, all

Box 35.1 Adductor muscle strain injury prevention programmes

Warm-up

- Bike
- Adductor stretching
- Sumo squats
- Side lunges
- Kneeling pelvic tilts

Strengthening programme

- Ball squeezes (legs bent to legs straight) with different ball sizes
- Concentric adduction with weight against gravity
- Adduction in standing on cable column or elastic resistance
- Seated adduction machine
- Standing with involved foot on sliding board moving in sagittal plane
- Bilateral adduction on sliding board moving in frontal plane (i.e. bilateral adduction simultaneously)
- Unilateral lunges with reciprocal arm movements

Sports-specific training

- On ice kneeling adductor pull together
- Standing resisted stride lengths on cable column to simulate skating
- Slide skating
- Cable column crossover pulls

Clinical goal

- Adduction strength at least 80% of the abduction strength

(From Tyler et al 2002.)

demonstrated good results without recurrence at 1 year (Schilders et al 2009).

Surgery may be warranted in cases of chronic adductor-related groin pain that do not improve. Due to limited outcomes with conservative management, surgical interventions should be considered if symptoms do not improve and there is no progression. Due to the complexity of the stresses that cause groin pain, the adductor muscle group, abdominal musculature, hip and pelvic floor should all be evaluated so as to determine the true cause of pain (Meyers et al 2000; Bedi et al 2011; Mei-Dan et al 2013). In particular, the adductor muscle group and rectus abdominis seem to be the commonest causes of abnormal stress through the groin (Bedi et al 2011). A study by Dojcinovic et al (2012) identified the presence of adductor tendinitis in 24% of cases with sports hernia. Adductor tenotomy, hernioplasty and pelvic floor repair have all been advocated to treat the associated pathology, with good outcomes, but again the identification of the true underlying cause of pathomechanics is paramount (Mei-Dan et al 2013).

Isolated adductor tenotomy has been demonstrated to yield good results in athletes suffering from chronic adductor-related pain (Akermark & Johansson 1992; Atkinson et al 2010; Robertson et al 2011). Schilders et al (2013) performed selective adductor release on 43 professional athletes (39 soccer players and 4 rugby players). After an average follow-up of 40 months, all but one returned to pre-injury level of sport an average of 9 weeks post-op (Schilders et al 2013). Bilateral tenotomies have also been shown to be effective in treating unilateral adductor-related groin pain. Maffulli et al (2012) performed bilateral adductor tenotomies on 29 athletes with unilateral adductor longus tendinopathy. At follow-up, 86% reported return to pre-injury activity level, or higher, with a median time to return at 11 weeks (Maffulli et al 2012).

If diagnosed quickly, conservative treatment may be effective for correcting muscle imbalances, especially adductor strength deficits, and allowing return to pre-injury activity (Tyler et al 2001; Machotka et al 2009; Weir et al 2010). Despite encouraging outcomes, long-term recurrence rates are high (25–50%) following conservative management (Verrall et al 2007b; Weir et al 2010). If conservative treatment fails, surgical management demonstrates excellent outcomes with >80% return to pre-injury levels within 3 months (Jansen et al 2008; Mei-Dan et al 2013).

Summary

Adductor tendinopathy is a common injury in sports, especially in ice hockey, Australian-rules football, soccer and rugby (Ekstrand & Gillquist 1983; Molsa et al 1997; Emery et al 1999; Tyler et al 2001; Kluin et al 2004; Crow et al 2010). Several risk factors including sport, mobility deficits, muscle imbalance and adductor weakness may lead to adductor-related groin pain (Ekstrand & Gillquist 1983; Molsa et al 1997; Emery et al 1999; Tyler et al 2001; Kluin et al 2004; Crow et al 2010). Adductor weakness in particular has been shown prior to and at the time of injury (Tyler et al 2001; Crow et al 2010). Non-operative management of adductor tendinopathy should be utilized to correct underlying impairments; however, recurrence is common, indicating the need for further research regarding pathomechanics and efficacious treatment strategies. If conservative management fails, surgical treatment has been shown to be effective in returning athletes to sport at pre-injury levels (Jansen et al 2008; Mei-Dan et al 2013). Further research is warranted to enhance preventative strategies and management of adductor tendinopathy and chronic groin pain.

Sports Hernia

Epidemiology

Sports hernia is a highly debated and controversial cause of lower abdominal and groin pain in athletes. The resulting chronic groin pain can lead to significant time away from work or participation in sports. Groin injuries account for 5% of all sports-related injuries (Moeller 2003). The incidence of sports hernia is reported to be between 0.5% and 6.2% (Campanelli 2010). In a retrospective review of 189 patients with chronic groin pain, Lovell (1995) reported that the condition was present in 50% of cases. Despite the reported prevalence of this condition, there is a lack of consistency of information regarding typical presentation, diagnosis and most effective treatment approach in this population (Kachingwe & Grech 2008).

The term 'athletic hernia' or 'sports hernia' has been used to describe the condition of a weakened posterior wall of the inguinal canal without palpable hernia, which results in chronic activity-related groin pain (Ahumada et al 2005; Swan & Wolcott 2007). The mechanism of injury, structures involved and terminology used to describe this condition vary among clinicians and within the literature (Swan & Wolcott 2007). There are numerous terms used to describe this condition, including footballers' hernia, inguinal insufficiency, conjoined tendon tear, hockey players' groin, Gilmore's groin and athletic pubalgia (Unverzagt et al 2008). The term athletic pubalgia has been used to describe this pathology owing to the absence of a palpable hernia. Pubalgia infers that there is an inconclusive physical exam with no identifiable cause of the persisting activity-related groin pain (Albers et al 2001; Kachingwe & Grech 2008). It is generally accepted that a sports hernia results from injury to muscular and / or fascial attachments at the anterior pubis, but there is much disagreement as to which specific anatomical structures are involved (Leblanc & Leblanc 2003; Ahumada et al 2005; Swan & Wolcott 2007). Groin pain related to sports hernia may be due to tears of the transversalis fascia, posterior inguinal wall, distal rectus abdominis insertion, conjoined tendon or external oblique aponeurosis (Albers et al 2001; LeBlanc & LeBlanc 2003; Kachingwe & Grech 2008) (Fig. 35.9). It was reported that only 6–8% of patients undergoing a sports hernia surgical repair had an isolated tear of the rectus abdominis (Meyers et al 2000; Ahumada et al 2005). Operative or surgical exploration commonly reveals multiple structures involved, all contributing to a weakened posterior inguinal wall (Diaco et al 2005; Van Veen et al 2007). For a more thorough review of the specific anatomical structures commonly involved in hip and groin injuries in an athletic population, readers are referred to the review 'Hip and groin injuries in athletes' by Anderson et al (2001).

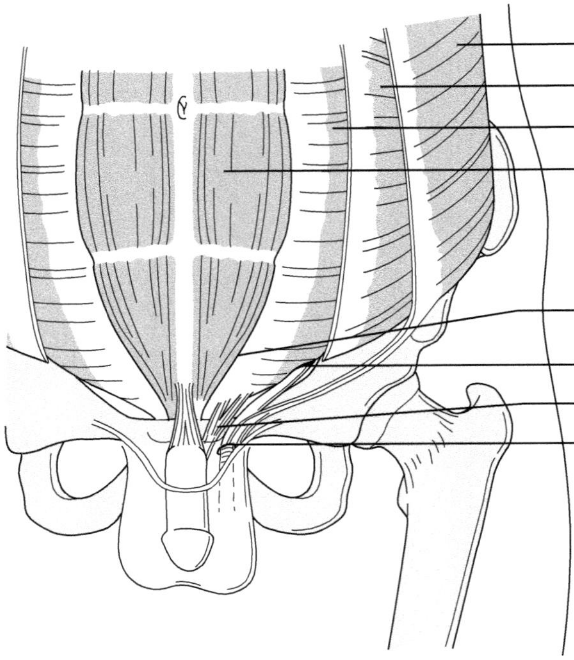

Figure 35.9 Different tissues related to the presence of sports hernia.

Pathomechanics

Overuse has been reported as the primary cause of sports hernia. Injury may occur from shearing forces that are produced at the pubic symphysis during sport-related activities, specifically those involving thigh hyperabduction and trunk hyperextension (Farber & Wilckens 2007). The resultant pelvic motion from higher intensity and increased range of motions involving hip adduction / abduction and flexion / extension produces shearing forces across the pubic symphysis, which leads to abnormal stresses on the soft tissues of the inguinal wall perpendicular to the fibres of the fascia and muscles (Anderson et al 2001). This may also help explain why osteitis pubis and adductor tenoperiostitis coexist in these patients (Hackney 1993). Muscular imbalances and decreased hip range of motion may increase the risk of injury in these individuals (Verrall et al 2007a).

Few studies look specifically at risk factors for sports hernia injuries; however, there have been several studies identifying potential risk factors for development of groin pain in athletes. A study performed by Engebretsen et al (2010) identified previous history of acute groin injury and weakness of the adductor muscle group as significant intrinsic risk factors for developing new groin injuries in male soccer players.

Patients presenting with sports hernia symptoms are typically males engaging in athletic-type activities (Albers et al 2001). Most patients will report unilateral deep groin, severe lower abdominal or pubic pain with exertion that is relieved by rest (Joesting 2002; Ahumada et al 2005; Kachingwe & Grech 2008). The pain is typically described as more proximal and deeper than a hip flexor or adductor muscle strain (Lynch & Renstrom 1999; Kachingwe & Grech 2008). The onset is more commonly insidious, but occasionally patients may report an acute event or specific movement that produced their symptoms once the pain was already present (Lynch & Renstrom 1999; Meyers et al 2002; Moeller 2007). Activities including kicking, sprinting, cutting and performing sit-up type motions are often reported to increase symptoms (Joesting 2002; Ahumada et al 2005; Kachingwe & Grech 2008). Occasionally, symptoms may be reproduced with coughing and sneezing (LeBlanc & LeBlanc 2003; Diaco et al 2005; Kachingwe & Grech 2008).

Diagnosis and clinical examination

The diagnosis of a sports hernia is made through exclusion without a definite diagnostic test. Patients will typically present with a normal physical exam, no palpable hernia and with all other pathologies ruled out (Joesting 2002; Ahumada et al 2005; Unverzagt et al 2008). The differential diagnosis of groin pain is challenging owing to the nature of overlapping symptoms and frequent coexisting conditions (Morelli & Smith 2001; Van Veen et al 2007; Kachingwe & Grech 2008). Numerous musculoskeletal conditions could produce anterior hip and groin pain. Differential diagnoses should include, but are not limited to: osteitis pubis, acetabular labral tears, adductor / hip flexor muscles tendinopathy and stress fracture of pubic ramus (Lacroix 2000; Anderson et al 2001; Johnson & Briner 2005; Unverzagt et al 2008). Possible nerve entrapment from the ilioinguinal, iliohypogastric, obturator, genitofemoral and lateral femoral cutaneous nerves could also produce deep groin pain in these individuals (Hackney 1993; Lacroix 2000; Anderson et al 2001; Unverzagt et al 2008). Urological diseases including prostatis, epididymitis, urethritis, hydrocoele and varicocoele can also refer pain to the inguinal region (Unverzagt et al 2008; Swan & Wolcott 2007). Further evaluation of female patients with similar symptoms often indicate gynaecological source of symptoms (Ahumada et al 2005; Moeller 2007; Kachingwe & Grech 2008). Once a thorough history and subjective description of the condition has been gathered from the patient and any possible systemic or non-musculoskeletal conditions have been considered, a more specific clinical exam can be completed.

Palpation should be used to exclude the presence of a true inguinal hernia (Minnich et al 2011). Resisted testing will often reproduce symptoms with resisted curl-up and resisted hip adduction at 0°, 45° and / or 90° of flexion (Minnich et al 2011). The clinician should include range of motion testing at both hips. As previously mentioned, reduced hip range of motion is a risk factor for developing chronic groin pain in athletes (Anderson et al 2001; Verrall et al 2007a). Hammoud et al (2012) reported a high incidence of sports hernia symptoms in athletes with femoroacetabular impingement (FAI). The authors recommend caution in diagnosing and treating an athlete for a sports hernia in isolation if signs or symptoms consistent with FAI are present (Hammoud et al 2012).

Specific muscle length and flexibility tests should be included in the clinical exam to identify muscular imbalances throughout the lumbopelvic region and lower extremities. The clinician should assess the length of the iliopsoas, adductors, tensor fasciae latae / iliotibial band and gluteal and piriformis muscles. Resisted testing will allow the clinician to eliminate or identify the presence of muscle strains or tendinopathy as a potential source of pain. The clinician should consider dynamometer testing of the hip adductors and abductors. The objective values allow the adductor-to-abductor strength ratio to be calculated; as previously discussed, a value of less than 80% increases an athlete's risk of groin strain (Tyler et al 2001).

Kachingwe and Grech (2008) clustered five signs and symptoms that were most indicative of sports hernia, including: subjective reports of deep groin or lower abdominal pain; pain that is worse with activity and relieved by rest; tenderness to palpation at the pubic ramus; insertion of the conjoined tendon or rectus abdominis; pain with resisted hip adduction at 0°, 45° and / or 90° of hip flexion; and pain with resisted curl-up.

Treatment

Initial management includes non-surgical modalities such as anti-inflammatory medications, soft tissue mobilization, ice and prolonged or relative rest from pain-provoking activities, followed by gradual return to and progression of activity. An initial trial of 6–8 weeks of physical therapy has been recommended to determine whether the patient will respond favourably without need for surgical intervention (Kachingwe & Grech 2008). There is little evidence in the literature to support conservative treatment including physical therapy in the management of sports hernia, however. The emphasis of an initial rehabilitation programme should be on core muscles strengthening and correction of any identified muscular imbalances throughout the hip, pelvis and lower extremities (Ahumada et al 2005; Farber & Wilckens 2007). Ekstrand and Ringborg (2001) performed a study on soccer players with sports hernia, who were randomized into four groups: a surgical group, physical therapy group, daily strength-training group and a control group. The physical therapy group received treatment three times a week for 4 weeks that included lower-abdominal-strengthening exercises and anti-inflammatory medications. The daily strength-training group participated in three lower-abdominal-strengthening exercises each day. The authors reported that only the surgical group had reduced symptoms during athletic activities at 6 months (Ekstrand & Ringborg 2001).

Surgical intervention is recommended when: (a) conservative management has failed, (b) the athlete can recall a specific acute tearing or ripping sensation in the pubic musculature and / or (c) the patient is a higher level athlete who is unable to have an extended time period to try a rehabilitation programme (Kachingwe & Grech 2008). A proposed algorithm for management of sports hernia published in 2008 stated that, if an athlete presented with the cluster of symptoms previously discussed, felt a tearing sensation during activity and is not expected to return to sport for 4 months, then the athlete should consider surgical repair. If the athlete is expected to return to participation within 4 months, a 3–4-week trial of physical therapy should be considered. After the 3–4-week trial period, if the athlete reports ≥80% subjective improvement, then the patient should continue with rehabilitation. If the athlete reports ≤80% improvement after the trial period then surgical consultation is recommended. If there was no tearing sensation felt by the athlete, then an initial 6-week trial of physical therapy is recommended (Kachingwe & Grech 2008).

Prognosis

Rehabilitation protocols and return to sport times vary, depending on the different structures repaired and surgical techniques used. Meyers et al (2008) reported that postoperative rehabilitation protocols recommend return to play at 3 days to 3 months, depending on the surgical technique, injured structures, sport and specific position of the athlete. The majority of athletes are able to return to sport participation 2–6 weeks after laparoscopic repair and between 1 and 4 weeks after the operation if an open surgical repair was performed (Farber & Wilckens 2007).

Summary

Sports hernia or athletic pubalgia is a disorder that affects athletes at all levels with increasing frequency, owing to increased sport participation. It is vital for the clinician to identify potential risk factors that can predispose an athlete to developing chronic groin pain, which could be potentially detrimental to an athlete's career. The diagnosis is generally made by excluding all other possible conditions, stressing the importance of completing a detailed and thorough history and examination of the athlete. With increasing awareness of the condition and greater amounts of literature available, it is important for any medical professional working with these athletes to identify symptoms promptly. Clinicians should understand the recommended best practices for management of this condition so as to return an athlete to activity safely and quickly, and without risk of further injury.

Conclusion

Injuries involving soft tissue structures supporting the hip and pelvis are common conditions seen by rehabilitation specialists. Increased understanding of the anatomical structures, mechanisms of injury and meaningful clinical examination findings has improved differential diagnosis in this region. As evidenced by this section, the most effective and efficient diagnosis / treatment of these conditions includes the expertise of a multidisciplinary team approach for appropriate management of these complex injuries.

References

Ahumada L, Ashruf S, Dspinosa-de-los-Monteros A, et al. 2005. Athletic pubalgia definition and surgical treatment. Annals Plastic Surg 55: 393–396.

Akermark C, Johansson C. 1992. Tenotomy of the adductor longus tendon in the treatment of chronic groin pain in athletes. Am J Sports Med 20: 640–643.

Albers S, Spritzer C, Garrett W Jr, et al. 2001. MR findings in athletes with pubalgia. Skelet Radiol 30: 270–277.

Anderson K, Strickland S, Warren R. 2001. Hip and groin injuries in athletes. Am J Sports Med 29: 521–533.

Arnason A, Sigurdsson SB, Gudmundsson A, et al. 2004. Risk factors for injuries in football. Am J Sports Med 32: 5S–16S.

Atkinson HD, Johal P, Falworth MS, et al. 2010. Adductor tenotomy: its role in the management of sports-related chronic groin pain. Arch Orthop Trauma Surg 130: 965–970.

Avrahami D, Choudur HN. 2010. Adductor tendinopathy in a hockey player with persistent groin pain: a case report. J Can Chiropr Assoc 54: 264–270.

Baker R, Souza R, Fredericson M. 2011. Iliotibial band syndrome: soft tissue and biomechanical factors in evaluation of treatment. Am Acad Phys Med Rehabil 6: 550–561.

Barber F, Sutker A. 1992. Iliotibial band syndrome. Sports Med 14: 144–148.

Bauer J, Duke L. 2012. Examining biomechanical and anthropometrical factors as contributors to iliotibial band friction syndrome. Sports Sci Rev 1–2: 39–53.

Bedi A, Dolan M, Leunig M, et al. 2011. Static and dynamic mechanical causes of hip pain. Arthroscopy 27: 235–251.

Bencardino JT, Kassarjian A, Palmer WE. 2003. Magnetic resonance imaging of the hip: sports-related injuries. Top Magn Imaging 14: 145–160.

Bewyer D, Bewyer K. 2003. Rationale for treatment of hip abductor pain syndrome. Iowa Orthopaedic J 23: 57–60.

Bird P, Oakley S, Shnier R, et al. 2001. Prospective evaluation of magnetic resonance imaging and physical examination findings in patients with greater trochanteric pain syndrome. Arthritis Rheum 44: 2138–2145.

Bolgla L, Uhl T. 2005. Electromyographic analysis of hip rehabilitation exercises in a group of healthy subjects. J Orthop Sports Phys Ther 35: 487–494.

Byrd JW. 2005. Snapping hip. Oper Tech Sports Med. 13: 46–54.

Campanelli G. 2010. Pubic inguinal pain syndrome: the so-called sports hernia. Hernia 14: 1–4.

Clohisy J, Knaus E, Hunt D, et al. 2009. Clinical presentation of patients with symptomatic anterior hip impingement. Clin Orthop Relat Res 467: 638–644.

Connell D, Bass C, Sykes C, et al. 2003. Sonographic evaluation of gluteus medius and minimus tendinopathy. Eur Radiol 13: 1339–1347.

Cook J, Purdam C. 2009. Is tendon pathology a continuum? A pathology model to explain the clinical presentation of load-induced tendinopathy. Br J Sports Med 43: 409–416.

Crow FJ, Pearce AJ, Veale JP, et al. 2010. Hip adductor strength is reduced in preceding and during the onset of groin pain in elite junior Australian football players. J Sci Med Sport 13: 202–204.

Delahunt E, Kennelly C, McEntree BL, et al. 2011. The thigh adductor test: 45° of hip flexion as the optimal test position for eliciting adductor muscle activity and maximum pressure values. Man Ther 16: 476–480.

Deslandes M, Guillin R, Cardinal E, et al. 2008. The snapping iliopsoas tendon: new mechanisms using dynamic sonography. AJR Am J Roentgenol 190: 576–581. doi: 10.2214/AJR.07.2375.

Diaco J, Diaco D, Lockhart L. 2005. Sports hernia. Oper Tech Sports Med 13: 68–70.

Docking S, Samiric T, Scase E, et al. 2013. Relationship between compressive loading and ECM changes in tendons. Muscles Ligaments Tendons J 3: 7–11.

Dojcinovic B, Sebecic B, Staresinic M, et al. 2012. Surgical treatment of chronic groin pain in athletes. Int Orthop 36: 2361–2365.

Ekstrand J, Gillquist J. 1983. The avoidability of soccer injuries. Int J Sports Med 4: 124–128.

Ekstrand J, Ringborg S. 2001. Surgery versus conservative treatment in soccer players with chronic groin pain: a prospective randomised study in soccer players. Eur J Sports Traumatol Related Res 23: 141–145.

Emery CA, Meeuwisse WH. 2001. Risk factors for groin injuries in hockey. Med Sci Sports Exerc 33: 1423–1433.

Emery CA, Meeuwisse WH, et al. 1999. Groin and abdominal strain injuries in the National Hockey League. Clin J Sport Med 9: 151–156.

Engebretsen A, Myklebust G, Holme I, et al. 2010. Intrinsic risk factors for groin injuries among male soccer players: a prospective cohort study. Am J Sports Med 38: 2051–2057.

Fairclough J, Hayashi K, Toumi H, et al. 2007. Is iliotibial band syndrome really a friction syndrome? J Sci Med Sport 10: 74–76.

Farber A, Wilckens J. 2007. Sports hernia: diagnosis and therapeutic approach. J Am Academy Orthop Surgeons 15: 507–514.

Flanum ME, Keene JS, Blankenbaker DG, et al. 2007. Arthroscopic treatment of the painful 'internal' snapping hip: results of a new endoscopic technique and imaging protocol. Am J Sports Med 35: 770–779.

Fredericson M, Cookingham C, Chaudhari A, et al. 2000a. Hip abductor weakness in distance runners with iliotibial band syndrome. Clin J Sport Med 10: 169–175.

Fredericson M, Guillet M, DeBenedictis L. 2000b. Quick solutions for iliotibial band syndrome. Phys Sports Med 28: 52–68.

Fredericson M, Weir A. 2006. Practical management of iiotibial band friction syndrome in runners. Clin J Sports Med 16: 261–268.

Fredericson M, Wolf C. 2005. Iliotibial band syndrome in runners: innovations in treatment. Sports Med 35: 451–459.

Fredericson M, White J, MacMahon J, et al. 2002. Quantitative analysis of the relative effectiveness of 3 iliotibial band stretches. Arch Phys Med Rehabil 83: 589–592.

Goom T. 2013. Gluteal tendinoathy. Running Physio 6 May. Online. Available: http://www.running-physio.com/gluteal-tendinopathy/. Accessed 19 Nov 2013.

Gruen GS, Scioscia TN, Lowenstein JE. 2002. The surgical treatment of internal snapping hip. Am J Sports Med 30: 607–613.

Grumet R, Frank R, Slabaugh M, et al. 2010. Lateral hip pain in an athletic population: differential diagnosis and treatment options. Sports Health 2: 191–196.

Hackney R. 1993. The sports hernia: a cause of chronic groin pain. Br J Sports Med 27: 58–62.

Hammoud S, Bedi A, Magennis E, et al. 2012. High incidence of athletic pubalgia symptoms in professional athletes with symptomatic femoroacetabular impingement. Arthroscopy 28: 1388–1395.

Hardcastle P, Nade S. 1985. The significance of the Trendelenburg test. J Bone Joint Surg 67: 741–746.

Herman K, Barton C, Malliaras P, et al. 2012. The effectiveness of neuromuscular warm-up strategies, that require no additional equipment, for preventing lower limb injuries during sports participation: a systematic review. BMC Med 10: 75.

Hollman J, Ginos B, Kozuchowski J et al. 2009. Relationship between knee valgus, hip muscle strength, and hip muscle recruitment during a single limb step down. J Sports Rehabil 18: 104–117.

Holmes J, Pruitt A, Whalen J. 1993. Iliotibial band syndrome in cyclists. Am J Sports Med 21: 419–424.

Holmich P, Holmich LR, Bjerg AM. 2004. Clinical examination of athlete with groin pain: an intra observer and inter-observer reliability study. Br J Sports Med 38: 446–451.

Holmich P, Uhrskou P, Ulnits L, et al. 1999. Effectiveness of active physical training as treatment for longstanding adductor-related groin pain in athletes: randomised trial. Lancet 6: 439–443.

Holmich P, Thorburg K, Dehlendorff C, et al. 2013. Incidence and clinical presentation of groin injuries in sub-elite male soccer. Br J Sports Med 48(16): 1245–1250. doi: 10.1136/bjsports-2013-092627.

Hoskins JS, Burd TA, Allen WC. 2004. Surgical correction of internal coxa saltans: a 20-year consecutive study. Am J Sports Med 32: 998–1001.

Hrysomallis C. 2009. Hip adductors' strength, flexibility, and injury risk. J Strength Cond Res.23: 1514–1517. doi: 10.1519/JSC.0b013e3181a3c6c4.

Ibrahim A, Murrell GA, Knapman P. 2007. Adductor strain and hip range of movement in male professional soccer players. J Orthop Surg 15: 46–49.

Ilizaliturri VM Jr, Villalobos FE Jr, Chaidez PA, et al. 2005. Internal snapping hip syndrome: treatment by endoscopic release of the iliopsoas tendon. Arthroscopy 21: 1375–1380.

Ilizaliturri VM, Chaidez PA, Villegas P, et al. 2009. Prospective randomized study of 2 different techniques for endoscopic iliopsoas tendon release in the treatment of internal snapping hip syndrome. J Arthro Relat Surg 25: 159–163.

Jacobson T, Allen WC. 1990. Surgical correction of the snapping iliopsoas tendon. Am J Sports Med. 18: 470–474.
Jansen JA, Mens JM, Backx FJ, et al. 2008. Treatment of longstanding groin pain in athletes: a systematic review. Scand J Med Sci Sports 18: 263–274.
Jansen JA, Poot B, Mens JM, et al. 2010. The effect of experimental groin pain on abdominal muscle thickness. Clin J Pain 26: 300–305.
Joesting D. 2002. Diagnosis and treatment of sportsman's hernia. Curr Sports Med Rep 1(2): 121–124.
Johnson J, Briner Jr W 2005. Primary care of the sports hernia: recognizing an often-overlooked cause of pain. Physician Sports Med 33: 35.
Kachingwe A, Grech S. 2008. Proposed algorithm for the management of athletes with athletic pubalgia (sports hernia): a case series. J Orthop Sports Phys Ther 38: 768–781.
Keskula DR, Lott J, Duncan JB. 1999. Snapping iliopsoas tendon in a recreation athlete: a case report. J Athl Train 34: 382–385.
Khaund R, Flynn S. 2005. Iliotibial band syndrome: a common source of knee pain. Am Fam Physician 71: 1545–1550.
Kingzett-Taylor A, Tirman P, Feller J, et al. 1999. Tendinosis and tears of gluteus medius and minimus muscles as a cause of hip pain: MR imaging findings. Am J Roentgenol 173: 1123–1126.
Kivlan G, Martin R. 2012. Functional performance testing of the hip in athletes: a systematic review for reliability and validity. Int J Sports Phys Ther 7: 402–412.
Klauser A, Martinoli C, Tagliafico A, et al. 2013. Greater trochanteric pain syndrome. Sem Musculoskel Radiol 17: 43–48.
Kluin J, den Hoed PT, van Linschoten R, et al. 2004. Endoscopic evaluation and treatment of groin pain in the athlete. Am J Sports Med. 32: 944–949.
Knapik JJ, Bauman CL, Jones BH, et al. 1991. Preseason strength and flexibility imbalances associated with athletic injuries in female collegiate athletes. Am J Sports Med 19: 76–81.
Konczak CR, Ames R. 2005. Relief of internal snapping hip syndrome in a marathon runner after chiropractic treatment. J Manipulative Physiol Ther 28: e1–e7.
LaBella CR, Huxford MR, Grissom J, et al. 2011. Effect of neuromuscular warm-up on injuries in female soccer and basketball athletes in urban public high schools: cluster randomized controlled trial. Arch Pediatr Adolesc Med 165: 1033–1040. doi: 10.1001/archpediatrics.2011.168.
Lacroix V. 2000. A complete approach to groin pain. Physician Sports Med 28: 66–86.
Lavine R. 2010. Iliotibial band friction syndrome. Curr Rev Musculoskelet Med 3: 18–22.
LeBlanc K, LeBlanc K. 2003. Groin pain in athletes. Hernia 7: 68–71.
Lequesne M, Mathieu P, Vuillemin-Bodaghi V, et al. 2008. Gluteal tendinopathy in refractory greater trochanter pain syndrome: diagnostic value of two clinical tests. Arthritis Rheum 59: 241–246.
Lewis CL. 2010. Extra-articular snapping hip: a literature review. Sports Health 2: 186–190.
Linderburg G, Pinshaw R, Noakes T. 1984. Iliotibial band syndrome in runners. Phys Sports Med 12: 118–130.
Lischuk AW, Dorantes TM, Wong W, et al. 2010. Imaging of sports-related hip and groin injuries. Sports Health 2: 252–261.
Little TL, Mansoor J. 2008. Low back pain associated with internal snapping hip syndrome in a competitive cyclist. Br J Sports Med 42: 308–309.
Lovell G. 1995. The diagnosis of chronic groin pain in athletes: a review of 189 cases. Aust J Sci Med Sport 27: 76–79.
Lustenberger D, Ng V, Best T, et al. 2011. Efficacy of treatment of trochanteric bursitis: a systematic review. Clin J Sports Med 21: 447–453.
Lynch S, Renstrom P. 1999. Groin injuries in sport: treatment strategies. Sports Med 28: 137–144.
Machotka Z, Kumar A, Perraton LG. 2009. A systematic review of the literature on the effectiveness of exercise therapy for groin pain in athletes. Sports Med Arthrosc Rehabil Ther Technol 1: 5.
Maffey L, Emery C. 2007. What are the risk factors for groin strain injury in sport?: a systematic review of the literature. Sports Med 37: 881–894.
Maffulli N, Loppini M, Longo UG, et al. 2012. Bilateral mini-invasive adductor tenotomy for the management of chronic unilateral adductor longus tendinopathy in athletes. Am J Sports Med 40: 1880–1886.
Magee D. 2002. Orthopedic physical assessment, 4th edn. Philadelphia: Elsevier.
Malliaras P, Hogan A, Nawrocki A, et al. 2009. Hip flexibility and strength measures: reliability and association with athletic groin pain. Br J Sports Med 43: 739–744.
McCulloch PC, Bush-Joseph CA. 2006. Massive heterotopic ossification complicating iliopsoas tendon lengthening: a case report. Am J Sports Med 34: 2022–2025.
Mei-Dan O, Lopez V, Carmont MR, et al. 2013. Adductor tenotomy as a treatment for groin pain in professional soccer players. Orthop 36: 1189–1197.
Meyers WC, Foley DP, Garrett WE, et al. 2000. Management of severe lower abdominal or inguinal pain in high- performance athletes. Am J Sports Med 28: 2–8.
Meyers W, Lanfranco A, Castellanos A. 2002. Surgical management of chronic lower abdominal and groin pain in high-performance athletes. Current Sports Med Reports 1: 301–305.
Meyers W, McKechnie A, Philippon M, et al. 2008. Experience with 'sports hernia' spanning two decades. Annals Surg 248: 656–665.
Micheli LJ. 1983. Overuse injuries in children's sports. Orthop Clin North Am 14: 337–360.
Minnich J, Hanks J, Muschaweck U, et al. 2011. Sports hernia diagnosis and treatment highlighting a minimal repair surgical technique. Am J Sports Med 39: 1341–1349.
Moeller J. 2003. Pelvic and hip apophyseal avulsion injuries in young athletes. Curr Sports Med Rep 2(2): 111–115.
Moeller, J. 2007. Sportsman's hernia. Curr Sports Med Rep 6(2): 111–114.
Molsa J, Airaksinen O, Näsman O, et al. 1997. Ice hockey injuries in Finland: a prospective epidemiologic study. Am J Sports Med 25: 495–499.
Morelli V, Smith V. 2001. Groin injuries in athletes. Am Family Physician 64: 1405–1414.
Neumann D, Cook T. 1985. Effect of load and carrying position on the electromyographic activity of the gluteus medius muscle during walking. Phys Ther 65: 305–311.
Orchard J, Marsden J, Lord S, et al. 1997. Preseason hamstring muscle weakness associated with hamstring muscle injury in Australian footballers. Am J Sports Med 25: 81–85.
Pelsser V, Cardinal E, Hobden R, et al. 2001. Extra-articular snapping hip: sonographic findings. AJR Am J Roentgenol 176: 67–73.
Pomeranz SJ, Heidt RS Jr. 1993. MR imaging in the prognostication of hamstring injury. Radiology 189: 897–900.
Poultsides L, Bedi A, Kelly B. 2012. An algorithmic approach to mechanical hip pain. HSS J 8: 213–224.
Robinson P, Barron DA, Parsons W, et al. 2004. Adductor-related pain in athletes: correlation of MR imaging with clinical findings. Skeletal Radiol 33: 451–457.
Robertson W, Gardner M, Barker J, et al. 2008. Anatomy and dimensions of the gluteus medius tendon insertion. Arthroscopy 24: 130–136.
Robertson IJ, Curran C, McCaffrey N, et al. 2011. Adductor tenotomy in the management of groin pain in athletes. Int J Sports Med. 32: 45–48.
Saikia S, Tepe R. 2012. Etiology, treatment, and prevention of iliotibial band syndrome: a literature review. Topics Integrative Healthcare 4(3): ID: 4.3004. Online. Available: http://www.tihcij.com/Articles/Etiology-Treatment-and-Prevention-of-ITB-Syndrome-A-Literature-Review.aspx?id=0000406.
Schaberg JE, Harper MC, Allen WC. 1984. The snapping hip syndrome. Am J Sports Med 12: 361–365.
Schilders E, Bismil Q, Robinson P, et al. 2007. Adductor-related groin pain in competitive athletes: role of the adductor enthesis, magnetic resonance magnetic and entheseal pubic cleft injections. J Bone Joint Surg 89: 2173–2178.
Schilders E, Tabot JC, Robinson P, et al. 2009. Adductor-related groin pain in recreational athletes: role of the adductor enthesis, magnetic resonance magnetic and entheseal pubic cleft injections. J Bone Joint Surg 91: 2455–2460.
Schilders E, Dimitrakopoulou A, Cooke M, et al. 2013. Effectiveness of selective partial adductor release for chronic adductor-related groin pain in professional athletes. Am Sport Med 41: 603–607.
Selkowitz D, Benneck G, Powers C. 2013. Which exercises target the gluteal muscles while minimizing activation of the tensor fascia lata? Electromyographic assessment using fine-wire electrodes. J Orthop Sports Phys Ther 43: 54–65.
Swan K JR, Wolcott M. 2007. The athletic hernia: a systematic review. Clin Orthop Related Res 455: 78–87.
Taylor GR, Clarke NM. 1995. Surgical release of the snapping iliopsoas tendon. J Bone Joint Surg Br. 77: 881–883.
Tegner Y, Lorentzon R. 1991. Ice hockey injuries: incidence, nature and causes. Br J Sports Med 25: 87–89.
Teitz CC, Garrett WE, Miniaci A, et al. 1997. Tendon problems in athletic individuals. J Bone Joint Surg Am 79: 138–152.
Tibor LM, Sekiya JK. 2008. Differential diagnosis of pain around the hip joint. Arthroscopy 24: 1407–1421.

Topol GA, Reeves KD. 2008. Regenerative injection of elite athletes with career-altering chronic groin pain who fail conservative treatment: a consecutive case series. Am J Phys Med Rehabil 87: 890–902.
Topol GA, Reeves KD, Hassanein KM. 2005. Efficacy of dextrose prolotherapy in elite male kicking-sport athletes with chronic groin pain. Arch Phys Med Rehabil 86: 697–702.
Tyler TF, Nicholas SJ. 2007. Rehabilitation of extra-articular sources of hip pain in athletes. North Am J Sport Phys Ther 2: 207–216.
Tyler T, Nicholas S, Campbell R, et al. 2001. The association of hip strength and flexibility with the incidence of adductor muscle strains in professional ice hockey players. Am J Sports Med 29: 124–128.
Tyler T, Nicholas S, Campbell R, et al. 2002. The effectiveness of a preseason exercise program to prevent adductor muscle strains in professional ice hockey players. Am J Sports Med 30: 680–683.
Unverzagt C, Schuemann T, Mathisen J. 2008. Differential diagnosis of a sports hernia in a high-school athlete. J Orthop Sports Phys Ther 38: 63–70.
Vaccaro JP, Sauser DD, Beals RK. 1995. Iliopsoas bursa imaging: efficacy in depicting abnormal iliopsoas tendon motion in patients with internal snapping hip syndrome. Radiology 197: 853–856.
Van der Worp M, van der Horst N, Wier A. 2012. Iliotibial band syndrome in runners: a systematic review. Sports Med 42: 969–992.
Van Veen, R, De Baat, P, Heijboer, M, et al. 2007. Successful endoscopic treatment of chronic groin pain in athletes. Surg Endoscop 21: 189–193.
Verrall G, Slavotinek J, Barnes P, et al. 2007a. Hip joint range of motion restriction precedes athletic chronic groin injury. J Sci Med Sport 10: 463–466.
Verrall GM, Slavotinek JP, Fon GT, et al. 2007b. Outcome of conservative management of athletic chronic groin injury diagnosed as pubic bone stress injury. Am J Sports Med 35: 467–474.
Wahl CJ, Warren RF, Adler RS, et al. 2004. Internal coxa saltans (snapping hip) as a result of overtraining: a report of 3 cases in professional athletes with a review of causes and the role of ultrasound in early diagnosis and management. Am J Sports Med 32: 1302–1309.
Weir A, Jansen J, van Keulen J, et al. 2010. Short and mid-term results of a comprehensive treatment program for longstanding adductor-related groin pain in athletes: a case series. Phys Ther Sport 11: 99–103.
Williams B, Cohen S. 2009. Greater trochanter pain syndrome: a review of anatomy, diagnosis and treatment. Anesth Analg 108: 1662–1670.
Winston P, Awan R, Cassidy JD, et al. 2007. Clinical examination and ultrasound of self reported snapping hip syndrome in elite ballet dancers. Am J Sports Med 35: 118–126.
Woodley S, Nicholson H, Livingstone V, et al. 2008. Lateral hip pain: findings from magnetic resonance imaging and clinical examination. J Orthop Sports Phys Ther 38: 313–328.
Youdas J, Mraz S, Norstad B, et al. 2007. Determining changes in pelvic on femoral position during the Trendelenburg test. J Sports Rehabil 16: 326–335.

Chapter 36

Postoperative Management of Hip Disorders

Robert C. Manske, Erik Meira

CHAPTER CONTENTS

Introduction and overview	413
Hip disorders and arthroscopic surgical procedures	413
Femoroacetabular impingement	413
Chondral defects	414
Capsular and ligamentous structures	414
Postoperative considerations	415
Precautions	415
Phases of rehabilitation of hip disorders	416
Maximum protection phase: day of surgery (day 0) to postoperative day 14	416
Moderate protection phase: 2–6 weeks postoperative	416
Minimal protection phase: 6–12 weeks postoperative	417
Return to sport or daily life activities phase: 12–24 weeks postoperative	418
An example acetabular labral repair with femoroplasty postoperative progression	418

Introduction and Overview

The hip joint has become the knee of the 1970s and 1980s – that is, due to advancement of arthroscopic instrumentation technique and recognition of intra-articular conditions, the incidence of hip arthroscopic procedures has surged (Boyd et al 1997; Byrd & Jones 2001, 2011; Byrd 2005, 2007). This is occurring in higher numbers especially in newly trained surgeons in the United States (Montgomery et al 2013). Bozic et al (2013) recently reported that the overall incidence of hip arthroscopy procedures performed by American Board of Orthopedic Surgeons Examinees has increased by around 600% over a 5-year period. Additionally, enhanced descriptions of patient indications as candidates for hip arthroscopy have been proposed (Farjo et al 1999; Philippon et al 2007a). Therefore, hip arthroscopic procedures have necessitated hip rehabilitation procedures required for optimal post-surgical results. The science of hip rehabilitation continues to evolve. However, there is still minimal high-level evidence to support rehabilitation guidelines. Just as post-surgical early rehabilitation procedures in the knee and shoulder have both seen dramatic developments, so too will early post-surgical rehabilitation for the hip. This chapter will be based upon the evidence to date; however, one needs to extrapolate from the basic science, biomechanical and cadaveric research and outcome studies to make clinical decisions regarding hip biomechanics and considerations related to soft tissue healing constraints. Additionally, guidelines and rehabilitation methods employed following minimally invasive procedures for the knee, shoulder, elbow and ankle will be applied to the management of post-surgical hip disorders when appropriate. The phases of rehabilitation can further be individualized based on patients' pre-surgical level of activity and fitness, age, previous medical and surgical history, other pathologies and, of course, their goals and preferences.

Hip Disorders and Arthroscopic Surgical Procedures

Femoroacetabular impingement

Several forms of pathology that may require surgical arthroscopy are related to bony overgrowth in the hip joint. These forms of pathology reflect the abutment of the acetabular rim and the femoral neck and are associated with abnormalities of the proximal femur and the acetabulum (Reynolds et al 1999; Ito et al 2001; Notzi et al 2002; Ganz et al 2003; Siebenrock et al 2003). The cam-type femoroacetabular impingement (FAI) occurs when there is a decrease in femoral head–neck offset. This offset will contribute to irregular abutment at the anterosuperior acetabular rim with repetitive activities. If this condition progresses, it can result in early chondral delamination and labral pathology (Beck et al 2005; Philippon et al 2007b; Ganz et al 2008; Byrd 2010a, 2010b). There are several types of FAI, including a pincer type, a cam type and a combined impingement (Ganz et al 2003).

Pincer-type impingement: definition and arthroscopic intervention

The pincer type of impingement is caused by an excessive prominence of the anterolateral rim of the acetabulum. Several causes of this impingement have been hypothesized, including a decreased amount of acetabular anteversion or relative retroversion of the acetabulum, where the face of the acetabulum tilts slightly backwards rather than adopting its normal anterior forward position (Ganz et al 2008). Pincer impingement can also occur from an overgrowth of the anterior edge of the acetabulum. The dominant feature with pincer impingement is that of a deep or retroverted socket in which the range of hip movement is limited by the overgrowing anterior acetabular rim. At the limit of movement the femoral neck abuts against the labrum, which acts like a bumper. The labrum is compressed between the underlying bone and the femoral neck and this force is transmitted further to the acetabular cartilage. The labrum will demonstrate intrasubstance fissuring and intrasubstance ganglion formation. With time, bone apposition occurs on the osseous rim next to the labrum, pushing the labrum forward. The labrum itself becomes progressively thinner until finally it is no longer distinguishable (Ganz et al 2008). The transmission force to the underlying articular cartilage is restricted to a narrow band along the acetabular rim. In pincer impingement, alterations of the labrum are more circumferential and are maximally between the 11 and 1 o'clock positions (Beck et al 2005).

The pincer-type impingement produces a rather slow process of degeneration that occurs more often in women between 30 and 40 years of age. Activities with high demands such as yoga and aerobics are likely to be those that create exacerbations (Ganz et al 2008).

The arthroscopic intervention for pincer lesions involves clear assessment of the anterior labral pathology. With good labral tissue, preservation is preferred. Once the labrum is detected, it can be dissected to expose the pincer lesion. Rim decompression can be performed in the central compartment or the peripheral compartment. The acetabulum can be recontoured with a motorized high-speed bur. Following recontouring of the acetabulum, the damaged labrum can be debrided or refixed with suture anchors if possible.

Cam-type impingement: definition and arthroscopic intervention

Cam-type impingement is caused by the cam effect of a non-spherical femoral head rotating inside the acetabulum (Ganz et al 2003). With motions such as flexion of the hip, the non-spherical portion of the head rotates into the acetabulum, thus creating a significant shear force on the anterolateral edge of the acetabulum. This repetitive activity can eventually lead to more significant delamination and articular cartilage breakdown than that found with pincer impingement (Byrd 2010a). With cam-type impingement most of the damage is located anterosuperiorly, at the 1 o'clock position according to previous arthroscopic studies demonstrating lesions in this area (Beyers et al 1970; Fitzgerald 1995; Byrd 1996; Lage et al 1996; McCarthy et al 2001). The cam-type impingement will typically be seen in athletic men whose average age is between 20 and 30 years. Unlike pincer-type impingement, symptoms of cam-type impingement may appear more acutely (Ganz et al 2008).

The arthroscopic management of cam impingement begins with careful evaluation of the anterolateral acetabulum. If overlying soft tissues, including fibrous and fibrocartilaginous, are found they are removed. The cam lesion is removed by reshaping the bone so recreating a more normal concave relationship at the junction of the articular surface, and eliminating the lesion (Byrd 2010a). The surgeon should resect only enough bone to relieve the FAI as determined by previous CT studies or periodic dynamic examination (Philippon et al 2007a). It is important not to resect more than 30% of the head–neck junction because the load-bearing capacity of the femoral neck needs to be preserved (Mardones et al 2005; Gaunche & Bare 2006; Sussmann et al 2007).

In some individuals a combined pincer and cam impingement can occur. In fact, Beck et al (2005) reported that rarely do these two lesions occur in isolation. In their study of 149 hips, only 26 presented with an isolated aspherical head, while just 16 presented with an isolated coxa profunda; most had a combination of the two basic types (Beck et al 2005). Any patient with both types is classified as mixed cam–pincer impingement.

Chondral defects

Chondral defects can occur on the acetabular side as the result of axial loading or shear injury of the cam-shaped head within the acetabulum. This can occur with subluxation or dislocation of the hip. One method of managing this arthroscopically is with micro-fracture techniques to exposed bone, and stabilization or debridement of loose articular cartilage, which is similar to procedures in the tibiofemoral joint.

A recent systematic review has indicated several findings when comparing different treatment approaches for FAI (Harris et al 2013); this demonstrated that, in most cases, surgical treatment for FAI was superior to non-operative treatment. Further, it found that there were differences in clinical outcomes between different surgical techniques. Two years following surgery, patients undergoing mini-open techniques and arthroscopy and mini-open techniques had significantly higher subjective scores than those undergoing arthroscopy. Labral refixation and repair resulted in better outcomes than labral debridement, and re-operations and complications were higher following open surgical dislocation and mini-open techniques compared with arthroscopic techniques (Harris et al 2013).

Capsular and ligamentous structures

The goal of arthroscopic treatment of hip instability due to capsular and ligamentous laxity is to reduce the volume of the hip joint capsule directly or to tighten lax ligaments so as to reduce capsular redundancy and enhance joint stability (Philippon 2001; Philippon & Schenker 2005; Philippon et al 2007c). Thermal capsulorraphy uses a flexible probe to move across the tissue in a striped, corn-row pattern, watching careful response and colour of tissue. It is very important not to exceed tissue-heating times or temperatures (Philippon 2006). When capsulorraphy is unable to correct the capsular redundancy, a capsular plication can be performed. Plication is done by passing a suture through more-proximal capsular tissue. The suture is grasped by piercing the distal capsular tissue, bringing the suture loop to the skin and passing anteriorly and or posteriorly through the tissue, resulting in capsular tightening (Philippon & Schenker 2005; Philippon et al 2007c).

Postoperative considerations

Complications after hip arthroscopy have been shown to be as low as 1.5% of cases (Lynch et al 2013). They typically involve traction-related nerve injuries, fluid management issues and iatrogenic chondral injuries. Heterotopic ossification frequency after hip arthroscopy has been historically observed to be as high as 1.6%, but prophylactic use of stronger non-steroidal anti-inflammatories such as indometacin postoperatively has been shown almost to eliminate the incidence (Randelli et al 2010).

When managing a patient after hip arthroscopy, it is important to take note of the structures that were involved during the surgery. It is always a good idea to have a copy of the full operative report before initiating care, as the patient is often unclear on the specific details of surgery. Since there are no randomized clinical trials published to date on postoperative management of hip arthroscopy, it is also a good idea for the medical, surgical and rehabilitation teams to discuss goals and concerns unique to their preferences, surgical technique and patient population to ensure that there is a consistent and agreed-upon plan of care among the providers and patients. Although there is some variation in provider preferences, there are some guidelines and precautions that can be followed for each procedure.

Precautions

Labral debridement with / without rim trimming and arthroscopy in general

A patient who has undergone debridement of the acetabular labrum with or without osteoplasty of the acetabulum (rim trimming) has no repair to protect. With this type of procedure, most activity is limited to that tolerated. The patient typically uses crutches for up to 2 weeks to allow the joint to recover from the trauma of surgery. Range of motion activities are permitted within pain-free positions to avoid irritation of the joint.

All patients who have undergone hip arthroscopy should be encouraged to minimize use of their hip flexor muscles during the first 6 weeks after surgery. Hip flexor recruitment applies pressure to the anterior hip joint where most surgeries are performed (Martin et al 2010). Since chronic anterior hip irritation is a common complication of hip arthroscopy, minimization discomfort in the early phases is ideal. Non-weight-bearing is rarely recommended in cases of hip arthroscopy as this encourages excessive use of the hip flexor.

Precautions for acetabular labral debridement

- Weight-bearing as tolerated (WBAT).
- Limit range of motion to 90° of flexion for the first 2 weeks. Do not push into other directions more than tolerated for the first 2 weeks.
- No active range of motion for the first 2 weeks. No active flexion for the first 6 weeks.

Femoroplasty

Removal of a cam lesion (femoroplasty) requires augmentation to the structure of the femoral neck. Historically there has been concern that this procedure would cause significant disruption to the vascular supply and / or the structural integrity of the femoral neck (Philippon et al 2007b) and, due to this, earlier recommendations have been for only partial weight-bearing (limiting it to 20 pounds / 9 kg) for up to 6 weeks after surgery (Philippon et al 2007b). However, this concern has not been supported by more recent literature. Fractures associated with normal activities of daily living after femoroplasty have been documented only in cases involving stumbling (Rothenfluh et al 2012).

Some surgeons recommend crutch use as tolerated for the first 1–2 weeks after surgery not only to reduce inflammation after surgery, but also to give early protection to the femoral neck. When patients can tolerate their full weight on the leg without the use of painkillers, crutches may be discontinued. Impact loads are typically permitted as tolerated after 8 weeks.

Precautions for femoroplasty

- 50% partial weight-bearing (PWB) for the first 2 weeks but may be WBAT.
- Limit range of motion to 90° of flexion for the first 2 weeks. Do not push into other directions more than tolerated for the first 2 weeks.
- No active range of motion for the first 2 weeks. No active flexion for the first 6 weeks.

Acetabular labral repair

In cases of acetabular labral repair, the repaired structure requires protection as biological healing is achieved. It has been suggested that the patient should be limited to partial weight-bearing for up to 6 weeks to protect the repaired labrum, but loads to the labral in patients without dysplasia have been shown to be only 1–2% of the total weight of the hip (Henak et al 2011). This small amount of load may actually be helpful for stimulating a stronger biological bond over time.

Since the anterior zone of the labrum contains the highest relative concentration of sensory fibres (Gerhardt et al 2012), some surgeons have felt that weight-bearing as tolerated should be adopted. Similar to femoroplasty, 1–2 weeks of crutch use may be helpful for reducing inflammation and allowing the involved structures to tolerate progressively heavier normal loads during typical activities of daily living. Impact activities typically begin as tolerated after 12 weeks.

Precautions for acetabular labral repair

- WBAT, but may be 50% PWB for first 2 weeks.
- Limit range of motion to 90° of flexion for the first 2 weeks. Do not push into other directions more than tolerated for the first 2 weeks.
- No active range of motion for the first 2 weeks. No active flexion for the first 6 weeks.
- No impact loading (jumping, running, swinging a racquet / club / bat, etc.) until at least 12 weeks post-op.

Capsular modification

Capsular modification to the hip joint almost always involves the anterior capsule or iliofemoral ligament (Domb et al 2013).

Hence limitation of extension and external rotation for the first 4 weeks is clearly recommended to avoid excessive tension to the affected capsular tissue. Patients are typically limited to partial weight-bearing for the first 2 weeks, but continuing to use crutches for another 2 weeks is also advised in order to assist the patient in adhering to the range of motion restriction.

After 4 weeks, progressive stretching to the anterior capsule is advised so as to achieve and maintain a normal range of motion. Impact activities typically begin as tolerated after 12 weeks.

Precautions for capsular modification

- PWB for first 2 weeks.
- Limit external rotation (ER) range of motion for 4 weeks.
- No active range of motion for the first 2 weeks. No active flexion for the first 6 weeks.
- No impact loading (jumping, running, swinging a racquet / club / bat, etc.) until at least 12 weeks post operation.

Micro-fracture

When micro-fracture is performed on a weight-bearing surface of the hip joint, touchdown weight-bearing (TDWB) is advised for 6 to 8 weeks to protect the newly forming fibrin clot (Byrd & Jones 2011). Typically, the presence of a micro-fracture will delay the rehabilitation progress by 6–8 weeks across all phases. Depending on surgeon preference, impact activities are permitted between 16 and 24 weeks.

Precautions for micro-fracture

- TDWB for the first 6–8 weeks.
- No impact loading (jumping, running, swinging a racquet / club / bat, etc.) until at least 18 weeks post-op.

Phases of Rehabilitation of Hip Disorders

Although there are specific concerns for each structure that could be involved, there are also some general guidelines that should be followed for all patients that have undergone hip arthroscopy. The rehabilitation can be divided into four phases: maximal protection, moderate protection, minimal protection and return to sport or daily activities. These phases follow a timeline based on tissue healing considerations of the involved structures. This section is a sample progression of an acetabular labral repair with femoroplasty, as this is the most commonly performed procedure under hip arthroscopy.

Maximum protection phase: day of surgery (day 0) to postoperative day 14

The goals of the phase are to control postoperative inflammation and pain, to limit weight-bearing so as to protect affected tissues while optimizing healing, to regain range of motion as tolerated and to begin hip isometrics.

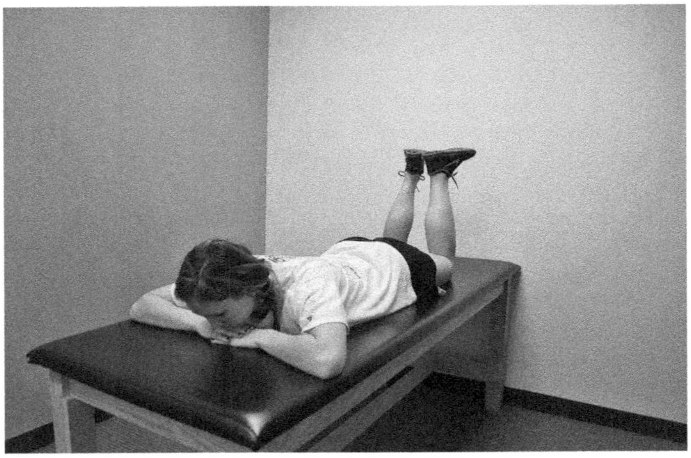

Figure 36.1 Prone heel squeeze. The patient lies prone with knees slightly apart and bent to 90°, heels touching, then pushes the heels together, creating an isometric contraction of the gluteus medius.

During the maximum protection phase, the focus should be on minimizing postoperative inflammation and discomfort. Special care should be taken to encourage rest, anti-inflammatory and cryotherapy use, and observance of weight-bearing restrictions. In fact, any increase in 'as-tolerated' activities is usually discouraged until after pain-killer use during normal activities of daily life has ceased.

The patient may begin gentle isometrics as tolerated as early as postoperative day two. Gluteal and quadriceps sets are encouraged, as is isometric adduction in a hook-lying position. The prone heel squeeze (Fig. 36.1) is an isometric exercise that generates high activity in the gluteus medius with low activity of the iliopsoas muscle (Philippon et al 2011).

Gentle passive range of motion may also start as early as postoperative day two, though the patient should be careful to avoid extremes of motion as this may stress involved structures (Enseki et al 2006). Passive flexion is usually limited to 90°. A caregiver may be trained to perform passive range of motion, but some patients may prefer to perform this themselves using a rope to achieve greater personal control. When tolerated, the patient may ride on an upright exercise bike with the seat elevated to avoid breaking the 90° of flexion restriction.

Since even high-load mobilizations have been shown to have very little mechanical effect on the hip joint (Loubert et al 2013), the focus of manual therapy interventions during this phase should be performed solely to help with discomfort. Anecdotally, patients typically prefer long distraction, posterior glides and lateral glides at 90° of flexion (Fig. 36.2). If these interventions are causing additional discomfort to the patient, however, they should be discontinued.

After 2 weeks have passed and all goals from the maximal protection phase have been achieved, the patient may progress to the moderate protection phase.

Moderate protection phase: 2–6 weeks postoperative

The goals of the phase are to achieve full weight-bearing as tolerated, to normalize gait, to restore full active range of

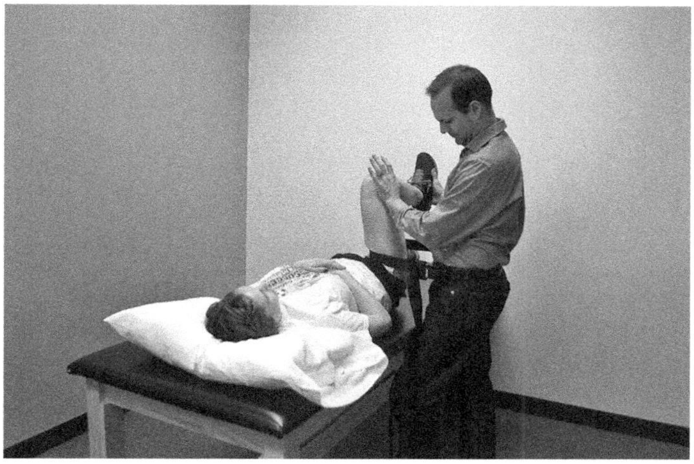

Figure 36.2 Lateral glide at 90° of flexion. With the patient in supine and their hip flexed to 90°, wrap a mobilization strap around the provider's body and the patient's proximal femur. A lateral force is applied to the hip by the provider shifting his/her weight back against the strap while applying a slight adduction force at the knee to stabilize.

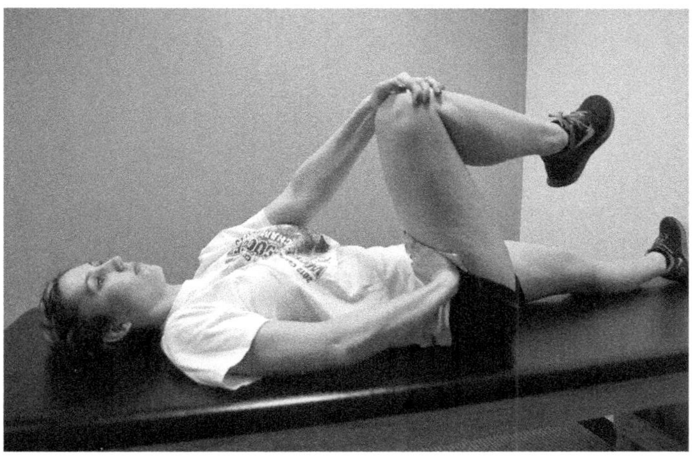

Figure 36.3 Caudal glide self-mobilization. The patient lies supine with the hip flexed as far as comfortably tolerated, and then places the ipsilateral hand into the proximal femur, applying a caudal glide with that hand while attempting additional hip flexion with the contralateral hand as tolerated.

motion as tolerated, to increase soft tissue flexibility / tolerance, to begin balance and proprioception activities and supported double-leg squatting as tolerated, and to maintain and / or improve muscle strength and coordination of trunk and lower leg.

During the moderate protection phase, the focus should be on normalizing gait mechanics and increasing muscle activation. Most activities of daily living can be safely resumed as tolerated during this phase, although the patient should take care to avoid impact loads, quick twisting motions and deep squatting.

Continue gentle passive range of motion exercise as tolerated. Anecdotally, when trying to progress passive hip flexion, the patient may tolerate further motion while performing a caudal glide self-mobilization (Fig. 36.3). Patients usually progress well with gentle stretching into external rotation and abduction if supported by a pillow to minimize muscle guarding of the joint. Gentle stretching to the hip flexors can be

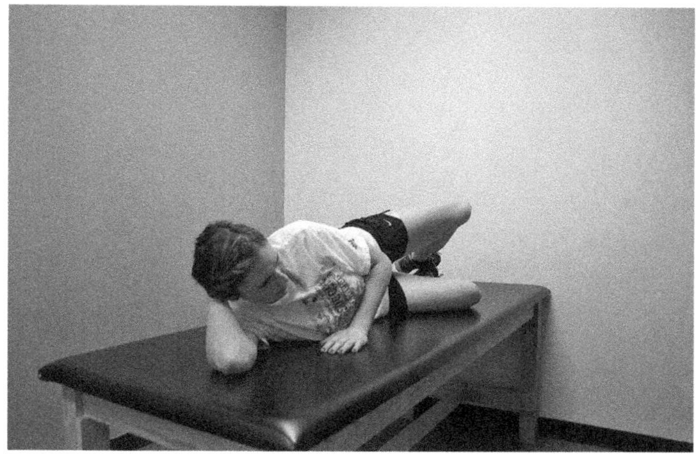

Figure 36.4 Clamshells. The patient is in side-lying, with knees bent to 90° and hips flexed to approximately 60°, then raises the top knee while externally rotating and abducting the top hip, and maintaining contact at the feet. The patient should avoid compensating by rotating the trunk posteriorly during the motion.

initiated at this point in the rehabilitation programme. Internal rotation movement may be slow to return as it places stress on the surgical repair and may not be well tolerated.

During this phase, full active range of motion should be encouraged with the exception of active hip flexion. Active hip flexion is unlikely to cause any damage to the surgical site, but it can commonly cause irritation to the anterior hip region. All other motions should be performed as tolerated.

Strengthening exercises should focus on activation of the hip abductors, specifically the gluteus medius (Philippon et al 2011). Clamshells (Fig. 36.4) and bridging have been shown to produce high activation of the gluteus medius with low activation of the tensor fascia lata (Selkowitz et al 2013). Clamshells are most effective at 60° of hip flexion while maintaining a neutral pelvis, and not allowing the top of the pelvis to roll back during the motion (Willcox & Burden 2013). Performance of standing open kinetic chain band exercises into extension, abduction and adduction can also be initiated during the beginning of this phase.

Towards the end of the moderate protection phase, the patient can begin band walking and single-leg bridging activities as tolerated. Ball squats can be initiated to progress squat depth in a safe, controlled manner while encouraging proper squat mechanics.

After 6 weeks have passed and all goals from the moderate protection phase have been achieved, the patient may progress to the minimal protection phase.

Minimal protection phase: 6–12 weeks postoperative

The goals of this phase are to achieve full squat depth as tolerated, to equalize strength between the involved and uninvolved limbs, to be able to perform single-leg squat, to maintain or improve muscle strength and coordination of the trunk and lower leg, and to be ready to initiate impact activities such as running and jumping.

During the minimal protection phase, the focus should be on returning the patient to equal limb strength. By the end of

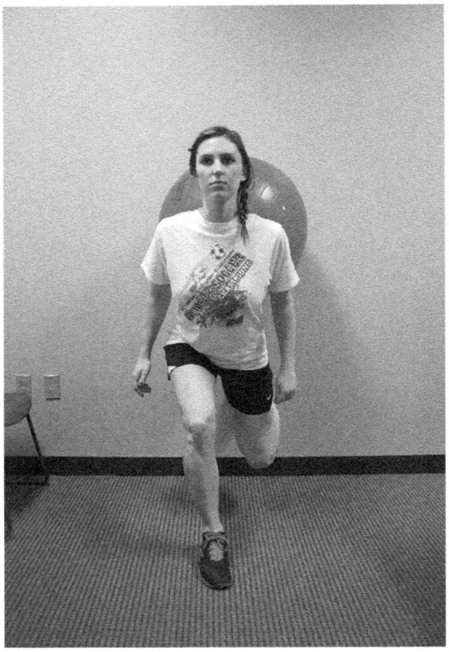

Figure 36.5 Single-leg squat with physioball. Standing upright on one leg while leaning back slightly on the physioball, the patient performs a squat while shifting the hips underneath the ball and while maintaining proper knee position. The patient should avoid excessive anterior knee translation, knee valgus, hip internal rotation and hip adduction.

the phase, the patient should be able to tolerate all activities of daily living and most weight-room activities that do not require impact loads or quick twisting movements.

Flexion, abduction, extension and external rotation range of motion should all be close to normal by 6 weeks. Any residual deficit into internal rotation can be pursued more aggressively at this point if tolerated. Also, if tolerated, active hip flexion strength can be progressed. Stretching to the hip flexors and adductors should be continued.

Once full-depth physioball squats are tolerated, the patient can be progressed to box squats from a bench or chair. Resistance can be added as needed. Athletes can then progress to front squats and deadlifts. Single-leg presses should also be initiated to encourage each lower extremity to function independently. When tolerated, single-leg squats can begin, using a physioball for support and taking care to avoid hip adduction, internal rotation or knee valgus (Fig. 36.5). These can be progressed with athletes in a Smith machine, increasing the resistance as tolerated.

After 12 weeks have passed and all goals from the minimal protection phase have been achieved, the patient may progress to the return to sport phase.

Return to sport or daily life activities phase: 12–24 weeks postoperative

The goals of this last phase are to be able to run as needed for training, to achieve hop performance in the affected limb at 90% that of the uninvolved limb, to return to full weight-room activities, and to return to sport participation

The focus of the return to sport phase is to increase tolerance of impact and other sport-specific activities. After 12 weeks, the surgically repaired structures have most likely achieved biological healing and can be tested against increasing loads. However, as all patients heal at different rates, care should nevertheless be taken to progress systematically only as per patient toleration.

Before passing into this phase, the patient should have already achieved symmetry in strength throughout the lower extremity. At this point, the patient can begin running as tolerated. As symptoms of limitations can appear several hours after running, we recommend starting with only 10 minutes and assessing the response of the joint over the next 24 hours. If there is no change in symptoms, running can then be increased by 5 minutes. As long as symptoms continue to remain under control, running may progress in 5-minute increments until the desired running time is achieved. If symptoms increase at any point, we recommend that the patient stop running until symptoms resolve, then continue without increasing the time. Progress may then continue as symptoms permit.

Once light running is tolerated, we advise progressing to a vertical drop jump, as failing this test has been shown to be a predictor of lower extremity injury in athletes (Hewett et al 2005; Paterno et al 2010). If this drop is tolerated, the patient can then progress to hop testing, as this has been shown to be a predictor of performance limitations in athletes returning from injury (Logerstedt et al 2012).

As the patient passes these tests, further testing specific to the patient's sports can be used. The patient can then return to sports in a graded fashion. If symptoms increase, we recommend holding further activity until the symptoms resolve.

An Example Acetabular Labral Repair with Femoroplasty Postoperative Progression

The clinician should always observe the above precautions for specific procedures. This section sets out an example rehabilitation programme following an acetabular labral repair procedure. Patients who have undergone only acetabular labral debridement may progress as tolerated once precautions have been met. In general, they should progress no faster than tolerated. For example, range of motion will usually progress well once inflammation is reduced.

Weeks 0–2

- Passive range of motion in all planes per precautions.
- Isometrics in all planes as tolerated.
- Exercise bike – upright bike only with seat elevated one step higher than normal. Begin at 5 minutes, then progress by 5 minutes each session as tolerated.
- Gait training as per precautions.
- Use ice and painkillers as needed.

Weeks 2–4

- Progress to full passive range of motion as tolerated.
- May begin full active range of motion.

- Begin stretching into ER, abduction and extension as tolerated.
- May add resistance to active range of motion if tolerated. Focus on hip abductor strength – *no resistance to hip flexion*.
- May begin double-leg bridging.
- Exercise bike – may bring seat back down to normal position. Up to 45 minutes as tolerated. No standing during pedalling.
- Continue gait training as per precautions.
- Continue using ice and painkillers as needed.

Weeks 4–6

- Full weight-bearing.
- Progress stretching into ER, abduction and extension.
- Balance training as tolerated.
- Begin ball-squats and other short-range closed kinetic chain exercises as tolerated.
- May begin elliptical exercise as tolerated.
- Progress hip abductor training.

Weeks 6–12

- Continue with elliptical training.
- Begin progressing squatting activities as tolerated – progress depth of squat before adding resistance.
- Progress toward single-leg activities.
- Progress proprioception activities as tolerated in a minimal impact environment.
- By the end of week 12, the patient should have strength in involved side within 90% that of uninvolved side.

Weeks 12–24

- May begin running activities as tolerated.
- Begin return to sport programme specific to the needs of the patient.
- Progressively return to impact activities (jumping, running, swinging a racquet / club / bat, etc.).
- Progress only as tolerated.

References

Beck M, Kalhor M, Leunig M, et al. 2005. Hip morphology influences the pattern of damage to the articular cartilage: femoroacetabular impingement as a cause of early osteoarthritis of the hip. J Bone Joint Surg 87: 1012–1018.

Beyers PD, Contepomi CA, Farkas TA. 1970. A post mortem study of the hip joint: including the prevalence of the features of the right side. Ann Rheum Dis 29:15–31.

Boyd KT, Peirce NS, Batt ME. 1997. Common hip injuries in sports. Sports Med 24: 273–280.

Bozic KH, Chan V, Valone FH 3rd, et al. 2013. Trends in hip arthroscopy utilization in the United States. J Arthroplasty 28: 140–143.

Byrd JW. 1996. Labral lesions: an elusive source of hip pain case reports and literature review. Arthroscopy 12: 603–612.

Byrd JW. 2005. Hip arthroscopy in athletes. Oper Tech Sports Med 13: 24–36.

Byrd JW. 2007. Hip arthroscopy in the athlete. North Am J Sports Phys Ther 2: 217–230.

Byrd JW. 2010a. Femoroacetabular impingement in athletes, part I: cause and assessment. Sports Health 2: 321–333.

Byrd JW. 2010b. Femoracetabular impingement in athletes, part II: treatment and outcomes. Sports Health 2: 403–409.

Byrd JW, Jones KS. 2001. Hip arthroscopy in athletes. Clin Sports Med 20: 749–762.

Byrd JW, Jones KS. 2011. Arthroscopic management of femoroacetabular impingement in athletes. Am J Sports Med 39: 7S–13S.

Domb BG, Phillippon MJ, Giordano BD. 2013. Arthroscopic capsulotomy, capsular repair, and capsular plication of the hip: relation to atraumatic instability. Arthroscopy 29: 162–173.

Enseki K, Martin R, Draovitch P, et al. 2006. The hip joint: arthroscopic procedures and postoperative rehabilitation. J Orthop Sports Phys Ther 36: 516–525.

Farjo LA, Glick JM, Sampson TG. 1999. Hip arthroscopy for acetabular labral tears. Arthroscopy 15: 132–137.

Fitzgerald RH Jr. 1995. Acetabular labrum tears: diagnosis and treatment. Clin Orthop 311: 60–68.

Ganz R, Parvizi J, Beck M, et al. 2003. Femoroacetabular impingement: a cause for osteoarthritis of the hip. Clin Orthop Rel Res 417: 112–120.

Ganz R, Leunig M, Leunig-Ganz K, et al. 2008. The etiology of osteoarthritis of the hip. An integrated mechanical concept. Clin Orthop 466: 264–272.

Gaunche CA, Bare A. 2006. Arthroscopic treatment of femoroacetabular impingement. Arthroscopy 22: 95–106.

Gerhardt M, Johnson K, Atkinson R, et al. 2012 Characterisation and classification of the neural anatomy in the human hip joint. Hip Int 22: 75–81.

Harris JD, Erickson BJ, Bush-Joseph CA, et al. 2013. Treatment of femoroacetabular impingement: a systematic review. Curr Rev Musculoskelet Med 6: 207–218.

Henak CR, Ellis BJ, Harris MD, et al. 2011. Role of the acetabular labrum in load support across the hip joint. J Biomech 44: 2201–2206.

Hewett TE, Myer GD, Ford KR, et al. 2005. Biomechanical measures of neuromuscular control and valgus loading of the knee predict anterior cruciate ligament injury risk in female athletes: a prospective study. Am J Sports Med 33: 492–501.

Ito K, Minka MA 2nd, Leunig M, Werlen S, et al. 2001. Femoracetabular impingement and the cam-effect: a MRA-based, quantitative anatomical study of the femoral head-neck offset. J Bone Joint Surg 83B: 171–176.

Lage LA, Patel JV, Villar RN. 1996. The acetabular labral tear: an arthroscopic classification. Arthroscopy 12:269–272.

Logerstedt D, Grindem H, Lynch A, et al. 2012. Single-legged hop tests as predictors of self-reported knee function after anterior cruciate ligament reconstruction. Am J Sports Med 40: 2348–2356.

Loubert PV, Zipple JT, Klobucher MJ, et al. 2013. In vivo ultrasound measurement of posterior femoral glide during hip joint mobilization in healthy college students. J Ortho Sports Phys Ther 43: 534–541.

Lynch TS, Terry MA, Bedi A, et al. 2013. Hip arthroscopic surgery: patient evaluation, current indications, and outcomes. Am J Sports Med 41: 1174–1189.

Mardones RM, Gonzalez C, Chen Q, et al. 2005. Surgical treatment of femoroacetabular impingement: evaluation of the effect of the size of resection. J Bone Joint Surg Am 87: 273–279.

Martin HD, Kelly BT, Leunig M, et al. 2010. The pattern and technique in the clinical evaluation of the adult hip: the common physical examination tests of hip specialists. Arthroscopy 26: 161–172.

McCarthy JC, Noble PC, Schuck M, et al. 2001. The role of labral lesions to development of early degenerative hip disease. Clin Orthop 393: 25–37.

Montgomery SR, Ngo SS, Hobson T, et al. 2013. Trends and demographics in hip arthroscopy in the United States. Arthroscopy 29: 661–665.

Notzi HP, Wyss TF, Stoecklin CH, et al. 2002. The contour of the femoral head-neck junction as a predictor for the risk of anterior impingement. J Bone Joint Surg 84B: 556–560.

Paterno MV, Schmitt LC, Ford KR, et al. 2010. Biomechanical measures during landing and postural stability predict second anterior cruciate ligament injury after anterior cruciate ligament reconstruction and return to sport. Am J Sports Med 38: 1968–1978.

Philippon MJ. 2001. The role of arthroscopic thermal capsulorrhaphy in the hip. Clin Sports Med 20:817–829.

Philippon MJ. 2006. New frontiers in hip arthroscopy: the role of arthroscopic hip labral repair and capsulorrhaphy in the treatment of hip disorders. AAOS Instructional Course Lectures 55: 33–55.

Philippon MJ, Schenker ML. 2005. Athletic hip injuries and capsular laxity. Oper Tech Orthop 15: 261–266.

Philippon M, Schenker M, Briggs K, et al. 2007a. Femoroacetabular impingement in 45 professional athletes: associated pathologies and return to sport following arthroscopic decompression. Knee Surg Sports Traumatol Arthrosc 15: 908–914.

Philippon MJ, Stubbs AJ, Schenker ML, et al. 2007b. Arthroscopic management of femoroacetabular impingement: osteoplasty technique and literature review. Am J Sports Med 35: 1571–1580.

Philippon MJ, Zehms CT, Briggs KK, et al. 2007c. Hip instability in the athlete. Oper Tech Sports Med 15: 189–194.

Philippon MJ, Decker MJ, Giphart JE, et al. 2011. Rehabilitation exercise progression for the gluteus medius muscle with consideration for iliopsoas tendinitis: an in vivo electromyography study. Am J Sports Med 39: 1777–1785.

Randelli F, Pierannunzii L, Banci L, et al. 2010. Heterotopic ossifications after arthroscopic management of femoroacetabular impingement: the role of NSAID prophylaxis. J Orthopaed Traumatol 11: 245–250.

Reynolds D, Lucas J, Klaue K. 1999. Retroversion of the acetabulum: a cause of hip pain. J Bone Joint Surg 81B: 281–288.

Rothenfluh E, Zingg P, Dora C, et al. 2012 Influence of resection geometry on fracture risk in the treatment of femoroacetabular impingement. Am J Sports Med 40: 2002–2008.

Selkowitz DM, Beneck GJ, Powers C. 2013. Which exercises target the gluteal muscles while minimizing activation of the tensor fascia lata? Electromyographic assessment using fine-wire electrodes. J Orthop Sports Phys Ther 43: 54–64.

Siebenrock KA, Schoeniger R, Ganz R. 2003. Anterior femoro-acetabular impingement due to acetabular retroversion: treatment with periacetabular osteotomy. J Bone Joint Surg 85A: 278–286.

Sussmann PS, Ranawat AS, Lipman J, et al. 2007. Arthroscopic versus open osteoplasty of the head-neck junction: a cadaveric investigation. Arthroscopy 23: 1257–1264.

Willcox EL, Burden AM. 2013. The influence of varying hip angle and pelvis position on muscle recruitment patterns of the hip abductor muscles during the clam exercise. J Orthop Sports Phys Ther 43: 325–331.

Chapter 37

Joint Mobilization and Manipulation of the Hip

Jack Miller, Wayne Hing

CHAPTER CONTENTS

Introduction 421
Joint mobilization/manipulation of the hip joint 421
Longitudinal traction mobilization/manipulation 422
Lateral distraction mobilization 422
Flexion/adduction mobilization: mobilization with movement internal rotation non-weight-bearing 423
Flexion/adduction mobilization: mobilization with movement internal rotation weight-bearing 423
Mobilization with movement in flexion 424
Mobilization with movement in extension weight-bearing 424

Introduction

The American Academy of Orthopaedic Surgeons (2008) ranks loss of mobility and degenerative changes of the hip joint as the most common cause of hip pain in older adults. The prevalence of hip pain appears to be population dependent, but it has been estimated to be as high as 27% (Dagenais et al 2009). Hip pain and dysfunction may result in significant personal mobility impairments and subsequent recreational, occupational and societal disabilities. A loss of hip range of motion, particularly internal rotation, has been identified as being highly predictive of hip osteoarthritis by Altman et al (1991), Sutlive et al (2008) and Birrell et al (2000, 2001). It is theorized that a loss of joint mobility impedes the normal compression–decompression cycle required to optimize joint cartilage synovial fluid exchange, thereby accelerating the degenerative process. Manual therapy has been demonstrated to increase joint space by up to 7 mm during the application of a lateral distraction procedure (Harding et al 2003) and to positively impact on hip pain, mobility and function (Hoeksma et al 2004; MacDonald et al 2006; Abbott et al 2013). Orthopaedic Manual Therapy (OMT) has been recognized to be of benefit to patient functional status and is included in the American Physical Therapy Association's Clinical Practice Guidelines for both arthritic and non-arthritic hip pain (Cibulka et al 2009; Keelan et al 2014).

This chapter focuses on restoration of lower limb functional tasks though a continuum of manual therapy interventions to the hip joint. Joint mobilizations including both arthrokinematics-based translatoric glides and function-based mobilizations with movement have been selected to provide clinicians with a repertoire of tools to use in clinical practice. The application of these techniques will be dependent on the individual clinical presentation of the patient and appropriate clinical reasoning on the part of the therapist.

Joint Mobilization/Manipulation of the Hip Joint

Manual therapy procedures to restore mobility and function of the pelvic girdle have been developed and described by a variety of authors (Kaltenborn et al 2002; Mulligan 2003; Hengeveld et al 2005). Translatoric accessory joint mobilization techniques are well established and form the basis of much of the curriculum of both entry level and postgraduate manual therapy training programmes internationally. Originally developed by contributors such as Kaltenborn and Evjenth from Norway (Kaltenborn et al 2002), OMT utilizes a clinical-reasoning paradigm based on the manual therapist's perception of joint restriction as revealed by passive movement examination and the application of the concave–convex rule. (See Ch 31 for further detail on OMT.)

Passive translatoric accessory mobilizations are performed parallel or perpendicular to the treatment plane as determined by the specific orientation of the joint surfaces. Mobilizations are graded in their range and sustained for specific durations according to their intended therapeutic goal(s) including pain relief and improving joint mobility. The theoretical conceptual model of OMT is the presence of joint capsule contracture, which must be passively elongated through tissue creep effected by sustaining the passive mobilization techniques; however, this hypothesis has not yet been scientifically confirmed. Technique repetition and an appropriate self-treatment regimen along with consideration of associated periarticular soft tissue dysfunction, neurophysiological and motor control factors are proposed to provide short- and long-term positive outcomes (Vicenzino et al 2007, 2011).

A growing body of evidence has demonstrated the value of combining traditional OMT manual therapy mobilizations concurrently with the patient's pain-limited physiological movements. Termed 'mobilization with movement' (MWM), this concept was developed by Brian Mulligan of New Zealand

(Mulligan 2003) and built on the foundations of OMT. Within the Mulligan concept, the management of the patient requires the identification of a comparable sign or client-specific impairment measure (CSIM) that is used to evaluate treatment effectiveness, often a limited functional activity. This clinically measurable functional deficit then becomes the benchmark against which the effectiveness of the intervention(s) is continually reassessed (Vicenzino et al 2007, 2011).

The clinical-reasoning paradigm of selection and progression of MWMs is based upon the patient's individual response to the selected mobilizations as measured by the pain-free improvement in the identified CSIM. The therapist must continuously monitor the patient's response to ensure that no pain is created. Utilizing his / her knowledge of joint arthrology, a well-developed sense of tissue tension and clinical reasoning, the therapist investigates various combinations of mobilization directions to find the correct treatment plane and grade of movement. While sustaining the pain-free accessory mobilization, the patient is requested to perform the previously identified pain-restricted CSIM. The CSIM should now be significantly improved – that is, increased range of motion, and a significant decrease in, or ideally absence of, the original pain. Failure to improve the CSIM would indicate that the therapist has not found the correct contact point, treatment plane, grade or direction of mobilization, or spinal segment, or that the technique is not indicated. The previously restricted and / or painful CSIM is repeated by the patient, initially as a trial treatment progressing up to sets of 10, while the therapist continues to maintain the appropriate accessory glide. Further gains are expected with repetition during a treatment session, which typically involves three to four sets of 10 repetitions. Repetition of the CSIM and pain-free end-range loading in the form of passive overpressure appears to be critical for achieving durable results (Miller 1999; Mulligan 2003; Hing et al 2008). As with all manual therapy concepts, a properly structured subjective and objective assessment of the patient and continuous reflective clinical reasoning (Jones & Rivett 2004) are mandatory both within the patient's assessment and during treatment sessions.

The theoretical model of the effect of MWMs is that either a positional fault of bony positional malalignment and / or a neuromechanical dysfunction is corrected by the mobilization component of the procedures (Vicenzino et al 2011). In place of the therapist's perception of passive accessory movement restriction and the concave–convex rule, the specific direction and grade of mobilization are determined by the patient reports of pain abolition and objective improvements in CSIM function (Miller 2006; Hing et al 2009; Vicenzino et al 2011). (See Ch 31 for further detail on MWM.)

Longitudinal traction mobilization / manipulation

The objective of this technique is to increase the available range of passive longitudinal caudal glide of the head of the femur and to reduce hip pain. The patient lies supine with the hip in the resting position of 30° of flexion, slight abduction and external rotation. The therapist is standing at end of bed in a walk / stride stance. The mobilization belt is looped over shoulders in a 'figure 8' position with hands inside the belt loop and placed over the ankle of the patient (Fig. 37.1). The

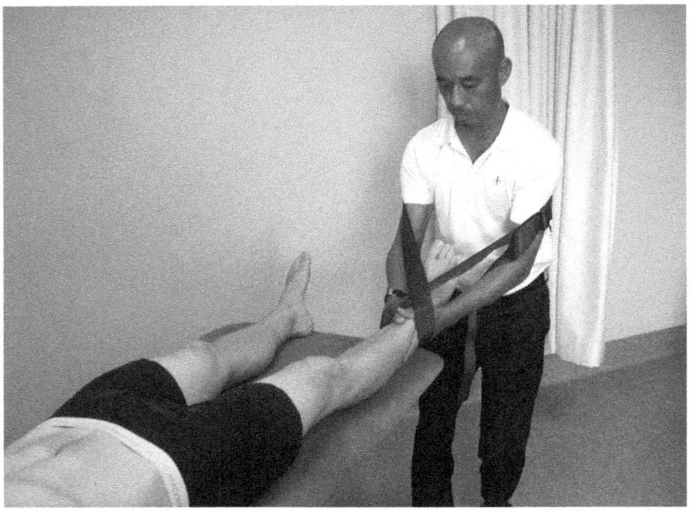

Figure 37.1 Longitudinal traction mobilization / manipulation from the ankle.

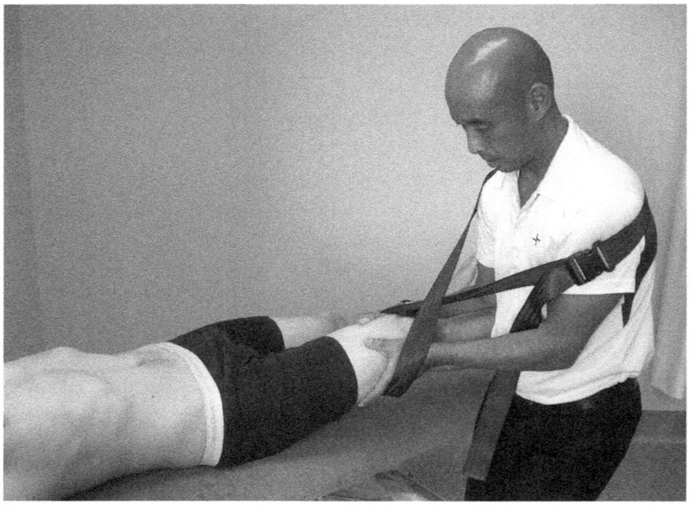

Figure 37.2 Longitudinal traction mobilization / manipulation from the knee.

mobilization consists of an inferior glide of the femur along the joint plane of the acetabulum. The therapist should allow the belt to perform the mobilization by relaxing arms and hands.

Note: A second belt or treatment table stabilization post can be placed in the groin and fixed to the bed to stabilize the pelvis. The belt can be put around the patient's lower leg above the ankle or, if the patient has knee pathology, above the knee (Fig. 37.2).

Lateral distraction mobilization

The objective of this technique is to increase the available range of passive lateral glide of the head of the femur and to decrease hip pain. The patient lies supine with the hip flexed to 90°, in neutral abduction / adduction and neutral internal / external rotation. The therapist stands at side of bed in a walk / stride stance. The mobilization belt is looped around the therapist's hips and inside the patient's upper thigh with padding as required for comfort (Fig. 37.3). The mobilization

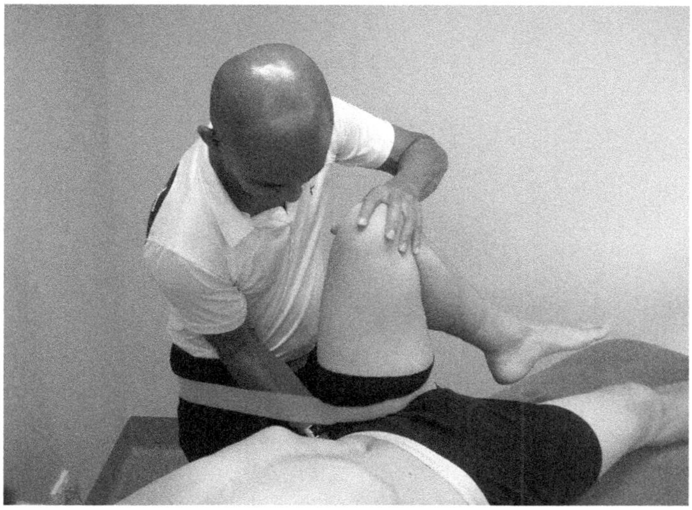

Figure 37.3 Lateral distraction mobilization of the hip.

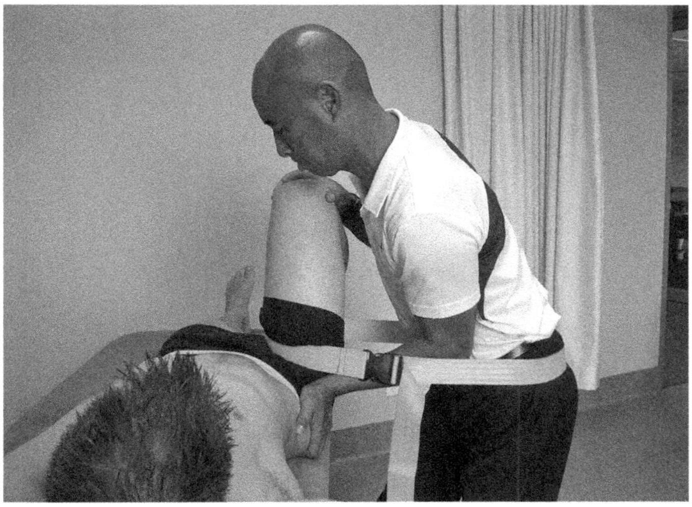

Figure 37.4 Lateral distraction mobilization of the hip. Lateral view showing the detail of the hand of the therapist on the lateral aspect of the pelvis.

consists of a lateral glide of the femur through the mobilization belt (Fig. 37.4).

Note: A treatment table stabilization post or second belt may be placed around the pelvis and fixated to the bed to stabilize the pelvis.

Flexion/adduction mobilization: mobilization with movement internal rotation non-weight-bearing

The objective of this technique is to reduce pain and to improve loss of hip internal rotation. The patient is supine with hip flexed to 90° and in neutral abduction / adduction. The therapist stands at side of bed in a walk / stride stance, placing the cephalic hand on the iliac crest of the patient inside the belt loop for lateral fixation of the pelvis (Fig. 37.5). The mobilization consists of a lateral glide of the femur through the mobilization belt. The internal hip rotation is imparted by the caudal hand of the therapist (Fig. 37.6).

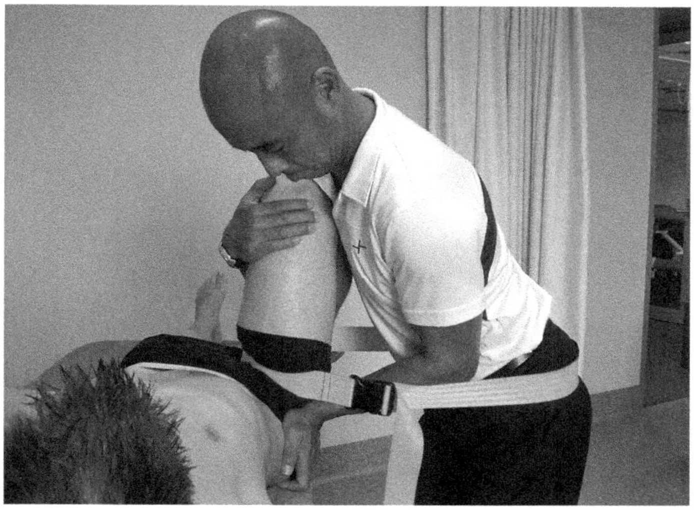

Figure 37.5 Flexion/adduction mobilization. Mobilization with movement internal rotation non-weight-bearing.

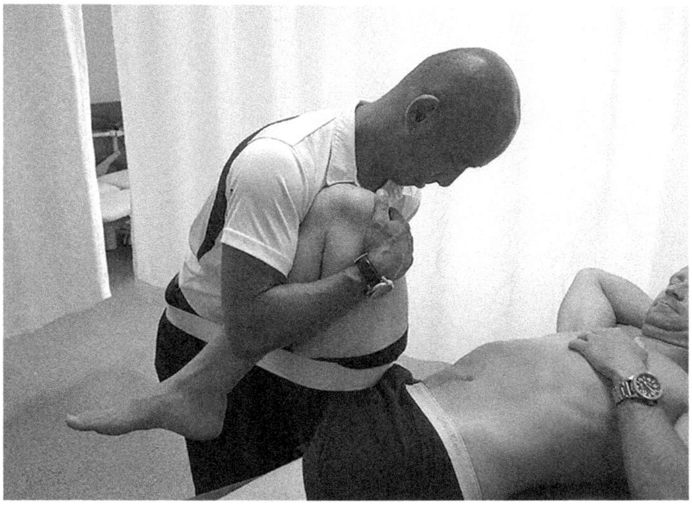

Figure 37.6 Flexion/adduction mobilization. Mobilization with movement internal rotation non-weight-bearing – lateral view showing the detail of the contact on the internal side of the knee of the patient.

Note: It is important to ensure that both mobilization and movement components are pain free during all end-range movement. The technique is held for 5–10 seconds and repeated in sets of 10 repetitions.

Flexion/adduction mobilization: mobilization with movement internal rotation weight-bearing

This technique is indicated when there is pain and / or loss of hip internal rotation and it should be considered as a progression of the previous one. The patient stands with the hip in neutral flexion / extension and neutral abduction / adduction. The patient can hold the treatment table for safety. The therapist stands in a walk / stride stance. The cephalic hand of the therapist is then placed on the iliac crest for lateral fixation of the pelvis. The mobilization consists of a lateral glide of the

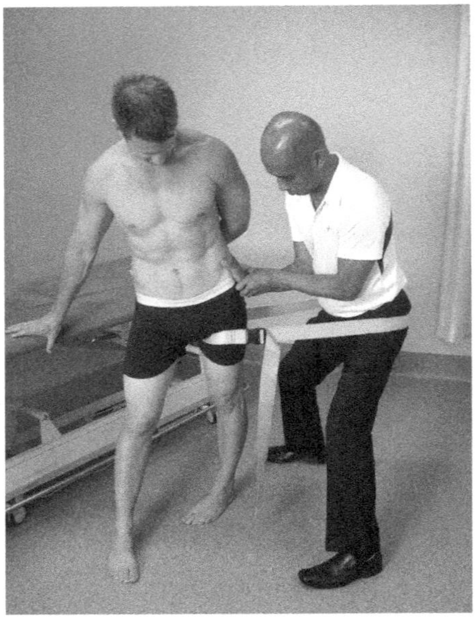

Figure 37.7 Flexion/adduction mobilization. Mobilization with movement internal rotation weight-bearing.

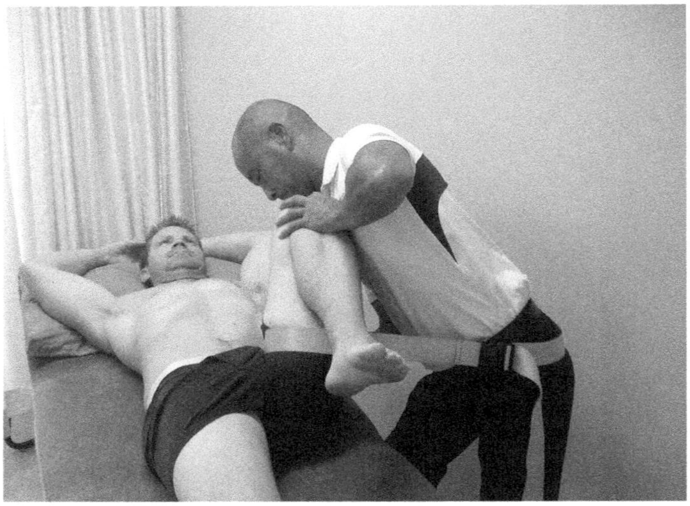

Figure 37.8 Mobilization with movement in flexion. Posterior view showing the detail of the belt position.

femur through the mobilization belt (Fig. 37.7). The technique focuses on internal hip rotation by the patient's rotation of the pelvis around the weight-bearing leg.

Note: It is important to ensure that both mobilization and movement components are pain free and to achieve maximum end-range movement. The technique is held for 5–10 seconds and repeated in sets of 10 repetitions.

Mobilization with movement in flexion

This technique is indicated when there is pain and / or loss of hip flexion. The patient lies supine with the hip flexed to 90° and in neutral abduction / adduction. The therapist stands at the side of bed in a walk / stride stance. The cephalic hand of the therapist is placed on the iliac crest of the patient inside the belt loop for lateral fixation of the pelvis (Fig. 37.8). The mobilization consists of a lateral glide of the femur through the mobilization belt. The flexion of the hip is imparted by the caudal hand of the therapist (Fig. 37.9).

Note: It is important to ensure that both mobilization and movement components are pain free and to achieve maximum end-range movement. The technique is held for 5–10 seconds and repeated in sets of 10 repetitions.

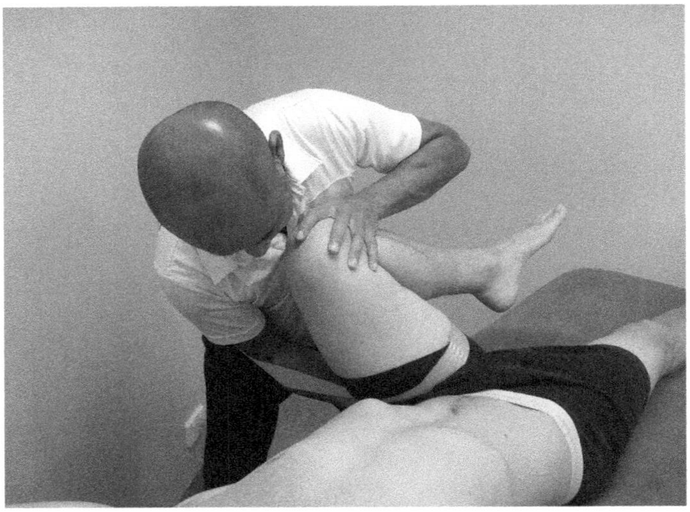

Figure 37.9 Mobilization with movement in flexion.

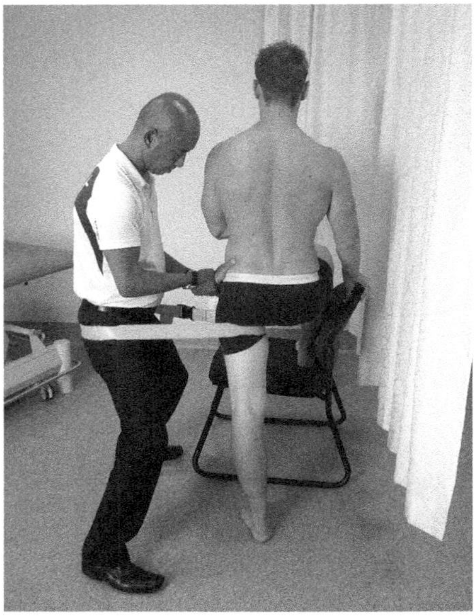

Figure 37.10 Mobilization with movement in extension weight-bearing. Posterior view showing the detail of both hands of the therapist on the lateral aspect of the pelvis.

Mobilization with movement in extension weight-bearing

This technique is indicated when there is pain and / or loss of hip extension. The patient is standing with contralateral hip

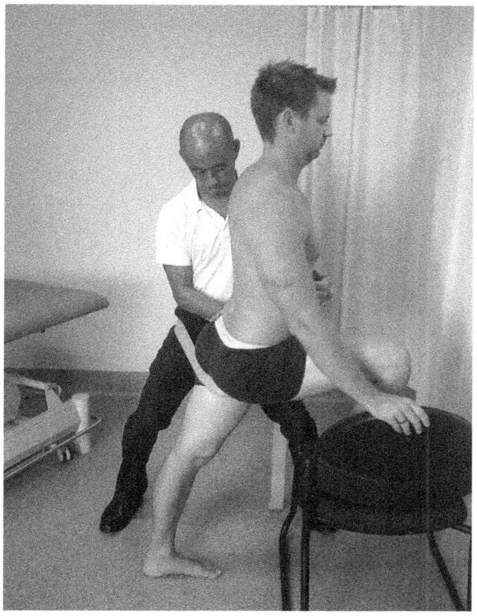

Figure 37.11 Mobilization with movement in extension weight-bearing. Lateral view.

and knee flexed via the foot on a chair, and in neutral abduction / adduction. The therapist stands at the side of the patient in a walk / stride stance, with both hands inside the belt loop fixating the lateral pelvis (Fig. 37.10). The mobilization consists of a lateral glide of femur through mobilization belt. The extension of the hip is performed via forward lunge of the patient (Fig. 37.11).

Note: It is important to ensure that both mobilization and movement components are pain free and to achieve maximum end-range movement. In addition, the patient should avoid an extension of the lumbar spine during the technique. The technique is held for 5–10 seconds and repeated in sets of 10 repetitions.

References

Abbott H, Robertson M, Chapple C, et al. 2013. Manual therapy, exercise therapy, or both, in addition to usual care, for osteoarthritis of the hip or knee: a randomized controlled trial. 1. Clinical effectiveness. Osteoarthritis Cartilage 21: 525–534.

Altman R, Alarcon G, Applerouth D, et al. 1991. The American College of Rheumatology criteria for the classification and reporting of osteoarthritis of the hip. Arthritis Rheum 34: 505–514.

American Academy of Orthopaedic Surgeons. 2008. Osteoarthritis of the hip: a compendium of evidence-based information and resources. Online. Available: www.aaos.org/home.asp.

Birrell F, Croft P, Cooper C, et al. 2000. Predicting radiographic hip osteoarthritis from range of movement. Rheumatology 40: 506–512.

Birrell F, Croft P, Cooper C, et al. 2001. Radiographic change is common in new presenters in primary care with hip pain. PCR Hip Study Group. Rheumatology 39: 772–775.

Cibulka M, White D, Woehrle J, et al. 2009. Hip pain and mobility deficits – hip osteoarthritis. Clinical practice guidelines linked to the the International Classification of Functioning, Disability and Health from the Orthopaedic Section of the American Physical Therapy Association. J Orthop Sport Phys Ther 39: A1–A25.

Dagenais S, Garbedian S, Wai EK. 2009. Systematic review of the prevalence of radiographic primary hip osteoarthritis. Clin Orthop Rel Res 467: 623–637.

Harding L, Barbe M, Shepard K, et al. 2003. Postero-antero glide of the femoral head in the acetabulum: a cadaver study. J Orthop Sport Phys Ther 33: 118–125.

Hengeveld E, Banks K, Maitland GD. 2005. Maitland's peripheral manipulation. Edinburgh: Elsevier Butterworth-Heinemann.

Hing WA, Biagalow R, Bremmer T. 2008. Mulligan's mobilisation with movement: a review of the tenets and prescription of MWMs. N Z Physiother J 36: 34–54.

Hing WA, Bigalow R, Bremner T. 2009. Mulligan's mobilisation with movement: a systematic review. J Manual Manipul Ther 17: E39–E66.

Hoeksma H, Dekker J, Ronday HK, et al. 2004. Comparison of manual therapy and exercise therapy of the hip: a randomized clinical trial. Arthritis Rheum 51: 722–729.

Jones MA, Rivett DA. 2004. Clinical reasoning for manual therapists. Edinburgh: Butterworth-Heinemann.

Kaltenborn FM, Evjenth O, Kaltenborn TB, et al. 2002. Manual mobilisation of the joints: the Kaltenborn method of joint examination and treatment: the extremities, 6th edn. Oslo: Olaf Norlis Bokhandel.

Keelna E, Harris-Hayes M, White D, et al. 2014. Nonarthritic hip joint pain, clinical practice guidelines linked to the International Classification of Functioning, Disability and Health from the Orthopaedic Section of the American Physical Therapy Association. J Orthop Sport Phys Ther 44: A1–A32.

MacDonald C, Whitman JM, Cleland JA, et al. 2006. Clinical outcomes following manual physical therapy and exercise for hip osteoarthritis: a case series. J Orthop Sport Phys Ther 36: 558–599.

Miller J. 1999. The Mulligan concept: the next step in the evolution of manual therapy. Canadian Physiotherapy Association Orthopaedic Division Review March / April: 9–13.

Miller J. 2006. The Mulligan concept: how: clinical application, when: clinical reasoning, why: clinical research. Canadian Physiotherapy Association Orthopaedic Division Review May / June: 45–46.

Mulligan BR. 2003. Manual therapy: 'NAGS', 'SNAGS', 'MWMS', 3rd edn. Wellington: Plane View Services.

Sutlive T, Lopez HP, Schnitker DE, et al. 2008. Development of a clinical prediction rule for diagnosing hip osteoarthritis in individuals with unilateral hip pain. J Orthop Sport Phys Ther 38: 542–555.

Vicenzino B, Paungmali A, Teys P. 2007. Mulligan's mobilization-with-movement, positional faults and pain relief: current concepts from a critical review of literature. Man Ther 12: 98–108.

Vicenzino B, Hing WA, Rivett D, et al. 2011. Mobilisation with movement: the art and the science. London: Elsevier.

38 Chapter

Therapeutic Exercises for the Lower Quadrant

Carol Kennedy, Lenerdene Levesque

CHAPTER CONTENTS

Introduction	426
Muscle performance: activation, endurance and strength	427
Neuromotor control: balance, proprioception, movement repatterning and functional integration	431
Mobility, myofascial and articular impairments	432
Designing an evidence-informed exercise programme	434
Mobility exercises	435
Muscle performance and neuromuscular control exercises	437
Exercise parameters	440
Conclusion	441

Introduction

Exercise prescription is an integral component of rehabilitation of lower extremity conditions. Optimal neuromuscular function is multifaceted and non-linear, as illustrated in Figure 38.1, and proper development of effective therapeutic exercise programmes must consider all these elements and their relationships. There is a growing body of evidence linking these various components and their effect on the biomechanics of the lower extremity. As it is impossible to describe all the possible exercises for the lower quadrant, this chapter will focus on exercise interventions to address hip dysfunction related to muscle imbalance, as demonstrated through a case-based presentation of a runner with anterior hip and posterolateral thigh pain.

First this chapter will explore the scientific evidence as it relates to exercises that can be used to address each of the individual elements required for optimal neuromuscular function. The second section will demonstrate how the evidence can inform our exercise prescription for this particular patient, remembering that evidence-informed practice also encompasses the patient's perspective and the clinical expertise of the clinician. The reader is directed to Chapter 23 for a detailed description of lumbopelvic exercises that would be incorporated into a lower quadrant exercise programme, particularly one focusing on the hip.

Case report

A 28-year-old physiotherapist presented with a 2-year history of right anterior hip and posterior–lateral thigh pain. He reported that the onset of the pain appeared to be related to an increase in his training volume for a half-marathon at that time. Running, squatting activities and cross-country skiing aggravated his current symptoms. The pain was alleviated when he discontinued the activity but it could take up to 2 days to resolve completely. His symptoms were limiting his ability to run and his goal was to be able to resume his previous training schedule. The patient rated his baseline pain on a numerical pain rating scale (NPRS) as 3 / 10 but it could reach as high as 8 / 10 after a 10 km run. The patient's score on the Lower Extremity Functional Scale was 60 / 80 with 80 representing maximum function (Binkley et al 1999).

Physical examination

- **Lumbar spine:** No articular restrictions were noted on biomechanical evaluation and neurological conduction and neural mechanosensitivity testing was normal.
- **Sacroiliac joint:** Laslett et al (2006) cluster of pain provocation tests was negative for reproduction of his symptoms.
- **Hip joint:** Decreased internal rotation at both 0° and 90° of hip flexion, hip flexion / adduction quadrant was positive for anterior hip pain and restriction of motion, flexion / abduction / extension / external rotation (FABER) test revealed a limitation of range of motion on the right with a myofascial end feel. Anterior translation of the femoral head was noted with a straight leg raise (SLR) manoeuvre – passive accessory testing revealed a reduced posterolateral glide of the femoral head with a capsular end feel.
- **Muscle strength:** Hip extensors grade 3+ / 5, hip abductors 3+ / 5, hip external rotators 4 / 5.
- **Muscle flexibility:** Modified Thomas test revealed tightness of the hip flexors and iliotibial band (ITB), Ober test was positive for decreased ITB length, hamstring muscle tightness was noted at 70° hip flexion – biasing with tibial medial rotation revealed greater tightness of biceps femoris, piriformis tightness was noted with internal rotation at both 0° and 90° hip flexion.

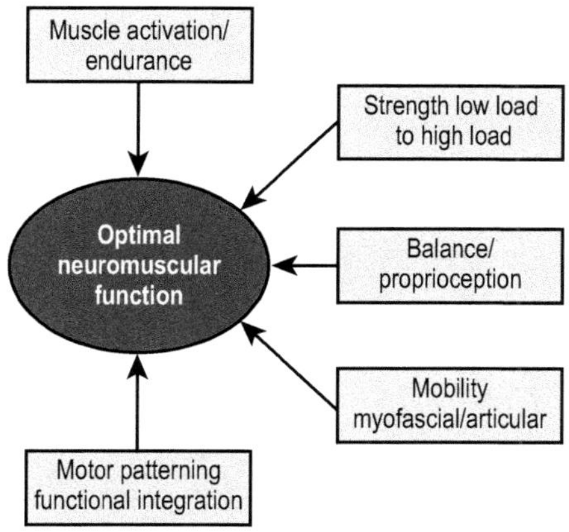

Figure 38.1 Optimal neuromuscular control.

Dynamic / functional assessment

Observation of the patient's gait revealed decreased hip extension at terminal stance, an increased hip adduction / internal rotation moment during the loading response and a slight trunk lean to the right during single leg support. A pattern of hamstring dominance relative to the gluteal muscles was noted during prone active leg extension. During the performance of a single-leg squat, a hip adduction / internal rotation moment was evident with poor control. During a step-down manoeuvre (Souza & Powers 2009), the patient revealed a contralateral pelvic drop and increased hip adduction and internal rotation. He also reported an increase in his symptoms (NPRS 6 / 10) during both the single-leg squat and the step-down.

Within the clinical decision-making process, the clinician may consider the following questions to guide the development of an individualized therapeutic exercise programme. The constructs within the bio-psychosocial framework must all be considered and how they inter-relate: the impairment addressed with exercise must be linked to an activity limitation or participation restriction, and consideration of the contextual factors (personal and environmental) is key to a successful outcome (Brody 2012). Designing an effective exercise programme requires 'equal parts science and art' (Brody 2012).

- What is the clinical hypothesis generated and what impairments need to be addressed with exercise?
- What muscles do we want to target initially in this rehabilitation programme?
- Are there certain muscle groups that will require lengthening procedures and others that will require activation, endurance, or strengthening?
- What is most important to this patient in relation to his activity limitation and participation restrictions and how do we incorporate this into his exercises?
- How can the evidence assist us in choosing the most appropriate exercises for this case?
- What are the parameters to consider in prescribing the exercises?
- How do we progress the exercises and incorporate motor retraining and functional integration into his rehabilitation programme?

Muscle Performance: Activation, Endurance and Strength

The gluteal muscles are important in stabilizing the pelvis and controlling femoral adduction and internal rotation during functional movements. Muscle weakness can contribute to lower extremity dysfunction and has been reported in patellofemoral pain, iliotibial band syndrome and chronic ankle instability (Baker et al 2011; Barton et al 2013; Webster & Gribble 2013; Noehern et al 2014). Hip abduction and external rotation weakness can lead to knee valgus, hip adduction and internal rotation creating stress on the joints in the lower extremity (Powers 2003).

Designing exercises for the gluteal muscles requires the therapist to consider carefully a number of factors including biomechanical principles, such as plane of the movement, patient positioning, effect of gravity, length of the moment arm, speed of the motion, base of support, load, volume and the type of muscle contractions (Reiman et al 2012). Exercises should progress from less challenging to more challenging, to functional integration and task specific.

Ward et al (2010) investigated the architecture of the gluteal muscles and the importance of considering this when assessing and targeting these muscles. The gluteus medius muscle (GMed) has a large physiological cross-sectional area and relatively short fibres and appears to be designed to stabilize the hip by generating large forces over a narrow range of lengths. It is capable of producing an exceptional amount of force given its size. It is not designed to produce very large forces over a wide range of lengths or hip positions. The gluteus maximus (GMax), on the other hand, has a large physiological cross-sectional area and long fibres – suggesting that it is capable of generating large forces over a wide range. The hamstrings have the potential to generate a major part of hip extensor torque.

The GMed consists of three distinct portions: anterior, middle and posterior, with separate innervation from the superior gluteal nerve. The primary role of this muscle is to stabilize the pelvis and control femoral motion during weight-bearing activities, with the greatest activation during the stance phase of gait (Gottschalk et al 1989; Gowda et al 2014). The phasic activity of the three parts is based on the fibre orientation. The anterior and middle portions of the muscle initiate hip abduction. Acting in isolation, the anterior portion abducts, medially rotates, assists with hip flexion and is active when the base of support is minimal (e.g. bridges, unilateral squat, lateral step-up) (Boudreau et al 2009). The posterior portion of the muscle extends, abducts and laterally rotates the hip. The posterior fibres have been described as the primary stabilizers of the femoral head in the acetabulum during weight transfer (Gottschalk et al 1989; Gowda et al 2014). The posterior segment of GMed is important in lunging and jumping tasks (Neumann 2010; Gowda et al 2014). With hip flexion angles greater than 60°, there is a shift of the anterior fibres of GMax anterior to the hip joint axis of rotation, turning it into an internal rotator; in this situation the posterior fibres of GMed act with the deep external rotators to provide control (Neumann 2010; Powers 2010; Gowda et al 2014).

A common exercise used in the early stages of hip abduction strengthening is the 'clam shell' (Fig. 38.2). Several studies

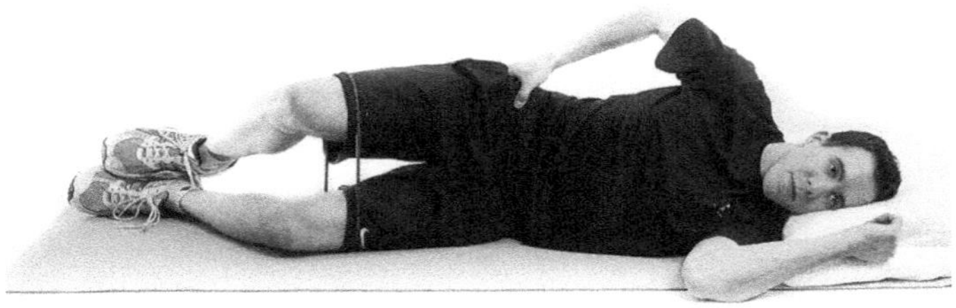

Figure 38.2 Clam shell. In the side-lying position with the knees flexed to 30° or 60°, the patient is instructed to raise his knee up and back while keeping the ankles together. He is cued to focus the motion at the hip (abduction and external rotation) and to avoid pelvis/trunk rotation. Elastic resistance can be added to increase the muscle demand.

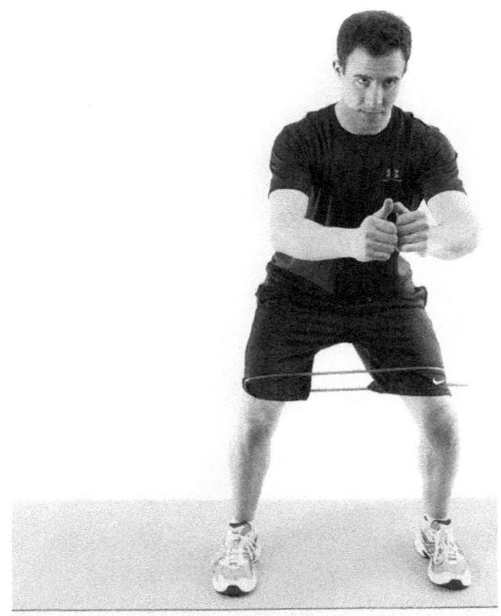

Figure 38.3 Lateral side-step. In a partial squat position with an elastic band around the thighs, the patient steps to the side maintaining good alignment of the knees over the toes. This can be done as single or multiple strides in one direction and then in the opposite direction, or performed as strides while walking forward.

have investigated the muscle activation of GMax and GMed during modifications to this exercise. Wilcox and Burden (2013) found that a neutral pelvis position optimized recruitment of both muscles and increasing the hip flexion angle increased the activation of GMed. The tensor fascia lata (TFL) activity was relatively low and unaffected by these variations to the exercise. Selkowitz et al (2013) wanted to determine which exercises were best for activating the GMed and the superior portion of GMax while minimizing the activity of the TFL. A common strategy utilized by patients with hip abductor weakness is to compensate with the TFL muscle, which contributes to excessive hip internal rotation. If the goal is to activate the gluteal muscles preferentially then these authors found that the clam shell, lateral side-step (Fig. 38.3), unilateral bridge and quadruped hip extension exercises with either the knee flexed or extended all achieved this.

O'Sullivan et al (2010) evaluated the activation of all three subdivisions of GMed during three weight-bearing exercises: the wall squat (Fig. 38.4), the pelvic drop (Fig. 38.5) and the wall press (Fig. 38.6) and found that the activation levels of GMed varied significantly across each of the subdivisions. All three exercises caused greater activation of the middle and posterior subdivisions than the anterior, with the wall press particularly increasing the activation of the posterior subdivision. Across all three subdivisions, the exercises were progressively more demanding from wall squat to pelvic drop to wall press. These authors proposed that the wall press exercise tends to cause hip internal rotation on the weight-bearing leg, thus increasing the hip external rotation force required to maintain pelvic and hip posture. Based on these results, the authors suggest that the wall press is an effective isometric strengthening exercise for the GMed, especially the posterior subdivision. The wall squat and pelvic drop may be useful in the early stages of rehabilitation to improve endurance, stability and motor control.

Table 38.1 summarizes the results of a systematic review by Reiman et al (2012) evaluating the activation of GMax and GMed muscles, as a percentage of the maximal voluntary contraction (MVC) during commonly prescribed rehabilitation

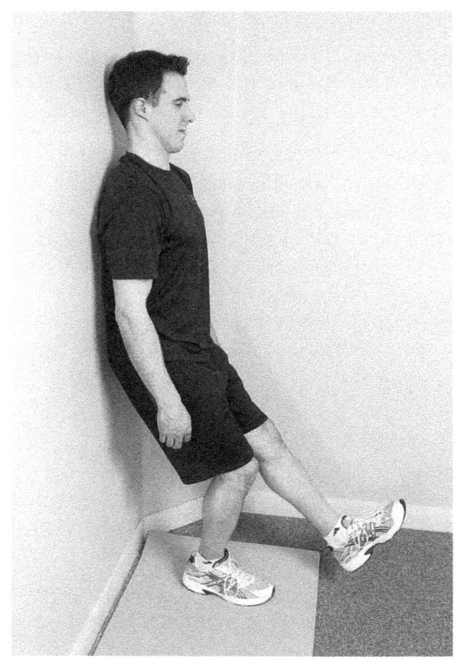

Figure 38.4 Single-leg wall squat. Standing on the affected leg with the back resting against the wall with hip and knee flexed to approximately 30°, the patient slowly lowers himself towards the ground. He is instructed to keep his knee over the second toe to prevent a valgus position of the knee.

exercises. It has been theorized that exercises requiring greater electromyographic (EMG) activity (>40% MVC) will result in strength gains and clinicians could apply this information when designing exercise programmes. Although the majority of the studies were conducted on samples of healthy subjects

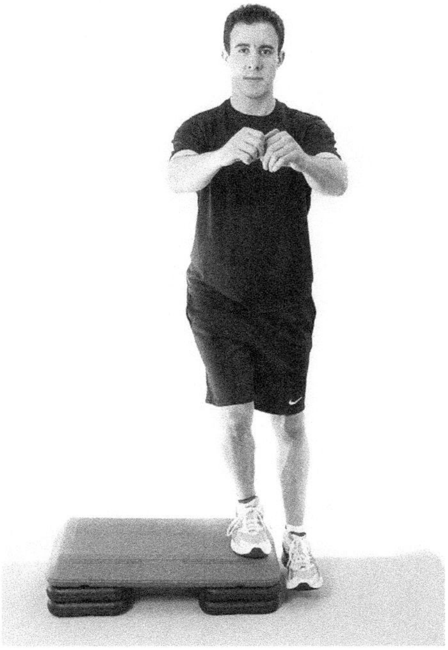

Figure 38.5 Pelvic drop. Standing with the affected leg on the edge of a step, maintaining a slightly flexed position of both knees, the patient slowly lowers one side of the pelvis towards the floor and then returns the pelvis to a level position.

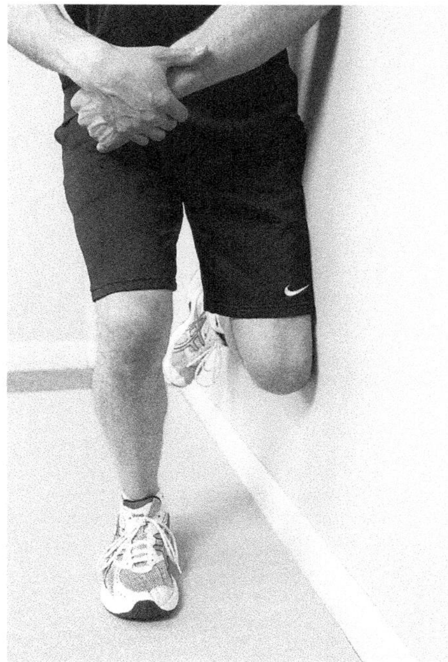

Figure 38.6 Wall press. Standing sideways to the wall on the affected leg in a single-leg stance position, the patient performs an isometric hip abduction/external rotation press against the wall with the unaffected non-weight-bearing leg, while maintaining proper alignment of the knee over the foot using hip external rotation of the stance leg. The trunk is kept vertical and the pelvis level throughout the exercise.

Table 38.1 Activation levels of gluteus medius and gluteus maximus during various therapeutic exercises

	Low-level activation (0–20% MVC)	Moderate-level activation (21–40% MVC)	High-level activation (41–60% MVC)	Very-high-level activation (>60% MVC)
Gluteus medius		Prone bridge plank (27%) Bridging on stable surface (28%) Lunge – neutral trunk position (34%) Unilateral mini-squat (36%) Retro step-up (37%) Clam shell at 60° (38%) Clam shell at 30° (40%) Sideways lunge (39%)	Lateral step-up (41%) Quadruped with contralateral arm and leg lift (42%) Forward step-up (44%) Unilateral bridge (47%) Transverse lunge (48%) Wall squat (52%) Side-lying hip abduction (56%) Pelvic drop (57%) Single-limb deadlift (58%)	Single-limb squat (64%) Side bridge to neutral spine position (74%)
Gluteus maximus	Prone bridge/plank (9%) Lunge with backward trunk lean (12%) Bridging on a Swiss ball (20%)	Side-lying hip abduction (21%) Lunge with forward trunk lean (22%) Bridging on a stable surface (25%) Clam shell with 30° hip flexion (34%) Lunge neutral trunk position (36%) Clam shell with 60° hip flexion (39%) Unilateral bridge (40%)	Sideways lunge (41%) Lateral step-up (41%) Transverse lunge (49%) Quadruped with contralateral arm/leg lift (56%) Unilateral mini-squat (57%) Retro step-up (59%) Wall squat (59%) Single-limb squat (59%) Single-limb dead-lift (59%)	Forward step-up (74%)

(From Reiman et al 2012.)

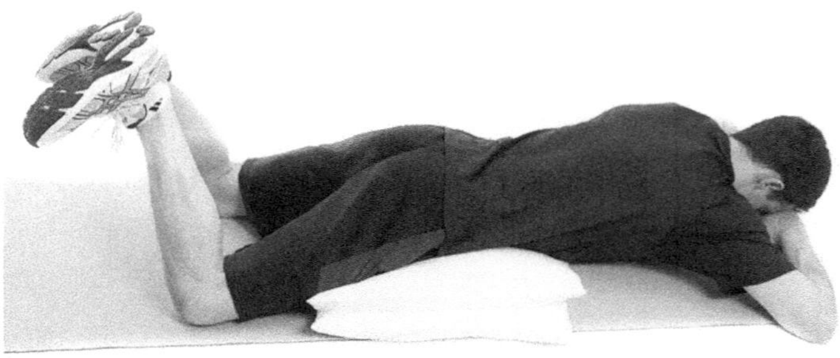

Figure 38.7 Prone heel squeeze. In prone lying with the hips slightly abducted and externally rotated, knees flexed to 45°–90° and heels touching, the patient presses the heels together. Slight hip extension can be added by raising the thighs off the table.

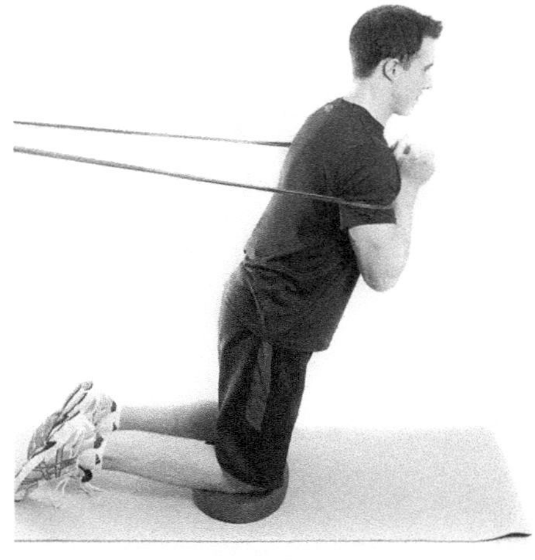

Figure 38.8 Eccentric lowers (Nordic hamstring). Starting in a kneeling position with the feet fixed, the patient falls forward using the hamstrings to control the descent and then catches himself with the hands. Initially assistance can be provided with an elastic band.

and the results may differ in people with musculoskeletal disorders, the knowledge of muscle activation during various exercises contributes to understanding neuromuscular control and is valuable information to consider when developing exercise programmes for individual patients.

Giphart et al (2012), using EMG, recorded the activation of pectineus and piriformis muscles during hip rehabilitation exercises in a group of 10 healthy volunteers. They found the highest activation of pectineus muscle was with supine active hip flexion (62.8% MVC concentrically, 55.4% eccentrically). Moderate to low activation was also recorded during both hip internal and external rotation. The single- and double-legged bridge exercises, which require static rotation stabilization in a neutrally positioned hip and incorporate weight-bearing, moderately activated the pectineus muscle. These authors propose that, functionally, pectineus is activated as a stabilizing muscle for rotational control of the hip in activities involving even slight weight-bearing. Based on their observations, the pectineus muscle probably stabilizes the hip in dynamic activities requiring pivoting movements and explosive accelerations (e.g. sprinting). High piriformis muscle activation was observed during resisted hip extension exercise, single-legged bridge, prone heel squeeze (Fig. 38.7) and side-lying abduction in external rotation, all of which require hip extension. They suggest that the most likely function of piriformis is as an external rotation stabilizer preventing internal rotation with the hip in a neutral-to-extended position. This would translate to activities such as jumping, skating stride or the toe-off phase of running, which require the muscle to produce a degree of external rotation to control hip internal rotation. Weakness of the piriformis could potentially result in increased valgus forces on the knee owing to the lack of stabilization needed to maintain hip external rotation. It would appear therefore that both of these deep hip muscles have an important role in hip stability in activities of daily living and sporting activities.

Comprehensive rehabilitation programmes should include both concentric and eccentric training, and clinicians should have an awareness of how to design exercises to have a greater eccentric emphasis and consider how eccentric exercise should be part of a systematic approach to post-injury retraining (Lorenz & Reiman 2011). Although not directly applicable to the case presented above, there is evidence in the literature for the use of eccentric exercise for the rehabilitation of lower extremity dysfunctions, mostly relating to rehabilitation after hamstring injuries or Achilles tendinopathy (Lorenz & Reiman 2011). (Readers are also referred to other chapters for exercises applied to particular disorders of the lower extremity.)

Several authors have proposed rehabilitation strategies to regain hamstring function, but most are related to recovery from muscle strain injuries (Comfort et al 2009; Heiderscheit et al 2010; Lorenz & Reiman 2011). Heiderscheit et al (2010) suggest that early rehabilitation consists of isometrics of the lumbopelvic musculature, single-limb balance exercises and short-stride frontal plane stepping drills while avoiding heavier isolated resistance training of the injured hamstring muscle. Hamstring-specific strengthening exercises can be implemented in non-weight-bearing and open kinetic chain, pain free and with intensity progressing from light to moderate as tolerated. Exercises would progress to low-velocity eccentric activities at low to middle ranges such as stiff leg deadlifts, walking lunges, eccentric hamstring lowers (also referred to as Nordic hamstring exercise) and split squats. Lorenz and Reiman (2011) recommend performing the eccentric lowers initially with elastic-band assistance (Fig. 38.8), as the elasticity of the band can assist in both the concentric and eccentric portions of the exercise. Finally, sport-specific exercises involving quick direction changes, functional movement patterns, plyometrics and eccentric exercises progressing to end range are added to complete the rehab. When considering intensity of hamstring muscle activity, McAllister et al (2014) found that, when comparing four exercises including the glute-ham raise, good morning, Roman deadlift and

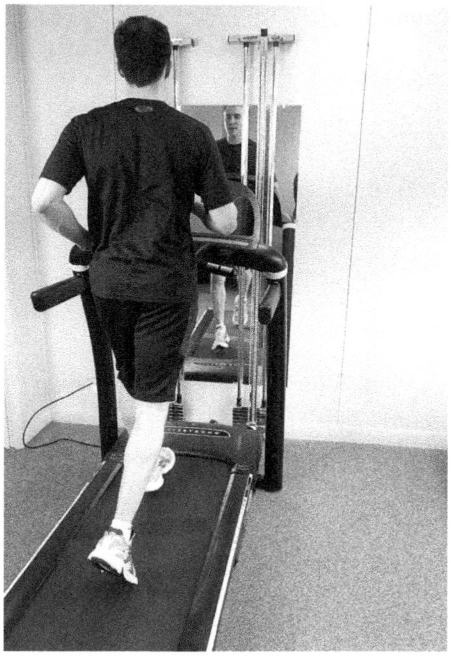

Figure 38.9 Treadmill running. Verbal and visual cues can be utilized as the patient runs on a treadmill with mirror feedback. This can improve transference of improvement in impairments to functional goals.

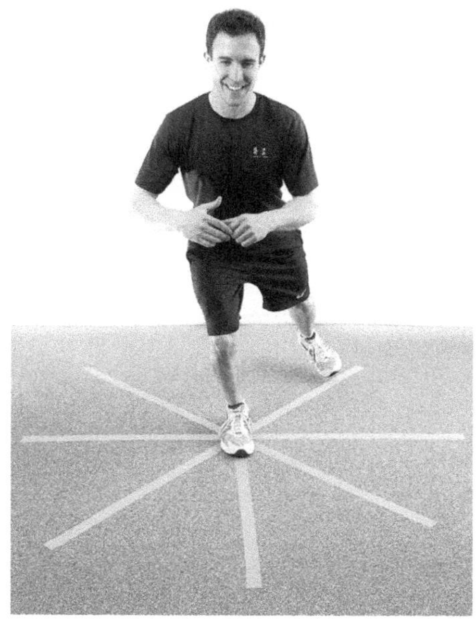

Figure 38.10 Star excursion balance exercise. In a partial single-leg squat, the patient is instructed to reach as far as possible with the contralateral limb in various directions (forward, forward diagonal, lateral, backward and backward diagonal).

prone leg curl exercises, the concentric activity was highest during the glute-ham raise and eccentric during the Roman deadlift.

Neuromotor Control: Balance, Proprioception, Movement Repatterning and Functional Integration

Willy and Davis (2011) conducted a randomized controlled trial to investigate whether a strengthening and movement education programme targeting the hip abductor and external rotator muscles altered hip mechanics during running and during a single-leg squat in a group of healthy females. They found improvement in the single-leg squat mechanics, but the training programme did not alter the abnormal hip mechanics during running. These authors therefore suggested that clinicians should consider incorporating activity-specific neuromuscular training into therapeutic programmes.

Willy et al (2012) evaluated a simple gait retraining technique using visual and verbal feedback in a group of female runners with patellofemoral pain and abnormal hip mechanics. The gait retraining consisted of providing visual feedback with a full-length mirror placed in front of the treadmill while running and verbal cueing – that is, 'run with your knees apart and your knee caps pointing straight ahead' and 'squeeze your buttocks' (Fig. 38.9). These authors found that the training was effective in improving mechanics during running and measures of pain and function. They also noted that the skill transferred to untrained tasks (i.e. squatting and step descent) and postulated that a higher level of motor learning had occurred.

Dynamic postural control is essential for return to function and sport after a lower extremity musculoskeletal injury / dysfunction. Unilateral weight-bearing exercises are often used to train dynamic postural control and proprioception. Proximal stability of the lumbopelvic region is required for coordinated movement in the lower extremity. The star excursion balance test (SEBT) is a test of dynamic postural control in which the individual balances on one leg while reaching with the other in eight different directions (Kinzey & Armstrong 1998; Hertel et al 2000). The SEBT is a useful tool for training dynamic balance and proprioception (Fig. 38.10). Neuromuscular control during the test is reflected by the distance reached in each direction, with an increase in the distance indicating greater neuromuscular control had been achieved. Norris and Trudelle-Jackson (2011) investigated activation of the proximal musculature (i.e. GMed, GMax, vastus medialis (VM)) during the eccentric phase of the lower extremity reaching in the anterior, medial and posteromedial directions of the SEBT. They found the level of GMed muscle recruitment to be greater in the anterior and medial directions (38% MVC and 48% MVC) and suggested that, when prescribing the SEBT as an exercise to address GMed specifically, the posterior–medial direction may be more appropriate during the early stages, progressing to the anterior direction and then, as motor control improves, the medial direction may be added as a strengthening stimulus. In their study, the GMax EMG amplitude was below the 40–60% threshold in all three directions, suggesting that the SEBT may not be an appropriate strengthening exercise for GMax; however, it may be used to promote muscle endurance in the early phases of rehabilitation before progressing to exercises requiring higher level of muscle activity. The VM amplitudes were above the 40–60% threshold suggesting that the three directions were equally effective for VM strengthening and, given the high level of recruitment, may be more appropriate in the later stages of rehabilitation for that muscle.

Altered frontal plane hip and knee mechanics may contribute to the aetiology of many common running injuries such as patellofemoral pain, tibial stress fractures and iliotibial band syndrome. Wouters et al (2012) hypothesized that hip muscle strengthening alone may not be sufficient to reduce hip or knee frontal plane motion and peak moments during the stance phase of running. These authors postulated that rehabilitation programmes should emphasize neuromuscular control elements, such as guided practice of movement performance and visual, verbal and tactile feedback, rather than hip strengthening alone. In their quasi-experimental design study, subjects participated in a 4-week movement-training programme using visual feedback (use of a mirror) and weekly instruction including cues such as keeping the knee in line with the hip and foot in the frontal plane, the pelvis parallel with the floor, increasing hip flexion to avoid anterior motion of the knee beyond the foot during the squat exercise and maintaining a neutral lumbar spine. Manual facilitation techniques such as tapping over the gluteal muscles or tactile feedback to the lateral knee to promote hip abduction were also used. The exercise progression utilized in their neuromotor-retraining programme is outlined in Table 38.2. At the end of the 4-week training programme, participants displayed reduced frontal plane hip and knee joints mechanics that may potentially contribute to and exacerbate running related injuries. These results support the concept that strategies to correct lower extremity alignment and motor patterning in functional movements are a crucial component in exercise programmes, in addition to strengthening.

Moreside and McGill (2012a) analysed the transference of increased passive hip range of motion (through stretching), motor control (through hip–spine dissociation exercises) and core endurance to functional movement in a cohort of 24 young healthy males with limited hip mobility. The dynamic activities that were analysed included active hip extension, lunge, a standing twist / reach manoeuvre and exercising on an elliptical trainer. They found that, although both flexibility and endurance improved over a 6-week intervention, there was minimal evidence that these changes transferred to functional movement patterns. The findings suggest that exercise programmes may require simultaneous movement repatterning and practising the desired movement patterning to ensure that the increased mobility and strength / endurance are incorporated into functional movement patterns.

Table 38.2 Neuromotor retraining programme

	Exercises	Volume (sets/reps)
Week 1	Wall squat	3/10
	Forward lunge	3/10
	Lateral step down (4"/10 cm)	3/10
	Single leg stance with ball toss	3/30 s hold
Week 2	Lateral step-down (7"/18 cm)	3/10
	Forward step-up (7"/18 cm)	3/10
	Single-leg dead-lift	3/10
	Lateral shuffles with band	3/40 feet (12 m)
Week 3–4	Forward step-down (7"/18 cm)	3/10
	Balance lunge	3/10
	Single-leg multidirectional reach	3/5
	Single-leg squat with band	3/10

(As per Wouters et al 2012.)

Mobility, Myofascial and Articular Impairments

It is difficult to obtain optimal function of the lower quadrant without adequate mobility, which can be reduced by a number of factors – including articular restriction and myofascial extensibility (length), as well as neuromeningeal mobility. A variety of manual therapy techniques can be utilized to regain articular mobility in the lower quadrant at the hip. It is then important to augment or maintain the gains achieved by utilizing joint mobility exercises. There is an absence of research regarding these types of hip exercises to guide that portion of the exercise design.

As suggested by Janda (1987), the following muscles tend to tighten around the hip: the hip flexors, hip adductors, hamstrings, deep hip external rotators and TFL / ITB; these should therefore be considered and addressed as required.

A systematic review by O'Sullivan et al (2012) concluded that there is consistent, strong evidence that eccentric training can improve lower extremity flexibility. This was true for the hamstrings, quadriceps and gastrocnemius–soleus musculature flexibility. Although eccentric training resulted in significant improvement in flexibility compared with controls, the one study that compared eccentric exercise with static stretching found similar gains in range of motion with either approach. One study within the review (Nelson & Bandy 2004) incorporated a static stretch at the end of range within low-load eccentric training and found this resulted in higher range gains than those found in other studies that utilized eccentric training alone. When comparing the effect of eccentric versus concentric exercises on muscle flexibility, two of the studies reported in the O'Sullivan et al (2012) review had different results – one favouring the eccentric mode and the other finding no difference. An additional randomized controlled trial conducted by Patel and Yadav (2013) reached the conclusion that, although both static stretching and eccentric exercise significantly improved hamstring flexibility, static stretching was statistically more effective. At this point in time, although it is impossible to say whether eccentric exercise training is as effective as static stretching in improving flexibility, as eccentric exercise also enhances other performance variables it should be considered an important component in a lower extremity exercise programme.

There are many different exercises designed to increase the length of the hamstring muscles. A systematic review by Decoster et al (2005) concluded that evidence supports the use of hamstring stretching for increasing flexibility, with a variety of stretching techniques, positions and durations. Ayala et al (2013) also found that improvement in hamstring length occurred with stretching in both those with normal (>80°) and those with limited hamstring length (<80°). Several of the parameters (i.e. position, mode, dosage) of various exercises have been investigated, with varying results. Although there do appear to be some consistent findings that might guide our choice of exercise, the specific patient presentation should be considered during the clinical-reasoning process to determine which exercise would be optimal for that particular patient.

Several studies have compared different types of hamstring stretching exercises: passive, active, static, dynamic and proprioceptive neuromuscular facilitation (PNF) / muscle energy techniques (MET). In a group of asymptomatic individuals, Fasen et al (2009) found that, at 4 weeks, active-stretching methods were significantly superior to passive, but this difference reversed at the 8-week point, at which the passive SLR stretch exercise resulted in the greatest improvement in hamstring length. Davis et al (2005) found static stretching to be superior at 4 weeks. Puentedura et al (2011) found that, although there was an immediate increase in hamstring length following both static and active (PNF) stretching, there was no difference between the two groups. Covert et al (2010) reported that both ballistic and static stretching increased hamstring length compared with controls, but the static group made significantly more gains. Because of these inconsistent results across studies, there is no clear indication as to which type of hamstring stretch is superior, although a static version seems to be preferred. Subjects did report that the active exercises were more engaging than passive exercises, which could be a factor in adherence (Fasen et al 2009).

There does not appear to be a clinically significant difference between a contract–relax exercise as compared with a reciprocal inhibition technique used during an MET / PNF stretching exercise (Youdas et al 2010). The duration of the passive stretch component (30 seconds versus 3 seconds) has no significant impact on the efficacy of MET / PNF for short-term increases in hamstring extensibility (Smith & Fryer 2008). Also, hamstring stretches appear to be equally effective regardless of the position: supine, sitting or standing (Decoster et al 2005; Borman et al 2011). Sairyo et al (2013), in a pilot study, found the standing jackknife hamstring stretch exercise to be effective for increasing hamstring length. Fasen et al (2009) compared various supine exercises and found that a passive straight leg stretch with the leg supported up the wall was superior to a 90 / 90 passive stretch with a strap; the active 90 / 90 stretch (Fig. 38.11) was superior to the passive 90 / 90 stretch, but not as effective in the longer term as the passive straight leg stretch up the wall (Fig. 38.12).

Subjects using an 'awareness through movement' exercise, consisting of controlled lengthening movements with no end-range stretch or hold, increased hamstring flexibility compared with controls (Stephens et al 2006). Ballantyne et al (2003) found that, although there was a significant increase in range to the point of discomfort following a MET stretch, there was no change in range when an identical force was used to retest the flexibility. They concluded that the differences in range found post stretch may be more related to an increase in stretch sensation tolerance than to any biomechanical or viscoelastic change in the muscle.

Incorporating a sciatic nerve 'slider' exercise in addition to either usual hamstring stretching and warm-up or sustained hamstring stretching may result in greater increase in lower quadrant flexibility (Fasen et al 2009; Mendez-Sanchez et al 2010; Castellote-Caballero et al 2013). (Readers are directed to

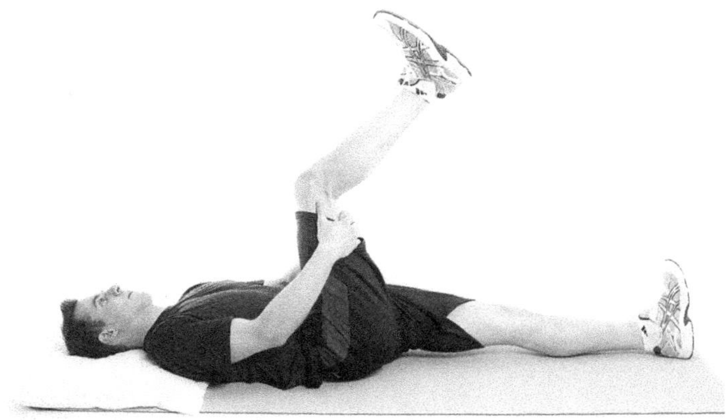

Figure 38.11 90/90 active hamstring muscle stretch. In supine the patient stabilizes the upper leg with his hands holding the hip at 90°. He then actively straightens the knee until a stretch discomfort is felt in the hamstrings muscles.

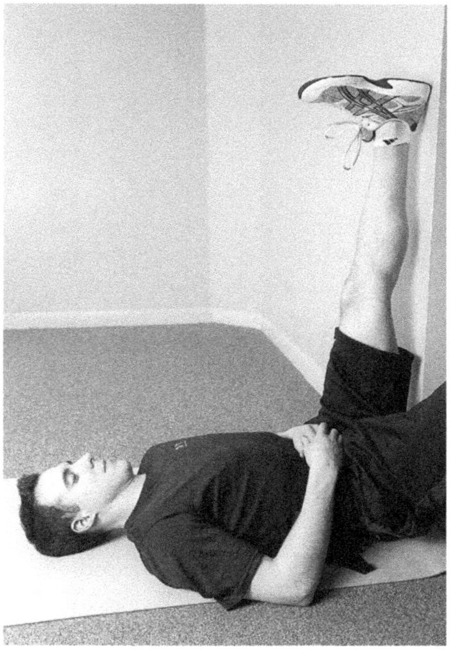

Figure 38.12 Hamstring muscle wall stretch. At a corner or through a door, the patient lies with the tight leg up the wall in a straight leg position to achieve a passive stretch. The stretch can be increased by bringing the hips closer to the wall.

Chapter 65 for more detailed information regarding neurodynamics in the lower quadrant.)

de Weijer et al (2003) found that the addition of a warm-up exercise prior to stretching did not significantly increase the effectiveness of static hamstring stretching. O'Sullivan et al (2009) found that, although an active aerobic warm-up significantly increased hamstring flexibility, the subsequent addition of static stretching further increased flexibility, whereas dynamic stretching reduced hamstring flexibility. Their conclusion was that if the aim was to increase hamstring length then static stretching should be employed. Further, a recent study found that dynamic hamstring stretching pre-activity reduced concentric and eccentric hamstring strength; this

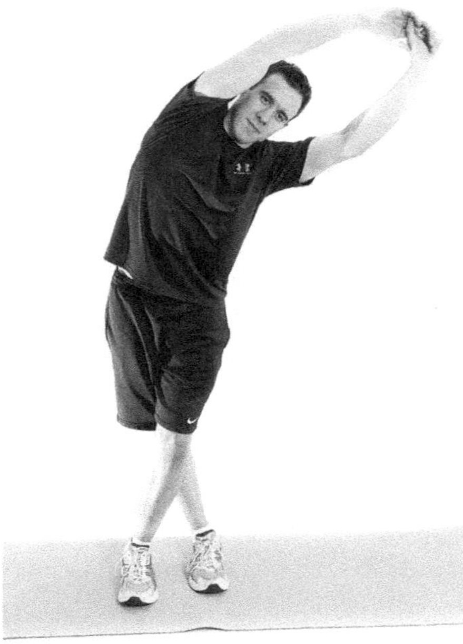

Figure 38.13 Standing iliotibial band stretch. The affected leg is extended and adducted behind the standing leg and then the patient reaches overhead side-flexing away from the stiff side.

suggests that clinicians need to be cautious when recommending dynamic rather than static stretching so as to prevent this post-stretch loss of muscle force (Costa et al 2014).

A stretch of the ITB can be achieved using either the flexed or the extended knee in Ober's side-lying position, with conflicting reports as to which position is more effective. Wang et al (2006) found that either position resulted in a similar stretch when the leg was dropped passively into adduction, but if a weight was added then the extended knee position resulted in more stretch. Conversely, Gajdosik et al (2003) found there was less range of adduction in the bent knee position compared with the extended position, which suggests that a stretch of the ITB would be amplified in the flexed position. Fredericson et al (2002) compared three standing stretches and found optimal ITB lengthening occurred when an overhead arm stretch was added to the traditional standing stretch of side-bending away with the tight leg extended and adducted behind the standing leg (Fig. 38.13).

The piriformis muscle is generally regarded as an external rotator of the hip, but it also acts as a hip abductor. As such, flexion / adduction / internal rotation of the hip would be considered the position of stretch for the piriformis (Hulbert & Deyle 2009; Fishman et al 2002). In contrast to this, Gulledge et al (2014) combined hip flexion, adduction and external rotation in their investigation into the optimal stretching protocol for the piriformis. They found that, at 90° hip flexion, piriformis elongation is similar (approximately 12%) regardless of the order of sequence of adding the two other movements (external rotation or adduction) to the stretch. We can infer from this that either of these stretches would be equally effective, and the choice of stretch would be best determined by the position with the strongest stretch sensation but also the most comfort. Through computer modelling these authors also determined that increasing the hip flexion component to 115° or to 120° elongates the piriformis muscle by approximately 15%, and so moving further into hip flexion could optimize the stretch as long as this does not cause symptoms of impingement.

Wright and Drysdale (2008) found that both contract–relax and reciprocal inhibition MET / PNF stretch techniques in prone resulted in significant increase in piriformis length, as measured by prone hip internal rotation range, but there was no difference between the two types of contraction used.

Winters et al (2004) found that a passive stretch exercise (lunge and propped prone hip extension) was equally effective as an active exercise (prone active hip extension with knee flexed and knee extended) in lengthening tight hip flexors in subjects with low back pain or lower extremity injuries. Godges et al (1989) found that three sets of a 2-minute static stretch of the hip flexors resulted in increased hip extension as well as improvement in gait (walking and running) economy as measured by submaximal oxygen consumption.

Moreside and McGill (2012b) proposed that stretching would be more effective in regaining hip mobility if the adjacent structures were incorporated into the stretch to tension the involved myofascial connections maximally, and that trunk stability might also influence flexibility of the lower extremity. They analysed the effect of three different exercise interventions: (1) stretching, (2) stretching with motor control exercises and (3) core endurance with motor control exercises (no stretching), versus a control group on passive hip range of motion, specifically extension and rotation. The stretching component included traditional exercises as well as whole-body myofascial lengthening, with an overhead arm position and trunk rotation added to optimize lengthening of adjacent tissues (Fig. 38.14). They also included a combination of static (30-second hold) and ballistic stretches. The motor control exercises focused on improving hip–spine dissociation, whereas the core endurance programme focused on trunk muscle activation. Hip extension and rotation mobility were dramatically improved in both groups 1 and 2, but the addition of the motor control exercises did not result in greater flexibility. A moderate increase in hip rotation range of motion was also noted in the group receiving core endurance and motor control exercises with no active stretching. As suggested by the authors, this highlights the role of including core stabilization in rehabilitation programmes for the lower extremity (see Ch 23).

Designing an Evidence-informed Exercise Programme

Considering both the subjective and objective data, our initial hypothesis is that the patient in the example Case Report demonstrated mobility and muscle performance impairments specific to the hip region. He presented with restricted hip joint mobility, decreased length of the ITB, hamstring and piriformis, weakness of the hip extensors, abductors and external rotators and an inability to control the hip and pelvis during functional movements of the lower extremity. Poor neuromuscular control and abnormal movement patterning contributed to the faulty lower limb mechanics during functional tasks (squat, step-downs). The patient's goal was to be able to return to running with minimal pain. Exercises increasing mobility of the hip joint, addressing the muscle imbalance (length and strength) around the hip, and correcting abnormal movement patterning of the lower extremity would therefore be the focus of the programme. Balance, proprioception, movement repatterning and functional integration exercises are critical to ensure transference of the improvement in individual impairments into functional activities, specifically the goal of running.

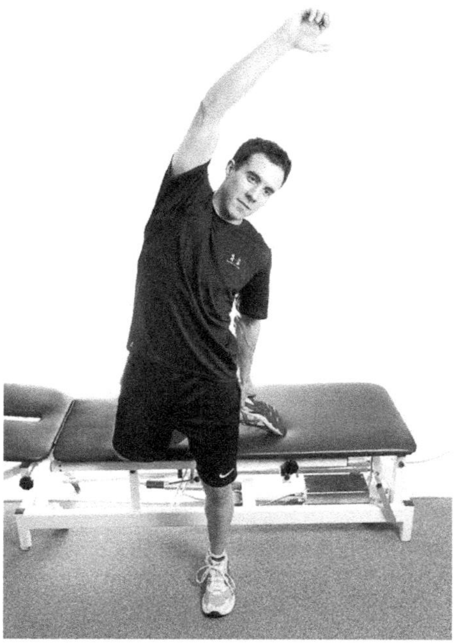

Figure 38.14 Hip myofascial stretch. In standing the patient places the foot onto a bench placing the hip in a FABER stretch position. An extended myofascial stretch of adjacent tissues is obtained by adding the ipsilateral overhead reach as well as incorporating trunk rotation and/or side-flexion.

The exercise progression model proposed by Brody (2012) and modified in Figure 38.15 provides a conceptual framework of the variables to consider in exercise programme design.

Mobility exercises

As is often seen clinically, the cause of reduced joint motion can be multifactorial. The restriction of hip mobility that this patient presents with may be related to articular hypomobility as indicated by the early capsular end feel with a posterolateral glide. It may also be a reflection of muscle imbalance, the lack of extensibility found on length testing as well as the weakness of the gluteal muscles and poor motor control. Addressing these impairments could potentially resolve hip hypomobility. In designing the therapeutic exercise programme, clinical reasoning must be used to determine when it would be most appropriate to add mobility exercises. In this case, a focus on the impairments of muscle performance and motor control would be a priority and may actually decrease the dominance of some of the tight muscle groups. Reassessment of length testing may well demonstrate normal muscle extensibility and, at that point, stretching exercises for muscles that continue to test short can be added.

In this particular case, the hip joint mobility restriction will have also been addressed with manual therapy to restore the posterolateral glide, and home exercises can then be given to maintain the range that has been gained with manual therapy. The quadruped sit-back exercise can be used to mobilize the hip, controlling lumbopelvic neutral and rocking back into hip flexion only as far as is pain free (Sahrmann 2002). This exercise encourages hip flexion, stretches the posterior hip musculature and encourages posterior glide of the femoral head, all issues that need to be addressed with this case. It also encourages a dissociation pattern between the hip and the lumbopelvic unit. If the patient finds it difficult to gain

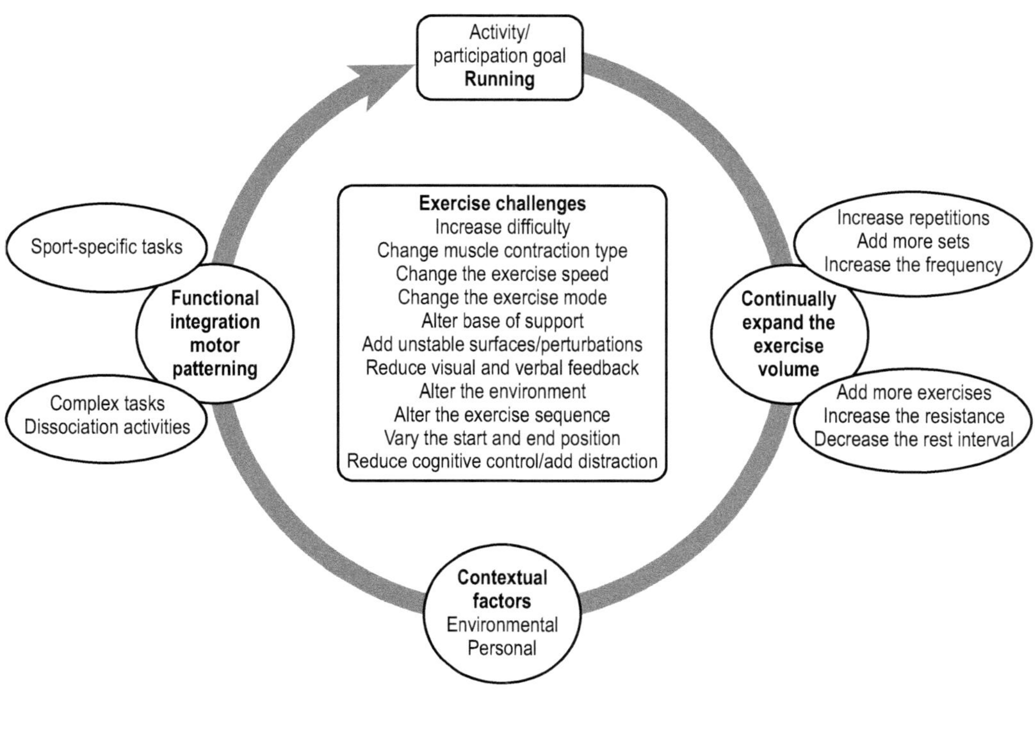

Figure 38.15 Exercise progression model. (Modified from Brody 2012.)

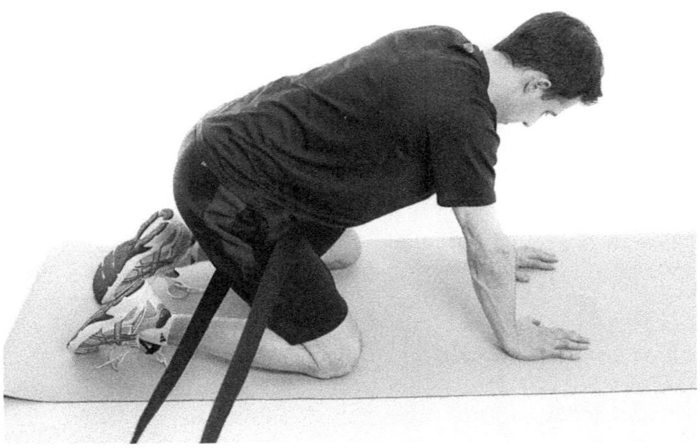

Figure 38.16 Quadruped sit-back exercise. In the quadruped position the patient adopts a neutral spine posture and maintains this throughout the exercise. Focusing on hip joint motion, the patient then sits back into hip flexion as far as he can without losing the neutral spine posture or experiencing any impingement at the anterior hip. A strap or heavy elastic band can be used to produce a lateral distraction to decrease impingement.

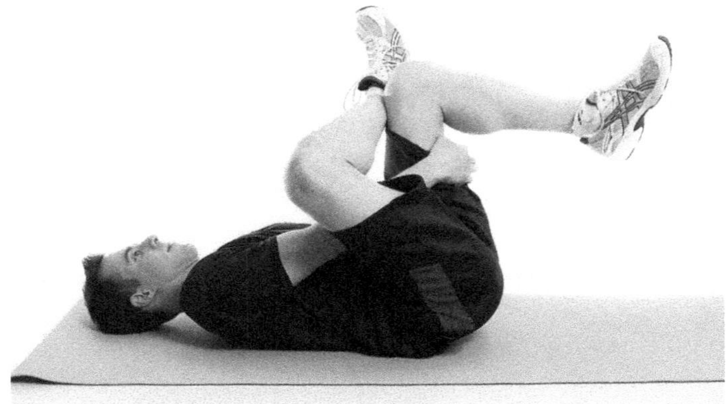

Figure 38.17 Figure 4 stretch. In supine the patient places the ankle of the affected side on the opposite knee and drops the affected leg into external rotation without allowing the pelvis to tilt. He then pulls the non-affected leg up towards the chest to produce the stretch.

range of motion without producing anterior impingement, a Mulligan mobilization with movement (MWM) technique can be modified to use as a home exercise (Mulligan 2004). A strap or heavy elastic band can be anchored on a post, looped around the right upper thigh as close to the groin as is comfortable and then used to apply either a lateral or posterior glide, while the subject moves into hip flexion in either quadruped or standing (Fig. 38.16). The patient is cautioned that there should be no reproduction of the anterior hip pain as he rocks back into flexion. One to three sets of 10 repetitions should be done daily (Hing et al 2008). (Readers are referred to Ch 37 for more manual therapies targeted to restore range of motion of the hip.)

In many cases there may be an overlap between exercises prescribed to increase joint range and those that stretch muscle. As there is often better adherence to exercise programmes when there are a limited number of exercises, it would be prudent to attempt to achieve both goals simultaneously (Medina-Mirapeix et al 2009). Lying prone with knees flexed to 90° and dropping the feet out to obtain end-range hip internal rotation is an exercise that will lengthen the articular capsule as well as obtain a stretch of piriformis and the other deep hip external rotators. This will also avoid the flexion–adduction position that is often used as a piriformis stretch as this position reproduced the anterior hip pain in this patient. Once the anterior impingement pain eases, the piriformis stretch can be progressed by moving into flexion in supine. As a similar intensity of stretch was found if external rotation was added prior to adduction, this might be the best sequence to minimize reproduction of pain (Gulledge et al 2014). A 'figure 4' position can be used to perform this stretch (Fig. 38.17). At a later point, it may be beneficial to include an internal rotation component via a cross-knees-to-chest or single-leg combined flexion / internal rotation / adduction stretch to ensure all portions of the deep lateral rotators along with portions of the gluteal muscles are lengthened.

The research has suggested that a PNF or active hamstring stretch may be more beneficial in the short term. Considering this, our patient could start with the 90 / 90 active knee extension exercise (see Fig. 38.11) and then include the passive SLR stretch up the wall (see Fig. 38.12), which has shown better long-term results (Davis et al 2005; Fasen et al 2009). Adding tibial medial rotation prior to knee extension may bias the stretch to the lateral hamstring, as was found on initial assessment. As there appears to be no superior position in which to stretch the hamstring, he would also benefit from instruction on the correct form of a standing stretch to use pre- and post-running (Decoster et al 2005; Borman et al 2011). The patient should also be educated that aggressive stretching pre-activity may negatively impact his performance; however, gentle stretching of 1–3 repetitions of a 30-second hold would be acceptable (Johnson et al 2014).

A FABER position stretch could be given in either supine or sitting position with the back against the wall, and the knees can be pushed down passively to increase the stretch. This is best performed bilaterally to prevent pelvic torsion. In supine or standing, additional stretch may be obtained by simultaneously elevating the right arm overhead and incorporating trunk rotation to expand the myofascial lengthening through adjacent structures (Moreside & McGill 2012b) (see Fig. 38.14).

The TFL / ITB can be stretched in side-lying, but the clinician should ensure verbal cueing is given to avoid compensatory motions through the lumbopelvic region. The pressure biofeedback unit can facilitate proper control, and this could be utilized to assist with this training in the clinic. Either the bent or extended knee position might be used, depending on which achieved the best stretch sensation. This position may be difficult to control, however, and a standing stretch may be preferred and also more easily performed pre- and post-running. The most effective stretch in standing has been shown to be the addition of a right-arm overhead stretch into side-flexion with the right leg back and crossed behind the left (see Fig 38.13). A foam roller may be used to achieve a more direct soft tissue release of the tight ITB.

Stretching the tight hip flexor muscles using hyperextension of the hip tends to create anterior translation of the femoral head and so should be avoided, at least initially. As motor control and repatterning improve, the hip flexors may in any case regain their normal length without the need for specific stretching exercises.

Muscle performance and neuromuscular control exercises

This portion of the patient's exercise programme will focus primarily on strengthening of the GMed and GMax muscles and neuromuscular retraining of proper lower extremity alignment during dynamic functional movements. Several authors have suggested progressing the exercises through three distinct phases: phase 1 – isolated muscle recruitment; phase 2 – weight-bearing strengthening; and phase 3 – functional training (Mascal et al 2003; Tonley et al 2010; Wagner et al 2010).

Phase 1

In the initial phase, non-weight-bearing recruitment exercises requiring moderate level activation of GMed and GMax muscles (see Table 38.1) with minimal TFL activation would be most appropriate. Lumbopelvic control would need to be established and emphasized during the performance of the lower extremity exercises. Possible options in this initial phase include the clam shell (see Fig. 38.2), bridging / unilateral bridging, side-lying leg lift with leg up against the wall, hip extension in prone lying (isometric with foot against the wall or concentric), resisted hip external rotation in sitting (Fig. 38.18) or quadruped hip extension. In selecting the exercises for this particular patient, consideration of the TFL and hamstring dominance and the anterior translation of the femoral head would influence the choices. The GMax and hamstring muscles are agonists and during the running cycle they decelerate the thigh during terminal swing and resist hip flexion during early stance (Lieberman et al 2006). Hamstring dominance was observed in our patient, along with weakness of the gluteal muscles, providing support for our decision to focus our interventions on strengthening and neuromuscular control. The exercises are initially performed without resistance and once the patient is able to perform three sets of 15 repetitions the exercises can be progressed by adding resistance with elastic tubing (Tonley et al 2010).

Neuromuscular control exercises in weight-bearing can be introduced in this initial phase to facilitate proper lower extremity alignment and promote activation of the target muscles in a more functional pattern. As recommended by O'Sullivan et al (2010), the wall press (see Fig. 38.6) is an effective isometric strengthening exercise for the posterior division of the GMed muscles; the wall squat (see Fig. 38.4) and pelvic drop (see Fig. 38.5) may also be useful in the early rehab stages. Wouters et al (2012) used the wall squat, forward lunge and step-downs (Fig. 38.19) early in their neuromotor retraining programme, while providing both visual and verbal feedback to monitor alignment and lower extremity pattern control.

Phase 2

Isolation exercises could be progressed to weight-bearing such as hip external rotation kneeling with the affected hip on a stool, which would also challenge balance and proprioception as well as dissociation (Fig. 38.20). Many exercise programmes incorporate squatting-based exercises as this

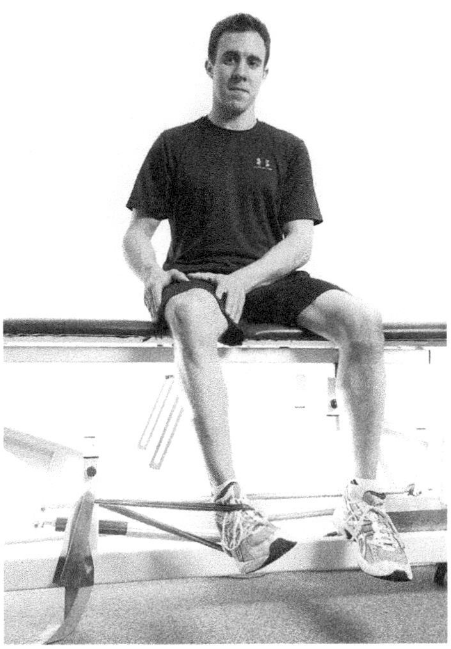

Figure 38.18 Resisted hip external rotation. The patient sits on the edge of the bed with the feet off the ground, holding the upper thigh to maintain control with an elastic band around the foot. Keeping the knee at 90°, he slowly moves the foot in against the elastic resistance. The patient is instructed to tighten his buttock muscles as he performs the movement.

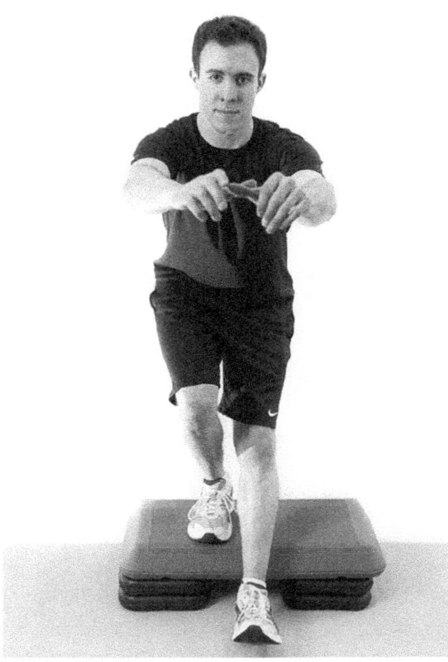

Figure 38.19 Forward step-down. The patient stands on the step and squats with the affected leg, slowly lowering the heel of the non-weight-bearing leg toward the floor while ensuring proper lower extremity alignment. This can be performed initially with upper extremity support if required.

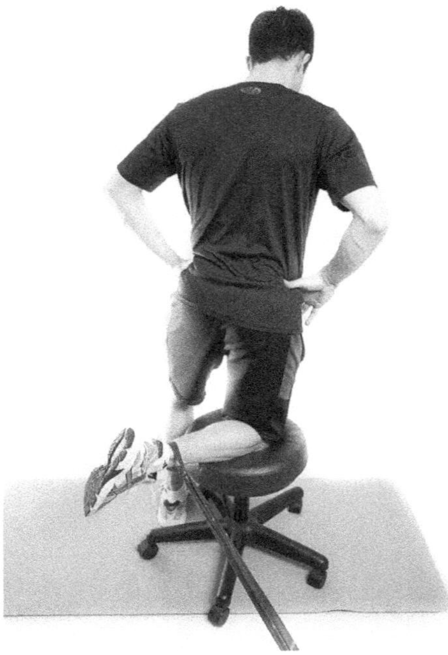

Figure 38.20 Weight-bearing resisted hip rotation. The patient stands with the affected knee on a swivel stool and elastic resistance is attached at the lower leg. Isolated hip external rotation is performed against the elastic resistance, ensuring good pelvic control.

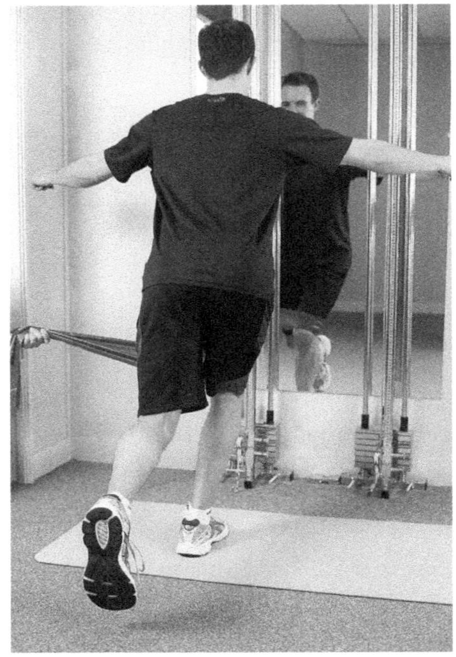

Figure 38.21 Single-leg squat with resistance. The patient stands on the affected leg, keeping the trunk and pelvis level with elastic resistance applied in the direction of hip adduction, requiring the patient to resist with hip abduction and external rotation while performing a single-leg squat.

movement strategy transfers to other functional activities such as descending stairs, sit to stand and running. Exercises in phase 2 can begin with double-leg weight-bearing and progress to single leg to increase the muscular demand as well as to challenge balance and proprioception. Squatting exercises can also be used to target other lower extremity musculature in addition to the gluteal muscles. Single-legged squat exercises produce a high level of GMax and GMed activation (>40% MVC) (see Table 38.1), and will therefore facilitate strength gains.

Single-leg squats can be progressed in front of a mirror, initially with one hand support if required, then unsupported, and finally further challenge to the hip abductors can be achieved by addition of a resistance band (Fig. 38.21) applied in the direction of hip adduction (Willy & Davis 2011). Proper lower extremity alignment should be emphasized during the weight-bearing exercises, and verbal cues such as 'keep the centre of the patella in line with both the anterior superior iliac spine proximally and with the second toe distally' or 'keep the patella pointing straight ahead to control hip internal rotation' can be used.

The forward step-down exercise can be progressed by adding 5 cm increments to the height of the step (see Fig. 38.19). Proper alignment of the lower extremity during the descent should be monitored to ensure control in the frontal and transverse planes. Controlled sit to stand is a functional movement that can be challenged by changing the base of support or adding resistance (Fig. 38.22). Multiplanar lunges or lateral, transverse or backward trunk lean (Fig. 38.23) can be added as all these exercises were shown to produce high activation of GMed and GMax muscles. The dynamic side step in a squat position with elastic resistance around the thighs (see Fig. 38.3) would be particularly beneficial for this

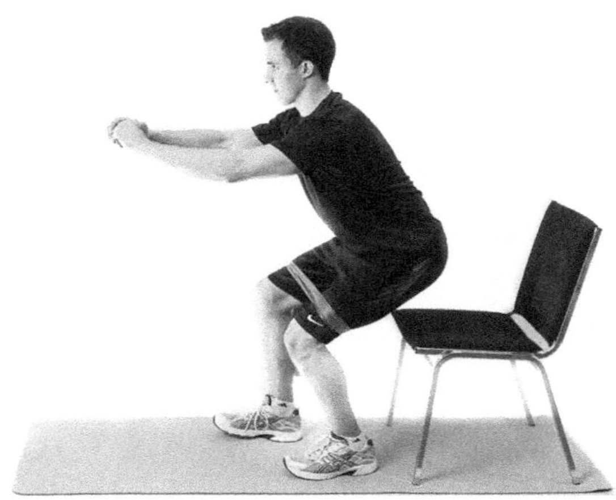

Figure 38.22 Controlled sit to stand. Starting in a stride foot position with elastic resistance around the lower legs, the patient rises from the sitting position, maintaining proper lower extremity alignment in the frontal and transverse planes. The exercise can be progressed by lowering the height of the sitting surface, increasing elastic resistance, adding an unstable surface under the foot or changing the base of support.

patient with a dominant TFL / ITB, as Selkowitz et al (2013) have found that this exercise produces high activation levels of GMed and the superior portion of GMax muscles while minimizing activation of the TFL. In the quadruped position, a triplanar exercise incorporating hip abduction, extension and external rotation against elastic resistance would target the GMed (Fig. 38.24). Challenges to forward and backward lunges can include adding an unstable base of support such as a BOSU® ball, or adding elastic resistance. Higher level activation exercises such as the side plank and front plank

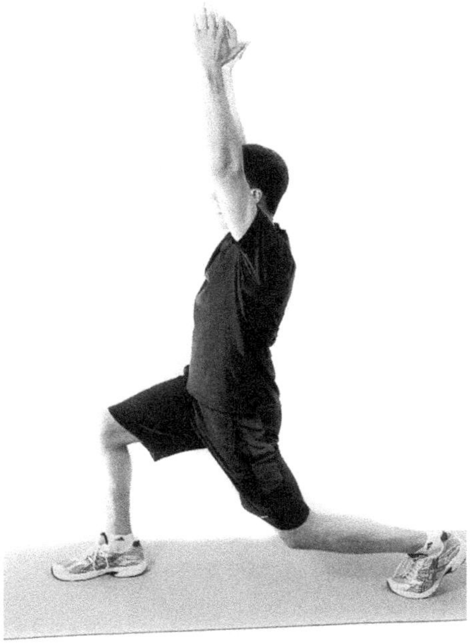

Figure 38.23 Lunge backward lean. Starting in standing with the hips and knees extended, arms overhead, leaning slightly backwards with the trunk and feet pointing straight forward, the patient lunges forward with the affected leg to a position of 90° of hip and knee flexion, with the other leg at 90° of knee flexion and 0° of hip extension.

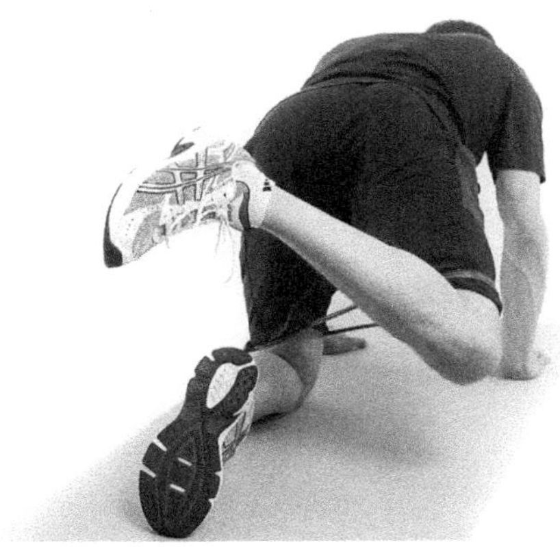

Figure 38.24 Quadruped gluteus medius strengthening. With the hip and knee in 90° of flexion, a triplanar movement of the hip into extension, abduction and external rotation is performed, while maintaining neutral spine and controlling compensatory rotation through pelvis. Elastic resistance can be used as a progression.

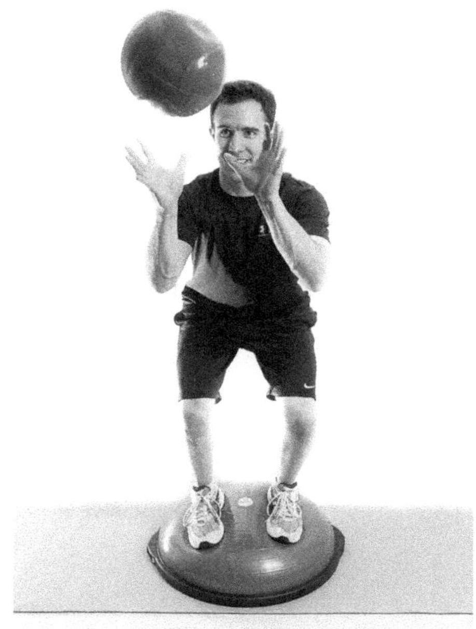

Figure 38.25 BOSU squat with ball toss. The patient stands on the BOSU® in a squat position, maintaining proper lower extremity alignment while the distraction of a ball toss is added.

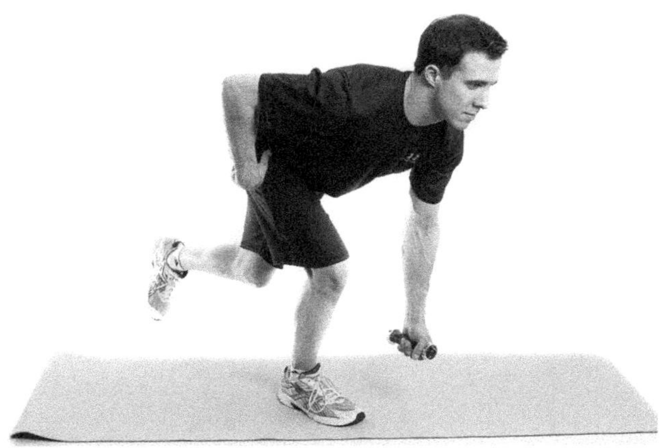

Figure 38.26 Single-leg dead lift. The patient balances on one leg with hip and knee flexed approximately 30°, slowly flexes the hip and trunk to touch down towards the ground beside the support foot and then returns to the starting position. The knee should be kept flexed at 30° to primarily obtain trunk and hip flexion and to keep the knee over the toes.

could be included in phase 2, and progressions for these specific exercises can be found in Chapter 23. From this patient's perspective, his activity limitation and goal is running, thus the choice of exercises and attention to motor patterning during the performance of these exercises in positions relevant to this specific task will be meaningful to him and facilitate transfer to his functional activities.

The star excursion balance exercise can be used as a dynamic motor control exercise that requires strength, flexibility and proprioception (see Fig 38.10). Other balance and proprioception challenges can include single- or double-leg stance on an unstable surface (BOSU®) with a ball toss (Fig. 38.25), single-leg dead lifts (Fig. 38.26) or the bowler's squat (Fig. 38.27).

Phase 3

Once adequate lower extremity alignment and control have been established, phase 3 emphasizes functional integration. Practising the movement patterns required for the individual's sport or specific tasks constitutes an essential element in this phase of the rehabilitation programme. Many of the

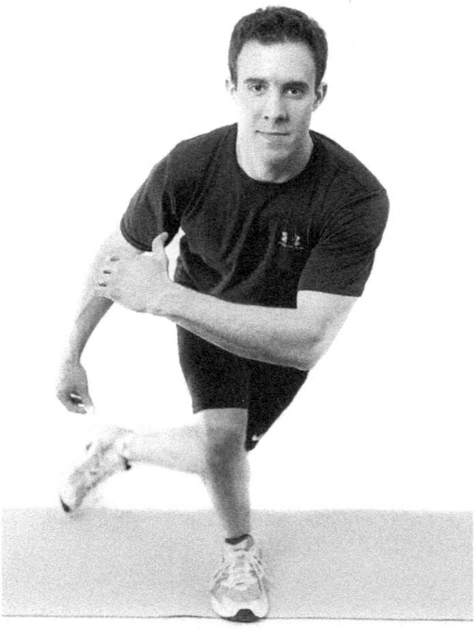

Figure 38.27 Bowler's squat. Standing on the affected leg in a semi-squat position, the patient reaches back with the opposite leg as he hinges forward at the hips, reaching forward and slightly across the body with the arm on the unaffected side. A light dumbbell can be added to that hand as a progression.

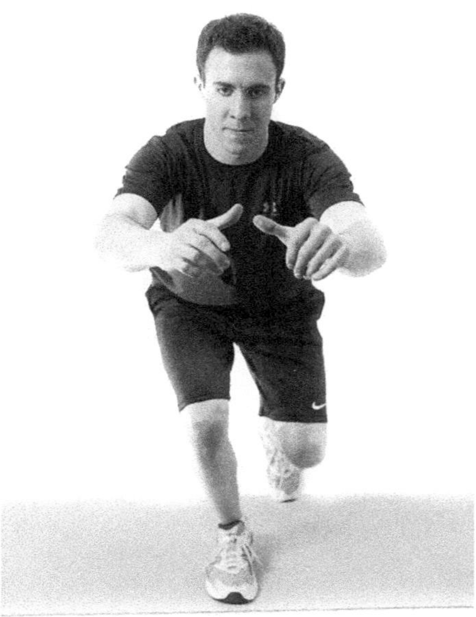

Figure 38.28 Single-leg vertical jump landing. The patient is instructed in proper single-leg landing technique, maintaining proper lower extremity alignment.

previously described proprioception / balance exercises can be integrated into sports-specific tasks and progressed by increasing the challenge through altering the base of support, adding resistance and removing visual cues. For this particular patient, exercises simulating the phases of the running cycle, double- and single-leg vertical jumping (Fig. 38.28), tasks involving quick multidirectional movements and dissociation tasks (Fig. 38.29) would be included. Increasing the speed, altering the base of support, adding plyometric activities and decreasing cognitive control could all be added elements to achieve progression.

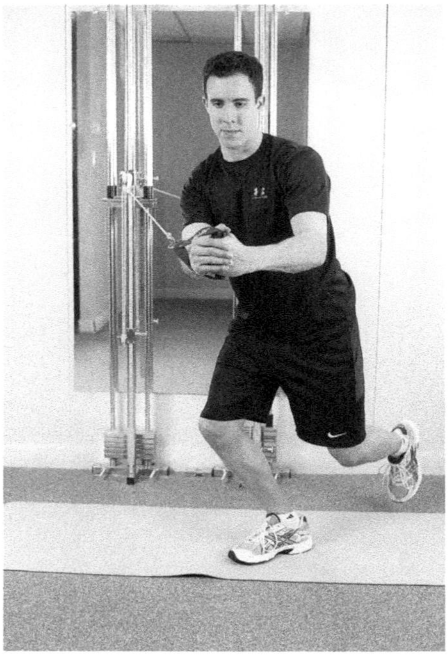

Figure 38.29 Functional integration / dissociation task. In a single-leg squat position, the patient maintains proper lower extremity alignment and lumbopelvic control while reaching and twisting with the thoracic spine against pulley resistance.

The ultimate goal from the patient's perspective is running, and treadmill running with mirror feedback is an excellent training device that encourages transference of gains made with specific strengthening exercises into more optimal lower extremity mechanics (see Fig. 38.9).

Exercise Parameters

Throughout the development and progression of the exercise programme, the dosage prescribed depends on several factors such as the aim of the exercise (recruitment / patterning, strength, endurance, mobility, stretching), the ability to perform the exercise properly, patient fitness level and tolerance, the presence of pain or swelling and the irritability of the condition.

In the first phase, with an emphasis on isolated muscle recruitment, 1–2 sets of 10 repetitions with a 2-minute rest would be completed daily, limiting the number to the amount that can be performed without substitution. As phase 2 focuses on weight-bearing strengthening, 2–4 sets of 8–12 repetitions would be indicated with 2–3 minute rest, performed at least 3 times a week. In the functional training phase 3, the endurance function would be achieved with 2 sets of 20 repetitions with a 2-minute rest. Neuromotor retraining, including balance and proprioception, would progress through graduated challenges for 1–3 repetitions of 30-second holds with 1-minute rest performed daily. Again, precision of movement pattern is a priority with all exercises and would assist

Table 38.3 **Exercise parameters**

Phase	Goal	Load	Sets x / reps	Rest	Frequency
Phase 1	Muscle recruitment	low	1–3 / 10	2 min	Multiple × / day
Phase 2	Muscle hypertrophy	60–70% MVC	2–4 / 8–12	2–3 min	2–3 × / week
Phase 3	Muscle endurance Neuromotor retraining Balance / proprioception	50% MVC Progressive challenge Progressive challenge	2 / 15–20 1–3 / 10 1–3 / 30 s hold	2–3 min 2 min 1 min	2–3 × / week Multiple × / day Daily
Mobility	Articular mobility	Stretch sensation	1 / 10–15 2/30 s hold		3–4 × / week
	Muscle lengthening	Stretch discomfort	2–4 / 30 s hold		Minimum 3–4 × / week

in determining the exact numbers of repetitions and load. Daily articular mobility (1×10–15 repetitions) and muscle extensibility (3×30-second hold) exercises would be included as required throughout these phases.

Table 38.3 provides a summary of suggested parameters for exercise prescription, but more detailed information is available from the American College of Sport Medicine's updated guidelines (Garber et al 2011) and can also be found in Chapter 23.

Conclusion

Therapeutic exercise is an integral component of rehabilitation of lower extremity conditions. The purpose of this chapter has been to present an evidence-informed approach to exercise prescription in the lower quadrant, focusing on hip dysfunction. Using sound clinical reasoning, the practitioner must utilize the available scientific research as well as clinical experience in designing effective exercise programmes. Overarching this is a continual consideration of the patient's individual perspective and their ultimate goals.

References

Ayala F, Sainz de Baranda P, De Ste Croix M. 2013. Comparison of active stretching technique in males with normal and limited hamstring flexibility. Phys Ther Sport 14: 98–104.

Baker R, Souza R, Fredericson M. 2011. Iliotibial band syndrome: soft tissue and biomechanical factors in evaluation and treatment. Phys Med Rehabil 3: 550–561.

Ballantyne F, Fryer G, McLaughlin P. 2003. The effect of muscle energy technique on hamstring extensibility: the mechanism of altered flexibility. J Osteopath Med 6: 59–63.

Barton C, Lack S, Malliaras P, Morrissey D. 2013. Gluteal muscle activity and patellofemoral pain syndrome: a systematic review. Br J Sports Med 47: 207–214.

Binkley JM, Stratford PW, Lott SA, et al. 1999. The Lower Extremity Functional Scale (LEFS): scale development, measurement properties, and clinical application. Phys Ther 79: 371–383.

Borman N, Trudelle-Jackson E, Smith S. 2011. Effect of stretch positions on hamstring muscle length, lumbar flexion range of motion, and lumbar curvature in healthy adults. Physiother Theor Practice 27:146–154.

Boudreau SN, Dwyer MK, Mattacola CG, et al. 2009. Hip-muscle activation during the lunge, single-leg squat, and step-up-and-over exercises. J Sport Rehabil 18: 91–103.

Brody LT 2012. Effective therapeutic exercise prescription: the right exercise at the right dose. J Hand Ther 25: 220–232

Castellote-Caballero Y, Valenza M, Martín-Martín L, et al. 2013. Effects of a neurodynamic sliding technique on hamstring flexibility in healthy male soccer players: a pilot study. Phys Ther Sport 14: 156–162.

Comfort P, Green CM, Matthews M. 2009. Training considerations after hamstring injury in athletes. J Strength Cond Res 31: 68–74.

Costa P, Herda J, Herda A, et al. 2014. Effects of dynamic stretching on strength, muscle imbalance, and muscle activation. Med Sci Sports Exerc 46: 586–593.

Covert C, Alexander M, Petronis J, et al. 2010. Comparison of ballistic and static stretching on hamstring muscle length using an equal stretching dose. J Strength Cond Res 24: 3008–3014.

Davis D, Ashby P, McCale KL, et al. 2005. The effectiveness of 3 stretching techniques on hamstring flexibility using consistent stretching parameters. J Strength Cond Res 19: 27–32.

de Weijer V, Gorniak G, Shamus E. 2003. The effect of static stretch and warm-up exercise on hamstring length over the course of 24 hours. J Orthop Sports Phys Ther 33: 727–733.

Decoster L, Cleland J, Altieri C, et al. 2005. The effects of hamstring stretching on range of motion: a systematic literature review. J Orthop Sports Phys Ther 35: 377–387.

Fasen J, O'Connor A, Schwartz S, et al. 2009. A randomized controlled trial of hamstring stretching: comparison of four techniques. J Strength Cond Res 23: 660–667.

Fishman L, Dombi G, Michaelsen C, et al. 2002. Piriformis syndrome: diagnosis, treatment and outcome: a 10-year study. Arch Phys Med Rehabil 83: 295–301.

Fredericson M, White J, MacMahon J, et al. 2002. Quantitative analysis of the relative effectiveness of 3 iliotibial band stretches. Arch Phys Med Rehabil 83: 589–592.

Gajdosik R, Sandler M, Marr H. 2003. Influence of knee positions and gender on the Ober test for length of the iliotibial band. Clin Biomech 18: 77–79.

Garber C, Blissmer B, Deschenes M, et al. 2011. Quantity and quality of exercise for developing and maintaining cardiorespiratory, musculoskeletal, and neuromotor fitness in apparently healthy adults: guidance for prescribing exercise. Med Sci Sports Exerc 43: 1334–1359.

Giphart JE, Stull JD, LaPrade RF, et al. 2012. Recruitment and activity of the pectineus and piriformis muscles during hip rehabilitation exercises: an electromyography study. Am J Sports Med 40: 1654–1663.

Godges J, MacRae H, Longdon C, et al. 1989. The effects of two stretching procedures on hip range of motion and gait economy. J Orthop Sports Phys Ther 10: 350–357.

Gottschalk F, Kourosh S, Leveau B. 1989. The functional anatomy of tensor fasciae latae and gluteus medius and minimus. J Anat 166: 179–189.

Gowda AL, Mease SJ, Donatelli R. 2014. Gluteus medius strengthening and the use of the Donatelli Drop Test in the athlete. Phys Ther Sport 15: 15–19.

Gulledge B, Marcellin-Little D, Levinea D, et al. 2014. Comparison of two stretching methods and optimization of stretching protocol for the piriformis muscle. Med Eng Phys 36: 212– 218.

Heiderscheit BC, Sherry MA, Slider A, et al. 2010. Hamstring strain injuries: recommendations for diagnosis, rehabilitation, and injury prevention. J Orthop Sports Phys Ther 40: 67–81.

Hertel J, Miller SJ, Denegar CR. 2000. Intratester and inter-tester reliability during the Star Excursion Balance Tests. J Sport Rehabil 9:104–116.

Hing W, Bigelow R, Bremner T. 2008. Mulligan's mobilisation with movement: a review of the tenets and prescription of MWMs. N Z J Physiother 36: 144–164.

Hulbert A, Deyle G. 2009. Differential diagnosis and conservative treatment for piriformis syndrome: a review of the literature. Current Orthop Practice 20: 313–319.

Janda V. 1987. Muscles and motor control in low back pain: assessment and management. In: Twomey LT (ed) Physical therapy of the low back. New York: Churchill Livingstone, pp 253–278.

Johnson A, Mitchell U, Meek K, et al. 2014. Hamstring flexibility increases the same with 3 or 9 repetitions of stretching held for a total time of 90s. Phys Ther Sport 15: 101–105.

Kinzey SJ, Armstrong CW. 1998. The reliability of the Star-Excursion Test in assessing dynamic balance. J Orthop Sports Phys Ther 27: 356–360.

Laslett M, Aprill CN, McDonald B. 2006. Provocation sacroiliac joint tests have validity in the diagnosis of sacroiliac joint pain. Arch Phys Med Rehabil 87: 874–875.

Lieberman DE, Raichlen DA, Pontzer H, et al. 2006. The human gluteus maximus and its role in running. J Exp Biol 209: 2143–2155.

Lorenz D, Reiman M. 2011. The role of implementation of eccentric training in athletic rehabilitation: tendinopathy, hamstring strains and ACL reconstruction. Int J Sports Phys Ther 6: 28–44.

Mascal CL, Landel R, Powers C. 2003. Management of patellofemoral pain targeting hip, pelvis, and trunk muscle function: 2 case reports. J Orthop Sports Phys Ther 33: 647–660.

McAllister M, Hammond K, Schilling B. 2014. Muscle activation during various hamstring exercises. J Strength Cond Res 28(6): 1573–1580. doi: 10.1519/JSC.0000000000000302.

Medina-Mirapeix F, Escolar-Reina P, Gascón-Cánovas J, et al. 2009. Predictive factors of adherence to frequency and duration components in home exercise programs for neck and low back pain: an observational study. BMC Musculoskel Dis 41: 347–352.

Mendez-Sanchez R, Alburquerque-Sendın F, Fernández-de-las-Peñas C, et al. 2010. Immediate effects of adding a sciatic nerve slider technique on lumbar and lower quadrant mobility in soccer players: a pilot study. J Altern Complement Med 16: 669–675.

Moreside JM, McGill SM. 2012a. Improvements in hip flexibility do not transfer to mobility in functional movement patterns. J Strength Cond Res 27: 2635–2643.

Moreside JM, McGill SM. 2012b. Hip joint range of motion improvements using three different interventions. J Strength Cond Res 26: 1265–1273.

Mulligan B 2004. Manual therapy nags, snags, MWMs etc., 5th edn. Wellington, NZ: Plain View Services.

Nelson R, Bandy W. 2004. Eccentric training and static stretching improve hamstring flexibility of high school males. J Athl Train 39: 254–258.

Neumann DA. 2010. Kinesiology of the hip: a focus on muscular actions. J Orthop Sports Phys Ther 40: 82–94.

Noehren B, Schmitz A, Hempel R. 2014. Assessment of strength, flexibility, and running mechanics in men with iliotibial band syndrome. J Orthop Sports Phys Ther 44: 217–222.

Norris B, Trudelle-Jackson E. 2011. Hip- and thigh-muscle activation during the star excursion balance test. J Sport Rehabil 20: 428–441.

O'Sullivan K, Murray E, Sainsbury D. 2009. The effect of warm-up, static stretching and dynamic stretching on hamstring flexibility in previously injured subjects. BMC Musculoskel Dis 10: 37.

O'Sullivan K, Smith SM, Sainsbury D. 2010. Electromyographic analysis of the three subdivisions of gluteus medius during weight-bearing exercises. Sports Med Arthrosc Rehabil Ther Technol 2: 17.

O'Sullivan K, McAuliffe S, DeBurca N. 2012. The effects of eccentric training on lower limb flexibility: a systematic review. Br J Sports Med 46: 838–845.

Patel P, Yadav A. 2013. Comparison of static stretching versus eccentric training to increase flexibility of hamstring muscle in healthy hospital nurses. Indian J Physiother Occupat Ther 7: 11–14.

Powers CM. 2003. The influence of altered lower-extremity kinematics on patellofemoral joint dysfunction: a theoretical perspective. J Orthop Sports Phys Ther 33: 639–646.

Powers CM. 2010. The influence of abnormal hip mechanics on knee injury: a biomechanical perspective. J Orthop Sports Phys Ther 40: 42–51.

Puentedura E, Huijbregts P, Celeste S, et al. 2011. Immediate effects of quantified hamstring stretching: hold–relax proprioceptive neuromuscular facilitation versus static stretching. Phys Ther Sport 12: 122–126.

Reiman MP, Bolgla LA, Loudon JK. 2012. A literature review of studies evaluation gluteus maximus and gluteus medius activation during rehabilitation exercises. Physiother Theory Pract 28: 257–268.

Sahrmann S. 2002. Diagnosis and treatment of movement impairment syndromes. St Louis, MO: Mosby.

Sairyo K, Kawamura T, Mase Y, et al. 2013. Jack-knife stretching promotes flexibility of tight hamstrings after 4 weeks: a pilot study. Eur J Orthop Surg Traumat 23: 657–663.

Selkowitz DM, Beneck GJ, Powers CM. 2013. Which exercises target the gluteal muscles while minimizing activation of the tensor fascia latae? Electromyographic assessment using fine-wire electrodes. J Orthop Sports Phys Ther 43: 54–64.

Smith M, Fryer G. 2008. A comparison of two muscle energy techniques for increasing flexibility of the hamstring muscle group. J Bodyw Mov Ther 12:312–317.

Souza RB, Powers CM. 2009. Differences in hip kinematics, muscle strength, and muscle activation between subjects with and without patellofemoral pain. J Orthop Sports Phys Ther 39: 12–19.

Stephens J, Davidson J, DeRosa J, et al. 2006. Lengthening the hamstring muscles without stretching using 'awareness through movement'. Phys Ther 86: 1641–1650.

Tonley JC, Yun SM, Kochevar RJ, et al. 2010. Treatment of an individual with piriformis syndrome focusing on hip muscle strengthening and movement reeducation: a case report. J Orthop Sports Phys Ther 40: 103–111.

Wagner T, Behnia N, Ancheta WK, et al. 2010. Strengthening and neuromuscular re-education of the gluteal maximus of a triathlete with exercise cramping of the hamstrings. J Orthop Sports Phys Ther 40: 112–119.

Ward SR, Winters TM, Blemker SS. 2010. The architectural design of the gluteal muscle group: implications for movement and rehabilitation. J Orthop Sports Phys Ther 40: 95–102.

Wang T, Jan M, Lin K, Wang HK. 2006. Assessment of stretching of the iliotibial tract with Ober and Modified Ober Tests: an ultrasonographic study. Arch Phys Med Rehabil 87: 1407–1411.

Webster KA, Gribble PA. 2013. A comparison of electromyography of gluteus medius and maximus in subjects with and without chronic ankle instability during two functional exercises. Phys Ther Sport 14: 17–22.

Wilcox EL, Burden AM. 2013. The influence of varying hip angle and pelvis position on muscle recruitment patterns of the hip abductor muscles during the clam exercise. J Orthop Sports Phys Ther 43: 325–331.

Willy RW, Davis IS. 2011. Effect of a hip-strengthening program on mechanics during running and during a single-leg squat. J Orthop Sports Phys Ther 41: 625–632.

Willy RW, Scholz JP, Davis IS. 2012. Mirror gait retraining for the treatment of patellofemoral pain in female runners. Clin Biomech 27: 1045–1051.

Winters M, Blake C, Trost J, et al. 2004. Passive versus active stretching of hip flexor muscles in subjects with limited hip extension: a randomized clinical trial. Phys Ther 84: 800–807.

Wouters, I, Almonroeder T, DeJarlais B, et al. 2012. Effects of a movement training program on hip and knee joint frontal plane running mechanics. Int J Sports Phys Ther 7: 638–646.

Wright P, Drysdale I. 2008. A comparison of post-isometric relaxation (PIR) and reciprocal inhibition (RI) muscle energy techniques applied to piriformis: British College of Osteopathic Medicine. Abstracts ICAOR 7. Int J Osteopath Med 11: 149–168.

Youdas J, Haeflinger K, Kreun M, et al. 2010. The efficacy of two modified proprioceptive neuromuscular facilitation stretching techniques in subjects with reduced hamstring muscle length. Physiother Theory Pract 26: 240–250.

PART 6

The Elbow Region In Upper Extremity Pain Syndromes

39 Elbow Tendinopathy: Lateral Epicondylalgia 445
Bill Vicenzino

40 Other Elbow Disorders: Elbow Instability, Arthritic Conditions 451
Chris A. Sebelski

41 Joint Mobilization and Manipulation of the Elbow 458
Helen Slater and César Fernández-de-las-Peñas

Chapter 39

Elbow Tendinopathy: Lateral Epicondylalgia

Bill Vicenzino

CHAPTER CONTENTS

Introduction 445
Diagnostic considerations 445
Pathological considerations 446
Prognostic considerations 447
Considerations in conservative treatment 447
Conclusion 448

Introduction

The common tendon of the extensor muscles of the wrist and fingers is the most frequently implicated tendon in elbow tendinopathy and will be the focus of this chapter. There is contention as to the correct nomenclature for the tendinopathy of the extensor muscles of the wrist and fingers. A number of terms are used in reference to this tendinopathy, such as tennis elbow, lateral epicondylitis, lateral epicondylosis and lateral epicondylalgia. 'Tennis elbow' is frequently used colloquially, but this term confuses many patients, as the condition is also very prevalent in those patients who do not play tennis. Further, 'epicondylitis' infers inflammation, which has long been shown not to be the case (Nirschl & Pettrone 1979; Regan et al 1992; Potter et al 1995; Kraushaar & Nirschl 1999; Alfredson et al 2000). 'Epicondylosis' or 'tendinosis' connotes a degenerative change – but, although elements of disarray, breakdown or degeneration of collagen fibrils have been identified in such tendons (Regan et al 1992; Kraushaar & Nirschl 1999), the relationship of these to presenting pain symptoms and associated clinical signs is not clear (Khan & Cook 2000).

'Lateral epicondylalgia' indicates that there is pain over the lateral epicondyle, which may be an accurate term to use for the patient presenting with pain over the lateral epicondyle; however, it provides little information about the underlying pathology. Recent reports of neovascularization and associated increased concentrations of algogenic mediators such as glutamate, substance P and calcitonin gene-related peptide (Ljung et al 1999, 2004; Alfredson et al 2000; Zeisig et al 2006; du Toit et al 2008) suggest that tendinopathy is far more complex than any of the above commonly used terms suggest. In this chapter, the term 'lateral epicondylalgia' will be used to describe the patient who attends the clinic with pain over the lateral epicondyle; as will be highlighted, this may be due to some pathology in the tendon (i.e. tendinopathy), but the pain may also be associated with other conditions, which need to be considered to rehabilitate the patient fully.

Although there is no definitive evidence, the incidence of lateral epicondylalgia varies from 1% to 3% in the general population (Allander 1974; Verhaar 1994), which contrasts with reports of prevalence rates as high as 35–64% in occupations requiring repetitive manual tasks (Kivi 1982; Dimberg 1987; Feuerstein et al 1998), where it is one of the most costly of all work-related injuries (Kivi 1982; Dimberg 1987; Feuerstein et al 1998). A survey of United States of America Department of Labor, Office of Worker's Compensation Programs, accepted claims of occupational upper extremity disorders demonstrated that lateral epicondylalgia was responsible for approximately 27% and 48% of all work-related claims for upper limb tendinopathies and enthesopathies, respectively (Feuerstein et al 1998). This chapter focuses on the most common tendinopathy about the elbow, lateral epicondylalgia, with specific consideration of the evidence in regards to diagnosis, pathology, conservative management and prognosis.

Diagnostic Considerations

Lateral epicondylalgia is usually identified or diagnosed on the basis of a clinical examination. Classically, the patient presents with pain over the lateral elbow and may spread into the dorsal forearm as far as the wrist, but no further than the wrist and not proximally to the elbow (see Slater et al (2003, 2005) for patterns of pain maps). Those with pain and symptoms into the hand and fingers or proximal to the elbow should be considered to have concomitant problems (e.g. cervical spine referral, neuropathy) in addition to, or instead of, lateral epicondylalgia. Patients with lateral epicondylalgia will have pain and weakness with tests that challenge the wrist extensor muscles – for example, muscle contraction tasks of gripping, wrist extension and middle finger extension (clinically described as a test of extensor carpi radialis brevis, largely due to the insertion of that tendon at the wrist). It is commonly reported that stretch of the wrist and finger extensors is present in these patients; however, although pain may be reproduced on stretching, it is not an uncommon observation by this author that patients exhibit increased length in these muscles (i.e. increased range of flexion of the wrist and fingers) associated with pain reproduction in those with chronic conditions. The pain reproduction is limited to the lateral epicondyle and, at most, some spread down into the dorsal forearm. Palpation will identify areas of hyperalgesia in and around the lateral epicondyle, at the site of the common extensor tendon as well as in some cases pain into the dorsal forearm muscles. These palpation findings need to be present with impairment in muscle contraction; otherwise it is more likely that the symptoms could be largely referred from other regions such as the cervical spine.

Typically, patients attending general practice with lateral epicondylalgia will be in their 4th or 5th decade of life. There is upper limb dominance bias, but no sex bias. Patients who perform repetitive tasks requiring sustained or repeated gripping of an implement or tool, such as those playing tennis or undertaking manual labour, may be younger than 40 years, but in such cases there should be a higher degree of suspicion of an alternative underlying cause and diagnosis. For example, in younger people consideration needs to be given to osteochondritis dissecans of the capitellum and radius in cases with insidious onset, and bursitis, radiohumeral joint synovitis and other soft tissue sprains where there is more acute onset pain and swelling; in more elderly patients the practitioner will need also to consider degenerative conditions of the radiohumeral joint and referral from the cervical spine (Brukner & Khan 2007).

Lateral epicondylalgia is by definition a clinical entity not usually requiring confirmatory diagnostic imaging or other medical pathology tests. Diagnostic imaging is likely more helpful for excluding differential diagnoses. For example, radiographs may be used to identify bone injuries, such as fractures, apophysitis and subchondral arthritic changes. Ultrasound has taken on a greater role in the direct identification of grey-scale hypoechoic lesions, which imply dysfunction in the connective tissues. These grey-scale changes are not necessarily linked to pain in the tendon (Cook et al 2001, 2004; du Toit et al 2008) and so they could be legitimately termed tendinopathy, meaning some pathology in the tendon, and are most likely due to degenerative breakdown of collagen fibrils (epicondylosis) – though fusiform swelling may be more indicative of cellular and matrix dysfunction (Cook & Purdam 2009). Increasing evidence points towards a link between neovascularization and symptoms such as pain (Cook et al 2001, 2004; du Toit et al 2008), with a recent study showing that, in a patient with longstanding lateral elbow pain that had failed to respond to treatment, the lack of neovascularization strongly indicated that the pain was not due to tendinopathy, prompting the practitioner to consider other diagnoses (du Toit et al 2008). Magnetic resonance imaging may be used to follow up recalcitrant cases where there are no radiographic or ultrasonographic changes present, but these cases will be in the minority.

Pathological Considerations

Nirschl and Pettrone (1979) described the underlying pathology of lateral epicondylalgia to be one of angiofibroblastic hyperplasia with the following identified histological changes: (a) proliferation in the number of cells and in ground substance, (b) neovascularization or vascular hyperplasia, (c) higher levels of algogenic substances, as well as (d) disorganized immature collagen (Nirschl & Pettrone 1979; Nirschl 1992; Regan et al 1992; Fredberg et al 2008). In an effort to explain different clinical presentations more adequately, Cook and Purdam (2009) have recently proposed a clinical model of histopathological changes across a continuum from: (a) reactive tendinopathy and (b) tendon disrepair, to (c) degenerative tendinopathy. A brief summary of their proposed clinical model follows and the reader is referred to their paper for more detail.

Reactive tendinopathy is a non-inflammatory proliferative cellular and matrix response to either an acute tensile overload, as may occur with a bout of unaccustomed physical activity, or a compressive overload, for instance that due to a direct contact injury. This is likely to occur in the younger athlete who rapidly increases the intensity or volume of physical activity and is managed well with a short period of absence from the increased loading activities before restoring pain-free function. Consequently the classic presentation of lateral epicondylalgia is not likely to fall into this category, though it is important to keep this category in mind for younger athletes such as tennis players or manual labourers, as well as patients who present with pain after an acute traumatic blow to the common extensor origin at the elbow. At the other end of the spectrum, the degenerative phase is characterized by angiofibroblastic hyperplasia changes, with considerable breakdown in the collagen framework and neovascularization. This tends to occur with chronic overloading in the older person; hence it more appropriately fits the likely presentation in a classical presentation of lateral epicondylalgia. There is a sound argument that exercises need to be a fundamental inclusion in the treatment plan for degenerative tendinopathy (Cook & Purdam 2009; Khan & Scott 2009).

As well as local tendon changes, clinicians need also to consider evidence that implicates the central nervous system in the clinical presentation of lateral epicondylalgia. This is especially important, as local tendon changes are not readily appreciated in the clinic, even with the assistance of diagnostic imaging. There are studies reporting widespread mechanical pain hyperalgesia – that is, reduced pressure pain threshold in the unaffected elbow and in the leg (Fernández-Carnero et al 2009a, 2009b; Coombes et al 2012), as well as evidence of spinal cord hyperexcitability – that is, reduced nociceptive flexion reflex threshold (Lim et al 2012) and reduced capacity to modulate nociceptive stimuli (Lim 2013). These findings implicate the central nervous system in the pain experienced in those patients with unilateral lateral epicondylalgia. Individuals with severe cases of unilateral epicondylalgia express cold hyperalgesia bilaterally (i.e. on the unaffected side as well) in addition to widespread mechanical pain hyperalgesia (Coombes et al 2012). This might have implications in the management approach for the more severe cases. As well as this sensory system involvement, there appear to be motor system changes. Patients with unilateral lateral epicondylalgia have bilaterally reduced reaction time of whole upper limb movements (Pienimaki et al 1997; Bisset et al 2009) and less extension on gripping (Bisset et al 2009). They also have weakness of most of the muscles on the affected upper limb, with the exception of the long finger extensors, which retain their strength (Alizadehkhaiyat et al 2009). It is interesting to speculate that the long finger extensors are increasingly used as wrist stabilizers when the wrist stabilizers (i.e. extensor carpi radialis brevis and longus) are impaired through the tendinopathy, which might explain the reduced extension on gripping. These sensory and motor system changes are important to consider when planning a physical therapy programme.

Prognostic Considerations

Lateral epicondylalgia is widely regarded as being self-limiting and resolving within 6 months to 2 years; however, this is low-level evidence as the natural history of this condition has not been definitively determined. Notwithstanding this, a number of randomized clinical trials have followed cases over 12 months (Smidt et al 2002; Bisset et al 2006, 2007; Smidt & van der Windt 2006) and provide data that may be used in determining prognosis.

The evidence from two randomized clinical trials (n=383) (Smidt et al 2002; Bisset et al 2006) that included randomizing a group of patients to following a wait-and-see policy indicates that 87% of patients self-reported being much improved or completely recovered 12 months after inclusion into the study (Bisset et al 2007). When considering that patients had on average approximately 6 months' duration of pain at inclusion into the study (Bisset et al 2007), an approximate indicative natural history of the condition is in the order of 18 months for the majority of sufferers. It is important to keep in mind that the patients allocated to the group following the wait-and-see policy were given advice on avoiding aggravating activities (e.g. ergonomic advice on how to lift objects and manipulate implements without aggravating pain) as well as being closely monitored in a clinical trial (and thereby prone to the Hawthorne effect), which is not necessarily the same as a person with lateral epicondylalgia not seeking out advice and doing nothing about the condition. Furthermore, Bisset et al (2006) reported that those in the group allocated to wait-and-see policy were 2.7 times more likely to seek out other treatments than those allocated to a mobilization with movement and exercise group (OR 4.7, 95% CI 2.1–10.3), which is not the same as doing nothing about the lateral epicondylalgia. On the contrary, it tends to indicate that, despite being recruited into a clinical trial and being closely monitored, patients do not feel comfortable doing nothing about their condition.

Smidt et al (2006) prospectively followed 349 patients from two randomized clinical trials (Hay et al 1999; Smidt et al 2002) over a 12-month period and found that those who had more severe pain of longer duration also had greater likelihood of a worse outcome (more severe pain) at 12 months. Another prognostic factor of poor outcome was concomitant neck pain (Smidt et al 2006). This finding is interesting because it indicates that the patient pool recruited in this study had a heterogenic pain presentation, including cases with more complex presentations (e.g. lateral epicondylalgia plus neck pain) and did not consist solely of patients with isolated lateral epicondylalgia.

Considerations in Conservative Treatment

A wide range of conservative treatments, such as medication, electrophysical agents, exercise and manual therapy, are advocated for lateral epicondylalgia, which is usually an indication that no one treatment has proven superiority, but also in part a product of an inconclusive understanding of the underlying pathology of the condition.

Corticosteroid injections are the most common conservative medical intervention for lateral epicondylalgia and accordingly they have been the most studied in high-quality rigorous clinical trials. There is level 1 evidence from a number of randomized clinical trials of short-term efficacy, with success rates over 80% in the first 4–6 weeks (Hay et al 1999; Smidt et al 2002; Bisset et al 2006, 2007; Smidt & van der Windt 2006), but this needs to be considered in light of post-6-weeks poorer outcomes in the form of lower success rates compared with the adoption of a wait-and-see policy (Smidt et al 2002; Bisset et al 2006, 2007; Smidt & van der Windt 2006), higher recurrence rates (70% versus 8%) and greater use of other not-per-protocol co-interventions (49% versus 21%) compared with those patients undergoing mobilization with movements and exercise intervention (Bisset et al 2006, 2007). The poorer downstream effects are sufficient to prompt caution in their use and some have advocated against their use in lateral epicondylalgia (Young et al 1954; Osborne 2010; Vicenzino 2009), at least in the first instance, without a concerted attempt at other interventions that do not have such a poor longer term effect on the condition. Other researchers have proposed combining the use of these injections with physiotherapy (Coombes et al 2009a; Olaussen et al 2009) in order to overcome the relatively poorer long-term effects. A recent randomized clinical trial evaluated the proposition of combining the mobilization with movement technique and exercise programme with a corticosteroid injection (Coombes et al 2013). However, this trial showed that this combination of therapies did not prevent the higher recurrence rates and delayed recovery following corticosteroid injections.

There is a sound level of evidence in support of exercise for treating lateral epicondylalgia; however, unlike in lower limb tendinopathy, eccentric exercise is not necessarily better than concentric exercise (Woodley et al 2007). Perhaps the most illustrative evidence comes from a randomized clinical trial comparing an exercise programme with ultrasound in a group of patients who had recalcitrant lateral epicondylalgia, having failed other treatments including corticosteroid injections and other common modalities (Pienimaki et al 1996). Follow-up some 3 years later revealed that the exercise group required fewer medical consultations, and had less surgery (NNT=3) and 586 fewer sick days than the group receiving ultrasound (Pienimaki et al 1998). The exercise programme was graduated and progressive from isometric to isotonic contractions of the wrist and forearm muscles, culminating in pragmatic exercises that replicated a patient's required function. It was supervised twice a week for approximately 8 weeks. A more-recent study has shown that supervision of the exercise programme returns superior effects compared with a home-based programme (Stasinopoulos et al 2010), which should be considered when prescribing exercise.

Electrophysical agents such as LASER, ultrasound and extracorporeal shock-wave therapy (ESWT) have attracted attention. Low-level LASER therapy has been shown to be effective in improving pain levels in the short term compared with control, but only at a wavelength of 908 nm (Bjordal et al 2008). There appears to be less conclusive evidence and some contention over the use of ultrasound and ESWT in the treatment of lateral epicondylalgia, perhaps because of a lack of specification and stratification of dosage parameters.

Elbow orthotics or tennis elbow bands that fit about the proximal forearm are frequently used, often on a self-selection basis by patients. However, systematic reviews have been unable to find sufficient high-quality clinical trials to support or refute their use (Struijs et al 2001, 2002, 2004).

Joint (high- and low-velocity) and soft tissue manipulations have been proposed for use in treatment of lateral epicondylalgia (Lee 1986; Vicenzino et al 2007a). The initial effects of elbow mobilizations with movement (Vicenzino 2003) used as a single modality have been shown in a number of studies (Vicenzino et al 1996, 2001, 2007b; Abbott et al 2001; Paungmali et al 2003) and been shown to be effective when used in combination with exercise (Kochar & Dogra 2002; Bisset et al 2006). There are conflicting interpretations of the literature regarding the use of Mill's manipulation and friction massage, also referred to as Cyriax physiotherapy (Vicenzino et al 2007a; Kohia et al 2008), which may be in part due to the lack of high-quality clinical trials (Bisset et al 2005). There is also a randomized clinical trial that has found wrist manipulation to be efficacious compared with ultrasound, friction massage and exercise (Struijs et al 2003).

As identified in a prognostic analysis, patients with neck pain as well as lateral epicondylitis have a poorer outcome (Smidt et al 2006), but as in this study the neck was not treated it is not possible to determine whether it would have been beneficial to have added neck treatment to the elbow treatment given. However, there are several other studies that show benefits of adding treatment of the cervical spine to elbow treatment (Gunn & Milbrandt 1976; Cleland et al 2004, 2005). Gunn and Milbrandt (1976) treated 50 recalcitrant cases of lateral epicondylalgia with non-thrust manipulation and traction of the cervical spine and showed an 86% success rate after treatment that persisted at 6 months. In a retrospective case audit of 112 cases, Cleland et al (2004) showed that significantly fewer treatments were required for those (n=51) who received additional manual therapy to the cervical spine in the form of non-thrust oscillatory manipulations, mobilization with movements and / or muscle energy techniques. More recently, in a pilot trial of 10 cases, Cleland et al (2005) reported a better result on pain-free grip force and the Disability of the Arm, Shoulder and Hand questionnaire. Furthermore, a number of studies show both high- and low-velocity manipulations of the cervical spine to produce an initial improvement in pain at the elbow (Vicenzino et al 1996, 1998; Fernández-Carnero et al 2008). This evidence provides a basis for the cervical spine to be treated if it is found on physical examination to be implicated, especially since there have been reported significant differences in pain provocation on manual examination of the cervical spine and significant reductions in sagittal plane motion in patients with lateral epicondylalgia when compared with age-matched controls (Waugh et al 2004; Berglund et al 2008).

The challenge facing the practitioner is how to best select a treatment approach for each individual patient, as each person is likely to be somewhat different in their individual clinical presentation. The continuum model of presentation of tendinopathy (Cook & Purdam 2009) outlined above along with the proposed integrative model of lateral epicondylalgia (Coombes et al 2009b) may provide some guidance on how the practitioner may wish to select from the many proposed treatments. In brief, Coombes et al (2009b) propose that each patient presents with a different proportional representation of dysfunction in the pain and motor systems as well as in tendon structure and physiology, which could be used to select specific interventions. For example, if a patient presents with relatively greater pain system impediment – as would be seen clinically with large deficits in pressure pain thresholds and high pain severity scores – then pain-relieving medications, electrophysical agents and manual therapy should be favoured. In contrast, a patient who presents with a progressed stage of degenerative tendinopathy with moderate to low levels of pain could be better managed more with specific exercise (Coombes et al 2009b; Khan & Scott 2009) and possibly injections of medication / materials (Rabago et al 2009) or glyceryl trinitrate transdermal patches (Paoloni et al 2003, 2009; Murrell 2007) that promote collagen synthesis. Further detail regarding the integrative model of lateral epicondylalgia can be found in Coombes et al (2009b).

Conclusion

Tendinopathy at the elbow is commonly experienced over the lateral epicondyle. Over the past decade there has been an increase in our knowledge and understanding of the underlying pathology, conservative management and prognosis of this pain condition. Although this has provided more information and data for practitioners to consider when treating patients with lateral epicondylalgia, the challenge still remains over how to apply specific treatments to individual patients in order to achieve optimal outcomes. This chapter provides a synopsis of the recent evidence and some indication of possible means by which to apply such evidence clinically.

References

Abbott JH, Patla CE, Jensen RH. 2001. The initial effects of an elbow mobilization with movement technique on grip strength in subjects with lateral epicondylalgia. Man Ther 6: 163–169.

Alfredson H, Ljung BO, Thorsen K, et al. 2000. In vivo investigation of ECRB tendons with microdialysis technique – no signs of inflammation but high amounts of glutamate in tennis elbow. Acta Orthop Scand 71: 475–479.

Alizadehkhaiyat O, Fisher AC, Kemp GJ, et al. 2009. Assessment of functional recovery in tennis elbow. J Electromyogr Kinesiol 19: 631–638.

Allander E. 1974. Prevalence, incidence, and remission rates of some common rheumatic diseases or syndromes. Scand J Rheumatol 3: 145–153.

Berglund KM, Persson BH, Denison E. 2008. Prevalence of pain and dysfunction in the cervical and thoracic spine in persons with and without lateral elbow pain. Man Ther 13: 295–339.

Bisset L, Paungmali A, Vicenzino B, et al. 2005. A systematic review and meta-analysis of clinical trials on physical interventions for lateral epicondylalgia. Br J Sports Med 39: 411–422.

Bisset L, Beller E, Jull G, et al. 2006. Mobilisation with movement and exercise, corticosteroid injection, or wait and see for tennis elbow: randomised trial. BMJ 333(7575): 939.

Bisset L, Smidt N, van der Windt DA, et al. 2007. Conservative treatments for tennis elbow do subgroups of patients respond differently? Rheumatology (Oxford) 46: 1601–1605.

Bisset LM, Coppieters MW, Vicenzino B. 2009. Sensorimotor deficits remain despite resolution of symptoms using conservative treatment in patients with tennis elbow: a randomized controlled trial. Arch Phys Med Rehabil 90: 1–8.

Bjordal JM, Lopes-Martins RA, Joensen J, et al. 2008. A systematic review with procedural assessments and meta-analysis of low level laser therapy in lateral elbow tendinopathy (tennis elbow). BMC Musculoskelet Disord 9: 75.

Brukner P, Khan K. 2007. Clinical sports medicine. Northe Ryde, NSW: McGraw-Hill.

Cleland JA, Whitman JM, Fritz JM. 2004. Effectiveness of manual physical therapy to the cervical spine in the management of lateral epicondylalgia: a retrospective analysis. J Orthop Sports Phys Ther 34: 713–722; discussion 722–714.

Cleland JA, Flynn T, Palmer J. 2005. Incorporation of manual therapy directed at the cervicothoracic spine in patients with lateral epicondylalgia: a pilot clinical trial. J Man Manip Ther 13: 143–151.

Cook JL, Purdam CR. 2009. Is tendon pathology a continuum? A pathology model to explain the clinical presentation of load-induced tendinopathy. Br J Sports Med 43: 409–416.

Cook JL, Khan KM, Kiss ZS, et al. 2001. Asymptomatic hypoechoic regions on patellar tendon ultrasound: a 4-year clinical and ultrasound follow-up of 46 tendons. Scand J Med Sci Sports 11: 321–327.

Cook JL, Malliaras P, De Luca J. 2004. Neovascularization and pain in abnormal patellar tendons of active jumping athletes. Clin J Sport Med 14: 296–299.

Coombes B, Bisset L, Connelly L, et al. 2009a. Optimising corticosteroid injection for lateral epicondylalgia with the addition of physiotherapy: a protocol for a randomised control trial with placebo comparison. BMC Musculoskelet Disord 10: 76.

Coombes B, Bisset L, Vicenzino B. 2009b. An integrative model of lateral epicondylalgia. Br J Sports Med 43: 252–258.

Coombes B, Bisset L, Vicenzino B. 2012. Thermal hyperalgesia distinguishes those with severe pain and disability in unilateral lateral epicondylalgia. Clin J Pain 28: 95–601.

Coombes B, Bisset L, Brooks P, et al. 2013. Effect of corticosteroid injection, physiotherapy, or both on clinical outcomes in patients with unilateral lateral epicondylalgia: a randomized controlled trial. JAMA 309: 461–469.

Dimberg L. 1987. The prevalence and causation of tennis elbow (lateral humeral epicondylitis) in a population of workers in an engineering industry. Ergonomics 30: 573–580.

Du Toit C, Stieler M, Saunders R, et al. 2008. Diagnostic accuracy of power-doppler ultrasound in patients with chronic tennis elbow. Br J Sports Med 42: 572–666.

Fernández-Carnero J, Fernández-de-las-Peñas C, Cleland JA. 2008. Immediate hypoalgesic and motor effects after a single cervical spine manipulation in subjects with lateral epicondylalgia. J Manipulative Physiol Ther 31: 675–681.

Fernández-Carnero J, Fernández-de-las-Peñas C, Ge H-Y, et al. 2009a. Widespread mechanical pain hypersensitivity as sign of central sensitization in unilateral epicondylalgia: a blinded, controlled study. Clin J Pain 25: 555–561.

Fernández-Carnero J, Fernández-de-las-Peñas C, Sterling M, et al. 2009b. Exploration of the extent of somato-sensory impairment in patients with unilateral lateral epicondylalgia. J Pain 10: 1179–1185.

Feuerstein M, Miller VL, Burrell LM, et al. 1998. Occupational upper extremity disorders in the federal workforce: prevalence, health care expenditures, and patterns of work disability. J Occup Environ Med 40: 546–555.

Fredberg U, Bolvig L, Andersen NT. 2008. Prophylactic training in asymptomatic soccer players with ultrasonographic abnormalities in Achilles and patellar tendons: the Danish Super League Study. Am J Sports Med 36: 451–460.

Gunn CC, Milbrandt WE. 1976. Tennis elbow and the cervical spine. CMAJ 114: 803–809.

Hay EM, Paterson SM, Lewis M, et al. 1999. Pragmatic randomised controlled trial of local corticosteroid injection and naproxen for treatment of lateral epicondylitis of elbow in primary care. BMJ 319: 964–968.

Khan KM, Cook JL. 2000. Overuse tendon injuries: where does the pain come from? Sports Med Arthrosc 8: 17–31.

Khan KM, Scott A. 2009. Mechanotherapy: how physical therapists' prescription of exercise affects tissue repair. Br J Sports Med 43: 247–252.

Kivi P. 1982. The etiology and conservative treatment of humeral epicondylitis. Scand J Rehabil Med 15: 37–41.

Kochar M, Dogra A. 2002. Effectiveness of a specific physiotherapy regimen on patients with tennis elbow. Physiotherapy 88: 333–341.

Kohia M, Brackle J, Byrd K, et al. 2008. Effectiveness of physical therapy treatments on lateral epicondylitis. Jo Sport Rehabil 17: 119–136.

Kraushaar BS, Nirschl RP. 1999. Tendinosis of the elbow (tennis elbow). Clinical features and findings of histological, immunohistochemical, and electron microscopy studies. J Bone Joint Surg Am 81: 259–278.

Lee D. 1986. Tennis elbow: a manual therapist's perspective. J Orthop Sports Phys Ther 8: 134–142.

Lim ECW. 2013. Towards a better understanding of the mechanisms underlying lateral epicondylalgia and its management. [PhD Thesis, St Lucia, Qld.]

Lim ECW, Sterling M, Pedler A, et al. 2012. Evidence of spinal cord hyperexcitability as measured with nociceptive flexion reflex (NFR) threshold in chronic lateral epicondylalgia with or without a positive neurodynamic test. J Pain 13: 676–684.

Ljung BO, Forsgren S, Friden J. 1999. Substance P and calcitonin gene-related peptide expression at the extensor carpi radialis brevis muscle origin: implications for the etiology of tennis elbow. J Orthop Res 17: 554–559.

Ljung BO, Alfredson H, Forsgren S. 2004. Neurokinin 1-receptors and sensory neuropeptides in tendon insertions at the medial and lateral epicondyles of the humerus: studies on tennis elbow and medial epicondylalgia. J Orthop Res 22: 321–327.

Murrell GAC. 2007. Using nitric oxide to treat tendinopathy. Br J Sports Med 41: 227–231.

Nirschl RP. 1992. Elbow tendinosis / tennis elbow. Clin Sports Med 11: 851–870.

Nirschl RP, Pettrone F. 1979. Tennis elbow: the surgical treatment of lateral epicondylitis. J Bone Surg 61: 832–839.

Olaussen M, Holmedal O, Lindbaek M, et al. 2009. Physiotherapy alone or in combination with corticosteroid injection for acute lateral epicondylitis in general practice: a protocol for a randomised, placebo-controlled study. BMC Musculoskelet Disord 10: 152.

Osborne H. 2010. Stop injecting corticosteroid into patients with tennis elbow, they are much more likely to get better by themselves! J Sports Sci Med 13 (4): 380–381.

Paoloni JA, Appleyard RC, Nelson J, et al. 2003. Topical nitric oxide application in the treatment of chronic extensor tendinosis at the elbow: a randomized, double-blinded, placebo-controlled clinical trial. Am J Sports Med 31: 915–920.

Paoloni JA, Murrell GA, Burch R, et al. 2009. Randomised, double blind, placebo controlled, multicentre dose-ranging clinical trial of a new topical glyceryl trinitrate patch for chronic lateral epicondylosis. Br J Sports Med 43: 299–302.

Paungmali A, O'Leary S, Souvlis T, et al. 2003. Hypoalgesic and sympathoexcitatory effects of mobilization with movement for lateral epicondylalgia. Phys Ther 83: 374–383.

Pienimaki TT, Tarvainen T, Siira P, et al. 1996. Progressive strengthening and stretching exercises and ultrasound for chronic lateral epicondylitis. Physiotherapy 82: 522–530.

Pienimaki TT, Kauranen K, Vanharanta H, 1997. Bilaterally decreased motor performance of arms in patients with chronic tennis elbow. Arch Phys Med Rehabil 78: 1092–1095.

Pienimaki T, Karinen P, Kemila T, et al. 1998. Long-term follow-up of conservatively treated chronic tennis elbow patients. A prospective and retrospective analysis. Scand J Rehabil Med 30: 159–166.

Potter HG, Hannafin JA, Morwessel RM, et al. 1995. Lateral epicondylitis: correlation of MR imaging, surgical, and histopathologic findings. Radiology 196: 43–46.

Rabago D, Best TM, Zgierska AE, et al. 2009. A systematic review of four injection therapies for lateral epicondylosis: prolotherapy, polidocanol, whole blood and platelet-rich plasma. Br J Sports Med 43: 471–481.

Regan W, Wold LE, Coonrad R, et al. 1992. Microscopic histopathology of chronic refractory lateral epicondylitis. Am J Sports Med 20: 746–749.

Slater H, Arendt-Nielsen L, Wright A, et al. 2003. Experimental deep tissue pain in wrist extensors – a model of lateral epicondylalgia. Eur J Pain 7: 277–288.

Slater H, Arendt-Nielsen L, Wright A, et al. 2005. Sensory and motor effects of experimental muscle pain in patients with lateral epicondylalgia and controls with delayed onset muscle soreness. Pain 114: 118–130.

Smidt N, van der Windt DAWM. 2006. Tennis elbow in primary care. BMJ 333: 927–928.

Smidt N, van der Windt D, Assendelft WJJ, et al. 2002. Corticosteroid injections, physiotherapy, or a wait-and-see policy for lateral epicondylitis: a randomised controlled trial. Lancet 359: 657–662.

Smidt N, Lewis M, Da VDW, et al. 2006. Lateral epicondylitis in general practice: course and prognostic indicators of outcome. J Rheumatol 33: 2053–2059.

Stasinopoulos D, Stasinopoulou K, Stasinopoulos I, et al. 2010. Comparison of effects of a home exercise programme and a supervised exercise programme for the management of lateral elbow tendinopathy. Br J Sports Med 44 (8): 579–583.

Struijs PAA, Smidt N, Arola H, et al. 2001. Orthotic devices for tennis elbow: a systematic review. Br J Gen Pract 51: 924–929.

Struijs PAA, Smidt N, Arola H, et al. 2002. Orthotic devices for the treatment of tennis elbow. Cochrane Database Syst Rev 1: CD001821.
Struijs PAA, Damen PJ, Bakker EWP, et al. 2003. Manipulation of the wrist for management of lateral epicondylitis: a randomized pilot study. Phys Ther 83: 608–616.
Struijs PAA, Kerkhoffs G, Assendelft WJJ, et al. 2004. Conservative treatment of lateral epicondylitis – brace versus physical therapy or a combination of both: a randomized clinical trial. Am J Sports Med 32: 462–469.
Verhaar JA. 1994. Tennis elbow. Anatomical, epidemiological and therapeutic aspects. Int Orthop 18: 263–267.
Vicenzino B. 2003. Lateral epicondylalgia: a musculoskeletal physiotherapy perspective. Man Ther 8: 66–79.
Vicenzino B. 2009. Time for a re-think on the role of corticosteroid injections? Rapid response to: Cohen SP et al, Comparison of fluoroscopically guided and blind corticosteroid injections for greater trochanteric pain syndrome: multicentre randomised controlled trial. BMJ 338: doi: 10.1136/bmj.b1088.
Vicenzino B, Collins D, Wright A. 1996. The initial effects of a cervical spine manipulative physiotherapy treatment on the pain and dysfunction of lateral epicondylalgia. Pain 68: 69–74.
Vicenzino B, Collins D, Benson H, et al. 1998. An investigation of the interrelationship between manipulative therapy induced hypoalgesia and sympathoexcitation. J Manip Physiol Ther 21: 448–453.
Vicenzino B, Paungmali A, Buratowski S, et al. 2001b. Specific manipulative therapy treatment for chronic lateral epicondylalgia produces uniquely characteristic hypoalgesia. Man Ther 6: 205–212.
Vicenzino B, Cleland J, Bisset L. 2007a. Joint manipulation in the management of lateral epicondylalgia. Clinical Commentary. J Man Manip Ther 15: 50–56.
Vicenzino B, Paungmali A, Teys P. 2007b. Mulligan's mobilization-with-movement, positional faults and pain relief: current concepts from a critical review of literature. Man Ther 12: 98–108.
Waugh EJ, Jaglal SB, Davis AM, et al. 2004. Factors associated with prognosis of lateral epicondylitis after 8 weeks of physical therapy. Arch Phys Med Rehabil 85: 308–318.
Woodley BL, Newsham-West RJ, Baxter GD, et al. 2007. Chronic tendinopathy: effectiveness of eccentric exercise. Br J Sports Med 41: 188–198.
Young HH, Ward LE, Henderson ED. 1954. The use of hydrocortisone acetate (compound F acetate) in the treatment of some common orthopaedic conditions. J Bone Joint Surg Am 36: 602–609.
Zeisig E, Ohberg L, Alfredson H. 2006. Extensor origin vascularity related to pain in patients with tennis elbow. Knee Surg Sports Traumatol Arthrosc 14: 659–663.

Chapter 40

Other Elbow Disorders: Elbow Instability, Arthritic Conditions

Chris A. Sebelski

CHAPTER CONTENTS

Introduction	451
Elbow instability	451
Anatomy review for elbow instability	451
General treatment planning guidelines for elbow instability	451
Lateral elbow instability	452
Medial elbow instability	454
Arthritic conditions	455
Anatomy review for arthritic conditions of the elbow	455
Incidence/prevalence of arthritic conditions of the elbow	455
Pathology/pathoanatomy of arthritic conditions of the elbow	456
Diagnosis of arthritic conditions of the elbow	456
Prognosis and treatment planning for patients with arthritic conditions of the elbow	456
Conclusion	457

Introduction

This chapter will present two specific conditions of the elbow: elbow instability and arthritic conditions. Each section presents a short introduction with relevant anatomy, incidence / prevalence, pathology, clinical examination information and, finally, non-operative treatment. The reader is encouraged to remember that elbow dysfunction rarely occurs in isolation (Royle 1991; Walker-Bone et al 2004). When approaching a clinical case involving elbow pathology, the clinician must determine the underlying primary aetiology, the potential secondary aetiologies, the associated impairments and finally the role of regional interdependence for determination of the appropriate plan of care.

Elbow Instability

Overall, the elbow is the second most commonly dislocated joint in adults, with posterior dislocation being the most common (Royle 1991). It is the most commonly dislocated joint in the paediatric age group (Kuhn & Ross 2008). In the very young or those of advanced age, associated injuries such as fractures occur, whereas non-complex dislocations most commonly occur within young athletic populations (Mehta & Bain 2004). There are five criteria (O'Driscoll et al 2001a) to assist in classifying elbow instability:

- the involved articulation(s)
- the direction of displacement
- the degree of displacement
- the duration (acute, chronic or recurrent)
- the presence / absence of associated fractures.

Injury progression is represented through the circle of Horii where the injury progresses from lateral to medial through soft tissue, bone or both. Due to the energy absorption by a fracture, one may see ligament sparing with a fracture of the radius or the coronoid. In the progression of stages, stage I demonstrates disruption of the lateral collateral ligament (LCL) with a presentation of posterolateral instability, stage II signifies disruption of the capsule with anterior and posterior instability and stage III demonstrates disruption of the portions of the medial collateral ligament. Stage III is further divided into subparts A, B and C (O'Driscoll et al 2001a).

Anatomy review for elbow instability

There are three primary constraints for elbow stability: the ulnohumeral joint, the medial collateral ligament and the lateral ulnar collateral ligament. Although O'Driscoll (2000) originally named the lateral ulnar collateral ligament as a primary constraint, there is controversy regarding its importance, as cadaver studies have demonstrated elbow posterolateral rotatory instability (PLRI) with artificially induced division of various ligaments in the LCL complex (Olsen et al 1996; Singleton & Conway 2004). Secondary constraints include: the radial head, the common flexor origin, the common extensor origin, and the joint capsule. Dynamic constraints produce compressive forces at the joint including the biceps brachii, triceps and anconeus (O'Driscoll 2000).

General treatment planning guidelines for elbow instability

Treatment varies according to the severity of the injury. In an acute dislocation without an associated elbow fracture, the recommended treatment is a closed reduction followed by bracing for a short period of time. The patient is typically directed to use the upper extremity for daily function within symptom tolerance after the brace is removed. Simple elbow dislocations have a good prognosis, with up to 95% of the persons affected returning to their previous level of activity (Hildebrand et al 1999). However, if symptoms persist, the intervention plan must be adapted according to the injury and the symptoms reported. The presence of fracture with a dislocation / subluxation changes the course of treatment, as typically there is surgical intervention for the fracture. If an acute ligament injury is sustained in conjunction with a fracture of the radius or the coronoid, a repair of that ligament is necessary to assist with the stability of the joint (O'Driscoll et al 2001a). In the sections that follow, elbow instability is further discussed by injury to the lateral or medial ligament structures.

Lateral elbow instability

Anatomy review for lateral elbow instability

The lateral collateral ligament (LCL) complex originates from the humerus at the trochlea and capitellum and continues distally to blend with the annular ligament inserting at the proximal ulna (Cohen & Bruno 2001). This complex consists of up to four structures: the annular ligament, the ulnar portion of the LCL, the radial portion of the LCL, and the accessory LCL (which is not always present). The lateral ligament complex is taut throughout elbow flexion and extension. Ligament tension is increased with the forearm positioned in supination.

Incidence / prevalence of lateral elbow instability

PLRI, an injury to the lateral collateral ligament and the soft tissue stabilizers, is the most common type of chronic instability at the elbow. In contrast, isolated varus instability from the laxity of the LCL is not as common as an isolated medial collateral ligament injury (Charalambous & Stanley 2008).

Pathology / pathoanatomy of lateral elbow instability

There are three typical scenarios that may lead to lateral collateral ligament injury: elbow dislocation, varus stress insufficiency / chronic attenuation and iatrogenic causes (Singleton & Conway 2004). Typically, elbow dislocation is an acute occurrence; O'Driscoll et al (1992) proposed that elbow PLRI may be the initial step towards elbow laxity. PLRI may present as an independent pathology, or it may be part of a continuum leading to dislocation (Smith et al 2001). PLRI has also been cited as the most common cause of recurrent symptoms following dislocation (O'Driscoll et al 2001a). Chronic attenuation and / or varus insufficiency may occur with overuse – such as in the cases of patients with significant weight-bearing activities on the upper extremities (e.g. crutch ambulation) – or in those persons with generalized ligament laxity. A causal relationship of cubitus varus and recurrent elbow instability in the form of PLRI has been reported by several authors, with symptoms that may not appear until more than two decades post injury (O'Driscoll et al 2001a, 2001b; Arrigoni & Kamineni 2009). It has been theorized that these symptoms may be secondary to the attenuation of the ligament from the repetitive torque on the LCL and the inappropriate pull of secondary stabilizers. Iatrogenic disruption of the integrity of the LCL may result from surgical approaches that involve the lateral elbow structures, such as a lateral epicondylar release procedure or an approach to access the radial head (O'Driscoll 2000).

PLRI affects the articulation between the ulna and the humerus while the proximal radioulnar joint remains intact. This differs from a simple posterior dislocation of the radial head, where the ulnohumeral joint remains intact and the proximal radioulnar joint is disrupted. With PLRI, the forearm externally rotates (supinates) away from the humerus, effectively 'pivoting' on the intact medial collateral ligaments and allowing the radial head to subluxate in a posterior direction.

These mechanics provide support for the use of orthopaedic tests that pay special attention to the position of the forearm. Traditionally, varus stress testing is utilized when examining a patient with probable disruption of the lateral ligaments of the elbow. Valgus stress testing is used to determine the laxity of the medial collateral ligament. Indications of probable medial collateral ligament laxity would be the presence of laxity / apprehension with the forearm in pronation and application of a valgus stress. The pronated forearm position and medially directed stress tension the medial collateral ligament. During forearm pronation, the lateral structures of the elbow are tensioned, stabilizing the radial head. However, if the forearm is positioned in supination and a valgus stress is applied, the lateral structures are unable to stabilize the radial head appropriately. Therefore, if the patient demonstrates laxity or appears apprehensive when the forearm is supinated and tensioned in the valgus direction, PLRI should be suspected (Smith et al 2001).

Diagnosis of lateral elbow instability

In a search for lateral collateral laxity, history taking should include inquiring about the three potential mechanisms, including both acute dislocations and a history of dislocation if a patient's report leads the tester to suspect chronic recurring instability. Questioning should include positions of the upper extremity that place the elbow at risk of chronic attenuation, including a history of elbow fracture as a youth. Additionally, a medical history that may contribute to generalized ligament laxity should be explored.

Patient concerns may include 'vague' aching about the elbow joint, pain, clicking, snapping or clunking that is worse with a supinated position of the forearm. Patients may comment on 'something not right' when extending their arm with the forearm in supination (Lee & Rosenwasser 1999; O'Driscoll 2000). Unless there is an associated traumatic event, however, the patient will only rarely be able to isolate the onset of the symptoms.

Physical exam measures include observation for a cubitus varus deformity, range of motion (ROM) and special orthopaedic testing (Table 40.1), which may be passive and / or active. Reporting of the statistical evidence for orthopaedic tests is limited and, due to the supportive roles of the secondary soft tissue constraints, it is often recommended that passive exam techniques be completed with the patient under

Table 40.1 **Orthopaedic examination techniques for lateral elbow instability**

Name of test	Physical exam technique	Outcome to indicate a positive test for pathology
Varus stress test	Application of a laterally directed force applied in both full extension and at approximately 30° of elbow flexion to allow the olecranon to move out of the olecranon fossa. It is recommended to perform this test with the humerus fully internally rotated (O'Driscoll et al 2001b).	Greater laxity is felt by therapist compared with the contralateral side.
Lateral pivot shift test	Patient lies supine with the shoulder passively flexed past 90°. With the elbow in extension, the examiner applies axial compression through the ulna and radius towards the humerus with a supination and valgus force, causing the elbow to subluxate at ~40–70° of elbow flexion. If the patient allows the passive examination to continue, an observable clunk occurs with continued flexion as the elbow reduces (O'Driscoll et al 1991, 1992; O'Driscoll, 2000).	Posterolateral displacement of radius occurs, followed by reduction as elbow flexion progresses to 90° (O'Driscoll et al 1991). The apprehension test would have the patient report apprehension prior to the subluxation.
Posterolateral instability test	The examiner flexes the elbow to 40°, with the forearm in external rotation; an anteroposterior force is applied to the ulna and radius (O'Driscoll et al 2001b).	Subluxation of the forearm away from the humerus.
Push-up sign (from floor) (Arvind & Hargreaves 2006)	Patient pushes up from the floor with shoulders in abduction, forearms supinated.	Apprehension and voluntary/involuntary guarding as involved elbow moves towards terminal extension.
Table-top relocation test (Arvind & Hargreaves 2006)	Three-step test: 1. Patient performs a press-up from a table top with the forearm in supination. 2. With onset of symptoms (approximately 40° of flexion) examiner applies a force through their thumb at the patient's radial head. 3. Then the examiner removes the force at the radial head.	First outcome: pain and apprehension. Second outcome: pain and apprehension are reduced. Third outcome: pain/apprehension returns.

anaesthesia for best results (O'Driscoll et al 2001b). In the case of a varus-directed stress test a false negative may be reported, as the ulnohumeral articulation is the main constraint to varus movements (Charalambous & Stanley 2008). As indicated above, the examination technique for medial collateral laxity via the valgus stress test may give the examiner clues to a potential PLRI pathology if completed with the forearm in supination (Olsen et al 1998). However, for detection of PLRI the most utilized examination technique is the PLRI test. It has also been advocated that the positive response of the PLRI test be changed to 'patient apprehension' rather than 'a visible clunk' has also been advocated (Charalambous & Stanley 2008). Suggested imaging includes stress radiographs, arthrogram or, for PLRI, MRI – for which a specific pulse sequence is described (Potter et al 1997).

Prognosis and treatment planning for patients with lateral elbow instability

Despite its high prevalence for dislocation, the elbow is considered to be one of the most stable joints in the body. The philosophy of treatment of elbow instability with associated fractures is first to stabilize the osseous–articular injuries. With the achievement of osseous stabilization, the next step is to address ligamentous injury. Although with more complex injuries the prognosis for full functional return declines, the intervention and management of a dislocation without fracture has demonstrated good outcomes overall (O'Driscoll et al 2001b; Kuhn & Ross 2008).

In general, non-operative care for patients who demonstrate symptom-producing recurrent instability, such as that found with PLRI or varus insufficiency, is not common. However, the use of bracing to assist in avoidance of forearm supination with valgus loading may be advocated for those patients with mild symptoms. In cases of recurrent symptoms, operative management may be undertaken via direct repair or reattachment of the ligament or in order to reconstruct the lateral ligament complex with a tendon graft reconstruction. The results following surgical reconstruction, though limited, are promising – with studies reporting resolution of symptoms, full range of motion and a return to activity (Nestor et al 1992; Lee & Teo 2003). Operative care may also be advocated for correction of cubitus varus in those patients who demonstrate positive physical exam signs for PLRI (O'Driscoll et al 2001a).

Medial elbow instability

Anatomy review for medial elbow instability

There are three ligaments of the medial collateral ligament (MCL) complex, namely the anterior oblique / bundle, the posterior oblique / band and the transverse ligament / band. The origin of the MCL is slightly posterior to the elbow joint, and so it demonstrates greater tension with increasing flexion. The anterior bundle of the MCL is the strongest of the three and it attaches the medial epicondyle to the medial coronoid process. Histologically, this bundle may be further divided into anterior and posterior bands (Safran & Baillargeon 2005). The anterior band is primarily taut from full extension to 60° of flexion, whereas the posterior band of the anterior bundle is taut from 60° to 120° of flexion (Cohen & Bruno 2001; Safran 2004; Safran & Baillargeon 2005). The posterior oblique portion of the MCL complex is a thickening of the capsule that has the greatest restraint at 90° of elbow flexion. It arises from the medial epicondyle and inserts onto the medial side of the semilunar notch. The third portion of the MCL is the transverse ligament, arising from the medial olecranon and the inferior medial coronoid process. It has limited impact, is not always present, and is often indistinguishable from the capsule (Cohen & Bruno 2001; Safran & Baillargeon 2005).

Additional stabilizers of the elbow include the radiocapitellar joint and the regional muscles. The radiocapitellar joint contributes up to 30% of the stability against valgus stress. The regional muscles of the pronator and the flexors may also have a role; however, the significance of their contribution is not yet completely understood (Cohen & Bruno 2001; Safran 2004).

Incidence / prevalence of medial elbow instability

Injury to the MCL is more common in the overhead-throwing athlete population than in the non-thrower population. In the throwing athlete, the consequences of such instability may include the inability to compete at the desired level. In the general population it rarely affects the activities of daily living (Grace & Field 2008), aside from particular job tasks within the work environment. Bennett et al (1992) provide one example, of industrial workers who demonstrated symptoms of chronic medial ligament instability during specific work tasks who eventually required surgical intervention in order to return to work.

Pathology / pathoanatomy of medial elbow instability

There are two mechanisms for MCL laxity: acute or spontaneous occurrence and chronic attenuation. The symptoms that the patient will report may differentiate the two incidences. A 'pop' may be heard in the more acute cases ,whereas there may be a report of vague elbow discomfort that becomes more prevalent over a length of time in a mechanism that involves chronic attenuation.

The mechanics of throwing have been studied to determine its contribution to medial collateral laxity. Of note, the MCL (primarily the anterior bundle) provides up to 54% of the varus torque to resist the valgus strain in the elbow during the late cocking and early deceleration phases of throwing (Fleisig et al 1995). The ultimate failure load of the MCL is calculated to be less (34 Nm) than the loads to which it is exposed during the majority of overhead sports (52–120 Nm) (Fleisig et al 1995). Therefore, it is hypothesized that there is a significant influence from the proximal segments and core of the upper extremity to generate secondary constraints for control of these forces (Kibler & Sciascia 2004); the suggestion is that an imbalance of the contribution from local structures and / or inadequate contribution from the proximal segments and core would create an environment of excessive strain, which would result in attenuation over time.

Typically with a chronic condition, the MCL laxity may represent only one aspect of a constellation of injuries that contribute to the medial elbow pain. For example, the ligament injury may be a part of valgus extension overload syndrome, which involves the compression of the olecranon of the ulna against the humerus with a valgus stress. Associated injuries may include: capitellar wear, posteromedial osteophytes, ulnar neuritis and degenerative or traumatic arthritis of the elbow. Furthermore, due to the dynamic nature of the population this pathology is often associated with, it is important to consider the influence of the kinetic chain. In two different reports, findings indicated that professional baseball players presenting with both medial elbow symptoms of insufficiency and significant glenohumeral internal rotation deficits demonstrate a kinetic chain relationship whereby impairments outside of the local region may have a causal relationship to the symptoms reported at the elbow (Kibler & Sciascia 2004; Dines et al 2009).

Diagnosis of medial elbow instability

The patient history should include not only location, duration of symptoms and the mechanism of injury but also the details of a throwing or overhead movement history if the patient is an athlete (Safran 2004). The patient presentation may be complicated by complaints from the secondary structures involved in the overload mechanism, including muscular strain, inflammation or tendinosis, that may be associated with the underlying instability.

Physical exam includes palpation, observation for a cubitus varus deformity, range of motion and special orthopaedic testing, which may be passive or active (Table 40.2). On palpation, the clinician may find tenderness approximately 2 cm distal from the medial epicondyle at the ulnar insertion of MCL. This tenderness has been reported in as many as 80% of those patients undergoing MCL reconstruction. ROM limitations may often include a flexion contracture (Thompson et al 2001).

For specific physical exam measures such as the valgus stress test and the milking manoeuvre statistical evidence is limited. Similar to the special testing of the lateral ligaments of the elbow, consideration must be paid to the supportive roles of the secondary soft tissue constraints. For example, during the valgus stress test, it has been stated that the position of supination for the forearm should provide a greater bias of the MCL over the contribution from the LCL (Smith et al 2001). However, in a cadaveric study by Safran et al (2005) where both the anterior and posterior bands of the anterior bundle of the MCL were sectioned and tested at various angles of flexion and forearm position, the neutral position of the forearm in relationship to the horizontal,

Table 40.2 **Orthopaedic examination techniques for medial elbow instability**

Name of test	Physical exam technique	Outcome to indicate a positive test for pathology
Valgus stress test	Application of a medial directed force applied at the elbow in both full extension and at 30–40° elbow flexion to allow the olecranon to move out of the olecranon fossa. The humeral position is suggested to be in external rotation.	Greater laxity is felt by therapist in comparison to contralateral side.
Milking test (Grace & Field 2008)	A valgus force is applied by the patient with the elbow flexed. This is done by the patient holding the thumb on the involved side with the contralateral upper extremity. The contralateral upper extremity must reach under the elbow of the involved side to grasp the thumb.	Medial elbow pain with this manoeuvre indicates a positive result.
Moving valgus stress test (O'Driscoll et al 2005)	Therapist passively moves the involved elbow through range of motion flexion to extension while simultaneously applying a valgus force.	The test is positive if the medial elbow pain is reproduced at the medial collateral ligament. Maximum symptoms should be felt at 120–70° during flexion and extension.

regardless of the degree of elbow flexion, assessed the integrity of the MCL more clearly than any other position. It should be noted, though, that this alteration in the procedure of the valgus stress test has not been tested in humans; therefore the information must be viewed cautiously.

For detection of medial ligament instability, such as commonly seen with partial tearing or attenuation in the throwing athlete, the moving valgus stress test as described by O'Driscoll et al (2005) is the most widely used, with supportive statistical evidence of sensitivity of 1.0 and specificity of 0.75. Imaging techniques such as static imaging, stress radiographs, MRI, CT scan and arthroscopic valgus stress testing have all been utilized with varying degrees of success (O'Driscoll et al 2005).

Prognosis and treatment planning for patients with medial elbow instability

Treatment of non-throwers and the general population is via a non-operative rehabilitation programme with reported successful return to the activities of daily living without symptoms (Grace & Field 2008). For that subset of patients wishing to return to high demand throwing, non-operative therapy is attempted initially and only with a failure to return is operative management considered.

In a single study by Rettig et al (2001), throwers with chronic medial instability were treated non-operatively. They achieved a 42% success rate in returning the athlete to sport within an average of 24.5 weeks. The rehabilitation was divided into two phases. The first phase involved a rest from throwing for up to 3 months, resolution of inflammation including wearing of a brace and achievement of full range of motion. The second phase included a progressive strengthening programme and stepwise progression towards a return to throwing.

Information gained from cadaveric studies can provide cues for rehabilitation. Armstrong et al (2000) studied the MCL in cadaveric elbows and concluded that active mobilization of the elbow in the vertical position with either a fully supinated or pronated forearm position is safe for decreased stress at the ligament. With tension in the medial structures, one might construct a rehabilitation programme that incorporates limited humeral external rotation in combination with neutral forearm positioning and avoidance of valgus stresses, especially during 70–120° of elbow flexion. In a cadaveric study by Bernas et al (2009), the immediate post-rehabilitative phase was concluded to be an appropriate time to introduce isometric flexion and extension below 90° of flexion and to limit motion from full extension to 50° of flexion to protect the MCL.

Arthritic Conditions

Anatomy review for arthritic conditions of the elbow

The elbow comprises three articulations: the ulna articulating with the humerus, the ulna articulating with the radius and the radius articulating with the humerus. There are two degrees of freedom in the elbow joint: flexion / extension and pronation / supination. The functional arc of motion of the elbow is 30–130°. A total range of less than 100° in the sagittal plane or the transverse plane will generate significant functional limitations (Morrey et al 1981).

Incidence/prevalence of arthritic conditions of the elbow

Arthritis of the elbow is relatively uncommon. It typically falls into three categories: rheumatoid arthritis (RA), post-traumatic arthritis or primary degenerative osteoarthritis (OA). In the patient population with RA, it has been found that 25–66% of the patients may have the presence of disease in one or both elbows (Porter et al 1974; Lehtinen et al 2001). Primary degenerative arthritis of the elbow has been reported to affect less

Table 40.3 Patient presentation with arthritic conditions of the elbow

Underlying disease	Patient report	Comments
Rheumatoid arthritis	Pain throughout the ROM	Loss of rotation Excessive motion in the coronal plane (Soojian & Kwon 2007) Possible underlying instability
Post-traumatic arthritis	Stiffness and pain with inadequate end ROM	History of trauma, surgery to joint Possible underlying instability
Primary degenerative osteoarthritis	Initially, pain only at the terminal ROM In later stages, pain throughout the ROM Catching/locking may be reported	Need to monitor progression of disease as this impacts treatment

than 2% of the population (Antuna et al 2002). Though the theory remains somewhat controversial, it is generally accepted that primary OA of the elbow affects males with a history of 'heavy use of the upper extremity' such as industrial labour, weightlifting, etc. (Gramstad & Galatz 2006; Kokkalis et al 2009). These patients are typically not less than 40 years of age (Gramstad & Galatz 2006).

Pathology/pathoanatomy of arthritic conditions of the elbow

RA is an inflammatory disease process that affects multiple joints. It is characterized by symmetric joint narrowing, disuse osteopenia and periarticular erosions, which will be seen on radiographic imaging (Kokkalis et al 2009). The course and natural history of OA are not well understood, however; it is typically characterized by destruction of the articular cartilage (Gramstad & Galatz 2006). Primary OA of the elbow demonstrates unique features such as sparing of the articular surfaces with preservation of the joint spaces and hypertrophic formation of osteophytes and capsular constriction (Cheung et al 2008). OA begins on the lateral aspect of the joint at the radiocapitellar joint (Goodfellow & Bullough 1967). In the younger population with a presentation of elbow stiffness, post-traumatic arthritis should be suspected. Associated disorders to this pathology include: trauma, osteochondritis dissecans, synovial chondromatosis and valgus extension overload syndrome (Gramstad & Galatz 2006).

Diagnosis of arthritic conditions of the elbow

Generally, patients report pain, stiffness and potential weakness. Functionally, they often have symptoms when attempting to carry a weighted object next to the body when the elbow is extended. Depending on the underlying cause of the arthritis, patient reports may vary, however. For example, a patient with elbow pain secondary to RA may complain of pain throughout the ROM (Soojian & Kwon 2007), a patient with OA may have concerns of 'pinching' or 'sharp pain' with terminal flexion or extension during the earlier stages of the disease (Cheung et al 2008), whereas patients with a diagnosis of post-traumatic arthritis may be younger and healthier than those with RA or OA, with less involvement of other body regions. The last group of patients may also possess an expectation of higher demand of the elbow (Amirfeyz & Blewitt 2009). In Table 40.3, specific features of each of the most common pathologies associated with elbow arthritis are highlighted.

A detailed interview of the patient to note the onset of symptoms, course of associated disease process or prior surgical / traumatic history is necessary. Prior treatment, either for the arthritic disease or specifically to the elbow, should be asked about, including the use of pharmacological therapies. Radiographs are the standard to determine the phase of the disease process and the potential plan of care. Of special note, one should recognize potential differential diagnoses that may produce similar patient concerns including septic arthritis, crystalline arthropathy, haemophilia and ochronosis (Soojian & Kwon 2007).

Prognosis and treatment planning for patients with arthritic conditions of the elbow

The underlying aetiology, functional limitations including the current ROM of the elbow and the age of the patient all significantly influence the treatment course. The current standard is non-operative treatment, which may include pharmacological management, corticosteroid injections, dynamic splinting and physical therapy (Gramstad & Galatz 2006; Kokkalis et al 2009). With the advent of improved and more aggressive treatment of RA, one report (Brasington 2009) stated that early management has the potential for complete resolution of symptoms in 10% of patients treated. For patients with primary OA at the elbow, activity modification is typically suggested, but with varying results.

If such non-operative measures fail to resolve the patient's functional limitations or symptoms, there is a wide variety of surgical options including arthroscopy and arthroplasty. The best results for management of OA and post-traumatic OA within the younger patient population have been reported after arthroscopy for a capsular release and clearing of osteophytes (Gramstad & Galatz 2006). The total elbow arthroplasty is typically reserved for the population of individuals over 60 years of age, who have lower physical demands and who are more likely to comply with the postoperative rehabilitative and long-term physical restrictions (Moro & King 2000).

Conclusion

In recent years, there has been a significant gain in understanding the anatomy and pathologies of the elbow that cause instability and stiffness. Building upon this new information, researchers now need to complete the development rehabilitation guidelines that will produce successful outcomes.

References

Amirfeyz R, Blewitt N. 2009. Mid-term outcome of GSB-III total elbow arthroplasty in patients with rheumatoid arthritis and patients with post-traumatic arthritis. Arch Orthop Trauma Surg 129(11): 1505–1510. doi:10.1007/s00402-009-0876-y.

Antuna SA, Morrey BF, Adams RA, et al. 2002. Ulnohumeral arthroplasty for primary degenerative arthritis of the elbow: long-term outcome and complications. J Bone Joint Surg Am 84A: 2168–2173.

Armstrong AD, Dunning CE, Faber KJ, et al. 2000. Rehabilitation of the medial collateral ligament-deficient elbow: an in vitro biomechanical study. J Hand Surg Am 25: 1051–1057.

Arrigoni P, Kamineni S. 2009. Uncovered posterolateral rotatory elbow instability with cubitus varus deformity correction. Orthopedics 32: 130.

Arvind CH, Hargreaves DG. 2006. Table top relocation test – new clinical test for posterolateral rotatory instability of the elbow. J Shoulder Elbow Surg 15: 500–501.

Bennett JB, Green MS, Tullos HS. 1992. Surgical management of chronic medial elbow instability. Clin Orthop Relat Res 278: 62–68.

Bernas GA, Ruberte Thiele R, Kinnaman KA, et al. 2009. Defining safe rehabilitation for ulnar collateral ligament reconstruction of the elbow: a biomechanical study. Am J Sports Med 37: 2392–2400. doi:10.1177/0363546509340658.

Brasington R. 2009. TNF-alpha antagonists and other recombinant proteins for the treatment of rheumatoid arthritis. J Hand Surg Am 34: 349–350.

Charalambous CP, Stanley JK. 2008. Posterolateral rotatory instability of the elbow. J Bone Joint Surg Br 90: 272–279.

Cheung R, Adams EV, Morrey BF. 2008. Primary osteoarthritis of the elbow: current treatment options. J Am Acad Orthop Surg 16: 77–87.

Cohen MS, Bruno RJ. 2001. The collateral ligaments of the elbow: anatomy and clinical correlation. Clin Orthop Relat Res 383: 123–130.

Dines JS, Frank JB, Akerman M, et al. 2009. Glenohumeral internal rotation deficits in baseball players with ulnar collateral ligament insufficiency. Am J Sports Med 37: 566–570.

Fleisig GS, Andrews JR, Dillman CJ, et al. 1995. Kinetics of baseball pitching with implications about injury mechanisms. Am J Sports Med 23: 233–239.

Goodfellow JW, Bullough PG. 1967. The pattern of ageing of the articular cartilage of the elbow joint. J Bone Joint Surg Br 49: 175–181.

Grace SP, Field LD. 2008. Chronic medial elbow instability. Orthop Clin North Am 39: 213–219.

Gramstad GD, Galatz LM. 2006. Management of elbow osteoarthritis. J Bone Joint Surg Am 88: 421–430.

Hildebrand KA, Patterson SD, King GJ. 1999. Acute elbow dislocations: simple and complex. Orthop Clin North Am 30: 63–79.

Kibler BW, Sciascia A. 2004. Kinetic chain contributions to elbow function and dysfunction in sports. Clin Sports Med 23: 545–552.

Kokkalis ZT, Schmidt CC, Sotereanos DG. 2009. Elbow arthritis: current concepts. J Hand Surg Am 34: 761–768.

Kuhn MA, Ross G. 2008. Acute elbow dislocations. Orthop Clin North Am 39: 155–161.

Lee BP, Teo LH. 2003. Surgical reconstruction for posterolateral rotatory instability of the elbow. J Shoulder Elbow Surg 12: 476–479.

Lee ML, Rosenwasser MP. 1999. Chronic elbow instability. Orthop Clin North Am 30: 81–89.

Lehtinen JT, Kaarela K, Ikavalko M, et al. 2001. Incidence of elbow involvement in rheumatoid arthritis. A 15 year endpoint study. J Rheumatol 28: 70–74.

Mehta JA, Bain GI. 2004. Posterolateral rotatory instability of the elbow. J Am Acad Orthop Surg 12: 405–415.

Moro JK, King GJ. 2000. Total elbow arthroplasty in the treatment of post-traumatic conditions of the elbow. Clin Orthop Relat Res 370: 102–114.

Morrey BF, Askew LJ, Chao EY. 1981. A biomechanical study of normal functional elbow motion. J Bone Joint Surg Am 63: 872–877.

Nestor BJ, O'Driscoll SW, Morrey BF. 1992. Ligamentous reconstruction for posterolateral rotatory instability of the elbow. J Bone Joint Surg Am 74: 1235–1241.

O'Driscoll SW. 2000. Classification and evaluation of recurrent instability of the elbow. Clin Orthop Relat Res 370: 34–43.

O'Driscoll SW, Bell DF, Morrey BF. 1991. Posterolateral rotatory instability of the elbow. J Bone Joint Surg Am 73: 440–446.

O'Driscoll SW, Morrey BF, Korinek S, et al. 1992. Elbow subluxation and dislocation. A spectrum of instability. Clin Orthop Relat Res 280: 186–197.

O'Driscoll SW, Jupiter JB, King GJ, et al. 2001a. The unstable elbow. Instr Course Lect 50: 89–102.

O'Driscoll SW, Spinner RJ, McKee MD, et al. 2001b. Tardy posterolateral rotatory instability of the elbow due to cubitus varus. J Bone Joint Surg Am 83A: 1358–1369.

O'Driscoll SW, Lawton RL, Smith AM. 2005. The 'moving valgus stress test' for medial collateral ligament tears of the elbow. Am J Sports Med 33: 231–239.

Olsen BS, Sojbjerg JO, Dalstra M, et al. 1996. Kinematics of the lateral ligamentous constraints of the elbow joint. J Shoulder Elbow Surg 5: 333–341.

Olsen BS, Sojbjerg JO, Nielsen KK, et al. 1998. Posterolateral elbow joint instability: the basic kinematics. J Shoulder Elbow Surg 7: 19–29.

Porter BB, Richardson C, Vainio K. 1974. Rheumatoid arthritis of the elbow: the results of synovectomy. J Bone Joint Surg Br 56B: 427–437.

Potter HG, Weiland AJ, Schatz JA, et al. 1997. Posterolateral rotatory instability of the elbow: usefulness of MR imaging in diagnosis. Radiology 204(1): 185–189.

Rettig AC, Sherrill C, Snead DS, et al. 2001. Nonoperative treatment of ulnar collateral ligament injuries in throwing athletes. Am J Sports Med 29: 15–17.

Royle SG. 1991. Posterior dislocation of the elbow. Clin Orthop Relat Res 269: 201–204.

Safran MR. 2004. Ulnar collateral ligament injury in the overhead athlete: diagnosis and treatment. Clin Sports Med 23: 643–663.

Safran MR, Baillargeon D. 2005. Soft-tissue stabilizers of the elbow. J Shoulder Elbow Surg 14: 179S–185S.

Safran MR, McGarry MH, Shin S, et al. 2005. Effects of elbow flexion and forearm rotation on valgus laxity of the elbow. J Bone Joint Surg Am 87: 2065–2074.

Singleton SB, Conway JE. 2004. PLRI: posterolateral rotatory instability of the elbow. Clin Sports Med 23: 629–642.

Smith JP 3rd, Savoie FH, Field LD. 2001. Posterolateral rotatory instability of the elbow. Clin Sports Med 20: 47–58.

Soojian MG, Kwon YW. 2007. Elbow arthritis. Bull N Y U Hosp Jt Dis 65: 61–71.

Thompson WH, Jobe FW, Yocum LA, et al. 2001. Ulnar collateral ligament reconstruction in athletes: muscle-splitting approach without transposition of the ulnar nerve. J Shoulder Elbow Surg 10: 152–157.

Walker-Bone K, Reading I, Coggon D, et al. 2004. The anatomical pattern and determinants of pain in the neck and upper limbs: an epidemiologic study. Pain 109: 45–51.

41 Chapter

Joint Mobilization and Manipulation of the Elbow

Helen Slater, César Fernández-de-las-Peñas

CHAPTER CONTENTS

Introduction 458
Evidence-based decision making 458
Definitions and clinical applications 459
Mobilization and manipulation techniques 460
Mobilization in extension combined with adduction (varus mobilization) 460
Mobilization in adduction and abduction (varus to valgus mobilization) 460
Mobilization in pronation/supination combined with flexion 461
Mobilization of the radiohumeral joint 461
Lateral glide mobilization with movement 462
Manipulation in lateral glide of the elbow (varus thrust manipulation) 462
Conclusion 462

Introduction

Mobilization and manipulation interventions of the elbow joint are frequently used in clinical practice, and although the evidence for their use is as yet insufficient, it is growing (Vicenzino et al 2007). Systematic reviews in relation to the elbow refer mainly to specific elbow conditions such as lateral epicondylalgia (Smidt et al 2003; Assendelft et al 2004; Vicenzino et al 2007). Despite the large number of studies, there is still insufficient evidence for most physiotherapy interventions owing to contradicting results, insufficient statistical power and the low number of studies per intervention (Smidt et al 2003). More-recent high-quality studies provide evidence that joint manipulation / mobilization directed at the elbow and wrist results in beneficial alterations in pain and the motor system (Vicenzino et al 2007). A meta-analysis of two randomized controlled trials showed that elbow mobilization improved pain-free grip strength and pressure pain threshold in comparison with placebo at short-term follow-up (Bisset et al 2005). A few cases reporting the use of specific mobilization interventions for elbow disorders have also been published, including a patient with ulnar tunnel syndrome (Lawrence & Humphreys 1997) and a patient with lateral epicondylalgia (Kaufman 2000). Given the low level of evidence for single case studies, clinicians are cautioned against making any conclusions from case studies alone.

Evidence-based Decision Making

In choosing joint mobilization as part of multimodal management, the therapist must give consideration to interpreting the clinical (patient) manifestations of peripheral and central sensitization processes involved in musculoskeletal disorders. For example, in patients with unilateral lateral epicondylalgia, evidence of bilateral manifestations of deep tissue hyperalgesia indicates that peripheral sensitization alone is unlikely to explain the clinical presentation (Slater et al 2005; Fernández-Carnero et al 2008, 2009). In the study by Slater et al (2005), evidence of widespread pain, referred pain and changes in somatosensory sensitivity raised the index of suspicion that patients with lateral epicondylalgia demonstrated alterations in the way that the nervous system processes nociceptive and non-nociceptive information. Therefore, clinical management of patients with lateral epicondylalgia may need to extend beyond local tissue-based pathology to incorporate strategies directed at normalizing nervous system sensitivity. Changes in somatosensory function, which are manifested clinically by persistent musculoskeletal pain (Graven-Nielsen 2006), also impact on motor systems as changes in the drive to muscle and altered motor control (Arendt-Nielsen & Graven-Nielsen 2008). Management cannot therefore focus just on the simple biomechanics of joint mobilization, but must also incorporate the more-recent findings on sensory–motor interactions in persistent musculoskeletal pain disorders.

In considering the choice of joint mobilization as an intervention, clinicians should also consider the potential neurophysiological and tissue mechanisms underlying the effects (positive and negative) of mobilization. Multiple interacting tissue and pain mechanisms are likely to contribute to the pain-modulatory effects of mobilization (Slater et al 2006; Vicenzino et al 2007). For a comprehensive review of putative mechanisms underlying the effects of mobilization, readers are referred to Paungmali et al (2003), Bisset et al (2006), Vicenzino et al (2007) and Chapter 39.

Where a patient's elbow disorder appears mediated primarily by peripheral nociceptive mechanisms (dominantly peripheral sensitization), early and appropriate physiological movements and functional activity should be encouraged. In such cases, although joint mobilization may offer benefits in terms of pain relief and restoration of joint mobility, the ultimate aim of such techniques is the restoration of function, limiting the chance of sustained central nervous system facilitation (central sensitization). Seldom in clinical practice would a unimodal approach using mobilization alone be considered appropriate for the management of elbow disorders. More commonly, mobilization would be incorporated into a multimodal approach. For example, depending on the chronicity of the disorder and the associated level of impairment and disability, patients would be educated about optimizing normal functional movements and undertaking active and specific exercises to maintain gains in pain-free joint ranges. The use of appropriate soft tissues techniques to address soft tissue contributions at the elbow may also be explored (see Chs 59–63). If required, help may be sought through the patient's doctor in regard to use of appropriate analgesics (e.g. acetaminophen, non-steroidal anti-inflammatories), the primary purpose of analgesia being to provide a therapeutic window for the patient to regain function.

Additional considerations may also be required when the elbow condition is compromised by contributing factors such as a loss of the normal dynamic control of the shoulder joint (see Chs 28, 29 and 32) or a compromise of wrist stability (see Ch 49). Such contributing factors need to be addressed in the overall management of the patient with elbow disorders if an optimal outcome is to be achieved. Equally, the possibility of intra-articular pathologies, including loose bodies, osteochondritis and other conditions such as osteoarthritis, valgus instability with ulnar nerve trauma in patients involved in throwing sports, or a covert posterolateral pathology following a fall onto an outstretched hand, should all be given due consideration prior to any decision that manual techniques are indicated in management (see Ch 40).

For all patients, reassessment of the outcome of any intervention, including joint mobilization, should include a subjective inquiry into the treatment effects (positive and negative), re-examination of key initial physical findings (e.g. loss of joint range and associated pain provocation, mechanical hyperalgesia) and functional limitations. Where possible, the parallel use of relevant outcome measures to assess the response to treatment is consistent with current best clinical practice. Examples of outcome measures that could be used for elbow disorders include the Patient-Specific Functional Scale (PSFS) and the Disability of Arm, Shoulder and Hand (DASH) tool.

Definitions and Clinical Applications

Joint mobilization is usually defined as low-velocity, high-amplitude passive motion inducing intracapsular movement at different amplitudes (Hengeveld et al 2005; Takei 2005), whereas joint manipulation is defined as a high-velocity, low-amplitude thrust motion. Maitland (1986) had described different grades of mobilization according to the amplitude of the motion and resistance offered by the surrounding tissues (Hengeveld et al 2005). In Maitland's (1986) classification, there were four different standard oscillatory grades of movement relating to amplitude, in which grades I and IV referred to small-amplitude oscillations, while II and III indicated large-amplitude oscillations. Conventionally, mobilizations of grades I–II are usually used in patients where the pain is the dominant symptom and a patient's disorder is considered irritable in nature. In contrast, grades III–IV are usually used in patients where the main symptom response relates to limitation of elbow joint range and this restriction is associated with some pain provocation. Grade V refers to high-velocity manipulation.

In order to regain range, joint mobilization is provided at the limit of the range, and the therapist expects a pain response; this should settle immediately after or within seconds of the mobilization being completed. In current clinical practice, the use of a grade I mobilization is rare. More commonly, acute nociceptive elbow pain is managed using a combination of simple analgesia if required and appropriate early active movement to regain function and minimize prolonged sensitization. If passive movement is indicated in such a presentation, then large-amplitude mobilization performed short of pain provocation (grade II or III^{-}) offers the patient the advantage of increasing range and reducing pain. Patients are encouraged to continue with appropriate analgesia and maintain gains in range with active movements. Where patients present with persistent elbow pain (e.g. tendinopathy or osteoarthritis), management will require a combined approach, with joint mobilization offering only limited benefit when used as a unimodal intervention. Treatment 'dose' (how long and how many) is decided based on the clinical presentation; 30–60 seconds followed by reassessment are typical for more acute disorders (2–3 repetitions), and 60–180 seconds (4–5 repetitions) for more chronic hypomobility disorders.

When choosing to mobilize the elbow joint, a skilled therapist typically uses a clinically reasoned process rather than a doctrinal or didactic approach. For example, the grade of a technique is typically guided by the patient's clinical presentation, with due consideration of irritability (i.e. severity of disorder; nature of associated pathology or systemic disease if appropriate; the acute, subacute or chronic stage of the disorder; how easy it is to trigger symptoms; how long these symptoms then take to resolve or reduce to baseline; and any precautions or contraindications to manual interventions such as posterolateral joint instability or significant neuropathic pain).

Typically, symptoms that are localized, mechanically patterned (nociceptive) and with clearly identifiable aggravating factors and easing factors appear to be the most amenable to mobilization techniques. In such presentations, the choice of the technique is made by considering which articulation of the elbow joint is problematic (radiohumeral, radioulnar or humeroulnar) and at what point in the joint range the symptoms occur. Most commonly, mobilization will be used at the point in range where loss of mobility occurs. Where an elbow disorder is more acute and hypomobility is evident through a large part of the joint range, physiological mobilization may be useful when performed throughout larger amplitudes of joint range. A good clinical example is the uncomplicated post-fracture (out-of-cast) elbow, where large-amplitude physiological joint mobilization helps to encourage joint mobility without compromising the fracture or exacerbating pain. Conversely, where joint mobility is lost at terminal extension or flexion, or into abduction or adduction at terminal elbow extension, passive accessory joint mobilization performed at the point in the range of restriction is most likely to be beneficial in restoring function. In summary, the use of clinical reasoning and current neurobiology of musculoskeletal pain to problem-solve and assist in decision making should be central to clinical practice. For a comprehensive review of clinical reasoning in physiotherapy practice see Jones et al (2004).

In the next part of the chapter, we will describe some of the more commonly performed elbow mobilization / manipulation interventions. For each technique, the optimal positions for patient relaxation and for the therapist are described; however, as with all manual techniques, appropriate positional modifications are to be considered and applied as required. For convenience, all technique descriptions relate to the right elbow. The combination of mobilization techniques with active movement (an approach described by Mulligan in 1989 as 'mobilization with movement' (MWM)) may also offer alternatives to or progressions of the basic techniques described here.

The techniques outlined are not exhaustive. As with any technique, modifications and variations are worthy of consideration if a logical and scientific rationale can be provided. Additionally, given the bony configuration of the elbow joint, most clinical presentations where joint mobilization is indicated as part of management involve pain provocation associated with hypomobility towards the end of joint ranges. These restrictions typically occur at terminal extension associated with a restriction of abduction and adduction, terminal extension with limitation of end-range supination or pronation, and flexion limitation with restriction of pronation and supination. Often these patterns of restriction are associated with soft tissue limitations or heightened deep tissue sensitivity or trigger points (see Ch 59). For example, in patients with lateral epicondylalgia, terminal extension and adduction / abduction can be provocative for pain; however, supination performed in extension is also frequently limited.

Careful examination may reveal a loss of tissue extensibility of the flexor and pronator muscle group, and trigger points may exist in these tissues as well as in the extensor muscles. Techniques directed at normalizing this soft tissue limitation or heightened sensitivity should assist in restoring supination in extension (see Chs 59–63). Given the intimate anatomical and functional relationships in the upper limb kinetic chain, the techniques described in this chapter are complemented by the techniques described in Chapters 31, 39 and 52.

Mobilization and Manipulation Techniques

Mobilization in extension combined with adduction (varus mobilization)

The aim of this mobilization technique is to improve the lateral glide of the elbow region, particularly of the radiohumeral joint, where pain or restriction is associated with active extension. Therefore, the clinical presentation would require limitation of terminal elbow extension and adduction; pain provocation in this position is also likely and probably

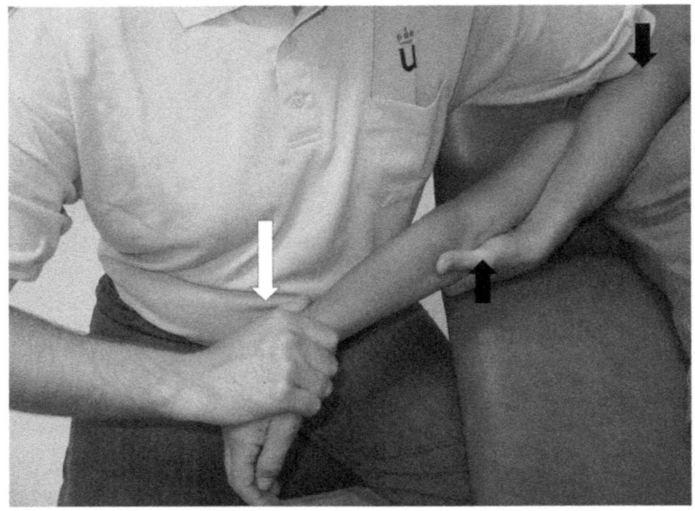

Figure 41.1 Mobilization in extension combined with adduction (varus mobilization). Black arrows show the stabilizations at the shoulder and the elbow of the patient; the white arrow shows the direction of the mobilization force.

most evident at the lateral elbow, although medial joint pain can also be elicited.

For this technique, the patient lies supine with the elbow extended (Fig. 41.1). To maximize stabilization, the therapist's left elbow contacts the anterior part of the patient's shoulder. Medial rotation of the whole arm allows the use of a gravity-assisted medial (varus) mobilization. The therapist's left hand supports the patient's elbow immediately proximal and medial to the elbow joint. The therapist's right hand grasps the patient's wrist, with the therapist's fingers placed over the dorsum of the hand. The technique consists of applying an appropriately graded oscillatory mobilization into adduction (varus). The technique would be performed at the point in the range prior to the onset of pain (acute, grade II or III) or at the limitation of range (chronic, grade III–IV). Symptoms should be monitored and the grade of movement adjusted if required.

Mobilization in adduction and abduction (varus to valgus mobilization)

The aim of this mobilization technique is to improve the lateral glide of the elbow region, specifically the radiohumeral and humeroulnar joints, at the limitation of extension range. Therefore, the clinical patient presentation would require limitation of terminal elbow extension and abduction. Pain provocation in this position is likely and probably most evident at the medial elbow, although lateral joint symptoms may also occur.

For this technique, the patient lies supine with the elbow extended (Fig. 41.2). The therapist with both hands grasps the forearm of the patient in close proximity to the elbow, with stabilization provided medially and laterally at the elbow; the tips of both thumbs are placed against the patient's radial head anteriorly, whereas the remaining fingers spread medially / laterally around the patient's forearm. The technique consists of applying a graded oscillatory lateral mobilization into abduction (valgus) or adduction (varus). The technique

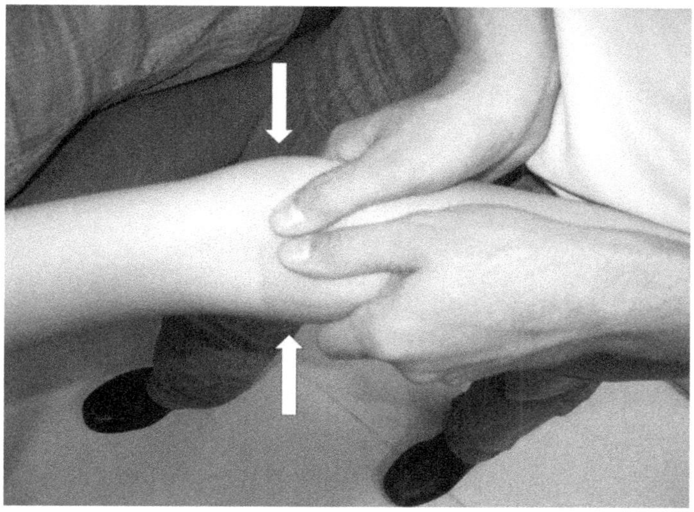

Figure 41.2 Mobilization in adduction and abduction (varus to valgus mobilization). White arrows show the direction of the medial or lateral mobilization force.

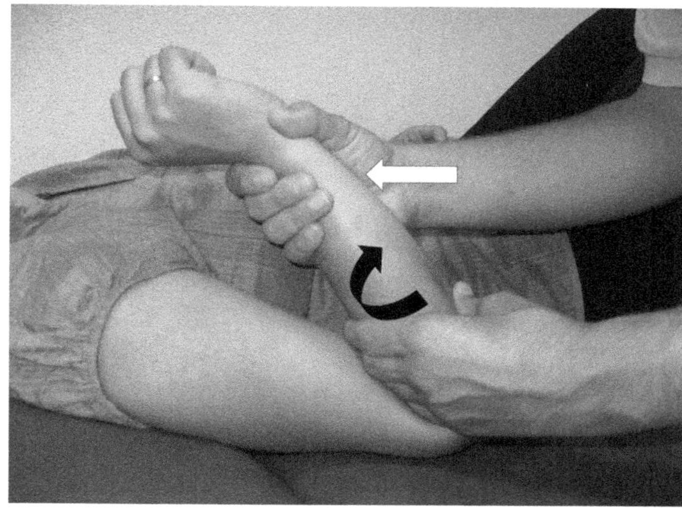

Figure 41.3 Mobilization in pronation combined with flexion. The white arrow shows the direction of the flexion force. A rotational mobilization in pronation of the forearm is applied with the other hand placed over the radiohumeral joint.

would be performed at the point in the range prior to the onset of pain (acute, grade II or III) or at the limitation of range (chronic, grade III–IV). Symptoms should be monitored as the grade of movement adjusted if required.

Mobilization in pronation/supination combined with flexion

The aim of this mobilization technique is to improve the pronation / supination rotational glide / spin of the radiohumeral joint where the limitation occurs in a flexion position. Therefore, the clinical presentation would require limitation of elbow flexion and pronation – which is functionally one of the most important positions to be able to attain. Pain provocation in this position is likely and is probably most evident at the radiohumeral joint laterally or at the anterior joint line (which is common post fracture).

For this technique, the patient lies supine with the right elbow flexed and the forearm pronated. The therapist's left hand is positioned with the dorsum of the fingers lying proximal to the elbow joint and the thumb distal to the elbow and making contact with the radial head. The proximal contact helps control the internal rotation of the patient's humerus that occurs with forearm pronation. The therapist's right hand grasps the patient's right wrist at the dorsum of the distal radioulnar joint. The technique consists of applying an oscillatory mobilization force combining pronation and flexion (Fig. 41.3). This technique may be also performed with the forearm in supination and at the limitation of flexion (Fig. 41.4), although this is less commonly used in clinical practice. Symptoms should be monitored and the grade of movement adjusted if required.

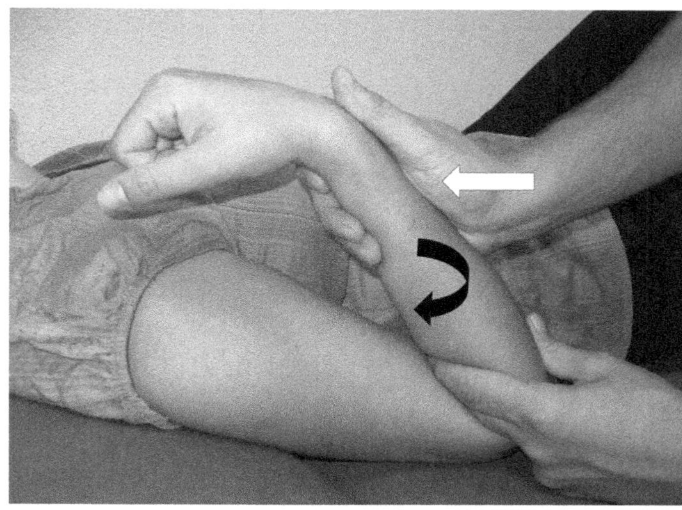

Figure 41.4 Mobilization in supination combined with flexion. The white arrow shows the direction of the flexion force. A rotational mobilization in supination of the forearm is applied with the other hand over the radiohumeral joint.

Mobilization of the radiohumeral joint

The aim of this technique is to improve the anterior glide of the radiohumeral joint (Edmond 2006) where there is associated joint restriction and pain provocation. Radioulnar joint mobilization in the posterior–anterior medial direction can be performed effectively at 60° to 90° of flexion.

For this technique, the patient is supine with the right elbow flexed to the point of restriction (Fig. 41.5). The forearm may be supinated or pronated at the point in the range where there is pain provocation or joint hypomobility. The therapist places the pads of both thumbs against the radial head posteriorly, whereas the remaining fingers spread comfortably proximally and distally around the patient's forearm. The technique consists of applying oscillatory posterior–anterior glides of the radial head using an appropriate grade of movement. Symptoms should be monitored and the grade of movement adjusted if required.

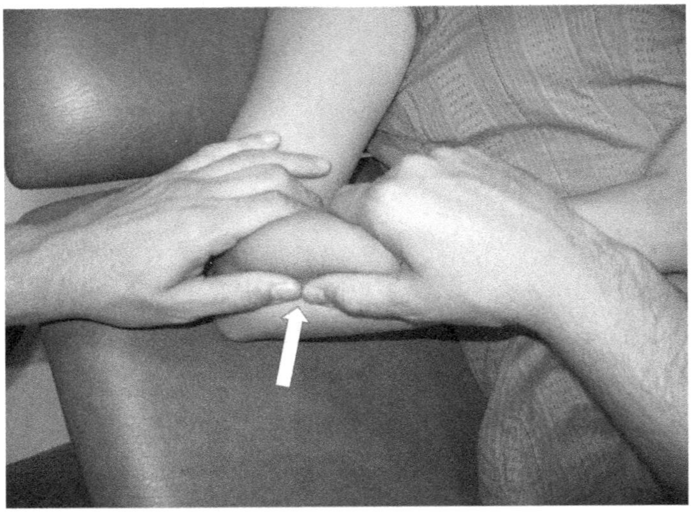

Figure 41.5 Mobilization of the radiohumeral joint. The white arrow shows the posteroanterior glide applied over the radial head laterally.

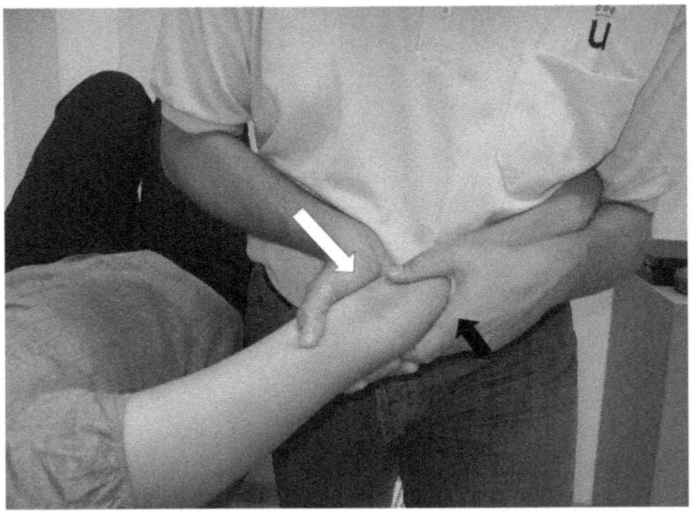

Figure 41.6 Manipulation in lateral glide of the elbow (varus thrust manipulation). The black arrow shows the therapist's lateral stabilizing hand placed distal to the radiohumeral joint. The white arrow shows the varus direction of the high-velocity low-amplitude thrust.

Lateral glide mobilization with movement

Despite the findings of human and animal studies, the specific mechanisms underlying the effects associated with the mobilization / manipulation techniques remain largely putative. The beneficial effects associated with the specific lateral glide MWM are likely to relate to multiple and potentially interacting mechanisms and these are discussed in more detail elsewhere (Slater et al 2006; Vicenzino et al 2007). (For a detailed description of this technique, see Ch 39.)

Manipulation in lateral glide of the elbow (varus thrust manipulation)

The patient is supine or seated with the elbow extended. For patients where no contraindications exist, joint manipulation can be an effective treatment progression. As with any manipulative technique, due care must be taken to exclude any contraindication to high-velocity thrust. Screening questions that contraindicate joint manipulation include evidence of, or suspicion of, intra-articular pathologies, fracture, compromised bone density, prolonged use of corticosteroids or anticoagulant medication, pain-dominant disorders and, in young children, incomplete bone maturity. Once the decision is made to proceed to manipulation, clear succinct information should be provided to the patient with risks and benefits discussed. As a minimum, verbal consent and a record in the patient notes indicating agreement to proceed with manipulation is recommended.

The therapist's left hand is placed just distal to the patient's right radiohumeral joint, extending over the lateral part of the elbow joint (Fig. 41.6). The therapist's right hand grasps the patient's forearm medially at the elbow. Slight external rotation of the patient's whole arm allows a gravity-assisted thrust. The therapist should ensure that the elbow joint is not locked in full extension but approximately 5° short of full extension, as this avoids a painful and unsuccessful thrust, and then examine the position of restriction to establish the direction that is restricted by gently guiding the joint laterally (varus force). It is important that the therapist's right (thrusting) arm is placed perpendicular to the patient's elbow joint. The therapist then informs the patient to soften the arm and relax, and that he / she will now provide a rapid thrust, which may be associated with an audible clicking or popping sound. Reassurance that this popping sound is expected and simply indicates a joint cavitation is helpful advice for patients. The technique then consists of applying a high-velocity low-amplitude thrust (grade V) force directed in a mediolateral direction. Post manipulation, joint range and pain provocation should be reassessed.

Conclusion

There is increasing evidence that, when used appropriately, joint mobilization and manipulation techniques can help to alleviate pain and assist in restoring function in patients with musculoskeletal elbow disorders. Clinicians need to understand the putative neurophysiological and tissue mechanisms underlying elbow joint mobilization (including placebo analgesia) and recognize that these techniques typically form only a small part of a more comprehensive evidence-based management approach.

References

Arendt-Nielsen L, Graven-Nielsen T. 2008. Muscle pain: sensory implications and interaction with motor control. Clin J Pain 24: 291–298.

Assendelft W, Green S, Buchbinder R, et al. 2004. Tennis elbow. Clin Evid 11: 1633–1644.

Bisset L, Paungmali A, Vicenzino B, et al. 2005. A systematic review and meta-analysis of clinical trials on physical interventions for lateral epicondylalgia. Br J Sports Med 39: 411–422.

Bisset L, Beller E, Jull G, et al. 2006. Mobilisation with movement and exercise, corticosteroid injection, or wait and see for tennis elbow: randomised trial. BMJ 333: 939.

Edmond SL. 2006. Joint mobilization / manipulation, 2nd edn. London: Mosby Elsevier, pp 86–87.

Fernández-Carnero J, Fernández de las Peñas C, de la Llave-Rincon AI, et al. 2008. Bilateral myofascial trigger points in the forearm muscles in patients with chronic unilateral lateral epicondylalgia: a blinded, controlled study. Clin J Pain 24: 802–807.

Fernández-Carnero J, Fernández de las Peñas C, de la Llave-Rincon AI, et al. 2009. Widespread mechanical pain hypersensitivity as sign of central sensitization in unilateral epicondylalgia: a blinded, controlled study. Clin J Pain 25: 555–561.

Graven-Nielsen T. 2006. Fundamentals of muscle pain, referred pain, and deep tissue hyperalgesia. Scand J Rheumatol 122: 1–43.

Hengeveld E, Banks K, Wells P. 2005. Maitland's peripheral manipulation, 4th edn. London: Elsevier Health Sciences.

Jones MA, Rivett DA, Twomey L. 2004. Clinical reasoning for manual therapists. London: Elsevier Science Ltd, Butterworth-Heinemann.

Kaufman RL. 2000. Conservative chiropractic care of lateral epicondylitis. J Manipulative Physiol Ther 23: 619–622.

Lawrence DJ, Humphreys CR. 1997. Cubital tunnel syndrome: a case report. Chiropractic Techniques 9: 27–31.

Maitland GD. 1986. Vertebral manipulation, 5th edn. London: Butterworth-Heinemann.

Mulligan B. 1989. Manual therapy 'NAGS', 'SNAGS', 'MWMs', etc. Wellington, NZ: Plane View Services.

Paungmali A, Vicenzino B, Smith M. 2003. Hypoalgesia induced by elbow manipulation in lateral epicondylalgia does not exhibit tolerance. J Pain 4: 448–454.

Slater H, Arendt-Nielsen L, Wright A, et al. 2005. Sensory and motor effects of experimental muscle pain in patients with lateral epicondylalgia and controls with delayed onset muscle soreness. Pain 114: 118–130.

Slater H, Arendt-Nielsen L, Wright A, et al. 2006. Effects of a manual therapy technique in experimental lateral epicondylalgia. Man Ther 11: 107–117.

Smidt N, Assendelft WJ, Arola H, et al. 2003. Effectiveness of physiotherapy for lateral epicondylitis: a systematic review. Ann Med 35: 51–62.

Takei H. 2005. Joint mobilization for bone and joint disease. Phys Ther Sci 20: 219–225.

Vicenzino B, Cleland JA, Bisset L. 2007. Joint manipulation in the management of lateral epicondylalgia: a clinical commentary. J Man Manip Ther 15: 50–56.

PART 7

The Knee Region In Lower Extremity Pain Syndromes

42 Ligamentous and Meniscal Injuries of the Knee 467
Carol A. Courtney and Craig P. Hensley

43 Knee Osteoarthritis 482
Lars Arendt-Nielsen and César Fernández-de-las-Peñas

44 Patellofemoral Pain Syndrome 493
Johnson McEvoy and Caroline MacManus

45 Postoperative Management of the Knee: Ligamentous, Meniscal and Total Joint Replacement 514
Jodi Young and Ellen Pong

46 Joint Mobilization and Manipulation of the Knee 525
Cody Weisbach, William Egan, Paul E. Glynn and Joshua A. Cleland

47 Tendinopathy of the Knee 531
Ellen Pong

Chapter 42

Ligamentous and Meniscal Injuries of the Knee

Carol A. Courtney, Craig P. Hensley

CHAPTER CONTENTS

Introduction	467
Anterior cruciate ligament	467
Anatomy	467
Biomechanics	467
Incidence/prevalence of injury	468
Biomechanical/neuromuscular risk factors	468
Posterior cruciate ligament	470
Anatomy	470
Biomechanics	470
Incidence/prevalence of injury	470
Mechanism of injury/risk factors	470
Lateral collateral ligament	471
Anatomy	471
Biomechanics	471
Incidence/prevalence of injury	471
Mechanism of injury/risk factors	471
Medial collateral ligament	471
Anatomy	471
Biomechanics	471
Incidence/prevalence of injury	471
Mechanism of injury/risk factors	471
Meniscus	471
Anatomy	471
Biomechanics	472
Incidence/prevalence of injury	472
Mechanism of injury/risk factors	472
Management of knee ligament rupture and meniscal tear	473
Conservative versus surgical management	473
Conservative management	474
Surgical management	477
Conclusion	477

Introduction

Articular structures of the knee, including ligaments and menisci, are commonly damaged during knee joint trauma. Considering the frequency of knee trauma in the human body (Louw et al 2008), and that post-traumatic knee osteoarthritis (OA) is often a consequence (Brown et al 2006), it is not surprising that considerable research has addressed the aetiology and management of knee injury. Three joints – the patellofemoral, the tibiofibular and tibiofemoral – encompass the knee, but acute injury usually occurs at the articular structures of the tibiofemoral joint. There are four major ligaments of the tibiofemoral joint: the anterior and posterior cruciate ligaments, and the medial and lateral collateral ligaments. Two fibrocartilaginous menisci are situated between the tibia and femur. These structures, in conjunction with the periarticular musculature, provide stability to the knee, yet allow multiplanar mobility required for static and dynamic responses. As a result, the human body is capable of remarkable bipedal agility and speed, and is also more susceptible to musculoskeletal insult.

Anterior Cruciate Ligament

Anatomy

The anterior cruciate ligament (ACL) consists of two functional units: the anteromedial and posterolateral bundles. It originates on the lateral intercondylar ridge on the medial wall of the lateral femoral condyle (Hensler et al 2012). The bundles travel parallel to each other anteriorly and medially, twisting to insert in a fossa anterolateral to the tibial spine, and blending with the anterior portion of the lateral meniscus (Markatos et al 2013). The ACL receives its nerve and blood supply from the tibial nerve and middle genicular artery from the popliteal artery respectively (Woo et al 2006).

Biomechanics

The ACL is generally considered to be isometric, meaning that it maintains a degree of tautness throughout the physiological knee range of motion (ROM) (Amis & Dawkins 1991). The two bundles work synergistically to control and limit anterior / posterior translation and rotation of the tibia as the knee flexes (Jordan et al 2007). In full knee extension, both bundles are under tension, with the posterolateral bundle under maximal lengthening (Hensler et al 2012). The anteromedial bundle achieves maximal tension between 45° and 90° of knee flexion (Jordan et al 2007; Markatos et al 2013). As the knee extends, the ACL assists in guiding the screw-home mechanism of the knee by internally rotating the femur and preventing internal rotation of the tibia in the closed chain (Pappas et al 2013). This function becomes critical in sporting events that require cutting and pivoting.

The maximum tensile strength of the ACL is approximately 1725±270 N, which is significantly less than the maximum forces occurring during vigorous athletic activities (Markatos et al 2013). However, other passive and dynamic stabilizers contribute to preventing injury. For muscles to assist in stabilization of the knee, effective proprioceptive feedback is required (Markatos et al 2013). Although it has been suggested that the ACL may play a role in proprioceptive feedback, owing to its rich supply of mechanoreceptors and free nerve endings (Markatos et al 2013), it is generally accepted that the muscle spindle is the main mediator of proprioceptive acuity (Gandevia & McCloskey 1976; Sharma 1999). Thus, although loss of proprioceptive acuity has been reported following ACL rupture (Barrack et al 1989; Roberts et al 2007), the mechanisms behind this somatosensory change are not fully understood and are probably more complex than simple peripheral receptor damage (Courtney et al 2013).

Incidence/prevalence of injury

Globally, the annual incidence of ACL injuries is estimated to be 0.01–0.05%, or 10–50 per every 100 000 people (Moses et al 2012), with approximately 70% sustained as non-contact injuries (Boden et al 2000; Hewett et al 2006a). Many potential risk factors for ACL injury have been identified (Box 42.1).

Biomechanical/neuromuscular risk factors

It has been suggested that ACL injury occurs within 10–40 ms of initial contact between the foot and the ground during movements such as cutting, landing, deceleration and pivoting (Krosshaug et al 2007; Koga et al 2010). A great deal of research has been conducted to elucidate the role of biomechanics and the neuromuscular system in risk for ACL injury, particularly that of non-contact origin. Findings lend support to the idea that poor control in all cardinal planes from the trunk to the ankle during dynamic movements is a major risk factor for developing ACL injury.

Trunk

Altered trunk position has a large impact on force attenuation and lower extremity kinematics. The performance of athletic manoeuvres, such as landing or cutting, with decreased trunk flexion is a risk factor for ACL injury, probably due to greater knee extensor effort (Kulas et al 2008) and rectus femoris activity (Zazulak et al 2005), which may increase anterior shear force on the knee and stress on the ACL (Mendiguchia et al 2011). Furthermore, it may lead to decreased hip extensor effort (Kulas et al 2008), gluteus maximus activity (Zazulak et al 2005) and shock absorption at the hip (Decker et al 2003). Females, who are at higher relative risk for ACL injury than males, tend to have higher knee-to-hip moment ratios during vertical drop jumps (Ford et al 2010), and those who exhibit higher knee valgus angles (Fig. 42.1) and moments have lower hip extensor moments and less shock absorption while decelerating from drop jumps (Pollard et al 2010), hence accentuating the risk of ACL injury.

In the coronal plane, trunk displacement has also been implicated with ACL injury. Placing the ground reaction force (GRF) lateral to the knee may increase knee valgus angle and torque (Pollard et al 2007; Dempsey et al 2009), a known risk factor for ACL injury (Fig. 42.2). In a prospective study, Zazulak et al (2007) found that increased lateral trunk displacement after a sudden force release predicted knee ligament injury. When coupling trunk displacement with poor

Box 42.1 Risk factors for anterior cruciate ligament or medial meniscus injury

Anterior cruciate ligament

- Competitive game (versus training)
- Playing surface
  - Dry surface
  - Cold temperature
  - Astroturf or rubber
- Athletes (versus non-athletes)
- Gender
  - Male: higher absolute risk
  - Female: higher injury rate
- Age: 15–25 years
- Elevated body mass
- Increased joint laxity
- Posture
  - Genu recurvatum
  - Navicular drop
  - Subtalar pronation
- Sex hormone variation
  - First half of menstrual cycle
  - During the menstrual cycle
- Fatigue
- Proprioceptive deficits knee
- Proprioceptive deficits lumbar spine
- Previous ACL injury
- Previous low back pain
- Genetics
  - *COL5A1* gene
  - Chromosomal region 11q22
- Range of motion limitations
  - Transverse plane: hip
  - Ankle dorsiflexion

Medial meniscus

- Increased body mass
- Caucasians/African
- Americans in US military
- Occupation
  - Sports requiring cutting and twisting
  - Prolonged kneeling
- Previous knee injury
- Generalized osteoarthritis
- Posture – knee varus

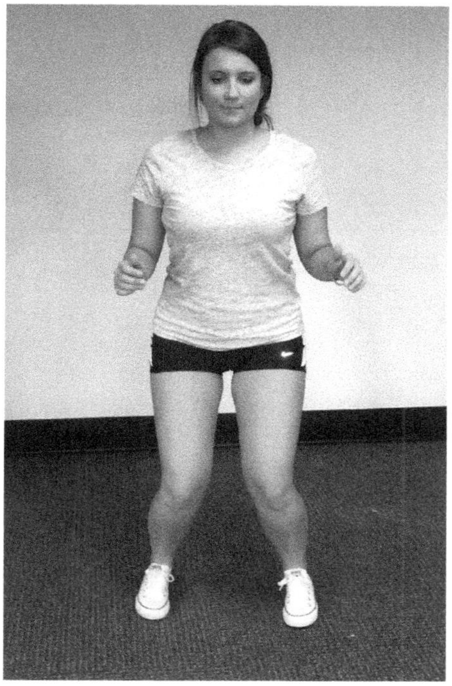

Figure 42.1 **Anterior cruciate ligament injury risk factor: increased knee valgus angle.**

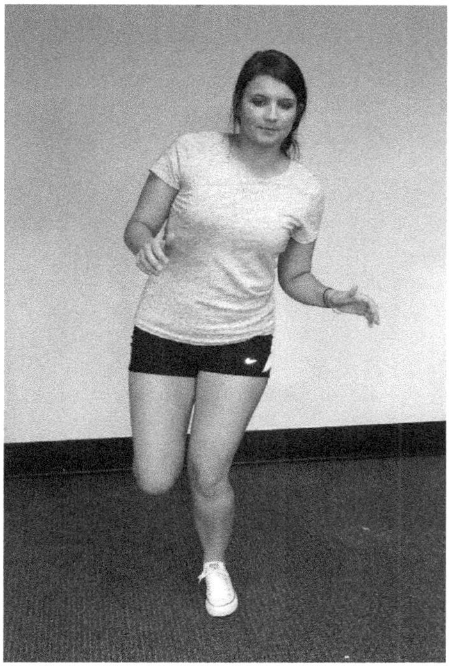

Figure 42.2 **Anterior cruciate ligament injury risk factor: lateral trunk displacement.**

trunk proprioception and history of low back pain, ACL injury was predicted with 91% accuracy in females. During in vivo analysis of ACL injury, Hewett et al (2009) found that females moved their trunks lateral to the ACL-injured limb, which was uncommon among males.

Limited research has been reported on the relationship between transverse plane trunk kinematics and ACL injury.

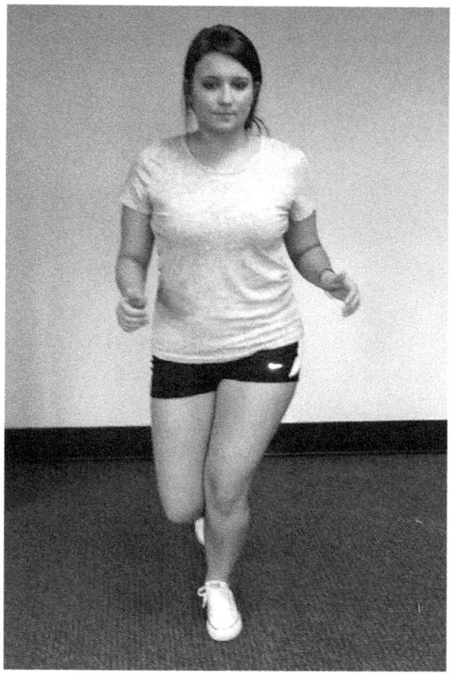

Figure 42.3 **Anterior cruciate ligament injury risk factor: increased hip adduction angle.**

Ireland (1999) described a 'position of no return' in which rotating the trunk to the opposite side potentially increases hip adduction and internal rotation angles, thereby leading to greater knee abduction angles and moments.

Hip

As with sagittal plane trunk posture, studies have demonstrated that females tend to land (Salci et al 2004; Schmitz et al 2007) and cut (Mclean et al 2004; Landry et al 2007) with lower hip flexion angles compared with males, resulting in ACL injury (Boden et al 2009) – although this evidence is controversial (Hewett et al 2006b).

In the coronal plane, peak hip adduction angles (Fig. 42.3) have been found to be greater in females during running (Chappell et al 2007; Chumanov et al 2008), single-leg hop tasks (Hewett et al 2006a) and cutting (McLean et al 2005; Landry et al 2007). The hip adduction angle was reported as the only significant predictor of higher knee abduction angle, a risk factor for ACL injury (Hewett et al 2005), during an unanticipated cutting manoeuvre (Imwalle et al 2009). Conversely, Sigward and Powers (2007) found that females with greater knee valgus moment during side-step cutting had larger hip abduction angles at initial contact; these authors speculated that this strategy moved the centre of pressure laterally to the centre of mass of the tibia, thus increasing the valgus moment.

Hip strength deficits have also been implicated with ACL injury. Weakness in both hip extension (Hollman et al 2013) and external rotation and abduction (Claiborne et al 2006) correlated with knee abduction angle and moment, although other studies have challenged this notion (Sigward & Powers 2006; Sigward et al 2008). In one study, deficits in hip external rotation torque during a landing task were independently predictive of ACL re-rupture (Paterno et al 2010). Lastly, Lawrence et al (2008) reported that the greatest knee anterior shear force in a landing task was demonstrated by the group with the weakest hip external-rotation strength.

Knee

Strain on the ACL has been shown to be highest when transverse and coronal plane loads at the knee are applied at less than 40° of knee flexion (Dürselen et al 1995; Markolf et al 1995). At lower knee flexion angles, the quadriceps exerts a higher anteriorly directed force on the tibia that is poorly counteracted by the ACL and hamstrings (Blackburn & Padua 2008). Therefore, it seems plausible that manoeuvres resulting in low knee flexion angles increase the risk of ACL injury. In a systematic review, Shimokochi and Schultz (2008) found that ACL injuries commonly occurred at or near full knee extension.

Altered quadriceps and hamstring muscle activation patterns may change anterior shear forces and knee extensor moments, hence making the individual more susceptible to ACL injury. Females tended to perform athletic manoeuvres with increased quadriceps activation (Malinzak et al 2001; Zazulak et al 2005; Sigward & Powers 2006; Yu et al 2006; Chappell et al 2007), producing greater anterior shear forces on the tibia and ACL (DeMorat et al 2004). Paterno et al (2010) found a 4.1 times greater asymmetry in knee extensor moment in those with re-ruptured ACLs in dynamic tasks. In a recent review, Hewett et al (2012) noted altered quadriceps and lowered hamstring activation strategies, along with lowered hamstring-to-quadriceps torque ratios in females.

Dynamic valgus torques on the knee may significantly increase anterior tibial translation and load on the ACL (Fukuda et al 2003). Females demonstrated more knee abduction moments and angles compared with males during athletic manoeuvres (Carson & Ford 2011). Hewett et al (2005) prospectively found that female athletes who suffered ACL injury had 2.5 times larger knee abduction moments, 8° more knee abduction angles at landing, and 20% higher GRF compared with uninjured athletes. Other studies have supported these findings (Olsen et al 2004; Paterno et al 2010).

Ankle / foot

In the sagittal plane, the ability of the ankle to absorb shock and prevent anterior tibial translation is critical to maintaining the stability of the ACL. Self and Paine (2001) found that landing with the largest ankle plantarflexion position at initial contact demonstrated the greatest shock absorption and least GRF. In preventing anterior tibial translation, the gastrocnemius and soleus provide a significant posterior force of the tibia during a landing task in healthy males (Mokhtarzadeh et al 2013).

Posterior Cruciate Ligament

Anatomy

The posterior cruciate ligament (PCL) consists of two bundles: an anterolateral and a posteromedial bundle (Mejia et al 2002). The PCL travels in a lateral-to-medial direction (Amis et al 2006; Bowman & Sekiya 2010) along the anterolateral aspect of the medial femoral condyle (Fanelli et al 2010) in the intercondylar notch. The PCL receives its nerve and blood supply from the popliteal plexus, derived from the posterior articular nerve off the tibial nerve and obturator nerve (Kennedy et al 1982) and middle genicular artery respectively.

Biomechanics

In cadaver studies the PCL has been shown to have the greatest tensile strength of the knee ligaments, the major contributor being the anterolateral bundle (Race & Amis 1996). The PCL's primary function is to resist posterior translation of the tibia, with the secondary function of limiting external rotation of the tibia (Butler et al 1980; Gollehon et al 1987; Grood et al 1988) and varus stress (Bowman & Sekiya 2010) in greater degrees of knee flexion. Whereas sectioning the PCL alone resulted in only a small amount of laxity in the coronal and transverse plane (Gollehon et al 1987; Grood et al 1988), cutting other posterolateral structures as well greatly increased the amount of laxity in these planes (Gollehon et al 1987; Grood et al 1988). This may be of clinical importance because posterolateral corner injuries may occur concurrently with PCL injury in up to 60% of injuries (Fanelli & Edson 1995). Posterolateral corner injuries may include the iliotibial band, biceps femoris tendon, quadriceps retinaculum, lateral patellofemoral ligament, lateral collateral ligament (LCL), popliteofibular ligament, popliteus muscle and tendon, arcuate ligament complex, posterolateral capsule and / or lateral capsular ligament (Quarles & Hosey 2004; Pacheco et al 2011).

Restraint of posterior translation by the PCL increases with increasing knee flexion, providing approximately 90–95% of posterior stability between 30° and 90° (Butler et al 1980; Race & Amis 1996; Covey et al 2008). Research has suggested that nearly 75% of posterior stability is accounted for by the anterolateral bundle between 40° and 120° knee flexion, but 57% is provided by the posteromedial bundle beyond 120° of flexion (Butler et al 1980). In PCL-deficient knees under loading with a leg press, the medial tibiofemoral contact point is more anterior than in healthy knees, a finding that hints at the importance of the PCL in sagittal plane biomechanics (Fukagawa et al 2010; Chandrasekaran et al 2012). Studies have also suggested that individuals with PCL injury typically have more medial femoral condyle cartilage degeneration (Strobel et al 2003).

Incidence / prevalence of injury

The reported incidence of PCL damage has ranged from 1% to 40% in acute knee injuries (O'Donoghue 1955; Degenhardt & Hughston 1981; Clancy et al 1983; Parolie & Bergfeld 1986; Fanelli 1993), with the vast majority of such damage occurring during trauma (Fanelli 1993; Fanelli et al 2010) and in combination with other ligamentous injury (48–94%) at the knee (Fanelli & Edson 1995, 2010; Schulz et al 2003).

Mechanism of injury / risk factors

The majority of PCL injuries occur in a hyperflexed knee from a posterior-directed force on the tibia, such as, for example, a dashboard injury during a motor vehicle accident, or a fall onto a flexed knee (Fanelli et al 2010).

Lateral Collateral Ligament

Anatomy

The extracapsular lateral collateral ligament (LCL), or fibular collateral ligament, extends approximately 6.5 cm in knee extension, connecting the posterior and superior aspect of the femoral lateral epicondylar ridge to the fibular head (Meister et al 2000; LaPrade et al 2004a). As the knee moves from extension to flexion, the trajectory of the ligament moves from an 11° posterior to a 19° anterior slope (Meister et al 2000). The biceps femoris bursa encapsulates the distal 25% of the LCL (LaPrade & Hamilton 1997). The average width of the LCL is 36.6 mm (Terry & LaPrade 1996; LaPrade et al 2003).

Biomechanics

With increasing knee flexion the LCL slackens (Meister et al 2000). The LCL serves as the primary limitation to varus opening (Sanchez et al 2006), particularly at 0–30° of knee flexion. LCL loading responses were found to be highest at 30° of knee flexion (Laprade et al 2004b), becoming slightly lax with flexion beyond 30° (LaPrade & Wentorf 2002).

In the transverse plane, the LCL is the primary restraint to external rotation of the tibia from 0° to 30° of knee flexion, with the popliteus muscle serving as the primary restraint beyond 60° (LaPrade et al 2004b). The LCL may also provide resistance to internal rotation of the tibia at 15° and beyond 60° of knee flexion (Meister et al 2000). Hence the LCL seems most susceptible to injury at 30° of knee flexion.

Incidence/prevalence of injury

Isolated injury to the LCL is rare. In patients with knee ligament injuries, only 7–16% had isolated LCL injury (DeLee et al 1983; Grana & Janssen 1987). Krukhaug et al (1998) reported that only 25–30% of lateral knee injuries were sports related, whereas 52% were due to traffic accidents. When the LCL is injured, other structures of the posterolateral corner are often damaged as well.

Mechanism of injury/risk factors

The most common cause of LCL and / or PLC injury in sport is a blow to the anteromedial knee near full extension, most typically in football, soccer or skiing on snow (Quarles & Hosey 2004). External rotation of the tibia while cutting or pivoting with hyperextension of the knee may increase the risk (Quarles & Hosey 2004).

Medial Collateral Ligament

Anatomy

The medial or tibial collateral ligament (MCL) is divided into two structural components: the superficial and the deep MCL. The superficial MCL attaches to the distal femur slightly proximal and posterior to the medial epicondyle (LaPrade & Wijdicks 2012) and has two tibial attachments: the proximal attachment, which blends with the semimembranosus tendon fascia and attaches 1 cm distal to the tibiofemoral joint line, and the distal, which attaches broadly to the posteromedial tibia 6 cm below the joint line (LaPrade & Wijdicks 2012; Schein et al 2012). Most of the distal attachment is within the pes anserine bursa and is the stronger of the two (Schein et al 2012). The deep MCL is a thickening of the joint capsule (LaPrade & Wijdicks 2012) and is attached to the medial meniscus (Laprade & Wijdicks 2012). A bursa lies between the deep and superficial MCL (Schein et al 2012).

Biomechanics

The MCL provides valgus stability to the knee. The proximal division of the superficial MCL has been shown to be the primary valgus stabilizer, whereas the deep MCL serves a secondary role (Griffith et al 2009; Wijdicks et al 2009). The MCL also contributes to transverse stability of the knee. The distal segment of the superficial MCL is critical for external rotation stability, particularly at 30° of knee flexion (LaPrade & Wijdicks 2012). The contribution of the superficial MCL to internal rotation stability is greatest at 45–90° of flexion (Kennedy et al 1976). One role of the deep MCL is to control anterior tibial translation when the knee is flexed and externally rotated (Griffith et al 2009).

Incidence/prevalence of injury

The MCL and associated medial knee stabilizers are the most frequently injured ligaments of the knee (Schein et al 2012). The majority of these tears are isolated injuries (LaPrade & Wijdicks 2012). The MCL is injured in at least 42% of knees with ligamentous injuries and the yearly incidence of medial knee injury in the USA is about 0.24 per 1000 people – roughly amounting to 74 000 injuries per year (Schein et al 2012).

Mechanism of injury/risk factors

The mechanism of MCL injury typically involves valgus knee loading, tibial external rotation or a combination of the two in knee flexion (Quarles & Hosey 2004), which may result from a contact injury such as a clip in American football. One study found that up to 70% of MCL injuries in professional soccer were contact injuries (Lundblad et al 2013). Medial knee injuries are more common in youth than in older age, and twice as likely in males as in females (LaPrade & Wijdicks 2012; Schein et al 2012).

Meniscus

Anatomy

The knee menisci are crescent-shaped fibrocartilaginous tissues located in the medial and lateral compartments of the tibiofemoral joint (Fox et al 2012). The peripheral 10–30% is vascularized and the remaining area receives nutrition via synovial fluid (Stärke et al 2009). The inner borders taper medially to a thin free edge (Fox et al 2012). The menisci are distally flat and proximally concave so as to accept the convex femoral condyles (Englund et al 2012). They are connected at their respective anterior horns via the transverse ligament. The nerve supply travels with the vasculature to the periphery and horns of the menisci (Kennedy et al 1982); hence pain is not typically elicited from mechanical stimulus of the inner region of the menisci (Dye et al 1998).

Medial meniscus

The medial meniscus is semicircular in shape, with the posterior horn broader in width than the anterior horn (Greis et al 2002). The horns demonstrate broader attachment compared with the lateral meniscus (Fox et al 2012). The coronary ligament is the tibial portion of the capsular attachment (Fox et al 2012). The medial meniscus is anchored at its midpoint to the femur via the deep MCL (Fox et al 2012).

Lateral meniscus

The lateral meniscus is nearly circular in shape. It covers a larger area of the tibia (Arnoczky & Warren 1982), and the anterior and posterior horns attach much closer to each other, compared with the medial meniscus (Fox et al 2012). The posterior horn attaches to the medial femoral condyle via anterior (Humphrey) and posterior (Wisberg) meniscofemoral ligaments that originate near the PCL attachment on the femur, although their presence is variable (Kusayama et al 1994) and their function unknown.

Biomechanics

Besides nutrition and lubrication to the joint (Renström & Johnson 1990), the primary functions of the menisci are to transmit load (Ahmed & Burke 1983) and absorb shock (Fithian et al 1990). The menisci transmit approximately 50% of the compressive load in knee extension, and 85% at 90° of flexion, mostly through the posterior horn (Walker & Erkman 1975). For every 30° of knee flexion, the contact surface between the tibiofemoral surfaces decreases by 4% (Walker & Hajek 1972), making compressive loads more focal. Removal of the menisci results in a significant reduction in femoral contact area (Ahmed & Burke 1983), increasing the risk of degenerative changes at the tibiofemoral joint (Englund et al 2012). It has been demonstrated that normal knees have a 20% greater capacity to absorb shock compared with those that undergone meniscectomy (Voloshin & Wosk 1983).

Studies have shown that, whereas the lateral meniscus moves anywhere from 9 mm to 11 mm in anterior–posterior displacement with knee flexion, the medial meniscus moves only about 2–5 mm (Thompson et al 1991). This lack of movement may place the medial meniscus at more risk of injury, particularly in the posteromedial corner, which moves the least (Thompson et al 1991). With the ACL intact, the medial meniscus has little effect on anterior–posterior translation; however, following ACL rupture the posterior horn of the medial meniscus becomes the most important anterior translation resistor (Shoemaker & Markolf 1986). Both menisci are important in knee joint stability (Levy et al 1989).

Incidence/prevalence of injury

In the US, meniscal injuries are the most common intra-articular knee lesions and are the most frequent cause of orthopaedic surgery (Salata et al 2010). The cumulative risk of meniscal injury that necessitates surgery in patients between the ages of 10 and 64 years is as high as 15% (Lohmander et al 2007). The mean annual incidence of meniscal lesions has been reported to be between 61 and 70 per 100 000, 61 of which result in meniscectomy (Baker et al 1985; Hede et al 1990; Nielsen & Yde 1991). Meniscal injury incidence rates in physically active populations have ranged between 0.33 and 0.61 per 1000 (Baker et al 1985; Lauder et al 2000). In one study in the US military, the medial meniscus was twice as likely to be injured relative to the lateral meniscus (Jones et al 2012).

The prevalence of meniscal lesions in patients with clinical and radiographic findings of OA is 68–90% (Bhattacharyya et al 2003; Englund et al 2007). The most frequent location is the posterior horn of the medial meniscus (Bhattacharyya et al 2003).

Mechanism of injury/risk factors

Gender

The ratio of male to female meniscal injury has ranged between 2.5:1 and 4:1 (Baker et al 1985; Steinbrück 1999). In a study in the US military, men were nearly 20% more likely than women to sustain a meniscal injury (Jones et al 2012); however, after adjusting for sports-related injury, males and females were shown to have similar risk. However, there is contradictory evidence suggesting that females are more likely than males to sustain medial meniscus injury, particularly at the posterior horn (Ozkoc et al 2008; Hwang et al 2012).

Age

Some studies have suggested that the injury risk peaks between the ages of 20 and 29 (Baker et al 1985; Steinbrück 1999). In the US military, increasing age was shown to be an independent risk factor, with those over the age of 40 having four times the risk compared with those younger than 20 (Jones et al 2012). Increasing age was also shown to be a risk factor in posterior horn medial meniscus tears (Ozkoc et al 2008; Hwang et al 2012). In professional basketball players, lateral meniscus tears were more common in those younger than 30, whereas in older players the medial meniscus injuries were more prevalent (Yeh et al 2012). In youth, 1 / 3 of meniscus injuries are sports related (Baker et al 1985); the mechanism of injury typically involves cutting or twisting movements with or without knee flexion (Greis et al 2002). Interestingly though, in professional basketball players the most common mechanism of injury is insidious (Yeh et al 2012). An increased incidence of meniscal tearing has been observed in skeletally immature children, as a growing number of individuals within this category are participating in athletics (Makris et al 2011). Motor vehicle accidents also account for a large majority of meniscal tears in the youngest age group (Baker et al 1985).

In middle-aged and elderly patients, meniscus tears are usually degenerative. In those aged 50–90 years, the prevalence of meniscal tears increases with age, ranging from 19% in women aged 50–59 years to over 50% in men aged 70–90 years (Englund et al 2008). It is important to note that many of these tears were asymptomatic. In a recent systematic review, age over 60 years was associated with increased risk for degenerative tears (Snoeker et al 2013). Other risk factors are noted in Box 42.1.

Management of Knee Ligament Rupture and Meniscal Tear

Proper management of knee joint trauma should entail a thorough subjective and objective examination, including a detailed account of the mechanism of injury when joint trauma has occurred. Previous medical history, including prior injuries, will aid in determining prognosis and treatment plan. Subjective screening for aberrant pain processing may help the clinician gain a more holistic understanding of the client's condition. Specifically, psychosocial 'drivers', such as depression, hypervigilance, catastrophization and fear avoidance may facilitate progression to chronic pain (Esteves et al 2013). In certain athletic settings, these contributing factors may be more prevalent because of the pressure or desire to return to sport (Clement et al 2013). Subjective questioning and use of written clinical outcome measures may help to determine functional deficits. Objectively, both physiological and accessory joint ROM should be examined to determine aberrant joint movement, including hypo- and hypermobility. Muscle performance assessment, including strength and motor control, is critical, with a strength at least 90% of that in the unaffected limb used as the typical standard for successful outcome (Thomeé et al 2012). Special tests aid in differential diagnosis, hence it is important to utilize tests that are both specific and sensitive (Table 42.1). Objective functional measures (Brumitt et al 2013) aid in determining prognosis and provide a baseline for developing return-to-sport skills and activities. Recent recommendations suggest restricting the use of diagnostic imaging to cases when fracture is suspected based on the Ottawa Knee rules, or when the physical examination is positive for meniscal or ligamentous damage (Jackson et al 2003). These guidelines have been confirmed by the American College of Radiology Appropriateness Criteria for acute knee injury (Tuite et al 2012).

Another clinical measure – quantitative sensory testing – may help to determine the effect of the joint trauma on nociceptive processing (Arendt-Nielsen & Yarnitzsky 2009; Courtney et al 2010a). The pressure pain threshold can provide an objective measure of musculoskeletal tissue tenderness (hyperalgesia) at the site of injury, such as the medial joint line; it also indicates expansion of nociceptive sensitivity through measurement at sites remote from the injury, such as the tibialis anterior muscle, the contralateral knee, or even sites in the upper extremity (Courtney et al 2010a; Graven-Nielsen & Arendt-Nielsen 2010). The cutaneous mechanical detection threshold and vibration detection threshold may be used to identify loss of sensory function or hypoaesthesia. Although loss of these modalities may occur with frank nerve injury, this sensory loss may also occur as a consequence of altered pain processing (Apkarian et al 1994). Clinically, proprioception is not commonly measured at the knee; however, deficits have been identified in individuals following ACL injury (Barrack et al 1989; Roberts et al 2007) and may contribute to the aberrant motor control that is sometimes demonstrated in this population (Hurley 1997).

Table 42.1 Special tests for ligament and meniscal injury

Test	Sensitivity (%)	Specificity(%)
Anterior cruciate ligament		
Lachman's test[a]	85	94
Pivot-shift[a]	24	98
Anterior drawer[a]	92	91
Posterior cruciate ligament		
Posterior drawer[b]	90	99
Posterior sag[b]	79	100
Quadriceps active[b]	98, 54	97–100
Meniscus		
Apley's[c]	60	70
McMurray's[c]	70	71
Joint line palpation[c]	63	77
Thessalys[d]	90	98
Ege's test[e]	67	81
Collateral ligaments		
Valgus stress test (MCL)[f]	86	Not reported
Varus stress test (LCL)[f]	25	Not reported

[a]Benjaminse et al 2006; [b]Malanga et al 2003; [c]Hegedus et al 2007; [d]Harrison et al 2009; [e]Akseki et al 2004; [f]Harilainen 1987.

Proprioceptive loss can be considered another example of hypoaesthesia, and may also be related to nociceptive sensitization (Courtney et al 2013); however, this has not been investigated.

Conservative versus surgical management

The data on the best therapeutic options following ACL injury are inconclusive. A Cochrane review concluded that there is insufficient evidence from randomized clinical trials to determine whether surgery or conservative management is best following ACL injury (Linko et al 2005). In a retrospective study, Streich et al (2011) found no differences in self-reported measures and the incidence of knee OA when comparing individuals undergoing ACL reconstruction with those receiving conservative physical therapy at 15-year follow-up. Similarly, Meuffels et al (2009) reported no statistical differences between conservative and operative treatment in those with ACL injury with respect to knee OA, meniscal lesions of the knee, activity level, or objective and subjective functional outcomes after 10 years; however, better mechanical stability was observed in the surgical group. It is important to remember that these studies utilized multimodal rehabilitation programmes including manual therapy and exercise programmes. Regarding the PCL, a Cochrane review found no randomized controlled clinical trials that compared operative and conservative interventions for PCL injury (Peccin et al 2012).

Meniscal injury has been implicated as a major contributor to early onset post-traumatic knee OA (Roos 2005). Some studies have suggested that early onset OA following ACL injury may be a consequence of the concomitant meniscal injury rather than ligamentous injury (Louboutin et al 2009). Nevertheless, a systematic review concluded that those individuals with an isolated ACL tear or an ACL tear with an associated meniscal injury reported good short- and long-term knee function with conservative treatment (Myklebust & Bahr 2005). Herrlin et al (2007) found that arthroscopic partial medial meniscectomy followed by supervised exercise was not superior to supervised exercise alone in terms of improvements in knee pain, knee function and quality of life in patients with non-traumatic medial meniscal tears. Similarly, a recent small randomized clinical trial also observed no differences between a conservative physical therapy programme (e.g. high-repetition, high-dosage exercises) and arthroscopic surgery in individuals with degenerative meniscus pathology (Østerås et al 2012).

Therefore, although patients may wish to return to their prior level of sport and request that everything possible be done to prolong their athletic careers, they should be informed that the risk of further knee lesions and knee OA remains high, whatever the treatment they receive, surgical or conservative (Delincé & Ghafil 2012).

Although conservative rehabilitation programmes and surgical procedures seem to be equally effective, up to one-third of the individuals receiving conservative treatment of ACL injury require late ligament reconstruction, approximately 20% return to their pre-injury level of activity without any restriction, and 35–68% require subsequent meniscal surgery (Ireland 2002). Therefore, despite all the data available for the management of knee joint injury, and particularly ACL injuries, a procedure for identifying which individuals may be better candidates for either conservative or surgical intervention is yet to be established. Nevertheless, some attempts have been made at categorizing those individuals with ACL injuries who will benefit from either intervention. For instance, '**copers**' are those individuals who are able to return to pre-injury activities, including sports, without episodes of the knee giving way and who do not require surgical management, whereas '**non-copers**' are those who either did not return to their previous activity level or experienced giving-way episodes on resumption of pre-injury activities (Kaplan 2011). Fithian et al (2005) suggested that copers are able to return to sports successfully for at least 6 months without ACL surgical intervention. However, this distinction seems to be arbitrary, since it is possible that a significant proportion of individuals who are initially considered as potential non-copers may, with proper rehabilitation programmes, be able to regain dynamic knee stability similar to that of potential copers (Muaidi et al 2007). Several studies have developed algorithms to identify those with the potential to return to pre-injury activity level (Kostogiannis et al 2007; Muaidi et al 2007; Hurd et al 2008); however, Eitzen et al (2010) suggested that conducting a screening examination after a series of rehabilitation sessions gave the best overall indications of functional outcomes following ACL injury.

Conservative management

The goals of conservative management following ligamentous or meniscal injury are to protect the joint from further structural damage, to delay knee osteoarthritic changes and to re-establish full ROM, muscle strength and neuromuscular control so as to return to pre-injury levels of function (Micheo et al 2010). Joint trauma is a known risk factor for knee OA (Felson 2004; Roos 2005), which may lead to a decrease in function and diminished quality of life. Surgery may be considered as a secondary insult to the joint, and thus it can promote knee OA disease progression. ACL reconstruction may aid in restoring mechanical stability to the joint and prevent meniscal damage that may occur due to excessive accessory joint motion in an ACL-deficient knee, although this premise has been questioned (Kaplan 2011). Therefore, a conservative approach is utilized when overall rehabilitative goals can be properly met and long-term prognosis is best enhanced.

Of all knee structures, the ACL has been researched by far the most extensively, including the efficacy of conservative rehabilitation. Strehl and Eggli (2007) found that all patients given successful conservative treatment were able to perform low-risk pivoting sports and that, in 1 / 3 of the individuals, conservative treatment led to good or very good clinical results. The goals of conservative treatment are achieved through a progressive rehabilitation programmes divided into acute, recovery and functional phases that could be perfectly applied either to treatment of individuals who do not undergo an operation or to those treated with surgical reconstruction. Other authors have suggested a six-stage rehabilitation programme through which an individual should progress following ACL reconstruction (Herrington et al 2013), and these stages can be also applied to conservative management of other joint injuries. Depending on whether or not the patient has received surgical treatment, the stages may include: preoperative, postoperative, progressive limb loading, unilateral load acceptance, sport-specific task training and unrestricted sport-specific training. Progression through a protocol should be guided by the patient's response to treatment, and treatment techniques should not elicit a flare-up of pain and inflammation. In this section we will focus on conservative treatment, and readers are referred to Chapter 45 for postoperative management of knee injuries.

Acute phase after ligamentous and meniscal injury

The overall goal throughout the rehabilitation process is to make steady progress in function while limiting concomitant pain and swelling, and to prevent re-injury. Whereas accelerated rehabilitation protocols have previously been deemed successful, recent research considering long-term outcomes has suggested that such protocols may, in part, promote osteoarthritic degeneration (Elsaid et al 2012). In the acute phase of rehabilitation, the goals therefore include the reduction of pain and swelling, regaining of the physiological ROM, in particular achievement of full knee extension and proper mobility of the patella, and early pain-free weight-bearing. In particular, regaining full knee extension is an important milestone in rehabilitation and is essential for normal gait. Hyperexcitability of central nociceptive processing has been demonstrated following ACL rupture (Courtney et al 2011), indicating that inflammation and pain should be carefully monitored to avoid facilitation of aberrant pain mechanisms. Although less researched in acute knee injury, manual therapy techniques applied at the joint may increase knee joint mobility, decrease pain and facilitate nociceptive processing (Deyle et al 2005; Courtney et al 2010b). Individuals should start with isometric and isotonic contraction of the quadriceps and hamstring muscles without resistance to prevent atrophy.

Recovery phase of ligamentous and meniscal injury

As pain and inflammation diminish, muscular strength, coordination and normalization of function can be addressed. Gait retraining, muscle activation and regaining of full pain-free physiological knee motion should be emphasized in this stage of the rehabilitation process. Also in this recovery phase, the goals are to achieve adequate motor control and strength in the lower extremity, improve proprioception and balance, and begin the integration of functional activities. Precautions at this stage of the rehabilitative process will depend upon the injured tissue, and may include avoidance of rotational stresses with meniscal injury or valgus stresses with MCL injury.

Quadriceps muscle strengthening is an important milestone in this stage and can be achieved through a combination of open kinetic chain exercises and closed kinetic chain exercises. Clinical guidelines on ACL injury from the Dutch Orthopaedic Association found moderate (level 2) evidence that open chain strength training had a positive effect on muscle strength of quadriceps and hamstring musculature and on knee functional recovery (Meuffels et al 2012). Knee extension in sitting is one of the most common open kinetic chain exercises used for strengthening the quadriceps muscle (Holm et al 1995). However, this exercise should be performed in a manner that avoids knee joint pain and inflammation. There is debate about which exercise prescription with respect to the number of repetitions and sets; it has been postulated that a high number of repetitions (25–30) of each set are more beneficial than sets containing a lower number of repetitions (12–15) (Østerås et al 2012). In clinical practice, a normal prescription includes three sets of 10–12 repetitions for each exercise, although this depends on the physical demands on the patient.

Closed kinetic chain exercises may be more beneficial than open kinetic chain exercises because they are thought to be more functional, provide knee compression forces and promote quadriceps / hamstrings co-contraction, thus reducing anterior tibial translation with activity. However, closed kinetic chain exercises should be used in a manner that minimizes stress on vulnerable tissues (Fig. 42.4). For example, greater angles of knee flexion can place increased stress on the menisci. Therefore, conservative rehabilitation programmes should incorporate both open kinetic chain and closed kinetic chain strength training as soon as the stability of the knee and pain permits this.

Most closed kinetic chain exercises are conducted in weight-bearing positions since weight-bearing is encouraged in rehabilitation programmes after knee injuries (Kvist 2004). The clinician must advance the patient through progressive lower limb loading from bilateral (Fig. 42.5) to unilateral (Fig. 42.6) load acceptance. During these exercises, careful monitoring of the patient's overall activity level is essential, as well as analysis of exercise performance and functional skills, so as to avoid the development of aberrant movement patterns. Subtle differences in weight-bearing may persist though unrecognized by the clinician. In fact, in ACL-deficient subjects (18±19 months since injury), significantly diminished weight-bearing was noted on the injured limb in normal stance as well as hyperexcitable nociceptive responses, even though all the individuals denied resting pain. It was hypothesized that this pain sensitivity may in part underlie asymmetries noted in functional activities post knee injury (Courtney et al 2011). (See Ch 38 for further information on exercises of the lower extremity.)

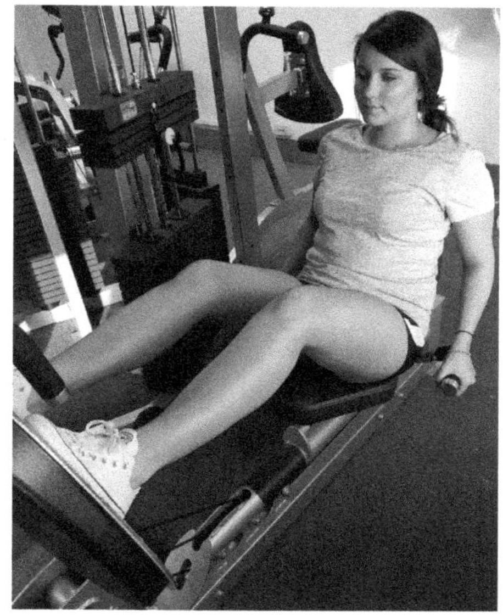

Figure 42.4 Leg press exercise for strengthening the quadriceps muscle.

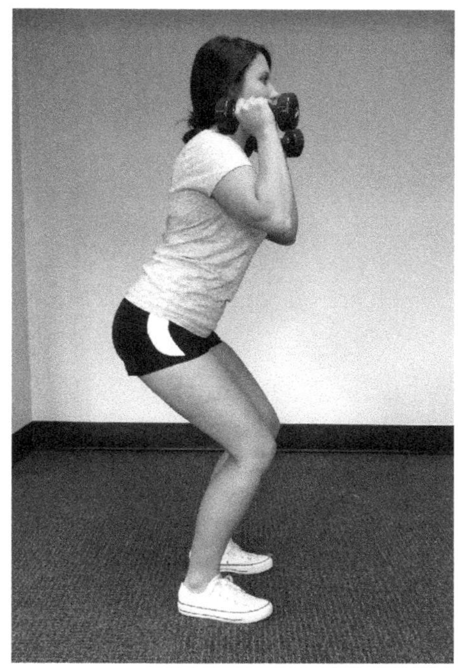

Figure 42.5 Bilateral squat exercise with less than 60° of knee flexion.

Finally, in addition to weight-bearing strengthening exercises, neuromuscular training programmes (i.e. proprioception programmes) have been shown to be superior to strength-training programmes alone for patients with ACL injuries (Risberg et al 2007). These exercises are used to decrease imbalances in quadriceps and hamstrings muscles'

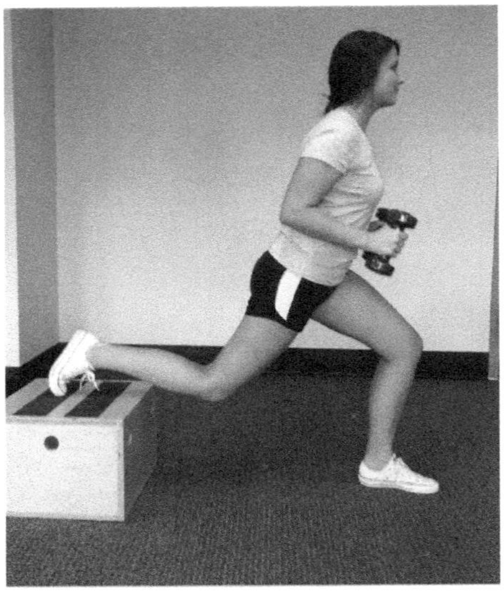

Figure 42.6 **Split squat exercise with less than 60° of knee flexion.**

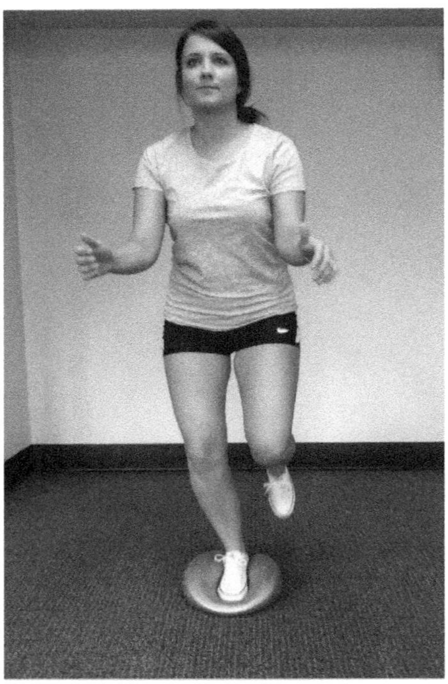

Figure 42.7 **Proprioceptive training on unstable surface in single-leg stance.**

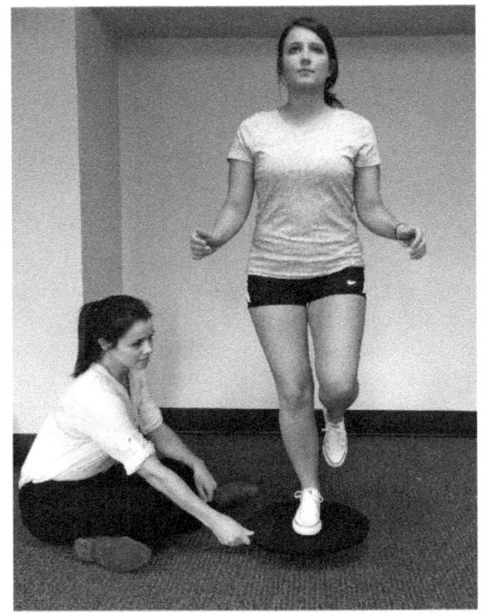

Figure 42.8 **Perturbation training induced by the therapist on unstable surface in single-leg stance.**

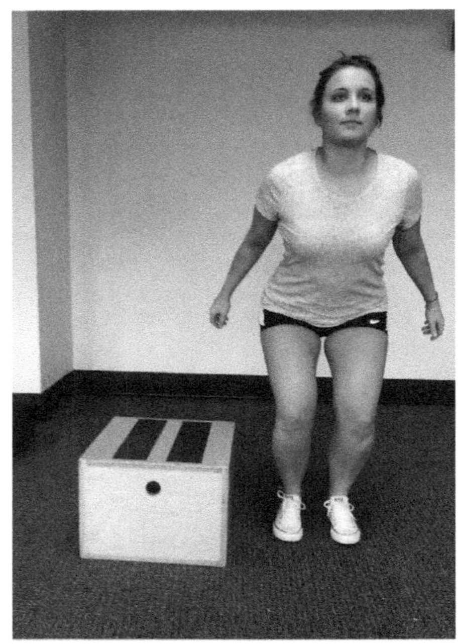

Figure 42.9 **Plyometric exercise: lateral box jumping.**

strength and to promote their coactivation for knee stabilization (Wilk et al 2003). Further, proprioceptive and neuromuscular interventions can be effective for the prevention of recurrent knee injuries (Zech et al 2009). Some exercises include weight shifts on stable and unstable surfaces (Fig. 42.7), perturbation training (Fig. 42.8), plyometric exercises (Fig. 42.9) and landing strategies (Wilk et al 2003). In fact, clinical guidelines on ACL injury from the Dutch Orthopaedic Association found level 1 evidence that balance and proprioception training has a positive effect on joint position sense, muscle strength, knee function, functional outcomes and return to full activity in individuals with ACL injury (Meuffels et al 2012).

During the recovery phase other functional exercises, such as cycling on a stationary bike or stair walking, should be progressively included. At the end of the recovery phase more functional weight-bearing exercises, such as jogging, jumping and landing, can also be initiated as tolerated.

Exercise programmes can be conducted in a clinical setting under the supervision of the physical therapist (clinic-based, supervised) or at home (home-based, self-monitored). Although there are no evidence-based arguments to recommend either one of these supervision regimens (Risberg et al 2007), the clinical guideline on ACL injury of the Dutch Orthopaedic Association supports supervised training as being more effective than non-supervised training (Meuffels et al 2012). In addition, supervised training programmes can lead to a lower risk of damage or excessive tension of the affected and surrounding structures.

Functional phase of ligamentous and meniscal injury

The goals of the functional phase include maximal strengthening, developing power and returning to sports. Clinical decision making on the return to normal sport-specific skills must include understanding of the physiological mechanisms behind healing of damaged and / or repaired tissues and the potential joint stresses involved in the activity. Safety in progression to more challenging weight-bearing tasks and sport-specific activities is essential. Motor-learning principles are carefully utilized in this phase of rehabilitation. Video analysis, for example, may aid in providing visual terminal feedback to the patient. Throughout the rehabilitation process, education on proper neuromuscular movement strategies that serve to prevent potential re-injury is necessary. A return to proper aerobic fitness should be emphasized throughout all phases (Della Villa et al 2012). Recent studies have recognized that the final stage of rehabilitation programmes is often limited or not included in the plan of care (Della Villa et al 2012; Herrington et al 2013). Notably, these studies emphasize the importance of sport-specific performance criteria since proper functional rehabilitation programmes may help prevent re-injuries in the future.

Surgical management

Anterior and posterior cruciate ligament

Unlike other ligaments of the knee, primary repair of the ACL, either surgical or non-surgical, has not been considered as a viable treatment option in recent years (Feagin & Curl 1976). Rather, the standard surgical management following ACL rupture has been the ACL reconstruction, which is performed on approximately 200 000 knees per year in the US (Brophy et al 2009). In this surgery, a 'new' ligament is harvested from the patient's middle third of their patellar tendon, hamstring tendon, cadaver graft, or another structure; however, the reported superior outcomes with any one of these surgical options is controversial (Foster et al 2010). The premise behind this surgical intervention is to promote return to function, prevent injury to other knee joint structures, in particular the menisci, and to impede the onset of post-traumatic OA (Fu & Lin 2013). However, recent estimates have suggested that 62% of individuals undergoing ACL reconstruction will nevertheless demonstrate osteoarthritic changes within 10–15 years following surgery (Oiestad et al 2010). A recent systematic review reported that, whereas ACL reconstruction offered greater objective tibiofemoral stability, there was only limited evidence demonstrating an increased benefit of either reconstruction or non-surgical management in terms of functional outcomes (Smith et al 2014).

Posterior cruciate ligament injuries are typically treated non-operatively when less severe, such as isolated grade I or II injury, with most patients returning to sport (Petrigliano & McAllister 2006). Surgical reconstruction of the PCL has been recommended in acute injuries with severe posterior tibia subluxation and instability (Margheritini et al 2002; Iwamoto et al 2004). The posterolateral corner injury can be easily missed on clinical exam, and surgical management has been the recommended course of treatment (Pacheco et al 2011). Peroneal nerve trauma may occur concomitantly with these injuries, so thorough neurological exam may be critical in these individuals. (See Ch 45 for post-surgery rehabilitation of ACL and PCL.)

Medial and lateral collateral ligament

Isolated MCL injuries are generally treated conservatively, and most have a successful outcome (LaPrade & Wijdicks 2012). Grade III injuries, defined as a complete tear of the ligament, are more likely than other grades to be associated with damage to other knee structures. For example, a general protocol for management of combined grade III MCL and ACL injury is to rehabilitate the medial knee injury first, allowing it to heal according to the guidelines for isolated medial knee injuries, and then to reconstruct the ACL 5–7 weeks after injury once there is good clinical and / or objective evidence of healing of the medial knee injury (Wijdicks et al 2010).

Typical management following LCL injury is directed toward conservative rather than surgical care. However, following high-impact injury, isolated LCL rupture is rare, indicating that surgical decision-making algorithms may change (Levy et al 2011). Bushnell et al (2010) studied LCL injuries in professional football players and found that non-operative management of isolated grade III injuries resulted in more rapid return to play and an equal likelihood of return to play at the professional level compared with operative management. (See Ch 45 for post-surgery rehabilitation.)

Meniscal injury

Meniscal surgery has a long history, with total meniscectomy serving as the treatment of choice until the latter part of the 20th century, until it was discovered that complete removal of the meniscus accelerated the rate of osteoarthritic degeneration (Englund et al 2012). Since then both partial meniscectomy, preserving as much tissue possible, and meniscal repair have been utilized in surgical management (Englund et al 2012). Repair of the meniscus has been advocated when the individual is in the second to fourth decade of life and can comply with postoperative precautions for the prescribed time frame, when the tear is symptomatic and greater than 10–12 mm in length, and when the tear is located in the peripheral aspect of the meniscus and is reducible (Noyes & Barber-Westin 2010). A systematic review has demonstrated better long-term outcomes with meniscal repair than with meniscectomy (Xu & Zhao 2013). (See Ch 45 for post-surgery rehabilitation of meniscal injuries.)

Conclusion

Knee joint trauma is common particularly in the young sporting population, and has been the topic of considerable research. Recent studies have suggested that specific exercise programmes may aid in preventing these injuries. In those individuals who have sustained joint injury, the goals of surgical and non-surgical management are to restore joint stability for the prevention of damage of other joint structures, to regain function and to prevent early onset of osteoarthritic degeneration at the joint. Recent evidence has placed a renewed focus on the importance of monitoring and limiting joint effusion, pain and inflammation during the rehabilitation process to prevent facilitation of aberrant pain mechanisms.

References

Ahmed AM, Burke DL. 1983. In-vitro measurement of static pressure distribution in synovial joints: Part I: Tibial surface of the knee. J Biomech Eng 105: 216–225.
Akseki D, Ozcan O, Boya H, et al. 2004. A new weight-bearing meniscal test and a comparison with McMurray's test and joint line tenderness. Arthroscopy 20: 951–958.
Amis AA, Dawkins G. 1991. Functional anatomy of the anterior cruciate ligament. J. Bone Joint Surg 73B: 260–267.
Amis AA, Gupte CM, Bull AM, et al. 2006. Anatomy of the posterior cruciate ligament and the meniscofemoral ligaments. Knee Surg Sports Traumatol Arthrosc 14: 257–263.
Apkarian AV, Stea RA, Bolanowski SJ. 1994. Heat-induced pain diminishes vibrotactile perception: a touch gate. Somatosens Mot Res 11: 259–267.
Arendt-Nielsen L, Yarnitsky D. 2009. Experimental and clinical applications of quantitative sensory testing applied to skin, muscles and viscera. J Pain 10: 556–572.
Arnoczky SP, Warren RF. 1982. Microvasculature of the human meniscus. Am J Sports Med 10: 90–95.
Baker BE, Peckham AC, Pupparo F, et al. 1985. Review of meniscal injury and associated sports. Am J Sports Med 13: 1–4.
Barrack RL, Skinner HB, Buckley SL. 1989. Proprioception in the anterior cruciate deficient knee. Am J Sports Med 17: 1–6.
Benjaminse A, Gokeler A, van der Schans CP. 2006. Clinical diagnosis of an anterior cruciate ligament rupture: a meta-analysis. J Orthop Sports Phys Ther 36: 267–288.
Bhattacharyya T, Gale D, Dewire P, et al. 2003. The clinical importance of meniscal tears demonstrated by magnetic resonance imaging in osteoarthritis of the knee. J Bone Surg Am 85A: 4–9.
Blackburn JT, Padua DA. 2008. Influence of trunk flexion on hip and knee joint kinematics during a controlled drop landing. Clin Biomech 23: 313–319.
Boden BP, Dean GS, Feagin JA Jr, et al. 2000. Mechanisms of anterior cruciate ligament injury. Orthopedics 23: 573–578.
Boden BP, Torg JS, Knowles SB, et al. 2009. Video analysis of anterior cruciate ligament injury: abnormalities in hip and ankle kinematics. Am J Sports Med 37: 252–259.
Bowman KF Jr, Sekiya JK. 2010. Anatomy and biomechanics of the posterior cruciate ligament, medial and lateral sides of the knee. Sports Med Arthrosc 18: 222–229.
Brophy RH, Wright RW, Matava MJ. 2009. Cost analysis of converting from single-bundle to double-bundle anterior cruciate ligament reconstruction. Am J Sports Med 37: 683–687.
Brown TD, Johnston RC, Saltzman CL, et al. 2006. Posttraumatic osteoarthritis: a first estimate of incidence, prevalence, and burden of disease. J Orthop Trauma 20: 739–744.
Brumitt J, Heiderscheit BC, Manske RC, et al. 2013. Lower extremity functional tests and risk of injury in division III collegiate athletes. Int J Sports Phys Ther 8: 216–227.
Bushnell BD, Bitting SS, Crain JM, et al. 2010. Treatment of magnetic resonance imaging-documented isolated grade III lateral collateral ligament injuries in National Football League athletes. Am J Sports Med 38: 86–91.
Butler DL, Noyes FR, Grood ES. 1980. Ligamentous restraints to anterior–posterior drawer in the human knee. A biomechanical study. J Bone Joint Surg Am 62: 259–270.
Carson DW, Ford KR. 2011. Sex differences in knee abduction during landing: a systematic review. Sports Health 3: 373–382.
Chandrasekaran S, Ma D, Scarvell JM, et al. 2012. A review of the anatomical, biomechanical and kinematic findings of posterior cruciate ligament injury with respect to non-operative management. Knee 19: 738–745.
Chappell JD, Creighton RA, Giuliani C, et al. 2007. Kinematics and electromyography of landing preparation in vertical stop-jump: risks for noncontact anterior cruciate ligament injury. Am J Sports Med 35: 235–241.
Chumanov ES, Wall-Scheffler C, Heiderscheit BC. 2008. Gender differences in walking and running on level and inclined surfaces. Clin Biomech 23: 1260–1268.
Claiborne TL, Armstrong CW, Gandhi V, et al. 2006. Relationship between hip and knee strength and knee valgus during a single leg squat. J Appl Biomech 22: 41–50.
Clancy WG Jr, Shelbourne KD, Zoellner GB, et al. 1983. Treatment of knee joint instability secondary to rupture of the posterior cruciate ligament: report of a new procedure. J Bone Joint Surg Am 65: 310–322.
Clement D, Granquist MD, Arvinen-Barrow MM. 2013. Psychosocial aspects of athletic injuries as perceived by athletic trainers. J Athl Train 48: 512–521.
Courtney CA, Kavchak AE, Lowry CD, et al. 2010a. Interpreting joint pain: quantitative sensory testing in musculoskeletal management. J Orthop Sports Phys Ther 40: 818–825.
Courtney CA, Witte PO, Chmell SJ, et al. 2010b. Heightened flexor withdrawal response in individuals with knee osteoarthritis is modulated by joint compression and joint mobilization. J Pain 11: 179–185.
Courtney CA, Durr RK, Emerson-Kavchak AJ, et al. 2011. Heightened flexor withdrawal responses following ACL rupture are enhanced by passive tibial translation. Clin Neurophysiol 122: 1005–1010.
Courtney CA, Rine R, Jenk DT, et al. 2013. Enhanced proprioceptive acuity at the knee in the competitive athlete. J Orthop Sports Phys Ther 43: 422–426.
Covey DC, Sapega AA, Riffenburgh RH. 2008. Effects of sequential sectioning of defined posterior cruciate ligament fiber regions on translational knee motion. Am J Sports Med 36: 480–486.
Decker MJ, Torry MR, Wyland DJ, et al. 2003. Gender differences in lower extremity kinematics, kinetics and energy absorption during landing. Clin Biomech 18: 662–669.
Degenhardt TC, Hughston JC. 1981. Chronic posterior cruciate instability: nonoperative management. Orthop Trans 5: 486–487.
DeLee JC, Riley MB, Rockwood CA Jr. 1983. Acute straight lateral instability of the knee. Am J Sports Med 11: 404–411.
Delincé P, Ghafil D. 2012. Anterior cruciate ligament tears: conservative or surgical treatment? A critical review of the literature. Knee Surg Sports Traumatol Arthrosc 20(1): 48–61.
Della Villa S, Boldrini L, Ricci M, et al. 2012. Clinical outcomes and return-to-sports participation of 50 soccer players after anterior cruciate ligament reconstruction through a sport-specific rehabilitation protocol. Sports Health 4: 17–24.
DeMorat G, Weinhold P, Blackburn T, et al. 2004. Aggressive quadriceps loading can induce noncontact anterior cruciate ligament injury. Am J Sports Med 32: 477–483.
Dempsey AR, Lloyd DG, Elliott BC, et al. 2009. Changing sidestep cutting technique reduces knee valgus loading. Am J Sports Med 37: 2194–2200.
Deyle GD, Allison SC, Matekel R, et al. 2005. Physical therapy treatment effectiveness for osteoarthritis of the knee: a randomized comparison of supervised clinical exercise and manual therapy procedures versus a home exercise program. Phys Ther 85: 1301–1317.
Dürselen L, Claes L, Kiefer H. 1995. The influence of muscle forces and external loads on cruciate ligament strain. Am J Sports Med 23: 129–136.
Dye SF, Vaupel GL, Dye CC. 1998. Conscious neurosensory mapping of the internal structures of the human knee without intraarticular anesthesia. Am J Sports Med 26: 773–777.
Eitzen I, Moksnes H, Snyder-Mackler L, et al. 2010. Functional tests should be accentuated more in the decision for ACL reconstruction. Knee Surg Sports Traumatol Arthrosc 18: 1517–1525.
Elsaid KA, Zhang L, Waller K, et al. 2012. The impact of forced joint exercise on lubricin biosynthesis from articular cartilage following ACL transection and intra-articular lubricin's effect in exercised joints following ACL transection. Osteoarthritis Cartilage 20: 940–948.
Englund M, Niu J, Guermazi A, et al. 2007. Effect of meniscal damage on the development of frequent knee pain, aching, or stiffness. Arthritis Rheum 56: 4048–4054.
Englund M, Germazi A, Gale D, et al. 2008. Incidental meniscal findings on knee MRI in middle-aged and elderly persons. N Engl J Med 359: 1108–1115.
Englund M, Roemer FW, Hayashi D, et al. 2012. Meniscus pathology, osteoarthritis and the treatment controversy. Nat Rev Rheumatol 8: 412–419.
Esteves JE, Wheatley L, Mayall C, et al. 2013. Emotional processing and its relationship to chronic low back pain: Results from a case–control study. Man Ther 18: 541–546.
Fanelli GC. 1993. Posterior cruciate ligament injuries in trauma patients. Arthroscopy 9: 291–294.

Fanelli GC, Edson CJ. 1995. Posterior cruciate ligament injuries in trauma patients: Part II. Arthroscopy 11: 526–529.

Fanelli GC, Beck JD, Edson CJ. 2010. Current concepts review: the posterior cruciate ligament. J Knee Surg 23: 61–72.

Feagin JA Jr, Curl WW. 1976. Isolated tear of the anterior cruciate ligament: 5-year follow-up study. Am J Sports Med 4: 95–100.

Felson DT. 2004. An update on the pathogenesis and epidemiology of osteoarthritis. Radiol Clin North Am 42: 1–9.

Fithian DC, Kelly MA, Mow VC. 1990. Material properties and structure–function relationships in the menisci. Clin Orthop Relat Res 252: 19–31.

Fithian DC, Paxton EW, Stone ML, et al. 2005. Prospective trial of a treatment algorithm for the management of the anterior cruciate ligament-injured knee. Am J Sports Med 33: 335–346.

Ford KR, Myer GD, Hewett TE. 2010. Longitudinal effects of maturation on lower extremity joint stiffness in adolescent athletes. Am J Sports Med 38: 1829–1837.

Foster TE, Wolfe BL, Ryan S, et al. 2010. Does the graft source really matter in the outcome of patients undergoing anterior cruciate ligament reconstruction? An evaluation of autograft versus allograft reconstruction results: a systematic review. Am J Sports Med 38: 189–199.

Fox AJ, Bedi A, Rodeo SA. 2012. The basic science of human knee menisci: structure, composition, and function. Sports Health 4: 340–351.

Fu RZ, Lin DD. 2013. Surgical and biomechanical perspectives on osteoarthritis and the ACL deficient knee: a critical review of the literature. Open Orthop J 7: 292–300.

Fukagawa S, Matsuda S, Tashiro Y, et al. 2010. Posterior displacement of the tibia increases in deep flexion of the knee. Clin Orthop Relat Res 468: 1107–1114.

Fukuda Y, Woo SL, Loh JC, et al. 2003. A quantitative analysis of valgus torque on the ACL: a human cadaveric study. J Orthop Res 21: 1107–1112.

Gandevia SC, McCloskey DI. 1976. Joint sense, muscle sense, and their combination as position sense, measured at the distal interphalangeal joint of the middle finger. J Physiol 260: 387–407.

Gollehon DL, Torzilli PA, Warren RF. 1987. The role of the posterolateral and cruciate ligaments in the stability of the human knee: a biomechanical study. J Bone Joint Surg Am 69: 233–242.

Grana WA, Janssen T. 1987. Lateral ligament injury of the knee. Orthopedics 10: 1039–1044

Graven-Nielsen T, Arendt-Nielsen L. 2010. Assessment of mechanisms in localized and widespread musculoskeletal pain. Nat Rev Rheumatol 6: 599–606.

Greis PE, Bardana DD, Holmstrom MC, et al. 2002. Meniscal injury: I. Basic science and evaluation. J Am Acad Orthop Surg 10: 168–176.

Grood ES, Stowers SF, Noyes FR. 1988. Limits of movement in the human knee: effect of sectioning the posterior cruciate ligament and posterolateral structures. J Bone Joint Surg Am 70: 88–97.

Griffith CJ, LaPrade RF, Johansen S, et al. 2009. Medial knee injury: Part 1, static function of the individual components of the main medial knee structures. Am J Sports Med 37: 1762–1770.

Harilainen A. 1987. Evaluation of knee instability in acute ligamentous injuries. Ann Chir Gynaecol 76: 269–273.

Harrison BK, Abell BE, Gibson TW. 2009. The Thessaly test for detection of meniscal tears: validation of a new physical examination technique for primary care medicine. Clin J Sport Med 19: 9–12.

Hede A, Jensen DB, Blyme P, et al. 1990. Epidemiology of meniscal lesions in the knee. 1,215 open operations in Copenhagen 1982–84. Acta Orthop Scand. 61:435–437.

Hegedus EJ, Cook C, Hasselblad V, et al. 2007. Physical examination tests for assessing a torn meniscus in the knee: a systematic review with meta-analysis. J Orthop Sports Phys Ther 37: 541–550.

Hensler D, Van Eck CF, Fu FH, et al. 2012. Anatomic anterior cruciate ligament reconstruction utilizing the double-bundle technique. J Orthop Sports Phys Ther 42: 184–195.

Herrington L, Myer G, Horsley I. 2013. Task based rehabilitation protocol for elite athletes following anterior cruciate ligament reconstruction: a clinical commentary. Phys Ther Sport 14: 188–198.

Herrlin S, Hållander M, Wange P, et al. 2007. Arthroscopic or conservative treatment of degenerative medial meniscal tears: a prospective randomised trial. Knee Surg Sports Traumatol Arthrosc 15: 393–401.

Hewett TE, Myer GD, Ford KR, et al. 2005. Biomechanical measures of neuromuscular control and valgus loading of the knee predict anterior cruciate ligament injury risk in female athletes: a prospective study. Am J Sports Med 33: 492–501.

Hewett TE, Myer GD, Ford KR. 2006a. Anterior cruciate ligament injuries in female athletes: Part 1, mechanisms and risk factors. Am J Sports Med 34: 299–311.

Hewett TE, Ford KR, Myer GD, et al. 2006b. Gender differences in hip adduction motion and torque during a single-leg agility maneuver. J Orthop Res 24: 416–421.

Hewett TE, Torg JS, Boden BP. 2009. Video analysis of trunk and knee motion during non-contact anterior cruciate ligament injury in female athletes: lateral trunk and knee abduction motion are combined components of the injury mechanism. Br J Sports Med 43: 417–422.

Hewett TE, Myer GD, Ford KR, et al. 2012. The 2012 ABJS Nicolas Andry Award: The sequence of prevention: a systematic approach to prevent anterior cruciate ligament injury. Clin Orthop Relat Res 470: 2930–2940.

Hollman JH, Hohl JM, Kraft JL, et al. 2013. Modulation of frontal-plane knee kinematics by hip-extensor strength and gluteus maximus recruitment during a jump-landing task in healthy women. J Sport Rehabil 22: 184–190.

Holm I, Hammer S, Larsen S, et al. 1995. Can a regular leg extension bench be used in testing deficits of the quadriceps muscle during rehabilitation? Scand J Med Sci 5: 29–35.

Hurd WJ, Axe MJ, Snyder-Mackler L. 2008. A 10-year prospective trial of a patient management algorithm and screening examination for highly active individuals with anterior cruciate ligament injury: Part 2, determinants of dynamic knee stability. Am J Sports Med 36:48–56.

Hurley MV. 1997. The effects of joint damage on muscle function, proprioception and rehabilitation. Man Ther 2: 11–17.

Hwang BY, Kim SJ, Lee SW, et al. 2012. Risk factors for medial meniscus posterior root tear. Am J Sports Med 40: 1606–1610.

Imwalle LE, Myer GD, Ford KR, et al. 2009. Relationship between hip and knee kinematics in athletic women during cutting maneuvers: a possible link to noncontact anterior cruciate ligament injury and prevention. J Strength Cond Res 23: 2223–2230.

Ireland ML. 1999. Anterior cruciate ligament injury in female athletes: epidemiology. J Athl Train 34: 150–154.

Ireland ML. 2002. The female ACL: why is it more prone to injury? Orthop Clin North Am 33: 637–651.

Iwamoto J, Takeda T, Suda Y, et al. 2004. Conservative treatment of isolated posterior cruciate ligament injury in professional baseball players: a report of two cases. Knee 11: 41–44.

Jackson JL, O'Malley PG, Kroenke K. 2003. Evaluation of acute knee pain in primary care. Ann Intern Med 139: 575–588.

Jones JC, Burks R, Owens BD, et al. 2012. Incidence and risk factors associated with meniscal injuries among active-duty US military service members. J Athl Train 47: 67–73.

Jordan SS, DeFrate LE, Nha KW, et al. 2007. The in vivo kinematics of the anteromedial and posterolateral bundles of the anterior cruciate ligament during weightbearing knee flexion. Am J Sports Med 35: 547–554.

Kaplan Y. 2011. Identifying individuals with an anterior cruciate ligament-deficient knee as copers and noncopers: a narrative literature review. J Orthop Sports Phys Ther 41: 758–766.

Kennedy JC, Hawkins RJ, Willis RB, et al. 1976. Tension studies of human knee ligaments. Yield point, ultimate failure, and disruption of the cruciate and tibial collateral ligaments. J Bone Joint Surg Am 58: 350–355.

Kennedy JC, Alexander IJ, Hayes KC. 1982. Nerve supply of the human knee and its functional importance. Am J Sports Med 10: 329–335.

Koga H, Nakamae A, Shima Y, et al. 2010. Mechanisms for noncontact anterior cruciate ligament injuries: knee joint kinematics in 10 injury situations from female team handball and basketball. Am J Sports Med 38: 2218–2225.

Kostogiannis I, Ageberg E, Neuman P, et al. 2007. Activity level and subjective knee function 15 years after anterior cruciate ligament injury: a prospective, longitudinal study of nonreconstructed patients. Am J Sports Med 35:1135–1143.

Krosshaug T, Nakamae A, Boden BP, et al. 2007. Mechanisms of anterior cruciate ligament injury in basketball: video analysis of 39 cases. Am J Sports Med 35: 359–367.

Krukhaug Y, Mølster A, Rodt A, et al. 1998. Lateral ligament injuries of the knee. Knee Surg Sports Traumatol Arthrosc 6: 21–25.

Kulas A, Zalewski P, Hortobagyi T, et al. 2008. Effects of added trunk load and corresponding trunk position adaptations on lower extremity biomechanics during drop-landings. J Biomech 41: 180–185.

Kusayama T, Harner CD, Carlin GJ, et al. 1994. Anatomical and biomechanical characteristics of human meniscofemoral ligaments. Knee Surg Sports Traumatol Arthrosc 2: 234–237.

Kvist J. 2004. Rehabilitation following anterior cruciate ligament injury: current recommendations for sports participation. Sports Med 34: 269–280.

Landry SC, McKean KA, Hubley-Kozey CL, et al. 2007. Neuromuscular and lower limb biomechanical differences exist between male and female elite adolescent soccer players during an unanticipated side-cut maneuver. Am J Sports Med 35: 1888–1900.

LaPrade RF, Hamilton CD. 1997. The fibular collateral ligament-biceps femoris bursa: an anatomic study. Am J Sports Med 25: 439–443.

LaPrade RF, Wentorf F. 2002. Diagnosis and treatment of posterolateral knee injuries. Clin Orthop Relat Res 402: 110–121.

LaPrade RF, Wijdicks CA. 2012. The management of injuries to the medial side of the knee. J Orthop Sports Phys Ther 42: 221–233.

LaPrade RF, Ly TV, Wentorf FA, et al. 2003. The posterolateral attachments of the knee: a qualitative and quantitative morphologic analysis of the fibular collateral ligament, popliteus tendon, popliteofibular ligament, and lateral gastrocnemius tendon. Am J Sports Med 31: 854–860.

LaPrade RF, Johansen S, Wentorf FA, et al. 2004a. An analysis of an anatomical posterolateral knee reconstruction: an in vitro biomechanical study and development of a surgical technique. Am J Sports Med 32: 1405–1414.

LaPrade RF, Tso A, Wentorf FA. 2004b. Force measurements on the fibular collateral ligament, popliteofibular ligament, and popliteus tendon to applied loads. Am J Sports Med 32: 1695–1701.

Lauder TD, Baker SP, Smith GS, et al. 2000. Sports and physical training injury hospitalizations in the army. Am J Prev Med 18: S118–S128.

Lawrence RK 3rd, Kernozek TW, Miller EJ, et al. 2008. Influences of hip external rotation strength on knee mechanics during single-leg drop landings in females. Clin Biomech 23: 806–813.

Levy IM, Torzilli PA, Gould JD, et al. 1989. The effect of lateral meniscectomy on motion of the knee. J Bone Joint Surg Am 71: 401–406.

Levy BA, Boyd JL, Stuart MJ. 2011. Surgical treatment of acute and chronic anterior and posterior cruciate ligament and lateral side injuries of the knee. Sports Med Arthrosc 19: 110–119.

Linko E, Harilainen A, Malmivaara A, et al. 2005. Surgical versus conservative interventions for anterior cruciate ligament ruptures in adults. Cochrane Database Syst Rev 2: CD001356.

Lohmander LS, Englund PM, Dahl LL, et al. 2007. The long-term consequence of anterior cruciate ligament and meniscus injuries: osteoarthritis. Am J Sports Med 35: 1756–1769.

Louboutin H, Debarge R, Richou J, et al. 2009. Osteoarthritis in patients with anterior cruciate ligament rupture: a review of risk factors. Knee 16: 239–244.

Louw QA, Manilall J, Grimmer KA. 2008. Epidemiology of knee injuries among adolescents: a systematic review. Br J Sports Med 42: 2–10.

Lundblad M, Waldén M, Magnusson H, et al. 2013. The UEFA injury study: 11-year data concerning 346 MCL injuries and time to return to play. Br J Sports Med 47: 759–762.

Margheritini F, Rihn J, Musahl V, et al. 2002. Posterior cruciate ligament injuries in the athlete: an anatomical, biomechanical and clinical review. Sports Med 32: 393–408.

Makris EA, Hadidi P, Athanasiou KA. 2011. The knee meniscus: structure-function, pathophysiology, current repair techniques, and prospects for regeneration. Biomaterials 32: 7411–7431.

Malanga GA, Andrus S, Nadler SF, et al. 2003. Physical examination of the knee: a review of the original test description and scientific validity of common orthopedic tests. Arch Phys Med Rehabil 84: 592–603.

Malinzak RA, Colby SM, Kirkendall DT, et al. 2001. A comparison of knee joint motion patterns between men and women in selected athletic tasks. Clin Biomech 16: 438–445.

Markatos K, Kaseta MK, Lallos SN, et al. 2013. The anatomy of the ACL and its importance in ACL reconstruction. Eur J Orthop Surg Traumatol 23(7): 747–752. doi: 10.1007/s00590-012-1079-8.

Markolf KL, Burchfield DM, Shapiro MM, et al. 1995. Combined knee loading states that generate high anterior cruciate ligament forces. J Orthop Res 13: 930–935.

McLean SG, Lipfert SW, van den Bogert AJ. 2004. Effect of gender and defensive opponent on the biomechanics of sidestep cutting. Med Sci Sports Exerc 36: 1008–1016.

McLean SG, Huang X, van den Bogert AJ. 2005. Association between lower extremity posture at contact and peak knee valgus moment during sidestepping: implications for ACL injury. Clin Biomech 20: 863–870.

Meister BR, Michael SP, Moyer RA, et al. 2000. Anatomy and kinematics of the lateral collateral ligament of the knee. Am J Sports Med 28: 869–878.

Mejia EA, Noyes FR, Grood ES. 2002. Posterior cruciate ligament femoral insertion site characteristics: importance for reconstructive procedures. Am J Sports Med 30: 643–651.

Mendiguchia J, Ford KR, Quatman CE, et al. 2011. Sex differences in proximal control of the knee joint. Sports Med 41: 541–557.

Meuffels DE, Favejee MM, Vissers M, et al. 2009. Ten year follow-up study comparing conservative versus operative treatment of anterior cruciate ligament ruptures: a matched-pair analysis of high level athletes. Br J Sports Med 43: 347–351.

Meuffels DE, Poldervaart MT, Diercks RL, et al. 2012. Guideline on anterior cruciate ligament injury. Acta Orthop 83: 379–386.

Micheo W, Hernández L, Seda C. 2010. Evaluation, management, rehabilitation, and prevention of anterior cruciate ligament injury: current concepts. PM R 2: 935–944.

Mokhtarzadeh H, Yeow CH, Hong Goh JC, et al. 2013. Contributions of the soleus and gastrocnemius muscles to the anterior cruciate ligament loading during single-leg landing. J Biomech 46: 1913–1920.

Moses B, Orchard J, Orchard J. 2012. Systematic review: annual incidence of ACL injury and surgery in various populations. Res Sports Med 20: 157–179.

Muaidi QI, Nicholson LL, Refshauge KM, et al. 2007. Prognosis of conservatively managed anterior cruciate ligament injury: a systematic review. Sports Med 37: 703–716.

Myklebust G, Bahr R. 2005. Return to play guidelines after anterior cruciate ligament surgery. Br J Sports Med 39: 127–131.

Nielsen AB, Yde J. 1991. Epidemiology of acute knee injuries: a prospective hospital investigation. J Trauma 31: 1644–1648.

Noyes FR, Barber-Westin SD. 2010. Repair of complex and avascular meniscal tears and meniscal transplantation. J Bone Joint Surg Am 92: 1012–1029.

O'Donoghue DH. 1955. An analysis of end results of surgical treatment of major injuries to the ligaments of the knee. J Bone Joint Surg Am 37: 1–13.

Oiestad BE, Holm I, Aune AK, et al. 2010. Knee function and prevalence of knee osteoarthritis after anterior cruciate ligament reconstruction: a prospective study with 10 to 15 years of follow-up. Am J Sports Med 38: 2201–2210.

Olsen OE, Myklebust G, Engebretsen L, et al. 2004. Injury mechanisms for anterior cruciate ligament injuries in team handball: a systematic video analysis. Am J Sports Med 32: 1002–1012.

Østerås H, Østerås B, Torstensen TA. 2012. Medical exercise therapy, and not arthroscopic surgery, resulted in decreased depression and anxiety in patients with degenerative meniscus injury. J Bodyw Mov Ther 16: 456–463.

Ozkoc G, Circi E, Gonc U, et al. 2008. Radial tears in the root of the posterior horn of the medial meniscus. Knee Surg Sports Traumatol Arthrosc 16: 849–854.

Pacheco RJ, Ayre CA, Bollen SR. 2011. Posterolateral corner injuries of the knee: a serious injury commonly missed. J Bone Joint Surg Br 93: 194–197.

Pappas E, Zampeli F, Xergia SA, et al. 2013. Lessons learned from the last 20 years of ACL-related in vivo-biomechanics research of the knee joint. Knee Surg Sports Traumatol Arthrosc 21: 755–766.

Parolie JM, Bergfeld JA. 1986. Long-term results of nonoperative treatment of isolated posterior cruciate ligament injuries in the athlete. Am J Sports Med 14: 35–38.

Paterno MV, Schmitt LC, Ford KR, et al. 2010. Biomechanical measures during landing and postural stability predict second anterior cruciate ligament injury after anterior cruciate ligament reconstruction and return to sport. Am J Sports Med 38: 1968–1978.

Peccin MS, Almeida GJ, Amaro JT, et al. 2012. Interventions for treating posterior cruciate ligament injuries of the knee in adults. Cochrane Database Syst Rev 3: CD002939.

Petrigliano FA, McAllister DR. 2006. Isolated posterior cruciate ligament injuries of the knee. Sports Med Arthrosc 14: 206–212.

Pollard CD, Sigward SM, Powers CM. 2007. Gender differences in hip joint kinematics and kinetics during side-step cutting maneuver. Clin J Sport Med 17: 38–42.

Pollard CD, Sigward SM, Powers CM. 2010. Limited hip and knee flexion during landing is associated with increased frontal plane knee motion and moments. Clin Biomech 25: 142–146.

Quarles JD, Hosey RG. 2004. Medial and lateral collateral injuries: prognosis and treatment. Prim Care 31: 957–975.

Race A, Amis AA. 1996. Loading of the two bundles of the posterior cruciate ligament: an analysis of bundle function in A-P drawer. J Biomech 29: 873–879.

Renström P, Johnson RJ. 1990. Anatomy and biomechanics of the menisci. Clin Sports Med 9: 523–538.

Risberg MA, Holm l, Myklebust G, et al. 2007. Neuromuscular training versus strength training during first 6 months after anterior cruciate ligament reconstruction: a randomized clinical trial. Phys Ther 87: 737–750.

Roberts D, Ageberg E, Andersson G, et al. 2007. Clinical measurements of proprioception, muscle strength and laxity in relation to function in the ACL-injured knee. Knee Surg Sports Traumatol Arthrosc 15: 9–16.

Roos EM. 2005. Joint injury causes knee osteoarthritis in young adults. Curr Opin Rheumatol 17: 195–200.
Salata MJ, Gibbs AE, Sekiya JK. 2010. A systematic review of clinical outcomes in patients undergoing meniscectomy. Am J Sports Med 38: 1907–1916.
Salci Y, Kentel BB, Heycan C, et al. 2004. Comparison of landing maneuvers between male and female college volleyball players. Clin Biomech 19: 622–628.
Sanchez AR 2nd, Sugalski MT, LaPrade RF. 2006. Anatomy and biomechanics of the lateral side of the knee. Sports Med Arthrosc 14: 2–11.
Schein A, Matcuk G, Patel D, et al. 2012. Structure and function, injury, pathology, and treatment of the medial collateral ligament of the knee. Emerg Radiol 19: 489–498.
Schmitz RJ, Kulas AS, Perrin DH, et al. 2007. Sex differences in lower extremity biomechanics during single leg landings. Clin Biomech 22: 681–688.
Schulz MS, Russe K, Weiler A, et al. 2003. Epidemiology of posterior cruciate ligament injuries. Arch Orthop Trauma Surg 123: 186–191.
Self BP, Paine D. 2001. Ankle biomechanics during four landing techniques. Med Sci Sports Exerc 33: 1338–1344.
Sharma L. 1999. Proprioceptive impairment in knee osteoarthritis. Rheum Dis Clin North Am 25: 299–314.
Shimokochi Y, Shultz SJ. 2008. Mechanisms of noncontact anterior cruciate ligament injury. J Athl Train 43: 396–408.
Shoemaker SC, Markolf KL. 1986. The role of the meniscus in the anterior–posterior stability of the loaded anterior cruciate-deficient knee. Effects of partial versus total excision. J Bone Joint Surg Am 68: 71–79.
Sigward SM, Powers CM. 2006. The influence of gender on knee kinematics, kinetics and muscle activation patterns during side-step cutting. Clin Biomech 21: 41–48.
Sigward SM, Powers CM. 2007. Loading characteristics of females exhibiting excessive valgus moments during cutting. Clin Biomech 22: 827–833.
Sigward SM, Ota S, Powers CM. 2008. Predictors of frontal plane knee excursion during a drop land in young female soccer players. J Orthop Sports Phys Ther 38: 661–667.
Smith TO, Postle K, Penny F, et al. 2014. Is reconstruction the best management strategy for anterior cruciate ligament rupture? A systematic review and meta-analysis comparing anterior cruciate ligament reconstruction versus non-operative treatment. Knee 21(2): 462–470. doi: 10.1016/j.knee.2013.10.009.
Snoeker BA, Bakker EW, Kegel CA, et al. 2013. Risk factors for meniscal tears: a systematic review including meta-analysis. J Orthop Sports Phys Ther 43: 352–367.
Stärke C, Kopf S, Petersen W, Becker R. 2009. Meniscal repair. Arthroscopy 25: 1033–1044.
Steinbrück K. 1999. Epidemiology of sports injuries: 25-year-analysis of sports orthopedic-traumatologic ambulatory care. Sportverletz Sportschaden 13: 38–52.
Strehl A, Eggli S. 2007. The value of conservative treatment in ruptures of the anterior cruciate ligament (ACL). J Trauma 62: 1159–1162.
Streich NA, Zimmermann D, Bode G, et al. 2011. Reconstructive versus non-reconstructive treatment of anterior cruciate ligament insufficiency: a retrospective matched-pair long-term follow-up. Int Orthop 35: 607–613.
Strobel MJ, Weiler A, Schulz MS, et al. 2003. Arthroscopic evaluation of articular cartilage lesions in posterior-cruciate-ligament-deficient knees. Arthroscopy 19: 262–268.
Terry GC, LaPrade RF. 1996. The biceps femoris muscle complex at the knee: its anatomy and injury patterns associated with acute anterolateral–anteromedial rotatory instability. Am J Sports Med 24: 2–8.
Thomeé R, Neeter C, Gustavsson A, et al. 2012. Variability in leg muscle power and hop performance after anterior cruciate ligament reconstruction. Knee Surg Sports Traumatol Arthrosc 20: 1143–1151.
Thompson WO, Thaete FL, Fu FH, et al. 1991. Tibial meniscal dynamics using three-dimensional reconstruction of magnetic resonance images. Am J Sports Med 19: 210–215.
Tuite MJ, Daffner RH, Weissman BN, et al. 2012. ACR appropriateness criteria(®) acute trauma to the knee. J Am Coll Radiol 9: 96–103. doi: 10.1016/j.jacr.2011.10.013.
Voloshin AS, Wosk J. 1983. Shock absorption of meniscectomized and painful knees: a comparative in vivo study. J Biomed Eng 5(2): 157–161.
Walker PS, Erkman MJ. 1975. The role of the menisci in force transmission across the knee. Clin Orthop Relat Res 109: 184–192.
Walker PS, Hajek JV. 1972. The load-bearing area in the knee joint. J Biomech 5: 581–589.
Wijdicks CA, Griffith CJ, LaPrade RF, et al 2009. Medial knee injury: part 2, load sharing between the posterior oblique ligament and superficial medial collateral ligament. Am J Sports Med 37: 1771–1776.
Wijdicks CA, Griffith CJ, Johansen S, et al. 2010. Injuries to the medial collateral ligament and associated medial structures of the knee. J Bone Joint Surg Am 92: 1266–1280.
Wilk KE, Reinold MM, Hooks TR. 2003. Recent advances in the rehabilitation of isolated and combined anterior cruciate ligament injuries. Orthop Clin North Am 34: 107–137.
Woo SL, Wu C, Dede O, et al. 2006. Biomechanics and anterior cruciate ligament reconstruction. J Orthop Surg Res 1: 2.
Xu C, Zhao J. 2015. A meta-analysis comparing meniscal repair with meniscectomy in the treatment of meniscal tears: the more meniscus, the better outcome? Knee Surg Sports Traumatol Arthrosc 23: 164–170.
Yeh PC, Starkey C, Lombardo S, et al. 2012. Epidemiology of isolated meniscal injury and its effect on performance in athletes from the National Basketball Association. Am J Sports Med 40: 589–594.
Yu B, Lin CF, Garrett WE. 2006. Lower extremity biomechanics during the landing of a stop-jump task. Clin Biomech 21: 297–305.
Zazulak BT, Ponce PL, Straub SJ, et al. 2005. Gender comparison of hip muscle activity during single-leg landing. J Orthop Sports Phys Ther 35: 292–299.
Zazulak BT, Hewett TE, Reeves NP, et al. 2007. Deficits in neuromuscular control of the trunk predict knee injury risk: a prospective biomechanical–epidemiologic study. Am J Sports Med 35: 1123–1130.
Zech A, Hübscher M, Vogt L, et al. 2009. Neuromuscular training for rehabilitation of sports injuries: a systematic review. Med Sci Sports Exerc 41: 1831–1841.

43 Chapter

Knee Osteoarthritis

Lars Arendt-Nielsen, César Fernández-de-las-Peñas

CHAPTER CONTENTS

Introduction	482
Sensory manifestations in osteoarthritis	482
Sensitization in osteoarthritis	483
Specific pain mechanisms in knee osteoarthritis	483
Pathophysiology and biochemistry of osteoarthritis	483
Biomechanics of knee osteoarthritis	484
Challenges in the management of osteoarthritis-related pain	484
Pharmacological management	484
Non-pharmacological management	485
Arthroplasty	488
Conclusion	489

Introduction

Osteoarthritis (OA) is the most frequent musculoskeletal diagnosis in the elderly population and the most common cause of disability (Peat et al 2001); 40% of females and 25% of males aged 60–70 years are diagnosed with OA (Van Saase et al 1989), in which knee OA is the most prevalent. With the expected global growth in the elderly population and concomitant rise in stationary lifestyle choices, the incidence of OA is predicted to increase in the coming years.

Sensory Manifestations in Osteoarthritis

At the individual patient level, severe knee joint damage may cause little pain, whereas that with minor / no radiological changes may cause severe pain (Davis et al 1992; Hannan et al 2000; Neogi et al 2009). However, at a population basis this discordance is less evident (Bedson & Croft 2008). A total of 10–20% of individuals with regional pain subsequently develop widespread pain (Mourão et al 2010; Atzeni et al 2011; Sarzi-Puttini et al 2011), as is often seen in musculoskeletal pain syndromes.

The subjective sensory manifestations of musculoskeletal pain in humans include cramp-like, diffuse aching pain and pain referred to distant somatic structures, as well as modifications in the superficial and deep pain sensitivity in the referred pain areas (Arendt-Nielsen & Graven-Nielsen 2002, 2003). These manifestations are different from cutaneous pain, which is normally superficial, localized around the injury and exhibits a sharp and burning quality. Pain localization is poor from musculoskeletal structures, and it is difficult to differentiate it from pain originating from tendons, ligaments and bones as well as from joints and their capsules.

Muscle-referred pain is typically described as a sensation from deep structures, in contrast to visceral-referred pain, which is both superficially and deeply located. Muscle-referred pain has been known and described for more than a century and it is used extensively as a diagnostic tool. The referred pain pattern more frequently follows the distribution of sclerotomes (muscle, fascia and bone) than that of the classical dermatomes. A distinction between spread of pain and referred pain is not possible, and these phenomena may share common pathophysiological mechanisms. Firm neurophysiologically based explanations for referred pain do not exist, but it has been shown that wide-dynamic-range neurons and nociceptive specific neurons in the spinal cord and the brainstem of animals receive convergent afferent inputs from the mucosa, skin, muscles, joints and viscera. This may cause a misinterpretation of the afferent information coming from muscle afferents and reaching high levels in the central nervous system, and hence it be one reason for the diffuse and referred characteristics.

Referred pain has been shown to be mainly a central phenomenon, as it is possible to induce referred pain to limbs with complete sensory loss due to spinal injury or anaesthetic blockade (Laursen et al 1997). The size of the referred pain area to experimental joint pain stimulation has been found to depend on both the intensity and the duration of the nociceptive musculoskeletal input (O'Neill et al 2009). OA patients demonstrating more than one location of pain often express pain symptoms extending from the knee to other locations (Thompson et al 2010), which supports the notion that spreading of pain and of sensitization are present in these patients (Arendt-Nielsen et al 2010b). Finally, animal models of OA (intra-articular injection of monosodium iodoacetate in the knee joint) have identified spreading sensitization through mitogen-activated protein kinases (MAPKs), specifically ERK and p38 phosphorylation (Lee et al 2011) with associated mechanical allodynia of the contralateral limb.

Sensitization in Osteoarthritis

Treating knee OA pain is challenging as the pathology is decoupled from the pain and (1) the underlying pain mechanisms are not fully understood and, hence, (2) efficient pharmacological and non-pharmacological treatments are not sufficiently developed. Pain in knee OA is highly individual and no features (e.g. on radiology) have demonstrated a robust correlation with pain manifestations. In recent years, a variety of new quantitative pain assessment tools have been developed for profiling of patients with OA according to the mechanisms involved, which in the future may help developing individualized pain management programmes (Malfait & Schnitzer 2013).

There is ample evidence that the sensitization in OA is caused by the nociceptive input from the joint, as successful joint replacement with total pain alleviation resets the sensitization (Graven-Nielsen et al 2012; Aranda-Villalobos et al 2013). The sensitization process in musculoskeletal pain is coded not only by pain intensity but also by pain duration, as a variety of studies have shown an association between pain duration and level of local and spreading sensitization (Arendt-Nielsen et al 2010a, 2010b). In knee OA, the pain intensity / duration codes for the degree of extrasegmental pressure pain hyperalgesia (Arendt-Nielsen et al 2010b), similar to temporomandibular joint disorder (TMD) (Fernández-de-las-Peñas et al 2009) and chronic tension-type headache (Fernández-de-las-Peñas et al 2008). Furthermore, the number of OA locations is important with respect to how diffusely the OA knee pain is perceived (Thompson et al 2010), and the more myofascial trigger points involved the more generalized is the sensitization (Xu et al 2010). Therefore, it has become increasingly evident that sensitization of the nociceptive pain system plays a role in the clinical presentation of knee OA pain (Kidd 2012). Peripheral and central sensitization mechanisms are present in patients with OA (Arendt-Nielsen et al 2010b), neuropathic descriptors apply to subunits of patients with OA (Finan et al 2013; Hochman et al 2013) and widespread hyperalgesia has been documented in a number of studies (Imamura et al 2008; Arendt-Nielsen et al 2010b; Graven-Nielsen et al 2012). Because of the role of sensitization, it has also been argued that patients with OA in will general benefit from 'desensitizing' drugs, such as duloxetine (Citrome & Weiss-Citrome 2012) or pregabalin, which have been shown efficacy in animal models of OA (Rahman et al 2009).

Specific Pain Mechanisms in Knee Osteoarthritis

If the anterior tibialis muscle in patients with OA is tested by pressure pain thresholds, this muscle shows pressure pain sensitization as a result of spreading sensitization (Suokas et al 2012). A method has been developed for mapping pressure pain sensitization in OA as a tool for monitoring, for example, disease progression or the effect of treatment. In this, pressure is applied to a number of predefined locations over the knee and the pressure pain thresholds are determined, which are, in turn, transferred onto a three-dimensional representation of individual knee surface contours estimated from MRI scans of the knee (Arendt-Nielsen et al 2010b). Courtney et al (2009) observed significantly reduced current amplitude and latency of reflex responses at flexion withdrawal reflexes threshold in individuals with knee OA, including those subjects without resting pain, compared with control subjects, which supports the presence of central sensitization in this population.

One factor suggested to be important for spreading of pain is the status of the descending pain control. In several chronic musculoskeletal pain conditions (e.g. OA, TMD, fibromyalgia) the potency of the descending inhibitory control is reduced, thus making the entire neuroaxis more vulnerable to pain (Arendt-Nielsen & Yarnitsky 2009).

Another factor that seems to play an important role in OA is central temporal summation (enhanced pain response to repeated experimental stimuli), which has been shown to be facilitated in patients with OA (Arendt-Nielsen et al 2010b) – and is similar to observations in many other patient populations with chronic musculoskeletal pain such as fibromyalgia (Sörensen et al 1998) and whiplash (Curatolo et al 2001). A recent large knee OA cohort study ($n=2126$) showed that the pressure pain threshold and the temporal summation were associated with OA-related pain intensity, but not with radiographic evidence of OA (Neogi et al 2013).

Finally, referred muscle pain areas evoked by intramuscular injection of hypertonic saline are significantly enlarged in patients with painful OA (Bajaj et al 2001), again supporting the conception that referred pain and central sensitization are closely related (Arendt-Nielsen & Graven-Nielsen 2002).

Pathophysiology and Biochemistry of Osteoarthritis

Pain is a central part of the clinical presentation of OA and the main reason for patients to seek consultation. Many and diverse structural features of the joint have been suggested to be involved in OA-associated pain including, but not limited to, the presence of osteophytes in the patellofemoral compartment, focal or diffuse cartilaginous abnormalities, subchondral cysts, bone marrow oedema, subluxation of the meniscus, meniscal tears and Baker cysts (Read & Dray 2008). However, pain perception is often highly individual, and so far none of these features have demonstrated a robust correlation with pain. It has always been a puzzle why radiological joint changes do not correlate with the clinical pain intensity (Lanyon et al 1998; Felson 2005), although a more-recent large clinical trial has shown a relationship between Kellgren and Lawrence severity of OA and the intensity of clinical pain (Laxafoss et al 2010).

Human articular cartilage has been thought to be avascular and aneural, but recently sympathetic and sensory nerves have been identified as present within vascular channels in the articular cartilage in both mild and severe OA. Perivascular and free nerve fibres and nerve trunks have also been observed both within the subchondral bone marrow and within the marrow cavities of osteophytes. The finding of nerve endings localized in damaged human articular cartilage by Suri et al (2007) suggests that vascularization and the associated innervation of articular cartilage may contribute to tibiofemoral pain in OA across a wide range of structural disease severity. The implications of these findings are that the musculoskeletal pain associated with OA may result from a combination of the hereto-accepted central and bone-derived effects. A hallmark of OA disease is progressive degeneration of articular cartilage and subsequent joint space narrowing. In the majority of patients, the aetiology of OA is not known. Among the known risk factors are age, significant trauma, obesity, altered gait, altered biomechanics (e.g. varus or valgus deformity) and excessive loading.

Experimental and clinical observations suggest that the structural integrity of articular cartilage is dependent on normal subchondral bone turnover, intact chondrocyte function and ordinary biomechanical stresses (Hayami et al 2004). An increasing line of evidence suggests that there is strong communication and interaction between the subchondral bone and the articular cartilage (Karsdal et al 2008). As bone and cartilage are closely inter-related, interventions affecting pain related to bone turnover might in addition be related to the OA relevant pain. Changes in the cartilage matrix turnover may reflect early alterations in cartilage structure accounting directly or indirectly for knee pain (Ishijima et al 2011). During early-stage OA, the presence and progression of osteophytosis are, for example, accompanied by increased levels of cartilage and inflammatory biomarkers (Attur et al 2013; Kumm et al 2013). Studies have indicated that specific pain mechanisms in OA may relate to biomarkers associated with cartilage and bone degradation (Kumm et al 2013). Articular cartilage and subchondral bone damage are key factors in OA and can be assessed by a variety of new biomarkers (Dam et al 2011) such as urinary C-terminal telopeptides of type I collagen (CTX-I), CTX-II, type III collagen *N*-propeptide (PIIINP), and matrix metalloproteinase (MMP)-mediated degradation fragments of type I, II and III collagen (C1M, C2M and C3M respectively) (Garnero 2001). Ishijima et al (2011) showed type II collagen degradation (sC2C and uCTX-II) and formation (sCPII), bone resorption (uNTx) and hence, for example, synovitis may contribute to joint pain.

Arthroscopic evaluations of knee joints reveal that about 25% of subjects with knee OA have inflamed synovial tissue (synovitis), resulting in symptomatic OA (i.e. joint swelling, pain and joint stiffness). These patients have increased risk of radiographic progression (Goldring & Otero 2011; Scanzello et al 2011). As inflammation is considered as one factor involved at some stages in the progression of OA, the inflammatory process may be associated with alterations in the profile of cytokines (e.g. interleukin-6, IL-6) (Livshits et al 2009). Some cytokines may act as biochemical markers of OA severity and pain (Saetan et al 2011) – the most commonly measured cytokines in knee OA are IL-6 and tumour necrosis factor α (TNF-α) (Pearle et al 2007; Livshits et al 2009; Scanzello et al 2009). Various studies have identified a correlation between knee OA severity and higher levels of serum cytokines, such as TNF-α soluble receptors sTNFR1 and sTNFR2, and C-reactive protein (CRP) (Pelletier et al 2001; Miller et al 2008). IL-1 and IL-1R inhibitors have been tested in clinical OA trials, but both anakinra and AMG-108 have been reported to have limited beneficial effects on symptoms and signs in knee OA (Chevalier et al 2009; Cohen et al 2011). However, these studies were done in a mixed population of OA patients. Similar effects on joint metabolism have been attributed to TNF-α, making it another target for anti-inflammatory treatment. Unfortunately none of these therapies has yet proven effective in OA, although a smaller study demonstrated trends towards improvement of joint health upon treatment with adalimumab (Magnano et al 2007). IL-6 is receiving increased interest in the OA field. TNF has been compared with other pro-inflammatory cytokines and has been shown to be elevated in elderly patients with knee OA (Stannus et al 2010).

Studies have described the association of disability (WOMAC) and higher levels of pro-inflammatory cytokines (Ferraro & Booth 1999; Ferrucci et al 2002; Miller et al 2008). In addition, specific cytokines may provoke damage of the extracellular matrix of the joint tissue (Goldring et al 2011). A novel biomarker specific to MMP cleavage is the CRPM, which reflects local inflammation, whereas circulating, uncleaved CRP reflects systemic inflammation (Vigushin et al 1993). It is therefore of relevance to investigate how joint damage, measured by these novel disease-related biomarkers, is related to pain mechanisms. Further, many authors have reported on the effects of different variables, such as functional performance (Ferrucci et al 2002), obesity (Miller et al 2008), clinical aspects (Penninx et al 2004) and radiological severity of OA (Livshits et al 2009) on the serum or intra-articular levels of cytokines. In obese patients, more and more studies have shown hypersensitivity to pain and also that these individuals are more vulnerable to developing pain, possibly owing to the low-level inflammatory processes initiated by cytokine release from adipose tissue (Deere et al 2012).

Biomechanics of Knee Osteoarthritis

Abnormal knee loading is an important factor in OA progression (Andriacchi et al 2004; Hunter & Felson 2006). The medial knee compartment is usually more affected than the lateral compartment as the medial part normally bears the majority of the loads across the knee during gait (Hurwitz et al 1998). Extrinsic measures of musculoskeletal loading during gait play a major role in the identification of injury mechanisms, as medial knee OA is associated with changes in gait patterns attributed to movement-induced nociception (Mündermann et al 2005; Henriksen et al 2006). The entire lower extremity acts as a linked kinetic unit with adaptations in distal body segments having significant effects on loading patterns throughout the extremity, including the knee (Mündermann et al 2005; Lidtke et al 2010). No correlation between plantar loading and Kellgren-Lawrence grade has been found (Lidtke et al 2010).

Few studies have investigated foot pronation in patients with knee OA, but they demonstrated that patients with medial knee OA exhibit a more pronated foot compared with controls (Reilly et al 2009; Barton et al 2010; Levinger et al 2010).

Challenges in the Management of Osteoarthritis-related Pain

Pharmacological management

For many years, oral analgesics such as acetaminophen and NSAIDs have been the mainstream treatment for symptomatic OA. In fact, pharmacological modalities conditionally recommended for the initial management of individuals with knee OA include acetaminophen, oral and topical NSAIDs, tramadol, and intra-articular corticosteroid injections, intra-articular hyaluronate injections and duloxetine, whereas opioids are conditionally recommended in patients who had an inadequate response to initial therapy (Hochberg et al 2012).

The increased awareness of NSAID toxicity has changed treatment recommendations to move away from the long-term use of these agents in symptomatic OA. Systematic reviews and meta-analyses of randomized placebo-controlled trials have been published to estimate the analgesic efficacy of NSAIDs, including selective cyclo-oxygenase-2 inhibitors (coxibs) in individuals with knee OA (Bjordal et al 2004, 2005, 2007b). The studies concluded that NSAIDs reduced short-term pain in OA of the knee slightly better than placebo. However, the subsequent analysis did not support long-term use of NSAIDs for this condition, as serious adverse effects can be associated with oral NSAIDs. Another meta-analysis evaluated randomized controlled trials of short-term (less than 4 weeks) efficacy of topical NSAIDs in OA and reported that after 2 weeks there was no evidence of their efficacy as being superior to placebo (Lin et al 2004).

Current recommendations for symptomatic treatment of OA list paracetamol (4 g per day) as the first-line analgesic despite its limited analgesic effect in this condition. It is obvious that current OA management regimens do not at all focus on possible peripheral and central manifestation of this chronic pain condition. One reason for this is the lack of understanding of the underlying causes of pain in OA in combination with a shortage of effective drug candidates.

Combination therapies are also used widely to treat pain in OA, as is the case in all other pain conditions. Stronger opioids such as oxycodone and transdermal fentanyl / buprenorphine have been shown to be effective in reducing pain scores and improving function in patients with knee and hip OA (Langford et al 2006; Breivik et al 2010). Overall, however, the relative lack of efficacy and the many safety issues surrounding both NSAIDs and opioids have led the pharmaceutical industry to invest in finding new and more effective compounds for managing OA pain, for example, and promising results have been published using, for example, monoclonal nerve growth factor (NGF) antibody in OA pain (Katz et al 2011; Seidel & Lane 2012; Sanga et al 2013). Unfortunately the anti-NGF treatment caused osteonecrosis in patients on additional NSAIDs, and hence the authorities temporarily terminated the clinical trials. However, the NGF target is of significant interest as a treatment for the future.

Other pharmacological approaches include the use of topical therapies such as NSAID creams and gels as they seem to show a better safety record (adverse events <1.5%) compared with oral administration. In a limited number of trials, topically applied capsaicin has been shown benefit for relieving pain in patients with OA (Mason et al 2004).

Intra-articular steroid injections are widely used to reduce OA pain, although the duration of relief may last only a few weeks (Bellamy et al 2005). Intra-articular hyaluronic acid (hyluronan) has symptomatic benefits similar to those of intra-articular steroids and, although the onset of action is delayed, the effect may last up to 12 months (Lo et al 2003). Glucosamine and chondroitin sulfate have been popular for the treatment of OA owing to the favourable early reports. However a large-scale multicentre and placebo-controlled trial could show no benefit over placebo (Clegg et al 2006).

The pharmaceutical industry has a strong interest in developing new analgesic compounds for OA pain. Compounds such as TrkA / B receptor blockers, anti-NGF monoclonal antibodies, CB2 agonists, FAAH inhibitors, different inhibitors of the prostaglandin cascade, different coxibs, P2X7 receptor antagonists and TRPV1 antagonists are currently under investigation in clinical trials for the treatment of pain in OA. The role of calcitonin in OA has also attracted renewed interest (Arendt-Nielsen et al 2009).

Non-pharmacological management

Several non-pharmacological modalities are clinically employed for rehabilitation of patients with knee OA. The American College of Rheumatology (ACR) recently concluded that non-pharmacological modalities strongly recommended for the management of knee OA pain include aerobic, aquatic and / or resistance exercise, as well as weight loss for overweight patients (Hochberg et al 2012). In addition, non-pharmacological modalities conditionally recommended for knee OA include medial wedge insoles for valgus knee OA, subtalar strapped lateral insoles for varus knee OA, medially directed patellar taping, manual physical therapy, walking aids, thermal agents, tai chi, self-management programmes and psychosocial interventions (Hochberg et al 2012). These recommendations have been further supported in other reviews (Roos & Juhl 2012; Segal 2012; Adams et al 2013; Uthman et al 2013). Further, the European League against Rheumatism (EULAR) has recently proposed 11 recommendations for the management of individuals with hip and knee OA including rehabilitation programmes as well as educational teaching activities to modify unhealthy lifestyle habits (Fernandes et al 2013). Nevertheless, clinicians should be aware that the choice of therapy should be determined by patient characteristics and patient choice.

Therapeutic exercise

Therapeutic exercise is probably the most recommended therapeutic intervention for individuals with knee OA, given its beneficial effects, ease of application, few adverse effects and relatively low costs. Regular exercise can reduce physical impairments, improve mobility, decrease the risk of falls, facilitate loss of body weight and improve quality of life by increasing participation in occupational, social and recreational activities (Roddy et al 2005; Bartels et al 2007; Fransen & McConnell 2008, 2009; Bennell & Hinman 2011). Beckwée et al (2013) suggested that exercise could achieve improvement in five categories: neuromuscular, periarticular, intra-articular, psychosocial components, and general fitness and health.

Several reviews and clinical guidelines recommend both strengthening and aerobic exercise, but there are multiple other approaches such as stretching / flexibility, endurance training, aquatic exercise and increasing general physical activity that have also shown promising results (Roddy et al 2005; Bartels et al 2007; Fransen & McConnell 2008, 2009; Bennell & Hinman 2011).

Fransen and McConnell (2008), in their Cochrane review, concluded that land-based therapeutic exercise had significant benefits in terms of pain (standardized mean difference (SMD) 0.40, 95% CI 0.30–0.50) and function (0.37, 95% CI 0.25–0.49) compared with a control group. This review did not find significant differences in the magnitude of treatment effects between difference types of exercise programmes, in agreement with other reviews (Roddy et al 2005; Bartels et al 2007; Jamtvedt et al 2008; Fransen & McConnell 2009). Another Cochrane review concluded that aquatic exercise interventions had small-to-moderate effects on function (SMD 0.26, 95% CI 0.11–0.42) and large effect on pain (0.86, 95% CI 0.25–1.47) for combined hip and knee OA (Bartels et al 2007). A more recent review found strong evidence for aerobic and strengthening exercise programmes, both land and water based, for improving pain and physical function in adults with mild-to-moderate knee and hip OA (Golightly et al 2012).

Contrary to previous reviews that concluded no clear superiority of one form of exercise over another in improving pain and function, a recent meta-analysis provided tentative evidence about the most effective exercise interventions for patients with lower limb OA (Uthman et al 2013). The overall difference between exercise and control in pain intensity was −2.03 cm (95% CI −2.82 to −1.26 cm, large effect size) for strengthening-only exercise, −1.26 cm (95% CI −2.12 to −0.40 cm, medium effect size) for flexibility plus strengthening exercise, −1.74 cm (95% CI −2.60 to −0.88 cm, medium effect size) for flexibility plus strengthening plus aerobic, −1.87 cm (95% CI −3.56 to −0.17, medium effect size) for aquatic strengthening, and −1.87 cm (95% CI −4.11 to −0.68 cm, large effect size) for aquatic flexibility plus strengthening exercise. The overall difference in function for the combination of strengthening, flexibility and aerobic exercise versus no control was −1.32 units (95% CI −2.44 to −0.21 units, medium effect size). This review concluded that exercise interventions combining strengthening with flexibility and aerobic exercise (either land or water based) seemed to be the most effective intervention when one considered measures of both pain and function in lower limb OA (SMD −0.63, 95% CI −1.16 to −0.10) (Uthman et al 2013).

Another recent systematic review concluded that muscle-strengthening exercises with / without weight-bearing and aerobic exercises are effective for pain relief in people with knee OA (Tanaka et al 2013). The most effective exercise of the three types is non-weight-bearing strengthening exercise (Tanaka et al 2013).

Based on available data, regular therapeutic exercise should be early included in the treatment of knee OA pain. Patients should progress from non-weight-bearing exercises without (Fig. 43.1) or with resistance to weight-bearing exercises, particularly those in close kinetic chain (Fig. 43.2). In fact, there is some evidence indicating the effectiveness of proprioceptive exercises conducted in close kinetic chain compared with general strengthening exercises in functional outcomes; however, more research in this area is clearly needed (Smith et al 2012).

Finally, areas related to exercise programmes as therapeutic interventions for knee OA that require further research include examination of the long-term effects of exercise programmes, balance training for OA, exercise programmes for severe knee OA, the effect of exercise programmes on progression of OA, the effectiveness of exercise for joint sites other than the knee or hip, and the effectiveness of exercise for OA by such factors as age, sex and obesity (Golightly et al 2012).

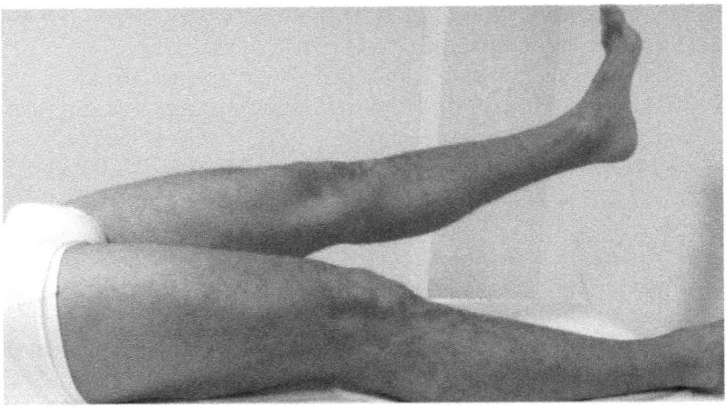

Figure 43.1 Active straight leg raise as non-weight-bearing exercise for strengthening the quadriceps muscle.

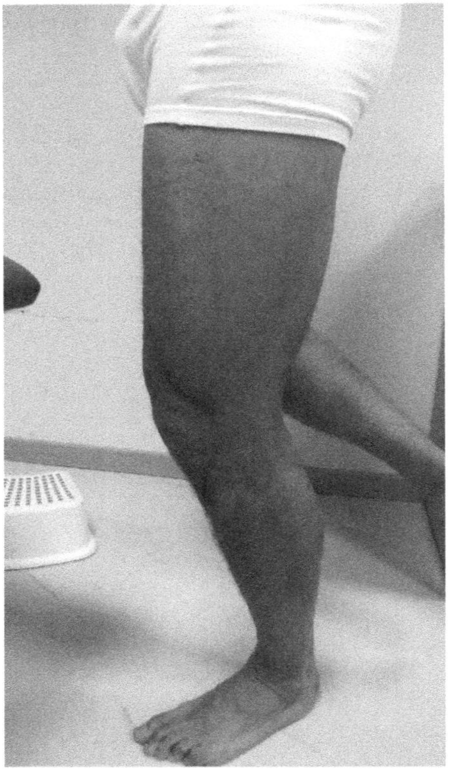

Figure 43.2 One-leg standing exercise with the knee bent for proprioceptive training in close kinetic chain.

Manual therapy

Some published clinical guidelines on the management of OA recommended manual therapy as an adjunctive therapy to exercise for OA (National Institute of Health and Clinical Excellence (NICE) 2008; Royal Australian College of General Practitioners (RACGP) 2009); however, these recommendations were based on limited evidence since few studies had been published at that time (French et al 2011). A questionnaire survey of physiotherapists based on clinical recommendations from NICE (2008) revealed that exercise was used by 100% of therapists, often supplemented with electrotherapeutic modalities (66%), manual therapy (64%) and acupuncture (60%) (Walsh & Hurley 2009). In fact, the application of exercise therapy or manual therapy was more cost effective than usual care at policy-relevant values of willingness-to-pay from the perspective of both the health system and society (Pinto et al 2013). Nevertheless, there is a lack of clear description of what constitutes manual therapy for knee OA in the literature, since it includes joint-biased techniques, soft-tissue-biased interventions, therapeutic exercise, postural corrections, etc.

Few systematic reviews on the effectiveness of manual therapy in knee OA have been published. French et al (2011) concluded that there is inconclusive (silver level) evidence that manual therapy is effective for decreasing pain and function in individuals with knee OA. Brantingham et al (2012) also found moderate evidence (level B) for short-term and inconclusive evidence (level C) for long-term treatment of knee OA with manipulative therapy.

The reasoning for including manual therapies into the management of patients with knee OA is that some studies have demonstrated analgesic effects and modulation of spinal excitability with use of manual therapy techniques, with clinical outcomes of improved gait and functional ability (Courtney et al 2011). Moss et al (2007) observed a decrease of pressure pain sensitivity both at the medial joint line and at a distal non-painful site (ankle) following a 9-minute bout of accessory mobilization of the tibiofemoral joint in patients with knee OA. Courtney et al (2010) reported diminished flexor withdrawal reflex responses following the application of a 6-minute bout of oscillatory joint mobilization in patients with knee OA, indicating that analgesic effects of knee mobilization include modulation of segmental spinal cord excitability or descending inhibition from the brainstem. This hypothesis is supported by an animal study where knee joint mobilization reduced capsaicin-induced hyperalgesia at the ankle (Sluka & Wright 2001). The mobilization interventions performed in these studies consists of large-amplitude, accessory mobilization technique to the knee in the posterior-to-anterior direction (Fig. 43.3). In these studies, the knee joint mobilization was applied at a rate of approximately 45 oscillations per minute for 6–9 minutes (Moss et al 2007; Courtney et al 2010).

Another manual therapy generally used in the management of chronic pain is massage. Perlman et al (2006) found that 8 weeks of massage therapy significantly improved pain and function in the short term in patients with knee OA; however, the authors recognized that the massage therapy was not standardized. In a follow-up study, the same authors standardized a protocol of massage for knee OA of 60-minute session including effleurage, petrissage, tapotement, vibration, friction and skin rolling applied mainly to the lower extremities (Fig. 43.4), but also to the upper extremity and discretionally (Ali et al 2012). A recent randomized controlled trial confirmed that this protocol of massage was effective for reducing pain and increasing function in patients with knee OA and that the best results were observed in those subjects receiving a greater dose (i.e. more sessions of 60 minutes) of massage (Perlman et al 2012).

Nevertheless, it has been suggested that manual therapy, although not to be used as a stand-alone treatment, may be

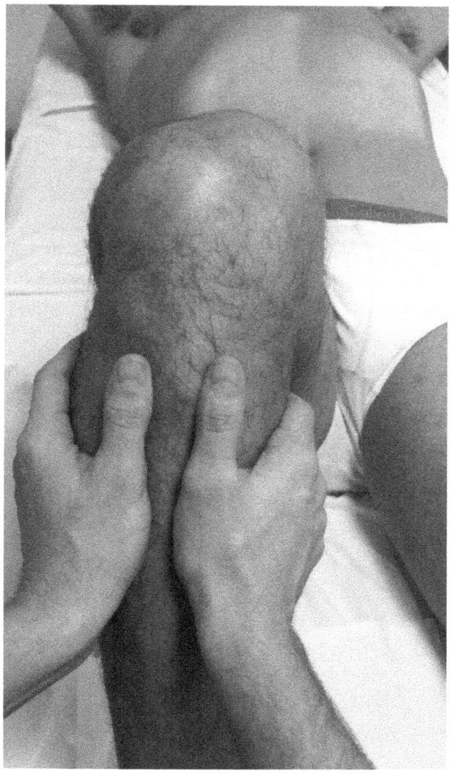

Figure 43.3 Posterior-to-anterior accessory mobilization technique applied on the tibiofemoral joint.

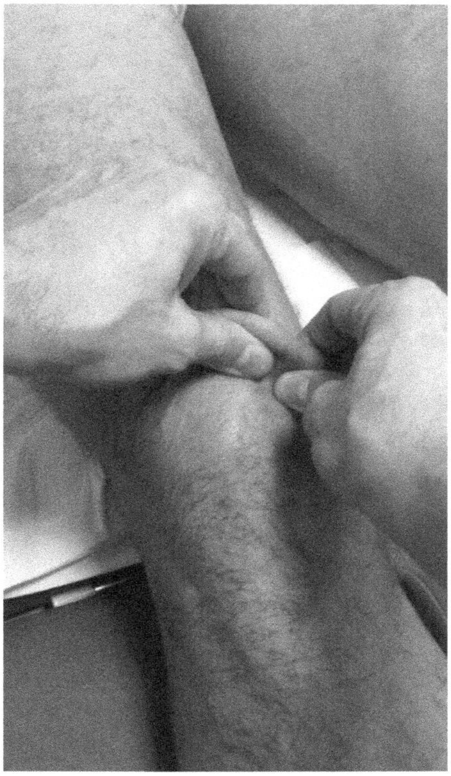

Figure 43.4 Skin rolling over the knee area as massage intervention.

beneficial for patients with knee OA (Page et al 2011). Deyle et al (2005) reported that adding some clinical visits for the application of manual therapy and supervised exercise adds greater symptomatic relief to home exercise programmes for knee OA. The systematic review conducted by Jansen et al (2011) found that exercise therapy plus manual mobilization showed a moderate effect size (0.69, 95% CI 0.42–0.96) on pain compared with the small effect sizes for strength training (0.38, 95% CI 0.23–0.54) or exercise therapy alone (0.34, 95% CI 0.19–0.49). In fact, a combination of exercise and manual therapy is recommended in the Dutch physiotherapy practice guideline in hip and knee OA (Peter et al 2011). However, these assumptions are not supported by a recent randomized controlled trial, which found that manual therapy was more effective than usual care at long-term follow-up (1 year) and was similarly effective as exercise for relief pain and to increase function in knee and hip OA, although there was no added benefit from a combination of manual therapy and exercise (Abbott et al 2013).

Inconsistency within the results of effectiveness of manual therapy or therapeutic exercise can be related to the fact that not all patients with knee OA will benefit from these interventions. In this line, Deyle et al (2012) suggested that the presence of patellofemoral pain, anterior cruciate ligament laxity and height >1.71 m were variables associated with non-successful outcomes after manual therapy in patients with knee OA (overall prognostic accuracy of 96%). It is therefore important that clinicians identify the clinical features of those patients with knee OA who will benefit from any particular intervention.

Acupuncture

Some clinical guidelines recommend acupuncture for individuals with knee OA, particularly for those patients with moderate-to-severe pain who are unable or unwilling to undergo knee arthroplasty (Zhang et al 2008; Hochberg et al 2012). However, other guidelines do not recommend its use (Jordan et al 2003; NICE 2008). A Cochrane review reported significant improvement in pain from acupuncture versus waiting list (SMD –0.96, 95% CI –1.19 to –0.72) or sham acupuncture (SMD –0.35, 95% CI –0.55 to –0.15) (Manheimer et al 2010); however, the authors of the review considered that the benefits were small, not clinically relevant and probably due, at least partially, to placebo effects from incomplete blinding. The most up-to-date meta-analysis concluded that acupuncture could be considered as a possible effective physical treatment for alleviating OA-related knee pain in the short term; however, much of the evidence in this area of research is of poor quality (Corbett et al 2013). In this meta-analysis, a sensitivity analysis of satisfactory- and good-quality studies revealed that most studies were of acupuncture (11 trials) or muscle-strengthening exercise (9 trials). The results showed that both interventions were significantly better than standard care treatment, with acupuncture being better than muscle-strengthening exercise (SMD 0.49, 95% CI 0.00–0.98).

Other therapeutic modalities

There are other therapeutic modalities that are currently used for knee OA including tai chi, neuromuscular electrical stimulation (NMES), transcutaneous electrical nerve stimulation (TENS) and short-wave diathermy (SWD).

A recent systematic review found moderate evidence for short-term improvement of OA-related pain, physical function and stiffness in patients with knee OA practising tai chi (Lauche et al 2013). The analysis revealed moderate evidence for short-term effects on pain (SMD –0.72, 95% CI –1.00 to –0.44), physical function (SMD –0.72, –1.01 to –0.44) and stiffness (SMD –0.59, –0.99 to –0.19). However, no evidence was found for long-term effects (Lauche et al 2013). The authors concluded that, assuming that tai chi is a short-term effective and safe intervention, it might be preliminarily recommended as an adjuvant treatment for individuals with knee OA; however, more high-quality randomized controlled trials are needed to confirm these results (Lauche et al 2013).

A recent systematic review showed moderate evidence in favour of NMES alone or combined with exercise for isometric quadriceps strengthening in elderly with OA (de Oliveira Melo et al 2013); however, the quality of the studies was low. In addition, variation in parameters (pulse frequencies, pulse duration, current type and time of application) makes it extremely difficult to reach any clinical conclusions. Despite this variation in parameters, the use of biphasic-pulsed currents of 100–400 ms delivered at stimulation frequencies ranging from 50 to 100 Hz at the highest tolerated current intensity are suggested as ideal for muscle strengthening, considering the individual variations within the population (de Oliveira Melo et al 2013).

The review conducted by Bjordal et al (2007a) concluded that TENS, electroacupuncture and low-level laser therapy were more effective than placebo for relieving pain in the management of knee OA. In a subgroup analysis of randomized clinical trials with assumed optimal doses, the short-term efficacy on pain was 22.2 mm (95% CI 18.1–26.3) for TENS and 24.2 mm (95% CI 17.3–31.3) for laser therapy (Bjordal et al 2007a). In contrast, the Cochrane review found little evidence for the use of TENS in individuals with knee OA (Rutjes et al 2009); this review observed a small SMD for pain intensity (SMD –0.07, 95% CI –0.46 to 0.32) in favour of TENS versus a control group.

Finally, the meta-analysis published by Laufer and Dar (2012) found small, significant effects on pain and muscle performance for SWD, but only when treatment evoked a local thermal sensation in the patient (SMD –0.334, 95% CI –0.643 to –0.0256).

Arthroplasty

Knee arthroplasty in one of the gold-standard surgical procedures for severe end-stage painful knee OA; however, approximately 13% of the patients after total knee replacement suffer from severe chronic postoperative pain (Harden et al 2003). For total hip replacement the range is 14–32% (Judge et al 2010). Further, 44% of fibromyalgia patients with significant signs of sensitization suffer from chronic postoperative pain after total knee replacement (D'Apuzzo et al 2012).

The possible importance of sensitization in total knee arthroplasty is supported by the findings that pre- and post-operative treatment of patients with OA with pregabalin reduces the development of chronic postoperative pain after knee replacement (Buvanendran et al 2010). In addition, as many patients with knee OA suffer from pain after total knee replacement, revisions are often performed even for unexplained pain. An early meta-analysis showed that the rate of revision of knee arthroplasty was 3.8% at a 4-year follow-up (Callahan et al 1994). Such revisions are associated with a low probability of success, often leaving the patients in more pain, with more impaired function (Brown et al 2006) and with more sensitization (Skou et al 2013).

Finally, it is important to consider that short-term and long-term outcomes after total knee replacement are related to the postoperative rehabilitation programmes that the patient will receive (Petterson et al 2009; Bade & Stevens-Lapsley 2011). The relevance of rehabilitation after total knee replacement is related to quadriceps weakness observed after the surgical procedure. In fact, quadriceps muscle strength is the strongest predictor of functional performance following total knee arthroplasty (Petterson et al 2009). Bade and Stevens-Lapsley (2012) suggested that use of NMES applied to the surgical limb's quadriceps muscle for the first 6 weeks following knee replacement improved the speed recovery of quadriceps muscle strength and led to long-term increases in strength and functional performance.

A recent systematic review identified four categories of postoperative rehabilitation interventions: (1) strengthening exercises, (2) aquatic therapy, (3) balance training and (4) clinical environment (e.g. group-based outpatient programme) (Pozzi et al 2013). This review concluded that outpatient rehabilitation under the supervision of trained physical therapists provides the best long-term outcome after total knee arthroplasty and should include individualized and progressive strengthening and functional exercises based on land-based or aquatic programmes (Pozzi et al 2013). In fact, the rehabilitation programmes should include higher intensity and progressive resistive exercises targeting all major muscle groups of the lower extremity (Bade & Stevens-Lapsley 2012). Nevertheless, information about the dose, frequency, intensity and duration of the rehabilitation protocols remains unknown.

Conclusion

Due to demographic and lifestyle changes, the prevalence of knee OA is forecast to increase dramatically in the future. Knee OA will eventually progress into a painful condition but, for the individual patient, no relationship can be established between joint damage and the intensity of the pain. In chronic OA pain patients, peripheral and spreading sensitization developed, causing the pain to be further facilitated. This can be mediated by factors such as localized inflammatory mechanisms, enhanced temporal integration, or impaired descending pain modulation. Due to safety issues and lack of long-term efficacy, there is a need to replace oral NSAIDs with new, better and safer pharmacological drugs. Several conservative interventions are claimed to be effective for knee OA, therapeutic exercise being the most effective one at both short- and long-term follow-up. Knee OA can develop into a disabling condition that requires total knee arthroplasty. Unfortunately many patients will experience chronic postoperative pain that is often further aggravated by repeated knee surgeries.

References

Abbott JH, Robertson MC, Chapple C, et al. 2013. Manual therapy, exercise therapy, or both, in addition to usual care, for osteoarthritis of the hip or knee: a randomized controlled trial. 1: clinical effectiveness. Osteoarthritis Cartilage 21: 525–534.

Adams T, Band-Entrup D, Kuhn S, et al. 2013. Physical therapy management of knee osteoarthritis in the middle-aged athlete. Sports Med Arthrosc 21: 2–10.

Ali A, Kahn J, Rosenberger L, et al. 2012. Development of a manualized protocol of massage therapy for clinical trials in osteoarthritis. Trials 13: 185.

Andriacchi TP, Mündermann A, Smith RL, et al. 2004. A framework for the in vivo pathomechanics of osteoarthritis at the knee. Ann Biomed Eng 32: 447–457.

Aranda-Villalobos P, Fernández-de-las-Peñas C, Navarro-Espigares JL, et al. 2013. Normalization of widespread pressure pain hypersensitivity in patients with hip osteoarthritis after total hip replacement is associated with clinical and functional improvements. Arthritis Rheum 65: 1262–1270.

Arendt-Nielsen L, Graven-Nielsen T. 2002. Deep tissue hyperalgesia. J Musculoskel Pain 10: 97–119.

Arendt-Nielsen L, Graven-Nielsen T. 2003. Central sensitization in fibromyalgia and other musculoskeletal disorders. Curr Pain Headache Rep 7: 355–361.

Arendt-Nielsen L, Yarnitsky D. 2009. Experimental and clinical applications of quantitative sensory testing applied to skin, muscles and viscera. J Pain 10: 556–572.

Arendt-Nielsen L, Hoeck HC, Karsdal MA, et al. 2009. Role of calcitonin in management of musculoskeletal pain. Rheumatol Rep 1: 39–42.

Arendt-Nielsen L, Graven-Nielsen T, Kidd B, et al. 2010a. From basic science to management of chronic musculoskeletal pain. In: Mogil JS (ed) An updated review: refresher course syllabus. Seattle: IASP Press, pp 73–83.

Arendt-Nielsen L, Nie H, Laursen MB, et al. 2010b. Sensitization in patients with painful knee osteoarthritis. Pain 149: 573–581.

Attur M, Krasnokutsky-Samuels S, Samuels J, et al. 2013. Prognostic biomarkers in osteoarthritis. Curr Opin Rheumatol 25: 136–144.

Atzeni F, Cazzola M, Benucci M, et al. 2011. Chronic widespread pain in the spectrum of rheumatological diseases. Best Pract Res Clin Rheumatol 25: 165–171.

Bade MJ, Stevens-Lapsley JE. 2011. Early high-intensity rehabilitation following total knee arthroplasty improves outcomes. J Orthop Sports Phys Ther 41: 932–941.

Bade MJ, Stevens-Lapsley JE. 2012. Restoration of physical function in patients following total knee arthroplasty: an update on rehabilitation practices. Curr Opin Rheumatol 24: 208–214.

Bajaj P, Bajaj P, Graven-Nielsen T, et al. 2001. Osteoarthritis and its association with muscle hyperalgesia: an experimental controlled study. Pain 93: 107–114.

Bartels EM, Lund H, Hagen KB, et al. 2007. Aquatic exercise for the treatment of knee and hip osteoarthritis. Cochrane Database Syst Rev 4: CD005523.

Barton CJ, Bonanno D, Levinger P, et al. 2010. Foot and ankle characteristics in patellofemoral pain syndrome: a case control and reliability study. J Orthop Sports Phys Ther 40: 286–296.

Beckwée D, Vaes P, Cnudde M, et al. 2013. Osteoarthritis of the knee: why does exercise work? A qualitative study of the literature. Ageing Res Rev 12: 226–236

Bedson J, Croft PR. 2008. The discordance between clinical and radiographic knee osteoarthritis: a systematic search and summary of the literature. BMC Musculoskelet Disord 9: 116–126.

Bellamy N, Campbell J, Robinson V, et al. 2005. Intraarticular corticosteroid for treatment of osteoarthritis. Cochrane Database Syst Rev 2: CD005328.

Bennell KL, Hinman RS. 2011. A review of the clinical evidence for exercise in osteoarthritis of the hip and knee. J Sci Med Sport 14: 4–9.

Bjordal JM, Ljunggren AE, Klovning A, et al. 2004. Non-steroidal anti-inflammatory drugs, including cyclo-oxygenase-2 inhibitors, in osteoarthritic knee pain: meta-analysis of randomised placebo controlled trials. BMJ 329: 1317.

Bjordal JM, Ljunggren AE, Klovning A, et al. 2005. NSAIDs, including coxibs, probably do more harm than good, and paracetamol is ineffective for hip OA. Ann Rheum Dis 64: 655–656.

Bjordal JM, Johnson MI, Lopes-Martins RA, et al. 2007a. Short-term efficacy of physical interventions in osteoarthritic knee pain. A systematic review and meta-analysis of randomised placebo-controlled trials. BMC Musculoskelet Disord 8: 51.

Bjordal JM, Klovning A, Ljunggren AE, et al. 2007b. Short-term efficacy of pharmacotherapeutic interventions in osteoarthritic knee pain: a meta-analysis of randomised placebo-controlled trials. Eur J Pain 11: 125–138.

Brantingham JW, Bonnefin D, Perle SM, et al. 2012. Manipulative therapy for lower extremity conditions: update of a literature review. J Manipulative Physiol Ther 35: 127–166.

Breivik H, Ljosaa TM, Stengaard-Pedersen K, et al. 2010. A 6-month, randomised, placebo-controlled evaluation of efficacy and tolerability of a low-dose 7-day buprenorphine transdermal patch in osteoarthritis patients naïve to potent opioids. Scand J Pain 1: 122–141.

Brown EC, Clarke HD, Scuderi GR. 2006. The painful total knee arthroplasty: diagnosis and management. Orthopedics 29: 129–136.

Buvanendran A, Kroin JS, Della Valle CJ, et al. 2010. Perioperative oral pregabalin reduces chronic pain after total knee arthroplasty: a prospective, randomized, controlled trial. Anesth Analg 110: 199–207.

Callahan CM, Drake BG, Heck DA, et al. 1994. Patient outcomes following tricompartmental total knee replacement. JAMA 271: 1349–1357.

Chevalier X, Goupille P, Beaulieu AD, et al. 2009. Intraarticular injection of anakinra in osteoarthritis of the knee: a multicenter, randomized, double-blind, placebo-controlled study. Arthritis Rheum 61: 344–352.

Citrome L, Weiss-Citrome A. 2012. A systematic review of duloxetine for osteoarthritic pain: what is the number needed to treat, number needed to harm, and likelihood to be helped or harmed? Postgrad Med 124: 83–93.

Clegg DO, Reda DJ, Harris CL, et al. 2006. Glucosamine, chondroitin sulfate, and the two in combination for painful knee osteoarthritis. N Engl J Med 354: 795–808.

Cohen SB, Proudman S, Kivitz AJ, et al. 2011. A randomized, double-blind study of AMG 108 (a fully human monoclonal antibody to IL-1R1) in patients with osteoarthritis of the knee. Arthritis Res Ther 13: R125.

Corbett MS, Rice SJ, Madurasinghe V, et al. 2013. Acupuncture and other physical treatments for the relief of pain due to osteoarthritis of the knee: network meta-analysis. Osteoarthritis Cartilage 21: 1290–1298.

Courtney CA, Lewek MD, Witte PO, et al. 2009. Heightened flexor withdrawal responses in subjects with knee osteoarthritis. J Pain 10: 1242–1249.

Courtney CA, Witte PO, Chmell SJ, et al. 2010. Heightened flexor withdrawal response in individuals with knee osteoarthritis is modulated by joint compression and joint mobilization. J Pain 11: 179–185.

Courtney CA, Clark JD, Duncombe AM, et al. 2011. Clinical presentation and manual therapy for lower quadrant musculoskeletal conditions. J Man Manip Ther 19: 212–222.

Curatolo M, Petersen-Felix S, Arendt-Nielsen L, et al. 2001. Central hypersensitivity in chronic pain after whiplash injury. Clin J Pain 17: 306–315.

Dam EB, Byrjalsen I, Arendt-Nielsen L, et al. 2011. Relationships between knee pain and osteoarthritis biomarkers based on systemic fluids and magnetic resonance imaging. J Musculoskelet Pain 19: 144–153.

D'Apuzzo MR, Cabanela ME, Trousdale RT, et al. 2012. Primary total knee arthroplasty in patients with fibromyalgia. Orthopedics 35: 175–178.

Davis MA, Ettinger WH, Neuhaus JM, et al. 1992. Correlates of knee pain among US adults with and without radiographic knee osteoarthritis. J Rheumatol 19: 1943–1949.

Deere KC, Clinch J, Holliday K, et al. 2012. Obesity is a risk factor for musculoskeletal pain in adolescents: findings from a population-based cohort. Pain 153: 1932–1938.

de Oliveira Melo M, Aragão FA, Vaz MA. 2013. Neuromuscular electrical stimulation for muscle strengthening in elderly with knee osteoarthritis – a systematic review. Complement Ther Clin Pract 19: 27–31.

Deyle GD, Allison SC, Matekel RL, et al. 2005. Physical therapy treatment effectiveness for osteoarthritis of the knee: a randomized comparison of supervised clinical exercise and manual therapy procedures versus a home exercise program. Phys Ther 85: 1301–1317.

Deyle GD, Gill NW, Allison SC, et al. 2012. Knee OA: which patients are unlikely to benefit from manual PT and exercise? J Fam Pract 61: E1–E8.

Felson DT. 2005. The sources of pain in knee osteoarthritis, Curr Opin Rheumatol 17: 624–628.

Fernandes L, Hagen KB, Bijlsma JW, et al. 2013. EULAR recommendations for the non-pharmacological core management of hip and knee osteoarthritis. Ann Rheum Dis 72: 1125–1135.

Fernández-de-las-Peñas C, Ge HY, Cuadrado ML, et al. 2008. Bilateral pressure pain sensitivity mapping of the temporalis muscle in chronic tension type headache. Headache 48: 1067–1075.

Fernández-de-las-Peñas C, Galán del Río F, Fernández Carnero J, et al. 2009. Bilateral widespread mechanical pain sensitivity in myofascial temporomandibular disorder: evidence of impairment in central nociceptive processing. J Pain 10: 1170–1178.

Ferraro KF, Booth TL. 1999. Age, body mass index, and functional illness. J Gerontol B Psychol Sci Soc Sci 54: S339–S348.

Ferrucci L, Penninx BWJH, Volpato S, et al. 2002. Change in muscle strength explains accelerated decline of physical function in older women with high interleukin-6 serum levels. J Am Geriatr Soc 50: 1947–1954.

Finan PH, Buenaver LF, Bounds SC, et al. 2013. Discordance between pain and radiographic severity in knee osteoarthritis: findings from quantitative sensory testing of central sensitization. Arthritis Rheum 65: 363–372.

Fransen M, McConnell S. 2008. Exercise for osteoarthritis of the knee. Cochrane Database Syst Rev 4: CD004376.

Fransen M, McConnell S. 2009. Land-based exercise for osteoarthritis of the knee: a meta-analysis of randomized controlled trials. J Rheumatol 36: 1109–1117.

French HP, Brennan A, White B, et al. 2011. Manual therapy for osteoarthritis of the hip or knee: a systematic review. Man Ther 16: 109–117.

Garnero P. 2001. Biochemical markers of bone remodeling. Ann Biol Clin 59: 298.

Goldring MB, Otero M. 2011. Inflammation in osteoarthritis. Curr Opin Rheumatol 23: 471–478.

Goldring MB, Otero M, Plumb DA, et al. 2011. Roles of inflammatory and anabolic cytokines in cartilage metabolism: signals and multiple effectors converge upon MMP-13 regulation in osteoarthritis. Eur Cell Mater 24: 202–220.

Golightly YM, Allen KD, Caine DJ. 2012. A comprehensive review of the effectiveness of different exercise programs for patients with osteoarthritis. Phys Sportsmed 40: 52–65.

Graven-Nielsen T, Wodehouse T, Langford RM, et al. 2012. Normalization of widespread hyperesthesia and facilitated spatial summation of deep-tissue pain in knee osteoarthritis patients after knee replacement. Arthritis Rheum 64: 2907–2916.

Hannan M, Felson D, Pincus T. 2000. Analysis of the discordance between radiographic changes and knee pain in osteoarthritis of the knee. J Rheumatol 27: 1513–1517.

Harden RN, Bruehl S, Stanos S, et al. 2003. Prospective examination of pain-related and psychological predictors of CRPS-like phenomena following total knee arthroplasty: a preliminary study. Pain 106: 393–400.

Hayami T, Pickarski M, Wesolowski GA, et al. 2004. The role of subchondral bone remodeling in osteoarthritis: reduction of cartilage degeneration and prevention of osteophyte formation by alendronate in the rat anterior cruciate ligament transection model. Arthritis Rheum 50: 1193–1206.

Henriksen M, Simonsen EB, Alkjær T, et al. 2006. Increased joint loads during walking: a consequence of pain relief in the knee osteoarthritis. Knee 13: 445–450.

Hochberg MC, Altman RD, April KT, et al. 2012. American College of Rheumatology 2012 recommendations for the use of nonpharmacologic and pharmacologic therapies in osteoarthritis of the hand, hip, and knee. Arthritis Care Res 64: 465–474.

Hochman JR, Davis AM, Elkayam J, et al. 2013. Neuropathic pain symptoms on the modified pain DETECT correlate with signs of central sensitization in knee osteoarthritis. Osteoarthritis Cartilage 21: 1236–1242.

Hunter DJ, Felson DT. 2006. Osteoarthritis. BMJ 332: 639–642.

Hurwitz DE, Sumner DR, Andriacchi TP, et al. 1998. Dynamic knee loads during gait predict proximal tibial bone distribution. J Biomech 31: 423–430.

Imamura M, Imamura ST, Kaziyama HH, et al. 2008. Impact of nervous system hyperalgesia on pain, disability, and quality of life in patients with knee osteoarthritis: a controlled analysis. Arthritis Rheum 59: 1424–1431.

Ishijima M, Watari T, Naito K, et al. 2011. Relationships between biomarkers of cartilage, bone, synovial metabolism and knee pain provide insights into the origins of pain in early knee osteoarthritis. Arthritis Res Ther 13: R22.

Jamtvedt G, Dahm K, Christie A, et al. 2008. Physical therapy interventions for patients with osteoarthritis of the knee: an overview of systematic reviews. Phys Ther 88: 123–136.

Jansen MJ, Viechtbauer W, Lenssen AF, et al. 2011. Strength training alone, exercise therapy alone, and exercise therapy with passive manual mobilisation each reduce pain and disability in people with knee osteoarthritis: a systematic review. J Physiother 57: 11–20.

Jordan KM, Arden NK, Doherty M, et al. 2003. EULAR Recommendations 2003: an evidence based approach to the management of knee osteoarthritis: report of a task force of the standing committee for international clinical studies including therapeutic trials (ESCISIT). Ann Rheum Dis 62: 1145–1155.

Judge A, Cooper C, Williams S, et al. 2010. Patient-reported outcomes one year after primary hip replacement in a European Collaborative Cohort. Arthritis Care Res 62: 480–488.

Karsdal MA, Leeming DJ, Dam EB, et al. 2008. Should subchondral bone turnover be targeted when treating osteoarthritis? Osteoarthritis Cartilage 16: 638–664.

Katz N, Borenstein DG, Birbara C, et al. 2011. Efficacy and safety of tanezumab in the treatment of chronic low back pain. Pain 152: 2248–2258
Kidd B. 2012. Mechanisms of pain in osteoarthritis. HSS J 8: 26–28.
Kumm J, Tamm A, Lintrop M, et al. 2013. The value of cartilage biomarkers in progressive knee osteoarthritis: cross-sectional and 6-year follow-up study in middle-aged subjects. Rheumatol Int 33: 903–911.
Langford R, McKenna F, Ratcliffe S, et al. 2006. Transdermal fentanyl for improvement of pain and functioning in osteoarthritis: a randomized, placebo-controlled trial. Arthritis Rheum 54: 1829–1837.
Lanyon P, O'Reilly S, Jones A, et al. 1998. Radiographic assessment of symptomatic knee osteoarthritis in the community: definitions and normal joint space. Ann Rheum Dis 57: 595–601.
Lauche R, Langhorst J, Dobos G, et al. 2013. A systematic review and meta-analysis of Tai Chi for osteoarthritis of the knee. Complement Ther Med 21: 396–406.
Laufer Y, Dar G. 2012. Effectiveness of thermal and athermal short-wave diathermy for the management of knee osteoarthritis: a systematic review and meta-analysis. Osteoarthritis Cartilage 20: 957–966.
Laursen RJ, Graven-Nielsen T, Jensen TS, et al. 1997. Referred pain is dependent on sensory input from the periphery: a psychophysical study. Eur J Pain 1: 261–269.
Laxafoss E, Jacobsen S, Gosvig KK, et al. 2010. Case definitions of knee osteoarthritis in 4,151 unselected subjects: relevance for epidemiological studies: The Copenhagen Osteoarthritis Study. Skeletal Radiol 39: 859–866.
Lee Y, Pai M, Brederson JD, et al. 2011. Monosodium iodoacetate-induced joint pain is associated with increased phosphorylation of mitogen activated protein kinases in the rat spinal cord. Mol Pain 7: 39.
Levinger P, Menz HB, Fotoohabadi MR, et al. 2010. Foot posture in people with medial compartment knee osteoarthritis. J Foot Ankle Res 3:1–8.
Lidtke RH, Muehleman C, Kwasny M, et al. 2010. Foot center of pressure and medial knee osteoarthritis. J Am Podiatr Med Assoc 100: 178–184.
Lin J, Zhang W, Jones A, et al. 2004. Efficacy of topical non-steroidal anti-inflammatory drugs in the treatment of osteoarthritis: meta-analysis of randomised controlled trials. BMJ 329: 324.
Livshits G, Zhai G, Hart DJ, et al. 2009. Interleukin-6 is a significant predictor of radiographic knee osteoarthritis: The Chingford Study. Arthritis Rheum 60: 2037–2045.
Lo GH, LaValley M, McAlindon T, et al. 2003. Intra-articular hyaluronic acid in treatment of knee osteoarthritis: a meta-analysis. JAMA 290: 3115–3121.
Magnano MD, Chakravarty EF, Broudy C, et al. 2007. A pilot study of tumor necrosis factor inhibition in erosive / inflammatory osteoarthritis of the hands. J Rheumatol 34: 1323–1327.
Malfait AM, Schnitzer TJ. 2013. Towards a mechanism-based approach to pain management in osteoarthritis. Nat Rev Rheumatol 9: 654–664.
Manheimer E, Cheng K, Linde K, et al. 2010. Acupuncture for peripheral joint osteoarthritis. Cochrane Database Syst Rev 1: CD001977
Mason L, Moore RA, Derry S, et al. 2004. Systematic review of topical capsaicin for the treatment of chronic pain. BMJ 328: 991.
Miller GD, Nicklas BJ, Loeser RF. 2008. Inflammatory biomarkers and physical function in older, obese adults with knee pain and self-reported osteoarthritis after intensive weight-loss therapy. J Am Geriatr Soc 56: 644–651.
Moss P, Sluka K, Wright A. 2007. The initial effects of knee joint mobilization on osteoarthritic hyperalgesia. Man Ther 12: 109–118.
Mourão AF, Blyth FM, Branco JC. 2010. Generalised musculoskeletal pain syndromes. Best Pract Res Clin Rheumatol 24: 829–840.
Mündermann A, Dyrby CO, Andriacchi TP. 2005. Secondary gait changes in patients with medial compartment knee osteoarthritis: increased load at the ankle, knee, and hip during walking. Arthritis Rheum 52: 2835–2844.
National Institute for Health and Clinical Excellence (NICE). 2008. Osteoarthritis: the care and management of osteoarthritis in adults. NICE Clin Guidel 59: 1–22.
Neogi T, Felson D, Niu J, et al. 2009. Association between radiographic features of knee osteoarthritis and pain: results from two cohort studies. BMJ 339: b2844.
Neogi T, Frey-Law L, Scholz J, et al. 2013. Sensitivity and sensitisation in relation to pain severity in knee osteoarthritis: trait or state? Ann Rheum Dis Dec 18. doi: 10.1136/annrheumdis-2013-204191. [Epub ahead of print.]
O'Neill S, Graven-Nielsen T, Manniche C, et al. 2009. Ultrasound guided, painful electrical stimulation of lumbar facet joint structures: an experimental model of acute low back pain. Pain 144: 76–83.
Page CJ, Hinman RS, Bennell KL. 2011. Physiotherapy management of knee osteoarthritis. Int J Rheum Dis 14: 145–151.
Pearle AD, Scanzello CR, George S, et al. 2007. Elevated high-sensitivity C-reactive protein levels are associated with local inflammatory findings in patients with osteoarthritis. Osteoarthritis Cartilage 15: 516–523.
Peat G, McCarney R, Croft P. 2001. Knee pain and osteoarthritis in older adults: a review of community burden and current use of primary health care. Ann Rheum Dis 60: 91–97.
Pelletier JP, Martel-Pelletier J, Abramson SB. 2001. Osteoarthritis, an inflammatory disease: potential implication for the selection of new therapeutic targets. Arthritis Rheum 44: 1237–1247.
Penninx BWJH, Abbas H, Ambrosius W, et al. 2004. Inflammatory markers and physical function among older adults with knee osteoarthritis. J Rheumatol 31: 2027–2031.
Perlman AI, Sabina A, Williams AL, et al. 2006. Massage therapy for osteoarthritis of the knee: a randomized controlled trial. Arch Intern Med 166: 2533–2538.
Perlman AI, Ali A, Njike VY, et al. 2012. Massage therapy for osteoarthritis of the knee: a randomized dose-finding trial. PLoS One 7: e30248.
Peter WF, Jansen MJ, Hurkmans EJ, et al. 2011. Physiotherapy in hip and knee osteoarthritis: development of a practice guideline concerning initial assessment, treatment and evaluation. Acta Rheumatol Port 36: 268–281.
Petterson SC, Mizner RL, Stevens JE, et al. 2009. Improved function from progressive strengthening interventions after total knee arthroplasty: a randomized clinical trial with an imbedded prospective cohort. Arthritis Rheum 61: 174–183.
Pinto D, Robertson MC, Abbott JH, et al. 2013. Manual therapy, exercise therapy, or both, in addition to usual care, for osteoarthritis of the hip or knee. 2: economic evaluation alongside a randomized controlled trial. Osteoarthritis Cartilage 21: 1504–1513.
Pozzi F, Snyder-Mackler L, Zeni J. 2013. Physical exercise after knee arthroplasty: a systematic review of controlled trials. Eur J Phys Rehabil Med 49(6):877–892.
Rahman W, Bauer CS, Bannister K, et al. 2009. Descending serotonergic facilitation and the antinociceptive effects of pregabalin in a rat model of osteoarthritic pain. Mol Pain 5: 45.
Read SJ, Dray A. 2008. Osteoarthritic pain: a review of current, theoretical and emerging therapeutics. Expert Opin Investig Drugs 17: 619–640.
Reilly K, Barker K, Shamley D, et al. 2009. The role of foot and ankle assessment of patients with lower limb osteoarthritis. Physiother 95: 164–169.
Roddy E, Zhang W, Doherty M, et al. 2005. Evidence-based recommendations for the role of exercise in the management of osteoarthritis of the hip or knee: the MOVE consensus. Rheumatology 44: 67–73.
Roos EM, Juhl CB. 2012. Osteoarthritis 2012 year in review: rehabilitation and outcomes. Osteoarthritis Cartilage 20: 1477–1483.
Royal Australian College of General Practitioners (RACGP). 2009. Guideline for the nonsurgical management of hip and knee osteoarthritis. Online. Available: http://www.racgp.org.au/your-practice/guidelines/musculoskeletal/hipandkneeosteoarthritis/.
Rutjes AW, Nüesch E, Sterchi R, et al. 2009. Transcutaneous electrostimulation for osteoarthritis of the knee. Cochrane Database Syst Rev 4: CD002823.
Saetan N, Honsawek S, Tanavalee A, et al. 2011. Association of plasma and synovial fluid interferon-γ inducible protein-10 with radiographic severity in knee osteoarthritis. Clin Biochem 44: 1218–1222.
Sanga P, Katz N, Polverejan E, et al. 2013. Efficacy, safety, and tolerability of fulranumab, an anti-nerve growth factor antibody, in the treatment of patients with moderate to severe osteoarthritis pain. Pain 154: 1910–1919.
Sarzi-Puttini P, Atzeni F, Mease PJ. 2011. Chronic widespread pain: from peripheral to central evolution. Best Pract Res Clin Rheumatol 25: 133–139.
Scanzello CR, Umoh E, Pessler F, et al. 2009. Local cytokine profiles in knee osteoarthritis: elevated synovial fluid interleukin-15 differentiates early from end-stage disease. Osteoarthritis Cartilage 17: 1040–1048.
Scanzello CR, McKeon B, Swaim BH, et al. 2011. Synovial inflammation in patients undergoing arthroscopic meniscectomy: molecular characterization and relationship to symptoms. Arthritis Rheum 63: 391–400.
Segal NA. 2012. Bracing and orthoses: a review of efficacy and mechanical effects for tibiofemoral osteoarthritis. PM R 4: S89–S96.
Seidel MF, Lane NE. 2012. Control of arthritis pain with anti-nerve-growth factor: risk and benefit. Curr Rheumatol Rep 14: 583–588.
Skou ST, Graven-Nielsen T, Rasmussen S, et al. 2013. Widespread sensitization in patients with chronic pain after revision total knee arthroplasty. Pain 154: 1588–1594.
Sluka K, Wright A. 2001. Knee joint mobilisation reduces secondary mechanical hyperalgesia induced by capsaicin injection into the ankle joint. Eur J Pain 5: 81–87.
Smith TO, King JJ, Hing CB. 2012. The effectiveness of proprioceptive-based exercise for osteoarthritis of the knee: a systematic review and meta-analysis. Rheumatol Int 32: 3339–3351.

Sörensen J, Graven-Nielsen T, Henrikson KG, et al. 1998. Hyperexcitability in fibromyalgia. J Rheumatol 25: 152–155.
Stannus O, Jones G, Cicuttini F, et al. 2010. Circulating levels of IL-6 and TNF-α are associated with knee radiographic osteoarthritis and knee cartilage loss in older adults. Osteoarthritis Cartilage 18: 1441–1447.
Suokas AK, Walsh DA, McWilliams DF, et al. 2012. Quantitative sensory testing in painful osteoarthritis: a systematic review and meta-analysis. Osteoarthritis Cartilage 20: 1075–1085.
Suri S, Gill SE, Massena de CS, et al. 2007. Neurovascular invasion at the osteochondral junction and in osteophytes in osteoarthritis. Ann Rheum Dis 66: 1423–1428.
Tanaka R, Ozawa J, Kito N, et al. 2013. Efficacy of strengthening or aerobic exercise on pain relief in people with knee osteoarthritis: a systematic review and meta-analysis of randomized controlled trials. Clin Rehabil 27: 1059–1071.
Thompson LR, Boudreau R, Newman AB, et al. 2010. The association of osteoarthritis risk factors with localized, regional and diffuse knee pain. Osteoarthritis Cartilage 18: 1244–1249.
Uthman OA, van der Windt DA, Jordan JL, et al. 2013. Exercise for lower limb osteoarthritis: systematic review incorporating trial sequential analysis and network meta-analysis. BMJ 347: f5555.
Van Saase J, Van Romunde L, Cats A, et al. 1989. Epidemiology of osteoarthritis: Zoetermeer survey. Comparison of radiological osteoarthritis in a Dutch population with that in 10 other populations. Ann Rheum Dis 48: 271–280.
Vigushin DM, Pepys MB, Hawkins PN. 1993. Metabolic and scintigraphic studies of radioiodinated human C-reactive protein in health and disease. J Clin Invest 91: 1351–1357.
Walsh NE, Hurley MV. 2009. Evidence based guidelines and current practice for physiotherapy management of knee osteoarthritis. Musculoskeletal Care 7: 45–56.
Xu YM, Ge HY, Arendt-Nielsen L. 2010. Sustained nociceptive mechanical stimulation of latent myofascial trigger point induces central sensitization in healthy subjects. J Pain 11: 1348–1355.
Zhang W, Moskowitz RW, Nuki G, et al. 2008. OARSI recommendations for the management of hip and knee osteoarthritis, part II: OARSI evidence-based, expert consensus guidelines. Osteoarthritis Cartilage 16: 137–162.

Chapter 44

Patellofemoral Pain Syndrome

Johnson McEvoy, Caroline MacManus

CHAPTER CONTENTS

Introduction	493
Anatomy of the patellofemoral joint	493
Patellofemoral pain	496
Pathophysiology of patellofemoral pain	498
Risk factors for patellofemoral pain	498
Remote and local factors in patellofemoral pain	499
Clinical assessment	499
Conservative treatment	502
Multimodal treatment	503
Balance training and neuromuscular control	506
Soft tissue massage and trigger point therapy	507
Trigger point dry needling and botulinum toxin injection	508
Selected electrophysical modalities	509
In-shoe orthoses	510
Conclusion	510

Introduction

Knee pain is common, accounting for approximately one-third of musculoskeletal presentations seen in primary care (Calmbach & Hutchens 2003). The 1-year prevalence of knee pain in athletes has been estimated to be as high as 54% (Rosenblatt et al 1983). In a study of adult recreational athletes (n=1089), knee pain accounted for the most common sports-related injury, at almost 25%, and was more common than shoulder, low back or ankle injuries, each of which accounts for approximately 10% of injuries (Ralph & Garrick 1996). Estimates of knee injury rates per 1000 hours of recreational sport are approximately 4.4 and 10.7 in non-running and running sports respectively (Ralph & Garrick 1996). The incidence of running-related knee injuries is estimated to be between 7.2% and 50%, and it is the most likely running-related injury (van Gent et al 2007). A 12-month study of athletes presenting to an Australian sports medicine centre (n=2429) reported knee injuries to be the most common condition (27.5%) (Baquie & Brukner 1997). Patellofemoral pain (PFP) was the most frequently presenting sports injury, followed by lumbar and shoulder rotator cuff conditions (Baquie & Brukner 1997). PFP has been estimated to affect 7–9% of the general population (Post 2005). (See Ch 2 for epidemiology.)

Anterior knee pain is a common subset of knee pain disorders and is a term used to group together a number of different potential conditions related to the anterior knee (Post 2005). The term **patellofemoral pain** is the preferred 'umbrella' term to describe pain in and around the patella in the absence of other pathologies (Crossley et al 2009), whereas the term **patellofemoral pain syndrome** (PFPS) is used in physical rehabilitation to describe pain or dysfunction of the patellofemoral joint (PFJ). Patellar nomenclature is varied and controversial, and consensus on definitions is lacking (Grelsamer 2005). This chapter offers a clinically focused evidenced-informed brief overview of PFP in terms of anatomy, pathophysiology, assessment and common physical treatments.

Anatomy of the Patellofemoral Joint

The patella is the largest sesamoid bone in the body and is embedded in the quadriceps tendon on the anterior knee (Williams et al 1995). The patella is an inverted triangular shaped bone with an anterior and posterior surface and a distal pointed apex. The patella articulates with the femoral condyles and forms the PFJ. The intrinsic bony structure of the patella consists of uniform dense trabecular bone covered by a thin lamina. The trabecular pattern is parallel on the anterior surface and radial on the articular surface (Williams et al 1995). Ossification develops from one to three centres between the third and sixth years of age (Prakask et al 1979).

The convex anterior surface is covered by the quadriceps tendon and prepatellar bursa and skin. Blood vessels pierce the anterior surface to supply the bone via vascular foramina (Williams et al 1995; Nemschak & Pretterklieber 2012). The thick superior border provides attachments for the rectus femoris and vastus intermedius muscles. The medial and lateral retinacula insert onto the medial and lateral borders of the patella bone. The retinacula are bands of fibrous tissue that assist in stabilizing the patella as part of the PFJ. The medial retinaculum expands from the vastus medialis muscle / tendon, the medial knee capsule and some transverse fibres of the medial femoral epicondyle. The lateral retinaculum arises from the vastus lateralis muscle / tendon, the lateral knee capsule and receives some expansion of fibres from the iliotibial tract laterally. Distally the patellar ligament arises from the apex of the patella and, in reality, it is a continuation of the quadriceps tendon and inserts into the tibial tuberosity of the tibia. The posterior surface articulates as part of the PFJ (Williams et al 1995). It has a smooth articular cartilage surface that contacts the femoral condyles with medial and lateral patellar facets, which are separated by a smooth ridge. The lateral facet is larger than the medial facet. Medial to the medial facet is a small semilunar area, which is termed the 'odd facet' (Goodfellow et al 1976; Williams et al 1995). The proximal attachment of the patellar ligament arises from the apex of the patella.

The patellofemoral joint is a synovial joint that makes up part of the knee joint (Williams et al 1995). The articular surface of the patella is adapted to fit the articular surfaces of the medial and lateral femoral condyles. The synovial membrane of the knee is the most extensive in the body. It extends above the patella to form the suprapatellar bursa between the quadriceps femoris and shaft of the femur; extending under the vastus medially and laterally and distal to the patella it lies underneath the infrapatellar fat pad (Fig. 44.1).

The arterial supply of the knee joint includes the descending genicular branches of the femoral artery, superior, middle and inferior genicular branches of the popliteal artery, anterior and posterior recurrent branches of the anterior tibial artery, the circumflex fibular artery and the descending branch of the lateral circumflex femoral artery (Williams et al 1995). The nerve supply to the knee includes the femoral, obturator, tibial and common peroneal nerves (Williams et al 1995).

The open-packed position of the PFJ is extension and the close-packed one is flexion (Houglum 2005). The patella increases the moment arm of the quadriceps and patellar complex (i.e. the bony congruence, muscles and retinacula) maintaining the quadriceps tendon in alignment (Oatis 2004; Houglum 2005). During knee flexion, the patella glides distally 5–7 cm (Hehne 1990). The PFJ can be subjected to loads estimated to be 0.5 to 8 times the body weight or more (Mathews et al 1977). As an example of functional activity, the PFJ loadings for walking, stair climbing and squatting are 0.5, 3.3 and 7.6 times the body weight respectively (Reilly & Martens 1972). For the straight leg raise exercise in full extension, the load estimate is 0.5 times the body weight (Reilly & Martens 1972). Proper movement of the PFJ is important for normal function of the knee, and an understanding of PFJ motion is clinically important and has been eloquently reviewed (Grelsamer & Klein 1998; Oatis 2004; Houglum 2005; Crossley et al 2009).

In full extension the patella has little contact with the femur and is therefore relatively mobile, and with relaxation the quadriceps muscle is restrained by the passive resistance of the retinacula (Grelsamer & Klein 1998; Oatis 2004). During initial flexion the patella enters the femoral trochlea and mobility becomes restricted. The area of contact on the patella increases and moves proximally as the knee flexes (Oatis 2004). Normal patellar motion is characterized by medial movement from 45° to 18° and lateral displacement from 18° to 0° at full extension (Powers et al 1998). Abnormal stresses during these movements, from local and remote kinetic chain influences, may lead to PFP (Oatis 2004; Crossley et al 2009; McConnell 2009).

Stability of the PFJ is dependent on passive and dynamic restraints. The quadriceps muscles attach to the patella and act to move and stabilize the patella locally on the femur, with the vastus medialis oblique (VMO) being an important influence on medial PFJ stability (Oatis 2004; Kendall et al 2005) (Fig. 44.2). The femur is influenced, stabilized and moved by many muscles, notably the hip abductors (gluteus medius, gluteus minimus and tensor fasciae latae) and the external rotators of the hip joint (piriformis, gemellus superior, obturator internus, gemellus inferior, obturator externus and quadratus femoris). These muscles play an important role in stability and control of the hip (Oatis 2004; Kendall et al 2005). Hip abductor and external rotator weakness are associated with PFP and therefore are of importance in rehabilitation (Lankhorst et al 2013).

The medial–lateral position of the patella is assessed in full extension and has been studied by magnetic resonance imaging (MRI) (Powers et al 1999). Clinical assessment

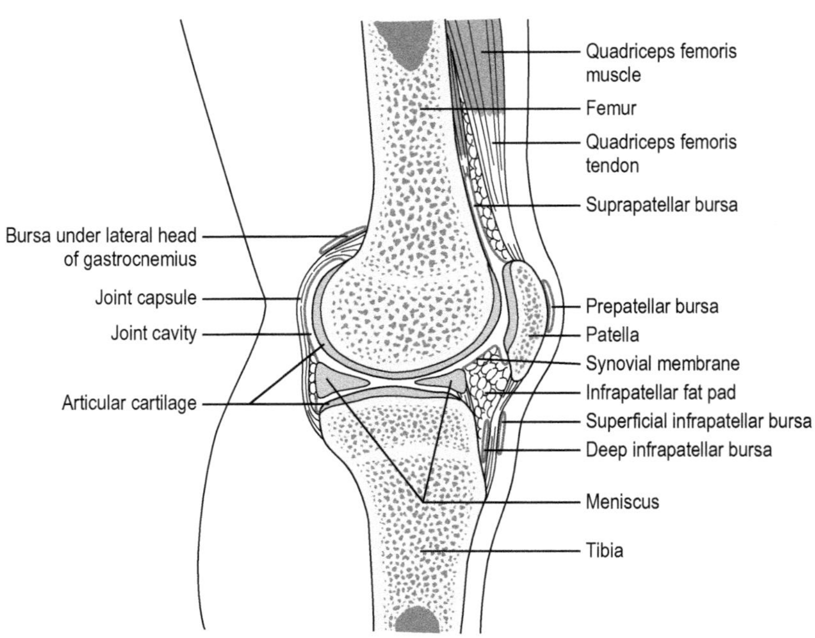

Figure 44.1 Lateral view of the knee.

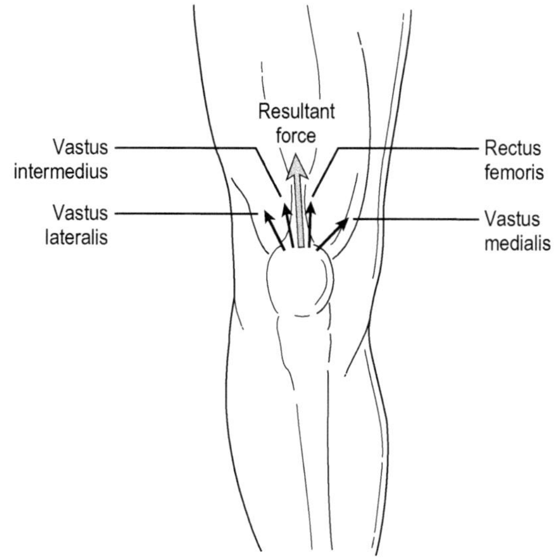

Figure 44.2 Muscular forces around the patella.

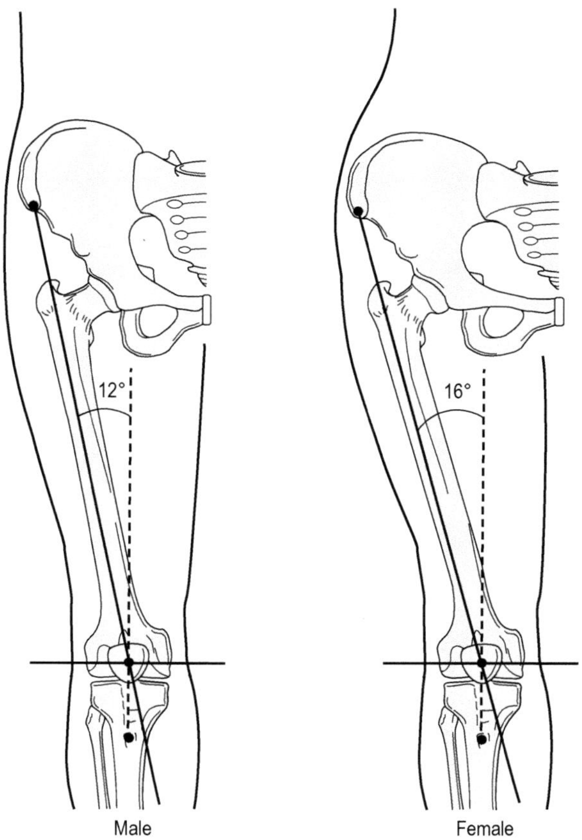

Figure 44.3 Q-angle of the knee. Comparison between male and female.

overestimates the medial–lateral position by more than twofold compared with MRI. Excessive medial, or more commonly lateral, position of the patella is termed medial or lateral tracking (Oatis 2004). The proximal–distal position of the patella is the ratio of the patellar tendon length and the length of the patella. This can be measured on lateral knee X-ray or MRI (Shabshin et al 2004). Patella *alta* (high) is determined as a ratio >1.5 and patella *baja* (low) as <0.74 (Shabshin et al 2004). Both patella *alta* and *baja* are related to PFP and abnormal patellar tracking, whereas patella *baja* is also associated with recurrent dislocations (Holmes & Clancy 1998; Oatis 2004).

The quadriceps angle (Q-angle) is the angle formed by a line from the anterior superior iliac spine to the middle patella and a line from the mid-patella to the tibial tuberosity (Houglum 2005). The Q-angle is often associated with PFP (Smith et al 2008). There is some disagreement as to the reliability and validity of the clinical measurement of the Q-angle (Smith et al 2008). Despite this controversy, the Q-angle is associated with PFP, but is not currently confirmed as a risk factor for future development (Lankhorst et al 2012, 2013). The Q-angle can vary, with estimates ranging from 10° to 15°, with a reported average of 12.73°, and with small variance from the left to the right side. The Q-angle is usually higher in females than in males (Fig. 44.3) and is an average of 20° in PFP patients (Aglietti et al 1983; Houglum 2005; Raveendranath et al 2011). The Q-angle can change from non-weight-bearing to weight-bearing owing to, for example, tibial rotation, pronation and weakness of the VMO especially (Houglum 2005), or possibly joint laxity. It is therefore important to assess the functional kinetic chain and responses to weight-bearing with such tests as the unilateral single-leg knee bend (Fig. 44.4), bilateral and unilateral knee-drop tests.

The patellar tilt angle (PT-angle) is the angle between a line drawn through the largest width of the patella and a line touching the most anterior surfaces of the medial and lateral femoral condyles (Fig. 44.5) and is associated with PFP (Oatis 2004; Lankhorst et al 2013). Assessment of the PT-angle by an experienced examiner has been shown to have strong criterion validity and intra-tester reliability (McEwan et al 2007). Normal individuals have a PT-angle of between 0° and 20° when moving from 0° to 60° of knee flexion (Pinar et al 1994). Quadriceps muscle contraction causes a slight increase in PT-angle, but this is not significant (Pinar et al 1994). In normal subjects, a clinically determined laterally tilted patella correlates well with MRI determination in extension (McEwan et al 2007). Subjects with a PT-angle <5° on clinical examination were assessed as having no degree of patellar tilt (McEwan et al 2007). Ultrasound imaging and MRI are reliable methods of assessing patellar position. Ultrasound has the added advantage of easier access and lower cost (Herrington et al 2006a). Taping, manual therapy and quadriceps muscle strengthening aim to influence PT-angle for therapeutic benefit.

The sulcus angle (S-angle) is the angle formed by lines drawn from the deepest point of the femoral sulcus to the highest point on the medial and lateral femoral condyles (Oatis 2004). Reported S-angle values range from 125° to 155°, with similar measurements reported in men and women (Oatis 2004). A shallow S-angle is associated with recurrent subluxation (Aglietti et al 1983). S-angle can be measured from radiographs.

The congruence angle (C-angle) is formed by a line bisecting the S-angle and a line from the base of the sulcus angle to the most prominent peak of the patellar ridge (Oatis 2004). The average C-angle has been reported as –8°, but is –2° in PFP patients and +16° in recurrent subluxation patients (Aglietti et al 1983). The C-angle is a determinant of the how well the patella sits into the femoral trochlear notch (Oatis 2004).

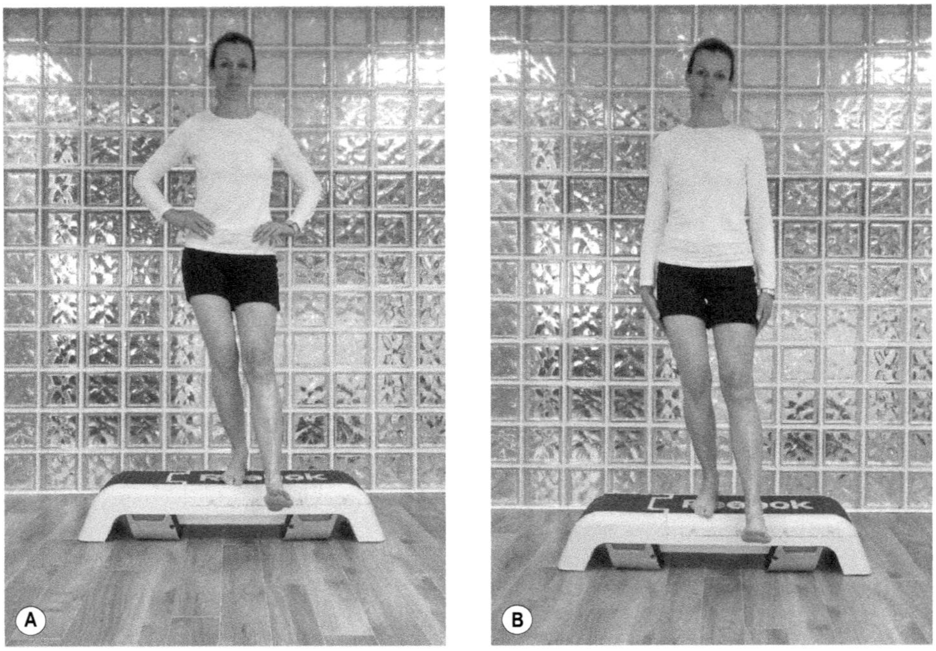

Figure 44.4 Dynamic Q-angle. step-down test or single-leg squat: (**A**) Positive test with valgus knee position with increased Q-angle during dynamic test. (**B**) Negative test with controlled and normal dynamic Q-angle. This can also be used as an exercise when appropriate.

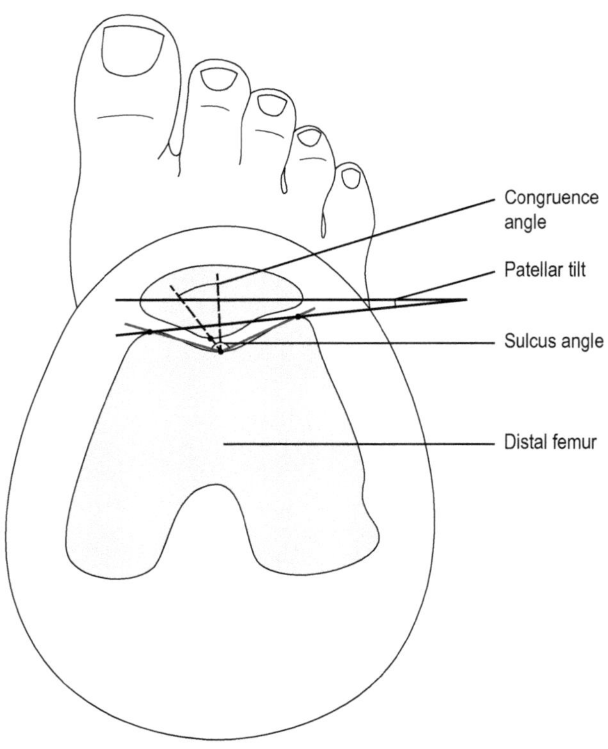

Figure 44.5 Patella angles. (See text for explanation of each angle.)

Patellofemoral Pain

PFP can arise from many structures including intra-articular or periarticular tissues – for example, the patella bone, retinacula, muscles, capsule, synovial membrane, infrapatellar fat pad, etc. (Houglum 2005; Crossley et al 2009). Sensitization of type IV receptor nerve endings may lead to the experience of pain (Wyke 1967; Warmerdam 1999). Patellar articular cartilage is not a source of pain (Dye et al 1998), but may indirectly affect other structures such as the synovial membrane owing to chemical or mechanical sensitization (Insall et al 1976; Warmerdam 1999; Fulkerson 2002; Crossley et al 2009).

Ultrasound imaging of the lateral retinaculum of PFP patients ($n=10$) and controls ($n=10$) revealed a trend towards a larger thickness and neovascularization as measured by colour Doppler ultrasound (Schoots et al 2013); the mean and standard deviation of PFP patients versus controls were 4.0 (1.4 mm, 95% CI 1.2–6.8) and 3.7 (0.8 mm, 95% CI 2.1–5.3) respectively, although this was not statistically significant. In the same study, Doppler ultrasound was positive in four out of ten of the PFP patients, but in none of the controls. The increased lateral retinaculum thickness was present in both knees of PFP patients compared with controls. Further research is required to identify the role of the lateral retinaculum in PFP.

In a novel approach, neurosensory mapping of the internal structures of the knee was carried out without intra-articular anaesthesia on the conscious senior author of the study (Dye et al 1998). Both asymptomatic knees were inspected arthroscopically with only local skin anaesthesia. Pressure was applied by way of a standard straight arthroscopic probe with a distal tip size of 1 × 3 mm attached to a spring-loaded device designed to measure force. Pain was graded 0–4 (no sensation to severe pain) and localized with A or B for accurate or poor spatial localization respectively. Results ranged from no sensation (0) on the patellar articular cartilage to 4A on the anterior synovial membrane, capsule and fat pad (Table 44.1). It must be noted that this study described the pain response in one subject of both asymptomatic knees only.

Referred pain from other structures should be considered in differential diagnosis such as low back, pelvic girdle, hip joint and structures, pubic and adductor areas, and also

Table 44.1 Neurosensory mapping of the human knee

Structure tested	Result*	Force (grams)	Summary
Patellar articular cartilage medial facet	0	500	No sensation
Patellar articular cartilage lateral facet	0	500	No sensation
Patellar articular cartilage central ridge**	0	500	No sensation
Patellar articular cartilage odd facet	1B	500	Non-painful awareness poorly localized
Menisci (medial and lateral) inner rims	1B	500	Non painful awareness poorly localized
Femoral condyles articular cartilage surface	1B–2B	500	Non-painful to slight discomfort poorly localized
Trochlea	1B–2B	500	Non-painful to slight discomfort poorly localized
Tibial plateau	1B–2B	500	Non-painful to slight discomfort poorly localized
ACL mid-region	1B–2B	500	Non-painful to slight discomfort poorly localized
PCL mid-region	1B–2B	500	Non-painful to slight discomfort poorly localized
Menisci (medial and lateral) capsular margin	2B–3B	300–500	Slight discomfort to moderate discomfort poorly localized
Menisci (medial and lateral) anterior/posterior horn	2B–3B	300–500	Slight discomfort to moderate discomfort poorly localized
ACL tibial and femoral ends	3B–4B	500	Moderate discomfort to servere pain poorly localised
PCL tibial and femoral ends	3B–4B	500	Moderate discomfort to servere pain poorly localized
Medial and lateral retinacula	3A–4A	<100	Moderate discomfort to severe pain accurately localized
Suprapatellar pouch synovial membrane	3A–4A	<100	Moderate discomfort to severe pain accurately localized
Capsule	3A–4A	<100	Moderate discomfort to severe pain accurately localized
Fat pad	4A		Severe pain accurately localized

*0: no sensation; 1: non-painful awareness; 2: slight discomfort; 3: moderate discomfort; 4: severe pain; A: accurate localization; B: poor localization.
**Central ridge asymptomatic grade II or III chondromalacia was identified on both patellas.
(Modified from Dye et al 1998.)

myofascial trigger points (TrPs), which are common in knee pain and other musculoskeletal conditions (Crossley et al 2009). (Readers are referred to other relevant chapters.)

Muscles that refer to the anterior knee area include, but are not limited to, the quadriceps, gluteus minimus and adductors amongst others (Travell & Rinzler 1952; Travell & Simons 1992; Dejung et al 2003). Reliable identification of TrPs depends on systematic palpation of accessible muscles by examiners who are knowledgeable and trained (McEvoy & Huijbregts 2011). (See Ch 59 for a review of myofascial pain in the lower extremity musculature.)

Additionally, several local knee conditions need also to be considered – such as osteoarthritis, rheumatoid and connective tissue disorders, bony lesions such as stress fractures, osteochondritis dissecans, bipartite patella, Perthes' disease and tumours, which though not common are more likely in the young (Goodman et al 2003; Crossley et al 2009; Boissonnault 2010).

Clinical classification systems for PFP have been presented, two of note being published simultaneously: those by Wilk et al (1998) and Holmes and Clancy (1998). Readers are encouraged to review these classification systems (available free at www.jospt.org). Holmes and Clancy (1998) selected a triclassification system: patellofemoral instability, patellofemoral pain with malalignment and patellofemoral pain without malalignment. In contrast, but with some similarities, Wilk et al (1998) opted for a wider eight-system classification (Table 44.2): patellar compression syndromes, patellar instability, biomechanical dysfunction, direct patellar trauma, soft tissue lesions, overuse syndromes, osteochondritis diseases and neurological disorders. Special consideration should be given to the child or adolescent patient owing to age-related conditions such as bipartite patella pain, growth plate issues of the hip and knee and Osgood–Schlatter disease, etc. (Holmes & Clancy 1998).

For clinicians, classification of PFP can assist in planning a treatment strategy pertinent to the needs of the individual patient identified from the assessment. Accuracy of the working diagnosis / classification is important for guiding safe and effective rehabilitation. It is therefore important to carry out a comprehensive assessment on each patient to guide the plan of care (see Clinical Assessment below).

Symptoms of PFP include pain around the patella or surrounding area, swelling, crepitus, catching of the knee and giving way (which may suggest patellar instability / subluxation). Pain can be mild to severe and can be local or diffuse. Behaviour of the symptoms often includes aggravation with loading of the joint such as stairs, knee bending, especially beyond 20–30° as the PFJ starts articulating, and sitting, especially with knee flexion. PFP is not a self-limiting condition and efforts to correct kinetic chain factors, both local and remote, are important (McConnell 2009).

Table 44.2 **Classification systems of patellofemoral pain disorders**

Holmes & Clancy (1998)	Wilk et al (1998)
1. Patellofemoral instability 2. Patellofemoral pain with malalignment 3. Patellofemoral pain without malalignment	1. Patellar compression syndromes 2. Patellar instability 3. Biomechanical dysfunction 4. Direct patellar trauma 5. Soft tissue lesions 6. Overuse syndromes 7. Osteochondritis diseases 8. Neurological disorders Special consideration for children or adolescents: Bipartite patella Growth plates (hip, knee) Osgood–Schlatter's

Pathophysiology of Patellofemoral Pain

The pathophysiology of PFP is not well understood and the general consensus is that the aetiology is multifactorial (Powers et al 2012). Tissue overload and stress may be induced by biomechanical alterations from local and remote areas, and passive and active kinetic chain influences (Crossley et al 2009). Such forces include joint shearing. There is a general consensus that pathomechanics contributes to pain and dysfunction of the PFJ and surrounding tissues via instability or malalignment (Holmes & Clancy 1998; Wilk et al 1998; Oatis 2004; Dye 2005; Houglum 2005; Crossley et al 2009). These stresses may induce symptomatic loss of tissue homeostasis (Dye 2005). As an example, PFJ pain has been associated with a change in PT-angle (Witonski & Goraj 1999) and increases in the C- and S-angles (Aglietti et al 1983), which is also linked with subluxations (Aglietti et al 1983). Pathomechanical stress on tissues, such as identified by Dye et al (1998) (see Table 44.1), may activate and sensitize group IV nociceptive nerve endings, resulting in altered motor patterning and dysfunction related to ongoing pain stimulus. This may induce peripheral and central sensitization and lead to hyperalgesia and allodynia.

Ischaemia has been proposed as a potential PFJ pain mechanism by inducing loss of tissue homeostasis (Selfe et al 2003; Dye 2005). Similar homeostatic mechanisms have been reported in muscle, tendon, bone and cartilage (Naslund et al 2007) and cardiac ischaemia, a well-recognized cause of cardiac pain. In chondromalacia patellae and knee osteoarthritis there is evidence of capillary ingrowth into the osteochondral junction and cartilage with coexisting increase of nerves containing substance P (Badalamente & Cherney 1989). Tissue hypoxia is a well-recognized trigger for substance P and neural growth factor leading to nerve hyperinnervation (Naslund et al 2007).

In a novel study, the pulsatile blood flow to the patella was measured by photoplethysmography in zero extension, 20° and 90° flexion in patients with PFP (n=22) and in controls (n=33) (Naslund et al 2007). The PFP patients had reduced blood flow after passive knee flexion of 20–90° whereas no such response was noted in the control group. This may, at least in part, explain the moviegoer's sign, which is seen often in PFP patients when sitting with knee flexion for sustained periods. Futhermore, patients' perception of coldness of their legs in warm surroundings correlated with a poor outcome in PFP rehabilitation (Selfe et al 2003), and females were more likely to be affected by cold (Selfe et al 2010). Selfe et al (2010) postulated that, in a subset of PFP patients, reflex sympathetic dystrophy (complex regional pain syndrome) may play a role.

In summary, there is a variable mosaic of processes affecting tissue homeostasis and neural activation (Dye 2005; Naslund et al 2007), with new evidence that ischaemia may play a role in PFP. Further research is clearly required. These findings may impact on the clinical management of patients.

Table 44.3 **Risk and associated factors for patellofemoral pain**

Risk factors for patellofemoral pain	Factors associated with patellofemoral pain
Knee extension strength	Q-angle
Female gender	S-angle
	Patellar tilt
	Reduced hip abduction strength
	Reduced hip external strength
	Reduced knee extension peak torque

Risk Factors for Patellofemoral Pain

The identification of risk factors is important in prevention and rehabilitation of musculoskeletal disorders. Risk factors can be considered intrinsic or extrinsic, and modifiable or non-modifiable. A recent systematic review of prospective risk factors for the development of PFP (Lankhorst et al 2012) reported that reduced knee extension strength and female gender were associated with development of PFP, although there was conflicting evidence on the onset timing of VMO versus vastus lateralis as a risk factor for future PFP based upon two studies. The Q-angle and the protective role of prior sport activity were not associated as a risk (Lankhorst et al 2012).

In a subsequent review of factors associated with PFP by the same researchers (Lankhorst et al 2013), 47 studies were evaluated with a staggering 523 variables. Pooling was possible for eight variables only and six of these were associated with PFP compared with controls – larger Q-angle, sulcus angle and patellar tilt, less hip abduction strength, weaker hip external rotation and less knee extension peak torque (Table 44.3) – whereas foot arch height and C-angle had no such association (Lankhorst et al 2013). Other factors were also related with PFP in the 47 studies reviewed, but pooling for analysis was not possible as these were were based upon single studies only. Readers are encouraged to refer to Lankhorst et al (2013) for further review of these factors.

In patients with PFP, the presence of anxiety and fear-avoidance beliefs about work and physical activity were associated with function, whereas only fear-avoidance beliefs about work and physical activity were associated with pain (Piva et al 2009a). Furthermore, in patients undergoing PFP rehabilitation (n=74), a change in fear-avoidance beliefs about physical activity was the strongest predictor of recovery in terms of both pain and function (Piva et al 2009b). This finding underpins the importance of strategies to target fear-avoidence beliefs in patients with PFP.

In general, lower extremity injury risk is often associated with neuromusclar kinetic chain dysfunction. The functional movement screen is a clinical assessment tool that assesses functional movement over seven movement tests, scored on a scale of 0–3 per test, to a maximum total of 21 (Cook 2010). Good to excellent reliability (intra-class correlation (ICC) 0.66–0.92) has been demonstrated with respect to intra-rater reliability; however, the test is poor for inter-rater reliability (ICC 0.38) (Shultz et al 2013). Preliminary moderate-quality evidence suggests that the functional movement screen can assist in accurately identifying individuals at greater risk of musculoskeletal injury amongst male professional football players, female collegiate basketball, soccer and volleyball players, and male marine trainee officers (Krumrei et al 2014). The functional movement screen may also be helpful in clinical practice for assessing motor skills, screening for risk of injury, measuring improvement and for return-to-play protocol.

An additional clinical tool is the star excursion balance test (SEBT), which assesses dynamic single-stance balance in eight-point reach or a modified three-point reach (Kinzey & Armstrong 1998; Hertel et al 2006) and has been shown to have good reliability (ICC 0.67–0.92) (Kinzey & Armstrong 1998; Plisky et al 2006; Munro & Herrington 2010; Gribble et al 2013). This test was a predictor of injury in high-school basketballer players (Plisky et al 2006) and is recommended as part of screening for predicting lower extremity injuries in team sports players (Dallinga et al 2012).

Remote and Local Factors in Patellofemoral Pain

When PFJ force application exceeds the capabilities of the joint and related structures, tissue stress leads to loss of homeostasis whereby activation of peripheral nociceptors leads to pain and dysfunction. Furthermore, PFJ pain and dysfunction influence movement in the local and kinetic chain. Force applications include tension, compression, shear and torsion. In reality, however, these force applications may act in more than one mode – for example, compresssion on the lateral joint due to increased tilt and tension in the lateral retinaculum with coexisting PFJ shear due to lack of VMO activation.

Loading can be sudden or accumulative. Acute loading is exemplified by a direct-blow injury to the anterior lateral patella, leading to shear–compression of the lateral patellar and tension application with physiological-stress-induced strain on the lateral retinaculum. An example of accumulative loading is a runner with increased weekly mileage superimposed upon kinetic chain factors such as increased valgus knee position, overpronation of the subtalar joint and weakness in the lateral hip rotators and hip abductors / stabilizers. In another example, accumulative loading may occur from static activities such as sitting for long periods with the knee in a bent position (compression–tension force). This may lead to loss of homeostasis and therefore pain. Ischaemia may play a role in this mode, as previously described, and further research is indicated (Naslund et al 2007).

Crossley et al (2009) suggested a useful strategy by considering local and remote factors identified in the assessment that may contribute to PFP. Such a tactic aims at designing individualized patient rehabilitation programmes. Clinicians should be aware of intrinsic (e.g. hip weakness) and extrinsic (e.g. playing surface) risk factors and whether these factors are modifiable (e.g. neuromuscular control or strength) or non-modifiable (e.g. age or sex). Local factors include patellar position, soft tissue and quadriceps neuromuscular control; remote factors include increased femoral internal rotation, increased knee valgus, subtalar pronation and muscle flexibility (Crossley et al 2009).

Clinical Assessment

There is no consensus gold standard or consistent usage of clinical or functional tests for the diagnosis of PFP (Cook et al 2012). Moreover, PFP is regarded as a multifactorial clinical diagnosis made by the clinical assessment of the presenting complaint, assessment of potential pain-producing structures, assessment of kinetic chain influences, functional tests and diagnostic imaging as appropriate (Cook et al 2012). In a systematic review, studies that used a diagnosis of exclusion as part of the definition of PFP were found to have the highest methodological quality (Naslund et al 2006; Cook et al 2012). The diagnosis of exclusion approach used imaging or arthroscopic surgery evaluation to eliminate competing diagnoses in patents with suspected PFP (Cook et al 2012). Cook et al (2010) considered this to improve the accuracy of diagnosis in suspected PFP. In summary, there is no current reference test(s) for the diagnosis of PFP. Clinical assessment, clinical reasoning and imaging coupled with patient response to rehabilitation are a reasonable clinical approach in practice.

The role of the assessment is to screen and identify a working diagnosis / classification with consideration of differential diagnosis. Subjective, history, objective and imaging (where indicated) data are gathered to assist in forming a working impression. Pertinent factors identified from the assessment drive the rehabilitation programme and goals of treatment. Due to multifactorial influences of local and remote contributors in PFP, the assessment needs to address the kinetic chain and also identify pertinent factors influencing the PFJ. Referred pain and dysfunction contributors, as exemplified by weakness of the hip, TrPs, benign hypermobility syndrome and sacroiliac joint dysfunction, and local factors, such as tightness of the retinaculum, VMO weakness, etc., require prioritization in the plan of care. Such a strategy is likely to optimize the outcomes. Principles of assessment have been presented in this book for other relevant areas. History taking for patients with lower extremity disorders, self-reported outcome measures for patients with lower extremity pain syndromes and red flags are presented in Chapter 4. Imaging is helpful for differential diagnosis and may include X-ray, ultrasound imaging, MRI, CT and bone scan. Blood tests may be required to assist in differential diagnosis of other systemic diseases (Crossley et al 2009; Boissonnault 2010).

The patient interview includes subjective presentation (Table 44.4), history of present complaint (Table 44.5), patient profile and medical history (Table 44.6). Objective assessment

Table 44.4 **Subjective complaint for patients with patellofemoral pain**

Reference to current complaint	Pertinent issues	Comments
What is the problem/are the symptoms?	Pain, stiffness, crepitus, clicking, giving way, swelling, weakness, functional changes. Nature of the complaint (e.g. pain – sharp, dull ache, throb, dull, etc.)?	Define what exactly are the symptoms and the nature.
Location of complaint?	Define the area. Local/diffuse/remote? Kinetic chain symptoms? Other limb or body symptoms? Unilateral/bilateral?	Local pain may suggest specific local cause (e.g. infrapatellar fat pad). Diffuse pain may suggest referral pain (e.g. L3 type referral may suggest referral from hip). Burning or electrical type pain may suggest neuropathy.
Characteristics of the complaint?	Intermittent/constant? Frequency? Irritability? Specific/local/diffuse?	This may allow an understanding of the dimensions of the problem.
Aggravating factors	Activities that provoke symptoms? Sitting, standing, walking, running, stairs (up & down). Sustained positions? Moviegoers sign?	Important as this may assist in an understanding of the potential tissues/stresses provoking the pain.
Relieving factors	What relieves the symptoms? Rest, exercise (specific or general), positions of comfort, heat, medications.	Important as assists in plan of care and management of symptoms and also an understanding of potential tissues/mechanisms/stresses involved in the complaint.
Response to exercise	Do the symptoms come on with exercise and what is the nature? None, warm up only, after activity, provokes but remains at tolerable level, gets worse and have to stop. Specific activities walk, run (up or down), jump, uneven ground, etc.	Improvement with warm up phase may suggest increased blood flow and gating of pain mechanisms for example. Pain that is severe and summates may suggest, for example, bone reaction.

Table 44.5 **History of complaint for patients with patellofemoral pain**

History of current complaint	Pertinent issues	Comments
When did the complaint start?	What was the date or time frame of the complaint? Is the complaint acute, subacute or chronic? Is the complaint recurring?	Often the longer the time frame the more complex due to movement pattern changes, for example. Acute symptoms may settle naturally. The focus of the plan of care may change in relation to acute or chronic presentation. When not settling in expected natural course, etc., imaging may play a role in assisting differential diagnosis.
Cause?	Was the complaint traumatic or non-traumatic? Specific incident remembered? Did complaint 'just come on'? What was the development of the complaint? Was there anything new or changed in the time frame before the start of the complaint?	Forces associated with specific trauma (e.g. kick to knee, knee impact to dashboard in road traffic accident) may require routine imaging X-ray or MRI. Was there any incident of subluxation, dislocation, traumatic or non-traumatic? Identifies the precipitating factor(s). Intrinsic, extrinsic and modifiable or non-modifiable factors. Identifies specific or overuse causality.

Table 44.6 **Patient profile, demographics and clinical history for patients with patellofemoral pain**

Patient demographics	Age, sex, etc. Weight, height, body mass index	Age and sex are non-modifiable factors. Chronological age may be different from functional/physiological age. If overweight or obese may influence kinetic chain forces. If underweight may influence repair capabilities. Female triad?
Medical history	Medical, surgical and sport injury history Presence of medical conditions may influence outcome and plan of care Pregnancy, children, etc.	The presence of comorbidities may influence plan of care and healing pathway (e.g. diabetes, obesity, vascular disease, osteoporosis, etc.). Previous sports injuries may influence plan of care, e.g. for previous ACL injury, Achilles rupture and surgical repair, etc.
Medication	Current and history	Medication may be used as part of the rehabilitation process with positive effects on pain control, especially in acute phase. Medication may lead to undesirable side effects (e.g. corticosteroid-injection-induced soft tissue atrophy, steroid induced myopathy, statin-induced muscle pain). Medication may draw awareness to a medical condition not reported, e.g. diabetes, etc.
Medical assessment/ tests	Has the patient had medical review with a specialist? Did the patient attend emergency room due to trauma or suspected dislocation? The patient may require physician follow-up or re-review? Blood tests?	The patient may require a medical review for medical disease, e.g. rheumatoid conditions (Reiter's syndrome, seronegative arthropathy, pigmented villonodular synovitis, neoplasm, etc.). Specialist review may be required with sports medicine, orthopaedic or rheumatology.
Imaging, special tests	X-ray, MRI, ultrasound, CT scan, bone scan, vascular	Imaging may assist in differential diagnosis and would be indicated especially with traumatic injury, dislocation and persistent problem not responding.
Red flags	Are red flags present? Current or past history of cancer Other medical condition Fatigue Malaise Acute medical condition Severe pain Pain unrelated to movement Unexplained weight loss/gain Bowel or bladder habit changes Numbness, loss of feeling Change in mood Cauda equina symptoms Suspected fracture or dislocation	Presence of red flags indicates referral to primary care physician or emergency room.
Employment/ lifestyle	What does the patient work at? Nature of work? Sitting, standing and occupational positions, e.g. kneeling, etc. What are the hobbies?	Habitual habits such as prolonged sitting or driving may require attention in the plan of care. Ergonomic assessment may be indicated. Change of habits, micro-breaks and rotation of activities may be required.
Sports and exercise	Ascertain sports demographics? Type of sport? Contact or non-contact? Specifics of sport? Biomechanics of sport? Equipment? Surface being used? Enquire about frequency of competition, training and periodicity, season and sports specific demands Consider overtraining	Know the sport, demands, biomechanics and requirements. Technique and coaching input may be required. Regulation of training frequency. Specialized equipment such as braces, orthotics may be required. Assess for overtraining.

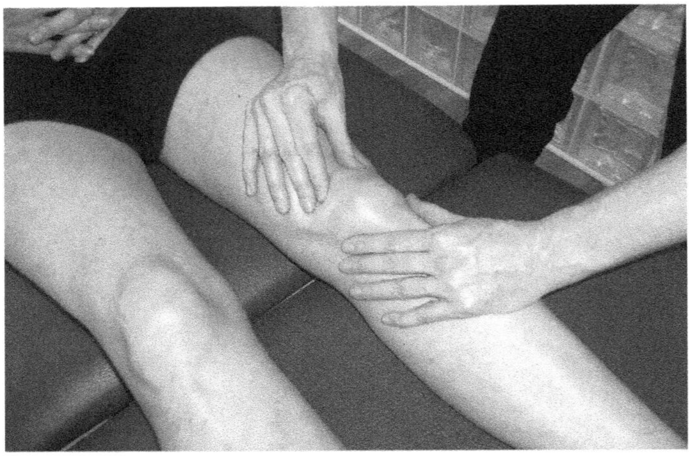

Figure 44.6 Patellar mobility tests. The patella is moved lateral to medial, superior to inferior and tilted from lateral to medial (lateral border lifted anteriorly). Palpate for mobility, end feel and pain. Compare with other side.

is important and includes local and remote kinetic chain contributing factors. A template for such an assessment is included in Table 44.7.

The overall diagnostic accuracy of patellar mobility and palpatory tests and the diagnostic accuracy of gross pain provocation measures were systematically reviewed by Cook et al (2012), who reported sensitivities, specificities, positive likelihood ratios (+LR) and negative likelihood ratios (–LR). Overall, results for most tests were low with respect to +LR and there was some variance of the tests across studies (Cook et al 2012). One of the reviewed studies reported higher +LR with positive pain on the Clarke grind test (+LR 7.4), pain during stair climbing (+LR 11.6) and pain with prolonged sitting or flexion (+LR 7.4) (Elton et al 1985; Cook et al 2012). It must be noted, however, that these results were in conflict with other studies that reported +LR of less than 2.0 (Cook et al 2012).

The assessment consists of elements as required, including observation, function, range of motion, flexibility, strength, inspection, palpation, PFJ mobility testing (Fig. 44.6), PFJ special tests, other factors and screening of kinetic chain as indicated (see Table 44.7). Clinical assessment is a dynamic process and not all tests may be necessary, or indeed appropriate. If the patient's pain is reproduced with a specific test, this is of significant value.

The evaluation process should direct the clinician to highlight specific concerns and needs of the individual patient. Plan of care should address these needs and monitor progress. Differential diagnosis should always be considered and, if appropriate, a multidisciplinary team approach may be required.

Conservative Treatment

There is evidence that multimodal physiotherapy programmes are effective for PFJ (Crossley et al 2009; McConnell 2009). The development of a plan of care for PFP is based upon the findings from the assessment. Differential diagnosis needs to be considered. Neuromuscular control deficits or dysfunctions

Table 44.7 **Objective assessment for patients with patellofemoral pain**

Observation of lower kinetic chain	Standing, walking, lying supine
Functional	Squat, step-up, step-down, single-leg squat Jump, drop jump, lunge Balance assessment (e.g. BESS, SEBT) Functional movement screen
Range of motion Accessory joint motion	Low back, hip, knee, ankle areas
Flexibility tests	Hip flexors (iliopsoas/rectus femoris) Thomas's test External and internal rotation Lateral hip (abductors/TFL) TFL/ITB – Ober's test Adductors, quadriceps, hamstring, calf muscles Ankle lunge test
Strength Manual muscle testing Dynamometery (handheld) Isokinetic	Hip abductors 0° and 30° (gluteus medius anterior and posterior fibres) External hip rotators, adductors, quadriceps, hamstrings Calf, trunk muscles
Inspection PFJ and knee	Swelling, temperature, deformity, congruency, colour
Palpation for tenderness	Borders of the patella Medial and lateral retinaculum Muscle attachments (vastus medialis and lateralis) Patellar tendon Knee joint Tibial tuberosity Palpation of medial and lateral under surface of patella (as accessible) Myofascial trigger points
PFJ Tenderness and pain provocation Mobility Compare left and right	Observation of position static position Passive mobility: medial glide, lateral glide, superior glide, inferior glide, tilt Patellar mobility with movement
PFJ special tests	Clarke's grind test Apprehension test Q-angle measurement (supine and observation in single leg squat)
Other	Knee joint assessment Low back screen (McKenzie assessment, sacroiliac joint, active straight leg raise) Hip Ankle Hypermobility scale test (Beighton) Functional test scales
Other special tests	Imaging (X-ray, ultrasound, MRI, CT, bone scan, etc.) Blood tests, etc.

in the remote or local kinetic chain need to be treated. Furthermore, treatment of identified painful structures should be considered, for example the synovial membrane, fat pad, TrPs, etc. Given the diverse nature of PFP, multimodal treatment, and especially exercise-based rehabilitation, is likely to potentiate outcomes as is similarly seen in conditions such as neck and low back pain (Boyling & Jull 2005; McConnell 2009). There is a general consensus that surgery should be avoided in PFP, especially when there is evidence of efficacy for conservative rehabilitation treatment (Crossley et al 2009; McConnell 2009). Nevertheless, there may be a role for surgery in a select cohort of PFP patients, but usually conservative measures should be exhausted first (Crossley et al 2009).

There is a plethora of treatments proposed for PFJ pain. Current best practice recommends a conservative multimodal rehabilitation approach for improved outcomes (McConnell 2009). Due to the multifactorial nature of PFJ, no one treatment is likely to be fully successful for PFP (McConnell 2009). Targeting of fear-avoidance beliefs may be an important treatment strategy and psychological intervention should be sought as required (Piva et al 2009a, 2009b).

Four clinical prediction rules (CPRs) for PFP have been reported in patellar taping (Lesher et al 2006), lumbar manipulation (Iverson et al 2008) and the use of orthotics (Sutlive et al 2004; Vicenzino et al 2008). The application of CPRs in clinical practice may help with decision making and should be used in conjunction with current existing evidence, patient preferences and clinical experience (Glynn & Weisbach 2011). Caution should be noted with CPRs, however, and they should not be used in isolation (Glynn & Weisbach 2011). (These CPRs are reported under each relevant treatment section.)

Patient lifestyle, ergonomic and sports factors should also be taken into account and may need to be addressed in the plan of care. Examples include habitual sitting postures with knees bent, use of high heels and sports footwear, and saddle height for cyclists. Ergonomic evaluation of the workplace and habitual postures or positions may require assessment, such as kneeling positions. Cyclists may require a professional bike-fitting and modification service. Sports-specific techniques may include coaching input and specialist equipment (e.g. kneepads, etc.). Advice and education is vital to the plan of care.

Multimodal treatment

Evidence is in favour of multimodal treatment for PFJ. McConnell (2009) reviewed studies ($n=8$) of therapies for PFJ and concluded that a multimodal physical therapy programme was effective. A McConnell-based multimodal physical therapy programme, consisting of patellar taping, patellar mobilizations, specific quadriceps and gluteal muscle exercises and stretching for the anterior hip and hamstrings, was found to be successful for the treatment of PFJ (Cowan et al 2002; Crossley et al 2002; McConnell 2009).

Patellar taping

The aim of taping is to improve patellar position. Evidence suggests an immediate effect on pain, and short-term effects on the onset timing of the VMO relative to the VL muscle and on the effect on functional gait, but the exact mechanism of effect is still under investigation (Crossley et al 2009; McConnell 2009). MRI assessment of lateral patellar displacement, with no tape versus tape, showed lateral patellar displacement reductions of 0.4 mm, 1.1 mm and 0.7 mm at 0°, 10° and 20° of knee flexion respectively (Herrington 2006). Though these changes are small, the question remains of whether they are statistically significant enough to be responsible for changes in pain and function.

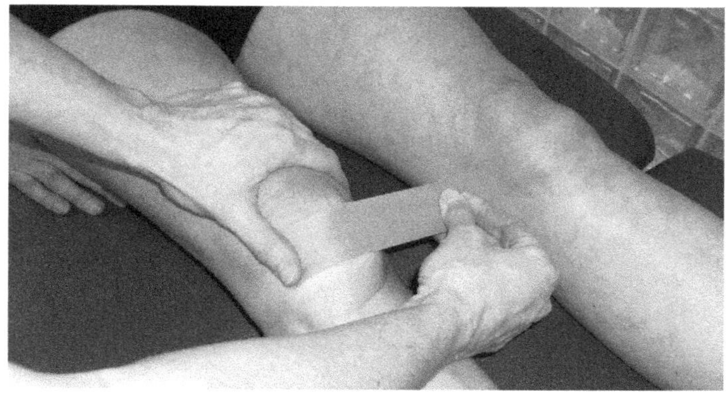

Figure 44.7 Patellar taping. The tape is placed in a direction to reduce lateral or lateral tilt position of the patella. This depends on the findings from the patellar mobility testing. Several layers of tape may be used and underlining tape may be required. Precautions for taping are noted.

Taping is recommended as a measure to relieve pain while strategies are applied to correct contributing factors and during exercises in the early stage (Crossley et al 2009; McConnell 2009). Rigid zinc oxide type tape with an underlining tape, to reduce allergic skin reaction, is applied on prepared shaved skin where appropriate with normal precautions. The tape is often applied with a medial glide, and the tape position varied so as to correct the abnormal tilt (e.g. lateral or inferior tilt) (Fig. 44.7).

A CPR for patellar taping for PFJ was developed with a methodological quality that was deemed acceptable (Lesher et al 2006; Glynn & Weisbach 2011). The presence of one or more of two predictor variables, including tibial varum >5° and positive patellar tilt test, led to a +LR of 4.4. This represents a small, but sometimes clinically important, shift in the probability of benefit from taping (Lesher et al 2006; Glynn & Weisbach 2011). Success was defined as perceived global improvement and / or a ≥50% reduction in pain with patellar taping (Lesher et al 2006).

Patellar mobilizations and lumbar manipulation

Manual therapy for PFP has evidence for improving pain, range of motion and function as part of a multimodal therapy programme. A literature review of the effects of manual therapy as part of a multimodal-based programme in individuals with lower kinetic chain disorders, including PFP, rated it as 'level B' (fair) evidence (Brantingham et al 2009). (For a more detailed discussion of manual therapy for PFP and example of mobilization glides (cephalad and caudal, lateral and medial) see Ch 46.)

A CPR for the use of lumbar manipulation in PFP has also been published (Iverson et al 2008). It encompassed the presence of three or more of five potential predictor variables – (1)

side-to-side hip internal rotation difference of >14°, (2) ankle dorsiflexion with knee flexed >16°, (3) navicular drop test >3°, (4) no self-reported stiffness with sitting >20 minutes and (5) squatting reported as the most painful activity – led to a +LR 18.4 of positive change (Iverson et al 2008; Glynn & Weisbach 2011). This was a large probability shift of success and was defined as a benefit in perceived global improvement and / or pain with functional testing and lumbar manipulation (Iverson et al 2008; Glynn & Weisbach 2011).

Stretching

There is little research on the effects of stretching alone as an intervention for PFP (Crossley et al 2009). One study assessed the effects of a 3-week weight-bearing (standing) static-stretching programme for the quadriceps muscle (Fig. 44.8) in patients with PFP (Peeler & Anderson 2007); the stretching improved PFP pain and function, but there was a poor correlation between quadriceps flexibility and the severity of knee pain.

The patella position (lateral displacement as described by McConnell) had a poor correlation with iliotibial band length as measured by Ober's test, but a moderate correlation with the modified Ober's test (Herrington et al 2006b). Muscle length tests from the assessment will reveal potential soft tissue length challenges to the kinetic chain. Muscles involved may include the anterior hip flexors (iliopsoas, rectus femoris), hip rotators, quadriceps (rectus femoris and vastus medialis and lateralis), hamstrings and lateral hip structures, particularly the tensor fasciae latae and the calf. A stretching programme may be of value to optimize kinetic chain influences; however, other aspects of the multimodal programme should not be neglected.

Overflexibility may be an issue and special consideration should be paid to individuals with a history of subluxation, dislocation and hypermobility syndromes so as to avoid inappropriate stretching. Prevalence estimates of hypermobility range from 4% to 7% in the normal population, 9.5% in ballet dancers and 11.7% in high-school students, and hypermobility is more common in girls and women than in boys and men (Klemp et al 1984; Alter 1996; Hakim & Grahame 2003; Seckin et al 2005). The Beighton score has been used to identify subjects with hypermobility and is commonly used in sports medicine, orthopaedics and rheumatology (Beighton et al 1973; Alter 1996).

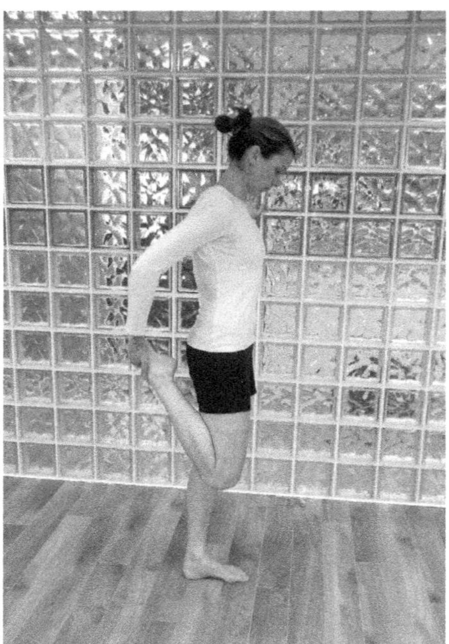

Figure 44.8 Standing quadriceps stretch. Stretches are held for 30 seconds for three repeats with normal precautions. Avoid anterior tilt of pelvis. Avoid pain and ensure safe stability.

Strengthening exercises

Strengthening is one of the main pillars of PFP rehabilitation. Local patellar stability is influenced by the quadriceps group, especially the VMO, which counteracts lateral patellar tilt. The main open chain kinetic exercises utilized are the isometric quadriceps set at 0°, terminal knee extension and the straight leg raise, with all three exercises working in less than 30° of knee flexion, therefore minimizing PFJ contact stress (McConnell 2009). These three open chain exercises do not preferentially activate the VMO, and variants of the exercises (e.g. external hip rotation during straight leg raise) do not confer greater VMO activity (Karst & Jewett 1993; Cerny 1995; Cuddeford et al 1996; Mirzabeigi et al 1999). There have been mixed results with respect to whether additional hip adduction influences VMO / VL activation (McConnell 2009).

In contrast, in one study closed chain kinetic exercises promoted balanced initial quadriceps activation and a larger amplitude of maximal voluntary contraction than did open chain exercises (Stensdotter et al 2003). In another, open chain kinetic exercises produced more rectus femoris activity whereas closed chain kinetic exercises produced more vastus muscle activity (Escamilla et al 1998). Furthermore, PFJ compressive force was greatest in closed chain exercises in near full flexion and in the mid-range knee-extending phase than in open chain kinetic exercises (Escamilla et al 1998).

These studies will influence the choice of exercises for PFP rehabilitation programmes. When patients are ready and it is appropriate, closed chain kinetic exercises should be initiated owing to the advantages of targeting the kinetic chain for floor-to-core and the additional neuromuscular balance aspect (McConnell 2009).

A comprehensive study of electromyographic (EMG) activity of eight kinetic chain core, trunk, hip and thigh muscles during nine rehabilitation exercises has been published (Ekstrom et al 2007). The results influence the choice of exercises in lower kinetic chain rehabilitation, including PFP. The nine exercises assessed were active hip abduction in side-lying, supine trunk bridge, unilateral bridge with one knee extended, side bridge, prone bridge, quadruped alternative arm and leg lift, lateral step-up to a 20 cm (8 inch) step, standing lunge and dynamic edge exercise machine. As part of the assessment, these exercises could be used as functional tests to examine the individual's neuromuscular control. This may be of importance in designing training programmes aimed at control of the active local and remote factors influencing the PFJ in individual patients. The muscles tested with EMG in the above study included the gluteus medius, gluteus maximus, VMO, hamstrings, longissimus thoracis, lumbar multifidus, external oblique and rectus abdominis (Table 44.8).

Table 44.8 **Exercises recommended for activation of selected hip and core muscles***

Exercise	Gluteus medius	Gluteus maximus	Vastus medialis	Hamstrings	Longissimus thoracis	Lumbar multifidus	External oblique	Rectus abdominis
Side bridge	1				2	3	1	2
Unilateral bridge	2	2		1	1	2		
Lateral step-up	3		1					
Quadruped arm/lower extremity lift	4	1		2	4	1		
Active hip abduction (side-lying)	5							
Lunge		3	2					
Bridge					3	4		
Prone bridge							2	1

*Numbering refers to priority of exercises based on EMG activation.
(Adapted from Ekstrom et al 2007.)

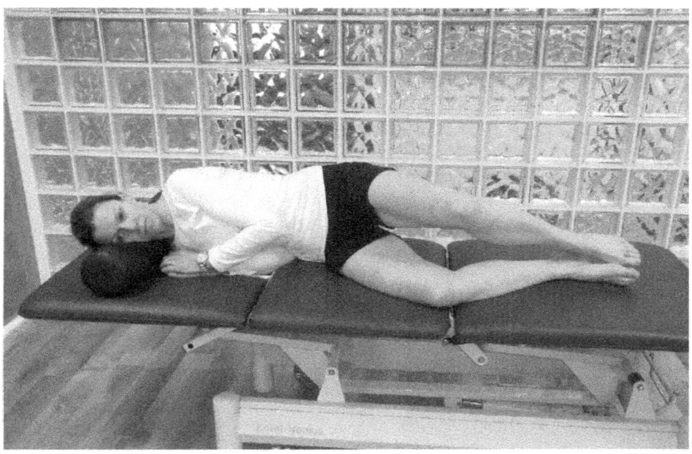

Figure 44.9 Clam exercise. An exercise to target the gluteus medius muscle especially. Make sure hips are stacked and avoid rotation of the trunk.

Other exercise regimens have been also recommended including VMO retraining, step-up / step-down, hip abduction and external rotation strengthening and lunges (Crossley et al 2009, McConnell 2009), and quadriceps and hamstring, wall squats, plies, lunges, mini-squats, step-up / step-down, lateral step-ups and machine and free-weight exercises (Houglum 2005). Caution should be noted when using exercises that cause pain, especially with excessive loading in flexion beyond 30° where PFJ forces increase substantially (Houglum 2005). The knee extension machine, which is an open chain kinetic exercise, should not be used or only be used with significant caution owing to potential for high PFJ compressive and shear forces (Houglum 2005).

Box 44.1 summarizes the types of exercise that target specific muscles, and Figures 44.9–44.15 present some examples of suitable exercises. As with any exercise programme, exercise prescription should be monitored for tolerance and appropriateness. (Readers are referred to other chapters for further information on therapeutic exercise principles.)

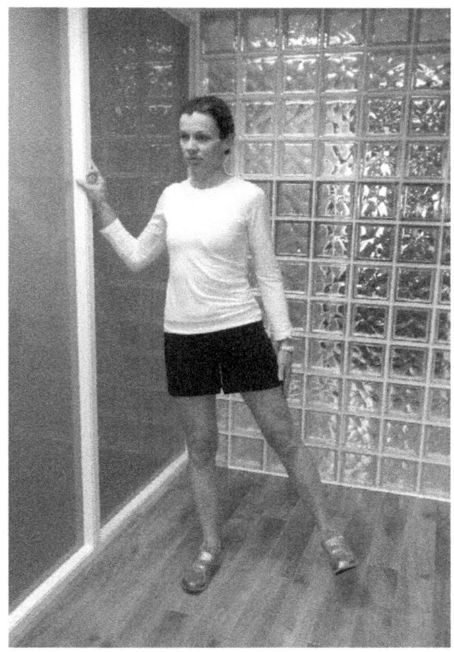

Figure 44.10 Standing hip abduction in 0° abduction and also with abduction in 30° extension to target the posterior gluteus medius muscle. Weight can be added for progression. Keep spine and trunk stable during exercise.

In a study that investigated the effect of low-load exercises targeting gluteal muscles on lower limb function / performance (Crow et al 2012), a neuromuscular warm-up routine was identified. It included seven exercises: the double-leg bridge, quadruped lower extremity lift, quadruped hip abduction, side-lying clam in 60° hip flexion, side-lying hip abduction, prone single-leg hip extension and double-leg stability ball squat. Although the precise mechanism for activation was not identified, the authors postulated that it might be a result of altered motor cortical activity. However, it was clear from the study that there was an increase in lower limb performance, a counter-movement jump increase resulting from the

Box 44.1 Examples of rehabilitation exercises*

Local knee open chain

Static quadriceps sets
Terminal knee extensions
Straight leg raises

Knee closed chain

Wall squats/mini-squats etc
Lateral step-up
Lunge
Step-downs/step-ups
Unilateral bridge

Hip

Clam exercise
Standing hip abduction 0° abduction and 30° abduction/extension (posterior gluteus medius)
Lying hip abduction 0° abduction and 30° abduction/extension (posterior gluteus medius)
External rotation of the hip in side-lying
Side bridge
Unilateral bridge
Lateral step-up
Quadruped arm/lower extremity lift
Step-downs/step-ups

Trunk

Side bridge
Unilateral bridge
Quadruped arm/lower extremity lift
Bridge
Prone bridge

Neuromuscular and balance

Single-leg stand
Single-leg stand foam/cushion/balance board, etc.
Single-leg stand with eyes closed
Single-leg stand foam/cushion/balance board, etc. with eyes closed
Star excursion balance exercise
Dynamic combined, e.g. balance cushion and medicine ball rebounder, shuttle balance
Step-down exercises
Multidirectional exercises (bounding, hopping, etc.)

Plyometric

Various as able and appropriate at end-stage rehabilitation and sports-specific exercises

*Exercises should be prescribed based upon individual needs and appropriateness. Monitor for ability to perform with good form and function and safety.

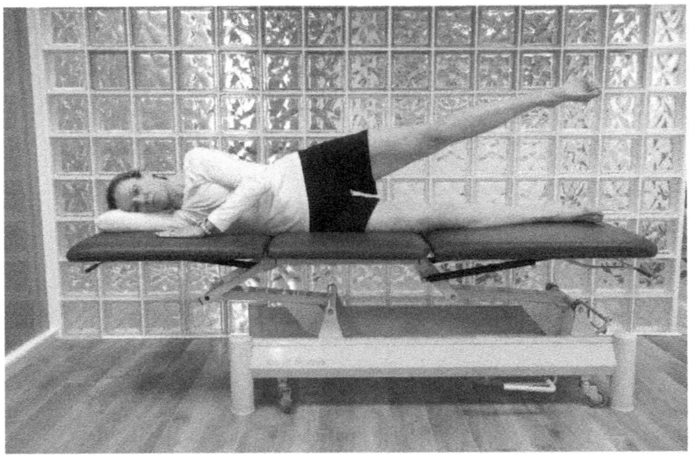

Figure 44.11 Side-lying hip abduction in 0° abduction and also with abduction in 30° extension to target the posterior gluteus medius muscle. Weight can be added for progression. Trunk should be stable during exercise with hips stacked.

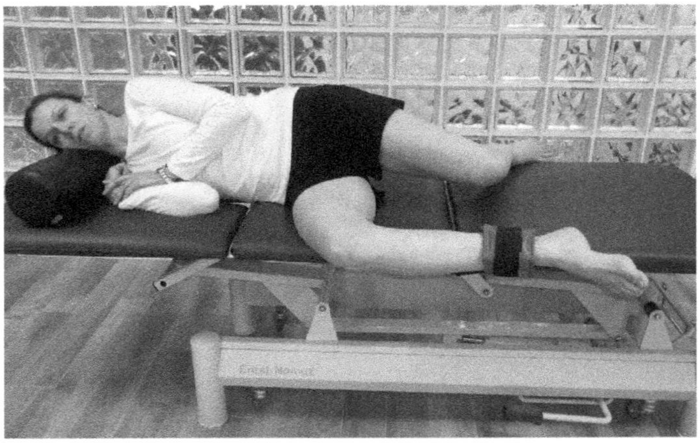

Figure 44.12 External rotation of the hip in side-lying. Target leg is lower leg on table. Rotate hip as foot moves up to ceiling in concentric mode and then lowers in eccentric. Weight can be added for progression. Trunk should be stable during exercise with hips stacked.

lower level gluteal activation exercises. There appears to be an expected transfer of muscle activation within the targeted muscle group, which further enhances activation down the kinetic chain. This does need validation with EMG, however. Extrapolating the results, these exercises may be an easy, non-fatiguing method of activating hip and thigh muscles before sports activity in patients presenting with PFPs, or when such patients are returning to sport.

Balance training and neuromuscular control

Neuromuscular control and balance training and retraining of the visual, vestibular and neuromuscular control systems should be considered in lower kinetic chain rehabilitation programmes (Houglum 2005; Kenji 2010). Proprioception impairment has been reported in PFP patients, most notably on the affected side but also on the uninvolved side, when compared with controls (Akseki et al 2008). One-leg static balance is decreased on the symptomatic side in PFP patients and a correlation with weakness of the quadriceps and hamstrings exists, with no correlation to severity of pain or lower extremity alignment and Q-angle (Citaker et al 2012). Various tools can be used to assess neuromuscular control and balance – for example, the balance error scoring system (BESS), which is an easy clinical test to administer and requires only a level

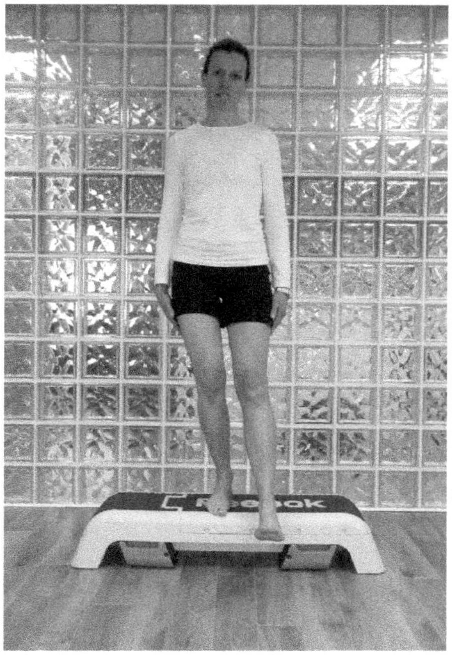

Figure 44.13 Step-down exercise. Dynamic lowering and raise from a step. Also use lateral step-up exercise as an alternative. Improve control and avoid increasing dynamic Q-angle by maintaining hip, knee and foot alignment.

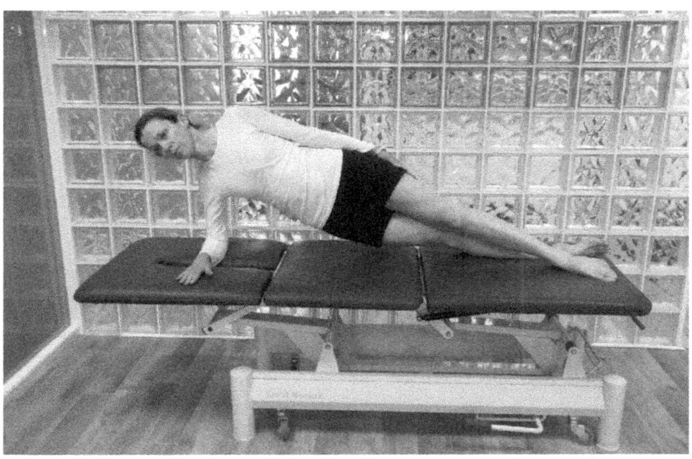

Figure 44.14 Side bridge. Trunk and hip muscle exercise. Hold for 5–10 seconds and repeat as indicated.

surface and piece of foam (Kenji 2010; Bell et al 2011). The average error score in controls is nine, where a low score signifies good neuromuscular control (Kenji 2010). The reliability of the BESS is reported as moderate to good, especially when large balance deficits exist in such cases as fatigue and concussion (Riemann & Guskiewicz 2000; Valovich et al 2003; Wilkins et al 2004; Docherty et al 2006; Bell et al 2011). When smaller subtle deficits are present the reliability will be lower (Bell et al 2011). BESS scores increase with age, ankle instability and external ankle bracing for 20 minutes after exertion and improve after neuromuscular control balance training (Riemann & Guskiewicz 2000; Susco et al 2004; Bell et al 2011). Whereas the BESS is a static balance test, the SEBT can be employed for dynamic clinical testing. Factors leading

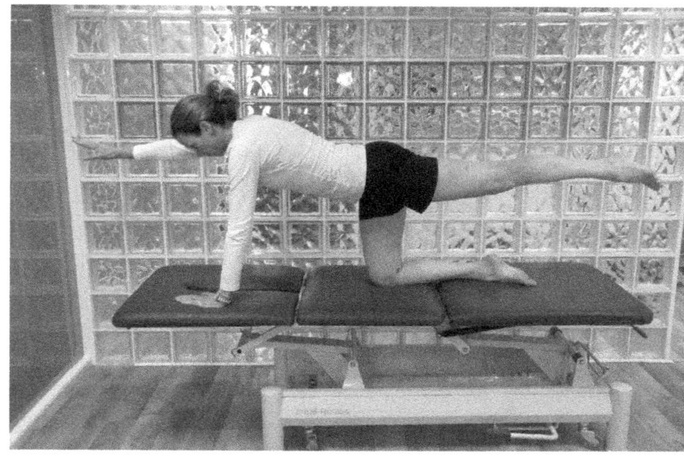

Figure 44.15 Quadruped arm/lower extremity lift. Maintain stability of trunk and avoid excessive trunk rotation.

to poor neuromuscular control and balance need to be identified. This will allow suitable rehabilitation exercise programmes to be properly designed. Closed chain kinetic exercises, as described above, may also assist in functional improvement of neuromuscular control, balance and strength in muscles related to the kinetic chain.

For treatment, balance retraining can consist of developing exercises based upon errors identified in the BESS test. The SEBT can also be adopted as an exercise. It is advised to start at the minimum challenging level and advance in a progressive graded manner. Balance exercise equipment can be employed to progress exercises, such as foam, air cushions, balance boards, beams and specialized equipment such as the Y-Balance System, Shuttle Balance System and a medicine ball rebounder, etc. Other treatment regimens include the Janda approach for muscle imbalance and sensorimotor training (Page et al 2010). A simple set of Janda balance sandals has been shown to facilitate volume and timing of EMG of gluteal muscles in normal subjects during walking (Bullock-Saxton et al 1993; Page et al 2010). Some examples of neuromuscular and balance exercises are shown in Figures 44.16–44.18.

Soft tissue massage and trigger point therapy

There is a lack of research on the effect of soft tissue massage for PFP. One trial reported higher bilateral prevalence of TrPs in the gluteus medius and quadratus lumborum muscles, with a corresponding lower hip abduction strength in PFP patients (n=26), compared with controls (n=26) (Roach et al 2013). However, TrP pressure release therapy had no effect on strength in the PFP subjects (Roach et al 2013). This study did not evaluate the vastus medialis or lateralis muscles (Fig. 44.19), which is a very clinically relevant group of muscles owing to their local effect on the PFJ, and especially the vastus lateralis and VMO, owing to their direct effect on lateral patellar tilt.

There are conflicting recommendations for soft tissue massage in other knee conditions such as osteoarthritis (Perlman et al 2006, 2012; Zhang et al 2007; Peter et al 2011; Atkins & Eichler 2013). Further research is needed to determine the effects, if any, of soft tissue technique including TrP therapy on PFP.

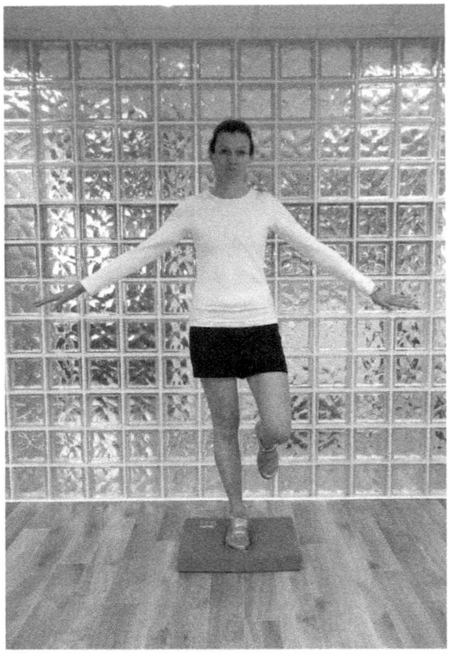

Figure 44.16 **Balance exercise.** Example of single-leg stand balance on foam. Maintain safety.

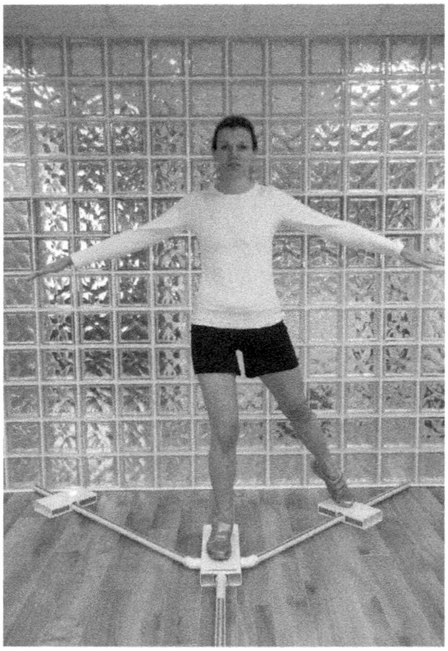

Figure 44.17 **Balance exercise.** Example of star excursion balance test used as an exercise. Here it is carried out on the Y-Balance tester. Reaching is carried out in anterior, lateral and medial direction repeated for 10–20 times in single-leg stand and repeated on opposite side.

Trigger point dry needling and botulinum toxin injection

Trigger point dry needling (TrP-DN) has become a common treatment in musculoskeletal and myofascial pain disorders (Dommerholt & Fernandez-de-las-Peñas 2013), and the

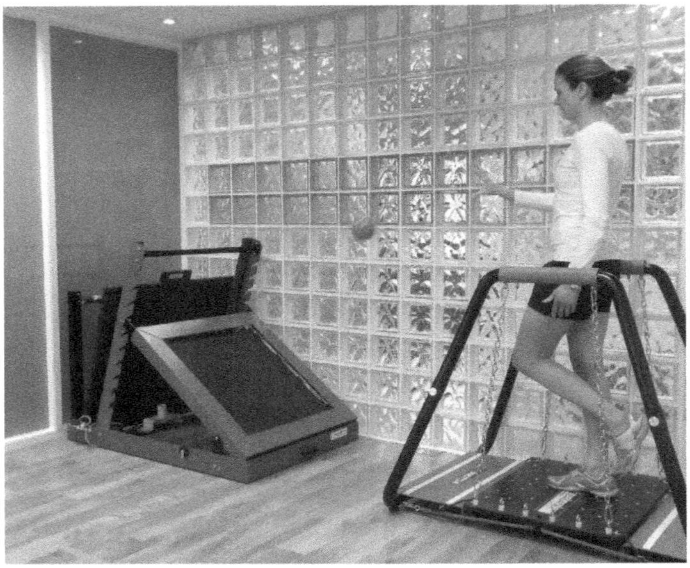

Figure 44.18 **Dynamic balance incorporating vestibular, visual and neuromuscular components carried out on the shuttle balance system with a medicine ball rebounder.** (Shuttle Balance Systems, WA, USA).

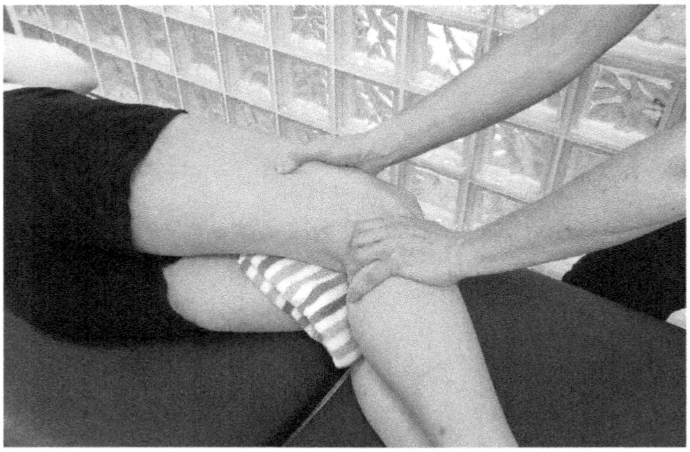

Figure 44.19 **Massage and myofascial trigger point release to the lateral thigh and vastus lateralis trigger points.**

American Academy of Orthopaedic Manual Therapists (AAOMPT) has published a support statement for TrP-DN (AAOMPT 2009). TrP-DN is a safe procedure when carried out by appropriately trained clinicians (Brady et al 2014), and guidelines for safe practice have been published (Irish Society of Chartered Physiotherapists (ISCP) 2012; McEvoy 2013).

Dry needling is a neurophysiological evidence-based treatment technique that requires effective manual assessment of the neuromuscular system. Physical therapists are well trained to utilize dry needling in conjunction with manual physical therapy interventions. Research supports the proposition that dry needling improves pain control, reduces muscle tension, normalizes biochemical and electrical dysfunction of motor end plates, and facilitates an accelerated return to active rehabilitation (AAOMPT 2009).

Readers are referred to Chapter 59 of this textbook for relevant review of TrPs. Although no study has assessed the effect of TrP-DN on PFP, TrP-DN targeted to muscles determined to contain clinically relevant TrPs such as the quadriceps, especially the vastus lateralis, gluteal muscles and quadratus lumborum, may be helpful as part of a multimodal programme. In patients with PFP, the gluteus medius and quadratus lumborum TrPs were more prevalent bilaterally, and corresponded to lower hip abduction strength (Roach et al 2013). Clinicians should be trained adequately to improve the accuracy of TrP palpation testing (McEvoy & Huijbregts 2011). Although needling therapies seem to be effective for pain control (Cummings & White 2001), no random placebo-controlled trial existed until recently (Mayoral et al 2013); in this trial, patients who would be receiving total knee arthroplasty were examined for TrPs before surgery (n=40). While under anaesthesia in the operating room, and before the surgery started, they were randomized to TrP-DN or placebo group and treated accordingly. Blinding was maintained by anaesthesia. The study authors concluded that a single TrP-DN treatment under anaesthesia reduced pain in the first month after total knee arthroplasty compared with placebo (Mayoral et al 2013). In another preliminary randomized controlled trial, older patients with knee osteoarthritis (n=30) were treated with TrP-DN, traditional acupuncture or sham at TrPs; the results demonstrated significant improvement with TrP-DN over acupuncture and sham for pain and function. (See Ch 61 for discussion on TrP-DN techniques.)

Botulinum toxin type A (Botox) has been tested in an open label pilot study of subjects with refractory anterior knee pain with relative overactivity of the VL, with encouraging results (Singer et al 2006). This initial study by a group of Australian researchers provoked interest. In a further study of Botox injection, for anterior knee pain associated with quadriceps muscles imbalance, subjects (n=24) were randomized to either Botox or saline injection to the vastus lateralis with all subjects prescribed a home programme for vastus medialis retraining (Singer et al 2011). Quadriceps muscle imbalance was assessed by EMG. Results at 12 weeks were significantly in favour of the Botox treatment group in terms of pain on kneeling, squatting and level walking and anterior knee pain scale. In a retrospective cohort study of subjects with refractory anterior knee pain, a single Botox injection to the VL resulted in relief of knee pain and improvement in function in 57 of 65 subjects, with an average benefit of 34 months in 44 out of the 57 cases (Silbert et al 2012).

In combination, these studies suggest that altering the vastus lateralis function by Botox injection has an effect on PFJ pain and dysfunction. This may act by altering vastus lateralis muscle activation, lateral knee tension and patellar tilt. This is similar in essence to the aim of other strategies such as manual therapy, soft tissue therapy and surgical release. It is worth noting that none of these studies strategically targeted TrP specifically, or compared TrP-DN with Botox. Areas of stiffness have been identified in TrP zones in studies using MRI elastography and ultrasound elastography (Chen et al 2007, 2008; Sikdar et al 2008, 2009). Furthermore, TrP-DN has been shown to reduce palpable muscle stiffness using ultrasound shear-wave elastography (Maher et al 2013) when tested using ultrasound. It is feasible that TrP-DN could be an effective adjunctive treatment to the multimodal programme in PFP rehabilitation. Further research is indicated to direct best practice.

Selected electrophysical modalities

A full discussion of electrophysical modalities is beyond the scope of this chapter; the main aim of this section is to stimulate the reader to consider electrophysical modalities as part of PFJ multimodal programme. Modalities may play a role for specific biological effects. The choice of modality will depend on clinical reasoning and evidence-informed research and goals. There is a lack of quality research on electrophysical modalities for PFJ. A systematic review of electrophysical modalities for PFP, based on 12 studies, concluded that some electrophysical modalities, when combined with other treatment, may confer an effect on pain, but when used alone had no beneficial effect (Lake & Wofford 2011). The electrophysical modalities reviewed were a combination study (ultrasound, ice massage, phonophoresis and iontophoresis), neuromuscular electrical stimulation, EMG biofeedback and low-intensity laser, and most studies were of low to moderate quality making conclusions difficult (Lake & Wofford 2011). Transcutaneous electrical nerve stimulation (TENS), interferential therapy and shockwave were not covered in this study. Future basic biological and randomized controlled trials are required to delineate best practice. Sluka and her group from the University of Iowa are investigating the peripheral and central mechanisms of chronic musculoskeletal pain and also the neurobiology of TENS analgesia in animal models with a focus on translating these studies to knee osteoarthritis in humans (Sluka 2014). Sluka has published a book on the mechanisms and management of pain for physical therapists and this is a valuable resource (Sluka 2009). Other helpful resources on electrophysical modalities and tissue repair are offered by Watson (2008).

Often modalities, such as superficial heat, TENS and interferential therapy, are employed as supportive treatments for musculoskeletal pain. As an example, interferential therapy has been reported to be helpful for knee osteoarthritis, with noxious and innocuous stimulation significantly decreasing chronic pain and morning stiffness, and significantly increasing pain threshold and range of motion compared with the control groups (Defrin et al 2005). In this study, noxious stimulation decreased pain intensity and increased pain threshold significantly more than innocuous stimulation. Modalities may help to reduce pain and medication use, as demonstrated in osteoarthritis knee pain and low back pain (Facci et al 2011; Atamaz et al 2012).

Shockwave is employed for effectively treating patellar tendon knee pain, amongst other pathologies (van Leeuwen et al 2009). There may be a role for shockwave therapy as a targeted therapy for structures involved in PFJ (see Table 44.1), such as the vastus lateralis tendon complex (Fig. 44.20), retinaculum and fat pad, though no studies have addressed this to date. In terms of TrPs, shockwave may be a promising therapy (Gleitz & Hornig 2012). It has efficiency for pain reduction and improving knee function over placebo in knee osteoarthritis patients (Zhao et al 2013). In animal studies, shockwave therapy has demonstrated a chondroprotective effect and regression of osteoarthritis in the rat knee (Wang et al 2011, 2013a, 2013b). In terms of peripheral and central pain effects, the application of shockwaves led to a significant decrease in the mean number of neurons immunoreactive for substance P within the dorsal root ganglion of L5 in rabbits exposed to high-energy shockwaves to the ventral side of the

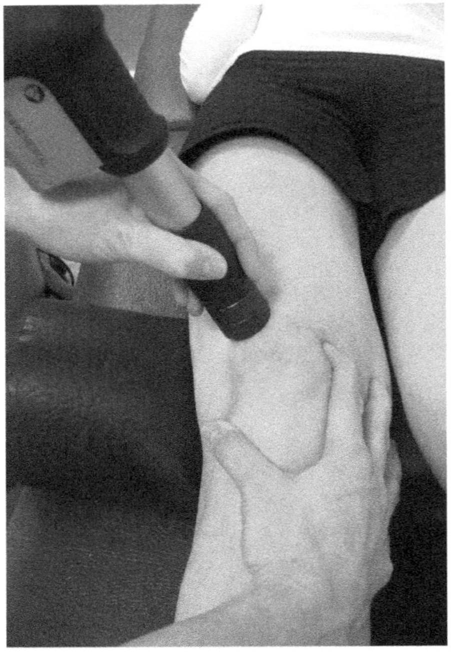

Figure 44.20 Shockwave therapy to the vastus lateralis muscle and tendon.

distal femur, whereas no such change was seen in the contralateral untreated side (Hausdorf et al 2008b). Additionally, shockwave therapy induced selective loss of unmyelinated nociceptive nerve fibres in a rabbit model (Hausdorf et al 2008a), a finding that may partially explain the reduction in pain by denervation of sensory nerves.

In summary, electrophysical modalities may play a role for pain relief in a multimodal programme for PFP. Clinicians are encouraged at least to consider these modalities as part of the plan of care for potential symptomatic relief. Future research is needed, however.

In-shoe orthoses

In-shoe foot orthoses are often prescribed for PFP to improve kinetic chain function through potential biomechanical and / or neuromuscular effects. Soft and hard orthoses may change foot biomechanics and ground reaction forces, but the effects on knee, hip and pelvic kinematics are generally limited (Nester et al 2003; Barton et al 2010). Orthoses may have an effect on the passive and active soft tissues (Nester et al 2003; McConnell 2009) and neuromuscular control (Crossley et al 2009).

Orthoses may be helpful for a select population, for example forefoot varus and excessive subtalar pronation, which can be associated with PFP (Eng & Pierrynowski 1993; Saxena & Haddad 2003; Johnston & Gross 2004; McConnell 2009; Munuera & Mazoteras-Pardo 2011; Rixe et al 2013). Foot orthoses may produce an improvement in pain symptoms when used as part of a multimodal programme (Barton et al 2010; Rixe et al 2013).

Two CPRs address orthoses and PFP. The first preliminary study (Vicenzino et al 2008) reported a +LR of 8.8 of 'marked improvement' on a 5-point Likert scale if three or more variables were present out of four predictor variables: (1) age >25 years, (2) height <165 cm, (3) worst pain <53.25 mm on 100 mm visual analogue scale, and (4) mid-foot width distance >10.96 mm. Caution should be exercised when applying this research, though, as it is a preliminary study and the methodological quality has been reported as below suggested standard (50%) (Vicenzino et al 2008; Glynn & Weisbach 2011).

The second preliminary study looked at prefabricated orthotics and modified activity for PFP patients, and the methodological score for this study was deemed acceptable (61%) (Sutlive et al 2004). The presence of one or more variables creates a small but sometimes clinically relevant shift in probability that patient's pain will decrease by ≥50%. The predictor variables and related positive likelihood ratios were reported as follows: (1) forefoot valgus ≥2° / +LR 4.0; (2) great toe extension ≤78° / +LR 4.0; and (3) navicular drop ≤3 mm / +LR 2.3 (Sutlive et al. 2004; Glynn & Weisbach 2011).

Conclusion

PFP is a common cause of musculoskeletal pain and is multifactorial in nature. Both local and remote kinetic chain influences can place stress on the PFJ and lead to pain and dysfunction. The pathophysiology of PFP is not fully understood, but tissue stress with loss of tissue homeostasis is thought to play a role in the development of pain and dysfunction. Recent evidence suggests that ischaemia may play a role in pain. Assessment of patients with PFP relies on a comprehensive assessment of the kinetic chain and local knee structures. Multimodal physiotherapy programmes appear to be effective in patients with PFP, whereas surgery should be avoided. Additional research is required to assist in further understanding of the mechanisms, causes, prevention of and optimum treatments for PFP patients.

References

AAOMPT. 2009. AAOMPT Position statements – dry needling. (2/3/2011 http://www.aaompt.org/about/statements.cfm).

Aglietti P, Insall JN, Cerulli G. 1983. Patellar pain and incongruence. I: Measurements of incongruence. Clin Orthop Relat Res 176: 217–224.

Akseki D, Akkaya G, Erduran M, et al. 2008. Proprioception of the knee joint in patello-femoral pain syndrome. Acta Orthop Traumatol Turc 42: 316–321.

Alter MJ. 1996. Science of flexibility. Champaign, IL: Human Kinetics.

Atamaz FC, Durmaz B, Baydar M, et al. 2012. Comparison of the efficacy of transcutaneous electrical nerve stimulation, interferential currents, and shortwave diathermy in knee osteoarthritis: a double-blind, randomized, controlled, multicenter study. Arch Phys Med Rehabil 93: 748–756.

Atkins DV, Eichler DA. 2013. The effects of self-massage on osteoarthritis of the knee: a randomized, controlled trial. Int J Ther Massage Bodywork 6: 4–14.

Badalamente MA, Cherney SB. 1989. Periosteal and vascular innervation of the human patella in degenerative joint disease. Semin Arthritis Rheum 18: 61–66.

Baquie P, Brukner P. 1997. Injuries presenting to an Australian sports medicine centre: a 12-month study. Clin J Sport Med 7: 28–31.

Barton CJ, Munteanu SE, Menz HB, et al. 2010. The efficacy of foot orthoses in the treatment of individuals with patellofemoral pain syndrome: a systematic review. Sports Med 40: 377–395.

Beighton P, Solomon L, Soskolne CL. 1973. Articular mobility in an African population. Ann Rheum Dis 32: 413–418.

Bell DR, Guskiewicz KM, Clark MA, et al. 2011. Systematic review of the balance error scoring system. Sports Health 3: 287–295.

Boissonnault WG. 2010. Primary care for the physical therapist: examination and triage. St Louis, MO: Elsevier / Saunders.

Boyling JD, Jull GA. 2005. The future scope of manual therapy. In: Boyling JD, Jull GA (eds) Grieve's modern manual therapy: the vertebral column, 3rd edn. Edinburgh: Churchill Livingstone, pp 367–380.

Brady S, McEvoy J, Dommerholt J, et al. 2014. Adverse events following trigger point dry needling: a prospective survey of chartered physiotherapists. J Man Manip Ther 22(3): 134–140. doi: 10.1179/2042618613Y.0000000044.

Brantingham JW, Globe G, Pollard H, et al. 2009. Manipulative therapy for lower extremity conditions: expansion of literature review. J Manipulative Physiol Ther 32: 53–71.

Bullock-Saxton JE, Janda V, Bullock MI. 1993. Reflex activation of gluteal muscles in walking. An approach to restoration of muscle function for patients with low-back pain. Spine 18: 704–708.

Calmbach WL, Hutchens M. 2003. Evaluation of patients presenting with knee pain: Part I. History, physical examination, radiographs, and laboratory tests. Am Fam Physician 68: 907–912.

Cerny K. 1995. Vastus medialis oblique / vastus lateralis muscle activity ratios for selected exercises in persons with and without patellofemoral pain syndrome. Phys Ther 75: 672–683.

Chen Q, Bensamoun S, Basford JR, et al. 2007. Identification and quantification of myofascial taut bands with magnetic resonance elastography. Arch Phys Med Rehabil 88: 1658–1661.

Chen Q, Basford J, An KN. 2008. Ability of magnetic resonance elastography to assess taut bands. Clin Biomech 23: 623–629.

Citaker S, Kaya D, Yuksel I, et al. 2012. Static balance in patients with patellofemoral pain syndrome. Sports Health 3: 524–527.

Cook G. 2010. Movement: functional movement systems: screening, assessment, and corrective strategies. Aptos, CA: On Target Publications.

Cook C, Hegedus E, Hawkins R, et al. 2010. Diagnostic accuracy and association to disability of clinical test findings associated with patellofemoral pain syndrome. Physiother Can 62: 17–24.

Cook C, Mabry L, Reiman MP, et al. 2012. Best tests / clinical findings for screening and diagnosis of patellofemoral pain syndrome: a systematic review. Physiotherapy 98: 93–100.

Cowan SM, Bennell KL, Crossley KM, et al. 2002. Physical therapy alters recruitment of the vasti in patellofemoral pain syndrome. Med Sci Sports Exerc 34: 1879–1885.

Crossley K, Bennell K, Green S, et al. 2002. Physical therapy for patellofemoral pain: a randomized, double-blinded, placebo-controlled trial. Am J Sports Med 30: 857–865.

Crossley KM, Cook J, Cowan S, et al. 2009. Anterior knee pain. In: Brukner P, Khan K (eds) Clinical sports medicine. New South Wales, Australia: McGraw Hill, pp 506–537.

Crow JF, Buttifant D, Kearny SG, et al. 2012. Low load exercises targeting the gluteal muscle group acutely enhance explosive power output in elite athletes. J Strength Cond Res 26: 438–442.

Cuddeford T, Williams AK, Medeiros JM. 1996. Electromyographic activity of the vastus medialis oblique and vastus lateralis muscles during selected exercises. J Man Manip Ther 1: 10–15.

Cummings TM, White AR. 2001. Needling therapies in the management of myofascial trigger point pain: a systematic review. Arch Phys Med Rehabil 82: 986–992.

Dallinga JM, Benjaminse A, Lemmink KA. 2012. Which screening tools can predict injury to the lower extremities in team sports? A systematic review. Sports Med 42: 791–815.

Defrin R, Ariel E, Peretz C. 2005. Segmental noxious versus innocuous electrical stimulation for chronic pain relief and the effect of fading sensation during treatment. Pain 115: 152–160.

Dejung B, Gröbli C, Colla F, et al. 2003. Triggerpunkttherapie. Bern: Hans Huber.

Docherty CL, Valovich McLeod TC, et al. 2006. Postural control deficits in participants with functional ankle instability as measured by the balance error scoring system. Clin J Sport Med 16: 203–208.

Dommerholt J, Fernandez de las Peñas C. 2013. Trigger point dry needling: an evidenced and clinical based approach. London: Churchill Livingstone.

Dye SF. 2005. The pathophysiology of patellofemoral pain: a tissue homeostasis perspective. Clin Orthop Relat Res: 100–110.

Dye SF, Vaupel GL, Dye CC. 1998. Conscious neurosensory mapping of the internal structures of the human knee without intraarticular anesthesia. Am J Sports Med 26: 773–777.

Ekstrom RA, Donatelli RA, Carp KC. 2007. Electromyographic analysis of core trunk, hip, and thigh muscles during 9 rehabilitation exercises. J Orthop Sports Phys Ther 37: 754–762.

Elton K, McDonough K, Savinar-Nogue E, et al. 1985. A preliminary investigation: History, physical, and isokinetic exam results versus arthroscopic diagnosis of chondromalacia patella. J Orthop Sports Phys Ther 7: 115–123.

Eng JJ, Pierrynowski MR. 1993. Evaluation of soft foot orthotics in the treatment of patellofemoral pain syndrome. Phys Ther 73: 62–68

Escamilla RF, Fleisig GS, Zheng N. et al. 1998. Biomechanics of the knee during closed kinetic chain and open kinetic chain exercises. Med Sci Sports Exerc 30: 556–569.

Facci LM, Nowotny JP, Tormem F, et al. 2011. Effects of transcutaneous electrical nerve stimulation (TENS) and interferential currents (IFC) in patients with nonspecific chronic low back pain: randomized clinical trial. Sao Paulo Med J 129: 206–216.

Fulkerson JP. 2002. Diagnosis and treatment of patients with patellofemoral pain. Am J Sports Med 30: 447–456.

Gleitz M, Hornig K. 2012. [Trigger points – diagnosis and treatment concepts with special reference to extracorporeal shockwaves]. Orthopade 41: 113–125.

Glynn PE, Weisbach PC. 2011. Clinical prediction rules: a physical therapy reference manual. Sudbury, MA: Jones and Bartlett.

Goodfellow J, Hungerford DS, Zindel M. 1976. Patello-femoral joint mechanics and pathology. 1. Functional anatomy of the patello-femoral joint. J Bone Joint Surg Br 58: 287–290.

Goodman CC, Boissonnault WG, Fuller K. 2003. Pathology: implications for the physical therapist. Philadelphia; London: WB Saunders.

Grelsamer RP. 2005. Patellar nomenclature: the tower of babel revisited. Clin Orthop Relat Res: 60–65.

Grelsamer RP, Klein JR. 1998. The biomechanics of the patellofemoral joint. J Orthop Sports Phys Ther 28: 286–298.

Gribble PA, Kelly SE, Refshauge KM, et al. 2013. Interrater reliability of the star excursion balance test. J Athl Train 48: 621–626.

Hakim A, Grahame R. 2003. Joint hypermobility. Best Pract Res Clin Rheumatol 17: 989–1004.

Hausdorf J, Lemmens MA, Heck KD, et al. 2008a. Selective loss of unmyelinated nerve fibers after extracorporeal shockwave application to the musculoskeletal system. Neuroscience 155: 138–144.

Hausdorf J, Lemmens MA, Kaplan S, et al. 2008b. Extracorporeal shockwave application to the distal femur of rabbits diminishes the number of neurons immunoreactive for substance P in dorsal root ganglia L5. Brain Res 1207: 96–101.

Hehne HJ. 1990. Biomechanics of the patellofemoral joint and its clinical relevance. Clin Orthop Relat Res: 73–85.

Herrington L. 2006. The effect of corrective taping of the patella on patella position as defined by MRI. Res Sports Med 14: 215–223.

Herrington L, McEwan I, Thom J. 2006a. Quantification of patella position by ultrasound scanning and its criterion validity. Ultrasound Med Biol 32: 1833–1836.

Herrington L, Rivett N, Munro S. 2006b. The relationship between patella position and length of the iliotibial band as assessed using Ober's test. Man Ther 11: 182–186.

Hertel J, Braham RA, Hale SA, et al. 2006. Simplifying the star excursion balance test: analyses of subjects with and without chronic ankle instability. J Orthop Sports Phys Ther 36: 131–137.

Holmes SW, Clancy WG. 1998. Clinical classification of patellofemoral pain and dysfunction. J Orthop Sports Phys Ther 28: 299–306.

Houglum PA. 2005. Therapeutic exercise for musculoskeletal injuries. Champaign, IL: Human Kinetics.

Insall J, Falvo KA, Wise DW. 1976. Chondromalacia patellae: a prospective study. J Bone Joint Surg Am 58: 1–8.

Irish Society of Chartered Physiotherapists (ISCP). 2012. Guidelines for dry needling practice. Dublin: ISCP.

Iverson CA, Sutlive TG, Crowell MS, et al. 2008. Lumbopelvic manipulation for the treatment of patients with patellofemoral pain syndrome: development of a clinical prediction rule. J Orthop Sports Phys Ther 38: 297–309

Johnston LB, Gross MT. 2004. Effects of foot orthoses on quality of life for individuals with patellofemoral pain syndrome. J Orthop Sports Phys Ther 34: 440–448.

Karst GM, Jewett PD. 1993. Electromyographic analysis of exercises proposed for differential activation of medial and lateral quadriceps femoris muscle components. Phys Ther 73: 286–295; discussion 295–289.

Kendall F, Kendall McCreary E, Provance P, et al. 2005. Muscles: testing and function with posture and pain. Baltimore, MD: Lippincott Williams & Wilkins.

Kenji C. 2010. Somatosensory, vestibular, and visual sensory integration: Implications for neuromuscular control and balance in orthopaedic practice. In: Donatelli R, Wooden MJ (eds) Orthopaedic physical therapy. Edinburgh: Churchill Livingstone, pp 641–671.

Kinzey SJ, Armstrong CW. 1998. The reliability of the star-excursion test in assessing dynamic balance. J Orthop Sports Phys Ther 27: 356–360.

Klemp P, Stevens JE, Isaacs S. 1984. A hypermobility study in ballet dancers. J Rheumatol 11: 692–696.

Krumrei K, Flanagan M, Bruner J, et al. 2014. The accuracy of the functional movement screen to identify individuals with an elevated risk of musculoskeletal injury. J Sport Rehabil 23(4): 360–364. doi: 10.1123/jsr.2013-0027.

Lake DA, Wofford NH. 2011. Effect of therapeutic modalities on patients with patellofemoral pain syndrome: a systematic review. Sports Health 3: 182–189.

Lankhorst NE, Bierma-Zeinstra SM, van Middelkoop M. 2012. Risk factors for patellofemoral pain syndrome: a systematic review. J Orthop Sports Phys Ther 42: 81–94.

Lankhorst NE, Bierma-Zeinstra S, van Middelkoop M. 2013. Factors associated with patellofemoral pain syndrome: a systematic review. Br J Sports Med 47: 193–206.

Lesher JD, Sutlive TG, Miller GA, et al. 2006. Development of a clinical prediction rule for classifying patients with patellofemoral pain syndrome who respond to patellar taping. J Orthop Sports Phys Ther 36: 854–866.

Maher RM, Hayes DM, Shinohara M. 2013. Quantification of dry needling and posture effects on myofascial trigger points using ultrasound shear-wave elastography. Arch Phys Med Rehabil 94: 2146–2150.

Mathews L, Sonstegard D, Henke J. 1977. Load-bearing characteristics of the patellofemoral joint. Acta Orthop Scand 48: 511–516.

Mayoral O, Salvat I, Martin MT, et al. 2013. Efficacy of myofascial trigger point dry needling in the prevention of pain after total knee arthroplasty: a randomized, double-blinded, placebo-controlled trial. Evid Based Complement Alternat Med 2013: 694941.

McConnell J. 2009. What are effective therapies for anterior knee pain? In: Wright JG (ed) Evidence-based orthopaedics: the best answers to clinical questions. Philadelphia: Saunders, pp 634–639.

McEvoy J. 2013. Trigger point dry needling: safety guidelines. In: Dommerholt J, Fernandez-de-las-Peñas C (eds) Trigger point dry needling: an evidenced and clinical based approach. London: Churchill Livingstone, pp 39–58.

McEvoy J, Huijbregts P. 2011. Reliability of myofascial trigger point palpation: a systematic review. In: Dommerholt J, Huijbregts P (eds) Myofascial trigger points: pathophysiology and evidenced-informed diagnosis and management. Sudbury: Jones and Bartlett, pp 65–88.

McEwan I, Herrington L, Thom J. 2007. The validity of clinical measures of patella position. Man Ther 12: 226–230.

Mirzabeigi E, Jordan C, Gronley JK, et al. 1999. Isolation of the vastus medialis oblique muscle during exercise. Am J Sports Med 27: 50–53.

Munro AG, Herrington LC. 2010. Between-session reliability of the star excursion balance test. Phys Ther Sport 11: 128–132.

Munuera PV, Mazoteras-Pardo R. 2011. Benefits of custom-made foot orthoses in treating patellofemoral pain. Prosthet Orthot Int 35: 342–349.

Naslund J, Naslund UB, Odenbring S, et al. 2006. Comparison of symptoms and clinical findings in subgroups of individuals with patellofemoral pain. Physiother Theory Pract 22: 105–118.

Naslund J, Walden M, Lindberg LG. 2007. Decreased pulsatile blood flow in the patella in patellofemoral pain syndrome. Am J Sports Med 35: 1668–1673.

Nemschak G, Pretterklieber ML. 2012. The patellar arterial supply via the infrapatellar fat pad (of Hoffa): a combined anatomical and angiographical analysis. Anat Res Int 2012: 713838.

Nester CJ, van der Linden ML, Bowker P. 2003. Effect of foot orthoses on the kinematics and kinetics of normal walking gait. Gait Posture 17: 180–187.

Oatis C. 2004. Kinesiology: the mechanics and pathomechanics of human movement. Philadelphia: Lippincott Williams & Wilkins.

Page P, Frank CC, Lardner R. 2010. Assessment and treatment of muscle imbalance: the Janda approach. Leeds: Human Kinetics.

Peeler J, Anderson JE. 2007. Effectiveness of static quadriceps stretching in individuals with patellofemoral joint pain. Clin J Sport Med 17: 234–241.

Perlman AI, Sabina A, Williams AL, et al. 2006. Massage therapy for osteoarthritis of the knee: a randomized controlled trial. Arch Intern Med 166: 2533–2538.

Perlman AI, Ali A, Njike V, et al. 2012. Massage therapy for osteoarthritis of the knee: a randomized dose-finding trial. PLoS One 7: e30248.

Peter WF, Jansen MJ, Hurkmans EJ, et al. 2011. Physiotherapy in hip and knee osteoarthritis: development of a practice guideline concerning initial assessment, treatment and evaluation. Acta Reumatol Port 36: 268–281.

Pinar H, Akseki D, Genc I, et al. 1994. Kinematic and dynamic axial computerized tomography of the normal patellofemoral joint. Knee Surg Sports Traumatol Arthrosc 2: 27–30.

Piva SR, Fitzgerald GK, Irrgang JJ, et al. 2009a. Associates of physical function and pain in patients with patellofemoral pain syndrome. Arch Phys Med Rehabil 90: 285–295.

Piva SR, Fitzgerald GK, Wisniewski S, et al. 2009b. Predictors of pain and function outcome after rehabilitation in patients with patellofemoral pain syndrome. J Rehabil Med 41: 604–612.

Plisky PJ, Rauh MJ, Kaminski TW, et al. 2006. Star Excursion Balance Test as a predictor of lower extremity injury in high school basketball players. J Orthop Sports Phys Ther 36: 911–919.

Post WR. 2005. Anterior knee pain: diagnosis and treatment. J Am Acad Orthop Surg 13: 534–543.

Powers CM, Shellock FG, Pfaff M. 1998. Quantification of patellar tracking using kinematic MRI. J Magn Reson Imaging 8: 724–732.

Powers CM, Mortenson S, Nishimoto D, et al. 1999. Criterion-related validity of a clinical measurement to determine the medial / lateral component of patellar orientation. J Orthop Sports Phys Ther 29: 372–377.

Powers CM, Bolgla LA, Callaghan MJ, et al. 2012. Patellofemoral pain: proximal, distal, and local factors, 2nd International Research Retreat. J Orthop Sports Phys Ther 42: A1–54.

Prakask S, Chopra S, Jit L. 1979. Ossification of the human patella. J Anat Soc India 28: 78–83.

Ralph R, Garrick J. 1996. Adult recreational fitness In: Caine D, Caine C, Koenraad L (eds) Epidemiology of sports injuries. Champaign: Human Kinetics.

Raveendranath R, Nachiket S, Sujatha N, et al. 2011. Bilateral variability of the quadriceps angle (Q angle) in an adult Indian population. Iran J Basic Med Sci 14: 465–471.

Reilly DT, Martens M. 1972. Experimental analysis of the quadriceps muscle force and patello-femoral joint reaction force for various activities. Acta Orthop Scand 43: 126–137.

Riemann BL, Guskiewicz KM. 2000. Effects of mild head injury on postural stability as measured through clinical balance testing. J Athl Train 35: 19–25.

Rixe JA, Glick JE, Brady J, et al. 2013. A review of the management of patellofemoral pain syndrome. Phys Sports Med 41: 19–28.

Roach S, Sorenson E, Headley B, et al. 2013. Prevalence of myofascial trigger points in the hip in patellofemoral pain. Arch Phys Med Rehabil 94: 522–526.

Rosenblatt RA, Cherkin DC, Schneeweiss R, et al. 1983. The content of ambulatory medical care in the United States. An interspecialty comparison. N Engl J Med 309: 892–897.

Saxena A, Haddad J. 2003. The effect of foot orthoses on patellofemoral pain syndrome. J Am Podiatr Med Assoc 93: 264–271.

Schoots EJ, Tak IJ, Veenstra BJ, et al. 2013. Ultrasound characteristics of the lateral retinaculum in 10 patients with patellofemoral pain syndrome compared to healthy controls. J Bodyw Mov Ther 17: 523–529.

Seckin U, Tur BS, Yilmaz O, et al. 2005. The prevalence of joint hypermobility among high school students. Rheumatol Int 25: 260–263.

Selfe J, Harper L, Pedersen I, et al. 2003. Cold legs: a potential indicator of negative outcome in the rehabilitation of patients with patellofemoral pain syndrome. Knee 10: 139–143.

Selfe J, Sutton C, Hardaker NJ, et al. 2010. Anterior knee pain and cold knees: a possible association in women. Knee 17: 319–323.

Shabshin N, Schweitzer ME, Morrison WB, et al. 2004. MRI criteria for patella alta and baja. Skeletal Radiol 33: 445–450.

Shultz R, Anderson SC, Matheson GO, et al. 2013. Test–retest and interrater reliability of the functional movement screen. J Athl Train 48: 331–336.

Sikdar S, Shah JP, Gilliams E, et al. 2008. Assessment of myofascial trigger points (MTrPs): a new application of ultrasound imaging and vibration sonoelastography. Conf Proc IEEE Eng Med Biol Soc 2008: 5585–5588.

Sikdar S, Shah JP, Gebreab T, et al. 2009. Novel applications of ultrasound technology to visualize and characterize myofascial trigger points and surrounding soft tissue. Arch Phys Med Rehabil 90: 1829–1838.

Silbert BI, Singer BJ, Silbert PL, et al. 2012. Enduring efficacy of Botulinum toxin type A injection for refractory anterior knee pain. Disabil Rehabil 34: 62–68.

Singer BJ, Silbert PL, Dunne JW, et al. 2006. An open label pilot investigation of the efficacy of Botulinum toxin type A [Dysport] injection in the rehabilitation of chronic anterior knee pain. Disabil Rehabil 28: 707–713.

Singer BJ, Silbert PL, Song S, et al. 2011. Treatment of refractory anterior knee pain using botulinum toxin type A (Dysport) injection to the distal vastus lateralis muscle: a randomised placebo controlled crossover trial. Br J Sports Med 45: 640–645.

Sluka K. 2009. Mechanisms and management of pain for the physical therapist. Seattle: IASP Press.

Sluka K. 2014. Summary statement: somatosensory system; neuropharmacology of pain. Online. Available: http://neuroscience.grad.uiowa.edu/faculty/kathleen-sluka.

Smith TO, Hunt NJ, Donell ST. 2008. The reliability and validity of the Q-angle: a systematic review. Knee Surg Sports Traumatol Arthrosc 16: 1068–1079.
Stensdotter AK, Hodges PW, Mellor R, et al. 2003. Quadriceps activation in closed and in open kinetic chain exercise. Med Sci Sports Exerc 35: 2043–2047.
Susco TM, Valovich McLeod TC, Gansneder BM, et al. 2004. Balance recovers within 20 minutes after exertion as measured by the balance error scoring system. J Athl Train 39: 241–246.
Sutlive TG, Mitchell SD, Maxfield SN, et al. 2004. Identification of individuals with patellofemoral pain whose symptoms improved after a combined program of foot orthosis use and modified activity: a preliminary investigation. Phys Ther 84: 49–61.
Travell JG, Rinzler SH. 1952. The myofascial genesis of pain. Postgrad Med 11: 425–434.
Travell JG, Simons DG. 1992. Myofascial pain and dysfunction: the trigger point manual (Vol II). Baltimore: Williams & Wilkins.
Valovich TC, Perrin DH, Gansneder BM. 2003. Repeat administration elicits a practice effect with the Balance Error Scoring System but not with the standardized assessment of concussion in high school athletes. J Athl Train 38: 51–56.
van Gent RN, Siem D, van Middelkoop M, et al. 2007. Incidence and determinants of lower extremity running injuries in long distance runners: a systematic review. Br J Sports Med 41: 469–480
van Leeuwen MT, Zwerver J, van den Akker-Scheek I. 2009. Extracorporeal shockwave therapy for patellar tendinopathy: a review of the literature. Br J Sports Med 43: 163–168.
Vicenzino B, Collins N, Cleland J, et al. 2008. A clinical prediction rule for identifying patients with patellofemoral pain who are likely to benefit from foot orthoses: a preliminary determination. Br J Sports Med 44: 862–866.
Wang CJ, Weng LH, Ko JY, et al. 2011. Extracorporeal shockwave shows regression of osteoarthritis of the knee in rats. J Surg Res 171: 601–608.
Wang CJ, Hsu SL, Weng LH, et al. 2013a. Extracorporeal shockwave therapy shows a number of treatment related chondroprotective effect in osteoarthritis of the knee in rats. BMC Musculoskelet Disord 14: 44.
Wang CJ, Sun YC, Siu KK, et al. 2013b. Extracorporeal shockwave therapy shows site-specific effects in osteoarthritis of the knee in rats. J Surg Res 183: 612–619.
Warmerdam A. 1999. Manual therapy: improve muscle and joint functioning. Wantagh: Pine Publications.
Watson T. 2008. Electrotherapy: evidence-based practice. Edinburgh: Churchill Livingstone.
Wilk KE, Davies GJ, Mangine RE, et al. 1998. Patellofemoral disorders: a classification system and clinical guidelines for nonoperative rehabilitation. J Orthop Sports Phys Ther 28: 307–322.
Wilkins JC, Valovich McLeod TC, Perrin DH, et al. 2004. Performance on the balance error scoring system decreases after fatigue. J Athl Train 39: 156–161.
Williams PL, Bannister LH, Berry MM, et al. 1995. The anatomical basis of medicine and surgery. In: Gray HA, Bannister L, Berry M (eds) Gray's anatomy: the anatomical basis of medicine and surgery. New York, Edinburgh: Churchill Livingstone, pp 1825–1861.
Witonski D, Goraj B. 1999. Patellar motion analyzed by kinematic and dynamic axial magnetic resonance imaging in patients with anterior knee pain syndrome. Arch Orthop Trauma Surg 119: 46–49.
Wyke B. 1967. The neurology of joints. Ann R Coll Surg Engl 41: 25–50.
Zhang W, Moskowitz RW, Nuki G, et al. 2007. OARSI recommendations for the management of hip and knee osteoarthritis, part I: critical appraisal of existing treatment guidelines and systematic review of current research evidence. Osteoarthritis Cartilage 15: 981–1000.
Zhao Z, Jing R, Shi Z, Zhao B, et al. 2013. Efficacy of extracorporeal shockwave therapy for knee osteoarthritis: a randomized controlled trial. J Surg Res 185: 661–666.

45 Chapter

Postoperative Management of the Knee: Ligamentous, Meniscal and Total Joint Replacement

Jodi Young, Ellen Pong

CHAPTER CONTENTS

Introduction 514
Anterior/posterior cruciate ligament reconstruction 514
Modalities 514
Bracing/weight-bearing 514
Range of motion exercises 515
Therapeutic exercise 516
Neuromuscular re-education 516
Medial collateral ligament repair/reconstruction 516
Bracing/weight-bearing 516
Range of motion exercises 516
Therapeutic exercise 516
Meniscus 517
Meniscal repair/transplantation 517
Partial meniscectomy 519
Total knee arthroplasty 520
Procedures 520
Treatment 521
Arthrofibrosis of the knee 522
Conclusion 523

Introduction

This chapter introduces evidence-based physical therapy interventions for patients undergoing surgery for ligamentous or meniscal injuries or total knee arthroplasty. Postoperative rehabilitation will vary depending on the severity of injury, the surgical approach and other tissues injured. The goals of rehabilitation after anterior cruciate ligament (ACL), posterior cruciate ligament (PCL) and medial collateral ligament (MCL) reconstruction, meniscal repair, transplantation and partial meniscectomy all include minimizing swelling and pain, restoring the knee range of motion and joint mobility, normalizing lower extremity strength, dynamic stability, gait and knee biomechanics, and enhancing proprioception and neuromuscular control (Logerstedt et al 2010b; Wijdicks 2010; Escamilla et al 2012; LaPrade & Wijdicks 2012; Noyes et al 2012; Rosenthal et al 2012; Yvas et al 2012). Provision of evidence-based interventions to address these goals will be the emphasis of this chapter. (See Ch 42 for further information on risk factors and conservative treatment of knee injuries.)

Anterior/Posterior Cruciate Ligament Reconstruction

Initial rehabilitation principles for ACL reconstruction emphasize full passive knee extension, immediate range of motion and partial weight-bearing (Wright et al 2008; Logerstedt et al 2010b; Wilk et al 2012). Autograft tissues, either bone–patellar, tendon–bone or hamstring tendon, are considered the gold standards in ACL reconstruction and have been shown to decrease time in surgery and reduce postoperative pain (Manske et al 2012; Nandra et al 2013). The most common autograft in PCL reconstruction is the bone–patellar–tendon–bone (Rosenthal et al 2012). Because current surgical practice favours the use of autografts, the focus on rehabilitation techniques after autograft surgical procedures for ACL/PCL reconstruction will be discussed. See Table 45.1 for rehabilitation goals.

Modalities

The use of cryotherapy, in conjunction with elevation and compression, should be utilized in patients immediately after surgery to assist in pain reduction and swelling (Logerstedt et al 2010b; Manske et al 2012; Rosenthal et al 2012; Wilk et al 2012). Patients can also be prescribed neuromuscular electrostimulation (NMES) for reduction of swelling and assistance of quadriceps facilitation (Manske et al 2012; Rosenthal et al 2012). In recent studies, those who received NMES two to three times per week for up to 12 weeks had improved quadriceps strength compared with those who did not receive the intervention (Logerstedt et al 2010b).

Bracing/weight-bearing

Hinged braces locked into 0° extension should be used during ambulation for up to 2 weeks after ACL or PCL reconstruction. Patients will often be allowed to unlock the brace while sitting, performing knee range of motion and strengthening

Table 45.1 ACL/PCL reconstruction rehabilitation goals

Time frame	Clinical goals
Weeks 0–2	**ACL** ROM 0–90° Quadriceps control Full weight-bearing
	PCL AROM/PROM: 90–0°/0–90° Quadriceps control
Weeks 2–6	**ACL** Knee flexion within 10° of uninvolved limb Implement neuromuscular re-education programme
	PCL ROM to 120° Full weight-bearing
Weeks 6–12	**ACL** Full ROM (by 8 weeks) Normal gait (by 8 weeks)
	PCL Full ROM (by 12 weeks) Normal gait (by 12 weeks) Implement closed kinetic chain exercises (week 6)
Weeks 12–16	**ACL** Begin sport-specific and agility exercises (week 12)
	PCL Begin basic agility exercises
Weeks 16–24	**ACL** Continue sport-specific, agility and plyometric training Return to sport (if cleared)
	PCL Begin sport-specific exercises/plyometrics
Weeks >24	PCL Return to sport

AROM=active range of motion; PROM=passive range of motion; ROM=range of motion.

exercises. Weight-bearing status will depend on surgeon specification and range from partial to total weight-bearing as tolerated (Rosenthal et al 2012; Wilk et al 2012). Individuals undergoing ACL reconstruction should be full weight-bearing by 2 weeks, whereas full weight-bearing may take up to 4–6 weeks after PCL reconstruction (Manske et al 2012; Rosenthal et al 2012; Wilk et al 2012). Depending on physician preference, the patient should continue to wear a brace for several weeks.

Range of motion exercises

Immediate mobilization for those undergoing ACL reconstruction is important so as to regain knee range of motion, and especially knee extension (Manske et al 2012). Early mobilization also helps to reduce pain and limit possible soft tissue restrictions (Logerstedt et al 2010b). Those who receive a PCL reconstruction may need to be immobilized for 2–4 weeks (Harner & Hoher 1998). Therapist interventions to assist with gaining full knee extension can include manual passive range of motion into hyperextension (Manske et al 2012), supine hamstring stretches with a wedge under the heel (Wilk et al 2012) or gravity-assisted extension (Manske et al 2012).

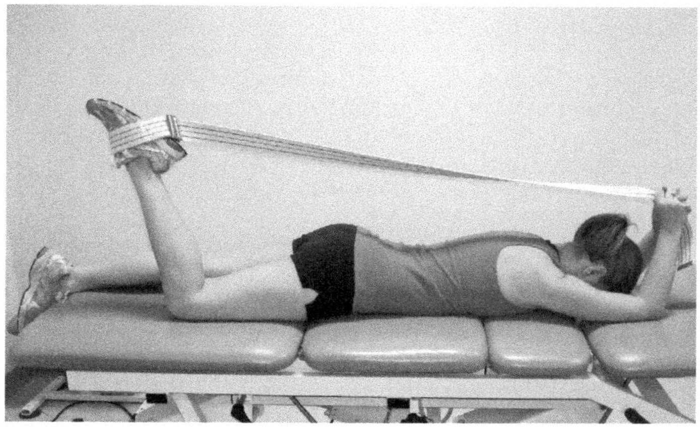

Figure 45.1 Passive knee flexion stretch with the patient prone.

To increase knee flexion, wall slides and active heels slides can be utilized. Active heel slides should not be performed for PCL reconstruction, or ACL reconstruction if a hamstring tendon graft was used (Manske et al 2012; Rosenthal et al 2012). Care should be taken in individuals undergoing PCL reconstruction to limit flexion to 90° until after week 2; this can be done through passive knee flexion with patients in a prone position, or with patients holding a strap and performing the stretch themselves (Fig. 45.1) (Rosenthal et al 2012). Progression past 90° of knee flexion can begin after 2 weeks, but should be restricted to 120° until 6 weeks after a PCL reconstruction (Wilk 1994; Rosenthal et al 2012).

Patellar mobilizations should be used immediately after surgery for those individuals who have undergone either an ACL or a PCL reconstruction. Superior, inferior, medial and lateral patellar mobilizations should be used both as a therapeutic intervention and as a home exercise programme (Rosenthal et al 2012; Wilk et al 2012). Tibiofemoral mobilizations can be performed with care to increase knee extension and flexion. Little has been studied on joint mobilizations in those undergoing ACL or PCL reconstruction, so therapist discretion is necessary when determining the type and grade of mobilization to utilize. Adams et al (2012) recommend the use of tibiofemoral joint mobilizations with rotation at 4 weeks, and Rosenthal et al (2012) advocate that tibiofemoral mobilizations be added immediately post surgery for PCL reconstruction. (See Ch 46 for a description of joint mobilization interventions of the knee joint.) Hunt et al (2010) described the use of one-time grade four anterior tibiofemoral joint mobilizations in 12 patients post ACL reconstruction. The results indicate that there was an increase in knee flexion after anterior glides; however, the results were temporary, so perhaps more than one session is appropriate.

Therapeutic exercise

Therapeutic exercise for those undergoing PCL reconstruction is similar to those undergoing ACL reconstruction, except for the use of active knee flexion and active hamstring-strengthening exercises in the latter. In PCL it is important to use passive knee flexion rather than active assisted or active knee flexion in the first 2 weeks after surgery so as to prevent posterior shear forces on the PCL from the hamstring (Rosenthal et al 2012).

General therapeutic exercises in the early stages of rehabilitation for both reconstructions should include isometric quadriceps sets, straight leg raises, weight shifts, leg press and squats in specific ranges of motion and open kinetic chain knee extension, with and without the use of weights (van Grinsven et al 2010; Manske et al 2012; Rosenthal et al 2012; Wilk et al 2012).

Closed kinetic chain exercises may begin at week 6 for those with a PCL reconstruction if performed in the range 0° to 45°, but resisted knee flexion or active hamstring contractions should not be performed until week 8 owing to posterior tibial shear (Wilk 1994; Pandy & Shelburne 1997). Closed kinetic chain exercises can begin earlier in the rehabilitation phase, between 1 and 4 weeks (Manske et al 2012). Typically, patients undergoing ACL reconstruction have been advised not to perform closed kinetic chain exercises from 0° to 45° and open kinetic chain exercises between 90° and 0°, but recent evidence indicates that there may be little harm in working in these ranges (Manske et al 2012). Eccentric strengthening has been studied in recent years, and the consensus is that physical therapists should integrate eccentric squats in PCL reconstruction rehabilitation and use an eccentric exercise ergometer for those following ACL reconstruction (Logerstedt et al 2010b).

Around week 6, patients can use a stair climber, elliptical or treadmill, as well as progress with balance / proprioception exercises (van Grinsven et al 2010; Manske et al 2012; Rosenthal et al 2012). This could include starting with squats on a stable surface and progressing to having the patient perform them on a rocker board, with the physical therapist providing manual pertubations (Manske et al 2012; Wilk et al 2012).

Starting around week 12, patients can incorporate functional dynamic balance activities, plyometrics, agility exercises and work on sport-specific activities (van Grinsven et al 2010; Adams et al 2012; Manske et al 2012). To assess for a patient's return to sport, activities such as side shuffling, cutting, start and stops, zig-zags, figure eights and cariocas can be integrated (Wilk et al 2012). It is recommended that those undergoing a PCL reconstruction wait until week 16 to begin sport-specific exercises and plyometrics (Rosenthal et al 2012).

Neuromuscular re-education

Neuromuscular re-education should be started when a patient is ambulating without an assistive device (van Grinsven et al 2010). DiStasi et al (2013) discussed the importance of neuromuscular training after ACL reconstruction to prevent a second injury. It has been found that muscle weakness, impaired neuromuscular control and deficits in a successful return to high-level sports remain after an initial ACL reconstruction (DiStasi et al 2013). Unidirectional single-leg activities, double- to single-leg exercises with decreasing base of support, perturbations during single-leg activities and multidirectional tasks needing plyometric and quick repetitions on unstable surfaces are just some of the activities that should be included (DiStasi et al 2013).

Medial Collateral Ligament Repair / Reconstruction

In patients with severe acute MCL injuries, surgery typically occurs only when there is a multiligament injury or knee dislocation involving the MCL. Direct repair with sutures, acute reconstruction or a repair with a hamstring graft may occur, but there is a risk for arthrofibrosis or heterotopic bone formation with these procedures (LaPrade & Wijdicks 2012). Patients with chronic medial knee injuries will have surgery when rotatory instability becomes an issue (LaPrade & Wijdicks 2012).

Bracing / weight-bearing

Individuals undergoing an MCL reconstruction will be non-weight-bearing or toe-touch weight-bearing and wear a brace for up to 6 weeks after surgery (LaPrade & Wijdicks 2012); those undergoing an MCL repair will be non-wearing for 3 weeks in a brace that allows 30–90° of motion (Quarles & Hosey 2004). The knee brace should be removed only when the patient is undergoing passive range of motion for the first 2 weeks after surgery; after that, the brace should be worn while sleeping or when the patient is moving around. When the patient achieves full weight-bearing status and has no gait deviation, the brace can be discontinued.

Range of motion exercises

Early range of motion is necessary to reduce the chances of arthrofibrosis or adhesions. Full knee extension is the goal by the end of 2 weeks, but care should be taken to avoid hyperextension, which would place tension on the graft (Wijdicks et al 2010). Passive or passive assisted knee flexion from 0° to 90° should occur within the first 2 weeks after surgery (LaPrade & Wijdicks 2012). Range of motion should improve to at least 130° flexion by 6 weeks after surgery. To assist in increasing the knee range of motion, patellofemoral joint mobilizations can be performed aggressively immediately after surgery.

Therapeutic exercise

Immediately following surgery, patients recovering from an MCL reconstruction can perform strengthening exercises such as quadriceps sets, straight leg raise, hip extension and abduction exercises (LaPrade & Wijdicks 2012), all while wearing a knee brace.

Closed kinetic chain exercises can be introduced at 6 weeks for functional strengthening, but if a leg press or double-limb squatting is performed then knee flexion should be limited to

70° to minimize extreme joint movement (Wijdicks et al 2010; LaPrade & Wijdicks 2012). It is also advised that no resistive or repetitive hamstring exercises be performed until 4 months after surgery (LaPrade & Wijdicks 2012).

Normalizing gait mechanics should be emphasized when incorporating closed kinetic chain exercises (Wijdicks et al 2010; LaPrade & Wijdicks 2012). Close attention should be paid to the individual's tolerance to full weight-bearing and gait to avoid joint effusion, which can affect quadriceps strength, range of motion and pain levels (Wijdicks et al 2010; LaPrade & Wijdicks 2012). The therapist should also observe the patient for a quadriceps avoidance gait, as it could cause knee hyperextension during stance (Wijdicks et al 2010). Lastly, patients should avoid any gait pattern that exhibits excessive knee valgus or internal or external rotation at the tibiofemoral joint so as to limit stress on grafts (LaPrade & Wijdicks 2012).

Sixteen weeks after surgery, the physical therapist may incorporate the use of plyometrics and agility training if the patient has progressed with strengthening, balance and proprioception (LaPrade & Wijdicks 2012). Examples of exercises may include multiplanar directional lunges (Fig. 45.2A–C), footwork drills for agility with a ladder, double-leg plyometric drills and manual perturbations from the physical therapist to challenge proprioception and balance. If the patient is able to tolerate 1–2 miles (≈1.5–3 km) of ambulating without antalgia at a brisk pace and shows controlled single-leg squatting, an interval-jogging programme may then be implemented (Wijdicks et al 2010; LaPrade & Wijdicks 2012). Return to sport or recreational activity may occur when the physician and physical therapist determine objectively that the patient is able to do so safely (LaPrade & Wijdicks 2012).

Meniscus

Meniscal injuries are often treated surgically with a partial meniscectomy or a meniscal repair, both of which are preferred to a total meniscectomy (Barber 1994). A newer surgical option is meniscal transplantation, which uses human allograft tissue (Heckmann et al 2006; Noyes et al 2012). Rehabilitation progression after meniscal repair, transplantation and total meniscectomy is slower than partial meniscectomy, but, as with every patient, the progression is dependent on many factors. Table 45.2 summarizes the postoperative management intervention strategies.

Meniscal repair/transplantation

Modalities

Early postoperative management includes cryotherapy and compression, with education of patients to elevate their lower extremity as often as possible (Heckmann et al 2006; Noyes et al 2012). NMES for pain management and quadriceps re-education for increasing quadriceps strength (Bax et al 2005; Heckmann et al 2006; Noyes et al 2012) can be incorporated.

Table 45.2 **Postoperative intervention strategies for meniscal repair/transplantation**

Intervention	Evidence-based recommendation
Modalities	Cryotherapy and compression (Heckmann et al 2006; Noyes et al 2012) NMES for pain management and quadriceps re-education (Bax et al 2005; Heckmann et al 2006; Noyes et al 2012)
Bracing/weight-bearing	Brace allowing 0–90° immediately after surgery but locked in 0° extension at night for the first 2 weeks (Heckmann et al 2006; Logerstedt et al 2010b; Noyes et al 2012) Immediate weight-bearing at tolerance (Shelbourne et al 1996a; Logerstedt et al 2010b)
Range of motion	Passive flexion and active/active assisted and passive knee extension from 0° to 90° immediately after surgery (Heckmann et al 2006; Cavanaugh & Killian 2012) Patellar mobilizations in superior, inferior, medial and lateral directions (Noyes et al 2012)
Therapeutic exercise	Early postsurgical quadriceps sets, straight leg raise and active assisted knee extension (Heckmann et al 2006; Cavanaugh & Killian 2012; Noyes et al 2012) Closed kinetic chain exercises when knee flexion improved to 85° and/or patients are 50% weight-bearing for meniscal repair and at weeks 7–8 for meniscal transplant (Heckmann et al 2006) Open kinetic chain non-weight-bearing exercises for those undergoing meniscal repair (Heckmann et al 2006; Noyes et al 2012) Step-up/step-down programme around weeks 6–14 depending on repair or transplant (Cavanaugh & Killian 2012) Plyometric/agility training at week 14 (Cavanaugh & Killian 2012) Return to sport activities at weeks 16–20 (Cavanaugh & Killian 2012) for repair and at 1 year for meniscal transplant
Neuromuscular re-education	Balance and proprioceptive exercises beginning when patient is 50% weight-bearing for meniscal repair (Heckmann et al 2006; Cavanaugh & Killian 2012; Noyes et al 2012) Rocker board, Airex, Bosu, mini trampoline, foam roll, BAPS or Biodex progressions for advanced neuromuscular re-education (Heckmann et al 2006; Noyes et al 2012)

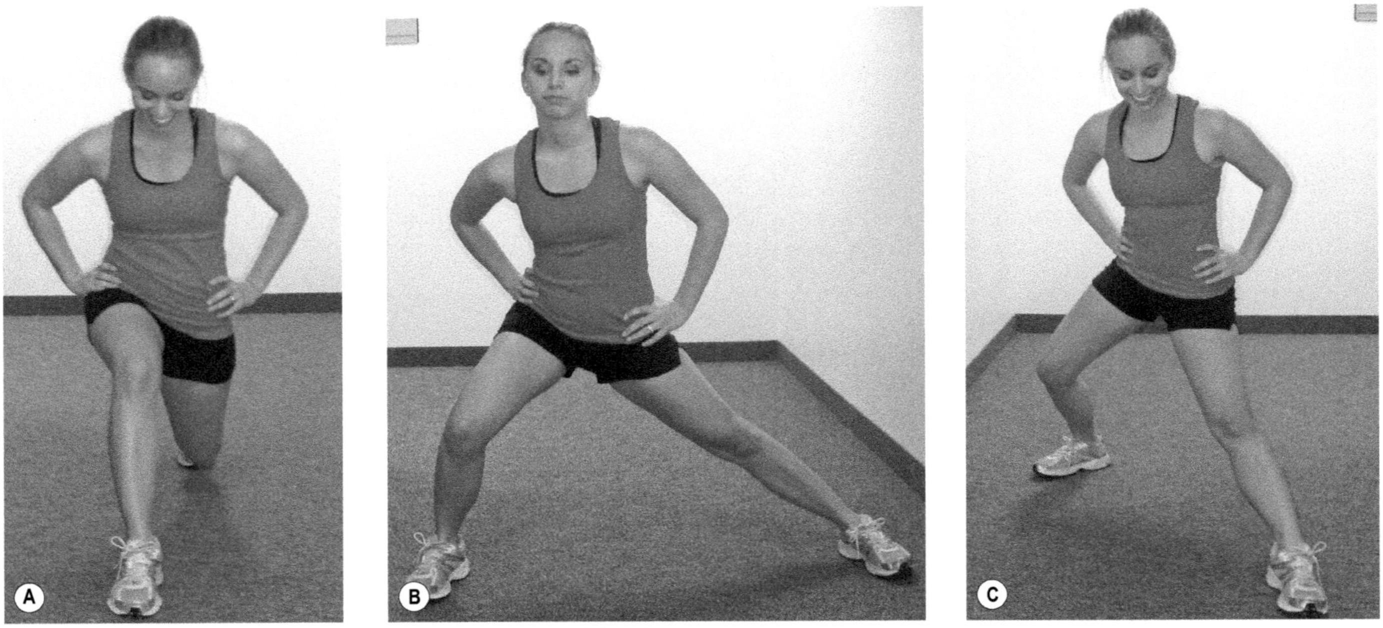

Figure 45.2 Multiplanar directional lunges: (**A**) anterior lunge; (**B**) lateral lunge; (**C**) posterior–lateral lunge.

Bracing / weight-bearing

To reduce effusion and pain, subjects undergoing meniscal repair / transplantation should wear a brace for up to 6 weeks after surgery, depending on the severity of the repair / transplant (Cavanaugh & Killian 2012; Noyes et al 2012). Subjects will be allowed range of motion from 0° to 90° immediately after surgery, but a brace should be locked at 0° extension for the first 2 weeks at night (Heckmann et al 2006; Logerstedt et al 2010a; Noyes et al 2012).

Weight-bearing status is dependent on the severity of the repair / transplant; however, individuals should be fully weight-bearing by 9 weeks after the operation (Heckmann et al 2006; Logerstedt et al 2010a; Noyes et al 2012). A study on accelerated rehabilitation allowed immediate weight-bearing at tolerance, early mobilization and a return to sport when a full range of motion had been regained. Individuals in the accelerated rehabilitation group had a full range of motion more quickly, with better quadriceps strength and an accelerated return to sport (Shelbourne et al 1996a; Logerstedt et al 2010a). Early mobilization may be the best option for those undergoing a meniscal repair.

Range of motion exercises

Heckmann et al (2006) and Cavanaugh and Killian (2012) recommend passive flexion and active / active assisted and passive knee extension exercises from 0° to 90° immediately after surgery. Overpressure for knee extension can be added through the use of a weight over the distal thigh and knee (Heckmann et al 2006) or by self-overpressure as educated by the physical therapist. Active knee flexion should be avoided immediately post surgery to reduce hamstring strain on the posterior–medial joint (Heckmann et al 2006), the semimembranosus medially and the popliteus laterally (Cavanaugh & Killian 2012).

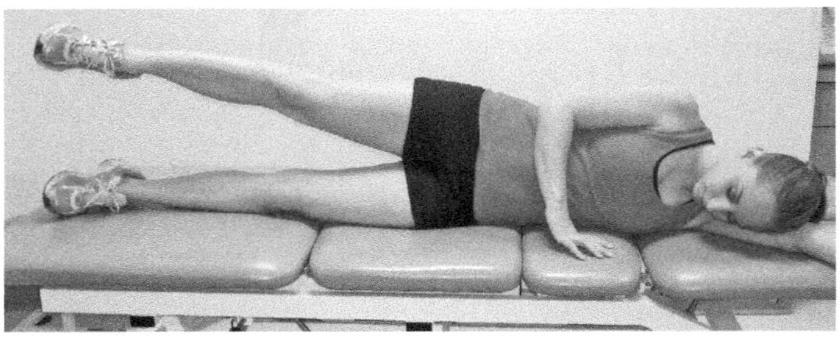

Figure 45.3 Straight leg hip abduction exercise.

Patellar joint mobilizations should begin in the first week of physical therapy after meniscal repair / transplant. Mobilizations in all directions should be performed (Noyes et al 2012). To assist in furthering the range of motion, hamstring and gastrocnemius / soleus stretching should be initiated 1 day postoperatively (Heckmann et al 2006; Noyes et al 2012).

Therapeutic exercise

Early strengthening exercises should include quadriceps sets, straight leg raise and active assisted knee extension (Heckmann et al 2006; Cavanaugh & Killian 2012; Noyes et al 2012). Straight leg raise should be performed in the sagittal plane only until any extensor lag is eliminated (Heckmann et al 2006; Noyes et al 2012); further straight leg raise for extension and abduction can be added (Fig. 45.3) when any lag is eliminated (Cavanaugh & Killian 2012).

When flexion improves to greater than 85° and / or patients are 50% weight-bearing (around 3–4 weeks postoperative) in those undergoing a meniscal repair, closed kinetic chain exercises can be added (Noyes et al 2012). Mini-squats, wall sits and bilateral leg presses can be incorporated within a 0° to 60° flexion range (Heckmann et al 2006; Cavanaugh & Killian

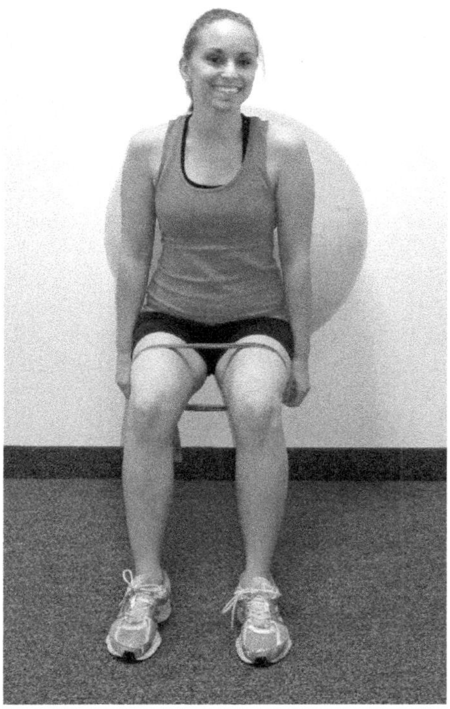

Figure 45.4 Squat with the use of a physioball and Theraband®.

2012). Individuals having a meniscal transplant must wait until weeks 7–8 to perform wall sits and mini-squats (Heckmann et al 2006). At 5–6 weeks after meniscal repair and 9–12 weeks after meniscal transplant, leg press exercises can be performed in the range of 70° to 10°. Open kinetic chain non-weight-bearing exercises can be utilized in those patients undergoing a meniscal repair around 5–6 weeks after surgery, including hamstring curls and quadriceps exercises without weight until the patient tolerates weight-bearing (Heckmann et al 2006; Noyes et al 2012).

As the patient resumes normal range of motion and demonstrates a normal gait pattern (around 6–14 weeks), further exercises can be added. Bilateral and unilateral eccentric leg press can be added when the knee flexion range of motion increases to greater than 120° (Cavanaugh & Killian 2012). Squats with progressive resistance with the use of a physioball initially and then Theraband® or tubing can be added (Fig. 45.4) (Heckmann et al 2006; Cavanaugh & Killian 2012). Four-inch (10 cm) step-ups progressing to 6 and then 8 inches (15 and 20 cm) are appropriate at this time, and should be implemented prior to a forward step-down programme (Cavanaugh & Killian 2012). The goal is to demonstrate a forward step-down on an 8-inch step without pain and any deviations in lower extremity control (Cavanaugh & Killian 2012). Noyes et al (2012) advocate the use of lateral step-ups at around 7–8 weeks. The stair climber, elliptical and retrograde treadmill can all be used in this phase, based on patient symptoms (Cavanaugh & Killian 2012).

The final phase of rehabilitation for meniscal repair involves optimization of function and preparation for a safe return to sport (Cavanaugh & Killian 2012). Running programmes can be implemented at 16–20 weeks postoperatively using retrograde running prior to forward running (Cavanaugh & Killian 2012). Individuals undergoing a meniscal transplant should wait until 1 year to start a running programme, and if a complex meniscal repair has been performed then approximately 30 weeks is appropriate (Noyes et al 2012).

Plyometric and agility training can begin at approximately week 14. Agility ladders can incorporate deceleration, cutting, sprinting, pivoting (Cavanaugh & Killian 2012) or lateral carioca or figure-of-eight exercises (Noyes et al 2012). To ensure that an individual is appropriate for return to sport, functional testing should be used. The single-limb single-hop test, the single-limb triple-hop test and the single-limb crossover-hop test have a reported reliability of 0.92, 0.88 and 0.84 for those having undergone an ACL reconstruction, but they can also be safely used in those undergoing meniscal repairs (Logerstedt et al 2010a). Cavanaugh and Killian (2012) report a goal of achieving an 85% limb symmetry score on the single-limb single-hop and single-limb crossover-hop tests before the patient returns to sport.

Neuromuscular re-education

Balance, proprioceptive and neuromuscular exercises can be added to the rehabilitation programme when patients are 50% weight-bearing (around 3–4 weeks postoperatively) after meniscal repair (Heckmann et al 2006; Cavanaugh & Killian 2012; Noyes et al 2012). Initial exercises should include simple weight shifts in the sagittal and frontal planes, tandem stance balance and cone walking (Heckmann et al 2006; Noyes et al 2012). Other progressions include using a rocker board with bilateral support for sagittal and coronal plane movements (Cavanaugh & Killian 2012), advancing to unilateral support on a rocker board. Single-leg balance is utilized for challenging the patient's proprioceptive capabilities (Heckmann et al 2006; Noyes et al 2012) with progression to manual perturbations by the physical therapist or single-leg balance performed on an Airex, Bosu, mini-trampoline, foam roll, biomechanical ankle platform system (BAPS) or a Biodex balance system.

Partial meniscectomy

Postoperative rehabilitation for partial meniscectomy has little evidence-based research to examine its efficacy, so there is controversy over what constitutes best practice (Kelln et al 2009). Dias et al (2013) recently conducted a systematic review on postoperative treatment for patients undergoing partial meniscectomy, and found that physical therapy with a home exercise programme is effective in improving self-reported knee function and range of motion; however, the quality of evidence analysed had a moderate to high risk of bias. Hence, this section will present the best-available evidence at this time.

Modalities

Cryotherapy, limb elevation and NMES, as discussed with previous surgical procedures, can be utilized for pain, oedema and quadriceps strength (Goodwin et al 2003; Bax et al 2005; Heckmann et al 2006; Noyes et al 2012).

Range of motion exercises

Weight-bearing status differs from meniscal repair / transplantation in that individuals are immediately weight-bearing at tolerance, starting with the use of two crutches but decreasing their use until there is full weight-bearing. Kelln et al (2009) studied cycle ergometry and its effect on several objective measures, including range of motion and gait; gait patterns and knee flexion range of motion values improved in the experimental group significantly compared with the control group, thus providing evidence that early range of motion is beneficial for those undergoing partial meniscectomy. Passive and active range of motion exercise is rarely limited in range, unlike in patients undergoing meniscal repair or transplantation (Brotzman & Wilk 2003). Early range of motion should include the emphasis of full knee extension and flexion to tolerance.

Manual therapy for patients following a partial meniscectomy can be more freely used than in meniscal repair or transplantation. Patellar mobilizations in all directions can be utilized, and tibiofemoral mobilizations in the cardinal plane directions, as well as combined motions, can also be implemented until patients are pain free and / or the full range of motion is achieved (Goodwin et al 2003).

Therapeutic exercise

Therapeutic exercise includes many of the previous described exercises for postoperative knee management, but can be utilized earlier on in the treatment phase than with other surgical procedures. Goodwin et al (2003) studied early physical therapy after an arthroscopic partial meniscectomy. The intervention group performed calf raises, step-ups, hip abductor, adductor and extensor exercises, bicycle ergometry and mini-trampoline and wobble-board activities. In the later phases of the study, the individuals performed bilateral lateral hops and zig-zag hops, then progressed to single-leg hops (Goodwin et al 2003). Although the individuals in the intervention group exhibited no significant difference from those in the control group, the information provided by this study does give rehabilitation ideas for clinical practice.

Lateral and front lunges, lateral step-ups, leg press and stair climber or the elliptical can be introduced around 2 weeks postoperatively. Return to sport / functional activities can occur around 4 weeks and may last up to 8 weeks, with similar exercises to those described above being used in this phase (Brotzman & Wilk 2003).

Total Knee Arthroplasty

The knee is a pivotal hinge joint, permitting flexion, extension and rotation with the knee flexed. Bipedal creatures, such as humans, load the weight of the entire body through the knee joints. It is therefore a site of frequent injury and degeneration. There are two types of cartilage in the knee joints: fibrous cartilage, contained in a large meniscus that separates the tibia and femur in weight-bearing to some degree, and hyaline cartilage, found on the bone ends. The meniscus protects the ends of the weight-bearing bones and prevents bone erosion. When the meniscus is torn or worn, the bone ends are exposed to degenerative forces and advanced joint arthrosis occurs. Osteoarthritis (OA), both primary and secondary, and rheumatoid arthritis (RA) are primary causes of joint destruction (Sarwark 2010). (See Ch 43 for further information on knee OA.) The total and partial (tricompartmental, bicompartmental and unicompartmental) knee arthroplasties are used to restore function and mobility in advanced cases.

Clinical symptoms of knee OA include pain with weight-bearing, pain at rest in advanced cases, buckling or giving way of the knee, difficulty in traversing stairs, and episodes of locking. Physical examination usually reveals a varus or valgus deformity of the knee. There may be diffuse tenderness along the joint lines. Loss of range of motion, both passive and active, as well as joint crepitus may be present (Sarwark 2010).

Diagnostic tests primarily include radiographs. A weight-bearing anteroposterior view of both knees in full available extension will show narrowing of the joint space. Degenerative arthritis will be evidenced as asymmetric joint narrowing, bone sclerosis, periarticular cysts and osteophytes. Inflammatory arthritis will demonstrate symmetric joint narrowing, disuse osteopenia and bony erosions at the articular margins. Lateral and axial patellofemoral view will further show the degeneration of the tibiofemoral joint and patellofemoral joint. The tunnel view will typically exhibit osteophytes and osteochondral loose bodies, if present (Sarwark 2010).

Procedures

The total knee arthroplasty (TKA) is indicated for disability, pain and limited function from OA, RA or any type of arthritic deformity about the knee. The goals of TKA include reducing pain, returning to activities of daily living, restoring mechanical alignment, preserving the joint line, balancing the ligaments and restoring a normal Q-angle (Van Manen et al 2012). There is no standard of severity indicated from radiographic findings because the decision to undergo the TKA is at least partially subjective, based on the patient's response to non-operative treatment, tolerance for pain and physical demand of daily activities (Van Manen et al 2012).

The unicompartmental arthroplasty is often presented as a means of transition between end-stage OA and TKA. Other physicians prefer use of the high tibial osteotomy for the same purpose. A comprehensive review of the literature in 2010 did not find marked advantages of one method over the other: 'With the correct indications, both treatments produce durable and predictable outcomes in the treatment of medial unicompartmental arthrosis of the knee. There is no evidence of superior results of one treatment over the other' (Dettoni et al 2010, p 131).

Indications for unicompartmental knee arthroplasty include unicompartmental OA, radiographic evidence of preservation of opposite compartment, absence of or only mild patellofemoral degeneration, a range of motion greater than 90°, flexion contracture <5°, angular deformity <15° and a relatively sedentary lifestyle (Iorio & Healy 2003; Borus & Thornhill 2008). Contraindications to the procedure are opposite compartment or patellofemoral arthritis, fixed varus or valgus deformity greater than 5°, significantly restricted range of motion including fixed contracture, ACL deficiency (relative contraindication for medial compartment, contraindication for lateral compartment) and symptomatic instability. Certain medical conditions may also be considered to be contraindications (Iorio & Healy 2003; Borus & Thornhill 2008).

Complications of all TKA procedures include tibial plateau fracture, medial collateral ligament avulsion / tear, stiffness or arthrofibrosis, infection, deep vein thrombosis / pulmonary embolism, and hardware failure. Complications unique to the unicompartment procedure include ACL rupture and adjacent compartment degeneration (Healy et al 2013).

Innovations in the arthroplasty procedure as a whole include minimally invasive surgery techniques, gender-specific prosthetics and computer-assisted navigation systems (Zanasi 2011).

Treatment

Minns Lowe et al (2007) compared outcomes of functional physical therapy exercises provided in clinic after acute care with simple at-home continuation of a basic exercise programme provided in acute care after primary elective knee arthroplasty. Their conclusion was that the clinically provided functional exercises subacutely had greater short-term benefit; however, there were no differences between the two programmes at 1 year after surgery (Minns Lowe et al 2007). Nevertheless, adequate and even intensive rehabilitation is commonly considered an important requirement for successful TKA outcomes (Kisner & Colby 2007; Lenssen et al 2008).

Physical therapy rehabilitation after TKA has five essential components: therapeutic exercise, manual therapy, transfer training, gait training and instruction in the activities of daily living. Rehabilitation varies as to where, how and when it is delivered. There is growing support for pre-rehabilitation – that is, physical therapy beginning weeks prior to the expected TKA (Desmeules et al 2013). Traditionally, the patient will receive basic physical therapy while in acute care, consisting of ambulation, transfer training and exercises for prevention of deep vein thrombosis as well as range of motion. After discharge from the acute care hospital, patients may receive more extensive inpatient physical therapy, which includes skilled nursing facilities and subacute rehabilitation facilities, or they may continue treatment on an outpatient basis, either at home or at an outpatient clinic (Health Quality Ontario 2005).

Modalities

Modalities such as ice, heat, and transcutaneous electric stimulation (TENS) are utilized to modulate pain and improve treatment tolerance (Kisner & Colby 2007). Continuous passive motion (CPM) is initiated in acute care and may or may not be continued after 3–5 days. Prolonged CPM use may increase short-term range of motion gains; however, long-term benefits to both range of motion and function have not been proven (Lenssen et al 2008).

Gait training and transfer training

Initially the patient learns to ambulate with a standard or rolling walker while in acute care (Beaupré et al 2001). Crutches may be used, but some patients, especially the elderly, may find a walker safer to handle (Kisner & Colby 2007). The type of prosthesis implanted, type of fixation used and other personal variables determine the progress of weight-bearing. With biological / cementless fixation, weight-bearing may vary from touch-down only for 4–8 weeks to weight-bearing as tolerated within a few days after surgery. Cemented fixation typically allows weight-bearing as tolerated with a walker or crutches, weaning the patient to full weight-bearing over 6 weeks (Kisner & Colby 2007).

When the patient is able to tolerate cane use with at least a fair gait pattern, the walker is gradually exchanged for a straight cane. Before discontinuing the assistive device altogether, the patient should be able to activate the lock-home mechanism of the knee with sufficient active extension, and demonstrate a good gait pattern without evidence of a painful limp or significant deficits in range of motion (Kisner & Colby 2007).

Manual therapy and range of motion expectations

Range-of-motion goals are progressive and may vary according to the surgeon's protocol. Generally, the expectations are 0–90° in weeks 1–4 and 0–110° or greater in weeks 4–8. After week 8 the goal is to obtain an easy and painless range of motion from 0° to 110° or more (Kisner & Colby 2007).

Patellar mobilizations begin at grades I and II during weeks 1–4. They are continued through to week 8 and after as needed. Tibiofemoral joint mobilization techniques, including holding a distraction force while performing passive or active assisted flexion, may be allowed. It is advisable to discuss this treatment with the surgeon before implementing this, however, as the design of the prosthetic component may prohibit mobilization of this type (Kisner & Colby 2007).

Therapeutic exercise

The patient is instructed in antithrombotic exercises acutely (Beaupré et al 2001). Ankle pumps, quadriceps setting and gluteal setting in repetition are performed for the first 2 weeks after surgery. With the leg elevated, and knee in extension, these exercises are also helpful for reducing swelling. In the subacute phase and beyond, exercises utilized to increase the range of motion, strength and function vary widely based on experience and preference of the physical therapist. Basic exercises include straight leg raises, heel slides, short-arc knee extensions, long arc knee extensions and hamstring curls (Beaupré et al 2001). Progressive resistance exercises may be initiated in the 4- to 8-week phase, depending upon the individual patient and surgeon. Cuff weights are often added to the basic exercises for progressive resistance exercises. Aquatic physical therapy may commence once the incision is fully closed. The recumbent bicycle may improve both range of motion and strength.

Several specific exercises are limited initially after knee arthroplasty. Side-lying straight leg raises (abduction / adduction) should be avoided early on owing to the varus and valgus stresses on the knee. The therapist should also delay initiation of unsupported weight-bearing exercises until there is sufficient strength in the quadriceps and hamstrings to stabilize the knee.

Activities of daily living: return to function

In addition to basic range of motion exercises and progressive resistance exercise, rehabilitation should include balance training, limited functional squatting, stabilization and proprioceptive exercises, step-ups / downs and stair training (Piva et al 2010). The patient should achieve sufficient easy knee flexion to allow normal functional activities such as tying of shoelaces, safe automobile transfers, and proper positioning of the leg and foot for sit-to-stand transfers.

Arthrofibrosis of the Knee

Arthrofibrosis is an abnormal proliferation of fibrotic tissue or scarring in and around a joint (Freeman et al 2009; Biggs-Kinzer et al 2010), and is often idiopathic. Idiopathic types may develop tissue metaplasia with abnormal formation of dense fibrous tissue, with surgical intervention and revision arthroplasty leading to worsening of the condition and disability (Freeman et al 2009). The incidence of arthrofibrosis of the knee is reported as 1.3–13.5% (Sharma et al 2008). However, a more blanket diagnosis of joint stiffness following surgery or trauma is purportedly as high as 54% (Sharma et al 2008). The aetiology of knee arthrofibrosis is multifactorial and may include infection, prolonged postoperative immobility of the knee, overly aggressive rehabilitation, incorrectly sized or placed components of the TKA, repeated surgeries, autoimmune diseases including diabetes, and preoperative deformities (Schiavone Panni et al 2009; Kim & Joo 2013).

Arthrofibrosis of the knee has no official classification system; however, it has been classified in individual studies (Shelbourne et al 1996b). An example of this is the four-type model used by Shelbourne et al (1996b): type 1, <10° extension loss and normal flexion; type 2, >10° extension loss and normal flexion; type 3, >10° extension loss and >25° flexion loss with a tight patella; and type 4, >10° extension loss, 30° or more flexion loss and patella infera with marked patellar tightness.

Arthrofibrosis demonstrates fibrogenesis which is characterized by fibroblast proliferation, excessive synthesis and accumulation of extracellular matrix components and reduced extracellular matrix remodelling (Bosch et al 2001; Freeman et al 2010; Monument et al 2012). Freeman et al (2010) suggested that tissue metaplasia in arthrofibrosis results from increased inflammation-associated oxidative stress, which initiates a chain of events including an accumulation of mast cells (secreting fibroblast growth factor), driving fibroblast proliferation and creating avascular regions of hypoxia. The hypoxia and associated oxidative stress together induce a metaplastic conversion of fibrotic tissue to fibrocartilage, and then, in instances of fibrosis of longer durations, subsequent bone formation by endochondral ossification.

In diagnosing knee arthrofibrosis, other causes of joint stiffness must be excluded, such as muscle inhibition, fluid in the joint (including infection), mechanical factors, such as a loose body or bucket-handle tear of the meniscus, joint bones out of alignment, interruption to the extensor mechanism, improperly placed ligament graft, and damaged nerves. However, these conditions may trigger or be present in combination with the arthrofibrosis (Noyes et al 1991).

There are no specific diagnostic tests for knee arthrofibrosis; rather, the medical team looks for inability to meet normal range of motion expectations, and alert signals such as flexed knee gait, worsening pain, persisting warmth in the joint and continued tissue swelling. Objective signs include restricted patellar mobility and / or downward migration of the patella, as well as restricted and / or worsening active and passive range of motion (Noyes et al 1991). Serial measurement of patellar height on a lateral plain film of both knees is recommended, as it has been shown that the progression of arthrofibrosis can trigger downward migration of the patella as early as a few weeks after the original tissue trauma (Noyes et al 1991).

Treatment of arthrofibrosis of the knee is extremely challenging and may utilize conservative and / or surgical techniques (Table 45.3).

Table 45.3 Treatment for arthrofibrosis of the knee after total knee arthroplasty

Conservative treatments	
Sustained low-load stretching recommended over high-load brief stretch (typical manual passive range of motion).	(Light et al 1984; Papotto & Mills 2012)
Home static and dynamic stretching devices recommended over serial casting.	(Jansen et al 1996; Biggs-Kinzer et al 2010; Papotto & Mills 2012)
Instrument-assisted soft tissue mobilization techniques for fibrosis outside of the joint, accompanying standard treatment.	(Black 2010)
Manual therapy, including mobilization, and mobilization with movement.	(Millett et al 2003)
Intra-articular injection of anakinra, an interleukin-1 (IL-1) antagonist targeting the inflammatory response mediated by IL-1.	(Brown et al 2010)
Surgical treatments	
Traditional surgical releases: quadricepsplasty, capsulotomy, excision of scar tissue in the patellofemoral joint and anterior part of the tibiofemoral joint, and release of the retinacula and the sliding mechanism on the medial and lateral sides of the joint.	(Farid et al 2013; Kim & Joo 2013)
Manipulation under anaesthesia (MUA), arthroscopic release (preferred by Kim and Joo), open surgical release (preferred by Ghani) and revision TKA.	(Ghani et al 2012; Farid et al 2013; Kim & Joo 2013)
Capsular distension with arthroscopic release.	(Millett & Steadman 2001)
Intra-articular injection of local anaesthetic and steroid given at the time of MUA.	(Sharma et al 2008)
Preoperative low-dose irradiation and constrained condylar or rotating-hinge revision for severe, idiopathic arthrofibrosis.	(Farid et al 2013)

Conclusion

Many of the interventions described in this chapter have been shown to be effective. Clinical practice guidelines continue to evolve and will change frequently. Thus, readers should note that best clinical practice encompasses using current evidence, as well as incorporating patient values and clinician experience, which will provide the best overall patient outcomes.

References

Adams D, Logerstedt D, Hunger-Giordano A, et al. 2012. Current concepts for anterior cruciate ligament reconstruction: a criterion-based rehabilitation program. J Orthop Sports Phys Ther 42: 601–614.

Barber FA. 1994. Accelerated rehabilitation for meniscus repairs. Arthroscopy 10: 206–210.

Bax L, Staes F, Verhagen A. 2005. Does neuromuscular electrical stimulation strengthen the quadriceps femoris? A systematic review of randomized controlled trials. Sports Med 35: 191–212.

Beaupré LA, Davies DM, Jones CA, et al. 2001. Exercise combined with continuous passive motion or slider board therapy compared with exercise only: a randomized controlled trial of patients following total knee arthroplasty. Phys Ther 81: 1029–1037.

Biggs-Kinzer A, Murphy B, Shelbourne KD, et al. 2010. Perioperative rehabilitation using a knee extension device and arthroscopic debridement in the treatment of arthrofibrosis. Sports Health 2: 417–423.

Black DW. 2010. Treatment of knee arthrofibrosis and quadriceps insufficiency after patellar tendon repair: a case report including use of the Graston Technique. Int J Therapeutic Massage Bodywork 3: 14–21.

Borus T, Thornhill T. 2008. Unicompartmental knee arthroplasty. J Am Acad Orthop Surg 16: 9–18.

Bosch U, Zeichen J, Skutek M, et al. 2001. Arthrofibrosis is the result of a T cell mediated immune response. Knee Surg Sports Traumatol Arthrosc 9: 282–289.

Brotzman SB, Wilk KE. 2003. Clinical orthopaedic rehabilitation. Philadelphia, PA: Mosby.

Brown CA, Toth AP, Magnussen B. 2010. Clinical benefits of intra-articular anakinra for arthrofibrosis. Orthopedics 33: 877.

Cavanaugh JT, Killian SE. 2012. Rehabilitation following meniscal repair. Curr Rev Musculoskelet Med 5: 46–58.

Desmeules F, Hall J, Woodhouse LJ. 2013. Pre-rehabilitation improves physical function of individuals with severe disability from hip or knee osteoarthritis. Physiother Can 65: 116–124.

Dettoni F, Bonasia DE, Castoldi F, et al. 2010. High tibial osteotomy versus unicompartmental knee arthroplasty for medial compartment arthrosis of the knee: a review of the literature. Iowa Orthop J 30: 131–140.

Dias JM, Mazuquin BF, Mostagi FQRC, et al 2013. The effectiveness of postoperative physical therapy treatment in patients who have undergone arthroscopic partial meniscectomy: systematic review with meta-analysis. J Orthop Sports Phys Ther 43: 560–576.

DiStasi S, Myer GD, Hewett TE. 2013. Neuromuscular training to target deficits associated with second anterior cruciate ligament injury. J Orthop Sports Phys Ther 43: 777–792.

Escamilla RF, Macleod TD, Wilk KE, et al. 2012. Anterior cruciate ligament strain and tensile forces for weight-bearing and non-weight bearing exercises: a guide to exercise selection. J Orthop Sports Phys Ther 42: 208–220.

Farid YR, Thakral R, Finn HA. 2013. Low-dose irradiation and constrained revision for severe, idiopathic, arthrofibrosis following total knee arthroplasty. J Arthroplasty 28: 1314–1320.

Freeman TA, Parvizi J, Della Valle CJ, et al. 2009. Reactive oxygen and nitrogen species induce protein and DNA modifications driving arthrofibrosis following total knee arthroplasty. Fibrogenesis Tissue Repair 2: 5. doi: 10.1186/1755-1536-3-17.

Freeman TA, Parvizi J, Dela Valle CJ, et al. 2010. Mast cells and hypoxia drive tissue metaplasia and heterotopic ossification in idiopathic arthrofibrosis after total knee arthroplasty. Fibrogenesis Tissue Repair 3: 17.

Ghani H, Maffulli N, Khanduja V. 2012. Management of stiffness following total knee arthroplasty: a systematic review. Knee 19: 751–759.

Goodwin PC, Morrissey MC, Omar RZ, et al. 2003. Effectiveness of supervised physical therapy in the early period after arthroscopic partial meniscectomy. Phys Ther 83: 520–535.

Harner CD, Hoher J. 1998. Evaluation and treatment of posterior cruciate ligament injuries. Am J Sports Med 26: 471–482.

Health Quality Ontario. 2005. Physiotherapy rehabilitation after total knee or hip replacement. Ont Health Technol Assess Ser 5: 1–91.

Healy WL, Della Valle CJ, Iorio R, et al. 2013. Complications of total knee arthroplasty: standardized list and definitions of the Knee Society. Clin Orthop Relat Res 471: 215–220.

Heckmann TA, Barber-Westin SD, Noyes FR. 2006. Meniscal repair and transplantation: indications, techniques, rehabilitation, and clinical outcome. J Orthop Sports Phys Ther 36: 795–814.

Hunt MA, DiCiacca SR, Jones IC, et al. 2010. Effect of anterior tibiofemoral glides on knee extension during gait in patients with decreased range of motion after anterior cruciate ligament reconstruction. Physiother Can 62: 235–241.

Iorio R, Healy WL. 2003. Unicompartmental arthritis of the knee. J Bone Joint Surg Am 85A: 1351–1364.

Jansen CM, Windau JE, Bonutti PM, et al. 1996. Treatment of a knee contracture using a knee orthosis incorporating stress-relaxation techniques. Phys Ther 76:182–186.

Kelln BM, Ingersoll CD, Saliba S, et al. 2009. Effect of early active range of motion rehabilitation on outcome measures after partial meniscectomy. Knee Surg Sports Traumatol Arthrosc 17: 607–616.

Kim YM, Joo YB. 2013. Prognostic factors of arthroscopic adhesiolysis for arthrofibrosis of the knee. Knee Surg Relat Res 25: 202–206.

Kisner C, Colby LA. 2007. Therapeutic exercise, 5th edn. Philadelphia, PA: FA Davis.

LaPrade RF, Wijdicks CA. 2012. The management of injuries to the medial side of the knee. J Orthop Sports Phys 42: 221–233.

Lenssen TA, van Steyn MJ, Crijns YH, et al. 2008. Effectiveness of prolonged use of continuous passive motion (CPM), as an adjunct to physiotherapy, after total knee arthroplasty. BMC Musculoskelet Disord 29: 60.

Light KE, Nuzik S, Personius W, et al. 1984. Low-load prolonged stretch vs. high-load brief stretch in treating knee contractures. Phys Ther 64: 330–333.

Logerstedt DS, Snyder-Mackler L, Ritter RC, et al. 2010a. Knee pain and mobility impairments: meniscal and articular cartilage lesions. J Orthop Sports Phys Ther 40: A1–A35.

Logerstedt DS, Snyder-Mackler L, Ritter RC, et al. 2010b. Knee stability and movement coordination impairments: knee ligament sprain. J Orthop Sports Phys Ther 40: A1–A37.

Manske RB, Prohaska D, Lucas B. 2012. Recent advances following anterior cruciate ligament reconstruction: rehabilitation perspectives. Curr Rev Musculoskelet Med 5: 59–71.

Millett PJ, Steadman JR. 2001. The role of capsular distention in the arthroscopic management of arthrofibrosis of the knee: a technical consideration. Arthroscopy 17: E31.

Millett PJ, Johnson B, Carson J, et al. 2003. Rehabilitation of the arthrofibrotic knee. Am J Orthopedics 32: 531–538.

Minns Lowe C, Barker KL, Dewey M, et al. 2007. Effectiveness of physiotherapy exercise after knee arthroplasty for osteoarthritis: systematic review and meta-analysis of randomised controlled trials. BMJ 15:812–815.

Monument MJ, Hart DA, Befus AD, et al. 2012. The mast cell stabilizer ketotifen reduces joint capsule fibrosis in a rabbit model of post-traumatic joint contractures. Inflamm Res 61: 285–292.

Nandra R, Matharu GS, Porter K, et al. 2013. Anterior cruciate ligament injuries and reconstructive techniques. Part 2: Treatment. Trauma 15: 116–127.

Noyes FR, Wojtys EM, Marshall MT. 1991. The early diagnosis and treatment of developmental patella infera syndrome. Clin Orthop 265: 241–252.

Noyes FR, Heckmann TP, Barber-Westin SD. 2012. Meniscus repair and transplantation: a comprehensive update. J Orthop Sports Phys Ther 42: 274–290.

Pandy MG, Shelbourne KD. 1997. Dependence of cruciate-ligament loading on muscle forces and external load. J Biomech 30: 1015–1024.

Papotto BA, Mills T. 2012. Treatment of severe flexion deficits following total knee arthroplasty: a randomized clinical trial. Orthop Nurs 31: 29–34.

Piva SR, Gill AB, Almeida GJM, et al. 2010. A balance exercise program appears to improve function for patients with total knee arthroplasty: a randomized clinical trial. Phys Ther 90:880–894.

Quarles JD, Hosey RG. 2004. Medial and lateral collateral injuries: prognosis and treatment. Primary Care 31: 957–975.

Rosenthal MD, Rainey CE, Tognoni A, et al. 2012. Evaluation and management of posterior cruciate ligament injuries. Phys Ther Sport 13: 196–208.

Sarwark JF (ed). 2010. Essentials of musculoskeletal care, 4th edn. Rosemont, IL: American Academy of Orthopaedic Surgeons.
Schiavone Panni A, Cerciello S, Vasso M, et al. 2009. Stiffness in total knee arthroplasty. J Orthop Traumatol 10: 111–118.
Sharma V, Maheshwari AV, Tsailas PG, et al. 2008. The results of knee manipulation for stiffness after total knee arthroplasty with or without an intra-articular steroid injection. Indian J Orthop 4: 314–318.
Shelbourne KD, Patel DV, Adsit WS, et al. 1996a. Rehabilitation after meniscal repair. Clin Sports Med 15: 595–612.
Shelbourne KD, Patel DV, Martini DJ. 1996b. Classification and management of arthrofibrosis of the knee after anterior cruciate ligament reconstruction. Am J Sports Med 24: 857–862.
Van Grinsven S, van Cingel REH, Holla CJM, et al. 2010. Evidence-based rehabilitation following anterior cruciate ligament reconstruction. Knee Surg Sports Traumatol Arthrosc 18: 1128–1144.
Van Manen MD, Nace J, Mont MA. 2012. Management of primary knee osteoarthritis and indications for total knee arthroplasty for general practitioners. J Am Osteopath Assoc 112: 709–715.
Wijdicks CA, Griffith CJ, Johansen S, et al. 2010. Injuries to the medial collateral ligament and associated medial structures to the knee. J Bone Joint Surg Am 92: 1266–1280.
Wilk KE. 1994. Rehabilitation of isolated and combined posterior cruciate ligament injuries. Clin Sports Med 13: 649–677.
Wilk KE, Macrina LC, Cain EL, et al. 2012. Recent advances in the rehabilitation of anterior cruciate ligament injuries. J Orthop Sports Phys Ther 42: 153–171.
Wright RW, Preston E, Fleming BC, et al. 2008. A systematic review of anterior cruciate ligament reconstruction rehabilitation: part II: open versus closed kinetic chain exercises, neuromuscular electrical stimulation, accelerated rehabilitation and miscellaneous topics. J Knee Surg 21: 225–234.
Yvas D, Rabuck SJ, Harner CD. 2012. Allograft anterior cruciate ligament reconstruction: indications, techniques and outcomes. J Orthop Sports Phys Ther 42: 196–207.
Zanasi S. 2011. Innovations in total knee replacement: new trends in operative treatment and changes in peri-operative management. Eur Orthop Traumatol 2(1–2): 21–31.

Chapter 46

Joint Mobilization and Manipulation of the Knee

Cody Weisbach, William Egan, Paul E. Glynn, Joshua A. Cleland

CHAPTER CONTENTS

Evidence of manual therapy in the knee 525
Mobilization interventions of the knee joint 527
Tibiofemoral posterior accessory glide 527
Tibiofemoral anterior accessory glide 527
Tibiofemoral knee flexion physiological mobilization 527
Tibiofemoral knee extension physiological mobilization 528
Tibiofemoral knee extension physiological mobilization variation 528
Tibiofemoral long-axis distraction manipulation 528
Tibiofemoral mobilization with movement 528
Proximal tibiofibular thrust manipulation 529
Patellofemoral mobilization: caudal and cephalad 529
Patellofemoral mobilization: medial and lateral 529

Evidence of Manual Therapy in the Knee

Disorders of the knee are a common reason for individuals to seek out the consultation of a physical therapist. Patellofemoral pain syndrome (PFPS) is estimated to affect 7–40% of adolescents and active young adults, making it a highly prevalent condition of the anterior knee (Almeida et al 1999). Knee osteoarthritis (OA) is another highly prevalent cause of knee pain for which individuals would seek consultation. It is estimated that, in adults aged over 45 years, the prevalence of radiographic knee OA is 28% and for symptomatic knee OA it is between 7% and 19%. With the ageing population and increasing obesity levels, these numbers are expected to continue to increase in the future (Nagoi 2013).

Manual therapy is one of many potential conservative treatment options that could be a part of the intervention package for individuals with knee pain. The goals of manual therapy are to improve range of motion and modulate pain through mechanical, neurophysiological and non-specific effects on the individual (Moss et al 2007; Bialosky et al 2009). Mobilization and manipulation are types of manual therapy that appear to have strong support for improving range of motion, pain and function for two of the more prevalent conditions of the knee: knee OA and PFPS. (These conditions are covered in Chs 43 and 44 respectively.)

Brantingham et al (2009) conducted a literature review on the effects of manual therapy with a multimodal care package in individuals with lower extremity disorders. In this review they judged that there was 'level B' evidence of manual therapy directed at the knee in patients with PFPS. The techniques most frequently used in this population tend to be directed at the patellofemoral joint and the proximal tibiofibular joint. Van den Dolder and Roberts (2006) sought to assess the efficacy of manual therapy in PFPS. They randomized 38 individuals with PFPS into two groups. The control group was put on a 2-week waiting list, while the intervention group received six sessions of manual therapy, including friction massage, patellar mobilizations and sustained medial glides with knee flexion and extension. After the six sessions, results indicated the experimental group had greater improvements compared with the waiting list group in pain, pain on stair climbing, knee flexion and the number of step-ups they were able to complete in 60 seconds. The researchers concluded that an approach incorporating manual therapy was superior to no treatment.

Crossley et al (2002) conducted a randomized controlled trial, building on the van den Dolder results by comparing the same intervention with a placebo treatment. They enrolled 67 individuals with PFPS and randomized them into two groups. The control group received placebo taping and subtherapeutic ultrasound. The treatment group received a multimodal treatment programme of lower body stretching, strengthening, patellar taping and medial patellar glides (60 seconds repeated three times). This group was seen once a week for 6 weeks. After treatment, the experimental group improved in pain and function, and was able to do more step-ups, step-downs and squats, in comparison with the placebo group.

Both the Crossley et al (2002) and van den Dolder and Roberts (2006) studies were constructed in such a way that all individuals received the same treatments regardless of examination findings, but interventions were selected clinically based on individual examination findings. Thereafter, Lowry et al (2008) published a case series to describe the examination and management of five individuals, aged between 14 and 50 years of age, who had been diagnosed with PFPS. Each patient underwent a detailed, individualized examination and received a customized treatment programme depending on the examination findings and responses to treatment. Treatments included manual therapy to the lumbar spine, hip, patellofemoral joint and proximal tibiofibular joint. Other components of the treatment programme included McConnell taping, custom orthoses, over-the-counter orthoses and an exercise programme for core, hip and knee stretching and strengthening with a progression from non-weight-bearing to weight-bearing exercise. Subjects were seen for between 8 and 14 treatments over a 6- to 14-week period. Outcomes of pain, self-report function of the lower extremity and global improvement were assessed at baseline, third visit, discharge and 6-month follow-up. The authors found that four of the five subjects had clinically meaningful improvements on all outcomes measured at discharge and 6-month follow-up.

As detailed by Brantingham et al (2009), 'level B' evidence exists for the use of manual therapy in the PFPS population and the discussion of the studies above will hopefully help the reader to understand better the current state of the evidence as well as providing ideas and clinical-reasoning approaches for these patients. Selected techniques from these studies are outlined later in this chapter.

Knee OA is another condition for which manual therapy has been proposed as an effective treatment approach. The literature review by Brantingham et al (2009) also found that 'level B' evidence existed for manual therapy in knee OA; since that review, additional studies have been published that further support the use of manual therapy in knee OA.

Several studies have been published that describe the use of manual therapy techniques to the tibiofemoral joint in subjects with knee OA as a stand-alone treatment (Hillerman et al 2006; Moss et al 2007; Pollard et al 2008; Takasaki et al 2013). French et al (2011) published a systematic review on the use of manual therapy only in patients with knee and hip OA; they found that employing manual therapy in isolation was not supported. Therefore, these studies are mentioned since the techniques described show promise; however, the majority of the discussion will focus on studies that include manual therapy as a part of a multimodal treatment plan, for which stronger evidence exists. Techniques such as long-axis tibiofemoral manipulation (Hillerman et al 2006), long-duration anterior–posterior tibiofemoral mobilizations (Moss et al 2007) and mobilization with movements applied in open or closed chain (Takasaki et al 2013) will all probably be useful in certain situations in the management of individuals with knee OA and are described in subsequent sections. However, in the authors' opinion, the techniques described in the studies below should make up the foundation of a manual therapy approach to this population, based on the strength of the best current evidence.

Deyle et al (2000) sought to investigate the effects of a multimodal physical therapy programme in patients with knee OA. They randomized 69 individuals with knee OA into a treatment and a placebo group. The treatment group received eight sessions of manual re-examination and manual therapy to the knee, hip, ankle and lumbar spine individualized to each patient based on the therapist's assessment. Manual therapy techniques used were similar to those described later in this chapter. Additionally this group participated in a standardized, supervised exercise programme, which consisted of knee active range of motion, aerobic exercise, lower extremity stretching plus hip and knee strengthening that progressed from open to closed chain. This group also performed a similar home exercise programme on off days. The placebo group received the same manual re-examination at each session as well as 10 minutes of detuned ultrasound. Outcomes were assessed with the Western Ontario and McMaster Universities Arthritis Index (WOMAC) and 6-minute walk test, at 4 weeks, 8 weeks and 1 year. They found significant improvements in both WOMAC and 6-minute walk test at 4 weeks and 8 weeks within the manual therapy group. At 1 year, subjects in the placebo group reported a higher incidence of knee surgery (20%) compared with the treatment group (5%).

Deyle et al (2005) performed a follow-up randomized controlled trial to expand on the results of their previous work. In this, 120 individuals with knee OA were randomized to a multimodal treatment group or a home exercise programme only group. The home exercise group received the same programme as the multimodal group, but with only one session of initial instruction, detailed handouts and one more session of instruction after 2 weeks. Again, the WOMAC and 6-minute walk test were assessed at 4 weeks, 8 weeks and 1 year. Results indicated that both groups improved at 4 and 8 weeks, but that the group that also received manual therapy improved significantly more than the exercise-only group. At 1 year, the difference in WOMAC scores was no longer significant between groups, but those in the manual therapy group reported significantly greater satisfaction with their treatment.

This line of inquiry was further pursued in 2012, when a secondary analysis of the data from both of the above trials was performed to create a clinical prediction rule (CPR) that would help determine which of the patients would not benefit from the manual therapy approach (Deyle et al 2012). This analysis found that three variables were included in the CPR and that individuals with two or more of those variables would be less likely to benefit from manual therapy. The variables were height greater than 5′ 7″(1.7 m), pain with patellar glides, and anterior cruciate ligament laxity. The authors noted that was a derivation-level CPR and that validation was necessary to increase the confidence that these findings are not due to chance, so an understanding of these design limitations should be understood prior to the routine application of these results in clinical practice.

Recent studies have studied the efficacy and cost-effectiveness of exercise and manual therapy in both hip and knee OA (Abbott et al 2013; Pinto et al 2013). They recruited 206 subjects, randomized to one of four arms. The first arm consisted of routine care, which was directed by the patient's general practitioner. The second arm was a manual therapy approach and a range-of-motion-based home programme adapted to the individual examination findings. The third arm was an exercise group where subjects received an individualized programme including strengthening and aerobic exercise. The fourth arm was a combination manual therapy and exercise approach. The primary outcome measure was the WOMAC score for the clinical effectiveness analysis. The Osteoarthritis Costs and Consequences Questionnaire, cost of care and quality of life measures were used in the economic analysis. The effectiveness analysis (Abbott et al 2013) found that, at 1 year, those who received manual therapy had significantly greater improvement on their WOMAC score compared with those who did not receive manual therapy. Those who received exercises were *not* significantly better than those who received manual therapy; interestingly though, they found an antagonistic effect in the manual therapy plus exercise group, indicating that this group actually fared worse than the others. Overall, those in the manual therapy group were significantly better compared with those in the general practitioner care group, exercise group or combination group at 1 year. These results were similar when hip OA and knee OA were considered individually. The economic analysis (Pinto et al 2013) found that those in the general practitioner group had more visits to the emergency department and rheumatologist, and received more meals on wheels, home health help and house-cleaning services. From a societal perspective, which takes into account cost of care and individual health, combination care was superior to usual care only in those who did not receive a joint replacement. They found that the exercise group was more costly than general practitioner care and that manual therapy was less costly than general practitioner care. Overall, this analysis seems to indicate that the approach in the manual therapy group led to the best balance between cost of care and health of individuals, regardless of whether or not they had a joint replacement.

The above indicates that manual therapy is well supported as a component of the care in patients with knee pain. What follows is the authors' interpretation of a selection of the techniques from the above studies.

Mobilization Interventions of the Knee Joint

Tibiofemoral posterior accessory glide

The patient's knee is placed in approximately at 20° of flexion. This can be accomplished using a rolled towel, a bolster or by resting the patient's knee over the clinician's knee. The clinician places one hand on the posterior aspect of the distal femur to stabilize and the web-space of the other hand on the anterior aspect of the proximal tibia to apply a graded, non-thrust oscillatory manipulation posteriorly (Fig. 46.1). This technique can be progressed by increasing the degree of knee flexion by positioning the patient in sitting with the legs off the side of the treatment table.

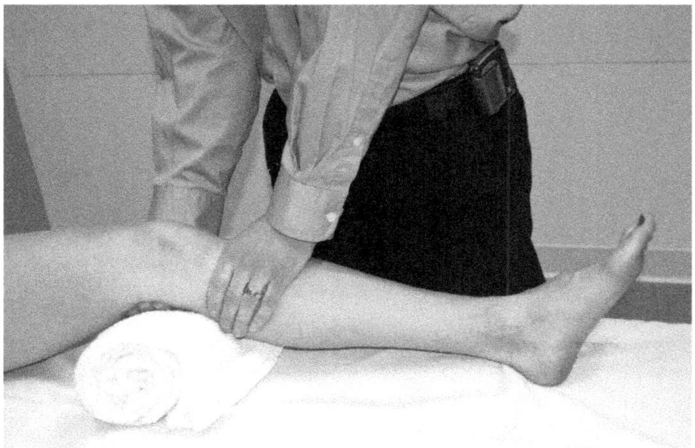

Figure 46.1 Tibiofemoral posterior accessory glide.

Tibiofemoral anterior accessory glide

The patient's knee is placed in approximately at 20° of flexion. The clinician places one hand on the anterior aspect of the distal femur to stabilize. The other hand is placed on the posterior aspect of the proximal tibia to apply a graded, non-thrust oscillatory manipulation anteriorly (Fig. 46.2). This technique can be progressed by increasing the amount of knee extension.

Tibiofemoral knee flexion physiological mobilization

The patient is positioned in supine. The clinician flexes the patient's hip to approximately 90° and places one hand on the lateral aspect of the femur to control its position. The other hand grasps the lower leg just proximal to the malleoli. The clinician stabilizes the femur and uses the other hand to flex the knee to the restrictive barrier (Fig. 46.3). Tibiofemoral internal rotation or external rotation can be added to refine the barrier. The clinician then uses the caudal hand

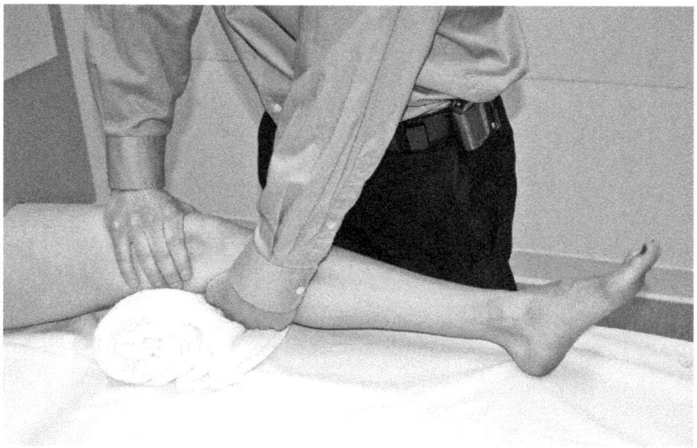

Figure 46.2 Tibiofemoral anterior accessory glide.

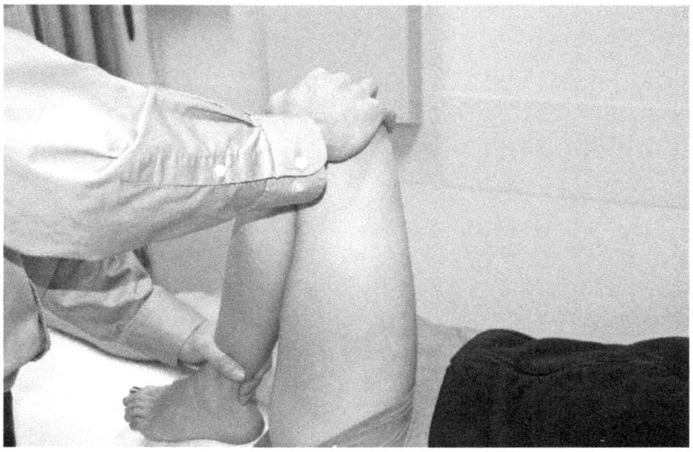

Figure 46.3 Tibiofemoral knee flexion physiological mobilization.

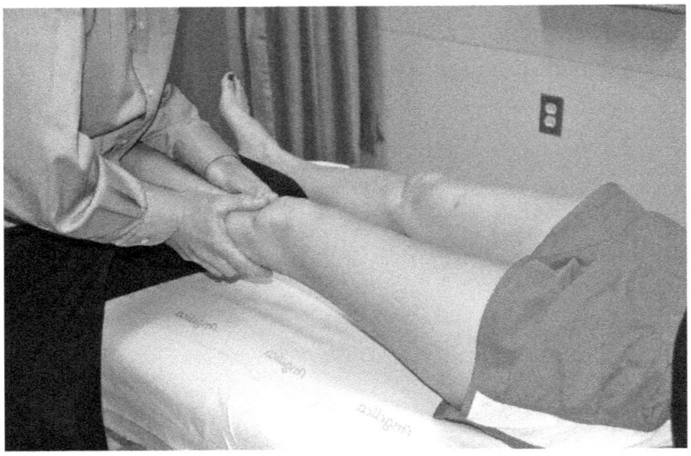

Figure 46.4 Tibiofemoral knee extension physiological mobilization.

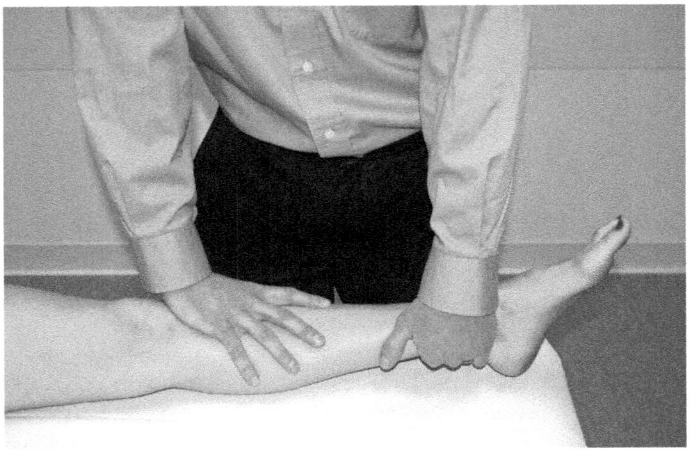

Figure 46.5 Tibiofemoral knee extension physiological mobilization variation.

to apply a graded, non-thrust oscillatory manipulation into flexion.

Tibiofemoral knee extension physiological mobilization

The patient is positioned in supine, with the patient's knee over the clinician's knee. The clinician grasps the patient's knee at the medial and lateral joint line while stabilizing the lower leg with the body and upper arm (Fig. 46.4). The clinician uses both hands to extend the patient's knee to the restrictive barrier. Varus or valgus forces can be added to refine the barrier. The clinician then uses the hands to apply a graded, non-thrust oscillatory manipulation into extension.

Tibiofemoral knee extension physiological mobilization variation

The patient is positioned in supine. The clinician grasps the patient's distal leg behind the malleoli with one hand to stabilize. The heel of the other hand is placed on the tibial tuberosity, the fingers facing distally and pressure is applied into extension to reach the restrictive barrier (Fig. 46.5). The clinician then applies a graded, non-thrust oscillatory manipulation into extension.

Tibiofemoral long-axis distraction manipulation

The patient is positioned in supine, near the edge of the table. The leg to be treated is off of the edge of the table. The clinician places the distal leg between his / her knees such that they hold the patient's lower leg just proximal to the malleoli. The clinician holds the knee at the joint line with both hands in slight flexion (Fig. 46.6), and then lets the knee drop into full extension while simultaneously performing rapid extension of the patient's knees to apply a high-velocity, low-amplitude thrust in the direction of tibiofemoral distraction. Varus or valgus forces can be added to refine induce lateral mobilization of the tibiofemoral joint.

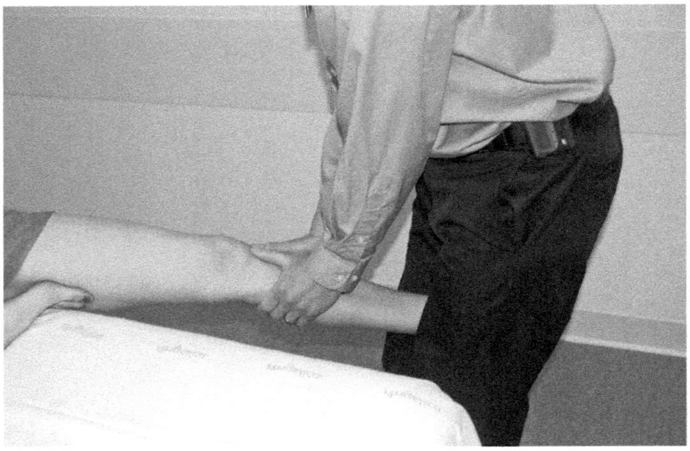

Figure 46.6 Tibiofemoral long-axis distraction manipulation.

Tibiofemoral mobilization with movement

The patient is positioned in supine and performs active knee extension and flexion. If either of those is painful, the clinician then applies test glides during active range of motion to determine the treatment direction. The test glides include medial, lateral, anterior, posterior, and medial and lateral rotation. For a lateral glide, the clinician stabilizes the proximal tibia medially, places the mobilizing hand on the lateral femur and applies a sustained force medially (relative tibiofemoral lateral glide; Fig. 46.7A) while the patient performs active knee flexion and extension motions. For a medial glide, the clinician stabilizes the proximal tibia laterally, places the mobilizing hand on the medial femur and applies a sustained force medially. For an anterior glide, the clinician stabilizes the posterior aspect of the proximal tibia, while the mobilizing hand is placed anteriorly on the distal femur with a sustained posterior force to create a tibiofemoral anterior glide. For a posterior glide, the clinician stabilizes the anterior aspect of the proximal tibia, while the mobilizing hand is placed posteriorly on the distal femur with a sustained anterior force to create a tibiofemoral anterior glide. For a medial and lateral rotational glide, the hands are placed on the medial and lateral

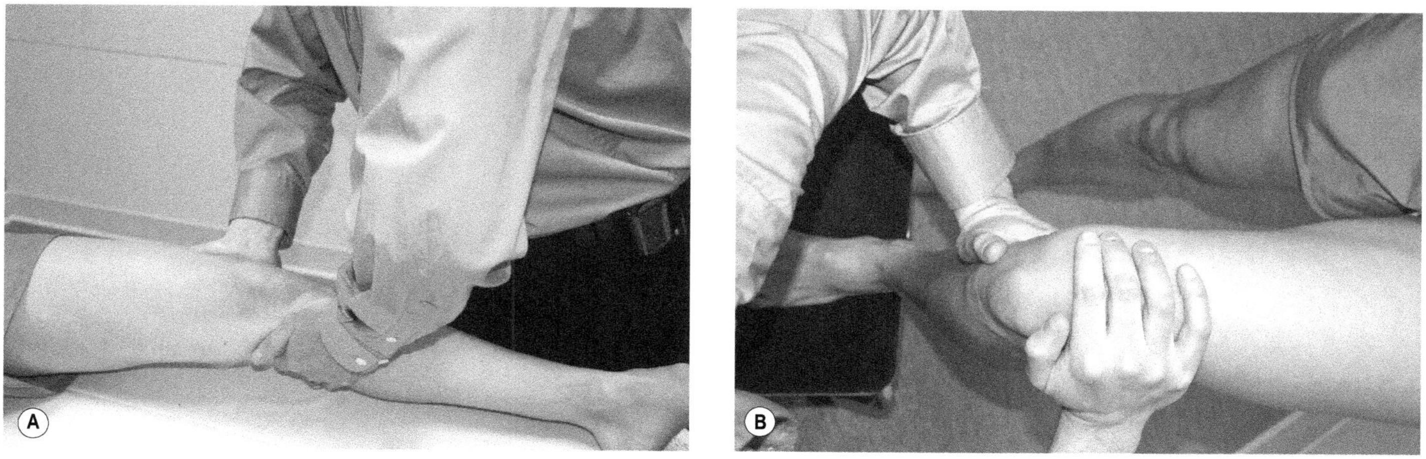

Figure 46.7 **Tibiofemoral mobilization with movement:** (**A**) in supine, and (**B**) in standing position with the knee over a supporting table.

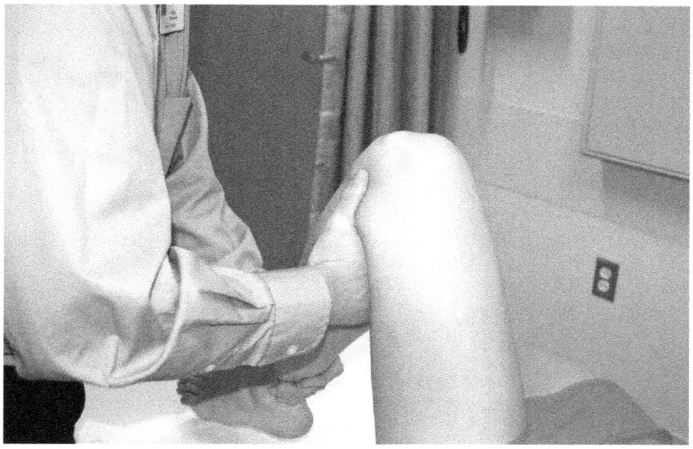

Figure 46.8 **Proximal tibiofibular thrust manipulation.**

aspect of the proximal tibia; to create a medial glide, a posterior force is applied medially and an anterior force is applied laterally; for a lateral glide, an anterior force is applied medially and a posterior force is applied laterally. The direction that creates the greatest pain relief is repeated for two sets of 10. If no pain is felt in the supine position, then the same procedure is followed with the patient in a standing position and the knee over a supporting table (Fig. 46.7B).

Proximal tibiofibular thrust manipulation

The clinician places his / her second metacarpophalangeal in the patient's popliteal fossa and pulls the soft tissue laterally until the metacarpophalangeal is firmly stabilized behind the patient's fibular head. The clinician uses the opposite hand to grasp the foot and ankle. The clinician externally rotates the leg and flexes the knee to the restrictive barrier (Fig. 46.8). Once the restrictive barrier is met, the clinician applies a high-velocity, low-amplitude force through the tibia (directing the patient's heel toward the ipsilateral buttock). Prior to performing this manipulation, the clinician should determine whether the patient can safely and comfortably achieve the degree of knee flexion required.

Patellofemoral mobilization: caudal and cephalad

The patient's knee is placed in approximately at 20° of flexion. This can be accomplished using a rolled towel or a bolster, or by resting the patient's knee over the clinician's knee. The clinician distracts the patella with the non-mobilizing hand by gently cupping around the patella with the palm. Using the heel of the other hand the clinician applies graded, oscillatory mobilizations in a caudal (Fig. 46.9A) or cephalad (Fig. 46.9B) direction. The clinician's forearm should be placed in line with the direction of the manipulation and care is taken to avoid compression of the patella into the femur. This technique can be progressed by increasing the degree of knee flexion either in supine or by having the patient sitting with the legs off the side of the treatment table.

Patellofemoral mobilization: medial and lateral

The patient's knee is placed in approximately at 20° of flexion. The clinician places the thumbs of both hands on the lateral side of the patellar and the second and third fingers of both hands on the medial side of the patella (Fig. 46.10). The clinician performs graded, oscillatory mobilizations of the patella on the femur in a medial or lateral direction. Care is taken to avoid compression of the patella into the femur. To progress the medial glide technique, the patient is positioned in side-lying. The clinician places the patient's top leg in approximately 10° of hip extension and adduction to put the lateral leg soft tissues, including the lateral patellar retinaculum, on stretch. Using the heel of the hand the clinician applies a graded, oscillatory, non-thrust mobilization of the patellar on the femur in a medial direction. The patient's top leg should be supported on the medial side to avoid placing a valgus stress on the knee during the manipulation.

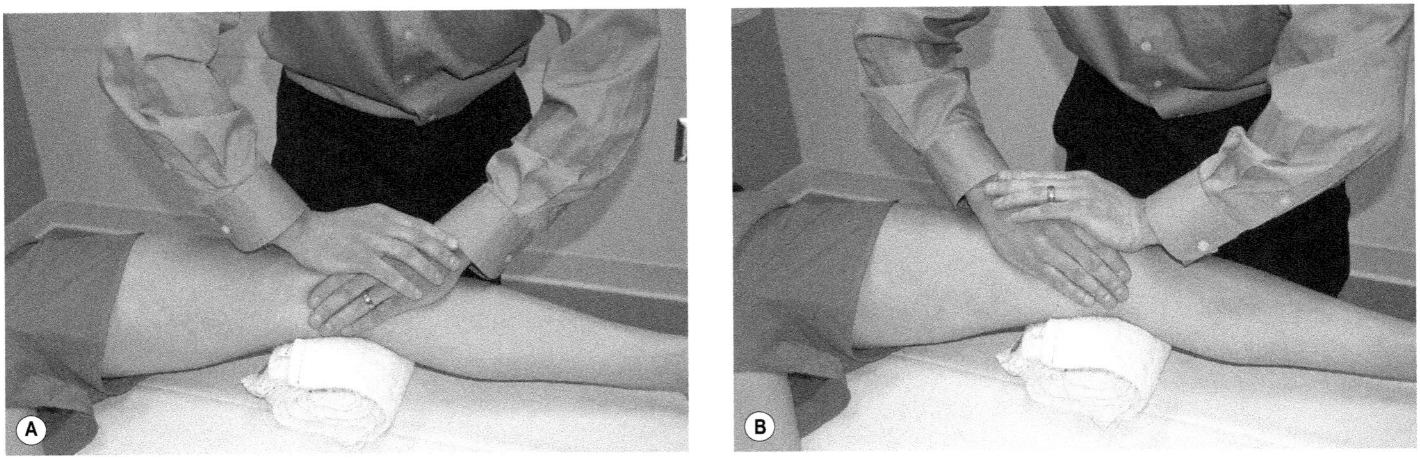

Figure 46.9 **Patellofemoral mobilization:** (**A**) in caudal, and (**B**) in cephalad, direction.

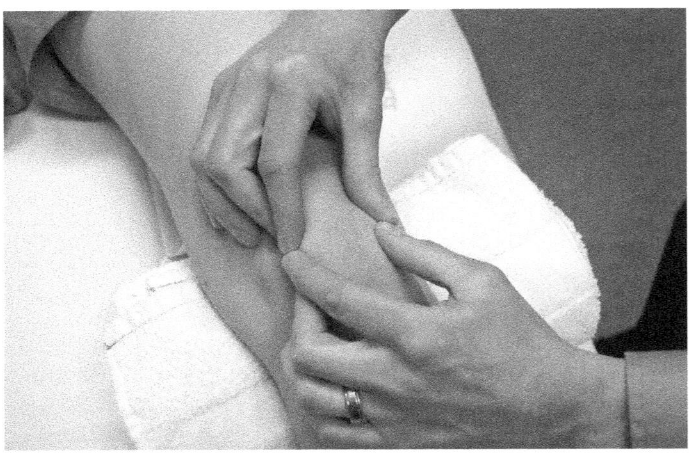

Figure 46.10 Patellofemoral mobilization in medial and lateral direction.

References

Abbott JH, Robertson MC, Chapple C, et al. 2013. Manual therapy, exercise therapy, or both, in addition to usual care, for osteoarthritis of the hip or knee: a randomized controlled trial. clinical effectiveness. Osteoarthritis Cartilage 21: 525–534.

Almeida SA, Williams KM, Shaffer RA, et al. 1999. Epidemiological patterns of musculoskeletal injuries and physical training. Med Sci Sports Exerc 31: 1176–1182.

Bialosky JE, Bishop MD, Price DD, et al. 2009. The mechanisms of manual therapy in the treatment of musculoskeletal pain: a comprehensive model. Man Ther 14: 531–538.

Brantingham JW, Globe G, Pollard H, et al. 2009. Manipulative therapy for lower extremity conditions: expansion of literature review. J Manipulative Physiol Ther 32: 53–71.

Crossley K, Bennell K, Green S, et al. 2002. Physical therapy for patellofemoral pain: a randomized, double-blinded, placebo-controlled trial. Am J Sports Med 30: 857–865.

Deyle GD, Allison SC, Matekel RL, et al. 2005. Physical therapy treatment effectiveness for osteoarthritis of the knee: a randomized comparison of supervised clinical exercise and manual therapy procedures versus a home exercise program. Phys Ther 85: 1301–1317.

Deyle GD, Henderson NE, Matekel RL, et al. 2000. Effectiveness of manual physical therapy and exercise in osteoarthritis of the knee: a randomized, controlled trial. Ann Int Med 132: 173–181.

Deyle GD, Gill NW, Allison SC, et al. 2012. Which patients are unlikely to benefit from manual PT and exercise? J Fam Pract 61: E1–E8.

French, HP, Brennan A, White B, et al. 2011. Manual therapy for osteoarthritis of the hip or knee: a systematic review. Man Ther 16: 109–117.

Hillermann B, Gomes AN, Korporaal C, et al. 2006. A pilot study comparing the effects of spinal manipulative therapy with those of extra-spinal manipulative therapy on quadriceps muscle strength. J Manipulative Physiol Ther 29: 145–149.

Lowry CD, Cleland JA, Dyke K. 2008. Management of patients with patellofemoral pain syndrome using a multimodal approach: a case series. J Orthop Sports Phys Ther 38: 691–702.

Moss P, Sluka K, Wright A. 2007. The initial effects of knee joint mobilization on osteoarthritic hyperalgesia. Man Ther 12: 109–118.

Nagoi T. 2013. The epidemiology and impact of pain in osteoarthritis. Osteoarthritis Cartilage 21: 1145–1153.

Pinto D, Robertson MC, Abbott JH, et al. 2013. Manual therapy, exercise therapy, or both, in addition to usual care, for osteoarthritis of the hip or knee: economic evaluation alongside a randomized controlled trial. Osteoarthritis Cartilage 21: 525–534.

Pollard H, Ward G, Hoskins W, et al. 2008. The effect of a manual therapy knee protocol on osteoarthritic knee pain: a randomized controlled trial. J Can Chiropr Assoc 52: 229–242.

Takasaki H, Hall T, Jull G. 2013. Immediate and short-term effects of Mulligan's mobilization with movement on knee pain and disability associated with knee osteoarthritis: a prospective case series. Phys Theory Pract 29: 87–95.

van den Dolder PA, Roberts DL. 2006. Six sessions of manual therapy increase knee flexion and improve activity in people with anterior knee pain: a randomised controlled trial. Aust J Physiother 52: 261–264.

Chapter 47

Tendinopathy of the Knee

Ellen Pong

CHAPTER CONTENTS

Introduction	531
Tendinopathies of the hamstrings	531
Background	531
Semimembranosus tendinopathy	532
Background	532
Anatomy	532
Pathology and patho-biomechanics	532
Diagnosis	532
Treatment and prognosis	532
Iliotibial band syndrome	532
Background	532
Anatomy	533
Pathology and patho-biomechanics	534
Diagnosis	534
Conservative treatment and prognosis	534
Patellar tendinopathy	535
Background	535
Anatomy	535
Pathology and patho-biomechanics	535
Diagnosis	535
Conservative treatment and prognosis	536
Popliteal tendinopathy	537
Background	537
Anatomy	537
Pathology and patho-biomechanics	538
Diagnosis	538
Conservative treatment and prognosis	538
Quadriceps tendinopathy	538
Background	538
Anatomy	538
Pathology and patho-biomechanics	538
Diagnosis	539
Conservative treatment and prognosis	539
Conclusion	539

Introduction

Tendinopathies of the knee can have devastating effects both functionally and financially whether the patient has a sedentary lifestyle or is a professional athlete. Basic causes such as overuse and failed healing, along with histopathology including hypovascularity and mucoid degeneration, are present in knee tendinopathies as they are present in tendinopathies throughout the body. Essential components of treatment are also similar: rest, physical modalities and particularly eccentric loading of the recovering tendon. Specific rehabilitation is tailored to fit the function and biomechanics of the pathological tendon. Although there is greater agreement on general characteristics of a tendinopathy in current literature, opinion and evidence still vary widely on anatomical variations, specific patho-biomechanics and components of treatment.

Tendinopathies of the Hamstrings

Background

Although a multitude of anecdotal information on tendinopathies of the biceps femoris and semitendinosus exists on sports medicine and fitness websites, and there is an occasional general reference to non-specific hamstring tendinopathies in textbooks, reports of these conditions in the peer-reviewed literature are extremely rare, and they generally discuss surgical management (Longo et al 2008). Information on injuries to the hamstrings is centred on muscle strain, tendon avulsion and rupture, which can be considered more-common injuries to these structures than tendinopathies (Voight et al 2007; Sarwark 2010; Kisner & Colby 2010). Snapping of the biceps femoris and semitendinosus tendons is described in the literature; however, this condition is normally treated surgically (Lyu & Wu 1989; Lokiec et al 1992; Bae & Kwon 1997; Karataglis et al 2008; Bernhardson & LaPrade 2010; Date et al 2012) and is not considered a degenerative or overuse tendinopathy, but rather a mechanical problem.

Semimembranosus Tendinopathy

Background

Semimembranosus tendinopathy (SMT) is a rare cause of pain in the posterior–medial knee. It was scantily addressed in the literature from the 1970s to the 1990s, but no new knowledge of the condition or how to treat it is in evidence today (Ray et al 1988; Safran & Fu 1995; Bylund & de Weber 2010). The incidence is unknown; however, it does appear to be more prevalent in older patients with additional knee pathologies than in young athletes as an overuse syndrome (Bylund & de Weber 2010). SMT usually presents as local tenderness at the distal semimembranosus tendon and patient complaints of aching posterior–medial knee pain (Bylund & de Weber 2010).

Anatomy

The semimembranosus muscle originates from the lateral aspect of the ischial tuberosity, follows a path down the posterior–medial aspect of the thigh and inserts at the posterior–medial aspect of the knee, where it acts as a knee flexor. The muscle forms a thick rounded tendon distally, which passes medial to the medial head of the gastrocnemius and lateral to the smaller semitendinosus tendon. The main insertions include the posterior–medial tibial plateau, just posterior to the medial collateral ligament (MCL), and the most anterior insertion (pars reflexa), which turns anteriorly almost 90° and passes beneath the MCL to insert on the tibia just distal to the medial joint line. A U-shaped bursa surrounds the distal semimembranosus tendon, which separates the distal aspects of the tendon from the medial tibial plateau, MCL and semitendinosus tendon. Tendinopathy normally develops at the main (direct) head, reflected insertions or distal tendon (Bylund & de Weber 2010).

Pathology and patho-biomechanics

The semimembranosus tendon is subjected to increased friction from the adjacent joint capsule, medial femoral condyle, medial tibial plateau and semitendinosus tendon during repetitive knee flexion. This overuse loading and friction are thought to produce degenerative changes in the tendon and its insertions, as well as irritation of the bursa (Bylund & de Weber 2010).

An important part of the cause of this tendinopathy may be the association with coexisting additional knee pathologies. The most frequently seen concomitant pathologies are chondromalacia and degenerative medial meniscal tears. Osteophytes from osteoarthritis may cause SMT when impinging on the nearby tendon at the joint line. Pes anserine tendonitis is an additional associated pathology. Impingement from total knee arthroplasty components may also cause secondary SMT. Other hypothesized influences on SMT development are increased knee valgus stress, increased Q-angle and overpronation of the foot – all of which may increase friction between the medial femoral condyle and the semimembranosus tendon (Bylund & de Weber 2010).

Diagnosis

The presentation of SMT can be variable and misdiagnosed because of the frequency of concomitant pathologies. On its own, presentation consists of an insidious, progressive ache in the posterior–medial knee area that may radiate proximally along the posterior–medial thigh or distally to the medial calf (Bylund & de Weber 2010).

Clinically, there is tenderness to palpation of the semimembranosus tendon, either near its tibial insertion site or slightly proximal to that. Passive deep flexion of the knee and passive internal tibial rotation of the knee while flexed to 90° may be used as provocative tests. As coexisting pathologies are common, the joints of the entire lower extremity should be evaluated for biomechanical features, such as those previously listed, that can contribute or predispose to semimembranosus tendon impingement or overuse (Bylund & de Weber 2010).

Imaging may be helpful in some cases. Bone scans can show increased radiotracer uptake at the area of tendinopathy. Magnetic resonance imaging (MRI) has poor ability to depict accurately any pathology of the posterior horn of the medial meniscus; however, it is useful for ruling out other causes of knee pain in this area. Visualization via ultrasound may assist diagnosis with findings of thickening of the tendon, degenerative tendinopathy at the site of clinical tenderness and surrounding bursal fluid (Bylund & de Weber 2010).

Treatment and prognosis

Conservative treatment should be attempted initially with relative rest, ice, modalities to reduce pain, possibly non-steroidal anti-inflammatory drugs and physical therapy. The exercises will focus on strengthening and stretching of the hamstrings, and addressing any causal factors that can be improved with therapy. As with all tendinopathies, the exercise programme should progress from concentric to eccentric contraction of the muscle. Prognosis for recovery with conservative treatment is good, based on the data currently available; in more than 90% of reported cases the condition resolves with treatment described above. If symptoms are not resolved or improved within at least 3 months, surgical rerouting of the tendon or other surgical techniques may be considered (Halperin et al 1987; Bylund & de Weber 2010).

Iliotibial Band Syndrome

Background

Iliotibial band syndrome (ITBS) (see also Ch 35) is an overuse injury most often occurring in the active athletic population (Hong & Kim 2013). Most patients complain of lateral side knee pain associated with repetitive activities. ITBS is cited as a common cause of lateral knee pain among runners, cyclists, rowers and other athletes, including military personnel, with a reported incidence ranging from 1.6% to 14% (van der Worp et al 2012; Hong & Kim 2013) to as great as 52% depending on the population studied (Kirk et al 2000).

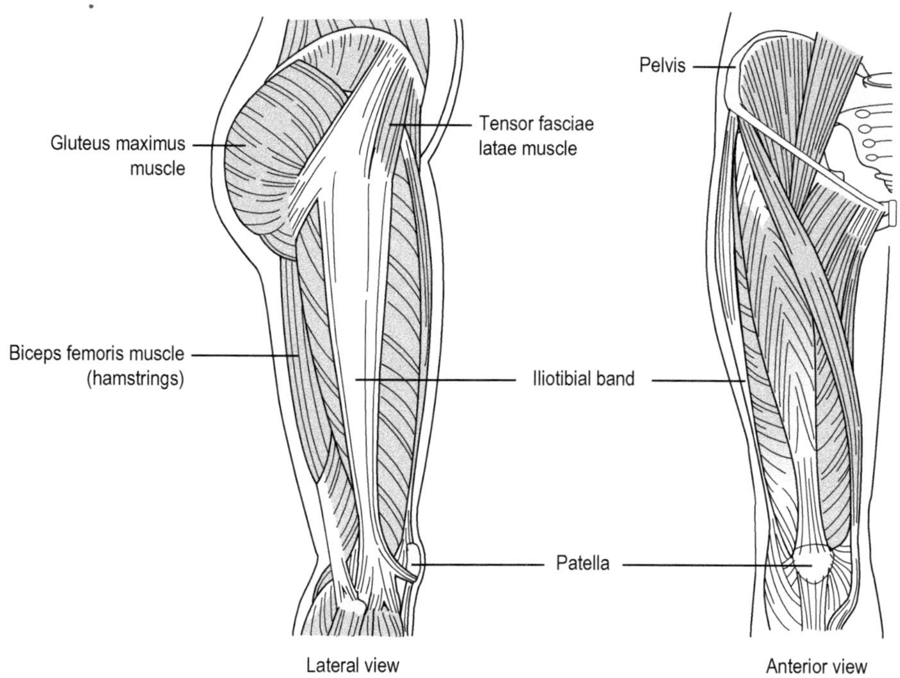

Figure 47.1 General anatomy of the iliotibial band.

Anatomy

The iliotibial band or tract (ITB) is a lateral thickening of the fascia lata in the thigh (Fig. 47.1). It originates along the margin of the iliac crest with dominant fibres condensing on the iliac tubercle (Sher et al 2011). The ITB splits into a superficial and a deep portion, which covers the tensor fasciae latae and anchors it to the iliac crest (Fairclough et al 2006). The tensor fasciae latae itself has an insertion on the ITB. Continuing in the distal direction along the femur, the ITB passes over the greater trochanter without developing a fixation to the bone (Birnbaum et al 2004). The ITB encompasses most of the tendon of the gluteus maximus (Birnbaum et al 2004; Fairclough et al 2006). It then passes over the vastus lateralis and inserts at the upper border of the lateral epicondyle through strong fibrous strands that are often obliquely orientated. These strands occasionally attach to the epicondyle itself; however, they are more usually attached immediately proximal to this site and fan out as they approach the bone. A region of adipose tissue is closely associated with the fibrous strands and intervenes between the ITB itself and the femur (Fairclough et al 2006). Distal insertions of the ITB include the transverse and longitudinal retinaculum of the patella, the infracondylar tubercle of the tibia or Gerdy's tubercle, the head of the fibula and the lateral intermuscular septum (Fairclough et al 2006; Vieira et al 2007).

Studies have differentiated two functional regions of the ITB: a tendinous part that is proximal to the lateral femoral epicondyle, and a ligamentous part that lies between the epicondyle and Gerdy's tubercle (Fig. 47.2) (Fairclough et al 2006). The ITB is tense when the limb is loaded, both in the neutral position and when the tibia is internally or externally rotated. As the knee flexes, tension shifts from the anterior to the posterior fibre bundles of the ITB. The bands of the fasciae latae, which are contiguous with the ITB and attached to the patella, come under tension as the patella moves around the femoral condyle, while the ligamentous part of the ITB is tensioned in turn as the tibia moves posteriorly (Fairclough et al 2006).

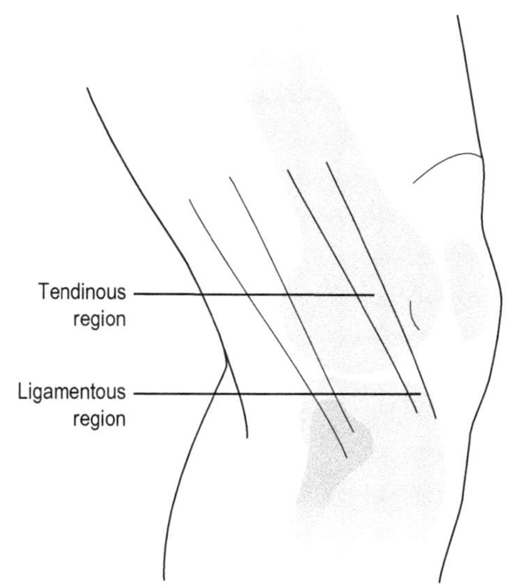

Figure 47.2 Two regions of the ITB tract: a tendinous part proximal to the lateral femoral epicondyle and a 'ligamentous' part between the epicondyle and Gerdy's tubercle.

In summary, there are several important considerations in the anatomy of the ITB that were previously overlooked. It is not a discrete structure, but rather a thickened part of the tensor fasciae latae that envelops the thigh. Additionally, it is connected to the linea aspera by an intermuscular septum and to the supracondylar region of the femur, including the epicondyle, by coarse fibrous bands that are not pathological adhesions. Finally, a bursa is rarely present, but this may be mistaken for the lateral recess of the knee (Fairclough et al 2007).

Pathology and patho-biomechanics

Several aetiologies have been considered and debated for ITBS, with little evidence that a pathological change such as inflammation takes place in the ITB itself (Hong & Kim 2013). In fact, the idea that 'friction' and 'inflammation' play a role in what some call 'iliotibial friction syndrome' is disputed based on current knowledge of the anatomy (Fairclough et al 2007). Proposed aetiologies include one subtype that involves irritation of a cyst, bursa or lateral synovial recess, and a second subtype arising from compression by the ITB of the connective tissues that underlie the portion of the band between the lateral epicondyle and the knee joint line (Lavine 2010; Strauss et al 2011). There may or may not be any actual anterior–posterior friction-producing motion of the ITB (Lavine 2010).

Patho-biomechanics of ITBS are also controversial. Some authors attribute ITBS to weakness of the hip abductors. Weak hip abductors could conceivably cause increased hip adduction during the stance phase of gait, with a consequent increase strain of the iliotibial band and a greater tendency for it to compress the tissues underneath (Lavine 2010). Indeed, some studies noted the presence of abductor weakness or increased hip adduction during the stance phase of gait, which could be interpreted as a result of abductor weakness (Fredericson et al 2000; MacMahon et al 2000; Noehren et al 2007). Grau et al (2008) reported different findings, however; hip abductor weakness, measured by a mechanically stabilized dynamometer, was not found in their study of 10 runners.

Tightness versus laxity of the ITB is another disputed factor in ITBS. Early studies (Gose & Schweizer 1989) correlated tightness of the ITB with ITBS, with the theory that a tighter band would lead to greater compression of the underlying tissues with each gait cycle. More recently researchers have shown that some runners with ITBS had a 'looser' ITB, exhibiting increased strain (i.e. it elongated more when subject to an external load) and a statistically significant increased strain rate (i.e. it elongated more rapidly) during running (Hamill et al 2008).

A predominance of studies assessing patho-biomechanical causes of ITBS had focused on the athletic runner population. Hence angle of knee flexion during stance phase (Orchard et al 1996), an increased angle of flexion of the knee at heel strike due to fatigue (Miller et al 2007), excessive rearfoot eversion (Busseuil et al 1998), reduced rearfoot eversion (Noehren et al 2007), increased landing forces, increased knee internal rotation, low hamstring to quadriceps strength ratio, genu recurvatum and a narrow step width are all thought to contribute to ITBS (Devan et al 2004; Noehren et al 2007; Meardon et al 2012).

Diagnosis

The case history and physical examination are usually sufficient for diagnosis, although refractory cases may indicate the need for an MRI scan to specify involved tissues or to rule out another disorder in the region (Lavine 2010). The patient usually, but not always, complains of pain in the area of the lateral femoral epicondyle or slightly below it, which presents after repetitive flexion and extension of the knee (Hong & Kim 2013).

Three special tests are used to evidence restriction of the iliotibial band or to reproduce the symptoms of ITBS: the Noble compression test, Ober's test and the Thomas test (Hong & Kim 2013). It should be noted that two of the tests indicate only ITB tightness; therefore, in patients with ITBS who do not have ITB tightness, the tests may give a false negative when used specifically for diagnosing ITBS (Hamill et al 2008).

In the Noble compression test, as described by Noble (1979), the patient lies in the supine position and the examiner brings the patient's knee into 90° of flexion with simultaneous hip flexion. The examiner then applies direct pressure over the lateral femoral epicondyle, or 1–2 cm proximal to it, while passively extending the knee. For a positive test, the patient's pain will be reproduced at the site of compression at approximately 30° of knee flexion (Magee 2008). The sensitivity and specificity of this test for detecting ITBS are not known.

Ober's test assesses tightness of the ITB (Magee 2008; Hong & Kim 2013). The examiner performs the test while standing behind the side-lying patient. The examiner manually stabilizes the patient's pelvis with one hand, passively flexes the patient's uppermost thigh and then brings it into maximal abduction. The examiner then maintains that abduction while passively moving the thigh into extension. The tested limb is then lowered into adduction until it stops, or until the pelvis starts to tilt. If tightness is present, the patient's thigh remains above the horizontal plane and does not reach the table (Magee 2008). The test, as originally described by Ober, was performed with the tested leg's knee flexed (Wang et al 2006). To avoid stress on the femoral nerve and to show the effect of greater stretch on the ITB, the test is now commonly performed as described above, with the knee extended (Wang et al 2006; Magee 2008). The sensitivity and specificity of this test to diagnose ITBS are not known.

The Thomas test is used to assess the tightness of iliopsoas muscle, rectus femoris and ITB. The patient lies supine while the examiner passively flexes the non-tested hip, bringing the knee to the patient's chest (Magee 2008). The patient then holds the knee to the chest. The tested straight leg will stay on the table; however, it will abduct at the hip. This is called the 'J' sign, and indicates tightness of the ITB (Magee 2008). The sensitivity and specificity of this test for determining ITBS are not known, however.

Conservative treatment and prognosis

Initially, in the acute phase, treatment will include activity modification, ice and non-steroidal anti-inflammatory medication (Fredericson & Wolf 2005; Fredericson & Weir 2006; Ellis et al 2007). Use of corticosteroid injection in cases of severe pain or swelling is debated. Although corticosteroid injections have been shown to reduce symptoms in the acute phase of ITBS, they may actually delay the eventual return to full pain-free activity because long-term cortisone effects include inhibition of collagen synthesis (Gunter et al 2004).

Most, if not all, published protocols appear to agree that treatment in the subacute phase entails a focus on stretching of the ITB and soft tissue therapy for any myofascial restrictions (Fredericson & Wolf 2005; Fredericson & Weir 2006; Ellis et al 2007). However, as research has shown that not all patients with ITBS have ITB tightness (Hamill et al 2008), a more individualized approach based on examination findings is recommended. (See also Ch 35 for further discussion on manual therapy approaches focusing on the role of the ITB in the hip.)

The recovery phase incorporates advanced exercises including eccentric muscle contractions to strengthen the hip abductors, as well as triplanar motions and integrated movement patterns (Fredericson & Weir 2006). For patients who are running athletes, the final return to running phase starts with easy sprints and avoidance of hill training, with a gradual increase in frequency and intensity (Fredericson & Weir 2006).

There is limited evidence of research quality to support that the conservative treatments discussed above offer any significant benefit in the management of ITBS (Ellis et al 2007). Despite this, the prognosis for recovery using a comprehensive conservative treatment plan is considered to be good and estimated to occur within 6 weeks of onset in most patients (Fredericson & Wolf 2005; Beers et al 2008).

Patellar Tendinopathy

Background

Patellar tendinopathy describes both acute and chronic anterior knee pain associated with tenderness at the inferior pole of the patella, in which ultrasound examination and MRI reveal abnormal signals at the junction of the patella and the patellar tendon (Khan et al 1998). Other names for this variable condition include 'jumper's knee', 'patellar tendinosis', 'patellar tendinitis', 'patellar tendonitis', 'patella tendon disorder', 'insertion tendinitis of the patellar tendon', 'partial rupture of the patellar tendon' and 'patellar apicitis' (Khan et al 1998). Patellar tendinopathy has an estimated incidence of 2.5% to 14% in athletes whose sports involve repetitive, sudden ballistic movements of the knee (Zwerver et al 2011; Ackermann & Renström 2012).

Both intrinsic and extrinsic factors contribute to patellar tendinopathy. Intrinsic factors include strength imbalance, postural alignment, foot structure, reduced ankle dorsiflexion and muscle weakness or tightness (Rutland et al 2010). The primary cause is attributed to the extrinsic factor of overuse (Rutland et al 2010; Rodriguez-Merchan 2013).

Anatomy

The patellar tendon, described by Khan et al (1998), is the extension of the common tendon of insertion of the quadriceps femoris muscle. It extends from the inferior pole of the patella to the tibial tuberosity. The patellar tendon is roughly 3 cm wide in the coronal plane and 4 to 5 mm deep in the sagittal plane.

The blood supply to the patellar tendon is thought to contribute to patellar tendinopathy. According to Khan et al (1998), an anastomotic ring that lies in the thin layers of loose connective tissue covering the dense fibrous expansion of the rectus femoris is responsible for vascularization of the patellar tendon. The main contributors to this ring are the medial inferior genicular, lateral superior genicular, lateral inferior genicular and anterior tibial recurrent arteries. The posterior aspect of the tendon is most commonly affected by tendinopathy, and it is here that the blood supply to the proximal portion of the patellar tendon enters (Khan et al 1998).

The quadriceps and patellar tendons are continuous with each other over the anterior surface of the patella (Toumi et al 2006). The deep surface of the patellar tendon is closely associated with the infrapatellar (Hoffa's) fat pad across its entire width, and the fat pad forms interdigitations with the proximal part of the tendon that are more obvious on the medial side than on the lateral side (Toumi et al 2006).

Pathology and patho-biomechanics

The patellar tendons of patients with chronic patellar tendinopathy contain mucoid degeneration and occasional hyaline degeneration, which is characterized by hardness rather than the softness normally inherent in mucoid degeneration (Khan et al 1998; Rutland et al 2010). There is abnormal collagen, tenocytes and vasculature (Kulig et al 2013). The tendon does not consist of tight parallel collagen bundles, as is normal, but rather appears disorganized with collagen replaced by degenerative and necrotic tissue. Micro-tearing in the collagen is suspected (Khan et al 1998; Kulig et al 2013).

The presence of inflammatory cells in the tendon is debated. One theory is that fibroblasts, more plentiful in the pathological tendon than in the normal, may have been mistaken for inflammatory cells early on (Khan et al 1998; Rutland et al 2010). Kulig et al (2013) found thicker proximal patellar tendons in both symptomatic and non-symptomatic basketball athletes compared with non-athletes, which they suggested was a normal adaptation to training loads. Inflammation was previously believed to be a central driving force to the pathological process; however, current histopathological evidence has not supported this, and affirmed that these conditions are instead due to a failed healing response (Kulig et al 2013; Rodriguez-Merchan 2013).

Excessive or inappropriate loading of the musculotendinous unit is believed to be a main factor in the disease process in the following manner. The normal crimped configuration of collagen fibres and fibrils in normal tendon at rest disappears when the tendon is stretched by about 2%. When the stretch reaches 5% elongation, tendon fibres become more parallel. Beyond 5% elongation, tendon micro-failures occur (Khan et al 1998; Rutland et al 2010). The vertical component of each ground reaction force in a jump is around six to eight body weights, and a basketball player jumps an average of 70 times per game. With the forces on the patellar tendon in activities ranging from level walking at 0.5 kN to 14.5 kN during competitive weightlifting, it is clear that sports activities impose stresses sufficient to cause tendon fibre failure (Khan et al 1998).

Diagnosis

Patellar tendinopathy is diagnosed clinically by history, knee examination and palpation of the tendon and its attachments (Cook et al 2001; Rutland et al 2010). An important physical finding in patellar tendinopathy is tenderness at the inferior pole of the patella or in the main body of the tendon when the knee is fully extended and the quadriceps is relaxed. Both patellae should be tested. The upper pole of the patella is grasped by the examiner so as to anteriorize the apex of the

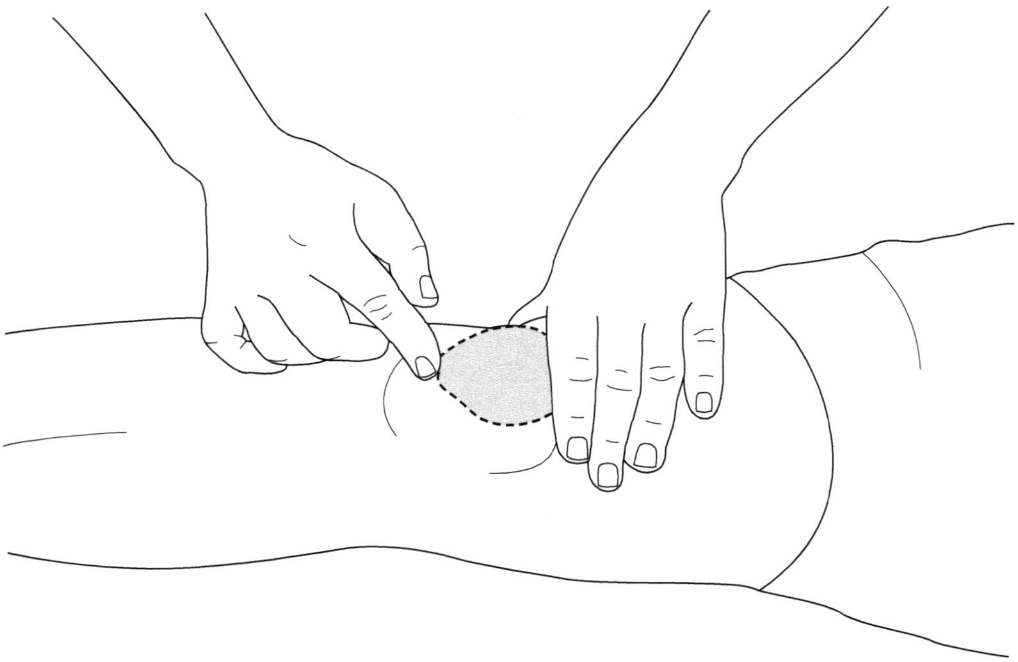

Figure 47.3 Palpation for tenderness of the inferior pole of the patella.

patella (Fig. 47.3). Using finger pressure on the patellar tendon immediately below the inferior pole of the patella, the examiner will elicit from the patient the test response of pain or no pain (Ramos et al 2009). The tenderness decreases or disappears when the knee is flexed to 90° (Khan et al 1998). Cook et al (2001) found palpation to be a moderately sensitive but not specific test in symptomatic tendons. Other researchers have reported high sensitivity and moderate specificity for diagnosing patellar tendinopathy (Ramos et al 2009).

The diagnosis may be confirmed with imaging, commonly ultrasonography and MRI (Khan et al 1998; Ramos et al 2009). Patellar tendon pain and tenderness, as well as imaging changes, are most often found to be present at the junction of the inferior pole of the patella and the tendon attachment (Cook et al 2001; Ramos et al 2009). Pain in the patellar tendon may also be reproduced with resisted knee extension and functional tests, including ascending or descending stairs, performing single-leg declining squats, and jumping or hopping (Rutland et al 2010).

There are several systems of grading jumper's knee according to the severity and timing of knee pain, including Blazina's knee scale, Kennedy's scale and the Victorian Institute of Sport Assessment (VISA) scale for patellar tendinopathy (VISA-P) and others. According to Khan et al (1998), the reliability of most of these scales has never been tested, and they may be incapable of discriminating between patients with widely differing symptoms. Some clinicians use the scales to determine when to advance the patient to the next stage of rehabilitation. For example, Blazina's scale presents the following stages (Panni et al 2000; Rutland et al 2010):

- **stage 1:** pain present only after athletic participation; no apparent functional impairment ($n=0$)
- **stage 2:** pain during and after activity; performance is still at a satisfactory level ($n=26$)
- **stage 3:** pain present during and after activity but is more prolonged; progressive difficulties with performing at a satisfactory level ($n=16$).

Of these scales, the VISA-P is the most well known and widely used. It is a short questionnaire assessing symptoms, simple tests of function and ability to play sport (Visentini et al 1998). Creators of the VISA-P scale reported excellent short-term test–retest and inter-tester reliabilities (both $r>0.95$), as well as good short-term (1-week) stability (Visentini et al 1998). More-recent various language translations of the VISA-P scale have also shown good test–retest reliability and valid use as a tool to evaluate symptoms, knee function and ability to play sports in athletes with patellar tendinopathy (Frohm et al 2004; Maffulli et al 2008; Zwerver et al 2009; Lohrer & Nauck 2011).

Conservative treatment and prognosis

Conservative treatment programmes for patellar tendinopathy are varied, and are often progressed in stages based on the patient's subjective report of pain, utilizing the scales discussed previously (Khan et al 1998; Panni et al 2000; Rutland et al 2010). Components of each stage are debated, and no single component has strong evidence-based support. Conservative treatment in general includes correction of any noted predisposing factors, relative or absolute rest from aggravating high-load activities (Bahr et al 2006; Frohm et al 2007; Rutland et al 2010) and stretching and strengthening. Eccentric loading is advocated by most (Panni et al 2000; Cannell et al 2001) but not all (Visnes et al 2005) clinicians. For advocates of eccentric loading, the eccentric decline squat, either bilateral (Fig. 47.4A) or unilateral (Fig. 47.4B), is specifically recommended (Purdam et al 2004; Young et al 2005; Rutland et al 2010). Recent research (Saithna et al 2012) has

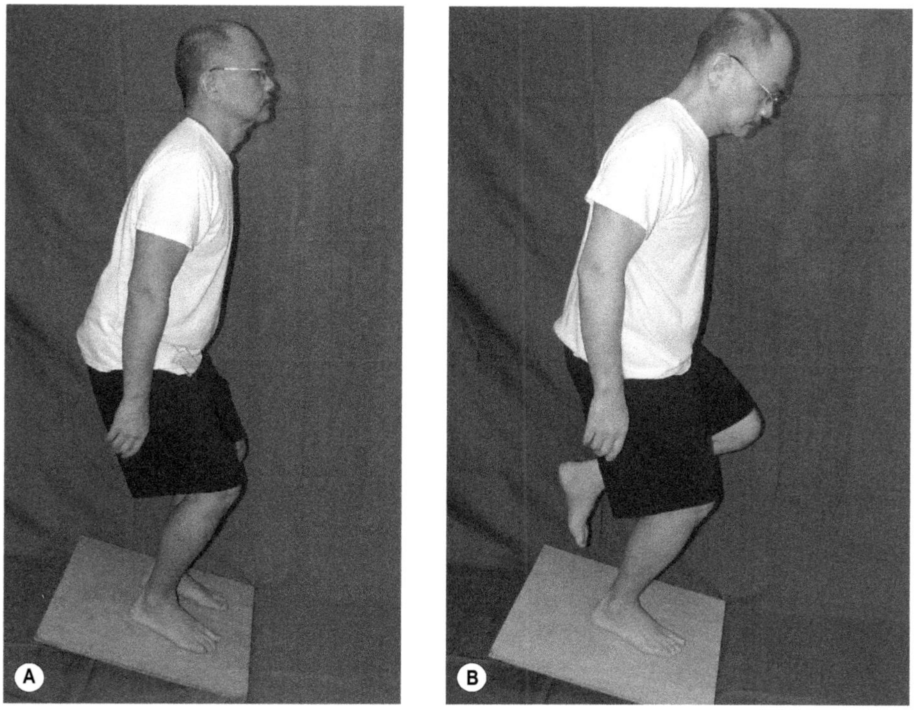

Figure 47.4 **Eccentric decline squat:** (**A**) bilateral, (**B**) unilateral.

disputed the practice of withdrawing the athlete from sport while engaged in eccentric exercise protocols, citing 'significant psychological, physiological and financial implications' (p 554), and referring to several studies in which athletes benefited from an eccentric exercise protocol while they continued to participate in sport.

Other conservative therapy treatments including transverse friction massage (Stasinopoulos & Stasinopoulos 2004), ice and NSAIDs or local anaesthetics (Gammaitoni et al 2013) with or without modalities may be helpful to reduce pain and any inflammation present, as well as increase treatment tolerance. Less frequently incorporated are bracing (Khan et al 1998), use of an infrapatellar strap (Lavagnino et al 2011) and novel modalities that have shown inconsistent clinical results, such as extracorporeal shockwave treatment (ESWT) (van der Worp et al 2013).

The most recent direction of treatment research for patellar tendinopathy is injection of the tendon with platelet-rich plasma (Ferrero et al 2012; Gosens et al 2012; Vetrano et al 2013) or with autologous bone marrow stem cells (Pascual-Garrido et al 2012). The reasoning is that traditional conservative treatment does not address the biological state of the condition, which is hypovascularity and programmed cell death (Gosens et al 2012). These treatments are recommended as an alternative treatment for those patients who have failed 6–8 months of non-operative treatment, but before surgical intervention is considered. Authors have reported significant long-term improvement of clinical symptoms, and the possibility of recovery of the tendon matrix (Ferrero et al 2012; Gosens et al 2012; Pascual-Garrido et al 2012; Vetrano et al 2013).

Prognosis for full recovery without symptom recurrence utilizing conservative treatment alone is poor. The natural history of patellar tendinopathy is that of chronic pain and reduced function, which often severely limits or even ends an athletic career. Significant pain and limitation will continue beyond 6 months after onset of pain in up to one-third of patients, while the majority of patients will have some level of symptoms for many years (Saithna et al 2012). Patients who continue to experience disabling symptoms after 6 months may elect surgery. Prognosis for full recovery without symptom recurrence after surgery is unknown, based on the variety of surgical methods available and postoperative protocols followed (Khan et al 1998; Cucurulo et al 2009; Maier et al 2013).

Popliteal Tendinopathy

Background

Popliteal tendinopathy is an uncommon cause of anterior–lateral knee pain and has been presented in the medical literature as rare cases of acute calcific tendonitis (Tibrewal 2002) and as popliteal tenosynovitis (Blake & Treble 2005). Rupture of the tendon is more common than tendinopathy.

Anatomy

The popliteus muscle originates from the lateral femoral condyle, the proximal fibula and the posterior horn of the lateral meniscus, although variations have been reported in the lateral meniscus point of origin. The femoral origin is considered to be the strongest point of origin. The popliteus muscle itself inserts into the posterior surface of the proximal tibia superior to the soleal line. The popliteus tendon lies deep to the lateral collateral ligament and passes through a hiatus in the coronary ligament to attach to the lateral femoral condyle (Nielsen & Helmig 1986; Blake & Treble 2005).

Pathology and patho-biomechanics

In the case of acute calcific tendonitis, the acutely painful phase is believed to occur as the organic matrix binding the calcific deposit disintegrates and stimulates an inflammatory response and phagocytosis (Tibrewal 2002). The mechanism of the origin and resolution of the calcium deposit may include response to tissue insult and healing by calcification, local stress necrosis and local hypoxia secondary either to mechanical factors or hypovascularity (Tibrewal 2002). It has been suggested that dystrophic calcification of degenerative tendon matrix is a different pathological entity from cell-mediated calcifying tendinitis (Tibrewal 2002). The exact pathogenesis remains uncertain, however: in tenosynovitis it is thought to involve inflammation within the tendon sheath (Vuillemin et al 2012), but in a reported case of popliteal tenosynovitis (Blake & Treble 2005) the pathogenesis was not described.

Although the primary function of the popliteus is to rotate the tibia medially on the femur, the popliteal tendon also effectively restrains varus instability from 0° to 90° of flexion (Nielsen & Helmig 1986; Blake & Treble 2005). It has also been stated that marked posterior–lateral instability is impossible with an intact popliteal tendon (Nielsen & Helmig 1986).

Diagnosis

In the case of acute calcific tendonitis, history and clinical examination may reveal an acute onset of pain, localized swelling with redness, and tenderness to palpation over the lateral side of the knee at the insertion of the popliteus tendon (Tibrewal 2002). A history of injury or predisposing factors may not be present. There will be difficulty or inability to bear weight on the affected leg. The knee cannot be fully extended owing to pain and possibly swelling or muscle spasm. There may be a palpable tender nodule at the site of the popliteus tendon (Tibrewal 2002). Calcific changes in the popliteal tendon may be noted on the plain radiograph and MRI (Tibrewal 2002).

In the case of popliteal tenosynovitis, there will be similar palpable tenderness and difficulty extending the knee. Arthroscopy has been utilized for both diagnosis and treatment (Blake & Treble 2005).

Conservative treatment and prognosis

Successful treatment of calcific tendonitis has been achieved by injection of 4 ml of 0.5% Marcaine and Depo-Medrone (20 mg) at the painful site, followed by anti-inflammatory medication (diclofenac 50 mg tds) for 2 weeks and physical therapy, as well as use of soft knee splints (Tibrewal 2002). Prognosis based on the little evidence available is good with conservative treatment as described (Tibrewal 2002).

Reported treatment for popliteal tenosynovitis other than arthroscopy is unknown; however, unreported cases may have been treated with a standard protocol for tenosynovitis consisting of corticosteroid injection and rest (Peters-Veluthamaningal et al 2009).

Quadriceps Tendinopathy

Background

Quadriceps tendinopathy is similar to that of the patellar tendon, which is mucoid degeneration in response to repetitive overload (Arumilli et al 2009). However, a significant difference is that, whereas patellar tendinopathy causes significant pain, quadriceps tendinopathy is often clinically silent until complete rupture occurs. Hence the first manifestation of quadriceps tendinopathy may be a rupture, although it may also coexist with symptomatic paratendinopathy (Arumilli et al 2009). Even the rupture itself is often misdiagnosed or diagnosed late owing to being mistaken for other pathologies such as stroke, rheumatoid arthritis, disc prolapse and neuropathy (Arumilli et al 2009). This is especially true in cases of bilateral spontaneous rupture.

Anatomy

It is commonly accepted that the four muscular elements of the quadriceps gather distally to create the quadriceps tendon in three layers that conjoin approximately 2 cm proximal to the patella. Some researchers, however, support the idea that the three layers of the quadriceps tendon remain distinct until their insertion into the patella (Waligora et al 2009). In addition, MRI has shown that the tendon has more lamination in its midline and medially than it does laterally. The quadriceps tendon is layered with a superficial contribution from the rectus femoris, intermediate additions from the vastus medialis and vastus lateralis, and deeply from the vastus intermedius. An additional deviation from the standard description of the quadriceps tendon is that apparently not all contain three fibre planes (Waligora et al 2009). Based on MRI study, it is possible that a significant proportion of quadriceps tendons contain only two fibre planes, with a smaller number of tendons classified as one layer or four layers (Waligora et al 2009). This may help to understand why there are cases reported of healthy active individuals, younger than the standard for this injury, who sustain seemingly spontaneous quadriceps tendon ruptures.

Pathology and patho-biomechanics

It is believed that, under normal conditions, the quadriceps tendon is resistant to tensile strain forces, and spontaneous ruptures occur only in abnormal tendons with evidence of hypovascular changes including narrowing and obliteration of small arteries, hypertrophy of the intima and media walls (Arumilli et al 2009; Maffulli et al 2012). Trobisch et al (2010) performed a histological analysis of ruptured quadriceps tendons and observed an increasing ratio of degenerative to non-degenerative tendons with increasing patient age. Maffulli et al (2012), however, reported a higher incidence of degenerative tendon changes in the ruptured quadriceps tendons of younger age patients, which disputes the notion that older patients are more prone to hypovascular quadriceps tendinopathy leading to rupture.

The common mechanisms of injury include forced contraction of the quadriceps with the knee flexed and the foot fixed to the ground; functionally speaking, this results from a stumble, a simple fall, or falling down the stairs or from a height (Arumilli et al 2009; Maffulli et al 2012). Quadriceps ruptures tend to occur commonly when the knee is flexed more than 60° owing to high forces transmitted through the extensor mechanism with an eccentric contraction of the quadriceps against the weight of the body (Maffulli et al 2012).

Pathogenesis is considered multifactorial, however, as a significant number of ruptures occur with no evidence of hypovascular tendinopathy, and many are associated with disorders such as renal insufficiency, primary or secondary hyperparathyroidism and other conditions that impair and weaken the osteotendinous junction (Arumilli et al 2009, Maffulli et al 2012). Obesity, repeated corticosteroid injections, and use of anabolic steroids or statins may also be predisposing factors (Maffulli et al 2012).

Diagnosis

Missed diagnosis and misdiagnosis are common both for quadriceps tendinopathy and for quadriceps tendon rupture (Arumilli et al 2009; Maffulli et al 2012; Volk et al 2014). Physical examination will reveal suprapatellar pain on palpation. In the case of a rupture, a suprapatellar gap may be palpated. There may be difficulty in achieving full knee extension against gravity. With a rupture there will be an inability to maintain full active extension. Gait abnormalities include stiff knee gait or exaggerated hip elevation for swing through circumduction when the quadriceps tendon is ruptured (Arumilli et al 2009; Volk et al 2014). In silent tendinopathies, there may be no clinical signs or symptoms. Radiographs reveal abnormal patella height (patella *baja*) in the case of quadriceps tendon rupture; MRI and ultrasound are useful for viewing degenerative changes in the unruptured tendon as well as for visualizing the ruptured tendon (Volk et al 2014).

In some cases the retinaculum is intact but the quadriceps tendon is ruptured. The patient is able to perform weak straight leg raise with the aid of the intact retinaculum; however, the quadriceps tendon is completely torn. Careful physical examination is recommended, including checking the extensor lag and, if necessary, aspirating blood from the knee and injecting with lidocaine before re-examining it (Volk et al 2014).

Conservative treatment and prognosis

Conservative treatment for quadriceps tendinopathy is not established in the literature as different to that for patellar tendinopathy. This may be due to the infrequent diagnosis and more common presentation as a rupture rather than a tendinopathy with an intact tendon. Rupture of the quadriceps is a surgical indication, and the best outcomes occur when surgery is performed quickly, followed by immobilization per protocol and intensive rehabilitation (Arumilli et al 2009; Grim et al 2010; Maffulli et al 2012; Saragaglia et al 2013; Boudissa et al 2014; Volk et al 2014).

Prognosis for full recovery from quadriceps tendinopathy is unknown; in fact, the evidence points to eventual rupture in most cases (Arumilli et al 2009; Maffulli et al 2012). Prognosis for functionally good recovery from a surgically repaired ruptured quadriceps tendon is considered good if the diagnosis and surgery are not delayed (Grim et al 2010; Saragaglia et al 2013; Boudissa et al 2014).

Conclusion

Clinicians and researchers continue to question previous assumptions regarding the cause, pathology, diagnosis and treatment of tendinopathies in the knee. The trend has moved away from viewing tendinopathy as an acute condition in which inflammation is the only pathological factor. Our current understanding of tendinopathy pathology is that of mucoid degeneration associated with hypovascularity and overuse with failed healing. Specific conservative treatments attempt to address replacement of the degeneration in the tendon with healthy collagen, often utilizing eccentric exercises to engender this transformation. At the same time, novel treatments, including injection of the tendon with platelet-rich plasma or with autologous bone marrow stem cells, attempt to address causative factors such as hypovascularity, while other proposed treatments such as extracorporeal shockwave treatment have not as yet proven themselves clinically. A conclusion across the span of knee tendinopathies is that early diagnosis and prompt, thorough, evidence-based treatments will provide the best possibility of a good prognosis for recovery.

References

Ackermann PW, Renström P. 2012. Tendinopathy in sport. Sports Health 4: 193–201.

Arumilli B, Adeyemo F, Samarji R. 2009. Bilateral simultaneous complete quadriceps rupture following chronic symptomatic tendinopathy: a case report. J Med Case Reports 3: 9031.

Bae DK, Kwon OS. 1997. Snapping knee caused by the gracilis and semitendinosus tendon: a case report. Bull Hosp Jt Dis 56:177–179.

Bahr R, Fossan B, Loken S, et al. 2006. Surgical treatment compared with eccentric training for patellar tendinopathy (jumper's knee): a randomized, controlled trial. J Bone Joint Surg Am 88: 1689–1698.

Beers A, Ryan M, Kasubuchi Z, et al. 2008. Effects of multi-modal physiotherapy, including hip abductor strengthening, in patients with iliotibial band friction syndrome. Physiother Can 60: 180–188.

Bernhardson AS, LaPrade RF. 2010. Snapping biceps femoris tendon treated with an anatomic repair. Knee Surg Sports Traumatol Arthrosc 18: 1110–1112.

Birnbaum K, Siebert CH, Pandorf T, et al. 2004. Anatomical and biomechanical investigations of the iliotibial tract. Surg Radiol Anat 26: 433–446.

Blake SM, Treble NJ. 2005. Popliteus tendon tenosynovitis. Br J Sports Med 39: e42.

Boudissa M, Roudet A, Rubens-Duval B, et al. 2014. Acute quadriceps tendon ruptures: a series of 50 knees with an average follow-up of more than 6 years. Orthop Traumatol Surg Res 100: 213–216.

Busseuil C, Freychat P, Guedj EB, et al. 1998. Rearfoot–forefoot orientation and traumatic risk for runners. Foot Ankle Int 19: 32–37.

Bylund WE, de Weber K. 2010. Semimembranosus tendinopathy: one cause of chronic posteromedial knee pain. Sports Health 2: 380–384.

Cannell LJ, Taunton JE, Clement DB, et al. 2001. A randomized clinical trial of the efficacy of drop squats or leg extension / leg curl exercises to treat clinically diagnosed jumper's knee in athletes: pilot study. Br J Sports Med 35: 60–64.

Cook JL, Khan KM, Kiss ZS, et al. 2001. Reproducibility and clinical utility of tendon palpation to detect patellar tendinopathy in young basketball players. Br J Sports Med 35: 65–69.

Cucurulo T, Louis ML, Thaunat M, et al. 2009. Surgical treatment of patellar tendinopathy in athletes: a retrospective multicentric study. Orthop Traumatol Surg Res 95: S78–S84.

Date H, Hayakawa K, Nakagawa K, et al. 2012. Snapping knee due to the biceps femoris tendon treated with repositioning of the anomalous tibial insertion. Knee Surg Sports Traumatol Arthrosc 20: 1581–1583.

Devan MR, Pescatello LS, Faghri P, et al. 2004. A prospective study of overuse knee injuries among female athletes with muscle imbalances and structural abnormalities. J Athl Train 39: 263–267.

Ellis R, Hing W, Reid D. 2007. Iliotibial band friction syndrome – a systematic review. Man Ther 12: 200–208.

Fairclough J, Hayashi K, Toumi H, et al. 2006. The functional anatomy of the iliotibial band during flexion and extension of the knee: implications for understanding iliotibial band syndrome. J Anat 208: 309–316.

Fairclough J, Hayashi K, Toumi H, et al. 2007. Is iliotibial band syndrome really a friction syndrome? J Sci Med Sport 10: 74–76.

Ferrero G, Fabbro E, Orlandi D, et al. 2012. Ultrasound-guided injection of platelet-rich plasma in chronic Achilles and patellar tendinopathy. J Ultrasound 15: 260–266.

Fredericson M, Weir A. 2006. Practical management of iliotibial band friction syndrome in runners. Clin J Sport Med 16: 261–268.

Fredericson M, Wolf C. 2005. Iliotibial band syndrome in runners: innovations in treatment. Sports Med 35: 451–459.

Fredericson M, Cookingham CL, Chaudhari AM, et al. 2000. Hip abductor weakness in distance runners with iliotibial band syndrome. Clin J Sport Med 10: 169–175.

Frohm A, Saartok T, Edman G, et al. 2004. Psychometric properties of a Swedish translation of the VISA-P outcome score for patellar tendinopathy. BMC Musculoskelet Disord 5: 49.

Frohm A, Saartok T, Halvorsen K, et al. 2007. Eccentric treatment for patellar tendinopathy: a prospective randomised short-term pilot study of two rehabilitation protocols. Br J Sports Med 41: e7.

Gammaitoni AR, Goitz HT, Marsh S, et al. 2013. Heated lidocaine / tetracaine patch for treatment of patellar tendinopathy pain. J Pain Res 6: 565–570.

Gose JC, Schweizer P. 1989. Iliotibial band tightness. J Orthop Sports Phys Ther 10: 399–407.

Gosens T, Den Oudsten BL, Fievez E, et al. 2012. Pain and activity levels before and after platelet-rich plasma injection treatment of patellar tendinopathy: a prospective cohort study and the influence of previous treatments. Int Orthop 36: 1941–1946.

Grau S, Krauss I, Malwald C, et al. 2008. Hip abductor weakness is not the cause for iliotibial band syndrome. Int J Sports Med 29: 579–583.

Grim C, Lorbach O, Engelhardt M. 2010. Quadriceps and patellar tendon ruptures. Orthopade 39: 1127–1134.

Gunter P, Schwellnus M, Fuller P. 2004. Local corticosteroid injection in iliotibial band friction syndrome in runners: a randomised controlled trial. Br J Sports Med 38: 269–272.

Halperin N, Oren Y, Hendel D, et al. 1987. Semimembranosus tenosynovitis: operative results. Arch Orthop Traum Surg 106: 281–284.

Hamill J, Miller R, Noehren B, et al. 2008. A prospective study of iliotibial band strain in runners. Clin Biomech 23: 1018–1025.

Hong JH, Kim JS. 2013. Diagnosis of iliotibial band friction syndrome and ultrasound guided steroid injection. Korean J Pain 26: 387–391.

Karataglis D, Papadopoulos P, Fotiadou A, et al. 2008. Snapping knee syndrome in an athlete caused by the semitendinosus and gracilis tendons: a case report. Knee 15: 151–154.

Khan KM, Maffulli N, Coleman BD, et al. 1998. Patellar tendinopathy: some aspects of basic science and clinical management. Br J Sports Med 32: 346–355.

Kirk KL, Kuklo T, Klemme W. 2000. Iliotibial band friction syndrome. Orthopedics 23: 1209–1214

Kisner C, Colby LA. 2010. Therapeutic exercise foundations and techniques, 5th edn. Philadelphia, PA: FA Davis.

Kulig K, Landel R, Chang YJ, et al. 2013. Patellar tendon morphology in volleyball athletes with and without patellar tendinopathy. Scand J Med Sci Sports 23: e81–e88.

Lavagnino M, Arnoczky SP, Dodds J, et al. 2011. Infrapatellar straps decrease patellar tendon strain at the site of the jumper's knee lesion: a computational analysis based on radiographic measurements. Sports Health 3: 296–302.

Lavine R. 2010. Iliotibial band friction syndrome. Curr Rev Musculoskelet Med 3: 18–22.

Lohrer H, Nauck T. 2011. Cross-cultural adaptation and validation of the VISA-P questionnaire for German-speaking patient with patellar tendinopathy. J Orth Sport Phys Ther 41: 180–190.

Lokiec F, Velkes S, Schindler A, et al. 1992. The snapping biceps femoris syndrome. Clin Orthop Relat Res 283: 205–206.

Longo UG, Garau G, Denaro V, et al. 2008. Surgical management of tendinopathy of biceps femoris tendon in athletes. Disabil Rehabil 30: 1602–1607.

Lyu SR, Wu JJ. 1989. Snapping syndrome caused by the semitendinosus tendon: a case report. J Bone Joint Surg Am 71: 303–305.

MacMahon JM, Chaudhari AM, Andriacchi TP. 2000. Biomechanical injury predictors for marathon runners: striding towards iliotibial band syndrome injury prevention. Conference of the International Society of Biomechanics in Sports, Hong Kong, June.

Maffulli N, Longo UG, Testa V, et al. 2008. VISA-P score for patellar tendinopathy in males: adaptation to Italian. Disabil Rehabil 30: 1621–1624.

Maffulli N, Del Buono A, Spiezia F, et al. 2012. Light microscopic histology of quadriceps tendon ruptures. Int Orthop 36: 2367–2371.

Magee DJ. 2008. Orthopedic physical assessment. London: Elsevier Health Sciences.

Maier D, Bornebusch L, Salzmann GM, et al. 2013. Mid- and long-term efficacy of the arthroscopic patellar release for treatment of patellar tendinopathy unresponsive to nonoperative management. Arthroscopy 29: 1338–1345.

Meardon SA, Campbell S, Derrick TR. 2012. Step width alters iliotibial band strain during running. Sports Biomech 11: 464–472.

Miller R, Lowry J, Meardon S, et al. 2007. Lower extremity mechanics of iliotibial band syndrome during an exhaustive run. Gait Posture 26: 407–413.

Nielsen S, Helmig P. 1986. The static stabilizing function of the popliteal tendon in the knee. Arch Orthop Trauma Surg 104: 357–362.

Noble CA. 1979. The treatment of iliotibial band friction syndrome. Br J Sports Med 13: 51–54.

Noehren B, Davis I, Hamill J. 2007. Prospective study of the biomechanical factors associated with iliotibial band syndrome. Clin Biomech 22: 951–956.

Orchard J, Fricker P, Abud A, et al. 1996. Biomechanics of iliotibial band friction syndrome in runners. Am J Sports Med 24: 375–379.

Panni AS, Tartarone M, Maffulli N. 2000. Patellar tendinopathy in athletes: outcome of nonoperative and operative management. Am J Sports Med 28: 392–397.

Pascual-Garrido C, Rolón A, Makino A. 2012. Treatment of chronic patellar tendinopathy with autologous bone marrow stem cells: a 5-year-followup. Stem Cells Int 2012: 953510. doi: 10.1155/2012/953510.

Peters-Veluthamaningal C, van der Windt DA, Winters JC, et al. 2009. Corticosteroid injection for de Quervain's tenosynovitis. Cochrane Database Syst Rev 3: CD005616.

Purdam CR, Jonsson P, Alfredson H, et al. 2004. A pilot study of the eccentric decline squat in the management of painful chronic patellar tendinopathy. Br J Sports Med 38: 395–397.

Ramos LA, de Carvalho RT, Garms E, et al. 2009. Prevalence of pain on palpation of the inferior pole of the patella among patients with complaints of knee pain. Clinics 64: 199–202.

Ray JM, Clancy WG Jr, Lemon RA. 1988. Semimembranosus tendinitis: an overlooked cause of medial knee pain. Am J Sports Med 16: 347–351.

Rodriguez-Merchan EC. 2013. The treatment of patellar tendinopathy. J Orthopaed Traumatol 14: 77–81.

Rutland M, O'Connell D, Brismée JM, et al. 2010. Evidence-supported rehabilitation of patellar tendinopathy. North Am J Sports Phys Ther 5: 166–178.

Safran MR, Fu FH. 1995. Uncommon causes of knee pain in the athlete. Orthop Clin North Am 26: 547–559.

Saithna A, Gogna R, Baraza N, et al. 2012. Eccentric exercise protocols for patella tendinopathy: should we really be withdrawing athletes from sport? A systematic review. Open Orthop J 6: S553–S557. doi: 10.2174/1874325001206010553.

Saragaglia D, Pison A, Rubens-Duval B. 2013. Acute and old ruptures of the extensor apparatus of the knee in adults (excluding knee replacement). Orthop Traumatol Surg Res 99: S67–S76.

Sarwark JF (ed). 2010. Essentials of musculoskeletal care, 4th edn. Rosemont, IL: American Academy of Orthopedic Surgeons.

Sher I, Umans H, Downie SA, et al. 2011. Proximal iliotibial band syndrome: what is it and where is it? Skeletal Radiol 40: 1553–1556.

Stasinopoulos D, Stasinopoulos I. 2004. Comparison of effects of exercise programme, pulsed ultrasound and transverse friction in the treatment of chronic patellar tendinopathy. Clin Rehabil 18: 347–352.

Strauss EJ, Kim S, Calcei JG, et al. 2011. Iliotibial band syndrome: evaluation and management. J Am Acad Orthop Surg 19: 728–736.

Tibrewal SB. 2002. Acute calcific tendinitis of the popliteus tendon: an unusual site and clinical syndrome. Ann R Coll Surg Engl 84: 338–341.

Toumi H, Higashiyama I, Suzuki D, et al. 2006. Regional variations in human patellar trabecular architecture and the structure of the proximal patellar tendon enthesis. J Anat 208: 47–57.

Trobisch PD, Bauman M, Weise K, et al. 2010. Histologic analysis of ruptured quadriceps tendons. Knee Surg Sports Traumatol Arthrosc 18: 85–88.

van der Worp MP, van der Horst N, de Wijer A, et al. 2012. Iliotibial band syndrome in runners: a systematic review. Sports Med 42: 969–992.

van der Worp H, van den Akker-Scheek I, van Schie H, et al. 2013. ESWT for tendinopathy: technology and clinical implications. Knee Surg Sports Traumatol Arthrosc 21: 1451–1458.

Vetrano M, Castorina A, Vulpiani MC, et al. 2013. Platelet-rich plasma versus focused shock waves in the treatment of jumper's knee in athletes. Am J Sports Med 41: 795–803.

Vieira El, Vieira EA, da Silva RT, et al. 2007. An anatomic study of the iliotibial tract. Arthroscopy 23: 269–274.

Visentini PJ, Khan KM, Cook JL, et al. 1998. The VISA score: an index of severity of symptoms in patients with jumper's knee (patellar tendinosis). J Sci Med Sport 1: 22–28.

Visnes H, Hoksrud A, Cook J, et al. 2005. No effect of eccentric training on jumper's knee in volleyball players during the competitive season: a randomized clinical trial. Clin J Sport Med 15: 227–234.

Voight ML, Hoogenboom BJ, Prentice WE. 2007. Musculoskeletal interventions. Techniques for therapeutic exercises. New York, NY: McGraw-Hill.

Volk WR, Yagnik GP, Uribe JW. 2014. Complications in brief: quadriceps and patellar tendon tears. Clin Orthop Relat Res 472: 1050–1057.

Vuillemin V, Guerini H, Bard H, et al. 2012. Stenosing tenosynovitis. J Ultrasound 15: 20–28.

Waligora AC, Johanson NA, Hirsch BE. 2009. Clinical anatomy of the quadriceps femoris and extensor apparatus of the knee. Clin Orthop Relat Res 467: 3297–3306.

Wang TG, Jan MH, Lin KH, et al. 2006. Assessment of stretching of the iliotibial tract with Ober and modified Ober tests: an ultrasonographic study. Arch Phys Med Rehabil 87: 1407–1411.

Young MA, Cook JL, Purdam CR, et al. 2005. Eccentric decline squat protocol offers superior results at 12 months compared with traditional eccentric protocol for patellar tendinopathy in volleyball players. Br J Sports Med 39: 102–105.

Zwerver J, Kramer T, van den Akker-Scheek I. 2009. Validity and reliability of the Dutch translation of the VISA-P questionnaire for patellar tendinopathy. BMC Musculoskelet Disord 10: 102.

Zwerver J, Bredeweg SW, van den Akker-Scheek I. 2011. Prevalence of jumper's knee among nonelite athletes from different sports: a cross-sectional survey. Am J Sports Med 39: 1984–1988.

PART 8

The Wrist and Hand Regions in Upper Extremity Pain Syndromes

48 Tendinopathies of the Wrist and Hand 545
C. Joseph Yelvington and Ellen Pong

49 Carpal Instability 558
Ellen Pong

50 Carpal Tunnel Syndrome 566
Luca Padua, Daniele Coraci and César Fernández-de-las-Peñas

51 Other Entrapment Neuropathies 575
Joy C. MacDermid and David M. Walton

52 Joint Mobilization and Manipulation 584
Peter A. Huijbregts, Freddy M. Kaltenborn and Traudi Baldauf Kaltenborn

53 Finger and Thumb Pathology 594
Joy C. MacDermid, Ruby Grewal and B. Jane Freure

Chapter 48

Tendinopathies of the Wrist and Hand

C. Joseph Yelvington, Ellen Pong

CHAPTER CONTENTS

Introduction	545
Definition of tendinopathy	545
Aetiology	546
Anatomy of the tendon	546
Basic components	546
Blood and nerve supply	546
Pathoanatomy	547
Tendinopathy classification	548
Tendinosis	548
Tendinitis	548
Paratenonitis	548
Combined paratenonitis and tendinosis	548
Examination and diagnosis	549
Clinical tests	549
Diagnostic imaging and invasive testing	549
Tendinopathic entities of the hand and wrist	550
Flexor carpi ulnaris	550
Extensor carpi ulnaris	550
Extensor carpi radialis longus and brevis (distal tendons)	551
Extensor indicis proprius	551
Extensor digiti minimi	551
Abductor pollicis longus and extensor pollicis brevis	552
Extensor pollicis longus	552
Flexor carpi radialis	553
Treatment and prognosis	553
Conservative treatment	553
Non-conservative treatment	554
Prognosis	555
Conclusion	555

Introduction

A large proportion of hand and wrist tendinopathies occur in individuals who perform highly repetitive and forceful jobs (Elder & Harvey 2005). The Department of Labor, Bureau of Labor Statistics (1999) reported incidence of hand and wrist tendinitis (tendinopathy not specified) as 3.66% of upper extremity workplace injuries recorded in 1999, resulting in a mean of 6 lost work days for all hand / wrist injuries.

Patients and practitioners had discovered that, once tendinopathy is established, resolving symptoms could be difficult. Treatment typically consists of resting in a splint, modifying activities for ergonomic correction, taking non-steroidal anti-inflammatory medications (NSAIDs), and receiving corticosteroid injections, often with positive results (Fredberg & Stengaard-Pedersen 2008). Deep tissue friction massage (DTFM), effleurage, connective tissue release and Rolfing have been utilized on tendons, with the premise that they will release scar tissue restrictions and allow improved collagen alignment. However, studies do not reliably confirm the positive benefit of these conservative treatments (Brousseau et al 2002). This demonstrates a typical problem: randomized clinical trials of manual therapy to the tendons of the hand and wrist are scarcely, if at all, available.

Investigators have continued to look more closely at tendons, discovering processes that may explain why outcomes are not more positive. Adequate animal models for in vivo studies have only recently been developed (Soslowsky et al 2000). Tendinopathy has been classified and redefined. Current studies attempt to explain why repetitive motion and strain cause tendon pathologies (Backman et al 2005). This developing knowledge of tendon pathology has shed new light on treatment rationale (Khan et al 2000).

This chapter follows the trend of current studies and expanding knowledge, including a review of the tendinopathy process from a molecular level. This review provides a knowledge base for the ensuing discussion of examination, diagnosis, categorization of tendinopathy and treatment.

Definition of Tendinopathy

The lack of more positive results with conservative treatment may be due to mislabelling tendinosis as tendinitis (Khan et al 2000). Tendinitis must be qualified. Studies are now consistently showing what was normally diagnosed as **tendonitis** may represent only one classification of **tendinopathy** (Futami & Itoman 1995). Tendinopathy represents histological findings that differ significantly from the generally accepted condition of tendonitis. This is due primarily to the lack of evidence of inflammatory precursors and cells in the tendon itself (Gabel et al 1994; Yuan et al 2003; Curwin 2005; Fredberg & Stengaard-Pedersen 2008). Khan et al (2006) supported Bonar's classification of tendinopathy, which defined four classifications, each with distinct histological findings. Clinicians have yet to apply this knowledge to support specific conservative treatment use (Cannon 2001). A fourth edition manual of upper extremity rehabilitation printed in 2001 did not use the words tendinosis or tendinopathy, but instead used the terms **tendinitis** and **paratendinitis** for all related conditions of upper extremity pain caused by tendon pathology (Cannon 2001).

One reason for the continued consideration of tendon pathologies as tendonitis may be the initially positive outcomes with corticosteroids in symptomatic tendons (Fredberg & Stengaard-Pedersen 2008). The presence of an '-itis' or inflammation in the form of neurogenic inflammation may also support persistence of the old terminology. Fredberg and Stengaard-Pedersen (2008) concluded that some combination of classic inflammation and neurogenic inflammation does mean that tendonitis is not a complete misnomer. It is the histological difference in tendinopathies stemming from tendinitis, tendinosis and paratenonitis that may dictate different treatments, particularly in manual therapy.

There continue to be areas of needed research into this subject. Findings from animal studies and from tendon studies performed on other areas of the body will be used in this chapter to provide data that may be extrapolated to apply to the hand and wrist, despite differences between weight-bearing versus positional tendons (Smith et al 1997).

Aetiology

Researchers report that knowledge of the aetiology of tendinopathy is evolving (Sharma & Maffulli 2005; Fredberg & Stengaard-Pedersen 2008). Many factors contribute to tendinopathy, both intrinsic and extrinsic (Riley 2004). Renstrom and Hach (2005) summarized extrinsic factors as: malalignments, reduced flexibility, muscle weakness or imbalance, overuse and excessive body weight. Hart et al (2005) added genetics, gender and fitness level, while Hammer (2007a) reported biomechanical faults. Intrinsic factors that affect apoptosis can lead to tendon degeneration. This process of programmed cell death can be exacerbated by intrinsic oxidative or mechanical stresses (Yuan et al 2003; Sharma & Maffulli 2005). Theories on tendon rupture have been separated into two categories: vascular and mechanical (Riley 2004). The reader is encouraged to read the work of Riley (2004) to explore this topic further.

Anatomy of the Tendon

Basic components

The tendon is the attachment site of a muscle to bone. It is designed to transfer tension from the muscle to the bone, thereby causing motion to take place (Kannus 2000).

The basic building block of the tendon, **tropocollagen**, is formed by fibroblasts (O'Brien 2005). These are assembled into **fibrils**, which are arranged into **fibres**, which are organized into **fascicles** and bound together with a loose connective tissue called **endotendon** (endotenon) (Kannus 2000; Sharma & Maffulli 2005). The endotendon is the pathway for blood vessels, nerves and lymphatics (Riley 2004). Bundles of fascicles are bound together by another layer of connective tissue called the **epitendon** (epitenon), which is continuous with the endotendon (Kannus 2000) (Fig. 48.1).

Synovial tendon sheaths, also called **paratendon** (paratenon), are found in areas subjected to increased mechanical stress, such as the tendons of the hands and feet, where efficient lubrication is required (Sharma & Maffulli 2005). Fibre bundles are predominantly aligned with the long axis of the tendon and these are responsible for the tensile strength of the tendon (Riley 2004). A small proportion of fibres run transversely, and there are even spirals and plait-like formations (Kannus 2000). This complex ultrastructure provides resistance against transverse, shear and rotational forces acting on the tendon (Riley 2004).

Blood and nerve supply

Tendon vascular support comes from three sources: at the myotendinous junction, the osteotendinous junction, and the extrinsic system through the paratendon (Benjamin & Ralphs 1996; Sharma & Maffulli 2005; Scott et al 2007). Innervation accompanies vascular pathways through the paratenon (Hart

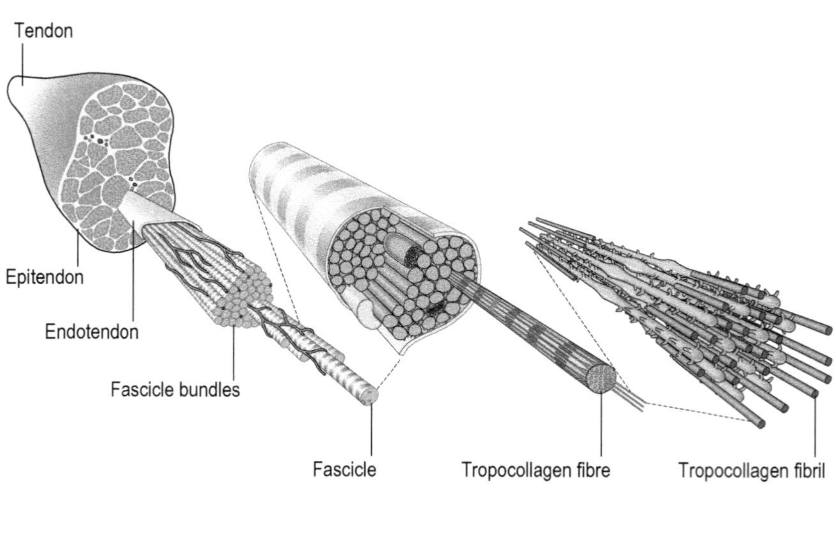

Figure 48.1 Basic tendon structure.

et al 2005). The nerve receptors that supply tendons can terminate in the vicinity of mast cells, where neuropeptides are involved in normal tendon regulatory control (Hart et al 2005).

Pathoanatomy

Tenocytes and **tenoblasts** are the cells involved in tendon healing (Sharma & Maffulli 2005, 2006). Tenocytes are sparse in tendon tissue but have extensions that create an extensive network inside the matrix (O'Brien 2005). They are responsible for maintenance of matrix and collagen (Harley & Bergman 2008). Tenocytes are crucially responsive to environmental conditions. Mechanical demands placed on tendon tissue will promote changes in the microarchitecture of the tissue (Magra et al 2007). Strain applied to a tendon can change its structure; these changes can be damaging, or they can be reparative if appropriately and purposefully applied in treatment.

Scott's research (Scott et al 2007) provided evidence that it is stimulation of the tenocytes rather than intrinsic inflammation that is associated with tendinosis. Alterations in cell activity lead to tendon changes from mechanical stress, rather than the converse (Riley 2004). The local stimulation of tenocytes, which is a load-driven cellular response, rather than inflammation or apoptosis, is the true mechanism in tendinosis (Scott et al 2007). Apoptosis plays a role later in the tendinopathic process (Scott et al 2007). Localized hypoxia from vigorous exercise can lead to tenocyte death (Sharma & Maffulli 2005) and tendinopathic changes.

Tenocyte metabolism is regulated partly by mechanical stimulation (Maeda et al 2009). Maeda et al (2009) showed that cyclic strain will change gene expression in tendon cells. Force applied to a tendon changes cellular process via mechanotransduction, the process in which a cell converts biomechanical stimuli into chemical signals (Maffulli & Longo 2008). Mechanotransduction utilizes gap junctions, stretch-activated channels (Wall & Banes 2005), voltage-operated calcium channels (VOCC) and tandem pore domain potassium channels (TPDPC) to communicate with adjoining tenocytes (Wall & Banes 2005; Magra et al 2007). Tension on surface proteins, called **integrins**, embedded in the cell membrane is transmitted to the cell's cytoskeleton. This force is transmitted via the intracellular network to the nucleus of the cell and can alter protein expression (Chiquet 1999). Huang et al (2004) observed that mechanical loading is essential for homeostasis of the bone, cartilage and skin. Additionally, external forces are capable of producing changes in intracellular reactions. Tenocytes are responsible for changing structure in response to demand by altering, 'gene expression patterns, protein synthesis and cell phenotype' (Maffulli & Longo 2008). This alteration is suspected of being the link to overuse and tendinopathic changes (Scott et al 2007). Importantly from a manual therapy perspective, Maffulli and Longo (2008) supported that an alteration of mechanical forces may augment the healing process. Conversely, understimulation can cause tendinopathic changes (Arnoczky et al 2006).

The tendon matrix is responsible for maintenance of the tendon. Its damage, according to Riley (2004), is the leading event in tendinopathy. The ground substance of the extracellular matrix network surrounding the collagen and the tenocytes contains proteoglycans, glycosaminoglycans, glycoproteins, as well as several other small molecules (O'Brien 2005). Water makes up 60–80% of the ground substance (O'Brien 2005). Proteoglycans are strongly hydrophilic, enabling rapid diffusion of water-soluble molecules and the migration of cells (Sharma & Maffulli 2005). They, along with glycoproteins, have a role in organization of collagen into fibrils and fibres (O'Brien 2005). When repetitive damage becomes extensive it overwhelms the ability to heal (Riley 2004). Arnoczky et al (2007) credited extracellular matrix degeneration as a precursor of tendon weakness. Riley (2004) described the possibility that changes in cellular activity in the matrix due to mechanical strain can influence the structural properties of tendons.

Tendon injury

Riley summarized overuse tendinopathy as the phenomenon caused by repeated strains below the failure threshold that outstrips the cell's ability to heal (Riley 2004). Tissue injury from repetitive strain is thought to be a cellular event (Arnoczky et al 2006). Recent studies in animal modelling have produced results of tendinopathy that correspond to those found in non-experimental tendinopathies in humans. Soslowky's model of repetitive motion identified tendinopathic changes in supraspinatus tendons in rats (Soslowsky et al 2000). These changes mimic those found in idiopathic tendinopathies in humans, including reduced mechanical properties (Lavagnino et al 2006; Arnoczky et al 2007). Glazebrook et al (2007) found similar changes in rats after overuse induced by repetitive running. Backman et al (2005) produced similar results with rabbits.

Post-injury disuse of a tendon, through immobilization or compensation, can also have detrimental effects. The concept of stress shielding can be applied to tendons. An example of this in terms of bone is the application of Wolff's law with reduced bone density following fracture immobilization. Woo et al (1981) observed that, after fracture healing, reapplied weight-bearing will increase bone density. Kannus and Jozsa (1991) showed that understimulation of tendon cells post-injury produced degenerative findings in the investigation of tendinopathy. De Boer et al (2007) supported this with his demonstration of tendon protein synthesis rates decreasing progressively through 10 days of immobilization. Lavagnino et al (2006) induced mechanical injury in rat-tail tendons, followed by immobilization, which revealed an up-regulation of collagenase mRNA and protein synthesis in this damaged area. Even undamaged fascicles showed similar up-regulation during the immobilization portion of this study. In an earlier study the same researchers found that these adverse effects could be controlled in vitro with cyclic stretching (Lavagnino et al 2003). Screen et al (2005) reported similar results with cyclic stretching in non-injured tendon fascicles. With regard to the treatment of tendinopathy, attempting to immobilize a tendinosis via splinting or casting thus appears to be detrimental.

Tendon healing

The phases of tendon healing following injury resemble that of other connective tissues in the body, that is: (1) acute inflammatory phase, lasting 1–2 days, (2) repair-regeneration or proliferative phase, lasting up to 6 weeks, and (3) maturation or remodelling phase, lasting 3 weeks to a year (Leadbetter 1992; Sharma & Maffulli 2005). Each of these phases in tendinopathy has unique cellular progression that should be considered when preparing a treatment plan. Tenocytes begin new collagen synthesis around day 5 after injury and continue synthesis for 5 weeks (Maffulli & Moller 2005). Intrinsic tenocytes begin proliferating at week 4 and are involved in remodelling through to week 8 (Maffulli & Moller 2005). Attempts to apply standard but specific treatments in a global fashion to all tendinopathies without addressing the stage of healing could be ineffective. Cook and Purdam (2009) recommended that interventions should be tailored to the suspected pathology.

Tendinopathy Classification

Tendinopathy actually represents several different mixed and sometimes overlapping degenerative processes. Histologically there are mixed findings. However, there is evidence of the absence of inflammatory cells, increased ground substance, increased vascularity and cellularity with collagen disorganization (Khan et al 2006). Each of these can disrupt some tendon fibres and weaken the remaining ones (Maffulli & Moller 2005). The role of the tenocyte in tendon changes has already been discussed. Murrell (2002) stated that apoptosis, or programmed cell death, may have a roll in tendinopathy. Oystein et al (2007) showed apoptosis to be enhanced in patellar tendinopathy biopsies compared with controls.

Inflammation is partially controlled by a neurogenic process. Substance P and calcitonin-related gene peptide are sensory neuropeptides (Hart et al 2005). These, among other substances, are found in symptomatic tendons (Andersson et al 2008) and directly stimulate nociceptor endings (Ueda 1999). Hart et al (2005) hypothesized that neuropeptides are involved via mast cells in tissue in normal tendon regulatory control; also, a dysfunctional regulatory loop produces an inadequate repair response. This differs from classic inflammation. Riley (2004, p 137) observed, 'nerve endings and mast cells may function as units to modulate tendon homeostasis and mediate adaptive responses to mechanical strain'. He also stated that 'excessive stimulation as a result of overuse may result in pathological changes to the tendon matrix'. There is a growing body of evidence that pain associated with tendinopathy may be neurogenic.

Tendinopathy severity is graded according to histological features distinguished under light microscopy (Maffulli et al 2008). Various scales have been proposed. Two early scales were originally developed for lower extremity research. The Movar scale and the Bonar scale have each since their development been applied successfully to research of the upper extremity (Maffulli et al 2008). Each scale considers the microscopic appearance of five to seven factors, and each factor is given a grade ranging from the lowest number (normal tendon) to the highest number (markedly abnormal tendon). The sample is graded cumulatively, with combined scores from each factor (Maffulli et al 2008). Scott et al (2007) used a modified Bonar scale to assess tendinosis specifically. This scale considers five histological changes: (1) tenocyte morphology, (2) tenocyte proliferation, (3) collagen changes, (4) glycosaminoglycans and (5) neovascularization (Scott et al 2007).

A lack of common description of these histological tissue changes, which vary from scale to scale to modified scale, has limited a clear classification and understanding of tendinopathy with its underlying causes. Khan et al (2006) cited Clancy as having initially made a classification of tendinopathy types, which was later modified by Bonar and now includes: **tendinosis**, **tendinitis** (tendonitis) or partial rupture, **paratenonitis** (paratendonitis / paratendinitis / tenosynovitis / tenovaginitis) and **paratenonitis with tendinosis**. The following sections provide details of these types.

Tendinosis

Tendinosis is defined by Maffulli et al (2003a) as intratendinous degeneration typical with ageing or devascularization. It is characterized by fibre disorientation, hypercellularity and focal necrosis and calcification (Maffulli et al 2003a). Kraushaar and Nirschl (1999) defined the three findings in tendinosis as fibroblastic hyperplasia, hypervascularity and abnormal collagen production, with the former being the first response. Kannus and Jozsa (1991) examined 891 spontaneously ruptured tendons in the upper and lower extremity. Histopathological examination showed that 97% of these had degenerative changes. These were subclassified into hypoxic degeneration (44%), mucoid degeneration (21%), tendolipomatosis (8%) and calcific tendinopathy (5%) (Kannus & Jozsa 1991) There is multiple cell / tissue involvement and this may be difficult to discern from other classifications.

Tendinitis

Tendinitis and partial rupture are grouped together in this classification. An active inflammatory response, symptomatic degeneration and true vascular disruption are characteristic findings (Khan et al 2006). Lymphocytes and neutrophils are seen (Kraushaar & Nirschl 1999). It has similar characteristics to tendinosis but histopathologically will also demonstrate fibroblastic proliferation, haemorrhage and granulation tissue (Maffulli et al 2003a). Hammer (2007a) stated that isolated active inflammation is not common but is usually associated with some degree of rupture, which implies that this classification is falsely overdiagnosed.

Paratenonitis

Paratenonitis, also termed paratendinitis or tenosynovitis, is evidenced as frank inflammation of the outer layer of the tendon (Khan et al 2006). Microscopically this will reveal infiltrate that possibly includes fibrin deposition, exudate and areolar tissue degeneration, which could explain the palpable crepitation at certain stages of its progression (Khan et al 2000; Maffulli et al 2003a).

Combined paratenonitis and tendinosis

This fourth classification (Khan et al 2006), originally described by Clancy, includes characteristics of tendinosis with an overlying paratenonitis as described above. Most clinicians, including primary care physicians, would not be able to differentiate which of these was most prominent in a patient presenting with general hand / wrist pain, as the signs and symptoms are similar to those of isolated paratenonitis.

Of the above categories, only tendinitis and paratenonitis have an inflammatory component and would conceivably respond to an anti-inflammatory regimen, and likewise would not logically respond to deep tissue friction massage.

Examination and Diagnosis

A comprehensive assessment is the most important step to determining appropriate treatment of most musculoskeletal disorders. History, clinical tests and imaging will contribute to a differential diagnosis. (See Chs 3–5 for a discussion of history taking and physical examination.) Clinical testing for tendinopathy can include palpation, selective tissue testing and provocation testing. It is theorized that clinical tests will help to differentiate the structure involved, yet reliability and validity are still being researched. Indeed, this is only one part of the diagnostic equation. Identifying the type of tendon involvement and stage of pathology is another factor of greater difficulty.

The diagnosis of tendinopathy will be the result from a comprehensive examination, but distinguishing between tendinosis and tendinitis can be difficult (Khan et al 2000). Maffulli et al (2003a) identified tendinopathy clinically as localized tendon swelling and pain with impaired function. Curwin (2005) stated that we must assume the level of tendon involvement can be correlated with the level of dysfunction and pain, although the degree of injury cannot be ascertained acutely. Elder and Harvey (2005) maintained that the specific area is usually easy to isolate when acute. Leadbetter (1992) defined acute injury as having a sudden specific onset followed by gradually decreasing pain. Identifying an acute onset during history taking should help to differentiate a current stage of acute or subacute inflammatory process from a chronic stage when inhibiting pain occurs during activity or afterwards (Leadbetter 1992), and will help guide treatment.

One complicating factor in isolating a specific involved structure is that most tendons to be identified will have anatomical variations or supernumerary insertions. These vary too much for inclusion here. Another complication is the possibility that a trigger point (TrP) is responsible for all or a portion of the symptoms. TrPs in the upper quarter can refer pain to the wrist area. The subscapularis, biceps brachii and brachialis are some of the muscles that can refer pain to the wrist (Finando & Finando 2005). Failure to clear these points / areas of potential contribution will delay appropriate treatment. It cannot be overemphasized that suspected TrPs should be cleared as part of the initial examination. (See Ch 59 for additional information on referred pain from muscle / myofascial trigger points in arm pain syndromes.)

Clinical tests

Regarding general palpation, evidence of oedema and hyperaemia of the paratenon may be found clinically. A fibrinous exudate accumulates within the tendon sheath, and crepitus may be felt on clinical examination (Khan et al 2000; Sharma & Maffulli 2005). This may be important in differentiating paratenonitis from tendinopathy; however, the presence of crepitis to palpation does not prove that paratenonitis is present (Khan et al 2000; Sharma & Maffulli 2005).

Palpation for tenderness is a common tool for clinical diagnosis and differential testing in tendinopathy. Cook et al (2001) assessed the value of palpation to identify patellar tendinopathy in a group of 326 young athletes. Intra-rater reliability was good at 82%. Palpation of tendons in patients with symptoms resulted in sensitivity of 68% and specificity of 9% (Cook et al 2001). However, applicability to the wrist is limited since the patellar tendon is larger than those of the hand / wrist.

Maffulli et al (2003b) found a high positive predictive value in palpation, when combined with the Royal London Hospital test and a painful arc sign to determine Achilles tendinopathy. The painful arc sign is theorized to differentiate pathology within the tendon itself versus that of the paratendon. If the pathology is confined to the tendon structure, a palpable area of thickness and tenderness will move with the tendon as the ankle is moved; if the painful, thickened area stays in a fixed position regardless of ankle movement then the pathology is within the paratendon (Easley & Le 2009). The sensitivity and specificity of this test were 52% and 83% respectively (Maffulli et al 2003b). The Royal London Hospital test identifies tendinopathy by eliciting local tenderness with palpation of the tendon in neutral or slightly on slack. The test is positive if the tenderness decreases significantly or disappears with the tendon on stretch. The sensitivity and specificity of this test were 54% and 91% respectively. The sensitivity and specificity of direct palpation were 58% and 74% respectively. When the three tests were combined, the sensitivity was 58% and the specificity was 83% (Maffulli et al 2003b). There is a dearth of evidence-based research application of these clinical tests to tendons of the wrist and hand.

Cyriax supported selective tissue tension testing (STT) (Hammer 2007b). STT is utilized to compare non-contractile with contractile tissue involvement (Hammer 2007b). The tendon is isolated as much as possible based on planes of motion performed: either isolated or overlapped with other tendons. The examiner attempts to administer a minimal isometric force to the tendon / muscle while the patient resists. Elicitation of pain is a positive test (Hammer 2007b). Hanchard et al (2005) found the agreement (0.71–0.79, kappa and 95% confidence interval) among Cyriax-trained assessors using STT combined with clinical history when assessing tendinopathy of the rotator cuff. Reliability has yet to be established for any upper extremity tendon application (Stasinopoulos & Johnson 2007).

Provocation tests (special tests) are used with varying evidence-based support of reliability, sensitivity and specificity. These tests are included, as available and relevant, in the outlined discussion of tendinopathies unique to specific tendons of the wrist and hand following diagnostic imaging and invasive testing.

Diagnostic imaging and invasive testing

Due to the difficulty in reliably diagnosing tendinopathy, Fredberg and Stengaard-Pedersen (2008) recommended ultrasound or magnetic resonance imaging (MRI) if there is no

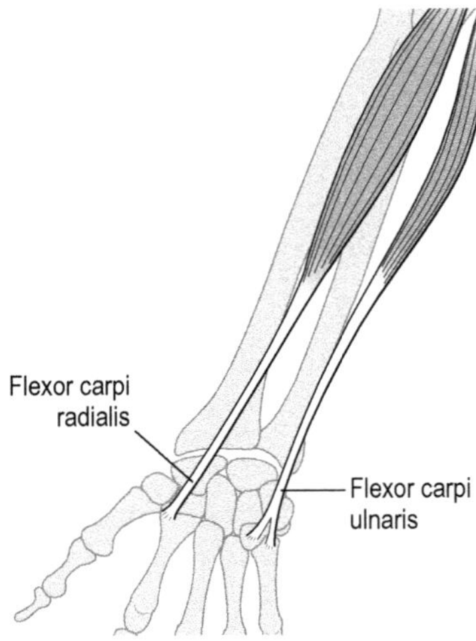

Figure 48.2 Tendiopathic entities: flexor tendons.

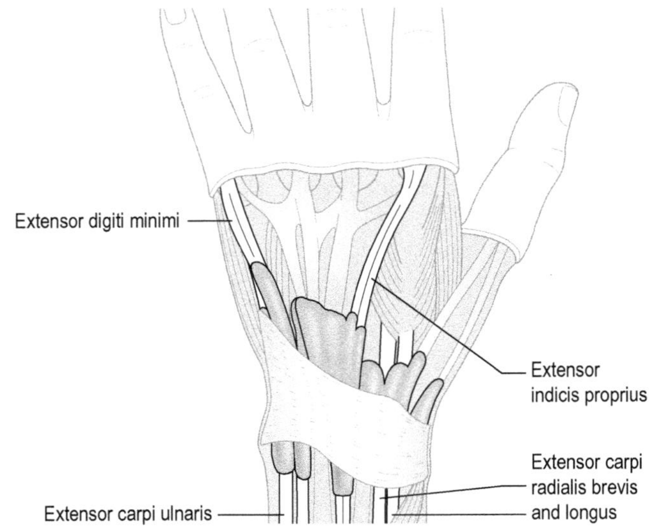

Figure 48.3 Tendiopathic entities: extensor tendons.

response to conservative treatment or if radicular pain is present. Fredberg and Stengaard-Pedersen (2008) described the efficacy of ultrasound versus MRI. These include more detailed visualization of tendon microstructure, better tendon border definition and its interactive nature. A focal thickening, visualized with ultrasound, is associated with tendinitis in tendons without sheaths. This may correspond to angiofibroblastic areas associated with micro-ruptures (Daenen et al 2003). Furthermore, the tendon or tendon sheath, as viewed via ultrasound, will be thickened on more chronically involved tendons (Daenen et al 2003). Ultrasound can be performed directly over the subjectively painful area and even during range of motion (Fredberg & Stengaard-Pedersen 2008). McNee and Teh (2007) considered ultrasound to be the 'investigation of choice' in tendon pathology. Beddi and Bagga (2007) stated that ultrasound is the gold standard for tendon examination.

Isolated identification of the involved structure can be assessed by removing sensation from specific areas, and continuing until the patient's symptoms are resolved. Selective anaesthetic injections, usually with lidocaine, are supported by Elder and Harvey (2005) as 'the best diagnostic test' for tendinopathy of the hand and wrist, but they offer no studies to back up this recommendation.

Tendinopathic Entities of the Hand and Wrist

This section will describe common areas of tendon pain in the wrist. Areas of rare involvement are not included.

Flexor carpi ulnaris

Pathology of the flexor carpi ulnaris (FCU) muscle (Fig. 48.2) may include tendinitis, tendinosis, or a combination of these two. This is the most common wrist flexor tendinopathy (Elder & Harvey 2005) and often occurs in those who play racquet sports and golf (Rettig 2001). The FCU inserts into the pisiform, the hook of the hamate and the fifth metacarpal (Moore 1992). It is not held in place by the flexor retinaculum, but instead relies on its own tendon sheath (Elder & Harvey 2005).

Testing

- Characterized by painful palpation of the pisiform and the FCU tendon, presence of angiofibroblastic hyperplasia is often evidenced by palpable swelling and thickening in symptomatic FCU tendons (Budoff et al 2005).
- Pain with resisted wrist flexion and ulnar deviation.
- Shuck test if pisotriquetral involvement is suspected (Rettig 2001).
- Passive wrist extension and radial deviation will provoke symptoms (Elder & Harvey 2005).

Differential diagnosis

Rettig (2001) recommended the pisotriquetral grind test to implicate the pisotriquetral joint pain over an FCU tendinopathy. Campbell (2001) and Burke (1996) describe the test as grasping the pisiform and compressing it onto the triquetrum and rotating the pisiform under pressure. Palpation alone may implicate the tendon with pain and crepitus, whereas pain with compression implicates the pisotriquetral joint. Pisotriquetral compression syndrome (Rettig 2001), arthritis, calcific tendonitis and ulnar neuritis, pisiform ligament complex syndrome, pisotriquetral arthrosis (Rayan 2005) and Guyon's canal syndrome (Elder & Harvey 2005) are additional differential diagnoses.

Extensor carpi ulnaris

Tendinopathy of the extensor carpi ulnaris (ECU) (Fig. 48.3) may commonly include a tendinitis, tendinosis, or a combination of these. The joint is also subject to subluxation (Elder & Harvey 2005). Activities such as racquet sports and baseball batting will cause rapid and repetitive supination, flexion and ulnar deviation, which have been cited as promoting factors (Elder & Harvey 2005; Hammer 2007c). Rettig (2001) noted that ECU tendinopathy often involved the non-dominant hand in tennis players who used a two-handed backhand stroke. Futami and Itoman (1995) found that, of 155 patients with dorsal wrist pain, 53 had pain possibly caused by tenovaginitis (paratenonitis) of the ECU induced by overuse. Bencardino and Rosenburg (2006) associated subluxations of the ECU with tenosynovitis and recommended testing supination and volar flexion for ulnar subluxation of the tendon. Montalvan et al (2007) studied 28 clinical cases of ECU-related pain with three clinical patterns described: (a) acute traumatic instability of the ECU in the fibro-osseus groove (12 cases); (b) tendinopathy (14 cases); and (c) complete ECU rupture (4 cases).

Testing

- Symptoms are provoked by combined active supination and wrist extension (Elder & Harvey 2005) and combined resisted ulnar deviation and extension (Elder & Harvey 2005; Young et al 2007).
- Dislocation can be reproduced by a clicking on supination and extension actively, but not passively (Elder & Harvey 2005).
- Tenderness to palpation over the sixth dorsal compartment (Rettig 2001) at the ECU tendon and ulnar head (Elder & Harvey 2005).

Differential diagnosis

Rupture, subluxation, dislocation, triangular fibrocartilage complex (TFCC) pain, triquetrum–lunate ligament lesion, pisiform–lunate joint pain, and fractures of the lunate, triquetrum and pisiform are differential diagnoses (Futami & Itoman 1995). Additional diagnoses to be excluded are extensor digiti minimi tenosynovitis, TFCC tears (Elder & Harvey 2005) and stenosing tenosynovitis in the ulnar wrist (Rettig 2001).

Extensor carpi radialis longus and brevis (distal tendons)

A common combined pathology of the extensor carpi radialis longus (ECRL) and brevis (ECRB) tendons (see Fig. 48.3) distally is known as intersection syndrome. This is also termed **peritendinitis crepitans** (Young et al 2007), **crossover tendinitis** and **squeaker's wrist** (Rettig 2001). The syndrome may include tendinitis, tendinosis and / or bursitis. It is common among racquet players, weightlifters and canoeists (Hammer 2007c). Ski pole and hammer usage can also provoke this particular syndrome (Elder & Harvey 2005).

Intersection syndrome is associated with friction from the crossing of the first dorsal compartment abductor pollicis longus (APL) and the extensor pollicis brevis (EPB) over the second dorsal compartment (ECRL and ECRB) (Young et al 2007). It is a paratenonitis (tenosynovitis) that can result in stenosis of the affected tendons.

Cvitanic (2007) noted a natural foramen between the extensor pollicis longus (EPL) and ECRB in cadavers at the site of the intersection. This could explain the areas of multiple symptoms in the dorsal forearm and could make differential diagnoses more complicated. Inflammatory conditions of the ECRB and ECRL at their insertions may be associated with bony protuberances at the capitate, second or third metacarpals, or trapezoid (Daenen et al 2003).

Testing

- Pain to palpation and visible swelling may be evidenced in the tendons proximal to the first compartment (Plancher et al 1996; Bencardino & Rosenburg 2006).
- Thickening and interstitial fluid collection around both tendons approximately 4 to 8 cm proximal to Lister's tubercle will show on MRI (Bencardino & Rosenburg 2006; Plancher et al 1996).
- Crepitation between the APL / EPB and ECRL / ECRB with wrist flexion or extension may be palpable (Elder & Harvey 2005).

Differential diagnosis

Finkelstein's test will be positive but in a more proximal region of the dorsal forearm than would be the case in De Quervain's tenosynovitis (Elder & Harvey 2005; Young et al 2007).

Extensor indicis proprius

Pain and swelling over the fourth dorsal compartment is the most common finding in extensor indicis proprius (EIP) (see Fig. 48.3) syndrome (Plancher et al 1996). This syndrome involves an irritation of the tenosynovium near the extensor retinaculum (Elder & Harvey 2005). Plancher et al (1996) attributed symptoms of EIP tendinopathy to overuse hypertrophy, or to synovitis secondary to overuse. The former could lead to the latter if symptoms were not addressed in a timely fashion. Anatomical variations (75%) are common, complicating the exact structure involved (Plancher et al 1996; Soejima et al 2002).

Testing

- Evidence of pain and swelling in the fourth dorsal compartment distal to the ulnar head with supination (Plancher et al 1996).
- Resisted index extension (Hammer 2007c) with the wrist fully flexed (Elder & Harvey 2005) provokes symptoms.

Differential diagnosis

Extensor digitorum communis (EDC) or EPL tenosynovitis, dorsoradial ganglion, Klebock's disease, extensor digitorum communis tendinopathy and fourth-compartment syndrome are diagnoses to be excluded (Elder & Harvey 2005).

Extensor digiti minimi

The extensor digiti minimi (EDM) (see Fig. 48.3) occupies the fifth dorsal compartment. The pathology most often occurring here is a tenosynovitis (Elder & Harvey 2005). Duplication of the tendon is common complicating implication of the proper structure (Young et al 2007). Elder and Harvey (2005) stated that continuous hand usage such as handwriting will provoke symptoms. Hammer (2007c) reported a lack of pain with resisted testing, which is unusual for tendinopathy, but no reason for this phenomenon was given.

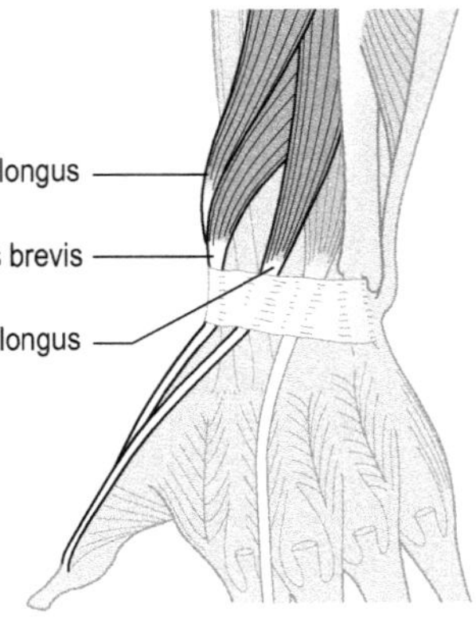

Figure 48.4 Tendiopathic entities: thumb tendons.

Testing

- Grip is painful (Elder & Harvey 2005).
- Limitation in fifth-digit extension is seen (Elder & Harvey 2005).
- Wrist flexion after fist closure or flexing a fist is painful (Elder & Harvey 2005).
- Tenderness to palpation is present just distal to the ulnar head (Plancher et al 1996).

Differential diagnosis

Extensor carpi ulnaris (ECU) tenosynovitis, TFCC pathology and ulnar impaction should be ruled out (Elder & Harvey 2005).

Abductor pollicis longus and extensor pollicis brevis

Together the abductor pollicis longus (APL) and extensor pollicis brevis (EPB) (Fig. 48.4) contribute to De Quervain's tenosynovitis. These tendons normally pass together through a single fibro-osseous tunnel to insert on the first metacarpal and first proximal phalanx respectively (Plancher et al 1996). De Quervain's tenosynovitis often results from excessive pinching or radial deviation (Hammer 2007c). This syndrome is a common occurrence in golf, racquet sports and fishing (Rettig 2001).

Testing

- Finkelstein's test (Fig. 48.5A): Ahuja and Chung (2004) detailed the true test and variations, as the test is misrepresented vigorously in the literature. The original test that Finkelstein (1930) described was completely passive: the clinician grasps the patient's thumb and quickly pulls the wrist into ulnar deviation via the thumb. A positive result is reproduction of pain at the ulnar styloid. The surgeon Eichhoff described a test for de Quervain's disease that is often mistaken for Finkelstein's test (Fig. 48.5B). His test consisted of the patient actively placing the thumb into the palm and folding the fingers down, holding the thumb in place while the clinician passively moves the wrist into ulnar deviation. A positive test is the same as described above for Finkelstein's test. This test, which many believe to be the Finkelstein test, has been criticized as giving false-positive results. Brunelli described a test in 2003 that he claimed was more accurate than the true Finkelstein's test. Brunelli criticized Finkelstein's test for false-positive results due to the stretch of the radial collateral ligament, the scaphotrapezial ligament, or the thumb carpometacarpal ligament caused by the APL and EPB tendons being moved away from the pulley, and described a test in which the wrist is held in radial deviation while forcibly abducting the thumb (Ahuja & Chung 2004). Psychometric properties of these tests have not been established (Elder & Harvey 2005).

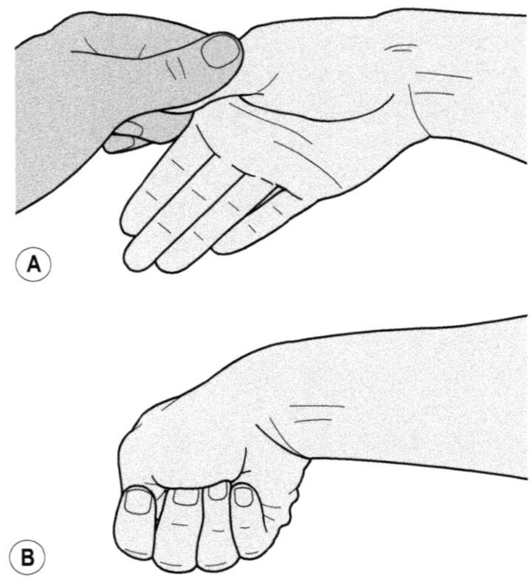

Figure 48.5 (A) Finkelstein's test. The clinician grasps the patient's thumb, uses it to quickly and passively place the wrist into ulnar deviation, causing pain at the radial styloid process. **(B) Eichhoff test.** The patient actively grips the thumb in the fist and then the clinician passively places the wrist into ulnar deviation, which causes pain at the radial styloid process (After Ahuja & Chung 2004.)

- The EPB entrapment test identifies separate compartments and resulting stenosis; this test was reported to have a sensitivity of 81% and specificity of 50% (Alexander et al 2002).
- Tenderness on palpation and swelling over the radial styloid (Elder & Harvey 2005) and first dorsal compartment (Rettig 2001) are present.
- Resisted thumb extension is painful (Elder & Harvey 2005).

Differential diagnosis

Intersection syndrome (Elder & Harvey 2005), scaphoid fracture, flexor carpi radialis (FCR) tendinopathy, first carpometacarpal (CMC) joint arthritis and Wartenburg's syndrome (Plancher et al 1996) are differential diagnoses.

Extensor pollicis longus

The extensor pollicis longus (EPL) (see Fig. 48.4) often exhibits a tenosynovitis common in racquet sports players. A history of repetitive trauma as occurs in racquet sports, pain, crepitus and swelling around Lister's tubercle will narrow the list of suspected diagnoses (Plancher et al 1996). Triggering of the thumb may be seen in severe cases.

Testing

- There is evidence of pain, swelling and crepitus along the EPL tendon at the third dorsal compartment (Plancher et al 1996) and at Lister's tubercle (Elder & Harvey 2005).
- Pain is elicited with resisted thumb extension or passive flexion (Elder & Harvey 2005).
- Passive interphalangeal joint flexion can reproduce the pain (Elder & Harvey 2005).

Differential diagnosis

Differential diagnoses have not been established as necessary for this tendon pathology.

Flexor carpi radialis

Flexor carpi radialis (FCR) (see Fig. 48.2) tendinopathy is common in people who play racquet sports, golf and baseball (Rettig 2001). Elder and Harvey (2005) reported an often-insidious onset without known trauma. A primary symptom is pain near the proximal aspect of the trapezium (Gabel et al 1994). This is often a result of overuse with repeated flexion of the wrist, of complication after scaphoid fracture or distal radius fracture, or of other direct trauma (Gabel et al 1994). The FCR is subject to traumatic injury owing to its position. The FCR lies in direct contact with the roughened surface of the trapezium. Its insertion onto the trapezium is only 20% of the entire insertion. Additional insertions include the second and third metacarpals (Bishop et al 1994) and the joint capsule of the trapezioscaphoid joint itself (Schmidt 1987). The tendon occupies 90% of the fibro-osseous tunnel, making it vulnerable to compression (Bishop et al 1994; Elder & Harvey 2005). FCR tendinopathy is also associated with scaphotrapezial joint osteoarthritis, malunion of the trapezium or a scaphoid cyst (Soejima et al 2002).

Testing

- Symptoms are exacerbated by resisted flexion and radial deviation of the wrist (Elder & Harvey 2005; Rayan 2005) and by resisted flexion (Rettig 2001); wrist hyperextension or resisted wrist flexion with radial deviation can reproduce symptoms (Young et al 2007).
- There is evidence of pain and notable swelling at the level of the distal wrist crease along its course (Elder & Harvey 2005) and near the fibro-osseous tunnel (Young et al 2007).

Differential diagnosis

Differential diagnoses include osteoarthritis of the first CMC joint, scaphoid cysts, fractures, ganglion cysts, De Quervain's syndrome and Lindburg's syndrome (Elder & Harvey 2005).

Treatment and Prognosis

Conservative treatment

Conservative treatment for tendinopathy includes modalities such as ultrasound, electric stimulation, ice and laser (Curwin 2005), as well as injections and splinting (Plancher et al 1996). Konijnenberg et al (2001) attempted a meta-analysis of outcomes of repetitive strain injuries. Many body areas were included in the analysis. They found no strong evidence for any conservative treatment option (Konijnenberg et al 2001). Conservative treatments included physiotherapy involving multiple types of interventions, but none included the hand or wrist.

Manual therapy, in particular deep tissue friction massage (DTFM), is a conservative treatment for tendinopathy that is utilized by some clinicians; however, efficacy has not been proven. This could be due at least in part to study design. DTFM for tendon pain was first popularized by James Cyriax. Cyriax did not perform outcome studies, but studies done by Stasinopoulos and Johnson (2007) concluded that effectiveness of DTFM for lateral epicondylitis could not be assessed from the studies they reviewed. Stasinopoulos did not study outcomes of the wrist.

Cyriax techniques of DTFM for treatment of soft tissue lesions are performed with direct pressure on the painful area. The clinician's finger rubs firmly transversely to the fibres of the tissue, which includes tendon. Recommended duration and frequency are 20-minute sessions for 6–12 treatments with at least 48 hours between treatments (Cyriax 1983). Cyriax (1983) theorized that the treatment eroded scar tissue between muscle fibres via abrasive contact; in tenosynovitis the rolling was theorized to smooth roughened synovial surfaces. More recent work has specified the optimal time of application for tendon strain based on the previously discussed stage of pathology. Research by Zeichen et al (2000) subjected fibroblasts to strain for varying times, monitoring for proliferation of fibroblasts as a response to a biaxial strain over subsequent hours. The results showed that 15 minutes of strain resulted in increased proliferation compared with controls at 6 and 24 hours (Zeichen et al 2000).

The 48 hours of recommended minimum accepted time frame between treatments roughly equals the ending of the acute stage of inflammation, when remodelling begins (Leadbetter 1992). The firmer pressure, as recommended by Cyriax (1983), may be justified by a study by Gehlsen et al (1999) showing that firmer pressure had more positive effects than lighter pressure.

Hammer (2007d) applied soft tissue mobilization with greater precision with respect to the stage of tendon pathology. Although he generally concurred with treatment in the 5–15-minute duration twice a week lasting 2 weeks to 2 months, he recommended no manual treatment until the proliferative phase, which was described as 7–14 days after original injury. Treatment during the acute phase when rest is recommended should be light, so as to aid fibroblastic proliferation and break down immature collagen. In the maturation phase the treatment could be more vigorous in order to reduce fibrosis (Hammer 2007c).

Khan and Scott (2009) and Kraushaar and Nirschl (1999) theorized that mechanical disruption may transform a failed intrinsic healing into a therapeutic extrinsic healing mechanism. The study by Brousseau et al (2002) on DTFM and tendinitis (not tendinosis) considered cross-friction treatment as only cross-friction and not other techniques, including a stroke along the muscle. This could be one explanation for the lack of more positive outcomes: improper or non-uniform direction of force. Another reason could be lack of proper selection of the subcategory of tendinopathy as classified earlier in this section. Some classifications, such as acute inflammation, in theory cannot be affected by manipulation.

Despite the lack of randomized controlled trials of tendon pain and DTFM, other research is emerging. These studies provide, on a small scale, a pathoanatomical link between manual therapy and reversal of tendinopathic changes. Meltzer and Standley (2007) demonstrated that a modelled indirect osteopathic manipulative technique (IOMT) significantly reduced pro-inflammatory secretions compared with controls 24 hours after application, and concluded that the modelled IOMT can reverse some of the effects of repetitive strain (Meltzer & Standley 2007). Standley and Meltzer (2008) studied the effect of modelled manual therapy on cellular response. Improved range of motion, reduced analgesic requirements and decreased oedema post-myofascial release was theorized to be a result of anti-inflammatory cytokines from strain inducement of myofascial release (Standley & Meltzer 2008).

Eccentric exercise is a more recently applied form of conservative treatment that is theorized as reversing degeneration via specific load application. This treatment has shown positive outcomes (Ohberg et al 2004). Eccentric exercise involves contraction of a muscle to control or decelerate a load while that muscle and tendon are lengthening or in a lengthened position. Eccentric exercises have been proven effective at changing ultrasonic findings in involved Achilles tendons within 12 weeks (Ohberg et al 2004); the study follow-up showed reduction in tendon diameter and return of normal tendon structure in a majority (19 of 26) of tendons. The unchanged tendons had undefined residual defects (Ohberg et al 2004).

Woodley et al (2006) reviewed 11 studies of eccentric exercises that met the inclusion criteria of methodological quality and levels of evidence. They covered both upper and lower extremity tendinopathies. Eccentric exercise was more effective than other treatments that included frictions, stretching, splinting and ultrasound in treating tendon pain and improving patient satisfaction and return-to-work outcomes (Woodley et al 2006).

Curwin (2005) outlined an eccentric programme that consisted of warm-up activities, stretching, three sets of 10 eccentric exercises, repeated stretching and ice application. This was continued for 6 weeks unless symptoms resolved before then. The protocol was performed by 200 patients with chronic tendinopathy that failed conservative therapy. Marked or complete relief of symptoms was reported in 90% of patients who completed the programme. However, despite the large sample size there was no control group or randomization (Curwin 2005).

Knobloch (2008) supported eccentric training on the wrist to be equally effective as that on the Achilles tendon in decreasing abnormal capillary tendon flow (angiogenesis) seen in tendinopathy. Khan and Scott (2009) promoted the theory that effects of eccentric muscle contraction on the tendon appear to stimulate tissue healing.

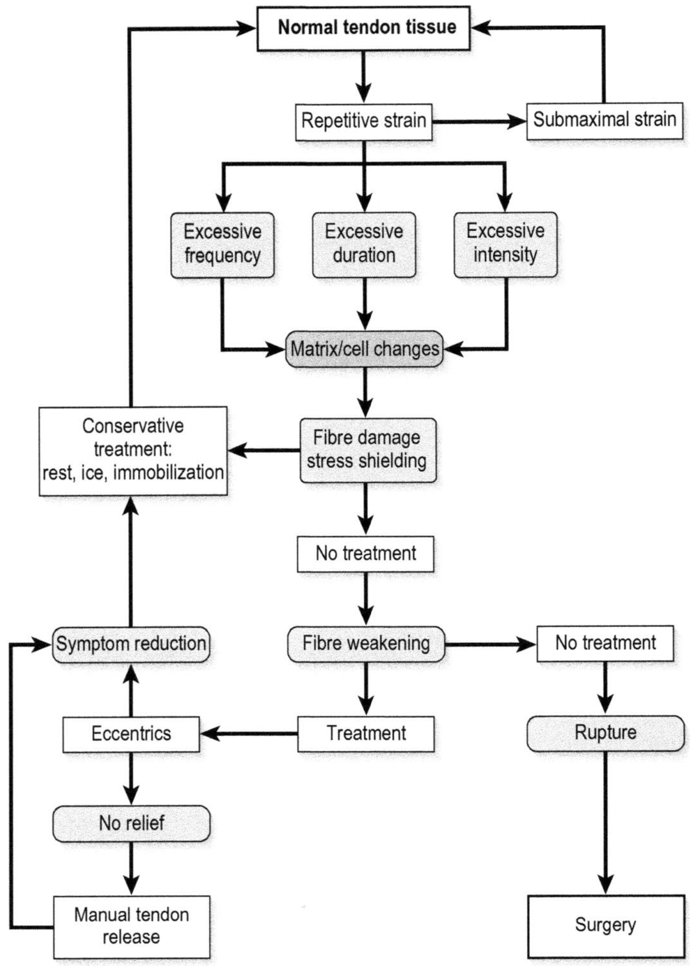

Figure 48.6 Selected treatment algorithm.

The research by Kannus and Josza (1991) illuminated how stress reduction can lead to degenerative changes in the tendon, including a reduction in mechanical properties. This may be why eccentric exercises are effective in some cases in reducing the effects of immobilization. Soft tissue mobilization along the tendon could also reduce the effects of immobilization, but only to a localized portion of that tendon. Any force, including eccentrics, will not affect the tendon equally. Undamaged fascicles will accept and transmit that force normally, while damaged fascicles, according to Arnoczky et al (2007), will not transfer that force to all fascicles, which leads to degeneration of the involved fascicles. This will be a necessary subject of future studies. An algorithm (Fig. 48.6) outlines a proposed pathway of manual treatment and eccentrics in tendinopathy.

Non-conservative treatment

Review of the recent literature on surgeries for wrist tendinopathy reveals a consistent use of the terms 'tendinitis' and 'tenosynovitis' in surgical cases. This usage is therefore continued in the report of surgical interventions.

De Quervain's tenosynovitis that does not respond to conservative therapy may undergo surgery. This involves decompression of the first dorsal compartment and is not without risks (Plancher et al 1996). Rettig (2001) reported that, after 7–10 days of splinting, return to sports can be expected in 6–9 weeks.

Flexor carpi ulnaris surgery often involves excision of the pisiform (Rettig 2001). The expected return to sports averages 8 weeks (Rettig 2001).

As the flexor carpi radialis occupies 90% of the available space in its synovial tunnel, surgery here involves decompression of the tunnel (Plancher et al 1996).

Plancher et al (1996) stated that extensor carpi ulnaris subluxation does not always respond to conservative care. The sixth dorsal compartment is released in extensor carpi ulnaris tendinitis. Due to the chance of subluxation, some authors recommend release of the fibro-osseus tunnel that it occupies (Plancher et al 1996). Rettig (2001) reported that, after 4–6 weeks of cast wearing, return to sports required a minimum of 8 weeks.

Surgery for intersection syndrome, according to Plancher et al (1996), involves release of the second compartment with synovectomy. Rettig (2001) mentioned bursectomy between the involved tendons. Release of the third dorsal compartment is also performed on non-responsive cases of extensor pollicis longus tendinitis.

Prognosis

Prognosis with conservative treatment for specific tendinopathies or syndromes is not widely available in evidence-based studies. Regarding conservative treatment for DeQuervain's tenosynovitis, Harvey et al (1990) reported 80% resolution of symptoms with injections alone. Lane et al (2001) concluded that classifying these patients before conservative treatment was initiated improved outcomes; 17 of 18 patients with classified mild symptoms improved with splinting and non-steroidal anti-inflammatory medications, whereas those with symptoms classified as moderate to severe responded most favourably to injections (76%). Richie and Briner (2003) reviewed seven descriptive studies comparing conservative treatments for De Quervain's tenosynovitis. They reported an overall cure rate of 83% for injection alone, 61% for injection and splint, 14% for splint alone and 0% for treatments that consisted solely of non-steroidal anti-inflammatory medications and rest. Tendinopathies of the other structures of the wrist have not been as widely studied.

Conclusion

Although much more is now known about tenocyte and matrix dysfunction, successful application of these concepts for treatment of tendinopathy in the wrist and hand has not been proven. Studies continue to be hampered by sample size, lack of meaningful outcomes, small population selection and lack of randomization. Adequate studies regarding conservative treatment of non-inflammatory tendinopathies do not appear to exist at present.

Eccentrics show promise for treating tendinopathy in a majority of weight-bearing tendons. Successful application of this into tendinopathies of the upper extremity has yet to be accomplished.

Manual therapy's place in treatment of wrist tendinopathy has not been established. If the efficacy of manual applied eccentrics or what some authors call 'active release' could be likewise established in the upper extremity, they could easily be performed adapting Curwin's (2005) guidelines for eccentric exercises. A study that reveals the effects of manual therapy on tendinopathy will require the following: (1) selection of appropriate tendon pathology, which will pose its own difficulties, (2) soft tissue mobilization such as 'active release' along the tendon fibres, (3) continued self-range of motion routinely for 48 hours, to reduce the effect of immobilization, and (4) the repetition of criteria (2) every 48 hours for up to 6 weeks until function has returned. A design incorporating these factors may be able to discern the true worth of DTFM in tendinopathy.

References

Ahuja NK, Chung KC. 2004. Fritz de Quervain, MD (1868–1940): stenosing tendovaginitis at the radial styloid process. J Hand Surg 29A: 1164–1170.

Alexander R, Catalano L, Barron O, et al. 2002. Extensor pollicis brevis entrapment test in the treatment of DeQuervain's disease. J Hand Surg 27: 813–816.

Andersson G, Danielson P, Alfredson H, et al. 2008. Presence of substance P and the neurokinin-1 receptor in tenocytes of the human Achilles tendon. Regul Pept 150: 81–87.

Arnoczky S, Lavagnino M, Egerbacher M. 2007. The mechanobiological aetiopathogenesis of tendinopathy: is it the over-stimulation or understimulation of tendon cells? Int J Exp Pathol 88: 217–226.

Arnoczky S, Tian T, Lavagnino M, et al. 2006. Activation of stress-activated protein kinases (SAPK) in tendon cells following cyclic strain: the effects of strain frequency, strain magnitude and cytosolic calcium. J Orthop Res 20: 947–952.

Backman C, Boquist L, Fridén J, et al. 2005. Chronic Achilles paratendonitis and tendinosis: an experimental model in the rabbit. J Orthop Res 8: 541–547.

Beddi TH, Bagga RN. 2007. Ultrasound in rheumatology. Indian J Radiol Imaging 17: 299–305.

Bencardino J, Rosenburg Z. 2006. Sports related injuries to the wrist: An approach to MRI interpretation. Clin Sports Med 25: 409–432.

Benjamin M, Ralphs J. 1996. Tendons in health and disease. Man Ther 1: 186–191.

Bishop A, Gabel G, Carmichael S. 1994. Flexor carpi radialis tendonitis I, operative anatomy. J Bone Joint Surg 76: 1009–1014.

Brousseau L Casimiro L, Milne S, et al. 2002. Deep transverse friction massage for treating tendinitis. Cochrane Database Syst Rev 4: CD003528.

Budoff J, Kraushaar B, Ayala G. 2005. Flexor carpi ulnaris tendinopathy. J Hand Surg 30: 125–129.

Burke FD. 1996. Pisotriquetral pathology: a differential diagnosis. In: Buchler U (ed) Wrist instability. London: CV Mosby, pp 213–217.

Campbell DA. 2001. How I examine the wrist. Curr Orthoped 14: 342–346.

Cannon N. 2001. Diagnosis and treatment manual for physicians and therapists: upper extremity rehabilitation, 4th edn. Indianapolis, IN: Hand Rehabilitation Center of Indiana.

Chiquet M. 1999. Regulation of extracellular matrix gene expression by mechanical stress. Matrix Biol 18: 417–426. [Abstract.]

Cook J, Purdam C. 2009. Is tendon pathology a continuum? A pathology model to explain the clinical presentation of load-induced tendinopathy. Br J Sports Med 43: 409–416.

Cook J, Khan K, Kiss Z. 2001. Reproducibility and clinical utility of tendon palpation to detect patellar tendinopathy in young basketball players. Br J Sports Med 35: 65–69.

Curwin SL. 2005. Rehabilitation after tendon injuries. In: Maffulli N, Renstrom P, Leadbetter W (eds) Tendon injuries: basic science and clinical medicine. London: Springer-Verlag, pp 242–266.

Cvitanic OA. 2007. Communicating foramen between tendon sheaths of the extensor carpi radialis brevis and extensor pollicis longus muscles: imaging of cadaver and patients. AJR Am J Roentgenol 18:9 1190–1197.

Cyriax J. 1983. Illustrated manual of orthopaedic medicine. London: Butterworth.

Daenen B, Houben G, Bauduin E, et al. 2003. Sonography in wrist pathology. J Clin Ultrasound 32: 462–469.

De Boer M, Selby A, Atherton P, et al. 2007. The temporal responses of protein synthesis, gene expression and cell signaling in human quadriceps muscle and patellar tendon to disuse. J Physiol 585: 241–251.

The Department of Labor, Bureau of Labor Statistics. 1999. Illnesses, Injuries and Fatalities Bureau of Labor Statistics. Washington, DC: United States Department of Labor. Online. Available: http://www.bls.gov./iff/home.htm (accessed 29.11.14.)

Easley M, Le I. 2009. Non-insertional achilles tendinopathy. In: Nunley J (ed) The Achilles tendon: treatment and rehabilitation. Durham, NC: Springer Science, pp 145–168.

Elder G, Harvey E. 2005. Hand and wrist tendinopathies. In: Maffulli N, Renstrom P, Leadbetter W (eds) Tendon injuries: basic science and clinical medicine. London: Springer-Verlag, pp 137–149.

Finando D, Finando S. 2005. Trigger point therapy for myofascial pain. Vermont: Healing Arts Press.

Finkelstein H. 1930. Stenosing tendovaginitis at the radial styloid process. J Bone Joint Surg 12: 509–540.

Fredberg U, Stengaard-Pedersen K. 2008. Chronic tendinopathy tissue pathology, pain mechanisms and etiology with a special focus on inflammation. Scand J Sports Med 18: 3–15.

Futami T, Itoman M. 1995. Extensor carpi ulnaris syndrome: findings in 43 patients. Acta Orthop Scand 66: 538–539.

Gabel G, Bishop AT, Wood MB. 1994. Flexor carpi radialis tendonitis II, results of operative treatment. J Bone Joint Surg 76: 1015–1018.

Gehlsen G, Ganion L, Helfst R. 1999. Fibroblast responses to variation in soft tissue mobilization pressure. Med Sci Sports Exerc 31: 531–555.

Glazebrook M, Wright J, Langman M, et al. 2007. Histological analysis of Achilles tendon in an overuse rat model. J Orthop Res 26: 840–846.

Hammer W. 2007a. Manual treatment methods. In: Hammer W (ed) Functional soft-tissue examination and treatment by manual methods, 3rd edn. Boston: Jones and Bartlett, pp 475–479.

Hammer W. 2007b. Basics of soft tissue examination. In: Hammer W (ed) Functional soft-tissue examination and treatment by manual methods, 3rd edn. Boston: Jones and Bartlett, pp 3–14.

Hammer W. 2007c. Wrist and hand. In: Hammer W (ed) Functional soft-tissue examination and treatment by manual methods, 3rd edn. Boston: Jones and Bartlett, pp 213–225.

Hammer W. 2007d. Combining friction massage with neuromuscular reeducation. In: Hammer W (ed) Functional soft-tissue examination and treatment by manual methods, 3rd edn. Boston: Jones and Bartlett, pp 563–589.

Hanchard N, Howe T, Gilbert M. 2005. Diagnosis of shoulder pain by history and selective tissue tension: agreement between assessors. J Orthop Sports Phys Ther 35: 147–153.

Harley B, Bergman J. 2008. Tendon and ligament anatomy, biology and biomechanics. In: P Toretta, T Einhorn (eds) Oncology and basic science. Philadelphia: Lippincott, Williams & Wilkins, pp 463–473.

Hart D, Cyrli B, Frank S, et al. 2005. Neurogenic, mast cell, and gender variables in tendon biology: potential role in chronic tendinopathy. In: Maffulli N, Renstrom P, Leadbetter W (eds) Tendon injuries: basic science and clinical medicine. London: Springer-Verlag, pp 40–48.

Harvey F, Harvey P, Horsley M. 1990. DeQuervain's disease: surgical or nonsurgical treatment. J Hand Surg Am 15: 83–87.

Huang H, Kamm R, Lee RT. 2004. Cell mechanics and mechanotransduction: pathways, probes, and physiology. Am J Physiol Cell Physiol 287: C1–C11.

Kannus P. 2000. Structure of the tendon connective tissue. Scand J Med Sci Sports 10: 312–320.

Kannus P, Jozsa L. 1991. Histopathologic changes preceding spontaneous rupture of a tendon. J Bone Joint Surg 73: 1507–1525.

Khan K, Scott A. 2009. Mechanotherapy: how physical therapists prescription of exercise promotes tissue repair. Br J Sports Med 43: 247–252.

Khan K, Cook J, Taunton J, et al. 2000. Overuse tendinosis not tendinitis: Part 1: a new paradigm for a difficult clinical problem. Phys Sportsmed 28(5): 38–48. doi: 10.3810/psm.2000.05.890.

Khan K, Cook J, Bonar F, et al. 2006. Histopathology of common tendinopathies: update and implications for clinical management. In: Khan K, Bruckner P (eds) Clinical sports medicine, 3rd edn. Sydney, NSW: McGraw-Hill Australia.

Knobloch K. 2008. The role of tendon microcirculation in achilles and patellar tendinopathy. J Orth Surg Res 3: 18. doi: 10.1186/1749-799X-3-18.

Konijnenberg H, deWilde N, Gerritsen A, et al. 2001. Conservative treatment for repetitive strain. Scand J Work Environ Health 27: 299–310.

Kraushaar B, Nirschl R. 1999. Tendinosis of the elbow. Clinical features and findings of histological, immunohistochemical, and electron microscopy studies. J Bone Joint Surg 81: 259–278.

Lane LB, Boretz RS, Stuchin SA. 2001. Treatment of DeQuervain's: role of conservative management. J Hand Surg Eur 26: 258–260.

Lavagnino M, Arnoczky S, Tian T, et al. 2003. Effect of amplitude and frequency of cyclic tensile strain on the inhibition of MMP1 mRNA expression in tendon cells: an in vitro study. Connect Tissue Res 44: 181–187.

Lavagnino M, Arnoczky SP, Egrebacher M, et al. 2006. Isolated fibular damage in tendons stimulates local collagenase mRNA expression and protein synthesis. J Biomech 39: 2355–2362.

Leadbetter W. 1992. Cell-matrix response in tendon injury. Clin Sports Med 11: 433–577.

Maeda E, Shelton JC, Bader DL, et al. 2009. Differential regulation of gene expression in isolated tendon fascicles exposed to cyclic strain in vivo. J Appl Physiol 106: 506–512. [Abstract.]

Maffulli N, Longo UG. 2008. How do eccentrics work in tendinopathy. Rheumatology 47: 1444–1445.

Maffulli N, Moller H. 2005. Optimization of tendon healing. In: Maffulli N, Renstrom P, Leadbetter W (eds) Tendon injuries: basic science and clinical medicine. London: Springer-Verlag, pp 204–206.

Maffulli N, Kenward M, Testa V, et al. 2003a. Clinical diagnosis of Achilles tendinopathy with tendinosis. Clin J Sports Med 13: 11–15. [Abstract.]

Maffulli N, Wong J, Almekinders LC. 2003b. Types and epidemiology of tendinopathy. Clin Sports Med 22: 675–692.

Maffulli N, Longo UG, Franceschi F. 2008. Movin and Bonar scores assess the same characteristics of tendon histology. Clin Orthop Relat Res 466: 1605–1611.

Magra M, Hughes S, El Haj AJ, et al. 2007. VOCC and TREK-1 ion channel expression in human tenocytes. Am J Physiol Cell Physiol 292: C1053–C1060.

McNee PA, Teh J. 2007. Imaging of the wrist. Imaging 19: 208–219.

Meltzer K, Standley P. 2007. Modeled repetitive motion strain and indirect osteopathic manipulative techniques in regulation of human fibroblast proliferation and interleukin secretion. J Am Osteopath Assoc 107: 527–536.

Montalvan B, Parier J, Brasseur J. 2007. Extensor carpi ulnaris injuries in tennis players: a study of 28 cases. Br J Sports Med 40 424–429.

Moore K. 1992. Clinically oriented anatomy, 3rd edn. Baltimore, MD: Williams & Wilkins, p 566.

Murrell G. 2002. Understanding tendinopathies. Br J Sports Med 36: 392.

O'Brien M. 2005. Anatomy of tendons. In: Maffulli N, Renstrom P, Leadbetter W (eds) Tendon injuries: basic science and clinical medicine. London: Springer-Verlag, pp 3–11.

Ohberg L, Lorentzon R, Alfredson H. 2004. Eccentric training in patients with chronic Achilles tendinosis: normalized tendons structure and decreased thickness at follow up. Br J Sports Med 38: 8–11.

Oystein L, Scott A, Engebretson L. 2007. Excessive apoptosis in patellar tendon in athletes. Am J Sports Med 35: 605–611.

Plancher KD, Peterson RK, Steichen JB. 1996. Compressive neuropathies and tendinopathies in athletic elbow and wrist. Clin Sports Med 15: 331–371.

Rayan G. 2005. Pisiform ligament complex syndrome and pisotriquetral arthrosis. Hand Clin 21: 507–517.

Renstrom P, Hach T. 2005. Insertional tendinopathy in sports. In: Maffulli N, Renstrom P, Leadbetter W (eds) Tendon injuries: basic science and clinical medicine. London: Springer-Verlag, pp 70–85.

Rettig A. 2001. Wrist and hand overuse syndromes. Clin Sports Med 20: 591–611.

Richie C, Briner W. 2003. Corticosteroid injection for treatment of DeQuervain's tenosynovitis: a pooled quantitative literature evaluation. J Am Board Fam Pract 16: 102–106. [Abstract.]

Riley G. 2004. The pathogenesis of tendinopathy a molecular perspective. Rheumatology 43: 131–142.

Schmidt H. 1987. Clinical anatomy of flexor carpi radialis tendon sheath. Acta Morphol Neerl Scand 25: 17–28.

Scott A, Cook J, Hart D, et al. 2007. Tenocyte response to mechanical load in vivo: a role for local insulin-like growth factor1 signaling in early tendinosis in rats. Arthritis Rheum 56: 871–881.

Screen H, Shelton J, Bader D. 2005. Cyclic tensile strain upregulates collagen synthesis in isolated tendon fascicles. Biochem Biophys Res Commun 336: 424–429.

Sharma P, Maffulli N. 2005. Tendon injury and tendinopathy: healing and repair. J Bone Joint Surg 87A: 187–202.

Sharma P, Maffulli N. 2006. Biology of tendon injury: healing, modeling and remodeling. J Musculoskelet Neuronal Interact 6: 181–190.

Smith R, Zunino L, Webbon P, et al. 1997. The distribution of cartilage oligomeric matrix protein (COMP) in tendon and its variation with tendon site, age and load. Matrix Biol 16: 255–271.
Soejima O, Iida H, Naito M. 2002. Flexor carpi radialis tendonitis caused by malunited trapezial ridge fracture in a professional baseball player. J Orthop Sci 7: 151–153.
Soslowsky L, Thomopoulos S, Tun S, et al. 2000. Overuse activity injuries in the supraspinatus tendon in an animal model: a histopathologic and biomechanical study. J Shoulder Elbow Surg 9: 79–84.
Standley P, Meltzer K. 2008. In vitro modeling of repetitive motion strain and manual medicine treatments: potential roles for pro- and anti-inflammatory cytokines. J Bodyw Mov Ther 12: 201–203.
Stasinopoulos S, Johnson M. 2007. It may be time to modify Cyriax's treatment for lateral epicondylitis. J Bodyw Mov Ther 11: 64–67.
Ueda H. 1999. In vivo molecular signal transduction of peripheral mechanisms of pain. Jpn J Pharmacol 79: 263–268.
Wall ME, Banes AJ. 2005. Early responses to mechanical load in tendon: role for calcium signaling, gap junctions and intracellular communication. J Musculoskelet Neuronal Interact 5: 70–84.
Woo SL, Kuei SC, Amiel D, et al. 1981. The effect of prolonged physical training on the properties of long bone. J Bone Joint Surg 63: 780–787.
Woodley B, Newsham-West R, Baxter GD. 2006. Chronic tendinopathy: effectiveness of eccentric exercise. Br J Sports Med 41: 188–198. [Abstract.]
Young D, Papp S, Biachino A. 2007. Physical exam of the wrist. Orthop Clin North Am 38: 149–165.
Yuan J, Wang MX, Murrel G. 2003. Cell death and tendinopathy. Clin Sports Med 22: 693–701.
Zeichen J, Griensven M, Bosch U. 2000. The proliferative response of isolated human tendon fibroblasts to cyclic biaxial mechanical strain. Am J Sports Med 28: 888–892.

49 Chapter

Carpal Instability

Ellen Pong

CHAPTER CONTENTS

Introduction to wrist instability 558
Functional stability 558
Defining wrist instability 558
Incidence and aetiology of carpal instability 558
Anatomy and biomechanics 559
Anatomy 559
Biomechanics 560
Aetiopathogenesis 560
Patterns and classification 560
Pathogenesis 561
Examination and diagnosis 561
Diagnostic considerations 561
Clinical tests 561
Radiological tests, diagnostic dynamic ultrasound and arthroscopy 563
Treatment and prognosis 563
Conservative treatment and prognosis 563
Surgical treatment and prognosis 564
Conclusion 564

Introduction to Wrist Instability

Functional stability

The human wrist is a necessary link between the power of the forearm and the precision of the hand. It has been proposed that there was a survival advantage in human evolution to having a carpus whose stability as a stationary platform enhanced precise use of instruments, weapons and tools (Wolfe et al 2006). Simple grasp of an object relies on at least four mechanisms of carpal stabilization. They include the proximal carpal row, the distal carpal row, the mid-carpal joint and the radiocarpal joint (Garcia-Elias 1997a). Although stability of the radial side is clearly a necessary component of opposable thumb use, stability of the distal radioulnar joint is just as important for provision of the rotational forearm in tool use and carrying (Dobbs 2003).

Defining wrist instability

Linscheid and associates are credited as the first to define carpal instability in 1972 (Schmitt et al 2006), but references to conditions of instability are recorded as early as 1923 (Linscheid et al 1972; Lichtman & Wroten 2006). Linscheid and Dobyns (2002) set forth specific concepts in defining types of instability as well as providing an overall definition; however, this definition has continued to evolve with time (Carlsen & Shin 2008).

There is disagreement among researchers regarding aetiology and pathomechanics, resulting in various accepted views of terminology and treatment for instability of the wrist and its specific joints (Lichtman & Wroten 2006). Linscheid and Dobyns (2002) defined wrist instability as a wrist having altered kinematics and / or being unable to support physiological loads. Taking this further, De Filippo et al (2006) specified: carpal instability occurs from all untreated dislocations and displaced or malunited fractures, integrity of interosseous ligaments and joint capsule determine stability, congenital ligamentous laxity (such as Ehlers–Danlos syndrome) is not considered to be pathological wrist / carpal instability, and pain may not be present as a diagnostic symptom in the initial stages of some carpal instabilities.

Four joints are grossly considered in the presentation of wrist instability: the carpometacarpal joint, the mid-carpal joint, the radiocarpal joint and the distal radioulnar joint (DRUJ), with DRUJ stability influenced by stability of the associated triangular fibrocartilage complex (TFCC) (Dumontier 1996). This chapter will focus on mid-carpal, radiocarpal and DRUJ instability.

Incidence and aetiology of carpal instability

Exact figures of carpal instability incidence and economic impact are difficult to obtain, primarily because many instabilities are not diagnosed early, or even revealed for treatment at all, owing to lack of pain in some cases and poor recognition and follow-up in others (Perron et al 2001; Dias & Garcia-Elias 2006).

The most widely recognized cause of carpal instability is trauma, with wrist hyperextension and various forearm rotations; however, the exact combination of joint position varies along with the resulting instability location (De Filippo et al 2006; Garcia-Elias 2006; Schmitt et al 2006). Linscheid et al (1972) found that instability was a complication in 10% of all reported carpal injuries. The most common carpal instability (up to 19% of wrist injuries) is within the mid-carpal joint, between the scaphoid and lunate (Bozentka 1999; Surdziel & Lubiatowski 2006).

The malunited distal radius fracture is recognized as a cause of carpal malalignment, developing during the period of immobilization and worsening gradually after fracture healing owing to continued stress and loading of the wrist (Gupta et al 2002). The incidence of carpal instability from this type of injury is possibly as high as 30% (Tang 1992). Rheumatoid arthritis and calcium pyrophosphate deposition disease (CPPD) are additional causes of wrist instability in the intercarpal, distal ulna and radiocarpal joints (Resnick & Niwayama 1977; Schmitt et al 2006). Avascular osteonecrosis, neurological disorders, neoplastic disease and specific congenital malformations have also been attributed as causes (De Filippo et al 2006; Schmitt et al 2006).

Anatomy and Biomechanics

Anatomy

This review is pertinent to wrist instability. The reader is encouraged to utilize other resources to revisit the basic anatomy of the distal forearm, wrist and hand, if needed.

Osseous anatomy

The osseous anatomy is important in considering carpal and wrist stability. Pathologies such as inflammatory arthritis, infection and fracture can change the shape of the carpal bones sufficiently to alter bony balance and produce instability (Garcia-Elias 2006). Yet, even after ligamentous injury, the bony anatomical features of the distal radius and proximal scaphoid have some ability to stabilize the carpus. Werner et al (2007) demonstrated this concept of bony geometry providing scapholunate stability in the presence of a torn scapholunate interosseous ligament.

Discussion begins with the distal radius and ulna. The radius widens distally to form a large articular surface for the scaphoid and lunate, creating the radiocarpal joint (Wadsworth 1988). The distal ends of the radius and ulna between them form the distal radioulnar joint. The distal ulna has an articular surface with the distal radius and another with the TFCC (Dobbs 2003). The articular surfaces of the DRUJ are incongruous and therefore vulnerable to translational dorsal and volar instability (Kleinman 2007).

The bones of the proximal carpal row are the scaphoid, lunate, triquetrum and pisiform. These carpals move with greater degrees of rotation to each other than do the carpals of the distal row. The lunate, which is coronally wedge shaped, has a tendency to dislocate into the dorsal direction from the scaphoid; it is additionally the most frequently dislocated carpal (Wadsworth 1988; Schmitt et al 2006).

The distal carpal row consists of the trapezium, trapezoid, capitate and hamate. This is a more solid functional unit than the proximal row, and with less intercarpal movement. The distal and proximal carpal rows articulate through the mid-carpal joint. The mid-carpal joint is a combination of three joints: the scaphotrapezoid–trapezial (STT) with scaphocapitate components in the lateral compartment, the capitolunate central compartment and the hamatotriquetral medial compartment (Schmitt et al 2006). Carlsen and Shin (2008) described the anatomy of the mid-carpal joint somewhat differently, in terms of the scaphocapitate / lunocapitate central articulation and the triquetrohamate medial articulation. This mid-carpal joint, as a whole, is compared to a ball and socket joint, with the capitate often intruding into the scapholunate gap (Schmitt et al 2006).

Ligamentous anatomy and stabilization

The ligaments of the wrist are classified as intra-articular or intracapsular. Intracapsular ligaments are integrated in the capsular sheaths and are either intrinsic or extrinsic to the carpus (Schmitt et al 2006). Schmitt et al (2006) described the interosseous scapholunate ligament (SLL, SLIL), interosseous lunotriquetral ligament (LTL) and mid-carpal ligaments as intra-articular. Carlsen and Shin (2008), in contrast, stated that all wrist ligaments are intracapsular with the exception of the transverse carpal ligament, the pisohamate ligament and the pisometacarpal ligament. They based this description on the intracapsular ligaments being contained in 'loose connective tissue and fat' (Carlsen & Shin 2008), which was previously poorly visualized with open surgical inspection.

The SLL (Fig. 49.1) is considered to be the most important and is the one most often injured. Each of the three SLL segments performs different biomechanical functions. It is centrally composed of fibrocartilage that merges with the articular cartilage of the scaphoid and the lunate (Linscheid & Dobyns 2002). The fibrocartilage section, or middle segment, lacks stabilizing function and is prone to degenerative injury (Ozcelik et al 2005; Schmitt et al 2006). It is the dorsal segment that is vital to scapholunate compartment stability. Rotary subluxation of the scaphoid and symptomatic scapholunate dissociation develops with the rupture of this segment (Schmitt et al 2006).

The LTL (see Fig. 49.1) plays a role in the stability of the lunotriquetral compartment similar to that of the SLL in the scapholunate compartment. It is smaller than the SLL but

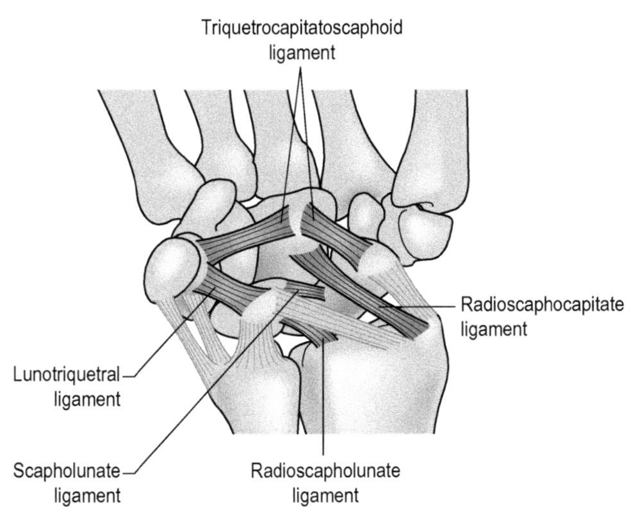

Figure 49.1 Critical volar stabilizing ligaments (right hand).

similarly shaped, and the central or middle segment, which is also prone to degeneration, has no stabilizing function. It is the volar segment, however, rather than the dorsal segment that maintains functional stability of the lunotriquetral compartment (Schmitt et al 2006).

Whereas the SLL and the LTL are intrinsic stabilizers of the proximal carpal row, three short extrinsic interosseous ligaments stabilize the scaphoid and lunate. The radioscapholunate ligament (RSLL) (see Fig. 49.1) is unique in that it has been proposed to carry an anterior interosseous nerve and artery to the proximal pole of the scaphoid (Schmitt et al 2006). These interosseous ligaments are deep and transverse, whereas the superficial and oblique complex is termed the **V-ligament** system (Schmitt et al 2006). This system includes the important volar support band or radioscaphocapitate ligament (RSCL) (see Fig. 49.1), which helps to stabilize the radiocarpal joint with an oblique orientation that prevents carpus translocation (Schmitt et al 2006). Disruption of the RSCL is a primary cause of scapholunate and capitolunate dissociation (Ozcelik et al 2005). The triquetrocapitatoscaphoid ligament (TCSL) (see Fig. 49.1) has a loose triquetrocapitate section, which is called the **ulnar link,** and a tight capitoscaphoid portion. This is an important stabilizer of the mid-carpal joint. The RSCL and TCSL together with others that make up the volar V-shaped complex are stronger and more supportive than the dorsal complex (Schmitt et al 2006). In the proximal portion of the volar V-ligament, disruption of the radiolunotriquetral ligament will result in lunotriquetral dissociation (Ozcelik et al 2005).

Prevention of axial (columnar) instability is the task of the transverse intercarpal ligaments and the flexor retinaculum (Schmitt et al 2006). These make up the support of the distal carpal row.

Stability of the DRUJ is minimally supported extrinsically by the interosseous mid-forearm ligament. The TFCC intrinsic radioulnar dorsal and palmer ligaments provide effective ligamentous stability (Kleinman 2007).

Muscular anatomy

The most relevant contribution of the muscular anatomy to stability of the carpus concerns the finding that both wrist flexors and extensors generate their maximum forces with the wrist fully extended (Lieber & Friden 1998). Indeed, there is an almost constant ratio of flexor to extensor torque over the wrist range of motion (Lieber & Friden 1998). This is possible, despite the flexors having a larger physiological cross-section area, because of the superior extensor moment over the flexor moment. Thus the wrist is most stable in extension and its design is biased towards balance and control instead of maximum torque (Lieber & Friden 1998).

Kleinman (2007) additionally described the tension of the extensor carpi ulnaris tendon across the ulna distal head with the superficial and deep heads of the pronator quadratus as important to dynamic stability of the DRUJ.

Biomechanics

An important consideration in understanding forces across the wrist is that there are no tendons attaching directly to the carpal bones, excluding the pisiform; however, the pisiform is a sesamoid bone within the tendon of the flexor carpi ulnaris, and this relationship is not considered to be significant in carpal stability (Bednar & Osterman 1993). The forces are summed across the carpus as the movement of the wrist begins distally with tendons inserted at the base of the metacarpals. The motion of the carpus is initiated at the distal row with forces proceeding from the distal to the proximal carpal row. The forces at the scaphoid–lunate–capitate compartment comprise 60% of the total force, with the remainder distributing at the radius–lunate joint and ulnocarpal compartment, according to Schmitt et al (2006). Thus movement of the proximal carpal row depends on the compressive forces of the distal row as well as the support of the ligamentous attachments (Bozentka 1999).

Flexion–extension and radial–ulnar deviation are the two planes of motion produced by the carpal joints. Flexion–extension total movement is an average of 121–150° (Bednar & Osterman 1993; De Filippo et al 2006). This motion is split between the radiocarpal and mid-carpal joints. The radial–ulnar deviation total movement is an average of 45–50°, with a distribution of 60% at the mid-carpal joint and 40% at the radiocarpal joint (Bednar & Osterman 1993; De Filippo et al 2006).

The scaphoid and lunate move dorsally and radially during wrist extension. Volar and ulnar movement of the scaphoid and lunate occur with wrist flexion. This scapholunate movement is three times greater than the lunotriquetral movement. With the scaphoid having the widest arc of rotation, both flexion and extension of the wrist effect a spatial change among the carpus elements. This intricate and specific mechanism must be intact to ensure carpal stability (De Filippo et al 2006).

The TFCC central articular disc reportedly bears the burden of load transmission from the medial carpus to the forearm when the wrist is ulnarly deviated (Kleinman 2007). With the forearm in neutral radioulnar deviation, the load passes from the mid-carpus to the distal radius interfossal ridge with a distribution of 84% to the radius and 16% to the TFCC disc (Kleinman 2007). The reader is referred to the work of Kleinman (2007) for an extensive discussion of DRUJ biomechanics.

Aetiopathogenesis

An understanding of patterns and classification of instability in the wrist is necessary to the discussion of aetiopathogenesis. Each advance in the evolving project of the classification of instability is accompanied by further understanding of common cause and effect on specific tissue or structure.

Patterns and classification

Recognized patterns and areas of carpal and wrist instability

There are three basic patterns of instability to consider, although each of these patterns has additional classification, which will be delineated later in this section. The patterns are based on radiological appearance. **Predynamic instability** refers to a clinical diagnosis without support of abnormalities seen on a radiograph. **Dynamic instability** has a clinical diagnosis plus altered kinematics viewed on special but not standard radiographs; it occurs, but inconsistently, when the carpals are loaded under certain conditions. **Static instability** is supported by clinical diagnosis and altered kinematics appearing on conventional radiographs; the malalignment is evident with any amount of load applied (Garcia-Elias 1997b; Van Rooyen 2005).

Classification of carpal and wrist instability

Linscheid et al (1972) are credited with the first classification of carpal instability. Their work identified two general types: dorsal and volar (Linscheid et al 1972), of which **dorsal intercalary segment instability** (DISI) is the more common. De Filippo et al (2006) attributed DISI to scaphotrapezoidal ligament injury, a non-union or badly healed trans-scaphoid fracture, or scapholunate ligament injury. DISI is detected with a lateral view plain film in which a dorsal tilt of the lunate is seen, along with aberrant capitolunate and scapholunate angles (De Filippo et al 2006). With the same plain film view, a **volar intercalary segment** (VISI) malalignment is evident with a volar tilt to the lunate (Garcia-Elias 1997a). VISI is described as caused by dissociation of the lunotriquetral, radiotriquetral or scaphotriquetral joints, as well as by badly healed and / or displaced fractures of these carpals (De Filippo et al 2006).

The Mayo Clinic system is currently the most widely known and used classification (Carlsen & Shin 2008). This system groups instabilities according to pattern: **carpal instability dissociative** (CID), **carpal instability non-dissociative** (CIND), **carpal instability combined** (CIC) and **adaptive carpal instability** (CIA).

Instability between individual carpals in the same row and involving the intrinsic ligaments is CID. An example of this is scapholunate dissociation. Progressive scapholunate dissociation (CID) becomes DISI before ending in severe degenerative arthritis, which is described as scapholunate advanced collapse (SLAC) (Bozentka 1999).

Instability that causes aberration of the entire proximal row at the radiocarpal and mid-carpal joints and involves the extrinsic ligaments is CIND (Garcia-Elias 1997b; Van Rooyen 2005). Perilunate instability results in CIND owing to the complex pathology at the radiocarpal and intercarpal levels.

Instability with combined involvement of the intra-row and inter-row intrinsic and extrinsic ligaments is CIC. De Filippo et al (2006) listed lunate dislocation as a typical example of CIC.

CIA is best described as instability of the carpals caused by pathology that is either distal or proximal to the carpals, but not within the wrist. An example of this is pathology at the distal radius from either a malunited fracture or Madelung's deformity (Van Rooyen 2005; Schmitt et al 2006; Carlsen & Shin 2008).

Discussion of DRUJ instability functionally includes the triangular fibrocartilage complex (TFCC). TFCC tears are classified by the Mayo Clinic system as traumatic tears and degenerative tears. Traumatic tears are classed as: (I) radial rim detachment, (II) central tears, (III) ulnar tears, and (IV) palmar tears. Degenerative tears are classed as: (I) central tears, (II) central tear with ulnocarpal impingement, (III) central tear with impingement and lunotriquetral ligament tear, and (IV) central tear, with impingement and lunotriquetral arthritis (Van Rooyen 2005). TFCC pathology can result from degenerative changes without causing DRUJ instability, however (Van Rooyen 2005).

Additional reading is recommended to follow the evolving classifications as knowledge of carpal biomechanics expanded, to include the views of Lichtman (Van Rooyen 2005; Lichtman & Wroten 2006) and Amadio (De Filippo et al 2006). Carlsen and Shin (2008) describe the Mayo system in greater detail, including the subdivisions.

Pathogenesis

Destruction of the wrist ligaments, through trauma or degeneration, and alteration of the bony articular surfaces are responsible for wrist instability. Two frequent types of instability due to malunited distal radius fractures are noted: mid-carpal and radiocarpal. Adaptive mid-carpal malalignments occur with the body's attempt to realign the hand to the malunion. Carpal ligaments and radiocarpal capsule are not disrupted. Pathological radiocarpal malalignments occur from injury to the radiocarpal ligaments and joint capsule during the fracture incident and result in instability of the radiolunate joint (Gupta et al 2002).

Pathological abnormalities of intra-articular ligaments in rheumatoid arthritis occur as a result of pannus invasion and destruction, while the abnormalities in calcium pyrophosphate deposition disease occur result from calcific deposition and cystic degeneration (Resnick & Niwayama 1977).

An additional cause of wrist instability at the scapholunate interval was reported by Mehdian and McKee (2005) to be excision of a dorsal wrist ganglion; the postulated reason for this occurring was that manipulation under anaesthesia of the wrist to recover from the ganglion-induced stiffness had triggered the instability.

Examination and Diagnosis

Diagnostic considerations

Cooney et al (1990) described an algorithm for diagnosis that included clinical examination, report of the patient's symptoms and use of provocative stress testing that would together determine, in absence of pathological standard radiographic examination results, an appropriate portal of entry for additional tests (e.g. arthrogram or arthroscopy). (See Chs 3–5 for the basic initial examination and history taking.)

Clinical tests

General mid-carpal tests

The mid-carpal shift test was described by Feinstein et al (1999) as a valid and useful clinical diagnostic test for indicating mid-carpal non-dissociative carpal instability. The examiner stabilizes the patient's forearm in pronation with one hand and, with the other, places a thumb over the patient's dorsal distal capitate. The thumb directs a palmar force via the capitate, allowing translation to occur. Maintaining this pressure, the examiner provides passive ulnar deviation to the patient's wrist. A positive test consists of a degree of clunking and / or laxity during the ulnar deviation. Dysfunction of stabilizing ligaments is thought to cause a loss of normal joint reaction forces between the proximal and distal carpal rows, resulting in loss of smooth translation (Feinstein et al 1999). The test was reviewed under videofluoroscopy, which showed that the proximal carpal row maintained a flexed volar position rather than moving smoothly from flexion to extension as the wrist was moved into ulnar deviation. Instead, the proximal row then suddenly snapped into extension once the ulnar deviation was achieved, hence the 'clunk' (Lichtman & Wroten 2006).

Scapholunate, second and third carpometacarpal joints and capitolunate tests

The scaphoid stress test (scaphoid shift test, Watson's test, SST, modified scaphoid shear test) is the most commonly used clinical test for the detection of scapholunate instability (Christodoulou & Bainbridge 1999). Rodner and Weiss (2008) noted that it might be difficult to perform the test well initially where there is swelling and pain. The examiner places a thumb on the scaphoid tubercle, applying pressure volar to dorsal, and passively moves the patient's wrist from ulnar deviation and slight extension into radial deviation with slight flexion (Fig. 49.2). The scaphoid will become prominent under the examiner's thumb with the movement to radial deviation. When the thumb pressure is removed, a positive test will demonstrate the scaphoid returning to position with an often painful and palpable 'clunk'. The clunk is thought to occur when, due to laxity or pathology, the proximal pole of the scaphoid shifts onto the dorsal rim of the radius with thumb pressure; then it returns with a clunk when the pressure is removed (Skirven 1996). The test is also meaningful when it reproduces pain over the scapholunate interval (Rodner & Weiss 2008). According to LaStayo and Howell (1995), this test was found to have a sensitivity of 69%, a specificity of 66%, a positive predictive value of 48% and a negative predictive value of 78% relative to arthroscopic findings in 50 painful wrists.

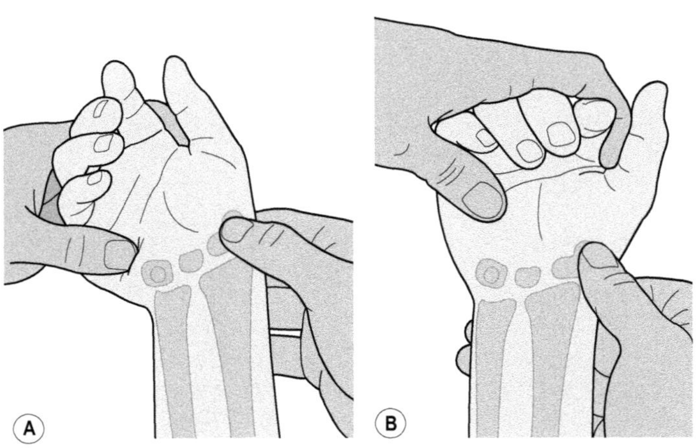

Figure 49.2 Scaphoid stress test: (**A**) The examiner applies pressure to scaphoid with wrist in ulnar deviation and extension. (**B**) The examiner maintains pressure while performing radial deviation and flexion of the wrist, noting any 'clunk' or pain.

Watson described the wrist-flexion finger-extension manoeuvre as an additional test of scapholunate instability (Skirven 1996). Truong et al (1994) included this test in their screening criteria that, in combination, had a sensitivity of 88.5% and a specificity of 84%. The patient's wrist is positioned in flexion while the examiner applies resistance against finger extension, the test being positive if this causes pain in the scapholunate region (Truong et al 1994).

The synovial irritation sign of the scaphoid has high sensitivity but low specificity for detecting scaphoid instability. Van Buul et al (1993) found that a positive synovial irritation sign test had significantly higher incidence in patients with suspected carpal instability. A positive test consists of pain elicited when the examiner provides pressure on the scaphoid through the anatomical snuffbox (van Buul et al 1993).

Still assessing the radial wrist, the Linscheid test produces pain in the second and third carpometacarpal joints when positive (Skirven 1996). The examiner supports the patient's metacarpal shafts while pressing into the distal metacarpal heads in both dorsal and volar directions (Skirven 1996).

The dorsal capitate–displacement test was found clinically to reproduce successfully a dorsal subluxation of the capitolunate or the capitolunate and radiolunate joints (Lichtman & Wroten 2006). A capitolunate instability pattern was described and tested in this way by Louis et al (1984) under videofluoroscopy in a series of 11 patients (Lichtman & Wroten 2006). The examiner applied pressure to the scaphoid tuberosity in a dorsal direction while simultaneously performing longitudinal traction and passive flexion to the patient's wrist. This produced nearly complete dorsal subluxation of the capitate from the lunate and reproduced the patient's pain in that area (Louis et al 1984). Instability was credited to dynamic laxity of the radiolunate ligaments and extrinsic scaphoid stabilizers, along with laxity of the dorsal capitolunate ligament complex (Louis et al 1984).

Lunotriquetral tests

The lunotriquetral (LT) ballottement test (Reagan's test) indicates LT instability with production of pain and / or excessive motion as the examiner translates the pisiform and triquetrum (together) volarly and dorsally relative to the stabilized lunate (Rodner & Weiss 2008). The test is performed with the examiner using the thumb and index finger of one hand to hold the patient's lunate while holding the triquetrum in the contralateral hand and providing simultaneous movement of the two bones against each other (Dobbs 2003) (Fig. 49.3). A positive result is where there is reproduction of pain, crepitus or excessive laxity. A sensitivity of 64%, a specificity of 44%, a positive predictive value of 24% and a negative predictive value of 81% were reported by LaStayo and Howell (1995) for this test, although Dobbs (2003) later described an inconsistent sensitivity of 33–100% (Dobbs 2003).

Kleinman's shear test does not stabilize the lunate but does, similarly to Reagan's test, apply dorsal translation to the pisiform and concurrent volar translation to the lunate for symptoms indicating LT instability, and it is one of three clinical tests that have been reported to be specific to LT injury (Dobbs 2003). The examiner places several fingers dorsal to the patient's lunate with a thumb on the latter's pisotriquetral joint (Skirven 1996), though other authors have described the use of the examiner's thumb on the lunate with the

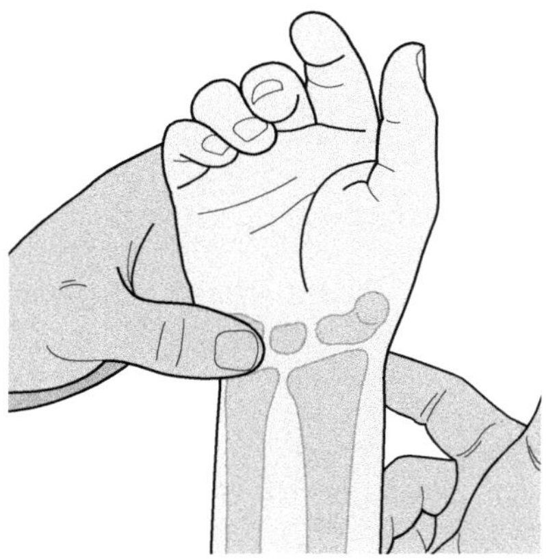

Figure 49.3 Lunotriquetral ballottement test. The examiner uses the thumb (not shown) and index finger of one hand to hold the patient's lunate while holding the triquetrum in the contralateral hand and providing simultaneous movement of these bones against one another, looking for pain, crepitus or excessive laxity.

contralateral thumb on the pisotriquetral joint (Dobbs 2003). While the lunate is stabilized, the thumb provides a volar-to-dorsal direction of force that creates a shear across the LT joint. The examiner then deviates the wrist first in the ulnar and then in the radial direction. Elicitation of pain or clicking demonstrates a positive test (Skirven 1996).

Dobbs (2003) also described the ulnar snuffbox compression test (Linscheid's test, LT compression test) as poorly specific for LT instability. The test is positive if pain is reproduced as the examiner pushes the patient's triquetrum into the lunate from the ulnar wrist, specifically in the sulcus, or snuffbox, which is formed by the extensor carpi ulnaris and flexor carpi ulnaris tendons (Skirven 1996; Rodner & Weiss 2008).

Distal radioulnar joint and triangular fibrocartilage complex tests

The piano-key test is a variation of the piano-key sign, and is used to assess for distal radioulnar joint DRUJ instability. The examiner stabilizes the radius with one hand while the other hand grasps the patient's distal ulna and moves it in dorsal and volar directions, with the forearm positioned in various degrees of pronation and supination. A positive test includes reproduction of pain, tenderness and hypermobility compared with the uninvolved side (Skirven 1996).

As mentioned earlier, the triangular fibrocartilage complex (TFCC) contributes to DRUJ stability, but it is not known whether clinical tests for DRUJ instability accurately demonstrate instability caused from tears of the triangular ligament of the TFCC (Moriya et al 2009). The biomechanical study of Moriya et al (2009), although limited, supported the DRUJ ballottement test but not the piano-key test or the ulnocarpal abutment test as having a statistically significant degree of accuracy in demonstrating this concept.

LaStayo and Howell (1995) examined the ulnomeniscotriquetral (UMT) dorsal glide test for pathology of the TFCC. The technique for this test has the patient's elbow resting on a table with forearm in neutral and vertical position. The patient's distal radius is stabilized by a golfer's grip of the examiner's hand. With the other hand, the examiner places his index finger (digit 2) curled such that the radial side of the proximal interphalangeal joint contacts the patient's volar pisotriquetral complex. With this finger providing dorsal pressure, the examiner simultaneously uses the thumb to apply volar pressure against the dorsal distal ulna, producing a dorsal glide of the pisotriquetral complex on the distal ulnar head. A positive test results in reproduction of the patient's pain and / or laxity in the UMT area (Hertling & Kessler 1996). LaStayo and Howell (1995) reported a sensitivity of 66%, a specificity of 64%, a positive predictive value of 58% and a negative predictive value of 69% for this test.

Radiological tests, diagnostic dynamic ultrasound and arthroscopy

Radiographic examination of the wrist ranges from standard static views to special dynamic positions and loading conditions, as well as complex films such as videofluoroscopy and arthrogram (Garcia-Elias 2006), in which the ultimate goal is to display the gap between dissociated bones. Toms et al (2009), in a small but relevant study, indicated that dynamic ultrasound may confirm mid-carpal instability via a triquetral catch-up clunk. However, it is wrist arthroscopy that is becoming the gold standard, although clinical tests are widely used to regionalize the pertinent area (Reynolds et al 1998; Garcia-Elias 2006). Arthroscopy versus open arthrotomy avoids suspension of the wrist under traction, enabling otherwise occult differences in ligament appearance to be revealed (Cooney et al 1990).

Treatment and Prognosis

Conservative treatment and prognosis

Additional research is needed to determine true efficacy of conservative treatment, including manual therapy of soft tissue and joint, for wrist instability. Most available information for manual therapy treatment of the wrist has focused on treatment of carpal tunnel syndrome, with positive outcomes noted (Burke et al 2007; O'Conner et al 2003).

The literature supports carpal manipulation for wrist instability as a diagnostic rather than a treatment tool. Manipulation is used to evoke signs whereas palpation is used to evoke symptoms during physical examination of the wrist (Dobbs 2003; Young et al 2007). Conservative treatment described in the literature has emphasized patient education, splinting and exercises (Hofmeister et al 2006; Lichtman & Wroten 2006; Prosser et al 2007).

Hofmeister et al (2006) reported temporary pain relief, at best, with conservative treatments including immobilization, splinting, non-steroidal medications and intra-articular injections. Most splinting consists of general immobilization after acute injury such as sprain or dislocation. Splints are often custom-made for best fit, and are dorsal or volar, thumb free or protected, depending on the location of the injured structure (Coppard & Lohman 2001).

Weiss et al (2000) recommended taping, splinting and anti-inflammatory medications for the athlete with a partial or complete membranous central tear of the LT ligament (with no VISI). The splint should be carefully moulded with a pad under the pisiform to attempt optimal alignment (Shin et al

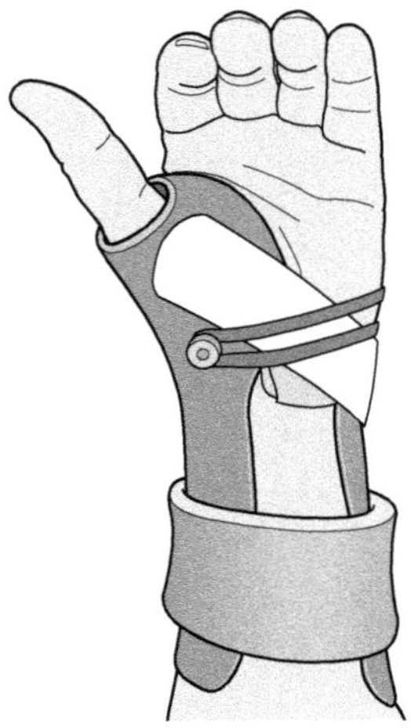

Figure 49.4 **DISI custom splint.**

2000). Patients with this type of injury and protocol are estimated to require 3–6 months for recovery (Weiss et al 2000).

Lichtman and Wroten (2006) supported a trial of conservative treatment as useful in only one of four instability types: that of dorsal mid-carpal instability. Garcia-Elias (1997a) concurred, with the added specification of a dorsal mid-carpal type termed the 'capitate lunate instability pattern' (CLIP), which is usually due to congenital laxity. A custom-made dorsal splint with a dynamic component, termed a **DISI splint** or **Lichtman splint** (Fig. 49.4), is the only orthotic specifically supported for this application (S. Kamal, personal communication, 2009).

Specific statistics for prognosis following conservative treatment are unavailable. The literature does agree, however, that prognosis has an increased chance of being favourable (not requiring surgery for restoration of function) if the injury is conservatively treated in the acute phase (Israeli et al 1981; Bednar & Osterman 1993; Garcia-Elias 1997a; Shin et al 2000; Lichtman & Wroten 2006). However, conservative treatment is not recommended for chronic wrist instability.

Surgical treatment and prognosis

Surgical interventions are performed when pain is intractable and affects quality of life. Carlsen and Shin (2008) listed the primary considerations that determine course of treatment as: arthritic changes, injury onset (chronicity), probability of the tissues, based on quality, to withstand surgical repair, and the ability of the surgeon to reduce the deformity. An ideal candidate for surgical repair would have an acute injury with reducible deformity and tissues of good quality (Carlsen & Shin 2008).

Decisions for choices of surgical procedure – such as Kirshner wire (K-wire), bone–ligament–bone graft, partial carpal fusion or arthrodesis, mid-carpal or four corner fusion and proximal row carpectomy – are based on the considerations above, as well as degree and location of injury (Garcia-Elias 2006). Other surgical options include: arthroscopic or open debridement including ligament and synovectomy, capsulodesis, and ligament repair or reconstruction; there is also anterior and posterior interosseous neurectomy (Hofmeister et al 2006; Johnston et al 2009). Prognosis is as widely varied as are the factors of cause, specific pathology, technique and skill of the surgeon.

Conclusion

Wrist instability is only now becoming accurately and successfully identified, classified and treated, owing to recent improvements in technology and a development of the knowledge base over the last 25 years. Arthroscopy in particular has allowed a relatively undisturbed view of the anatomy, biomechanics and pathology of the wrist that has been incorporated into the body of classifications, clinical tests, formal diagnoses and treatments.

The current literature supports manual interventions by the clinician for clinical tests, but not for conservative treatment in chronic wrist instability. Conservative treatment, consisting primarily of patient education, splinting and exercises is most efficacious when applied acutely.

Additional research is necessary to improve the reliability and validity of clinical testing as the aforementioned knowledge base of wrist anatomy and biomechanics improves. Tailoring of splint applications to specific pathological and functional needs will probably improve conservative treatment outcomes, but this must be diligently pursued and recorded in order to develop evidence-based treatment.

References

Bednar JM, Ostermann AL. 1993. Carpal instability: evaluation and treatment. J Am Acad Orthop Surg 1: 10–17.

Bozentka DJ. 1999. Scapholunate instability. Univ Penn Orthop J 12: 27–32.

Burke J, Buchberger DJ, Carey-Loghmani MT, et al. 2007. A pilot study comparing two manual therapy interventions for carpal tunnel syndrome. J Manipulative Physiol Ther 30: 50–61.

Carlsen BT, Shin AY. 2008. Wrist instability. Scand J Surg 97 324–332.

Christodoulou L, Bainbridge LC. 1999. Clinical diagnosis of triquetrolunate ligament injuries. J Hand Surg Br 24B: 598–600.

Cooney WP, Dobyns JH, Linscheid, RL. 1990. Arthroscopy of the wrist: anatomy and classification of carpal instability. Arthroscopy 6: 133–140.

Coppard BM, Lohman H. 2001. Introduction to splinting. A clinical-reasoning and problem-solving approach, 2nd edn. St Louis, MO: Mosby, pp 139–241.

De Filippo M, Sudberry JJ, Lombardo E, et al. 2006. Pathogenesis and evolution of carpal instability: imaging and topography. Acta Biomed 77: 168–180.

Dias JJ, Garcia-Elias M. 2006. Hand injury costs. Injury 37: 1071–1077.

Dobbs A. 2003. The ulnar side of the wrist. Eugene, OR: North American Institute of Orthopaedic Manual Therapy 8: pp 1–5.

Dumontier C. 1996. Physical examination of wrist instabilities. Maitrise Orthop 49. [Online orthopedic journal.]

Feinstein WK, Lichtman DM, Noble PC, et al. 1999. Quantitative assessment of the midcarpal shift test. J Hand Surg Am 24: 977–983.

Garcia-Elias M. 1997a. The treatment of wrist instability. J Bone Joint Surg 79B (4): 684–690.

Garcia-Elias M. 1997b. Kinetic analysis of carpal stability during grip. Hand Clin 13: 151–158.

Garcia-Elias M. 2006. Treatment of scapholunate instability. Ortop Traumatol Rehabil 2: 160–168.

Gupta A, Batra S, Jain P, et al. 2002. Carpal alignment in distal radius fractures. BMC Musculoskelet Disord 3: 14.

Hertling D, Kessler RM. 1996. Management of common musculoskeletal disorders: physical therapy principals and methods, 3rd edn. Philadelphia: Lippincott-Raven, p 278.

Hofmeister EP, Moran SL, Shin AY. 2006. Anterior and posterior interosseous neurectomy for the treatment of chronic dynamic instability of the wrist. Hand 1: 63–70.

Israeli A, Ganel A, Engel J. 1981. Post traumatic ligamentous instability of the wrist. Br J Sports Med 15: 17–19.

Johnston K, Durand D, Hildebrand KA, et al. 2009. Chronic volar distal radioulnar joint instability: joint capsular placation to restore function. Can J Surg 52: 112–118.
Kleinman WB. 2007. Stability of the distal radioulnar joint: biomechanics, pathophysiology, physical diagnosis, and restoration of function what we have learned in 25 years. J Hand Surg 32A: 1086–1106.
LaStayo P, Howell J. 1995. Clinical provocative tests used in evaluating wrist pain: a descriptive study. J Hand Ther 8: 10–17.
Lichtman DM, Wroten ES. 2006. Understanding midcarpal instability. J Hand Surg 31A: 491–498.
Lieber RL, Friden J. 1998. Musculoskeletal balance of the human wrist elucidated using intraoperative laser diffraction. J Electromyogr Kinesiol 8: 93–100.
Linscheid RL, Dobyns JH. 2002. Dynamic carpal stability. Keio J Med 51: 140–147.
Linscheid RL, Dobyns JH, Beabout JW, et al. 1972. Traumatic instability of the wrist: diagnosis, classification and pathomechanics. J Bone Joint Surg Am 54: 1612–1632.
Louis DS, Hankin FM, Greene TL, et al. 1984. Central carpal instability – capitate lunate instability pattern: diagnosis by dynamic displacement. Orthopedics 7: 1693–1696.
Mehdian H, McKee D. 2005. Scapholunate instability following dorsal wrist ganglion excision: a case report. Iowa Orthop J 25: 203–206.
Moriya T, Aoki M, Iba K, et al. 2009. Effect of triangular ligament tears on distal radioulnar joint instability and evaluation of three clinical tests: a biomechanical study. J Hand Surg Eur 34E: 219–223.
O'Conner D, Marshall SC, Massey-Westropp N. 2003. Non-surgical treatment (other than steroid injection) for carpal tunnel syndrome. Cochrane Database Syst Rev 1: CD0033219. doi: 10.1002/14651858.CD003219.
Ozcelik A, Gunal I, Kose N, et al. 2005. Wrist ligaments: their significance in carpal instability. TJTES 11: 115–120.
Perron AD, Brady WJ, Keats TE, et al. 2001. Orthopedic pitfalls in the ED: lunate and perilunate injuries. Am J Emerg Med 19: 157–162.
Prosser R, Herbert R, LaStayo PC. 2007. Current practice in the diagnosis and treatment of carpal instability – results of a survey of Australian hand therapists. J Hand Ther 20: 239–242.
Resnick D, Niwayama G. 1977. Carpal instability in rheumatoid arthritis and calcium pyrophosphate deposition disease. Pathogenesis and roentgen appearance. Ann Rheum Dis 36: 311–318.
Reynolds RAK, Johnston GHF, Friedman L, et al. 1998. The carpal stretch test. Can J Surg 41: 119–126.
Rodner CM, Weiss APC. 2008. Acute scapholunate and lunotriquetral dissociation. Fractures of the upper extremity: a master skills publication. Chicago, IL: American Society for Surgery of the Hand, Ch 10, pp 155–171.
Schmitt R, Froehner S, Coblenz G, et al. 2006. Carpal instability. Eur Radiol 16: 2161–2178.
Shin AY, Battaglia MJ, Bishop AT. 2000. Lunotriquetral instability: diagnosis and treatment. J Am Acad Orthop Surg 8: 170–179.
Skirven T. 1996. Clinical examination of the wrist. J Hand Ther 9: 96–107.
Surdziel P, Lubiatowski P. 2006. Scapholunate instability: natural history, diagnostics and therapeutic algorithm. Ortop Traumatol Rehabil 8: 115–121.
Tang JB. 1992. Carpal instability associated with fracture of the distal radius. Incidence, influencing factors and pathomechanics. Chin Med J 105: 758–765.
Toms A, Chojnowski A, Cahir J. 2009. Midcarpal instability: a diagnostic role for dynamic ultrasound? Ultraschall Med 30: 286–290.
Truong NP, Mann FA, Gilula LA, et al. 1994. Wrist instability series: increased yield with clinical–radiologic screening criteria. Radiology 192: 481–484.
van Buul MM, Bos KE, Dijkstra PF, et al. 1993. Carpal instability, the missed diagnosis in patients with clinically suspected scaphoid fracture. Injury 24 257–262.
Van Rooyen C. 2005. Radiologic evaluation of the hand and wrist. In: McKinnis LN (ed) Fundamentals of musculoskeletal imaging, 2nd edn. Philadelphia: FA Davis, pp 509–521.
Wadsworth C. 1988. Manual examination and treatment of the spine and extremities. Philadelphia: Williams & Wilkins, p 154.
Weiss LE, Taras JS, Sweet S, et al. 2000. Lunotriquetral injuries in the athlete. Hand Clin 16: 433–438.
Werner FW, Short WH, Green JK, et al. 2007. Severity of scapholunate instability is related to joint anatomy and congruency. J Hand Surg Am 32: 55–60.
Wolfe SW, Crisco JJ, Orr CM, et al. 2006. Clinical perspective: the dart-throwing motion of the wrist: is it unique to humans? J Hand Surg 31A: 1429–1437.
Young D, Papp S, Giachino A. 2007. Physical examination of the wrist. Orthop Clin North Am 38: 149–165.

50 Chapter

Carpal Tunnel Syndrome

Luca Padua, Daniele Coraci, César Fernández-de-las-Peñas

CHAPTER CONTENTS

Introduction	566
Anatomy	566
Patho-biomechanism of carpal tunnel syndrome	567
Sensory and motor aspects in carpal tunnel syndrome	568
Diagnosis of carpal tunnel syndrome	568
Clinical examination	568
Questionnaires	569
Electrodiagnostic evaluation	569
Ultrasound assessment	569
Prognosis	570
Prognosis of untreated carpal tunnel syndrome	570
Therapy	571
Carpal tunnel syndrome and pregnancy	571
Conclusion	572

Introduction

Carpal tunnel syndrome (CTS) is characterized by compression of the median nerve in the carpal tunnel. It is a common pathology affecting an estimated 10% of the population, according to the American Academy of Neurology (AAN 1993a, 1993b; Olney 2001). It is considered the most common nerve compression disorder of the arm, with reported prevalence rates of 3.8% (95% confidence interval (CI) 3.1–4.6%) for women and 2.7% (95% CI 2.1–3.4%) for men (Atroshi et al 1999). Bland and Rudolfer (2003) found an annual incidence of 139.4 cases per 100 000 females and 67.2 cases per 100 000 males, with a female: male ratio of 2:1. Bongers et al (2007) have reported an incidence rate of CTS of 1.8 / 1000 (95% CI 1.7–2.0). In females the incidence was 2.8 (95% CI 2.6–3.1) and in males 0.9 (95% CI 0.8–1.0), showing a female: male ratio of 3:1 (Bongers et al 2007). Additionally, this study showed that in 2001 the incidence of CTS was calculated to be 1.5 times higher than in 1987 (however, this difference disappeared after subdividing patients by age and sex) (Bongers et al 2007). A more recent study has reported an annual prevalence of 3.1% for CTS on active workers, representing 4.8 million people in the United States (USA) (Luckhaupt et al 2013). This study also found an overall lifetime prevalence of CTS of 6.7% in workers (Luckhaupt et al 2013). Dale et al (2013) pooled the epidemiological data of CTS and reported an overall prevalence rate of 7.8% and an incidence rate of 2.3 / 100 persons / year. Analysis of the literature raises the difficulty of accurately estimating the incidence and prevalence of CTS because it is a common pathology and, as we discuss below, can be associated with manual and repetitive work. This last controversial association means that the incidence and prevalence of CTS are often calculated in a specific work population, as in the study by Luckhaupt et al (2013). Moreover, another confounding factor could be the method used to diagnose CTS, as Atroshi et al (1999) reported; in their study, the combination of clinical and neurophysiological evaluations contributed to physicians diagnosing CTS in one of five symptomatic subjects from the general population.

Two decades ago, it was been estimated that in the USA around 1 million people required care for CTS, around 200 000 surgical interventions were needed and that the social costs were in the range of millions of dollars (Tanaka et al 1995). A decade later, a study by Stapleton (2006) found that CTS aggregated health costs of approximately US$ 2 billion annually in the USA.

Anatomy

In the carpal tunnel the median nerve is surrounded by bones on three sides with the transverse carpal ligament on the top. The transverse carpal ligament is a fibrous structure constituted by dense connective tissue (Fig. 50.1), with a clear predominance of transverse fibres (61%) in the pisiform–trapezium and scaphoid–hamate direction (Prantil et al 2012). Furthermore, the transverse carpal ligament exhibits high neural nociceptive innervation (Mashoof et al 2001). The median nerve lies within the nine flexor tendons of the hand, and supplies function, feeling and movement to the first three digits of the hand and one-half of the ring finger (Fig. 50.2).

The median branches for the finger and wrist flexors originate in the forearm, whereas the motor branches that control the thumb flexor and adductor muscles, and the sensory branches that provide over half the hand with the sense of touch, usually originate at the end of the tunnel. Compression of the nerve can be due to a decrease in the size of the canal, an increase of the size of tendons, or both.

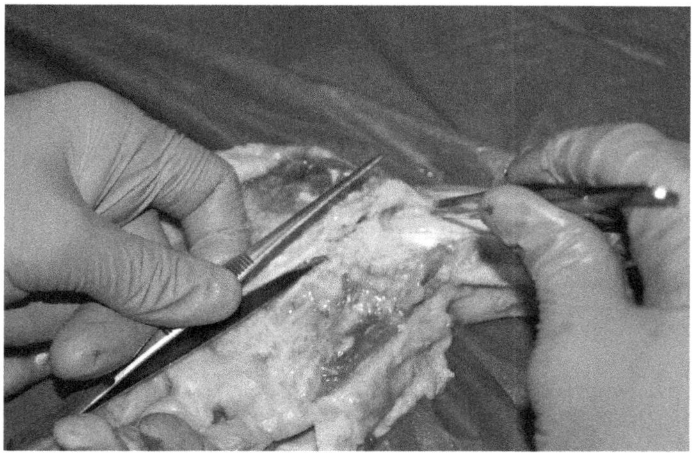

Figure 50.1 Dissection of a right hand in a human cadaver. The figure shows the connective tissue of the transverse carpal ligament and the transverse disposition of the fibres.

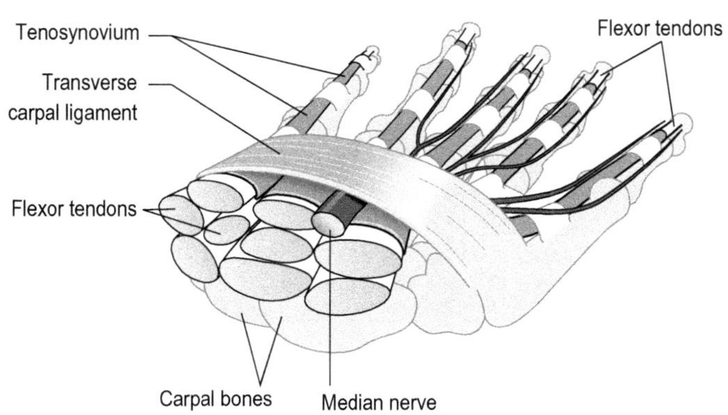

Figure 50.2 Scheme of the carpal tunnel.

Patho-biomechanism of Carpal Tunnel Syndrome

In most cases CTS is idiopathic (Sternbach 1999) but sometimes it is associated with trauma, pregnancy, hypothyroidism, multiple myeloma, amyloidosis, rheumatoid arthritis or acromegaly (Stevens et al 1992). Some risk factors include female gender (odds ratio (OR) 3.7, 95% CI 2.6–5.2), middle age (OR 2.2, 95% CI 0.9–4.9), diabetes mellitus (OR 5.3, 95% CI 1.6–16.8) and excessive alcohol abuse (OR 2.3, 95% CI 0.7–2.3) (Spahn et al 2012). Perumal and Stringer (2014) have recently reported that right hands from female cadavers exhibited significant reduction in the intrinsic arterial vascularity of the median nerve at the entrance to the carpal tunnel. Gender differences in the intrinsic arterial supply of the median nerve may be a factor predisposing to CTS (Perumal & Stringer 2014). Obesity has been also found to be a risk factor (OR 2.7, 95% CI 1.9–3.9) for impaired median nerve function (Coggon et al 2013). For instance, a BMI of >29 (obese subjects) increases the risk by 2.5 compared with a BMI of <20 (slender individuals) (Werner et al 1994).

As discussed above, anatomical changes occurring in the carpal tunnel due to underlying medical conditions are responsible for the median compression. For example:

- Rheumatoid arthritis causes inflammation of the flexor tendons determining median nerve compression (Karadag et al 2012).
- Pregnancy and hypothyroidism cause fluid retention in tissues, which swells the tenosynovium (we discuss the role of pregnancy in more details later in this chapter).
- Acromegaly causes the compression of the nerve because of the abnormal growth of bones around the hand and wrist.
- Tumours (usually benign), such as a ganglion or a lipoma, can protrude into the carpal tunnel, reducing the amount of space, although this is exceedingly rare (<1%). Carpal tunnel tumours can mimic CTS (Padua et al 2006) and in these cases the use of ultrasound evaluation has been crucial. This topic will be discussed in further detail below (Granata et al 2008).
- Double-crush syndrome is a speculative and debated theory, which postulates that, when there is compression or irritation of nerve branches contributing to the median nerve in the neck or anywhere above the wrist, this increases the liability of the nerve to become compressed in the wrist. Pierre-Jerome and Bekkelund (2005) reported that patients with CTS experienced a higher incidence of narrowing of the cervical foramen compared with controls; these authors hypothesized that the compromised neural foramen could potentially lead to nerve compression and possibly a double-crush syndrome in patients with CTS. However, there is a little evidence that this syndrome actually exists in CTS (Wilbourn & Gilliatt 1997; Russell 2008).
- There are a great number of traumatic injuries of the forearm causing CTS (Colles fracture, dislocation of one of the carpal bones of the wrist, haematoma forming inside the wrist, etc.) (Zyluk & Waśków 2011).
- A recent study has demonstrated that the presence of the Val158Met (rs4680) polymorphism in the *COMT* gene that codes the enzyme catechol-*O*-methyltransferase seems not to be a risk factor for development of CTS; however, Val158Met (rs4680) polymorphism was associated with increased perception of pain and higher disability scores, suggesting a potential genetic effect in clinical manifestations of this syndrome (Fernández-de-las-Peñas et al 2013).
- The role of manual activities and CTS is still a matter of debate. A number of authors found that there is strong relationship between hand positions and increased pressure on the carpal tunnel (Keir et al 1998; Luchetti et al 1998) and this strongly supports the hypothesis that forceful use of the hands, repetitive use of the hands and hand–arm vibration may all cause or contribute to CTS. However, other studies do not support the relationship between manual activity and CTS (Chiang et al 1993; Moore & Garg 1994) and so, despite researchers' efforts, the debate is still far from over. Readers are referred to other texts for a greater understanding of these

mechanisms (Werner 2006; van Rijn et al 2009; Jenkins et al 2013).

Sensory and Motor Aspects in Carpal Tunnel Syndrome

Although the aetiology of CTS is not completely understood, there is some evidence involving the whole nociceptive system (De-la-Llave-Rincón et al 2012). Previous studies have investigated the function of nociceptive thermoreceptive fibres in CTS. Different studies found elevated thermal pain thresholds in the fingers and the palm within the affected hand in patients (Arendt-Nielsen et al 1991; Westerman & Delaney 1991; Goadsby & Burke 1994). Lang et al (1995) suggested that pain intensity in CTS depends on alterations of peripheral and central nervous function.

More recent studies found that 45% of patients with CTS also reported spreading proximal symptoms, which might be related to central nervous system mechanisms (Zanette et al 2006, 2007). Chow et al (2005) found that neck pain was present in 14% of patients with CTS. Tucker et al (2007) found bilateral generalized increases in vibration thresholds in CTS, which suggested a generalized disturbance of somatosensory functions rather than the existence of an isolated peripheral neuropathy. In fact, two imaging studies have shown cortical remapping in the primary somatosensory cortex (S1) in patients with CTS, supporting the possible involvement of central mechanisms in CTS (Tecchio et al 2002; Napadow et al 2006).

Additionally, different clinical studies also support the presence of both peripheral and central sensitization mechanisms in CTS. Fernández-de-las-Peñas et al (2009a) found bilateral widespread decrease in pressure pain thresholds (PPT) in women suffering from unilateral CTS (clinically and neurophysiological) compared with healthy controls. This study reported bilateral lower PPTs over the median, radial and ulnar nerve, the carpal tunnel, the C5–C6 zygapophyseal joint and the tibialis anterior muscle. A significant decrease in PPT over the C5–C6 joint may represent the existence of segmental sensitization of the nociceptive system in CTS, whereas a bilateral decrease in PPT over the tibialis anterior muscle may indicate multisegmental sensory sensitization or sensitization of the central nervous system in CTS patients (Fernández-de-las-Peñas et al 2009a). Another study has revealed that bilateral pressure pain hypersensitivity was heterogeneously distributed over the hand region in CTS, with some areas being more sensitive to pressure than others (Fernández-de-las-Peñas et al 2010a). Zanette et al (2010) observed that individuals with CTS with extramedian symptoms exhibited pressure pain hyperalgesia and enhanced wind-up pain in the territories innervated by the median, ulnar and radial nerves, which further confirms a widespread sensitization process. All these studies support the concept that pain sensitivity to pressure is a feature of CTS. This hypothesis has been confirmed in a study where women with minimal, moderate or severe CTS exhibited similar widespread pressure pain hyperalgesia (De-la-Llave-Rincón et al 2011a).

Similar results have also been reported for thermal pain sensitivity in CTS. De-la-Llave Rincón et al (2009) found that women with unilateral moderate CTS exhibit bilaterally thermal hyperalgesia (reduced heat and cold thermal pain threshold), but not hypo-aesthesia (normal heat and cold thermal detection thresholds) compared with healthy controls. Zanette et al (2010) also showed that subjects with CTS with extramedian symptoms exhibit thermal hyperalgesia in the territories related to the median, ulnar and radial nerves. Bilateral sensory changes in individuals with unilateral diagnosis (clinical and neurophysiological) of CTS reflect the presence of central sensitization mechanisms. As with pressure pain sensitivity, heat and cold thermal hyperalgesia, but not hypo-aesthesia, was similar in women with minimal, moderate or severe CTS (De-la-Llave-Rincón et al 2011a). These clinical findings are supported by animal studies where peripheral neural pathology in one local area causes widespread effects including in the uninvolved limbs (Koltzenburg et al 1999; Kleinschnitz et al 2005).

In addition to sensory symptoms, including pain and numbness, patients with CTS usually describe self-perceived pinch-strength deficits, sensations of clumsiness during their activities of daily living and some difficulty in grasping small objects. Some studies have also demonstrated the relevance of motor disturbances in this population. A study investigating impairments in fine motor control skills revealed bilateral deficits in fine motor control ability and pinch-grip force in women with unilateral CTS (Fernández-de-las-Peñas et al 2009b). The presence of bilateral motor impairments and pinch-grip force deficits in patients with unilateral sensory symptoms reflects a reorganization of the motor control strategy of the central nervous system that occurs as a consequence of the pain (Tamburin et al 2008). In fact, another study confirmed also that the deficits in fine motor control and pinch-grip force were similar in patients with minimal, moderate or severe CTS; this result suggests that motor disturbances may be present from the onset of the pain condition (De-la-Llave-Rincón et al 2011b).

Finally, these studies also demonstrated that bilateral sensory and motor deficits were related to the intensity and duration of pain symptoms, supporting the theory that the peripheral nervous system has a role in initiating and maintaining the central sensitization mechanism (De-la-Llave-Rincón et al 2009, 2011a, 2011b; Fernández-de-las-Peñas et al 2009a, 2009b). Gracely et al (1992) proposed a model of neuropathic pain in which an ongoing nociceptive afferent input from a peripheral nociceptive focus dynamically maintains altered central processing. In fact, Tecchio et al (2002) suggested that the continuous sensory bombardment from the median nerve might trigger cortical plastic changes found in these patients. In such instances, it can be suggested the painful condition – that is, the ischaemia of the **nervi nervorum** (Watkins & Maier 2004) (the nerves innervating the connective tissue layers of the nerve itself) sensitized by the compression of the median nerve in the carpal tunnel (Hall & Elvey 1999) – may as such act as a trigger for gradual sensitization of nociceptive pathways in CTS patients. New studies should investigate the role of these sensitization mechanisms in the evolution of CTS.

Diagnosis of Carpal Tunnel Syndrome

Clinical examination

The gold standard for the diagnosis of CTS is considered to be the following clinical presentation, according to the AAN

(1993a, 1993b) diagnostic criteria: paraesthesia, pain, swelling, weakness or clumsiness of the hand provoked or worsened by sleep, sustained hand or arm position, repetitive action of the hand or wrist that is mitigated by changing postures or by shaking of the hand, sensory deficits in the median innervated region of the hand and motor deficits in, or hypotrophy of, the median innervated thenar muscles. Wainner et al (2005) developed a clinical prediction rule for the diagnosis of CTS. The rule identified consisted of one question (does shaking hands give symptom relief?), a wrist-ratio index >0.67, a symptom severity scale score >1.9, a reduced median sensory field of the first digit, and age >45 years (LR 18.3).

Some studies have identified the relationship between the distribution of sensory symptoms and the severity of CTS according to the neurophysiological classification. Patients with lower severity of pathology complain of sensory symptoms with a glove distribution, whereas patients with higher severity of pathology complain of sensory symptoms with the 'classical' median distribution (Caliandro et al 2006).

The patient history is extremely important for the differential diagnosis, especially as CTS can be secondary to endocrinal and metabolic pathologies, and so therapy for the primary pathology can produce CTS remission. In the clinical examination, it is additionally possible to use a subjective and objective scale of CTS that includes two measures (Giannini et al 2002). The first measure (historical–objective, or Hi-Ob) includes a clinical history and the following objective subscores: (1) nocturnal paraesthesia only, (2) nocturnal and diurnal paraesthesia, (3) sensory deficit, (4) hypotrophy or motor deficit of the median innervated thenar muscles and (5) plegia of the median thenar eminence muscles. The second measure evaluates categorically, by patient questioning, the presence or absence of pain with a forced-choice answer (i.e. 'yes' or 'no'). Therefore, the historical–objective–distribution (Hi-Ob-Db) score comprises a number (Hi-Ob) with or without the variable measuring pain or the distribution of paraesthesiae (Db) (Giannini et al 2002; Caliandro et al 2010).

The physical examination includes the Phalen test (Fig. 50.3), performed by a prolonged (1-minute) passive forced flexion of the wrist, the Tinel test, consisting of a percussion of the median nerve trophism of the thenar eminence, and evaluations of motor function of the median innervated muscles and the sensory function (cotton wool is used as a standard material for skin stimulation). Bilkis et al (2012) developed a modified Phalen test, which has shown a higher sensitivity (84.4%) than the traditional Phalen test (50%); this test combines the classic Phalen test, obtained by wrist flexion

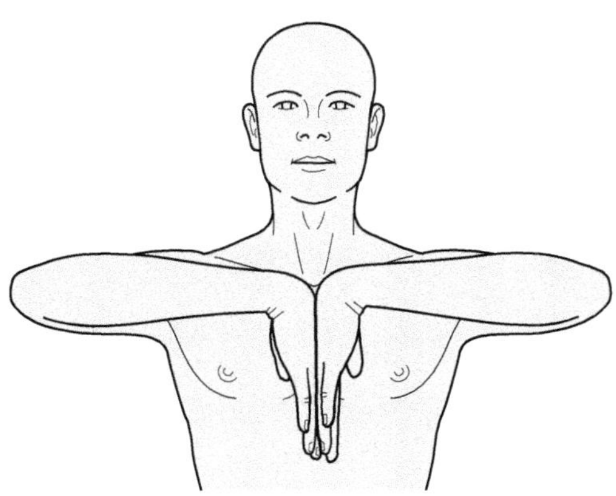

Figure 50.3 The Phalen test.

for 1 minute, with the application of a Semmes–Weinstein 2.83-unit monofilament to the palmar and lateral surface of the five fingers. The test is positive if the subject does not refer to the touch in at least one finger of the median nerve territory.

Questionnaires

As doctors want to help patients, the assessment of the patient's perspective is also useful in the comprehensive evaluation of CTS. The most commonly used questionnaire is the Boston Carpal Tunnel Questionnaire (BCTQ) (Levine et al 1993). The BCTQ evaluates two domains of CTS: 'symptoms' (SYMPT=patient-oriented symptom), assessed on an 11-step scale, and 'functional status' (FUNCT=patient-oriented function), assessed on an 8-step scale. Each item includes five possible responses, and the score for each section (SYMPT or FUNCT) is calculated as the mean of the responses to the individual items. The use of this questionnaire in several multicentre studies on CTS showed interesting results; whereas function has a linear significant correlation when assessed both by physicians and patients, the symptoms do not demonstrate a clear linear correlation (Padua et al 2002). Patients with mild-to-moderate CTS seemed to function well, although severe symptoms may be reported by the patient. However, when nerve impairment becomes severe, the patient's hand function is extremely impaired although symptoms may be milder. The data also show that the patient's point of view is reliable (Padua et al 2002).

Electrodiagnostic evaluation

Electrodiagnostic evaluation is very important to define the impairment of the median nerve. It is now accepted that, in order to increase the sensitivity of conventional nerve conduction studies (sensory digit–wrist and motor wrist–thenar), segmental nerve assessment and / or comparative tests should be used (see below) as stated in AAN and AAEM recommendations (AAN 1993a, 1993b). When the standard tests yield normal results ('standard negative' hands), the following studies increase the electrodiagnostic sensitivity:

- segmental motor or sensory conduction tests in the palm–wrist segment
- comparative studies (median–ulnar or median–radial)
- segmental / comparative studies (as distal : proximal ratio).

A study conducted on patients with CTS showed that the sensitivity of standard tests can reach 83.5%, and comparative / segmental tests can disclose abnormal findings in a further 11.4% of cases, providing CTS electrodiagnosis in about 7 of 10 'standard negative' cases. The overall sensitivity of the protocol thus reaches 94.9% (Padua et al 1999). The severity of neurophysiological CTS impairment can be assessed and scored according to a published neurophysiological classification (Padua et al 1997a, 1997b).

Ultrasound Assessment

Thanks to the advances in technology (refinement of high-frequency broadband linear-array transducers, and sensitive

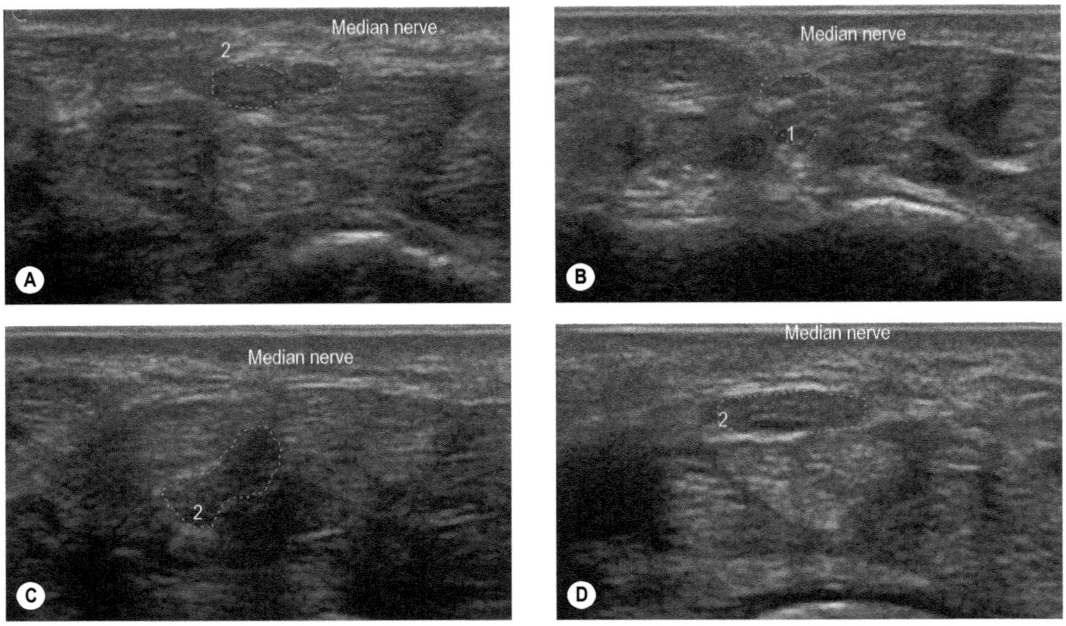

Figure 50.4 The median nerve at the wrist (in the carpal tunnel). Note the change in shape and position between the nerve and the tendons (1, 2) in relation to the different wrist angle: (**A**) neutral position, (**B**) 45° wrist flexion, (**C**) 90° wrist flexion, and (**D**) maximal wrist extension.

colour and power Doppler technology), low cost, wide availability and ease of use, ultrasound (US) has recently been applied to the study of tendons and nerves.

In tendon and nerve imaging, US can assess a great number of pathologies such as dislocations, degenerative changes and extrinsic or intrinsic focal compression. Moreover, it can support clinical and electrophysiological testing and, in most cases, a focused US examination can be performed more rapidly and efficiently than MRI (Martinoli et al 2002).

From a technical point of view, although tendons and nerves share similar characteristics (dimensions, tubular conformation and striated appearance), US can easily differentiate them. Tendons have a fibrillar pattern of parallel hyperechoic lines in the longitudinal plane because of the collagen bundles and endotendineum septa, with a hyperechoic round-to-ovoid image containing bright dots (Fornage & Rifkin 1988; Martinoli et al 1993); in contrast, nerves have a fascicular pattern due to hypoechoic parallel linear areas – the neuronal fascicles – separated by hyperechoic bands (the interfascicular epineurium) (Graif et al 1991; Silvestri et al 1995). On transverse scans, nerves assume a honeycomb-like appearance, with hypoechoic dots surrounded by a hyperechoic background (Fig. 50.4).

Ultrasound has been mainly tested in the evaluation of CTS because of the complementary perspective it provides (Beekman & Visser 2003; Hobson-Webb & Padua 2009; Smith et al 2009; Karadağ et al 2010). CTS can be assessed using the following measures: cross-sectional area (CSA), swelling ratio, retinacular bowing, retinacular thickness and flattening ratio. Several studies have shown that the most useful diagnostic criterion is the CSA, which is the area of median nerve calculated at the wrist, either by using the ellipse formula or by manual tracing; the best cut-off value is a CSA of ≥9.875 mm^2 at the pisiform level (Wang et al 2008). A meta-analysis concluded that a CSA of the median nerve between 9.5 and 10.5 mm^2 has a pooled sensitivity of 0.84 (95% CI 0.81–0.87), a specificity of 0.78 (95% CI 0.69–0.88), a likelihood ratio for a negative test of 0.21 (95% CI 0.17–0.27), and a likelihood ratio for a positive test of 3.74 (95% CI 2.30–6.10) (Descatha et al 2012).

More sensitive tests have been developed in order to obtain the best sensitivity and specificity. For example, the wrist-to-forearm ratio of the median nerve area can be considered more sensitive than a measure of median nerve area at the wrist alone (Hobson-Webb et al 2008). The sensitivity of the combination of US and neurophysiology is higher than that of either neurophysiology or US alone. Ultrasound is therefore a potential useful complementary tool for CTS assessment, with positive correlation between US findings and conventional measures of CTS severity (clinical, neurophysiological and patient oriented) (Padua et al 2008).

Ultrasound allows clinicians to collaborate efficiently with surgeons because it is able to show the anatomy before the surgery (e.g. showing bifid median nerve). Furthermore, with respect to decision making, US is able to show extrinsic (anatomical variant as muscles) or intrinsic (nerve tumour) nerve compression, providing crucial information for the choice of treatment.

In conclusion, there is increasing evidence that US is a useful complement in a neurophysiology laboratory; it greatly increases the diagnostic power and therapeutic work-up of patients with mononeuropathies (Padua et al 2007), and the morphological evaluation of nerves helps the clinician to avoid severe misdiagnoses (e.g. a median nerve tumour that may mimic CTS), especially in cases with atypical neurophysiological findings (Padua & Martinoli 2008).

Prognosis

Prognosis of untreated carpal tunnel syndrome

The knowledge and evolution of untreated CTS is very important in order to administer the best therapeutic approach.

Only a few studies have evaluated this topic (Padua et al 1998, 2001; Resende et al 2003; Ortiz-Corredor et al 2008; Pensy et al 2011) and all agreed that many patients improve spontaneously. When the evolution is analysed according to the initial clinical picture, it is observed that CTS hands with initial low severity tend to get worse while CTS hands with initial high severe impairment tend to improve (this is observed in all CTS measurements, either patient oriented or neurophysiological). However, Kiylioglu et al (2009) found that treatment was superior to spontaneous improvement in subjects with idiopathic CTS.

The factor that is most predictive of untreated CTS evolution is the duration of symptoms. In particular, a long duration of symptoms is a poor prognostic factor according to all patient-oriented measurements. Conversely, a long duration of symptoms is not significantly associated with a bad neurophysiological or clinical examination outcome. With regard to the positive prognostic value of hand stress at the baseline, it should be noted that this value is probably due to the interruption of the stress. In this sense, it is interesting to note that in the entrapment syndrome the 'natural history' can be influenced by the physician giving an explanation of the pathophysiology of CTS. Therefore if doctors, while giving patients this diagnosis, also provide practical information about the hand positions to be avoided, they can alter the natural course of the pathology.

Therapy

Scientific evidence for the management of CTS is conflicting. With regard to the conservative options of CTS therapy, a review by Piazzini et al (2007), including 33 randomized controlled trials, showed that there is a strong evidence (level 1) for the efficacy of local and oral steroids; moderate evidence (level 2) that vitamin B_6 is ineffective but that splints are effective, and limited and / or conflicting evidence that NSAIDs, diuretics, yoga, laser and US are effective, whereas exercise therapy and botulinum toxin B injection are ineffective. An additional systematic review, which focused on neural mobilization interventions for the management of CTS, included six studies and found weak-to-strong effects of neural-gliding exercises, with benefits seen across different outcome measures (Medina McKeon & Yancosek 2008). Nevertheless, the authors proposed that the benefit of neural gliding may be best identified within a specific subpopulation of patients with CTS – that is, it is possible that neural gliding may be more effective in those with minimal or mild CTS or with lower central sensitization. Fernández-de-las-Peñas et al (2010b) found that peripheral sensitization, rather than central sensitization, was related to a positive physical therapy response in women with CTS. These authors found that pressure hyperalgesia over the cervical spine and heat hyperalgesia over the carpal tunnel, but not widespread pressure pain or cold pain hyperalgesia, were associated with a successful outcome after the application of physical therapy (Fernández-de-las-Peñas et al 2010b). In a follow-up review, Huisstede et al (2010) found strong and moderate evidence for the effectiveness of oral steroid, steroid injections, US, electromagnetic field therapy, nocturnal splinting, and traditional cupping versus heat pads in the short term but sparse evidence on their benefits in the mid- and long-term management of CTS. Nevertheless, the most recent Cochrane review concluded that there is only limited and low-quality evidence of benefit for interventions such as exercise and mobilization in CTS (Page et al 2012).

Regarding surgical intervention, the Cochrane review concluded that surgical treatment relieves symptoms significantly better than splinting, but further research is needed to determine whether this conclusion applies to individuals with mild symptoms and or whether surgical treatment is better than steroid injection (Verdugo et al 2008). In fact, a randomized controlled trial demonstrated that hand surgery and physical therapy exhibited similar pain relief in patients with CTS, and that 61% of patients with CTS will try to avoid surgery (Jarvick et al 2009). The most updated review analysing surgical versus conservative management in CTS showed that both interventions had benefits for CTS but that surgical treatment had a superior benefit, in terms of reduction of symptoms and function, at 6 and 12 months compared with conservative treatment (Shi & MacDemid 2011). In addition, this review concluded that patients with surgical release were twice as likely to have normal nerve conduction studies, but also experienced more complications and side effects than those receiving conservative treatment (Shi & MacDemid 2011).

A number of studies have been performed analysing the factors that influence the surgical results in different populations; for example, the results of surgical decompression were found to be similar in men and women (Mondelli et al 2004a). Furthermore, elderly patients showed less improvement compared with younger patients, which was presumably due to greater preoperative damage and a reduced repair capacity of the compressed nerve, although this aspect was not a contraindication for surgical release in elderly patients (Mondelli et al 2004b). The presence of comorbidity has also been investigated; for example, patients with diabetes have the same probability of positive surgical outcome as those with idiopathic CTS (Mondelli et al 2004a).

Along the same lines, an analysis of the cost-effectiveness of non-surgical versus surgical treatment has shown that surgery, rather than non-surgical care, should be considered as the initial form of treatment when patients are diagnosed with CTS (confirmed by nerve conduction studies), as this option provides symptom resolution at a favourable cost–benefit (Pomerance et al 2009).

Carpal Tunnel Syndrome and Pregnancy

Carpal tunnel syndrome is frequent during pregnancy (PRCTS) but can be considered as a distinct entity. The incidence of CTS in pregnant women reported in the literature ranges from 2% up to 70% (Padua et al 2010; Zyluk 2013). Hormonal fluctuation, fluid accumulation with tendency to oedema, nerve hypersensitivity and fluctuations in blood glucose level are factors that predispose pregnant women to the development of symptoms. Studies have shown that PRCTS does not disappear after delivery (it may improve, but on the contrary may also persist, and the prolonged compression can result in median nerve defect) so CTS symptoms must be accurately assessed in pregnant women. When present they must be monitored either clinically or neurophysiologically (also, the role of US in PRCTS is not well known and this must be assessed as it could be a non-invasive monitoring tool). In fact, most cases with pregnancy-related CTS usually improve spontaneously without treatment, but symptoms can persist in more than 50% of the patients after 1 year and in about 30% after 3 years (Pazzaglia et al 2005; Padua et al 2010).

In cases of early CTS appearance (i.e. before the last trimester), the median compression must be thoroughly assessed as it may result in acute or disabling CTS, in which improvement is less frequent. In cases of severe CTS with early onset, surgical decompression during pregnancy may prevent nerve damage and a negative psychological influence after delivery.

Appearance of CTS symptoms in the last trimester is the more usual occurrence and has a higher probability of improvement after delivery; nevertheless, around half of these women may complain of CTS symptoms for a long time post partum, so clinical and neurophysiological monitoring is advised. Note that in one study (Mondelli et al 2007), despite improvement of symptoms, the distal sensory conduction velocity of the median nerve improved but remained delayed in 84% of women well after the delivery.

Apart from acute CTS, which may be an emergency (with the need for rapid surgical decompression), the first line in approaching PRCTS should be conservative therapy. But in absence of improvement and the presence of severe neurophysiological CTS (disappearance of sensory or motor responses), or disabling symptoms, surgical decompression before delivery must be considered in order to prevent not only median nerve damage (Osterman et al 2012) but also deterioration of quality of life due to difficulty and anxiety in handling the baby.

Conclusion

Although CTS has been defined as 'complex issues with a "simple" condition' (Olney 2001), and this has been confirmed by the high number of publications concerning all aspects of CTS, in recent years there have been many efforts to improve knowledge of this condition. Tools imported from other fields, such as ultrasound, have been commonly accepted as methods to improving the diagnostic accuracy, although the gold standard for diagnosis remains the clinical presentation. The natural history of the pathology shows that some untreated patients with CTS can improve, but this is probably due to the doctor explaining to the patient how to avoid wrong hand postures and thus reduce the stresses on the neural tissues. Conservative therapies are often used for the management of CTS and have been demonstrated to be effective, but surgical decompression, also used in elderly or diabetic patients, remains a definite cure and is efficient from the cost-effectiveness point of view. Nevertheless, it is possible that patients with minimal or mild CTS can benefit from conservative intervention, particularly physical therapy, as a first therapeutic option.

The opinion of the authors concerning surgical decompression, based on clinical experience and on unpublished data on the natural history of CTS, is that surgery may be suggested in severe cases (either neurophysiologically or clinically) with duration of symptoms longer than 1 year and for patients over 50 years of age. A brief period of conservative therapy can be tried in cases of acute CTS, but in cases where we suspect acute CTS that is not secondary to a particularly stressing event – a very rare but very severe condition – urgent decompression must be considered, together with a comprehensive assessment of a possible primary subclinical cause.

References

AAN [no authors listed] 1993a. American Academy of Neurology, American Association of Electrodiagnostic Medicine, American Academy of Physical Medicine and Rehabilitation. Practice parameter for electrodiagnostic studies in carpal tunnel syndrome (summary statement). Neurology 43: 2404–2405.

AAN [no authors listed] 1993b. American Academy of Neurology, American Association of Electrodiagnostic Medicine, American Academy of Physical Medicine and Rehabilitation. Practice parameter for carpal tunnel syndrome (summary statement). Neurology 43: 2406–2409.

Arendt-Nielsen L, Gregersen H, Toft E, et al. 1991. Involvement of thin afferents in carpal tunnel syndrome: evaluated quantitatively by argon laser stimulation. Muscle Nerve 14: 508–514.

Atroshi I, Gummesson C, Johnsson R, et al. 1999. Prevalence of carpal tunnel syndrome in a general population. JAMA 282: 153–158.

Beekman R, Visser LH. 2003. Sonography in the diagnosis of carpal tunnel syndrome: a critical review of the literature. Muscle Nerve 27: 26–33.

Bilkis S, Loveman DM, Eldridge JA, et al. 2012. Modified Phalen's test as an aid in diagnosing carpal tunnel syndrome. Arthritis Care Res 64: 287–289.

Bland JD, Rudolfer SM. 2003. Clinical surveillance of carpal tunnel syndrome in two areas of the United Kingdom, 1991–2001. J Neurol Neurosurg Psychiatry 74: 1674–1679.

Bongers FJ, Schellevis FG, van den Bosch WJ, et al. 2007. Carpal tunnel syndrome in general practice (1987 and 2001): incidence and the role of occupational and non-occupational factors. Br J General Pract 57: 36–39.

Caliandro P, La Torre G, Aprile I, et al. 2006. Distribution of paresthesias in carpal tunnel syndrome reflects the degree of nerve damage at wrist. Clin Neurophysiol 117: 228–231.

Caliandro P, Giannini F, Pazzaglia C, et al. 2010. A new clinical scale to grade the impairment of median nerve in carpal tunnel syndrome. Clin Neurophysiol. 121(7): 1066–1171. doi: 10.1016/j.clinph.2010.02.002.

Chiang HC, Ko YC, Chen SS, et al. 1993. Prevalence of shoulder and upper-limb disorders among workers in the fish-processing industry. Scand J Work Environ Health 19: 126–131.

Chow CS, Hung LK, Chiu CP, et al. 2005. Is symptomatology useful in distinguishing between carpal tunnel syndrome and cervical spondylosis? Hand Surg 10: 1–5.

Coggon D, Ntani G, Harris EC, et al. 2013. Differences in risk factors for neurophysiologically confirmed carpal tunnel syndrome and illness with similar symptoms but normal median nerve function: a case-control study. BMC Musculoskelet Disord 14: 240.

Dale AM, Harris-Adamson C, Rempel D, et al. 2013. Prevalence and incidence of carpal tunnel syndrome in US working populations: pooled analysis of six prospective studies. Scand J Work Environ Health 39: 495–505.

De-la-Llave-Rincón AI, Fernández-de-las-Peñas C, Fernández-Carnero J, et al. 2009. Bilateral hand / wrist head and cold hyperalgesia, but not hypoesthesia, in unilateral carpal tunnel syndrome. Exp Brain Res 198: 455–463.

De-la-Llave-Rincón AI, Fernández-de-las-Peñas C, Laguarta-Val S, et al. 2011a. Increased pain sensitivity is not associated with electrodiagnostic findings in women with carpal tunnel syndrome. Clin J Pain 27: 747–754.

De-la-Llave-Rincón AI, Fernández-de-las-Peñas C, Pérez-de-Heredia-Torres M, et al. 2011b. Bilateral deficits in fine motor control and pinch grip force are not associated with electrodiagnostic findings in women carpal tunnel syndrome. Am J Phys Med Rehabil 90: 443–451.

De-la-Llave-Rincón AI, Puentedura EJ, Fernández-de-las-Peñas C. 2012. New advances in the mechanisms and etiology of carpal tunnel syndrome. Discov Med 13: 343–348.

Descatha A, Huard L, Aubert F, et al. 2012. Meta-analysis on the performance of sonography for the diagnosis of carpal tunnel syndrome. Semin Arthritis Rheum 41: 914–922.

Fernández-de-las-Peñas C, De-la-Llave-Rincón AI, Fernández-Carnero J, et al. 2009a. Bilateral widespread mechanical pain sensitivity in carpal tunnel syndrome: evidence of central processing in unilateral neuropathy. Brain 132: 1472–1479.

Fernández-de-las-Peñas C, Pérez-de-Heredia M, Martínez-Piédrola R, et al. 2009b. Bilateral deficits in fine motor control and pinch grip force in patients with unilateral carpal tunnel syndrome. Exp Brain Res 194: 29–37.

Fernández-de-las-Peñas C, Madeleine P, Martínez-Pérez A, et al. 2010a. Pressure pain sensitivity topographical maps reveal bilateral hyperalgesia of the hands in patients with unilateral carpal tunnel syndrome. Arthritis Care Res 62: 1055–1064.

Fernández-de-las-Peñas C, Cleland JA, Ortega-Santiago R, et al. 2010b. Central sensitization does not identify patients with carpal tunnel syndrome who are likely to achieve short-term success with physical therapy. Exp Brain Res 207: 85–94.

Fernández-de-las-Peñas C, Ambite-Quesada S, Ortega-Santiago R, et al. 2013. Catechol-O-methyltransferase val158met polymorphism is associated with pain and disability, but not widespread pressure pain sensitivity, in women with carpal tunnel syndrome. Pain Phys 16: 591–600.

Fornage BD, Rifkin M. 1988. Ultrasound examination of tendons. Radiol Clin North Am 6: 87–107.

Giannini F, Cioni R, Mondelli M, et al. 2002. A new clinical scale of carpal tunnel syndrome: validation of the measurement and clinical-neurophysiological assessment. Clin Neurophysiol 113:71–77.

Goadsby P, Burke D. 1994. Deficit in the function of small and large afferent fibres in confirmed cases of carpal tunnel syndrome. Muscle Nerve 17: 614–622.

Gracely RH, Lynch SA, Bennett GJ. 1992. Painful neuropathy: altered central processing maintained dynamically by peripheral input. Pain 51: 175–194.

Graif M, Seton A, Nerubali J, et al. 1991. Sciatic nerve: sonographic evaluation and anatomic–pathologic considerations. Radiology 18:405–408.

Granata G, Martinoli C, Pazzaglia C, et al. 2008. Letter to Editor: carpal tunnel syndrome due to an atypical deep soft tissue leiomyoma: the risk of misdiagnosis and mismanagement. World J Surg Oncol 6: 22.

Hall TM, Elvey RL. 1999. Nerve trunk pain: physical diagnosis and treatment. Man The 4: 63–73.

Hobson-Webb LD, Massey JM, Juel VC, et al. 2008. The ultrasonographic wrist-to-forearm median nerve area ratio in carpal tunnel syndrome. Clin Neurophysiol 119:1353–1357.

Hobson-Webb LD, Padua L. 2009. Median nerve ultrasonography in carpal tunnel syndrome: findings from two laboratories. Muscle Nerve 40: 94–97.

Huisstede BM, Hoogvliet P, Randsdorp MS, et al. 2010. Carpal tunnel syndrome. Part I: effectiveness of nonsurgical treatments-a systematic review. Arch Phys Med Rehabil 91: 981–1004.

Jarvik JG, Comstock BA, Kliot M, et al. 2009. Surgery versus non-surgical therapy for carpal tunnel syndrome: a randomised parallel-group trial. Lancet 374: 1074–1081.

Jenkins PJ, Srikantharajah D, Duckworth AD, et al. 2013. Carpal tunnel syndrome: the association with occupation at a population level. J Hand Surg Eur 38: 67–72.

Karadağ YS, Karadağ O, Çiçekli E, et al. 2010. Severity of carpal tunnel syndrome assessed with high frequency ultrasonography. Rheumatol Int 30: 761–765.

Karadag O, Kalyoncu U, Akdogan A, et al. 2012. Sonographic assessment of carpal tunnel syndrome in rheumatoid arthritis: prevalence and correlation with disease activity. Rheumatol Int 32: 2313–2319.

Keir PJ, Bach JM, Rempel DM. 1998. Effects of finger posture on carpal tunnel pressure during wrist motion. J Hand Surg Am 23: 1004–1009.

Kiylioglu N, Bicerol B, Ozkul A, et al. 2009. Natural course and treatment efficacy: one-year observation in diabetic and idiopathic carpal tunnel syndrome. J Clin Neurophysiol 26: 446–453.

Kleinschnitz C, Brinkhoff J, Sommer C, et al. 2005. Contra-lateral cytokine gene induction after peripheral nerve lesions: dependence on the mode of injury and NMDA receptor signalling. Mol Brain Res 136: 23–28.

Koltzenburg M, Wall PD, McMahon SB. 1999. Does the right side know what the left is doing? Trends Neurosci 22: 122–127.

Lang E, Claus D, Neundörfer B, et al. 1995. Parameters of thick and thin nerve-fibres functions as predictors of pain in carpal tunnel syndrome. Pain 60: 295–302.

Levine DW, Simmons BP, Koris MJ, et al. 1993. A self-administered questionnaire for the assessment of severity of symptoms and functional status in carpal tunnel syndrome. J Bone Joint Surg Am 75: 1585–1592.

Luchetti R, Schoenhuber R, Nathan P. 1998. Correlation of segmental carpal tunnel pressures with changes in hand and wrist positions in patients with carpal tunnel syndrome and controls. J Hand Surg 23: 598–602.

Luckhaupt SE, Dahlhamer JM, Ward BW, et al. 2013. Prevalence and work-relatedness of carpal tunnel syndrome in the working population, United States, 2010 National Health Interview Survey. Am J Ind Med 56: 615–624.

Martinoli C, Derchi LE, Pastorino C, et al. 1993. Analysis of echotexture of tendons with US. Radiology 186: 839–843.

Martinoli C, Bianchi S, Dahmane M, et al. 2002. Ultrasound of tendons and nerves. Eur Radiol 12: 44–55.

Mashoof AA, Levy HJ, Soifer TB, et al. 2001. Neural anatomy of the transverse carpal ligament. Clin Orthop Relat Res 386: 218–221.

Medina McKeon JM, Yancosek KE. 2008. Neural gliding techniques for the treatment of carpal tunnel syndrome: a systematic review. J Sports Rehabil 17: 324–341.

Mondelli M, Padua L, Reale F, et al. 2004a. Outcome of surgical release among diabetics with carpal tunnel syndrome. Arch Phys Med Rehabil 85: 7–13.

Mondelli M, Padua L, Reale F. 2004b. Carpal tunnel syndrome in elderly patients: results of surgical decompression. J Peripher Nerv Syst 9:168–176.

Mondelli M, Rossi S, Monti E, et al. 2007. Long term follow-up of carpal tunnel syndrome during pregnancy: a cohort study and review of the literature. Electromyogr Clin Neurophysiol 6: 259–271.

Moore JS, Garg A. 1994. Upper extremity disorders in a pork processing plant: relationships between job risk factors and morbidity. Am Ind Hyg Assoc J 55: 703–715.

Napadow V, Kettner N, Ryan A, et al. 2006. Somatosensory cortical plasticity in carpal tunnel syndrome: a cross-sectional fMRI evaluation. Neuroimage 31: 520–530.

Olney RK. 2001. Carpal tunnel syndrome. Complex issues with a 'simple' condition. Neurology 56: 1431–1432.

Ortiz-Corredor F, Enríquez F, Díaz-Ruíz J, et al. 2008. Natural evolution of carpal tunnel syndrome in untreated patients. Clin Neurophysiol 119: 1373–1378.

Osterman M, Ilyas AM, Matzon JL. 2012. Carpal tunnel syndrome in pregnancy. Orthop Clin North Am 43: 515–520.

Padua L, Martinoli C. 2008. From square to cube: ultrasound as a natural complement of neurophysiology. Clin Neurophysiol 119: 1217–1218.

Padua L, Lo Monaco M, Padua R, et al. 1997a. Neurophysiological classification of carpal tunnel syndrome: assessment of 600 symptomatic hands. Ital J Neurol Sci 18: 145–150.

Padua L, Lo Monaco M, Gregori B, et al. 1997b. Neurophysiological classification and sensitivity in 500 carpal tunnel syndrome hands. Acta Neurol Scand 96: 211–217.

Padua L, Padua R, Lo Monaco M, et al. 1998. Natural history of carpal tunnel syndrome according to the neurophysiological classification. Ital J Neurol Sci 19: 357–361.

Padua L, Giannini F, Girlanda P, et al. 1999. Usefulness of segmental and comparative tests in the electrodiagnosis of carpal tunnel syndrome: the Italian multicenter study. Italian CTS Study Group. Ital J Neurol Sci 20: 315–320.

Padua L, Padua R, Aprile I, et al. 2001. Italian CTS Study Group. Carpal tunnel syndrome. Multi-perspective follow-up of untreated carpal tunnel syndrome: a multicenter study. Neurology 56: 1459–1466.

Padua L, Padua R, Aprile I, et al. 2002. Carpal tunnel syndrome: relationship between clinical and patient-oriented assessment. Clin Orthop Relat Res 395: 128–134.

Padua L, Pazzaglia C, Insola A, et al. 2006. Schwannoma of the median nerve (even outside the wrist) may mimic carpal tunnel syndrome. Neurol Sci 26: 430–434.

Padua L, Aprile I, Pazzaglia C, et al. 2007. Contribution of ultrasound in a neurophysiological lab in diagnosing nerve impairment: a one-year systematic assessment. Clin Neurophysiol 118: 1410–1416.

Padua L, Pazzaglia C, Caliandro P, et al. 2008. Carpal tunnel syndrome: ultrasound, neurophysiology, clinical and patient-oriented assessment. Clin Neurophysiol 119: 2064–2069.

Padua L, Di Pasquale A, Pazzaglia C, et al. 2010. Systematic review of pregnancy-related carpal tunnel syndrome. Muscle Nerve 42: 697–702.

Page MJ, O'Connor D, Pitt V, et al. 2012. Exercise and mobilisation interventions for carpal tunnel syndrome. Cochrane Database Syst Rev 6: CD009899.

Pazzaglia C, Caliandro P, Aprile I, et al.; Italian CTS and others entrapment Study Group. 2005.

Pensy RA, Burke FD, Bradley MJ, et al. 2011. A 6-year outcome of patients who cancelled carpal tunnel surgery. J Hand Surg Eur 36(8): 642–647. doi: 10.1177/1753193411410155.

Perumal V, Stringer MD. 2014. The intrinsic arterial vascularity and morphology of the median nerve within the carpal tunnel: a microscopic study. Anat Sci Int 89: 28–33.

Piazzini DB, Aprile I, Ferrara PE, et al. 2007. A systematic review of conservative treatment of carpal tunnel syndrome. Clin Rehabil 21: 299–314.

Pierre-Jerome C, Bekkelund SI. 2005. Magnetic resonance assessment of the double-crush phenomenon in patients with carpal tunnel syndrome: a bilateral quantitative study. Scand J Plast Reconstr Surg Hand Surg 37: 46–53.

Pomerance J, Zurakowski D, Fine I. 2009. The cost-effectiveness of nonsurgical versus surgical treatment for carpal tunnel syndrome. J Hand Surg Am 7: 1193–1200.

Prantil RK, Xiu K, Kim KE, et al. 2012. Fiber orientation of the transverse carpal ligament. Clin Anat 25: 478–482.

Resende LA, Tahara A, Fonseca RG, et al. 2003. The natural history of carpal tunnel syndrome. A study of 20 hands evaluated 4 to 9 years after initial diagnosis. Electromyogr Clin Neurophysiol 43: 301–304.

Russell BS. 2008. Carpal tunnel syndrome and the 'double crush' hypothesis: a review and implications for chiropractic. Chiropr Osteopat 16: 2.

Shi Q, MacDemid JC. 2011. Is surgical intervention more effective than non-surgical treatment for carpal tunnel syndrome? A systematic review. J Orthop Surg Res 6: 17.

Silvestri E, Martinoli C, Derchi LE, et al. 1995. Echotexture of peripheral nerves: correlation between US and histologic findings and criteria to differentiate tendons. Radiology 197: 291–296.

Smith C, O'Neill J, Parasu N, et al. 2009. The role of ultrasonography in the assessment of carpal tunnel syndrome. Can Assoc Rad J 60: 279–280.

Spahn G, Wollny J, Hartmann B, et al. 2012. [Metaanalysis for the evaluation of risk factors for carpal tunnel syndrome (CTS) Part I. General factors]. Z Orthop Unfall 150: 503–515. [Article in German.]

Stapleton MJ. 2006. Occupation and carpal tunnel syndrome. A NZ J Surg 76: 494-496.

Sternbach G. 1999. The carpal tunnel syndrome. J Emerg Med 17: 519–523.

Stevens JC, Beard CM, O'Fallon WM, et al. 1992. Conditions associated with carpal tunnel syndrome. Mayo Clin Proc 67: 541–548.

Tamburin S, Cacciatori C, Marani S, et al. 2008. Pain and motor function in carpal tunnel syndrome: A clinical, neurophysiological and psychophysical study. J Neurol 255: 1636–1643.

Tanaka S, Wild DK, Seligman PJ, et al. 1995. The U.S. prevalence of self-reported carpal tunnel syndrome: 1988 national health interview survey data. Am J Indirect Med 27: 451–470.

Tecchio F, Padua L, Aprile I, et al. 2002. Carpal tunnel syndrome modifies sensory hand cortical somatotopy: a MEG study. Hum Brain Mapp 17(1): 28–36.

Tucker AT, White PD, Kosek E, et al. 2007. Comparison of vibration perception thresholds in individuals with diffuse upper limb pain and carpal tunnel syndrome. Pain 127: 263–269.

van Rijn RM, Huisstede BM, Koes BW, et al. 2009. Associations between work-related factors and the carpal tunnel syndrome: a systematic review. Scand J Work Environ Health 35:19–36.

Verdugo RJ, Salinas RA, Castillo JL, et al. 2008. Surgical versus non-surgical treatment for carpal tunnel syndrome. Cochrane Database Syst Rev 4: CD001552.

Wainner RS, Fritz JM, Irrgang JJ, et al. 2005. Development of a clinical prediction rule for the diagnosis of carpal tunnel syndrome. Arch Phys Med Rehabil 86: 609–618.

Wang LY, Leong CP, Huang YC, et al. 2008. Best diagnostic criterion in high-resolution ultrasonography for carpal tunnel syndrome. Chang Gung Med J 31: 469–476.

Watkins L, Maier S. 2004. Neuropathic pain: the immune connection. Pain: Clinical Update 12(1): 1–4. Online. Available: http://iasp.files.cms-plus.com/Content/ContentFolders/Publications2/PainClinicalUpdates/Archives/PCU04-1_1390264782800_34.pdf. (Accessed 2.12.14.)

Werner RA. 2006. Evaluation of work-related carpal tunnel syndrome. J Occup Rehabil 16: 207–222.

Werner RA, Albers JW, Franzblau A, et al. 1994. The relationship between body mass index and the diagnosis of carpal tunnel syndrome. Muscle Nerve 17: 632–636.

Westerman RA, Delaney CA. 1991. Palmar cold threshold test and median nerve electromyography in carpal tunnel compression neuropathy. Clin Exp Neur 28: 154–167.

Wilbourn AJ, Gilliatt RW. 1997. Double-crush syndrome: a critical analysis. Neurology 1: 21–27.

Yugueras P, Berger RA. 2006. Anatomy of the carpal tunnel. In: Luchetti R, Amadio P (eds) Carpal tunnel syndrome. Berlin: Springer-Verlag, Ch 2, pp 10–12.

Zanette G, Marani S, Tamburin S. 2006. Extra-median spread of sensory symptoms in carpal tunnel syndrome suggests the presence of pain-related mechanisms. Pain 2122: 264–270.

Zanette G, Marani S, Tamburin S. 2007. Proximal pain in patients with carpal tunnel syndrome: a clinical neuro-physiological study. J Periph Nerv Syst 12: 91–97.

Zanette G, Cacciatori C, Tamburin S. 2010. Central sensitization in carpal tunnel syndrome with extraterritorial spread of sensory symptoms. Pain 148: 227–236.

Zyluk A. 2013. Carpal tunnel syndrome in pregnancy: a review. Pol Orthop Traumatol 78: 223–227.

Zyluk A, Waśków B. 2011. [Symptoms of the compression of median nerve in patients after fractures of the distal radius treated operatively]. Chir Narzadow Ruchu Ortop Pol 76: 189–192. [Article in Polish.]

Chapter 51

Other Entrapment Neuropathies

Joy C. MacDermid, David M. Walton

CHAPTER CONTENTS

Epidemiology	575
Anatomy	575
Ulnar nerve	575
Radial nerve	576
Median nerve	577
Pathology	577
Diagnosis	577
Ulnar nerve	578
Radial nerve	580
Median nerve	580
Prognosis	581
Conservative treatment	581
General treatment principles	581
Ulnar nerve	581
Radial nerve	582
Median nerve	582
Conclusion	582

Epidemiology

Compression neuropathy can exist anywhere along the course of a nerve, although all reported sites are uncommon compared with the carpal tunnel. The second most common site of upper extremity compression involves the ulnar nerve at the cubital tunnel (Mondelli et al 2005). The ulnar nerve may also be compromised at Guyon's canal. The annual incidence of cubital tunnel compression in workers performing repetitive work has been estimated at 0.8% per person-year (Descatha et al 2004). A single large study (Pascarelli & Hsu 2001) suggested that the rate of electrophysiological abnormality in the median nerve at the upper extremity is twice that of the ulnar nerve, and affected median nerves are twice as likely to be symptomatic, thus resulting in a ratio of carpal to cubital tunnel syndromes of 4:1(Seror & Nathan 1993).

Entrapment of the median nerve in the proximal forearm is relatively uncommon, but is an important component of differential diagnosis and a potential explanation for failed treatment of carpal tunnel syndrome. The most-reported compression syndromes are pronator teres syndrome and anterior interosseous nerve (Kiloh–Nevin) syndrome. In a large series, these contributed 1% of the compression syndromes of the upper limb (Pascarelli & Hsu 2001).

The radial nerve has multiple sites of compression in the forearm, with 'radial tunnel' the most common. Since there is little agreement on diagnostic approaches or criteria for radial nerve compressions of the forearm, incidence / prevalence rates have not been clearly defined. In a large series of patients with work-related upper extremity disorders, 7% were diagnosed as having radial tunnel syndrome (Pascarelli & Hsu 2001).

Risk factors for developing nerve compression in the forearm are related to both activity and the individual. 'Holding a tool in position' was predictive of risk for cubital tunnel (odds ratio (OR) 4.1). Obesity (OR 4.3) had a similar risk, and the presence of concomitant upper extremity tendinosis also increased the risk (Descatha et al 2004). A gender effect has been established for cubital tunnel syndrome with males at greater risk (Richardson et al 2001). A systematic review examined the exposure–response relationships between work-related physical and psychosocial factors including cubital tunnel syndrome and radial tunnel syndrome in occupational populations (van Rijn et al 2009). The occurrence of cubital tunnel syndrome was associated with the factor 'holding a tool in position' (OR 3.5), whereas handling loads >1 kg (OR 9), static work of the hand during the majority of the cycle time (OR 5.9) and full extension (0–45°) of the elbow (OR 4.9) were associated with radial tunnel syndrome. Roquelaure et al (2000) had previously found similar risk factors: exertion of force of over 1 kg (OR 9.1), prolonged static loading of the hand (OR 6) and working with the elbow extended (OR 5).

Anatomy

Ulnar nerve

The ulnar nerve is vulnerable because of its location, its path through the forearm and the effects of position and movement. The C8 and T1 nerve roots give rise to the medial cord of the brachial plexus, which branches into the ulnar nerve and the medial component of the median nerve. The ulnar nerve travels on the medial side of the brachial artery in the upper arm, and at the mid upper arm it pierces the intermuscular septum to continue on the medial head of the triceps. At the elbow, it passes through the cubital tunnel, a groove between the medial humeral epicondyle and the olecranon. The nerve then travels between the two heads of the flexor carpi ulnaris and down the forearm between the deep and superficial finger flexors. Just below the elbow, it sends branches to the **flexor carpi ulnaris** and the ulnar half of the **flexor digitorum profundus**. There are five potential entrapment sites:

1. The arcade of Struthers, a fibrous band from the medial head of the triceps to the medial intermuscular septum (the fibrous band occurs in only 70% of people)
2. The medial intermuscular septum
3. The cubital tunnel (most common site) where the medial collateral ligament of the elbow forms the floor and the arcuate ligament (cubital tunnel retinaculum) the roof
4. The aponeurosis between the two heads of the flexor carpi ulnaris (Osborne band)
5. The aponeurotic covering between the flexors digitorum profundus and superficialis, which is occasionally a site of compression. Anatomical variants are commonly reported in case studies as unusual causes of nerve compression.

An average of 5 mm of ulnar nerve excursion is required at the elbow to accommodate shoulder motion from 30° to 110° of abduction, or elbow motion from 10° to 90°. When the wrist is moved from 60° of extension to 65° of flexion, 14 mm excursion of the ulnar nerve are required at the wrist. When all the motions of the wrist, fingers, elbow and shoulder are combined, 22 mm of ulnar nerve excursion are required at the elbow and 23 mm at the wrist. Ulnar nerve strain of 15% or more occurs at the elbow with elbow flexion and at the wrist with wrist extension and radial deviation (Wright et al 2001). Ultrasonography of 200 normal individuals revealed that the ulnar nerve changes its course at the fibrous band region 11.5 mm distal to the medial epicondyle. Dynamic studies showed that, during elbow flexion, the nerve moved to the tip of the epicondyle in 27% of individuals, whereas it dislocated anteriorly in 20% (Okamoto et al 2000). Some believe that subluxation of the nerve during movement can contribute to cubital tunnel syndrome.

At the wrist, the ulnar nerve runs above the flexor retinaculum lateral to the flexor carpi ulnaris tendon and medial to the ulnar artery. At the proximal carpal bones, it courses between the pisiform and the hook of the hamate at the entrance to the Guyon canal (the roof of the canal is formed by an extension of the **transverse carpal ligament**, which links these two bones). Three zones of the ulnar nerve within the distal ulnar tunnel have been defined, as follows:

- **zone 1:** ulnar nerve proximal to the bifurcation
- **zone 2:** the deep branch
- **zone 3:** the superficial branch or branches.

The deep (motor) branch supplies the abductor digiti minimi (ADM), then crosses under one head of the flexor digiti minimi (FDM), supplies this muscle and then crosses over to supply the opponens digiti minimi (ODM) before rounding the hook of the hamate bone to enter the mid-palmar space and supply other hand muscles. These anatomical zones correlate with the clinical symptomatology. After zone 1 the nerve bifurcates into superficial and deep branches. These **terminal branches** include the superficial cutaneous branch to the ulnar portion of the palm and volar surfaces of ulnar 1½ fingers, the deep motor branch that passes adjacent to the hook of hamate bone, and the deep branch that innervates the hypothenar muscles, third and fourth lumbricales, adductor pollicis, all the interossei and deep head of the **flexor pollicis brevis**. Depending on the exact site of compression within the Guyon canal, the ADM or both the ADM and the FDM may be spared. The ODM is always affected, together with the interossei, lumbricals 3 and 4, and the adductor pollicis. Patients with zone 1 compression can present with motor, sensory or mixed lesions, those with zone 2 only motor lesions, and zone 3 only sensory lesions. Compression of the deep branch is the most common and usually occurs at the level of the fibrous arch of the hypothenar muscles. The distal canal is also the commonest site for ganglions arising from the wrist.

Radial nerve

The radial nerve is the largest branch of the brachial plexus (posterior cord) and receives fibres from C6, C7 and C8 (sometimes T1). Its crosses the latissimus dorsi deep to the axillary artery, passes the inferior border of the teres major, winds around the humerus and then enters the triceps muscle between the long and medial heads. It progresses along the spiral groove of the humerus to pierce the lateral intermuscular septum and runs between the brachialis and brachioradialis to lie anterior to the lateral condyle of the humerus. Branches to the brachioradialis and extensor carpi radialis longus are given off just proximal to the elbow. The anconeus receives a branch, and the nerve then divides into a superficial branch and a deep branch. The extensor carpi radialis brevis (ECRB) receives its innervation either from the radial nerve proper or from the posterior interosseous nerve. The superficial branch, which is purely sensory, runs under the cover of the brachioradialis in the forearm. Eight centimetres proximal to the tip of the radial styloid, the nerve pierces the fascia medial to the brachioradialis to lie dorsal to the extensor tendons. It divides into a medial branch and a lateral branch to innervate the radial wrist (with some variable overlap from the lateral antebrachial cutaneous nerve), dorsal radial hand, and dorsum of the radial 3½ digits to approximately the middle phalanx level.

The deep branch, or posterior interosseous nerve (PIN), winds to the dorsum of the forearm, around the lateral side of the radius and through the muscle fibres of the supinator. It then divides into medial and lateral branches, each of which supplies different extensor muscles. The PIN supplies the ECRB and supinator before entering the arcade of Frohse. This arcade is a fibrotendinous structure at the proximal origin of the supinator and the most common site for entrapment of the radial nerve. In 25% of individuals, the PIN actually touches the dorsal aspect of the radius opposite the bicipital tuberosity; thus fracture fixation (plates) placed high on the dorsal surface of radius may trap the nerve underneath. The most common compression site is at the supinator muscle. However, proximal lesions should be suspected with humeral fractures. Radial nerve palsy associated with fracture is more common after fracture of the middle third of the humerus (Holstein–Lewis fracture) or at the junction of the middle and distal thirds. The nerve also can be compressed by the lateral intermuscular septum. Less-common compression sites include the fibrous arch of the lateral head of the triceps muscle and the accessory subscapularis–teres–latissimus muscle.

The aetiology of PIN syndrome is similar to that of radial tunnel syndrome. PIN compression is most commonly associated with tendinous hypertrophy of the arcade of Frohse and fibrous thickening of the radiocapitellar joint capsule. Lesions, such as lipoma, synovial cyst, rheumatoid synovitis or vascular aneurysm, may be causative and should be considered where symptoms do not respond predictably to mechanical forces. Hobbies or occupations associated with repetitive and forceful supination predispose the individual to PIN neuropathy. Chronic trauma to the flexion surface of the forearm can also create problems. Crutches that include forearm rings, inappropriately placed forearm braces (e.g. for tennis elbow) or tight clothing can provide such external compression.

Compression affects branches innervating the radial wrist extensors and the radial sensory nerve (RSN). After emerging from the supinator, the nerve may be compressed before it bifurcates into medial and lateral branches, causing a complete paralysis of the digital extensors and dorsoradial deviation of the wrist secondary to paralysis of the **extensor carpi ulnaris** (ECU). If compression occurs after the nerve bifurcates, selective paralysis of muscles occurs, depending on which branch is involved. Compression of the medial branch causes paralysis of the ECU, **extensor digitorum minimi** (EDM), and **extensor digitorum communis** (EDC). Compression of the lateral branch causes paralysis of the **abductor pollicis longus**, **extensor pollicis longus** and **extensor indices**. Other possible aetiologies for posterior interosseous nerve dysfunction include trauma (Monteggia fractures), synovitis (rheumatoid), tumours and iatrogenic injuries.

Wartenberg syndrome, or RSN entrapment, is unique in that it has isolated sensory symptoms. Insidious onset may occur in association with de Quervain tenosynovitis. Acute onset can occur following post-surgical injury, external compression or trauma on the radial aspect of the wrist. The anatomical site of compression corresponds to the transit of the nerve from its submuscular position beneath the brachioradialis to its subcutaneous position on the ECRL. With pronation, these two muscles can create a scissor-like effect, compressing the RSN.

Median nerve

The median nerve arises from both the lateral and medial cords of the brachial plexus and travels with the brachial artery on the medial side of the arm between the biceps brachii and brachialis. In the upper arm it is lateral to the artery, but then crosses anteriorly to run medial to the artery inside the cubital fossa, in front of the point of insertion of the brachialis muscle and deep to the biceps. The median nerve gives off an articular branch in the upper arm as it passes the elbow joint, and then passes between the two heads of pronator teres. It innervates the **pronator teres** (PT), **flexor carpi radialis** (FCR) and **flexor digitorum superficialis** (FDS), then travels between the FDS and **flexor digitorum profundus** (FDP) before emerging between the FDS and FCR. The median nerve gives off two branches as it courses through the forearm: the anterior interosseous branch courses with the anterior interosseous artery and innervates the flexor pollicis longus (FPL), the FDP to the second and third fingers and ends with its innervation of pronator quadratus. The palmar cutaneous branch of the median nerve arises at the distal part of the forearm and supplies sensory innervation to the lateral aspect of the skin of the palm (but not the digits).

Compression of the median nerve in the forearm can arise as a result of anatomical variations (supracondylar process, Struthers ligament, lacertus fibrosus) at the biceps brachii, or overuse / tightness of the pronator teres muscle or flexor superficialis. With lower frequency, an anomalous accessory head of the flexor pollicis longus (Ganzer's muscle) or persistent median artery can be found. Rarer causes of extrinsic compression of the median nerve are chronic compartment syndrome or partial rupture of the distal biceps tendon (or bicipital tendon bursitis). The most common site of compression of the median nerve is the tendinous origin of deep head of pronator teres.

Pathology

Nerve compression can occur directly from anatomical structures, as highlighted above. Also, repetitive or acute trauma to a nerve may result in microvascular (ischaemic) changes, oedema, or injury to the myelin sheath and structural alterations in membranes in both the myelin sheath and the nerve axon. Wallerian degeneration of the axons and permanent fibrotic changes in the neuromuscular junction may prevent full re-innervation after compression is relieved. Seddon has classified nerve injuries into three categories:

- **Neuropraxia:** A transient episode without disruption of the nerve or its sheath – complete recovery is expected.
- **Axonotmesis:** Disruption of the axon but maintenance of the Schwann sheath. In this case, motor, sensory and autonomic effects are expected and recovery may be complete or incomplete.
- **Neurotmesis:** Nerve and sheath damage and incomplete recovery are usual.

Nerve fibres are not affected uniformly but according to their proximity to the source of compression. Superficially located fibres tend to bear the brunt of compression, whereas central fibres are relatively spared. As large-diameter, heavily myelinated fibres are more sensitive to compression than poorly myelinated fibres, they are more affected. This explains the earlier and more pronounced impairment of light touch (vibration) sensibility in nerve compression disorders. Mild compression produces a transient conduction and disruption of axoplasmic flow that may be evident only with provocative manoeuvres. In chronic compression, segmental demyelination results in slowing of conduction and more persistent symptoms. With progression, axolysis occurs in compressed segments and Wallerian degeneration occurs distally. The critical threshold pressure for initiating changes in nerve has been reported to be 30 mmHg (Mackinnon 2002).

Diagnosis

Nerve compression presents with loss of sensory and motor function where mixed nerves are involved. Radial tunnel and distal sensory nerve compressions are examples of where these symptoms may occur separately. In general, progression of motor symptoms may start with a feeling of clumsiness or aching, then progress to substantial loss of muscular strength and endurance. By the time that patients have identified weakness a substantial loss in grip strength is usually measurable. Muscle atrophy is typically a late finding. Sensory abnormalities tend to progress from positional- or activity-based paraesthesiae, which be associated with pain, to persistent symptoms. In later stages, numbness may be so profound that neither pain nor paraesthesiae is as pronounced as earlier. Sensory abnormalities are first detected in vibration or touch thresholds and later appear in discriminative touch tests, such as two-point discrimination. Tables 51.1–51.3 show respectively the clinical signs, the special tests and common differential diagnosis depending on the site of nerve entrapment.

Ulnar nerve

The presenting symptoms with ulnar nerve are numbness and / or tingling, most noted by the patient in the little finger,

Table 51.1 **Symptoms and signs depending on the site of nerve entrapment**

	Ulnar nerve		Median nerve		Radial nerve	
	Cubital tunnel syndrome	*Guyon's tunnel syndrome*	*Anterior interosseus nerve syndrome*	*Radial tunnel syndrome*	*Posterior interosseus nerve syndrome*	*Distal sensory radial nerve syndrome (Wartenberg's syndrome)*
Area of symptoms	Medial elbow All of 5th and ulnar half of 4th digits	Palmar aspect of 4th and 5th digits only – sensation should be spared over dorsal aspect	Poorly localized to the volar proximal forearm	Approximately 5 cm (2″) distal to the lateral epicondyle	Over arcade of Frohse	Dorsal aspect of the radial 3½ digits, as far distally as the proximal interphalangeal joints. The subungual region[a] should be spared
Nature of symptoms	Pain, numbness or tingling, weakness	Could be any or all of pain, numbness or tingling, weakness	Pain and/or weakness	Pain and fatigue, weakness	Weakness	Pain, numbness or tingling
Motor signs	Grip and/or pinch weakness Possible Froment's sign[b] Possible Wartenberg's sign[c] May have difficulty crossing 2nd and 3rd digits Specific weakness of 1st dorsal interosseous, abductor digiti minimi and flexor digitorum profundus of the 4th and 5th digits	Froment's sign[b] Wartenberg's sign[c] Weakness of the dorsal and palmar interossei and hypothenar muscles[d]	Weakness of flexor pollicis longus and flexor digitorum profundus of the 2nd digit Affected individuals will be unable to form a circle by pinching the tips of the thumb and 2nd digit together	No obvious muscle weakness in early stages[e]	With complete palsy, patients will be unable to extend the thumb or fingers at the metacarpophalangeal joints Will also have difficulty or be unable to extend the wrist in neutral or ulnar positions[f]	No obvious muscle weakness should be present

[a]The region directly under the nail.
[b]Usually tested by asking the patient to pinch a piece of paper between the thumb and index finger, then the examiner pulls it away. Inability to hold the paper, or excessive flexion of the median innervated flexor pollicis longus (flexion of the 1st interphalangeal joint) is considered positive for ulnar nerve palsy.
[c]Abduction and extension of the 5th digit.
[d]Opponens digiti minimi, abductor digiti minimi, flexor digiti minimi brevis.
[e]Prolonged compression of the radial nerve may lead to weakness of the radially innervated muscles of the forearm including extensor digitorum, extensor pollicis longus and brevis and extensor carpi ulnaris. If weakness is present the condition is usually referred to as posterior interosseous nerve syndrome.
[f]Branches supplying ECRB and ECRL usually come off the radial nerve prior to entering the arcade of Frohse and therefore are spared.

Table 51.2 **Special tests depending on the site of nerve entrapment**

Ulnar nerve		Median nerve		Radial nerve	
Cubital tunnel syndrome	*Guyon's tunnel syndrome*	*Anterior interosseus nerve syndrome*	*Radial tunnel syndrome*	*Posterior interosseus nerve syndrome*	*Distal sensory radial nerve syndrome (Wartenberg's syndrome)*
Positive upper limb neurodynamic testing with ulnar nerve bias Positive Tinel's sign at the cubital tunnel[a] Positive elbow flexion test[b] Tenderness or hyperalgesia over the cubital tunnel[c]	Positive upper limb neurodynamic testing with ulnar nerve bias Positive Tinel's sign over Guyon's tunnel	Positive upper limb neurodynamic testing with median nerve bias May reproduce symptoms with deep palpation of the two heads of pronator teres	Positive upper limb neurodynamic testing with radial nerve bias Tenderness over the radial tunnel[d] Pain with resisted extension of the 3rd digit Pain may be reproduced with active or resisted forearm supination with wrist flexion	Positive upper limb neurodynamic testing with radial nerve bias Pain with extreme pronation Tenderness over the radial tunnel Pain with resisted extension of the 3rd digit Pain may be reproduced with active or resisted forearm supination with wrist flexion	Positive upper limb neurodynamic testing with radial nerve bias Positive Tinel's sign over the site of exit of the SRN[e] Symptoms increase when tightly pinching the thumb and 2nd digit together Pain may be reproduced with extreme pronation

[a]Positive Tinel's sign at the cubital tunnel is not an uncommon finding in asymptomatic people.
[b]Flex elbow past 90°, supinate forearm and extend wrists. Positive test is reproduction of pain or discomfort within 60 seconds. Shoulder abduction can be added to increase the symptoms.
[c]Between the medial epicondyle and olecranon.
[d]Approximately 5 cm (2″) distal to the lateral epicondyle.
[e]Between the brachioradialis and extensor carpi radialis tendons, approximately two-thirds of the way down the forearm. SRN=sensory radial nerve branch.

Table 51.3 **Common differential diagnosis depending on the site of nerve entrapment**

Ulnar nerve		Median nerve		Radial nerve	
Cubital tunnel syndrome	*Guyon's tunnel syndrome*	*Anterior interosseus nerve syndrome*	*Radial tunnel syndrome*	*Posterior interosseus nerve syndrome*	*Distal sensory radial nerve syndrome (Wartenberg's syndrome)*
C8/T1 root lesions Guyon's tunnel syndrome Thoracic outlet syndrome Valgus ligament instability Systemic – diabetes, alcoholism Pancoast tumour Medial epicondyle fracture	C8/T1 root lesions Carpal tunnel syndrome Thoracic outlet syndrome Systemic – diabetes, alcoholism Pancoast tumour	Flexor digitorum profundus avulsion Lateral cord lesion C8 radiculopathy (rare) Parsonage–Turner syndrome	Lateral epicondylitis Brachial plexus injury C5–C6 radiculopathy	C5–C8 radiculopathy Lateral epicondylitis Extensor digitorum rupture	De Quervain's tenosynovitis Brachial plexus injury C5–C8 radiculopathy

but a loss of sensory function throughout the nerve distribution. Aching pain and loss of hand function are usually reported. Symptoms are aggravated in positions of flexion (and at night). Sensory and motor impairments can be variable, and electrodiagnosis is recommended before proceeding to surgery (Nakazumi & Hamasaki 2001). Patients with an ulnar neuropathy with a gradual non-traumatic onset may report a history of repetitive elbow flexion or prolonged resting of the elbow on a hard surface. Elbow flexion creates narrowing of the cubital tunnel as a result of traction on the arcuate ligament and bulging of the medial collateral ligament. Elbow flexion may also contribute to the injury by increasing the intraneural pressure. With scarring and adhesion of the epineurium, elongation accentuates the tethering effect on the axons. These effects may be accentuated at night when the patient sleeps with the elbow in flexion.

Sensory and motor examinations of the hand reveal weakness of grip, atrophy of the thenar muscles and weakness of pinch (adductor pollicis muscle). Atrophy of affected muscles is most easily observable in the first dorsal interosseous area. Inability to cross fingers may indicate interosseous weakness, although manual muscle testing may also be used. The FCU and FDP to the ring and little finger are usually not affected. Special tests include Froment's sign, where pronounced thumb interphalangeal (IP) flexion is observed when grasping a piece of paper between thumb and index finger, as the FPL is used to stabilize the paper substituting for the absent adductor force. If the ulnar nerve is affected below the mid-forearm, an ulnar claw (hand of benediction) deformity may be produced, as the metacarpophalangeal joints of the fourth and fifth fingers are hyperextended by the long extensors (owing to a lack of balance because of weak lumbricals to these fingers) with a length-residual FDP tension producing flexion of the IP joints. If the ulnar nerve is compromised above the mid-forearm, clawing does not occur because the FDP is also affected. Deformity usually indicates more profound compression.

Sensory evaluation should include touch threshold or vibration examination to detect milder compression. A Tinel's (percussion) test can also be used, but, given the superficial nature of the nerve, a positive test in isolation should not be considered definitive proof of ulnar neuropathy as it has been reported in 24% of asymptomatic people (Rayan et al 1992). A compression test (fingertip pressure over the ulnar nerve) may be more accurate, although evidence is limited. In a small study, it was reported that the most sensitive provocative test in the diagnosis of cubital tunnel syndrome was elbow flexion when combined with pressure on the ulnar nerve. Provocative tests include sustained elbow flexion, which is positive if it reproduces symptoms within 1 minute. A study of the elbow flexion test in 216 elbows using Rayan's four positions indicated that the false positive rate was 3.6% at 1 minute and 16.2% at 3 minutes (Rosati et al 1998).

If the ulnar nerve is compromised at the wrist then a Tinel's response (electrical, shooting or tingling into the nerve distribution) may be obtained by percussing at Guyon's canal. A wrist flexion test (usually used for carpal tunnel syndrome) that produces paraesthesiae in the ring and small fingers is also a positive finding. Both palpation and observation should be used to look for abnormalities at the hamate hook or for swelling that indicates ganglia or masses. A history of 'hammering' or repeated trauma to the palm is not uncommon. The classic presentation is a young man with painless atrophy of the hypothenar muscles and interossei with sparing of the thenar group. Sensory loss and pain involving the ulnar 1½ digits may be present. Distal ulnar compression can be differentiated as the dorsum of the hand is spared, whereas in cubital tunnel compression sensation is affected over both the dorsum of the ulnar half of the ring finger and the little finger. This is because the dorsal cutaneous branch, which leaves the ulnar nerve prior to entering Guyon canal, would be spared if the compression were in Guyon's canal alone.

Radial nerve

Radial tunnel syndrome is characterized by pain over the anterolateral proximal forearm in the region of the radial head that can be aggravated by repetitive elbow extension or forearm rotation. The symptoms of radial tunnel syndrome can appear similar to those of lateral epicondylitis (Henry & Stutz 2006), although the maximum tenderness is usually located four fingerbreadths distal to the lateral epicondyle, as opposed to directly over the top of it. Based on a cadaveric study, a clinical test for radial tunnel was proposed that involved constructing nine equal squares on the anterior aspect of the forearm, and noting squares in which tenderness is elicited; in radial tunnel syndrome the tenderness (due to PIN compression) is confined to the lateral column (crossing two or three of the lateral squares) (Loh et al 2004). Symptoms can be reproduced by extending the elbow and pronating the forearm. In addition, resisted active supination and extension of the long finger cause pain (middle finger test). A compression test, where the thumb is used to compress over the radial tunnel (similar to that used for carpal compression), is positive if it reproduces symptoms or aching muscle pain. This has been reported as the most consistent finding in radial tunnel syndrome (Rinker et al 2004).

Posterior interosseous nerve syndrome presents with weakness or paralysis of the wrist and digital extensors. Pain may be present, but usually is not a primary symptom. Attempts at active wrist extension often result in weak dorsoradial deviation, owing to preservation of the radial wrist extensors but involvement of the ECU muscle and extensor digitorum communis. These patients do not have a sensory deficit. Muscle testing should include extension of the metacarpophalangeal joints, which will be weak, whereas IP extension remains intact because innervation to the lumbricals will be spared (ulnar nerve). Since the extensor indicis proprius (EIP) and EDM are independent from the EDC and separately innervated, the index and small fingers are less affected than the extension of the third and fourth digits. An extension lag in the middle two fingers, whereas the index and little fingers extend ('sign of horns') is suggestive of PIN compression.

Patients with compression of the RSN complain of pain over the distal radial forearm associated with paraesthesiae over the dorsal radial hand. They frequently report symptom magnification with wrist movement or when tightly pinching the thumb and index digit. These individuals demonstrate a positive Tinel sign over the RSN as well as local tenderness. Hyperpronation of the forearm can cause a positive Tinel sign. A high percentage of these patients reveal examination findings consistent with de Quervain tenosynovitis, and the synovitis may be a contributing factor in the compression of the nerve. Thus careful examination is required to distinguish isolated diagnosis of either condition from coexistent pathology. Finkelstein's test may be positive in both cases, but quantitative sensory testing will reveal deficit when the RSN has been compromised.

Median nerve

Patients with pronator syndrome usually complain of pain in the anterior forearm aggravated by forearm rotation. Unlike carpal tunnel patients, the symptoms are not worse at night. Compression of the median nerve is indicated by sensory motor disturbances affecting the thumb, index and long fingers, and occasionally 'ring-splitting' phenomena, where the lateral side of the ring finger is noted as different from the medial side. If the palm is also affected then confidence is increased that compression is proximal to the carpal tunnel. Muscle testing should attempt to differentiate between potential compressive structures including the lacertus fibrosus (resisted supination and flexion), FDS (independent flexion of the middle finger localizes the level of entrapment to the fibrous arcade of the FDS) and pronator teres (pronation and wrist flexion). A compression test where the thumb is used to create pressure over the pronator muscle that reproduces paraesthesia within 30 seconds is diagnostic. A differential diagnosis for C6 / C7 radiculopathy can be determined by examining the function of the muscles innervated by the C6 / C7 portions of the radial nerve (i.e. the wrist extensors and the triceps).

Involvement of the anterior interosseous nerve (AIN) can be distinguished from the median nerve proper because it is primarily a motor nerve except for some sensory branches to the distal radioulnar and carpal joints. The latter may contribute to pain in the wrist with this syndrome; however, paraesthesia is absent. The AIN supplies the FPL, the lateral half of the FDP, and the pronator quadratus. A more common misdiagnosis is FDP avulsion, as loss of terminal joint flexion may be interpreted as a loss of tendon integrity. Patients with AIN syndrome primarily complain of weakness, whereas those with pronator syndrome may present with symptoms of pain and paraesthesia that can be confused with those in carpal tunnel syndrome.

Prognosis

The extent of nerve damage affects symptoms and prognosis as discussed above. In general, severe compression detected by electrodiagnosis, atrophy, changes in two-point discrimination and persistent numbness indicates more-severe nerve damage and thus poorer prognosis. Dellon et al (1993) followed a cohort of 128 patients treated non-operatively for cubital tunnel syndrome. At 5 years, 89% of patients with symptoms only, 67% of those with abnormal sensorimotor thresholds and 38% of those with abnormal sensorimotor innervation density had not progressed to surgery. A history of elbow injury significantly worsened outcome ($p<0.02$), but the results of the pretreatment electrodiagnosis did not. For patients who do proceed to cubital tunnel release, outcomes are better if physical therapy is initiated within 3 days rather being delayed for 14 days (Warwick & Seradge 1995).

Conservative Treatment

General treatment principles

As the majority of nerve compression syndromes discussed in this chapter are rare, specific high-quality evidence on best management approaches is virtually lacking. Therefore, extrapolation of the efficacies of specific techniques studied in the commoner compression neuropathies (e.g. carpal tunnel syndrome) has of necessity been used, resulting in lower confidence in these recommendations. A treatment programme generally selects a variety of techniques that address specific objectives such as: to alter factors that are contributing to compression or compromise of the nerve, to promote nerve recovery, to enhance nerve gliding and to facilitate normalized cortical reorganization.

Techniques are routinely used to reduce static (compressive) postures, repetitive trauma or external forces. The specific positions / activities to avoid are discussed by each syndrome below. Careful examination of contractile versus insert structures may delineate the source of compression. Where musculotendinous hypertrophy is a contributing factor, strengthening of these muscles may worsen symptoms. However, strengthening of muscles for postural realignment is needed to reduce positional nerve compression. Muscle endurance may be important to prevent oedema with activity or abnormal movement patterns that contribute to compression. Rest may be required to reduce compression related to inflammation, but lack of muscle extensibility is likely to worsen symptoms. Therefore, careful examination of potential sites / aetiologies is required so as to customize the rest / mobilization / realignment strategy for each patient. A generalized progression of activity would move from rest and gentle nerve-gliding exercises to reduce symptoms, to treatment focusing on restoring muscle and nerve length extensibility, and finally to functional / postural restrengthening / rebalancing. An important goal throughout treatment is to ensure that proper body mechanics and muscle recruitment are used during functional and occupational tasks.

Nerve recovery is primarily promoted by removal of compromising / compressive forces and allowing the body to heal nerve fibres that remain viable. Facilitation of this recovery with adjunctive physical agents may promote this process or be used to facilitate mobilization of the nerve. Low-dose ultrasound (1.0 W / cm^2), of long duration (15-minute sessions – 5× / week for 2 weeks, then 2× / week for 5 weeks), resulted in better nerve conduction velocity in carpal tunnel syndrome patients both immediately after the end of treatment and 6 months later (Ebenbichler et al 1998). In contrast, higher doses at shorter intervals have not shown effectiveness. Iontophoresis with dexamethasone and lidocaine was used in one small trial of patients who failed splinting for patients with carpal tunnel syndrome, and 11 / 19 recovered (Banta 1994). Another trial suggested that, in mild to moderate cases, 10 treatments of iontophoresis and ultrasound was effective in reducing symptoms (Dakowicz & Latosiewicz 2005).

The ability of the nerve to glide between different structures in the forearm has been highlighted in the section above on anatomy. Consequently, there have been suggestions that 'nerve-sliding' techniques may enhance the mobility of the nerve, while producing less strain (Coppieters & Alshami 2007). An approach that encourages nerve mobility has been suggested as beneficial, but current clinical trials are limited to those using such exercises as an adjunct to splinting and these trials tend to be underpowered (Coppieters et al 2004; Pinar et al 2005; Baysal et al 2006; Svernlov et al 2009). (See Ch 64 for a discussion of nerve neurodynamics.) There is rationale (level 5 evidence) to suggest that a detailed examination of muscle mobility, activation and positional effects on symptoms that are characteristic of physical therapy expertise may identify structures that require specific mobilization, although this will remain inherently difficult to study in clinical trials.

Ulnar nerve

The mainstay of treating cubital tunnel syndrome has been night positioning, activity modification (Padua et al 2002), splinting the elbow in extension and nerve-gliding exercise.

Although custom-made hard thermoplastic splints are common, compliance can be a problem and soft versions that restrict full flexion may be more acceptable to patients. These can range from inexpensive off-the shelf (neoprene and other materials) or homemade approaches (e.g. a pair of socks used to create a sleeve and flexion block) to custom-made individual padded orthoses.

Behavioural changes should include avoiding compression (e.g. resting on the elbows, elbow flexion, external pressure on the elbows) and repetitive flexion or any activity in extremes of position. Office workers may need work-station evaluation, and postural and ergonomic training.

Nerve mobilization if slowly progressed may be useful, but care should be taken to avoid overaggressive mobilization that contributes to the problem through tractioning the ulnar nerve. There is empirical evidence that 'sliding techniques' result in a substantially larger excursion of the ulnar nerve at the elbow than 'tensioning techniques' (8.3 mm versus 3.8 mm) and that this larger excursion is associated with a much smaller change in strain (Coppieters & Butler 2008). Differential stretching of specific muscles (FDS) may also increase mobility. Although strength may be compromised, and functional goals may suggest the need for improved strength, therapists should exercise caution as strengthening exercise has the potential to increase compressive factors.

The evidence for conservative management is sparse and inconclusive. A recent small trial suggested that 75% of patients with mild to moderate ulnar neuropathy improve within 6 months, but that splinting and nerve gliding provide no additional benefit over activity modification (Svernlov et al 2009); the potential for lack of power in this trial of 70 patients is substantial, but it does indicate the need for more evidence. The potential for natural history of recovery with minor changes (Szabo & Kwak 2007) suggests that activity modification and evaluation of a recovery pathway should be implemented as a first approach. Failure to respond to a more comprehensive physical therapy programme indicates a need for surgical release (Robertson & Saratsiotis 2005; Lund & Amadio 2006).

Radial nerve

Evidence for the effectiveness of conservative management and radial tunnel is lacking (Huisstede et al 2008). Mobilization of the potential compressive structures and differential movement of both muscle and tendon may be useful. Ergonomic changes to workstations may include tilting / split or modified keyboards to reduce excessive rotation or extreme wrist positioning. Tissue pressures suggest that positions of elbow flexion, supination and wrist extension place the least stress and strain on the radial tunnel. This is not functional, but patients may benefit from a wrist support that places the wrist in moderate wrist extension and being given advice on avoiding forearm rotation and elbow-extended positions during activity. Given that radial nerve symptoms can be confused with lateral epicondylitis, patients whose symptoms are unimproved or are worsened by a tennis elbow counterforce bracing should be re-evaluated for potential radial tunnel syndrome and switched if necessary to a wrist extension splint.

Median nerve

Changes in activity to reduce median nerve irritation include prevention of repetitive forearm rotation and excessive forceful grip. A rest splint that maintains mid-rotation is sometimes used for a short period, although the necessity of this has not been proven (Lee & LaStayo 2004). The natural history of compressive disorders would suggest that activity modification is more important. Stretching of the pronator teres and nerve gliding may be useful.

Conclusion

Nerves can be compromised in the forearm as a result of anatomic, biomechanical or external forces. Muscle testing and sensory examination should reveal the nerve affected and the most likely site of compression. Quantitative measures of muscle strength and sensory detection threshold are imperative for accurate diagnosis and monitoring progress in treatment. A treatment programme that mitigates the compressive forces, facilitates nerve healing, restores normal gliding, uses postural and cortical retraining to normalize anatomical balance and interpretation of nerve responses, and teaches patients to be proactive in identifying potential sources of compression in their work and behaviour (and how to modify these appropriately) should be successful for mild to moderate cases of nerve compression. Advanced compression may require surgical release, with early physical therapy being indicated. Both the quality and quantity of evidence on physical therapy techniques or programmes are insufficient, and studies that look at the immediate impact of specific interventions on nerve function and the more global functional impacts of physical therapy programmes over the longer term are needed.

References

Banta CA. 1994. A prospective, nonrandomized study of iontophoresis, wrist splinting, and anti-inflammatory medication in the treatment of early-mild carpal tunnel syndrome. J Occup Med 36: 166–168.

Baysal O, Altay Z, Ozcan C, et al. 2006. Comparison of three conservative treatment protocols in carpal tunnel syndrome. J Clin Prac 60: 820–828.

Coppieters MW, Alshami AM. 2007. Longitudinal excursion and strain in the median nerve during novel nerve gliding exercises for carpal tunnel syndrome. J Orthop Res 25: 972–980.

Coppieters MW, Butler DS. 2008. Do 'sliders' slide and 'tensioners' tension? An analysis of neurodynamic techniques and considerations regarding their application. Man Ther 13: 213–221.

Coppieters MW, Bartholomeeusen KE, Stappaerts KH. 2004. Incorporating nerve-gliding techniques in the conservative treatment of cubital tunnel syndrome. J Manipulative Physiol Ther 27: 560–568.

Dakowicz A, Latosiewicz R. 2005. The value of iontophoresis combined with ultrasound in patients with the carpal tunnel syndrome. Rocz Akad Med Bialymst 50: 196–198.

Dellon AL, Hament W, Gittelshon A. 1993. Nonoperative management of cubital tunnel syndrome: an 8-year prospective study. Neurology 43: 1673–1677.

Descatha A, Leclerc A, Chastang JF, et al. 2004. Incidence of ulnar nerve entrapment at the elbow in repetitive work. Scand J Work Environ Health 30: 234–240.

Ebenbichler GR, Resch KL, Nicolakis P, et al. 1998. Ultrasound treatment for treating the carpal tunnel syndrome: randomised 'sham' controlled trial. BMJ 316: 731–735.

Henry M, Stutz C. 2006. A unified approach to radial tunnel syndrome and lateral tendinosis. Tech Hand Up Extrem Surg 10: 200–205.

Huisstede B, Miedema HS, van Opstal T, et al. 2008. Interventions for treating the radial tunnel syndrome: a systematic review of observational studies. J Hand Surg Am: 33 72–78.

Lee MJ, LaStayo PC. 2004. Pronator syndrome and other nerve compressions that mimic carpal tunnel syndrome. J Orthop Sports Phys Ther 34: 601–609.

Loh YC, Lam WL, Stanley JK, et al. 2004. A new clinical test for radial tunnel syndrome, the Rule-of-Nine test: a cadaveric study. J Orthop Surg 12: 83–86.

Lund AT, Amadio PC. 2006. Treatment of cubital tunnel syndrome: perspectives for the therapist. J Hand Ther 19: 170–178.

Mackinnon E. 2002. Pathophysiology of nerve compression. Hand Clin 18: 231–241.

Mondelli M, Giannini F, Ballerini M, et al. 2005. Incidence of ulnar neuropathy at the elbow in the province of Siena (Italy). J Neurol Sci 234: 5–10.

Nakazumi Y, Hamasaki M. 2001. Electrophysiological studies and physical examinations in entrapment neuropathy: sensory and motor functions compensation for the central nervous system in cases with peripheral nerve damage. Electromyogr Clin Neurophysiol 41: 345–348.

Okamoto M, Abe M, Shirai H, et al. 2000. Morphology and dynamics of the ulnar nerve in the cubital tunnel. Observation by ultrasonography. J Hand Surg Br 25: 85–89.

Padua L, Aprile I, Caliandro P, et al. 2002. Natural history of ulnar entrapment at elbow. Clin Neurophysiol 113: 1980–1984.

Pascarelli EF, Hsu YP. 2001. Understanding work-related upper extremity disorders: clinical findings in 485 computer users, musicians, and others. J Occup Rehabil 11: 1–21.

Pinar L, Enhos A, Ada S, et al. 2005. Can we use nerve gliding exercises in women with carpal tunnel syndrome? Adv Ther 22: 467–475.

Rayan GM, Jensen C, Duke J. 1992. Elbow flexion test in the normal population. J Hand Surg Am 17: 86–89.

Richardson JK, Green DF, Jamieson SC, et al. 2001. Gender, body mass and age as risk factors for ulnar mononeuropathy at the elbow. Muscle Nerve 24: 551–554.

Rinker B, Effron CR, Beasley RW. 2004. Proximal radial compression neuropathy. Ann Plast Surg 52: 174–180.

Robertson C, Saratsiotis J. 2005. A review of compressive ulnar neuropathy at the elbow. J Manipulative Physiol Ther 28: 345

Roquelaure Y, Raimbeau G, Dano C, et al. 2000. Occupational risk factors for radial tunnel syndrome in industrial workers. Scand J Work Environ Health 26: 507–513.

Rosati M, Martignoni R, Spagnolli G, et al. 1998. Clinical validity of the elbow flexion test for the diagnosis of ulnar nerve compression at the cubital tunnel. Acta Orthop Belg 64: 366–370.

Seror P, Nathan PA. 1993. Relative frequency of nerve conduction abnormalities at carpal tunnel and cubital tunnel in France and the United States: importance of silent neuropathies and role of ulnar neuropathy after unsuccessful carpal tunnel syndrome release. Ann Chir Main Memb Super 12: 281–285.

Svernlov B, Larsson M, Rehn K, et al. 2009. Conservative treatment of the cubital tunnel syndrome. J Hand Surg Eur 34: 201–207.

Szabo RM, Kwak C. 2007. Natural history and conservative management of cubital tunnel syndrome. Hand Clin 23: 311–313.

van Rijn RM, Huisstede BM, Koes BW, et al. 2009. Associations between work-related factors and specific disorders at the elbow: a systematic literature review. Rheumatology (Oxford) 48(5): 528–536. doi: 10.1093/rheumatology/kep013.

Warwick L, Seradge H. 1995. Early versus late range of motion following cubital tunnel surgery. J Hand Ther 8: 245–248.

Wright TW, Glowczewskie F, Cowin D, et al. 2001. Ulnar nerve excursion and strain at the elbow and wrist associated with upper extremity motion. J Hand Surg Am 26: 655–662.

52 Chapter

Joint Mobilization and Manipulation

Peter A. Huijbregts, Freddy M. Kaltenborn, Traudi Baldauf Kaltenborn

CHAPTER CONTENTS

Introduction 584
Scientific evidence for mobilization of the wrist and hand 585
Mobilization/manipulation of the wrist and hand 586
Distal radioulnar joint dorsal glide radius 587
Distal radioulnar joint ventral glide radius 587
Distal radioulnar joint MWM 587
Radiocarpal traction 587
Radiocarpal palmar glide 588
Radiocarpal dorsal glide 588
Radiocarpal radial glide 588
Radiocarpal ulnar glide 588
Radiocarpal MWM 589
Opponens roll 589
Transverse carpal extension 589
Radial carpal palmar glides 589
Central carpal palmar glides 590
Ulnar carpal palmar glides 590
Radial carpal dorsal glides 590
Central carpal dorsal glides 590
Ulnar carpal dorsal glides 590
Carpal glide manipulation with proximal fixation 590
Carpal glide manipulation with distal fixation 591
Carpometacarpal I traction 591
Carpometacarpal I glides 592
Metacarpophalangeal I MWM 592
Finger joint traction 592
Finger-joint glides 592
Finger joint MWM 592

Introduction

Therapists use mobilization and manipulation techniques to reduce pain and increase range of motion (ROM) (Kaltenborn et al 2007). Kaltenborn et al (2007) classify joint restrictions as periarticular, extra-articular, intra-articular, or combined in aetiology. Periarticular restrictions due to adaptive shortening of neuromuscular and inert structures (including skin, retinacula and scar tissue) and extra-articular structures (capsule and ligaments) are best treated with sustained mobilization techniques, whereas periarticular restriction due to muscle hypertonicity responds best to neurophysiological inhibitory techniques. Intra-articular restrictions are best treated with (traction) manipulation initiated from the actual resting position (Kaltenborn et al 2008).

Guiding both diagnosis and management, Kaltenborn et al (2007) have described grades of movement (Fig. 52.1):

- **Grade I** is a very small traction force that eliminates the normal compressive forces across the joint.
- **Grade II** takes up the slack with initially very little resistance to passive movement (slack zone), then more resistance as tissues are tightened (transition zone), and finally a marked resistance called the first stop.
- **Grade III** occurs after the first stop: as tissues become taut, resistance to movement rapidly increases within this range.

In joint dysfunction both the expected normal excursion and resistance to movement for the various grades will be altered. Grade I traction movements facilitate gliding movements used during examination, mobilization and manipulation and are applied during all techniques described later. Treatment to relieve pain occurs in the grade I and grade II slack zone ranges. Limited movement in the absence of shortened tissues can be treated by joint mobilization techniques throughout grade II (Kaltenborn et al 2007). Extra-articular restrictions due to capsuloligamentous connective tissue shortening are best treated with non-thrust grade III mobilization techniques. Thrust manipulation techniques are used both for diagnosis and for management of intra-articular restrictions (Kaltenborn et al 2008). To date, the specific nature of these intra-articular restrictions remains unknown but clinically they may present with restricted ROM, an earlier first stop, abnormal end feel and altered through-range resistance (perhaps due to small positional faults or synovial fluid changes with resultant alterations in cohesion and adhesion) with traction and gliding joint play motions, and pain on compression due to possible intra-articular entrapment of sensitive structures.

Without proposing the location of the tissue at fault, Mulligan (2004) has suggested 'minor positional faults' as an alternate aetiology for joint dysfunction that will respond to mobilization with movement (MWM). With an MWM the therapist applies a sustained accessory glide, long-axis

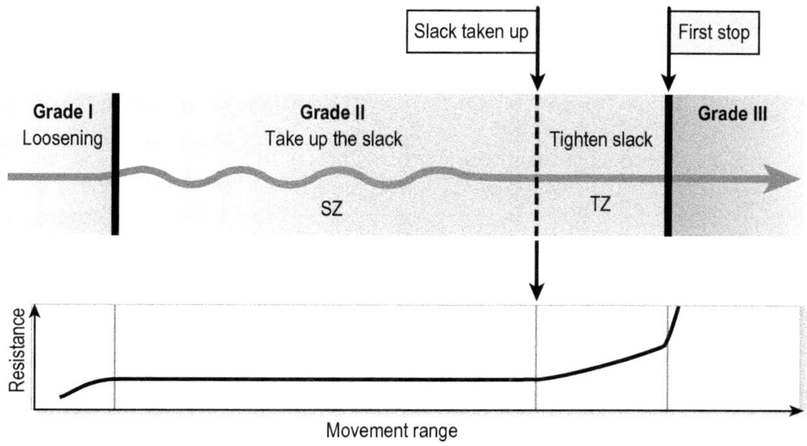

Figure 52.1 Kaltenborn grades of movement. SZ=slack zone; TZ=transition zone. (Redrawn from Kaltenborn et al 2007, with permission.)

rotation, or combination of these while the patient actively performs a previously painful movement. (See Ch 31 for further discussion of MWM in the shoulder.) Central to both the Kaltenborn and the Mulligan approach is the emphasis on restoration of the gliding component of the normal joint roll-gliding movement (Exelby 1996). Central also to both is the treatment plane defined as the plane across the concave joint surface. Translatoric techniques encompassing traction, compression and gliding techniques, traction and compression are performed perpendicular to this treatment plane, whereas gliding techniques induce movement parallel to this plane (Kaltenborn et al 2007).

The difference between the Kaltenborn and Mulligan techniques is that, whereas Kaltenborn emphasizes gliding techniques in the direction normally associated with the restricted physiological motion, Mulligan often starts with a sustained glide at a right angle to this physiological glide. An iterative process then tests glides in different directions or long-axis rotation before settling on the most effective direction allowing for pain-free active range of motion or isometric muscle contraction constituting the MWM (Exelby 1996; Hsieh et al 2002). Two to three sets of 6–10 repetitions are performed, supported by a home programme of self-mobilization and corrective taping (Mulligan 2004). An additional difference between the two techniques is that the Kaltenborn concept uses only straight-lined (linear) gliding techniques parallel to the treatment plane for joint mobilization, whereas Mulligan adapts continuously to the contour of the joint surface with curvilinear gliding techniques. It should be noted, though, that the Kaltenborn technique has also traditionally used curvilinear gliding techniques, albeit for assisted active movements and solely according to the convex–concave rule.

Scientific Evidence for Mobilization of the Wrist and Hand

Research evidence for the use of mobilization and manipulation techniques in the wrist and hand region is limited but emerging. Using animal research, Olson (1987) showed increased passive ROM and ROM during gait in dogs with immobilization-induced radiocarpal hypomobility receiving end-range oscillatory traction and gliding mobilization, compared with controls not receiving this intervention.

Sucher (1994) provided preliminary clinical evidence for manual therapy for patients with carpal tunnel syndrome (CTS) in the form of an uncontrolled case series showing decreased severity of symptoms and normalization of electrodiagnostic findings. Sucher et al (2005) also provided basic science evidence in cadavers for the use of sustained manual techniques, including variations of the opponens roll and transverse carpal extension manoeuvres intended to stretch the flexor retinaculum. However, although noting significant within-group improvement for self-reported physical and mental distress, nerve conduction studies and finger sensation for both study groups, Davis et al (1998) found no significant between-group differences in their randomized controlled trial (RCT) of 91 subjects with CTS treated either with 16 sessions over 9 weeks of chiropractic cervicothoracic spine and upper extremity joint and soft tissue manipulation, ultrasound and night splinting or with medical management consisting of ibuprofen and splinting. In 21 patients with CTS scheduled for surgery, Tal-Akabi and Rushton (2000) compared 3 weeks of treatment using neurodynamic mobilization or palmar and dorsal carpal gliding mobilization and flexor retinaculum stretching with a control group. They reported significant within-group improvements with regard to pain and active wrist extension ROM for both mobilization groups and significant between-group differences favouring both experimental groups over the control group with regard to pain. Six of seven subjects in the control group proceeded with surgery, whereas 11 of 14 in the mobilization groups cancelled surgery. Two systematic reviews (O'Connor et al 2003; Muller et al 2004) have recommended carpal bone mobilization for the management of patients with CTS.

In an RCT with 52 patients, Taylor and Bennell (1994) compared management of patients suffering from Colles fracture consisting of advice, heat and a home programme with the same programme plus manual mobilization; they reported no between-group difference in wrist extension ROM. In an RCT with 32 patients, McPhate and Robertson (1998) looked at the effects of a home programme with or without manual mobilization and also found no between-group difference for wrist extension ROM or grip strength, but they did note significantly lower pain scores in the mobilization group. Kay et al (2000) randomly assigned 39 patients with cast and / or internal fixation post-Colles fracture to a home programme with or without Maitland grade 1–2 accessory mobilization of the distal radioulnar and carpal joints, progressing to grade 3–4 physiological techniques. They reported significant within-group differences on pain, ROM, grip strength and function for both groups, but only one statistically (but not clinically) significant difference in wrist flexion ROM favouring the mobilization group. Using a single-subject design for eight subjects with stable (type I or III) Colles fractures, Coyle and Robertson (2002) compared six sessions of various combinations of two 60-second end-range oscillatory and sustained palmar gliding radiocarpal mobilization in maximum pain-free extension; they noted improvement in wrist extension ROM in both groups. They also noted that oscillation was most effective in increasing ROM if used first in treatment session and in the presence of pain, whereas the sustained technique was more effective in later treatment sessions and when used as a second technique for increasing ROM. A systematic review reflected these equivocal findings in stating that manual mobilization for Colles fracture was not supported by an RCT, but did show positive outcomes in a case series design (Michlovitz et al 2004).

Randall et al (1992) randomly assigned 18 subjects after at least 2 weeks of immobilization for a metacarpal fracture to an active ROM home programme or a home programme combined with three sessions of end-range oscillatory metacarpophalangeal (MCP) traction and gliding mobilization. Over the course of 1 week, the mobilization group improved significantly with regard to joint stiffness and ROM compared with the control group. Two case reports have also lent support to the use of long-axis rotation MWM in post-fall MCP I dysfunction, although one report using MRI did not support Mulligan's hypothesis of resolution of a 'minor positional fault' (Folk 2001; Hsieh et al 2002).

One case report indicated the possible benefit of a multimodal management approach in a patient with de Quervain syndrome consisting of neural mobilization and joint mobilization of the cervicothoracic spine, shoulder and wrist including palmar and dorsal gliding mobilization of the capitate and lunate bone (Anderson & Tichenor 1994). Backstrom (2002) reported positive outcomes in a patient with de Quervain syndrome using a multimodal programme including palmar manipulation of the capitate, 'conventional' joint mobilization and MWM techniques including radial glide of the proximal carpal row during thumb and wrist motion and ulnar glide of the trapezium and trapezoid bones during active thumb motion.

Reflecting the role of the wrist in the upper extremity kinetic chain, Struijs et al (2003) compared (a maximum of) nine treatments over 6 weeks of 15–20 minutes of repeated palmar scaphoid gliding manipulation and passive wrist ROM with a control treatment of friction massage, ultrasound and strengthening in an RCT on 28 patients with lateral epicondylalgia. They reported a significant between-group difference on a global measure of improvement at 3 weeks and on pain at 6 weeks, both results being in favour of the manipulation group.

Mobilization / Manipulation of the Wrist and Hand

In the Kaltenborn concept, traction mobilization and manipulation are specific translatoric techniques always performed perpendicular to the treatment plane. When choosing a translatoric gliding mobilization technique, clinicians need to consider the Kaltenborn convex–concave rule describing the arthrokinematic roll-gliding combinations (Kaltenborn et al 2007). When the moving joint partner has a convex joint surface, gliding mobilization occurs in the direction opposite to the direction of restricted bone movement. When the moving joint partner has a concave joint surface, gliding mobilization (in both cases with concurrent grade I traction) occurs in the same direction as the restricted bone movement. Knowledge of joint surface geometry (Mink et al 1990) is, therefore, a necessary prerequisite for appropriate gliding mobilization technique choice. It should be noted that Mulligan MWM techniques generally apply glides perpendicular to, or even opposite to, the directions proposed by the convex–concave rule – assuming the presence of undefined 'minor positional faults' interfering with normal arthrokinematic movement behaviour. Unless otherwise indicated, all techniques described in this section are taken from Kaltenborn et al (2007).

In the distal radioulnar joint, the radius is the concave joint partner and the ulna has the convex joint surface. Supination requires a dorsal glide of the distal radius and pronation a palmar glide in relation to the distal ulna.

The proximal row of carpal bones offers a convex articular surface to the concave radius–triangular fibrocartilage complex. This means that roll and glide occur in opposite directions during radiocarpal movements.

The situation is more complex in the articulation between the proximal and distal carpal row. The concave surface on trapezium and trapezoid articulates with a convex surface on the (biconvex) scaphoid. This means that, during wrist extension, the trapezium and trapezoid roll dorsally and also glide in a dorsal direction and that, during wrist flexion, roll and glide of the trapezium and trapezoid are both in a palmar direction. In addition, with the trapezium–trapezoid complex able to assume a more dorsal position, radial deviation is made possible. In the central (lunate / capitate) and ulnar (triquetrum and hamate) carpal bones, the proximal row has the concave joint surfaces, whereas the distal carpals have convex joint surfaces. That means that during wrist extension the roll of the capitate and hamate is dorsal, but their glides are in a palmar direction. During wrist flexion, the hamate and capitate roll palmar, but glide dorsally. During wrist extension, the radial carpal bones lock early, but an additional 52° occurs lunate and capitate. This requires the presence of a large amount of mobility between the scaphoid and the adjacent lunate.

The carpometacarpal (CMC) II–IV joints are almost flat joints but the CMC V joint is a sellar joint. The concave surface on the fifth metacarpal runs medial–lateral and the convex surface runs dorsal–palmar. The CMC I joint is also a sellar joint. The concave distal surface is involved in flexion and extension of the thumb; the convex distal surface is involved in abduction and adduction of the thumb (i.e. roll and glide are in the same direction for flexion and extension), whereas for abduction and adduction the roll is in the same direction to and the glide is in the opposite direction to the bone movement.

The distal end of the metacarpals I–V is biconvex; the proximal end of the proximal phalanx is biconcave. Therefore, in the MCP II–V joints, roll and glide of the proximal phalanx are in the same direction, with both flexion–extension and

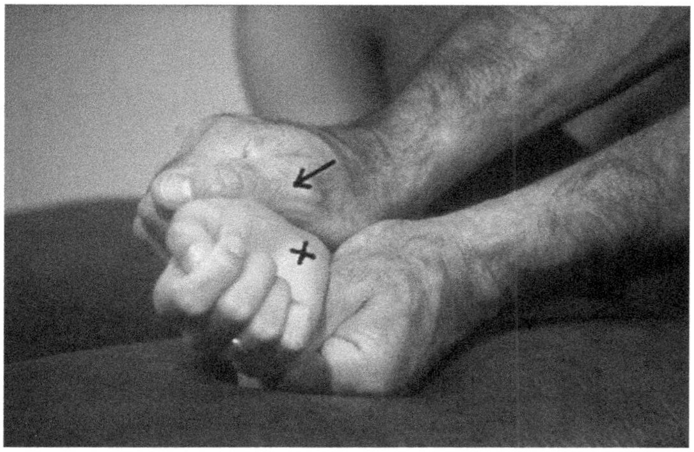

Figure 52.2 Distal radioulnar joint dorsal glide radius.

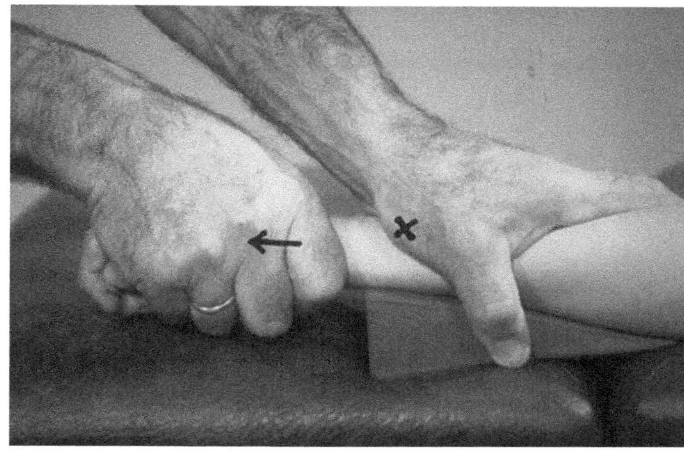

Figure 52.3 Radiocarpal traction.

radial–ulnar deviations. The interphalangeal joints I–V are hinge joints with the convexity proximal and the concavity distal, resulting in roll and glide in the same direction during flexion and extension.

Distal radioulnar joint dorsal glide radius (Fig. 52.2)

This technique is indicated in patients with restricted supination. The patient is sitting with the arm by the side, and the forearm supported on table and supinated. The therapist stands facing the palmar side of the patient's forearm. The stabilizing hand of the therapist fixates the distal ulna on its palmar aspect with the thenar and on its dorsal aspect with the fingertips. The thenar portion of therapist's mobilizing hand provides dorsal gliding mobilization to the distal radius. This technique can be performed in various positions of supination up to pathological end range.

Distal radioulnar joint ventral glide radius

This technique is indicated in patients with restricted pronation. The patient is sitting with arm abducted at shoulder, forearm supported on the table and pronated. The therapist stands facing the dorsal side of the patient's forearm. The stabilizing hand of the therapist fixates the distal ulna on its palmar aspect with the fingertips and on its dorsal aspect with thenar or thumb. The thenar portion of therapist's mobilizing hand provides ventral gliding mobilization to the distal radius. This mobilization can be performed in various positions of pronation up to the pathological end range.

Distal radioulnar joint MWM (Mulligan 2004)

This technique is indicated in patients with restricted supination due to a minor positional fault (note that the direction of glide is *opposite* to normal arthrokinematic gliding). The patient is sitting, shoulder flexed, elbow bent and forearm supinated. The therapist is standing dorsal to the hand. The therapist places the fingers of the ipsilateral hand on the palmar aspect of the distal radius and then covers these with the fingers of the contralateral hand. The ipsilateral thumb is placed over the contralateral thumb on the distal dorsal aspect of the radius. The fingers apply dorsal gliding to ulna and, maintaining this, the patient actively supinates (with therapist-applied overpressure).

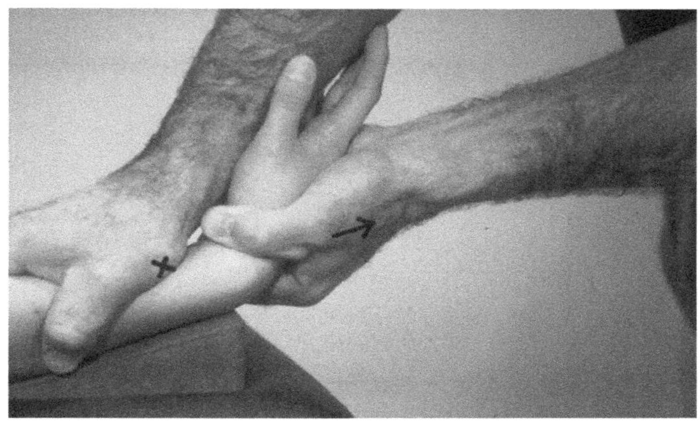

Figure 52.4 Radiocarpal traction in flexion.

Radiocarpal traction

This technique serves as a non-specific joint mobilization. The patient is sitting, with arm pronated and resting on wedge or table. The therapist stands distal to patient's wrist. The distal forearm is fixated against a wedge by the therapist's stabilizing hand; the thenar portion stabilizes just proximal to the wrist. The mobilizing hand grasps the carpal bones just distal to the wrist joint and performs traction (Fig. 52.3).

This technique can be made more effective by various degrees of wrist flexion (Fig. 52.4), extension (Fig. 52.5), radial deviation or ulnar deviation; shifting the stabilizing and mobilizing hands distally allows for traction between the distal and proximal carpal rows. This mobilization can be made more specific when the mobilizing hand grasps one carpal bone with the thumb dorsal and index fingertip ventral.

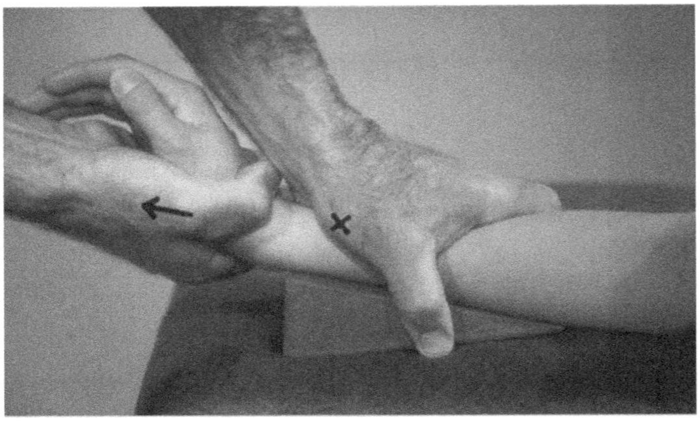

Figure 52.5 Radiocarpal traction in extension.

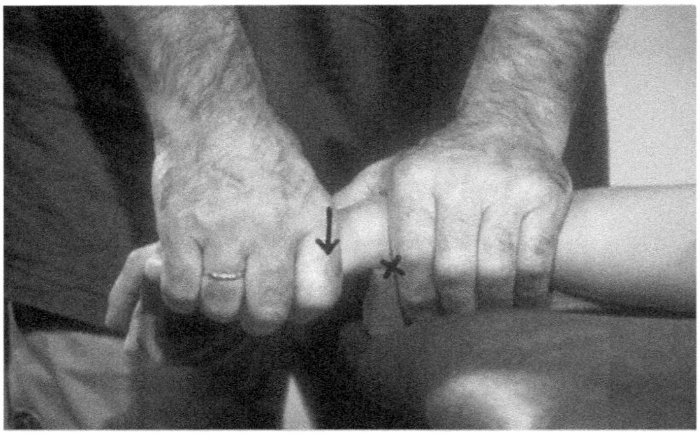

Figure 52.6 Radiocarpal palmar glide.

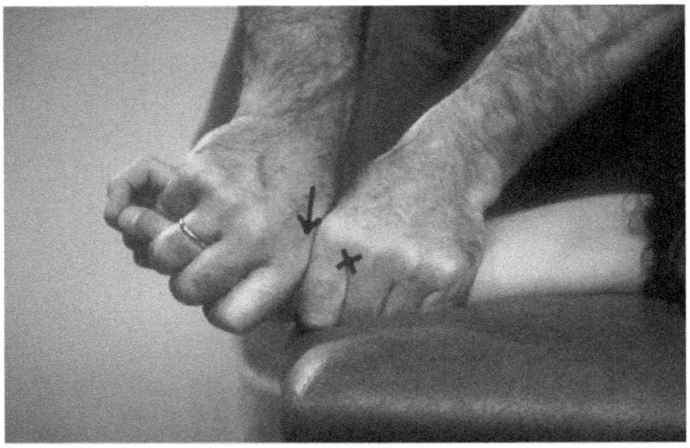

Figure 52.7 Radiocarpal palmar glide in extension.

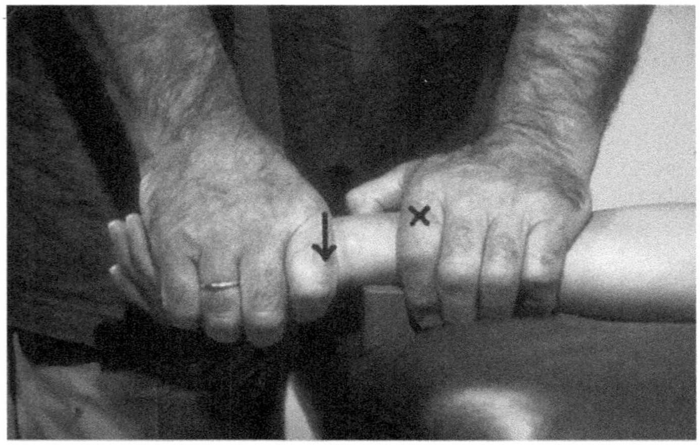

Figure 52.8 Radiocarpal dorsal glide.

Radiocarpal palmar glide

This technique is indicated in patients with restricted wrist extension. The patient is sitting, with arm pronated and resting on a wedge or table. The therapist is standing at the ulnar side of the patient's wrist. The distal forearm is fixated against a wedge by the therapist's stabilizing hand; the thenar portion stabilizes just proximal to the wrist. The mobilizing hand grasps the patient's carpal bones just distal to the wrist joint and performs the palmar glide (Fig. 52.6).

This mobilization can be also done in various degrees of wrist extension (Fig. 52.7); shifting stabilizing and mobilizing hands distally allows for glide between the distal and proximal carpal rows. It can be made more specific when the head of metacarpal II of the mobilizing hand is placed on one carpal bone.

Radiocarpal dorsal glide

This technique is indicated in patients with restricted wrist flexion. The patient is sitting, with arm supinated and resting on a wedge. The therapist is standing at the radial side of the wrist. The distal forearm is fixated against the wedge by the therapist's stabilizing hand; the thenar portion stabilizes just proximal to the wrist. The mobilizing hand grasps the carpal bones just distal to wrist joint and performs the dorsal glide (Fig. 52.8).

This technique can be also done in various degrees of wrist flexion (Fig. 52.9); shifting stabilizing and mobilizing hands distally allows for glide between the distal and proximal carpal row.

Radiocarpal radial glide (Fig. 52.10)

This technique is indicated in patients with restricted ulnar deviation. The patient is sitting, with shoulder abducted, forearm pronated and resting on a wedge, or can be also supine, with shoulder elevated and externally rotated. The therapist is standing at the palmar side of the wrist. The patient's distal forearm is fixed against a wedge by the therapist's stabilizing hand just proximal to wrist. The mobilizing hand grasps the carpal bones from the ulnar side, just distal to the wrist joint, and performs the radial glide. This mobilization can be done in various degrees of wrist ulnar deviation.

Radiocarpal ulnar glide (Fig. 52.11)

This technique is indicated in patients with restricted radial deviation. The patient is sitting, with arm supinated and resting with the ulnar aspect on a wedge. The therapist is

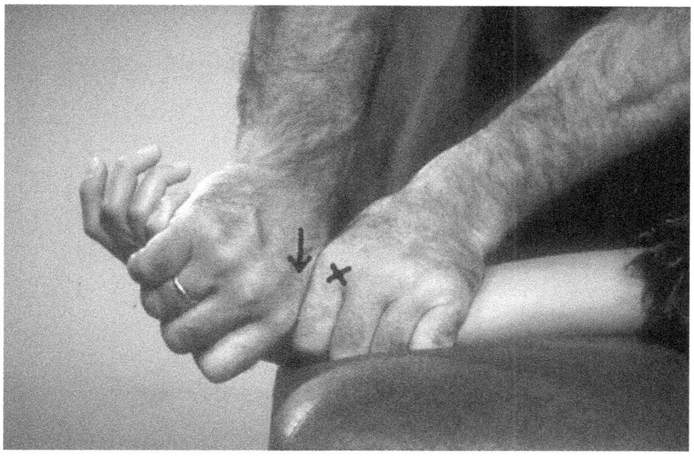

Figure 52.9 Radiocarpal dorsal glide in flexion.

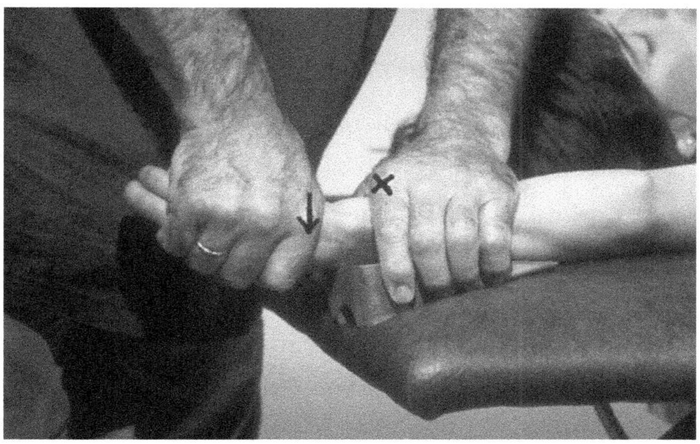

Figure 52.10 Radiocarpal radial glide.

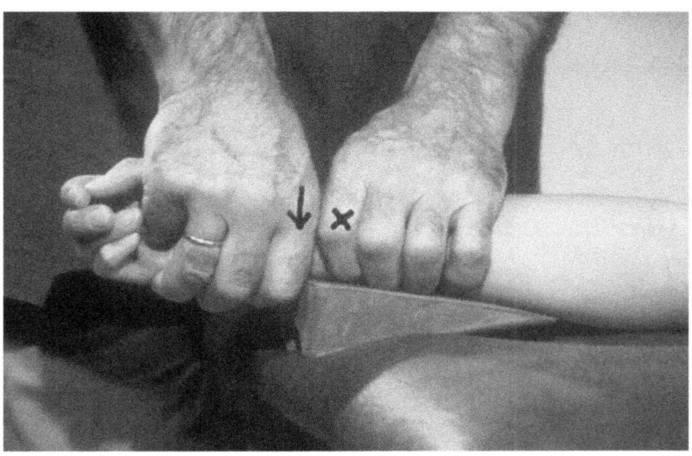

Figure 52.11 Radiocarpal ulnar glide.

standing at the dorsal side of the wrist. The distal forearm is fixated against the wedge by the therapist's stabilizing hand just proximal to the wrist. The mobilizing hand grasps the carpal bones from the radial side just distal to the wrist joint and performs the ulnar glide. The mobilization can be also done in various degrees of wrist radial deviation.

Radiocarpal MWM (Mulligan 2004)

This technique is indicated in patients with restricted wrist extension or flexion due to a minor positional fault (note the direction of glide is perpendicular to normal arthrokinematic gliding). The patient is sitting. The therapist is standing proximal to the patient's wrist, and grasps the latter's distal forearm with one hand so that the web between index finger and thumb lies over the distal radius. The other hand grasps the proximal carpal row from the ulnar aspect so that the web space is now over the triquetrum. Radial translation is applied to the proximal carpal row until a direction is found that allows the patient to perform previously painful active wrist flexion or extension.

Opponens roll (Sucher 1994)

This technique is indicated in patients with decreased length of the flexor retinaculum implicated in the aetiology of CTS. The patient is sitting, with arm supinated and resting on the table. The therapist is standing distal to patient's hand. The thumb and thenar portion of the ipsilateral hand stabilize the ulnar palmar aspect of the hand. The thumb is then brought into abduction with slight extension and supination along the axis of the first metacarpal bone by the contralateral hand of the therapist.

Transverse carpal extension (Sucher et al 2005)

This technique is indicated in patients with decreased length of the flexor retinaculum implicated in the aetiology of CTS. The patient is sitting, with arm supinated and resting on the table. The therapist is standing distal to the patient's hand. The mobilization consists of a three-point bending technique whereby the therapist hooks his / her thumbs on the inner palmar edge of the carpal bones (trapezium and hamate distally, scaphoid and pisiform proximally) while his / her fingers wrap around dorsally to converge on the centre of the patient's wrist, providing a counterforce. The technique can be done combined with passive thumb and little finger abduction and extension or with the opponens roll technique. Similar three-point techniques over the metacarpal bones causing concave and convex movements of the metacarpal arch can be done as a general mobilization for the intermetacarpal connections.

Radial carpal palmar glides

This technique is indicated in patients with restricted wrist extension and radial deviation. The patient is sitting, with arm pronated and resting on a wedge. The therapist is standing at the ulnar side of the patient's wrist, and the distal radius is fixed against the wedge by the therapist's stabilizing hand; the thenar portion stabilizes dorsally just proximal to wrist with the fingers palmar. The mobilizing hand grasps the patient's hand from the radial side; with the thenar eminence dorsal against the scaphoid, the therapist glides the scaphoid palmar. Movement of the fixation distally to include the scaphoid and mobilization of the trapezium and trapezoid in

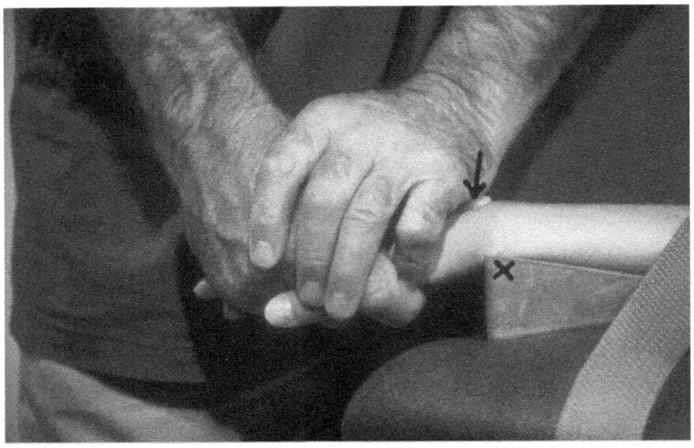

Figure 52.12 Central carpal palmar glides.

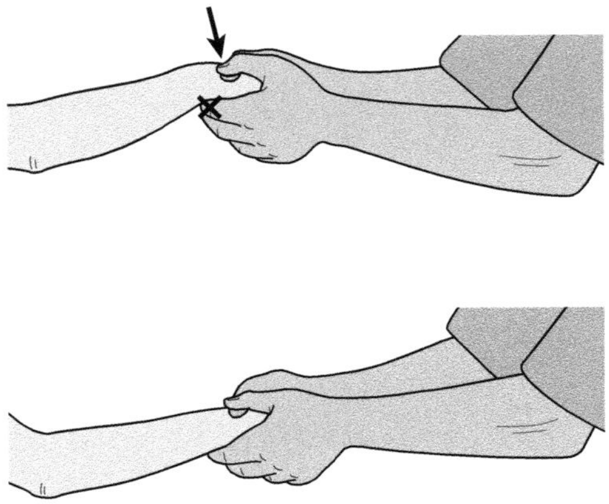

Figure 52.13 Carpal glide manipulation with proximal fixation.

a palmar direction increase restricted flexion and ulnar deviation.

Central carpal palmar glides (Fig. 52.12)

This technique is indicated in patients with restricted wrist extension. The patient is sitting, with arm pronated and resting on a wedge. The therapist is standing distal to the patient's wrist, and the distal radius is fixed against the wedge by a fixation belt. The therapist, with one hand, grasps the patient's hand from the radial side with the thumb dorsal and index finger palmar over the lunate; the hypothenar of the other hand placed over his / her own thumb glides the lunate palmar. Movement of the fixation distally to include the lunate and mobilization of the capitate in a palmar direction increase restricted extension.

Ulnar carpal palmar glides

This technique is indicated in patients with restricted wrist extension. The patient is sitting, with arm pronated and resting on a wedge. The therapist is standing distal to the patient's wrist, and the distal ulna is fixed against the wedge by a fixation belt. The therapist grasps the patient's hand from the ulnar side with the thumb dorsal and index finger palmar over the triquetrum; the hypothenar of the other hand placed over his / her own thumb glides the triquetrum palmar. Movement of the fixation distally to include the triquetrum and mobilization of the hamate in a palmar direction increase restricted extension.

Radial carpal dorsal glides

This technique is indicated in patients with restricted wrist flexion and ulnar deviation. The patient is sitting, with arm supinated and resting on a wedge. The therapist stands distal to the patient's wrist, and the distal radius is fixated dorsally against the wedge by a fixation belt. With one hand the therapist grasps the patient's hand from the radial side with the thumb palmar on the scaphoid and fingers dorsal; the hypothenar of the other hand is placed on his / her own thumb and produces the dorsal glide. Movement of the fixation distally to include the scaphoid and then mobilization of the trapezium and trapezoid in a dorsal direction will increase restricted extension and radial deviation. With all carpal dorsal glides, the therapist may need to 'soften' contact on the often-painful palmar aspect of the carpal bones, for example by using the head of the second metacarpal rather than the thumb as a palmar contact.

Central carpal dorsal glides

This mobilization is indicated in patients with restricted wrist flexion. The patient is sitting, with arm supinated and resting on a wedge. The therapist stands distal to the patient's wrist, and the distal radius is fixated dorsally against the wedge by a fixation belt. The therapist with one hand grasps the hand from the radial side with the thumb (or 'softer' contact) palmar on the lunate and the index finger dorsal; the other hand places the hypothenar on his / her own thumb and produces a dorsal glide. Movement of the fixation distally to include the lunate and mobilization of the capitate in a dorsal direction increase restricted flexion.

Ulnar carpal dorsal glides

This mobilization is indicated in patients with restricted wrist flexion. The patient is sitting, with arm supinated and resting on a wedge. The therapist stands distal to the patient's wrist, and the distal ulna is fixated dorsally against the wedge by a fixation belt. The therapist's hand grasps the hand from the ulnar side with thumb (or 'softer' contact) palmar on the triquetrum and index finger dorsal; the other hand places the hypothenar on his / her own thumb and produces a dorsal glide. Movement of the fixation distally to include the triquetrum and mobilization of the hamate in a dorsal direction increase restricted flexion.

Carpal glide manipulation with proximal fixation (Fig. 52.13)

This manipulation is indicated in patients with restricted wrist extension (in the presence of normal radial and ulnar deviation). The patient stands with the arm flexed forward at the shoulder. The therapist stands in front of the patient and grips the latter's hand from both sides. The index fingers on top of each other stabilize the lunate on its palmar aspect. The capitate bone is contacted with the pads of thumbs on top of each other on its dorsal aspect. Slack is taken up and tightened between the index fingers and thumbs. The impulse consists of a quick downward movement of the patient's arm and wrist from a slightly flexed position. The movement stops suddenly, when the wrist is in the zero position (not in extension). A traction component is maintained throughout the whole procedure. This technique can be applied for wrist extension restrictions resulting from joint restrictions between radius and lunate, lunate and capitate (described above) and radius and scaphoid. The site of restriction in case of restricted extension and radial deviation is mostly between the radius and scaphoid, and / or the scaphoid and trapezoid–trapezium complex. (A manipulation to restore movement between the scaphoid and trapezoid–trapezium complex in case of restricted extension and radial deviation is described not here but under the next technique.) Note that proximal fixation on the palmar aspect of the scaphoid with a thrust applied to the dorsal aspect of the trapezoid–trapezium complex serves to increase wrist flexion.

Carpal glide manipulation with distal fixation (Fig. 52.14)

This manipulation is indicated in patients with restricted wrist flexion. The patient stands with the arm flexed forward at the shoulder. The therapist stands in front of the patient and grips the latter's hand from both sides. The index fingers on top of each other stabilize the capitate on its palmar aspect. The lunate is contacted with the pads of the thumbs on top of each other on its dorsal aspect. Slack is taken up and tightened between the index fingers and thumbs. The impulse consists of a quick downward movement of the patient's arm and wrist from a slightly flexed position. The movement stops suddenly, when the wrist is in the zero position (not in extension). A traction component is maintained throughout the whole procedure. Often the palmar aspects of the carpal bones are too sensitive to have a thrust applied to them. Therefore, with distal fixation, the distal bone is stabilized and the proximal bone is moved in a palmar direction, resulting in relative dorsal movement of the distal bone. This technique can be used for all bones in the proximal and distal row. Note that carpal glide manipulation of the scaphoid with distal fixation of the trapezoid–trapezium complex is used for restricted wrist extension and radial deviation.

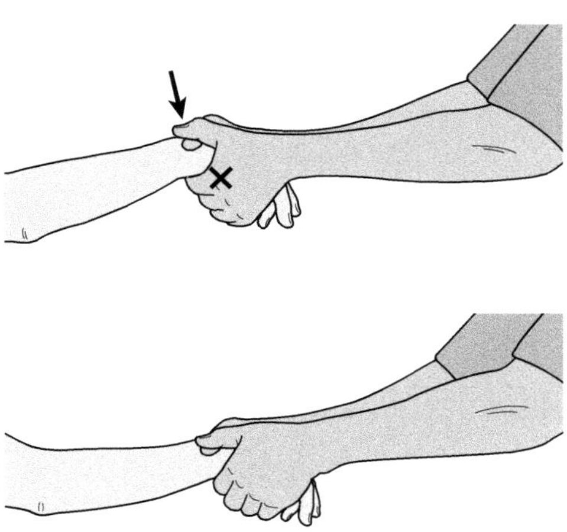

Figure 52.14 Carpal glide manipulation with distal fixation.

Carpometacarpal I traction

The patient is sitting, with the arm stabilized with its ulnar aspect against the table. The therapist is standing proximal to the patient's hand. The stabilizing hand of the therapist fixates the trapezium with the thumb palmar and fingers dorsal. The therapist's mobilizing hand grasps the first metacarpal with the thenar dorsal (radial) and finger palmar and applies traction (Fig. 52.15). Similar techniques with the hand pronated on the table, the proximal joint partner stabilized, and the metacarpal bone tractioned can be used for the CMC II–V joints (Fig. 52.16).

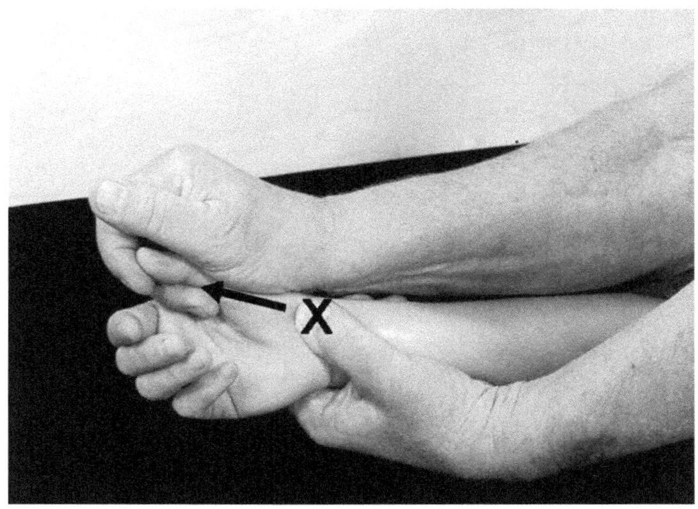

Figure 52.15 Carpometacarpal I traction.

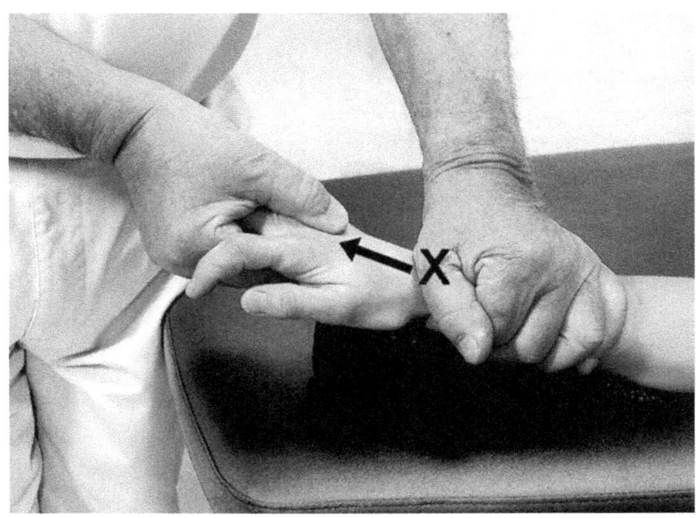

Figure 52.16 Carpometacarpal II–V traction.

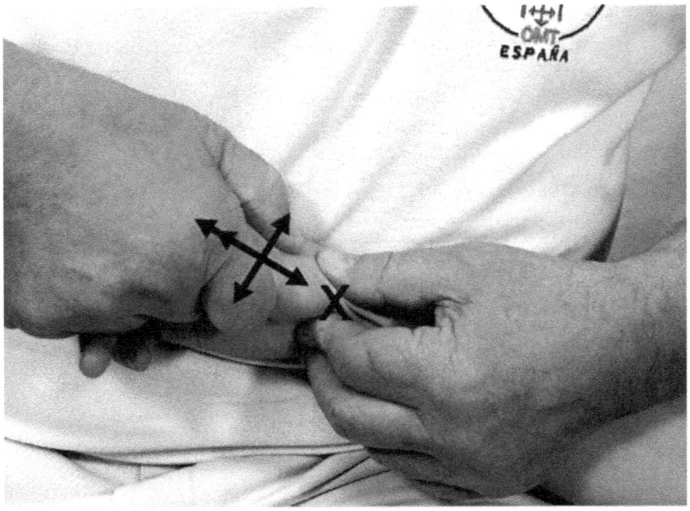

Figure 52.17 Carpometacarpal I glides.

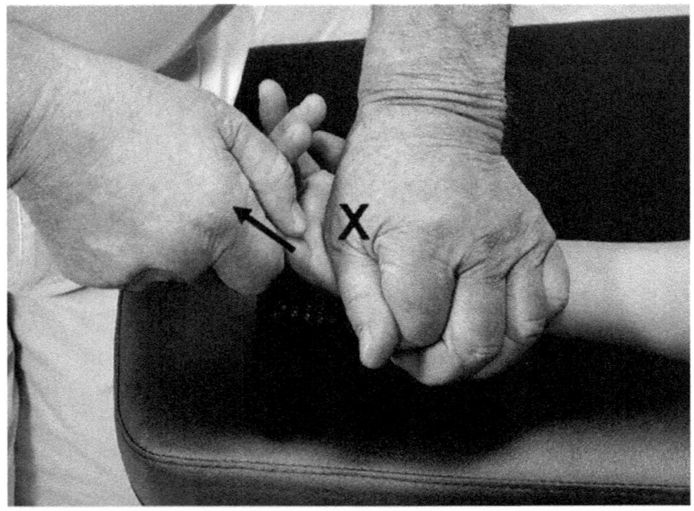

Figure 52.18 Finger-joint traction.

Carpometacarpal I glides
(Fig. 52.17)

These techniques are indicated in patients with restricted thumb movements. The stabilizing hand grasps the trapezium with the thumb dorsal and index finger palmar, and fixes it in a position maximally rotated towards the palm. The mobilizing hand grasps the first metacarpal just distal to the CMC I joint space and applies the glides:

1. For restricted abduction and adduction, the patient sits with the ulnar side of the hand against the therapist's body (Fig. 52.17). For restricted abduction, the glide is in a dorsal direction. For restricted adduction, the glide is in a palmar direction (convex rule).
2. For restricted extension and flexion, the patient's hand is turned, so that the dorsal side is against the therapist's body (not pictured). For restricted extension, the glide is in a radial direction. For restricted flexion, the glide direction is ulnar (concave rule).

Metacarpophalangeal I MWM (Folk 2001; Hsieh et al 2002)

This mobilization in indicated in patients with restricted MCP I motion due to a minor positional fault (medial or lateral glide is perpendicular to normal arthrokinematic gliding). The patient is sitting, with elbow bent and forearm supinated. The therapist is standing or sitting at the radial aspect of the patient's wrist. The therapist stabilizes the first metacarpal bone between index finger and thumb and applies a lateral or medial glide or long-axis rotation that allows the patient to perform a previously painful motion.

Finger joint traction (Fig. 52.18)

The patient is sitting, with arm supinated, with the dorsum of his / her hand resting on a wedge or table. The therapist is sitting or standing at the distal aspect of the patient's hand. The thenar eminence of the therapist's stabilizing hand fixates the proximal joint partner; the mobilizing hand then grips the distal joint partner and applies traction. The technique can be done in various finger joint positions; shifting fixation distally allows for traction to first MCP, then proximal interphalangeal (PIP), then distal interphalangeal (DIP) joints.

Finger-joint glides

This technique in indicated in patients with restricted MCP, PIP or DIP extension. The patient is sitting, with arm supinated, and the dorsum of his / her hand resting on the wedge or table. The therapist is sitting or standing at ulnar aspect of the patient's hand. The thenar eminence of the therapist's stabilizing hand fixates the proximal joint partner; the mobilizing hand then grips the distal joint partner and applies a dorsal glide. With the hand pronated, a palmar glide can be applied to mobilize flexion. Radial and ulnar glides can also be used at the MCP joints to restore radial and ulnar deviation, respectively.

Finger joint MWM (Mulligan 2004)

This technique is indicated in patients with restricted PIP or DIP flexion due to minor positional fault (the direction of glide is perpendicular to normal arthrokinematic gliding). The patient is sitting, and the therapist is standing to the side of the patient. The therapist fixes the proximal partner between the thumb and index finger. A medial or lateral glide is applied to the distal joint partner until a direction is found that allows the patient to perform previously painful active PIP or DIP finger flexion.

Acknowledgements

The authors would like to gratefully acknowledge the librarian of the Physical Therapy Association of British Columbia, Ms. Deb Monkman, MLS, BSc, for her help in retrieving the references used in this chapter.

References

Anderson M, Tichenor CJ. 1994. A patient with De Quervain's tenosynovitis: a case report using an Australian approach to manual therapy. Phys Ther 74: 314–326.

Backstrom KM. 2002. Mobilization with movement as an adjunct intervention in a patient with complicated De Quervain's tenosynovitis: a case report. J Orthop Sports Phys Ther 32: 86–97.

Coyle JA, Robertson VJ. 2002. Comparison of two passive mobilizing techniques following Colles' fracture: a multi-element design. Man Ther 3: 34–41.

Davis PT, Hulbert JR, Kassak KM, et al. 1998. Comparative efficacy of conservative medical and chiropractic treatments for carpal tunnel syndrome: a randomized clinical trial. J Manipulative Physiol Ther 21: 317–326.

Exelby L. 1996. Peripheral mobilisations with movement. Man Ther 1: 118–126.

Folk B. 2001. Traumatic thumb injury management using mobilization with movement. Man Ther 6: 178–182.

Hsieh CY, Vicenzino B, Yang CH, et al. 2002. Mulligan's mobilization with movement for the thumb: a single case report using magnetic resonance imaging to evaluate the positional fault hypothesis. Man Ther 7: 44–49.

Kaltenborn FM, Evjenth O, Baldauf Kaltenborn T, et al. 2007. Manual mobilization of the extremity joints: joint examination and basic treatment. Vol. I: The extremities, 6th revised edn. Oslo: Norli.

Kaltenborn FM, Baldauf Kaltenborn T, Vollowitz E, et al. 2008. Manual mobilization of the joints: joint examination and basic treatment. Vol. III: Traction-manipulation of the extremities and spine, basic thrust techniques. Oslo: Norli.

Kay S, Haensel N, Stiller K. 2000. The effect of passive mobilization following fractures involving the distal radius: a randomised study. Aust J Physiother 46: 93–101.

McPhate M, Robertson VJ. 1998. Physiotherapy treatment of Colles fractures: hands off or hands on? Proceedings of the fifth international Australian Physiotherapy Association congress. Hobart: APA, p 235.

Michlovitz SL, Harris BA, Watkins MP. 2004. Therapy interventions for improving joint range of motion: a systematic review. J Hand Ther 17: 118–131.

Mink AJF, Ter Veer HJ, Vorselaars JACT. 1990. Extremiteiten: functie-onderzoek en manuele therapie. Houten: Bohn Stafleu Van Loghum.

Muller M, Tsui D, Schnurr R, et al. 2004. Effectiveness of hand therapy interventions in the primary management of carpal tunnel syndrome: a systematic review. J Hand Ther 17: 210–228.

Mulligan BR. 2004. Manual therapy: 'NAGS', 'SNAGS', 'MWMS' etc., 5th edn. Wellington: Plane View Services.

O'Connor D, Marshall SC, Massy-Westropp N. 2003. Non-surgical treatment (other than steroid injection) for carpal tunnel syndrome. Cochrane Database Syst Rev 1: CD003219.

Olson VL. 1987. Evaluation of joint mobilization treatment. Phys Ther 67: 351–356.

Randall T, Portney L, Harris BA. 1992. Effects of joint mobilization on joint stiffness and active motion of the metacarpal–phalangeal joint. J Orthop Sports Phys Ther 16: 30–36.

Struijs PAA, Damen PJ, Baller EWP, et al. 2003. Manipulation of the wrist for management of lateral epicondylitis: a randomized pilot study. Phys Ther 83: 608–616.

Sucher BM. 1994. Palpatory diagnosis and manipulative management of carpal tunnel syndrome. J Am Osteopath Assoc 94: 647–663.

Sucher BM, Hinrichs RN, Welcher RL, et al. 2005. Manipulative treatment of carpal tunnel syndrome: biomechanical and osteopathic intervention to increase the length of the transverse carpal ligament: Part 2. Effect of sex differences and manipulative 'priming. J Am Osteopath Assoc 105: 135–143.

Tal-Akabi A, Rushton A. 2000. An investigation to compare the effectiveness of carpal bone mobilization and neurodynamic mobilization as methods of treatment for carpal tunnel syndrome. Man Ther 5: 214–222.

Taylor NF, Bennell KL. 1994. The effectiveness of passive joint mobilisation on the return of active wrist extension following Colles' fracture: a clinical trial. N Z J Physiother 22: 24–28.

53 Chapter

Finger and Thumb Pathology

Joy C. MacDermid, Ruby Grewal, B. Jane Freure

CHAPTER CONTENTS

Introduction	594
Digital fractures	594
Epidemiology: incidence, prevalence, economic impact	594
Anatomy	594
Pathology	595
Diagnosis of digital fractures	596
Prognosis for digital fractures	596
Conservative treatment of digital fractures	596
Ulnar collateral ligament injury of the thumb	598
Epidemiology	598
Anatomy	598
Pathology	599
Diagnosis	599
Prognosis	600
Conservative treatment of UCL injury	600
Other digital tendon injuries	600
Osteoarthritis of the digits	600
Epidemiology	600
Anatomy	600
Pathology	600
Diagnosis	601
Prognosis	601
Conservative treatment of digital arthritis	601
Rheumatoid arthritis affecting the digits	601
Conclusion	601

Introduction

Physical therapy for the hand must embrace an understanding of the hand as an 'organ' that interfaces the person with their world by bringing in sensory information, and allowing the person to engage in activity that determines function and quality of life. The hand has intricate anatomical structures in close proximity that contract, glide and heal following injury. Maintenance of joint mobility and stability while the structures in the proximity remain free to glide and resist contractile forces is critical to hand motor performance. Issues of motor control and sensory motor integration are critical to the functionality of the hand. Exquisitely innervated, the hand can serve as a sensory organ or contribute painful stimuli that alter the cortex and produce chronic pain. Manual therapy techniques can contribute to normalizing the neurosensorimotor function of the hand, in combination with other techniques. In this chapter we highlight the most prevalent conditions affecting the digits.

Digital Fractures

Epidemiology: incidence, prevalence and economic impact

Hand fractures are common traumatic injuries, usually arising during workplace, sporting or recreational activities. Fractures of the metacarpals and phalanges are most common (Hove 1993; van Onselen et al 2003; Aitken & Court-Brown 2008; Feehan & Sheps 2008), and in particular the outer digits (i.e. thumb / small finger). The majorities are treated conservatively (Feehan & Sheps 2008). Metacarpal fractures represent 35% of hand fractures.

Anatomy

To understand hand fractures better, one must first understand the relationship between soft tissue and bony factors that contribute to both soft tissue and skeletal stability. We suggest that readers consult a standard anatomy text or *The electronic textbook of hand surgery* (http://www.eatonhand.com/hom/hom033.htm) website for details of hand / wrist anatomy as this chapter will highlight only the key elements. The website has primal pictures (used with permission), some radiographic images of anatomy and pathology and information on various bony and soft tissues, providing accessible and clearly visualized aspects of key anatomical features. More-detailed descriptions of anatomical features are available in the classic anatomy textbooks.

Pathology

Bone fractures result from excessive force, in comparison to bone strength. Fracture angulation is determined by the forces exerted by the soft tissues on both the proximal and the distal fragments. Movement recovery following fracture can be affected by the nature and severity of the original fracture, associated soft tissue injuries and the extent of malalignment in bony structure that occurs following bone healing.

The mechanism of injury plays a role in the type of fractures that should be anticipated. A direct blow will result in a transverse fracture, a twisting injury will cause a spiral fracture and combination of torque and axial force will result in a short oblique fracture. Fractures are further classified according to the location (e.g. head, neck, shaft or base of a specific hand bone) and any associated soft tissue injury.

All fractures are associated with soft tissue injury. The nature of these injuries can be difficult to determine even with imaging and clinical examination. Muscle and ligament injuries can be important aspects of the fracture and may become more evident as the fracture heals and swelling subsides, or when movement is initiated. Scar healing of injured soft tissue can be a substantial component of active movement limitation.

Metacarpal fractures

The metacarpal bones have intrinsic stability provided by strong interosseus ligaments binding them to the carpal bones, and proximally by the transverse metacarpal ligament, which links all the metacarpal heads. The ligaments tend to prevent excessive displacement with injury. The fifth metacarpal is commonly fractured during a 'punch' mechanism (the majority of these injuries occur in males) and is treated conservatively since full motion / function is often obtained despite malrotation. There is generally a good blood supply, which supports high rates of healing, usually within 4–6 weeks. The most important soft tissue concerns are to preserve middle phalanx (MP) joint flexion and maintain extensor digitorum communis (EDC) glide.

Fractures of the base of metacarpals are intra-articular fractures that usually result from high forces disrupting the rigid carpal ligaments of the index and middle finger or overwhelming the normal flexibility of the ulnar metacarpals. Shaft fractures are extra-articular fractures that usually arise during a fall or blow and usually angulate dorsally (with components of shortening or rotation). They are described as transverse, oblique or spiral. Intrinsic muscle tension will cause both ends of the metacarpal bone to flex into an apex dorsal presentation. This causes a shortening, which compromises the extensor mechanism by altering the muscle length relationship. Metacarpal neck fractures are the most common metacarpal fracture ('boxer's fracture'). The impact of a closed fist causes a break at the extra-articular neck. If associated with a bite, infection is a potential complication that can substantially increase tissue damage. Metacarpal head fractures are intra-articular fractures caused by high axial loading that may involve collateral ligaments and substantial comminution. These fractures can lead to chronic pain and joint instability.

Phalangeal fractures

Phalangeal fractures have greater tendency towards instability as the phalanges lack intrinsic muscle support and are adversely affected by the mechanical forces of the extrinsic flexors and extensors. However, these fractures are also more likely to become stiff with immobilization (Shehadi 1991); the predicted motion return is 84%, but if the period of immobilization is longer than 4 weeks, the predicted motion is 66%.

Intra-articular fractures of the base of the proximal phalanx (PP) usually occur following an abduction force, which is most commonly seen in sports injuries or a fall. Displaced fractures may not be reducible conservatively because of collateral ligament avulsion, which worsens the fracture displacement with MP flexion. This can lead to higher rates of non-union if managed conservatively (Shewring & Thomas 2006). PP shaft fractures have the poorest prognosis for regaining of full ability as they occur in flexor zone II. As 90% of the PP surface is covered by gliding structures, these can easily become adhered to the fracture callus. PP condyle fractures usually occur with the lateral deviation force and may be associated with collateral ligament injury. This is a common sports injury, and a commonly missed diagnosis.

The interossei and lumbricals muscles are the prime MCP flexors. The lumbricals originate from the tendons of the flexor digitorum profundus tendon, and the three palmar and four dorsal interossei muscles originate from the volar and dorsal surfaces of the metacarpal respectively (Smith 1975). The interossei insert onto the anterolateral base of the PP and the extensor mechanism forming part of the lateral band with the lumbricals, which also inserts dorsally into the extensor apparatus. These intrinsic muscles, along with the extrinsic flexor tendons, create deforming forces on the fractured metacarpal shaft that result in apex dorsal angulation (Flatt 1996). A PP fracture will typically angulate with an apex volar deformity because the interossei will flex the proximal fragment, owing to their insertion at the PP base, while the distal fragment is pulled into hyperextension by the central slip, which inserts at the base of the middle phalanx and acts to extend the distal fragment.

Fractures of the shaft of the MP occur less commonly, and may displace either dorsally or volarly. Intra-articular fractures at the base of the MP occur commonly from a fall or direct force. These may be associated with proximal interphalangeal (PIP) joint dislocation and damage to the volar plate and / or central slip. If the compression trauma is severe, a comminuted fracture of the articular surface occurs, with depression of the fragments into the bone shaft or 'pilon' fracture. MP fractures of the distal third tend to angulate with an apex volar deformity as the flexor digitorum superficialis (FDS) acts to flex the proximal fragment. A proximal third fracture usually angulates with an apex dorsal deformity as the FDS will flex the distal fragment while the central slip extends the proximal fragment.

Distal phalanx (DP) fractures are common during crush injuries and may not displace significantly because the presence of a rigid nail plate dorsally helps to preserve alignment. However, due to the space restrictions inherent in the fingertip anatomical structures and their dense innervations, these injuries can be particularly painful. The DP accounts for 50% of hand fractures, which may be attributed to its vulnerability as the fingertip. Tendon avulsion can occur either alone or with a variable amount of the articular surface 'chip fracture'. This commonly occurs in sports and hence the existence of sport-related names for these injuries ('jersey'=flexor avulsed from the volar base of the DP; 'baseball'=avulsion of the terminal extensor tendon from the DP). PP shaft fractures are proximal to the nail bed and usually result from direct trauma. PP tuft fractures are the most distal fracture and can be quite painful and difficult to manage since union may be slow.

Thumb fractures

The first carpometacarpal (CMC) joint is a double saddle-joint, which allows movement both in the flexion / extension plane and in abduction / adduction. Because of the wide range of motion (ROM) present at the thumb CMC joint, angulation of up to 30° is well tolerated, allowing full function to be achieved in rehabilitation even when pre-morbid joint mobility is not attained. In extra-articular fractures, dorsal angulation occurs because the abductor pollicus brevis, adductor pollicis and flexor pollicis brevis muscles attaching at the base of the PP act to flex the distal fragment while the abductor pollicus longus muscle (which attaches to the metacarpal base) extends the proximal fragment. A Bennett fracture is an intra-articular fracture involving the metacarpal base. The fracture fragment involves the volar–ulnar portion of the metacarpal base. This fragment is held undisplaced by the anterior oblique ligament. The remainder of the thumb metacarpal usually subluxes radially, proximally and dorsally by the forces exerted by the abductor pollicus longus.

Diagnosis of digital fractures

The focus of assessment depends on the stage of healing. Clinical and radiographic assessment of fracture union should be performed until union is established. Clinical signs of non-union include exquisite local pain at the fracture site and movement of the fractured components. Computed tomography can be a useful adjunct to radiographs as it can help to delineate accurately the degree of articular displacement and can identify other associated injuries. Radiographs are routinely used to identify fractures and to determine the degree of displacement; however, X-ray cannot be used to rule out a rotational deformity. Patients can be asked to flex their digits actively to determine whether there is any scissoring of the digits (i.e. overlap). If pain from the acute injury precludes an active flexion effort, passive wrist flexion and extension will place a flexion moment across the fingers, with the tenodesis effect allowing an assessment of rotation to be made. A thorough clinical assessment should be made to determine whether there is any associated soft tissue or neurovascular injury and to identify any rotational deformity. Assessment should include evaluation of impairments and disabilities arising from fracture complications or treatment sequelae. A summary of these and potential treatment approaches are described in Table 53.1.

Prognosis for digital fractures

Prognosis varies according to the outcome of interest. Successful union of the fracture and restoration of normal anatomy, pre-injury movement / grip strength and function are typical goals and outcomes evaluated. Union is dependent on the person's individual capacity for bone healing and is thus affected by prognostic factors that affect bone healing in a generic sense, including individual physical factors (nutrition, comorbidity, age, bone quality), the bone affected (composition, blood supply, biomechanics), behaviour (compliance with fixation, immobilization, remobilization, rehabilitation, activity levels), injury (type of fracture, size of defect, soft tissue components, associated injuries) and complications (nerve compression, infection, loss of reduction).

Optimal anatomical outcomes and functional outcomes are moderately related, in that malunion can lead to decreased pain, grip strength, scissoring, or loss of joint motion (Synn et al 2009). However, poor functional outcomes can occur in the presence of good anatomical restoration, particularly where pronounced joint stiffness, chronic pain, or chronic regional pain syndrome exist (Field et al 1992; Field & Atkins 1997). Conversely, adequate functional outcomes are attained in older sedentary individuals despite lack of restoration of normal anatomy (Grewal & MacDermid 2007). When fracture malunion results in scissoring, a corrective rotational osteotomy may be required.

Evidence on prognosis and fractures is generally sparse and of poor quality (level IV studies). One study found that functional (DASH), aesthetic and fracture union outcomes in metacarpal shaft and neck fractures were not affected by palmar angular deformity, but functional and aesthetic outcomes were better in non-operatively managed patients (Westbrook et al 2008). Spiral / long oblique fractures of the shaft of the metacarpal are at risk of shortening and resultant extension lag and reduced grip strength. However, there may be progressive recovery of the extension lag by 1 year and a mean of 94% of the contralateral hand motion by 1 year after injury (Al-Qattan 2008). In 51 unstable metaphyseal MP and PP fractures where fixation was maintained with miniature titanium plates union, the final range of total active motion (% TAM) was excellent (>85%) for 26, good (70–84%) for 17, fair (50–69%) for 5, and poor (<49%) for 3 (Omokawa et al 2008). Postoperative complications included loss of reduction (2 cases), condylar head collapses (2 cases) and one superficial infection. Plates were removed in 30 cases, and additional surgery was required in 20 cases. Postoperative grip strength averaged 87% that of the contralateral side. Older age, intra-articular fracture, phalangeal bone involvement and soft tissue injury were associated with a poorer range of finger motion following fracture (Omokawa et al 2008). A level IIb study of 120 MC and PP emergency room fractures indicated that infection, increased bony defect and associated soft tissue injury increased the risk of non-union (Ali et al 2007). In another study, 36% of MC or PP fractures showed different complications; PP and open fractures were at higher risk for stiffness, non-union, plate prominence, infection and tendon rupture (Page & Stern 1998).

Conservative treatment of digital fractures

The general principles of fracture management are to reduce the fracture (open or closed) in a manner that will restore normal anatomy and to maintain the reduced position through an immobilization / fixation technique that is sufficient to withstand the potential for loss of reduction through

Table 53.1 Summary of treatment problems and associated treatment techniques for hand fractures

Problem	Physiotherapeutic treatment strategies
Fracture protection (Fess et al 2004)	Custom-made or off-the-shelf orthoses
Pain	Frequent, low-intensity active exercise of unaffected joints and affected joints when stable Adequate fracture protection and oedema management Desensitization programme Electrothermal agents Coordinate pharmacological management and therapy
Nerve irritation/neuroma	Desensitization programme (Robinson & McPhee 1986; Waylett-Rendall 1988) Iontophoresis with lidocaine – evidence in other conditions (Fedorczyk 1997; Baskurt et al 2003; Bolin 2003; Yarrobino et al 2006; Polomano et al 2008) Mirror box therapy (Altschuler & Hu 2008; Ezendam et al 2009) – limited evidence Visualization exercises – limited evidence Nerve-gliding/neurodynamic techniques focused on at-risk or symptomatic nerve bias
Oedema	Exercise in elevation Compression (compressive gloves, retrograde massage, Coban wrap, string wrapping (Flowers 1988) (especially for digits) Thermal agents (cold in acute stages for those who can tolerate; heat should be used only in elevation with monitoring of volume) Physical agents (high-voltage stimulation) (Stralka et al 1998)
Loss of joint motion (Michlovitz et al 2004)	Active exercise of affected joints (stable fixation or healed) Physiological and accessory joint mobilization Static progressive splinting Dynamic splinting Continuous passive motion (Soffer & Yahiro 1990) (low evidence in other upper extremity joints) Constrained movement therapy (blocking or casting of adjacent mobile digits to enforce movement of stiff joints)
Loss of power	Progressive resisted exercise (Hostler et al 2001; Bautmans et al 2009)
Loss of endurance	Progressive resisted exercise Progressive functional activity
Scissoring	Buddy tape to adjacent digit May require osteotomy
Joint Instability	Buddy taping, taping, custom or premade orthoses Activity modification to avoid lateral stress
Non-union	Low-dose ultrasound (Busse et al 2002; Griffin et al 2008)
Abnormal sensorimotor integration or motor control	Sensorimotor retraining (focused, progressive retraining of normal sensory responses) Motor control exercises Dexterity training/functional activity
Prevention of future fractures	Assess risk for future fracture (based on age mechanism of injury and comorbid status) Manage modifiable risk factors (safety training, activity modification, protective devices, fall prevention, balance training as needed)
General	In simple, closed metacarpal fractures, early motion has the potential to result in earlier recovery of mobility and strength, facilitate an earlier return to work, and not affect fracture alignment (Feehan & Bassett 2004)
Dorsal skin scar contracture	Silicone gel/topical agents to superficial scars Scar massage/mobilization for adherence Simultaneous heat, stretch and tendon-gliding exercises (Wehbe 1987) Scar mobilization with hand-held suction device Ultrasound Laser
MP joint contracted an extension	Early positioning MP joint at 70° Later dynamic or static progressive splinting of MP

Continued

Table 53.1 Summary of treatment problems and associated treatment techniques for hand fractures—cont'd

Problem	Physiotherapeutic treatment strategies
Intrinsic muscle contracture	Early – active intrinsic minus exercises; blocking exercise Later – dynamic splinting; muscle stimulation
Absence of MP head	Educate patient about shortening of metacarpal; assess whether any functional implications (may not affect functional outcome) Assess functionality of extensors; if redundancy is apparent splinting extension at night and strengthen intrinsic Assess alignment – volar prominence = volar angulation and may require adaptive padding/gloves/positioning or osteotomy Communicate with health care team
Loss of IP extension	Blocking exercises MP block extension splint during the day PIP extension splint thing at night Neuromuscular stimulation to EDC and inter-rossei Joint mobilizations
Loss of IP flexion	FDP/FDS tendon glide exercises Daytime MP flexion blocks blunting Dynamic or static progressive nights splinting Heat and composite stretching Joint mobilizations Stretch of oblique retinacular ligament
Boutonniere deformity	Early – DIP active flexion to maintain length of lateral bands Later – splinting
Swan neck deformity	Orthotic to hold MP joint in flexion

(From: Freeland et al 2003; Hardy 2004.)

deforming or external forces. Since immobilization leads to comorbid stiffness / weakness, early mobilization is preferable where it does not compromise reduction. In keeping with these goals (Fig. 53.1), the general principles of rehabilitation of fractures are divided into two stages (MacDermid 2004):

- **Stage 1 – early rehabilitation,** which includes protecting the healing fracture, minimizing pain and oedema, restoring normal motion and tissue extensibility, monitoring patients for associated injuries or complications, preventing therapy-induced complications, assisting patients in dealing with their injury using appropriate coping mechanisms and avoidance of patterns that increase the risk of developing chronic pain / disability syndromes and helping patients to understand their injury, the role of healthcare providers, and how to take an active role in their rehabilitation.
- **Stage 2 – later rehabilitation,** which includes amelioration of joint contracture, restoration of hand and arm strength, adaptation to residual physical impairments, transition into normal work or activity and teaching prevention strategies to reduce the risk of further fracture.

There is a lack of clinical trials comparing different treatment approaches for digital fractures. A single small low-quality trial suggested that the use of a compression glove avoided the loss of function imposed by splinting and was associated with a greater range of movement during the second and third weeks following a metacarpal fracture (McMahon et al 1994). Management is based on the stage of bone healing and presenting fracture sequelae (see treatments based on presenting problems in Table 53.1). Poor-quality studies support the use of metacarpal bracing for early mobilization.

Ulnar Collateral Ligament Injury of the Thumb

Epidemiology

Ulnar collateral ligament (UCL) injuries can be acute or chronic. Acute injuries are much more common and are the result of an acute valgus stress rupturing the ligament. Chronic injuries are referred to as 'gamekeeper's thumb', as it was traditionally noticed in Scottish gamekeepers who fractured the necks of the rabbits between their thumbs and index fingers. This is also an injury of the UCL; however, it is the result of attenuation of the ligament due to a chronic, repetitive radially directed force on the ulnar side of the thumb.

Anatomy

The thumb MP joint has both static and dynamic stabilizers. The static restraints include the volar plate and the proper and accessory collateral ligaments. The proper collateral ligament acts as the primary stabilizer of the MP joint in flexion; in

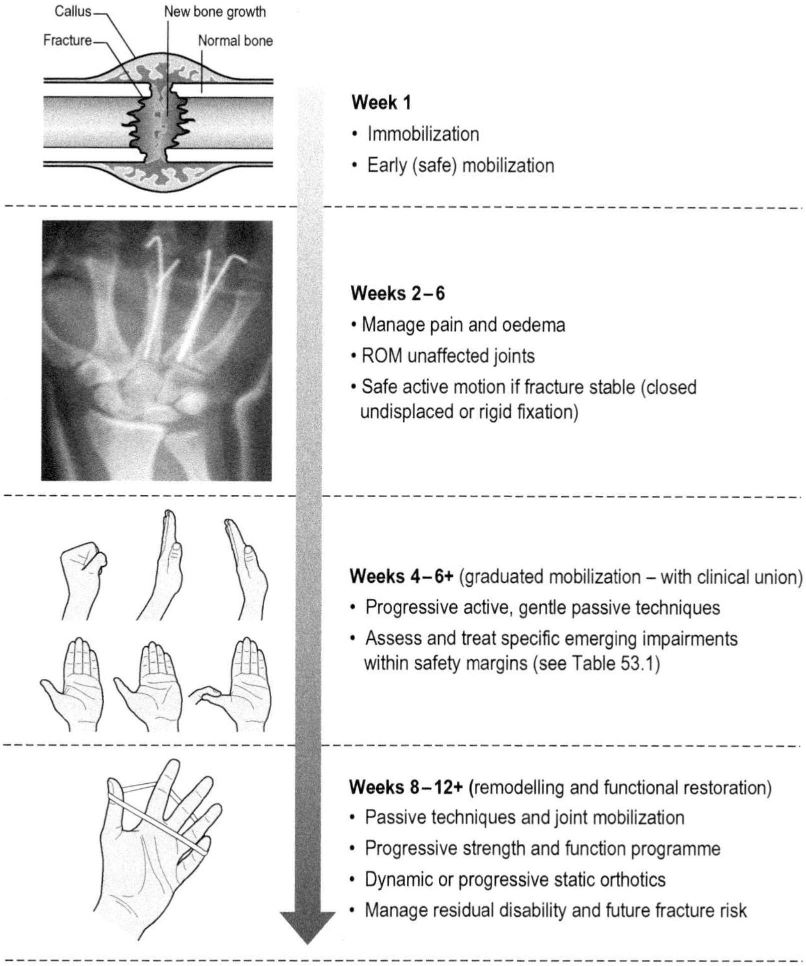

Figure 53.1 **Progression in the rehabilitation process.**

extension, the accessory collateral ligament and the volar plate are the primary joint stabilizers (Minami et al 1984; Heyman et al 1993). The dynamic stabilizers include both the thumb extrinsic (EPL, EPB and FPL) and the intrinsic (APB, FPB and adductor pollicis muscles) structures. The adductor pollicis is the most important dynamic stabilizer of the thumb MP joint. It inserts into the extensor hood (through its aponeurosis) and lies superficial to the joint and the UCL.

Pathology

When a valgus stress is applied to the thumb (i.e. a fall onto the abducted thumb) the dynamic and static stabilizers fail sequentially depending on the magnitude of the force. When the injury is limited to the dynamic stabilizers, the thumb will be stable on valgus stress testing. When the proper collateral ligament ruptures valgus instability will be present in MP flexion. When the accessory collateral is also torn, there will be valgus instability in both flexion and extension, indicating a complete tear (Heyman et al 1993). At times, the ruptured distal end of the ligament can become displaced such that it lies superficial and proximal to the adductor aponeurosis; this entity was first described in 1962 by Stener and so the lesion bears his name (Stener 1962). Due to interposition of the adductor aponeurosis, this injury will not heal without operative intervention.

Diagnosis

Patients will report a history of a valgus injury and complain of pain and swelling over the ulnar aspect of the MP joint. Pain will be exacerbated by forceful pinch and activities such as unscrewing jar tops and holding large objects because of a lack of power due to the thumb's inability to generate counterpressure on the object. Occasionally a Stener lesion may be evident, as a palpable mass on the ulnar aspect of the joint; however, lack of such a mass does not rule out a Stener lesion. Radiographs should be obtained and viewed prior to stress testing of the ligament to rule out an avulsion fracture, thereby avoiding potential displacement of the fracture fragment. Stress testing of the UCL is performed by placing a valgus stress across the MP joint in 30° of flexion and then in extension. If there is more than 30° of laxity (or 15° more than the contralateral side) in flexion (30° of MP flexion) then rupture of the proper collateral ligament is likely. The valgus stress is then applied in extension; if there is less than 30° of valgus laxity then the accessory collateral is intact, precluding a Stener lesion. If there is greater than 30° of laxity in both flexion and extension, the accessory collateral ligament is also ruptured and the probability of an underlying Stener lesion is then approximately 80% (Stener 1962). Radiographs demonstrate radial deviation at the MP joint and possible volar subluxation.

Prognosis

There are no specific prognostic studies on this topic. Inadequate mobilization or failure to detect a Stener lesion can lead to chronic instability and pain.

Conservative treatment of UCL injury

Management consists primarily of immobilization that is sufficient to permit ligament reattachment / healing. Although biomechanical evidence suggests early control of mobilization might be feasible (Harley et al 2004), this has not been tested in clinical trials. Casting or customized splinting can be used for mobilization, but removable splints are best reserved for compliant patients. A Stener lesion or failure to achieve a stable thumb with minimal pain during pinch is an indication for surgery (Dinowitz et al 1997) – that is, early repair or late ligament reconstruction. Progressive strengthening and protection from lateral stress (functional splinting / taping) will allow remodelling of the collagen fibres to ligament orientations that provide tensile strength. Stretching the UCL prematurely can lead to chronic instability, however.

Other Digital Tendon Injuries

Other tendon injuries that affect the digits can occur through lacerations, avulsion injuries (e.g. mallet / jersey finger), acute boutonniere and pulley ruptures. Lacerations of the flexor tendons that rupture in zones I or II require surgical repair and specific tendon rehabilitation protocols (Groth 2005; Newport & Tucker 2005; Libberecht et al 2006; Koul et al 2008; Soni et al 2009). These may involve active (protected) early mobilization in specially selected cases where repair strength is sufficient. Early passive mobilization protocols remain more common. Consultation with the referring surgeon and awareness of hand therapy rehabilitation protocols are required (Klein 2003; Chai & Wong 2005; Sueoka & LaStayo 2008; Yen et al 2008). Extensor tendon rupture or lacerations in the digits require extension splinting (4–6 weeks), and in some cases surgical repair. Gradually progressed, protected active ROM protocols instituted within the safety margins allowable by the specific repair are required to ensure that tendon glide is restored without compromising repair (tendon rupture or gapping). Active motion with differential gliding is emphasized during rehabilitation. When tendon scarring limits differential gliding, tenolysis may be required.

Osteoarthritis of the Digits

Epidemiology

Digital osteoarthritis (OA) is the most prevalent form of degenerative arthritis, although functional consequences vary (Doherty et al 2000; Hunter et al 2004). The distal interphalangeal (DIP) joint is the most affected, although functional consequences tend to be more severe in the CMC joint of the thumb, which affects 1 in 4 women and 1 in 12 men. In patients older than 75 years the prevalence of radiographic CMC degeneration increases to 40% in women and 25% in men (Armstrong et al 1994; Doherty et al 2000; Caspi et al 2001).

Anatomy

The CMC joint acts as a universal joint, allowing motion in extension, flexion, adduction and abduction. Together, these movements allow the complex movements of the thumb such as opposition, retropulsion, palmar and radial abduction, and adduction. The CMC joint has little intrinsic stability and relies on static ligamentous restraints to limit translation of the metacarpal base during these movements. There are three ligaments that help to stabilize the CMC joint. The primary stabilizer is the anterior oblique ligament, or volar beak ligament. It is an intracapsular structure that originates from the palmar tubercle of the trapezium and inserts on the ulnar side of the metacarpal base, along the articular margin. It resists abduction, extension and pronation forces. The secondary stabilizers include the dorsoradial and intermetacarpal ligaments. The dorsoradial ligament resists dorsal and radial translation of the CMC joint and is the most robust of the CMC joint ligaments. The intermetacarpal ligament lies between the base of the first and second metacarpals and prevents radial translation of the base of the first metacarpal (Bettinger et al 1999). The thenar muscles also play a role as dynamic stabilizers of the CMC joint. These muscles work in concert, stabilizing the thumb in position to allow activities such as pinching.

Pathology

OA is a degenerative condition characterized by pain, intermittent inflammation and cartilage degeneration. The pathological processes that underlie this degeneration are multifactorial and not fully defined, but include both genetic and biomechanical factors. Loss of joint space, subchondral sclerosis, loss of cartilage, osteophytes and joint deformities occur. The DIP joint can also be affected with mucous cysts that occur during the early stages of degenerative joint disease.

Doerschuk et al (1999) conducted a cadaveric study and demonstrated that the degree of degeneration in the anterior oblique ligament was correlated with the stage of the OA. Eaton and Littler (1973) also demonstrated a strong association between excessive laxity at the thumb CMC joint and premature degenerative changes. Laxity combined with repetitive loading may predispose certain individuals to synovitis and, with continued loading, the articular surfaces gradually wear resulting in joint space narrowing and OA. Orsoradial subluxation occurs at the base of the thumb metacarpal, while distally the adductor pollicis pulls the thumb into an adducted position (Blank & Feldon 1997). This adducted posturing of the thumb leads to difficulty in spreading the hand around objects for grasping and leads to compensatory, progressive hyperextension of the MP joint. The aetiology of CMC joint laxity has been attributed to hormonal influences (i.e. prolactin, relaxin and oestrogen), which potentially explains the increased incidence of CMC OA seen in women.

Diagnosis

Hand OA is diagnosed by its clinical features along with radiographic substantiation (Zhang et al 2009). Heberden and Bouchard nodes are clinically defined posterolateral firm / hard swellings of the IP and PIP joints respectively. Nodal OA exists in the presence of these nodes, plus underlying IP joint arthritis defined clinically and / or radiologically. Non-nodal OA is defined by IP joint OA in the absence of nodes. Erosive OA is defined radiographically by subcortical erosion, cortical destruction and subsequent reparative change, and may include bony ankylosis. Generalized OA is hand arthritis existing in combination with OA at other sites. Thumb base OA is when the first CMC joint is involved and the scaphotrapezial joint.

Typical hand OA symptoms are pain on use, mild morning pain and inactivity stiffness, particularly when affecting only single or a few consistent joints. Lateral deviation of IPs, subluxation and adduction of the thumb base are the common deformities.

The diagnosis of CMC OA is based on history and clinical exam. The typical presentation is a woman in her 50s to 70s with radial-sided hand or thumb pain. Clinical examination will reveal tenderness localized to the CMC joint, with a positive grind test (axial compression of the thumb) reproducing pain and crepitus. Radiographs are used to confirm the diagnosis. Various stages of joint involvement can be seen, ranging from a widened joint space (joint effusion or synovitis) to joint space narrowing, subluxation, sclerosis and osteophyte formation. The differential diagnosis includes psoriatic arthritis, rheumatoid arthritis, gout and haemochromatosis, each of which tends to have different target sites of involvement that can be used to assist with differentiation (Zhang et al 2009).

Prognosis

Genetic factors, female gender, age over 40, menopausal status, obesity, higher bone density, greater forearm muscle strength, joint laxity, prior hand injury and higher occupational recreational use are all associated with increased risk of hand OA and its severity and progression (Zhang et al 2009).

Conservative treatment of digital arthritis

Hand OA is a multijoint problem and treatment approach. European League Against Rheumatism (EULAR) evidence-based recommendations for management suggest that a combination of pharmacological and non-pharmacological treatment be individualized to the patient (Klein 2003; Chai & Wong 2005; Sueoka & LaStayo 2008; Yen et al 2008). Education about joint protection and exercise are recommended for all patients. Local application of heat, especially prior to exercise, splints for thumb OA and orthotics to prevent or correct lateral angulation flexion deformities are also recommended. Local treatments are preferred over systemic ones for mild to moderate pain and when only a few joints are affected. Topical NSAIDs and capsaicin are effective and safe treatments. Pharmacological and surgical interventions should be considered in patients with marked pain or disability, or when conservative treatments have failed. There is insufficient evidence to choose between different orthotics options (off-the-shelf / custom fit, long / short opponens, dorsal / volar, thermoplastic / neoprene / other materials). Orthotics should be customized according to the joint deformity / damage, functional requirements and patient preferences. It is common for patients with hand arthritis to have multiple orthoses to suit different activities or levels of disease activity. Exercise and education have been shown to be more efficacious than OA information alone (Moe et al 2009).

Rheumatoid Arthritis Affecting the Digits

Rheumatoid arthritis is an inflammatory arthritis that has diffuse digital and other involvement. In the past, severe hand deformities were common, but are now uncommon because of pharmacological advances in the management of the disease. However, older patients may continue to present with severe deformity and for surgical reconstruction. Rheumatoid arthritis hand deformity can include boutonniere, swan neck, ulnar drift, caput ulna, tendon rupture and sagittal band / tendon subluxation.

Conclusion

Injuries to the joints, tendons, ligaments and nerves in the digits are common and attention to detail is required during rehabilitation so as to restore the fine precision movement that is essential to their function. Rehabilitation principles suggest that the requirements include protected motion during healing / joint irritability, progressive active movement and strengthening that incorporates functional activities and selected use of joint mobilization techniques to enhance joint kinematics. Oedema management and integration of sensory and motor assessment / retraining are particularly important. Reliance on these principles is essential, given the dearth of physical therapy evidence for digital disorders and the specific lack of attention to this area within manual therapy literature.

References

Aitken S, Court-Brown CM. 2008. The epidemiology of sports-related fractures of the hand. Injury 39: 1377–1383.

Al-Qattan MM. 2008. Outcome of conservative management of spiral / long oblique fractures of the metacarpal shaft of the fingers using a palmar wrist splint and immediate mobilisation of the fingers. J Hand Surg 33: 723–727.

Ali H, Rafique A, Bhatti M, et al. 2007. Management of fractures of metacarpals and phalanges and associated risk factors for delayed healing. J Pak Med Assoc 57: 64–67.

Altschuler EL, Hu J. 2008. Mirror therapy in a patient with a fractured wrist and no active wrist extension. Scand J Plast Reconstr Surg Hand Surg 42: 110–111.

Armstrong AL, Hunter JB, Davis TR. 1994. The prevalence of degenerative arthritis of the base of the thumb in post-menopausal women. J Hand Surg Br 19: 340–341.

Baskurt F, Ozcan A, Algun C. 2003. Comparison of effects of phonophoresis and iontophoresis of naproxen in the treatment of lateral epicondylitis. Clin Rehabil 17: 96–100.

Bautmans I, Van PK, Mets T. 2009. Sarcopenia and functional decline: pathophysiology, prevention and therapy. Acta Clin Belg 64: 303–316.

Bettinger PC, Linscheid RL, Berger RA, et al. 1999. An anatomic study of the stabilizing ligaments of the trapezium and trapeziometacarpal joint. J Hand Surg Am 24: 786–798.

Blank J, Feldon P. 1997. Thumb metacarpophalangeal joint stabilization during carpometacarpal joint surgery. Atlas Hand Clin 2: 217–225.

Bolin DJ. 2003. Transdermal approaches to pain in sports injury management. Curr Sports Med Rep 2: 303–309.

Busse JW, Bhandari M, Kulkarni AV, et al. 2002. The effect of low-intensity pulsed ultrasound therapy on time to fracture healing: a meta-analysis. CMAJ 166: 437–441.

Caspi D, Flusser G, Farber I, et al. 2001. Clinical, radiologic, demographic, and occupational aspects of hand osteoarthritis in the elderly. Semin Arthritis Rheum 30: 321–331.

Chai SC, Wong CW. 2005. Dynamic traction and passive mobilization for the rehabilitation of zone II flexor tendon injuries: a modified regime. Med J Malaysia 60: 59–65.

Dinowitz M, Trumble T, Hanel D, et al. 1997. Failure of cast immobilization for thumb ulnar collateral ligament avulsion fractures. J Hand Surg Am 22: 1057–1063.

Doerschuk SH, Hicks DG, Chinchilli VM, et al. 1999. Histopathology of the palmar beak ligament in trapeziometacarpal osteoarthritis. J Hand Surg Am 24: 496–504.

Doherty M, Spector TD, Serni U. 2000. Epidemiology and genetics of hand osteoarthritis. Osteoarthritis Cartilage 8: 14S–15.

Eaton RG, Littler JW. 1973. Ligament reconstruction for the painful thumb carpometacarpal joint. J Bone Joint Surg Am 55: 1655–1666.

Ezendam D, Bongers RM, Jannink MJ. 2009. Systematic review of the effectiveness of mirror therapy in upper extremity function. Disabil Rehabil 31: 2135–2149.

Fedorczyk J. 1997. The role of physical agents in modulating pain. J Hand Ther 10: 110–121.

Feehan LM, Bassett, K. 2004. Is there evidence for early mobilization following an extraarticular hand fracture? J Hand Ther 17: 300–308.

Feehan LM, Sheps SS. 2008. Treating hand fractures: population-based study of acute health care use in British Columbia. Can Fam Physician 54: 1001–1007.

Fess EE, Philips CA, Gettle K, et al. 2004. Hand and upper extremity splinting: principles and methods. Philadelphia, PA: Elsevier Health Sciences.

Field J, Atkins RM. 1997. Algodystrophy is an early complication of Colles' fracture. What are the implications? J Hand Surg Br 22: 178–182.

Field J, Warwick D, Bannister GC. 1992. Features of algodystrophy ten years after Collees' fracture. J Hand Surg Br 17B: 318–320.

Flatt AE. 1996. Closed and open fractures of the hand: fundamentals of management. Postgrad Med 39: 17–26.

Flowers KR. 1988. String wrapping versus massage for reducing digital volume. Phys Ther 68: 57–59.

Freeland AE, Hardy MA, Singletary S. 2003. Rehabilitation for proximal phalangeal fractures. J Hand Ther 16: 129–142.

Grewal R, MacDermid JC. 2007. The risk of adverse outcomes in extra-articular distal radius fractures is increased with malalignment in patients of all ages but mitigated in older patients. J Hand Surg Am 32: 962–970.

Griffin XL, Costello I, Costa ML. 2008. The role of low intensity pulsed ultrasound therapy in the management of acute fractures: a systematic review. J Trauma 65: 1446–1452.

Groth GN. 2005. Current practice patterns of flexor tendon rehabilitation. J Hand Ther 18: 169–174.

Hardy MA. 2004. Principles of metacarpal and phalangeal fracture management: a review of rehabilitation concepts. J Orthop Sports Phys Ther 34: 781–799.

Harley BJ, Werner FW, Green JK. 2004. A biomechanical modeling of injury, repair, and rehabilitation of ulnar collateral ligament injuries of the thumb. J Hand Surg Am 29: 915–920.

Heyman P, Gelberman RH, Duncan K, et al. 1993. Injuries of the ulnar collateral ligament of the thumb metacarpophalangeal joint – biomechanical and prospective clinical-studies on the usefulness of valgus stress-testing. Clin Orthop Relat Res 292: 165–171.

Hostler D, Crill MT, Hagerman FC, et al. 2001. The effectiveness of 0.5-lb increments in progressive resistance exercise. J Strength Cond Res 15: 86–91.

Hove LM. 1993. Fractures of the hand. Distribution and relative incidence. Scand J Plastic Reconstr Surg Hand Surg 27: 317–319.

Hunter DJ, Demissie S, Cupples LA, et al. 2004. A genome scan for joint-specific hand osteoarthritis susceptibility: the Framingham Study. Arthritis Rheum 50: 2489–2496.

Klein L. 2003. Early active motion flexor tendon protocol using one splint. J Hand Ther 16: 199–206.

Koul AR, Patil RK, Philip V. 2008. Complex extensor tendon injuries: early active motion following single-stage reconstruction. J Hand Surg Eur 33: 753–759.

Libberecht K, Lafaire C, Van HR. 2006. Evaluation and functional assessment of flexor tendon repair in the hand. Acta Chir Belg 106: 560–565.

MacDermid JC. 2004. Hand therapy management of intra-articular fractures with open reduction and pi plate fixation: a therapist's perspective. Tech Hand Up Extrem Surg 8: 219–223.

McMahon PJ, Woods DA, Burge PD. 1994. Initial treatment of closed metacarpal fractures. A controlled comparison of compression glove and splintage. J Hand Surg Br 19: 597–600.

Michlovitz SL, Harris BA, Watkins MP. 2004. Therapy interventions for improving joint range of motion: a systematic review. J Hand Ther 17: 118–131.

Minami A, An K, Cooney WI, et al. 1984. Ligamentous structures of the metacarpophalangeal joint: a quantitative anatomic study. J Orthop Res 1: 361–368.

Moe RH, Kjeken I, Uhlig T, et al. 2009. There is inadequate evidence to determine the effectiveness of nonpharmacological and nonsurgical interventions for hand osteoarthritis: an overview of high-quality systematic reviews. Phys Ther 89: 1363–1370.

Newport ML, Tucker RL. 2005. New perspectives on extensor tendon repair and implications for rehabilitation. J Hand Ther 18: 175–181.

Omokawa S, Fujitani R, Dohi Y, et al. 2008. Prospective outcomes of comminuted periarticular metacarpal and phalangeal fractures treated using a titanium plate system. J Hand Surg Am 33: 857–863.

Page SM, Stern PJ. 1998. Complications and range of motion following plate fixation of metacarpal and phalangeal fractures. J Hand Surg Am 23: 827–832.

Polomano RC, Rathmell JP, Krenzischek DA, et al. 2008. Emerging trends and new approaches to acute pain management. Pain Manag Nurs 9: S33–S41.

Robinson SM, McPhee SD. 1986. Treating the patient with digital hypersensitivity. Am J Occup Ther 40: 285–287.

Shehadi SI. 1991. External fixation of metacarpal and phalangeal fractures. J Hand Surg Am 16: 544–550.

Shewring DJ, Thomas RH. 2006. Collateral ligament avulsion fractures from the heads of the metacarpals of the fingers. J Hand Surg Br 31: 537–541.

Smith R. 1975. Intrinsic muscles of the fingers: function, dysfunction, and surgical reconstruction. Instr Course Lect 24: 200–220.

Soffer SR, Yahiro MA. 1990. Continuous passive motion after internal fixation of distal humerus fractures. Orthop Rev 19: 88–93.

Soni P, Stern CA, Foreman KB, et al. 2009. Advances in extensor tendon diagnosis and therapy. Plast Reconstruct Surg 123: 727–728.

Stener B. 1962. Displacement of the ruptured ulnar collateral ligament of the metacarpo-phalangeal joint of the thumb: a clinical and anatomical study. J Bone Joint Surg Br 44: 869–879.

Stralka SW, Jackson JA, Lewis AR. 1998. Treatment of hand and wrist pain. A randomized clinical trial of high voltage pulsed, direct current built into a wrist splint. AAOHN J 46: 233–236.

Sueoka SS, LaStayo PC. 2008. Zone II flexor tendon rehabilitation: a proposed algorithm. J Hand Ther 21: 410–413.

Synn AJ, Makhni EC, Makhni MC, et al. 2009. Distal radius fractures in older patients: Is anatomic reduction necessary? Clin Orthop Relat Res 467: 1612–1620.

van Onselen EB, Karim RB, Hage JJ, et al. 2003. Prevalence and distribution of hand fractures. J Hand Surg Br 28: 491–495.

Waylett-Rendall J. 1988. Sensibility evaluation and rehabilitation. Orthop Clin North Am 19: 43–56.

Wehbe MA. 1987. Tendon gliding exercises. Am J Occup Ther 41: 164–167.

Westbrook AP, Davis TR, Armstrong D, et al. 2008. The clinical significance of malunion of fractures of the neck and shaft of the little finger metacarpal. J Hand Surg Eur 33: 732–739.

Yarrobino TE, Kalbfleisch JH, Ferslew KE, et al. 2006. Lidocaine iontophoresis mediates analgesia in lateral epicondylalgia treatment. Physiother Res Int 11: 152–160.

Yen CH, Chan WL, Wong JW, et al. 2008. Clinical results of early active mobilisation after flexor tendon repair. Hand Surg 13: 45–50.

Zhang W, Doherty M, Leeb BF, et al. 2009. EULAR evidence-based recommendations for the diagnosis of hand osteoarthritis: report of a task force of ESCISIT. Ann Rheum Dis 68: 8–17.

PART 9

The Foot and Ankle in Lower Extremity Pain Syndromes

54 Ankle Sprains 605
Thomas Denninger and Gary Austin

55 Plantar Heel Pain 616
Matthew P. Cotchett

56 Postoperative Management of Foot and Ankle Disorders 623
Stephanie Albin, Mark W. Cornwall and Thomas G. McPoil

57 Manipulation of the Foot and Ankle 637
William Egan, Wayne Hing, Jack Miller and Joshua A. Cleland

58 Tendinopathy of the Foot and Ankle 646
Ellen Pong

Chapter 54

Ankle Sprains

Thomas Denninger, Gary Austin

CHAPTER CONTENTS

Introduction	605
Anatomy and physiology	605
Distal tibiofibular joint	605
Talocrural joint	606
Subtalar joint	606
Biomechanics of the ankle	606
Lateral ankle sprains	607
Medial ankle sprains/syndesmotic injuries	607
Chronic ankle instability	608
Examination	608
Ottawa ankle rules	608
Subjective history	608
Ankle range of motion	609
Anterior drawer test	609
Medial talar tilt test	609
Figure-of-eight test	609
Functional testing	610
Conservative treatment	610
Thrust and non-thrust joint mobilization	610
Therapeutic exercise	613

Introduction

Approximately 10% to 34% of all sports injuries are related to the ankle (Surve et al 1994; Tropp & Gillquist 1985), with lateral ankle sprains accounting for 77–83% of these injuries (Broglio et al 2009). A review of emergency department records in the United States between 2002 and 2006 estimated the incidence of an ankle sprain to be 2.15 per 1000 person-years in the general population (Waterman et al 2010). This incidence, however, is most probably underestimated as McKay et al (2001) found that 56.8% of basketball players who sustained an ankle sprain did not seek treatment. Nearly half of all ankle sprains (49.3%) occurred during athletic activity, with baseball (41.1%), football (9.3%) and soccer (7.9%) associated with the highest percentages of ankle sprains (Waterman et al 2010). In dynamic sports, ankle sprains represent 25% of all lost-time injuries (Reid 1992). The incidence rate of ankle sprains for male soccer players is 0.46 for every 1000 hours of playing time and 0.86 for every 1000 hours of playing time for those with a previous history of an ankle sprain (Surve et al 1994). In other dynamic sports, such as basketball, a previous history of ankle injury resulted in a re-occurrence rate of five times the normal sprain rate of 3.85 per 1000 participants (McKay et al 2001). Ankle sprains have been shown to be 2.4 times more common in the dominant leg, and they have a high (73.5%) prevalence of reoccurrence (Yeung et al 1994).

Most basketball players who sustained an ankle sprain employed some form of self-treatment, such as ice, compression and / or elevation (McKay et al 2001). Among those who sought professional treatment, 62.5% received medical attention and 56.3% saw a physical therapist (McKay et al 2001). This is of concern as the clinical course of ankle sprains suggests that, although there is a rapid reduction in pain during the first 14 days, up to 33% of patients still experience persistent pain and instability at 1 year (Gerber et al 1998; Van Rijn et al 2008).

Anatomy and Physiology

Distal tibiofibular joint

The ankle joint complex encompasses multiple joints including the distal tibiofibular joint, talocrural joint, subtalar joint and talonavicular joint. The distal tibiofibular joint is the syndesmotic union of the distal extents of the tibia and fibula. The syndesmosis is created by the following ligaments: the anterior inferior tibiofibular ligament (AITFL), the posterior inferior tibiofibular ligament (PITFL), the interosseus ligament and the transverse ligament.

The PITFL runs from the posterior tibial malleolus to the posterior tubercle of the fibula. It is dense and strong and when stressed is more likely to result in an avulsion fracture than in failure (Van de Perre et al 2004). The inferior transverse ligament is located posteriorly and deep to the PITFL, and often blending with the PITFL to form the intermalleolar ligament and forming a labral-like structure (Hermans et al 2010). The intermalleolar ligament may contribute to posterior impingement syndrome in patients who frequently perform extreme plantarflexion (Rosenberg et al 1995; Oh et al 2006). The AITFL is the weakest of the syndesmotic ligaments, and is the first to fail under external rotation forces

(Hermans et al 2010). Distal to the AITFL is the intra-articular accessory anterior–inferior tibiofibular ligament, also known as Bassett's ligament, which contacts the lateral aspect of the trochlea during ankle dorsiflexion (Hermans et al 2010), possibly contributing to anterolateral ankle impingement.

The interosseous membrane courses between the length of the tibia and fibula, and the distal aspect transitions into the interosseous ligament, ultimately blending with the AITFL and PITFL (Hermans et al 2010). The interosseous ligament, along with fatty and synovial tissue, may add a spring-like effect to the mortise, accommodating the wedge-shaped talus during ankle dorsiflexion (Hermans et al 2010). Furthermore, the interosseous ligament appears to play a role in stabilizing the talocrural joint during loading (Hermans et al 2010).

Talocrural joint

The talocrural joint is the articulation between the body of the talus, including the trochlear surface, and the malleoli of the tibia and fibula. The slightly concave tibial surface articulates with the plane to convex (Dutton 2004) triangular-shaped distal end of the fibula. The structure of the mortise consists of the tibia superiorly, the medial malleolus medially and the lateral malleolus of the fibula laterally. The medial surface of the fibular malleolus articulates with the lateral facet of the talar body to create the fibulotalar joint. Similarly, the lateral surface of the tibial malleolus articulates with the medial facet of the talar body to create the tibiotalar joint (Moore 1985).

The mortise functions as a concave surface to accept the convex surface of the talar body. The trochlea of the talus is up to 6 millimetres (mm) wider anteriorly than posteriorly, causing the talus to act as a wedge within the ankle mortise, enhancing the congruence and static stability of the talocrural joint in dorsiflexion. The tibiotalar joint, fibulotalar joint and distal position of the tibiofibular joint reside in the same capsule and make up the synovial hinge joint known as the talo-crural joint (Moore 1985).

Ligaments supporting the talocrural joint include the anterior and posterior talofibular ligaments (ATFL and PTFL respectively), calcaneofibular ligament laterally and the deltoid ligament medially. The ATFL is frequently sprained during an uncontrolled inversion movement, typically in the plantarflexed position (Hosea et al 2000). When compared with other ligaments, ATFL sprains occur relatively easily secondary to low load to failure and high sprain to failure rates (Attarian et al 1985).

Subtalar joint

The subtalar joint is irregularly shaped and can be classified as a synovial bicondylar joint. There are two articulating surfaces between the talus and the calcaneus. The anterior articulation is convex on the talus and concave on the calcaneus, whereas the posterior articulation is concave on the talus and convex on the calcaneus. Between these two articulations is the interosseus membrane, also referred to as the axial ligament, which assists in stabilization of an eversion movement (Kapanji 1970). With the anterior articulation lying medial to the posterior articulation and with irregular joint surfaces, the subtalar joint will move in opposite directions during functional weight-bearing (Dutton 2004).

Ligaments are present to maintain integrity of the subtalar joint. They include the medial and lateral interosseus, the calcaneofibular ligaments (CFL), the deltoid ligaments (DL) and the lateral talocalcaneal ligaments (LTCL). The medial talocalcaneal interosseus ligaments project from the medial tubercle of the talus posteriorly to just behind the sustentaculum tali of the calcaneus and serves to protect the talus from anterior translation on the calcaneus. The lateral talocalcaneal interosseus ligaments (cervical ligaments) project from the sinus tarsi posteriorly to the calcaneus and serve to prevent the excess separation of the talus from the calcaneus during inversion moments. These ligaments are typically injured when an excessive moment is applied in inversion and coupled with dorsiflexion (Dutton 2004). The cervical ligament is further fortified in preventing subtalar inversion by the deep fibres of the extensor retinaculum. Medially, the deltoid and calcaneonavicular ligaments prevent excessive eversion. Laxity of the ligaments in the lateral compartments is implicated frequently in lateral instability owing to an excess of active and passive ranges of motion. Laxity in the medial compartment is predominately less frequent, but may be functionally more problematic since this type of sprain is associated with a higher incidence of cartilage damage and concomitant lateral ligamentous damage (Cook 2007). Table 54.1 summarizes the role of the ligaments in ankle stability.

Biomechanics of the ankle

As in all joints, the ankle complex has two types of possible motion: translator movement, also known as arthrokinematic movement, and rotational movement, also known as osteokinematic movement. Osteokinematic movement incorporates translatory motion in order to stabilize the instantaneous axis of rotation. This is important to translate forces over a larger surface area within the joint, as well as to prevent unnatural forces during the end ranges, which may damage the passive structures of the joint.

The collective movement patterns and passive and active control of ankle motion allow for transfer of force throughout the ankle complex during functional movement. This process involves the individual range of motions provided at each articulation.

Table 54.1 **Role of collateral ligaments in ankle stability**

Movement	Controlled by
Abduction of the talus	Tibiocalcaneal and tibionavicular bands
Adduction of the talus	Calcaneofibular ligament
Plantarflexion	ATFL and anterior tibiotalar ligament
Dorsiflexion	Posterior tibiotalar band and PTFL
External rotation of the talus	Anterior tibiotalar and tibionavicular bands
Internal rotation of the talus	ATFL, anterior tibiotalar and tibionavicular bands

Although the talocrural joint is typically described as a uniplanar ginglymus or hinge joint, the anatomy would suggest otherwise.

Range of motion

The talocrural joint demonstrates approximately 50° of plantarflexion and 20° of dorsiflexion. The subtalar joint is reported to have 40° of inversion and 20° of eversion. The tarsal joints are reported to have 10° of pronation and 20° of supination (Cook 2007).

Open-packed and closed-packed positions

The terms open-packed and closed-packed positions of the ankle refer to the theoretical supposition that selected movements will increase the compression (closed-packed) or distraction (open-packed) between the joints of the ankle. With respect to the mechanics of articulation, the closed-packed position refers to the specific joint position when the articular surfaces are at the maximum point of congruency, whereas the open-packed position is the opposite of this situation. Unfortunately, no studies yet exist to support this assumption, and hence the validity behind the theory of open- and closed-packed positions is essentially unknown (Cook 2007).

Axes of rotation / osteokinematics

The talocrural joint axis travels predominately in the medial–lateral direction, with smaller components in the anterior–posterior and superior–inferior directions. The longer and more posterior lateral malleolus contributes to the departure of the talocrural joint axis from a pure medial–lateral axis in the frontal plane (about 10°) and transverse plane (about 6°). Such an orientation allows for large amounts of motion in the sagittal plane (dorsiflexion / plantarflexion) and smaller amounts of motion in the frontal (inversion / eversion) and transverse (abduction / adduction) planes. The subtalar joint axis is oriented 42° from the transverse plane, travelling nearly midway between anterior–posterior and superior–inferior directions, with a minor component in the medial–lateral direction. It has been described that the axis of rotation is 42° from the horizontal plane and 16° from the sagittal plane, running in an anterior, medial and superior direction. Such an orientation allows for large amounts of motion in the frontal (inversion / eversion) and transverse (abduction / adduction) planes and smaller amounts of motion in the sagittal plane (dorsiflexion / plantarflexion). At the ankle, most motions are coupled and triplanar in nature. At the talocrural joint smaller but significant amounts of eversion and abduction accompany dorsiflexion (pronation), whereas smaller but significant amounts of inversion and adduction accompany plantarflexion (supination). At the subtalar joint, larger amounts of eversion and abduction are accompanied by small but significant amounts of dorsiflexion, whereas inversion and adduction are accompanied by small but significant amounts of plantarflexion.

The closed- and open-packed positions in the hindfoot work in concert with the axes of motion to create coupled and functional movement patterns in the lower extremity (Dutton 2004). Subtalar joint supination assists in locking the mid-tarsal joint, creating a mechanically advantageous rigid lever during propulsion. Pronation at the subtalar joint unlocks the mid-tarsal joint, promoting a flexible foot that is able to accommodate uneven surfaces and absorb the shock of ground reaction forces.

Arthrokinematics

During dorsiflexion at the talocrural joint, the superior surface of the talus rolls anteriorly within the mortise while simultaneously sliding posteriorly. During plantarflexion, the talus rolls posteriorly while simultaneously sliding anteriorly (Dutton 2004). The motion, however, is not purely in the sagittal plane as it has smaller, but important, movements in the frontal and transverse planes.

The articulation of the subtalar joint is more complex, with pronation and supination resulting, primarily, from relative sliding motions between the calcaneus and talus at the subtalar facets (anterior, medial and posterior) (Cook 2007). The relative sliding motion can occur from a mobile calcaneus moving on a fixed talus, a mobile talus moving on a fixed calcaneus or motion between a mobile talus and calcaneus.

Lateral Ankle Sprains

Acute lateral ankle sprains are often described according to the severity of the injury. Traditionally, lateral ankle sprains are assigned grades of I to III to represent the extent and severity of ligament damage, with grade I being the least involved and grade III being the most severe type of injury (Martin et al 2013). Grading scales often incorporate multiple static and dynamic measures to describe the severity of the injury. Static measures include an assessment of ligament laxity, haemorrhaging, swelling and tenderness. Dynamic measures have included range of motion, strength and ability to perform functional tests.

A commonly utilized method to grade acute lateral ankle sprains has been defined as follows (Hockenbury & Sammarco 2001):

- **grade I:** no loss of function, no ligamentous laxity, little or no haemorrhaging, no point tenderness, decreased total ankle motion of ≤5°, and swelling ≤0.5 cm or less
- **grade II:** some loss of function, positive anterior drawer test (ATFL), negative talar tilt (CFL), haemorrhaging, point tenderness, decrease in total ankle motion between 5° and 10° and swelling between 0.5 and 2.0 cm
- **grade III:** near-total loss of function, positive anterior drawer test (ATFL) and talar tilt tests (CFL), haemorrhaging, extreme point tenderness, decreased total ankle motion >10° and swelling >2.0 cm. Grade III injuries have been further divided according to stress radiograph results, with anterior drawer movement of ≤3 mm being IIIA and >3 mm of movement being IIIB.

Medial Ankle Sprains / Syndesmotic Injuries

Medial ankle sprains occur much less frequently than lateral ankle sprains, accounting for approximately 5–10% of all ankle sprains (Broglio et al 2009). The DL is often not injured secondary to its strong internal structure and ligamentous connections. Isolated DL injury is rare, typically occurring with an avulsion fracture of the medial malleolus (Pott fracture). The mechanism of injury for an isolated deltoid injury is plantarflexion and eversion. Individuals with this rare injury will report pain on the medial aspect of the foot and reproduction of pain upon subtalar inversion and eversion. Syndesmotic injuries can occur concomitantly to medial ankle sprains secondary to gapping of the distal tibiofibular joint due to wedging to the talus that occurs with dorsiflexion eversion and rotation injuries. This can include injury to the anterior tibiofibular ligament, interosseus membrane and DL. This can result in widening of the ankle mortise as a result of damage to the tibiofibular ligaments (Brosky et al 1995).

Initial management of medial ankle sprain and syndesmotic injury is more conservative than with lateral ankle sprains, often requiring a longer period of immobilization with non-weight-bearing. Progressive weight-bearing and rehabilitation are suggested for gradual resumption of normal and ultimately athletic activity (Lin et al 2006).

Chronic Ankle Instability

When symptoms of instability continue after a lateral ankle injury, patients are commonly diagnosed as having mechanical or functional ankle instability. Chronic ankle instability has been defined as the presence of persistent post-acute symptoms such as occasional swelling, impaired strength, instability and impaired balance responses. This has been operationalized as symptoms of giving way for greater than 6 months following the initial injury (O'Loughlin et al 2009) This diagnosis has been further broken down in to patients with functional ankle instability and those with mechanical ankle instability.

Functional ankle instability has been defined as recurrent ankle sprains or ongoing sensations of the ankle giving way with normal ankle motion and the absence of objective joint laxity. In a study of 80 individuals with functional ankle instability, side-to-side comparisons of ankle laxity were made between the ankle with functional ankle instability and the uninvolved ankle (Hirai et al 2009). This study suggests that functional ankle instability is not associated with joint laxity. Factors that may contribute to functional ankle instability appear to include muscle weakness, muscle recruitment patterns, decreased ankle range of motion, balance deficits and joint proprioception. A meta-analysis concluded that patients with functional ankle instability have poor balance compared with subjects without ankle instability (Arnold et al 2009). Additionally there are documented deficits in sensorimotor performance in subjects with functional ankle instability (Konradsen et al 1998; O'Driscoll & Delahunt 2011). Patients with functional ankle instability have demonstrated improved balance and reductions in disability through balance programmes utilizing stable and unstable surfaces.

Mechanical ankle instability is distinguished from functional ankle instability by the presence of ankle ligamentous laxity (Caulfield 2000). Persistent ligamentous laxity occurs in approximately 30% of patients post inversion ankle sprain 1 year after initial injury (Hubbard et al 2004). Rehabilitation of mechanical instability does not differ from that of functional ankle instability. For most patients, rehabilitation including bracing and functional training leads to recovery (Broglio et al 2009; Hale et al 2007; de Vries et al 2011). Persistent findings of unilateral ligamentous laxity via clinical or radiographic examination may be associated with worse prognosis, and if complaints persist following a comprehensive conservative treatment approach then the literature suggests that surgical intervention may be required (Hintermann et al 2002). It is important to note that dichotomizing ankle instability into mechanical or functional is difficult, as patients may present with a mixture of mechanical and functional instability.

Examination

Ottawa ankle rules

The Ottawa ankle rules were developed in 1992 to reduce the frequency of radiographic imagery following ankle sprain. Prior to the onset of these rules, plain radiographs were customarily ordered for suspected ankle sprains, even though less than 15% of ankle sprains result in a fracture (Bachmann et al 2003). The rules dictate that, in the presence of a traumatic injury to the foot and / or ankle, there is a need for an ankle radiographic series if a patient demonstrates: (1) tenderness at the posterior edge or tip of the lateral malleolus, (2) tenderness at the posterior edge or tip of the medial malleolus, and / or (3) inability to bear weight both immediately post injury and in the emergency room for four steps (including limping). The rules also dictate the need for a foot radiographic series if the patient demonstrates: (1) tenderness at the base of the fifth metatarsal bone, (2) tenderness at the navicular, and / or (3) inability to bear weight immediately post injury and in the emergency room for four steps (including limping). A summary of several studies demonstrated that the absence of these factors is excellent in ruling out the presence of fracture (–LR 0.07; 95% CI 0.03–0.18) (Bachmann et al 2003) and can support a decision to proceed with treatment without obtaining radiographs. The rules lack sufficient specificity and positive likelihood ratios (LRs) to rule in a fracture; thus the presence of these factors prevents the ability to rule out a fracture, and a plain foot or ankle radiograph is suggested. The specificity and positive likelihood ratio are sufficiently diagnostic with the addition of a tuning fork applied to the distal fibula shaft (Dissman & Han 2006).

Subjective history

Important history items collected during the subjective examination include the presence of comorbidities, any relevant past history of ankle disorders (including the number and degree of previous ankle sprains), a history of previous surgery, and occupational and avocational demands. The mechanism of injury can assist in determining the likelihood of the presence of a fracture. High-impact injuries or profound ankle sprains should automatically initiate the assessment of the Ottawa ankle rules.

The behaviour of the symptoms may help to outline the cause of the disorder and to rule out more serious pathology. Locking disorders that exhibit an intermittent pattern may be indicative of osteochondritis dissecans of the talar dome

(Cook 2007). Pain associated with osteochondritis dissecans should be represented so as to differentiate from anterior impingement at the anterolateral ankle joint line; anterior impingement is consistently triggered during dorsiflexion at end range, whereas osteochondritis dissecans may occur intermittently and during different planes of motion. Significant dorsolateral ankle pain may suggest cuboid syndrome. Paraesthesiae along the dorsum or dorsolateral aspect of the foot may indicate potential neurodynamic involvement of the peroneal and sural nerves respectively (Jennings & Davies 2005).

Ankle range of motion

Goniometric measurement of passive and active ankle range of motion in the non-weight-bearing position has been used to assess physiological motion of the ankle joint. Common measurements are dorsiflexion measured in prone both with the knee extended and with it flexed to 45°, plantarflexion in supine, and eversion / inversion in supine. A reliability is established for intra-tester reliability of >0.90 and an inter-tester reliability of 0.70 (Martin & McPoil 2005; Menadue et al 2006). The reliability of plantarflexion is consistently lower than that for dorsiflexion. Ankle dorsiflexion can also be reliably measured in a weight-bearing lunge position using either an inclinometer or a tape measure (Bennell et al 1998).

Anterior drawer test

The anterior drawer test is utilized to assess the integrity of the ATFL. The amount of anterior talar translation in relation to the ankle mortise is quantified (Croy et al 2013). The patient is sitting in 90° of knee flexion, with the leg relaxed and unsupported and with the ankle positioned in 10–20° of plantar flexion. One hand of the examiner is placed on the distal tibia while palpating the articulation between the lateral surface of the talus and the anterior aspect of the distal fibula. The second hand grasps the posterior aspect of the calcaneus. The test is performed by pulling the calcaneus and subsequently the talus in an anterior direction with the distal tibia stabilized (Fig. 54.1). To assess the ATFL properly in the presence of an intact anterior tibiotalar and tibionavicular ligaments and avoid a false negative, the examiner then introduces abduction of the foot (Tohyama et al 2003). The diagnostic accuracy was established in one study (Croy et al 2013) as: sensitivity 0.74 (95% CI 0.58–0.86), specificity 0.38 (95% CI 0.24–0.56), +LR 1.2–1.4 and –LR 0.41–0.60. In another study (van Dijk et al 1996), the combination of pain with palpation of the ATFL, lateral haematoma and a positive anterior drawer on examination 5 days after injury had a sensitivity of 100%, specificity of 75%, +LR of 4.13 and –LR of 0.01 for identifying lateral ligament ruptures. However, the same test performed less than 48 hours following injury was not informative, showing a sensitivity of 0.71, specificity of 0.33, –LR of 1.06 and +LR of 0.88. Inter-tester reliability ranged between 0.5 and 1.0. The test is most useful for both ruling in and ruling out anterior talofibular ligament laxity when performed at least 5 days following injury.

Medial talar tilt test

The medial talar tilt test is utilized to assess the amount of talar inversion occurring within the ankle mortise, testing the integrity of the CFL. The test is performed with the patient sitting in 90° of knee flexion, with the leg relaxed and unsupported. One hand of the examiner grasps the distal tibia and fibula while the second hand grasps the calcaneus, holding the ankle in a neutral position. The test is performed by inverting the calcaneus and subsequently the talus, relative to the ankle mortise. Variations of the test have been described in supine, side-lying (Fig. 54.2) and prone. Diagnostic accuracy has been established with sensitivity of 0.50 (95% CI 0.25–0.75), specificity of 0.88 (95% CI 0.53–0.98), +LR of 4.00 (95% CI 0.59–27.25) and –LR of 0.57 (95% CI 0.31–1.07) (Hertel et al 1999). The test is most useful for ruling in CFL laxity.

Figure-of-eight test

The figure-of-eight test has been utilized to measure ankle circumference as an indication of the amount of ankle oedema following traumatic injury (Mawdsley et al 2000). The ankle

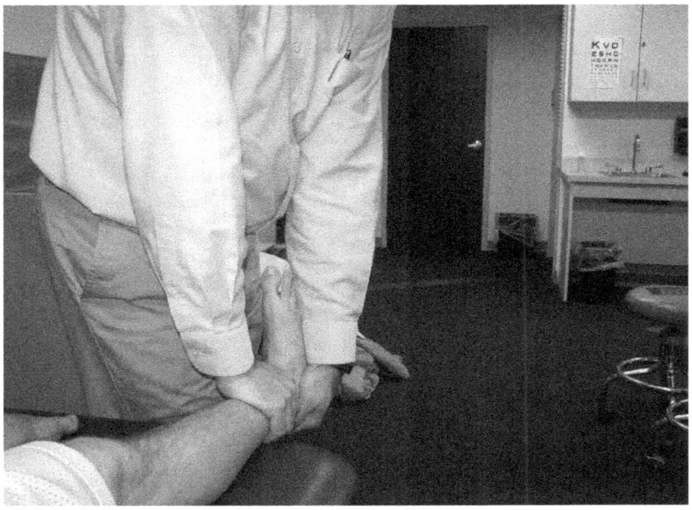

Figure 54.1 Anterior drawer test.

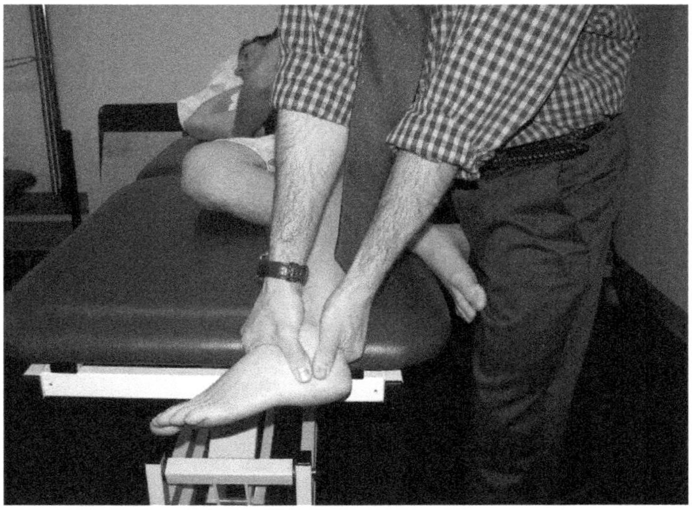

Figure 54.2 Talar tilt test with the patient in side-lying.

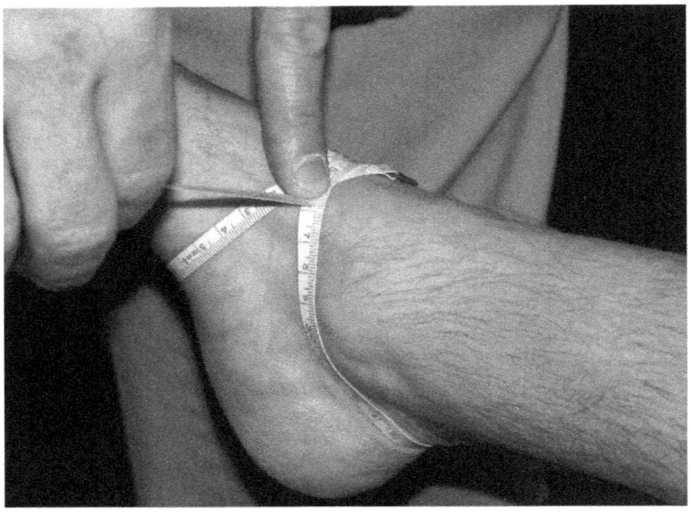

Figure 54.3 Figure-of-eight test.

is positioned in either neutral comfortable or 20° of plantarflexion. The zero end point of a tape measure is positioned at the groove on the edge of the lateral malleolus, midway between the prominence of the lateral malleolus and tibialis anterior tendon. The tape is drawn medially around the foot to cross the plantar aspect to and behind the base of the fifth metatarsal. The tape is then drawn towards and under the medial malleolus, across the Achilles tendon, to and under the lateral malleolus of the fibula, and finally to meet the original zero point (Fig. 54.3). Inter-tester reliability has been found to be excellent (intraclass correlation coefficients (ICC) 0.93–0.99) with a minimal detectable change of 6.8 mm when measured in 20° (Rohner-Spengler et al 2007).

Functional testing

Single-limb balance

Single-limb balance should be assessed as a baseline measure of functional ankle stability prior to the progression to dynamic activity (Akbari et al 2006). Testing should be completed with patient safety in mind and therefore should either be guarded or have a close hand-hold to guard against loss of balance. Timed duration of single limb stance should be completed with eyes open and eyes closed, on both the affected and unaffected limbs. Alternatively, patients may be timed for 1-minute durations in both testing conditions, counting the number of touches with the contralateral leg or upper extremity. Normative data (Bohannon et al 1984) suggest that the average limb balance time for individuals between 20 and 49 years of age ranges between 29.76 and 30.0 seconds with eyes open and between 24.2 and 28.8 seconds with eyes closed; for those between the ages of 50 and 79 years of age the average times decrease to between 14.2 and 29.4 seconds with eyes open and 4.3 to 21.0 seconds with eyes closed.

Star excursion balance test

The star excursion balance test layout consists of eight lines from a centre point arranged at 45° angles. The lines can be labelled according to their position in a counterclockwise direction with reference to the tested limb as follows: anterior, anterolateral, lateral, posterolateral, posterior, posteromedial, medial and anterior–medial. The test consists of having the subject stand with the lower extremity being tested in the centre while the examiner measures the maximum reach distance of the contralateral lower extremity achieved along each of the directions. Patients are not allowed to move the support foot and should keep their hands on hips. The reach distance can be normalized by dividing the excursion distance by the lower extremity length. The test–retest reliability in healthy individuals has been found to be good (ICC 0.67–0.96) (Buchanan et al 2008), whereas inter-tester reliability has been demonstrated as poor to excellent (ICC 0.35–0.94) (Hertel et al 2009). The Y-Balance test is an adaptation of the star excursion balance test that is instrumented and involves only three directions (anterior, posterolateral and posteromedial) (Hertel et al 2006; Plisky et al 2006).

Conservative Treatment

Mobility is essential in the recovery of lateral ankle sprains. For grade I and grade II injuries, early mobilization has been shown to be more effective than immobilization. In a group of 82 patients with lateral ankle sprains, 87% who were immobilized with a plaster cast for 10 days reported the presence of pain at 3 weeks. This compared with 57% of patients who received early mobilization in the form of an elastic strap followed by a functional brace for 8 days (Eiff et al 1994). Studies generally favour mobilization, compared with immobilization, in outcome measures reflecting return to sport (weighted mean difference 4.6 days; 95% CI 1.5–7.6 days), return to work (weighted mean difference 2.1 days; 95% CI 5.6–8.7 days) and instability (weighted mean difference 2.5 days; 95% CI 1.3–3.6 days) (Kerkhoffs et al 2001). There were also small effect sizes of treatment that favoured the early mobilization group for ankle range of motion and swelling.

Thrust and non-thrust joint mobilization

Several studies have demonstrated the effectiveness of early manual therapy in decreasing pain, decreasing oedema and reducing recovery time (Nield et al 1993; Green et al 2001; Pellow & Brantingham 2001; Fryer et al 2002; Eisenhart et al 2003; Whitman et al 2005; van der Wees et al 2006). Most recently, Cleland et al (2013) demonstrated superior short- and long-term outcomes in a group receiving manual therapy and exercise as compared with a group receiving home exercise programme in isolation. Other studies have demonstrated similar results compared with true control and in-clinic exercise alone. Whitman et al (2009) developed a clinical prediction rule for patients likely to respond to manual therapy directed at the foot–ankle complex for patients post lateral ankle sprain. Predictors of success included symptoms worse while standing, symptoms worse in the evening, navicular drop test greater than 5 mm and distal tibiofibular hypomobility. Presence of three of the predictors was associated with a positive likelihood of 5.90 (95% CI 1.08–41.60), increasing post-test probability of success to 95%. It is worthwhile noting that 75% of the patients had a successful outcome with the treatment, questioning whether a clinical prediction rule is needed to determine the efficacy of manual therapy directed to the foot and ankle for patients post lateral ankle sprain. Here we summarize some of the most commonly used techniques for ankle sprains. (See also Ch 57 for more joint mobilization and manipulation techniques targeted to the ankle.)

Anterior–posterior non-thrust mobilization (see Fig. 57.2)

The therapist uses one hand to stabilize the lower leg firmly at the level of the malleoli. The therapist grasps the anterior, medial and lateral talus with the mobilizing hand, just distal to the malleoli, being careful to avoid painful and sensitive injured tissues. The therapist then applies a low-velocity, anterior–posterior oscillatory force to the talus. The therapist may use his / her thigh to stabilize the foot and progressively increase the amount of ankle dorsiflexion. Fine adjustments in supination and pronation may help optimize the technique. Lastly, the introduction of an anterior roll may improve the arthrokinematics and facilitate the restoration of ankle dorsiflexion range of motion (Maitland 2005).

Lateral–medial non-thrust mobilization (see also Figs 57.3–57.5)

Talocrural joint lateral glide

The therapist grasps the malleoli just proximal to the talocrural joint with the index finger / thumb of the cephalad hand and uses the forearm to stabilize the patient's leg against the table. The therapist places the thenar eminence on the talus just distal to the malleoli and grasps the rearfoot. The therapist then uses his / her body to impart a low-velocity oscillatory force to the talus through the extended arm and thenar eminence (Maitland 2005).

Subtalar joint lateral glide

The therapist shifts the cephalad hand / forearm distally and grasps the talus with the index finger / thumb. The therapist places the thenar eminence on the patient's medial aspect of the calcaneus and grasps the rearfoot (Fig. 54.4). The therapist uses his / her body to impart a low-velocity oscillatory force to the calcaneus through the extended arm and thenar eminence (Maitland 2005).

Rearfoot distraction thrust manipulation (see also Fig. 57.1)

The therapist grasps the dorsum of the patient's foot immediately distal to the talocrural joint line with interlaced fingers and places the foot into dorsiflexion. Firm pressure, with both thumbs, is applied to the middle of the plantar surface of the foot (Fig. 54.5). The therapist engages the restrictive barrier by passively dorsiflexing and everting the ankle (protecting the injured ATFL) and applying a long-axis distraction. The therapist everts and dorsiflexes the foot to fine-tune the barrier. The therapist applies a high-velocity, low-amplitude force in the caudal direction (Fig. 54.6) (Whitman et al 2009).

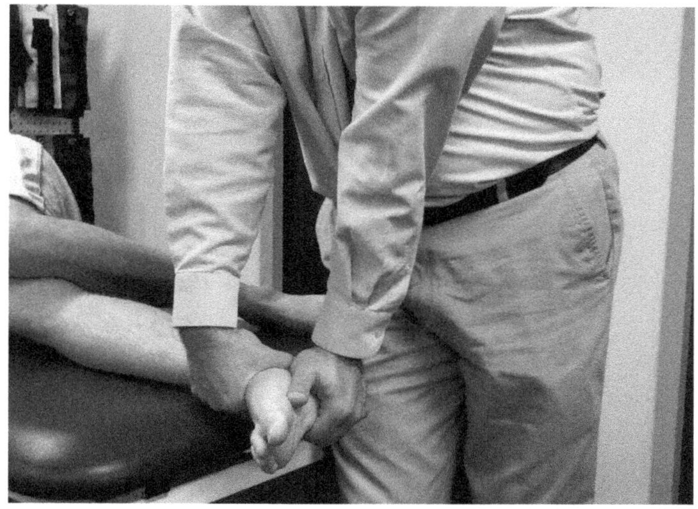

Figure 54.4 Non-thrust lateral glide mobilization of the subtalar joint.

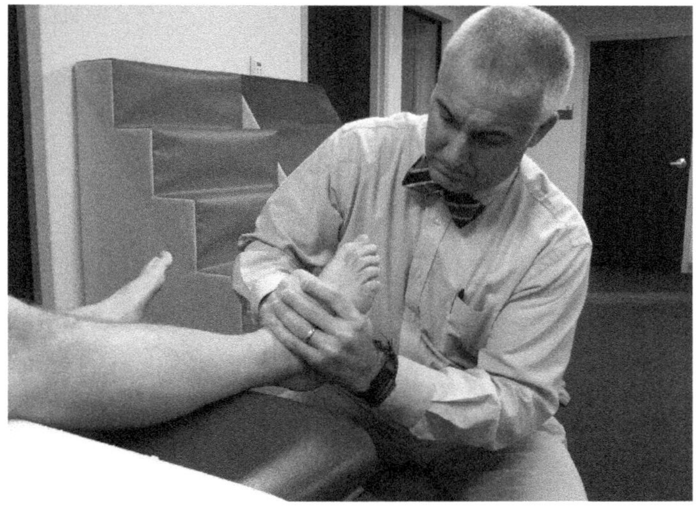

Figure 54.5 Rearfoot (subtalar) distraction thrust manipulation set-up.

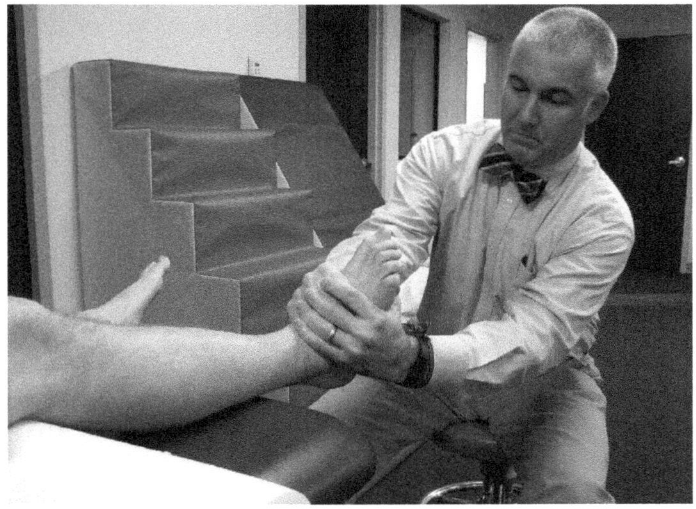

Figure 54.6 Rearfoot (subtalar) distraction thrust manipulation.

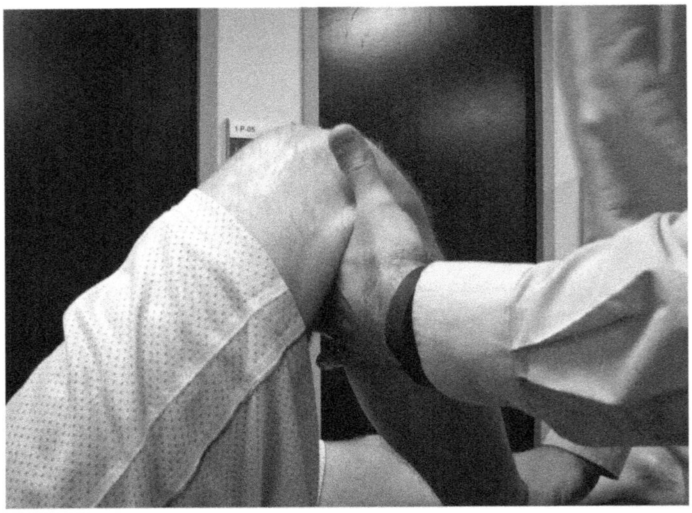

Figure 54.7 **Proximal tibiofibular joint thrust manipulation set-up.**

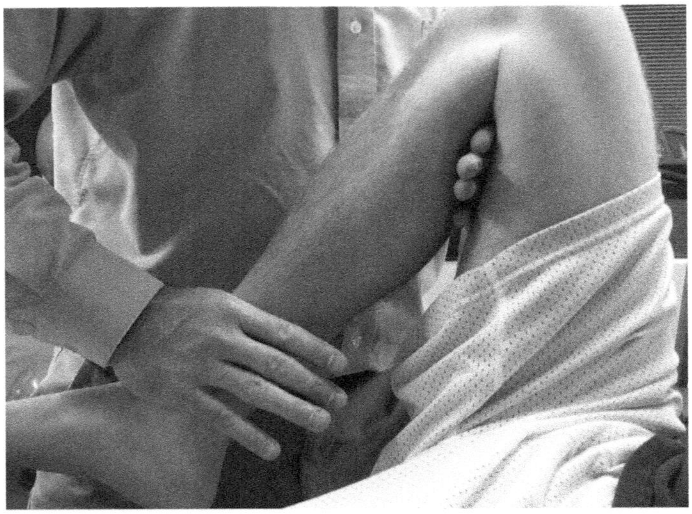

Figure 54.8 **Proximal tibiofibular joint thrust manipulation.**

Distal tibiofibular joint non-thrust mobilization (see Fig. 57.7)

The therapist grasps and stabilizes the distal tibia with one hand placed posterior to the medial malleolus. The therapist then places the thenar eminence of the opposite hand over the anterior aspect of the lateral malleolus and uses his / her body to impart a low-velocity, oscillatory, anterior-to-posterior force to the fibula on the tibia (Mulligan 1995).

Proximal tibiofibular joint thrust manipulation (see also Fig. 57.6)

The therapist places the second metacarpophalangeal joint in the popliteal fossa, pulling the soft tissue laterally until the metacarpophalangeal joint is firmly stabilized behind the patient's fibular head (Fig. 54.7). The therapist uses the opposite hand to grasp the foot and ankle. The therapist externally rotates the leg and flexes the knee to the restrictive barrier (Fig. 54.8). The therapist delivers a high-velocity, low-amplitude force through the tibia, directing the patient's heel to the ipsilateral buttock (Whitman et al 2009; Beazell et al 2012).

Weight-bearing dorsiflexion mobilization with movement (see also Fig. 57.4B)

The therapist supports the arch of the foot with the medial hand and applies a stabilizing force (anterior–posterior) over the anterior talus. A belt is placed around the patient's distal posterior tibia and fibula and around the therapist's buttock region. The patient is guided into dorsiflexion of the involved ankle while the therapist applies a posterior-to-anterior-directed force to the distal leg by leaning backward / pulling on the belt. As the patient dorsiflexes more, the therapist squats down while leaning back in order to maintain a perpendicular orientation to the lower leg and thus apply a direct posterior–anterior force at the talocrural joint (Fig. 54.9) (Mulligan 1995; Collins et al 2004; Vincenzino et al 2006).

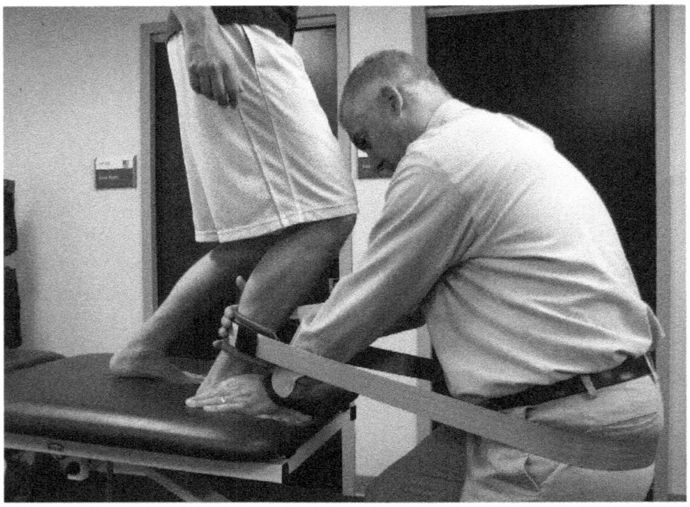

Figure 54.9 **Weight-bearing dorsiflexion mobilization with movement.**

Cuboid whip thrust manipulation (see also Fig. 57.8)

Patients post inversion ankle sprain with persistent pain located over the lateral dorsum of the foot associated with mid-foot hypomobility may benefit from a cuboid whip technique. Care should be taken with use of the technique in patients with high acuity and injury of the ATFL, given the end position of the technique. The patient is positioned in prone. The examiner grasps the patient's foot with the knee positioned in flexion. The therapist interlocks the fingers of both hands over the dorsum of the foot, with both thumbs applying firm pressure to the plantar surface of the cuboid directed in a dorsal and slightly lateral direction (Fig. 54.10). The therapist then applies a high velocity, low-amplitude force, moving the ankle in the plantarflexed and inverted position with simultaneous knee extension (Jennings & Davies 2005).

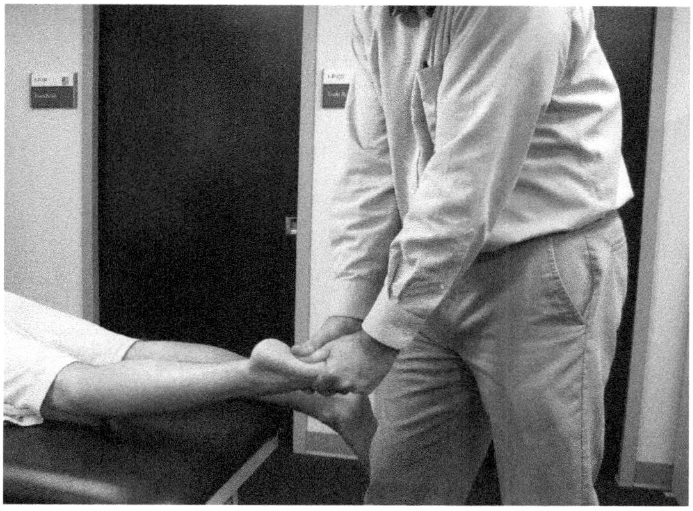

Figure 54.10 Cuboid whip thrust manipulation.

Therapeutic exercise

Mobility exercise

After initial ankle sprain with respect to protection, early active mobilization is recommended for increasing extracellular fluid exchange, decreasing swelling, increasing range of motion, decreasing stiffness and restoring normal joint mechanics (van der Wees et al 2006). For lateral ankle sprains, emphasis is placed on restoration of motion to pre-existing or contralateral measures; however, particular note is placed on restoration of subtalar eversion and dorsiflexion given the tendency for reductions in range, which may play a role in recurrence or other lower extremity injury (Denegar et al 2002).

This can include static and dynamic stretching of the ankle plantarflexor and also non-weight-bearing and weight-bearing mobilizations into combined pronation (Etnyre & Abraham 1986). An example of this is a split kneel into weight-bearing dorsiflexion; this may be combined with an elastic posteriorly directed force to serve as a self-mobilization similar to the weight-bearing dorsiflexion mobilization with movement.

Strengthening

Early strengthening exercises for patients recovering from ankle sprains often include isometric or concentric and / or eccentric contractions, using elastic resistance in non-weight-bearing positions. Cardinal planes of movements should be utilized including dorsiflexion, plantarflexion, inversion and eversion (Uh et al 2000; Bassett & Prapavessis 2007; Kemler et al 2011).

In order to avoid exercise tolerance, patients should transition to weight-bearing exercises as pain and swelling decrease with respect to physiological healing times, especially in cases of more severe ligamentous injury. This may include weight-shifting and progression to active heel rising through partial and eventually full ranges of motion. Gentle and gradual progressive squatting can promote talocrural and subtalar joint pronation. Gait-restorative exercises utilizing the full functional range of motion of the ankle should be implemented early on so as to prevent compensatory patterns (Wilson & Gansneder 2000).

Proprioceptive exercises

Proprioceptive exercises have well-established importance for patients returning to previous function. Deficits related to joint proprioception are thought to be associated with chronic ankle instability and recurrence (Lentell et al 1995). Proprioceptive exercises have taken many forms: on stable versus unstable surfaces, open versus closed eye circumstances, single- versus double-limb stance, and static versus dynamic activities. Common examples of these exercises include static single-limb stance with the degree of difficulty progressed with the addition of decreased visual input, an unstable surface, or contralateral lower extremity and upper extremity motion (Hess et al 2001; Osborne et al 2001). These advances serve to challenge the neuromusculoskeletal system to improve joint proprioception and muscle recruitment and reaction times (Han et al 2009; Wester et al 1996).

More-advanced modifications include the addition of ball throwing with a partner or on a trampoline. Especially in return-to-sport cases, jumping and bounding exercises are essential for restoring function and decreasing the likelihood of recurrence (Holme et al 1999; Hupperets et al 2009). Uniplanar motion should begin with an emphasis on repetitions and speed of landing to take off, with progressions made by increasing height or distance, and incorporating multiple directions in a pattern or at random. Readers are referred to other chapters of the current textbook for further discussion and progression of exercises in relation to proprioceptive rehabilitation.

References

Akbari M, Karimi H, Farahini H, et al. 2006. Balance problems after unilateral lateral ankle sprains. J Rehabil Res Dev 43: 819–824.

Arnold BL, De La Motte S, Linens S, et al. 2009. Ankle instability is associated with balance impairments: a meta-analysis. Med Sci Sports Exerc 41: 1048–1062.

Attarian DE, McCrackin HJ, DeVito D, et al. 1985. Biomechanical characteristics of human ankle ligaments. Foot Ankle 6: 54–58.

Bachmann LM, Kolb E, Koller MT, et al. 2003. Accuracy of Ottawa ankle rules to exclude fractures of the ankle and mid-foot: systematic review. BMJ 326: 417.

Bassett SF, Prapavessis H. 2007. Home-based physical therapy intervention with adherence-enhancing strategies versus clinic-based management for patients with ankle sprains. Phys Ther 87: 1132–1143.

Beazell JR, Grindstaff TL, Sauer LD, et al. 2012. Effects of a proximal or distal tibiofibular joint manipulation on ankle range of motion and functional outcomes in individuals with chronic ankle instability. J Orthop Sports Phys Ther 42: 125–134. doi: 10.2519/jospt.2012.3729.

Bennell KL, Talbot RC, Wajswelner H. 1998. Intra-rater and inter-rater reliability of a weight bearing lunge measure of ankle dorsiflexion. Aust J Physiother 44: 175–180.

Bohannon RW, Larkin PA, Cook AC, et al. 1984. Decrease in timed balance scores with aging. Phys Ther 64: 1067–1070.

Broglio SP, Monk A, Sopiarz K, et al. 2009. The influence of ankle support on postural control. J Sci Med Sport 12: 388–392.

Brosky T, Nyland A, Nitz A. 1995. The ankle ligaments: consideration of syndesmotic injury and implications for rehabilitation. J Orthop Sports Phys Ther 21: 197–205.

Buchanan AS, Docherty CL, Schrader J. 2008. Functional performance testing in participants with functional ankle instability and in a healthy control group. J. Athl Train 43: 342–346.

Caulfield B. 2000. Functional instability of the ankle joint. Physiother 86: 401–411.

Cleland JA, Mintken P, McDevitt A, et al. 2013. Manual physical therapy and exercise versus supervised home exercise in the management of patients with inversion ankle sprain: a multicenter randomized clinical trial. J Orthop Sports Phys Ther 43: 443–455.
Collins N, Teys P, Vincenzino B. 2004. The initial effects of a Mulligan's mobilization technique on dorsiflexion and pain in subacute ankle sprains. Man Ther 9: 77–82.
Cook CE. 2007 Orthopedic manual therapy: an evidence based approach. Upper Saddle River, NJ: Pearson Prentice Hall.
Croy T, Koppenhaver S, Saliba S, et al. 2013. Anterior talocrural joint laxity: diagnostic accuracy of the anterior drawer test of the ankle. J Orthop Sports Phys Ther 43: 911–919.
de Vries JS, Krips R, Sierevelt IN, et al. 2011. Interventions for treating chronic ankle instability. Cochrane Database Syst Rev 8: CD004124.
Denegar CR, Hertel J, Fonseca J. 2002. The effect of lateral ankle sprain on dorsiflexion range of motion, posterior talar glide, and joint laxity. J Orthop Sports Phys Ther 32: 166–173.
Dissman PD, Han KH. 2006. The tuning fork test– a useful tool for improving specificity in 'Ottawa positive' patients after ankle inversion injury. Emerg Med J 23: 788–790.
Dutton M. 2004. Orthopedic examination, evaluation, and intervention. New York: McGraw-Hill.
Eiff MP, Smith AT, Smith GE. 1994. Early mobilization versus immobilization in the treatments of lateral ankle sprains. Am J Sports Med 22: 83–88.
Eisenhart AW, Gaeta TJ, Yeus DP. 2003. Osteopathic manipulative treatment in the emergency department for patients with acute ankle sprains. J Am Osteopath Assoc 103: 417–421.
Etnyre BR, Abraham LD. 1986. Gains in range of ankle dorsiflexion using three population stretching techniques. Am J Phys Med 65: 189–196.
Fryer GA, Mudge JM, McLaughlin PA. 2002. The effect of talocrural joint manipulation on range of motion at the ankle. J Manipulative Physiol Ther 25: 384–390.
Gerber JP, Williams GH, Scoville CR, et al. 1998. Persistent disability associated with ankle sprains: a prospective examination of an athletic population. Foot Ankle Int 19: 653–660.
Green T, Refshauge K, Crosbie J, et al. 2001. A randomized controlled trial of a passive accessory joint mobilization on acute ankle inversion sprains. Phys Ther 81: 984–994.
Hale SA, Hertel J, Olmstead-Kramer LC. 2007. The effect of a 4-week comprehensive rehabilitation program on postural control and lower extremity function in individuals with chronic ankle instability. J Orthop Sports Phys Ther 37: 303–311.
Han KM, Ricard MD, Fellingham GW. 2009. Effects of a 4-week exercise program on balance using elastic tubing as a perturbation force for individuals with history of ankle sprains. J Orthop Sports Phys Ther 39: 246–255.
Hermans JJ, Beumer A, de Jong TA, et al. 2010. Anatomy of the distal tibiofibular syndesmosis in adults: a pictorial essay with a multimodality approach. J Anat 217: 633–645.
Hertel J, Braham RA, Hale SA. 2006. Simplifying the star excursion balance test: analyses of subjects with and without chronic ankle instability. J Orthop Sports Phys Ther 36: 131–137.
Hertel J, Denegar CR, Monroe MM, et al. 1999. Talocrural and subtalar joint instability after lateral ankle sprain. Med Sci Sports Exerc 31: 1501–1508.
Hertel J, Miller SJ, Denegar CR. 2009. Intra-tester and inter-tester reliability during the Star Excursion Balance Tests. J Sport Rehabil 9: 104–116.
Hess DM, Joyce CJ, Arnold BL, et al. 2001. Effect of a 4-week agility training program on postural sway in the functionally unstable ankle. J Sport Rehabil 10: 24–35.
Hintermann B, Boss A, Shäfer D. 2002. Arthroscopic findings in patients with chronic ankle instability. Am J Sports Med 30: 402–409.
Hirai D, Docherty CL, Schrader J. 2009. Severity of functional and mechanical ankle instability in an active population. Foot Ankle Int 30: 1071–1077.
Hockenbury RT, Sammarco GJ. 2001. Evaluation and treatment of ankle sprains – clinical recommendations for a positive outcome. Phys Sports Med 24: 57–64.
Holme E, Magnusson SP, Becher K, et al. 1999. The effect of supervised rehabilitation on strength, postural sway, position sense and re-injury risk after acute ankle ligament sprain. Scand J Med Sci Sports 9: 104–109.
Hosea TM, Carey CC, Harrer MF. 2000. Epidemiology of ankle injuries in athletes who participate in basketball. Clin Orthop 372: 45–49.
Hubbard TJ, Kaminski TW, Van der Griend RA, et al. 2004. Quantitative assessment of mechanical laxity in the functionally unstable ankle. Med Sci Sports Exer 36: 760–766.
Hupperets MDW, Verhagen EALM, van Mechelen W. 2009. Effects of unsupervised home based proprioceptive training on reoccurrence of ankle sprain: randomized clinical trial. BMJ 339: 2684.
Jennings J, Davies GJ. 2005. Treatment of cuboid syndrome secondary to lateral ankle sprains: a case series. J Orthop Sports Phys Ther 35: 409–415.
Kapanji IA. 1970. Physiology of the joints. Vol II. The lower limb. London: Churchill Livingstone.
Kemler E, van de Port I, Backx F, et al. 2011. A systematic review on the treatment of acute ankle sprain: brace versus other functional treatment types. Sports Med 41: 185–197.
Kerkhoffs GM, Rowe BH, Assendelft WJ, et al. 2001. Immobilization for acute ankle sprain: a systematic review. Arch Orthop Trauma Surg 121: 462–471.
Konradsen L, Olesen S, Hansen HM. 1998. Ankle sensorimotor control and eversion strength after acute ankle inversion injuries. Am J Sports Med 26: 72–78.
Lentell G, Bass B, Lopez D, et al. 1995. The contributions of proprioceptive deficits, muscle function, and anatomic laxity to functional instability of the ankle joint. J Orthop Sports Phys Ther 21: 206–215.
Lin CF, Gross ML, Weinhold P. 2006. Ankle syndesmosis injuries: anatomy, biomechanics, mechanism of injury, and clinical guidelines for diagnosis and intervention. J Orthop Sports Phys Ther 36: 372–384.
Maitland GD. 2005. Peripheral manipulation, 4th edn. Oxford: Butterworth-Heinemann.
Martin RL, McPoil TG. 2005. Reliability of ankle goniometric measurements: a literature review. J Am Podiatr Med Assoc 95: 564–572.
Martin RL, Davenport TE, Paulseth S, et al. 2013. Ankle stability and movement coordination impairments: ankle ligament sprains. J Orthop Sports Phys Ther 43: A1–40.
Mawdsley RH, Hoy DK, Erwin PM. 2000. Criterion-related validity of the figure-of-eight method of measuring ankle edema. J Orthop Sports Phys Ther 30: 149–153
McKay GD, Goldie PA, Payne WR, et al. 2001. Ankle injuries in basketball: injury rate and risk factors. Br J Sports Med 35: 103–108.
Menadue C, Raymond J, Kilbreath SL, et al. 2006. Reliability of two goniometric methods of measuring active inversion and eversion range of motion at the ankle. BMC Musculoskelet Disord 7: 60.
Moore K. 1985. Clinically oriented anatomy. Baltimore: Williams & Wilkins.
Mulligan BR. 1995. Manual therapy 'nags', 'snags', 'mwms', etc. Wellington, NZ: Plain View Services.
Nield S, Davis K, Latimer J, et al. 1993. The effect of manipulation on range of movement at the ankle joint. Scand J Rehabil Med 25: 161–166.
O'Driscoll J, Delahunt E. 2011. Neuromuscular training to enhance sensorimotor and functional deficits in subjects with chronic ankle instability: a systematic review and best evidence synthesis. Sports Med Arthrosc Rehabil Ther Technol 3: 3–19
O'Loughlin PF, Murawski CD, Egan C, et al. 2009. Ankle instability in sports. Phys Sport Med 37: 93–103.
Oh CS, Won HS, Hur MS. 2006. Anatomic variations and MRI of the intermalleolar ligament. Am J Roentgenol 186: 943–947.
Osborne MDCL, Laskowski ER, Smith J, et al. 2001. The effect of ankle disk training on muscle reaction time in subjects with a history of ankle sprain. Am J Sports Med 29: 627–632.
Pellow JE, Brantingham JW. 2001. The efficacy of adjusting the ankle in the treatment of subacute and chronic grade I and grade II ankle inversion sprains. J Manipulative Physiol Ther 24: 17–24.
Plisky PJ, Rauh MJ, Kaminski TW, et al. 2006. Star Excursion Balance Test as a predictor of lower extremity injury in high school basketball players. J Orthop Sports Phys Ther 36: 911–919.
Reid DC. 1992. Sports injury assessment and rehabilitation. London: Churchill Livingstone.
Rohner-Spengler M, Mannion AF, Babst R. 2007. Reliability and minimal detectable change for the figure-of-eight-20 method of measurement of ankle edema. J Orthop Sports Phys Ther 37: 199–205.
Rosenberg ZS, Cheung YY, Beltran J. 1995. Posterior intermalleolar ligament of the ankle: normal anatomy and MR imaging features. Am J Roentgenol 165: 387–390.
Surve I, Schwellnus MP, Noakes T, et al. 1994. A fivefold reduction in the incidence of recurrent ankle sprains in soccer players using the sport-stirrup orthosis. Am J Sports Med 22: 601–606.
Tohyama H, Yasuda K, Ohkoshi Y, et al. 2003. Anterior drawer test for acute anterior talofibular ligament injuries of the ankle: how much load should be applied during the test? Am J Sports Med 31: 226–232.
Tropp ACH, Gillquist J. 1985. Prevention of ankle sprains. Am J Sports Med 13: 259–261.

Uh BS, Beynnon BD, Helie BV, et al. 2000. The benefit of a single-leg strength training program for the muscles around the untrained ankle: a prospective, randomized, controlled study. Am J Sports Med 28: 568–573.

Van de Perre S, Vanhoenacker FM, De Vuyst D. 2004. Imaging anatomy of the ankle. JBR-BTR 87: 310–314.

van der Wees PJ, Lenssen AF, Hendricks EJ, et al. 2006. Effectiveness of exercise therapy and manual mobilization in ankle sprain and functional instability: a systematic review. Aust J Physiother 52: 27–37.

van Dijk CN, Lim LS, Bossuyt PM, et al. 1996. Physical examination is sufficient for the diagnosis of sprained ankle. J Bone Joint Surg Br 78: 958–962.

Van Rijn RM, van Os AG, Bernsen RM, et al. 2008. What is the clinical course of acute ankle sprains? A systematic literature review. Am J Med 121: 324–331.

Vincenzino B, Branjerdporn M, Teys P, et al. 2006. Initial changes in posterior talar glide and dorsiflexion of the ankle after mobilization with movement in individuals with recurrent ankle sprain. J Orthop Sports Phys Ther 36: 464–471.

Waterman BR, Owens B, Davey D, et al. 2010. The epidemiology of ankle sprains in the United States. J Bone Joint Surg Am 92: 2279–2284.

Wester JU, Jespersen SM, Nielsen KD, et al. 1996. Wobble board training after partial sprains of the lateral ligaments of the ankle: a prospective randomized study. J Orthop Sports Phys Ther 23: 332–336.

Whitman JM, Childs JD, Walker V. 2005. The use of manipulation in a patient with an ankle sprain injury not responding to conventional management: a case report. Man Ther 10: 224–231.

Whitman JM, Cleland JA, Mintken P, et al. 2009. Predicting short-term response to thrust and non-thrust manipulation and exercise in patients post inversion ankle sprain. J Orthop Sports Phys Ther 39: 188–200.

Wilson RW, Gansneder BM. 2000. Measures of functional limitation as predictors of disablement in athletes with acute ankle sprains. J Orthop Sports Phys Ther 30: 528–535.

Yeung MS, Chan KM, So CH, et al. 1994. An epidemiological survey on ankle sprains. Br J Sports Med 28: 112–116.

55 Chapter

Plantar Heel Pain

Matthew P. Cotchett

CHAPTER CONTENTS

Introduction 616
Prevalence 616
Origin of plantar heel pain 616
Anatomical considerations 616
Pathology of plantar heel pain 616
Diagnosis 617
Symptoms 617
Signs 617
Imaging 617
Risk factors 618
Prognosis 618
Management strategies for plantar heel pain 618
Non-invasive manual therapy for plantar heel pain 618
Invasive manual therapy for plantar heel pain – dry needling 620
Conclusion and recommendations 621

Introduction

Prevalence

Plantar heel pain is a common source of pain and disability, with an estimated prevalence of 3.6–7.5% in the general population (Dunn et al 2004; Menz et al 2006; Hill et al 2008). In the United States, an estimated 1 million patient visits to office-based physicians and hospital outpatient departments per year were for plantar heel pain (Riddle & Schappert 2004). Plantar heel pain predominantly affects middle-aged as well as older adults (Dunn et al 2004), and is estimated to contribute 8.0% of all running-related injuries (Taunton et al 2002). The disorder appears to be more common in females (Davis et al 1994; Rano et al 2001; Landorf et al 2006; Radford et al 2006, 2007; Cleland et al 2009, Kalaci et al 2009; Labovitz et al 2011; Renan-Ordine et al 2011; McMillan et al 2012; Saban et al 2014), although there are few high-quality epidemiological studies available. The high prevalence of plantar heel pain is associated with a large economic burden to the community. Tong & Furia (2010) projected that in 2007 the annual economic cost of plantar heel pain was between $US192 and $US376 million to third party payers.

Origin of plantar heel pain

Pain beneath the heel can be neurological, vascular, arthritic, neoplastic or traumatic in origin (Thomas et al 2010). However, it is generally accepted that a mechanical overload of the plantar fascia is the most common source of pain in this region. An overload of the plantar fascia, and associated changes to its connective tissue structure, is most often referred to as **plantar fasciitis** (McPoil et al 2008). The term **plantar heel pain** is also used frequently in the literature, as it highlights the involvement of other structures and tissues (e.g. muscle and bone), which might be associated with an overload of the plantar fascia in people with plantar fasciitis.

Anatomical considerations

The plantar heel region comprises the calcaneus, muscle and tendons (spread over two layers) and three neurovascular bundles. Overlying and intertwined within the plantar heel intrinsic muscles is a thickened band of connective tissue called the plantar fascia (Fig. 55.1). The central band of the plantar fascia attaches to the medial tubercle of the plantar surface of the calcaneus and is adjacent to other structures that attach to this region, including the muscles and tendons of abductor hallucis, flexor digitorum brevis and quadratus plantae (Fig. 55.2). Evidence from comparative cross-sectional studies reports that the thickness of the plantar fascia ranges from 2.4 mm to 3.6 mm (Crofts et al 2014).

Pathology of Plantar Heel Pain

Pathological changes within the plantar fascia are common in people with plantar heel pain. Histological examination of specimens obtained from the proximal attachment of the plantar fascia in people with plantar heel pain shows collagen necrosis, increased mucoid ground substance, angiofibroblastic hyperplasia, chondroid metaplasia and matrix calcification (Wearing et al 2006). Such findings suggest a loss of organized tissue structure, which is consistent with a degenerative fasciosis (Lemont et al 2003), although some studies have reported evidence of local non-specific inflammatory changes.

Pathological changes within the plantar intrinsic musculature have also been reported in people with plantar heel pain.

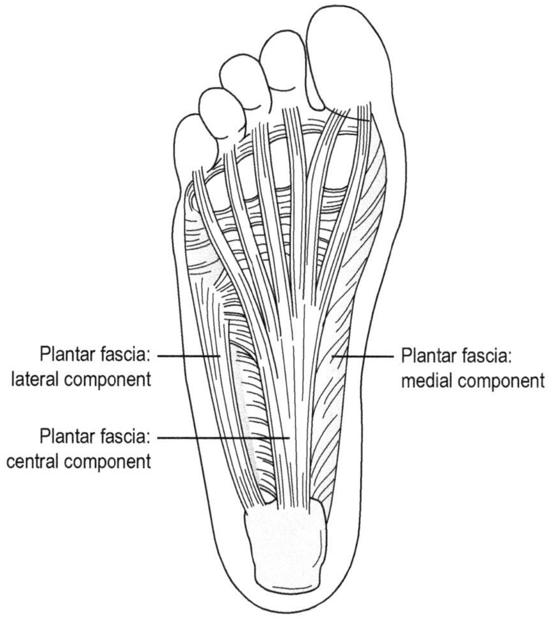

Figure 55.1 Anatomical diagram highlighting the various bands of the plantar fascia.

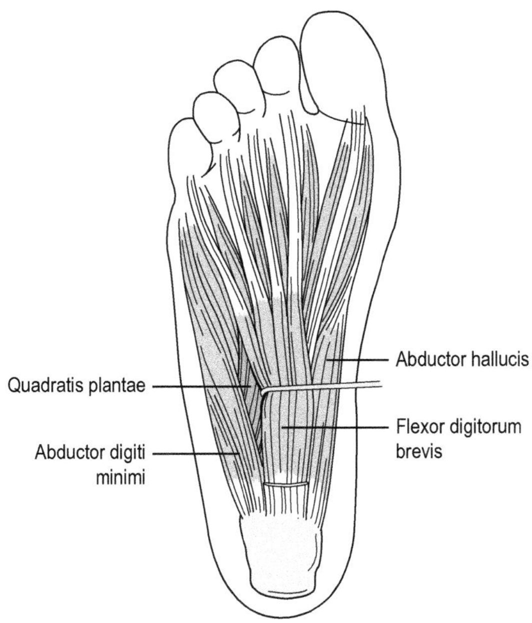

Figure 55.2 Anatomical diagram highlighting the intrinsic muscles within layers one and two of the heel.

Cross-sectional studies have revealed atrophy of the abductor digiti minimi (Chundru et al 2008) and atrophy of the forefoot intrinsic muscles (Chang et al 2012), findings that have been hypothesized to exacerbate the load placed on a swollen or degenerative plantar fascia (Chang et al 2012).

Diagnosis

A diagnosis of plantar heel pain is usually made on the basis of a thorough history and physical examination. This section will highlight the key symptoms and signs of plantar heel pain. The reader is also referred to an excellent review on the differential diagnosis of pain beneath the heel (Buchbinder 2004).

Symptoms

Patients with plantar heel pain typically present with an insidious onset of pain in the medial plantar heel region. Symptoms are usually unilateral, but they can present bilaterally in approximately 40% of cases (Lapidus & Guidotti 1965; Landorf et al 2006; Radford et al 2006, 2007; Labovitz et al 2011). Bilateral symptoms should raise suspicion of a spondyloarthropathy (e.g. Reiter's syndrome, psoriatic arthropathy, ankylosing spondylitis) (Buchbinder 2004). The type of pain can vary from symptoms that are initially sharp and localized to pain that is deep, dull and poorly localized. Symptoms are worse upon weight-bearing after periods of rest and often improve with initial activity, although it is also common for symptoms to be worse at the end of the day, particularly following prolonged periods of standing and walking. Nocturnal symptoms are uncommon, and should alert the clinician to other conditions including cancer, infection and neuropathic pain (Buchbinder 2004). The onset of plantar heel pain often coincides with a change in the type and level of activity, or a change in footwear (McPoil et al 2008).

Signs

The physical examination should be conducted with the patient both non-weight-bearing and weight-bearing and include active and passive movements, muscle tests, nerve tests, palpation and other special tests, for example the tarsal tunnel syndrome test, the windlass test, medial and lateral squeeze test of the calcaneus, and an assessment of foot posture using a reliable and valid measure such as the Foot Posture Index (Redmond et al 2006). The key diagnostic feature of plantar heel pain is localized tenderness at the proximal insertion of the plantar fascia (McPoil et al 2008).

Imaging

Diagnostic imaging for plantar heel pain is generally used only when the assessment is inconclusive. Diagnostic musculoskeletal ultrasound (MSKUS) is the modality of choice for the assessment of soft tissue structures beneath the heel, although magnetic resonance imaging (MRI) and plain radiographs can be used when there is a need to rule out other possible causes of heel pain (McPoil et al 2008). MSKUS often reveals fusiform swelling of the plantar fascia that is greater than 4 mm in thickness (McMillan et al 2009) with surrounding local or diffuse areas of hypoechogenicity. MRI often shows increased intrafascial oedema on T1- and T2-weighted images, and perifascial oedema at the insertion of the plantar fascia, which is more common in patients with longstanding symptoms (Chimutengwende-Gordon et al 2010). Finally, it is common to identify subcalcaneal spurs on plain radiographs in patients with plantar heel pain (McMillan et al 2009). The presence of a spur is of no diagnostic value, although it might alert the clinician to the possibility of an underlying spondyloarthropathy if the spur is ill defined (Buchbinder 2004).

Risk Factors

Despite the prevalence of plantar heel pain, the aetiology remains uncertain. The highest level of evidence, which has evaluated physical and functional associates of plantar heel pain, is derived from a systematic review by Irving et al (2006) that found increased body weight in a non-athletic population to have a strong association with plantar heel pain. Weak evidence was also found for an association between plantar heel pain and increased body mass index in an athletic population, as well as increased age, decreased ankle dorsiflexion, decreased first metatarsophalangeal joint dorsiflexion and prolonged standing. The association between plantar heel pain and foot posture, foot motion and foot function was inconclusive, however (Irving et al 2006).

Prognosis

Plantar heel pain is considered a self-limiting condition (Buchbinder 2004). This statement is supported by the fact that symptoms normally resolve within 12 months regardless of the intervention implemented (Lapidus & Guidotti 1965; Davis et al 1994; Wolgin et al 1994; Martin et al 1998; Crawford & Thomson 2003). An increased risk of persistent pain has been reported in those patients that are obese, and have bilateral symptoms (Wolgin et al 1994).

Management Strategies for Plantar Heel Pain

Numerous interventions are used to treat plantar heel pain; however, two systematic reviews have concluded that there are few interventions that are supported by good evidence (Crawford & Thomson 2003; Landorf & Menz 2008). An evidenced-based management algorithm provided by the American College of Foot and Ankle Surgeons (ACFAS) recommends a multifaceted, tiered treatment approach (Thomas et al 2010). Initial options include padding and strapping, stretching exercises, over-the-counter foot orthoses, shoe recommendations, and oral and / or injectable anti-inflammatories. Second-tier options for patients with minimal improvement at 6 weeks include night splints, custom orthoses, cast or boot immobilization, or a programme of manual therapy for a further 4–6 weeks. Surgery is recommended as a last resort and usually only after failure of at least 6 months of conservative therapy (Thomas et al 2010).

The purpose of the following section is to review the evidence for the effectiveness of manual therapy for plantar heel pain under the categories of non-invasive manual therapy and invasive manual therapy (i.e. dry needling). The focus will be on studies that have used randomized controlled trial methodology, which is considered the gold standard for a clinical trial to evaluate the effectiveness of an intervention (Portney & Watkins 2009).

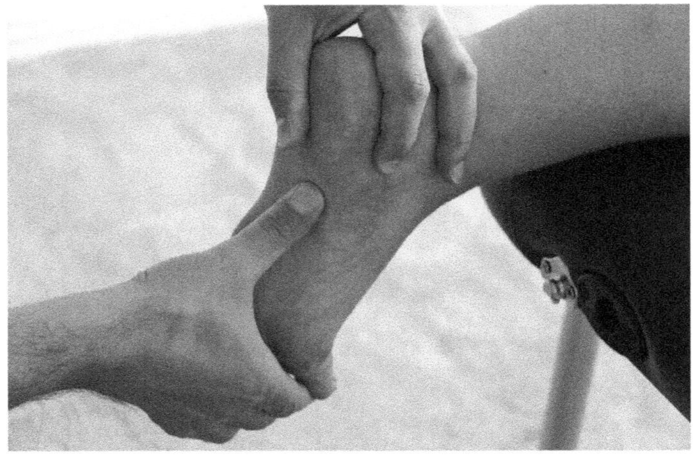

Figure 55.3 Soft tissue mobilization of the plantar fascia. The patient is prone with the knee extended. With the ankle and first metatarsophalangeal joints in dorsiflexion, the clinician applies deep pressure along the length of the plantar fascia. The technique is performed for approximately 3 minutes, and the depth of mobilization is dependent on the patient's tolerance.

Non-invasive manual therapy for plantar heel pain

Three randomized controlled trials have evaluated the effectiveness of manual therapy for plantar heel pain, although each trial differed in regards to the type of manual therapy implemented, comparator intervention, outcome measures, follow-up and frequency of treatment. As such, each trial will be discussed separately below, and all are summarized in Table 55.1.

Cleland et al (2009) evaluated the effectiveness of manual therapy and exercise in comparison to electrophysical agents and exercise. A sample size of 60 participants was randomly allocated to two equal groups: one group receiving electrophysical agents (iontophoresis and dexamethasone) and the other group receiving manual therapy (i.e. 5 minutes of aggressive soft tissue mobilization of the Achilles and insertion of the plantar fascia (Fig. 55.3), and rearfoot eversion mobilization). In addition, participants in the manual therapy group received joint mobilization and / or manipulation of the foot and ankle, depending on the presentation of that patient. Such motions included subtalar joint lateral glides, talocrural anterior–posterior glides, rearfoot distraction manipulation, cuboid manipulation, intertarsal mobilization and distal tibiofibular mobilization. Manual therapy techniques were also applied to the hip and knee at the discretion of the clinician. The manual therapy group was also advised to perform self-mobilization of the subtalar joint, and passive manual soft tissue mobilization of the plantar fascia at home. Both groups undertook a programme of calf and plantar fascia stretching. Participants in both groups received six treatments over a 4-week period. Changes in physical function were assessed at baseline, at 4 weeks and at 6 months, using the Lower Extremity Function Scale (LEFS), while foot pain was assessed using the Numeric Pain Rating Scale (NPRS). At 4 weeks and 6 months, significant effects favoured the group receiving manual therapy. For lower extremity function, the between-group difference was 13.5 points (95% CI 6.3–20.8) at 4 weeks and 9.9 points (95% CI 1.2–18.6) at

Table 55.1 **Evidence for the effectiveness of non-invasive manual therapy for plantar heel pain**

Author(s)	Primary intervention(s)	Comparator intervention(s)	Major results
Renan-Ordine et al (2011)	Trigger point pressure release technique of the gastrocnemius (usually 3 repetitions by 90 seconds) – 4 days a week for 4 weeks Three longitudinal strokes (distal to proximal) over the gastrocnemius – 4 days a week for 4 weeks Self-stretching of the calf and plantar fascia (20-second holds followed by 20 seconds rest for a total of 3 minutes, 2× / day)	Self-stretching of the calf and plantar fascia (20-second holds followed by 20 seconds rest for a total of 3 minutes, 2× a day)	At 4 weeks, significant reductions in pain favoured the group receiving trigger point pressure release (between-group difference 7.8 points, 95% CI 2.5–13.3, $p<0.05$) At 4 weeks, significant improvements in physical function favoured the group receiving trigger point release (between-group difference 9.3, 95% CI 3.9–14.8, $p<0.05$)
Saban et al (2014)	10 minutes of deep, forceful massage to painful incompliant areas of the calf (1–2 times a week for 6 weeks – total of 8 treatments) Passive straight leg raise exercise (20 seconds by 5 repetitions, 3× a day) Self-stretching of the calf (20 seconds by 5 repetitions, 3× a day)	Self-stretching of the calf (20 seconds by 5 repetitions, 3× a day) Ultrasound (1 MHz; 1.0 W/cm^2, continuous dose) – (1–2 times a week for 6 weeks for a total of 8 treatments)	At 6 weeks, physical function improved significantly more in the group receiving deep massage therapy (between-group difference 9, 95% CI 0.7–16, $p=0.034$). No significant differences *between* groups for pain
Cleland et al (2009)	5 minutes of aggressive soft tissue mobilization of the Achilles and insertion of the plantar fascia, and rearfoot eversion mobilization (6 treatments over 4 weeks) Impairments based manual therapy approach (subtalar joint lateral glides, talocrural anterior/posterior glides, rearfoot distraction manipulation, cuboid manipulation, intertarsal mobilization, distal tibiofibular mobilization, hip, knee, patellofemoral and fibula–tibia joint mobilization) – (6 treatments over 4 weeks) Self-mobilization of the plantar fascia and subtalar joint into eversion Self-stretching of the calf and plantar fascia	Ultrasound followed by: electrophysical agents (iontophoresis and dexamethasone) and ice application post treatment (6 treatments over 4 weeks) Intrinsic foot strengthening Self-stretching of the calf and plantar fascia	At 4 weeks, physical function was significantly improved in favour of the group receiving manual therapy (between-group difference 13.5 points, 95% CI 6.3–20.8, $p=0.001$). Foot pain was significantly more reduced in the manual therapy group (between-group difference −1.5, 95% CI −0.4 to −2.5, $p=0.008$). At 6 months, physical function was significantly more reduced in the manual therapy group (between-group difference 9.9, 95% CI 1.2–18.6), $p=0.027$). No significant between-group difference in pain was reported at 6 months

6 months. At both time points, the between-group difference was greater than the minimal important difference of 9 points, which suggests that the results are of clinical importance. For pain, the group receiving manual therapy had significantly larger improvements in pain at 4 weeks with a between-group difference of −1.5 points (95% CI −0.4 to −2.5). There were no significant findings for pain at 6 months. Although these findings are promising for the use of manual therapy for plantar heel pain, it is not possible to ascertain which component(s) of this multimodal treatment programme were responsible for the improvement in pain and function (Cleland et al 2009).

Renan-Ordine et al (2011) conducted a randomized controlled trial to evaluate the effectiveness of trigger point therapy for plantar heel pain. Sixty participants were randomly allocated to a group that received either self-stretching of the plantar fascia and calf muscles (soleus and gastrocnemius specific stretches) or to one that received the same stretching programme in conjunction with manual therapy (trigger point pressure release of the gastrocnemius muscle and a neuromuscular technique involving longitudinal strokes directed over the calf musculature). The exact mechanism for the efficacy of trigger point manual therapy is uncertain, although trigger points in the soleus muscle have been proposed as a source of pain in people with plantar heel pain (Travell & Simons 1992). In this regard, trigger point manual therapy might deactivate trigger points by normalizing the length of contracted sarcomeres in the affected region. All participants in the trial were treated four times a week for 4 weeks. The primary outcome measures included the bodily pain and physical function domains of the Short-Form 36 Health Survey (SF-36) and were recorded at baseline and at 4 weeks. Both groups showed decreased pain at 4 weeks; however, there were significant between-group effects that favoured the group receiving trigger point manual therapy. For bodily pain, the between-group difference was 7.8 points (95% CI 2.5–13.3), whereas for physical function the between-group difference was 9.3 points (95% CI 3.9–14.8). For both outcomes, the results were also clinically significant. It is important to note, however, that the methodological quality of the trial might have been compromised as there was no evidence that the allocation sequence was concealed or whether the data was analysed on an intention-to-treat basis. In addition, the follow-up period was short (i.e. 4 weeks) so it is unclear whether the treatment is effective in the long term (Renan-Ordine et al 2011).

In a similar study that evaluated manual therapy for plantar heel pain, Saban et al (2014) investigated whether deep massage of the calf, neural mobilization exercises and a self-stretch programme was more effective than ultrasound therapy plus the same self-stretch programme. Sixty-nine participants with a diagnosis of plantar heel pain were randomly allocated to two groups; one group received 10 minutes of forceful, deep massage therapy to painful incompliant areas of the calf. The technique was applied using the clinician's thumb or elbow in a medial and lateral direction, across the fibres of the gastrocnemius and soleus. In addition, this group performed a passive straight leg raise exercise, with dorsiflexion of the ankle, using a long belt. Each exercise was held for 20 seconds, repeated five times, and conducted three times a day. In comparison, the stretching and ultrasound group received 3 minutes of ultrasound (frequency of 1 MHz and intensity of 1.0 W / cm^2, continuous dose). Both groups were asked to perform gastrocnemius and soleus specific stretches, at the same dosage as in the neural mobilization exercise group. All patients were treated twice a week, with a total of eight treatments over a 6-week period. Outcome measures included functional status, assessed using the Foot and Ankle Computerized Adaptive Test (CAT), as well as the change in foot pain determined with a 10 cm visual analogue scale. All outcome measures were assessed at baseline and at 6 weeks. At the 6-week follow-up, both groups reported a significant improvement in function and pain. However, significant effects favoured the group receiving deep massage therapy, with a between-group difference in function of 9 points (95% CI 0.7–16), a result that was also clinically important (Saban et al 2014). Changes in foot pain were less convincing, with between-group differences of −0.1 cm (95% CI −0.7, 1.7) that were not statistically significant. It is important to note, however, that a large percentage of patients dropped out in the study (28% in the deep massage therapy group, 24% in the stretching and ultrasound group), which might have yielded biased estimates of treatment effects (Bell et al 2013). In addition, the short-term outcomes preclude any assumption about the long-term effectiveness of deep massage therapy for plantar heel pain (Saban et al 2014).

In summary, the evidence for the effectiveness of manual therapy for plantar heel pain is limited to three studies with substantial methodological heterogeneity. Nevertheless, there is moderate evidence that: (i) a multimodal manual physical therapy approach that combines soft tissue mobilization of the plantar fascia, mobilization and / or manipulation of lower extremity joints and self-stretching is superior to a combination of iontophoresis, ultrasound and self-stretching exercises, (ii) myofascial trigger point manual therapy of the calf, in combination with self-stretching of the calf and plantar fascia, is superior to the sole application of self-stretching, and (iii) deep massage therapy of the calf in combination with neural mobilization exercises and calf stretching is superior to a combination of ultrasound and calf stretching. Future work is required to: (i) determine whether trigger point manual therapy, deep massage therapy or aggressive soft tissue mobilization of the plantar fascia is more effective than a sham treatment, (ii) determine the amount of force that needs to be applied during manual therapy of the calf or plantar fascia to obtain a clinically worthwhile improvement, (iii) determine which specific joint mobilization techniques, or combination of techniques, is most effective for plantar heel pain, and (iv) compare the effectiveness of non-invasive manual therapy techniques against other common treatments for plantar heel pain (e.g. foot orthoses).

Invasive manual therapy for plantar heel pain – dry needling

In addition to standard therapies, dry needling is increasingly used by practitioners to treat myofascial pain within all parts of the body, including the plantar heel region. Dry needling for plantar heel pain is most often guided by the trigger point model (Cotchett et al 2011), which involves the insertion of needles into a trigger point to reduce pain and improve function (Dommerholt & Fernández-de-las-Peñas 2013). The muscles most commonly dry needled, when guided by the trigger point model for plantar heel pain, include the soleus, gastrocnemius, quadratus plantae (Fig. 55.4), abductor hallucis and flexor digitorum brevis (Cotchett et al 2011), although it is also not uncommon for some practitioners to dry-needle the gluteus medius, gluteus minimus and erector spinae if their treatment is guided by the radiculopathy model (i.e. a model that suggests myofascial pain is secondary to a spinal nerve dysfunction) (Cotchett et al 2011).

Evidence to support the use of dry needling for plantar heel pain is limited to two case series and a single randomized controlled trial (Cotchett et al 2010). Tillu and Gupta (1998) found a significant improvement in 18 adults with plantar heel pain (68% improvement) after 2 weeks (1 treatment per week) of dry needling of the calf and heel regions, following a 4-week period of traditional Chinese acupuncture. Perez-Millan and Foster (2001) also demonstrated a

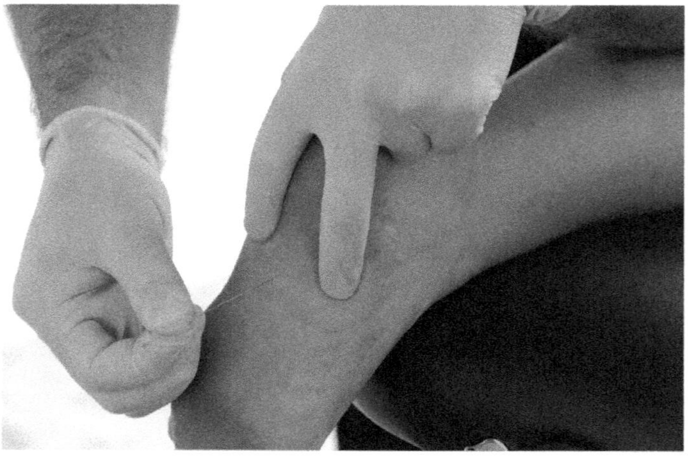

Figure 55.4 Trigger point dry needling of the quadratus plantae muscle.

significant reduction in pain (46% improvement) in 18 participants with plantar heel pain after a 6-week (1 treatment per week) programme of traditional Chinese acupuncture and dry needling of the heel and arch. However, these trials were case series of poor methodological quality, which lacked control groups. Therefore, the effects of the trigger point treatment are likely to have been overestimated owing to confounding and possible bias.

Based on the results of the systematic review, a trial to evaluate the effectiveness of trigger point dry needling for plantar heel pain was conducted (Cotchett et al 2014). The protocol, including needling details and treatment regimen, was formulated by general consensus (using the Delphi research method) using 30 experts worldwide who commonly use dry needling for plantar heel pain (Cotchett et al 2011a). Readers are referred to another text for more details on dry needling of these muscles (Dommerholt & Fernández-de-las-Peñas 2013).

The results of the randomized controlled trial revealed that, at the primary end-point (i.e. 6 weeks), significant effects favoured real dry needling over sham dry needling for pain (adjusted mean difference: visual analog first-step pain −14.4 mm, 95% CI −23.5 to −5.2, p=0.002; Foot Health Status Questionnaire foot pain 10.0 points, 95% CI 1.0 to 19.1, p=0.029), although the between-group difference was lower than the minimal important difference. The number needed to treat at 6 weeks was 4 (95% CI 2 to 12) (Cotchett et al 2014).

Conclusion and Recommendations

Plantar heel pain is one of the most common musculoskeletal disorders of the lower extremity and has a negative impact on health-related quality of life. The condition primarily effects middle-aged and older adults, and is a common source of pain in athletes. Plantar heel pain is not considered an inflammatory condition but rather a degenerative fasciosis. The disorder is diagnosed based on a thorough history and physical examination to help distinguish the condition from pain beneath the heel that might be arthritic, neurological, traumatic or the result of other systemic conditions. Key diagnostic features include pain in the plantar medial heel region that is worse upon weight-bearing after periods of rest, and pain upon palpation of the plantar fascia insertion.

Numerous interventions are used to manage plantar heel pain, although there are few interventions that are supported by good evidence. Despite the limited evidence, clinical practice guidelines, written by the ACFAS in 2011, recommend an initial low cost and minimal risk approach, which includes padding and strapping, calf and plantar fascia stretching, footwear advice, over-the-counter arch supports, activity modification and oral or injectable anti-inflammatories. Second-tier options include night splints, cast and boot immobilization, a repeat cortisone injection and a course of manual therapy. Surgery should be considered only after 6 months of failed conservative care.

The recommendation by the ACFAS to include manual therapy as a second-tier option may need to be revised based on recent evidence published after the ACFAS guidelines were written. This chapter has highlighted that there is moderate evidence to recommend the inclusion of non-invasive manual therapies for plantar heel pain in the short term, particularly as a first-tier option. Such manual therapy techniques include: (i) trigger point manual therapy and longitudinal massage strokes of the calf in combination with calf and plantar fascia stretching, (ii) deep massage to the calf in combination with neural mobilization exercises and calf stretching, and (iii) a multimodal manual therapy programme including aggressive soft tissue mobilization of the plantar fascia, joint mobilization within the foot and lower extremity, and calf stretching.

Whereas there is moderate evidence from three trials recommending non-invasive manual therapies for plantar heel pain, there is only moderate evidence from a single randomized controlled trial supporting the use of invasive manual therapies (i.e. dry needling) for plantar heel pain.

Despite the promising evidence for the use of manual therapies for plantar heel pain, more rigorous randomized controlled trials are needed. Future trials should evaluate these interventions when used alone, and in comparison with a sham intervention, including appropriate blinding procedures. Furthermore, it is recommended that future trials compare manual therapy techniques against other common treatments for plantar heel pain.

References

Bell ML, Kenward MG, Fairclough DL, et al. 2013. Differential dropout and bias in randomised controlled trials: when it matters and when it may not. BMJ 346: e8668.

Buchbinder R. 2004. Plantar fasciitis. N Engl J Med 350: 2159–2166.

Chang R, Kent-Braun JA, Hamill J. 2012. Use of MRI for volume estimation of tibialis posterior and plantar intrinsic foot muscles in healthy and chronic plantar fasciitis limbs. Clin Biomech 27: 500–505.

Chimutengwende-Gordon M, O'Donnell P, Singh D. 2010. Magnetic resonance imaging in plantar heel pain. Foot Ankle Int 31: 865–870.

Chundru U, Liebeskind A, Seidelmann F, et al. 2008. Plantar fasciitis and calcaneal spur formation are associated with abductor digiti minimi atrophy on MRI of the foot. Skel Radiol 37: 505–510.

Cleland JA, Abbott JH, Kidd MO, et al. 2009. Manual physical therapy and exercise versus electrophysical agents and exercise in the management of plantar heel pain: a multicenter randomized clinical trial. J Orthop Sports Phys Ther 39: 573–585.

Cotchett MP, Landorf KB, Munteanu SE, et al. 2010. Effectiveness of dry needling and injections of myofascial trigger points associated with plantar heel pain: a systematic review. J Foot Ankle Res 3: 18.

Cotchett MP, Landorf KB, Munteanu SE, et al. 2011. Consensus for dry needling for plantar heel pain (plantar fasciitis): a modified Delphi study. Acupunct Med 29: 193–202.

Cotchett MP, Munteanu SE, Landorf KB. 2014. Effectiveness of trigger point dry needling for plantar heel pain: a randomized controlled trial. Phys Ther 94(8): 1083–1094. doi: 10.2522/ptj.20130255.

Crawford F, Thomson CE. 2003. Interventions for treating plantar heel pain. Cochrane Database Syst Rev 3: CD000416.

Crofts G, Angin S, Mickle KJ, et al. 2014. Reliability of ultrasound for measurement of selected foot structures. Gait Posture 39: 35–39.

Davis PF, Severud E, Baxter DE. 1994. Painful heel syndrome: results of non-operative treatment. Foot Ankle Int 15: 531–535.

Dommerholt J, Fernández-de-las-Peñas C. 2013. Trigger point dry needling: an evidence and clinical- based approach. London: Churchill Livingstone Elsevier.

Dunn JE, Link CL, Felson DT, et al. 2004. Prevalence of foot and ankle conditions in a multiethnic community sample of older adults. Am J Epidemiol 159: 491–498.

Hill CL, Gill T, Menz HB, et al. 2008. Prevalence and correlates of foot pain in a population-based study: the North West Adelaide health study. J Foot Ankle Res 1: 2.

Irving DB, Cook JL, Menz HB. 2006. Factors associated with chronic plantar heel pain: a systematic review. J Sci Med Sport 9: 11–22.

Kalaci A, Çakici H, Hapa O, et al. 2009. Treatment of plantar fasciitis using four different local injection modalities: a randomized prospective clinical trial. J Am Podiatr Med Assoc 99: 108–113.

Labovitz JM, Yu J, Kim C. 2011. The role of hamstring tightness in plantar fasciitis. Foot Ankle Spec 4: 141–144.
Landorf KB, Menz HB. 2008. Plantar heel pain and fasciitis. Clin Evid 2: 1–16.
Landorf KB, Keenan AM, Herbert RD. 2006. Effectiveness of foot orthoses to treat plantar fasciitis. Arch Intern Med 166: 1305–1310.
Lapidus PW, Guidotti FP. 1965. Painful heel: report of 323 patients with 364 painful heels. Clin Orthop Relat Res 39: 178–186.
Lemont L, Ammirati KM, Usen N. 2003. Plantar fasciitis: a degenerative process (fasciosis) without inflammation. J Am Podiatr Med Assoc 93: 234–237.
Martin RL, Irrgang JJ, Conti SF. 1998. Outcome study of subjects with insertional plantar fasciitis. Foot Ankle Int 19: 803–811.
McMillan AM, Landorf KB, Barrett JT, et al. 2009. Diagnostic imaging for chronic plantar heel pain: a systematic review and meta-analysis. J Foot Ankle Res 2: 32.
McMillan AM, Landorf KB, Gilheany MF, et al. 2012. Ultrasound guided corticosteroid injection for plantar fasciitis: randomised controlled trial. BMJ 344: 3260.
McPoil TG, Martin RL, Cornwall MW, et al. 2008. Heel pain–plantar fasciitis: clinical practice guidelines linked to the international classification of function, disability, and health from the orthopaedic section of the American Physical Therapy Association. J Orthop Sports Phys Ther 38: A1–A18.
Menz HB, Tiedemann A, Kwan MMS, et al. 2006. Foot pain in community-dwelling older people: an evaluation of the Manchester Foot Pain and Disability Index. Rheumatol 45: 863–867.
Perez-Millan R, Foster L. 2001. Low frequency electroacupuncture in the management of refractory plantar fasciitis. Med Acupunct 13: 1–6.
Portney LG, Watkins MP. 2009. Foundations of clinical research. Applications to practice, 3rd edn. New Jersey: Julie Levin Alexander.
Radford JA, Landorf KB, Buchbinder R, et al. 2006. Effectiveness of low-dye taping for the short-term treatment of plantar heel pain: a randomised trial. BMC Musculoskelet Disord 7: 64.
Radford JA, Landorf KB, Buchbinder R, et al. 2007. Effectiveness of calf muscle stretching for the short term treatment of plantar heel pain: a randomised trial. BMC Musculoskelet Disord 8: 36.
Rano JA, Fallat LM, Savoy-Moore RT. 2001. Correlation of heel pain with body mass index and other characteristics of heel pain. J Foot Ankle Surg 40: 351–356.
Redmond AC, Crosbie J, Ouvrier RA. 2006. Development and validation of a novel rating system for scoring standing foot posture: the Foot Posture Index. Clin Biomech 21: 89–98.
Renan-Ordine R, Alburquerque-Sendín F, de Souza DP, et al. 2011. Effectiveness of myofascial trigger point manual therapy combined with a self-stretching protocol for the management of plantar heel pain: a randomized controlled trial. J Orthop Sports Phys Ther 41: 43–50.
Riddle DL, Schappert SM. 2004. Volume of ambulatory care visits and patterns of care for patients diagnosed with plantar fasciitis: a national study of medical doctors. Foot Ankle Int 25: 303–310.
Saban B, Deutscher D, Ziv T. 2014. Deep massage to posterior calf muscles in combination with neural mobilization exercises as a treatment for heel pain: a pilot randomized clinical trial. Man Ther 19(2): 102–108. doi: 10.1016/j.math.2013.08.001.
Taunton JE, Ryan MB, Clement DB, et al. 2002. A retrospective case–control analysis of 2002 running injuries. Br J Sports Med 36: 95–101.
Thomas JL, Christensen JC, Kravitz SR, et al. 2010. The diagnosis and treatment of heel pain: a clinical practice guideline-revision 2010. J Foot Ankle Surg 49: S1–S19.
Tillu A, Gupta S. 1998. Effect of acupuncture treatment on heel pain due to plantar fasciitis. Acupunct Med 16: 66–68.
Tong KB, Furia J. 2010. Economic burden of plantar fasciitis treatment in the United States. Am J Orthop 39: 227–231.
Travell JG, Simons DG. 1992. Myofascial pain and dysfunction. The trigger point manual. The lower extremities. Vol 2. Baltimore: Williams & Wilkins.
Wearing SC, Smeathers JE, Urry SR, et al. 2006. The pathomechanics of plantar fasciitis. Sports Med 36: 585–611.
Wolgin M, Cook C, Graham C, et al. 1994. Conservative treatment of plantar heel pain: long-term follow-up. Foot Ankle Int 15: 97–102.

Chapter 56

Postoperative Management of Foot and Ankle Disorders

Stephanie Albin, Mark W. Cornwall, Thomas G. McPoil

CHAPTER CONTENTS

Introduction	623
Total ankle arthroplasty	623
Introduction	623
Ankle arthrodesis versus arthroplasty	624
Surgical procedures	624
Postoperative rehabilitation treatment	625
Efficacy of rehabilitation treatment	627
Achilles tendon ruptures	628
Introduction	628
Epidemiology	629
Risk factors	629
Diagnosis	629
Surgical versus non-surgical treatment	630
Early range of motion versus immobilization	631
Early weight-bearing versus late weight-bearing	632
Post-surgical rehabilitation treatment	632
Conclusion	635

Introduction

The effectiveness of manual therapy has been documented in patients with acute and chronic foot and ankle conditions (Vicenzino et al 2006; Cleland et al 2009, 2013; Whitman et al 2009; Hensley & Kavchak 2012). However, literature assessing the effectiveness after surgical procedures is somewhat rare, and almost non-existent in the foot and ankle. This chapter focuses on manual therapy and rehabilitation after surgical repair of the Achilles tendon and after total ankle arthroplasty. As literature is sparse in these areas, much of the treatment recommendations are based on clinical experience and principles of best practice. A proper description procedure and clinical outcomes have been provided for both surgical procedures so as to provide insight into areas where we could potentially improve treatment and the potential for manual therapy to serve as an adjunct in the management of these patient populations.

Total Ankle Arthroplasty

Introduction

Total ankle arthroplasty began increasing in popularity in the 1970s with approximately 23 different procedures being developed during the 1970s and 1980s (Gittins & Mann 2002; Hintermann & Valderrabano 2003; Claridge & Sagherian 2009). By the mid 1980s, arthroplasty for end-stage arthritis of the ankle was nearly abandoned owing to high failure rates of these early-prosthetic-generation designs. These first-generation ankle prostheses did not fully take into account the biomechanics of the ankle joint (Gittins & Mann 2002). Poor outcomes of these early prosthetic designs led some authors to question whether it was even possible to replicate the ankle joint (Hintermann & Valderrabano 2003). However, due to the high success rates of total hip and total knee replacements along with new prosthetic designs, ankle arthroplasty is again regaining popularity. These new prostheses currently being developed do account for the complexity of ankle biomechanics and assist with preserving more bone stock than did the previous generations of replacements (Gittins & Mann 2002).

As with other joint replacement surgeries, osteoarthritis (OA) is the main reason for joint replacement. OA of the ankle joint leads to joint stiffness, pain, decreases in physical and sporting activities, and limitations in activities of daily living, and often restricts work-related activities (Claridge & Sagherian 2009; Horisberger et al 2009). During normal daily activities, extreme compressive loads are placed on the talocrural joint. For example, during normal gait, compressive forces through the talocrural joint reach 5.5 times the body weight (Hintermann & Valderrabano 2003). Surprisingly though, less than 1% of the general population suffers from ankle OA (Horisberger et al 2009). Primary OA occurs predominately in the hip and knee, and only rarely in the ankle joint (Hintermann & Valderrabano 2003). About 65–80% of ankle OA occurs secondary to a traumatic event (Hintermann & Valderrabano 2003; Horisberger et al 2009; Hubbard et al 2009). In comparison, only about 9.8% of knee OA and 1.6% of hip OA occur after a traumatic event (Horisberger et al

2009). Patients with ankle OA are often younger than those with hip and/or knee OA (Hintermann & Valderrabano 2003; Horisberger et al 2009).

The exact mechanism of the development of post-traumatic ankle OA is unclear. Possible causes include severity or type of fracture, the amount of cartilage damage related to the injury, age, obesity and joint congruency after reduction (Horisberger et al 2009). Fracture type has been related to the onset of post-traumatic OA, with malleolar fractures being the most common fracture type causing ankle OA, followed by pilon fractures and then talus fractures (Horisberger et al 2009). Malleolar fractures occur much more frequently than pilon fractures, which account for less than 1% of all lower extremity fractures, and may lead to the increased rate of OA (Horisberger et al 2009).

The average latency time between fractures and the development of end-stage ankle OA has been reported to be, on average, between 10 and 20 years (Horisberger et al 2009). Coetzee (2010) found 39% of patients with pilon fractures developed ankle arthritis, demonstrated radiographically, within 2–3 years of the time of injury. Another study reported that the incidence rate of post-traumatic OA after talar fractures ranged from 47% to 97% (Thomas & Daniels 2003). Patients with intra-articular fractures develop end-stage ankle arthritis more quickly than do those with extra-articular fractures (Horisberger et al 2009). In addition, it appears the older a patient is at the time they sustain an ankle fracture, the more quickly this end-stage OA progresses (Horisberger et al 2009). Due to the trauma involved, it is believed that the soft tissue envelope around the ankle is involved in the process (Hintermann & Valderrabano 2003). This thin soft tissue envelope becomes scarred and elasticity is compromised (Hintermann & Valderrabano 2003). In addition to bony injuries, ligamentous injuries are also a significant cause of post-traumatic OA, with 66–78% of patients with chronic ankle instability eventually developing ankle OA (Hubbard et al 2009). Surgeries more proximal to the ankle, such as a total knee replacement, that change the alignment at the talocrural joint have been shown to increase the incidence of ankle OA (Lee & Jeong 2012).

Studies have demonstrated gait deviations between patients with ankle arthritis compared with a group of age- and gender-matched controls (Dyrby et al 2004). Patients with ankle arthritis demonstrate decreased walking speeds, decreased stride length and increased cadence (Dyrby et al 2004). Similarly, patients post ankle arthrodesis demonstrated a decreased gait velocity of 16%, an increase in oxygen consumption of 3% and significant differences in static balance variables compared with matched controls (Hintermann & Valderrabano 2003; Hubbard et al 2009). Subjects with ankle OA reported significantly more centre of pressure total displacement and centre of pressure total velocity (Hubbard et al 2009).

Patients with end-stage OA are often managed conservatively with bracing, assistive devices, anti-inflammatories, shoe modifications (such as a rocker-bottom shoe) and foot orthoses (Claridge & Sagherian 2009). In addition, physical therapy may be prescribed to assist with stretching, joint mobilization and strengthening as indicated, although research on the benefits of physical therapy in this patient population is limited (Claridge & Sagherian 2009). Although the authors could find no research on manual therapy techniques in the management of patients with ankle OA, joint mobilizations may benefit this population since manual therapy techniques have been found to be beneficial in other populations with lower extremity OA (Deyle et al 2005; MacDonald et al 2006; Hando et al 2012). If conservative treatment fails, the two most commonly performed operative procedures for end-stage ankle arthritis are arthrodesis and arthroplasty (Claridge & Sagherian 2009).

Ankle arthrodesis versus arthroplasty

Ankle arthrodesis was first introduced in 1879, and has long since been considered the gold standard for treatment of ankle OA (Coester et al 2001). However, this procedure is not without shortcomings. Problems after fusion include subtalar and midfoot arthritis, pain with weight-bearing activities, the long-term need for assistive devices, permanent shoe modifications and decreased functional ability (Thomas & Daniels 2003). Stress fractures of the tibia, nonunion, malunion, infection and neurovascular injury are other complications associated with ankle fusion (Thomas & Daniels 2003). In response, arthroplasty was introduced as an alternative. Due to the lack of consistently good long-term patient outcomes following arthroplasty, appropriate patient selection is critical and should be considered only after conservative treatment has failed. Unlike patients undergoing total knee and total hip surgery, the ideal candidate for a total ankle is not completely understood. Indications for arthroplasty are surgeon dependent, but generally include normal vascular status, good hindfoot–ankle alignment, no immunosuppression, well-preserved ankle joint motion, sufficient medial and lateral ankle stability and low-demand sporting activities (cycling, swimming, walking, golfing) (Hintermann & Valderrabano 2003). In addition, individuals with bilateral ankle arthritis would benefit from arthroplasty, as bilateral ankle fusions often exhibit poor functional outcomes (Saltzman et al 2000). Some contraindications for receiving an ankle arthroplasty include neuroarthropathic degenerative disease (Charcot arthropathy), avascular necrosis of the talus, non-reconstructable misalignment, severe joint hypermobility, active or recurrent infection, sensory or motor dysfunction of the foot or leg, and high-demanding sport activities (running, contact sports) (Hintermann & Valderrabano 2003; Thomas & Daniels 2003).

Surgical procedures

Total ankle arthroplasty surgical procedures are complex and dependent upon the type of prosthesis used. Details of each procedure are beyond the scope of this chapter. However, some of the procedures and prostheses used affect rehabilitation and are therefore worth mentioning here. In the United States, three main prosthetic devices are used: the Agility Ankle® (dePuy Inc., Wausau, IN), the STAR® (Link Inc., Hamburg, Germany) and the Salto-Talaris® (Tornier, Grenoble, France). All of these prosthetic devices rely on bony ingrowth for stability of the implant instead of cement (Saltzman et al 2000). The advantages of relying on bony ingrowth rather than cement are threefold. First, less bone resection is needed owing to a decrease in the space between the bone and the implant needed for cement. Secondly, the damage to soft tissue structures is minimized as high levels of heat produced from the exothermic process of curing the acrylic cement are decreased. Lastly, the risk of inadvertent spillage or displacement of the cement is eliminated (Saltzman et al 2000). Bony ingrowth of the prosthesis occurs as a result of a beaded surface along the interface with the bone, a hydroxyapatite layer, or a combination of the two (Saltzman et al 2000). The ingrowth for the beaded surface occurs over a 6–12-week period, during which time any motion should be limited, as it is believed that motion between the prosthesis and bone can disrupt the bony ingrowth, which may lead to migration of the prosthesis and failure of the implant. The hydroxyapatite coating takes only 3–6 weeks to become bonded. However, this layer eventually resorbs, creating potential long-term fixation issues (Saltzman et al 2000). Currently, the main prosthetic devices used in the United States all use a beaded surface for fixation. Implications of the beaded prosthetic devices should be incorporated into an early rehabilitation protocol. For example, talocrural joint mobilization may be best implemented at 12 weeks postoperatively to ensure that bony ingrowth has occurred.

Postoperative rehabilitation treatment

History and physical examination

A thorough patient history is critical after total ankle arthroplasty since it will guide patient management. To begin, it is important to identify whether there is a history of previous trauma. For example, a stable ankle after arthroplasty is imperative for preserving the life of the implant; therefore it would be important to know whether the patient has a history of chronic ankle instability. Another important question to ask the patient is how long symptoms have persisted prior to receiving total ankle arthroplasty. Patients with previous history of ankle arthritis will often exhibit gait deviations and, with time, muscle atrophy (Valderrabano et al 2007). The process of rehabilitation for these patients may therefore be more extensive. Therapy will thus need an increased focus on balance and proprioceptive retraining after ankle replacement to ensure that the patient is safe with weight-bearing precautions early in the post-surgical phase (Coetzee 2010). Finding out whether a patient has a history of diabetes is also important to the rehabilitation process, as many patients present with neuropathies and impaired proprioceptive awareness. It is also important to ask the patients whether they currently smoke cigarettes, as additional attention will need to be devoted to wound complications in this population (Saltzman et al 2000). Probably one of the most important questions after ankle arthroplasty deals with the patient's long-term expectations, and setting realistic obtainable goals in this population is crucial to help preserve the life of the implant.

Immediate postoperative phase (weeks 0–6)

Postoperative protocols vary based on surgeon preference, the type of prosthetic implant used and the concurrent procedures performed. Physical therapy is often seen as a necessary adjunct to patients receiving total hip and total knee replacements; however, this has not historically been the case after total ankle arthroplasty. Valderrabano et al (2007, p 290) state that patients who have undergone a total ankle arthroplasty 'should have an intensive physiotherapeutic rehabilitation programme and be encouraged to perform regular muscle strengthening and stretching exercises even 1 year after ankle arthroplasty'. Saltzman et al (2000, p 66), however, stated 'in our current practice, approximately 20% of patients require physical therapy to make satisfactory postoperative progress'. The evidence for formal rehabilitation after total ankle arthroplasty is lacking and future studies are needed to assess the effect on patient outcomes.

Addressing comorbid deformities either prior to or at the time of total ankle arthroplasty is crucial for preserving the component and decreasing premature wear. Some additional procedures commonly performed in this patient population include osteotomies, tendon transfers, tendon- or muscle-lengthening procedures and fusions (e.g. midfoot, subtalar joint or triple arthrodesis). Intraoperative fractures (particularly those involving the medial malleolus) are not uncommon during ankle replacement surgery. Due to these aforementioned issues, obtaining an operative report is highly recommended before initiating any physical therapy programme following total ankle arthroplasty.

In the initial postoperative phase, wound healing without complication, solid fixation of the implant and adequate ankle motion are the main goals (Saltzman et al 2000). The patient is often placed in a splint for the first 2–3 weeks after surgery until the sutures are removed (Coetzee 2010). The patient is splinted in a neutral position so as to avoid plantarflexion contracture, and the splint typically remains on the full 2–3 weeks to minimize the chance of infection. After sutures are removed, the patient is often placed in a removable walking boot, which again helps to prevent plantarflexion contractures, and is encouraged to wear the boot as much as possible until beginning active range of motion. If procedures such as a midfoot fusion are done in concurrence with the total ankle arthroplasty, the patient may be casted for the first 6 weeks after surgery. Patients typically remain non-weight-bearing for approximately 3–6 weeks to ensure bony fixation of the implant. Patients with an Agility® implant are often held to 6 weeks of non-weight-bearing due to the syndesmotic fusion at the time of the replacement. Patients receiving a Salto-Talaris® implant are often allowed to begin partial weight-bearing approximately 3 weeks after surgery. Again, these guidelines assume no other procedures such as subtalar joint or midfoot fusions have been performed.

Approximately 25–30° of total dorsiflexion and plantarflexion range of motion can be expected after total ankle arthroplasty. Due to the motion limitations of the arthritic talocrural joint, this amount of motion is often more than patients had prior to total ankle arthroplasty. Most of the range of motion will be gained in the first 3 months after surgery, but patients can expect to continue to gain more range of motion for up to 12 months after surgery (Saltzman et al 2000). There is current debate amongst surgeons regarding whether to allow early initiation of range of motion after total ankle arthroplasty, because this may inhibit solid bony fixation of the implant (Saltzman et al 2000). Active dorsiflexion range of motion is limited for the first 6 weeks after surgery as the extensor retinaculum is cut at the time of the joint replacement (Fig. 56.1). Future studies are needed to assess the effects of early range of motion following total ankle arthroplasty.

During the first 6 weeks after surgery, the main goals of rehabilitation are to maintain the patient's weight-bearing

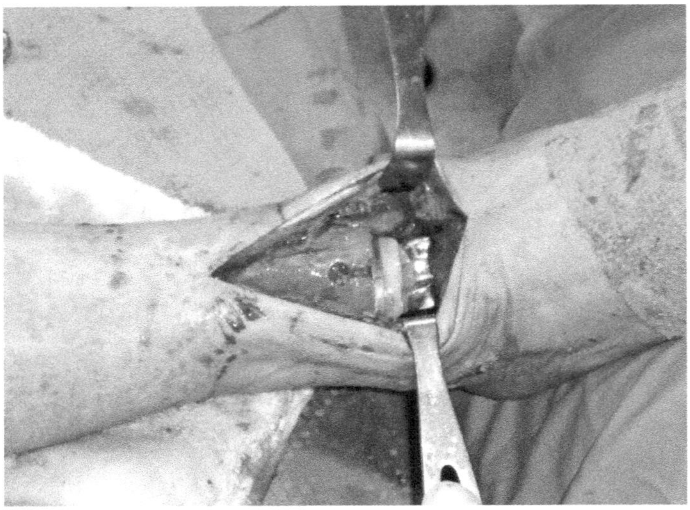

Figure 56.1 Right total ankle using Salto-Talaris® implant visible through transected extensor retinaculum.

status, prevent any wound complications, prevent plantarflexion contractures and manage swelling. Elevation is crucial for these patients in order to minimize swelling, as the use of cryotherapy is limited for the first 2–3 weeks while wearing the splint. Also, addressing proximal strength is important at this stage in the rehabilitation process. Muscles such as the gluteus medius act as dynamic stabilizers of the pelvis; however, during this non-weight-bearing period they tend to atrophy. Addressing such issues early on in rehabilitation can help to decrease common problems such as hip and low back pain as the patient begins weight-bearing in the boot. (See other chapters for details on strengthening of the hip muscles.)

Intermediate postoperative phase (weeks 6–12)

Around 6 weeks after surgery, the extensor retinaculum should be healed enough to begin active dorsiflexion range of motion. Early in this process, it is important to educate patients regarding how much range of motion they can expect in the long term. After ankle arthroplasty, it is often felt that stability is more important than mobility of the foot and ankle. However, the art in the rehabilitation process is to achieve a balance of stability with mobility. For this reason, subtalar joint mobility should possibly be limited in order to create a stable base for the implant, potentially increasing the longevity of the total ankle arthroplasty. After the wound is completely healed and bony fixation of the implant has occurred (around week 12), posterior glides of the talocrural joint may be initiated (see Ch 57). Previous literature in a non-operative patient population demonstrates that posterior glides of the talus improve dorsiflexion range of motion (Loudon et al 2014). Many patients will complain of metatarsal–phalangeal joint pain after being immobilized in the walking boot. Since joints receive their nutrition through motion, manual therapy techniques addressing the impairments at the metatarsal–phalangeal joints may improve patient's pain levels while wearing the boot and also aid a more normal gait pattern as the patient transitions out of the boot. Again, the importance of knowing about concurrent surgical procedures that were performed is imperative before initiating any manual therapy programmes.

From weeks 6 to 12, the patient progresses to full weight-bearing and then from wearing the boot, with pain as the ultimate guide. Gait training should be emphasized in this period of rehabilitation process as patients with ankle arthritis have demonstrated altered gait patterns (Horisberger et al 2009). Because such individuals typically developed abnormal gait patterns prior to their ankle arthroplasty, correcting these patterns can be challenging, especially in light of additional surgical procedures such as a triple arthrodesis or midfoot fusion. After nearly full ankle motion is restored, strengthening exercises can be initiated. Many of these patients receive a tendo-Achilles lengthening concurrently with the ankle replacement, so aggressive muscular strengthening should be avoided for approximately 12 weeks after a tendo-Achilles lengthening procedure. In addition, if the patient has had an Agility® ankle replacement where the syndesmosis is fused, it is critical to avoid forced dorsiflexion activities at an early stage, so as to encourage healing of the fusion. Several previous studies have demonstrated changes in balance and proprioception after manual therapy technique (López-Rodriguez et al 2007; Alburquerque-Sendin et al 2009; Hoch & McKeon 2011); however, these studies were done in non-surgical patient populations, and so future research is needed to examine the effectiveness of manual therapy techniques in patients with ankle arthroplasty. Nevertheless, once the patient is weight-bearing, balance and proprioception exercises should be initiated.

Pain management is an important component during this phase of the rehabilitation process. Patient education regarding activities that do not increase pain can aid in improving long-term outcomes. Again, manual therapy may play a role in aiding in pain management. One study of non-surgical patients has suggested that posterior glides of the talus for 1 minute repeated three times with a 30-second rest interval improve pain tolerance (Yeo & Wright 2011). As such, although not substantiated in a post-surgical population, manual therapy techniques may play a beneficial role during this phase of rehabilitation.

Later postoperative phase (weeks 12–24)

From 3 to 6 months, although an emphasis should still be placed on continued compliance with a home programme, patients should begin transitioning to a more independent therapy programme. At this stage, the balance and proprioception should be similar to that on the contralateral side. Gait patterns should be similar to age- and gender-matched norms, though this will depend on the additional surgical procedures performed. More work- and sport-specific activities should be incorporated into the rehab programme at this stage. Nevertheless, avoidance of high-impact activities should be stressed in order to preserve the integrity of the implant. Cycling, swimming, hiking and golfing are all safe activities for clinicians to encourage patients to undertake (Valderrabano et al 2006; Bonnin et al 2009). As patients become more active, they should also be educated about signs of component loosening. Similar to component loosening at the hip and knee, patients will often describe start-up pain, or pain with the first few steps after prolonged periods of inactivity. The pain is typically described as 'deep in the joint'. If component loosening is suspected, the patient should be referred back to the surgeon for follow-up radiographs. Box 56.1 provides a guide for rehabilitation of individuals following total ankle arthroplasty. It is important to bear in mind, however, that rehabilitation is patient specific and depends on several factors. These include, but are not limited to, concomitant surgical procedures, type of implant used, patient history, functional deficits and patient goals. A definite need exists for additional cohort studies and clinical trials examining the role of rehabilitation programmes after total ankle arthroplasty, and the most effective treatments.

Efficacy of rehabilitation treatment

As previously mentioned, appropriate patient selection for an ankle arthroplasty is crucial to achieving successful outcomes. The number of long-term outcome studies after total ankle arthroplasty is relatively limited compared with knee and total hip replacements.

Changes in range of motion

Although a full ankle range of motion is not restored after ankle arthroplasty, patients often have an increase in motion compared with before surgery. Several studies have compared the total dorsiflexion-to-plantarflexion range of motion prior to surgery versus after ankle replacement. Preoperatively, total ankle range of motion ranges from 15.2° to 23° (Wood & Deakin 2003; Bonnin et al 2004; San Giovanni et al 2006; Doets et al 2007; Valderrabano et al 2007). Postoperatively, the total ankle range of motion ranges from 23° to 36° (Pyevich et al 1998; Buechel et al 2003; Wood & Deakin 2003; Bonnin et al 2004; San Giovanni et al 2006; Doets et al 2007; Valderrabano et al 2007).

Gait

Historically, patients with ankle arthrodesis have problems with stair climbing, getting up from a chair and walking on uneven ground. As motion is lost at the talocrural joint after ankle fusion, the adjacent joints are under increased stresses to make up for some of the lost motion. A total ankle arthroplasty, in theory, should decrease the stress of the adjacent joints and create a more normal walking pattern. After fusion, it has been shown that gait velocity decreases by approximately 16% (Valderrabano et al 2003). However, after ankle arthroplasty the gait velocity decreases by only 6% (Doets et al 2007). During gait, the range of motion of the normal ankle joint has been reported to be 14.7° + 0.9° of dorsiflexion and 28.2° + 0.8° of plantarflexion (Valderrabano et al 2003). Patients who had undergone ankle fusion exhibited only 4.4° + 0.4° of dorsiflexion and 8.1° + 0.2° of plantarflexion, although this motion originated from the subtalar joint and not from the talocrural joint. Patients with arthroplasty, in contrast, demonstrated 10.0–11.1° of dorsiflexion and 22.7–30.0° of plantarflexion (Valderrabano et al 2003). Although patients with a fusion compensated with some motion, this slight amount of motion would make activities such as going down stairs difficult.

Overall, it appears that total ankle arthroplasty reproduces a more-normal ankle range of motion compared with an ankle fusion, which in turn should lead to less stress through

Box 56.1 Rehabilitation protocol for total ankle arthroplasty

0–6 weeks post-op

Goals

1. Minimize swelling.
2. Prevent wound complications.
3. Prevent plantarflexion contractures.
4. Patient avoiding weight-bearing status.

Treatment

1. Elevation/compression stockings.
2. Suture removal at 2–3 weeks after surgery.
3. Patient placed in walking boot at 2–3 weeks after surgery in neutral position (unless casting for midfoot fusion, etc. required).

6–12 weeks post-op

Goals

1. Active range of motion.
2. Full weight-bearing and out of boot.
3. Work toward symmetrical balance and proprioception.
4. Normalize gait pattern.

Treatment

1. Initiate active range of motion at 6 weeks (goal: 80% of operative range of motion by 3 months after surgery).
2. Manual therapy (assess based on limitations and concomitant procedures. Avoid talocrural joint mobilization for 12 weeks after surgery).
3. Progress to full weight-bearing and weaning the patient out of boot during this time based on type of implant – Agility® implant will be slower, due to time for syndesmotic fusion.
4. Balance and proprioception retraining.
5. Gait training (may be modified based on additional surgical procedures).
6. May initiate light strengthening avoiding aggressive gastrocnemius strengthening.

3–6 months post-op

Goals

1. Increase functional strength.
2. Normal or near-normal proprioception and balance.
3. Initiate work or sport-specific activities.
4. Begin transition to an independent programme.

Treatment

1. Ensure dorsiflexion and plantarflexion range of motion is near 25–30°.
2. Progress balance and proprioception exercises so that balance is symmetrical or near-symmetrical to contralateral side.
3. Increase functional strength; may now begin increasing intensity of gastrocnemius strengthening if TAL performed.
4. Begin work-/sport-specific training with an emphasis on avoiding high-impact activities.
5. Set up long-term independent programme to meet patient's goals/expectations. Emphasis on continued functional strengthening for at least 12 months after surgery.

adjacent joints. Further, in arthroplasty the increased weight-bearing motion may lead to improvements in functional activities compared with patients undergoing an ankle fusion.

Balance and proprioception

There is no consistent scale for assessing balance and proprioception after total ankle arthroplasty reported in the literature; however, both static proprioception (the ability to sense joint position) and kinaesthesia (the ability to sense joint movement) seem to play a critical role in successful outcome after ankle arthroplasty (Conti et al 2008).

Prior to total ankle replacement, individuals with ankle arthritis demonstrate limitations in both mechanical and sensorimotor characteristics (Hubbard et al 2009). Patients demonstrate significant increases in mechanical stiffness and increases in centre-of-pressure displacement (Hubbard et al 2009). These changes are consistent with patients who have knee OA and demonstrate increased postural sway (Masui et al 2006). Conti et al (2008) reported that, 2 years after ankle arthroplasty, there were no significant differences in joint position sense for the surgical ankle versus the unaffected side. It is possible that the addition of manual therapy may accelerate this normalization of joint position sense after total ankle arthroplasty; however, future research in this area is warranted.

Self-reported outcomes

Self-reported functional outcomes following a total ankle arthroplasty seem promising. Patients consistently report decreases in pain as well as improved function. Valderrabano et al (2006) reported, at a 3-year follow-up, that 70% of patients reported no pain after their ankle arthroplasty. However, other studies have stressed that individuals report a decrease in pain after ankle arthroplasty, but not necessarily a resolution of their pain (Kim et al 2013). Kim et al (2013) stated that it was important, both for the patients and for the surgeons, to understand that some residual pain is to be expected. Table 56.1 provides a summary of the literature regarding functional outcomes. As can be seen in the table, of 778 patients from 9 different studies, the mean AOFAS (American Orthopaedic Foot and Ankle Society) score prior to surgery was 41 / 100 and it increased to 81 / 100 following surgery (mean follow-up of 4.3 years).

Achilles Tendon Ruptures

Introduction

Formed by the gastrocnemius and soleus muscles, the Achilles tendon is the largest and strongest tendon in the human body and is a trademark of the bipedal human (Deangelis et al 2009; Jiang et al 2012). Although the Achilles tendon is the largest and strongest tendon in the human body, it is also the most frequently ruptured tendon (Kongsgaard et al 2005; Maffulli et al 2011; Maquirriain 2011; Garras et al 2012; Hando et al 2012; Horstmann et al 2012; Jiang et al 2012). Unlike other tendons, which are surrounded by a synovial sheath, the Achilles tendon is encased by a thinner paratenon (Mortensen et al 1999; Strom & Casillas 2009). The middle layer of the paratenon, the mesotenon, supplies most of the blood to the tendon. During a muscle contraction, the blood flow to the tendon is greatly diminished or can even cease completely (Strom & Casillas 2009). When damaged, the Achilles tendon is slow to heal, as it is a hypocellular and hypovascular tissue (Godbout et al 2006). These anatomical and physiological features create significant challenges in the management of Achilles tendon ruptures.

With ageing, lower rates of collagen regeneration and replacement occur, along with decreases in vascular supply and reduced water content. These changes can result in alterations to the molecular properties of the collagen, which is responsible for withstanding the tensile forces placed on the Achilles tendon (White et al 2007; Strom & Casillas 2009). As the collagen becomes stiffer, the tensile strength of the tendon decreases, making it more susceptible to tears (White et al 2007). In addition, as a person ages, the blood supply to the extremities decreases and collagen regeneration may be unable to occur at an adequate rate, thereby leaving the tendon susceptible to failure (Deangelis et al 2009; Strom & Casillas 2009). Tendon failures can also occur as a result of chronic degeneration of the tendon or failure of the inhibitory mechanism of the musculotendinous unit (Deangelis et al 2009; Strom & Casillas 2009; Jiang et al 2012). Finally, tendon failures may also occur as the result of direct or indirect trauma (Strom & Casillas 2009). Approximately 80% of Achilles tendon ruptures occur 3–6 cm above the insertion of the Achilles tendon onto the calcaneus, which is the smallest

Table 56.1 **Functional outcomes before and after total ankle arthroplasty**

Study (year)	Number of patients	Mean follow-up years (range)	AOFAS score pre-surgery	AOFAS score post-surgery (range)
Pyevich et al (1998)	85	4.8 (2.8–12.3)	NA	85 (40–100)
Bonnin et al (2004)	91	3.9 (2–5.6)	32.3	83.1
Doets et al (2006)	93	7.2 (0.4–16.3)	NA	77 (73.2–80.8)
San Giovanni et al (2006)	28	8.3 (5–12.2)	NA	81 (40–92)
Valderrabano et al (2006)	147	2.8 (2–4)	36 (10–74)	84 (28–100)
Claridge & Sagherian (2009)	28	1.8	34.9	76.4
Kim et al (2013)	120	3.3 (1.2–7)	59.3 (21–89)	83 (49–100)
Sproule et al (2013)	85	3.3 (2.5–5)	38.2 (12–59)	74.8 (46–100)

cross-sectional area of the tendon (Deangelis et al 2009; Maquirriain 2011).

Epidemiology

It is well documented that the incidence of Achilles tendon ruptures is steadily increasing (Suchak et al 2005; Costa et al 2006; Clayton & Court-Brown 2008; Deangelis et al 2009; Mullaney et al 2011; Garras et al 2012; Jiang et al 2012). Suchak et al (2005) reported that the total incidence increased from 5.5 ruptures per 100 000 in 1998 to 9.9 ruptures per 100 000 in 2002. Clayton and Court-Brown (2008) reported an increase in incidence rates in Denmark between 1984 and 1996 of 18.2 per 100 000 to 37.3 per 100 000. In addition, incidence rates differ based on gender, with males ranging from 8.8 to 14 ruptures per 100 000 males, and females ranging from 2.1 to 6.1 ruptures per 100 000 females (Suchak et al 2005). The male to female ratio for these ruptures is reported to be 4 : 1 (Suchak et al 2005; White et al 2007; Jiang et al 2012). The increased rate of ruptures during participation in athletic activities by middle-aged individuals is felt to contribute to the increasing incidence of Achilles ruptures (Suchak et al 2005; Deangelis et al 2009). Achilles tendon ruptures are most frequently seen in males aged 30–39 years (Owens et al 2007; Jiang et al 2012).

Risk factors

Several risk factors have been implicated in Achilles tendon ruptures. These include: previous Achilles tendon changes due to tendinopathy, participation in athletic activities involving repetitive loading of the tendon, medication use, hereditary factors and race (Deangelis et al 2009).

It has been suggested that people with a history of Achilles tendinopathy are more susceptible to Achilles rupture, since a pathological continuum exists from a healthy tendon to a thickened tendon associated with neovascularization and neoneuralization (Kraemer et al 2012). Perhaps this deteriorated tendon is more susceptible to complete rupture than a healthy tendon to stresses that would otherwise not result in injury (Strom & Casillas 2009; Kraemer et al 2012).

Studies have reported that 60–75% of all Achilles tendon ruptures occur during athletic activities, with the greatest risk for athletes who participate in jumping, cutting and/or making quick acceleration or deceleration movements (Suchak et al 2005; Deangelis et al 2009; Maffulli et al 2011; Kearney & Costa 2012). On the other hand, it has been estimated that 11% of Achilles ruptures occur from accidents, and approximately 5% occur from activities of daily living (Suchak et al 2005). Suchak et al (2005) reported that patients between the ages of 20 and 30 years were more likely to rupture the Achilles tendon during sporting activities, whereas older patients (50–60 years) were more likely to rupture it during activities of daily living such as tripping on the stairs or stepping in a hole. Deangelis et al (2009) estimate that most tendons in the human body have a failure stress point of 100 MPa and that the typical stress placed upon them is below 30 MPa. The Achilles tendon, however, often experiences up to 70 MPa of stress during a maximal eccentric plantarflexion contracture (Deangelis et al 2009). This increased stress placed on the Achilles may therefore play a role in the ultimate failure of the tendon.

Medications such as fluoroquinolone antibiotics have been implicated in increased Achilles tendon rupture rates (Deangelis et al 2009; Kraemer et al 2012). These medications are often used in the treatment of serious bacterial infections, especially hospital-acquired infections such as pneumonia. It is theorized the fluorinated quinolone compounds may alter the collagenases and matrix metalloproteinases, which could lead to an increased risk of tendon rupture (White et al 2007).

Hereditary factors may also play a role in the incidence of Achilles tendon ruptures. Individuals who have sustained a previous Achilles tendon rupture are 200 times more likely to rupture the contralateral one (Kongsgaard et al 2005; Deangelis et al 2009). In addition, in one study (Deangelis et al 2009) individuals with ABO blood group O have been linked to a higher risk of Achilles tendon ruptures, although other studies failed to demonstrate such an association (Owens et al 2007).

In a study done looking at tendon ruptures in US service members, the adjusted rate ratio for African-American service members compared with Caucasian service members for Achilles tendon ruptures was 3.85 (95% CI 3.31–3.88) (Owens et al 2007). The authors of this study offered a potential biomechanical explanation, citing studies that showed the viscoelastic properties of the Achilles tendon had a higher stiffness in African-American athletes. The increased stiffness may result in tendon rupture with sufficient trauma (Owens et al 2007).

Diagnosis

The mechanism of an Achilles tendon rupture generally occurs from a sudden plantarflexion or 'pushing off' from a weight-bearing forefoot with the knee extended, or from unexpected dorsiflexion of the ankle, for example stepping in a hole (Strom & Casillas 2009; Jiang et al 2012). Some studies suggest misdiagnosis of an Achilles tendon rupture occurs in 20% to 36% of all cases (Deangelis et al 2009; Garras et al 2012). A delay in the diagnosis, and therefore treatment, of an Achilles rupture (be it surgical or non-surgical) can result in an unfavourable outcome (Deangelis et al 2009; Garras et al 2012). As such, making an accurate diagnosis early on can have a significant impact on patient outcomes.

Subjectively, individuals will often report they heard or felt a loud 'pop'. In addition, individuals will also report feeling like they were kicked or hit in the back of the leg (Deangelis et al 2009; Kearney & Costa 2012). Many of these subjects report difficulty in walking immediately after the injury. Clinically, three main tests are used to diagnosis a rupture of the Achilles tendon: the Thompson test, the Matles test and the presence of a palpable defect. An abnormal Thompson test is described as diminished or absent plantarflexion of the ankle joint when the examiner squeezes the patient's calf muscle, indicating an Achilles rupture. The sensitivity and specificity of the Thompson test are 0.96 and 0.93 respectively (Garras et al 2012). The Matles test assesses the normal resting tension of the Achilles tendon. The normal resting tension of the ankle is approximately 20° to 30° of plantarflexion (Garras et al 2012). The patient is tested in prone with the knee bent to 90°. If the affected side has an increased dorsiflexion angle

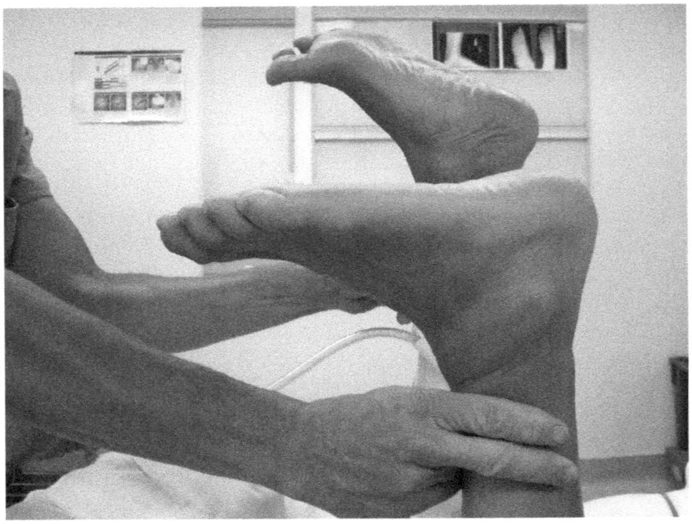

Figure 56.2 Positive Matles test. Increased resting dorsiflexion of right ankle after Achilles tendon rupture.

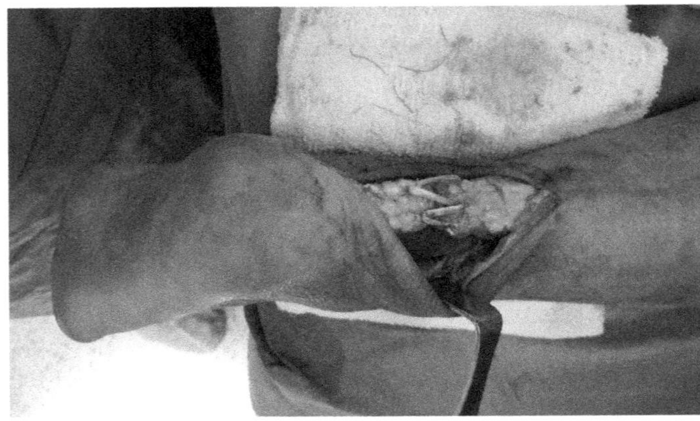

Figure 56.3 Right chronic Achilles tendon repair with plantaris tendon transfer.

compared with the unaffected side, this constitutes a positive test (Fig. 56.2). The sensitivity and specificity of the Matles test are 0.88 and 0.85 respectively (Garras et al 2012). The third test is defined as being able to palpate a gap in the Achilles tendon. The sensitivity of this test is 0.73 and the specificity is 0.85 (Deangelis et al 2009; Garras et al 2012).

Garras et al (2012) reported that the combination of these three clinical tests was more accurate than MRI in diagnosing an Achilles tendon rupture. In addition, those patients in this study who underwent MRI had delayed times between initial injury and time to surgical intervention. The mean time between rupture and surgery was 12.4 days (95% CI 10.5–14.3) for the group of patients receiving MRI compared with 5.6 days (95% CI 5.0–6.2) for the group of patients who received only the three clinical tests to make the diagnosis of Achilles tendon rupture (Garras et al 2012). As previously mentioned, patients with longer times between diagnosis and surgical repair of the Achilles tendon often present with inferior outcomes The patients in this study who were diagnosed with clinical tests required no additional procedures, whereas almost 30% of the patients who were in the MRI group received additional surgical procedures such as a flexor hallucis longus transfer (Garras et al 2012). Therefore, it would seem that MRI should be used judiciously in the diagnosis of Achilles tendon rupture. One reason a delayed diagnosis makes surgical repair more challenging is that, like rotator cuff tears, the Achilles tendon will start to retract and adhere to underlying structures with scar tissue, requiring additional procedures such as tendon transfers (Fig. 56.3). Other medical imaging such as a plain radiograph is indicated if an avulsion fracture is suspected (Deangelis et al 2009).

Surgical versus non-surgical treatment

There is controversy surrounding the best management of Achilles tendon ruptures. With a majority of US states having direct access, physical therapists are often the first medical providers to counsel patients with an Achilles tendon repair on the various options that are available. These injuries can be managed both surgically and non-surgically. Surgical repair for Achilles tendon ruptures accounts for approximately 40% of all operatively repaired tendons (Garras et al 2012). Currently, there is no clear consensus on the best management strategy. Some considerations for surgical versus non-surgical management include: age, associated medical conditions and athletic activity (Strom & Casillas 2009). As previously discussed, ageing directly affects the healing process at a cellular level and less-aggressive forms of treatment may be indicated (Strom & Casillas 2009). Associated medical conditions include smoking, as it leads to impedance of cutaneous blood flow, decreased proliferation of red blood cells, fibroblasts and macrophages, which are essential to the healing process. Also systemic diseases such as rheumatoid arthritis and systemic lupus erythematosus can weaken collagen and damaged joint surfaces, impeding the healing of the Achilles tendon (Strom & Casillas 2009). It is also speculated that patients who are more active may achieve better outcomes owing to increased self-motivation (Strom & Casillas 2009).

There are several different ways to repair an Achilles tendon rupture surgically, including: open repair, percutaneous repair and mini-open procedures. Each of these procedures has its advantages and disadvantages. For example, some studies report increased wound complications in open repairs compared with percutaneous procedures; however, studies also demonstrate that percutaneous procedures present with more sural nerve injuries (Deangelis et al 2009). Different suture techniques such as the Kessler, Bunnell and Krackow techniques have been studied in the literature, and the Krackow suturing technique appears to have a biomechanical advantage over both the Bunnell and Kessler techniques (Deangelis et al 2009). Epitendinous suturing plays two important roles. First, it increases the resistance to gapping and, secondly, it improves the load to failure compared with suturing of just the core of the Achilles tendon (Deangelis et al 2009; Maquirriain 2011).

Surgical repair of the Achilles tendon leads to shorter sick-leave duration, decreased re-rupture rate and higher rates of infections. However, patients treated operatively also have higher risks of developing wound complications than patients who are managed conservatively (Deangelis et al 2009; Maquirriain 2011; Kearney & Costa 2012). The most common wound problems following an Achilles tendon repair include infection, wound dehiscence and scarring. Wound complications greatly increase in this population if patients are diabetic, or use tobacco or steroids (Deangelis et al 2009). The chance of developing a wound complication after an Achilles tendon repair is around 6%; however, if one or more of the above risk factors is present, the chance of developing a wound complication increases to 40% (Deangelis et al 2009).

Patients undergoing surgical repair of the Achilles tendon return to work more quickly and have a shorter mean sick time than do those treated non-operatively. A meta-analysis published by Jiang et al (2012) reported that patients undergoing surgically treated Achilles ruptures returned to work on average of 23.8 days (95% CI –41.6 to –5.9) sooner than those who were treated non-surgically. This is consistent with another study that reported an average of 19.2 days (95% CI 3.9 to 34.0) less days for return to work (Soroceanu et al 2012).

Re-rupture rates for patients with surgically repaired tendons are also lower compared with patients treated non-surgically (Maquirriain 2011). A recent meta-analysis found that patients treated surgically had 8.8% less risk of re-rupture, and that the number of patients needed to treat in order to prevent one re-rupture was 12 (Soroceanu et al 2012). In the meta-analysis performed by Jiang et al (2012), 4.3% (19 of 441) of patients in the operative group re-ruptured the Achilles tendon whereas 9.7% (44 of 453) in the non-operative group reported re-rupture of this tendon (relative risk (RR) 0.44, 95% CI 0.26–0.74). Interestingly, some research suggests that patients treated conservatively who begin an early functional rehabilitation programme, may have similar re-rupture rates to those treated operatively (Soroceanu et al 2012). Historically, patients treated conservatively were often casted (Strom & Casillas 2009). More recent protocols are now allowing for earlier functional rehabilitation in this conservative population, which may result in re-rupture rates similar to those in patients treated operatively.

Early range of motion versus immobilization

Two main concerns of early range of motion after an Achilles tendon repair include increased incidence of re-rupture and overstretching of the repaired tendon, making it difficult to regain functional strength (Sorrenti 2006; Deangelis et al 2009; Strom & Casillas 2009). Immobilization usually includes placing the patient in a cast with the foot placed in equinus as the tendon repair heals for 6–8 weeks (Strom & Casillas 2009). This immobilization period is often followed by a supervised rehabilitation programme (Strom & Casillas 2009). Early mobilization often includes placing the patient in a removable walking boot. Again, the foot is initially positioned in equinus to place less tension on the healing tendon. Although there are several benefits to a removable boot compared with a cast with respect to performing activities of daily living such as bathing, a removable device relies heavily on patient compliance in order to prevent complications and delayed healing.

Prolonged immobilization is associated with joint stiffness, muscle atrophy, soft tissue adhesions, deep venous thrombosis and ulceration of joint cartilage (Sorrenti 2006). An immobilized joint undergoes degradative and destructive changes to the joint surfaces (Sorrenti 2006; Strom & Casillas 2009). In an immobilized tendon, the newly formed collagen fibrils may not be remodelled properly (Sorrenti 2006). In a similar vein, one study looking at Achilles tendon ruptures in rats found that prolonged immobilization impeded the healing process, because it compromised the up-regulation of repair gene expression in the healing Achilles tendon (Bring et al 2010). The authors of this study suggested that a shorter period of immobilization, such as 1 week, would not impair the healing process of the tendon. In addition, these authors found that early mobilization post Achilles tendon rupture induced a higher density of blood vessels. Further, fibroblasts were more differentiated and there was a higher degree of collagen organization compared with an immobilized group (Bring et al 2010).

The concern for tendon elongation after Achilles repair prohibits some therapists from allowing early range of motion. This elongation often occurs as a result of gapping between the ends of the tendon after surgical fixation. If a gap is present then granulation tissue, adhesions and delayed collagen maturation may occur, resulting in a weaker repair (Maquirriain 2011). Kangas et al (2007) assessed differences in tendon separation between a group of patients beginning early range of motion and those placed in a below-knee cast with the foot in a neutral position for 6 weeks. Early range of motion allowed for full plantarflexion range of motion, but dorsiflexion only to a neutral position. Both groups were allowed full weight-bearing by 3 weeks postoperatively (Kangas et al 2007). Markers were placed within the tendon and plain radiographs were taken at follow-up visits to measure the amount of separation. At a mean of 60 weeks postoperatively, the authors found that elongation occurred to a lesser extent in the group starting early range of motion (2 mm) than in the immobilized group (5 mm) (Kangas et al 2007). Mortensen et al (1999) found similar results; they also compared a group of patients beginning early range of motion with a group immobilized in a cast for 8 weeks and found no significant difference in separation of the intratendinous markers in the Achilles tendon at 12 weeks postoperatively. In addition, patients who were in the early mobilization group were able to return to work more quickly compared with the group that was immobilized (Mortensen et al 1999).

The second concern with initiating early mobilization after an Achilles repair is re-rupture. A meta-analysis performed by Suchak et al (2006) indicated that no significant difference in re-rupture existed between patients who initiated early mobilization and those subjects who were immobilized after Achilles tendon repair. Individuals who initiated early mobilization incurred a re-rupture rate of 2.5%, whereas those who were immobilized reported a re-rupture rate of 3.8% (Suchak et al 2006).

Based on the literature, it therefore appears that early functional rehabilitation does not increase the risk of re-rupture after surgical repair of the Achilles tendon, nor does it increase the length of the tendon after the repair. In addition, wound complications (superficial or deep infections) were not more prominent in those who initiated early mobilization compared with those who were immobilized. The average infection rates for the early mobilization group versus the immobilization group were 2.6% and 3.9% respectively (Suchak et al 2006). Finally, patients who initiated early mobilization also reported greater satisfaction than patients who were immobilized after surgery (88% and 62% respectively)

(Suchak et al 2006). Based on these findings, early mobilization after Achilles tendon rupture can be considered beneficial to this patient population.

Early weight-bearing versus late weight-bearing

It was formerly common practice for clinicians to advise 6–8 weeks of non-weight-bearing after an Achilles tendon repair. However, more-recent studies have suggested that early weight-bearing is not detrimental to the repair and indeed may have several benefits. Suchak et al (2008) found early benefits for a group of patients who initiated weight-bearing as tolerated at the first postoperative visit 2 weeks after surgery compared with a group of patients who remained non-weight-bearing until 6 weeks after surgery. At 6 weeks after surgery, the early-weight-bearing group reported significantly improved outcomes on physical functioning, vitality, social functioning and role-emotional measures (Suchak et al 2008). By 6 months, differences no longer existed between the two groups and there were no re-ruptures in either group (Suchak et al 2008). Costa et al (2006) found similar results in a study comparing immediate weight-bearing versus a group that was initially non-weight-bearing. Patients initiating immediate weight-bearing returned to normal walking and stair climbing more quickly (12.5 versus 18 weeks for walking and 13 versus 22 weeks for stair climbing). Two patients re-ruptured in the immediate weight-bearing group; however, both of these were performing strenuous activities in breach of the study's protocol at the time of re-rupture (Costa et al 2006). It appears from the current literature that functional advantages exist for patients who initiate early weight-bearing after a surgical repair of an Achilles tendon rupture. Patients who bore weight early also reported feeling that they could perform activities that were not in line with accepted principles of tissue healing, indicating the importance of stressing protocol compliance.

Post-surgical rehabilitation treatment

The first clinical guidelines for the treatment of acute Achilles tendon rupture were published in 2010 by the American Academy of Orthopaedic Surgeons and the American Foot and Ankle Society (Kearney & Costa 2012). The guidelines were as follows: (1) the use of early postoperative weight-bearing (within 2 weeks) and (2) the use of a 'protective device' allowing for early mobilization (Kearney & Costa 2012). It seems a 'protective device' should be used with this patient population; however, there is no consensus on which devices should be used, and what degree of ankle plantarflexion the patient should be in. There is also a lack of evidence for the optimal time these devices should be worn. Rehabilitation protocols appear to follow this trend of uncertainty; controversy still exists on an optimal physical therapy protocol for Achilles tendon ruptures, whether managed surgically or conservatively (Deangelis et al 2009).

The phases of tendon healing should be kept in mind when designing a rehabilitation protocol. The three phases of tendon healing are inflammation (occurs during the first week), proliferation (occurs between weeks 2 and 8), and remodelling (can take up to 12 months) (Kearney & Costa 2012). When developing a protocol for treatment of Achilles tendon ruptures, early limited range of motion and weight-bearing are beneficial. As previously discussed, the range of motion should be in a protected range so as to avoid tendon elongation. Most of the immediate weight-bearing protocols involve using a removable protective device such as a walking boot. Further, studies consistently demonstrate that one main goal in recovering strength after an Achilles tendon rupture is to prevent tendon elongation. However, the optimal time to begin functional strengthening or balance and proprioception exercises after an Achilles tendon rupture is also unclear.

Rupture of the Achilles tendon can result in permanent loss of plantarflexion strength, gait deviations, and difficulties with activities of daily living such as stair climbing and return to sports (Garras et al 2012). After an Achilles tendon rupture, it is often difficult to achieve full function as only minor improvements are seen after the first 12 months following surgery (Maquirriain 2011). For example, approximately 30% of US National Football League players are unable to return to professional football after an Achilles rupture (Kraemer et al 2012). Therefore, regardless of the lack of our complete understanding of tendon healing, it is clear that tendon-training exercises should be part of the rehabilitation protocol. Repetitive loading of the Achilles tendon orients the collagen fibres parallel to the longitudinal axis of the tendon, which increases tendon strength, improves vascularity and increases the number of collagen filaments (Sorrenti 2006). One such exercise includes plantarflexion with an elastic band (Fig. 56.4). However, care should be taken when performing such plantarflexion to prevent the ankle dorsiflexion going past neutral, which would place undue stress on the Achilles tendon. Cycling is another tendon-training exercise. Early in the rehabilitation process, patients can begin cycling out of the walking boot and in a shoe with heel lifts to maintain the plantarflexed position of the foot and reduce strain on the Achilles tendon. This again allows the patient to begin tendon training early on in the rehabilitation process. The exact time frame, however, is surgeon dependent. There is no research to support duration or frequency of these tendon-training exercises after Achilles tendon repairs, but it seems prudent to let pain be a guide. Patients often report minimal pain after an Achilles tendon rupture, so it is important to stress not pushing into pain during this phase of the rehabilitation process.

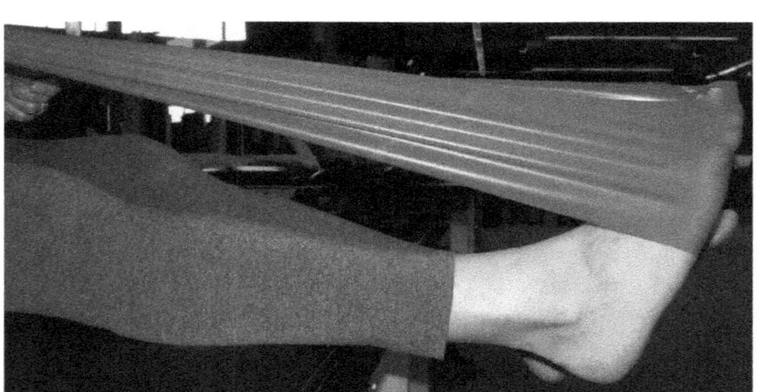

Figure 56.4 Tendon training exercise with elastic band after Achilles tendon repair, avoiding stretching into dorsiflexion.

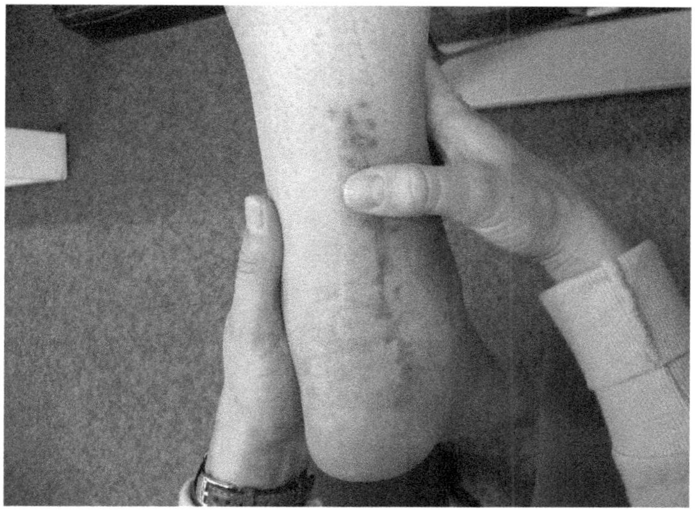

Figure 56.5 Scar tissue mobilization after Achilles tendon incision has healed.

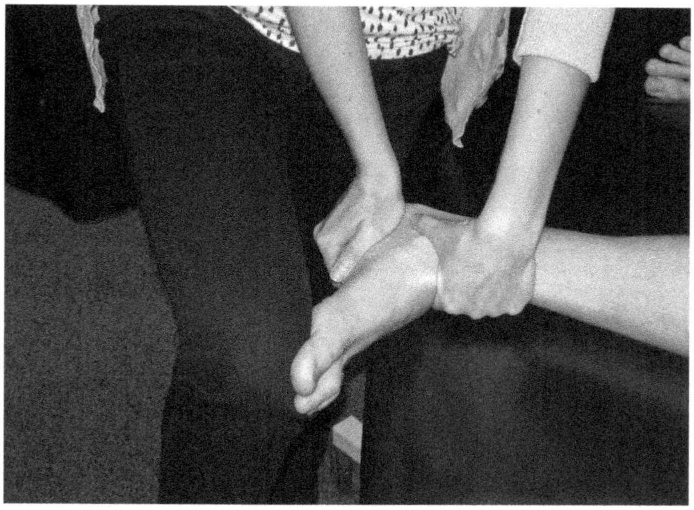

Figure 56.6 Subtalar lateral glide joint mobilization.

Scar tissue builds rapidly in patients who have had a surgical repair of an Achilles tendon rupture. The literature suggests that patients will ultimately end up with a tendon that is 45–50% thicker than the unaffected side (Mortensen et al 1999). Once the incision is healed, scar tissue mobilization should be initiated to decrease adhesions (Fig. 56.5). Patients initiating range of motion early tend to develop fewer scar adhesions than those who are immobilized or casted (Mortensen et al 1999).

Swelling should be addressed early after an Achilles tendon ruptures. Swelling can be managed in a variety of ways including cryotherapy, elevation and compression stockings. Manual therapy techniques aimed at decreasing swelling, such as effleurage, can be implemented immediately after the patient is out of the splint and placed into a removable walking boot. Care should be taken to avoid stressing the incision site.

Long-term limitations in proprioception persist after Achilles tendon ruptures. Bressel et al (2004) conducted a study of proprioception in patients 5.8 years after Achilles tendon injury by measuring the errors in matching joint position. Errors for the involved limb and uninvolved limb were measured and compared with an age- and gender-matched control group. The results of the study indicated that significantly greater errors existed for both the involved (27%) and uninvolved (31%) limbs compared with the control group (Bressel et al 2004). However, as patients were analysed only after Achilles rupture, it is not possible to know whether there were deficits prior to Achilles injury that may have made them more susceptible to tearing the Achilles. It should be noted that only 45% of patients in this study reported they were prescribed an organized physical therapy programme (Bressel et al 2004). As such, when clinicians are designing a rehabilitation programme for patients after an Achilles tendon rupture, addressing proprioception for both the ipsilateral and contralateral sides is warranted; however, no clear consensus exists for the ideal time to initiate balance and proprioception exercises after an Achilles tendon rupture. Studies utilizing electromyographic (EMG) analysis have shown that some balance exercises activate the gastrocnemius less than simple plantarflexion using an elastic band (Mullaney et al 2011). Therefore, initiation of balance exercises early in the rehabilitation process while the patient is in the boot seems to be a safe and beneficial activity after an Achilles repair. Although there is currently no research to support the effectiveness of manual therapy techniques aimed at the talocrural joint to improve balance and proprioception in this population, it may be a useful adjunct once the tendon has adequately healed.

Although the trend is for starting early range of motion exercises, patients typically spend approximately 10–12 weeks in a walking boot after Achilles tendon ruptures and joint stiffness often persists. Since joints receive nutrition through movement, the thousands of steps we take throughout the day provide this nutrition. However, being immobilized in a walking boot does not allow for the same motion of the joints as normal gait. As such, patients often complain of metatarsal–phalangeal joint stiffness along with subtalar joint stiffness. Manual therapy may play an important role in improving joint mobility prior to the patient beginning to be weaned out of the walking boot in order to decrease gait deviations, although care should be taken not to stress the incision site. Sorrenti (2006) published a typical physical therapy protocol. This protocol included joint mobilization to the subtalar joint (Fig. 56.6) and the forefoot beginning as early as 2–6 weeks postoperatively After a period of weight-bearing in the boot with heel lifts, patients commonly complain of low back pain, hip and knee pain. Manual therapy techniques aimed at proximal structures seem to benefit this patient population. Although there are currently no research studies at this time specifically addressing the effectiveness of manual therapy after Achilles tendon ruptures, clinical experience suggests a benefit for many of the patients who struggle with joint stiffness after a period of immobilization. Future research should examine the effects of incorporating manual therapy into a postoperative rehabilitation protocol following Achilles tendon repair.

Although no evidence-based protocols exist when rehabilitating patients after surgical repair of an Achilles rupture, consideration of the forces applied to the Achilles tendon during common activities or exercises is pertinent to safely progress these patients. This tendon transmits more force than any other tendon in the human body, and studies suggest that its repair may fail at forces ranging from 45 to

Table 56.2 EMG activity of the triceps surae muscle for healthy individuals

Task	MVIC (%)
Balance board	23.4
Ankle pumps	36.7
Plantarflexion red elastic band	43.2
Walking	43.2
Lateral step-up	59
Heel rise	112.6
Hopping	128.9

MVIC: maximal voluntary isometric contractions.

250 Newtons (N) (Maquirriain 2011; Mullaney et al 2011). Mullaney et al (2011) performed a study on healthy individuals assessing the percentage of maximal voluntary isometric contractions (MVICs) of the calf during commonly prescribed therapeutic exercises. A single-limb heel rise and hopping elicited the highest percentages of MVIC (112.6% and 128.9% respectively), whereas balance and ankle pumps elicited lower percentages of MVIC compared with walking (23.4% and 36.7% respectively) (Mullaney et al 2011). The results are summarized in Table 56.2.

Patients immobilized in a walking boot after an Achilles tendon rupture are often placed in plantarflexion to reduce stress on the tendon as it heals. This is usually done with heel lifts. Approximately 80% of normal plantarflexion contractile activity is exerted during walking with the foot immobilized in a neutral position (Maquirriain 2011). However, adding a 1-inch (2.5 cm) heel lift reduces the plantarflexion contractile activity to 57% (Maquirriain 2011). As the tendon heals, the lifts are gradually removed from the boot in order to prepare the tendon to accept tensile stress during walking out of the boot. There appears to be a subset of patients who naturally stretch out the repaired tendon more quickly compared with others. These patients present with a decreased resting plantarflexion position of the foot with the knee bent to 90°. It may therefore be beneficial for this subset of patients to wean themselves off of the heel lifts more slowly. These patients may also benefit from a small lift in the shoe when transitioning out of the walking boot. The larger the degree of plantarflexion the ankle is immobilized in, the greater is the resultant atrophy (Maquirriain 2011). However, too much stress on the tendon during weight-bearing activities in the boot may jeopardize the repair and impede functional outcomes. The goal of the therapist managing patients after an Achilles tendon repair is to find the balance between limiting muscle atrophy and unduly stressing the healing tendon. This goal is more easily accomplished when the clinician understands the stresses placed on the healing tendon with various activities. Strengthening the plantarflexed muscles in a range that avoids increased dorsiflexion of the ankle is therefore prudent so as to avoid overlengthening of the tendon (Maquirriain 2011). Serial sarcomere adaptation during this phase of rehabilitation can be improved by combining eccentric exercises while avoiding the end range of dorsiflexion (Maquirriain 2011).

Available rehabilitation protocols provide only a general guideline and should be modified based on the patient's goals and ability. Protocols should also be developed or modified in consultation with surgeons based on several factors. First, it is important to consider the nature of the rupture. The time from initial diagnosis until surgery is an important factor to consider. Patients who present with chronic ruptures often have additional procedures such as a flexor hallucis longus augmentation or plantaris tendon transfer (see Fig. 56.3). Another important factor to consider is whether the rupture was primary or recurrent. Re-ruptures are difficult injuries to manage owing to wound complications. Therefore, therapy should be modified to reflect these additional considerations. The age and health of the patient will reflect patient goals and ultimately rehabilitation considerations. For example, patients who present with diseases such as diabetes will have special wound- and tissue-healing considerations. In addition, high-level recreational athletes should be moved through a protocol very differently to a non-athletic population.

Manual therapy techniques may be of benefit in order to improve mobility to joints more proximal and distal to the ankle joint, to decrease swelling and to improve balance and proprioception. Assessment of the benefits of incorporating manual therapy techniques into rehabilitation protocols after Achilles tendon ruptures still requires future research. A general protocol for patients undergoing Achilles tendon repair, which should be modified based on the above factors, has been included in Table 56.3.

It has been demonstrated that, after Achilles tendon repair, elongation of the tendon occurs, resulting in suboptimal outcomes including both muscle weakness and permanent functional impairment (Mortensen et al 1999; Maquirriain 2011; Mullaney et al 2011; Horstmann et al 2012; Silbernagel et al 2012). This lengthening has two primary causes: first is a lack of proper tensioning at the time of operative repair, and second is a progressive tendon lengthening during the postoperative period (Maquirriain 2011), since the lengthened Achilles tendon has a compromised capacity to produce force at a given ankle angle (Horstmann et al 2012). Silbernagel et al (2012) found significant side-to-side differences in heel-rise height and tendon length at 6 months and 12 months. The authors of this study found that the majority of the tendon elongation occurred during the first 3 months after surgery. Although the sample size was small, a significant negative correlation was still found between the degree of tendon elongation and the side-to-side difference in heel-rise height at 6 months and 12 months after surgical repair (Silbernagel et al 2012). So, as tendon elongation increased, patients' ability to perform plantarflexion at end range of motion diminished (Silbernagel et al 2012). Clinical outcomes also significantly correlate with tendon elongation; Maquirriain (2011) showed that patient outcomes improved as tendon elongation decreased and stated that gapping greater than 5 mm was considered to be a clinical failure. Managing these patients becomes much more difficult once the elongation becomes permanent (Maquirriain 2011).

Both calf muscle strength and endurance are limited after Achilles tendon rupture. On average, at 1 year after injury, muscle endurance recovers to only 52–88% of the unaffected side as measured by the maximum number of heel raises performed in a full-weight-bearing position (Bostick et al

Table 56.3 Achilles tendon repair rehabilitation protocol

Time period (postoperatively)	Treatment
0–6 weeks	Ankle pumps (limited dorsiflexion to neutral) Weight-bearing with crutches in walking boot with ankle in plantarflexion (should be full weight-bearing by 6 weeks postoperatively) Swelling management (ice, elevation, compression stocking, manual therapy techniques) Plantar flexion against light resistance for tendon training Bilateral balance and proprioception in the boot Joint mobilization (subtalar joint, forefoot, metatarsal–phalangeal joints, and proximal joints as needed)
6–12 weeks	Scar tissue mobilization (once wound is healed) Continue swelling management Continue joint mobilization as needed Slowly reduce heel lifts in boot until in neutral position Balance and proprioception (progressing to unilateral on both contralateral and ipsilateral sides) Stationary bike (in shoe with heel lifts to maintain plantarflexion) At 10–12 weeks – wean patient out of boot Gait training Bilateral heel raise (starting with increased weight on contralateral side and increasing to equal weight bilaterally)
12–16 weeks	Increased plantarflexion strength – adding in eccentric work in weight-bearing Progress to unilateral heel raise Focus on end range of motion plantarflexion strength Continue balance and proprioception exercises
16 weeks	May begin jogging if able to perform unilateral heel raise with only 2-finger light touch for balance at 75% of endurance of contralateral side (measured by number of unilateral heel raises)
6 months	Progress to sprinting and plyometric work in order to return to full sport activity

2010). Permanent strength deficits of 10–30% can commonly be seen after Achilles tendon ruptures (Silbernagel et al 2012). One study showed that calf circumference remains significantly smaller even 10 years after Achilles tendon rupture (Horstmann et al 2012). In addition, the authors of this study reported significantly decreased heel raise height compared with the contralateral limb. Patients in this 10-year follow-up study had decreased eccentric plantarflexion strength and increased muscle activation compared with the contralateral limb, owing to the decreased force production of the plantarflexors (Horstmann et al 2012). It is of note that only about two-thirds of patients in this study received formal physical therapy (Horstmann et al 2012).

Two years after an Achilles rupture, patients typically still have gait deviations (Silbernagel et al 2012). Strength deficits of the calf muscles may help to explain these deviations in the normal gait pattern, which in turn may increase stress on the Achilles (Horstmann et al 2012).

Conclusion

Although the effectiveness of manual therapy has been shown to be of benefit to patients with acute and chronic foot and ankle conditions, little evidence supports the use of manual therapy in a population of patients who have undergone surgery to the foot or ankle. There is great potential for future research supporting the judicious use of manual therapies in patients who have undergone a total ankle arthroplasty or who have sustained an Achilles tendon rupture.

References

Alburquerque-Sendin F, Fernandez-de-las-Peñas C, Santos-del-Rey M, et al. 2009. Immediate effects of bilateral manipulation of talocrural joints on standing stability in healthy subjects. Man Ther 14: 75–80.

Bonnin M, Judet T, Colombier JA, et al. 2004. Midterm results of the Salto Total Ankle Prosthesis. Clin Orthop Relat Res 424: 6–18.

Bonnin MP, Laurent JR, Casillas M. 2009. Ankle function and sports activity after total ankle arthroplasty. Foot Ankle Int 30: 933–944.

Bostick GP, Jomha NM, Suchak AA, et al. 2010. Factors associated with calf muscle endurance recovery 1 year after Achilles tendon rupture repair. J Orthop Sports Phys Ther 40: 345–351.

Bressel E, Larsen BT, McNair PJ, et al. 2004. Ankle joint proprioception and passive mechanical properties of the calf muscles after an Achilles tendon rupture: a comparison with matched controls. Clin Biomech 19: 284–291.

Bring D, Reno C, Renstrom P, et al. 2010. Prolonged immobilization compromises up-regulation of repair genes after tendon rupture in a rat model. Scand J Med Sci Sports 20: 411–417.

Buechel FF Sr, Buechel FF Jr, Pappas MJ. 2003. Ten-year evaluation of cementless Buechel-Pappas meniscal bearing total ankle replacement. Foot Ankle Int 24: 462–472.

Claridge RJ, Sagherian BH. 2009. Intermediate term outcome of the agility total ankle arthroplasty. Foot Ankle Int 30: 824–835.

Clayton RA, Court-Brown CM. 2008. The epidemiology of musculoskeletal tendinous and ligamentous injuries. Injury 39: 1338–1344.

Cleland JA, Abbott JH, Kidd MO, et al. 2009. Manual physical therapy and exercise versus electrophysical agents and exercise in the management of plantar heel pain: a multicenter randomized clinical trial. J Orthop Sports Phys Ther 39: 573–585.

Cleland JA, Mintken PE, McDevitt A, et al. 2013. Manual physical therapy and exercise versus supervised home exercise in the management of patients with inversion ankle sprain: a multicenter randomized clinical trial. J Orthop Sports Phys Ther 43: 443–455.

Coester LM, Saltzman CL, Leupold J, et al. 2001. Long-term results following ankle arthrodesis for post-traumatic arthritis. J Bone Joint Surg Am 83A: 219–228.

Coetzee J. 2010. Arthritis and arthroplasty: the foot and ankle. Philadelphia, PA: Saunders.

Conti SF, Dazen D, Stewart G, et al. 2008. Proprioception after total ankle arthroplasty. Foot Ankle Int 29: 1069–1073.

Costa ML, MacMillan K, Halliday D, et al. 2006. Randomised controlled trials of immediate weight-bearing mobilisation for rupture of the tendo Achillis. J Bone Joint Surg Br 88: 69–77.

Deangelis JP, Wilson KM, Cox CL, et al. 2009. Achilles tendon rupture in athletes. J Surg Orthop Adv 18: 115–121.

Deyle GD, Allison SC, Matekel R, et al. 2005. Physical therapy treatment effectiveness for osteoarthritis of the knee: a randomized comparison of supervised clinical exercise and manual therapy procedures versus a home exercise program. Phys Ther 85: 1301–1317.

Doets HC, Brand R, Nelissen RG. 2006. Total ankle arthroplasty in inflammatory joint disease with use of two mobile-bearing designs. J Bone Joint Surg Am 88: 1272–1284.

Doets HC, van Middelkoop M, Houdijk H, et al. 2007. Gait analysis after successful mobile bearing total ankle replacement. Foot Ankle Int 28: 313–322.

Dyrby C, Chou LB, Andriacchi TP, et al. 2004. Functional evaluation of the Scandinavian total ankle replacement. Foot Ankle Int 25: 377–381.

Garras DN, Raikin SM, Bhat SB, et al. 2012. MRI is unnecessary for diagnosing acute Achilles tendon ruptures: clinical diagnostic criteria. Clin Orthop Relat Res 470: 2268–2273.

Gittins J, Mann RA. 2002. The history of the STAR total ankle arthroplasty. Foot Ankle Clin 7: 809–816, vii.

Godbout C, Ang O, Frenette J. 2006. Early voluntary exercise does not promote healing in a rat model of Achilles tendon injury. J Appl Physiol 101: 1720–1726.

Hando BR, Gill NW, Walker MJ, et al. 2012. Short- and long-term clinical outcomes following a standardized protocol of orthopedic manual physical therapy and exercise in individuals with osteoarthritis of the hip: a case series. J Man Manip Ther 20: 192–200.

Hensley CP, Kavchak AJ. 2012. Novel use of a manual therapy technique and management of a patient with peroneal tendinopathy: a case report. Man Ther 17: 84–88.

Hintermann B, Valderrabano V. 2003. Total ankle replacement. Foot Ankle Clin 8: 375–405.

Hoch MC, McKeon PO. 2011. Joint mobilization improves spatiotemporal postural control and range of motion in those with chronic ankle instability. J Orthop Res 29: 326–332.

Horisberger M, Valderrabano V, Hintermann B. 2009. Posttraumatic ankle osteoarthritis after ankle-related fractures. J Orthop Trauma 23: 60–67.

Horstmann T, Lukas C, Merk J, et al. 2012. Deficits 10-years after Achilles tendon repair. Int J Sports Med 33: 474–479.

Hubbard TJ, Hicks-Little C, Cordova M. 2009. Mechanical and sensorimotor implications with ankle osteoarthritis. Arch Phys Med Rehabil 90: 1136–1141.

Jiang N, Wang B, Chen A, et al. 2012. Operative versus nonoperative treatment for acute Achilles tendon rupture: a meta-analysis based on current evidence. Int Orthop 36: 765–773.

Kangas J, Pajala A, Ohtonen P, et al. 2007. Achilles tendon elongation after rupture repair: a randomized comparison of 2 postoperative regimens. Am J Sports Med 35: 59–64.

Kearney RS, Costa ML. 2012. Current concepts in the rehabilitation of an acute rupture of the tendo Achillis. J Bone Joint Surg Br 94: 28–31.

Kim BS, Choi WJ, Kim J, et al. 2013. Residual pain due to soft-tissue impingement after uncomplicated total ankle replacement. Bone Joint J 95B: 378–383.

Kongsgaard M, Aagaard P, Kjaer M, et al. 2005. Structural Achilles tendon properties in athletes subjected to different exercise modes and in Achilles tendon rupture patients. J Appl Physiol 99: 1965–1971.

Kraemer R, Wuerfel W, Lorenzen J, et al. 2012. Analysis of hereditary and medical risk factors in Achilles tendinopathy and Achilles tendon ruptures: a matched pair analysis. Arch Orthop Trauma Surg 132: 847–853.

Lee JH, Jeong BO. 2012. Radiologic changes of ankle joint after total knee arthroplasty. Foot Ankle Int 33: 1087–1092.

López-Rodriguez S, Fernandez de-las-Peñas C, Alburquerque-Sendin F, et al. 2007. Immediate effects of manipulation of the talocrural joint on stabilometry and baropodometry in patients with ankle sprain. J Manipulative Physiol Ther 30: 186–192.

Loudon JK, Reiman MP, Sylvain J. 2014. The efficacy of manual joint mobilisation / manipulation in treatment of lateral ankle sprains: a systematic review. Br J Sports Med 48(5): 365–370. doi: 10.1136/bjsports-2013-092763.

MacDonald CW, Whitman JM, Cleland JA, et al. 2006. Clinical outcomes following manual physical therapy and exercise for hip osteoarthritis: a case series. J Orthop Sports Phys Ther 36: 588–599.

Maffulli N, Longo UG, Maffulli GD, et al. 2011. Achilles tendon ruptures in elite athletes. Foot Ankle Int 32: 9–15.

Maquirriain J. 2011. Achilles tendon rupture: avoiding tendon lengthening during surgical repair and rehabilitation. Yale J Biol Med 84: 289–300.

Masui T, Hasegawa Y, Yamaguchi J, et al. 2006. Increasing postural sway in rural-community-dwelling elderly persons with knee osteoarthritis. J Orthop Sci 11: 353–358.

Mortensen HM, Skov O, Jensen PE. 1999. Early motion of the ankle after operative treatment of a rupture of the Achilles tendon. A prospective, randomized clinical and radiographic study. J Bone Joint Surg Am 81: 983–990.

Mullaney M, Tyler TF, McHugh M, et al. 2011. Electromyographic analysis of the triceps surae muscle complex during Achilles tendon rehabilitation program exercises. Sports Health 3: 543–546.

Owens B, Mountcastle S, White D. 2007. Racial differences in tendon rupture incidence. Int J Sports Med 28: 617–620.

Pyevich MT, Saltzman CL, Callaghan JJ, et al. 1998. Total ankle arthroplasty: a unique design. Two to twelve-year follow-up. J Bone Joint Surg Am 80: 1410–1420.

Saltzman CL, McIff TE, Buckwalter JA, et al. 2000. Total ankle replacement revisited. J Orthop Sports Phys Ther 30: 56–67.

San Giovanni TP, Keblish DJ, Thomas WH, et al. 2006. Eight-year results of a minimally constrained total ankle arthroplasty. Foot Ankle Int 27: 418–426.

Silbernagel KG, Steele R, Manal K. 2012. Deficits in heel-rise height and Achilles tendon elongation occur in patients recovering from an Achilles tendon rupture. Am J Sports Med 40: 1564–1571.

Soroceanu A, Sidhwa F, Aarabi S, et al. 2012. Surgical versus nonsurgical treatment of acute Achilles tendon rupture: a meta-analysis of randomized trials. J Bone Joint Surg Am 94: 2136–2143.

Sorrenti SJ. 2006. Achilles tendon rupture: effect of early mobilization in rehabilitation after surgical repair. Foot Ankle Int 27: 407–410.

Sproule JA, Chin T, Amin A, et al. 2013. Clinical and radiographic outcomes of the mobility total ankle arthroplasty system: early results from a prospective multicenter study. Foot Ankle Int 34: 491–497.

Strom AC, Casillas MM. 2009. Achilles tendon rehabilitation. Foot Ankle Clin 14: 773–782.

Suchak AA, Bostick G, Reid D, et al. 2005. The incidence of Achilles tendon ruptures in Edmonton, Canada. Foot Ankle Int 26: 932–936.

Suchak AA, Spooner C, Reid DC, et al. 2006. Postoperative rehabilitation protocols for Achilles tendon ruptures: a meta-analysis. Clin Orthop Relat Res 445: 216–221.

Suchak AA, Bostick GP, Beaupre LA, et al. 2008. The influence of early weight-bearing compared with non-weight-bearing after surgical repair of the Achilles tendon. J Bone Joint Surg Am 90: 1876–1883.

Thomas RH, Daniels TR. 2003. Ankle arthritis. J Bone Joint Surg Am 85-A: 923–936.

Valderrabano V, Hintermann B, Nigg BM, et al. 2003. Kinematic changes after fusion and total replacement of the ankle: part 1: range of motion. Foot Ankle Int 24: 881–887.

Valderrabano V, Pagenstert G, Horisberger M, et al. 2006. Sports and recreation activity of ankle arthritis patients before and after total ankle replacement. Am J Sports Med 34: 993–999.

Valderrabano V, Nigg BM, von Tscharner V, et al. 2007. Total ankle replacement in ankle osteoarthritis: an analysis of muscle rehabilitation. Foot Ankle Int 28: 281–291.

Vicenzino B, Branjerdporn M, Teys P, et al. 2006. Initial changes in posterior talar glide and dorsiflexion of the ankle after mobilization with movement in individuals with recurrent ankle sprain. J Orthop Sports Phys Ther 36: 464–471.

White DW, Wenke JC, Mosely DS, et al. 2007. Incidence of major tendon ruptures and anterior cruciate ligament tears in US Army soldiers. Am J Sports Med 35: 1308–1314.

Whitman JM, Cleland JA, Mintken PE et al. 2009. Predicting short-term response to thrust and nonthrust manipulation and exercise in patients post inversion ankle sprain. J Orthop Sports Phys Ther 39: 188–200.

Wood PL, Deakin S. 2003. Total ankle replacement. The results in 200 ankles. J Bone Joint Surg Br 85: 334–341.

Yeo HK, Wright A. 2011. Hypoalgesic effect of a passive accessory mobilisation technique in patients with lateral ankle pain. Man Ther 16: 373–377.

Chapter 57

Manipulation of the Foot and Ankle

William Egan, Wayne Hing, Jack Miller, Joshua A. Cleland

CHAPTER CONTENTS

Introduction	637
Manipulation/mobilizations	637
Ankle sprains	637
Ankle fractures	638
Plantar heel pain	638
Cuboid syndrome	638
Foot and ankle tendinopathies	639
Other disorders of the forefoot	639
Clinical decision making for manipulation of foot and ankle disorders	639
Passive joint manipulation/mobilization techniques of the talocrural joint	639
Talocrural distraction thrust manipulation	639
Talocrural posterior glide non-thrust manipulation	640
Talocrural lateral glide non-thrust manipulation	640
Mobilization with movement techniques of the talocrural joint	640
Non-weight-bearing talocrural posterior glide mobilization with movement	641
Weight-bearing talocrural posterior glide mobilization with movement	641
Passive manipulation/mobilization techniques of other ankle and foot joints	641
Subtalar joint lateral glide non-thrust manipulation	641
Proximal tibiofibular thrust manipulation	642
Distal tibiofibular non-thrust manipulation	642
Cuboid thrust manipulation	642
First metatarsal phalangeal non-thrust and thrust manipulation	643
Distal tibiofibular mobilization with movement: 'sprained ankle'	643
Self-mobilization interventions	643
Weight-bearing dorsiflexion mobility assessment	643
Talocrural dorsiflexion self-mobilization	644
Subtalar lateral glide self-mobilization	644

Introduction

Disorders involving the ankle and foot are common in both athletic and non-athletic populations. Patients with these disorders often present with joint mobility impairments that are potentially amenable to joint mobilization or manipulation. Practitioners of manual therapy and manual therapy textbooks have described techniques of manipulation for foot and ankle disorders for some time (Hengeveld & Banks 2005; Mulligan 2010; Boyles et al 2013). However, manipulation for foot and ankle disorders is an area that has only recently become more studied in the literature. Emerging, high-quality evidence suggests that manipulation can be an effective intervention as part of a multimodal programme involving education and therapeutic exercise for several different foot and ankle disorders (Brantingham et al 2012). These disorders include: ankle sprains, ankle fractures, plantar heel pain and forefoot pain. In this chapter we will first provide an overview of the evidence and rationale for manipulation in the management of foot and ankle disorders. Following this, descriptions and figures of the more commonly used foot and ankle manipulation techniques will be provided, based on the literature and the authors' clinical experience. (For information concerning differential diagnosis and further management of foot and ankle disorders, the reader is directed to other chapters in this book that cover these topics in detail.)

Manipulation/Mobilizations

Ankle sprains

Lateral ankle sprains are one of the most common traumatic lower extremity injuries in athletic and active populations. Individuals with acute to chronic lateral ankle sprains often present with impairments in ankle mobility. The most commonly reported mobility impairment is a limitation in ankle dorsiflexion mobility (Denegar et al 2002). A limitation of the accessory joint glide of the talus within the ankle mortise has been proposed to lead to a limitation in ankle dorsiflexion mobility. Specifically the talus is proposed to glide posteriorly within the mortise during ankle dorsiflexion and a limitation of this glide could lead to a reduction in dorsiflexion mobility. Motion occurring at the proximal and distal articulation between the fibula and tibia also contributes to ankle dorsiflexion mobility. Limitations in mobility at these articulations resulting from the consequences of an ankle sprain injury could also theoretically lead to a decrease in ankle dorsiflexion mobility. As a result of these impairments, manual therapy techniques for individuals with ankle sprains have often been directed towards the talocrural joint and the proximal and distal tibiofibular joints in attempts to improve ankle joint dorsiflexion range of motion. Evidence from several studies, summarized in a systematic review by Loudon et al (2014), indicates that manipulation leads to an improvement in ankle joint range of motion including dorsiflexion. In addition to an improvement in ankle dorsiflexion mobility, manipulation, combined with an impairment-based exercise programme, leads to a clinically meaningful improvement in self-reported function and a decrease in pain for individuals with acute, subacute and chronic lateral ankle sprains (Brantingham et al 2012; Loudon et al 2014).

In one of the best-quality studies to date, Cleland et al (2013) reported the results of eight sessions of manual therapy and supervised exercise compared with a control programme of four sessions of therapist-taught home exercises for 74 individuals with inversion ankle sprain injuries. Individuals between the ages of 16 and 60 years who had sustained a grade I or II inversion ankle sprain and who reported at least a 3 out 10 on the Numerical Rating of Pain Scale (NRPS) were included. Individuals with fractures, grade III sprains or contraindications to manual therapy were excluded. The manual therapy techniques included the following: ankle distraction thrust manipulation (see Fig. 57.1), talocrural posterior glide non-thrust manipulation (weight-bearing and non-weight-bearing; see Figs 57.2–57.4), talocrural and subtalar lateral glide non-thrust manipulation (see Figs 57.3–57.5), a proximal tibiofibular thrust manipulation (see Fig. 57.6) and a distal tibiofibular anterior–posterior non-thrust manipulation (see Fig. 57.7). The manipulations were delivered once per session and the non-thrust manipulation were typically dosed as Maitland grades III–IV and provided for five bouts of 30 seconds each. Individuals in the manual therapy group were also provided with self-mobilization exercises targeting the talocrural (see Fig. 57.12) and subtalar joints (see Fig. 57.13). The exercise programme was identical for both groups and consisted of mobility, strengthening, balance and coordination exercises that were progressed over time. Both groups reported decreased pain and improved function at 4-week and 6-month follow-up. However, the manual therapy group reported a clinically significant difference in pain and function compared with the control group at 4-week and 6-month follow-ups. Although there were some limitations, including a potential attention bias for the manual therapy group, this study adds to the evidence for the effectiveness of manipulation for individuals with lateral ankle sprains. (See Ch 54 for more discussion on management of ankle sprains.)

Ankle fractures

Ankle fractures are a common disorder leading to significant loss of function and disability. Similar to and more severe than ankle sprains, ankle fractures often result in a loss of ankle mobility as a result of the prolonged immobilization following the fracture and / or surgery (Lin et al 2010). Manual therapy in the management of ankle fractures has not been well studied, but some literature does exist. In a randomized clinical trial, Lin et al (2008) reported that grade III anterior–posterior talocrural joint non-thrust manipulation combined with a supervised exercise programme did not enhance patient outcomes compared with exercise alone for patients who were post immobilization for ankle fractures of varying severity. In a pilot study involving 10 patients, Wilson (1991) reported that adding a variety of non-thrust manipulation techniques targeting the talocrural, subtalar and additional lower extremity joints to a standard exercise programme led to an improvement in ankle dorsiflexion range of motion, but not function, compared with exercise alone. Additional research investigating the use of a variety of manipulation techniques for individuals with ankle fractures is required before definitive conclusions can be reached.

Plantar heel pain

Plantar heel pain is a very common non-traumatic foot disorder. Typical treatment involves rest, medication, stretching exercises, soft tissue mobilization, electrothermal modalities and foot orthotics (McPoil et al 2008). Plantar heel pain can be associated with mobility impairments in the ankle and foot joints, and a limitation in ankle dorsiflexion is a risk factor for developing plantar heel pain. Given these mobility impairments, manipulation could potentially have a role in the management of plantar heel pain. In a case series by Young et al (2004) and in randomized clinical trials by Cleland et al (2009) and Dimou et al (2004), manual therapy directed to the foot and ankle was shown to lead to both short- and long-term improvement in pain and self-reported function. In the Cleland et al (2009) study, patients were randomized to receive either six treatments of manual therapy, including soft tissue mobilization and impairment-based lower extremity joint manipulation combined with exercise, or electrothermal modalities and exercise. At 4-week and 6-month follow-up there was a clinically meaningful difference in pain and patient-reported function in favour of the manual therapy intervention. Manipulation techniques common to all of these studies included talocrural joint distraction thrust manipulation (see Fig. 57.1), talocrural joint posterior glide non-thrust manipulation (see Fig. 57.2) and subtalar lateral glide non-thrust manipulation (see Fig. 57.5). Proposed mechanisms for manipulation in the management of plantar heel pain include biomechanical, with an increase in ankle and rearfoot mobility, and neurophysiological, via descending pain modulation (Bialosky et al 2009). (See Ch 55 for more discussion on the management of plantar heel pain.)

Cuboid syndrome

Cuboid syndrome is an uncommon but potentially very painful and disabling disorder (Jennings & Davies 2005; Adams & Madden 2009). It is proposed to be caused by a forceful contraction of the fibularis longus tendon pulling on the cuboid bone, either in reaction to an inversion ankle sprain or during an end-range plantar flexion manoeuvre such as in ballet dancing. The result is plantar–lateral foot pain located in the vicinity of the cuboid bone and its articulations. Clinical examination findings include point tenderness on the dorsal, lateral or plantar aspect of the cuboid bone along with symptom reproduction during manual accessory gliding of the cuboid. It is proposed that the cuboid mobility becomes limited, particularly in a plantar to dorsal direction, and that manipulation of the cuboid (see Fig. 57.8) can be effective in relieving pain from this disorder. Observational case series studies have reported an immediate and lasting improvement in pain and function following a plantar–dorsal cuboid manipulation.

Foot and ankle tendinopathies

There is no current evidence that manipulation can be effective in the management of foot or ankle tendinopathies such as Achilles tendon or posterior tibial tendinopathy. However, using an impairment-based approach the clinician may find a limitation in ankle and foot joint mobility, such as limited ankle dorsiflexion, and use manipulation as part of an intervention programme in the management of these disorders. Further research is needed to investigate this proposal.

Other disorders of the forefoot

Common disorders of the forefoot include metatarsalgia, hallux valgus and hallux rigidus. These disorders may involve mobility restrictions of the ankle, rearfoot, midfoot, and inter-metatarsal and metatarsal phalangeal joints. In a systematic review, Brantingham et al (2012) reported that there was grade C or limited evidence for manipulation in the management of these disorders based on poor-to-moderate-quality studies. Du Plessis et al (2011) described a progressive manipulation technique directed to the first metatarsal phalangeal joint in the management of hallux valgus (see Fig. 57.9). Additional high-quality research is needed to investigate the use of manipulation in the management of forefoot disorders.

Clinical Decision Making for Manipulation of Foot and Ankle Disorders

When determining which techniques or what grades of manipulation to apply in a patient with a foot or ankle disorder, the authors recommend that clinicians take into account all relevant variables that may affect clinical decision making. The clinician should also consider any contraindications to manipulation for patients with foot and ankle disorders. For example, in the Cleland et al (2013) study on manipulation for patients with inversion ankle sprains, the following were exclusion criteria for being enrolled in the study: grade III sprain, tumour, fracture, rheumatoid arthritis, osteoporosis, prolonged history of steroid use, and severe vascular disease. Selection of the techniques is based on the relevant impairments found by the clinician during the physical examination. For example, a therapist may decide to utilize a talocrural posterior glide non-thrust manipulation technique for a patient with an acute ankle sprain who has a limitation in ankle dorsiflexion with a restricted posterior talar glide. Dosage of the manual therapy technique, including the grade of mobilization, duration, frequency and number of bouts, will depend on the patient's response in addition to the clinician's determination of the patient's irritability (Hengeveld & Banks 2005). It is suggested that clinicians attempt to use the most comfortable technique with the least amount of force to accomplish the desired goal and to progress the vigour of any technique over time using the patient's response as a guide. The use of a functional asterisk or concordant sign can be very helpful in guiding technique selection and progression. An example of a commonly used functional asterisk sign is a lunge (see Fig. 57.11), which gauges the patient's ability to perform weight-bearing ankle dorsiflexion (Chisholm et al 2012). The clinician could utilize this as a functional assessment before and after manipulation to determine whether a within-session change in that functional impairment has occurred. Techniques proven to be successful within session should then be augmented with a specific exercise that targets the same impairment as the manual therapy technique. For example, if a talocrural posterior glide non-thrust manipulation led to a within-session improvement in weight-bearing dorsiflexion such as during a lunge, the patient would be instructed in an ankle dorsiflexion self-mobilization (see Fig. 57.12). Another self-mobilization technique common among several of the research studies described in this chapter is the subtalar lateral glide self-mobilization (see Fig. 57.13). It is important to reiterate that manipulation would form only a single part of a comprehensive rehabilitation programme for patients with foot and ankle disorders. It has been proposed that manual therapy leading to decreased pain and improved mobility serves as a catalyst to the patient actively engaging in rehabilitation (Bialosky et al 2009). The following sections of this chapter describe some of the more commonly utilized manipulation techniques, based on research evidence and clinical experience. For additional techniques and detailed information, readers are referred to various manual therapy texts (e.g. Hengeveld & Banks 2005; Mulligan 2010; Boyles et al 2013).

Passive Joint Manipulation/Mobilization Techniques of the Talocrural Joint

Talocrural distraction thrust manipulation (Fig. 57.1)

This technique is indicated when there is limited ankle dorsiflexion and restricted posterior accessory glide of the talus. The patient is supine-lying, with the ankle off the end of the treatment table. The therapist is standing at end of bed in a walk / stride stance. The clinician uses both hands to grasp the patient's ankle / foot with the fingers interlaced around the dorsum of the foot and the thumbs on the plantar aspect. The therapist induces pronation and dorsiflexion of the patient's foot and takes up the slack in a caudal / distraction direction. The clinician applies a high-velocity, low amplitude force in a caudal direction.

Notes: For individuals with lateral ankle sprains, the lateral ligaments and soft tissue structures are protected by dorsiflexion and eversion / pronation of the foot / ankle. The manipulation should not be performed if a patient reports an increase in pain during the set-up. A modification where the thrust is delivered in a combined caudal and posterior direction (J-stroke) may be useful if initial attempts do not achieve an improvement in ankle dorsiflexion.

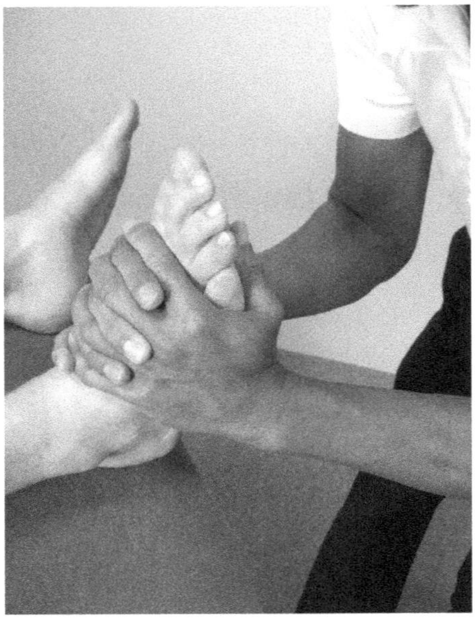

Figure 57.1 Talocrural distraction thrust manipulation.

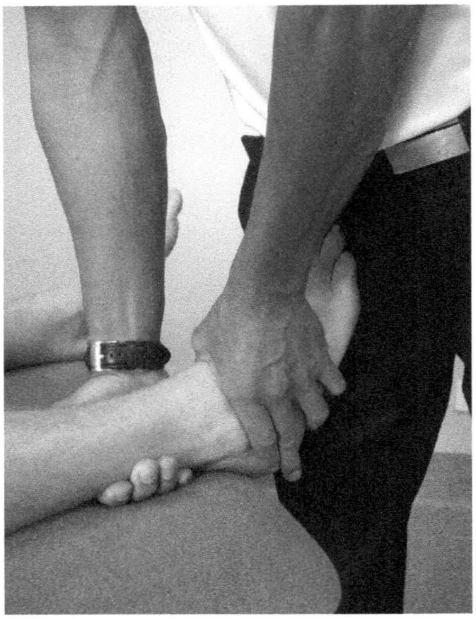

Figure 57.2 Talocrural posterior glide non-thrust manipulation.

Talocrural posterior glide non-thrust manipulation (Fig. 57.2)

This technique is indicated when the patient exhibits limited ankle dorsiflexion, and restricted posterior accessory glide of the talus. The patient is supine-lying, with the ankle off the end of the treatment table. The therapist is standing at end of bed in a walk / stride stance. The clinician uses one hand to stabilize the lower leg firmly at the malleoli and grasps the anterior, medial and lateral talus with the web space of the opposite hand. The therapist now applies a low-velocity, anterior–posterior oscillatory force to the talus.

Notes: The clinician can use his / her thigh to help stabilize the foot and to increase the amount of ankle dorsiflexion progressively, and may need to adjust the amount of foot / ankle supination / pronation to optimize the technique.

Talocrural lateral glide non-thrust manipulation (Fig. 57.3)

This technique is indicated when the patient exhibits restricted talocrural inversion or eversion. The patient is side-lying on the involved side, with the ankle / foot off the end of the treatment plinth. The therapist is standing over the patient's ankle / foot. The clinician grasps the patient's medial malleoli just proximal to the talocrural joint with the index finger / thumb and uses the forearm to stabilize the patient's leg against the table. The clinician also places the thenar eminence of the opposite hand on the talus just distal to the medial malleoli and grasps the rearfoot. The clinician uses his / her body to impart a low-velocity oscillatory force to the talus through the arm and thenar eminence.

Notes: It may be useful for the therapist to apply slight distraction of the talus with the mobilizing hand prior to applying the lateral glide. The patient's ankle / foot can be stabilized in neutral by the therapist's thigh.

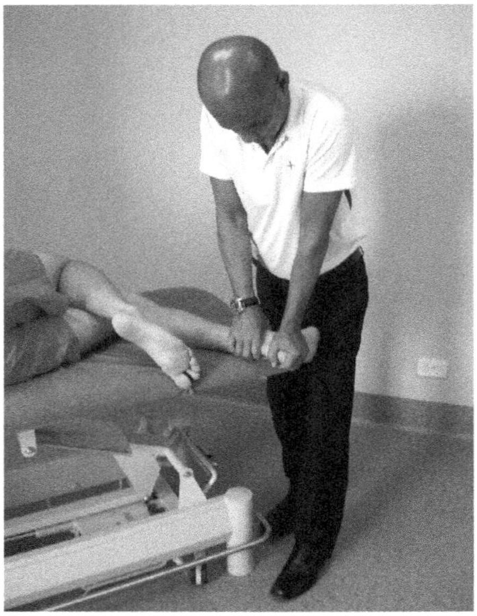

Figure 57.3 Talocrural lateral glide non-thrust manipulation.

Mobilization with Movement Techniques of the Talocrural Joint

Both weight-bearing and non-weight-bearing mobilization with movement techniques have been demonstrated to be of significant value in the restoration of ankle dorsiflexion range when measured in functional weight-bearing (Collins et al 2004; Reid et al 2007). Early research indicates that mobilization with movement may also be effective in the management of a distal tibia–fibular derangement post ankle inversion sprain (Hubbard et al 2006; Vincenzino et al 2006; Hubbard & Hertel 2008).

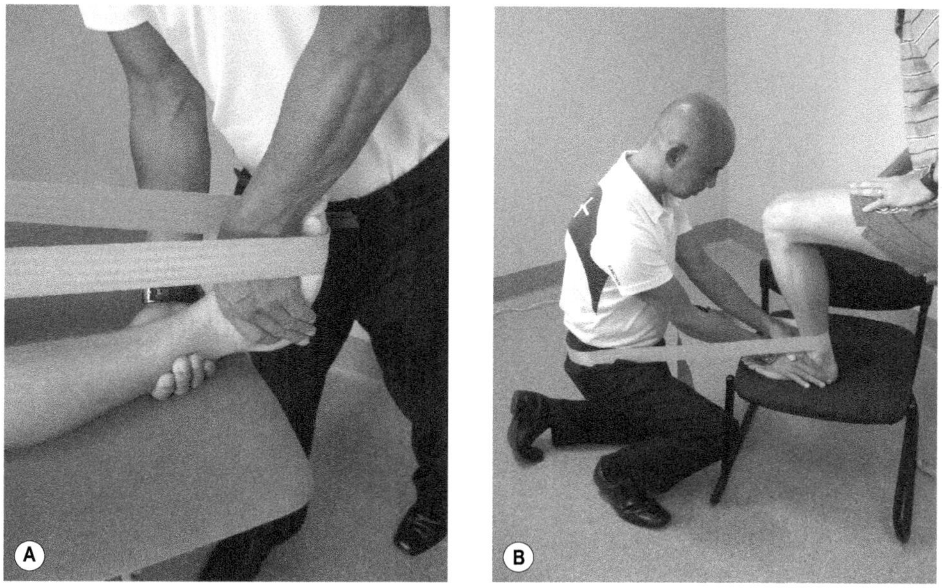

Figure 57.4 **Talocrural posterior glide mobilization with movement:** (**A**) non-weight-bearing, (**B**) weight-bearing.

Non-weight-bearing talocrural posterior glide mobilization with movement (Fig. 57.4A)

This technique is indicated when the patient exhibits limited ankle dorsiflexion and restricted posterior accessory glide of the talus. The patient is supine-lying, with the ankle off the end of the treatment table. The therapist is standing at end of bed in a walk / stride stance. The clinician grasps the talus with one hand and the calcaneus with the other. The talus is glided posterior–medially in the plane of the ankle joint with no pain reproduction. While maintaining the posterior glide, the patient is requested to assist in the performance of ankle dorsiflexion through the pull of a mobilization belt, but not active dorsiflexion.

Note: If this passive dorsiflexion is also pain free, overpressure of dorsiflexion may be applied by pressure from the therapist's thigh on the sole of the foot.

Weight-bearing talocrural posterior glide mobilization with movement (Fig. 57.4B)

This technique is indicated when there is limited ankle dorsiflexion and restricted posterior accessory glide of the talus. The patient is in step-kneeling on the treatment plinth. The therapist stands at the end of the treatment plinth with a mobilization belt looped around the therapist's hips and around the patient's posterior tibia. The patient's talus and midfoot are stabilized by the therapist's hands. The clinician uses a mobilization belt applied to the posterior tibia to effect a pain-free anterior, lateral glide of the tibia. The patient is requested to lunge forwards, effecting passive pain-free ankle dorsiflexion. The therapist must perform a partial squat to maintain the belt parallel to the dynamic tibial joint treatment plane.

Note: Pain-free passive overpressure may be applied by the patient's hands on the knee.

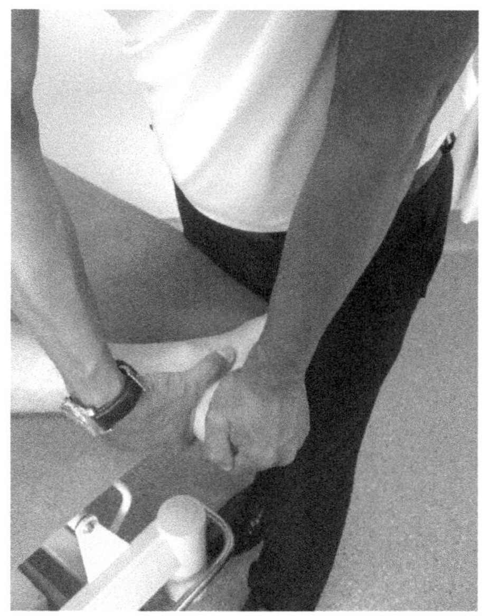

Figure 57.5 **Subtalar joint lateral glide non-thrust manipulation.**

Passive Manipulation / Mobilization Techniques of Other Ankle and Foot Joints

Subtalar joint lateral glide non-thrust manipulation (Fig. 57.5)

This technique is indicated when the patient exhibits restricted talocalcaneal (subtalar) inversion or eversion. The patient is side-lying on the involved side, with the ankle / foot off the end of the treatment plinth. The therapist is standing over the

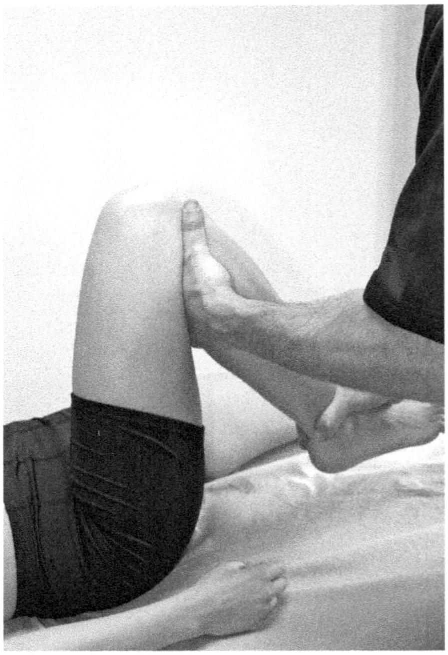

Figure 57.6 Proximal tibiofibular thrust manipulation.

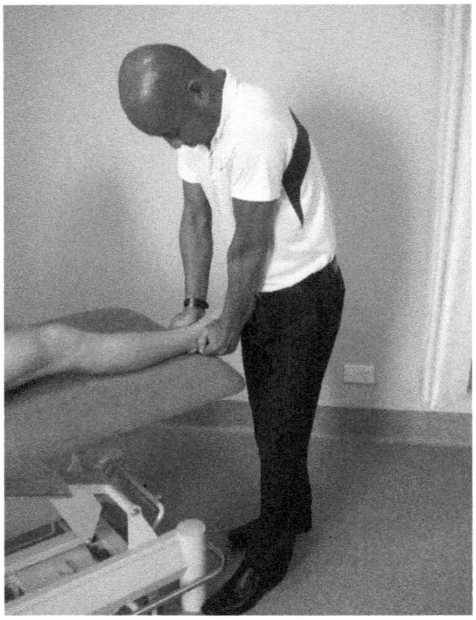

Figure 57.7 Distal tibiofibular non-thrust manipulation.

patient's ankle / foot, then grasps the patient's talus just proximal to the subtalar joint with the index finger / thumb and uses the forearm to stabilize the patient's leg against the table. The clinician places the thenar eminence of the opposite hand on the calcaneus just distal to the talus. The clinician then uses his / her body to impart a low-velocity oscillatory force to the calcaneus through the arm and thenar eminence.

Notes: It may be useful for the therapist to apply slight distraction of the calcaneus with the mobilizing hand prior to applying the lateral glide. The patient's ankle / foot can be stabilized in neutral by the therapist's thigh. The therapist reassesses the patient's rearfoot range of motion pre and post manipulation to determine which of the previous two techniques (talocrural versus subtalar) creates the greatest change in rearfoot mobility.

Proximal tibiofibular thrust manipulation (Fig. 57.6)

This technique is indicated when there is restricted ankle dorsiflexion and restricted accessory glide of the proximal tibiofibular joint. The patient is supine lying with the involved leg flexed at the knee. The therapist stands at the side of the treatment plinth in a walk / stride stance. The clinician places his / her second metacarpophalangeal in the popliteal fossa and pulls the soft tissue laterally until the metacarpophalangeal is firmly stabilized behind the patient's fibular head. The clinician uses the opposite hand to grasp the foot and ankle. The clinician externally rotates the leg and flexes the knee to the restrictive barrier. Once the restrictive barrier is met, a high-velocity, low-amplitude force is applied through the tibia (directing the patient's heel toward his/her ipsilateral buttock).

Note: If the patient has a knee disorder, the clinician should use caution when considering applying this technique, although it can also be used in the treatment of patients with knee pain.

Distal tibiofibular non-thrust manipulation (Fig. 57.7)

This technique is indicated when there is restricted ankle dorsiflexion and restricted accessory glide of the distal tibiofibular joint. The patient is supine-lying, with the involved ankle / foot off the end of the treatment plinth. The therapist is standing at the end of the treatment plinth, then grasps and stabilizes the distal tibia with one hand and places the thenar eminence over the lateral malleolus. The clinician uses his / her body to impart a low-velocity, oscillatory, anterior–posterior force to the fibula on the tibia.

Notes: If the lateral malleolus is tender the clinician can use a towel or foam padding over the lateral malleolus for patient comfort. The clinician can progress the technique by using his / her thigh to dorsiflex the patient's ankle.

Cuboid thrust manipulation (Fig. 57.8)

This technique is indicated when there is cuboid syndrome and restricted accessory glide of the cuboid. The patient lies prone and the therapist stands at the end of the treatment plinth. The clinician places the tips of the thumbs over the medial plantar surface of the patient's cuboid. The patient's knee is flexed to 90°, with the ankle in neutral. The patient's knee is then passively extended as the ankle is plantarflexed with slight supination of the subtalar joint. The therapist applies a high-velocity thrust force to the cuboid with both thumbs in a dorsal lateral direction.

Note: For patients with concomitant lateral ankle sprains, it is important to avoid placing the ankle in end-range plantarflexion and inversion during the manipulation.

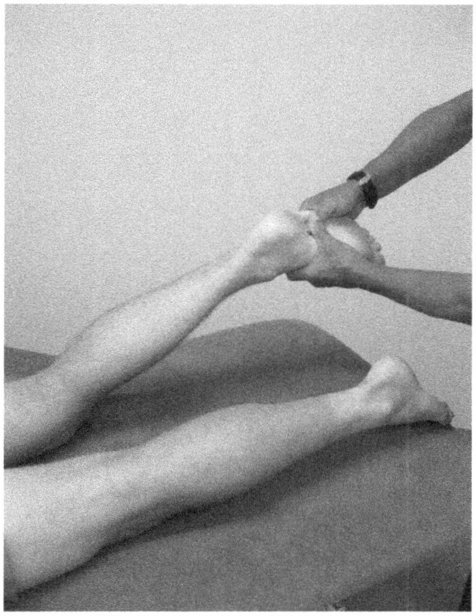

Figure 57.8 Cuboid thrust manipulation.

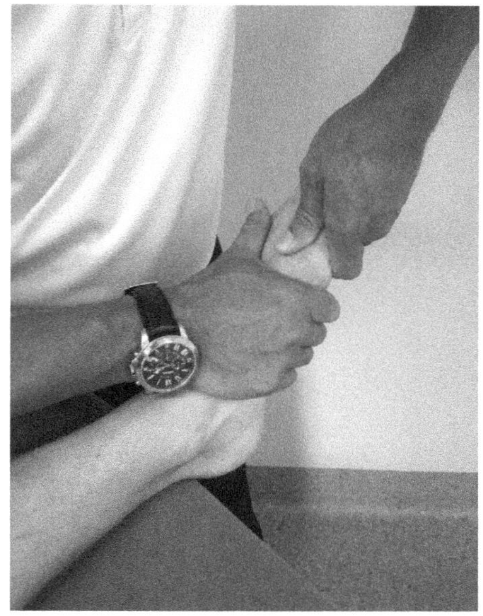

Figure 57.9 First metatarsal phalangeal non-thrust and thrust manipulation.

First metatarsal phalangeal non-thrust and thrust manipulation (Fig. 57.9)

This technique is indicated when the patient exhibits restricted first metatarsal phalangeal joint extension. The patient is supine-lying, with the ankle / foot off the end of treatment plinth. The therapist stands at the end of the treatment plinth. He / she stabilizes the patient's foot and first metatarsal with one hand then, using the second and third fingers of the opposite hand, grasps the patient's first proximal phalanx on the plantar and dorsal aspects. The clinician uses graded, low-velocity oscillatory force in a direction of longitudinal traction.

Notes: For patients with hallux valgus, traction force can be combined a slight medial glide / adduction of the phalanx and lateral glide / abduction of the first metatarsal. Based on the patient's tolerance and response to the non-thrust manipulation, the clinician may impart a high-velocity thrust.

Distal Tibiofibular Mobilization with Movement: 'Sprained Ankle' (Fig. 57.10)

This technique is indicated in lateral ankle sprains and painful / restricted ankle plantar flexion and inversion. The patient is supine-lying with the involved ankle / foot off the end of the treatment plinth. The therapist is standing at the end of the treatment plinth, then contacts the lateral malleolus of the patient with his / her thenar eminence and stabilizes the distal tibia with the other hand. The therapist uses the thenar eminence contact on the lateral malleolus to glide the fibula posteriorly in relation to the stabilized tibia. The foot / ankle will passively dorsiflex and evert during this mobilization secondary to the increased tension in the anterior tibiofibular ligament. While maintaining the pain-free posterior fibular glide, the patient is requested to perform combined plantarflexion and inversion that should now be fully pain free.

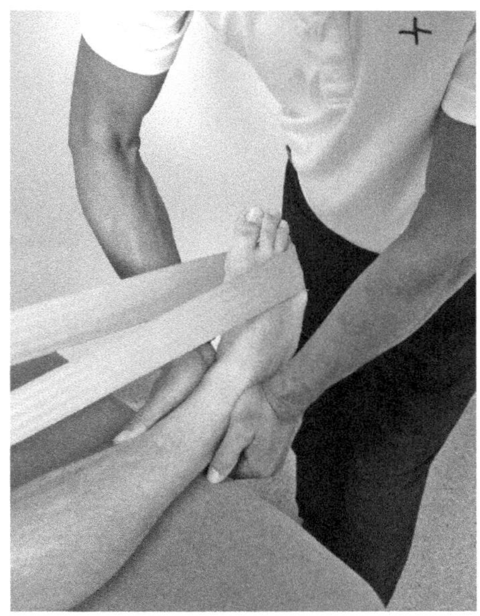

Figure 57.10 Distal tibiofibular mobilization with movement: 'sprained ankle'.

Notes: If the lateral malleolus is tender, the clinician can use a towel or foam padding over the lateral malleolus for patient comfort. Pain-free passive overpressure of the inversion force may be provided by the patient pulling on a mobilization belt and / or the therapist's manual force.

Self-mobilization Interventions

Weight-bearing dorsiflexion mobility assessment (Fig. 57.11)

The patient faces a wall in a lunge position with the involved foot forward. The clinician instructs the patient to lunge

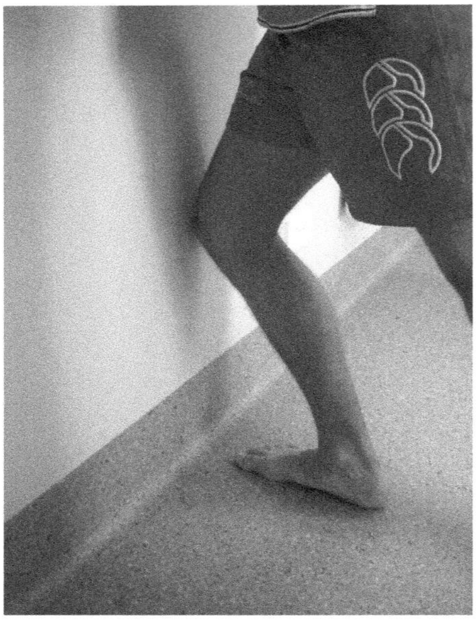

Figure 57.11 **Weight-bearing dorsiflexion mobility assessment.**

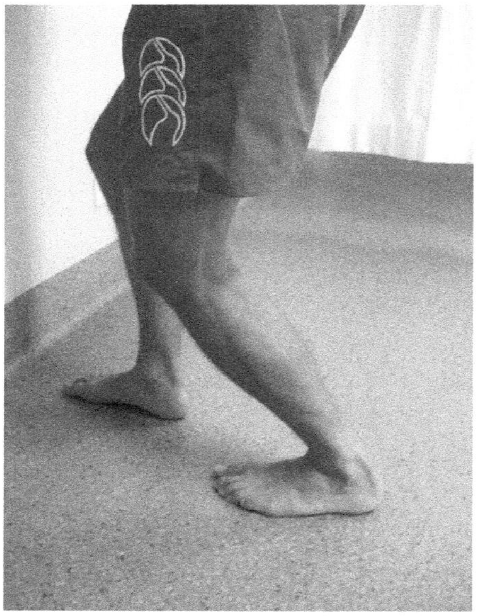

Figure 57.12 **Talocrural dorsiflexion self-mobilization.**

forwards while attempting to touch the knee of the involved side to the wall. The maximum distance between the first toe and the wall in which the patient is able to contact the knee to the wall is recorded. The clinician should ensure that the patient lunges forwards through the talocrural joint and does not compensate by utilizing midfoot pronation.

Talocrural dorsiflexion self-mobilization (Fig. 57.12)

The patient faces a wall with the hands on the wall and places the foot / ankle to be mobilized behind the other, as shown in Figure 57.12. With the foot pointing straight forwards, the patient is instructed to bring the knee forwards while 'driving' the heel down and back. The heel should be kept in contact

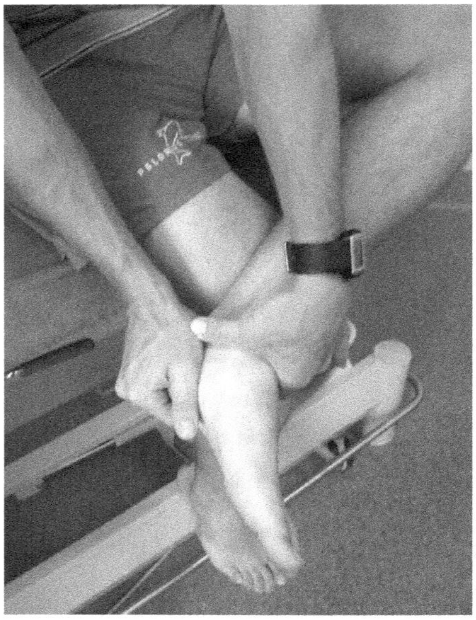

Figure 57.13 **Subtalar lateral glide self-mobilization.**

with the floor. If the patient reports pain in the anterior area of the ankle, he/she can adjust the foot position to minimize the pain and maximize the stretch. The patient is instructed to perform the exercise in an oscillatory fashion for 30 seconds repeating up to three times.

Subtalar lateral glide self-mobilization (Fig. 57.13)

The patient sits and crosses the involved leg over the opposite leg. The patient stabilizes the talus with one hand and grasps the calcaneus with the other hand. The patient is instructed to push the calcaneus towards the floor, and is also instructed to perform the exercise in an oscillatory fashion for 30 seconds, repeating up to three times.

References

Adams E, Madden C. 2009. Cuboid subluxation: a case study and review of the literature. Curr Sports Med Rep 8: 300–307.

Bialosky JE, Bishop MD, Price DD, et al. 2009. The mechanisms of manual therapy in the treatment of musculoskeletal pain: a comprehensive model. Man Ther 14(5): 531–538. doi: 10.1016/j.math.2008.09.001.

Boyles R, Flynn T, Whitman J, et al. 2013. Spinal and extremity manipulation: the basic skill set, 2nd edn. Louisville, KY: Evidence in Motion.

Brantingham JW, Bonnefin D, Perle SM, et al. 2012. Manipulative therapy for lower extremity conditions: an update of a literature review. J Manipulat Physiol Ther 35: 128–166.

Chisholm MD, Birmingham TB, Brown J, et al. 2012. Reliability and validity of a weight-bearing measure of ankle dorsiflexion range of motion. Physiother Can 64: 347–355.

Cleland JA, Mintken PE, McDevitt A, et al. 2013. Manual physical therapy and exercise versus supervised home exercise in the management of patients with inversion ankle sprain: a multicenter randomized clinical trial. J Orthop Sports Phys Ther 43: 443–455.

Cleland JA, Abbott JH, Kidd MO, et al. 2009. Manual physical therapy and exercise versus electro-physical agents and exercise in the management of plantar heel pain: a multicenter randomized clinical trial. J Orthop Sports Phys Ther 39: 573–585.

Collins N, Teys P, Vincenzino B. 2004. The initial effects of a Mulligan's Mobilization with Movement technique on dorsiflexion and pain in sub acute ankle sprains. Man Ther 9: 77–82.

Denegar CR, Hertel J, Fonseca J. 2002. The effect of lateral ankle sprain on dorsiflexion range of motion, posterior talar glide, and joint laxity. J Orthop Sports Phys Ther 32: 166–173.
Dimou E, Brantingham J, Wood T. 2004. A randomized controlled trial (with blinded observer) of chiropractic manipulation and Achilles stretching vs. orthotics for the treatment of plantar fasciitis. J Am Chiropr Assoc 41: 32–42.
du Plessis M, Zipfe B, Brantingham JW. 2011. Manual and manipulative therapy compared to night splint for symptomatic hallux abductor valgus: an exploratory randomised clinical trial. Foot 21: 71–78.
Hengeveld E, Banks K. 2005. Maitland's peripheral manipulation, 4th edn. Edinburgh: Elsevier Butterworth-Heinemann.
Hubbard T, Hertel J. 2008. Anterior positional fault of the fibula after sub-acute lateral ankle sprains. Man Ther 13: 63–67.
Hubbard T, Hertel J, Sherbondy P. 2006. Fibular position in individuals with self-reported chronic ankle instability. J Orthop Sports Phys Ther 36: 3–9.
Jennings J, Davies GJ. 2005. Treatment of cuboid syndrome secondary to lateral ankle sprains: a case series. J Orthop Sports Phys Ther 35: 409–415.
Lin CW, Moseley AM, Haas M, et al. 2008. Manual therapy in addition to physiotherapy does not improve clinical or economic outcomes after ankle fracture. J Rehabil Med 40: 433–439.
Lin CW, Hiller CE, de Bie R. 2010. Evidence-based treatment for ankle injuries: a clinical perspective. J Man Manip Ther 18: 22–28.
Loudon JK, Reiman MP, Sylvain J. 2014. The efficacy of manual joint mobilisation / manipulation in treatment of lateral ankle sprains: a systematic review. Br J Sports Med 48(5): 365–370. doi: 10.1136/bjsports-2013-092763.
McPoil TG, Martin RL, Cornwall MW, et al. 2008. Heel pain-plantar fasciitis: clinical practice guidelines linked to the international classification of function, disability, and health from the orthopaedic section of the American Physical Therapy Association. J Orthop Sports Phys Ther 38: A1–A18.
Mulligan BR. 2010. Manual therapy, NAGS, SNAGS, MWM, etc., 6th edn. Minneapolis, MN: Orthopedic Physical Therapy Products.
Reid A, Brimingham T, Alcock G. 2007. Efficacy of mobilization with movement for patients with limited dorsiflexion after ankle sprain: a crossover trial. Physiother Can 59: 166–172.
Vincenzino B, Branjerdporn M, Teys P, et al. 2006. Initial changes in posterior talar glide and dorsiflexion of the ankle after mobilization with movement in individuals with recurrent ankle sprain. J Orthop Sports Phys Ther 36: 464–471.
Wilson F. 1991. Manual therapy versus traditional exercises in mobilization of the ankle post fracture: a pilot study. NZ J Physiother 19: 11–16.
Young B, Walker MJ, Strunce J, et al. 2004. A combined treatment approach emphasizing impairment-based manual physical therapy for plantar heel pain: a case series. A combined treatment approach emphasizing impairment-based manual physical therapy for plantar heel pain: a case series. J Orthop Sports Phys Ther 34: 725–733.

58 Chapter

Tendinopathy of the Foot and Ankle

Ellen Pong

CHAPTER CONTENTS

Introduction	646
Achilles tendinopathy	646
Background	646
Anatomy	647
Pathology and patho-biomechanics	647
Diagnosis	647
Treatment and prognosis	648
Peroneal tendinopathy	649
Background	649
Anatomy	649
Pathology and patho-biomechanics	650
Diagnosis	650
Treatment and prognosis	651
Tibialis anterior tendinopathy	651
Background	651
Anatomy	652
Pathology and patho-biomechanics	652
Diagnosis	652
Treatment and prognosis	652
Tibialis posterior tendinopathy	653
Background	653
Anatomy	653
Pathology and patho-biomechanics	653
Diagnosis	653
Treatment and prognosis	654
Other tendinopathies of the foot and ankle	654
Background	654
Anatomy	654
Pathology and patho-biomechanics	654
Diagnosis	654
Treatment and prognosis	655
Conclusion	655

Introduction

Tendinopathies of the foot and ankle represent an incredibly diverse and complex group of pathologies. The causes include systemic disease causing pathological tissue changes, intrinsic faulty biomechanics of the individual patient causing improper use, and daily habits and activities causing overuse or acute trauma The spectrum of tendinopathies commonly seen in the foot and ankle includes inflammatory and degenerative insults to the tendon and, with seemingly greater frequency than anywhere else in the body, tendon ruptures. These pathologies can end an athlete's career, or create a number of fall hazards in an elderly person's daily routine. The proportion of tendinopathies requiring surgical intervention either outright or after failed conservative treatment appears highest in the foot and ankle. It is important to know the specific characteristics of each tendon's pathological presentation and needs in treatment in order to best serve this patient population.

Achilles Tendinopathy

Background

Achilles tendinopathy is a prevalent condition in sports involving running and jumping (van Sterkenburg & van Dijk 2011). The risk of long-distance runners for developing an Achilles tendinopathy is estimated to be 52% (van Sterkenburg & van Dijk 2011). The risk is not confined to athletes, however. One-third of patients with Achilles tendinopathies have sedentary lifestyles (van Sterkenburg & van Dijk 2011; Papa 2012). People in their middle years (aged 30–50), regardless of physical activity level, are the most affected (van Sterkenburg & van Dijk 2011; Papa 2012). Physical deconditioning, acute injury, repeated overuse, comorbidities, corticosteroid injection and intrinsic risk factors are all implicated in development of Achilles tendinopathies (Hart 2011; van Sterkenburg & van Dijk 2011; Papa 2012).

Achilles tendinopathies are represented in the literature under a confusion of names. Van Dijk et al (2011) proposed a new terminology with specific locations, symptoms, clinical findings and histopathology; mid-portion Achilles tendinopathy; Achilles paratendinopathy, acute and chronic; insertional Achilles tendinopathy; retrocalcaneal bursitis involving the anterior inferior aspect of the Achilles tendon; and superficial calcaneal bursitis comprise the list of currently preferred terminology. Additionally, there is also a recommendation to abandon previous terms such as Haglund's disease, Haglund's syndrome, Haglund's deformity, and pump bump (calcaneus altus, high-prow heels, knobbly heels, cucumber heel) (van Dijk et al 2011).

Anatomy

The Achilles tendon is a combined tendon of two muscle origins: the soleus and the gastrocnemius (van Sterkenburg & van Dijk 2011). Both the gastrocnemius and the soleus form an aponeurosis, from which the two tendons of the combined Achilles tendon originate. The gastrocnemius muscle originates from the posterior medial and lateral femoral condyles, crosses the knee, subtalar and ankle joints, and inserts within the combined tendon onto the calcaneus. The soleus muscle originates from the proximal tibia, fibula and interosseous membrane, crosses the ankle and subtalar joints, and also inserts within the combined tendon onto the calcaneus (van Sterkenburg & van Dijk 2011).

The Achilles tendon begins to rotate and becomes more marked 2–7 cm proximal to its insertion. Within the tendon, the gastrocnemius fibres rotate to the lateral side and the soleus fibres are rotated to the medial side of the tendon's insertion. The Achilles tendon, via the gastrocnemius and soleus muscles, is the primary plantarflexor of the ankle. Insertional shapes for the Achilles tendon have been described as 'oval' in many anatomy texts. Lohrer et al (2008) viewed images of the insertion from the transverse plane, and reported a slightly bent or unbowed tendon insertion.

Pathology and patho-biomechanics

Basic representation of the pathogenesis of Achilles tendinopathy begins with a change in the mode, intensity or duration of physical activity that imposes an abnormal biomechanical demand (Papa 2012). Usually a combination of intrinsic and extrinsic factors is found. Malalignment of the foot and hyperpronation place abnormal strains on the tendon (van Sterkenburg & van Dijk 2011) Chronic disease produces blood flow changes to the tendon and fibres of the tendon itself. Additionally, the elastic properties of the tendon decrease with age; this demands more work of the muscle and results in local temperature increase and subsequent pathological tendon changes (van Sterkenburg & van Dijk 2011).

Incomplete recovery time engenders breakdown of the tendon at a cellular level (van Sterkenburg & van Dijk 2011; Papa 2012); this incomplete healing response may be due to hypovascularity and / or continued mechanical forces on the tendon. Degenerative changes to the tendon include fibrin deposition, reduction of neutrophils and macrophages, neovascularization and collagen fibre disorganization (van Sterkenburg & van Dijk 2011; Papa 2012). The neovascularization within the pathological tendon is believed to cause, at least in part, the pain of this condition, which results from ingrowth of nerve fascicles (Papa 2012). Van Sterkenburg and van Dijk (2011), however, make a distinction between the aetiology of degenerative changes described above and tendon neovascularization specific to mid-portion Achilles tendinopathy. The full aetiology of pain accompanying neovascularization is not fully known. An additional consideration to this aetiology is the recent finding of nerves accompanying the peritendinous neovascularization from the paratenon into the tendon itself. These nerves contain high concentrations of nociceptive substances (glutamate, substance P, calcitonin gene-related peptide) (van Sterkenburg & van Dijk 2011). The healthy Achilles tendon has superficial innervations by the paratenon, but is normally considered a non-neuronal tissue. Chronically painful tendons, however, demonstrate this new ingrowth of nerve fibres along with the pathological changes of neovascularization (van Sterkenburg & van Dijk 2011).

Diagnosis

The diagnosis of Achilles tendinopathy is made based on history and physical examination; however, specification of the type of tendinopathy is assisted by magnetic resonance imaging (MRI) and ultrasonography (Scott et al 2011; van Sterkenburg & van Dijk 2011; Hutchison et al 2013).

The most valid clinical diagnostic tests for Achilles tendinopathies are: pain with palpation of the tendon (sensitivity 84%, specificity 73%) and subjective localization of pain 2–6 cm above the insertion into the calcaneus (sensitivity 78%, specificity 77%) (Hutchison et al 2013). Yet patients with Achilles tendinopathy may or may not exhibit and report pain (van Sterkenburg & van Dijk 2011). Tendinopathy and paratendinopathy may coexist, with the paratendinopathy producing pain while the intratendinous changes remain silent. A palpable swelling, usually located 2–7 cm from the insertion on the calcaneus medially, may be painless or painful; this may be the only clinical physical finding (Figs 58.1–58.2). Ankle dorsiflexion and plantarflexion will produce movement of the swollen area if tendinopathy is present without involvement of the paratenon. There is local thickening of the paratenon, which will not move with ankle dorsiflexion and plantarflexion if tendinopathy is not also present (van Sterkenburg & van Dijk 2011).

Painful peritendinous crepitus may be present as the tendon glides within the inflamed sheath in acute conditions (van Sterkenburg & van Dijk 2011). The clinician may also note localized heat, increased erythema and palpable tendon nodules. In chronic conditions, these signs of inflammation diminish, but pain is reproduced with active plantarflexion of the ankle (van Sterkenburg & van Dijk 2011).

The Victorian Institute of Sports Assessment – Achilles (VISA-A) questionnaire is used to determine clinical severity

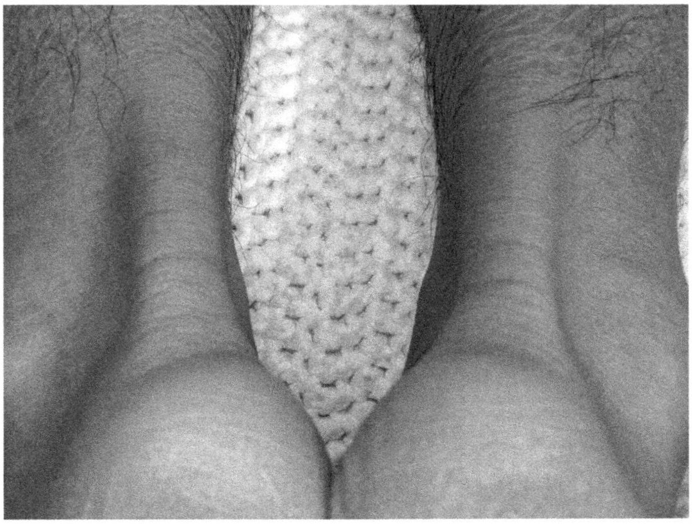

Figure 58.1 Seemingly normal appearance of Achilles tendinosis from bilateral tendon width comparison.

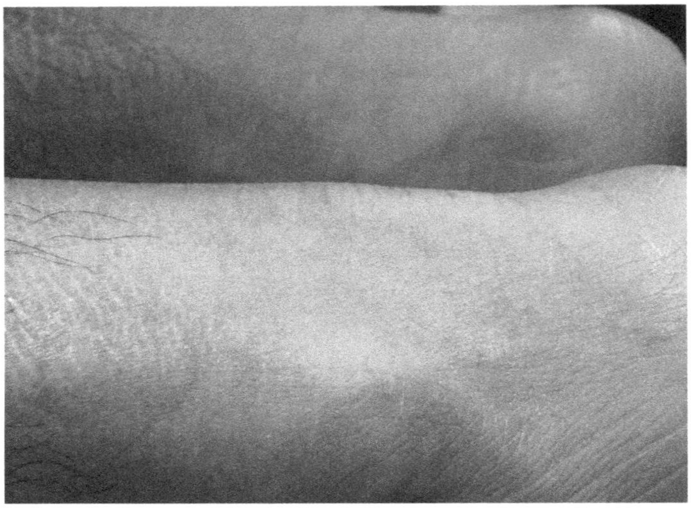

Figure 58.2 Pathological nodule on the Achilles tendon revealed with ankle dorsiflexed.

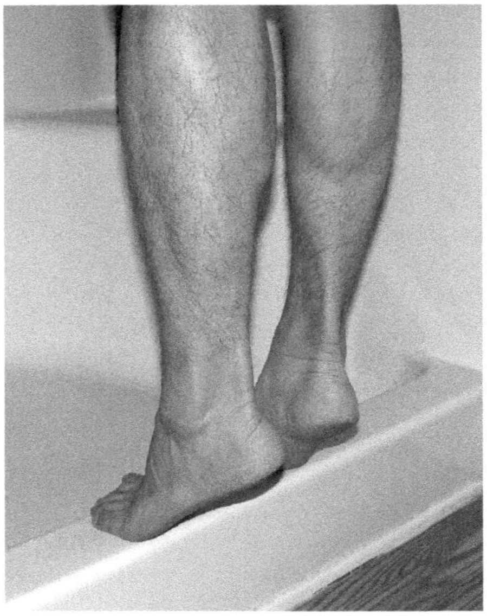

Figure 58.3 The concentric portion of bilateral eccentric heel raises. The patient pushes up into full plantarflexion using either the unaffected leg or both legs to perform this concentric portion of the exercise.

of the condition and provide a guideline for treatment, as well as monitor the effect of treatment. Currently, the VISA-A is considered the only valid, reliable and disease-specific assessment tool for measuring the condition of the Achilles tendon (Lohrer & Nauck 2009).

Treatment and prognosis

Conservative and surgical treatment options for Achilles tendinopathies are widely varied (van Sterkenburg & van Dijk 2011; Wiegerinck et al 2013). Both treatment types normally address the intratendinous degenerative changes when they are present (van Sterkenburg & van Dijk 2011). Non-insertional Achilles tendinopathies are most often managed conservatively (Wiegerinck et al 2013). Although conservative treatment is recommended as the initial treatment for insertional Achilles tendinopathies, it is generally recognized that surgical treatments may be more successful (Wiegerinck et al 2013). Both conservative and surgical treatment outcomes are less favourable in non-athletic populations and in those with insertional tendinopathy versus mid-portion tendinopathy (Papa 2012).

Surgical procedures may be open or minimally invasive with both types attempting debridement of the tendon or tenotomy (van Sterkenburg & van Dijk 2011). This also involves release or removal of the paratenon. Although paratendinopathy and tendinopathy often coexist, some surgical procedures address only the peritendinous structures. Examples of this are the open or minimally invasive paratenectomy as well as Achilles tendoscopy, in which the paratenon is released and the plantaris tendon is cut to relieve symptoms (van Sterkenburg & van Dijk 2011). The prognosis for good recovery after surgical treatment in 6 weeks to 6 months is good. When the surgery addresses the tendon itself rather than the paratenon in isolation, the tendon is initially weakened. Recovery from this procedure may require 3–18 months before sports and running / jumping activities can be resumed again (van Sterkenburg & van Dijk 2011).

Most conservative treatments for Achilles tendinopathies, like other tendinopathies, do not demonstrate strong evidence of a treatment effect in randomized controlled trials (Magnussen et al 2009; Scott et al 2011). Extracorporeal shockwave therapy, local corticosteroid treatments, injections of sclerosing agents, polidocanol, glycosaminoglycan polysulfate, platelet-rich plasma or deproteinized haemodialysate, as well as topical glyceryl nitrate application, may be part of a conservative treatment protocol for Achilles tendinopathies; however, further investigation is needed in order to ascertain their efficacy (Magnussen et al 2009; Scott et al 2011).

Ice, transverse friction massage, therapeutic ultrasound, medical acupuncture and the Graston Technique® of soft tissue treatment are utilized and regarded as beneficial by physical therapists and chiropractors; however, these treatments have a similar lack of evidence base at this time (Magnussen et al 2009; Scott et al 2011; Papa 2012). Although custom orthotics may be helpful when accompanied by other forms of treatment, to be of benefit the patient must have an identifiable malalignment that the orthotic corrects (Scott et al 2011). Air braces and night splints are not supported as effective treatments for Achilles tendinopathy (Scott et al 2011).

The single conservative intervention with strong supporting evidence in the medical literature is heavy-load exercise, usually in the form of eccentric exercise (Magnussen et al 2009; Scott et al 2011; Papa 2012). For example, bilateral and unilateral eccentric heel raises or drops are performed for both the soleus muscle and the gastrocnemius muscle actions. For bilateral eccentric heel raises, the patient pushes up into full plantarflexion using the unaffected leg or both legs to perform this concentric portion of the exercise (Fig. 58.3). The affected foot is then placed on the ground in the same position next to the unaffected side, and both limbs perform the slow, controlled eccentric lowering the ankle into neutral. If this exercise is performed from the edge of a step this changes the heel raise to a heel drop, with the eccentric portion continuing past neutral and into ankle dorsiflexion. Unilateral heel raises / drops are performed in a similar fashion, with the exception that the affected lower extremity alone performs the

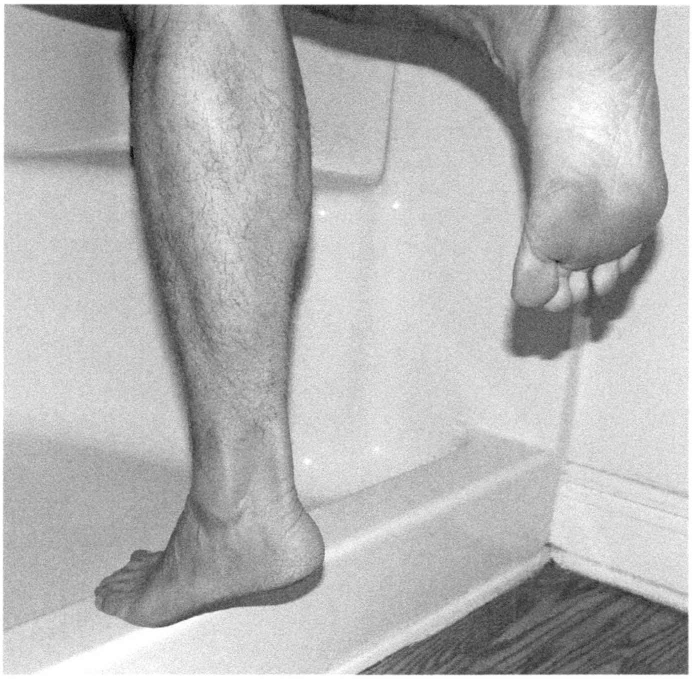

Figure 58.4 When performing unilateral heel raises/drops, the affected lower extremity alone controls the eccentric lowering portion of the exercise.

eccentric portion of the exercise (Papa 2012) (Fig 58.4). (See Ch 38 for further exercises for the lower extremity.)

Prognosis for recovery from chronic Achilles tendinopathies, like chronic tendinopathies located elsewhere in the body, remains poor to fair with conservative treatment (Magnussen et al 2009; Scott et al 2011). Long-term prognosis for recovery from acute to subacute Achilles tendinopathies is reportedly more favourable, however, as 71–100% of patients are able to return to their prior level of function with minimal to no complaints (Papa 2012).

Peroneal Tendinopathy

Background

Peroneal tendinopathy is a common cause of lateral ankle pain when ankle trauma has occurred that is often misdiagnosed as a lateral ligament injury (Scanlan & Gehl 2002). Peroneal tendinopathies may occur as a result of direct or indirect trauma or overuse. Direct trauma produces acute conditions, such as cutting with a sharp object, whereas mechanisms of indirect injury, including overuse, are multifactorial (Palmanovich et al 2012). Anatomical location, vascularity, skeletal maturity and the magnitude of forces are factors that produce peroneal tendinopathies (Scanlan & Gehl 2002; Palmanovich et al 2012).

Peroneal longus and brevis injury may appear together or separately. Stenosing tenosynovitis may occur in the peroneus brevis tendon, in isolation of any injury to the peroneus longus (Boya & Pinar 2010). Reports of chronic tendinitis and stenosing tenosynovitis occurring without a tear of the peroneus longus tendon are more common than presentation of non-traumatic ruptures (Simpson & Howard 2009; Palmanovich et al 2012). Traumatic ruptures at the musculotendinous junction and avulsion fractures are more common than mid-substance tendon ruptures. The estimated incidence of peroneal tendon tears ranges from 11% to 37%, based on cadaver dissection findings (Palmanovich et al 2012). Peroneal tendon tears are also associated with significant lateral ankle instability. Tears of the peroneus longus usually occur in three anatomical zones: the lateral malleolus, the peroneal tubercle of the calcaneus and the cuboid notch (Palmanovich et al 2012). The most common tears occur in the first three peroneals: the longus, the brevis and the tertius. Often there are existing tears of the longus and the brevis at the same time. Another mode of tendinopathy is tendon subluxation, which is also termed dislocation, of the peroneus longus and brevis tendons snapping over the lateral malleolus (Oliva et al 2006). More rarely, intrasheath peroneal tendon subluxation occurs (Michels et al 2013).

Anatomy

The middle third of the lateral surface of the calcaneus features a bony protrusion inferiorly, called the eminentia retrotrochearis (retrotrochearis eminence) (Palmanovich et al 2012). The peroneal tubercle, which is reportedly found in 50–90% of the population, lies anterior to this structure (Hyer et al 2005; Saupe et al 2007; Heller & Robinson 2010; Palmanovich et al 2012). This tubercle, when present, separates the peroneus longus tendon from the peroneus brevis tendon (Palmanovich et al 2012); it is situated below the angle formed by the lateral border of the sinus tarsi and the lateral border of the posterior articular facet on the talus. The peroneal tubercle shape is classified into three groups: group α is an oval form, group β is a ridge form, and group γ is an imperfectly developed form (Palmanovich et al 2012).

Specific location of the tubercle is represented in four classifications; however, these were formed long ago from the findings of a single study. Type I has a single peroneal tubercle located anteroinferior to the tubercle of insertion, the calcaneofibular ligament, type II consists of a single peroneal tubercle incompletely divided into anterior and posterior parts by a smooth groove, type III features two peroneal tubercles completely separated by a roughened area in the middle and type IV is a null classification in which the peroneal tubercle is completely absent (Agarwal et al 1984).

The dimensions of the peroneal tubercle are important, as hypertrophy of this structure is repeatedly associated with peroneal tendinopathy (Ochoa & Banerjee 2007; Taki et al 2007; Boya & Pinar 2010; Taneja et al 2013). The peroneal tubercle on average measures from 2 to 17 mm in length, from 2 to 10 mm in base width and from 1 to 7 mm in height (Saupe et al 2007; Palmanovich et al 2012). Another important bony feature predisposing to the development of peroneal tendinopathy near the cuboid tunnel is the os perineum, which is present in roughly 20% of the population. This ossified sesamoid bone, when present, lies near the calcaneocuboid joint.

Both peroneal tendons are guided by the inferior retinaculum, which is attached to the calcaneus both superior and inferior to the trochlear process. The muscle of the peroneus longus tendon originates from the lateral condyle of the tibia, and the head of the fibula then turns at the cuboid groove before inserting into the plantar–lateral aspect of the first metatarsal and medial cuneiform. Originating from the middle third of the fibula, the peroneus brevis muscle inserts into the base of the fifth metatarsal bone. Both tendons have musculotendinous junctions proximal to the superior peroneal retinaculum.

The peroneus tertius is a unique muscle, which is present only in humans and varies in its specific course and attachments (Joshi et al 2006; Ellis 2007). It originates from the distal third of the anterior surface of fibula, the interosseous margin, and is often fused with the distal portion of the extensor digitorum longus. The peroneus tertius inserts on the dorsal surface of the base of the fifth metatarsal, although there are variants of this. The peroneus quartus is a normal variant that can occur in 13–25% of patients and has been associated with chronic pain and swelling at the lateral ankle / foot (Murlimanju et al 2012). Some authors feel that it may be symptomatic because of the mass effect of the muscle. It can be confused with a soft tissue mass, or the third tendon may mimic the appearance of a split tear in the peroneus brevis (Bilgili et al 2014). Its origin may include the distal lateral portion of the fibula as well as the peroneus brevis or longus muscle. Insertion locations of the peroneus quartus include the phalanges or metatarsal bone of the fifth toe, the calcaneus, the cuboid bone and the lateral retinaculum of the ankle (Murlimanju et al 2012; Bilgili et al 2014).

The innervation of the peroneus brevis and longus is via the superficial peroneal nerve, and both receive their blood supply from the posterior peroneal artery and branches of the medial tarsal artery (Palmanovich et al 2012). Avascular zones correspond with frequent locations of tendinopathy. The peroneus longus has an avascular zone around the lateral malleolus, which extends to the peroneal tubercle, and another avascular zone around the cuboid (Petersen et al 2000; Palmanovich et al 2012).

Pathology and patho-biomechanics

Tendinopathy of the peroneal tendons occurs as a result of many factors, both acute and chronic. Peroneal tendinopathy has been associated with occurrence of the variant peroneus quartus muscle, osteochondroma, fracture, flatfoot, pes cavus, congenital deficiency of the superior peroneal retinaculum and a shallow fibular groove (Oliva et al 2006; Lee et al 2013).

The peroneus longus together with the peroneus brevis provide lateral ankle stability in addition to the lateral ligaments, especially during the mid-stance and heel rise of the gait cycle (Palmanovich et al 2012). Musculotendinous junction tears often occur owing to an acute, violent contraction beneath the superior peroneal retinaculum or at its distal edge (Palmanovich et al 2012). Subluxation represents another tendinopathy. The peroneus longus and brevis share a common tendon sheath proximally, whereas each tendon lies distally in its own sheath (Oliva et al 2006). The common sheath is proximal to the distal tip of the fibula and contains the peroneus brevis lying medial and anterior to the peroneus longus. The fibular groove on the posterior–lateral aspect of the fibula contains the common sheath. Along with the superior peroneal retinaculum, the groove prevents subluxation of the common tendon sheath. The fibular groove is normally 5–10 mm wide and 3 mm deep. The superior peroneal retinaculum originates on the posterior–lateral aspect of the fibula and inserts onto the lateral aspect of the calcaneus. Acute subluxation is less common than chronic subluxation (Oliva 2006).

Mechanically, the cavovarus foot is identified as a predisposing factor for peroneal longus tendinopathy (Redfern & Myerson 2004; Lee et al 2006). The altered placement, and therefore reduction of the moment arm of the tendon in conditions of the cavernous foot, increases frictional forces on the tendon in three locations; the peroneal longus tendon is at high risk for pathological friction at the level of the lateral malleolus, at the peroneal tubercle and at the cuboid notch (Redfern & Myerson 2004; Lee et al 2006).

Another source of mechanically induced tendinopathy is the presence of an enlarged peroneal tubercle (Boya & Pinar 2010; Heller & Robinson 2010; Schubert 2013). An enlarged or hypertrophied peroneal tubercle can produce chronic friction at the anterior aspect of the peroneus longus tendon as it passes over the bony prominence of the enlarged tubercle. The normal function of the peroneal tubercle includes: (1) insertion of the inferior peroneal retinaculum, (2) physical separation of the common peroneal sheath into separate sheaths for the peroneus longus and brevis, and (3) serving as second fulcrum or pulley for the peroneal tendons (Heller & Robinson 2010; Schubert 2013). Alterations of the peroneal tubercle's normal morphology could affect any or all of these functions, hence putting the tendons at risk of injury (Schubert 2013).

Diagnosis

Diagnosis of peroneal tendinopathies varies as the specific disorders present in variable ways. Tendinopathy without tendon subluxation, rupture, longitudinal tear, stenosing tenosynovitis and subluxation may each present differently, with the potential for any one or more of four tendon involvements (Table 58.1). A full medical history must also include comorbidities affecting tissue, such as rheumatoid arthritis or diabetes. The examiner must also note patient reports of any local steroid injections or trauma to the area, including previous sprains or fractures (Palmanovich et al 2012).

Peroneal tendinitis presents as patient reports of a gradual onset of pain, swelling and warmth in the posterior–lateral ankle (van Dijk & Kort 1998). There may be a decline in function due to the pain (van Dijk & Kort 1998; Palmanovich et al 2012). This pain is reproduced with passive hindfoot inversion, with ankle plantarflexion and by active hindfoot eversion and ankle dorsiflexion (Karageanes 2005; Magee 2008). Physical examination may reveal swelling posterior to the lateral malleolus. Tenderness to palpation may exist along the peroneal tendon trajectory. Pain or tendon rupture may produce a marked loss of strength; however, a tendon tear or rupture can exist even in the presence of a seemingly strong plane of movement, such as eversion. The examiner should note a probable dysfunction of the peroneus longus tendon in the presence of limited plantarflexion of the first ray. Weakness and symptoms of chronic tendinopathy could represent a longitudinal tear of the peroneus longus. An apparent tenosynovitis that does not respond to conservative treatment could instead be a partial tear of the tendon (Palmanovich et al 2012).

Special tests specific to peroneal tendon dysfunction are few, and those described closely resemble one another. The

Table 58.1 **Presentation of pain and dysfunction in peroneal tendinopathies**

Peroneal tendinopathy type	Presentation of pain and dysfunction
Peroneal tendinitis	Symptoms of pain behind and distal to the lateral malleolus when the patient returns to activity after a period of rest. Swelling and tenderness may also be present.
Peroneal tendon subluxation	A painful snapping along the lateral ankle is present, with a sense of weakness or pain. Pain at the lateral ankle when walking on the toes. In acute injury, pain and swelling are present over the posterior–lateral aspect of the ankle. In chronic injury, subluxation may be present, along with lateral ankle instability.
Peroneal tendon tears	In acute injury, there is a decrease in strength as well as pain and swelling located inferior and posterior to the lateral malleolus. Chronic injury demonstrates a subtle, insidious onset of pain at the posterior to lateral malleolus. This condition progressively worsens in both pain and decreased function.
Anomalous peroneus brevis muscle injury	The patient may report acute or chronic debilitating pain while performing the push-off portion of the stance, with or without a history of ankle injury.

(Adapted from van Dijk & Kort 1998.)

test for peroneal dislocation is performed with the patient positioned in prone, with the knee flexed to 90°. The examiner first inspects the posterior–lateral region of the ankle for swelling. The patient is then asked to dorsiflex actively and plantarflex with eversion while the examiner provides a resisting force. Subluxation of the tendon from behind the lateral malleolus is considered to be a positive test (Magee 2008). The peroneal tendon stability test is performed with the patient sitting, with legs hanging over the edge of the table and knee flexed to 90°. The examiner holds the patient's foot with one hand, while using the opposite hand gently to locate the peroneal tendons just posterior to the lateral malleolus. The examiner moves the foot into end-range inversion, and then asks the patient to evert against resistance. If the examiner feels a palpable snap or translation of the tendon, the test is considered positive (Karageanes 2005). Reliability, specificity and sensitivity are not currently established for these tests.

Radiography or computed tomography (CT) in the Harris heel view can demonstrate the peroneal tubercle, which may be hypertrophied, as well as associated fractures and the os perineum. Recent reports indicate that three-dimensional colour volume-rendered imaging provides superior diagnostic results compared with traditional CT (Ohashi et al 2015). Ultrasound is reportedly both accurate (90–94%) and specific (85–90%) in diagnosis of peroneal tendinopathies (Park et al 2010; Vuillemin et al 2012). MRI may indicate tenosynovitis, tendinosis or a tear with areas of increased signal on T2-weighted and STIR images, as well as loss of homogeneous signal. Researchers have agreed that, although MRI is a useful tool for revealing peroneal tendinopathies, it is often vague and should be utilized only as an adjunct to a thorough physical examination (Park et al 2010).

Treatment and prognosis

Although acute peroneal tendinopathies may be conservatively treated, chronic tendon injuries have demonstrated poor response to conservative treatment and are often considered surgical indications (Scanlan & Gehl 2002). Conservative treatment for peroneal tendon subluxation, even when acute, has a low rate of success for the prevention of recurrent subluxation (Roth et al 2010). A classification system based on the transverse (cross-sectional) area of viable tendon that remains after debridement of the damaged portion of the tendon may be used to guide surgical decision making in cases of peroneal tendon tears, assuming that the retained portion of the tendon has no split tears (Krause & Brodsky 1998). Tendon repair is indicated with grade I lesions, which are less than 50% of the cross-sectional area, whereas tenodesis is recommended with grade II lesions, which are more than 50% of the tendon's cross-sectional area (Krause & Brodsky 1998). Postoperative treatment protocols are based on the type of surgery performed, and may include non-weight-bearing, casting, range of motion and initiation of physical therapy at 6 weeks (Palmanovich et al 2012).

Anti-inflammatory treatment, rest, activity modification and cast immobilization are attempted in conservative treatment (Palmanovich et al 2012; Tzoanos et al 2012). Exercises and manual therapy techniques, including the lateral calcaneal glide, are recommended as part of a comprehensive physical therapy programme (Hensley & Kavchak 2012). (See Ch 57 for further information on manual therapies targeted to the ankle and foot.)

With such a varied list of pathologies encompassed in peroneal tendinopathies, the majority of which are considered to be surgical indications, a single statement of prognosis is not feasible. If the pathology is well matched to the surgical technique, and the patient is compliant, it is generally considered that return to maximum activity after surgery is prolonged, but that good-to-excellent results can be expected (Krause & Brodsky 1998; Dombek et al 2001; Scanlan & Gehl 2002). Prognosis for conservative treatment in chronic conditions is considered to be often poor, and in acute conditions fair to variable (Roth et al 2010; Hensley & Kavchak 2012; Palmanovich et al 2012; Tzoanos et al 2012).

Tibialis Anterior Tendinopathy

Background

Spontaneous rupture of the tibialis anterior tendon is considered to be well recognized by some and an unusual occurrence by others (Negrine 2007; Beischer et al 2009). Tendinopathy of the tibialis anterior tendon, however, is generally acknowledged to be a rare clinical presentation (Beischer et al 2009; Waizy et al 2011). Injury to the tibialis anterior tendon occurs with forced dorsiflexion against resistance of a plantarflexed foot (eccentric stress on tibialis anterior tendon), usually in running athletes, or minimal to normal stresses on a degenerated tendon, owing to chronic overuse, in elderly patients (Simpson & Howard 2009). Degenerative tendinosis is more prevalent in elderly, overweight females, whereas spontaneous tendon rupture is found more often in elderly males with a history of minor trauma (Negrine 2007; Beischer et al 2009).

Anatomy

The tibialis anterior muscle has four common points of origin: the lateral condyle and upper half to two-thirds of the lateral surface of the body of the tibia, the adjoining part of the interosseous membrane, the deep surface of the fascia, and the intermuscular septum that separates it from the extensor digitorum longus (Wheeless 2011).

The tibialis anterior tendon, viewed prominently on the anterior–medial dorsal aspect of the foot close to the ankle, provides an insertion for the muscle at the medial surface and undersurface of the medial cuneiform bone and the base of the first metatarsal bone (Wheeless 2011).

Pathology and patho-biomechanics

The tibialis anterior tendon passes through three tunnels, formed by the superior extensor retinaculum, oblique superomedial and oblique inferomedial limbs of the inferior extensor retinaculum (Lee et al 2006). In partial tears, the level of the tear corresponds to the approximate level of the oblique superior–medial limb. In complete tears, the proximal ends of torn tendons are retracted so as to lie below the oblique superior–medial limb. In all tears, the oblique superior–medial limb surrounding the torn tendon is thickened, and there is a fluid collection within the tendon sheath in tendon tears (Lee et al 2006).

Tendinosis of the tibialis anterior is described as typical of a degenerative tendinosis with macroscopic thickening and loss of normal fibrillary appearance (Beischer et al 2009). Swelling over the tibialis tendon is present, and longitudinal split tears are often found. Chondral thinning, and / or osteophyte formation at the first tarsometatarsal or medial naviculocuneiform joints, is observed in some cases (Beischer et al 2009; Waizy et al 2011).

Tibialis anterior tendinopathy has been linked to systemic disease (e.g. diabetes), mechanical stress (e.g. tight shoelaces), accumulated overuse trauma and both forceful dorsiflexion and passive hyper-plantarflexion (Beischer et al 2009; Grundy et al 2010; Hart 2011; Negrine 2007).

Diagnosis

The presenting patient is usually elderly, and sometimes overweight, with often a history of minor trauma to the tendon. Burning medial midfoot pain that is worse at night is often reported (Grundy et al 2010). There will be tenderness with direct palpation over the tendon, and a gap may be found in the case of complete ruptures (Grundy et al 2010). Pain and / or weakness with resisted dorsiflexion and inversion may indicate a tendinopathy or tear. In chronic cases, active dorsiflexion may lack 10–15° from normal. The examiner can ask the patient to perform a heel walk (toes lifted) in order to demonstrate the degree of defect and disability (Jerome et al 2010). A steppage-type gait is apparent in complete rupture, with active dorsiflexion demonstrating concurrent eversion as the peroneus tertius provides assistance (Wheeless 2011). A classic triad in the presentation of tibialis anterior tendon rupture includes: (1) pseudotumour at the anterior part of the ankle that corresponds with the ruptured tendon end, (2) loss of the normal contour of the tendon and (3) weak dorsiflexion (Sammarco et al 2009).

Additional diagnostic tests include ultrasound and MRI (Lee et al 2006; Jerome et al 2010). MRI findings will show discontinuity of the tendon, thickening of the retracted portion of the tendon, and excess fluid in the tendon sheath in the case of complete ruptures. Tendinopathies including partial tears will manifest as an attenuated tendon with increased surrounding fluid (Lee et al 2006; Jerome et al 2010).

Treatment and prognosis

In cases of rupture, partial tear and tendinosis, conservative treatment is recommended and may be successful; however, it may not restore complete function, especially in cases of chronic complete rupture and elderly patient (Jerome et al 2010; Waizy et al 2011). With conservative treatment attempted first, conditions of partial tear may demonstrate good functional outcomes while complete ruptures reveal themselves with poor response. Research has shown, however, that conservatively treated patients may develop late sequelae such as foot drop, mild-to-moderate flatfoot deformity and ankle arthrosis (Jerome et al 2010).

Conservative treatment is not detailed in the literature; however, the standard treatment appears to be a protocol similar to that for degenerative tendinopathies in other tendons of the lower extremities (Simpson & Howard 2009). Tibialis anterior eccentric exercises may provide a challenge regarding loading technique, owing to the functional use of the muscle in normal activity. Tools that provide elastic resistance in both isotonic and eccentric movements of ankle dorsiflexion with inversion are recommended (Simpson & Howard 2009). When surgery is not an option for high-risk patients, an ankle–foot orthosis can mechanically support the foot during gait in order to prevent or reduce risk of falls due to foot drop (Negrine 2007). Other standard treatment may include any of the following: short-term immobilization, protection, relative rest, ice, compression, elevation, medication and rehabilitative exercise modalities (Beischer et al 2009; Simpson & Howard 2009; Grundy et al 2010).

Surgical options for advanced tendinosis and tendon tears include simple tendon debridement and reinforcement with a suture anchor (Grundy et al 2010; Waizy et al 2011). Chronic complete ruptures of the tibialis anterior tendon may be augmented with an extensor hallucis longus transfer into the medial cuneiform (Grundy et al 2010; Jerome et al 2010). This procedure can engender some symptomatic hallux interphalangeal joint extensor lag and / or unsafe toe-catching when the patient is ambulating without shoes (Grundy et al 2010; Waizy et al 2011).

Postoperative prognosis for functional recovery is reported to be good to excellent. Patients with a low-demand lifestyle may demonstrate a good outcome with conservative treatment alone, with tendinosis, partial tear and complete rupture (Jerome et al 2010). Acute rupture surgical treatment will have the optimal outcome when provided without delay (Grundy et al 2010; Jerome et al 2010).

Tibialis Posterior Tendinopathy

Background

Tibialis posterior tendinopathy is a common and well-recognized source of pain and walking dysfunction, and is cited as one of the leading causes of acquired flatfoot deformity in the adult population (Kulig et al 2009; Simpson & Howard 2009). Factors associated with tibialis posterior tendinopathy include age-related degeneration, inflammatory arthritis, hypertension, diabetes mellitus, obesity, valgus flat-feet and, less frequently, acute traumatic rupture (Simpson & Howard 2009; Burks 2014). Specific tendinopathies include chronic tendinosis with progressive rupture, tenosynovitis, tendon dislocation and acute ruptures (Lhoste-Trouilloud 2012).

Anatomy

The tibialis posterior is the largest, most anterior-lying tendon on the medial aspect of the ankle. The tibialis posterior tendon muscle originates at three locations: the tibia, the interosseous membrane and the fibula (Lhoste-Trouilloud 2012). It descends within the posterior compartment of the leg, between the flexor digitorum longus and the flexor hallucis longus muscles, with a central lamina that continues downwards with the distal tendon. The distal tendon terminates at ankle level with a nearly 90° change in direction around the medial malleolus. The insertion on the plantar foot is complex; there are multiple insertions on the navicular tuberosity as well as main tendon insertions on all of the tarsal bones, with the exception of the astragalus, and the second, third and fourth metatarsals (Lhoste-Trouilloud 2012). The tibialis posterior tendon, along with the calcaneonavicular ligament, provides significant support for the medial arch of the foot. It is also a powerful plantar and supinator of the ankle (Lhoste-Trouilloud 2012).

Pathology and patho-biomechanics

The tibialis posterior muscle and tendon together as a unit provide the primary stabilization of the medial longitudinal arch (Bek et al 2012; Lhoste-Trouilloud 2012). They achieve this by lifting the medial longitudinal arch with its active plantarflexion and inversion movement, thus locking the mid-tarsal articulation and stabilizing the hindfoot (Bek et al 2012). When the middle and posterior foot are stable in this manner, the gastrocnemius and soleus muscles are effectively activated. However, when the middle foot cannot be locked in the forward phase of walking, excessive force is applied on the mid-tarsal joint by the gastrocnemius and soleus muscles. In turn, this causes a collapse of the medial arch and eversion of the subtalar articulation. Tibialis posterior tendinopathy with strength insufficiency causes a posterior shift of the centre of gravity of the foot and produces an abnormal load on its medial structures (Bek et al 2012).

The pathological process leading to chronic tendinopathies of the tibialis posterior develops as a result of degenerative or inflammatory causes or repeated micro-trauma. Different stages of this process may produce rigid structural foot deformities and degenerative changes (Bek et al 2012). Previous reports suggested that the dysfunction arises from an inflammatory process such as tendinitis or tenosynovitis; however, current histological studies show that the changes associated with this tendinopathy are more consistent with a degenerative process as described above (Bek et al 2012; Lhoste-Trouilloud 2012).

Diagnosis

Three stages, also termed ‘grades’, of tibialis posterior tendinopathy are described in the literature, and treatment decisions are based upon this classification (Kulig et al 2009; Simpson & Howard 2009; Bek et al 2012; Lhoste-Trouilloud 2012). Stage 1 is characterized by mild swelling, medial ankle pain and normal but possibly painful single heel raise, but no deformity. Stage 2 features progressive flattening of the arch, pes planus and midfoot abduction; however, the subtalar joint is still flexible. The tendon at this point is functionally incompetent or ruptured; the patient is unable to perform a heel raise. Stage 3 incorporates all of the features of stage 2, except that the subtalar joint has become fixed (Kulig et al 2009; Simpson & Howard 2009; Bek et al 2012; Lhoste-Trouilloud 2012). A fourth stage was later added to encompass progression to valgus tilt of the talus in the ankle mortise, leading to lateral tibiotalar degeneration (Kulig et al 2009).

An excellent physical examination will include a number of tests, including the single-limb rise, first-metatarsal rise sign and the ‘too-many-toes’ sign (Churchill & Sferra 1998; Simpson & Howard 2009). The first-metatarsal rise test has excellent sensitivity, but unknown specificity, for diagnosis of tibialis posterior tendon dysfunction. Patients are tested while in standing with full weight-bearing bilaterally. The examiner holds the shank of the affected foot with one hand and externally rotates it, or, when the heel of the affected foot is held by the examiner’s hand and brought passively into a varus position, the head of the first metatarsal lifts or raises in the case of tibialis posterior tendon dysfunction but remains on the floor when the tendon is functioning normally (Churchill & Sferra 1998).

The too-many-toes sign, with a reported sensitivity of 65–80%, is a commonly used test to identify tibialis posterior tendon tendinopathy (Churchill & Sferra 1998; Simpson & Howard, 2009). To perform this test, the examiner will view the patient’s foot from behind; a positive test will be indicated by the examiner viewing more toes exposed on the lateral aspect of the involved foot, along with flattening of the arch (Churchill & Sferra 1998; Kulig et al 2009; Simpson & Howard 2009).

Other physical findings include excessive pronation of the injured foot, relative weakness of the posterior tibial tendon and abnormal heel varus when the patient is asked to stand on tiptoe (Churchill & Sferra 1998; Simpson & Howard, 2009). The patient will have difficulty and pain when performing a single-leg heel raise (Churchill & Sferra 1998; Kulig et al 2009; Simpson & Howard 2009). Frank rupture of the tibialis posterior tendon is indicated by an inability to initiate and maintain plantarflexion with a single-leg heel raise or the presence of abnormal heel varus with this manoeuvre (Kulig et al 2009).

Ultrasound and will reveal a thickened retinaculum and / or tendon. The classic picture consists of an irregular cortical bone profile, heterogeneity of the tendon insertion and hyperaemia on colour Doppler ultrasound (Premkumar et al 2002; Lhoste-Trouilloud 2012). The sensitivity and specificity of ultrasound for diagnosing tibialis posterior tendinopathy are 80% and 90% respectively; for diagnosing tibialis posterior peritendinosis they are 90% and 80% respectively (Premkumar et al 2002). High-resolution sonography with colour and power Doppler imaging is nearly as accurate as MRI for diagnosing tibialis posterior tendinopathy (Premkumar et al 2002).

Treatment and prognosis

There is no agreement or strong evidence in the literature regarding the efficacy of conservative treatment approaches for tibialis posterior tendinopathy (Bowringa & Chockalingam 2010). General recommendations are for relative rest, pain medication, physical therapy and walking cast or ankle foot orthosis in stage 1, with the addition of referral to an orthopaedic surgeon in stage 2 (Kulig et al 2009; Simpson & Howard 2009). Surgical repair is the prescribed treatment for stage 3 or 4 (Kulig et al 2009; Simpson & Howard 2009).

Focusing on the supposed tendon pathogenesis of degeneration, physical therapy programmes in the early stages of tibialis posterior tendinopathy attempt to support the flattened arch mechanically so as to prevent further tendon lengthening and foot deformity (Kulig et al 2009). Exercises to strengthen the weakened tibialis posterior musculotendinous complex, albeit in the presence of painful tendon dysfunction, are strongly recommended (Simpson & Howard 2009); a closed-chain resisted foot adduction exercise performed barefoot most effectively and selectively activated the tibialis posterior muscle in people with a normal arch index. Gastrocnemius and soleus muscle stretching and the addition of eccentric tendon loading when tolerated are additional details of rehabilitation strategies (Kulig et al 2009).

Surgical options, which are preferred in the later stages of tendinopathy, include tendon transfers, osteotomies, arthrodeses and their various combinations. Overcorrection and undercorrection are complications specific to the tendon-transfer procedure (Bek et al 2012).

Prognosis for full functional recovery after conservative treatment or surgery is based on treatment options according to the tendon's pathological stage. Provided that the recommendations for treatment are followed according to the stage as discussed above, outcomes of both options are good to excellent (Kulig et al 2009; Bek et al 2012).

Other Tendinopathies of the Foot and Ankle

Background

Most tendinopathies in the foot and ankle other than those discussed earlier in this chapter involve the flexor hallucis longus (FHL) tendon, although literally any tendon in the foot and ankle could present pathologically. Restricted movement of the FHL tendon causes tendinopathies most often in runners, ballet dancers and other athletes; however, this condition presents in the sedentary population as well. Tendinopathy of the flexor FHL tendon is often misdiagnosed as plantar fasciitis, which then proves recalcitrant to treatment (Michelson & Dunn 2005; Simpson & Howard 2009). Chronic tendinopathy of the FHL causes chronic pain, early arthritis, fibrosis with decreased range of motion, and possibly an early end to a dancer's or athlete's career (Simpson & Howard 2009).

Anatomy

The FHL originates from at least four sites: the inferior two-thirds of the posterior surface of the body of the fibula, the lower part of the interosseous membrane, an intermuscular septum between it and the peroneals laterally, and the fascia covering the tibialis posterior medially (Magee 2008). The tendon of the FHL occupies nearly the entire length of the posterior surface of the muscle. Grooves on the talus and calcaneus contain the FHL tendon. The groove crosses the posterior surface of the distal tibia, the posterior talus and undersurface of the sustentaculum tali of the calcaneus. The tendon passes between the medial and lateral sesamoid bones at the metatarsophalangeal joint, then runs forwards in the sole of the foot between the two heads of the flexor hallucis brevis muscle, and finally inserts into the base of the last phalanx of the great toe (Magee 2008; Wheeless 2012).

Pathology and patho-biomechanics

The FHL tendon movement can be restricted at the level of the posterior ankle and at its passage between the two sesamoids (Michelson & Dunn 2005; Simpson & Howard 2009). This is not always a stenosing type of tenosynovitis. Tendinopathy of the FHL is also caused by posterior impingement by the talus. In some cases, however, the mechanism of injury is trauma that may or may not be compounded later with chronic degeneration (Michelson & Dunn 2005; Simpson & Howard 2009; Corte-Real et al 2012).

Diagnosis

Patients may report pain with palpation at the posterior–medial ankle, the plantar heel, the plantar midfoot, and multiple other locations (Michelson & Dunn 2005; Simpson & Howard 2009). In short, the pain may manifest itself anywhere from the posterior leg to the plantar foot and the hallux. Length testing of the FHL muscle and tendon reveals restriction by limited hallux metatarsophalangeal joint dorsiflexion when the ankle is dorsiflexed (Michelson & Dunn 2005). MRI of the FHL may reveal synovitis, degenerative tendon changes, or tears (Michelson & Dunn 2005; Corte-Real et al 2012).

Treatment and prognosis

Conservative treatment includes stretching, short-term immobilization and modalities for pain. Surgery including open or arthroscopic release of the FHL tendon yields good results when conservative treatment fails (Corte-Real et al 2012). Information on prognosis is limited. An estimated 50–64% of those treated conservatively will have successful results. Prognosis reported for surgical intervention is excellent (Michelson & Dunn 2005; Simpson & Howard 2009; Corte-Real et al 2012).

Conclusion

Tendinopathies of the ankle and foot vary widely and often require surgical intervention for rupture or severe degradation. Conservative treatments, both novel and traditional, are largely unsupported by reports of efficacy in the medical literature (Magnussen et al 2009; Bowringa & Chockalingam 2010; Papa 2012; Scott et al 2013). A general rehabilitation plan may be followed, but with less than optimal results (Bek et al 2012). The development of an effective rehabilitation treatment plan for confirmed symptomatic tendinopathy requires not only cognizance of evidence-based treatment but also pathoanatomical knowledge, as well as complex clinical reasoning (Kulig et al 2009; Hensley & Kavchak 2012). Tendon pathology in the foot and ankle varies greatly from tendon to tendon and according to the mechanism of injury. Conservative treatment should be tailored to the site of pathology, the stage of the tendinopathy, the functional assessment, the activity status of the person, any contributing issues throughout the kinetic chain and comorbidities (Scott et al 2011, 2013; Papa 2012). Neither evidence-based medicine nor the practitioner's clinical reasoning and experience should stand alone as 'best practice' for the treatment of tendinopathies in the foot and ankle (Kulig et al 2009; Scott et al 2011, 2013; Papa 2012).

References

Agarwal AK, Jeyasingh P, Gupta SC, et al. 1984. Peroneal tubercle and its variations in the Indian calcanei. Anat Anz 156: 241–244.

Beischer AD, Beamond BM, Jowett AJ, et al. 2009. Distal tendinosis of the tibialis anterior tendon. Foot Ankle Int 30: 1053–1059.

Bek N, Simşek IE, Erel S, et al. 2012. Home-based general versus center-based selective rehabilitation in patients with posterior tibial tendon dysfunction. Acta Orthop Traumatol Turc 46: 286–292.

Bilgili MG, Kaynak G, Botanlıoğlu H, et al. 2014. Peroneus quartus: prevalence and clinical importance. Arch Orthop Trauma Surg 134(4): 481–487. doi: 10.1007/s00402-014-1937-4.

Bowringa B, Chockalingam N. 2010. Conservative treatment of tibialis posterior tendon dysfunction: a review. Foot 20: 18–26.

Boya H, Pinar H. 2010. Stenosing tenosynovitis of the peroneus brevis tendon associated with hypertrophy of the peroneal tubercle. J Foot Ankle Surg 49: 188–190.

Burks J. 2014. When conservative treatment fails for posterior tibial tendon dysfunction. Podiatry Today 27(1): npn. Online. Retrieved from http://www.podiatrytoday.com/when-conservative-treatment-fails-posterior-tibial-tendon-dysfunction.

Churchill RS, Sferra JJ. 1998. Posterior tibial tendon insufficiency. Its diagnosis, management, and treatment. Am J Orthop 27: 339–347.

Corte-Real NM, Moreira RM, Guerra-Pinto F. 2012. Arthroscopic treatment of tenosynovitis of the flexor hallucis longus tendon. Foot Ankle Int 33: 1108–1112.

Dombek MF, Orsini R, Mendicino RW, et al. 2001. Peroneus brevis tendon tears. Clin Podiatr Med Surg 18: 409–427.

Ellis H. 2007. Morphology of peroneus tertius muscle. Clin Anat 20: 230.

Grundy JRB, O'Sullivan RM, Beischer AD. 2010. Operative management of distal tibialis anterior tendinopathy. Foot Ankle Int 31: 212–219.

Hart L. 2011. Corticosteroid and other injections in the management of tendinopathies: a review. Clin J Sport Med 21: 540–541.

Heller E, Robinson D. 2010. Traumatic pathologies of the calcaneal peroneal tubercle. Foot 20: 96–98.

Hensley CP, Kavchak AJ. 2012. Novel use of a manual therapy technique and management of a patient with peroneal tendinopathy: a case report. Man Ther 17: 84–88.

Hutchison AM, Evans R, Bodger O, et al. 2013. What is the best clinical test for Achilles tendinopathy? Foot Ankle Surg 19: 112–117.

Hyer CF, Dawson JM, Philbin TM, et al. 2005. The peroneal tubercle: description, classification, and relevance to peroneus longus tendon pathology. Foot Ankle Int 26: 947–950.

Jerome JTJ, Varghese M, Sankaran B, et al. 2010. Tibialis anterior rupture: a missed diagnosis. Foot Ankle Online J 3: 2.

Joshi SD, Joshi SS, Athavale SA. 2006. Morphology of peroneus tertius muscle. Clin Anat 19: 611–614.

Karageanes SJ. 2005. Principles of manual sports medicine. Baltimore: Lippincott Williams & Wilkins.

Krause JO, Brodsky JW. 1998. Peroneus brevis tendon tears: pathophysiology, surgical reconstruction, and clinical results. Foot Ankle Int 19(5): 271–279.

Kulig K, Reischl SF, Pomrantz AB, et al. 2009. Nonsurgical management of posterior tibial tendon dysfunction with orthoses and resistive exercise: a randomized controlled trial. Phys Ther 89: 26–37.

Lee MH, Chung CB, Cho JH, et al. 2006. Tibialis anterior tendon and extensor retinaculum: imaging in cadavers and patients with tendon tear. AJR Am J Roentgenol 187: W161–W168.

Lee SJ, Jacobson JA, Kim SM, et al. 2013. Ultrasound and MRI of the peroneal tendons and associated pathology. Skeletal Radiol 42: 1191–1200.

Lhoste-Trouilloud A. 2012. The tibialis posterior tendon. J Ultrasound 15: 2–6.

Lohrer H, Nauck T. 2009. Cross-cultural adaptation and validation of the VISA-A questionnaire for German-speaking Achilles tendinopathy patients. BMC Musculoskelet Disord 10: 134.

Lohrer H, Arentz S, Nauck T, et al. 2008. The Achilles tendon insertion is crescent-shaped: an in vitro anatomic investigation. Clin Orthop Relat Res 466: 2230–2237.

Magee DJ. 2008. Orthopedic physical assessment. London: Elsevier Health Sciences.

Magnussen RA, Dunn WR, Thomson AB. 2009. Non-operative treatment of mid-portion Achilles tendinopathy: a systematic review. Clin J Sport Med 19: 54–64.

Michels F, Jambou S, Guillo S, et al. 2013. Endoscopic treatment of intrasheath peroneal tendon subluxation. Case Rep Med 2013: 274685.

Michelson J, Dunn L. 2005. Tenosynovitis of the flexor hallucis longus: a clinical study of the spectrum of presentation and treatment. Foot Ankle Int 26: 291–303.

Murlimanju BV, D'Souza PS, Prabhu LV, et al. 2012. Peroneus quartus, an accessory muscle in human: case report and its clinical importance. Clin Ter 163: 307–309.

Negrine JP. 2007. Tibialis anterior rupture: acute and chronic. Foot Ankle Clinics 12: 569–572.

Ochoa LM, Banerjee R. 2007. Recurrent hypertrophic peroneal tubercle associated with peroneus brevis tendon tear. J Foot Ankle Surg 46: 403–408.

Ohashi K, Sanghvi T, El-Khoury GY, et al. 2015. Diagnostic accuracy of 3D color volume-rendered CT images for peroneal tendon dislocation in patients with acute calcaneal fractures. Acta Radiol 56(2): 190–195.

Oliva F, Ferran N, Maffulli N. 2006. Peroneal retinaculoplasty with anchors for peroneal tendon subluxation. Bull Hosp Jt Dis 63: 113–116.

Palmanovich E, Laver L, Brin YS, et al. 2012. Peroneus longus tear and its relation to the peroneal tubercle: a review of the literature. Muscles Lig Tendons J 1: 153–160.

Papa JA. 2012. Conservative management of Achilles tendinopathy: a case report. J Can Chiropr Assoc 56: 216–224.

Park HJ, Cha SD, Kim HS, et al. 2010. Reliability of MRI findings of peroneal tendinopathy in patients with lateral chronic ankle instability. Clin Orthop Surg 2: 237–243.

Petersen W, Bobka T, Stein V, et al. 2000. Blood supply of the peroneal tendons: injection and immunohistochemical studies of cadaver tendons. Acta Orthop Scand 71: 168–174.

Premkumar A, Perry MB, Dwyer AJ, et al. 2002. Sonography and MR imaging of posterior tibial tendinopathy. AJR Am J Roentgenol 178: 223–232.

Redfern D, Myerson M. 2004. The management of concomitant tears of the peroneus longus and brevis tendons. Foot Ankle Int 25: 695–707.

Roth JA, Taylor WC, Whalen J. 2010. Peroneal tendon subluxation: the other lateral ankle injury. Br J Sports Med 44: 1047–1053.

Sammarco VJ, Sammarco GJ, Henning C, et al. 2009. Surgical repair of acute and chronic tibialis anterior tendon ruptures. J Bone Joint Surg Am 91A: 325.

Saupe N, Mengiardi B, Pfirrmann CW, et al. 2007. Anatomic variants associated with peroneal tendon disorders: MR imaging findings in volunteers with asymptomatic ankles. Radiology 242: 509–517.

Scanlan RL, Gehl RS. 2002. Peroneal tendon injuries. Clin Podiatr Med Surg 19: 419–431.

Schubert R. 2013. MRI of peroneal tendinopathies resulting from trauma or overuse. Br J Radiol 86: 20110750.

Scott A, Huisman E, Khan K. 2011. Conservative treatment of chronic Achilles tendinopathy. CMAJ 183: 1159–1165.

Scott A, Docking S, Vicenzino B, et al. 2013. Sports and exercise-related tendinopathies: a review of selected topical issues by participants of the Second International Scientific Tendinopathy Symposium (ISTS) Vancouver 2012. Br J Sports Med 47: 536–544.

Simpson MR, Howard TM. 2009. Tendinopathies of the foot and ankle. Am Fam Physician 80: 1107–1114.

Taki K, Yamazaki S, Majima T, et al. 2007. Bilateral stenosing tenosynovitis of the peroneus longus tendon associated with hypertrophied peroneal tubercle in a junior soccer player: a case report. Foot Ankle Int 28: 129–132.

Taneja AK, Simeone FJ, Chang CY, et al. 2013. Peroneal tendon abnormalities in subjects with an enlarged peroneal tubercle. Skeletal Radiol 42: 1703–1709.

Tzoanos G, Manidakis N, Tsavalas N, et al. 2012. Non-operative treatment of peroneal split syndrome: a case report. Acta Orthop Belg 78: 804–807.

van Dijk CN, Kort N. 1998. Tendoscopy of the peroneal tendons. Arthroscopy 14: 471–478.

van Dijk CN, van Sterkenburg MN, Wiegerinck JI, et al. 2011. Terminology for Achilles tendon related disorders. Knee Surg Sports Traumatol Arthrosc 19: 835–841.

van Sterkenburg MN, van Dijk CN. 2011. Mid-portion Achilles tendinopathy: why painful? An evidence-based philosophy. Knee Surg Sports Traumatol Arthrosc 19: 1367–1375.

Vuillemin V, Guerini H, Bard H, et al. 2012. Stenosing tenosynovitis. J Ultrasound 15: 20–28.

Waizy H, Goede F, Plaass C, et al. 2011. Tendinopathy of the tibialis anterior tendon: surgical management. Orthopade 40: 630–632.

Wheeless CR. 2011. Tibialis anterior. Wheeless' textbook of orthopaedics. Online. Retrieved from http://www.wheelessonline.com/ortho/tibialis_anterior.

Wheeless CR. 2012. Flexor hallucis longus. Wheeless' textbook of orthopaedics. Online. Retrieved from http://www.wheelessonline.com/ortho/flexor_hallucis_longus.

Wiegerinck JI, Kerkhoffs GM, van Sterkenburg MN, et al. 2013. Treatment for insertional Achilles tendinopathy: a systematic review. Knee Surg Sports Traumatol Arthrosc 21: 1345–1355.

PART 10

Soft Tissues in the Upper and Lower Quadrants

59 Referred Pain from Myofascial Trigger Points 659
César Fernández-de-las-Peñas, Hong-You Ge, Lars Arendt-Nielsen and Jan Dommerholt

60 Manual Treatment of Myofascial Trigger Points 678
César Fernández-de-las-Peñas, Jaime Salom-Moreno, Hong-You Ge and Jan Dommerholt

61 Dry Needling of Trigger Points 690
Jan Dommerholt and Erik H. Wijtmans

62 Muscle Energy Approaches 710
Gary Fryer

63 Myofascial Induction Approaches 729
Andrzej Pilat

Chapter 59

Referred Pain from Myofascial Trigger Points

César Fernández-de-las-Peñas, Hong-You Ge, Lars Arendt-Nielsen, Jan Dommerholt

CHAPTER CONTENTS

Introduction 659
Myofascial trigger points 660
Definition of a trigger point 660
Characteristics of the referred pain elicited by muscle trigger points 660
Manual identification of myofascial trigger points 660
Neurophysiological basis of trigger points 661
Exploration of trigger points related to upper quadrant pain syndromes 662
Neck–shoulder muscles 662
Scalene muscles 663
Pectoralis minor muscle 663
Supraspinatus muscle 664
Infraspinatus muscle 664
Teres minor and major muscles 665
Subscapularis muscle 665
Pectoralis major muscle 665
Deltoid muscle 666
Biceps brachii muscle 666
Triceps brachii muscle 666
Brachioradialis muscle 667
Supinator muscle 667
Wrist/hand extensor muscles 667
Pronator teres muscle 669
Wrist/hand flexor muscles 669
Other muscles of the upper quadrant 670
Exploration of trigger points related to lower quadrant pain syndromes 670
Quadratus lumborum muscle 670
Psoas major muscle 670
Piriformis muscle 671
Gluteus medius muscle 671
Gluteus minimus muscle 671
Quadriceps muscle 672
Adductor muscles 672
Gastrocnemius and soleus muscles 672
Tibialis anterior, extensor digitorum longus and extensor hallucis longus muscles 673
Other muscles of the lower quadrant 673
Conclusion 673

Introduction

Referred pain (pain felt in a region remote from the source of pain) has been known and described for more than a century and has been used extensively as a diagnostic clinical tool. In clinical practice, it is very common to see patients with neck or shoulder pain that refers to the upper arm, the forearm or hand, or patients with low back or hip pain that spreads to the thigh, knee or leg. Occasionally, pain may refer to the contralateral side (Carli et al 2002). Pain from deep tissues, such as muscles, joints, ligaments, tendons and viscera is often described as deep and diffuse and difficult to locate precisely (Mense 1994). The term 'referred pain' is actually only partially correct, however, as referred pain is not necessarily limited to pain but can also include other referred sensations or paraesthesiae. Referred pain symptoms can be involved in upper and lower quadrant pain syndromes in which there is no clear diagnosis (Gerwin 1997). For instance, patients with deep pain in the shoulder and posterior deltoid region spreading to the upper arm may be diagnosed as a non-specific arm pain syndrome, since they complain of diffuse arm pain and tenderness with loss of function but lack objective physical signs (Macfarlane et al 2000). Simons et al (1999) described common referred pain patterns from the infraspinatus trigger points (TrPs), which may resemble the clinical picture of these patients. What was considered to be a non-specific arm pain syndrome may in fact originate from infraspinatus TrPs. Another example would be a patient with deep pain in the posterior part of the leg spreading to the posterior part of the knee or the lower leg. In this case, the patient may be diagnosed with sciatic nerve pain. However, TrPs within the piriformis muscle can mimic similar symptoms (Simons et al 1999). Similarly, what was considered to be sciatic nerve compression may in fact originate from piriformis TrPs.

An additional clinical reasoning challenge is that, in individuals with musculoskeletal pain, the symptoms may be the summation of referred pain from multiple muscle TrPs and from joints and viscera, making it more difficult to establish the proper diagnosis. This chapter will describe the clinical and the neurophysiological basis of myofascial TrPs with referred pain patterns spreading to the upper and lower quadrants.

Myofascial Trigger Points

Definition of a trigger point

Although there are different definitions of TrPs, the most commonly accepted definition states that a TrP is a hyperirritable spot within a taut band of a skeletal muscle that is painful on compression, stretch, overload or contraction, which causes a referred pain that is perceived distant from the spot (Simons et al 1999). From a clinical point of view, we can distinguish between active and latent TrPs. Active TrPs are those in which local and referred pain reproduce sensory or motor symptoms reported by the patient, and the pain is recognized by the patient as a usual pain (Simons et al 1999). Latent muscle TrPs are those in which local and referred pain do not reproduce any symptom that is familiar or usual for the subject (Simons et al 1999). Active and latent TrPs have similar physical findings. The difference is that latent TrPs do not reproduce any spontaneous symptoms. In addition, active TrPs are bigger and induce larger referred pain areas and higher pain intensities than do latent TrPs (Hong et al 1997; Ballyns et al 2011). For instance, a patient with lateral epicondylalgia can have active TrPs, which reproduce the symptoms within the affected arm (Fernández-Carnero et al 2007), but this patient may also have latent TrPs on the non-affected side, as the local and referred pain is not usually perceived in this arm (Fernández-Carnero et al 2008). Similarly, Ge et al (2008a) found that individuals with unilateral shoulder pain exhibit active TrPs in the infraspinatus muscle within the symptomatic side, but also latent TrPs in the same muscle on the non-symptomatic side. Additionally, both active and latent TrPs provoke motor dysfunctions, for example muscle weakness, inhibition, increased motor irritability, muscle imbalance and altered motor recruitment (Lucas et al 2004), in either the affected muscle or in functionally related muscles (Simons et al 1999). Lucas et al (2010) demonstrated that latent TrPs were associated with an impaired motor activation pattern and that the elimination of these latent TrPs induces normalization of the impaired motor activation pattern. During the past decade, an increasing number of researchers have shown an interest in the aetiology and clinical relevance of latent TrPs (Ge & Arendt-Nielsen 2011).

Characteristics of the referred pain elicited by muscle trigger points

- The duration of referred pain could last for as short as a few seconds or as long as a few hours, days, weeks or sometimes indefinitely, depending upon the TrP activity.
- The referred pain is described as deep, diffuse, burning, tightening or pressing pain, which is completely different from neuropathic or superficial (skin) pain.
- The referred pain can spread cranial / caudal or ventral / dorsal, depending on the TrP.
- The referred pain intensity and spreading area are positively correlated with the degree of TrP activity (irritability of the nervous system).
- The referred pain can be accompanied by other symptoms, such as numbness, coldness, stiffness, weakness, fatigue and motor dysfunction, which suggests that the term 'referred sensation' may be a more appropriate and accurate description.
- Inactivation of active TrPs should effectively relieve the referred pain.
- TrP referred pain patterns may be similar to joint referred pain patterns (Bogduk 2004).

Manual identification of myofascial trigger points

Competent TrP diagnosis requires adequate manual skills, training and clinical practice to develop a high degree of reliability in the examination (Gerwin et al 1997; Simons et al 1999; Sciotti et al 2001). There are several signs and symptoms that may be used for the TrP diagnosis: (a) presence of a palpable taut band in a skeletal muscle when accessible to palpation, (b) presence of a hyperirritable spot in the taut band, (c) palpable local twitch response on snapping palpation (or needling) of the TrP, and (d) presence of referred pain elicited by stimulation or palpation of the hyperirritable spot (Simons et al 1999). Additional helpful signs for diagnosis are muscle weakness, pain on contraction in the shortened or lengthening position, or a jump sign. However, different reviews investigating the reliability of TrP diagnosis have concluded that further high-quality investigations are needed of the currently used clinical diagnostic criteria in different populations (Tough et al 2007; Myburgh et al 2008; Lucas et al 2009). Factors that may have contributed to the varying reliability of the results from studies are lack of identification of taut bands, inexperienced examiners in assessing muscle TrPs, incorrect positioning of the patient or the assessor, incorrect palpation techniques, and variations in the amount of manual force exerted on the palpated point and the duration of force applied. Nevertheless, it has been reported that in some muscles a TrP may consistently be more reliably examined than others (Gerwin et al 1997; Sciotti et al 2001). Readers are referred to other texts for discussion on the reliability of diagnosing TrP (Tough et al 2007; Myburgh et al 2008; Fernández-de-las-Peñas et al 2009b; Lucas et al 2009; Bron & Dommerholt 2012).

In clinical practice, Simons et al (1999) and Gerwin et al (1997) recommend that the *minimum* acceptable criteria for TrP diagnosis are the presence of a hyperirritable spot within a palpable taut band of a skeletal muscle combined with the patient's recognition of the referred pain elicited by the TrP. When applied by an experienced assessor, these criteria have obtained good inter-examiner reliability (kappa) ranging from 0.84 to 0.88 (Gerwin et al 1997). More-recent studies found that taut bands and TrPs can be visualized using magnetic resonance and sonographic elastography (Chen et al 2007, 2008; Sikdar et al 2008, 2009), although future studies are needed to optimize these procedures. These studies have demonstrated that taut bands exhibit higher stiffness (Chen et al 2007), reduced vibration amplitude (Sikdar et al 2009), higher peak systolic velocities and negative diastolic velocities (Sikdar et al 2010) compared with normal muscle sites.

Neurophysiological basis of myofascial trigger points

TrP referred pain is a process of central sensitization, which is mediated by peripheral nociceptive activity and which can be facilitated by sympathetic activity or altered descending inhibition.

TrPs: are they a focus of peripheral sensitization?

Muscle pain is dependent upon activation of muscle nociceptors by endogenous substances (e.g. neuropeptides or inflammatory mediators). Different algogenic substances are commonly used in experimental pain models for eliciting both local and referred pain from muscle tissues, including hypertonic saline (Arendt-Nielsen & Svensson 2001; Graven-Nielsen 2006), bradykinin and serotonin (Babenko et al 1999a), capsaicin (Witting et al 2000), substance P (Babenko et al 1999b), glutamate (Svensson et al 2003a), nerve growth factor (Svensson et al 2003b) and acidic saline (Sluka et al 2001). It is interesting to note that the referred pain patterns reported with injection of these substances are similar to the referred pain patterns described in the trigger point manuals (Simons et al 1999).

The pressure sensitivity is lower at TrPs than at control points suggesting an increased nociceptive sensitivity at TrPs and peripheral sensitization. In fact, active TrPs and their overlying cutaneous and subcutaneous tissues are usually more sensitive to pressure and electrical stimulation than are latent TrPs (Vecchiet et al 1990, 1994).

Microdialysis studies showed that the concentrations of bradykinin, calcitonin gene-related peptide, substance P, tumour necrosis factor-α, interleukin-1β, serotonin and norepinephrine were significantly higher in active muscle TrPs compared with latent TrP or control non-TrP points (Shah et al 2005, 2008). A more recent animal rabbit study confirmed the increased concentrations of β-endorphin, substance P, tumor necrosis factor α (TNF-α), cyclo-oxygenase-2 (COX-2), hypoxia-inducible factor 1α, inducible nitric oxide synthase, and vascular endothelial growth factor (Hsieh et al 2012).

These studies establish the presence of nociceptive hypersensitivity in active TrPs and validate that TrPs are a focus of persistent peripheral sensitization. Li et al (2009) reported nociceptive (hyperalgesia) and non-nociceptive (allodynia) hypersensitivity at TrPs, suggesting that TrPs sensitize both nociceptive and non-nociceptive nerve endings. Nevertheless, painful stimulation induces higher pain response than non-noxious stimulation at TrPs (Li et al 2009). Additionally, Wang et al (2010) observed that ischaemic compression, which mainly blocked large-diameter myelinated muscle afferents, induced increased pressure pain and referred pain thresholds at the TrP, but not at non-TrP regions. All these studies support the idea that TrPs constitute a focus of sensitization of both nociceptive and non-nociceptive nerve endings.

TrPs and central sensitization mechanisms

When muscles are in a state of sensitization, muscle nociceptors are more easily activated and may respond to normal innocuous or weak stimuli such as light pressure and muscle movement. The presence of multiple TrPs (spatial summation), or of TrPs during prolonged periods of time (temporal summation), would sensitize the spinal cord and supraspinal structures by continued nociceptive afferent barrage into the central nervous system (Fernández-de-las-Peñas et al 2009a). In these sensitization mechanisms, new receptive fields would appear and cause referred pain (Mense 1994).

Emerging research suggests a physiological link between the clinical manifestations of TrPs, such as hyperalgesia and consistently referred pain, and the phenomenon of central sensitization, although the causal relationships and mechanisms are still unclear (Fernández-de-las-Peñas & Dommerholt 2014). Several studies have confirmed that the area of referred pain correlates with the intensity and duration of the muscle pain (Graven-Nielsen et al 1997; Laursen et al 1997). These studies suggest that muscle-referred pain is maintained by peripheral sensitization mechanisms. Kuan et al (2007) reported that spinal cord connections of TrPs were more effective than non-TrPs in inducing neuroplastic changes in the dorsal horn neurons. Imaging studies have demonstrated that active TrP pain is, at least partially, processed at supraspinal levels as TrP hyperalgesia is processed in various brain areas; enhanced somatosensory activity was observed in the primary and secondary somatosensory cortex, inferior parietal, mid-insula and limbic system (Niddam et al 2007, 2008; Niddam, 2009).

Some clinical studies have demonstrated that sensitization mechanisms related to TrPs may be reversible with proper management (Mellick & Mellick 2003; Hsieh et al 2007). For instance, dry needling inactivation of primary TrPs inhibits the activity in satellite TrPs situated in their zone of referred pain (Hsieh et al 2007). TrP injection into neck muscles produces rapid relief of palpable scalp or facial tenderness and also alleviates associated symptoms of nausea, photophobia and phonophobia in migraine (Carlson et al 1993; Mellick & Mellick 2003). Anaesthetic injections of active TrPs have been shown to decrease mechanical hyperalgesia, allodynia and referred pain significantly in patients suffering from migraine (Giamberardino et al 2007), fibromyalgia (Affaitati et al 2011) and whiplash (Freeman et al 2009). It is conceivable that the degree of central sensitization may influence whether a patient will respond to TrP treatment. In fact, in clinical practice it is common that individuals with less central sensitization require fewer treatments. Multiple factors can hence influence the degree of sensitization, including altered descending inhibitory systems, sympathetic activity and neuropathic activation, and therefore increase the likelihood that myofascial pain syndromes may be reversible.

TrPs and the sympathetic nervous system

There is a growing interest in the association between muscle TrPs and the sympathetic nervous system. Studies in rabbits (Chen et al 1998b) and humans (McNulty et al 1994; Chung et al 2004) have shown evidence of a sympathetic contribution to the modulation of spontaneous electrical activity at TrPs. In these studies, increased sympathetic efferent discharge increased both the frequency and the amplitude of spontaneous electrical activity of muscle TrPs, whereas sympathetic blockers decreased the frequency and amplitude of spontaneous electrical activity. Ge et al (2006) found increased referred pain intensity and tenderness with sympathetic hyperactivity at TrPs, which suggests a sympathetic contribution to the mechanisms responsible for the generation of referred pain. A later study found an attenuated skin blood flow response after painful stimulation of latent muscle TrPs compared with control non-TrPs, suggesting that there was increased sympathetic vasoconstriction activity at latent TrPs (Zhang et al 2009).

Since both peripheral and central sensitization mechanisms participate in the development of muscle-referred pain (for a more complete review see Arendt-Nielsen et al 2000), sympathetic facilitation can involve peripheral, spinal and / or supraspinal sympathetic structures. The interactions between sympathetic and central nervous systems, and between the sympathetic–sensory and sympathetic–motor coupling at TrPs, are still unknown (for a review see Arendt-Nielsen & Ge 2009). Gerwin et al (2004) suggested that the presence of α- and β-adrenergic receptors at the end plate might provide a possible mechanism for autonomic interaction (Maekawa et al 2002). Stimulation of the α- and β-adrenergic receptors stimulated the release of ACh (acetylcholine) in the phrenic nerve of rodents (Bowman et al 1988).

TrPs: the integrated hypothesis

To explain the various potential hypotheses of the pathogenesis of TrPs is beyond the scope of this chapter, but a summary of current data will be reviewed. The activation of a TrP may result from a variety of factors (e.g. repetitive muscle overuse, acute or sustained overload, psychological stress or other key myofascial TrPs). Particular attention has been paid to injured or overloaded muscle fibres in the pathogenesis of TrPs (Chen et al 2000; Gerwin et al 2004; Itoh et al 2004; Treaster et al 2006). Some authors have hypothesized that muscle trauma, repetitive low-intensity muscle overload or intense eccentric contractions may create a vicious cycle of events. Damage to the sarcoplasmic reticulum or the cell membrane may lead to an increase of the calcium concentration, an activation of actin and myosin filaments, a relative shortage of adenosine triphosphate (ATP) and an impaired calcium pump (Simons et al 1999; Gerwin et al 2004).

Based on these events, Simons and Travell proposed the so-called 'energy crisis hypothesis' introduced in 1981 and enhanced by subsequent research, leading to the **integrated hypothesis** (Simons 2004). This hypothesis proposes that abnormal depolarization of the post-junctional membrane of motor end plates enhanced by sustained muscular contraction gives rise to a localized hypoxic energy crisis associated with sensory and autonomic reflex arcs that are sustained by sensitization mechanisms (McPartland & Simons 2006). The notion that damage to the sarcoplasmic reticulum would be an initiating event has now been abandoned in favour of less biomechanical explanations. Hypoxia reduces the pH of muscle tissue, which will activate acid-sensing ion channels and transient receptor potential vanilloid receptors, which in turn leads to the antidromic release of multiple sensitizing chemicals (Dommerholt 2011). Qerama et al (2004) found higher pain intensity and pain characteristics similar to muscle TrPs when noxious stimuli were applied to motor end-plate regions, compared with silent muscle sites. Further, end-plate noise and end-plate spikes (EMG signals from dysfunctional motor end-plate regions) have been significantly associated with muscle TrPs in both human and animal studies (Chen et al 1998a; Hong & Yu 1998; Couppé et al 2001; Simons 2001; Kuan et al 2002; Macgregor et al 2006; Chang et al 2008). Findings from these studies support the theory that TrPs are subsequently associated with dysfunctional motor end plates (Simons et al 2002). Although there is evidence to support the integrated hypothesis as an aetiological pathogenesis of TrPs, the hypothesis still has some weak links that need to be addressed in future studies to solidify the theoretical foundations further. As new research is published, the hypothesis of the formation of TrPs is becoming increasingly complex (Gerwin 2005; Dommerholt et al 2006; McPartland & Simons 2006; Bron & Dommerholt 2012). Additionally, although current evidence supports the theory that dysfunctional motor end plates are clearly associated with TrPs, preliminary evidence suggests that muscle spindles may also be involved in this complex process (Ge et al 2009).

Exploration of Trigger Points Related to Upper Quadrant Pain Syndromes

Clinical history, examination of active and passive movement patterns, quality and area of pain and symptoms, and consideration of referred pain patterns assist clinicians in determining which muscles may be clinically relevant for upper quadrant pain syndromes. There are currently no laboratory or imaging tests available that can confirm the presence of TrPs; however, new emerging imaging techniques are promising (Sikdar et al 2009).

TrP palpation starts with the identification of a taut band within the skeletal muscle by palpating perpendicular to the fibre direction. Patients may be asked to contract the muscle so as to locate the fibres better. Muscles may be placed in a relaxed or slightly pre-stretched position for palpation, depending on the patient's clinical presentation. Once the taut band is located, a hypersensitive spot within that band is identified, which by definition is a TrP. If the examiner manually strums the taut band, a local twitch response (LTR) can be elicited, which is a sudden involuntary contraction of the taut band. The LTR and referred pain increase the certainty of the TrP diagnosis. Clinicians should be wary of preconceived expectations of the location and referred pain patterns of TrPs, although most textbooks will use some kind of standard marks for didactic purposes.

TrP can be identified through (a) flat palpation, in which the therapist applies finger or thumb pressure to the muscle against underlying bone tissue (Fig. 59.1), and (b) pincer palpation, where the muscle is rolled between the tips of the digits (Fig. 59.2). In the following section, we will describe the muscles most commonly involved in the genesis of upper quadrant pain syndromes.

Neck–shoulder muscles

There are several neck–shoulder muscles (i.e. the upper trapezius, sternocleidomastoid, levator scapulae, rhomboid, serratus posterior superior, splenius capitis and splenius cervicis) from which TrP-referred pain can contribute to arm pain syndromes (Skubick et al 1993; Simons et al 1999). For instance, Fernández-de-las-Peñas et al (2007a) demonstrated that the referred pain elicited by the upper trapezius,

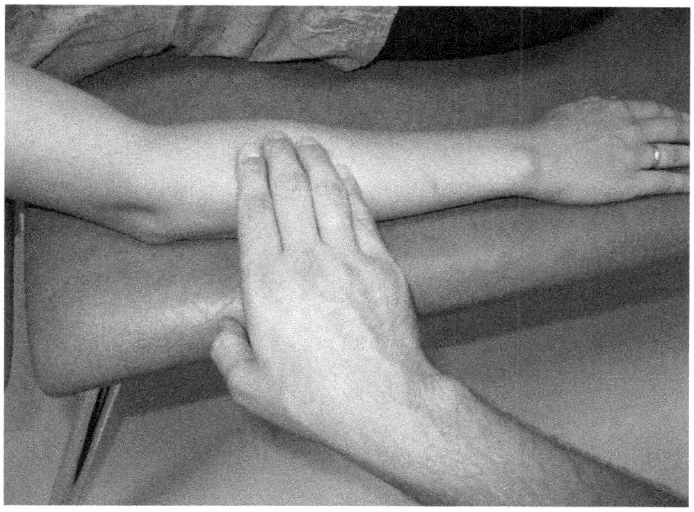

Figure 59.1 Flat palpation of a taut band within the extensor wrist muscles.

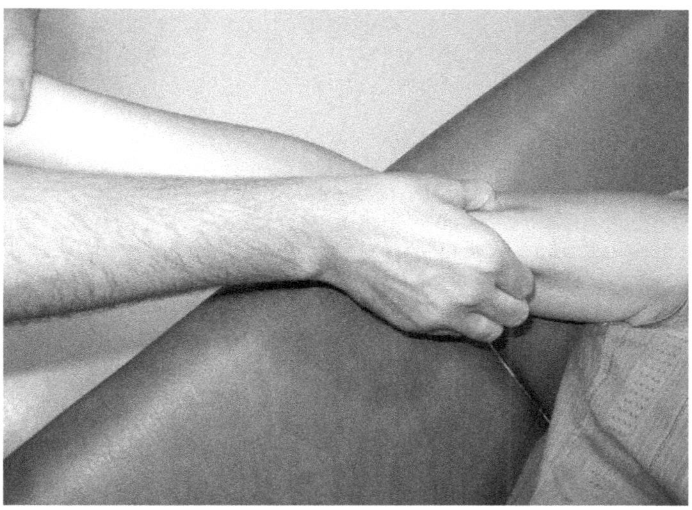

Figure 59.2 Pincer palpation of a taut band within the biceps brachii muscle.

sternocleidomastoid, suboccipital and levator scapulae TrPs reproduced the pain pattern in patients with idiopathic neck pain. The referred pain from these muscles often spreads to the head and the neck, for instance the upper trapezius (Fernández-de-las-Peñas et al 2007b) or sternocleidomastoid (Fernández-de-las-Peñas et al 2006) in individuals with chronic tension-type headache. The levator scapulae and rhomboid TrPs refer pain to the angle of the neck, along the vertebral border of the scapula bone and to the posterior part of the shoulder (Simons et al 1999). Readers are referred to other texts for the exploration of neck–shoulder muscles from which TrPs refer pain to the head and the neck (Simons et al 1999; Gerwin 2005; Fernández-de-las-Peñas et al 2009c).

Scalene muscles

TrPs may be located in either the anterior, medial or posterior scalene muscle. The referred pain spreads anteriorly to the chest (over the pectoral region), to the anterior shoulder

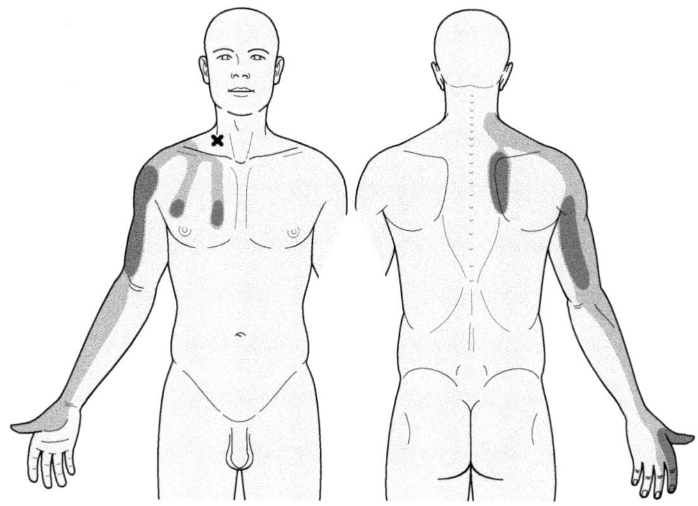

Figure 59.3 Referred pain elicited by myofascial trigger points in the scalene muscle.

area, to the lateral (radial) border of the upper extremity reaching the thumb and / or index finger, and posteriorly to the medial scapular border and interscapular region (Fig. 59.3). Spanos (2005) suggested that scalene muscle TrPs are one of the most ignored causes of interscapular dorsal pain. Active TrPs within the scalene muscle have been found in patients with mechanical neck pain (Muñoz-Muñoz et al 2012), whiplash neck pain (Fernández-Pérez et al 2012), non-specific arm pain (Fernández-de-las-Peñas et al 2012), breast cancer (Fernández-Lao et al 2010) and fibromyalgia (Alonso-Blanco et al 2011). Further, since the brachial plexus anatomically runs between the anterior and the medial scalene muscles, TrPs in either scalene muscle may be related to entrapment of peripheral nerves (Chen et al 1998a), contributing to different arm pain syndromes, for example carpal tunnel syndrome (Simons et al 1999) and thoracic outlet syndrome (Ferguson & Gerwin 2005). In addition, shortening of these muscles induced by TrP taut bands may be related to upward dysfunctions of the first rib (Ferguson & Gerwin 2005). It seems that scalene muscle TrPs can have repercussions in both neural and joint tissues in upper quadrant pain syndromes.

Pectoralis minor muscle

The pectoralis minor muscle pulls the coracoid process anterior and downwards, producing a protracted shoulder position (Ferguson & Gerwin 2005). TrPs within the pectoralis minor muscle refer pain to the anterior part of the chest, the anterior part of the shoulder (coracoid process) and usually to the ulnar aspect of the arm and forearm (Fig. 59.4). Lawson et al (2011) demonstrated that active TrPs in the pectoralis minor muscle could mimic angina symptoms. In addition, since the brachial plexus runs anatomically under the pectoralis minor muscle, an increased tension of this muscle can trap the lower trunk (C7–C8 nerve trunks) of the brachial plexus, resulting in an ulnar radiculopathy (Simons 1991; Vemuri et al 2013). Langley (1997) suggested that patients exhibiting symptoms of brachial plexus irritation and other compression neuropathies should be examined for the

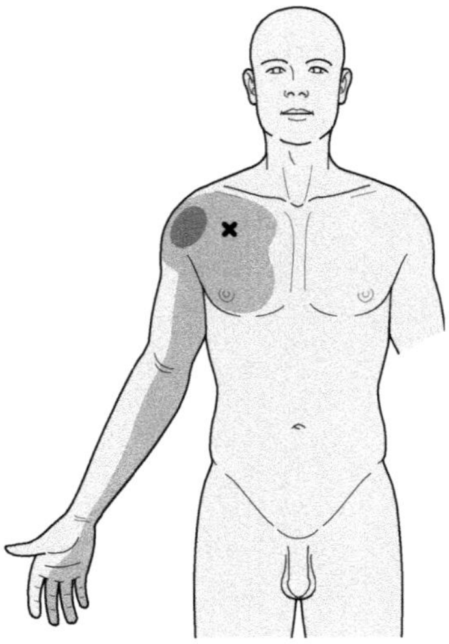

Figure 59.4 Referred pain elicited by myofascial trigger points in the pectoralis minor muscle.

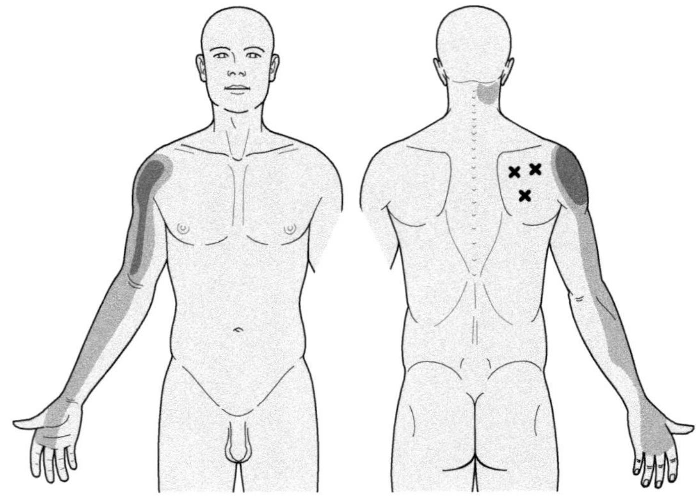

Figure 59.6 Referred pain elicited by myofascial trigger points in the infraspinatus muscle.

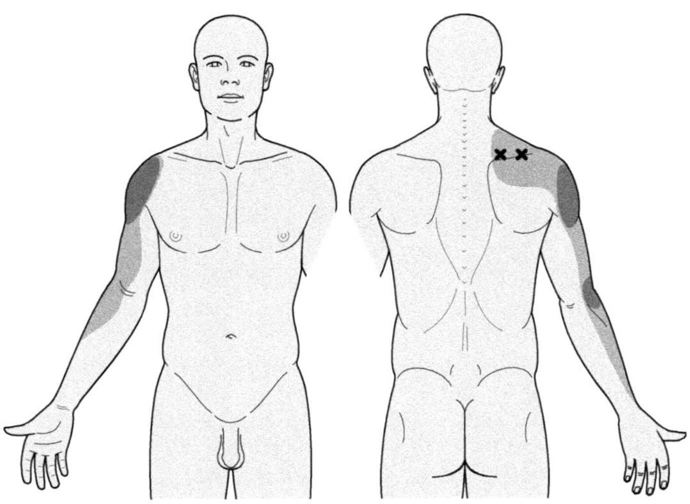

Figure 59.5 Referred pain elicited by myofascial trigger points in the supraspinatus muscle.

presence of TrPs within the pectoralis minor muscle. Hong and Simons (1993) demonstrated that patients with chronic whiplash exhibit active TrPs in the pectoralis minor reproducing their arm pain symptomatology.

Supraspinatus muscle

The supraspinatus muscle assists abduction of the arm and stabilization of the humeral head during arm movements. Stability prevents superior translation of the humeral head and is accomplished through compressive forces applied to the convex humeral head into the concave glenoid fossa. TrPs within the supraspinatus muscle elicit a referred pain that is felt as deep pain in and around the shoulder, particularly over the mid-deltoid region. Deep pain over the mid-deltoid area may be mistaken for subdeltoid bursitis (Simons et al 1999). The referred pain may also spread down to the arm and the forearm, and sometimes over the lateral epicondyle (Fig. 59.5).

Active TrPs in the supraspinatus muscle have been found in patients with shoulder impingement (Hidalgo-Lozano et al 2010), shoulder pain (Bron et al 2011) and non-specific arm pain (Fernández-de-las-Peñas et al 2012). Jacobson et al (1989) reported that repetitive strain injury over the shoulder joint may be a precipitating factor for supraspinatus TrPs. Chaitow and Delany (2008) suggested that supraspinatus TrPs may lead to imbalance or dysfunction of this muscle, inducing non-proper functioning of the humeral head stabilization during arm elevations. This situation could lead to a compression of supraspinatus tendon against the acromion (Chaitow & Delany 2008). Empirically, TrPs in the supraspinatus muscle can contribute to muscle imbalances observed in individuals with subacromial pain syndrome.

Srbely et al (2008) reported that treatment of the infraspinatus TrPs reduced the sensitivity of the supraspinatus TrP, which probably occurs because both muscles receive their innervation from the suprascapular nerve (C5 nerve root). This study supported the suggestion that all scapular girdle muscles may contribute to symptoms of shoulder / arm pain.

Infraspinatus muscle

The infraspinatus muscle assists external rotation of the arm and stabilization of the humeral head during arm movements. Simons et al (1999) suggested that TrPs in the infraspinatus muscle may be among the most ignored causes of shoulder and arm pain. Lucas et al (2004) found that the presence of latent TrPs within the infraspinatus muscle induced early activation of the muscle, although the authors recognized that the group muscle activation pattern was inconsistent in that study.

The referred pain from this muscle is perceived as deep joint pain in the anterior part of the shoulder area and downwards to the anterior–lateral (radial) aspect of the arm, forearm and fingers (Fig. 59.6). Infraspinatus muscle TrPs can induce restriction of shoulder internal rotation (Simons et al 1999). Bron et al (2007) found that infraspinatus muscle TrPs showed a better inter-rater reliability (pair-wise agreement 69–80%) than either the biceps or the deltoid muscles.

Qerama et al (2009) demonstrated that 49% of subjects with normal electrophysiological findings of the median nerve, but symptoms mimicking carpal tunnel syndrome, presented with active TrP in the infraspinatus muscle associated with paraesthesia and referred pain to the arm and fingers. In the same study, patients with mild electrophysiological signs of carpal tunnel syndrome showed a significantly higher occurrence of infraspinatus muscle TrPs within the symptomatic arm, compared with patients with moderate to severe electrophysiological signs (33% versus 20%).

Ge et al (2008a) found multiple, rather than single, active TrPs in the infraspinatus muscle on the painful side in patients with shoulder–arm pain, with the majority of TrPs located in the mid-fibre region of the muscle belly. Active TrPs in the infraspinatus muscle have also been found in subjects with shoulder impingement (Hidalgo-Lozano et al 2010), shoulder pain (Bron et al 2011) and non-specific arm pain (Fernández-de-las-Peñas et al 2012). Ohmori et al (2013) recently reported that TrPs in the supraspinatus and infraspinatus muscles contributed to shoulder pain with ipsilateral upper extremity elevation after muscle-sparing thoracotomy.

Hong (1994) suggested that infraspinatus muscle TrPs may be considered as primary (key) TrPs of deltoid muscle TrPs. Hsieh et al (2007) confirmed that treating infraspinatus TrPs can inactivate TrPs in the anterior deltoid muscle, whereas other authors have observed electromyographically that infraspinatus TrPs can inhibit use of the anterior deltoid muscle, with full functional recovery after inactivation of these TrP. Infraspinatus TrPs are the most important TrPs to consider in patients with upper quadrant pain syndromes, particularly scapular girdle pain.

Teres minor and major muscles

TrPs in the teres minor muscle elicit referred pain in the posterior part of the deltoid region, mimicking a 'painful bursitis' in the posterior part of the shoulder joint (Escobar & Ballesteros 1988) (Fig. 59.7A). TrPs within the teres major refer pain to the posterior deltoid area and shoulder joint, which can occasionally spread to the dorsal forearm (Fig 59.7B). Active TrPs in the teres minor and major muscles have been found in patients with non-specific shoulder pain (Bron et al 2011).

Subscapularis muscle

Subscapularis TrPs cause severe pain at rest and during motion. The referred pain spreads to the posterior aspect of the shoulder joint and the scapula, extending down to the posterior aspect of the arm and the volar surface of the wrist (Fig. 59.8). The insertion of the subscapularis tendon is usually described on the lesser tuberosity of the humerus; however, it seems that this muscle also expands its insertion to the anterior part of the shoulder joint (Cash et al 2009). In addition, the subscapularis muscle has a destabilizing inferior shear potential over the shoulder joint (Ackland & Pandy 2009). Therefore, shortening of this muscle may be implicated in shoulder retraction pathologies such as the 'frozen shoulder' (Simons et al 1999; Ferguson & Gerwin 2005); Jankovic and Van Zundert (2006) reported that five patients with frozen shoulder syndrome experienced pain relief after injections into TrPs in the subscapularis muscle. This muscle is one of the most commonly involved muscles in shoulder dysfunction and pain syndromes and, as it serves as an antagonist to most of the other shoulder joint stabilizers, its dysfunction encourages the development of TrPs in other musculature. In fact, TrPs in the subscapularis muscle have been found to be involved in elite swimmers with shoulder pain (Hidalgo-Lozano et al 2013). Therefore, this muscle should not be overlooked in TrP examination, which does require considerable manual skill.

Pectoralis major muscle

Shortening of the pectoralis major muscle has been linked clinically to the upper cross syndrome (Janda 1996). TrPs within the pectoralis major muscle refer pain particularly to the anterior part of the chest and to the ulnar aspect of the arm (Fig. 59.9). Active TrPs in the pectoralis major muscle have been studied in different populations and were found to reproduce non-specific arm pain in blue-collar and white-collar workers (Fernández-de-las-Peñas et al 2012), as well as in women with fibromyalgia (Alonso-Blanco et al 2011). The

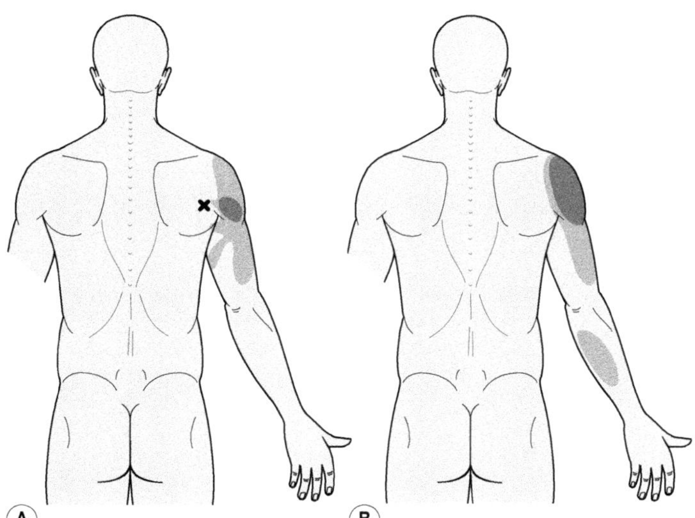

Figure 59.7 Referred pain elicited by myofascial trigger points in the teres minor (A) and major (B) muscles.

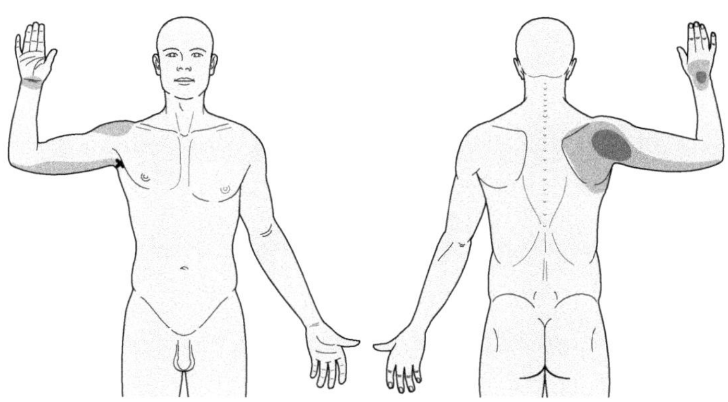

Figure 59.8 Referred pain elicited by myofascial trigger points in the subscapularis muscle.

referred pain from the left pectoralis major muscle may simulate angina pectoris (Simons et al 1999). Further, it is conceivable that angina pectoris may be a precipitating factor for activation of pectoralis major TrPs. In fact, individuals with known or suspected angina pectoris usually present with pain and tenderness in this muscle (Kumarathurai et al 2008). Rinzler and Travell (1948) reported that patients with pain complaints of coronary insufficiency with no history or evidence of cardiac disease are often afflicted with active pectoralis major TrPs. Some studies have found that post-mastectomy pain is also related to active TrPs in the pectoralis major, latissimus dorsi and serratus anterior muscles (Fernández-Lao et al 2010; Torres Lacomba et al 2010). Active TrPs in the right pectoralis major have also been described in patients with tachycardia (Simons et al 1999).

Deltoid muscle

The deltoid is a muscle that commonly develops TrPs in any of its bellies (anterior, middle or posterior). The middle and anterior parts of this muscle can contribute significantly to superior shear forces of the humeral head (Ackland & Pandy 2009); therefore, deltoid muscle TrPs may contribute to shoulder muscle imbalance (Simons et al 1999). Ibarra et al (2011) found that the presence of latent TrPs in the posterior deltoid muscle reduced antagonist reciprocal inhibition during arm elevation. TrPs in the deltoid muscle could contribute to a delayed and incomplete muscle relaxation following exercise, disordered fine movement control and unbalanced motor activation of the shoulder girdle complex. Deltoid TrPs typically refer a burning and deep pain to the region where the muscle is located: (a) TrPs in the anterior part of the deltoid refer pain to the anterior and middle shoulder regions (Fig. 59.10A), (b) TrPs in the middle part of the muscle refer pain over the middle and posterior areas (Fig. 59.10B) and (c) TrPs in the posterior part refer pain to the posterior area of the shoulder (Fig. 59.10C). Hsueh et al (1998) reported that C5–C6 disc lesions were associated with active TrPs in the deltoid muscle, suggesting the clinical relevance of assessing cervical segments related to the innervation of the affected muscle.

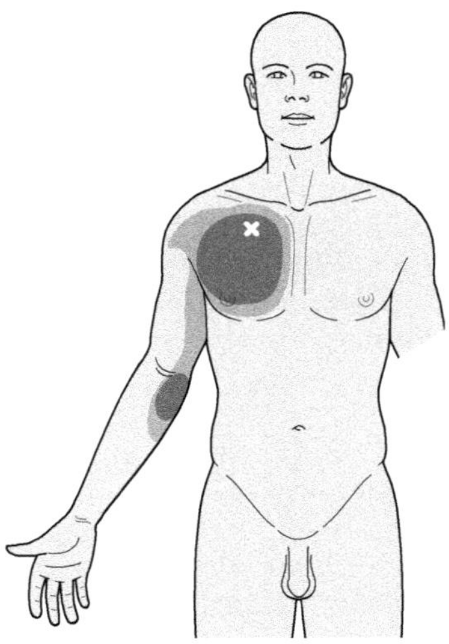

Figure 59.9 Referred pain elicited by myofascial trigger points in the pectoralis major muscle.

Biceps brachii muscle

The referred pain elicited by TrPs in the biceps brachii muscle spreads up the muscle into the anterior region of the shoulder. Referred pain in the region of the biceps tendon can be misdiagnosed as bicipital tendonitis (Simons et al 1999). The referred pain can also spread down the muscle to the anterior area of the elbow region (Fig. 59.11). It is important to note that the median nerve runs anatomically medial to the muscle belly of the biceps brachii (Maeda et al 2009). Therefore, tension induced by TrP taut bands or abnormal muscle bands (Paraskevas et al 2008) located over the biceps brachii muscle may lead to median nerve tension.

Triceps brachii muscle

As the radial nerve runs deep to the lateral head of the triceps muscle (Rezzouk et al 2002), TrPs in this muscle may contribute to radial nerve entrapment (Simons et al 1999). TrPs can be located in any of the heads of this muscle: (a) TrPs within

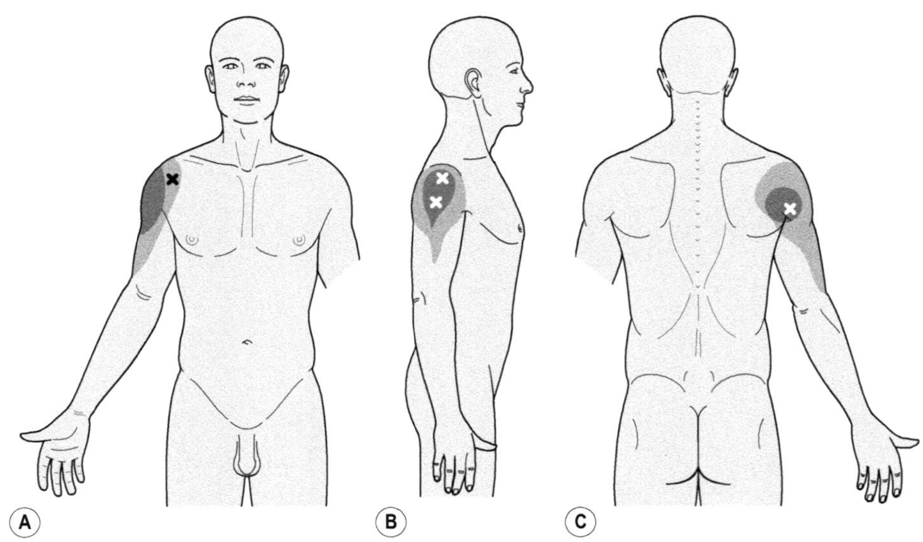

Figure 59.10 Referred pain elicited by myofascial trigger points in the anterior (A), middle (B) and posterior (C) deltoid muscle.

the long head of the muscle refer pain upwards to the posterior area of the shoulder joint, spreading occasionally to the upper trapezius region, and sometimes down the dorsum of the forearm, skipping the elbow (Fig. 59.12A, right arm); (b) TrPs over the lateral head of the muscle refer pain to the posterior part of the arm, sometimes spreading to the dorsum of the forearm or the fourth and fifth digits (Fig. 59.12B, right arm); (c) the referred pain elicited by TrPs within the medial head of the muscle is projected to the lateral epicondyle and to the olecranon process (Fig. 59.12B, left arm). Janssens (1991) found, in a study with dogs, that treatment of TrPs in the triceps brachii muscle was critical for the recovery of normal walking and running.

Brachioradialis muscle

The brachioradialis is an elbow flexor muscle with the forearm in neutral position inducing symptoms in the forearm or wrist (Simons et al 1999). A recent case report demonstrated that the radial nerve could become trapped at the humeral origin of the brachioradialis muscle (Cherchel et al 2013).

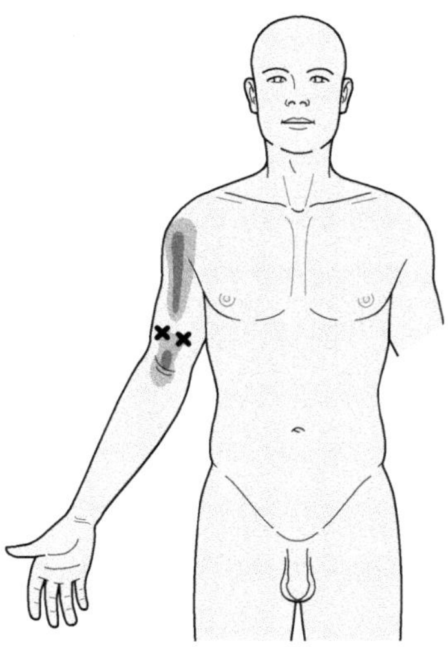

Figure 59.11 Referred pain elicited by myofascial trigger points in the biceps brachii muscle.

Brachioradialis TrPs project their referred pain to the lateral epicondyle, the radial aspect of the forearm, the wrist and the base of the thumb, in the web between the thumb and index finger (Fig. 59.13). Referred pain from TrPs in this muscle can mimic de Quervain's syndrome. Some studies have observed that the brachioradialis muscle was more irritable than other elbow muscles, owing to the presence of latent TrPs in both children (Han et al 2012) and adults (Kao et al 2007).

Fernández-Carnero et al (2007) found that 50% of patients with unilateral lateral epicondylalgia showed active TrPs within the brachioradialis muscle, which supports its role in this pain condition. Finally, shortening of the brachioradialis may cause an entrapment of the radial nerve (Mekhail et al 1999).

Supinator muscle

The supinator muscle is extremely important for a properly functioning elbow joint. It is known that the radial nerve crosses the fibrous arch of the supinator muscle, called the arcade of Frohse, the main region of entrapment of this nerve (Tatar et al 2009; Tubbs et al 2013). Therefore, muscle tension induced by TrP taut bands in this muscle can trap the radial nerve, particularly its motor branch (posterior interosseus) (Simons et al 1999; Schneider 2005). TrPs in the supinator muscle refer pain to the lateral epicondyle, the lateral area of the elbow, and sometimes can project spillover pain to the dorsal aspect of the web of the thumb (Fig. 59.14).

Simons et al (1999) suggested that supinator muscle TrPs simulate symptoms experienced by individuals with lateral epicondylalgia. Slater et al (2003) confirmed that hypertonic saline injected into the supinator muscle simulated sensory and motor manifestations of lateral epicondylalgia patients. In a subsequent study, Slater et al (2005) found that the injection of hypertonic saline into the supinator muscle in patients with lateral epicondylalgia increased the referred pain areas and motor disturbances.

Wrist/hand extensor muscles

The wrist extensor musculature is located over the radial aspect of the forearm. These muscles have complex

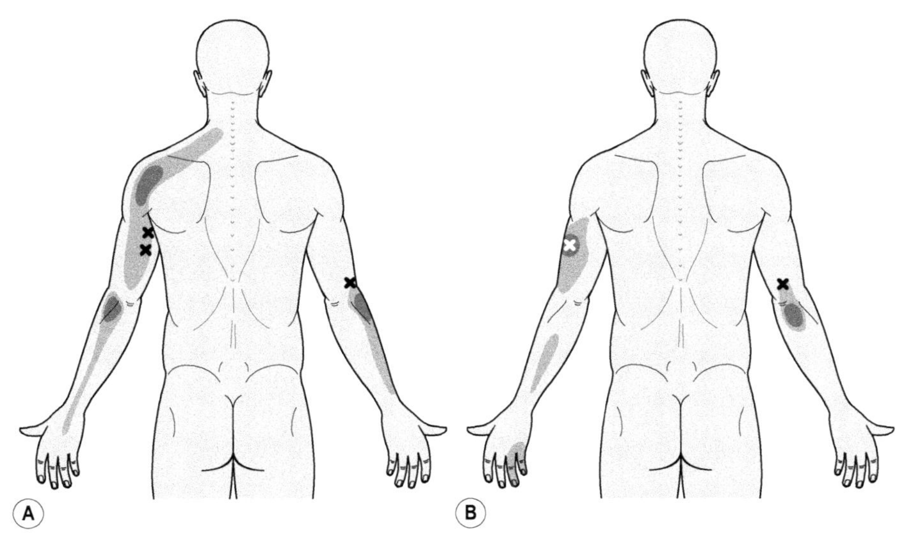

Figure 59.12 Referred pain elicited by myofascial trigger points in the triceps brachii muscle.

agonist–antagonist function, which makes them vulnerable for repetitive strain and overload situations. For instance, the extensor carpi radialis longus muscle induces wrist extension and radial deviation and the extensor carpi ulnaris muscle exerts wrist extension and ulnar deviation (Livingston et al 2001). Chen et al (2000) found that piano students exhibited significantly decreased pressure thresholds over latent TrPs in the wrist extensor muscles after only 20 minutes of piano playing. Latent TrPs may transition into active TrPs and compromise motor function. The wrist extensor musculature is innervated by the deep branch of the radial nerve (posterior interosseous nerve). The radial nerve may become trapped in the superior–lateral aspect of the extensor carpi radialis brevis muscle (Clavert et al 2009; Cho et al 2013).

In general, referred pain patterns elicited by wrist extensor muscle TrPs spread upwards to the lateral epicondyle and downwards along the muscle belly towards their insertion in the wrist / hand: (a) TrPs in the **extensor carpi radialis longus** muscle refer pain to the lateral epicondyle and to the dorsum of the hand next to the thumb (Fig. 59.15A), (b) TrPs in the **extensor carpi radialis brevis** muscle project pain to the radial and posterior aspects of the hand and the wrist (Fig. 59.15B), (c) **extensor digitorum communis** TrPs refer pain downwards to the forearm, reaching the same digit that the fibres activate (Fig. 59.15C), and (d) referred pain from the **extensor carpi ulnaris muscle** TrPs is perceived on the ulnar side of the back of the wrist (Fig. 59.15D).

Fernández-Carnero et al (2007) found that active TrPs within these muscles (65% extensor carpi radialis brevis, 55% extensor carpi radialis longus and 25% extensor digitorum communis) reproduced the pain pattern experienced by individuals with lateral epicondylalgia. Interestingly, these same muscles developed latent TrPs on the non-symptomatic side in individuals with unilateral elbow pain (Fernández-Carnero et al 2008). It is remarkable to note that the extensor carpi radialis brevis, the muscle most affected by active TrPs in subjects with lateral epicondylalgia, seems to be the most relevant for tendon changes in elbow pain (Ljung et al 1999). Therefore, clinicians should examine the wrist extensor muscles in patients with lateral epicondylalgia.

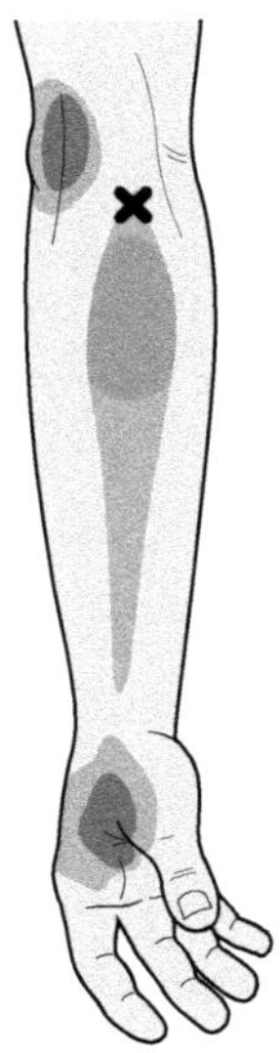

Figure 59.13 Referred pain elicited by myofascial trigger points in the brachioradialis muscle.

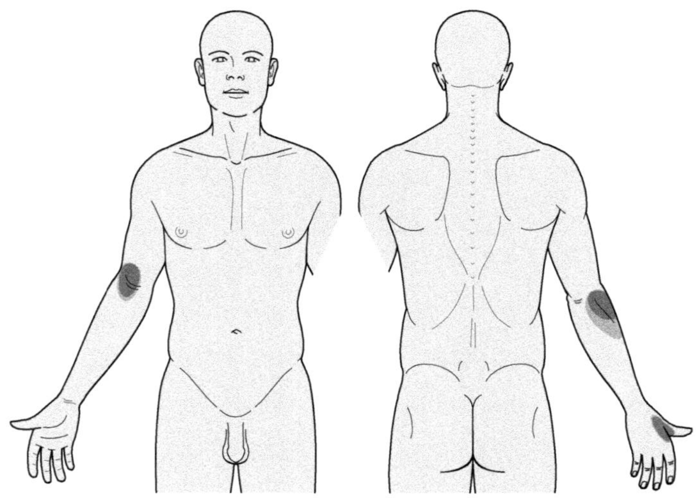

Figure 59.14 Referred pain elicited by myofascial trigger points in the supinator muscle.

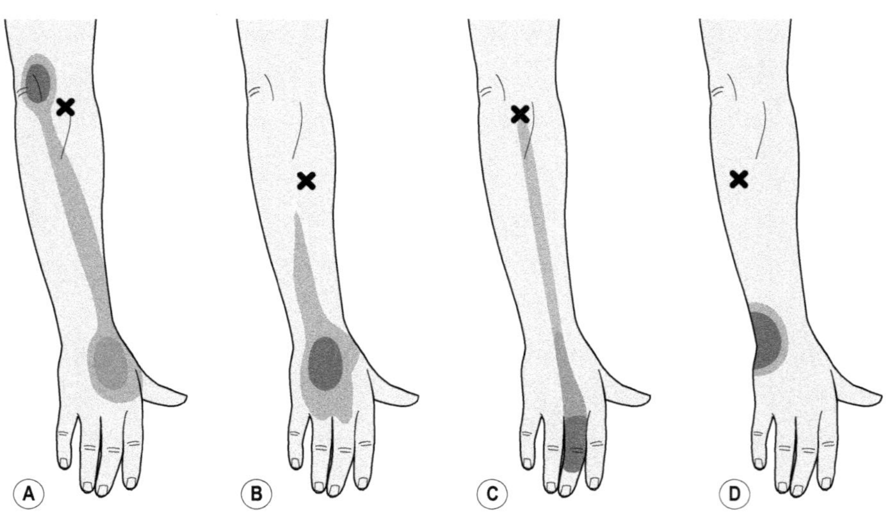

Figure 59.15 Referred pain elicited by myofascial trigger points in the extensor carpi radialis longus (A), extensor carpi radialis brevis (B), the extensor digitorum communis (C) and extensor carpi ulnaris (D) muscles.

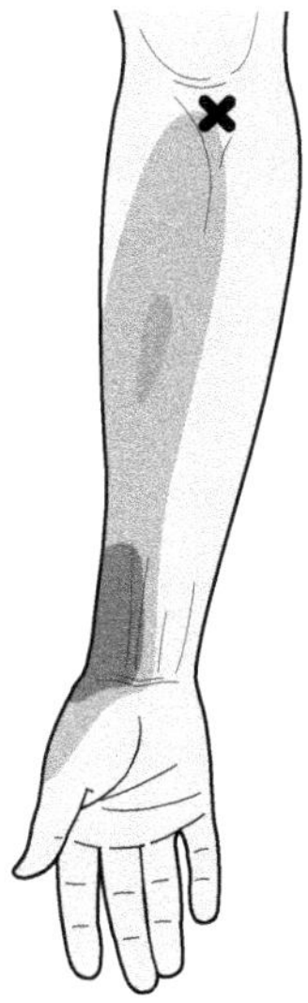

Figure 59.16 Referred pain elicited by myofascial trigger points in the pronator teres muscle.

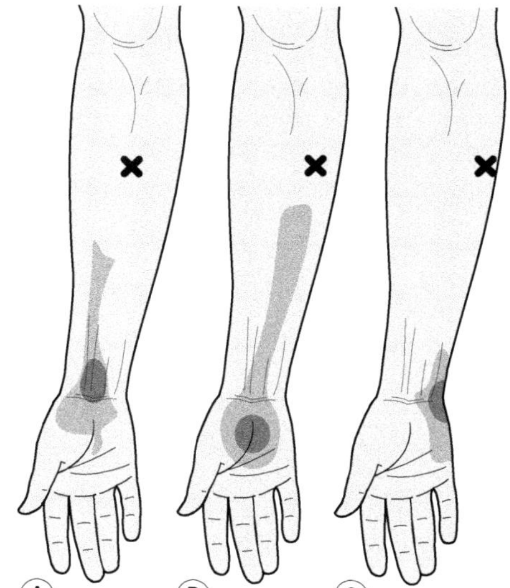

Figure 59.17 Referred pain elicited by myofascial trigger points in the flexor carpi radialis (A), palmaris longus (B) and flexor carpi ulnaris (C) muscles.

Pronator teres muscle

The pronator teres muscle is the main pronator of the forearm. The median nerve passes between the two heads of the pronator teres muscle, making this muscle a common entrapment region of the nerve (Bilecenoglu et al 2005; Demirci et al 2007). An entrapment of the median nerve in the pronator teres muscle is known as pronator syndrome (Lee & LaStayo 2004). Tension induced by TrP taut bands in this muscle may be relevant for symptoms associated with median nerve compression (Simons et al 1999). Pronator teres TrPs refer pain downwards to the forearm and the volar radial region of the wrist (Fig. 59.16). Hains et al (2010) found that compression at TrPs located in the pronator teres muscle was effective for reducing symptoms in patients with carpal tunnel syndrome.

Wrist/hand flexor muscles

The wrist flexor musculature has a similar complex agonist–antagonist function as the wrist extensors. For instance, the flexor carpi radialis induces wrist flexion and radial deviation, whereas the flexor carpi ulnaris muscle exerts wrist flexion and ulnar deviation. In general, referred pain patterns elicited from wrist flexor muscle TrPs usually spread downwards along the muscle belly towards their insertion in the wrist: (a) TrPs in the **flexor carpi radialis** refer pain to the volar aspect of the wrist (Fig. 59.17A); (b) **palmaris longus muscle** TrPs project superficial, needle-like pain over the volar area of the palm (Fig. 59.17B), though the palmaris longus muscle is not present in all subjects; (c) referred pain from the **flexor carpi ulnaris muscle** TrPs is perceived in the ulnar side of the volar aspect of the wrist (Fig. 59.17C). Finally, no easy distinction can be made between referred pain patterns of the **flexors digitorum superficialis** and those of the **profundus** muscles (Simons et al 1999) as, in these muscles, TrPs will refer pain to the same digit that the fibres activate (Fig. 59.18). For instance, TrPs in the fibres of the middle finger flexor muscle refer pain through the length of the middle finger, similarly to the extensor digitorum communis muscle.

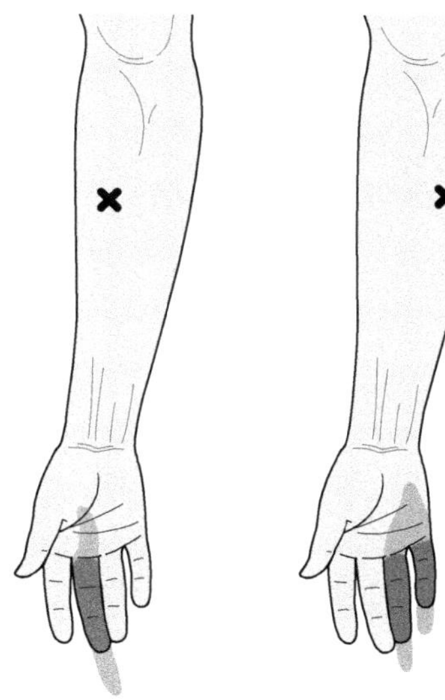

Figure 59.18 Referred pain elicited by myofascial trigger points in the flexors digitorum superficialis and profundus muscles.

Wrist flexor muscles are innervated by the median and ulnar nerves. Due to their anatomical relationships, the median nerve can become trapped by the flexor digitorum profundus and superficialis muscles, whereas the ulnar nerve can become trapped by the flexor carpi ulnaris and flexor digitorum profundus muscles (Chaitow & Delany 2008; Pappas et al 2010). Clinicians should examine and treat TrPs in this musculature in patients with pain symptoms in either ulnar or median nerve territories, for example carpal tunnel syndrome or ulnar neuropathy (Ferguson & Gerwin 2005).

Other muscles of the upper quadrant

Finally, clinicians should be aware that there is a greater number of muscle TrPs with their own specific referred pain patterns contributing to upper quadrant pain syndromes. For example, the brachialis, coracobrachialis, latissimus dorsi, serratus anterior and subclavius muscles also refer pain to the arm or the forearm (Simons et al 1999). Several studies have described referred pain from other muscles, such as the pronator quadratus (Hwang et al 2005a) or the abductor pollicis longus (Hwang et al 2005b), which were included in the comprehensive book by Simons et al (1999). In this chapter we have also not included any hand musculature, such as the flexor pollicis longus, adductor pollicis, abductor pollicis, opponens pollicis, thumb flexor or interosseous muscles, which also can be involved in hand pain syndromes (Simons et al 1999).

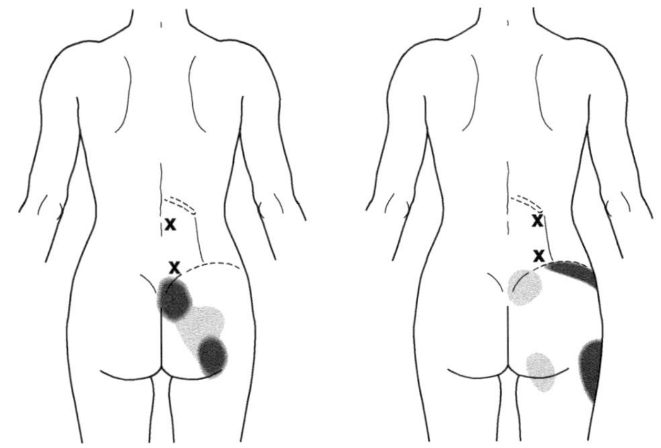

Figure 59.19 Referred pain elicited by myofascial trigger points in the quadratus lumborum muscle.

Exploration of Trigger Points Related to Lower Quadrant Pain Syndromes

The clinical examination of TrPs in patients with lower quadrant syndromes, particularly those with low back pain, can be complex. There is a considerable overlap of referred pain patterns and, because many of the muscles are deep, palpation of the taut band and the ability to elicit a local twitch response are more difficult. Clinicians should be wary of preconceived expectations of the location and referred pain patterns of TrPs, although most textbooks use some kind of standard marks for didactic purposes. In this section, we will describe the muscles most commonly involved in the genesis of lower quadrant pain syndromes.

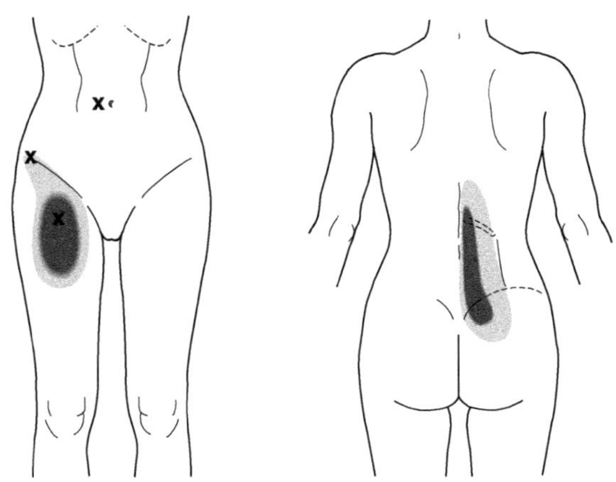

Figure 59.20 Referred pain elicited by myofascial trigger points in the iliopsoas muscle.

Quadratus lumborum muscle

The quadratus lumborum muscle is the main stabilizer of the twelfth rib and the lower attachments of the diaphragm. It assists with inspiration, but its main role is related to movement of the spine. When the muscle contracts unilaterally, it controls contralateral side-bending (eccentric contraction) and it performs ipsilateral side-bending of the spine (when the pelvis is fixed). When acting bilaterally, it assists with facilitation of spine extension. The referred pain can spread to the iliac crest, the greater trochanter, the lateral thigh, the lower portion of the abdomen, the sacroiliac joint, the lower buttock (Fig. 59.19) and, sometimes, to the groin, labia and testicles.

Several studies have demonstrated that active TrPs in the quadratus lumborum muscle are present in patients with low back pain. Teixera et al (2011) identified that active TrPs within the quadratus lumborum and gluteus medius muscles were present in 85.7% of patients with post-laminectomy pain syndrome. Chen and Nizar (2011) found that 63.5% of patients with chronic back pain exhibited TrPs in the piriformis and quadratus lumborum muscles, and these patients experienced a favourable outcome following TrP-dry-needling intervention. A recent study (Iglesias-González et al 2013) supported the role of active TrPs in non-specific low back pain, as the presence of TrPs in the quadratus lumborum, iliocostalis lumborum and gluteus medius muscles was associated with higher pain intensity and worse sleep quality. It is possible that the presence of active TrPs in this muscle can be related to the muscle atrophy found in patients with degenerative disc disease (Ploumis et al 2011), or with the changes in motor control strategies observed in patients with low back pain (Park et al 2013).

Psoas major muscle

The psoas major muscle is one of the main stabilizers of the lumbar spine (Penning 2000). TrPs in the psoas major muscle refer pain to the groin area, superior part of the thigh and lumbar spine (Fig. 59.20). This is an important muscle since it is anatomically related to several urogenital structures and the lumbar plexus (Stepnik et al 2006; Petchprapa et al 2010). Entrapment of the femoral nerve in the psoas major muscle can induce paralysis of the quadriceps muscle (Lefevre et al 2015). Similarly, the lateral femoral cutaneous nerve emerges from the lateral border of the psoas and crosses the iliacus muscles before emerging from the pelvis medial to the anterior superior iliac spine under the inguinal ligament and so it is especially vulnerable to injury in this area (Craig 2013). Therefore, taut bands in the psoas major muscle can contribute to possible entrapments of the lumbar plexus. Cummings (2003) described a case where TrPs in the iliopsoas muscle reproduced knee pain symptoms.

Patients with low back pain exhibit increased activity during functional tasks (Arbanas et al 2013) and decreased muscle size at the lumbar level (Lee et al 2011) of the psoas major muscle. TrPs in this muscle may be also related to the muscle activity changes observed in patients with low back pain. One of the problems with identifying TrPs in this muscle is that it is not easily accessible to proper palpation, as the reliability of TrP identification is low (Hsieh et al 2000).

Piriformis muscle

The piriformis muscle is the main stabilizer between the sacrum and the femur. The sciatic nerve anatomically runs deep to the piriformis; however, variations exist and the nerve may exit either above or through the muscle (Natsis et al 2014). The referred pain travels along the path of the sciatic nerve, which may include the sacroiliac region and the proximal two-thirds of the thigh (Fig. 59.21). Due to the anatomical relationship between the sciatic nerve and the piriformis muscle, TrPs in this muscle may be related to entrapment of the nerve, which is commonly referred to as piriformis syndrome. Piriformis syndrome continues to be a somewhat controversial diagnosis for sciatic pain (Jankovic et al 2013). Active TrPs in the piriformis muscle have been found in patients with non-specific low back pain (Iglesias-González et al 2013) and with fibromyalgia syndrome (Alonso-Blanco et al 2011).

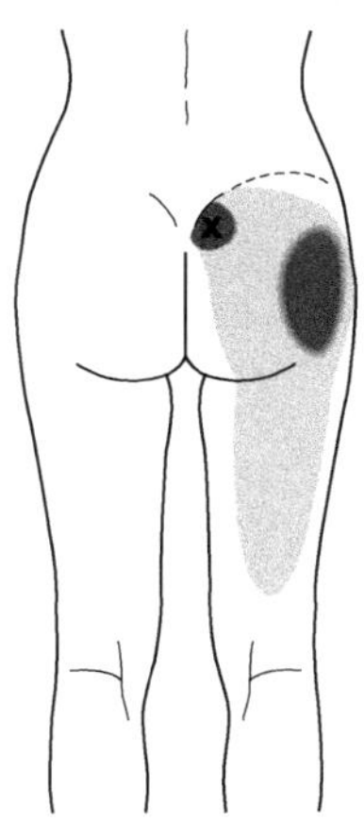

Figure 59.21 Referred pain elicited by myofascial trigger points in the piriformis muscle.

Gluteus medius muscle

The gluteus medius is the main hip abductor and lateral stabilizer of the pelvis. Insufficiency of this muscle results in a positive Trendelenburg test. Burnet and Pidcoe (2009) observed that lower isometric gluteus medius torque was a poor predictor of frontal plane pelvic drop during running. TrPs in this muscle mainly refer pain to the sacroiliac joint, gluteal and lumbosacral regions (Fig. 59.22). Since it is not possible to separate referred pain pattern from the gluteus minimus muscle in the area where the two muscles overlap, it is likely that gluteus medius TrPs also refer pain to the iliotibial tract, the posterior thigh and posterior lower leg.

Active TrPs in the gluteus medius muscle have been found in patients with non-specific low back pain (Iglesias-González et al 2013), lumbar disc prolapse (Samuel et al 2007) and fibromyalgia syndrome (Ge et al 2011). Samuel et al (2007) found that active TrPs in the gluteus medius muscle were related to an L5–S1 disc prolapse. It is possible that TrPs in this muscle are intrinsically related to disc prolapses at the innervation-related segment. Additionally, a recent study found that patients with patellofemoral pain syndrome also exhibited bilateral TrPs in the gluteus medius muscle (Roach et al 2013). Rainey (2013) reported that management of TrPs in the gluteus medius and maximus muscles were effective for a single patient with chronic low back pain.

Gluteus minimus muscle

This muscle is found deep to the gluteus medius. It has a bursa between the tendon and its insertion at the greater trochanter (Flack et al 2012). The gluteus minimus assists the gluteus medius with hip abduction and it is a lateral stabilizer of the hip. It supports the body in single-leg stance with the tensor fascia lata muscle (Bewyer & Bewyer 2003). Referred pain from gluteus minimus muscle TrPs spreads to the iliotibial tract, gluteal region, posterior thigh and posterior third of the lower leg (Fig. 59.23). It is not possible to separate its

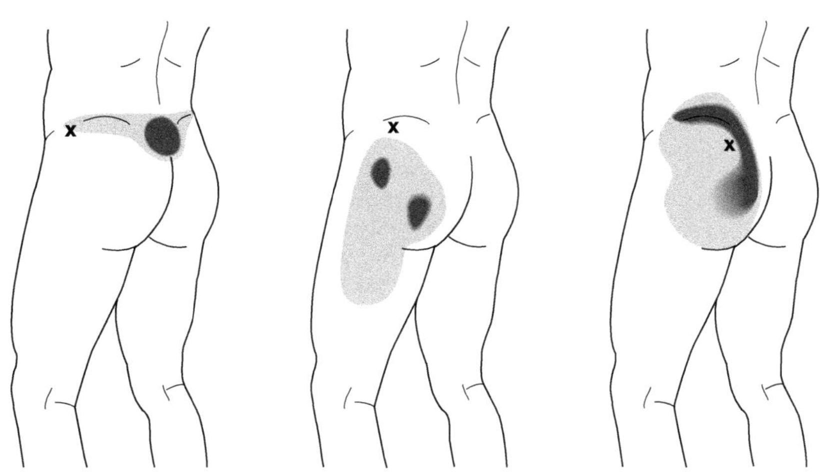

Figure 59.22 Referred pain elicited by myofascial trigger points in the gluteus medius muscle.

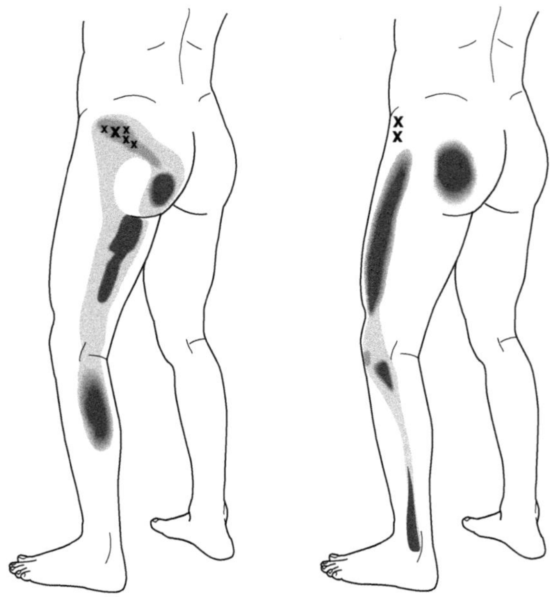

Figure 59.23 Referred pain elicited by myofascial trigger points in the gluteus minimus muscle.

referred pain patterns from those of the gluteus medius muscle in the area where the two muscles overlap.

Quadriceps muscle

This muscle is formed by four main bellies: the rectus femoris, vastus medialis, vastus lateralis and vastus intermedius muscles. The muscles insert at the base of the patella via the thick flat quadriceps femoris tendon. The patellar tendon is a continuation of the quadriceps femoris main tendon and connects the muscle to the tibial tuberosity.

The primary function of the quadriceps muscle is knee extension. The rectus femoris also assists with hip flexion, whereas the vastus lateralis and vastus medialis muscles play an important role in maintaining patella tracking. The referred pain elicited by TrPs in the quadriceps muscle spreads to the anterior thigh and knee pain (**rectus femoris**; Fig. 59.24A), to the lateral side of the thigh from the iliac crest to midway down the lower leg (**vastus lateralis**), and to the anterior–medial aspect of the thigh down to the medial aspect of the knee area (**vastus medialis**; Fig. 59.24B). Active TrPs in any of these muscles may induce motor disturbances and pain in the knee area. Henry et al (2012) reported that patients with knee osteoarthritis awaiting knee arthroplasty exhibited TrPs in the vastus medialis and gastrocnemius muscles. In addition, Huang et al (2013) demonstrated in an animal model that active TrPs in the vastus medialis muscle could be provoked by repeated blunt injury. Additionally, active TrPs in these muscles can be present after knee surgery (e.g. restoration of anterior cruciate ligament or arthroscopy after a meniscectomy).

Adductor muscles

The adductor group includes the adductor longus, adductor brevis and adductor magnus muscles. Their main function is adduction and medial rotation of the thigh as well as hip

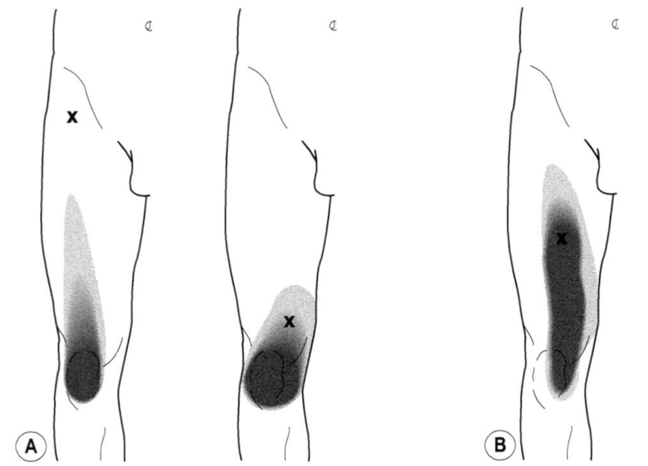

Figure 59.24 Referred pain elicited by myofascial trigger points in the rectus femoris (A) and vastus medialis (B) muscles.

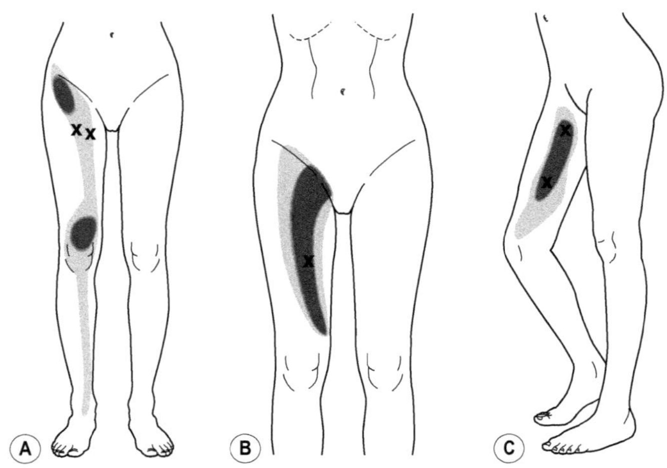

Figure 59.25 Referred pain elicited by myofascial trigger points in the adductor longus and brevis (A), adductor magnus (B) and gracilis (C) muscles.

flexion when the hip is extended. TrPs can be located in any of these muscles along their muscle bellies. The referred pain extends from the femoral triangle to the knee (**adductor longus and brevis**; Fig. 59.25A), from the pelvic floor and genitals to the internal side of the leg (**adductor magnus**; Fig. 59.25B), and along a line within the medial aspect of the thigh (**gracilis**; Fig. 59.25C). TrPs from the adductor muscles can also refer pain to the intrapelvic area (Longbottom 2009). Kim et al (2013) have recently demonstrated that TrP injection of the hip flexors, adductors and lower abdominal muscles resulted in excellent outcomes relative to groin pain in patients with chronic prostatitis / chronic pelvic pain syndrome. Finally, since the obturator nerve merges several motor and sensory branches to the adductor group muscles, this nerve can become trapped as it enters the thigh in the adductor canal (Craig 2013).

Gastrocnemius and soleus muscles

The gastrocnemius and the soleus muscles insert into the Achilles tendon, which attaches to the posterior surface of the

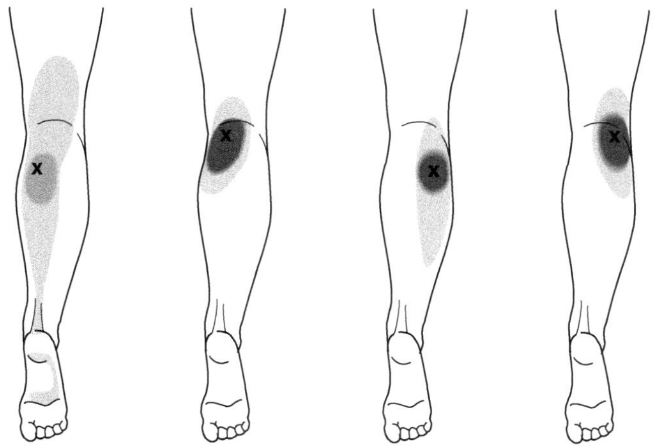

Figure 59.26 Referred pain elicited by myofascial trigger points in the gastrocnemius muscles.

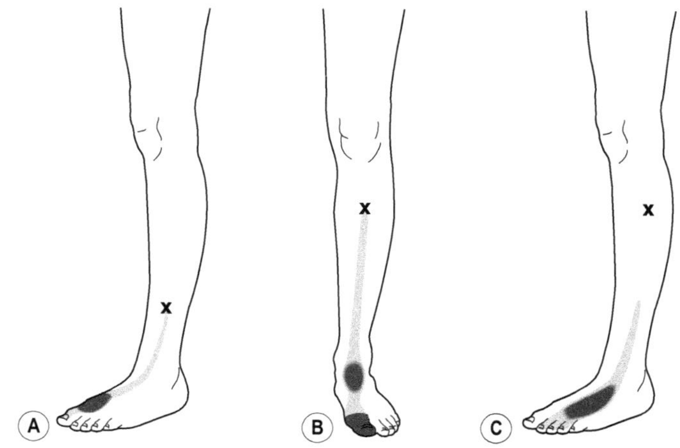

Figure 59.27 Referred pain elicited by myofascial trigger points in the extensor hallucis longus brevis (A), tibialis anterior (B) and extensor digitorum longus (C) muscles.

calcaneus bone. Their main function is plantar flexion and stabilization of the knee (gastrocnemius) and ankle. Most TrPs in the **gastrocnemius muscles** refer pain locally deep in the leg (Fig. 59.26). TrPs in the belly of the medial head tend to refer pain to the instep of the foot, sometimes spreading to the lower posterior thigh, the back of the knee and the posterior–medial aspect of leg and ankle. The **soleus muscle** refers pain to the distal part of the Achilles tendon and the posterior and plantar surfaces of the heel. TrPs in the proximal part of the gastrocnemius muscles are responsible for posterior knee pain in patients before (Mayoral et al 2013) and after (Henry et al 2012) total knee replacement surgery, and after knee arthroscopy (Rodríguez et al 2005). These TrPs can also contribute to calf pain (Grieve et al 2013). Indeed, TrPs in the gastrocnemius muscles seem to be important contributors to muscle cramps (Ge et al 2008b). In a small clinical trial, Prateepavanich et al (1999) demonstrated that injections of gastrocnemius muscle TrPs resulted in better long-term efficacy on calf cramps compared with oral quinine.

Plantar heel pain, which is often diagnosed as plantar fasciitis, can be also related to TrPs in the calf and foot musculature. Several reports have demonstrated that conservative treatment of TrPs in calf muscles is useful in the treatment of plantar heel pain and plantar fasciitis (Nguyen 2010; Renan-Ordine et al 2011). Although there is no solid evidence of the effectiveness of invasive treatments (Cotchett et al 2010), some reports suggest that needling and injections of TrPs in the calf and foot muscles can help the management of this condition (Imamura et al 1998; Kushner & Ferguson 2005; Sconfienza et al 2011).

Tibialis anterior, extensor digitorum longus and extensor hallucis longus muscles

These muscles have their insertion in the anterior–lateral part of leg between the tibia and the fibula. Their combined main function is ankle dorsal flexion and stabilization. Of course, the extensor muscles are also responsible for extension of the toes. The extensor **hallucis longus brevis** muscle spreads pain to the distal aspect of the dorsum of the first metatarsal, sometimes spreading distally to the tip of the great toe (Fig. 59.27A); the **tibialis anterior muscle** refers pain to the anterior–medial aspect of the ankle and over the great toe (Fig. 59.27B); the **extensor digitorum longus muscle** refers pain to the dorsum of the foot and toes (Fig. 59.27C).

There is general agreement that active TrPs in the tibialis anterior and intrinsic foot muscles can contribute to heel pain (Cotchett et al 2011). In addition, Samuel et al (2007) found an association between the presence of TrPs in the muscles innervated by the corresponding affected segmental level – for example L4–L5 disc lesion and tibialis anterior TrPs – in individuals with lumbar disc prolapse.

Other muscles of the lower quadrant

Finally, clinicians should be aware that there are many more TrPs with referred pain patterns contributing to lower quadrant pain syndromes. For instance, the gluteus maximus, tensor fascia lata, biceps femoris, sartorius, tibialis posterior, peroneus longus and intrinsic foot muscles also refer pain to the thigh, knee, leg or foot (Simons et al 1999).

Conclusion

In summary, there are numerous muscles of the neck / upper extremity and the trunk / lower extremity with TrPs and specific referred pain patterns that can contribute to the initiation and maintenance of symptoms in several upper and lower quadrant pain syndromes. Clinicians should examine clinically relevant muscles and TrPs to characterize and manage better the various upper and lower quadrant pain syndromes. Although much progress has been made, further studies are required in order to elucidate further the role of muscle TrPs in the clinical evolution of these syndromes.

References

Ackland DC, Pandy MG. 2009. Lines of action and stabilizing potential of the shoulder musculature. J Anat 215: 184–197.

Affaitati G, Costantini R, Fabrizio A, et al. 2011. Effects of treatment of peripheral pain generators in fibromyalgia patients. Eur J Pain 15: 61–69.

Alonso-Blanco C, Fernández-de-las-Peñas C, Morales-Cabezas M, et al. 2011. Multiple active myofascial trigger points reproduce the overall spontaneous pain pattern in women with fibromyalgia and are related to widespread mechanical hypersensitivity. Clin J Pain 27: 405–413.

Arbanas J, Pavlovic I, Marijancic V, et al. 2013. MRI features of the psoas major muscle in patients with low back pain. Eur Spine J 22:1965–1971.

Arendt-Nielsen L, Ge HY. 2009. Pathophysiology of referred muscle pain. In: Fernández-de-las-Peñas C, Arendt-Nielsen L, Gerwin RD (eds) Tension type and cervicogenic headache: pathophysiology, diagnosis and treatment. Boston: Jones & Bartlett Publishers, pp 51–59.

Arendt-Nielsen L, Svensson P. 2001. Referred muscle pain: basic and clinical findings. Clin J Pain 17: 11–19.

Arendt-Nielsen L, Laursen RJ, Drewes AM. 2000. Referred pain as an indicator for neural plasticity. Prog Brain Res 129: 343–356.

Babenko V, Graven-Nielsen T, Svensson P, et al. 1999a. Experimental human muscle pain and muscular hyperalgesia induced by combinations of serotonin and bradykinin. Pain 82: 1–8.

Babenko V, Graven-Nielsen T, Svensson P, et al. 1999b. Experimental human muscle pain induced by intra-muscular injections of bradykinin, serotonin, and substance P. Eur J Pain 3: 93–102.

Ballyns JJ, Shah JP, Hammond J, et al. 2011. Objective sonographic measures for characterizing myofascial trigger points associated with cervical pain. J Ultrasound Med 30: 1331–1340.

Bewyer DC, Bewyer KJ. 2003. Rationale for treatment of hip abductor pain syndrome. Iowa Orthop J 23: 57–60.

Bilecenoglu B, Uz A, Karalezli N. 2005. Possible anatomic structures causing entrapment neuropathies of the median nerve: an anatomic study. Acta Orthopaedica Belgica 71: 169–176.

Bogduk N. 2004. The neck and headaches. Neurol Clin North Am 22: 151–171.

Bowman WC, Marshall IG, Gibb AJ, et al. 1988. Feedback control of transmitter release at the neuromuscular junction. Trends Pharmacol Sci 9: 16–20.

Bron C, Dommerholt JD. 2012. Etiology of myofascial trigger points. Curr Pain Headache Rep 16: 439–444.

Bron C, Franssen J, Wensing M, et al. 2007. Inter-rater reliability of palpation of myofascial trigger points in three shoulder muscles. J Manual Manipul Ther 15: 203–215.

Bron C, Dommerholt J, Stegenga B, et al. 2011. High prevalence of shoulder girdle muscles with myofascial trigger points in patients with shoulder pain. BMC Musculoskelet Disord 12: 139.

Burnet EN, Pidcoe PE. 2009. Isometric gluteus medius muscle torque and frontal plane pelvic motion during running. J Sports Sci Med 8: 284–288.

Carli G, Suman AL, Biasi G, et al. 2002. Reactivity to superficial and deep stimuli in patients with chronic musculoskeletal pain. Pain 100: 259–269.

Carlson CR, Okeson JP, Falace DA, et al. 1993. Reduction of pain and EMG activity in the masseter region by trapezius trigger point injection. Pain 55: 397–400.

Cash CJ, MacDonald KJ, Dixon AK, et al. 2009. Variations in the MRI appearance of the insertion of the tendon of subscapularis. Clin Anat 22: 489–494.

Chaitow L, Delany J (eds). 2008. Clinical application of neuromuscular techniques: the upper body, 2nd edn. Shoulder, arm and hand. London: Elsevier, p 445.

Chang CW, Chen YR, Chang KF. 2008. Evidence of neuroaxonal degeneration in myofascial pain syndrome: a study of neuromuscular jitter by axonal micro- stimulation. Eur J Pain 12: 1026–1030.

Chen CK, Nizar AJ. 2011. Myofascial pain syndrome in chronic back pain patients. Korean J Pain 24: 100–104.

Chen D, Fang Y, Li J, et al. 1998a. Anatomical study and clinical observation of thoracic outlet syndrome. Zhonghua Wai Ke Za Zhi 36: 661–663.

Chen JT, Chen SM, Kuan TS, et al. 1998b. Phentolamine effect on the spontaneous electrical activity of active loci in a myofascial trigger spot of rabbit skeletal muscle. Arch Phys Med Rehabil 7: 790–794.

Chen SM, Chen JT, Kuan TS, et al. 2000. Decrease in pressure pain thresholds of latent myofascial trigger points in the middle finger extensors immediately after continuous piano practice. J Musculoskelet Pain 8: 83–92.

Chen Q, Bensamoun S, Basford JR, et al. 2007. Identification and quantification of myofascial taut bands with magnetic resonance elastography. Arch Phys Med Rehabil 88: 1658–1661.

Chen Q, Basford JR, An KN. 2008. Ability of magnetic resonance elastography to assess taut bands. Clin Biomech 23: 623–629.

Cherchel A, Zirak C, De Mey A. 2013. The humeral origin of the brachioradialis muscle: an unusual site of high radial nerve compression. J Plast Reconstr Aesthet Surg 66: 325–327.

Cho H, Lee HY, Gil YC, et al. 2013. Topographical anatomy of the radial nerve and its muscular branches related to surface landmarks. Clin Anat 26: 862–869.

Chung JW, Ohrbach R, McCall WD Jr. 2004. Effect of increased sympathetic activity on electrical activity from myofascial painful areas. Am J Phys Med Rehabil 83: 842–850.

Clavert P, Lutz JC, Adam P, et al. 2009. Frohse's arcade is not the exclusive compression site of the radial nerve in its tunnel. Orthopaed Traumatol Surg Res 95: 114–118.

Cotchett MP, Landorf KB, Munteanu SE. 2010. Effectiveness of dry needling and injections of myofascial trigger points associated with plantar heel pain: a systematic review. J Foot Ankle Res 3: 18.

Cotchett MP, Landorf KB, Munteanu SE, et al. 2011. Consensus for dry needling for plantar heel pain (plantar fasciitis): a modified Delphi study. Acupunct Med 29: 193–202.

Couppé C, Midttun A, Hilden J, et al. 2001. Spontaneous needle electromyographic activity in myofascial trigger points in the infraspinatus muscle: a blinded assessment. J Musculoskelet Pain 9: 7–16.

Craig A. 2013. Entrapment neuropathies of the lower extremity. PM R 5: S31–S40.

Cummings M. 2003. Referred knee pain treated with electroacupuncture to iliopsoas. Acupunct Med 21: 32–35.

Demirci SM, Alp M, Marur T, et al. 2007. Innervation pattern of the pronator teres muscle. Saudi Med J 28: 838–840.

Dommerholt J. 2011. Dry needling: peripheral and central considerations. J Man Manip Ther 19: 223–227.

Dommerholt J, Bron C, Franssen JLM. 2006. Myofascial trigger points: an evidence-informed review. J Manual Manipul Ther 14: 203–221.

Escobar PL, Ballesteros J. 1988. Teres minor: source of symptoms resembling ulnar neuropathy or C8 radiculopathy. Am J Phys Med Rehabil 67: 120–122.

Ferguson L, Gerwin R. 2005. Shoulder dysfunction and frozen shoulder. In: Ferguson L, Gerwin R (eds) Clinical mastery in the treatment of myofascial pain. Baltimore: Lippincott Williams & Wilkins, pp 91–121.

Fernández-Carnero J, Fernández-de-las-Peñas C, De-la-Llave-Rincón AI, et al. 2007. Prevalence of and referred pain from myofascial trigger points in the forearm muscles in patients with lateral epicondylalgia. Clin J Pain 23: 353–360.

Fernández-Carnero J, Fernández-de-las-Peñas C, De-la-Llave-Rincón AI, et al. 2008. Bilateral myofascial trigger points in the forearm muscles in chronic unilateral lateral epicondylalgia: a blinded controlled study. Clin J Pain 24: 802–807.

Fernández-de-Las-Peñas C, Dommerholt J. 2014. Myofascial trigger points: peripheral or central phenomenon? Curr Rheumatol Rep 16: 395.

Fernández-de-las-Peñas C, Alonso-Blanco C, Cuadrado M, et al. 2006. Myofascial trigger points and their relationship with headache clinical parameters in chronic tension type headache. Headache 46:1264–1272.

Fernández-de-las-Peñas C, Alonso-Blanco C, Miangolarra J. 2007a. Myofascial trigger points in subjects presenting with mechanical neck pain: a blinded, controlled study. Man Ther 12: 29–33.

Fernández-de-las-Peñas C, Ge H, Arendt-Nielsen L, et al. 2007b. Referred pain from trapezius muscle trigger point shares similar characteristics with chronic tension type headache. Eur J Pain 11: 475–482.

Fernández-de-las-Peñas C, Caminero AB, Madeleine P, et al. 2009a. Multiple active myofascial trigger points and pressure pain sensitivity maps in the temporalis muscle are related in chronic tension type headache. Clin J Pain 25: 506–512.

Fernández-de-las-Peñas C, Ge HY, Dommerholt J. 2009b. Manual identification of trigger points in the muscles associated with headache. In: Fernández-de-las-Peñas C, Arendt-Nielsen L, Gerwin RD (eds) Tension type and cervicogenic headache: pathophysiology, diagnosis and treatment. Boston: Jones & Bartlett, pp 183–194.

Fernández-de-las-Peñas C, Simons DG, Gerwin RD. 2009c. Muscle trigger points in tension type headache. In: Fernández de las Peñas C, Arendt-Nielsen L, Gerwin RD (eds) Tension type and cervicogenic headache: pathophysiology, diagnosis and treatment. Boston: Jones & Bartlett, pp 61–76.

Fernández-de-las-Peñas C, Gröbli C, Ortega-Santiago R, et al. 2012. Referred pain from myofascial trigger points in head, neck, shoulder, and arm muscles reproduces pain symptoms in blue-collar (manual) and white-collar (office) workers. Clin J Pain 28: 511–518.

Fernández-Lao C, Cantarero-Villanueva I, Fernández-de-las-Peñas C, et al. 2010. Myofascial trigger points in neck and shoulder muscles and widespread pressure pain hypersensitivity in patients with postmastectomy

pain: evidence of peripheral and central sensitization. Clin J Pain 26: 798–806.
Fernández-Pérez AM, Villaverde-Gutiérrez C, Mora-Sánchez A, et al. 2012. Muscle trigger points, pressure pain threshold, and cervical range of motion in patients with high level of disability related to acute whiplash injury. J Orthop Sports Phys Ther 42: 634–641.
Flack NA, Nicholson HD, Woodley SJ. 2012. A review of the anatomy of the hip abductor muscles, gluteus medius, gluteus minimus, and tensor fascia lata. Clin Anat 25: 697–708.
Freeman MD, Nystrom A, Centeno C. 2009. Chronic whiplash and central sensitization; an evaluation of the role of a myofascial trigger points in pain modulation. J Brachial Plex Peripher Nerve Inj 4: 2.
Ge HY, Arendt-Nielsen L. 2011. Latent myofascial trigger points. Curr Pain Head Rep 15: 386–392.
Ge HY, Fernández-de-las-Penas C, Arendt-Nielsen L. 2006. Sympathetic facilitation of hyperalgesia evoked from myofascial tender and trigger points in patients with unilateral shoulder pain. Clin Neurophysiol 117: 1545–1550.
Ge HY, Fernández-de-las-Peñas C, Madeleine P, et al. 2008a. Topographical mapping and mechanical pain sensitivity of myofascial trigger points in the infraspinatus muscle. Eur J Pain 12: 859–865.
Ge HY, Zhang Y, Boudreau S, et al. 2008b. Induction of muscle cramps by nociceptive stimulation of latent myofascial trigger points. Exp Brain Res 187: 623–629.
Ge HY, Serrao M, Andersen OK, et al. 2009. Increased H-reflex response induced by intramuscular electrical stimulation of latent myofascial trigger points. Acupunct Med 27: 150–154.
Ge HY, Wang Y, Fernández-de-las-Peñas C, et al. 2011. Reproduction of overall spontaneous pain pattern by manual stimulation of active myofascial trigger points in fibromyalgia patients. Arthritis Res Ther 13: R48.
Gerwin RD. 1997. Myofascial pain syndromes in the upper extremity. J Hand Ther 10: 130–136.
Gerwin RD. 2005. Headache. In: Ferguson L, Gerwin RD (eds) Clinical mastery in the treatment of myofascial pain. Baltimore: Lippincott Williams & Wilkins, pp 1–24.
Gerwin RD, Shannon S, Hong CZ, et al. 1997. Inter-rater reliability in myofascial trigger point examination. Pain 69: 65–73.
Gerwin RD, Dommerholt D, Shah JP. 2004. An expansion of Simons' integrated hypothesis of trigger point formation. Curr Pain Head Rep 8: 468–475.
Giamberardino M, Tafuri E, Savini A, et al. 2007. Contribution of myofascial trigger points to migraine symptoms. J Pain 8: 869–878.
Graven-Nielsen T. 2006. Fundamentals of muscle pain, referred pain, and deep tissue hyperalgesia. Scand J Rheumatol 122: 1–43.
Graven-Nielsen T, Arendt-Nielsen L, Svensson P, et al. 1997. Quantification of local and referred muscle pain in humans after sequential intra-muscular injections of hypertonic saline. Pain 69: 111–117.
Grieve R, Barnett S, Coghill N, et al. 2013. Myofascial trigger point therapy for triceps surae dysfunction: a case series. Man Ther 18: 519–525.
Hains G, Descarreaux M, Lamy AM, et al. 2010. A randomized controlled (intervention) trial of ischemic compression therapy for chronic carpal tunnel syndrome. J Can Chiropr Assoc 54: 155–163.
Han TI, Hong CZ, Kuo FC, et al. 2012. Mechanical pain sensitivity of deep tissues in children possible development of myofascial trigger points in children. BMC Musculoskelet Disord 13: 13.
Henry R, Cahill CM, Wood G, et al. 2012. Myofascial pain in patients waitlisted for total knee arthroplasty. Pain Res Manag 17: 321–327.
Hidalgo-Lozano A, Fernández-de-las-Peñas C, Alonso-Blanco C, et al. 2010. Muscle trigger points and pressure pain hyperalgesia in the shoulder muscles in patients with unilateral shoulder impingement: a blinded, controlled study. Exp Brain Res 202: 915–925.
Hidalgo-Lozano A, Fernández-de-las-Peñas C, Calderón-Soto C, et al. 2013. Elite swimmers with and without unilateral shoulder pain: mechanical hyperalgesia and active / latent muscle trigger points in neck-shoulder muscles. Scand J Med Sci Sports 23: 66–73.
Hong CZ. 1994. Considerations and recommendations regarding myofascial trigger point injection. J Musculoskelet Pain 2: 29–59.
Hong CZ, Simons DG. 1993. Response to treatment for pectoralis minor myofascial pain syndrome after whiplash. J Musculoskelet Pain 1: 89–131.
Hong CZ, Yu J. 1998. Spontaneous electrical activity of rabbit trigger spot after transection of spinal cord and peripheral nerve. J Musculoskelet Pain 6: 45–58.
Hong CZ, Kuan TS, Chen JT, et al. 1997. Referred pain elicited by palpation and by needling of myofascial trigger points: a comparison. Arch Phys Med Rehabil 78: 957–960.
Hsieh CY, Hong CZ, Adams AH, et al. 2000. Interexaminer reliability of the palpation of trigger points in the trunk and lower limb muscles. Arch Phys Med Rehabil 81: 258–264.
Hsieh YL, Kao MJ, Kuan TS, et al. 2007. Dry needling to a key myofascial trigger point may reduce the irritability of satellite MTrPs. Am J Phys Med Rehabil 86: 397–403.
Hsieh YL, Yang SA, Yang CC, et al. 2012. Dry needling at myofascial trigger spots of rabbit skeletal muscles modulates the biochemicals associated with pain, inflammation, and hypoxia. Evid Based Complement Alternat Med 2012: 342165.
Hsueh TC, Yu S, Kuan TS, et al. 1998. Associations of active myofascial trigger points and cervical disc lesions. J Formosan Med Ass 97: 174–180.
Huang QM, Ye G, Zhao ZY, et al. 2013. Myoelectrical activity and muscle morphology in a rat model of myofascial trigger points induced by blunt trauma to the vastus medialis. Acupunct Med 31: 65–73.
Hwang M, Kang YK, Kim DH. 2005a. Referred pain pattern of the pronator quadratus muscle. Pain 116: 238–242.
Hwang M, Kang YK, Shin JY, et al. 2005b. Referred pain pattern of the abductor pollicis longus muscle. Am J Phys Med Rehabil 84: 593–597.
Ibarra JM, Ge HY, Wang C, et al. 2011. Latent myofascial trigger points are associated with an increased antagonistic muscle activity during agonist muscle contraction. J Pain 12: 1282–1288.
Iglesias-González JJ, Muñoz-García MT, Rodrigues-de-Souza DP, et al. 2013. Myofascial trigger points, pain, disability, and sleep quality in patients with chronic nonspecific low back pain. Pain Med 14: 1964–1970.
Imamura M, Fischer AA, Imamura ST, et al. 1998. Treatment of myofascial pain components in plantar fasciitis speeds up recovery: documentation by algometry. J Musculoskelet Pain 6: 91-110.
Itoh K, Okada K, Kawakita K. 2004. A proposed experimental model of myofascial triggers points in human muscle after slow eccentric exercise. Acupunct Med 22: 2–13.
Jacobson EC, Lockwood MD, Hoefner VC Jr, et al. 1989. Shoulder pain and repetition strain injury to the supraspinatus muscle: etiology and manipulative treatment. J Am Osteopath Assoc 89: 1037–1045.
Janda V. 1996. Upper cross syndrome. In: Liebenson C (ed) Rehabilitation of the spine: a practitioner manual. Baltimore: Williams & Wilkins, pp 97–112.
Jankovic D, Van Zundert A. 2006. The frozen shoulder syndrome. Description of a new technique and five case reports using the subscapular nerve block and subscapularis trigger point infiltration. Acta Anaesthesiol Belgica 57: 137–413.
Jankovic D, Peng P, van Zundert A. 2013. Brief review: piriformis syndrome: etiology, diagnosis, and management. Can J Anaesth 60: 1003–1012.
Janssens LA. 1991. Trigger points in 48 dogs with myofascial pain syndromes. Vet Surg 20: 274–278.
Kao MJ, Han TI, Kuan TS, et al. 2007. Myofascial trigger points in early life. Arch Phys Med Rehabil 88: 251–254.
Kim DS, Jeong TY, Kim YK, et al. 2013. Usefulness of a myofascial trigger point injection for groin pain in patients with chronic prostatitis / chronic pelvic pain syndrome: a pilot study. Arch Phys Med Rehabil 94: 930–936.
Kuan TS, Chen JT, Chen SM, et al. 2002. Effect of botulinum toxin on endplate noise in myofascial trigger spots of rabbit skeletal muscle. Am J Phys Med Rehabil 81: 512–520.
Kuan TS, Hong CZ, Chen JT, et al. 2007. The spinal cord connections of the myofascial trigger spots. Eur J Pain 11: 624–634.
Kumarathurai P, Faroog MK, Christensen HW, et al. 2008. Muscular tenderness in the anterior chest wall in patients with stable angina pectoris is associated with normal myocardial perfusion. J Manipul Physiol Ther 31: 344–347.
Kushner RM, Ferguson LW. 2005. Heel and arch pain. In: Ferguson LW, Gerwin RD (eds) Clinical mastery in the treatment of myofascial pain. Baltimore: Lippincot Williams & Wilkins, pp 391-413.
Langley P. 1997. Scapular instability associated with brachial plexus irritation: a proposed causative relationship with treatment implications. J Hand Ther 10: 35-40.
Laursen RJ, Graven-Nielsen T, Jensen TS, et al. 1997. Quantification of local and referred pain in humans induced by intramuscular electrical stimulation. Eur J Pain 1: 105–113.
Lawson GE, Hung LY, Ko GD, et al. 2011. A case of pseudo-angina pectoris from a pectoralis minor trigger point caused by cross-country skiing. J Chiropr Med 10: 173–178.
Lee MJ, LaStayo DC. 2004. Pronator syndrome and other nerve compressions that mimic carpal tunnel syndrome. J Orthop Sports Phys Ther 34: 601–609.

Lee HI, Song J, Lee HS, et al. 2011. Association between cross-sectional areas of lumbar muscles on magnetic resonance imaging and chronicity of low back pain. Ann Rehabil Med 35: 852–859.

Lefevre N, Bohu Y, Klouche S, et al. 2015. Complete paralysis of the quadriceps secondary to post-traumatic iliopsoas hematoma: a systematic review. Eur J Orthop Surg Traumatol 25: 39–43.

Li LT, Ge HY, Yue SW, et al. 2009. Nociceptive and non-nociceptive hypersensitivity at latent myofascial trigger points. Clin J Pain 25: 132–137.

Livingston BP, Segal RL, Song A, et al. 2001. Functional activation of the extensor carpi radialis muscles in humans. Arch Phys Med Rehabil 82: 1164–1170.

Ljung BO, Lieber RL, Friden J. 1999. Wrist extensor muscle pathology in lateral epicondylitis. J Hand Surg Br 24B: 177–183.

Longbottom J. 2009. The treatment of pelvic pain with acupuncture: Part 1. J Chinese Med 91: 1–15.

Lucas KR, Polus BI, Rich PA. 2004. Latent myofascial trigger points: their effects on muscle activation and movement efficiency. J Bodyw Mov Ther 8: 160–166.

Lucas N, Macaskill P, Irwig L, et al. 2009. Reliability of physical examination for diagnosis of myofascial trigger points: a systematic review of the literature. Clin J Pain 25: 80–89.

Lucas KR, Rich PA, Polus BI. 2010. Muscle activation patterns in the scapular positioning muscles during loaded scapular plane elevation: the effects of latent myofascial trigger points. Clin Biomech 25: 765–770.

Macfarlane GJ, Hunt IM, Silman AJ. 2000. Role of mechanical and psychosocial factors in the onset of forearm pain: prospective population based study. BMJ 321: 676–679.

Macgregor J, Graf von Schweinitz D. 2006. Needle electromyographic activity of myofascial trigger points and control sites in equine cleidobrachialis muscle: an observational study. Acupuncture Medicine 24: 61–70.

Maeda S, Kawai K, Koizumi M, et al. 2009. Morphological study of the communication between the musculo-cutaneous and median nerves. Anat Sci Int 84: 34–40.

Maekawa K, Clark GT, Kuboki T. 2002. Intramuscular hypoperfusion, adrenergic receptors, and chronic muscle pain. J Pain 3: 251–260.

Mayoral O, Salvat I, Martín MT, et al. 2013. Efficacy of myofascial trigger point dry needling in the prevention of pain after total knee arthroplasty: a randomized, double-blinded, placebo-controlled trial. Evid Based Complement Alternat Med 2013: 694941.

McNulty WH, Gevirtz R, Hubbard D, et al. 1994. Needle electromyographic evaluation of trigger point response to a psychological stressor. Psychophysiology 31: 313–316.

McPartland JM, Simons DG. 2006. Myofascial trigger points: translating molecular theory into manual therapy. J Manual Manipul Ther 14: 232–239.

Mekhail AO, Checroun AJ, Ebraheim NA, et al. 1999. Extensile approach to the anterolateral surface of the humerus and the radial nerve. J Shoulder Elbow Surg 8: 112–118.

Mellick GA, Mellick LB. 2003. Regional head and face pain relief following lower cervical intramuscular anesthetic injection. Headache 43: 1109–1111.

Mense S. 1994. Referral of muscle pain. Am Pain Society J 3: 1–9.

Muñoz-Muñoz S, Muñoz-García MT, Alburquerque-Sendín F, et al. 2012. Myofascial trigger points, pain, disability, and sleep quality in individuals with mechanical neck pain. J Manipulative Physiol Ther 35: 608–613.

Myburgh C, Larsen AH, Hartvigsen J. 2008. A systematic, critical review of manual palpation for identifying myofascial triggers points: evidence and clinical significance. Arch Phys Med Rehabilitation 89: 1169–1176.

Natsis K, Totlis T, Konstantinidis GA, et al. 2014. Anatomical variations between the sciatic nerve and the piriformis muscle: a contribution to surgical anatomy in piriformis syndrome. Surg Radiol Anat 36(3): 273–280. doi:10.1007/s00276-013-1180-7.

Nguyen BM. 2010. Trigger point therapy and plantar heel pain: a case report. Foot 20: 158–162.

Niddam DM. 2009. Brain manifestation and modulation of pain from myofascial trigger points. Curr Pain Headache Rep 13: 370–375.

Niddam DM, Chan RC, Lee SH, et al. 2007. Central modulation of pain evoked from myofascial trigger point. Clin J Pain 23: 440–448.

Niddam DM, Chan RC, Lee SH, et al. 2008. Central representation of hyperalgesia from myofascial trigger point. Neuroimage 39: 1299–1306.

Ohmori A, Iranami H, Fujii K, et al. 2013. Myofascial involvement of supra- and infraspinatus muscles contributes to ipsilateral shoulder pain after muscle-sparing thoracotomy and video-assisted thoracic surgery. J Cardiothorac Vasc Anesth 27: 1310–1314.

Pappas N, Baldwin K, Keenan MA. 2010. Efficacy of median nerve recurrent branch neurectomy as an adjunct to ulnar motor nerve neurectomy and wrist arthrodesis at the time of superficialis to profundus transfer in prevention of intrinsic spastic thumb-in-palm deformity. J Hand Surg Am 35: 1310–1316.

Paraskevas G, Natsis K, Ioannidis O, et al. 2008. Accessory muscles in the lower part of the anterior compartment of the arm that may entrap neurovascular elements. Clin Anat 21: 246–251.

Park RJ, Tsao H, Cresswell AG, et al. 2013. Changes in direction-specific activity of psoas major and quadratus lumborum in people with recurring back pain differ between muscle regions and patient groups. J Electromyogr Kinesiol 23: 734–740.

Penning L. 2000. Psoas muscle and lumbar spine stability: a concept uniting existing controversies: critical review and hypothesis. Eur Spine J 9: 577–585.

Petchprapa CN, Rosenberg ZS, Sconfienza LM, et al. 2010. MR imaging of entrapment neuropathies of the lower extremity. Part 1: the pelvis and hip. Radiographics 30: 983–1000.

Ploumis A, Michailidis N, Christodoulou P, et al. 2011. Ipsilateral atrophy of paraspinal and psoas muscle in unilateral back pain patients with monosegmental degenerative disc disease. Br J Radiol 84: 709–713.

Prateepavanich P, Kupniratsaikul V, Charoensak T. 1999. The relationship between myofascial trigger points of gastrocnemius muscle and nocturnal calf cramps. J Med Assoc Thai 82:451–459.

Qerama E, Fuglsang-Frederiksen A, et al. 2004. Evoked pain in motor endplate region of the brachial biceps muscle: an experimental study. Muscle Nerve 29: 393–400.

Qerama E, Kasch H, Fuglsang-Frederiksen A. 2009. Occurrence of myofascial pain in patients with possible carpal tunnel syndrome: a single-blinded study. Eur J Pain 13: 588–591.

Rainey CE. 2013. The use of trigger point dry needling and intramuscular electrical stimulation for a subject with chronic low back pain: a case report. Int J Sports Phys Ther 8: 145–161.

Renan-Ordine R, Alburquerque-Sendín F, de Souza DP, et al. 2011. Effectiveness of myofascial trigger point manual therapy combined with a self-stretching protocol for the management of plantar heel pain: a randomized controlled trial. J Orthop Sports Phys Ther 41: 43–50.

Rezzouk J, Durandeau A, Vital JM, et al. 2002. Long head of the triceps brachii in axillary nerve injury: anatomy and clinical aspects. Rev Chir Orthop Reparatrice Appar Mot 88: 561–564. [Article in French.]

Rinzler SH, Travell J. 1948. Therapy directed at the somatic component of cardiac pain. Am Heart J 35: 248–268.

Roach S, Sorenson E, Headley B, et al. 2013. Prevalence of myofascial trigger points in the hip in patellofemoral pain. Arch Phys Med Rehabil 94: 522–526.

Rodríguez Fernández AL, Bartolomé Martín JL, Martínez Cepa CB, et al. 2005. Dolor miofascial tras la artroscopia de rodilla: estudio de la prevalencia y de los posibles factores de activación. Fisioterapia 27: 201–209. [Article in Spanish.]

Samuel S, Peter A, Ramanathan K. 2007. The association of active trigger points with lumbar disc lesions. J Musculoskelet Pain 15 (2): 11–18.

Schneider M. 2005. Tennis elbow. In: Ferguson L, Gerwin R (eds) Clinical mastery in the treatment of myofascial pain. Baltimore: Lippincott Williams & Wilkins, pp 122–144.

Sciotti VM, Mittak VL, DiMarco L, et al. 2001. Clinical precision of myofascial trigger point location in the trapezius muscle. Pain 93: 259–266.

Sconfienza LM, Lacelli F, Bandirali M, et al. 2011. Long-term survey of three different ultrasound guided percutaneous treatments of plantar fasciitis: results of a randomized controlled trial. Ultraschall Med 32: 99–100. [Abstract.]

Shah JP, Phillips TM, Danoff JV, et al. 2005. An in vitro microanalytical technique for measuring the local biochemical milieu of human skeletal muscle. J Appl Physiol 99: 1977–1984.

Shah JP, Danoff JV, Desai MJ, et al. 2008. Biochemicals associated with pain and inflammation are elevated in sites near to and remote from active myofascial trigger points. Arch Phys Med Rehabil 89: 16–23.

Sikdar S, Shah JP, Gilliams E, et al. 2008. Assessment of myofascial trigger points (TrPs): a new application of ultrasound imaging and vibration sonoelastography. Conf Proc IEEE Eng Med Biol Soc 2008: 5585–5588. doi:10.1109/IEMBS.2008.4650480.

Sikdar S, Shah JP, Gebreab T, et al. 2009. Novel applications of ultrasound technology to visualize and characterize myofascial trigger points and surrounding soft tissue. Arch Phys Med Rehabil 90: 1829–1838.

Sikdar S, Ortiz R, Gebreab T, et al. 2010. Understanding the vascular environment of myofascial trigger points using ultrasonic imaging and computational modeling. Conf Proc IEEE Eng Med Biol Soc 1: 5302–5305.

Simons DG. 1991. Symptomatology and clinical pathophysiology of myofascial pain. Brachial Schmerz 5: S29–S37.

Simons DG. 2001. Do endplate noise and spikes arise from normal motor endplates? Am J Phys Med Rehabil 80: 134–140.
Simons DG. 2004. Review of enigmatic MTrPs as a common cause of enigmatic musculoskeletal pain and dysfunction. J Electromyograph Kinesiol 14: 95–107.
Simons DG Travell JG, Simons LS. 1999. Travell & Simons' Myofascial pain and dysfunction: the trigger point manual. Vol. 1, 2nd edn. Baltimore: Lippincott William & Wilkins, pp 278–307.
Simons DG, Hong CZ, Simons L. 2002. Endplate potentials are common to midfiber myofascial trigger points. Am J Phys Med Rehabil 81: 212–222.
Skubick DL, Clasby R, Donaldson CC, et al. 1993. Carpal tunnel syndrome as an expression of muscular dysfunction in the neck. J Occupational Rehab 3: 31–43.
Slater H, Arendt-Nielsen L, Wright A, et al. 2003. Experimental deep tissue pain in wrist extensors: a model of lateral epicondylalgia. Eur J Pain 7: 277–288.
Slater H, Arendt-Nielsen L, Wright A, et al. 2005. Sensory and motor effects of experimental muscle pain in patients with lateral epicondylalgia and controls with delayed onset muscle soreness. Pain 114: 118–130.
Sluka KA, Kalra A, Moore SA. 2001. Unilateral intramuscular injections of acidic saline produce a bilateral, long-lasting hyperalgesia. Muscle Nerve 24: 37–46.
Spanos T. 2005. Inter-scapular pain: a myofascial composite syndrome. In: Ferguson L, Gerwin R (eds) Clinical mastery in the treatment of myofascial pain. Baltimore: Lippincott Williams & Wilkins, pp 213–226.
Srbely JZ, Dickey JP, Lowerison M, et al. 2008. Stimulation of myofascial trigger points with ultrasound induces segmental anti-nociceptive effects: a randomized controlled study. Pain 139: 260–266.
Stepnik MW, Olby N, Thompson RR, et al. 2006. Femoral neuropathy in a dog with iliopsoas muscle injury. Veterinarian Surg 35: 186–190.
Svensson P, Cairns BE, Wang K, et al. 2003a. Glutamate-evoked pain and mechanical allodynia in the human masseter muscle. Pain 101: 221–227.
Svensson P, Cairns BE, Wang K, et al. 2003b. Injection of nerve growth factor into human masseter muscle evokes long-lasting mechanical allodynia and hyperalgesia. Pain 104: 241–247.
Tatar I, Kocabiyik N, Gayretli O, et al. 2009. The course and branching pattern of the deep branch of the radial nerve in relation to the supinator muscle in fetus elbow. Surg Radiol Anat 31: 591–596.
Teixeira M, Yeng LT, Garcia OG, et al. 2011. Failed back surgery pain syndrome: therapeutic approach descriptive study in 56 patients. Rev Assoc Med Bras 57: 282–287.
Torres-Lacomba M, Mayoral-del-Moral O, Coperias-Zazo JL, et al. 2010. Incidence of myofascial pain syndrome in breast cancer surgery: a prospective study. Clin J Pain 26: 320–325.
Tough EA, Write AR, Richards SS, et al. 2007. Variability of criteria used to diagnose myofascial trigger point pain syndrome: evidence from a review of the literature. Clin J Pain 23: 278–286.
Treaster D, Marras W, Burr D, et al. 2006. Myofascial trigger point development from visual and postural stressors during computer work. J Electromyograph Kinesiol 16: 115–124.
Tubbs RS, Mortazavi MM, Farrington WJ, et al. 2013. Relationships between the posterior interosseous nerve and the supinator muscle: application to peripheral nerve compression syndromes and nerve transfer procedures. J Neurol Surg A Cent Eur Neurosurg 74: 290–293.
Vecchiet L, Giamberardino MA, Dragani L. 1990. Latent myofascial trigger points: changes in muscular and subcutaneous pain thresholds at trigger point and target level. J Man Med 5: 151–154.
Vecchiet L, Giamberardino MA, Bigontina P. 1994. Comparative sensory evaluation of parietal tissues in painful and nonpainful areas in fibromyalgia and myofascial pain syndrome. In: Gebhart GB, Hammond DL, Jensen JS (eds) Proceedings of the 7th World Congress on Pain: progress in pain research and management. Seattle: IASP Press, pp 177–185.
Vemuri C, Wittenberg AM, Caputo FJ, et al. 2013. Early effectiveness of isolated pectoralis minor tenotomy in selected patients with neurogenic thoracic outlet syndrome. J Vasc Surg 57: 1345–1352.
Wang YH, Ding X, Zhang Y, et al. 2010. Ischemic compression block attenuates mechanical hyperalgesia evoked from latent myofascial trigger point. Exp Brain Res 202: 265–267.
Witting N, Svensson P, Gottrup H, et al. 2000. Intramuscular and intra-dermal injection of capsaicin: a comparison of local and referred pain. Pain 84: 407–412.
Zhang Y, Ge HY, Yue SW, et al. 2009. Attenuated skin blood flow response to nociceptive stimulation of latent myofascial trigger points. Arch Phys Med Rehabil 90: 325–332.

60 Chapter

Manual Treatment of Myofascial Trigger Points

César Fernández-de-las-Peñas, Jaime Salom-Moreno, Hong-You Ge, Jan Dommerholt

CHAPTER CONTENTS

Introduction 678
Treatment interventions for myofascial trigger points 678
Best evidence of manual therapies for myofascial trigger points 679
Manual therapies for the management of myofascial trigger points 679
Compression interventions 679
Massage therapies 680
Stretching interventions 680
Dynamic interventions 680
Clinical applications of manual therapies over myofascial TrPs 681
Stretching compression of levator scapulae muscle taut band 681
Longitudinal strokes of scalene muscle taut band 681
Compression and contraction of supraspinatus muscle 681
Stretching strokes of infraspinatus muscle taut band 682
Stretching longitudinal strokes of infraspinatus muscle taut band 682
Stretching compression of teres major muscle taut band 682
Stretching compression of subscapularis muscle taut band 683
Dynamic transverse strokes of deltoid muscle trigger points 683
Dynamic longitudinal strokes of biceps/triceps brachii muscle taut band 683
Dynamic longitudinal strokes of hand/wrist extensor muscle taut band 684
Transverse massage of hand/wrist flexor muscle trigger points 684
Stretching compression of thumb muscles taut bands 684
Transverse massage of quadratus lumborum muscle taut bands 685
Post-isometric relaxation of quadratus lumborum muscle taut bands 685
Stretching compression of psoas major muscle taut bands 686
Stretching longitudinal stroke/dynamic longitudinal stroke of gluteus medius muscle taut bands 686
Stretching longitudinal stroke of quadriceps muscle taut bands 687
Stretching longitudinal massage of adductor muscle taut bands 687
Stretching compression of gastrocnemius muscle taut bands 687
Compression and contraction of anterior–lateral leg muscles 687
Conclusion 688

Introduction

Treatment interventions for myofascial trigger points

In clinical practice, there are several intervention modalities aimed at eliminating myofascial trigger points (TrPs): dry needling therapies (Cummings & White 2001; Dommerholt et al 2006a; Tough et al 2009; Dommerholt & Fernández-de-las-Peñas 2013; Kietrys et al 2013), ultrasound (Gam et al 1998; Majlesi & Unalan 2004; Srbely & Dickey 2007; Srbely et al 2008; Kim et al 2014), thermotherapy (Lee et al 1997), laser therapy (Pöntinen & Airaksinen 1995; Altan et al 2005; Dundar et al 2007; Uemoto et al 2013), electrotherapy (Tanrikut et al 2003), magnetic therapy (Brown et al 2002; Smania et al 2005), extracorporeal shockwave therapy (Gleitz & Hornig 2012; Jeon et al 2012) and manual therapies (Simons et al 1999; Lewit 1999). Among these interventions, manual therapies are the basic treatment options (Dommerholt et al 2006b).

This chapter will focus on different manual approaches that can be used for inactivating myofascial TrPs. Several manual therapies are suggested in the literature: massage (Simons et al 1999), ischaemic compression or TrP pressure release (Hong et al 1993; Simons et al 1999; Fryer & Hodgson 2005; Fernández-de-las-Peñas et al 2006b; Gemmell et al 2008; Dommerholt & McEvoy 2011; Bodes-Pardo et al 2013), myofascial induction (Pilat 2009), spray and stretch (Jaeger & Reeves 1986; Hong et al 1993; Simons et al 1999), passive stretching (Hanten et al 2000), muscle energy or post-isometric relaxation techniques (Lewit 1999; Rodríguez-Blanco et al 2006; Oliveira-Campelo et al 2013), neuromuscular approaches (Ibáñez-García et al 2009), active head retraction–extension (Hanten et al 1997), strain/counterstrain (Dardzinski et al 2000) and spinal manipulation (Ruiz-Sáez et al 2007; Fernández-de-las-Peñas 2009; Srbely et al 2013).

Best evidence of manual therapies for myofascial trigger points

The first systematic review of manual therapies in the management of TrPs found inconclusive evidence since few studies had investigated manual therapy approaches for the management of TrPs (Fernández-de-las-Peñas et al 2005a). Later studies reported that the ischaemic compression technique is effective in reducing pain sensitivity of latent (Fryer & Hogson 2005) and active (Fernández-de-las-Peñas et al 2006b) TrPs. No significant differences were found between ischaemic compression and transverse friction massage in the reduction of self-perceived pain and pressure pain sensitivity over the upper trapezius muscle TrPs (Fernández-de-las-Peñas et al 2006b). A later systematic review analysing the effectiveness of non-invasive treatments for active TrPs revealed that there is evidence of the short-term effectiveness of manual therapies, but no conclusions can be made relating to medium- and long-term follow-ups (Rickards 2006). One study not included in these reviews found that neuromuscular approaches were also effective for reducing pressure pain sensitivity of latent TrPs (Ibáñez-García et al 2009). Other studies reported improvements in range of motion after treatment with ischaemic compression (Fernández-de-las-Peñas et al 2004) or post-isometric relaxation technique of latent TrPs in the masseter muscle (Rodríguez-Blanco et al 2006; Heredia-Rizo et al 2013). A subsequent review summarized moderately strong evidence supporting the use of ischaemic pressure for immediate pain relief of TrPs, but only limited evidence for long-term pain relief (Vernon & Schneider 2009). A recent meta-analysis concluded that muscle manual therapies had a favourable effect on pressure pain thresholds when compared with no-treatment and sham / inert groups and comparable effects were also observed when compared with those of other active treatments (Gay et al 2013).

Further, there is preliminary evidence investigating changes in muscle sensitivity after spinal manipulations. Ruiz-Sáez et al (2007) showed that a manipulation directed at the C3–C4 segment evoked changes in pressure pain sensitivity of latent TrPs in the upper trapezius muscle. A recent study has observed that spinal manipulation evokes short-term regional increases in pressure pain thresholds within myofascial tissues in healthy young adults (Srbely et al 2013). Nevertheless, although a clinical relationship between myofascial TrPs and joint impairments has been suggested by some authors (Lewit 1999; Fernández-de-las-Peñas et al 2005b, 2006a; Fernández-de-las-Peñas 2009), the clinical effects of spinal manipulations on active TrP sensitivity remain unclear.

Therefore, it is difficult to draw clinical conclusions from current scientific evidence as most studies had investigated single modalities, whereas multimodal approaches are usually practised by many clinicians. Clinical studies investigating multimodal interventions including the treatment of myofascial TrPs with manual therapies are needed. There are some clinical studies demonstrating the effectiveness of the inclusion of myofascial TrP techniques into multimodal manual therapy protocol for the management of heel pain (Renan-Ordine et al 2011), shoulder pain (Bron et al 2011), ankle sprain (Truyols-Domínguez et al 2013) or chronic pelvic pain (Anderson et al 2005). The inclusion of manual therapies targeted at inactivating TrPs can potentiate the therapeutic effects of other physical therapy interventions.

Manual Therapies for the Management of Myofascial Trigger Points

Compression interventions

There are different compression techniques depending on the amount of pressure applied, the duration of application, the position of the tissue (shortened / lengthened) and the presence / absence of pain. In clinical practice, the pressure level, duration of application and position of the muscle are determined based on the sensitization mechanisms of the patient and the degree of irritability of the tissue.

Simons (2002) proposed that compression of the sarcomeres by direct pressure in a vertical or perpendicular manner combined with active contraction of the involved muscle may equalize the length of the muscle sarcomeres in the involved TrP and consequently decrease the pain; however, this notion has not been scientifically investigated (Dommerholt & Shah 2010). Other authors have suggested that pain relief from direct pressure may result from reactive hyperaemia within the TrP or a spinal reflex mechanism for the relief of muscle tension (Hou et al 2002).

One of the compression techniques applied over TrPs is the so-called **ischaemic compression technique** (Simons et al 1999). In this technique, with the muscle in a lengthened position, the therapist gradually applies manual pressure to the TrP until the sensation of pressure becomes painful, at which moment the pressure is maintained until the discomfort / pain is eased by around 50–75% as perceived by the patient under treatment; at that point the pressure is increased once more until the discomfort / pain reappears. This process is usually repeated for 90 seconds (Simons et al 1999), with two or three repetitions (Hains et al 2010).

Fryer and Hodgson (2005) recommended compression up to 7 / 10 on a Numerical Pain Rating Scale; however, particularly for patients with chronic pain, this level of pain may be excessive. Hou et al (2002) provided alternative compression approaches using either low pressure below the pain threshold for prolonged periods (90 seconds) or high pressure above the pain threshold (pain tolerance) for a short period (30 seconds). In clinical practice, the pressure level depends on the mechanisms of pain sensitization in the individual patient and the degree of irritability of the TrP. For instance, in the case of a high-level athlete, the technique can include short-duration high pressure, whereas in a patient diagnosed with fibromyalgia it would be preferable to use prolonged low pressure.

The ischaemic compression technique has now been replaced by the **TrP pressure release technique**, which consists of an application of pressure over the TrP until an increase in muscle resistance (tissue barrier) is perceived by the therapist (Lewit 1999). That pressure is then maintained until the therapist perceives a release of the taut band. At this stage the pressure is increased to return the patient to the previous level of muscle tension; the above process is then repeated for 90 seconds (usually there are two to three repetitions). In most patients the moment of increased muscle tension is not painful, but in some the increase in tissue resistance may correlate with moderate discomfort (Grieve et al 2011).

Another compression intervention that can be applied to a TrP is the **strain/counterstrain technique** (Jones 1981; D'Ambrogio & Roth 1997). In this technique, the therapist applies pressure until reaching the patient's pain threshold. At that moment, the patient's involved body part is passively placed in a position that reduces the tension under the palpating fingers and causes a subjective reduction of pain by around 90–100%. This position is maintained for 90 seconds (Jones 1981). This technique was designed for the management of tender points; however, there is no evidence that these tender points as described by Jones (1981) are indeed the same entity as TrPs. The relationship between tender points and TrPs has not been investigated. Dardzinski et al (2000) reported a positive immediate improvement in symptoms of 50–75% in a patient after the application of a protocol including strain / counterstrain interventions and body exercises. Rodríguez-Blanco et al (2006) demonstrated that the application of a single session of strain / counterstrain technique over latent TrPs in the masseter muscle produced a small increase in active mouth opening.

Massage therapies

The application of massage for inactivating TrPs was discussed by Simons (2002). Buttagat et al (2011) showed that traditional Thai massage increased heart rate variability and improved stress-related parameters in patients presenting with back pain associated with TrPs. Massage can be done along the taut band (longitudinal strokes) or across the taut band (transverse massage or strokes). Hong et al (1993) reported that deep tissue massage was more effective in decreasing pressure pain sensitivity than spray and stretch and other manual therapies. Ibáñez-García et al (2009) showed that neuromuscular approaches were effective for reducing pressure pain sensitivity in latent muscle TrPs. Fernández-de-las-Peñas et al (2006b) found that transverse massage was as effective as the ischaemic compression for reducing TrP pressure pain sensitivity. FitzGerald et al (2012) observed that application of TrP massage therapy was more effective than global therapeutic massage in women with interstitial cystitis / painful bladder syndrome.

Simons (2002) and Hong et al (1993) have proposed that massage may exert a lengthening effect similar to compression techniques. For instance, transverse friction massage may offer a transverse mobilization to the taut band, whereas stroking may offer a longitudinal mobilization of the taut band. In some muscles, particularly those where clinicians can use pincer palpation, the therapist's fingers can grasp the taut band from both sides of the muscle TrP, stroking it centrifugally and elongating it away from the TrP (Simons 2002). Bodes-Pardo et al (2013) recently demonstrated that massage therapy targeted to active TrPs in the sternocleidomastoid muscle was effective for reducing headache and neck pain intensity and for increasing motor performance of the deep cervical flexors, pressure pain thresholds and active cervical range of motion in individuals with cervicogenic headache.

Stretching interventions

There are several applications of stretching approaches: passive stretching (where the therapist passively stretches the muscle without participation of the patient), active stretching (where the patient actively stretches the muscle without the participation of the therapist), spray and stretch (Hong et al 1993; Simons et al 1999) and post-isometric relaxation (Lewit 1999). Fryer (2000) suggested that the therapeutic mechanism of stretching interventions may be the combination of 'creep' (i.e. temporary elongation of connective tissue during the stretch) and plastic changes in the connective tissues caused by the stretch. There is, however, little evidence showing that stretching is beneficial for TrP treatment. Further, patients with benign hypermobility or Ehlers–Danlos syndrome should not partake in any stretching exercises, as stretching will most likely contribute to increased laxity of connective tissues and ligaments without any positive effect on muscles, taut bands and TrPs.

Jaeger and Reeves (1986), in a low-quality study, found that spray and stretch was effective for reducing pain sensitivity and symptoms in active TrPs. Hong et al (1993) demonstrated that spray and stretch showed immediate positive effects on pressure pain sensitivity and was more effective when combined with deep pressure massage. Hou et al (2002) found that the application of spray and stretch in combination with other modalities was more effective than hot-packs for inactivating TrPs. Emad et al (2012) showed that TrP injections plus stretching were significantly more effective in reducing pain than TrP injections alone. It should be noted, however, that the commercially available sprays have a considerable environmental impact, including ozone depletion and increased global warming.

Dynamic interventions

As myofascial TrPs are located in muscle tissue, it is important to include dynamic interventions, in which clinicians apply manual techniques, such as TrP pressure release or longitudinal stroking, combined with contraction or stretching of the affected muscle. For instance, during TrP manual compression, the patient is asked to contract the affected muscle actively through a small range of motion (Gröbli & Dommerholt 1997; Gröbli & Dejung 2003). The active muscle contraction is thought to stretch the shortened sarcomeres against the compression (Simons 2002). The mechanisms of these techniques are still unknown, but may be related to activation of the intrafascial pacinian / paciniform and Ruffini mechanoreceptors, which are found in all types of dense proper connective tissues (Schleip 2003). Ruffini endings are especially responsive to tangential forces and lateral stretch (Kruger 1987), and stimulation of Ruffini corpuscles is assumed to result in a lowering of sympathetic nervous system activity (Van den Berg & Cabri 1999). During manual compression or longitudinal stroking, the patient may also be asked to move the segment actively through a particular range (Gröbli & Dejung 2003).

Clinical Applications of Manual Therapies over Myofascial TrPs

In this section, different manual TrP therapies are described in muscles with referred pain patterns into the upper and lower quadrants. The featured techniques are not exclusive and are not the only possible options. Clinicians are encouraged to develop other techniques based on established principles. The selection of techniques will depend partially on the irritability of TrPs and the sensitization of the patient's central nervous system.

Stretching compression of levator scapulae muscle taut band

A stretching compression technique combines compression (TrP pressure release or ischaemic compression) with passive or active stretching of the TrP taut band. In our clinical practice, we apply this technique for inactivating levator scapulae TrPs located at the angle of the neck where the levator scapulae muscle emerges from the anterior border of the upper trapezius. For this technique, the patient is seated with the torso resting against the backrest. The therapist brings the upper trapezius muscle in a relaxed position to achieve good contact with the levator scapulae TrP. In that position, a compression technique is applied. When the therapist perceives a slight relaxation of the TrP, the patient's neck is gently turned, either passively or actively, towards the opposite side to increase the tension within the taut band (Fig. 60.1). This procedure is repeated until a relaxation within the taut band is perceived or until the referred pain disappears.

Longitudinal strokes of scalene muscle taut band

TrP taut bands in the anterior or medial scalene muscles can trap the brachial plexus (Chen et al 1998). In addition, tension induced by TrP taut bands within the scalene muscles may be related to upward dysfunctions of the first rib (Ferguson & Gerwin, 2005). In our clinical practice, the application of longitudinal strokes to both anterior and medial scalene muscles is useful for relaxing TrP taut bands without increasing tension within the brachial plexus.

The anterior scalene is easily palpated below the posterior border of the clavicular division of the sternocleidomastoid muscle. The medial scalene lies deep and lateral to the anterior scalene and anterior to the deep fibres of the levator scapulae muscle.

Longitudinal strokes are usually performed using one thumb in a cranial–caudal direction (Fig. 60.2). The degree of pressure applied is determined by the feedback reported by the patient, or the tension felt within the patient's tissue.

Compression and contraction of supraspinatus muscle

This technique combines a manual compression with an active contraction of the compressed muscle (Gröbli & Dejung 2003). For the technique, the patient lies prone with the shoulder abducted 90°. The therapist places the upper trapezius muscle in a relaxed position to approximate the supraspinatus fossa of the scapula. In that position, he / she applies manual compression over the supraspinatus TrPs with both thumbs. When the therapist perceives a slight relaxation of the tissue, the patient is asked to contract the muscle abducting the

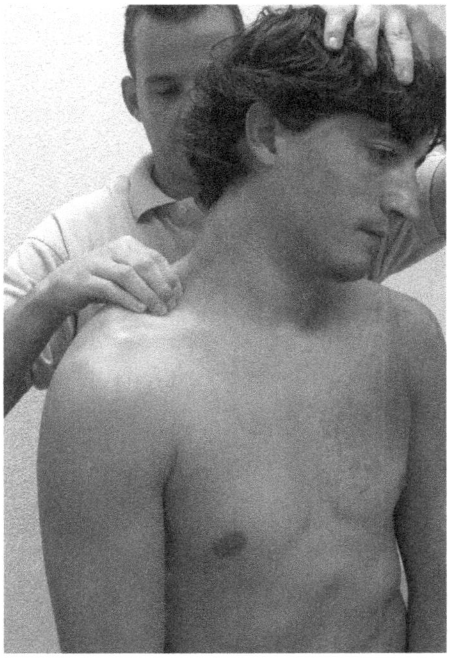

Figure 60.1 Stretching compression of levator scapulae muscle taut band.

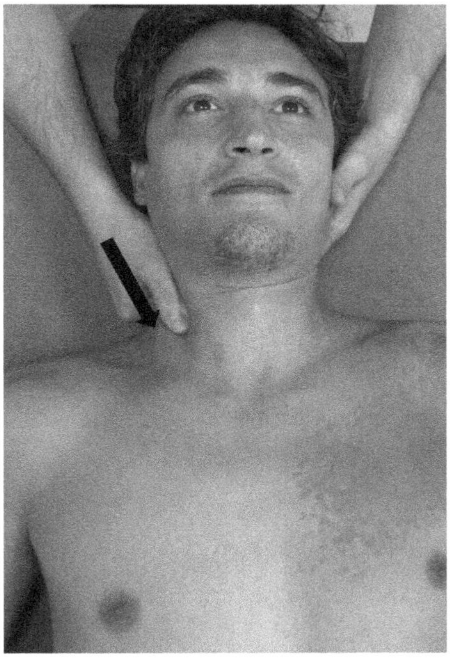

Figure 60.2 Longitudinal stroke of scalene muscle taut band. The black arrow shows the direction of the stroke.

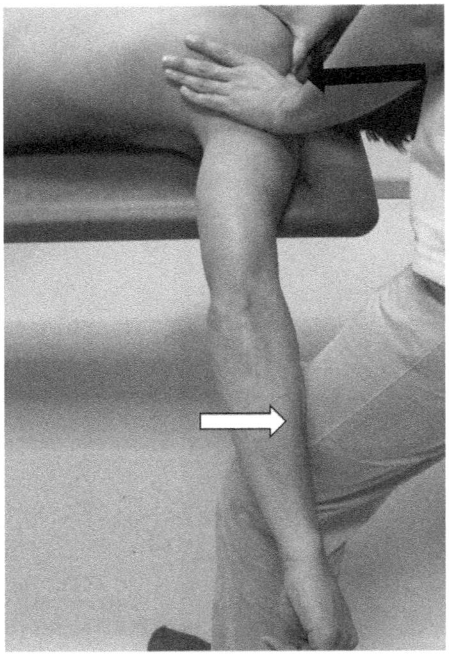

Figure 60.3 Compression and contraction of supraspinatus muscle. The black arrow shows the compression of the therapist and the white arrow shows the direction of the contraction force by the patient (abduction).

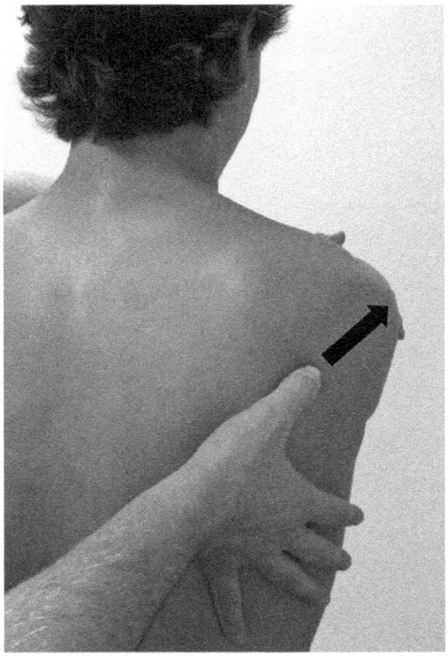

Figure 60.4 Stretching strokes of infraspinatus muscle taut band. The black arrow shows the direction of the stroke.

shoulder for 5 seconds. The therapist offers resistance with the leg pushing against the patient's arm in order to achieve an isometric contraction (Fig. 60.3). This technique is repeated until the referred pain disappears.

Stretching strokes of infraspinatus muscle taut band

A stretching stroke consists of a longitudinal stroke applied over a muscle placed in a stretched position. With the patient seated, the infraspinatus muscle is stretched by bringing the hand and the arm across the front of the chest to grasp the far armrest of the chair. In this stretched position, the therapist performs longitudinal strokes using one thumb in a medial (thoracic spine) to lateral (spine of the scapula) direction (Fig. 60.4).

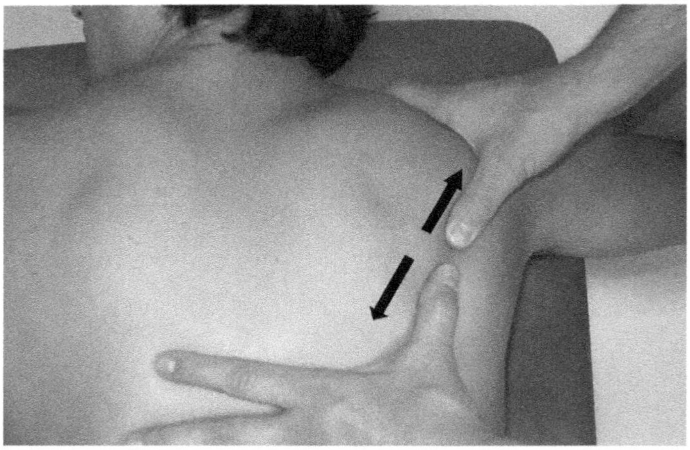

Figure 60.5 Stretching longitudinal strokes of infraspinatus muscle taut band. The black arrows show the centrifugal direction of the stroke.

Stretching longitudinal strokes of infraspinatus muscle taut band

This technique consists of a combination of compression and longitudinal strokes along the TrP taut band. The patient lies prone with the shoulder in 90° of abduction. The fingers of the therapist compress the infraspinatus TrPs, grasp the taut band from both sides of the TrP and stroke centrifugally away from the TrP (Fig. 60.5).

Stretching compression of teres major muscle taut band

With the patient lying on the opposite side, the teres major muscle can be easily located by pincer palpation. Using pincer palpation of the axillary fold a few centimetres below the arm, the therapist locates the teres major muscle and the lateral border of the scapula. With one hand he / she then pinches the teres major TrP and with the other hand grasps the forearm of the patient. The therapist passively abducts the patient's shoulder until a tension within the TrP taut band is perceived (Fig. 60.6). The tension is usually perceived when the shoulder joint reaches approximately 60° of abduction. The therapist should avoid any compensatory movement of the scapula. The technique is rhythmically repeated until a relaxation in the teres major muscle taut band is perceived.

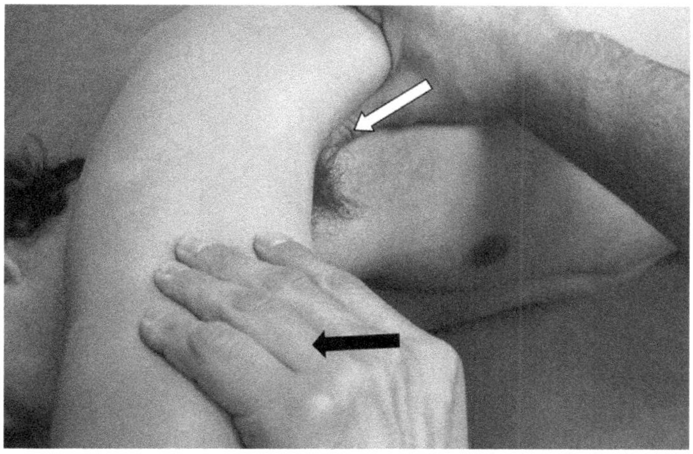

Figure 60.6 Stretching compression of teres major muscle taut band. The black arrow shows the shoulder abduction and the white arrow shows the stabilization force of the therapist.

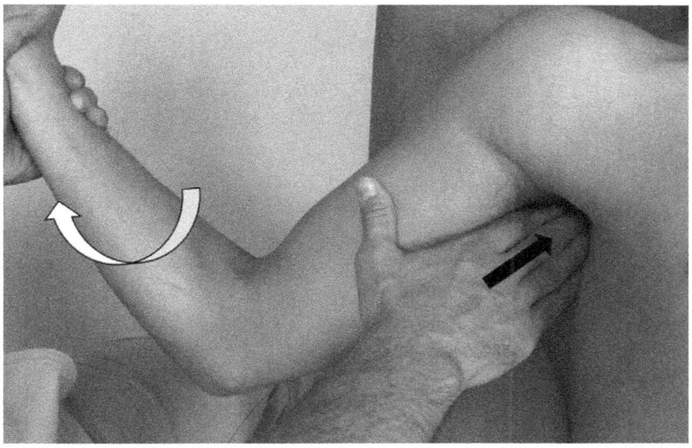

Figure 60.7 Stretching compression of subscapularis muscle taut band. The black arrow shows the compression over the subscapularis whereas the white arrow shows the external rotation and abduction movement.

Stretching compression of subscapularis muscle taut band

The patient is supine with the shoulder abducted between 30° and 60°. The therapist holds on to the medial border of the scapula and manually moves the scapula laterally. Manual compression is applied cephalad and towards the spine of the scapula. From that position, the therapist dynamically externally rotates and abducts the patient's shoulder until muscle tension is perceived (Fig. 60.7).

Dynamic transverse strokes of deltoid muscle trigger points

This technique combines a transverse stroke with passive rotation of the shoulder joint. With the patient supine and the shoulder in 90° of abduction, the therapist grasps the anterior or posterior part of the deltoid muscle. The thumb of the therapist's hand should be placed over the TrP taut band. The

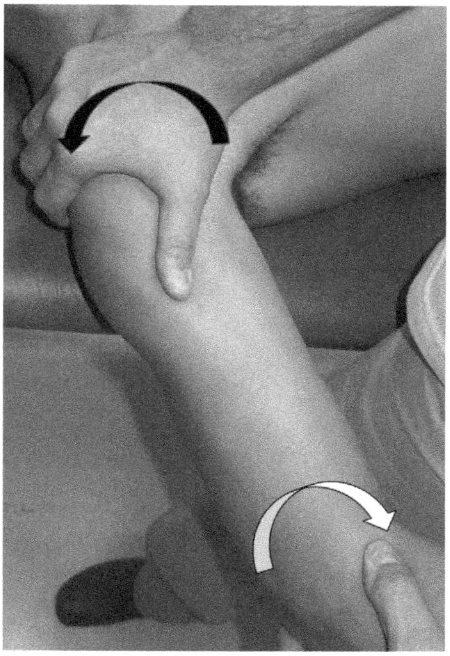

Figure 60.8 Dynamic transverse strokes of anterior deltoid muscle trigger points. The black arrow shows the anterior to posterior stroke of the deltoid and the white arrow shows the internal rotation movement.

therapist's other hand grasps the forearm. In order to rotate the shoulder joint, the patient's elbow should be extended. For anterior deltoid muscle TrP, the therapist passively internally rotates the shoulder joint and at the same time introduces an anterior–posterior transverse stroke to the anterior part of the deltoid muscle (Fig. 60.8). For posterior deltoid muscle TrPs, the therapist passively externally rotates the shoulder and at the same time introduces a posterior–anterior transverse stroke to the posterior part of the muscle (Fig. 60.9).

Dynamic longitudinal strokes of biceps/triceps brachii muscle taut band

This technique combines longitudinal manual strokes with the patient being asked to contract the muscle and move the forearm through its range of motion. For the biceps brachii muscle, the patient lies supine with the shoulder flat on the table, the elbow extended (if possible) and the forearm supinated. The therapist applies longitudinal strokes over the TrP taut band with both thumbs from a cranial (shoulder) to caudal (elbow) direction and at the same time the patient flexes the elbow by contracting the biceps brachii muscle (Fig. 60.10).

For the triceps brachii muscle, the patient lies prone with the shoulder flat on the table, the elbow flexed (if possible) and the hand in neutral position. The therapist applies longitudinal strokes over the taut band with both thumbs from a cranial (shoulder) to caudal (olecranon) direction and at the same time the patient extends the elbow by contracting the triceps brachii (Fig. 60.11). It is perceived clinically that the strokes should be applied simultaneously with the muscle contraction.

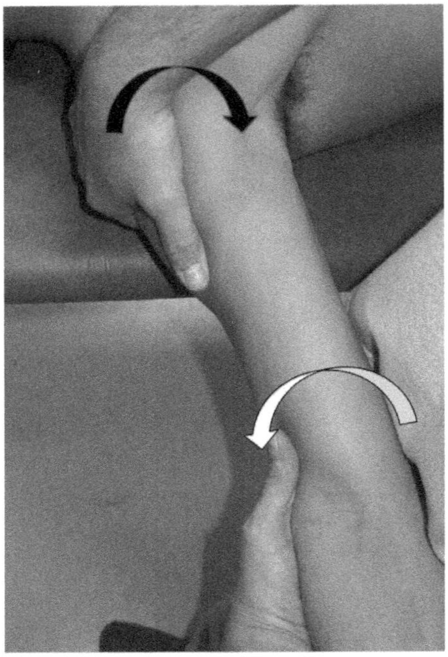

Figure 60.9 Dynamic transverse strokes of posterior deltoid muscle trigger points. The black arrow shows the posterior to anterior stroke of the deltoid and the white arrow shows the external rotation movement.

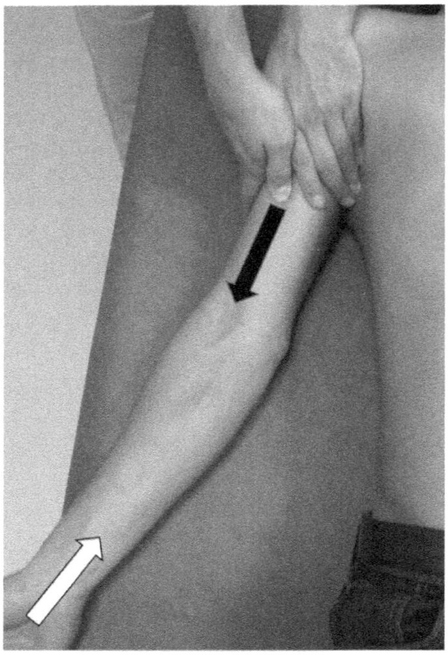

Figure 60.10 Dynamic longitudinal strokes of biceps brachii muscle taut band. The black arrow shows the longitudinal stroke and the white arrow shows the elbow flexion motion.

Dynamic longitudinal strokes of hand / wrist extensor muscle taut band

This technique is the same as that described for the biceps / triceps brachii muscle. The patient is seated with the elbow at 90° of flexion, and the hand pronated and closed.

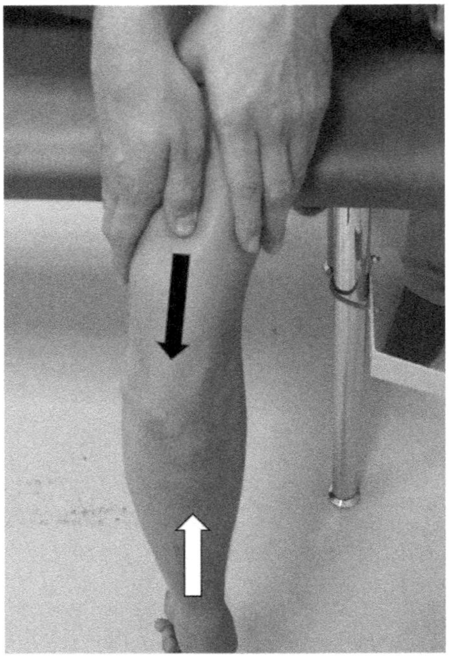

Figure 60.11 Dynamic longitudinal strokes of triceps brachii muscle taut band. The black arrow shows the longitudinal stroke and the white arrow shows the elbow extension motion.

The therapist applies longitudinal strokes over TrP taut bands with both thumbs from a cranial (elbow) to caudal (wrist) direction and at the same time the patient extends the wrist by contracting the hand / wrist extensor muscles. Since these muscles run longitudinally along the forearm, the therapist can focus the stroke over each hand / wrist extensor muscle (i.e. extensor carpi radialis longus or brevis, extensor digitorum communis or extensor carpi ulnaris muscle).

Transverse massage of hand / wrist flexor muscle trigger points

This technique combines a transverse massage with or without the patient moving the forearm through its range of motion. The patient is asked to actively contract the hand / wrist flexor muscles. The patient is seated with the elbow at 90° of flexion, and the hand supinated and opened. The therapist applies a transverse friction massage over the TrP taut band of the affected muscle. The patient has two options: (a) to open and close the hand by contracting the hand flexor muscles (Fig. 60.12); (b) to close the hand and to flex the wrist by contracting both the hand and wrist flexors (Fig. 60.13). Since these muscles also run longitudinally along the forearm, the therapist can focus the transverse massage over the taut band of each hand / wrist flexor muscle (i.e. the palmaris longus, flexor carpi radialis or ulnaris, flexor digitorum superficialis or profundus muscle).

Stretching compression of thumb muscles taut bands

Any muscle located in the thenar eminence can develop TrPs. For instance, a TrP within the adductor pollicis muscle refers

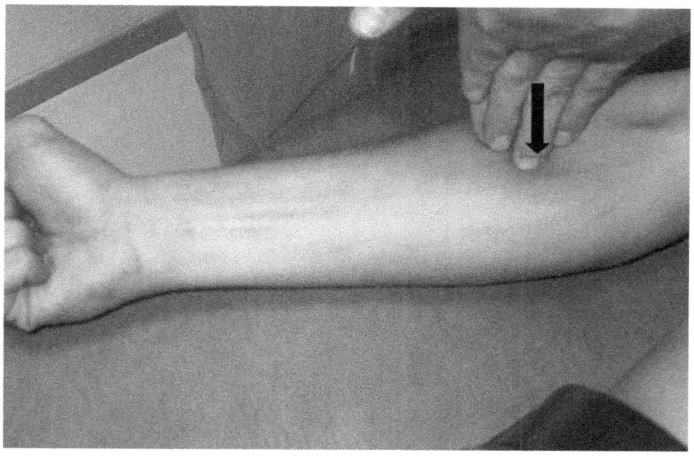

Figure 60.12 **Transverse massage of hand flexor muscle trigger points.**

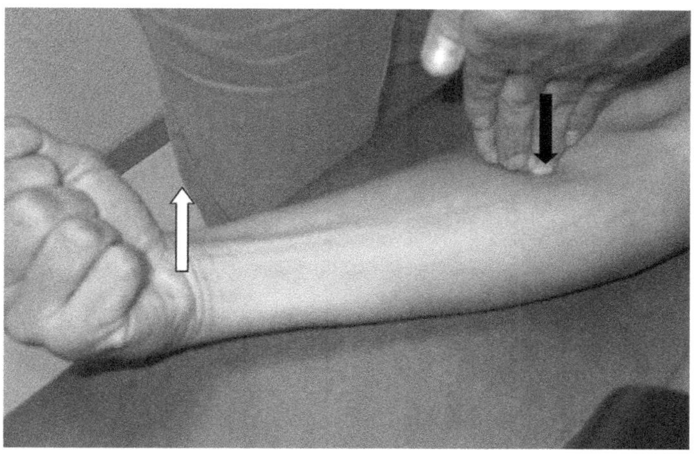

Figure 60.13 **Transverse massage of hand/wrist flexor muscle trigger points.** The black arrow shows the transverse friction massage and the white arrow shows the wrist and finger flexion motion.

an aching and deep pain along the thumb and to the radial styloid. TrPs in the opponens pollicis muscle refer pain to the palmar surface of the thumb and to the radial side of the palmar aspect of the wrist.

The stretching compression technique for thenar eminence muscle TrPs consists of the therapist applying compression to the TrP with the thumb whilst passively and rhythmically stretching the muscle. Figure 60.14 shows the technique applied over the opponens pollicis muscle TrPs.

Transverse massage of quadratus lumborum muscle taut bands

This technique combines a transverse massage with or without moving the legs of the patient to induce lateral flexion of the body. The patient is lying on the unaffected / non-symptomatic side with the therapist standing in front of the patient. The ulnar aspect of the therapist's forearm should be placed over the taut band of the muscle. The technique consists of applying a smooth and slow transverse massage over the TrP taut

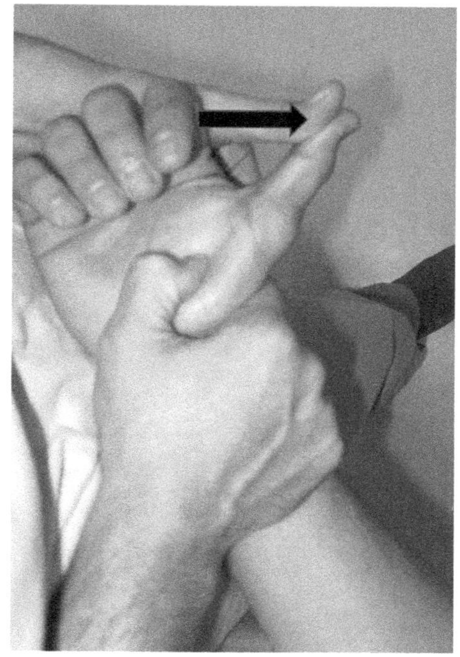

Figure 60.14 **Stretching compression of opponens pollicis muscle.**

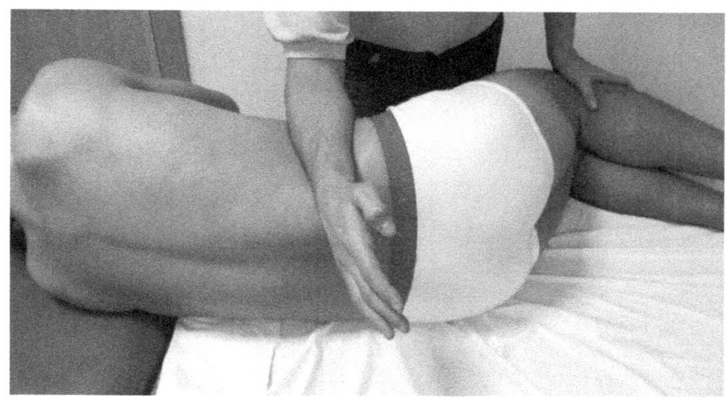

Figure 60.15 **Transverse massage of quadratus lumborum muscle taut bands.**

band (Fig. 60.15). If the therapist wants to conduct a dynamic intervention, the feet of the patient are placed outside of the table and the patient lifts the feet to the horizontal level. This action provokes an isometric contraction of the quadratus lumborum muscle by inducing side-bending of the trunk.

Post-isometric relaxation of quadratus lumborum muscle taut bands

This technique can be applied when the muscle is very tight and direct palpation of the muscle is too painful for the patient. The patient is side-lying on the unaffected / non-symptomatic side with the superior leg arranged in front of the other leg. A pillow can be placed under the waist to increase the lateral convexity of the lumbar spine. The therapist's caudal hand stabilizes the iliac bone, and the cranial hand is placed on the rib cage of the patient. The rib cage is

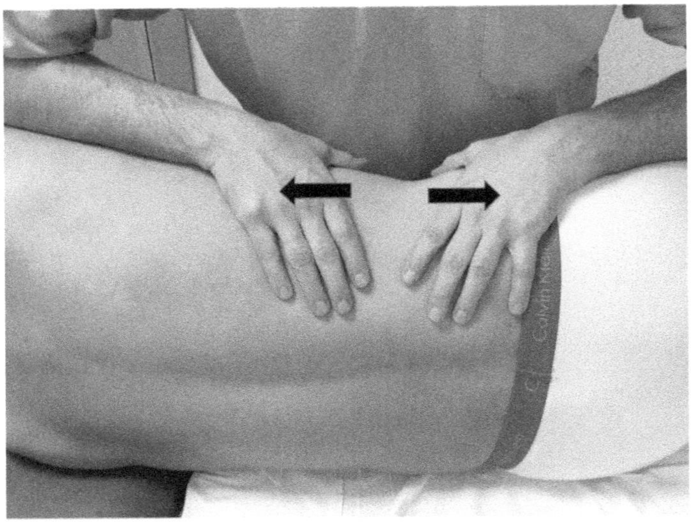

Figure 60.16 **Post-isometric relaxation of quadratus lumborum muscle taut bands.** The black arrows show the centrifugal direction of the stroke.

stretched away from the iliac bone until tension is perceived (Fig. 60.16).

In that position, the patient actively contracts the muscle by lifting the leg for 4–8 seconds, and then releases it. When the therapist feels that the contraction has ceased and the muscle is becoming more relaxed, an increase in muscle stretch is slowly introduced. The patient can actively participate by gently lengthening the leg at the start of the stretch.

Stretching compression of psoas major muscle taut bands

Management of the psoas major muscle is important since this muscle is anatomically related to several urogenital structures and the lumbar plexus (Stepnik et al 2006). A stretching compression technique combines a compression intervention with passive or active stretching of the TrP taut band. The patient is supine with the knee and hip flexed, and the foot on the table. The therapist compresses the TrP (which is usually located within the muscle belly, reached through the overlying abdominal muscles) with the tips of the fingers of one or both hands (Fig. 60.17). At the time that he / she perceives a relaxation of the taut band, the patient is asked to straighten the knee and the hip, either passively or actively, to increase the tension in the taut band (Fig. 60.18). The aim of this technique is for the patient to achieve pain-free extension of the hip and knee at the same time that the therapist maintains the compression.

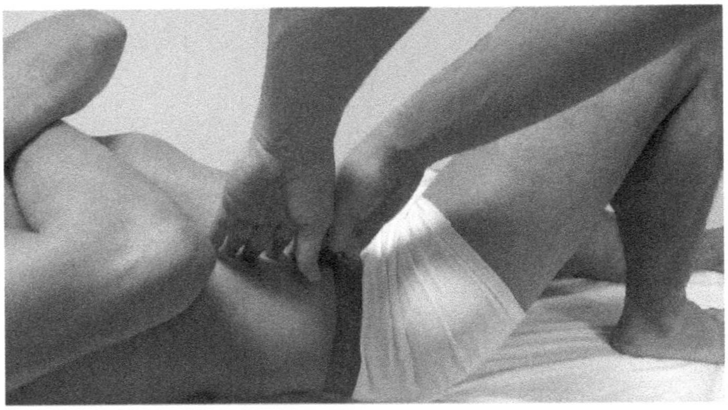

Figure 60.17 **Stretching compression of psoas major muscle taut bands in flexion.**

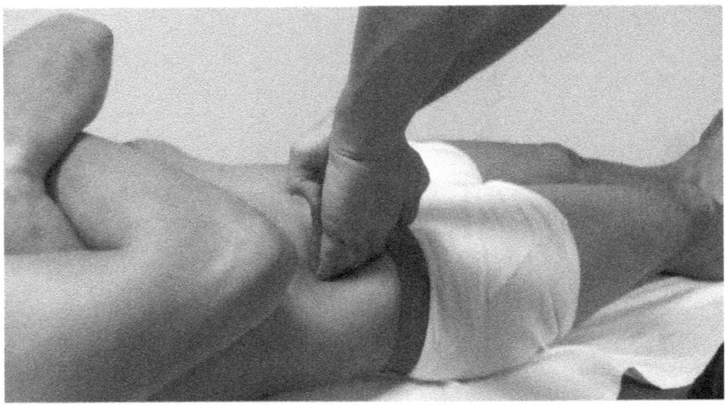

Figure 60.18 **Stretching compression of psoas major taut bands in extension.**

Stretching longitudinal stroke / dynamic longitudinal stroke of gluteus medius muscle taut bands

A stretching stroke consists of a longitudinal stroke applied over a muscle taut band placed in a stretched position. With the patient side-lying, the gluteus medius can be stretched by adduction of the leg with the knee flexed. In this stretched position, longitudinal strokes can be performed with the ulnar aspect of the therapist's forearm, from a posterior to an anterior direction (Fig. 60.19). When the patient lifts the knee, the technique will be converted into a dynamic longitudinal stroke of the gluteus medius muscle.

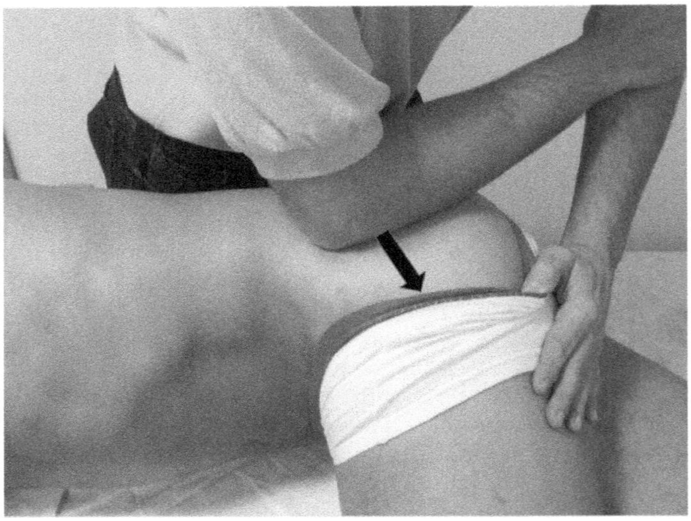

Figure 60.19 **Stretching longitudinal stroke / dynamic longitudinal stroke of gluteus medius muscle taut bands.** The black arrow shows the direction of the stroke.

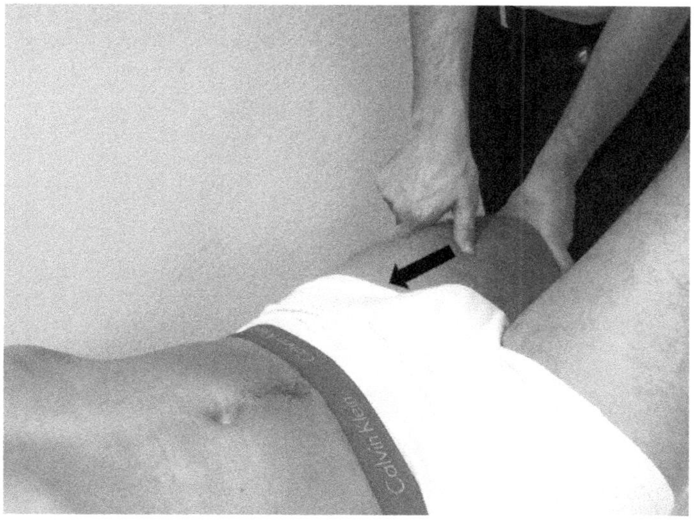

Figure 60.20 Stretching longitudinal stroke of quadriceps muscle taut bands. The black arrow shows the direction of the stroke.

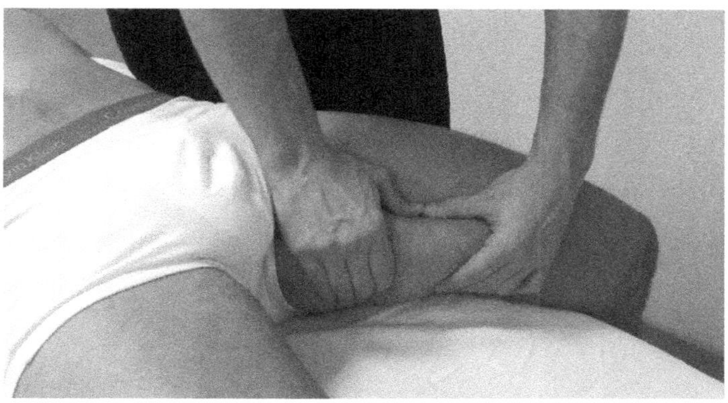

Figure 60.21 Stretching longitudinal massage of adductor muscle taut bands.

Stretching longitudinal stroke of quadriceps muscle taut bands

With the patient in supine, the quadriceps muscle can be stretched by flexing the knee with the hip extended. In this stretched position, longitudinal strokes can be performed with the therapist's thumb–index fingers or knuckles, from a caudal to a cranial direction (Fig. 60.20). When the patient lifts the knee, the technique will be converted into a dynamic longitudinal stroke of the quadriceps muscle.

Stretching longitudinal massage of adductor muscle taut bands

The aim of this technique is lengthen the muscle taut band by applying a pincer stroke. The patient is supine or side-lying. Once the therapist locates a TrP in any of the adductor muscles, a pincer palpation of the TrP taut band is firmly applied. The therapist's fingers grasp the taut band from both sides, and strokes are applied centrifugally away from the TrP. This technique is particularly effective for the adductor magnus and longus muscles (Fig. 60.21).

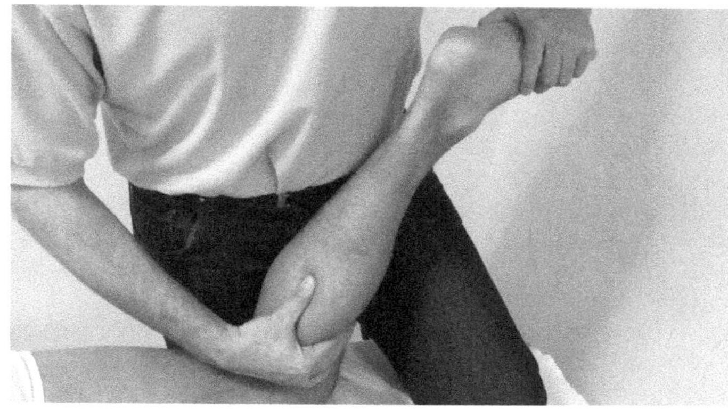

Figure 60.22 Stretching compression of gastrocnemius and soleus muscles taut bands.

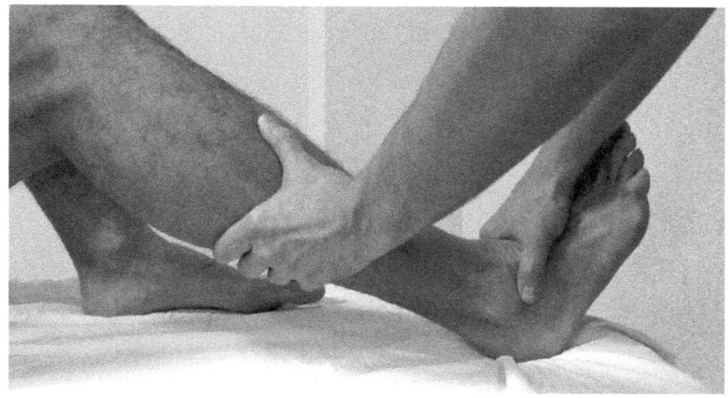

Figure 60.23 Compression and contraction of anterior–lateral leg muscles.

Stretching compression of gastrocnemius muscle taut bands

The stretching compression technique combines any TrP compression with passive or active stretching of the TrP taut band. The patient lies prone with the knee at 90° of flexion. The stretching compression technique for gastrocnemius muscle TrPs consists of compression of the TrP with a pincer palpation, which the therapist can combine with passive and rhythmical stretching of the muscle by inducing passive ankle dorsiflexion (Fig. 60.22). The procedure is repeated until a relaxation within the taut band is perceived or until the referred pain disappears.

Compression and contraction of anterior–lateral leg muscles

For this technique, the patient is supine. With the thumb, the therapist compresses the TrP on the anterior–lateral leg muscles (tibialis anterior, extensor digitorum longus or extensor hallucis longus muscle). When the therapist perceives a slight relaxation of the tissue, the patient is asked to contract the muscles by inducing active dorsiflexion and plantar flexion of the ankle (Fig. 60.23). This technique is repeated until the referred pain disappears, which usually happens within 10–12 repetitions.

Conclusion

There are several manual therapies that can be used for inactivating muscle TrPs in the upper and lower quadrant musculature. Current scientific evidence has investigated single applications of a few manual therapies (i.e. ischaemic contraction, neuromuscular approach and muscle energy); however, manual therapies are usually part of a multimodal approach for pain relief. Some clinical studies have demonstrated the effectiveness of the inclusion of TrP manual therapies into different multimodal approaches for the management of lower quadrant pain syndromes, such as heel pain or ankle sprains. New studies are needed to elucidate the neurophysiological mechanisms of manual therapies applied to myofascial TrPs. In addition, the inclusion of manual therapies aimed at inactivating TrPs in multimodal approaches of patients with different upper quadrant pain syndromes should be investigated.

References

Altan L, Bingol U, Aykac M, et al. 2005. Investigation of the effect of Ga-As laser therapy on cervical myofascial pain syndrome. Rheumatol Int 25: 23–27.

Anderson RU, Wise D, Sawyer T, et al. 2005. Integration of myofascial trigger point release and paradoxical relaxation training treatment of chronic pelvic pain in men. J Urol 174: 155–160.

Bodes-Pardo G, Pecos-Martín D, Gallego-Izquierdo T, et al. 2013. Manual treatment for cervicogenic headache and active trigger point in the sternocleidomastoid muscle: a pilot randomized clinical trial. J Manipulative Physiol Ther 36: 403–411.

Bron C, de Gast A, Dommerholt J, et al. 2011. Treatment of myofascial trigger points in patients with chronic shoulder pain; a randomized controlled trial. BMC Med 9: 8.

Brown CS, Ling FW, Wan JY, et al. 2002. Efficacy of static magnetic field therapy in chronic pelvic pain: a double-blind pilot study. Am J Obstet Gynecol 187: 1581–1587.

Buttagat V, Eungpinichpong W, Chatchawan U, et al. 2011. The immediate effects of traditional Thai massage on heart rate variability and stress-related parameters in patients with back pain associated with myofascial trigger points. J Bodyw Mov Ther 15: 15–23.

Chen D, Fang Y, Li J, et al. 1998. Anatomical study and clinical observation of thoracic outlet syndrome. Zhonghua Wai Ke Za Zhi 36: 661–663.

Cummings TM, White AR. 2001. Needling therapies in the management of myofascial trigger point pain: a systematic review. Arch Phys Med Rehabil 82: 986–992.

D'Ambrogio KJ, Roth GB. 1997. Positional release therapy. St Louis: Mosby.

Dardzinski JA, Ostrov BE, Hamann LS. 2000. Myofascial pain unresponsive to standard treatment: successful use of a strain and counter-strain technique with physical therapy. J Clin Rheumatol 6: 169–174.

Dommerholt J, McEvoy J. 2011. Myofascial trigger point release approach. In: Wise CH (ed) Orthopaedic manual physical therapy: from art to evidence. Philadelphia: FA Davis.

Dommerholt J, Shah J. 2010. Myofascial pain syndrome. In: Fishman SM, Ballantyne JC, Rathmell JP (eds) Bonica's management of pain. Baltimore: Lippincott, Williams & Williams, pp 450–471.

Dommerholt J, Mayoral-Del-Moral O, Gröbli C. 2006a. Trigger point dry needling. J Man Manipul Ther 14: E70–E87.

Dommerholt J, Bron C, Franssen JLM. 2006b. Myofascial trigger points: an evidence informed review. J Man Manipul Ther 14: 203–221.

Dommerholt J, Fernandez-de-las-Peñas C. 2013. Trigger point dry needling: an evidence and clinical-based approach, 1st edn. London: Churchill Livingstone Elsevier.

Dundar U, Evcik D, Samli F, et al. 2007. The effect of gallium arsenide aluminum laser therapy in the management of cervical myofascial pain syndrome: a double blind, placebo-controlled study. Clin Rheumatol 26: 930–934.

Emad MR, Roshanzamir S, Ghasempoor MZ, et al. 2012. Effectiveness of stretching after trigger point injections. J Musculoskel Res 14: ID 1250002.

Ferguson L, Gerwin R. 2005. Shoulder dysfunction and frozen shoulder. In: Ferguson L, Gerwin R (eds) Clinical mastery in the treatment of myofascial pain. Baltimore: Lippincott Williams & Wilkins, pp 91–121.

Fernández-de-las-Peñas C. 2009. Interaction between trigger points and joint hypo-mobility: a clinical perspective. J Man Manipul Ther 17: 74–77.

Fernández-de-las-Peñas C, Fernández-Carnero J, Galán-del-Río F, et al. 2004. Are myofascial trigger points responsible of restricted range of motion? A clinical study. J Musculoskelet Pain 12 (Suppl 9): 19. [Abstract.]

Fernández-de-las-Peñas C, Sohrbeck-Campo M, Fernández J, et al. 2005a. Manual therapies in the myofascial trigger point treatment: a systematic review. J Bodyw Mov Ther 9: 27–34.

Fernández-de-las-Peñas C, Fernández-Carnero J, Miangolarra-Page JC. 2005b. Musculoskeletal disorders in mechanical neck pain: myofascial trigger points versus cervical joint dysfunctions: a clinical study. J Musculoskelet Pain 13: 27–35.

Fernández-de-las-Peñas C, Alonso-Blanco C, Alguacil-Diego IM, et al. 2006a. Myofascial trigger points and posterior–anterior joint hypomobility in the mid-cervical spine in subjects presenting with mechanical neck pain: a pilot study. J Man Manipul Ther 14: 88–94.

Fernández-de-las-Peñas C, Alonso-Blanco C, Fernández J, et al. 2006b. The immediate effect of ischemic compression technique and transverse friction massage on tenderness of active and latent myofascial triggers points: a pilot study. J Bodyw Mov Ther 10: 3–9.

FitzGerald MP, Payne CK, Lukacz ES, et al. 2012. Randomized multicenter clinical trial of myofascial physical therapy in women with interstitial cystitis / painful bladder syndrome and pelvic floor tenderness. J Urol 187: 2113–2118.

Fryer G. 2000. Muscle energy concepts: a need for change. J Osteopath Med 3: 54–59.

Fryer G, Hodgson L. 2005. The effect of manual pressure release on myofascial trigger points in the upper trapezius muscle. J Bodyw Mov Ther 9: 248–255.

Gam AN, Warming S, Larsen LH, et al. 1998. Treatment of myofascial trigger points with ultrasound combined with massage and exercise: a randomised controlled trial. Pain 77: 73–79.

Gay CW, Alappattu MJ, Coronado RA, et al. 2013. Effect of a single session of muscle-biased therapy on pain sensitivity: a systematic review and meta-analysis of randomized controlled trials. J Pain Res 6: 7–22.

Gemmell H, Miller P, Nordstrom H. 2008. Immediate effect of ischaemic compression and trigger point pressure release on neck pain and upper trapezius trigger points: a randomized controlled trial. Clin Chiropractic 11: 30–36.

Gleitz M, Hornig K. 2012. Trigger points: diagnosis and treatment concepts with special reference to extracorporeal shockwaves. Orthopäde 41: 113–125.

Grieve R, Clark J, Pearson E, et al. 2011. The immediate effect of soleus trigger point pressure release on restricted ankle joint dorsiflexion: a pilot randomised controlled trial. J Bodywork Mov Ther 15: 42–49.

Gröbli C, Dejung B. 2003. Nichtmedikamentöse Therapie myofaszialer Schmerze. Schmerz 17: 475–480.

Gröbli C, Dommerholt J. 1997. Myofasziale Triggerpunkte; Pathologie und Behandlungsmöglichkeiten. Manuelle Med 35: 295–303.

Hains G, Descarreaux M, Hains F. 2010. Chronic shoulder pain of myofascial origin: a randomized clinical trial using ischemic compression therapy. J Manipulative Physiol Ther 33: 362–369.

Hanten WP, Barrett M, Gillespie-Plesko M, et al. 1997. Effects of active head-retraction with retraction / extension and occipital release on the pressure pain threshold of cervical and scapular trigger points. Physiother Theory Pract 13: 285–291.

Hanten WP, Olson SL, Butts NL, et al. 2000. Effectiveness of a home program of ischemic pressure followed by sustained stretch for treatment of myofascial trigger points. Phys Ther 80: 997–1003.

Heredia-Rizo AM, Oliva-Pascual-Vaca A, Rodríguez-Blanco C, et al. 2013. Immediate changes in masticatory mechanosensitivity, mouth opening, and head posture after myofascial techniques in pain-free healthy participants: a randomized controlled trial. J Manipulative Physiol Ther 36: 310–318.

Hong CZ, Chen YC, Pon CH, et al. 1993. Immediate effects of various physical medicine modalities on pain threshold of an active myofascial trigger point. J Musculoskelet Pain 1: 37–53.

Hou CR, Tsai LC, Cheng KF, et al. 2002. Immediate effects of various physical therapeutic modalities on cervical myofascial pain and trigger-point sensitivity. Arch Phys Med Rehabil 83: 1406–1414.

Ibáñez-García J, Alburquerque-Sendín F, Rodríguez-Blanco C, et al. 2009. Changes in masseter muscle trigger points following strain-counter / strain or neuro-muscular technique. J Bodyw Mov Ther 13: 2–10.

Jaeger B, Reeves JL. 1986. Quantification of changes in myofascial trigger point sensitivity with the pressure algometer following passive stretch. Pain 27: 203–210.

Jeon JH, Jung YJ, Lee JY, et al. 2012. The effect of extracorporeal shock wave therapy on myofascial pain syndrome. Ann Rehabil Med 36: 665–674.

Jones LN. 1981. Strain and counter-strain. Newark, OH: American Academy of Osteopathy.

Kietrys DM, Palombaro KM, Azzaretto E, et al. 2013. Effectiveness of dry needling for upper quarter myofascial pain: a systematic review and meta-analysis. J Orthop Sports Phys Ther 43: 620–634.

Kim Y, Yang HR, Lee JW, et al. 2014. Effects of the high-power pain threshold ultrasound technique in the elderly with latent myofascial trigger points: a double-blind randomized study. J Back Musculoskelet Rehabil 27(1): 17–23. doi: 10.3233/BMR-130414.

Kruger L, 1987. Cutaneous sensory system. In: Adelman G (ed) Encyclopedia of neuroscience. Vol. 1. Boston: Birkhäuser, pp 293–294.

Lee JC, Lin DT, Hong CZ. 1997. The effectiveness of simultaneous thermotherapy with ultrasound and electrotherapy with combined AC and DC current on the immediate pain relief of myofascial trigger points. J Musculoskelet Pain 5: 81–90.

Lewit K. 1999. Manipulative therapy in rehabilitation of the locomotor system, 3rd edn. Oxford: Butterworth Heinemann.

Majlesi J, Unalan H, 2004. High-power pain threshold ultrasound technique in the treatment of active myofascial trigger points: a randomized, double-blind, case-control study. Arch Phys Med Rehabil 85: 833–836.

Oliveira-Campelo NM, de Melo CA, Alburquerque-Sendin F, et al. 2013. Short- and medium-term effects of manual therapy on cervical active range of motion and pressure pain sensitivity in latent myofascial pain of the upper trapezius muscle: a randomized controlled trial. J Manipulative Physiol Ther 36: 300–309.

Pilat A. 2009. Myofascial induction approaches for patients with headache. In: Fernández-de-las-Peñas C, Arendt-Nielsen L, Gerwin R (eds) Tension type and cervicogenic headache: pathophysiology, diagnosis and treatment. Boston: Jones & Bartlett, pp 339–367.

Pöntinen PJ, Airaksinen O. 1995. Evaluation of myofascial pain and dysfunction syndromes and their response to low level laser therapy. J Musculoskeletal Pain 3: 149–154.

Renan-Ordine R, Alburquerque-Sendín F, Rodrígues-de-Souza D, et al. 2011. Effectiveness of myofascial trigger point manual therapy combined with a self-stretching protocol for the management of plantar heel pain: a randomized controlled trial. J Orthop Sports Phys Ther 41: 43–50.

Rickards LD. 2006. The effectiveness of non-invasive treatments for active myofascial trigger point pain: a systematic review of the literature. Int J Osteopathic Med 9: 120–136.

Rodríguez-Blanco C, Fernández-de-las-Peñas C, Hernández-Xumet JE, et al. 2006. Changes in active mouth opening following a single treatment of latent myofascial trigger points in the masseter muscle involving post-isometric relaxation or strain / counter-strain. J Bodyw Mov Ther 10: 197–205.

Ruiz-Sáez M, Fernández-de-las-Peñas C, Rodríguez-Blanco C, et al. 2007. Changes in pressure pain sensitivity in latent myofascial trigger points in the upper trapezius muscle following a cervical spine manipulation in pain-free subjects. J Manipul Physiol Ther 30: 578–583.

Schleip R. 2003. Fascial plasticity: a new neurobiological explanation. J Bodyw Mov Ther 7: 11–19.

Simons DG, 2002. Understanding effective treatments of myofascial trigger points. J Bodyw Mov Ther 6: 81–88.

Simons D, Travell J, Simons P. 1999. Travell & Simons' myofascial pain & dysfunction: the trigger point manual: the upper half of body. Baltimore: Williams & Wilkins.

Smania N, Corato E, Fiaschi A, et al. 2005. Repetitive magnetic stimulation: a novel approach for myofascial pain syndrome. J Neurol 252: 307–314.

Srbely JZ, Dickey JP. 2007. Randomized controlled study of the anti-nociceptive effect of ultrasound on trigger point sensitivity: novel applications in myofascial therapy? Clin Rehabil 21: 411–417.

Srbely JZ, Dickey JP, Lowerison M, et al. 2008. Stimulation of myofascial trigger points with ultrasound induces segmental anti-nociceptive effects: a randomized controlled study. Pain 139: 260–266.

Srbely JZ, Vernon H, Lee D, et al. 2013. Immediate effects of spinal manipulative therapy on regional antinociceptive effects in myofascial tissues in healthy young adults. J Manipulative Physiol Ther 36: 333–341.

Stepnik MW, Olby N, Thompson RR, et al. 2006. Femoral neuropathy in a dog with iliopsoas muscle injury. Vet Surg 35: 186–190.

Tanrikut A, Ozaras N, Ali-Kaptan H, et al. 2003. High voltage galvanic stimulation in myofascial pain syndrome. J Musculoskelet Pain 11: 11–15.

Tough EA, White AR, Cummings TM, et al. 2009. Acupuncture and dry needling in the management of myofascial trigger point pain: a systematic review and meta-analysis of randomised controlled trials. Eur J Pain 13: 3–10.

Truyols-Domínguez S, Salom-Moreno J, Abian-Vicent J, et al. 2013. Efficacy of thrust and nonthrust manipulation and exercise with or without the addition of myofascial therapy for the management of acute inversion ankle sprain: a randomized clinical trial. J Orthop Sports Phys Ther 43: 300–309.

Uemoto L, Garcia MA, Gouvêa CV, et al. 2013. Laser therapy and needling in myofascial trigger point deactivation. J Oral Sci 55: 175–181.

Van den Berg F, Cabri J. 1999. Angewandte Physiologie – Das Bindegewebe des Bewegungsapparates verstehen und beeinflussen. Stuttgart, Germany: Georg Thieme Verlag.

Vernon H, Schneider M. 2009. Chiropractic management of myofascial trigger points and myofascial pain syndrome: a systematic review of the literature. J Manipul Physiol Ther 32: 14–24.

61 Chapter

Dry Needling of Trigger Points

Jan Dommerholt, Erik H. Wijtmans

CHAPTER CONTENTS

Introduction to trigger point dry needling	690
Scientific evidence of dry needling	691
General guidelines for dry needling	692
Dry needling of selected neck, shoulder and arm muscles	693
Scalene muscles	693
Pectoralis minor muscle	693
Pectoralis major muscle	693
Supraspinatus muscle	693
Infraspinatus/teres major/teres minor muscles	694
Rhomboid major and minor muscles	694
Subscapularis muscle	694
Latissimus dorsi muscle	695
Deltoid muscle	695
Biceps brachii muscle	696
Brachialis muscle	696
Brachioradialis muscle	696
Supinator muscle	696
Wrist and finger extensor muscles	697
Dry needling of selected trunk muscles	697
Thoracic and lumbar multifidus muscles	697
Longissimus thoracis muscle	698
Quadratus lumborum muscle	698
Rectus abdominis muscle	698
External and internal oblique muscles	699
Dry needling of selected hip and leg muscles	700
Gluteus maximus muscle	700
Gluteus medius muscle	700
Gluteus minimus muscle	700
Piriformis muscle	700
Adductor longus muscle	701
Adductor brevis muscle	701
Adductor magnus muscle	701
Pectineus muscle	702
Psoas major muscle	702
Iliacus muscle	703
Quadriceps femoris muscle group	703
Biceps femoris muscle	704
Semimembranosus muscle	705
Semitendinosus muscle	705
Tibialis anterior muscle	705
Gastrocnemius muscle	705
Soleus muscle	706
Flexor digitorum longus muscle	706
Fibularis (peroneus) longus and brevis muscles	707

Introduction to Trigger Point Dry Needling

Treating clinically relevant trigger points (TrPs) with invasive procedures requires a thorough knowledge of the functional anatomy of muscles and their direct environment. TrPs are identified with manual palpation using either a flat or a pincher palpation technique (see Ch 59). TrPs feature increased muscle tension (Buchmann et al 2014) and can be palpated accurately in most muscles. Once a TrP is identified, the clinician must visualize its location in a three-dimensional perspective and appreciate the depth and presence of neighbouring structures, including arteries, veins, nerves and internal organs. For most muscles, the needle should not be used to locate the TrP, as this would make inactivating TrPs a rather random process (Dommerholt et al 2006). Most muscles can be palpated manually, but there are several exceptions. Parts of the subscapularis and serratus anterior muscles, for example, are partially in between the scapula and the rib cage. The iliacus muscle is on the inside of the pelvis and the muscle is inaccessible to manual palpation. In those cases, the clinician can use a needle to locate and treat these TrPs approaching the muscles from the medial border of the scapula and directly over the edge of the ilia respectively. Inactivating TrPs with a needle requires an excellent kinaesthetic sense and awareness, based on training, experience and anatomical knowledge (Noë 2004). At any time, the clinician must know whereabouts in the body the tip of the needle is and which structures will be encountered. Well-developed kinaesthetic perception makes needling procedures safe and accurate, as the clinician will be able to appreciate changes in structures and accurately identify when the needle penetrates the skin, the subcutaneous connective tissue and fascial layers, the muscle, and ultimately the taut band and the TrP (Mayoral del Moral 2005).

Invasive TrP therapies can be divided into injections and dry needling. TrP injections are administered with a hypodermic syringe; TrP dry needling is administered with a solid filament needle. Dry needling can be divided into superficial and deep dry needling (Dommerholt et al 2006). Some older studies suggested that dry needling would cause more post-needling soreness (Hong 1994; Kamanli et al 2005), but in these studies injections were compared with dry needling using a syringe. In a more recent study comparing injections with dry needling using a solid filament needle, there was no significant difference between the two approaches (Ga et al 2007). Dry needling provided longer-lasting relief, however (Ga et al 2007). This chapter focuses on deep dry-needling techniques and does not include specific information about superficial dry needling or TrP injections, although injection techniques are not all that different from deep dry needling. Readers are referred to other textbooks for this information (Dommerholt & Fernández-de-las-Peñas 2013). The chapter also does not include any information about dry needling of other structures, such as ligaments, tendons and tendon–bone attachments, scar tissue or fascial adhesions. In clinical practice, dry needling can be applied to any of these entities (Lewit 1979).

Dry needling is within the scope of practice of medicine, acupuncture, physical therapy, chiropractic, veterinary medicine, dentistry and myotherapy, depending on local jurisdiction. Each practitioner will use discipline-specific philosophy and management approaches to determine when and how dry needling techniques will be applied. Acupuncture practitioners may refer to dry needling as 'TrP acupuncture', but this does not imply that dry needling would be in the exclusive domain of any discipline (Association of Social Work Boards et al 2006). Although dry needling is generally performed with the same needle used in acupuncture, it does not require any knowledge of traditional acupuncture theory or Chinese medicine (Baldry 2005; Amaro 2007; White 2009). Currently, there are several commercially available needles designed specifically for the practice of dry needling. As early as the 19th century, physicians used needles, including ladies' hat-pins, to treat tender points in the low back region (Churchill 1821, 1828; Elliotson 1827; Osler 1912). Dry needling is an expansion of the TrP injection techniques promoted by Travell, Simons and others and is based on the observation that the actual mechanical stimulation of a TrP by the needle may be responsible for the therapeutic benefits (Steinbrocker 1944; Travell & Simons 1992; Simons et al 1999).

However, dry needling is not without risk (Dommerholt et al 2006; Lee et al 2011; McCutcheon & Yelland 2011; Usman et al 2011). Due to the invasive nature of the procedure, there is a risk of penetrating vital organs and other body structures, such as the lungs, intestines, kidneys, urethra, nerves and arteries, and the brainstem through the foramen magnum, among others. While the incidence of acupuncture-induced pneumothorax is less than 1/10000, the incidence of dry needling-induced pneumothorax is unknown. A prospective study of the risk of adverse events of dry needling showed that the risk of a significant adverse event was less than 0.04% in nearly 8000 dry-needling treatments by Irish physiotherapists (Brady et al 2014). Dry needling should always be anatomy driven; a thorough knowledge of anatomical relations is required for the technique (Peuker & Gronemeyer 2001; Yang & Mullan 2011). In addition, clinicians must follow established protocols for preventing the spread of blood-borne pathogens and maintain sound guidelines for safe dry-needling practice, which includes hand washing and other hygienic measures (McEvoy et al 2011; Australian Society of Acupuncture Physiotherapists (ASAP) 2013).

Scientific Evidence of Dry Needling

One of the first prospective scientific studies of dry needling was published in 1980 and showed its effectiveness in the treatment of injured workers with low back pain (Gunn et al 1980). An authoritative Cochrane review found that dry needling was a potentially useful adjunct in the treatment of individuals with chronic low back pain, but agreed that more high-quality studies are needed (Furlan et al 2005). A study of the effects of latent TrPs on muscle activation patterns in the shoulder region demonstrated that a combination of TrP dry needling and passive stretching restored normal muscle activation patterns (Lucas et al 2004). A prospective, open-label, randomized study on the effect of deep dry needling on shoulder pain in 101 patients following a cerebrovascular accident showed that, after only four dry needling treatments, patients who were treated with dry needling reported significantly less pain during sleep and during physical therapy treatments, had more restful sleep and experienced significantly less frequent and less intense pain. They reduced their use of analgesic medications and demonstrated increased compliance with the rehabilitation programme compared with patients who received the regular rehabilitation programme (Dilorenzo et al 2004). A few studies confirmed the positive effects of dry needling on temporomandibular pain (Fernández-Carnero et al 2010; Dıraçoğlu et al 2012; Gonzalez-Perez et al 2012; Itoh et al 2012).

A recent meta-analysis of the effectiveness of dry needling for upper-quarter myofascial pain concluded that dry needling is an effective treatment modality (Kietrys et al 2013). Another study found that dry needling produced an improvement in pain intensity, pain pressure thresholds and scores on the Disabilities of the Arm, Shoulder and Hand (DASH) test and may be prescribed for subjects with TrPs in the upper trapezius muscles (Ziaeifar et al 2014). Maher et al (2013) established objective improvements in posture and pain following dry needling using ultrasound shear-wave elastography. Dry needling can improve both muscle blood flow and oxygenation (Cagnie et al 2012).

Single-case reports also suggested that dry needling was useful in the treatment of: plantar fasciitis (Akhbari et al 2014), chest wall pain (Westrick et al 2012), posterior knee pain (Mason et al 2014), adhesive capsulitis (Clewley et al 2014), hamstrings tendinopathy (Jayaseelan et al 2014), shoulder injuries (Osborne & Gatt 2010), temporomandibular disorder when combined with other interventions (González-Iglesias et al 2013), low back pain (Rainey 2013) and groin pain (Paantjens 2013). A fear of needles does not seem to impact the clinical outcome (Joseph et al 2013).

In one study (Hsieh et al 2007), TrP dry needling of the infraspinatus muscle decreased the pain intensity of the shoulder, and increased active and passive shoulder internal rotation and the pressure pain threshold of TrPs in the ipsilateral anterior deltoid and extensor carpi radialis longus muscles. In another (Tsai et al 2010), dry needling of TrPs in the extensor carpi radialis longus reduced the irritability of TrPs in the ipsilateral trapezius muscle and the overall pain intensity, and improved cervical range of motion. A similar study (Chou et al 2009) of the effect of needling two acupuncture points in the extensor carpi radialis longus and extensor indices muscles reduced the pain intensity and end-plate noise associated with a TrP in the trapezius muscle; the authors compared the results with a sham-needling procedure whereby a needle was inserted into a rubber connector with direct contact on the skin. Subjects could feel the sharp needle tip, however, which makes it questionable whether this was a true sham procedure. Tekin et al (2013) demonstrated the positive effects of dry needling, but in this study the sham needling procedure was in fact a variation on superficial dry needling. Any needling is likely to have a physiological effect, such as a release of endorphins, a change in pain thresholds or an expectancy of a positive outcome (Pariente et al 2005; Birch 2006; Lund & Lundeberg 2006; Wang et al 2008). Both actual needling and so-called sham procedures can activate brain areas involved in sensorimotor processing, and deactivate brain regions more active during rest than during other tasks. Interestingly though, in one study the areas associated with cognitive functioning were activated by both real and sham needling, but actual needling evoked a stronger response. The authors noted that some of the differences could be due to atypical stimuli from deeper, subdermal receptors being stimulated by needling, as opposed to the cutaneous receptors stimulated by sham procedures (Napadow et al 2009). Likewise, a light touch of the skin has been shown to be able to stimulate mechanoreceptors coupled to slow conducting unmyelinated C-fibre afferents, which in turn can activate the insular region, but not necessarily the somatosensory cortex (Olausson et al 2002). Kong et al (2006) confirmed that mild and moderate pain stimuli were more effective at activating particular areas of the brain than strong pain stimuli. The only true double-blind study of the effectiveness of dry needling involved TrP dry needling prior to total knee replacement (Mayoral et al 2013). Forty subjects scheduled for a total knee replacement with TrPs in either the tensor fascia lata, hip abductors, hamstrings, quadriceps, gastrocnemius or popliteus muscles were randomly allocated to either an intervention group, who received TrP dry needling, or a placebo-needling group. After each subject was anaesthetized, dry needling was performed. Obviously, the subjects were blinded to the procedure. The study demonstrated that a single treatment of TrPs produced a significant decrease in pain intensity over and above placebo 1 month after knee replacement surgery (Mayoral et al 2013).

Dry needling may reduce end-plate noise at TrPs (Chen et al 2001) and the chemical concentrations of several nociceptive substances found in the immediate environment of active TrPs (Shah et al 2005, 2008). A recent rabbit study showed that the effects on chemical concentrations with dry needling of TrPs were actually dose dependent (Hsieh et al 2012). Short-term dry needling modulated the biochemicals associated with pain and inflammation, such as substance P, β-endorphin and tumour necrosis factor α (TNF-α). Immediately after dry needling the levels of β-endorphin and TNF-α increased, whereas the levels of substance P decreased. The longer term needling also caused changes in the levels of cyclo-oxygenase-2 (COX-2), vascular endothelial growth factor (VEGF), inducible nitric oxide synthase (iNOS), and hypoxia-inducible factor 1α (HIF-1α). The increase in substance P, COX-2 and TNF-α levels may be associated with more tissue damage (Hsieh et al 2012). Up-regulation of HIF-1α may be associated with hypoxia, as seen in TrPs, but can also be associated with mechanical stress. It should be noted that the expression of HIF-1α, iNOS and VEGF proteins may be important factors in improving the local circulation after intensive dry needling.

Individuals with active TrPs demonstrated abnormal central processing and hyperalgesia in response to electrical stimulation and compression of the TrP (Niddam et al 2007, 2008). Enhanced brain activity was observed in the somatosensory and limbic regions, and suppressed activity was noted in the hippocampus (Niddam et al 2008). There is increasing evidence that TrPs contribute to the development of central sensitization (Fernández-de-las-Peñas et al 2007, 2009; Giamberardino et al 2007; Fernández-Carnero et al 2008). There is also some evidence from animal studies that needling therapies involve the descending pain inhibitory system (Takeshige et al 1992a, 1992b). It is likely that dry needling influences both peripheral and central pain mechanisms (Dommerholt 2011; Fernández-de-las-Peñas & Dommerholt 2014). The tissue damage caused by dry needling lasts only a few days in a dry-needling model in mice (Domingo et al 2013).

General Guidelines for Dry Needling

This following section provides basic guidance to needling TrPs in the neck, shoulder, arm, trunk, hip and leg muscles. It should be noted that the skills needed to use these techniques safely and accurately can be learned only through attending hands-on courses offered by qualified and experienced tutors. Reading this chapter does not constitute any qualification to use dry needling in clinical practice. There are general guidelines, however, which should be adhered to. It is recommended that patients are lying down during any needling procedures, because of the risk of vasodepressive syncope. For every muscle, anatomical landmarks should be identified, including the margins of the muscle and any relevant bony structures (e.g. the medial and lateral borders of the scapula and the scapular spine when needling the supraspinatus muscle). Once a TrP is identified, the landmarks are once again verified to assure safe needling. There is ongoing debate over whether disinfection of the skin is necessary, and guidelines vary in different countries and regions. For TrP dry needling, use of needles in tubes is recommended (White et al 2008). The tube is placed on the skin overlying the TrP and the needle is quickly tapped into the skin. The tube is removed, and the needle is moved in and out into the region of the TrP by drawing the needle back to the subcutaneous tissue and redirecting it. If the needle is not withdrawn sufficiently, the needle will follow the same pathway and the clinician will not be able to alter its direction. The objective of needling is to elicit so-called local twitch responses, which are an indication that the TrP is indeed inactivated (Hong 1994). Following needling procedures, haemostasis must be accomplished to prevent or minimize local bleeding, help restore and maintain range of motion, and facilitate a return to normal function.

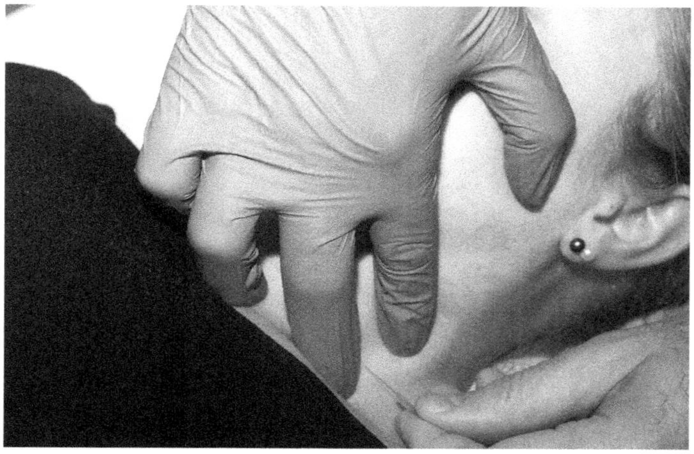

Figure 61.1 **Dry needling of TrPs in the anterior scalene muscle.**

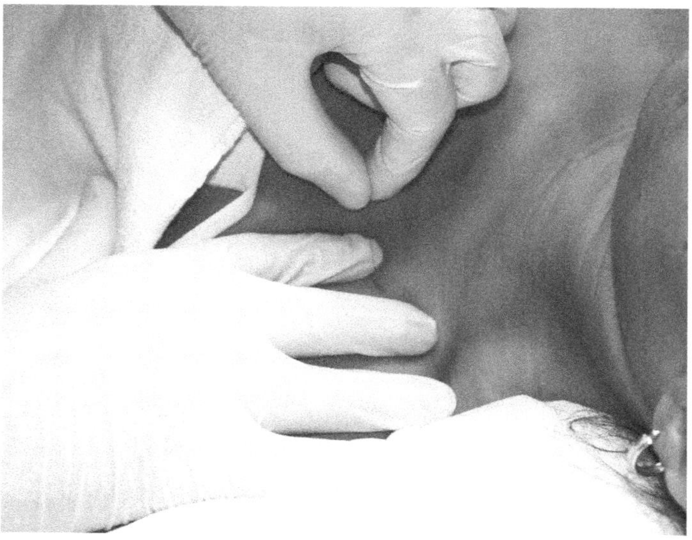

Figure 61.2 **Dry needling of TrPs in the pectoralis minor muscle.**

Only very experienced clinicians should use needling procedures with patients who routinely take warfarin or anticoagulants. Muscles that are inaccessible to manual palpation and therefore to haemostasis should be avoided, such as the psoas major, iliacus, lateral pterygoid, and parts of the subscapularis and serratus muscles, among others. The use of platelet inhibitors is generally not an absolute contraindication to needling, but the therapist needs to be careful to achieve haemostasis.

Dry Needling of Selected Neck, Shoulder and Arm Muscles

Scalene muscles

Anatomy: The anterior and middle scalene muscles originate from the first rib; the posterior scalene muscle comes from the second rib. The muscles insert at the transverse processes of cervical vertebrae C3–C8.

Needling technique: The patient is lying either supine or in the lateral decubitus position. The medial scalene muscle lies anterior to the transverse processes of the cervical spine. The needle is inserted into the belly of the muscle (Fig. 61.1). The anterior scalene muscle is identified by asking the patient to sniff sharply (Katagiri et al 2003). The muscle is approached lateral to the clavicular head of the sternocleidomastoid muscle. The posterior scalene muscle is not needled, owing to its close proximity to the apex of the lungs.

Precautions: The jugular vein should be identified and avoided. The scalene muscles cannot be needled towards the lungs, because of the high risk of causing a pneumothorax.

Pectoralis minor muscle

Anatomy: The muscle originates from the third, fourth and fifth ribs near their costal cartilages and inserts at the coracoid process of the scapula.

Needling technique: The patient lies supine. The coracoid process should be identified first. The needle is inserted through the pectoralis major muscle and directed either upwards towards the coracoid process (Fig. 61.2) or toward the thumb of the palpating hand using a pincer palpation.

Precautions: Care must be taken to avoid pneumothorax. Also, the neurovascular bundle of the arm lies under the pectoralis minor muscle close to the coracoid process.

Pectoralis major muscle

Anatomy: The pectoralis major muscle has four separate origins: the first arises from the clavicle, the second from the sternum, the third from the ribs, and the fourth is an abdominal attachment via the aponeuroses of the external abdominal oblique and rectus abdominis muscles. The muscle inserts over the greater tubercle of the humerus along the lateral lip of the bicipital groove.

Needling technique: The patient lies supine. When treatment is over the chest wall, needling is always directed towards a rib with the therapist's index and middle fingers placed in the intercostal space to avoid causing pneumothorax (Fig. 61.3). Other portions of the muscle can be needled via a pincer palpation, with the needle directed towards the fingers. The clavicular part of the muscle can be needled either with a pincer palpation or shallowly towards the humerus.

Precautions: The ribs must be palpated and used as a guideline to avoid pneumothorax.

Supraspinatus muscle

Anatomy: The muscle arises from the supraspinatus fossa and attaches to the upper part of the greater tubercle of the humeral head.

Needling technique: The patient is in side-lying. The needle is directed slightly posteriorly towards the upper border of the scapula and scapular spine (Fig. 61.4).

Precautions: If the needle is directed towards the anterior wall of the supraspinatus fossa, there is a considerable risk of causing a pneumothorax.

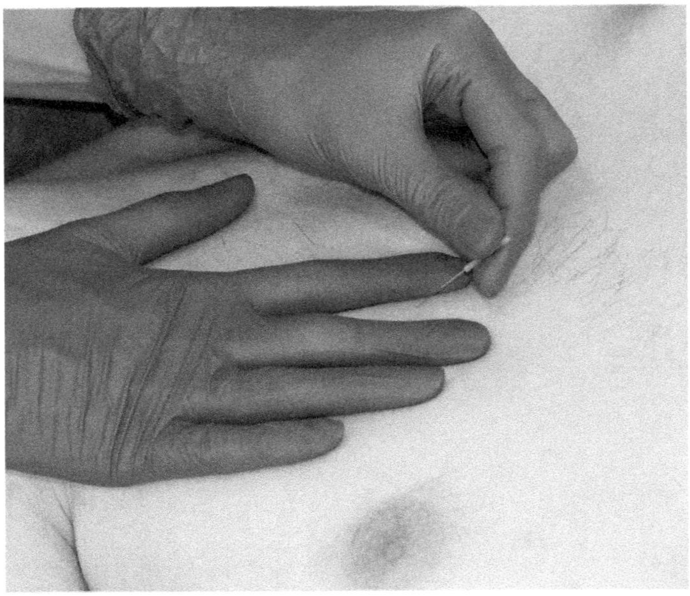

Figure 61.3 **Dry needling of TrPs in the pectoralis major muscle.** (Modified from Dommerholt J, Fernández-de-las-Peñas C 2013.)

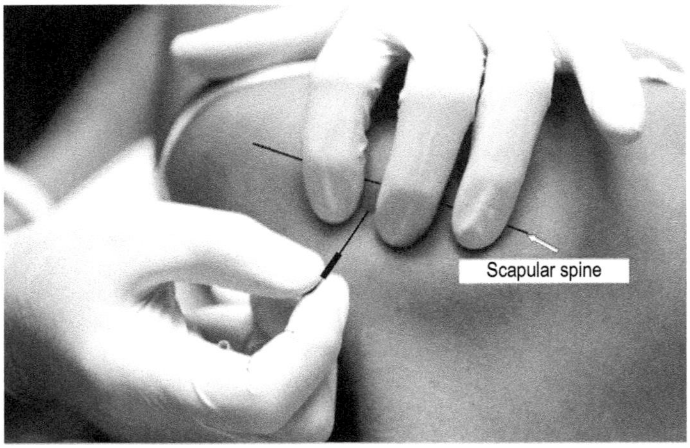

Figure 61.4 **Dry needling of TrPs in the supraspinatus muscle.**

Infraspinatus/teres major/teres minor muscles

Anatomy: The three muscles originate from different aspects of the posterior surface of the scapula below the scapular spine. The teres major originates at the inferior angle of the scapula and inserts in front of the humerus to its lesser tubercle. The teres minor originates from a higher and more lateral point than the teres major muscle near the axillary border of the scapula. The teres minor inserts behind the humerus to the greater tubercle.

Needling technique: The patient lies in the prone position or in side-lying with the arm supported with a pillow. Body landmarks must be palpated before each needle insertion. The medial and lateral border of the scapula should be palpated prior to the needle insertion. For the infraspinatus, the needle

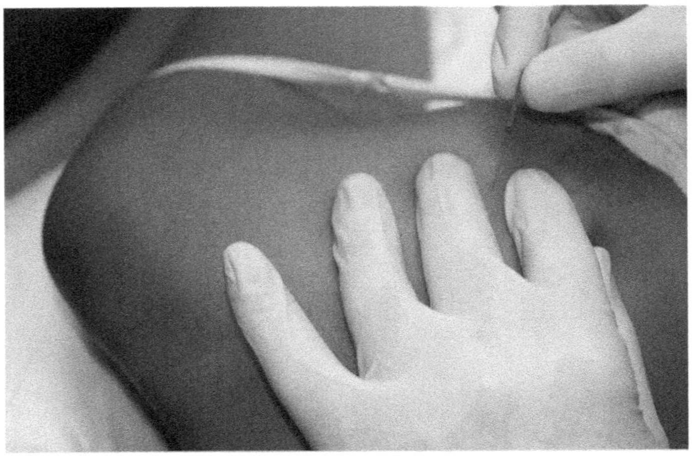

Figure 61.5 **Dry needling of TrPs in the infraspinatus muscle.**

is inserted directly into the TrP (Fig. 61.5). When possible, the teres major and minor are grasped between the thumb and the index finger and the needle is inserted towards the finger or the scapula. If the muscles cannot be held in a pincer palpation, careful needling in a lateral direction tangential to the curvature of the rib cage is indicated.

Precautions: Individuals with osteoporosis may present with thin and fenestrated scapulae. By developing a good kinaesthetic awareness of needling, clinicians should notice when the needle leaves the muscle.

Rhomboid major and minor muscles

Anatomy: The rhomboid minor attaches from the spinous processes of C7–T1 and reaches inferolaterally to the medial scapular border at the level of its spine. The rhomboid major muscle originates from the spinous processes of T2–T5 and inserts over the medial border of the scapula into its inferior angle. Both muscles also attach to the serratus anterior muscle.

Needling technique: The muscle is needled in side-lying or prone position. When needling over the chest wall, the therapist should always direct the needle towards a rib, with the index and middle fingers placed in the intercostal space so as to avoid causing a pneumothorax. The needle is inserted in a shallow angle towards the rib in order to avoid penetrating the lung (Fig. 61.6).

Precautions: The rhomboid muscle poses a relatively high risk for pneumothorax. The ribs must be palpated and the needle should always be directed towards the ribs.

Subscapularis muscle

Anatomy: The muscle lies over the anterior surface of the scapula. It originates from the inner surface of the scapula and attaches to the lesser tuberosity of the humerus.

Needling technique I: To treat the more medial TrPs, the patient is placed in a side-lying position on the side that needs to be treated. The patient's trunk is positioned in such a way that there is winging of the scapula, which makes it possible to needle trigger points in the subscapularis muscle. The needle is directed towards the undersurface of the scapula tangential over the rib cage (Fig. 61.7).

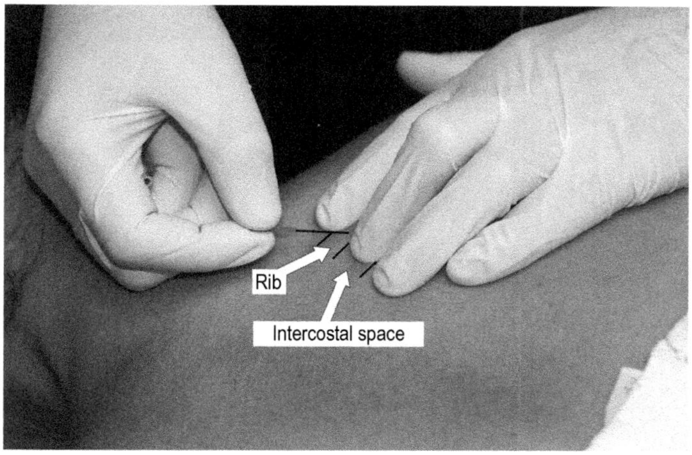

Figure 61.6 Dry needling of TrPs in the rhomboid muscle.

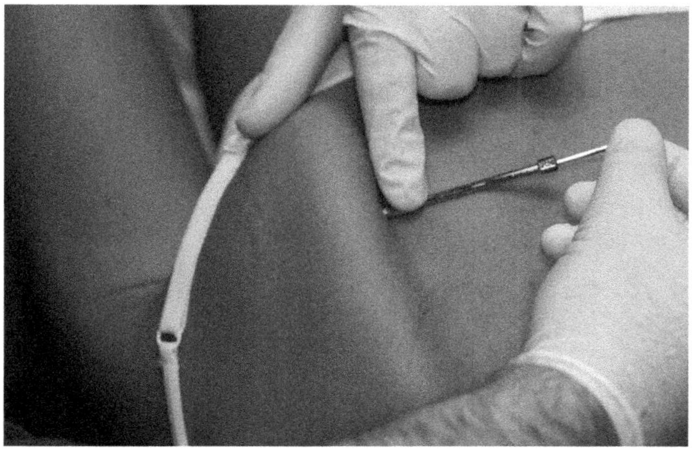

Figure 61.7 Dry needling of TrPs in the subscapularis muscle.

Needling technique II: The patient lies supine with the arm held in approximately 90° of abduction with the elbow bent. The clinician manually brings the scapula into a protracted and laterally displaced position, which will provide greater access to the lateral aspect of the muscle. The palpating hand is placed against the rib cage and rests on the muscle. The needle is inserted between the palpating fingers towards the undersurface of the scapula (similar to Fig. 61.8).

Precautions: When needling the lateral aspect of the muscle, the therapist should protect the lungs by keeping the palpating fingers against the chest wall to locate the rib cage accurately. Needling towards the ribs must be avoided for both needle techniques.

Latissimus dorsi muscle

Anatomy: The muscle originates from the spinous process of the lower six thoracic vertebrae, the thoracolumbar fascia, iliac crest and inferior three or four ribs. The insertion of the muscle is into the inter-tubercular groove of the humerus.

Needling technique: The muscle can be needled with the patient in supine, prone or side-lying. To needle the latissimus dorsi in the axilla, the patient lies supine with the arm abducted at shoulder level. The muscle is then palpated with

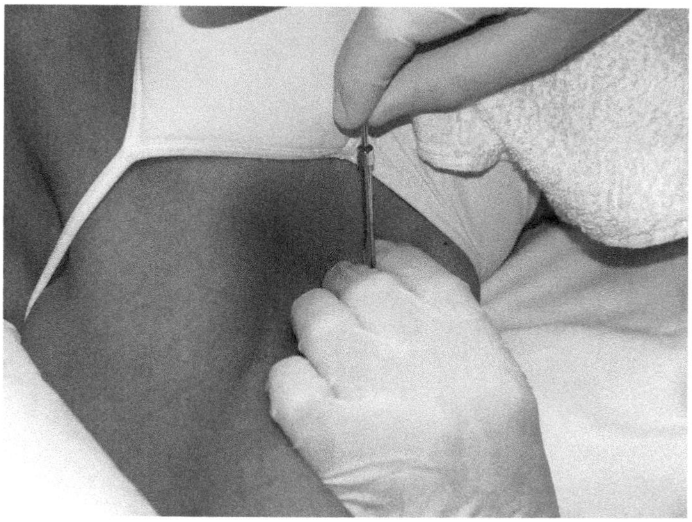

Figure 61.8 Dry needling of TrPs in the latissimus dorsi muscle in the axilla.

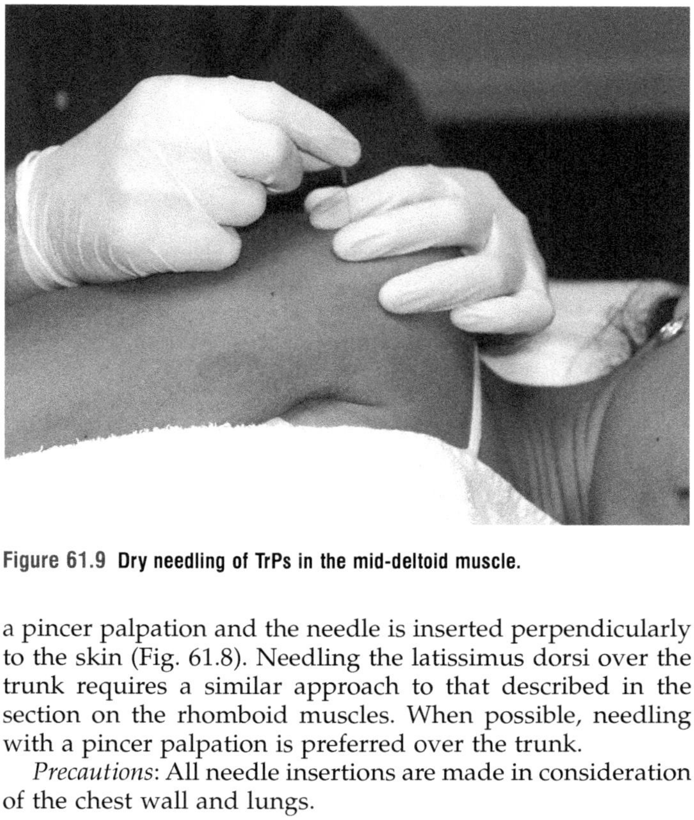

Figure 61.9 Dry needling of TrPs in the mid-deltoid muscle.

a pincer palpation and the needle is inserted perpendicularly to the skin (Fig. 61.8). Needling the latissimus dorsi over the trunk requires a similar approach to that described in the section on the rhomboid muscles. When possible, needling with a pincer palpation is preferred over the trunk.

Precautions: All needle insertions are made in consideration of the chest wall and lungs.

Deltoid muscle

Anatomy: The muscle originates from the anterior border of the lateral third of the clavicle, the lateral border of the acromion, the lower lip of scapular spine and the fascia over the infraspinatus muscle. The insertion is over the deltoid tuberosity at the humerus.

Needling technique: The patient is either in supine or side-lying position. The needle is inserted perpendicularly through the skin directly into the taut band (Fig. 61.9).

Precautions: None.

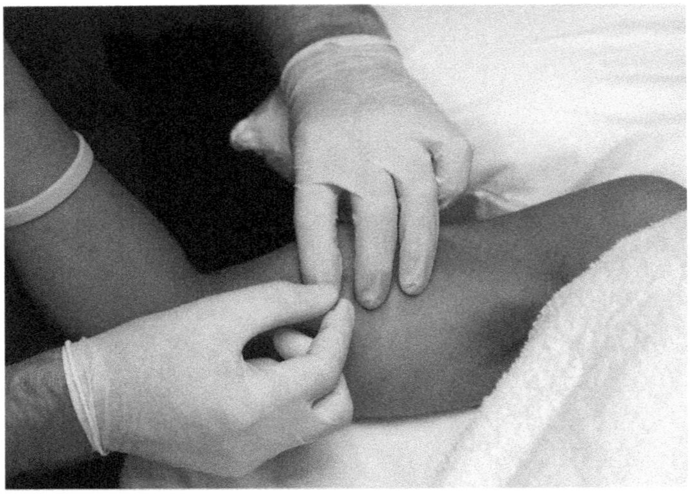

Figure 61.10 **Dry needling of TrPs in the biceps brachii muscle.**

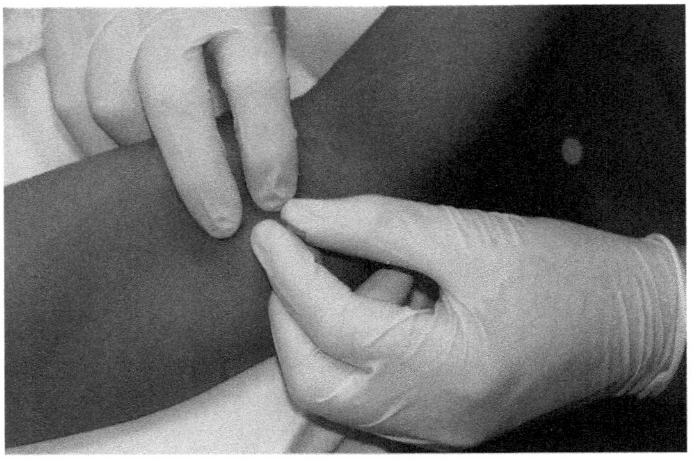

Figure 61.11 **Dry needling of TrPs in the brachialis muscle.**

Biceps brachii muscle

Anatomy: The long head of the biceps brachii muscle originates from the glenoid fossa with its tendon passing through the glenohumeral joint. The short head originates from the coracoid process without passing through the glenohumeral joint. Both heads attach distally to the lesser tuberosity of the radius.

Needling technique: The patient lies in supine. The muscle is palpated and picked up via a pincer palpation. The needle is inserted perpendicular to the skin and directed towards the clinician's finger (Fig. 61.10).

Precautions: The neurovascular bundle, including the median nerve, the musculocutaneous nerve, the ulnar nerve and the brachial artery, is located medial to the biceps brachii muscle and must be avoided.

Brachialis muscle

Anatomy: The muscle originates from the distal two-thirds of the humerus and inserts at the coronoid process of the ulnar tuberosity. The muscle extends into the joint capsule of the elbow.

Needling technique: The patient lies supine with the elbow supported and relaxed in a slight flexion. The muscle is palpated with a flat palpation technique. The muscle is needled from the lateral aspect of the arm only so as to avoid hitting the neurovascular bundle. The needle is directed medially (Fig. 61.11).

Precautions: The neurovascular bundle should be avoided over the medial head of the muscle.

Brachioradialis muscle

Anatomy: The muscle starts from the upper two-thirds of the supracondylar ridge of the humerus and attaches over the distal radius at the styloid process.

Needling technique: The patient lies in supine position. The TrPs are identified via pincer palpation. The needle is inserted and directed towards the practitioner's finger (Fig. 61.12).

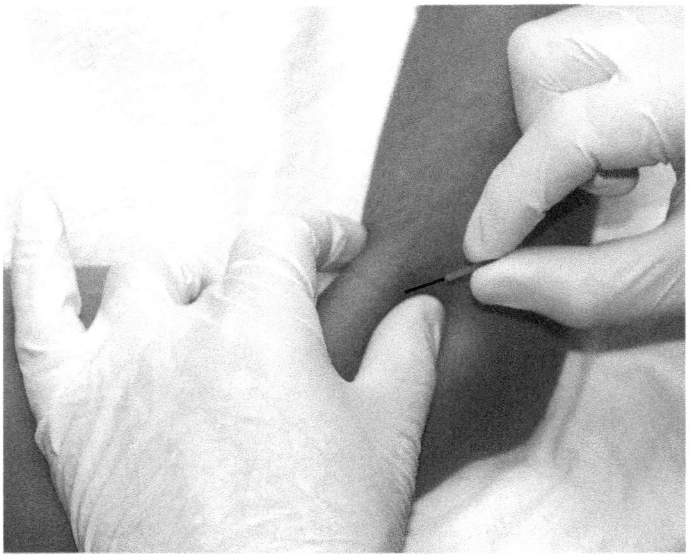

Figure 61.12 **Dry needling of TrPs in the brachioradialis muscle.**

Precautions: The brachioradialis muscle is the most superficial muscle over the lateral elbow. The radial nerve passes close to it and should be avoided.

Supinator muscle

Anatomy: The muscle originates from the lateral humeral epicondyle, and radial collateral ligament, the annular ligament and the supinator crest of the ulna. The muscle inserts over the radial tuberosity and upper third of the radial shaft.

Needling technique: The patient is in supine with the arm supinated. Flat palpation against the radial bone on the volar side of the arm is used to identify the muscle. The needle is inserted pointing proximally towards the humerus (Fig. 61.13). It is possible to needle the supinator muscle at the dorsal aspect of the forearm, but there is a risk of hitting the superficial radial nerve, which lies over the muscle, or the posterior interosseus nerve, which lies in between the two heads of the muscle.

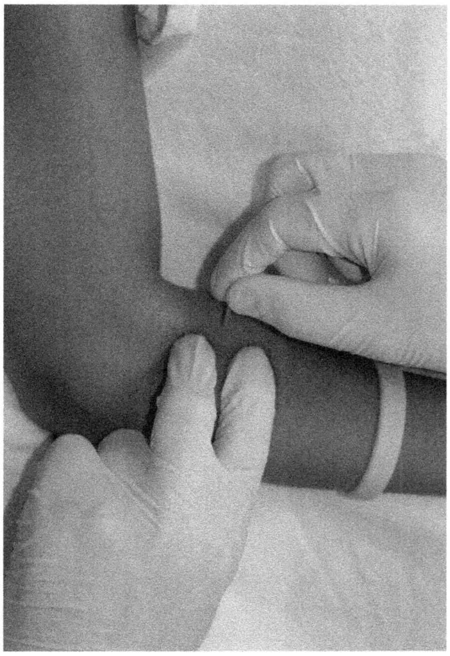

Figure 61.13 Dry needling of TrPs in the supinator muscle.

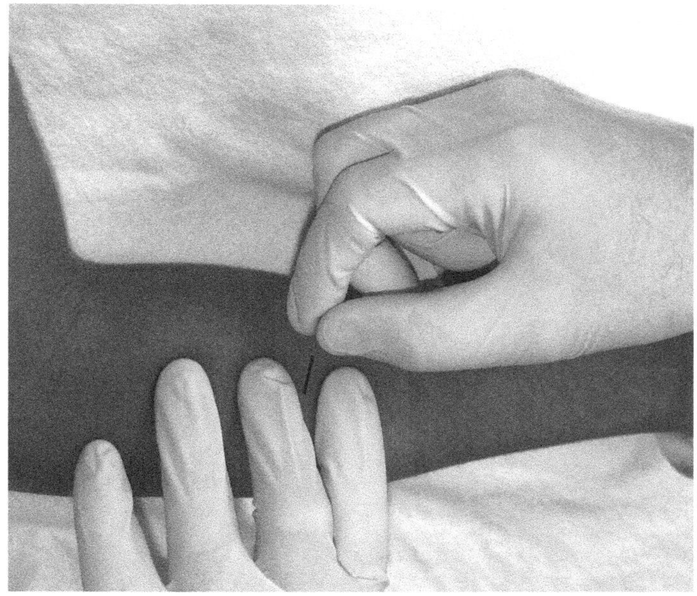

Figure 61.14 Dry needling of TrPs in the extensor digitorum muscle.

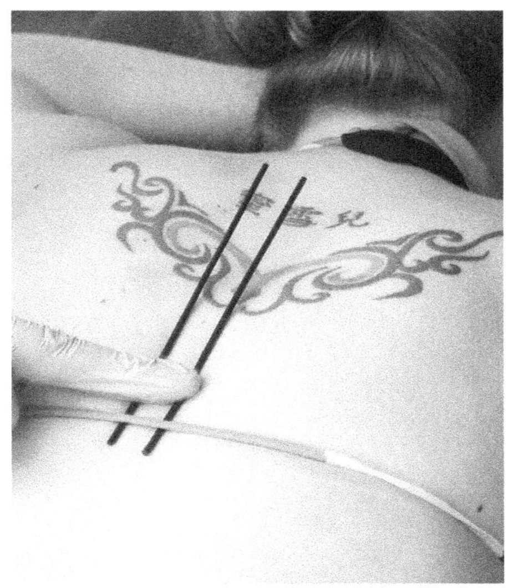

Figure 61.15 The spinal safe-needling zone. (Modified from Dommerholt J, Fernández-de-las-Peñas C 2013.)

Precautions: With the posterior approach, there is a risk of hitting the sensory and motor branches of the radial nerve.

Wrist and finger extensor muscles

Anatomy: The wrist extensors (extensor carpi radialis longus and brevis muscles) originate from the lateral supracondylar ridge of the humerus, the lateral epicondyle, the radial ligament of the elbow and the intermuscular septa through a common tendon, which is shared with the extensor carpi ulnaris muscle and the extensor digitorum muscle. The attachments are at the base of the second and third metacarpal bone, the ulnar side of the base of the fifth metacarpal bone and the distal phalanx of the fingers respectively.

Needling technique: The extensor carpi radialis longus and brevis can be needled with the muscles held in a pincer palpation. The extensor carpi ulnaris and extensor digitorum muscles are treated with a flat palpation (Fig. 61.14).

Precautions: The radial nerve crosses over the extensor digitorum muscle.

Dry Needling of Selected Trunk Muscles

Thoracic and lumbar multifidus muscles

Anatomy: These muscles form the deeper paraspinal muscles and consist of fasciculi, which in the sacral area originate from the lower portion of the dorsal sacrum, the posterior–superior iliac spine and the deep surface of tendinous origin of the erector spinae, in the lumbar spine from the mammillary processes of all lumbar vertebrae, and in the thoracic spine from the transverse processes of all thoracic vertebrae. Each fasciculus runs superior and medially to the base or the tip of the spinous process above. In the lumbar spine they attach to the adjacent vertebra; in the thoracic spine they can skip one to three segments.

Needling technique: The patient lies prone. Using a flat palpation technique, the muscle is identified just lateral of the spinous processes. For needling in the thoracic spine, it is important to stay within the so-called 'safe needling zone', which is defined as the areas approximately one finger-breath on each side of the spinous processes (Fig. 61.15). The needle is inserted perpendicular to the skin and directed in an inferior (caudal)–medial direction towards the lamina (Fig. 61.16).

Precautions: Stay within the safe needling zone to avoid the possibility of a pneumothorax in the thoracic spine. Direct the needle in a caudal–medial direction along the entire spine to avoid penetrating the epidural space.

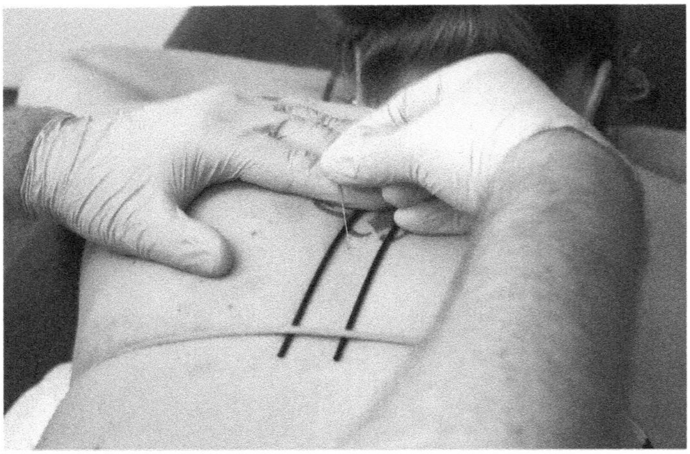

Figure 61.16 Dry needling of TrPs in the multifidus muscle. (Modified from Dommerholt J, Fernández-de-las-Peñas C 2013.)

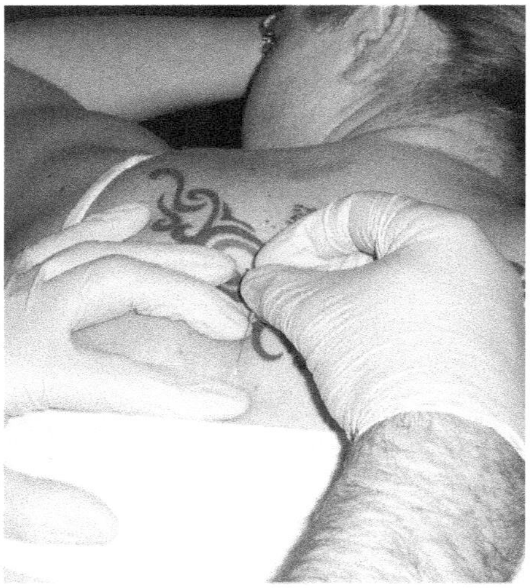

Figure 61.17 Dry needling of TrPs in the longissimus muscle. (Modified from Dommerholt J, Fernández-de-las-Peñas C 2013.)

Longissimus thoracis muscle

Anatomy: The muscle originates from a common tendinous origin in the sacrum, the iliac crest, and the spinous processes of lower thoracic and most lumbar vertebrae. In the lumbar region, the muscle blends with the iliocostalis lumborum muscle. It attaches to the tips of the transverse processes of all thoracic vertebrae and ribs 3 or 4 to 12 between their tubercles and angles. Some of its fibres are attached to the entire posterior surface of the transverse processes, to the accessory processes of the lumbar vertebrae and to the middle layer of the thoracolumbar fascia.

Needling technique: The patient is prone. The taut band is identified using a flat palpation perpendicular to the direction of the muscle fibres. The needle is inserted perpendicular to the skin between two fingers, just superior to the trigger point. The needle is then directed towards the TrP longitudinally in a shallow angle (Fig. 61.17).

Precautions: Maintain a shallow angle in order to avoid the possibility of a pneumothorax.

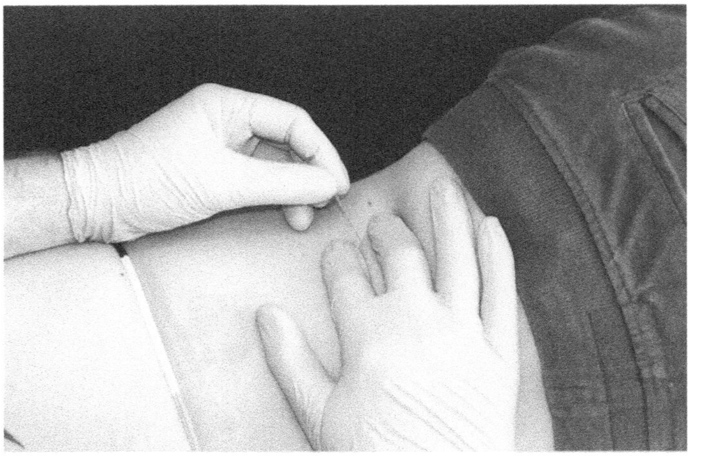

Figure 61.18 Dry needling of TrPs in the quadratus lumborum muscle. (Modified from Dommerholt J, Fernández-de-las-Peñas C 2013.)

Quadratus lumborum muscle

Anatomy: The muscle originates from the medial half of the lower border of the 12th rib, the transverse processes of L1–4, and occasionally the transverse process or body of T12. It inserts by aponeurotic fibres to the iliolumbar ligament and the adjacent portion of the internal lip of the iliac crest. Occasionally a second muscle layer is present; this attaches superiorly to the medial lower border of the 12th rib, and inferiorly to the transverse processes of the lower three or four lumbar vertebrae.

Needling technique: The patient lies in the side-lying position with the affected side up. The muscle is identified by flat palpation just posterior to the midline between the 12th rib and the iliac crest. If needed, the therapist can increase the space between the 12th rib and the iliac crest by placing a towel under the patient, by raising up the patient's arm, or by extending the upper leg. The needle must be long enough to reach the depth of the transverse process. While giving adequate compression to the subcutaneous tissue, the needle is inserted between two fingers straight lateral–medially, and is directed towards the transverse process (Fig. 61.18).

Precautions: Needle below L2 in order to avoid the kidney, the pleura and the diaphragm. Do not needle in a cephalic direction so as to avoid the pleura.

Rectus abdominis muscle

Anatomy: The muscle originates inferiorly from the pubic crest and the pubic tubercle, and interlaces with the contralateral muscle on the symphysis pubis. Superiorly it inserts on the costal cartilages of ribs 5–7 and the xiphoid process. The paired recti are separated by the linea alba in the midline, and are interrupted by three or four more or less complete transverse tendinous inscriptions.

Needling technique: The patient lies supine. For superior and inferior TrPs, the taut band and TrP are located using flat palpation. The needle is inserted perpendicular to the skin and then directed in a very shallow angle towards the costal cartilage (Fig. 61.19), or to the pubic bone (Fig. 61.20). For TrPs in the muscle belly, the operator sits on the contralateral side of the patient, and the TrP is identified with flat palpation.

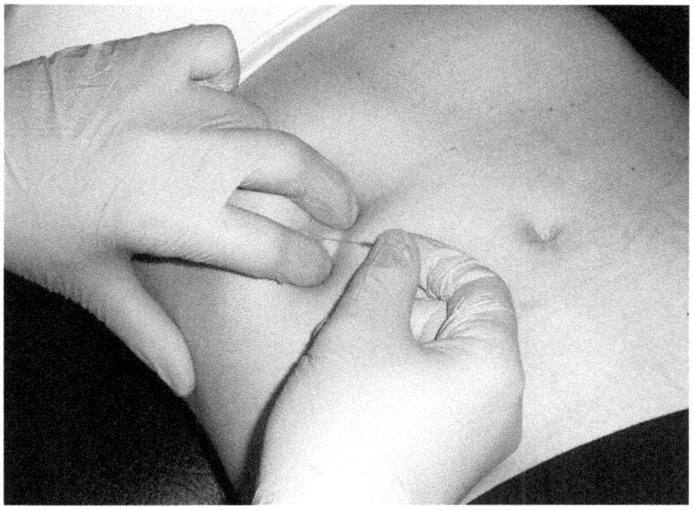

Figure 61.19 Dry needling of TrPs in the rectus abdominis muscle (at the rib cage). (Modified from Dommerholt J, Fernández-de-las-Peñas C 2013.)

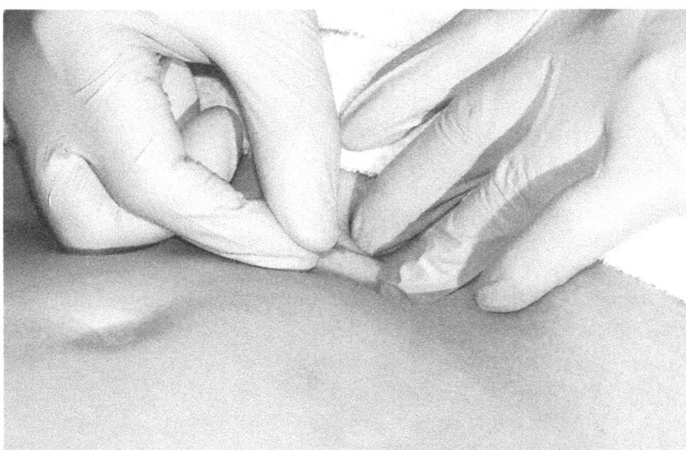

Figure 61.20 Dry needling of TrPs in the rectus abdominis muscle (at the pubic bone). (Modified from Dommerholt J, Fernández-de-las-Peñas C 2013.)

The therapist depresses the abdominal wall just lateral of the taut band and pulls it medially with the TrP fixated between two fingers, thus creating a 'wall', or a 'shelf'; the needle is inserted perpendicular to the (now vertically oriented) skin, and is directed medially, thus staying in the frontal plane (Fig. 61.21).

Precautions: Maintain a shallow angle in order to avoid entering the abdominal cavity; keep the needle parallel to the rib margin in order to avoid entering the pleural cavity and thereby possibly causing a pneumothorax.

External and internal oblique muscles

Anatomy: The external oblique is the most superficial of the lateral abdominal muscles. It originates from eight digitations from the external surfaces and inferior borders of ribs 5–12 near to where they meet the cartilages. The superior five digitations interdigitate with the serratus anterior, and the lower three with the latissimus dorsi. The fibre direction is from almost vertical in the lateral fibres, to more and more oblique

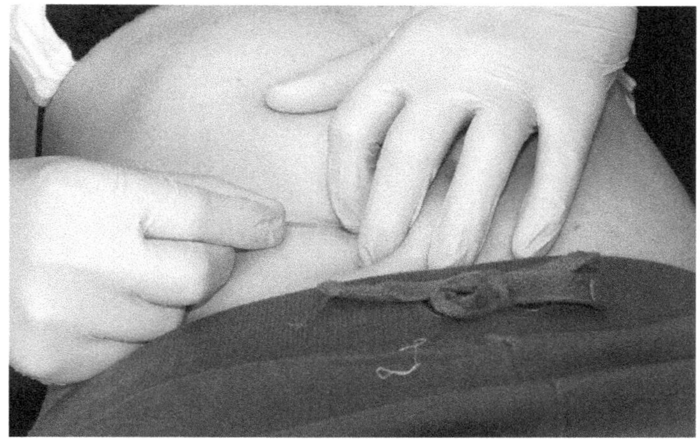

Figure 61.21 Dry needling of TrPs in the rectus abdominis muscle (shelf technique). (Modified from Dommerholt J, Fernández-de-las-Peñas C 2013.)

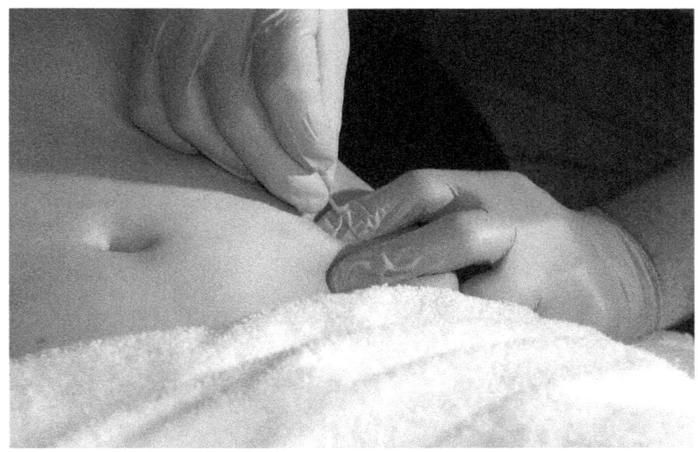

Figure 61.22 Dry needling of TrPs in the oblique abdominal muscles. (Modified from Dommerholt J, Fernández-de-las-Peñas C 2013.)

in the more-medial fibres, all of which extend caudally. The more-lateral fibres attach to the anterior half of the iliac crest, whereas the medial fibres join the abdominal aponeurosis, which attaches to the linea alba.

The internal oblique lies underneath the external oblique muscle, and the fibre direction is often more or less perpendicular to the fibre direction of the latter. It originates on the lower portion of the thoracolumbar fascia, the anterior two-thirds of the iliac crest, and the lateral half of the inguinal ligament. The fibre direction is from nearly vertical in the lateral fibres, to more and more oblique in the more-medial fibres, all of which extend cephalically. The more-lateral fibres attach to the cartilages of the lower three or four ribs. The more-medial fibres attach to the linea alba via the anterior and posterior rectus sheath, and the most-medial fibres run more horizontally and attach as a common tendon with the transverse abdominis to the pubic crest and pectineal line.

Needling technique: The patient is in supine or in side-lying with the affected side up. Using a pincher palpation, the lateral portion of the abdominal muscles is grasped and pulled away from the abdomen. The therapist needles the TrP between two fingers towards the opposite thumb or finger while holding a firm grip (Fig. 61.22).

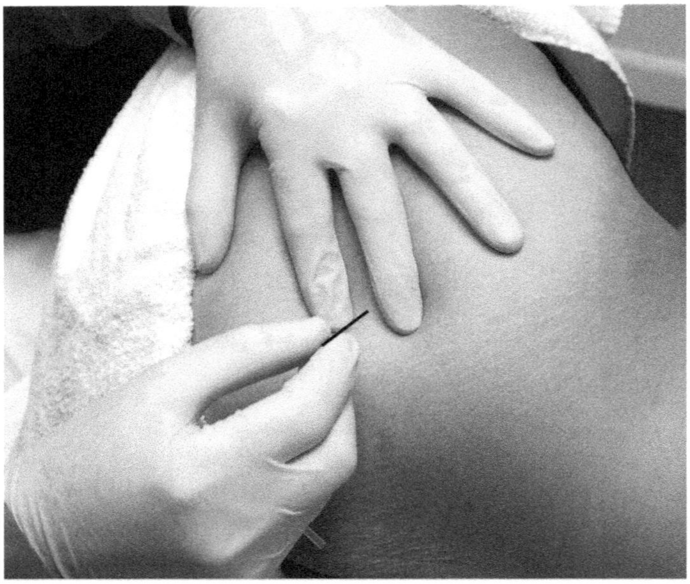

Figure 61.23 **Dry needling of TrPs in the gluteus maximus muscle.**

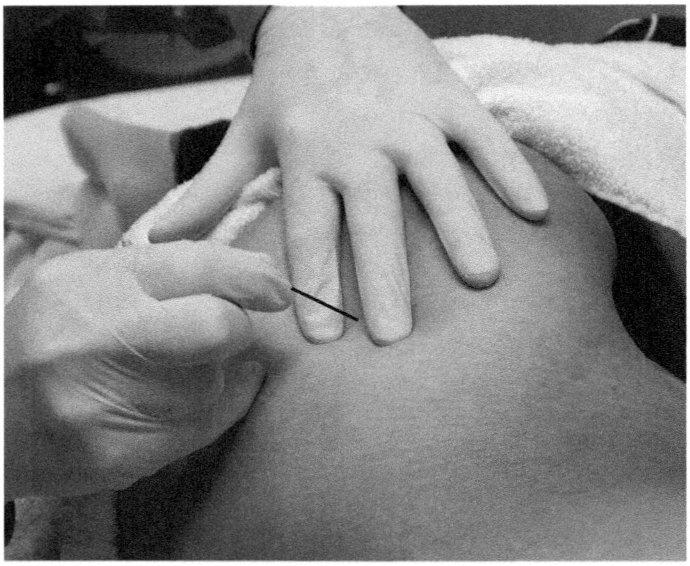

Figure 61.24 **Dry needling of TrPs in the gluteus medius muscle.**

Precautions: Use of a pincer palpation will avoid the needle going into the abdominal cavity.

Dry Needling of Selected Hip and Leg Muscles

Gluteus maximus muscle

Anatomy: The muscle originates from the posterior iliac crest, the lateral sacrum and the coccyx. The fibres run diagonally inferolaterally and insert onto the iliotibial band of the tensor fasciae latae and the gluteal tuberosity on the femur between the vastus lateralis and adductor magnus.

Needling technique: The patient is in prone position with a pillow under the abdomen, or in side-lying with the affected side up. TrPs can be located and needled using flat palpation perpendicular to the muscle, while the subcutaneous tissue is compressed adequately (Fig. 61.23). If the TrP is located in the inferior part of the muscle, often a pincer palpation can be used: while fixating the taught band between the fingers and the thumb, the therapist directs the needle towards the opposite finger.

Precautions: Avoid needling the sciatic nerve by needling away from the nerve. The depth of penetration is also dependent on the amount of subcutaneous tissue.

Gluteus medius muscle

Anatomy: The muscle is found between the gluteus maximus and the tensor fasciae latae. It originates from the anterior three-quarters of the iliac crest and inserts onto the greater trochanter. The posterior fibres have a diagonal direction towards the inferior–lateral sides, while the more-anterior fibres have a more vertical course.

Needling technique: The patient is in prone position or in side-lying position with the affected side up. TrPs are identified with flat palpation perpendicular to the muscle fibres (Fig. 61.24). Strong depression of the subcutaneous tissue is required. The needle direction is posterior to anterior. Needle contact at the periosteum is common.

Precautions: Avoid needling the sciatic nerve by needling away from the nerve. The depth of penetration is also dependent on the amount of subcutaneous tissue. In addition, there are deep branches of the superior gluteal vessels and nerve between the gluteus medius and minimus, which should be avoided.

Gluteus minimus muscle

Anatomy: The muscle is found deep to the gluteus medius. It originates between the anterior and inferior gluteal lines on the posterior (dorsal) aspect of the ilium. It inserts onto the anterior aspect of the greater trochanter.

Needling technique: The patient is in prone or in side-lying position with the affected side up. TrPs are identified with flat palpation perpendicular to the muscle fibres (Fig. 61.25). Strong depression of the subcutaneous tissue is required. The needle direction is posterior to anterior. Needle contact at the periosteum is common.

Precautions: There are deep branches of the superior gluteal vessels and nerve between the gluteus medius and minimus, which should be avoided. The depth of penetration is also dependent on the amount of subcutaneous tissue.

Piriformis muscle

Anatomy: The muscle originates from the anterior surface of the sacrum at S2–S4. It exits the pelvis through the greater sciatic foramen. It inserts onto the upper border of the greater trochanter of the femur.

Needling technique: The patient is in prone or in side-lying position with the affected side up. The bony landmarks of S2–S4 and the greater trochanter are recognized. TrPs are identified with flat palpation perpendicular to the muscle

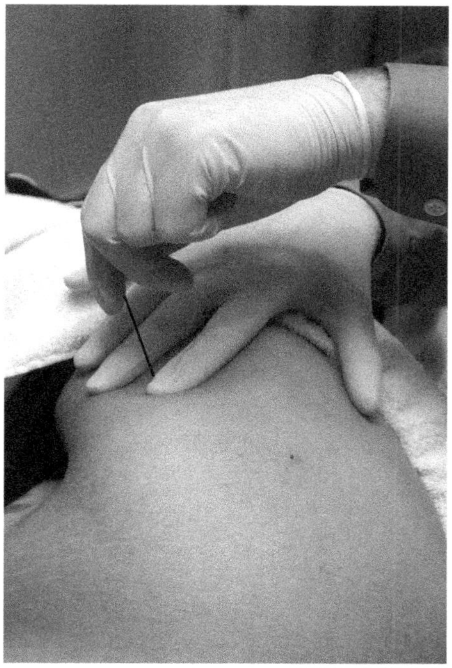

Figure 61.25 Dry needling of TrPs in the gluteus minimus muscle.

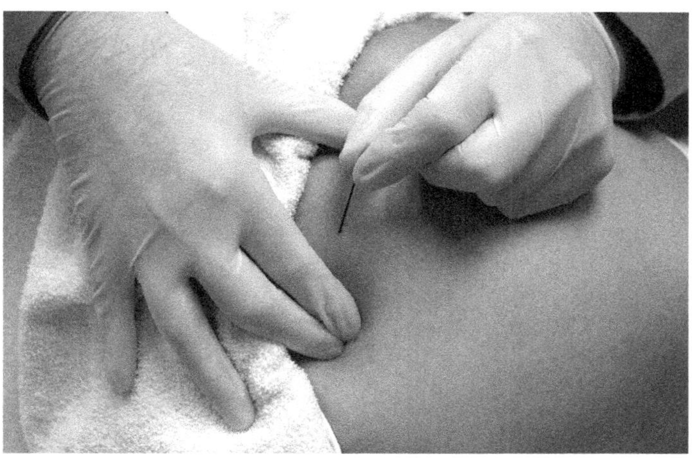

Figure 61.26 Dry needling of TrPs in the piriformis muscle.

fibres. The needle direction is directly into the muscle through the gluteus maximus muscle (Fig. 61.26).

Precautions: Avoid needling the sciatic nerve by needling away from the nerve, which is located in the middle third of the muscle. If needling over the sciatic nerve is indicated, advance the needle very slowly to identify the exact location of the nerve. The depth of penetration is also dependent on the amount of subcutaneous tissue.

Adductor longus muscle

Anatomy: The muscle originates from the superior pubic ramus between the crest and the symphysis, and inserts onto the linea aspera in the middle third of the femur.

Needling technique: The patient is in supine, with the knee flexed and the hip flexed and externally rotated. Using a firm

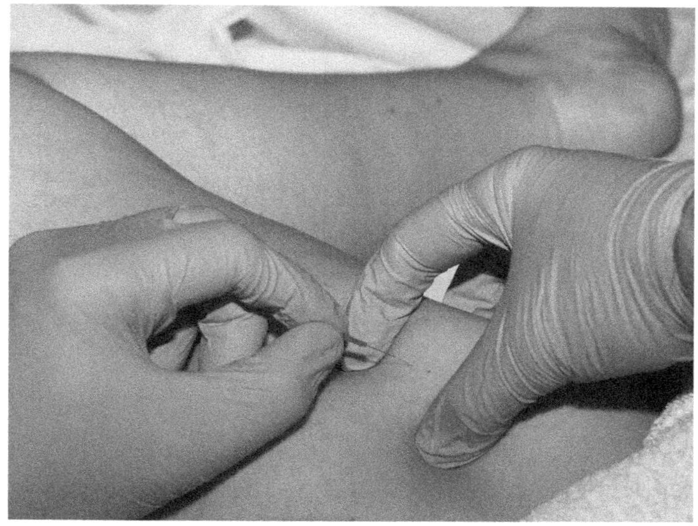

Figure 61.27 Dry needling of TrPs in the adductor longus and brevis muscles. (Modified from Dommerholt J, Fernández-de-las-Peñas C 2013.)

pincer palpation, the taut band and the TrP are identified. The needle direction is anterior to posterior, perpendicular to the muscle surface (Fig. 61.27). Sometimes, the adductor longus and brevis can be needled at the same time.

Precautions: Avoid needling the femoral nerve, artery and vein, and the sciatic nerve.

Adductor brevis muscle

Anatomy: The muscle originates from the anterior surface of the inferior pubic ramus, inferior to the origin of the adductor longus. It inserts onto the femur at the pectineal line and the superior part of the medial lip of the linea aspera.

Needling technique: The patient is in supine position, with the knee flexed and the hip flexed and externally rotated. Using a flat palpation or a firm pincer palpation, the therapist identifies the taut band and the TrP in the upper part of the thigh between the adductor longus and the pectineus. The needle direction is anterior–posterior, perpendicular to the muscle surface and towards the buttock crease. Sometimes the adductor longus and brevis can be needled at the same time (see Fig. 61.27).

Precautions: Avoid needling the femoral nerve, artery and vein, and the sciatic nerve.

Adductor magnus muscle

Anatomy: The muscle is a large fan-shaped muscle with three different fibre directions. It originates from the inferior ramus of the pubis, the conjoined ischial ramus, and the inferior–lateral aspect of the ischial tuberosity. The short horizontal fibres insert onto the rough line of the femur leading from the greater trochanter to the linea aspera, medial to the gluteus maximus. The oblique fibres are oriented inferior–lateral and insert by means of a broad aponeurosis into the linea aspera and the upper part of its medial prolongation below. The most medial portion, which is also called the ischiocondylar portion, has a vertical fibre direction, inserts into the adductor tubercle on the medial condyle of the femur and is connected by a

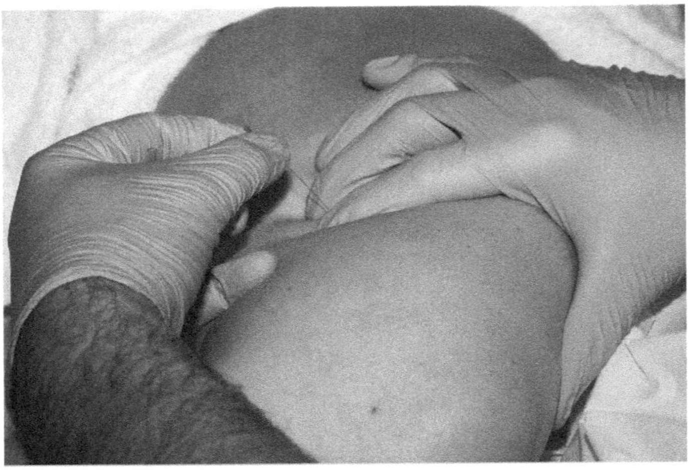

Figure 61.28 **Dry needling of TrPs in the adductor magnus muscle (supine).** (Modified from Dommerholt J, Fernández-de-las-Peñas C 2013.)

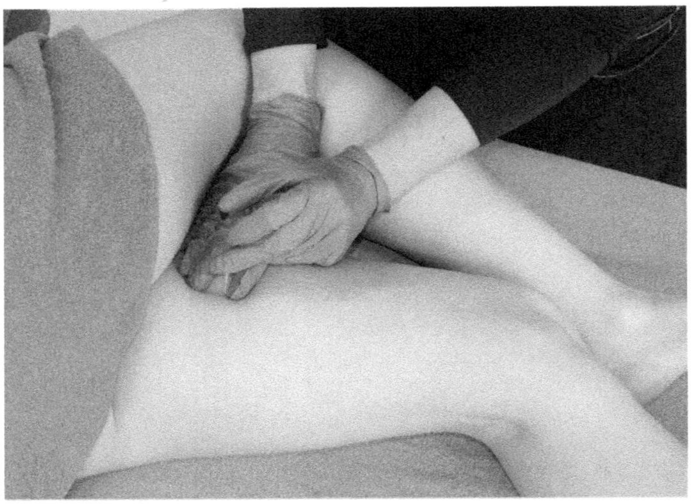

Figure 61.29 **Dry needling of TrPs in the adductor magnus muscle (side-lying).** (Modified from Dommerholt J, Fernández-de-las-Peñas C 2013.)

fibrous expansion to the line leading upwards from the tubercle to the linea aspera.

Needling technique: The patient is in supine position with the knee flexed and the hip flexed and externally rotated (Fig. 61.28), or in side-lying position with the side to be treated underneath while the upper leg is flexed in front of the lower leg (Fig. 61.29) TrPs are identified via flat palpation and the needle is inserted perpendicular to the muscle surface. The needle direction is medial–lateral.

Precautions: Avoid needling the femoral nerve, artery and vein along the adductor canal, and the sciatic nerve.

Pectineus muscle

Anatomy: The muscle is a flat, quadrangular muscle. It originates from the pectin pubis (the pectineal line) and from the surface of the bone just anterior to it. It inserts at the lesser trochanter distally of the iliopsoas. The fibre direction is inferior–lateral.

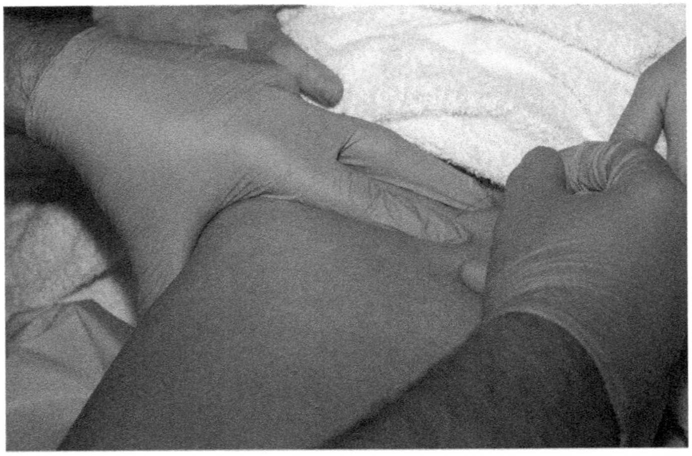

Figure 61.30 **Dry needling of TrPs in the pectineus muscle.** (Modified from Dommerholt J, Fernández-de-las-Peñas C 2013.)

Needling technique: The patient is in supine position, with the knee flexed and the hip flexed and slightly externally rotated. The therapist should first identify the femoral artery lateral of the muscle and then, while holding a finger on this, identify the TrP via flat palpation just medial of the neurovascular bundle. The needle is inserted perpendicular to the muscle surface (Fig. 61.30). The needle direction is anterior–posterior.

Precautions: Avoid needling the femoral artery, vein and nerve lateral to the muscle. Avoid needling the obturator nerve medially, which lies deep under the muscle next to the tendon of the adductor longus muscle.

Psoas major muscle

Anatomy: The psoas major attaches at the 12th thoracic and all lumbar vertebral bodies, intervertebral discs, and the anterior and inferior portions of the lumbar transverse processes. It passes anterior to the sacroiliac joint. The muscle shares a common tendinous insertion with the iliacus muscle at the lesser trochanter on the posteromedial surface of the femur.

Needling technique: Needling of the belly of the psoas muscle is accomplished with the patient in the side-lying position. There are two approaches. In the lateral approach, the quadratus lumborum serves as the anatomical landmark. The needle technique is similar to the technique used for the quadratus lumborum, but the needle is directed at an anterior angle of approximately 10–30° into the psoas muscle (Fig. 61.31). A 75 mm needle may be used in most individuals of average build, but more-obese individuals may require a 90 mm needle.

In the posterior approach, the muscle is approached at the level of L3–L5, well below the kidney, which is usually at L1–L2. Palpate the spinal processes of L3–L5 and the adjacent longissimus muscle. The needle is placed just lateral to the lumbar longissimus muscle into the iliocostalis muscle. The psoas lies alongside the vertebrae anterior to the transverse processes. The needle is directed parallel to the table with the patient in the side-lying position (Fig. 61.32). If the needle hits the transverse process, the needle placement was too medial. A 75 mm needle may be used in most individuals of average

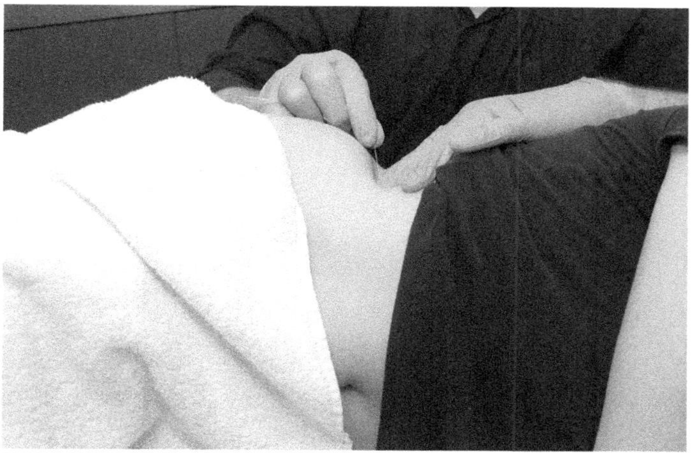

Figure 61.31 Dry needling of TrPs in the psoas major muscle (lateral approach).

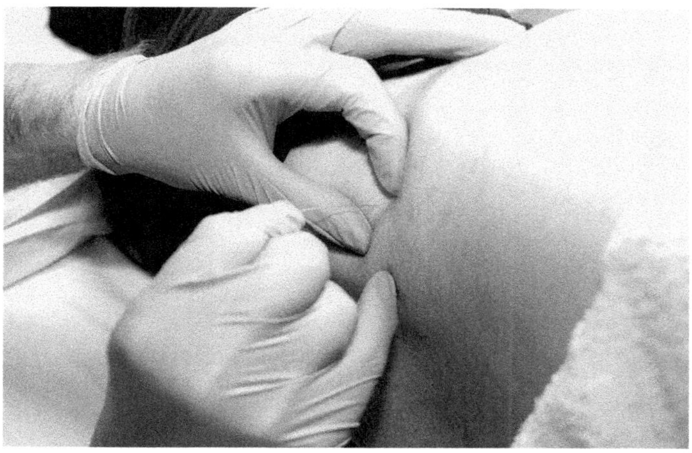

Figure 61.32 Dry needling of TrPs in the psoas major muscle (posterior approach). (Modified from Dommerholt J, Fernández-de-las-Peñas C 2013.)

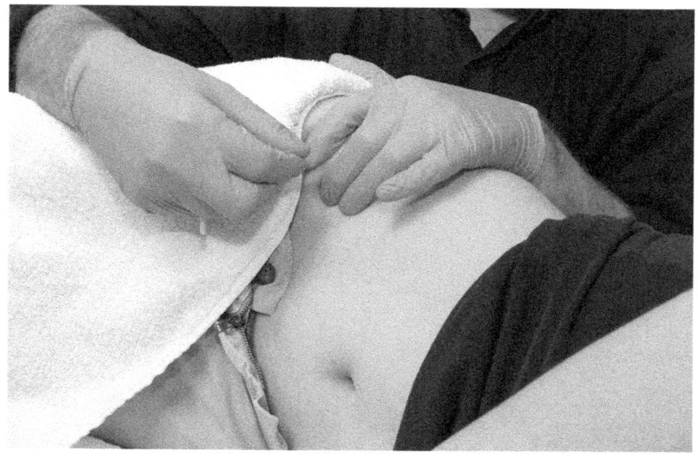

Figure 61.33 Dry needling of TrPs in the iliacus muscle. (Modified from Dommerholt J, Fernández-de-las-Peñas C 2013.)

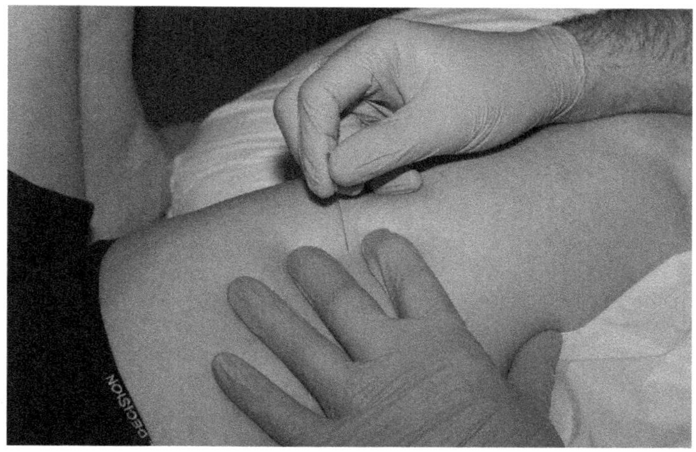

Figure 61.34 Dry needling of TrPs in the rectus femoris muscle. (Modified from Dommerholt J, Fernández-de-las-Peñas C 2013.)

build, but more-obese individuals will require a 90 mm needle.

Precautions: To avoid penetration of the kidney, as well as the more cephalic diaphragm and pleura, needle below the level of L2.

Iliacus muscle

Anatomy: The iliacus muscle comes from the superior half of the iliac fossa, the inner lip of the iliac crest, the anterior ligaments of the sacroiliac joint and the superior surface of the lateral portion of the sacrum filling the lateral pelvic wall. It shares a common tendinous insertion with the psoas major muscle at the lesser trochanter on the posteromedial surface of the femur, while some fibres pass below the trochanter onto the medial surface of the proximal femur.

Needling technique: The iliacus muscle may be approached below the crest of the iliac bone with the patient in the side-lying position. The therapist wraps the fingers of the non-needling hand around the iliac crest to 'hook on' to the bone, and inserts the needle approximately 5 mm from the bone into the abdominal external oblique muscle. The needle is directed towards the ilium and kept close to the inner surface of the ilium so as to avoid penetrating the abdominal contents (Fig. 61.33). For most patients, a 50–60 mm solid filament needle is sufficient, although this may be difficult to do in obese individuals. Use of a spinal needle or a 50–75 mm needle allows the deeper parts of the iliacus to be reached from the iliac crest.

Precautions: To avoid penetration of the peritoneum, direct the needle towards the inner surface of the ilium.

Quadriceps femoris muscle group

Rectus femoris muscle

Anatomy: The muscle originates from the anterior–inferior iliac spine and the upper margin of the acetabulum. It inserts as a flat thick tendon at the base of the patella, which eventually terminates via the patellar ligament on the tibial tuberosity.

Needling technique: The patient is in supine position. The needle is inserted perpendicular to the muscle surface directly into the taut band, as identified by flat palpation (Fig. 61.34).

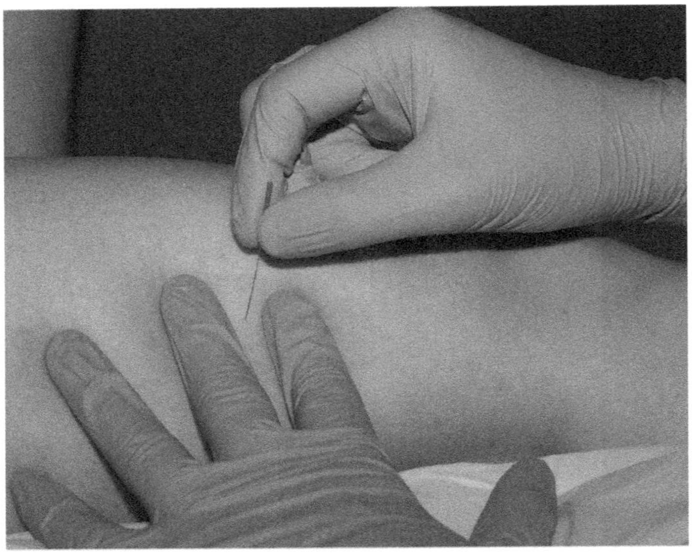

Figure 61.35 Dry needling of TrPs in the vastus lateralis muscle (supine). (Modified from Dommerholt J, Fernández-de-las-Peñas C 2013.)

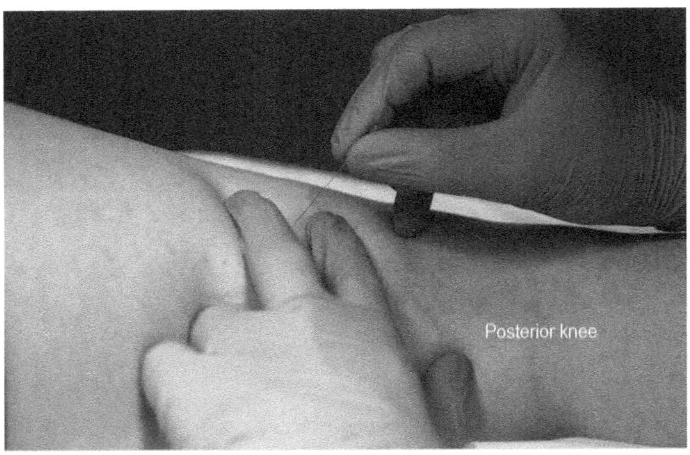

Figure 61.36 Dry needling of TrPs in the vastus lateralis muscle (side-lying). (Modified from Dommerholt J, Fernández-de-las-Peñas C 2013.)

Precautions: Avoid needling the lateral circumflex artery by not needling through the muscle.

Vastus lateralis muscle

Anatomy: The muscle originates from a broad aponeurosis, which is attached to the upper part of the intertrochanteric line, to the anterior and inferior borders of the greater trochanter, to the lateral lip of the gluteal tuberosity and to the upper half of the lateral lip of the linea aspera; this aponeurosis covers the upper three-quarters of the muscle, and many fibres originate from its deep surface. It inserts via the common flat tendon to the base and lateral border of the patella. It is the largest muscle of the quadriceps femoris.

Needling technique: TrPs in the anterior aspect of the muscle are needled with the patient in supine position (Fig. 61.35); TrPs in the lateral aspect of the muscle and in the part of the muscle that is posterior of the iliotract band are needled with the patient in side-lying or in prone position (Fig. 61.36). The

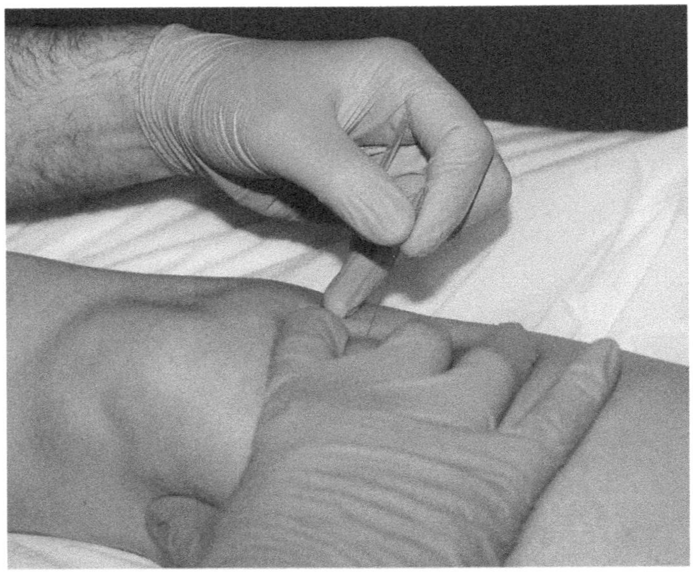

Figure 61.37 Dry needling of TrPs in the vastus medialis muscle. (Modified from Dommerholt J, Fernández-de-las-Peñas C 2013.)

needle is inserted perpendicular to the muscle surface directly into the taut band, as identified by flat palpation.

Precautions: None.

Vastus medialis muscle

Anatomy: The muscle originates from the front and middle sides of the intertrochanteric line of the femur, traversing the pectineal line, the medial lip of the linea aspera, and the medial supracondylar line of the femur. It inserts as all the fibres converge onto the medial part of the quadriceps femoris tendon and the medial border of the patella.

Needling technique: The patient is in supine position. The needle is inserted perpendicular to the muscle surface directly into the TrP, as identified by flat palpation (Fig. 61.37).

Precautions: None, although it is possible to get close to the saphenous nerve and popliteal artery.

Biceps femoris muscle

Anatomy: The muscle is composed of two heads. The long head originates from the upper part of the ischial tuberosity via a tendon it shares with the semitendinosus muscle, and from the lower parts of the sacrotuberous ligament. The short head of the muscle comes from the lateral lip of the linea aspera, but it may be totally absent. The two heads merge at the distal end of the muscle and attach to the fibular head, the lateral condyle of the tibia and the fibular collateral ligament.

Needling technique: The patient is in prone position, with the knee slightly flexed and the lower leg supported by a pillow. The needle is inserted perpendicular to the muscle surface directly into the TrP, as identified by flat palpation (Fig. 61.38).

Precautions: Avoid needling the sciatic nerve, which lies in the midline of the posterior thigh, by inserting the needle medially when needling the proximal part of the muscle, and laterally when needling the distal part of the muscle. When

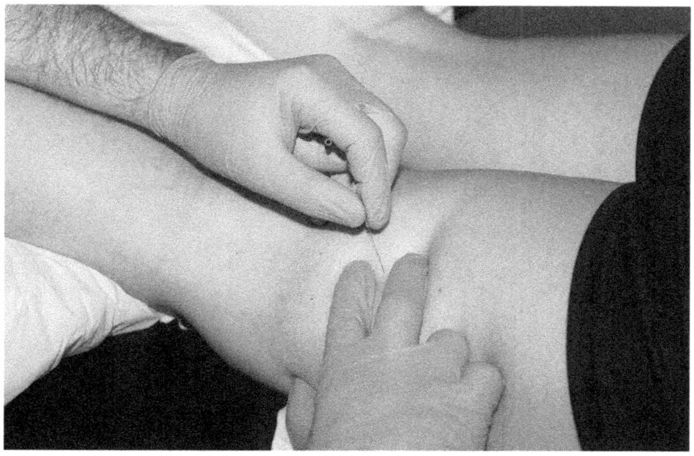

Figure 61.38 Dry needling of TrPs in the biceps femoris muscle. (Modified from Dommerholt J, Fernández-de-las-Peñas C 2013.)

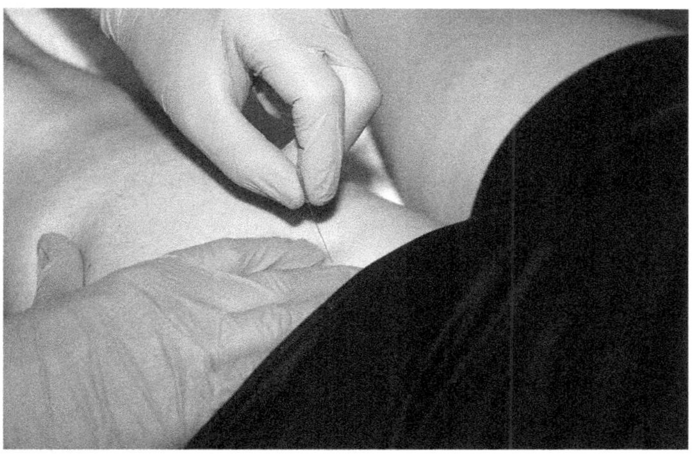

Figure 61.39 Dry needling of TrPs in the semi hamstrings muscle. (Modified from Dommerholt J, Fernández-de-las-Peñas C 2013.)

needling directly over the nerve, careful exploration of the region with the needle will easily identify the exact location of the nerve.

Semimembranosus muscle

Anatomy: The muscle originates, with a flat tendon it shares with the biceps femoris and the semitendinosus muscles, from the superior–lateral aspect of the ischial tuberosity. It then travels deep to the semitendinosus muscle and inserts at the tubercle of the medial tibial condyle, the medial margin of the tibia, the fascia over the popliteus muscle and the lateral femoral condyle where it forms much of the oblique popliteal ligament.

Needling technique: The patient is in prone position, with the knee slightly flexed and the lower leg supported by a pillow. The needle is inserted perpendicular to the muscle surface directly into the TrP, as identified by flat palpation (Fig. 61.39).

Precautions: Avoid the sciatic nerve by needling in a medial direction.

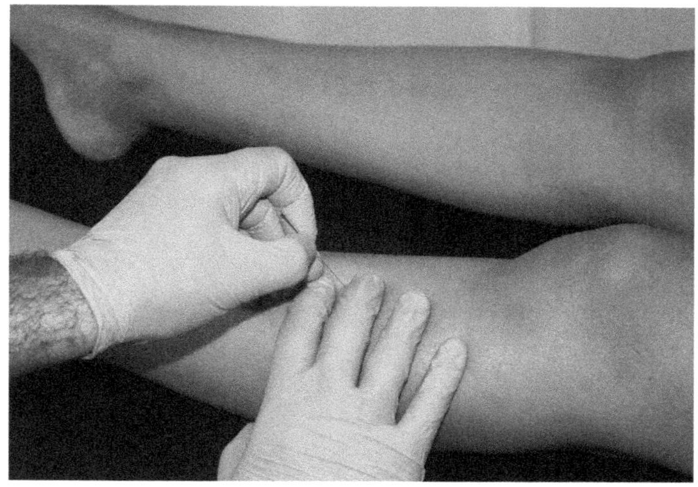

Figure 61.40 Dry needling of TrPs in the anterior tibialis muscle. (Modified from Dommerholt J, Fernández-de-las-Peñas C 2013.)

Semitendinosus muscle

Anatomy: The semitendinosus muscle originates from the inferomedial part of the ischial tuberosity via a tendon it shares with the biceps femoris and the semimembranosus muscles, and from an aponeurosis connecting the muscles. It inserts via a long tendon overlying the semimembranosus muscle at the upper part of the medial surface of the tibia behind the insertion of the sartorius and distal to the insertion of the gracilis (pes anserine).

Needling technique: The patient is in prone position, with the knee slightly flexed and the lower leg supported by a pillow. The needle is inserted perpendicular to the muscle surface directly into the TrP, as identified by flat palpation, similarly to needling the semimembranosus muscle (see Fig. 61.39).

Precautions: Avoid needling the sciatic nerve by needling in a medial direction.

Tibialis anterior muscle

Anatomy: The muscle originates from the lateral condyle of the tibia and upper two-thirds of the lateral surface of the tibia. It inserts into the plantar and medial aspects of the medial cuneiform and the medial aspect of the base of the first metatarsal bones.

Needling technique: The patient is in supine position. The needle is inserted perpendicular to the muscle surface, and the needle is directed slightly medial to the tibia into the TrP, as identified by flat palpation (Fig. 61.40).

Precautions: Avoid needling the neurovascular bundle, which is composed of the anterior tibial artery and vein and the deep fibular nerve, and which runs directly behind the lateral aspect of the muscle, by needling medially towards the tibia or by initially needling superficially with deeper advances with each needle movement until the trigger point has been reached.

Gastrocnemius muscle

Anatomy: The muscle is composed of two heads. The medial and lateral heads originate from each respective condyle of

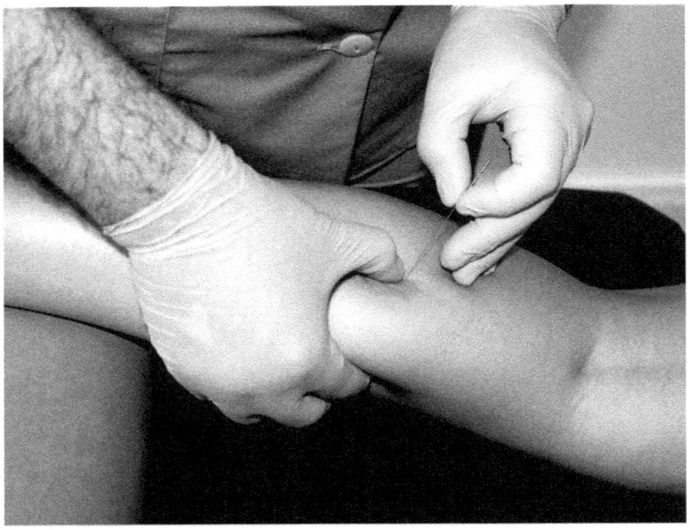

Figure 61.41 Dry needling of TrPs in the gastrocnemius muscle (medial head). (Modified from Dommerholt J, Fernández-de-las-Peñas C 2013.)

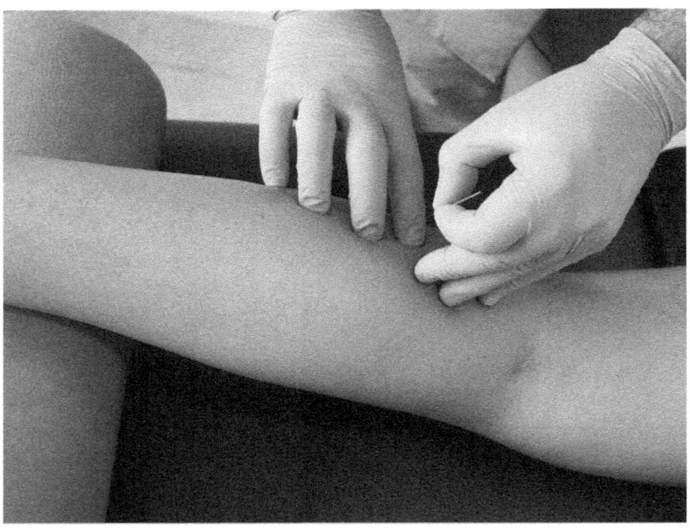

Figure 61.42 Dry needling of TrPs in the gastrocnemius muscle (lateral head). (Modified from Dommerholt J, Fernández-de-las-Peñas C 2013.)

the femur and attach to the capsule of the knee joint. Distally, the muscle fibres end on an aponeurosis that joins the soleus muscle to form the Achilles tendon, which subsequently attaches to the posterior surface of the calcaneus.

Needling technique: The patient is prone, with the knee slightly flexed and the lower leg supported by a pillow. For TrPs in the central part of the medial head, a pincer palpation is used to locate and fix the taut band and the TrP. The needle is angled medially, towards the finger located at the opposite side (Fig. 61.41). For TrPs in the central part of the lateral head, a flat palpation is more commonly used to locate and fix the taut band and the TrPs. The needle is directed perpendicular to the muscle surface, aiming towards the TrP in a posterior–anterior direction with a slightly lateral angulation (Fig. 61.42).

Precautions: When needling the proximal heads of the muscle, care must be taken not to needle the neurovascular

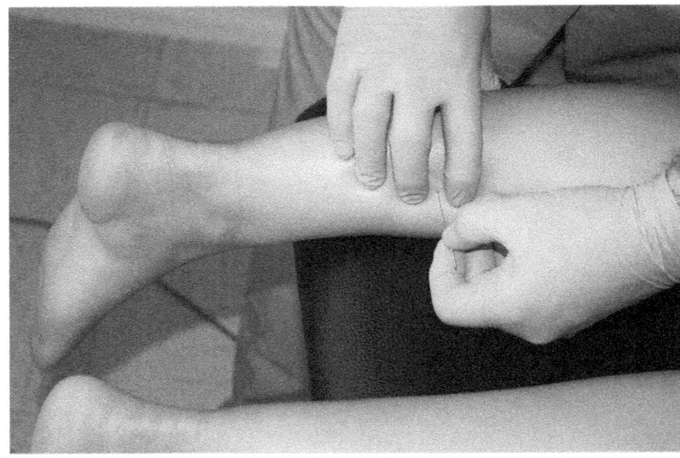

Figure 61.43 Dry needling of TrPs in the soleus muscle. (Modified from Dommerholt J, Fernández-de-las-Peñas C 2013.)

bundle, which is composed of the tibial nerve and the popliteal artery and vein in the midline of the popliteal fossa. In addition, care must be taken to avoid needling the fibular nerve when needling the lateral head, which lies just medial to the biceps femoris tendon. There are many anatomical variations with regards the location and splits of the nerves. It is therefore imperative that clinicians use good clinical skills and judgements in order to needle the TrPs in this area safely. Furthermore, the posterior capsule of the knee should be avoided. Lastly, when needling the central bellies of both heads, the neurovascular bundle in the midline should be avoided by needling medially when needling the medial head, and by needling laterally when needling the lateral head.

Soleus muscle

Anatomy: The muscle originates from the posterior aspect of the head and the middle third of the posterior border of the fibula and the soleal line, from the middle third of the medial border of the tibia, and from the tendinous arch spanning between the two bones. Distally, the muscle fibres attach to the aponeurosis and join the gastrocnemius muscle to form the Achilles tendon, which subsequently attaches to the posterior surface of the calcaneus.

Needling technique: Proximal TrPs can be needled towards the fibula with the patient lying on the uninvolved side. The needle is inserted perpendicular to the muscle surface directly into the TrP, as identified by flat palpation. For distal medial or lateral TrPs, the whole muscle can be held in a pincer between the thumb and two fingers, with the patient either in a prone or in a side-lying position. The needle is directed towards the opposite finger or thumb (Fig. 61.43).

Precautions: When needling the medial part of the muscle, care must be taken to avoid needling the posterior tibial nerve, by avoiding needling the midline.

Flexor digitorum longus muscle

Anatomy: The muscle originates from the posterior surface of the middle two-quarters of the tibia below the attachment of

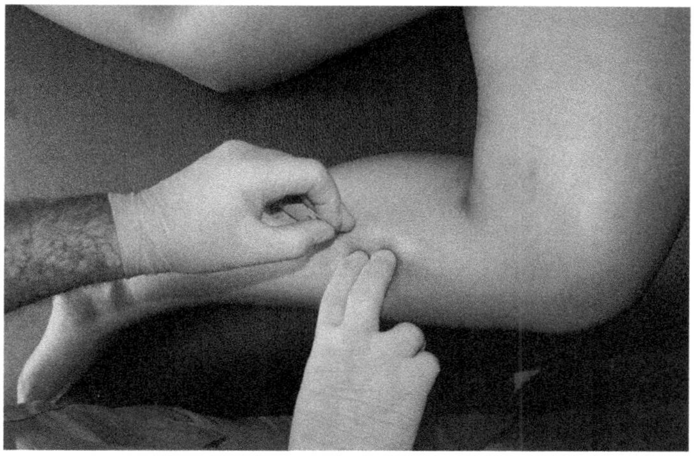

Figure 61.44 Dry needling of TrPs in the flexor digitorum longus muscle. (Modified from Dommerholt J, Fernández-de-las-Peñas C 2013.)

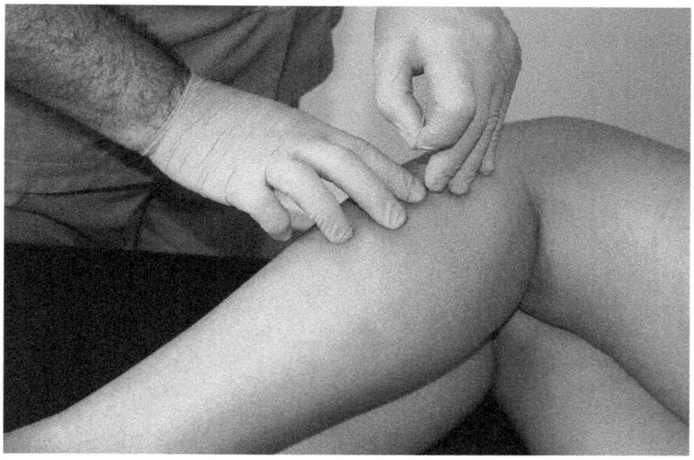

Figure 61.45 Dry needling of TrPs in the fibularis longus and brevis muscles. (Modified from Dommerholt J, Fernández-de-las-Peñas C 2013.)

the soleus muscle, and the deep layer of the intermuscular septum shared with the tibialis posterior muscle. Distally, each of the four tendons attaches to the corresponding base of the distal phalanx of the second, third, fourth and fifth toes.

Needling technique: The patient lies on the involved side, with the hips and knees bent at 90°. TrPs are identified by flat palpation directly behind the posterior surface of the tibia. The needle is inserted perpendicular to the muscle surface and is directed mainly in a lateral but also slightly anterior direction (Fig. 61.44). The needle should be kept close to the posterior aspect of the tibia. Alternatively, the muscle can be treated with the patient in the prone position.

Precautions: Avoid needling the neurovascular bundle, which is composed of the tibial nerve, the posterior tibial artery and vein, and which lies directly behind the muscle, by keeping the needle close to the tibia.

Fibularis (peroneus) longus and brevis muscles

Anatomy: The fibularis longus muscle originates from the fibular head, from the proximal two-thirds of the lateral aspect of the fibula, and from the adjacent muscular septa. It inserts onto the dorsal and lateral sides of the medial cuneiform and the first metatarsal bones. The fibularis brevis originates from the lower two-thirds of the lateral aspect of the fibula and from the adjacent muscular septa. It inserts onto the lateral side of the base of the fifth metatarsal bone. The fibularis brevis is partially covered by the longus.

Needling technique: The patient lies on the uninvolved side, with the hips and knees bent to 90°. TrPs are identified by flat palpation. The needle is inserted laterally perpendicular to the muscle surface and is directed in a medial direction towards the fibula (Fig. 61.45).

Precautions: Avoid needling the common fibular nerve, which lies deep to the proximal third of the fibularis longus muscle. Avoid needling the superficial fibularis nerve, which lies just anterior of the fibularis brevis muscle, by avoiding needling in an anterior direction, but instead directing the needle away from the nerve.

References

Akhbari B, Salavati M, Ezzati K, et al. 2014. The use of dry needling and myofascial meridians in a case of plantar fasciitis. J Chiropr Med 13: 43–48.

Amaro JA, 2007. When acupuncture becomes 'dry needling'. Acupuncture Today 33: 43. Online. Available: http://www.iama.edu/Articles/DryNeedling.htm.

Association of Social Work Boards, Federation of State Boards of Physical Therapy, et al. 2006. Changes in healthcare professions scope of practice: legislative considerations. Washington, DC: ASWB.

Australian Society of Acupuncture Physiotherapists (ASAP). 2013. Guidelines for safe acupuncture and dry needling practice. Available: http://www.dryneedling.com.au/wp-content/uploads/2013/08/ASAP_Guidelines_2013.pdf.

Baldry PE, 2005. Acupuncture, trigger points and musculoskeletal pain. Edinburgh: Churchill Livingstone.

Birch S, 2006. A review and analysis of placebo treatments, placebo effects, and placebo controls in trials of medical procedures when sham is not inert. J Altern Complement Med 12: 303–310.

Brady S, McEvoy J, Dommerholt J, et al. 2014. Adverse events following trigger point dry needling: a prospective survey of chartered physiotherapists. J Manual Manip Ther 22(3): 134–140. doi: 10.1179/2042618613Y.0000000044.

Buchmann J, Neustadt B, Katharina Buchmann-Barthel K, et al. 2014. Objective measurement of tissue tension in myofascial trigger point areas before and during the administration of anesthesia with complete blocking of neuromuscular transmission. Clin J Pain 30: 191–198.

Cagnie B, Barbe T, De Ridder E, et al. 2012. The influence of dry needling of the trapezius muscle on muscle blood flow and oxygenation. J Manipulative Physiol Ther 35: 685–691.

Chen JT, Chung KC, Hou CR, et al. 2001. Inhibitory effect of dry needling on the spontaneous electrical activity recorded from myofascial trigger spots of rabbit skeletal muscle. Am J Phys Med Rehabil 80: 729–735.

Chou LW, Hsieh YL, Kao MJ, et al. 2009. Remote influences of acupuncture on the pain intensity and the amplitude changes of endplate noise in the myofascial trigger point of the upper trapezius muscle. Arch Phys Med Rehabil 90: 905–912.

Churchill JM. 1821. A treatise on acupuncturation being a description of a surgical operation originally peculiar to the Japanese and Chinese, and by them denominated zin-king, now introduced into European practice, with directions for its performance and cases illustrating its success. London: Simpkins & Marshall.

Churchill JM. 1828. Cases illustrative of the immediate effects of acupuncturation in rheumatism, lumbago, sciatica, anomalous muscular diseases and in dropsy of the cellular tissues, selected from various sources and intended as an appendix to the author's treatise on the subject. London: Simpkins & Marshall.

Clewley D, Flynn TW, Koppenhaver S. 2014. Trigger point dry needling as an adjunct treatment for a patient with adhesive capsulitis of the shoulder. J Orthop Sports Phys Ther 44: 92–101.

Dilorenzo L,Traballesi M, Morelli D, et al. 2004. Hemiparetic shoulder pain syndrome treated with deep dry needling during early rehabilitation: a prospective, open-label, randomized investigation. J Musculoskeletal Pain 12(2): 25–34.
Dıraçoğlu D, Vural M, Karan A, et al. 2012. Effectiveness of dry needling for the treatment of temporomandibular myofascial pain: a double-blind, randomized, placebo controlled study. J Back Musculoskelet Rehabil 25: 285–290.
Domingo A, Mayoral O, Monterde S, et al. 2013. Neuromuscular damage and repair after dry needling in mice. Evid Based Complement Alternat Med 2013: 260806.
Dommerholt J. 2011. Dry needling: peripheral and central considerations. J Manual Manipul Ther 19: 223–237.
Dommerholt J, Fernandez-de-las-Peñas C. 2013. Trigger point dry needling: an evidence and clinical-based approach, 1st edn. London: Churchill Livingstone Elsevier.
Dommerholt J, Mayoral O, Gröbli C. 2006. Trigger point dry needling. J Manual Manipulative Ther 14: E70–E87.
Elliotson J. 1827. The use of the sulphate of copper in chronic diarrhoea together with an essay on acupuncture. Med Chir Trans 13 (Pt 2): 451–467.
Fernández-Carnero J, Fernández-de-las-Peñas C, de-la-Llave-Rincón AI, et al. 2008. Bilateral myofascial trigger points in the forearm muscles in patients with chronic unilateral lateral epicondylalgia: a blinded, controlled study. Clin J Pain 24: 802–807.
Fernández-Carnero J, La Touche R, Ortega-Santiago R, et al. 2010. Short-term effects of dry needling of active myofascial trigger points in the masseter muscle in patients with temporomandibular disorders. J Orofac Pain 24: 106–112.
Fernández-de-las-Peñas C, Dommerholt J. 2014. Myofascial trigger points: peripheral or central phenomenon? Curr Rheumatol Rep 16: 395.
Fernández-de-las-Peñas C, Cuadrado ML, Arendt-Nielsen L, et al. 2007. Myofascial trigger points and sensitization: an updated pain model for tension-type headache. Cephalalgia 27: 383–393.
Fernández-de-las-Peñas C, Galán-del-Rio F, Fernández-Carnero J, et al. 2009. Bilateral widespread mechanical pain sensitivity in women with myofascial temporomandibular disorder: evidence of impairment in central nociceptive processing. J Pain 10: 1170–1178.
Furlan A, Tulder M, Cherkin D, et al. 2005. Acupuncture and dry-needling for low back pain: an updated systematic review within the framework of the Cochrane Collaboration. Spine 30: 944–963.
Ga H, Koh HJ, Choi JH, et al. 2007. Intramuscular and nerve root stimulation vs lidocaine injection to trigger points in myofascial pain syndrome. J Rehabil Med 39: 374–378.
Giamberardino MA, Tafuri E, Savini A, et al. 2007. Contribution of myofascial trigger points to migraine symptoms. J Pain 8: 869–878.
González-Iglesias J, Cleland JA, Neto F, et al. 2013. Mobilization with movement, thoracic spine manipulation, and dry needling for the management of temporomandibular disorder: a prospective case series. Physiother Theory Pract 29: 586–595.
Gonzalez-Perez LM, Infante-Cossio P, Granados-Nuñez M, et al. 2012. Treatment of temporomandibular myofascial pain with deep dry needling. Med Oral Patol Oral Cir Bucal 17: e781–785.
Gunn CC, Milbrandt WE, Little AS, et al. 1980. Dry needling of muscle motor points for chronic low-back pain: a randomized clinical trial with long-term follow-up. Spine 5: 279–291.
Hong CZ. 1994. Lidocaine injection versus dry needling to myofascial trigger point. The importance of the local twitch response. Am J Phys Med Rehabil 73: 256–263.
Hsieh YL, Kao MJ, Kuan TS, et al. 2007. Dry needling to a key myofascial trigger point may reduce the irritability of satellite MTrPs. Am J Phys Med Rehabil 86: 397–403.
Hsieh YL, Yang SA, Yang CC, et al. 2012. Dry needling at myofascial trigger spots of rabbit skeletal muscles modulates the biochemicals associated with pain, inflammation, and hypoxia. Evid Based Complement Alternat Med 2012: 342165.
Itoh K, Asai S, Ohyabu H, Imai K, et al. 2012. Effects of trigger point acupuncture treatment on temporomandibular disorders: a preliminary randomized clinical trial. J Acupunct Meridian Stud 5: 57–62.
Jayaseelan DJ, Moats N, Ricardo CR. 2014. Rehabilitation of proximal hamstring tendinopathy utilizing eccentric training, lumbopelvic stabilization, and trigger point dry needling: 2 case reports. J Orthop Sports Phys Ther 44: 198–205.
Joseph L, Mohd Ali K, Ramli A, et al. 2013. Fear of needles does not influence pain tolerance and sympathetic responses among patients during a therapeutic needling. Pol Ann Med 20: 1–7.
Kamanli A, Kaya A, Ardicoglu O, et al. 2005. Comparison of lidocaine injection, botulinum toxin injection, and dry needling to trigger points in myofascial pain syndrome. Rheumatol Int 25: 604–611.
Katagiri M, Abe T, Yokoba M, et al. 2003. Neck and abdominal muscle activity during a sniff. Respir Med 97: 1027–1035.
Kietrys DM, Palombaro KM, Azzaretto E, et al. 2013. Effectiveness of dry needling for upper quarter myofascial pain: a systematic review and meta-analysis. J Orthop Sports Phys Ther 43: 620–634.
Kong J, White NS, Kwong KK, et al. 2006. Using fMRI to dissociate sensory encoding from cognitive evaluation of heat pain intensity. Hum Brain Mapp 27: 715–721.
Lee JH, Lee H, Jo DJ. 2011. An acute cervical epidural hematoma as a complication of dry needling. Spine 36: E891–E893.
Lewit K. 1979. The needle effect in the relief of myofascial pain. Pain 6: 83–90.
Lucas KR, Polus BI, Rich PA. 2004. Latent myofascial trigger points: their effect on muscle activation and movement efficiency. J Bodyw Mov Ther 8: 160–166.
Lund I, Lundeberg T. 2006. Are minimal, superficial or sham acupuncture procedures acceptable as inert placebo controls? Acupunct Med 24: 13–15.
Maher RM, Hayes DM, Shinohara M. 2013. Quantification of dry needling and posture effects on myofascial trigger points using ultrasound shear-wave elastography. Arch Phys Med Rehabil 94: 2146–2150.
Mason JS, Tansey KA, Westrick RB. 2014. Treatment of subacute posterior knee pain in an adolescent ballet dancer utilizing trigger point dry needling: a case report. Intern J Sports Phys Ther 9: 116–124.
Mayoral del Moral O. 2005. Fisioterapia invasiva del síndrome de dolor miofascial. Fisioterapia 27: 69–75.
Mayoral O, Salvat I, Martín MT, et al. 2013. Efficacy of myofascial trigger point dry needling in the prevention of pain after total knee arthroplasty: a randomized, double-blinded, placebo-controlled trial. Evid Based Complement Alternat Med 2013: 694941.
McCutcheon L, Yelland M. 2011. Iatrogenic pneumothorax: safety concerns when using acupuncture or dry needling in the thoracic region. Phys Ther Rev 16: 126–132.
McEvoy J, Dommerholt J, Rice D, et al. 2011. Guidelines for safe dry needling practice for chartered physiotherapists. Dublin. [Electronic guideline.]
Napadow V, Dhond RP, Kim J, et al. 2009. Brain encoding of acupuncture sensation–coupling on-line rating with fMRI. Neuroimage 47: 1055–1065.
Niddam DM, Chan RC, Lee SH, et al. 2007. Central modulation of pain evoked from myofascial trigger point. Clin J Pain 23: 440–448.
Niddam DM, Chan RC, Lee SH, et al. 2008. Central representation of hyperalgesia from myofascial trigger point. Neuroimage 39: 1299–1306.
Noë A. 2004. Action in perception. Cambridge, MA: MIT Press.
Olausson H, Lamarre Y, Backlund H, et al. 2002. Unmyelinated tactile afferents signal touch and project to insular cortex. Nat Neurosci 5: 900–904.
Osborne NJ, Gatt IT. 2010. Management of shoulder injuries using dry needling in elite volleyball players. Acupunct Med 28: 42–45.
Osler W. 1912. The principles and practice of medicine. New York: Appleton.
Paantjens MA. 2013. Dry needling en adductorenmanipulatie voor de behandeling van een voetballer met adductorgerelateerde liespijn. Nederlands Militair Geneeskundig Tijdschrift 66–61–68: 64–70.
Pariente J, White P, Frackowiak RS, et al. 2005. Expectancy and belief modulate the neuronal substrates of pain treated by acupuncture. Neuroimage 25: 1161–1167.
Peuker E, Gronemeyer D. 2001. Rare but serious complications of acupuncture: traumatic lesions. Acupunct Med 19: 103–108.
Rainey CE. 2013. The use of trigger point dry needling and intramuscular electrical stimulation for a subject with chronic low back pain: a case report. Int J Sports Phys Ther 8: 145–161.
Shah JP, Phillips TM, Danoff JV, et al. 2005. An in-vivo microanalytical technique for measuring the local biochemical milieu of human skeletal muscle. J Appl Physiol 99: 1977–1984.
Shah JP, Danoff JV, Desai MJ, et al. 2008. Biochemicals associated with pain and inflammation are elevated in sites near to and remote from active myofascial trigger points. Arch Phys Med Rehabil 89: 16–23.
Simons DG, Travell JG, Simons L. 1999. Travell and Simons' myofascial pain and dysfunction; the trigger point manual. Baltimore: Williams & Wilkins.
Steinbrocker O. 1944. Therapeutic injections in painful musculoskeletal disorders. JAMA 125: 397–401.
Takeshige C, Kobori M, Hishida F, et al. 1992a. Analgesia inhibitory system involvement in nonacupuncture point-stimulation-produced analgesia. Brain Res Bull 28: 379–391.

Takeshige C, Sato T, Mera T, et al. 1992b. Descending pain inhibitory system involved in acupuncture analgesia. Brain Res Bull 29: 617–634.
Tekin L, Akarsu S, Durmuş O, et al. 2013. The effect of dry needling in the treatment of myofascial pain syndrome: a randomized double-blinded placebo-controlled trial. Clin Rheumatol 32: 309–315.
Travell JG, Simons DG. 1992. Myofascial pain and dysfunction: the trigger point manual. Baltimore: Williams & Wilkins.
Tsai CT, Hsieh LF, Kuan TS, et al. 2010. Remote effects of dry needling on the irritability of the myofascial trigger point in the upper trapezius muscle. Am J Phys Med Rehabil 89: 133–140.
Usman F, Bajwa A, Shujaat A, et al. 2011. Retrosternal abscess after trigger point injections in a pregnant woman: a case report. J Med Case Rep 5: 403.
Wang SM, Kain ZN, White PF. 2008. Acupuncture analgesia: II. Clinical considerations. Anesth Analg 106: 611–621.
Westrick RB, Zylstra E, Issa T, et al. 2012. Evaluation and treatment of musculoskeletal chest wall pain in a military athlete. Intern J Sports Phys Ther 7: 323–332.
White A. 2009. Western medical acupuncture: a definition. Acupunct Med 27: 33–35.
White A, Cummings M, Filshie J. 2008. An introduction to Western medical acupuncture. Edinburgh: Churchill Livingstone.
Yang L, Mullan B. 2011. Reducing needle stick injuries in healthcare occupations: an integrative review of the literature. ISRN Nurs 2011: 315432.
Ziaeifar M, Arab AM, Karimi N, et al. 2014. The effect of dry needling on pain, pressure pain threshold and disability in patients with a myofascial trigger point in the upper trapezius muscle. J Body Movement Ther 18: 298–305.

62 Chapter

Muscle Energy Approaches

Gary Fryer

CHAPTER CONTENTS

Introduction 710
Evidence of effectiveness 710
Physiological mechanisms 711
An integrated approach to muscle energy 711
Principles of muscle energy application 712
General principles 712
Cautions and contraindications 712
Techniques for the spine, rib cage and pelvis 712
Principles of application of muscle energy to the joints of the spine 713
Cervical spine 714
Thoracic spine 716
Rib cage 718
Lumbar spine 720
Pelvic girdle 721
Techniques for myofascial tissues 723
Principles of application of muscle energy to myofascial tissues 723
Muscles of the upper quadrant 724
Muscles of the lower quadrant 726

Introduction

Muscle energy technique (MET) is a system of manual procedures that utilizes active muscle contraction effort from the patient, usually against a controlled matching counterforce from the practitioner. The MET system was developed by osteopathic physician Fred Mitchell Sr in the 1950s, although techniques using resisted muscle effort to increase range of motion were documented as early as 1919 (Swart 1919). The evolution of MET continued with contributions from Fred Mitchell Jr, who systematized and further developed the methods in technique manuals (Mitchell Jr & Mitchell 1995). The MET approach has benefited from contributions by many individuals and is practised by clinicians in different manual therapy disciplines. MET has been used to lengthen shortened muscles, mobilize articulations with restricted mobility, strengthen weakened muscles and reduce localized oedema and passive congestion (Mitchell Jr & Mitchell 1995; Goodridge & Kuchera 1997; Chaitow 2013).

The most commonly described MET is the post-isometric relaxation (or 'contract–relax') technique, which is used particularly when increasing muscle length or joint range of motion. The number of repetitions is influenced by the response of the involved tissues, but three to five repetitions have been recommended (Mitchell Jr & Mitchell 1995; Goodridge & Kuchera 1997; Chaitow 2013). The force and duration of isometric effort can vary, depending on the aim of the technique and the tissues involved. A gentle, controlled isometric effort is usually suitable for treatment of specific joint dysfunctions, myofascial trigger points (TrPs), or acute myofascial pain; a stronger contraction can be employed for fibrotic, shortened muscles. Other variations of this technique exist, such as the use of concentric contractions against a yielding resistance to increase strength and recruitment of a muscle, or reciprocal inhibition techniques that facilitate relaxation of a muscle when applied to the antagonist muscle, but these techniques will not be detailed in this chapter.

Similarities exist between MET and other forms of post-isometric stretching, such as proprioceptive neuromuscular facilitation techniques, particularly when the techniques are applied to facilitate the lengthening of muscle. However, MET was developed along biomechanical principles for the treatment of spinal and pelvic joint dysfunction, which is evident in many MET texts (Mitchell Jr & Mitchell 1995). Thus, it is very different from other treatment systems that use isometric contraction.

Evidence of effectiveness

As with many manual therapy approaches, robust, high-quality research investigating the clinical effectiveness of MET is lacking (Fryer 2013). More research is needed for using MET in patients with spinal pain and disability, but a number of small randomized controlled trials offer low-quality support for the effectiveness of MET for acute and chronic low back pain (LBP) and for neck pain. Additionally, evidence suggests there are short-term increases in spinal range of motion and muscle extensibility following treatment.

Regarding acute LBP, researchers have found that MET applied to spinal and pelvic joint or muscle dysfunctions improved pain and disability. Wilson et al (2003) assigned 19 patients with acute LBP to an MET group (for treatment of a specific lumbar joint dysfunction) or to a matched control group that received a sham treatment (side-lying passive motion); both groups also undertook a home exercise programme. The MET patients showed a significantly higher change in disability scores than did the control patients, and every MET patient had a greater improvement than control patients. Selkow et al (2009) applied MET to innominate dysfunction in patients with a recent acute episode of lumbopelvic pain and reported a significant decrease in pain severity in the MET group 24 hours after treatment compared with a sham control group.

Several studies reported improvements in acute LBP following MET applied to the lumbar and pelvic musculature. Salvador et al (2005) compared MET applied to the paraspinal, quadratus lumborum, hamstrings and piriformis muscles with transcutaneous nerve stimulation in 28 garbage workers with acute LBP. The authors reported significant pain reduction and increased extensibility of muscles in the MET group. Similarly, Patil et al (2010) randomized 20 subjects with acute LBP pain into two groups; both received interferential therapy but the MET group also received MET to stretch the quadratus lumborum muscle. Although pain decreased in both groups, a significant decrease in disability and increase in spinal range of motion was reported for the MET group.

Studies also suggest benefits of MET for patients with chronic LBP. Rana et al (2009) reported large improvements in pain and disability in LBP patients who underwent six sessions of MET or passive mobilization applied to specific pelvic dysfunctions, but not in the control group. Dhinkaran et al (2011) reported greater improvements in pain and disability in the group that received MET to a diagnosed pelvic dysfunction compared with those who received transcutaneous electrical stimulation. These studies used small sample sizes, however, and the statistical analysis procedures were unclear.

MET has been reported as helpful for neck pain. Gupta et al (2008) found that MET (referred to as post-isometric relaxation) produced a greater improvement in pain, disability and motion in 38 patients with non-specific neck pain compared with isometric exercises over 3 weeks. In a case series, Murphy et al (2006) reported positive results using muscle energy or cervical manipulation in 27 patients with neck and / or arm pain with findings of cervical spinal cord encroachment. Regardless of the treatment, these patients reported substantial improvement in neck pain and disability without any major complications associated with the treatment.

MET (or similar isometric stretching techniques) has increased the extensibility of muscles more than by passive stretching alone (Fryer 2013). MET has also increased the range of neck and trunk motion (Schenk et al 1994, 1997; Lenehan et al 2003; Fryer & Ruszkowski 2004; Burns & Wells 2006). However, these motion and flexibility studies have examined only the immediate or short-term effect of treatment, often in healthy pain-free patients, but little evidence links improvements in flexibility and mobility to positive patient outcomes. Altogether, the research on MET supports its use for improving clinical outcomes, such as pain, disability and restricted motion, but the studies are generally of low quality and further investigation is required that uses robust methodology and larger sample sizes, including measures of the longevity of these effects, in order to verify the clinical benefit of MET.

Physiological mechanisms

Although the mechanisms by which MET produces therapeutic benefit are speculative, MET may produce neurological and biomechanical effects, but possibly through mechanisms not typically described in MET texts (Fryer & Fossum 2010; Fryer 2013). Traditionally, MET was thought to produce muscle relaxation via Golgi tendon organ and muscle spindle reflexes (Kuchera & Kuchera 1992; Mitchell Jr & Mitchell 1995), but this explanation seems unlikely as studies had reported increases in electromyographic activity following post-isometric stretching techniques (Osternig et al 1987, 1990). MET has also been proposed to reset the neurological resting length of muscles, but it appears that motor activity does not play a significant role in limiting passive stretch of a muscle, at least in healthy, uninjured individuals (Magnusson et al 1996a).

Increased flexibility of muscle groups following isometric contraction is largely attributable to an increase in an individual's tolerance to stretch, rather than to lasting biomechanical change in the tissue (Magnusson et al 1996b; Fryer 2013). Increased stretch tolerance may be a result of a decrease in pain perception (hypoalgesia) through the activation of muscle and joint mechanoreceptors involving centrally mediated pathways, such as the periaqueductal grey in the midbrain region and non-opioid serotonergic and noradrenergic descending inhibitory pathways (Souvlis et al 2004; Fryer & Fossum 2010). Additionally, MET produces hypoalgesia via peripheral mechanisms associated with increased fluid drainage. Rhythmic muscle contractions increase muscle blood and lymph flow rates (Coates et al 1993; Havas et al 1997). Mechanical forces, such as loading and stretching, acting on fibroblasts in connective tissues may affect fibroblast mechanical signal transduction processes (Langevin et al 2004), thus changing the interstitial pressure and increasing transcapillary blood flow (Langevin et al 2005). These factors may play a role in the tissue response to injury and inflammation; MET may support these processes by reducing the concentrations of pro-inflammatory cytokines, resulting in decreased sensitization of peripheral nociceptors.

In addition to hypoalgesia, MET may involve neurological mechanisms to enhance proprioception and motor control in patients with pain. Patients with spinal pain have decreased awareness of the direction of spinal motion and position (Leinonen et al 2002; Grip et al 2007; Lee et al 2007) and changes in paraspinal muscle motor strategies (Fryer et al 2004). For instance, high-velocity spinal manipulation improves head re-positioning in chronic neck pain patients (Rogers 1997; Palmgren et al 2006) and motor recruitment strategies in LBP patients (Ferreira et al 2007). Malmstrom et al (2010) found that a prolonged unilateral neck muscle contraction task increased the accuracy of head repositioning. Although the suggestion is speculative, MET may enhance proprioception, motor control and motor learning because it involves active and precise recruitment of muscle activity. This area deserves further investigation.

An integrated approach to muscle energy

MET was developed to be applied in a holistic manner, consistent with osteopathic principles. The osteopathic discipline emphasizes the unity and interconnectedness of the body, the inter-relationship of structure and function, and the influence of the musculoskeletal system on other systems and general health. The MET approach was based on a specific diagnostic model that emphasized a global view of body biomechanics and included screening and scanning of global posture, movement patterns and gross and segmental range of motion (Mitchell Jr & Mitchell 1995). For example, in patients presenting with neck and arm pain, the body may be examined from head to toe (posture, static and dynamic symmetry, and active and passive range of motion), and treatment may be directed at any or all of the regions that are believed to be problematic – lower limb, pelvic, lumbar, thoracic, rib cage, neck, head and upper extremity. Implicit in this approach are the concepts that dysfunction in one region may cause compensation and strain in other regions and that treatment that addresses only the symptomatic site is likely to achieve only short-term relief. In recent years, researchers have reported that manipulative treatment produces remote and systemic effects; for instance, cervical treatment improves shoulder symptoms (Aparicio et al 2009) and thoracic treatment improves neck pain (Cleland et al 2005; González-Iglesias et al 2009) and shoulder pain and disability (Boyles et al 2009).

Assessment and treatment of the thorax – including the spinal joints, ribs, and muscles – are extremely important for patients with neck and arm complaints. Treatment of this region should precede treatment of the neck and upper extremity because (in the author's experience) it often produces improvement of symptoms and physical findings in the neck and extremities.

MET may be applied in combination with other manual techniques, such as soft tissue manipulation, passive joint articulation, high-velocity thrust, and gentle indirect techniques such as functional technique and counterstrain (where tissues are held in a position of ease). There is no universal agreement on the criteria for selection of a particular technique for a given condition or patient, but practitioner and patient preferences are significant determinants. Little evidence is available to guide clinicians regarding the most effective combination of techniques. However, Trampas et al (2010) found that the combination of cross-fibre massage with a contract–relax technique produced significant improvements in pressure pain sensitivity of a TrP, which supports personal experience that soft tissue techniques work well with MET for treating muscle dysfunction.

Techniques may be selected based on their likely therapeutic mechanisms, despite the speculative nature of those mechanisms. For example, MET may be used where fluid drainage and improved proprioception are desired, high-velocity thrust may be used where joint end feel is particularly hard, end-range articulation may be used where joint motion appears to be restricted by fibrotic changes in periarticular tissues, and indirect approaches may be used where significant inflammation and pain are present. The integration of these different techniques may involve intuitive cues from palpation and the pragmatic use of alternative techniques if the initial techniques fail to achieve the intended tissue and motion changes.

Principles of Muscle Energy Application

General principles

The elements comprising the application of MET – restrictive barrier engagement, force of contraction, duration of contraction and post-isometric stretch, number of repetitions – can be varied according to the tissue or joint, the aim of the technique and the response of tissues to treatment. In general, the precise localization of leverages in one or more planes to a restrictive joint barrier with a gentle contraction effort is important for the application of MET to a single joint dysfunction. These principles may also be applied to irritable or painful myofascial tissues, and the force of stretch and contraction intensity may be progressively increased for muscles that are short and fibrotic without substantial tenderness. In all cases, the practitioner should have a well-balanced posture to provide control and resistance to the isometric effort in an economical manner. The patient should always be comfortable; the procedures should not be painful even when the therapist is using a moderate stretching force for large muscles. This chapter describes techniques for a number of commonly encountered joint and muscle dysfunctions; however, the practitioner with a clear understanding of muscle anatomy, joint biomechanics and the principles of MET should be able to modify the techniques to address any joint restriction or shortened muscle.

Cautions and contraindications

MET is a safe technique, and no reports of serious adverse reactions have been found in the literature. Typically, very gentle to moderate applications of stretch or isometric contraction are performed, so MET is also perceived as a technique with little risk of serious injury. The cautions and contraindications for MET are similar to those of other soft tissue techniques and include caution with the use of force and leverage when dealing with acute pain conditions and individuals with weakened bone. When applied to previously injured, healing tissues, the forces of contraction or stretch should be matched to the stage of healing and repair in order to avoid further tissue damage and to promote optimal healing (Lederman 2005).

Cerebrovascular accidents following high-velocity manipulation to the cervical spine have been reported as rare complications (Di Fabio 1999; Haldeman et al 2001). Although no such incidents have been reported for MET, caution should be taken when treating the cervical spine. Fortunately, the leverages advocated for MET applied to the cervical spine are subtle and minimal, and the avoidance of end-range rotation and extension leverages may further reduce risks posed by MET.

All techniques should be applied slowly and carefully with patient feedback. If the patient experiences discomfort or anything other than a pleasant stretching sensation, the practitioner should stop the procedure immediately and reassess the patient. The technique should also be stopped and the patient reassessed if there are any signs of vertebrobasilar insufficiency (Gibbons & Tehan 2006) such as vertigo, visual disturbances, dysphagia, dysarthria, hoarseness, facial numbness, paraesthesia, confusion or syncope (drop attacks).

Techniques for the Spine, Rib Cage and Pelvis

The following are descriptions of techniques that illustrate the application of MET to address motion restrictions at various spinal segments and to the joints of the rib cage and pelvis.

The techniques are intended to address specific physical diagnostic findings, and a brief description of diagnostic approaches is provided. It is beyond the scope of this chapter to describe assessment procedures thoroughly and it is assumed that the clinician will already be skilled in assessing the spine and pelvis. The listed techniques and descriptions are not intended to be exhaustive, but rather to illustrate the application in different regions. Once the reader understands the principles of application, techniques can be adapted for any combination of motion restrictions at any motion segment.

Principles of application of muscle energy to the joints of the spine

The application of MET to the intervertebral joints of the spine differs from its application to large muscles in terms of the need for localization, control and force (Mitchell Jr & Mitchell 1995). The basic principles of application to intervertebral segments to increase range of motion include:

1. **Localization:** Careful attention is required to engage the restrictive barrier accurately at the involved level using the initial sense of increasing resistance to motion ('first' or 'feather edge' of barrier) (Mitchell Jr & Mitchell 1995). The primary plane of motion restriction should be engaged first, after which 'fine-tuning' can be performed using secondary planes of motion restriction (if detected) and / or translation. The patient must be relaxed, so that active muscle contraction is not helping or hindering the engagement of the restrictive barrier.
2. **Contraction and control:** The patient is instructed to push actively but using a very gentle force away from the restrictive barrier against the practitioner's controlled, unyielding counterforce for 3–5 seconds. Too strong a contraction will recruit larger, multisegmental muscles and create difficulty in maintaining accurate localization. The practitioner should give clear instructions to the patient and be relaxed in order to facilitate patient relaxation.
3. **Relaxation:** The patient should be allowed to relax fully for several seconds.
4. **Re-engage the barrier:** Usually the restrictive barrier is perceived to change or recede, and the practitioner should take up the slack to re-engage this barrier.
5. **Repetition:** The procedure is typically performed 2–4 times.
6. **Re-examination:** This will determine whether the range or quality of motion has improved.

Box 62.1 shows common errors in MET application.

Box 62.1 Common errors in muscle energy application

- Joint barrier is overlocked.
- Patient pushes too hard.
- Patient's contraction duration is too short.
- The use of too few repetitions (wait for tissue change).
- Patient does not relax.
- Practitioner does not offer stable support of limb, region or patient.
- Practitioner allows movement during contraction phase.
- Practitioner is uncomfortable, awkward, poorly positioned, unbalanced or tense.

Spinal coupled motion

Many texts on MET emphasize the coupled motions that are common in different spinal regions and describe a diagnostic and treatment approach to address the planes of restricted motion in a segment (Mitchell Jr & Mitchell 1995; Greenman 2003). The traditional MET approach was based on the biomechanical principles of spinal coupled motion proposed by Fryette (1954), where type 1 'neutral' coupled motion was described as contralateral coupling of rotation and lateral flexion, and type 2 'non-neutral' coupled motion involved ipsilateral coupling of rotation and lateral flexion when the spine was in a non-neutral (flexed or extended) posture. Some authors advocate that the clinician should assess the spine for asymmetry of the transverse processes while the spine is in different postures (neutral, flexed or extended) and make inferences about motion restrictions from the relative position of these landmarks (Mitchell Jr & Mitchell 1995; Greenman 2003).

Nevertheless, the use of this model has been criticized for its prescriptive diagnostic labelling, which allows only three possible combinations of triplanar motion restriction: one type 1 (side-bending and rotation to opposite sides) and two type 2 combinations (side-bending and rotation to the same side with either flexion or extension), and has questionable inferences from static positional assessment (Gibbons & Tehan 1998; Fryer 2000, 2009). Spinal coupled motion in the lumbar region appears to be unpredictable, with variability between spinal levels and between individuals (Gibbons & Tehan 1998; Legaspi & Edmond 2007), and there is little evidence to indicate consistent patterns of thoracic motion coupling, although more rigorous studies are required (Sizer et al 2007). The original Fryette model described the cervical spine (C2–C7) as having only type 2 coupled motion. This notion is consistent with recent studies (Cook et al 2006; Ishii et al 2006), but others suggest that variability in the amount and direction of these movements is influenced by gender, age and cervical posture (Edmondston et al 2005; Malmstrom et al 2006).

Due to the unpredictability of coupled motions in the lumbar and thoracic regions and the possibility of variability in the cervical spine, this author recommends addressing motion restrictions that present on motion testing, rather than relying on assumptions based on coupled motion and static palpatory findings. If motion is introduced in the primary plane of restricted motion, spinal coupling will occur automatically and without the intervention of the practitioner. Therefore, the author recommends a pragmatic approach for addressing the primary motion restriction (in one or more planes) and suggests that associated coupled motions will occur without the practitioner intentionally addressing them.

Variations of application

The common application of MET previously described is a post-isometric technique primarily used to increase range of motion in a spinal segment. The author has used variations of MET to promote fluid drainage and pain relief in the acute joint and to promote proprioception and motor control.

Applications for acute dysfunctions

For an acutely painful joint with markedly restricted motion, the typical application of MET – where a restrictive barrier is engaged and an attempt is made to increase range of motion after each isometric effort – may be difficult because of patient apprehension and fear of pain. Further, such conditions may involve minor trauma to the spinal segment and inflammation of the joint capsule and surrounding tissues (Fryer 2003, 2011), although evidence of inflammation or effusion in the spinal joint is lacking (Fryer & Adams 2011). In acute conditions, the author has found it effective to use gentle isometric contraction against the resistance of the practitioner, alternating the contraction from right to left, with the joint in the neutral region of motion. Thus the joint is not near the painful barrier, and the patient can be relaxed and not fearful of experiencing pain. The repetitive contraction and relaxation phases are theorized to promote trans-synovial flow (moving fluid out of the effused joint by changing pressure gradients) and drainage of tissue fluid from around the joint. Additionally, the muscle contraction may stimulate muscle and joint mechanoreceptors to promote descending inhibition of pain, as previously discussed. As the patient becomes less fearful, the joint can be progressively positioned towards the restrictive barrier, and decrease in pain may allow a standard end-range MET to be performed.

Applications to promote proprioception and control

For a chronically painful joint or region, many patients appear to lose optimal positional sense and control and have difficulty in allowing the region to relax fully for passive motion to be applied. The author has used variations of MET that may be effective in promoting improved proprioception and motor control, and promoting confidence in contracting the muscles and moving the joint where patients are fearful because of ongoing or episodic pain. Initially, motion restrictions should be treated using conventional MET. A plane of motion should be chosen that is easy to manage and control (usually rotation is suitable) and gentle isometric contraction efforts towards neutral are performed through 'stages' of ranges of motion (e.g. in neutral, at 20°, at 40°, etc.). The patient should be relaxed so that the contraction phases and positions do not cause any pain.

Following successful (and painless) application as described above, gentle controlled isotonic (i.e. concentric, allowing motion and muscle shortening) contraction phases can be employed. Initially, the joint is placed at the end range (in one of the cardinal planes of rotation, lateral flexion, flexion or extension) and the patient is instructed to push gently *towards the end-range barrier* against the resistance of the practitioner. The first contraction is an isometric contraction, where no movement is allowed to occur. The joint is then repositioned approximately one-third of the range towards neutral and away from the barrier. The patient is requested a gain to push gently towards the barrier against the resistance of the practitioner and also to move slowly towards the end range under the control of the practitioner. This process is then repeated with the starting position in neutral. Repetitions can be performed with the patient progressively producing stronger contraction efforts. The procedure should cause no pain and produce a comfortable, consistent contraction and movement, and the patient should be relaxed and not apprehensive. The aim of the technique is for the patient to perform isotonic contractions of progressively increasing intensity against resistance through the full range of motion without pain, apprehension or fear.

Cervical spine

Assessment of the cervical region should include inspection of neck posture and head carriage, active and passive range of motion, palpation, orthopaedic tests where appropriate, and examination for segmental pain and dysfunction. Segmental examination may include palpation for tenderness, tissue abnormality and segmental motion. Passive lateral translation (an accessory motion analogous to the primary motion of lateral flexion or side-bending) is a useful diagnostic procedure to identify segmental motion restriction. Palpation of tenderness, restricted motion and abnormal end feel will all help to determine segmental side-bending restriction. Some authors recommend assessing lateral translation when the cervical spine is passively flexed and extended to assess the contribution of flexion and extension restriction; however, these motions can be assessed independently. In addition to motion assessment, translation may provoke tenderness and familiar pain from a symptomatic joint, so care should be taken to avoid aggravating a symptomatic segment.

For treatment, side-bending muscle activation force is easily controlled by the practitioner, although other directions can be used at the practitioner's discretion. Many authors recommend engaging the restrictive barriers in either cervical flexion or extension first, and then localizing side-bending (depending on whether lateral translation is most restricted in either of these positions during assessment) because this order of motion introduction is easily controlled and localized.

Typical cervical (C2–C7) segments

Although MET texts traditionally describe only type 2 multiplanar restrictions, procedures may be adapted and applied to restrictions in a single plane (side-bending, rotation, flexion or extension) or in multiple planes, depending on the clinical findings. In general, the practitioner should treat the typical cervical segments before the upper cervical complex (C0–C2).

Procedure for restriction of flexion, side-bending and rotation (Fig. 62.1, main photo)

1. The patient is in supine position. Stand or sit at the head of the table.
2. Place the 1st–3rd fingertips of both hands on the right and left articular pillars of the upper segment (e.g. the C3 pillars for a C3–C4 dysfunction).
3. Flex the neck to the level of dysfunction. Introduce side-bending / lateral translation until the first barrier at that segment is engaged. Fine-tune with very subtle additional leverage (i.e. rotation, more / less flexion or extension) as required.

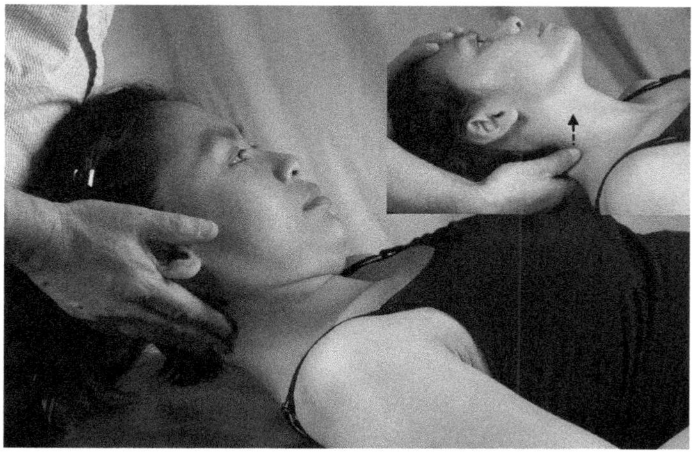

Figure 62.1 **Muscle energy technique for the typical cervical (C2–C7) segments.** *Main photo:* for restriction of flexion, side-bending and rotation. The restricted motion barriers are engaged in one or more planes, and the patient gently pushes the head back towards the midline against the unyielding counterforce of the practitioner. *Inset photo:* for restriction of extension, side-bending and rotation. Note pincer hold on articular pillars producing segmental extension (dotted arrow).

4. Request the patient to push the head gently towards the midline (side-bending away from the restrictive barrier) *or* extend against your unyielding resistance for 3–5 seconds.
5. Allow the patient to relax for a few seconds.
6. Re-engage the new barrier by taking up any slack in side-bending or extension that has developed since the contraction and relaxation phases.
7. Repeat 2–4 times.
8. Re-examine.

Procedure for restriction of extension, side-bending and rotation (Fig. 62.1, inset photo)

1. The patient is in supine position. Stand or sit at the head of the table.
2. Two hand positions are suitable for introducing segmental extension:
   a. Place the fingertips (1st–3rd) of both hands on the right and left articular pillars of the upper segment (e.g. the C3 pillars for a C3–C4 dysfunction).
   b. Place the index and middle finger of one hand on one articular pillar, with the thumb on the opposite pillar of the lower segment. The other hand contacts the patient's head. This 'pincer' hold is useful for introducing highly localized extension (without the need to extend the neck) and lateral translation, as well as for creating a local fulcrum for lateral flexion.
3. Extend the segment by lifting the fingertips on the pillars until the extension barrier is palpated. Introduce side-bending (using the cephalic hand to introduce motion and the fingers or thumb of the pincer hand as a fulcrum) and / or lateral translation (using the pincer contact) until the barrier is engaged. Fine-tune with very subtle additional leverage (i.e. rotation, more / less flexion or extension) as required.

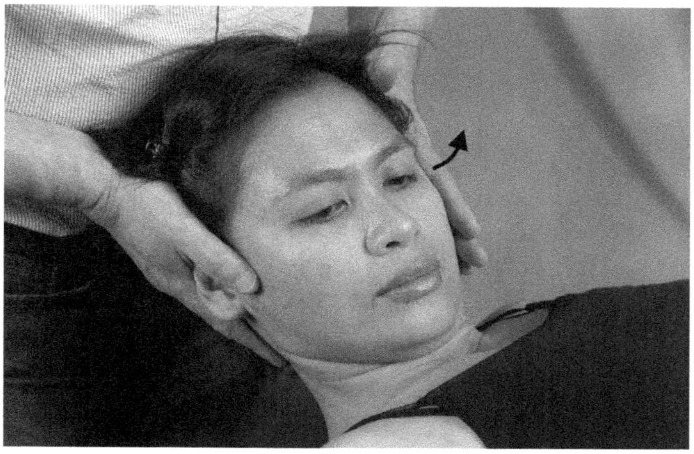

Figure 62.2 **Muscle energy technique for the C1–C2 segment.** The neck is flexed to minimize rotation below C1, and the C1 segment is rotated to the restrictive barrier. The patient is instructed to rotate gently towards the midline (arrow) against the unyielding counterforce of the practitioner.

4. Request the patient to push the head gently towards the midline (side-bending away from the restrictive barrier) *or* flex against your unyielding resistance for 3–5 seconds.
5. Allow the patient to relax for a few seconds.
6. Re-engage the new barrier by taking up any slack in side-bending or extension that has developed since the contraction and relaxation phases.
7. Repeat 2–4 times.
8. Re-examine.

Atlanto-axial (C1–C2) segment

The primary movement at the C1–C2 segment is rotation and, although some authors advocate addressing additional planes (Mitchell Jr & Mitchell 1995), in the experience of the author the engagement of rotation alone is highly effective. For examination and treatment, the neck can be placed in full flexion, which relatively 'locks' the lower cervical joint segments and localizes available rotation to the atlanto-axial segment (Oginee et al 2006).

Procedure for restricted C1–C2 rotation (Fig. 62.2)

1. The patient is in supine position. Stand or sit at the head of the table.
2. The fingertips of both hands are placed on the articular pillars of the upper segment, with palms cradling the head. The chest or abdomen can also be used to support your hands.
3. Flex the patient's neck fully (until a sense of resistance) to 'lock' the middle and lower cervical spine. Maintain the flexion and rotate the neck until the barrier of restricted rotation is engaged. Fine-tune with additional leverages (i.e. side-bending, flexion, extension) as determined with palpation.

4. Request the patient to rotate the head gently towards the midline (rotating away from the restrictive barrier) against your unyielding resistance for 3–5 seconds.
5. Allow the patient to relax for a few seconds.
6. Re-engage the new barrier by taking up any slack in rotation that has developed since the contraction and relaxation phases.
7. Repeat 2–4 times.
8. Re-examine.

Occipito-atlanto (C0–C1) segment

The primary movements at the C0–C1 segment are flexion and extension, but examination and treatment of the restricted side-bending and rotation can be clinically rewarding. Techniques can be used to address a single plane (usually flexion or extension) or multiple plans (contralateral side-bending and rotation, with flexion or extension).

Procedure for single-plane restricted flexion (or extension) (Fig. 62.3, main photo)

1. The patient is in supine position. Stand or sit at the head of the table.
2. Place one hand under the occiput with the fingertips palpating the suboccipital tissues close to the occipito-atlanto joint line and the other hand resting on the patient's forehead.
3. Gently flex (or extend) the head without engaging movement in the cervical spine until the initial sense of barrier at the C0–C1 segment is palpated.
4. Request the patient to extend (or flex) the head gently by stating the instruction to 'nod the head upwards' or 'look upwards' (or downwards) against your unyielding resistance for 3–5 seconds.
5. Allow the patient to relax for several seconds.
6. Re-engage the new barrier by taking up any slack in flexion (or extension) that has developed since contraction and relaxation phases.
7. Repeat 2–4 times.
8. Re-examine.

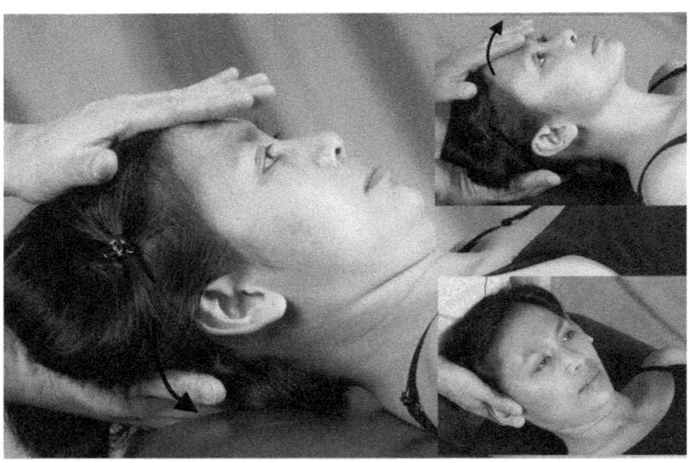

Figure 62.3 Muscle energy technique for the C0–C1 segment. *Main photo:* treatment of single-plane restricted flexion. The practitioner carefully flexes the head to the barrier, and the patient gently extends the head (arrow) against the unyielding counterforce of the practitioner. *Inset photo above:* treatment of single-plane restriction, extension. The practitioner carefully extends the head to the barrier, and the patient gently flexes the head (arrow). *Inset photo below:* multiple plane restriction, emphasizing side-bending. The practitioner carefully flexes (or extends) the head to the barrier, and then introduces side-bending, lateral translation and/or rotation to address the motion barriers. The patient gently pushes away from the barrier in side-bending, flexion or extension.

Procedure for multiple-plane restriction: flexion (or extension), lateral flexion and contralateral rotation (Fig. 62.3, inset photo below)

1. The patient is in supine position. Stand or sit at the head of the table.
2. Cradle the occiput and head using both hands, with the fingertips palpating the suboccipital muscles near the occipito-atlanto joint line.
3. Gently flex (or extend) the head until the initial sense of barrier is palpated.
4. Introduce side-bending by a combination of gentle side-bending and lateral translation of the head on the neck until the barrier is engaged. Fine-tune with subtle contralateral rotation, if required.
5. Request the patient to push the head gently towards the midline (side-bending away from the restrictive barrier) against your unyielding resistance for 3–5 seconds. Alternatively, a flexion (or extension) activating force can be used.
6. Allow the patient to relax for several seconds.
7. Re-engage the new barrier by taking up any slack in flexion (or extension) or side-bending that has developed since the contraction and relaxation phases.
8. Repeat 2–4 times.
9. Re-examine.

Thoracic spine

Assessment of the thoracic region should include inspection of trunk posture when standing and seated, active and passive gross motion, palpation for tenderness and tissue texture abnormality, orthopaedic tests where appropriate and examination for segmental pain and dysfunction. Assessment of segmental motion can include short-lever, posterior–anterior accessory motion (vertebral 'springing' with the patient prone), as well as assessment of cardinal plane motion (flexion, extension, rotation, side-bending), which can be performed with the patient seated. When seated, the patient should sit upright because a slumped posture will restrict passive rotation and side-bending.

The techniques described below illustrate MET applications to the thoracic spine for segmental motion restriction, but the principles can be applied to any combination of motion restriction by modifying the technique. Although only seated techniques are illustrated in this section, MET can also be applied with the patient in the lateral recumbent, prone or supine positions.

For mid–low thoracic techniques, the patient's arms are best if folded with the hands on the opposite shoulders. Lateral and anterior–posterior translation of the patient's body is useful for precise localization and fine-tuning of side-bending, flexion and extension barriers. For upper thoracic segments (T1–T4), the patient's head and neck or the hands interlocked around the patient's neck are often used as levers to produce localization of motion in the upper thoracic segments. Many cervical techniques can be modified for the upper thoracic region.

Restriction of flexion combinations

Procedure for restriction of flexion, with or without concurrent restrictions of rotation and side-bending (Fig. 62.4, mid–low thoracic segments; inset: upper thoracic segments)

1. The patient is seated with arms folded; stand behind the patient. Palpate the involved segment.
2. For mid–low thoracic segments, contact the patient's arms or elbows and gently guide the patient into trunk flexion until the involved segment starts to flex. For upper thoracic segments, gently flex the head and neck until the involved segment starts to flex. Subtle posterior translation of the trunk may be used to localize flexion motion further to the involved segment. Side-bending and rotation to restricted barriers can also be introduced using a small amount of lateral translation.
3. Request the patient to try to straighten or extend the trunk (mid–low thoracic) or neck (upper thoracic) gently against your unyielding resistance for 3–5 seconds. Alternatively, a side-bending activating force can be used when side-bending restriction is apparent.
4. Allow the patient to relax for several seconds.
5. Re-engage the new barrier by taking up any slack in flexion or side-bending that has developed since the contraction and relaxation phases.
6. Repeat 2–4 times.
7. Re-examine.

Restriction of extension combinations

Procedure for restriction of extension, with or without concurrent restrictions of rotation and side-bending (Fig. 62.5, mid–low thoracic segments; inset: upper thoracic segments)

1. For mid–low thoracic segments, the patient is seated with the arms crossed and hands resting on the opposite shoulders. For upper thoracic segments, the patient is seated with the hands interlocked around the neck. Stand behind the patient and palpate the involved segment.
2. Using the patient's elbows as a lever, gently extend the trunk until the involved segment starts to extend. Subtle anterior translation may be used to localize extension to the involved segment. Side-bending and rotation to restricted barriers can be introduced by using the head and neck leverage, or by introducing a small amount of lateral translation.
3. Request the patient to push the trunk gently forwards (flexion) against your unyielding resistance for 3–5 seconds.
4. Allow the patient to relax for several seconds.
5. Re-engage the new barrier by taking up any slack in extension and side-bending that has developed since the contraction and relaxation phases.
6. Repeat 2–4 times.
7. Re-examine.

Alternative procedure for restriction of extension, with or without concurrent restrictions of rotation and side-bending (Fig. 62.6, mid–low thoracic segments; inset: upper thoracic segments)

This procedure is useful when the patient is bigger than the practitioner and when the upper thoracic region is stiff and flexed and requires stronger leverage to produce extension.

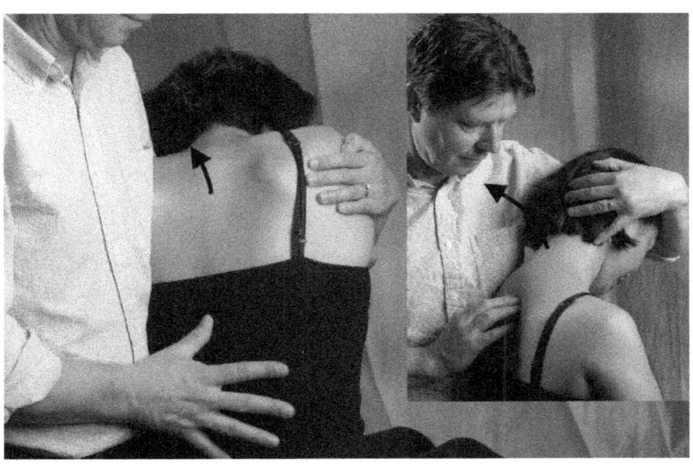

Figure 62.4 Muscle energy technique for restricted flexion in the thoracic spine. *Main photo:* treatment in the mid-low thoracic region. The practitioner carefully flexes the trunk to the barrier, and the patient gently extends (arrow) against the unyielding counterforce of the practitioner. *Inset photo:* treatment of the upper thoracic region. The practitioner carefully flexes the head until motion is palpated at the restricted segment, and the patient gently extends the neck (arrow) against the unyielding counterforce of the practitioner.

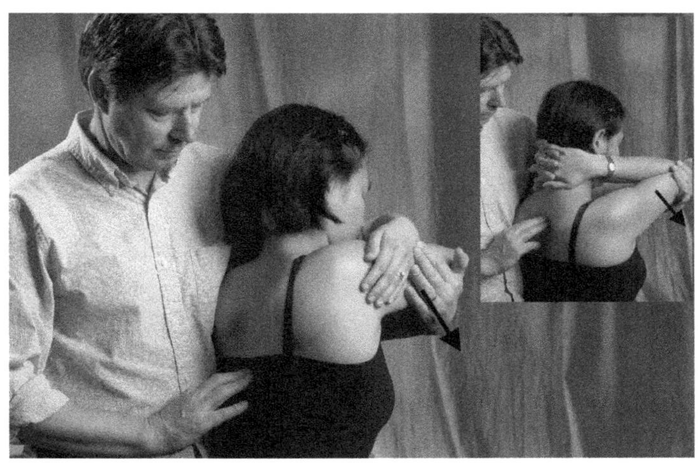

Figure 62.5 Muscle energy technique for restricted extension in the thoracic spine. *Main photo:* treatment in the mid–low thoracic region. The practitioner carefully extends the trunk to the barrier, and the patient gently flexes (arrow) against the unyielding counterforce of the practitioner. *Inset photo:* treatment of the upper thoracic region. The practitioner carefully extends the head and neck until motion is palpated at the restricted segment, and the patient gently flexes the neck (arrow) against the unyielding counterforce of the practitioner. Note the different hand holds for each region.

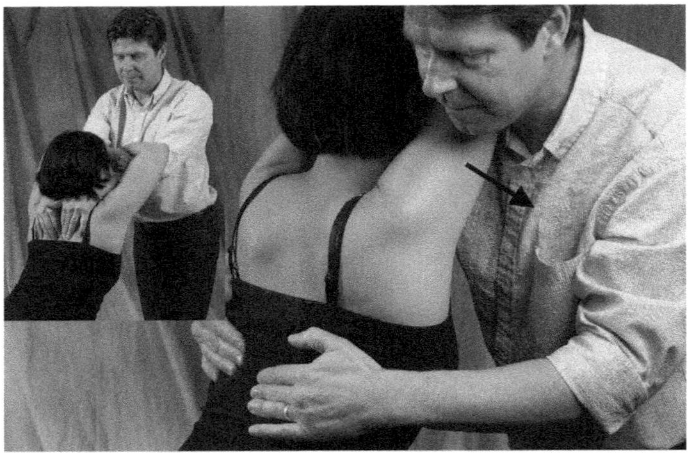

Figure 62.6 Muscle energy technique for restricted extension in the thoracic spine (alternative procedure). This technique is useful for small practitioners and/or large patients. *Main photo:* treatment in the mid–low thoracic region. The practitioner carefully extends the trunk to the barrier by drawing the segment anteriorly, and the patient gently flexes (arrow) against the unyielding counterforce of the practitioner. *Inset photo:* treatment of the upper thoracic region. The practitioner carefully extends the upper thoracic segment by drawing the segment anteriorly and elevating until extension motion is palpated at the restricted segment, and the patient gently flexes the neck against their arms and the unyielding counterforce of the practitioner. Note the different hand holds for each region.

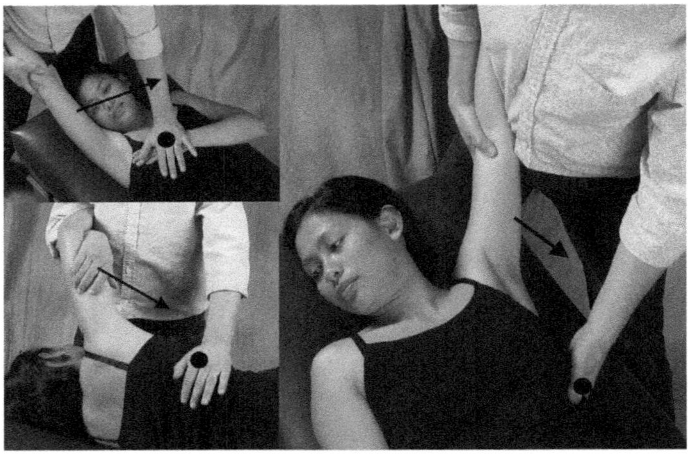

Figure 62.7 Muscle energy technique for restricted rib inhalation or exhalation motion. *Main photo:* treatment of mid–low ribs in supine. The practitioner stabilizes (circle) either the rib below for inhalation restrictions or the involved rib for exhalation restrictions. The patient's arm is abducted and elevated until the tension is palpated at the rib and intercostal and associated muscles are stretched. The patient pushes the arm down against the unyielding counterforce of the practitioner (arrow) against the unyielding counterforce of the practitioner. *Inset photo below:* treatment of mid–low ribs in lateral recumbent position. *Inset photo above:* treatment of upper ribs in supine.

1. For mid–low thoracic treatment, the patient is seated on a table facing the practitioner with the arms either folded or resting on a pillow over the practitioner's shoulder. Your arms should link around the patient so that your fingers contact each side of the involved segment (Fig. 62.6, main photo).
2. For upper thoracic segment treatment, the patient is seated on a low table or chair with the arms folded and head resting on the forearms. Stand in front of patient and thread your arms under the patient's forearms so that your fingers contact each side of the involved segment (Fig. 62.6, inset photo).
3. Gently raise your arms and shift your weight onto your back leg to translate the patient forward and produce localized extension at the involved segment. Your fingers can be used as a fulcrum to assist this localization. Subtle side-bending and rotation to restricted barriers can be introduced by shifting your stance.
4. Request the patient to push the head or trunk gently forwards (flexion) against your unyielding resistance for 3–5 seconds.
5. Allow the patient to relax for several seconds.
6. Re-engage the new barrier by taking up any slack in extension and side-bending that has developed since the contraction and relaxation phases.
7. Repeat 2–4 times.
8. Re-examine.

Rib cage

Assessment of the rib cage involves inspection for thoracic cage deformity, palpation for thoracic cage contour and symmetrical expansion during full inhalation and assessment of rib mobility by accessory motion or gentle 'springing' techniques. Some authors divide rib dysfunction into two categories: 'respiratory' dysfunctions, which are restrictions of inhalation or exhalation motion, and 'structural' dysfunctions, which are claimed to be rib 'subluxation' and associated with considerable pain and limited motion (Mitchell Jr & Mitchell 1998; Greenman 2003). The proposed aetiology of these structural dysfunctions is dubious, but may involve sprain of the costovertebral or costotransverse joints. In clinical practice, MET is often effective in reducing pain and improving motion. With the exception of an acutely painful rib dysfunction, rib dysfunctions should be treated following treatment of thoracic spine dysfunction, as rib restrictions may occur secondarily to thoracic dysfunction.

Restriction of inhalation

The following technique is based on the principle of stretching the intercostal muscles below the restricted rib to promote greater movement of that rib during inhalation. Arm flexion is used to encourage pump handle motion of the upper ribs, and arm abduction is used to encourage bucket-handle motion of the middle and lower ribs. The technique can also be performed with the patient sitting or in the lateral recumbent position.

Procedure for restricted inhalation motion (Fig. 62.7)

1. The patient is in supine position. Stand at the side of the table.
2. Fix on the anterior or lateral shaft of the rib below the affected rib (i.e. rib 9 when rib 8 is restricted) with the thenar or hypothenar part of your hand (broad contact is most comfortable; a towel can be used for padding).
3. Elevate the rib using leverage on the patient's ipsilateral arm (upper ribs arm flexion; middle and lower ribs –

arm abduction) to a position of comfortable stretch, while maintaining tension on the lower rib.

4. Request the patient to inhale fully and hold, and then to push the arm gently down against your unyielding resistance for 3–5 seconds.
5. Allow the patient to breathe out and relax for several seconds.
6. Re-engage the new barrier by taking up any slack in abduction and tension on the lower rib that has developed since the contraction and relaxation phases.
7. Repeat 2–4 times.
8. Re-examine.

Restriction of exhalation

This technique uses a myofascial approach based on the principle of stretching the intercostal muscles *above* the restricted rib (in contrast to *below* the rib for restrictions of inhalation) so as to promote greater movement of that rib during exhalation. The same technique is used to treat restricted inhalation (see above), except that for exhalation restriction the practitioner fixes the shaft of the involved rib to encourage rib depression and stretch the intercostal muscles superior to it (see Fig. 62.7).

Elevated first rib

Techniques have been described for an elevated first rib, in which the rib is held in an elevated position, has restriction of exhalation motion and is associated with marked tissue hypertonicity and tenderness (Mitchell Jr & Mitchell 1998; Greenman 2003). This dysfunction has been postulated to involve a superior subluxation of the joint with shortening of the attaching scalene muscles, but this aetiology is purely speculative. The following technique is proposed to operate by reciprocal inhibition of the scalene muscles, but the guiding downward pressure on the rib during patient relaxation may contribute to the success of the technique. It is helpful to alternate the isometric contraction with the patient taking a deep breath, an exhalation and then relaxation.

Procedure for elevated first rib (Fig. 62.8)

1. The patient is seated. Stand behind the patient. Alternatively, this technique may be performed with the patient supine and the practitioner sitting at the head of the table.
2. Contact the posterior shaft of the first rib through the trapezius muscle with the thumb and the superior aspect of the shaft with the first phalange or fingers. Exert a caudal and anterior force on the posterior rib shaft to guide it downwards.
3. Side-bend the patient's neck to the side of the involved rib just before the motion of the rib is sensed.
4. Request the patient to push the head gently towards the midline (side-bending away from the side of the rib) against your unyielding resistance for 3–5 seconds.
5. Allow the patient to relax for a few seconds.
6. Re-engage the new barrier by taking up any slack in rib depression or side-bending while maintaining the caudal and anterior force on the posterior rib shaft.

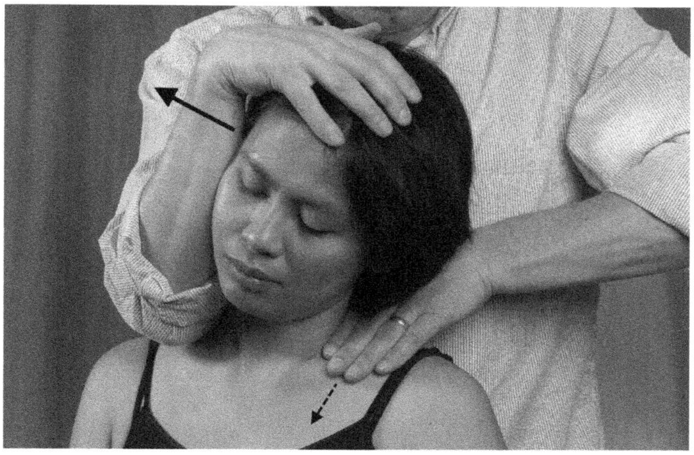

Figure 62.8 Muscle energy technique for an elevated first rib. Note the caudal and anterior pressure applied to the posterior shaft of the first rib (dotted arrow) and the side-bending of the patient's neck to relax the tissues around the rib. The patient uses a gentle side-bending contraction away from the side of the rib (arrow) against the unyielding counterforce of the practitioner.

7. Repeat 2–4 times.
8. Re-examine.

Acute rib dysfunction

Muscle energy authors have described a number of 'structural' rib dysfunctions that are proposed to be 'subluxations' where the normal joint apposition is disrupted (Mitchell Jr & Mitchell 1998; Greenman 2003). The author suggests that the underlying process may in fact be joint sprain, effusion and tissue inflammation. An acute rib dysfunction may present with pain around the costotransverse joint that becomes intense on trunk rotation and inhalation effort. There is often tissue hypertonicity and tenderness of the iliocostalis muscles around the rib angle, and there may be pain and restricted motion on accessory movement testing ('springing') of the rib.

In the author's experience, structural rib techniques are useful for acutely painful rib dysfunction. These techniques may activate descending pain inhibition pathways and improve tissue drainage around the inflamed joint (Fryer 2011). The author often combines indirect techniques (Greenman 2003) with MET when the joint is acutely painful. The following procedure is a modification of the 'posteriorly subluxed' rib dysfunction technique (Mitchell Jr & Mitchell 1998; Greenman 2003) (Fig. 62.9):

1. The patient is seated with the hand of the involved side resting on the opposite shoulder. Stand behind the patient with one hand on the patient's elbow and the other palpating the angle of the involved rib through the iliocostalis muscles.
2. Elevate the patient's elbow until localization of motion is palpated at the rib angle. Then apply moderately firm pressure to the rib angle in a medial and anterior direction.
3. Request the patient to push the elbow gently laterally against your unyielding resistance for 3–5 seconds. Alternatively, the direction may be upward or medially,

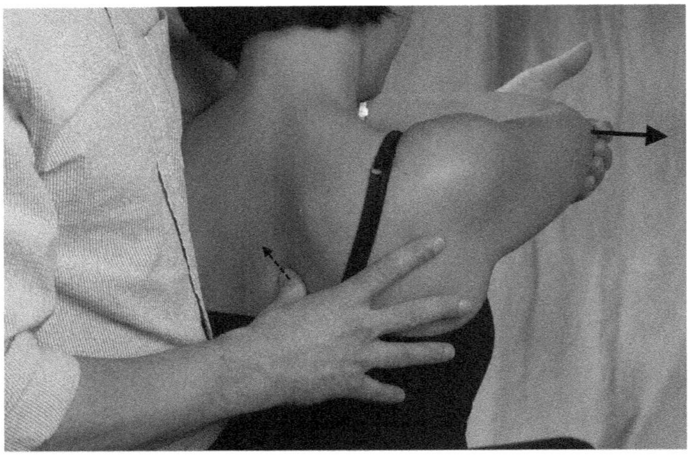

Figure 62.9 Muscle energy technique for an acutely painful rib dysfunction. The practitioner elevates the patient's elbow until localization of motion is palpated at the posterior rib angle of the involved rib. Moderately firm pressure is maintained over the rib angle in a medial and anterior direction (dotted arrow). The patient gently pushes the elbow laterally against the unyielding counterforce of the practitioner (arrow).

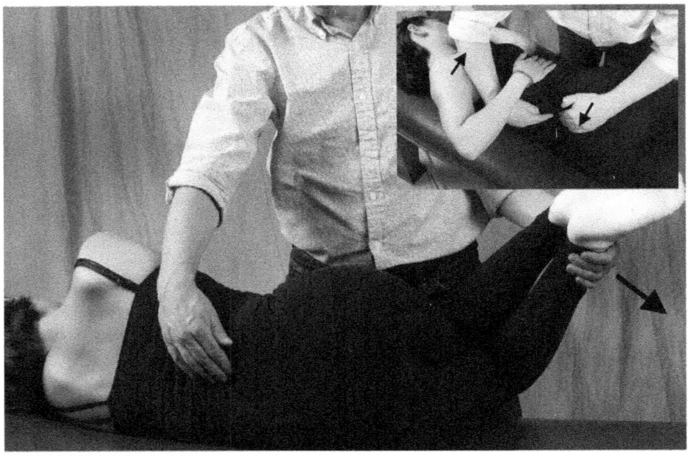

Figure 62.10 Muscle energy technique for restriction of uniplanar motions in the lumbar spine. Using the patient's legs as a lever, the lumbar spine can be positioned at the barrier of flexion, extension, or side-bending motion restrictions. *Main photo:* treatment of restricted right side-bending. The patient is instructed to push the legs gently down (arrow) against the unyielding resistance of the practitioner. *Inset photo:* treatment of rotation restriction. The restricted segment is positioned at the motion barrier, and the patient is instructed to 'untwist' gently (arrows).

depending on which direction creates a sense of tissue contraction and localization.

4. Allow the patient to relax for several seconds.
5. Re-engage the new barrier or tissue tension that has developed since the contraction and relaxation phases.
6. Repeat 2–4 times.
7. Re-examine.

Lumbar spine

Assessment of the lumbar region should include inspection of trunk posture when the patient is standing and seated, active motion to determine range and pain, orthopaedic and neurological tests where appropriate and examination for segmental pain and dysfunction with palpation. Segmental motion testing is often performed with the patient in the lateral recumbent position, and with the practitioner using the flexed hips and legs as levers for flexion and extension. In the author's experience, assessment of accessory motion or facet glide using posterior–anterior overpressure when the patient is in the 'sphinx' position (i.e. prone, with the upper body resting on the elbows or straightened arms to extend the lumbar spine) can also be useful to confirm segmental restriction of extension.

The techniques below illustrate MET applications to the lumbar spine for segmental motion restrictions of flexion and extension, but the principles can be applied to any combination of motion restriction by modification of the technique. Although only lateral recumbent techniques are illustrated in this section, MET can be applied with the patient in the seated, prone or supine position.

Restriction of uniplanar motion

Although most MET texts describe techniques for combinations of motion restriction based on the Fryette model of coupled motion, joint restrictions may be detected in only a single plane; however, techniques are easily developed for these situations based on the principles of application described above (Fig. 62.10).

Restriction of flexion combinations

The following technique is for restriction of flexion, with concurrent restrictions of ipsilateral rotation and side-bending. Although the technique may appear awkward, with practice it is comfortable for both patient and practitioner, and allows good control and localization of flexion and side-bending of a lumbar segment. The technique may be useful to promote optimal flexion (upward and forward gliding) of the involved facet joint.

Procedure for restriction of flexion, rotation and side-bending (Fig. 62.11)

1. The patient is in the prone position. Stand to the side of the patient, bend the patient's knees, and move and rotate the patient's hips to a semi-Sims position.
2. Using the thighs and pelvis as levers, flex and extend the spine until the involved segment starts to flex. Carefully lower the legs to localize side-bending to the segment (be careful to support the patient's thigh with your thigh to avoid discomfort against the edge of the table).
3. Request the patient to lift the legs gently against your unyielding resistance for 3–5 seconds.
4. Allow the patient to relax for several seconds.
5. Re-engage the new barrier by taking up any slack in flexion or side-bending that has developed since the contraction and relaxation phases.
6. Repeat 2–4 times.
7. Re-examine.

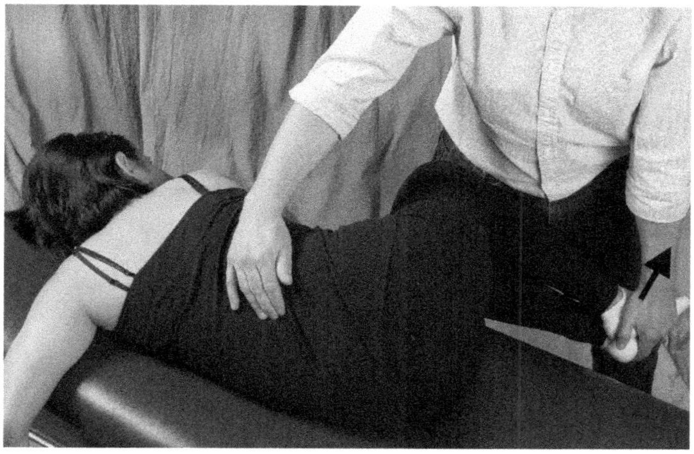

Figure 62.11 **Muscle energy technique for restriction of flexion combinations in the lumbar spine.** The technique illustrated is for restriction of segmental flexion, left rotation and left side-bending. The patient is repositioned from the prone position to the semi-Sims position by flexion of the knees and rotation of the pelvis. Flexion motion is localized to the involved segment by flexing the hips, followed by side-bending by carefully lowering the legs. The patient gently lifts the legs (arrow) against the unyielding counterforce of the practitioner.

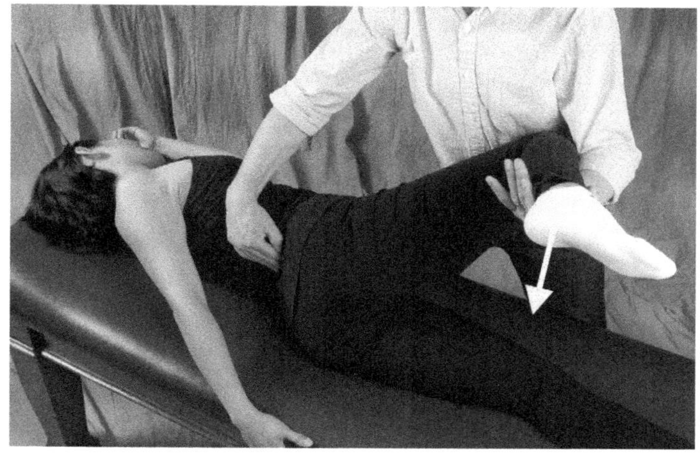

Figure 62.12 **Muscle energy technique for restriction of extension combinations in the lumbar spine.** Localization of lumbar extension is produced by extension of the leg and upper body, with further extension obtained by translating the segment anteriorly; localization of rotation is achieved by moving the shoulder posteriorly to rotate the trunk, with the patient anchoring the shoulder by holding the table; localization of side-bending is created by lifting the leg, being careful not to lose extension of the spine. The patient gently pushes the leg toward the floor (arrow) against the unyielding counterforce of the practitioner.

Restriction of extension combinations

Restriction of segmental extension in the lumbar spine is considered clinically relevant because it reverses the normal lumbar lordosis and shock absorption of the region. The following technique is a procedure for restriction of extension, with or without concurrent restrictions of rotation and side-bending. Lifting the patient's leg may sometimes be awkward, so it may be helpful for the practitioner to hold the leg close to their body (without allowing hip and lumbar flexion) while positioning the patient in a degree of side-bending with an adjustable table or pillows.

Procedure for restriction of extension, rotation and side-bending (Fig. 62.12)

1. The patient is in the lateral recumbent position on the side of the uninvolved facet. Stand in front of the patient.
2. Palpate the involved segment and localize extension by extending the leg on the table and gliding the upper body posteriorly. Using the fingertips of both hands (sliding around the patient's waist), the involved segment can be translated anteriorly using the fingertips to localize extension further.
3. Rotation can be localized to the segment by posterior translation of the shoulder. If possible, the patient can hold the edge of the table to maintain the rotated position.
4. Side-bending can be localized to the segment by lifting the patient's leg to produce motion in the pelvis and then side-bending of the lumbar spine.
5. Request the patient to press the leg gently downward against your unyielding resistance for 3–5 seconds.
6. Allow the patient to relax for several seconds.
7. Re-engage the new barriers by taking up any slack in extension or side-bending that has developed since the contraction and relaxation phases.
8. Repeat 2–4 times.
9. Re-examine.

Pelvic girdle

Authors of traditional MET texts described a large range of pelvic somatic dysfunctions – subdivided into pubic, sacroiliac and iliosacral dysfunctions – based on a biomechanical pelvic model proposed by Mitchell Sr (Mitchell Jr & Mitchell 1999; Greenman 2003). The biomechanical model and associated dysfunctions were developed largely through clinical observation and have been a catalyst for the development of MET. However, the validity of these dysfunctions as real clinical entities is dubious, and these dysfunctions may instead reflect the individual variability of sacroiliac joint anatomy and the small motions available (Fryer 2000, 2011). Furthermore, the reliability and validity of most motion and static symmetry diagnostic tests used to detect pelvic dysfunctions are dubious. For instance, pelvic girdle symmetry may be influenced by pelvic muscle tone (Bendova et al 2007), and many techniques purported to address articular dysfunction might improve pelvic girdle symmetry through stretching or activating myofascial tissues.

The traditional MET approach involves systematically detecting and treating pubic, sacroiliac and iliosacral dysfunctions to improve motion and symmetry of the pelvis. The focus has been on improving motion in dysfunctions with restricted motion; however, hypermobility of sacroiliac joints and lack of stabilizing mechanisms may be a greater contributor to pelvic pain (Hossain & Nokes 2005). The author therefore recommends a three-tiered approach to treating the pelvic region: (1) treating myofascial imbalance (treating muscles for length and strength and deactivating TrPs), (2) treating articular dysfunction (when the joint appears to be hypomobile or painful, guided by the plane of the joint as assessed with palpation) and (3) improving pelvic stability (strength and control of pelvic muscles). It is beyond the scope of this chapter to explore these issues and treatment approaches, however.

Several techniques are described below to correct apparent articular dysfunction (that may also be acting on myofascial tissues), which the author has found useful in clinical practice. It should be noted that static pelvic torsion is common and is typically unrelated to dysfunction or pain; restriction of motion should be considered only where there are clinical signs suggesting dysfunction other than asymmetry.

Restriction of innominate anterior rotation

A restriction of anterior rotation of the innominate might be considered when pelvic torsion is identified with signs of dysfunction (asymmetrical motion on springing and accessory motion tests, pain and positive pain provocation tests) and when the involved side appears to be posteriorly rotated (superior anterior superior iliac spine (ASIS) and medial malleoli relative to the other side with the patient supine; inferior posterior superior iliac spine (PSIS) with the patient prone). MET authors refer to this dysfunction as a 'posterior innominate,' but the author recommends avoiding terminology that promotes obsolete 'bone-out-of-place' concepts because such terminology may promote inappropriate beliefs, fear and dependence on treatment in susceptible patients.

Careful localization of motion to the sacroiliac joint is recommended for the success of the technique and may stimulate joint proprioceptors and subsequent neurological effects. However, in cases of long-term, pain-free stiffness, the author uses stronger end-range mobilizing forces. The technique can also be performed with the patient in the lateral recumbent or supine position.

Procedure for restriction of innominate anterior rotation (Fig. 62.13)

1. The patient is in the prone position. Stand on the side to be treated.
2. Monitor the sacroiliac joint using three fingers (one on the PSIS and two medial to it to cover the sacrum).
3. Slightly abduct the thigh (to promote a loose-packed position), and then extend the thigh until localization is palpated at the sacroiliac joint. Localize the motion to the point just before the sacrum begins to move.
4. Request the patient to push the thigh gently back to the table against your unyielding counterforce for 3–5 seconds.
5. Allow the patient to relax for a few seconds.
6. Re-engage the new barrier by taking up any slack in hip extension that has developed since contraction and relaxation phases to localize to the sacroiliac joint again.
7. Repeat 2–4 times.
8. Re-examine.

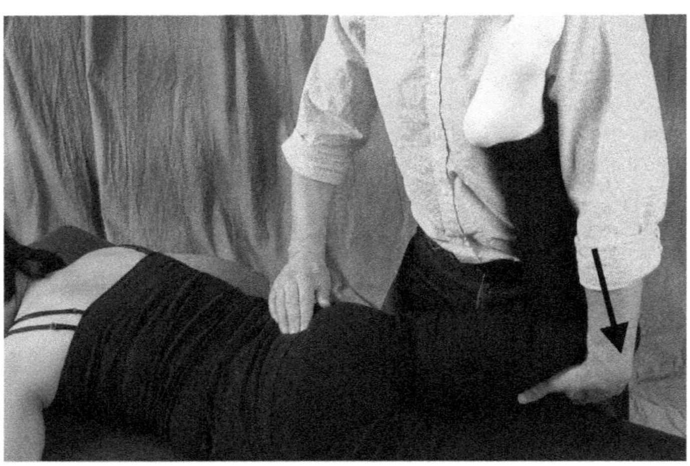

Figure 62.13 Muscle energy technique for restriction of innominate anterior rotation. The practitioner abducts the thigh slightly and then extends until localization of motion is palpated at the sacroiliac region (before the sacrum starts to move). The patient gently pushes the thigh towards the table (arrow) against the unyielding counterforce of the practitioner.

Restriction of innominate posterior rotation

A restriction of posterior rotation of the innominate might be considered when pelvic torsion (static asymmetry) is identified with other signs of dysfunction (e.g. regional pain, positive pain provocation tests, asymmetrical motion on springing, and accessory motion tests) and when the involved side appears to be anteriorly rotated (inferior ASIS and medial malleoli relative to the other side with the patient supine; superior PSIS with the patient prone). This dysfunction may be clinically relevant because posterior rotation of the innominate is an important adaptation to the forces of gravity during one-legged stance and contributes to the self-locking mechanism of the pelvis (Hungerford et al 2004). MET authors refer to this dysfunction as an 'anterior innominate', but the author recommends avoiding this terminology for the reasons explained above. Careful localization of motion to the sacroiliac joint may be important for the success of the technique, but, in cases of long-term, pain-free stiffness, the author uses stronger end-range mobilizing forces. The technique can also be performed with the patient in the prone or supine position.

Procedure for restriction of innominate posterior rotation (Fig. 62.14)

1. Patient is laterally recumbent, lying on the uninvolved side. Stand facing the patient.
2. Monitor the sacroiliac joint using three fingers of one hand (one on the PSIS and two medial to it to cover the sacrum).
3. Slightly abduct the thigh (to promote a loose-packed position), and then flex the hip and knee until localization is palpated at the sacroiliac joint (being careful not to lose the slight abduction). Monitor the joint while fine-tuning hip flexion and extension to localize the motion to the point just before the sacrum begins to move. The patient's knee or foot can be stabilized against your hip or stomach.
4. Request the patient to push the thigh gently back against your unyielding resistance to extend the hip for 3–5 seconds.
5. Allow the patient to relax for a few seconds.
6. Re-engage the new barrier by taking up any slack in hip flexion that has developed since contraction and relaxation phases to localize to the sacroiliac joint again.
7. Repeat 2–4 times.
8. Re-examine.

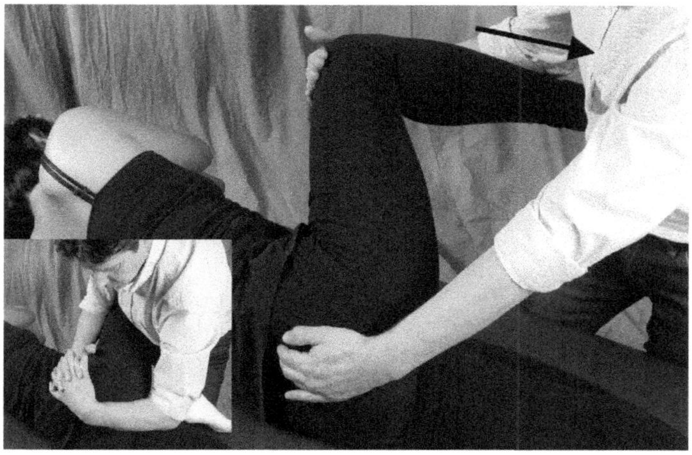

Figure 62.14 Muscle energy technique for restriction of innominate posterior rotation. The practitioner flexes the hip until motion is localized at the sacroiliac joint (before the sacrum starts to move). *Main photo:* the patient gently produces an extension effort of the hip by pushing the foot or thigh (arrow) against the unyielding counterforce of the practitioner. *Inset photo:* alternative hand hold to produce stronger articulatory forces for posterior rotation.

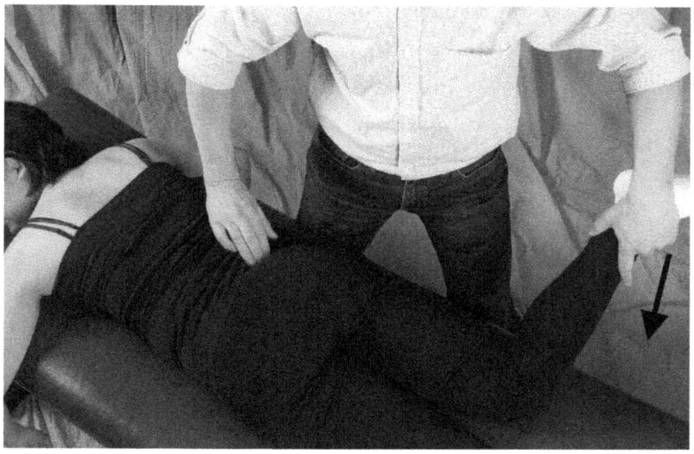

Figure 62.15 Muscle energy sacroiliac 'gapping' technique. The practitioner palpates the sacroiliac region and internally rotates the hip until motion is localized at the joint (just before the sacrum starts to move). The patient gently pushes the foot and leg into external rotation (arrow) against the unyielding counterforce of the practitioner.

Sacroiliac 'gapping' technique

This technique has been used to promote motion and tissue relaxation around the sacroiliac joint. It is unlikely that true joint gapping or separation is possible using manual techniques, but, in the author's experience, this technique appears to have clinical utility and may cause tissue relaxation and pain reduction by activating joint and muscle mechanoreceptors and descending pain inhibitory pathways. The technique utilizes the leverage of hip internal rotation to 'gap' the posterior aspect of the joint (Fig. 62.15).

Techniques for Myofascial Tissues

The following sections describe MET for lengthening and desensitizing myofascial tissue. Due to space limitations of this chapter, techniques will be described only for muscles that are, in the opinion of the author, most clinically relevant. However, the reader will be able to apply the principles of MET to any muscle that warrants treatment. (See Ch 59 for detailed descriptions of myofascial TrPs and associated diagnostic findings.)

Principles of application of muscle energy to myofascial tissues

MET can be applied to muscles and soft tissues to stretch and lengthen the tissues, to deactivate muscle TrPs and to improve lymphatic drainage. The main principles for application of MET are described below:

1. **Stretch the involved muscle:** The muscle should be stretched to its barrier (sense of palpated resistance or end range):
   a. light stretching force to the initial or 'first barrier' if the muscle is acutely painful
   b. moderate stretching force to a comfortable sensation of stretch experienced by the patient if the muscle is mildly painful or not painful.
2. **Isometric contraction:** Request the patient to contract the targeted muscle (push away from the barrier) against your controlled, unyielding resistance for 3–5 seconds:
   a. light contraction force if the muscle is painful or contains active TrPs
   b. moderate contraction force for pain-free, fibrotic muscles.
3. **Muscle relaxation:** The patient should fully relax for several seconds, with the stretch maintained. A deep inhalation or exhalation may assist relaxation. Chaitow (2013) recommends maintaining this stretch for up to 60 seconds for chronically shortened muscles (removing the muscle from stretch for a rest period), but this long period of stretch is probably appropriate only for larger muscle groups. A stretch maintained for approximately 10 seconds is recommended for neck, shoulder and upper limb muscles that are shortened and fibrotic and are not provoked by stretching. A stretch maintained for only a few seconds is appropriate for tender and irritable muscles.
4. **Re-engage barrier:** The slack that has developed in the tissues following the contraction and relaxation phases is taken up, and usually the muscle can then be stretched to a new barrier without using increased force.
5. **Repetition:** This process is repeated 2–4 times, or until a change in length and tissue texture is noted.
6. **Re-examine:** To determine whether the tissues have changed.

For optimal localization and effectiveness, many of the muscle stretches require subtle fine-tuning for each patient. Practitioners are encouraged to experiment with small amounts of additional leverage – flexion, rotation, side-bending and traction – using palpation of tissue stretch and patient feedback to maximize the localization of the techniques.

Muscles of the upper quadrant

Many of the muscles of the chest and neck are susceptible to shortening and dysfunction and may adversely affect posture, causing abnormal stress and strain on other structures that aggravate neck and upper extremity symptoms. Additionally, two muscles – the scalenes and pectoralis minor – may compress, trap and compromise neurovascular structures that pass by these muscles and aggravate upper extremity symptoms (Simons et al 1999).

Upper trapezius and levator scapulae muscles

TrPs are commonly reported in the upper trapezius muscle and are an overlooked source of neck pain and headaches (Simons et al 1999; Fernández-de-las-Peñas et al 2007). The levator scapulae muscle, which produces local pain in the ipsilateral neck, will also be stretched during treatment of the trapezius. These muscles can be stretched together, but cervical rotation may selectively stretch particular fibres. There are different views about the amount and direction of rotation that is needed to select specific parts of the muscle (Liebenson 2007; Chaitow 2013), so the author recommends subtle fine-tuning of rotation using palpatory and patient feedback to determine the most effective position for each individual (Fig. 62.16).

Scalene muscles

The scalene muscles (anterior, middle and posterior) are a commonly overlooked source of back, shoulder and arm pain. TrPs in these muscles may contribute to symptoms in patients with cervicogenic headache (Simons et al 1999). Stretching involves depression of the shoulder and lateral flexion of the neck (Fig. 62.17). Opinions differ on the degree and direction of rotation required to stretch the scalene muscles (Gerwin 2005; Liebenson 2007; Chaitow 2013), so the author recommends experimentation using palpatory and patient feedback.

Pectoralis major muscle

TrPs in the pectoralis major muscle typically refer pain to the chest and arm (Simons et al 1999), and shortened muscles can produce a round-shouldered, head-forward posture that may lead to ongoing strain in the shoulder and neck regions. Treatment of this muscle should be reinforced by exercises and regular stretching at home to correct the head-forward posture. This technique is enhanced by the practitioner carefully anchoring the fascia over the sternum and applying traction through the length of the humerus (Fig. 62.18).

Caution: This technique is not suitable for any patient with an unstable shoulder joint, a previous shoulder injury, or limited shoulder movement due to pain. Do not use external rotation as the primary leverage because this will cause pain and discomfort even in the healthy shoulder joint.

Pectoralis minor muscle

The pectoralis minor muscle may refer pain to the anterior deltoid region or to the ulnar side of the arm, hand and fingers; it may trap the axillary artery and brachial plexus to mimic cervical radiculopathy (Simons et al 1999). Like the pectoralis major muscle, shortened pectoralis minor muscles may affect posture, producing rounded shoulders and a head-forward posture, which may place strain on these structures. A small towel can be folded and placed on the patient's anterior shoulder to cushion the practitioner's hand if the patient

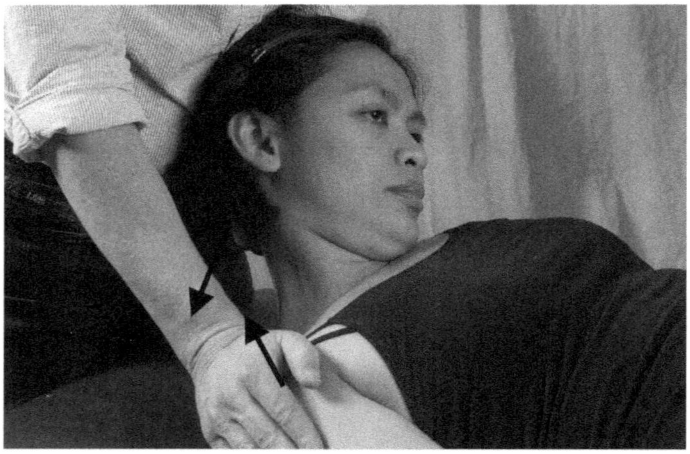

Figure 62.16 Muscle energy technique to lengthen the upper trapezius and levator scapulae muscles. The shoulder is firmly depressed and stabilized, and the neck is flexed and side-bent away from the involved side, with rotation of the neck dependent on the fibre direction and sense of stretch. The patient's isometric effort is either neck extension with side-bending towards the involved side (arrow) or elevation of the shoulder (arrow) against the unyielding counterforce of the practitioner.

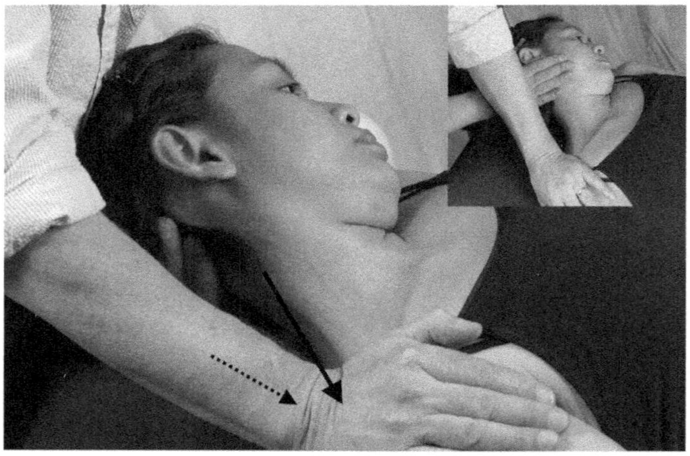

Figure 62.17 Muscle energy technique to lengthen the scalene muscles. *Main photo:* the shoulder and upper ribs are stabilized by downward pressure on the shoulder and clavicle (dotted line). Alternatively, the hand and thenar eminence can be placed below the medial clavicle to stabilize the first and second ribs. The neck is slightly extended, laterally flexed, and rotated away from the involved side. The patient gently performs an isometric effort in lateral flexion towards the involved side (arrow) against the unyielding counterforce of the practitioner. *Inset photo:* alternative hold in which the arms are crossed.

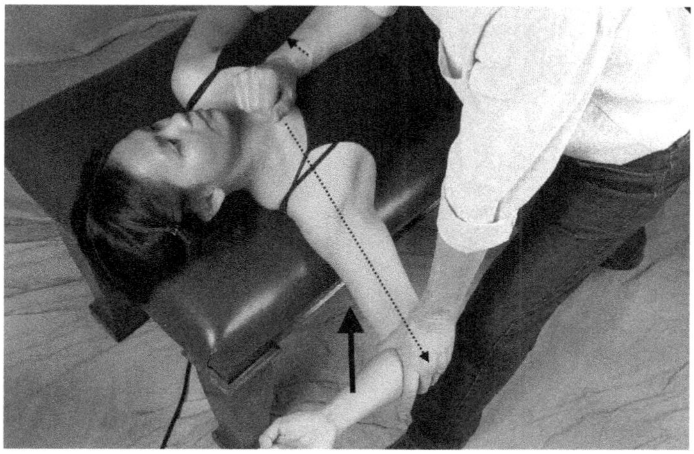

Figure 62.18 Muscle energy technique to lengthen the pectoralis major muscle. Note that the chest is firmly stabilized by the practitioner's forearm and the leverages applied to the shoulder are chiefly horizontal extension and traction (long dotted arrow). Pre-tension on the fascia over the sternum using a light compressive and lateral force (small dotted arrow) will help to minimize the amount of leverage necessary for the shoulder. The patient lifts the arm (arrow) against the unyielding counterforce of the practitioner. Note also that the applicator arm is straight and the isometric force is easily resisted by the practitioner's body weight.

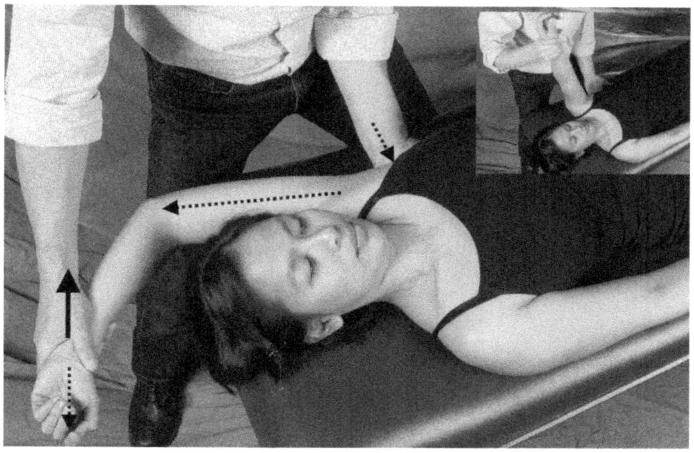

Figure 62.20 Muscle energy technique to lengthen the subscapularis muscle. *Inset photo:* the arm is first lifted to allow the practitioner's hand to contact and stabilize the lateral border of the scapula. *Main photo:* the scapula is firmly stabilized using medial compression against the border of the scapular (small dotted arrow) to prevent upward rotation. The shoulder is then abducted and externally rotated with slight traction through the arm and wrist (dotted arrows). The patient provides isometric effort by lifting the arm (arrow) against the practitioner's unyielding counterforce.

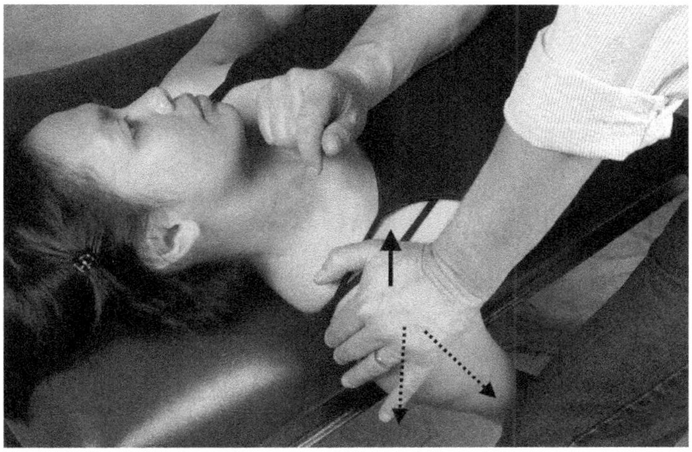

Figure 62.19 Muscle energy technique to lengthen the pectoralis minor muscle. The tissues over the sternum are firmly stabilized by the practitioner's forearm, and a posterior and lateral force is applied to the anterior shoulder (dotted arrows). A small towel may be used for padding if the contact on the shoulder is uncomfortable. The patient attempts to lift the shoulder (arrow) against the unyielding counterforce of the practitioner. Note that the applicator arm is straight and the isometric force is easily resisted by the practitioner's body weight.

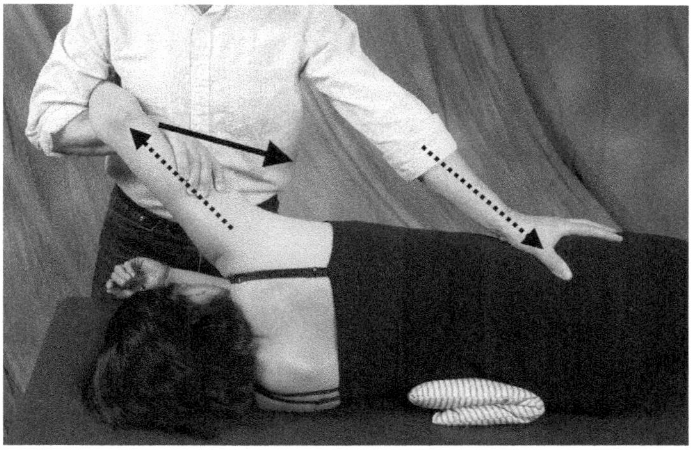

Figure 62.21 Muscle energy technique to lengthen the latissimus dorsi muscle. The patient is positioned on the unaffected side with a pillow under the waist region to promote lumbar side-bending. The patient's iliac crest is stabilized with one hand (dotted arrow), while the other hand links through the patient's arm to apply an abduction and traction force (dotted arrow). The patient produces an isometric effort by attempting to push the arm down (arrow) against the unyielding counterforce of the practitioner.

experiences discomfort from the pressure of the contact (Fig. 62.19).

Subscapularis muscle

TrPs in the subscapularis muscle may present as deep anterior shoulder pain and may produce substantial limitation of external rotation, thus mimicking adhesive capsulitis (Simons et al 1999). Effective stretch of this muscle requires firm stabilization of the scapula and may be performed with the patient in a supine or lateral recumbent position (Fig. 62.20).

Caution: This technique is contraindicated if the patient has an unstable shoulder.

Latissimus dorsi muscle

The latissimus dorsi is a large superficial muscle that may refer pain to the inferior scapula, the medial arm and forearm, and the flank and lumbar regions (Simons et al 1999). Additionally, shortening of this muscle may restrict full arm elevation, and patients characteristically compensate when performing bilateral arm elevation by overextension of the lumbar spine to achieve full elevation (Fig. 62.21).

Muscles of the lower quadrant

Assessment of the key muscles of the lower body by palpation for TrPs and assessment of shortness and strength should be part of the physical examination of any patient with lower back or lower extremity pain. In addition, shortness of some muscles may affect pelvic tilt and spinal curvature and therefore have potential to disturb the static and dynamic equilibrium of other regions. In the case of back and lower extremity pain, referral from TrPs in these muscles should be carefully differentiated from other causes of referred pain, such as radicular pain.

Quadratus lumborum muscle

The quadratus lumborum muscle is a deep muscle and a frequently overlooked source of LBP. Referred pain typically spreads to the iliac crest, sacral region and the greater trochanter. The author finds this muscle to be frequently involved in chronic LBP, which may be present concurrently with disc and facet joint pain. The addition of slight traction through the leg often increases the effectiveness of the stretch (Fig. 62.22).

Hip flexor muscle group

The flexor muscles of the hip that commonly present with shortness or TrPs are the iliopsoas, rectus femoris, pectineus and tensor fascia lata muscles. The iliopsoas, rectus femoris and pectineus may refer pain to the anterior thigh and groin, whereas the tensor fascia lata refers pain to the lateral thigh. Additionally, the iliopsoas may produce ipsilateral lumbar pain (Travell & Simons 1992). When shortened, these muscles restrict hip extension and promote pelvic anteversion, which may lead to further strain on the lumbar spine. These muscles can be treated in the Thomas test position, using extension and fine-tuning of knee flexion, adduction or abduction to localize the stretch to each muscle (Fig. 62.23).

Gluteus medius and gluteus minimus muscles

The gluteus medius and minimus muscles are important hip abductors and they stabilize the pelvis during single-limb stance. TrPs in these muscles may produce local pain in the sacroiliac and hip region (medius), or may refer pain down the posterior or lateral thigh and leg (minimus) (Travell & Simons 1992). For treatment, the muscle can be divided into posterior, middle and anterior portions. Stretching requires the primary leverage of hip adduction, with hip flexion or extension to localize the stretch to the posterior and anterior portions, respectively. These muscles often have TrPs in patients with low back or sacroiliac pain and instability, and they probably become a secondary source of noxious input in these cases. The muscles can be stretched and treated in different positions, but the techniques that the author finds most efficient are illustrated in Figure 62.24.

Piriformis muscle

The piriformis may be a common cause of pain and distress, and TrPs may refer pain to the sacroiliac region, laterally across the buttock and over the hip region posteriorly, and to the proximal two-thirds of the posterior thigh (Travell & Simons 1992). Additionally, the piriformis may produce an entrapment syndrome of the neurovascular structures against the rim of the greater sciatic foramen, although true entrapment may actually be rare. This muscle acts as an external rotator of the hip when the hip is in a neutral position, but

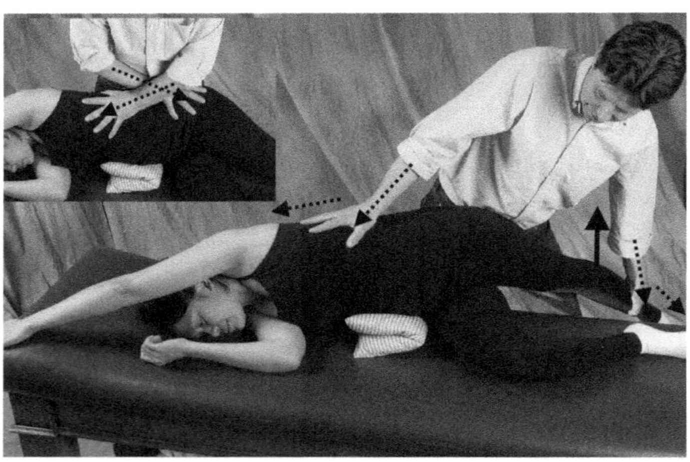

Figure 62.22 Muscle energy technique to lengthen the quadratus lumborum muscle. *Main photo:* the patient is positioned on the unaffected side with a pillow under the waist region to promote side-bending of the trunk and stretch of the quadratus lumborum on the upper side. The leg on the upper side can be extended slightly and adducted to assist this stretch, and the practitioner's hip may contact the patient to stabilize the pelvis to avoid rotation. One hand is used to fix the lower ribs with a comfortable broad contact (dotted arrows), while the other hand contacts the leg to produce further hip adduction and traction (dotted arrows). The patient provides isometric effort by attempting to lift the leg (arrow) or hitch up the hip against the unyielding counterforce of the practitioner. *Inset photo:* alternative hand contact on the iliac crest, which will avoid stretching the hip adductors.

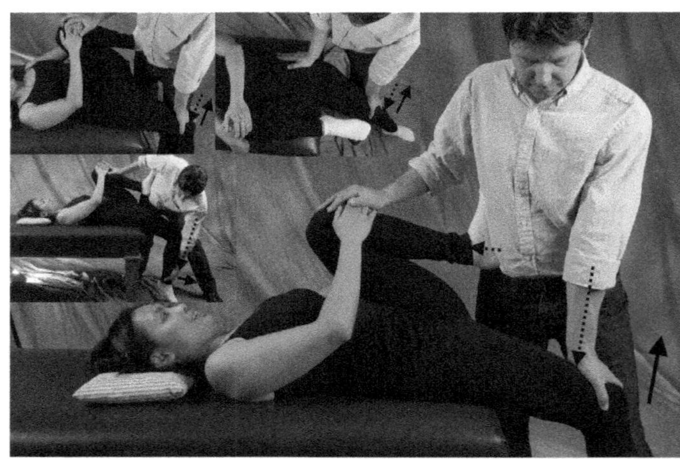

Figure 62.23 Muscle energy technique to lengthen the hip flexor muscle group. Patients are most effectively treated in the Thomas test position, where they are supine with the pelvis just on the end of the table. The untreated leg should be fully flexed, held by the patient and stabilized by the practitioner's body (dotted arrow) to ensure stability of the pelvis and lumbar spine. *Main photo:* treatment of iliopsoas muscle. An extension force is applied to the treated thigh (dotted arrow) until a barrier is palpated or a moderate stretching force is perceived by the patient. The patient pushes the thigh up (arrow) against the unyielding counterforce of the practitioner. *Inset top left photo:* addition of abduction will localize the stretch to the pectineus and short abductor muscles. *Inset top right photo:* addition of adduction will localize the stretch to the tensor fascia lata muscle. *Inset bottom photo:* addition of knee flexion will localize the stretch to the rectus femoris muscle.

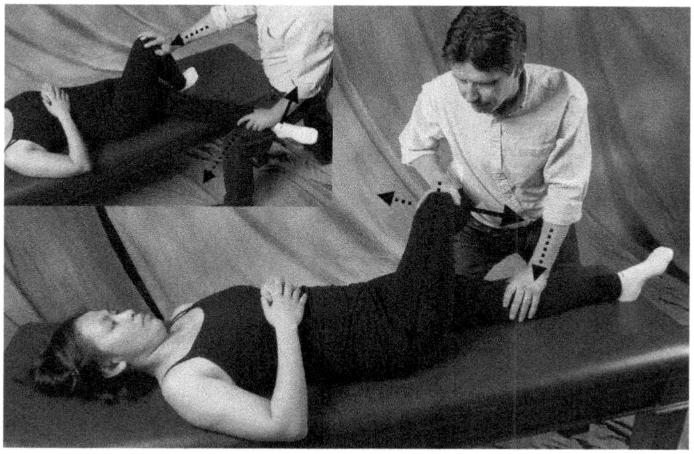

Figure 62.24 Muscle energy technique to lengthen the gluteus medius and gluteus minimus muscles. These two muscles are treated as one muscle, but they can also be treated as posterior, middle and anterior portions. The anterior division can be treated in the same way as the tensor fascia lata in Fig. 62.23. *Main photo:* the posterior division requires hip flexion and adduction. The practitioner position illustrated permits a very effective stretch that requires little effort to maintain. The hip is flexed to approximately 30° and is then slightly adducted. A mild compressive force is placed down the axis of the femur (long dotted arrow) to stabilize the pelvis. Minor shifts in weight by the practitioner produce further adduction (short dotted arrow) for a localized and effective stretch. The patient provides isometric effort by attempting to push the leg back to midline (arrow) against the unyielding counterforce of the practitioner. *Inset photo:* treatment of the middle fibres of the left hip using adduction. The uninvolved hip is flexed to create room for the adducted treated leg and stabilized by the practitioner (dotted arrow). The treated leg is abducted using the practitioner's thigh (dotted arrow) and the patient gently pushes the thigh in adduction (arrow).

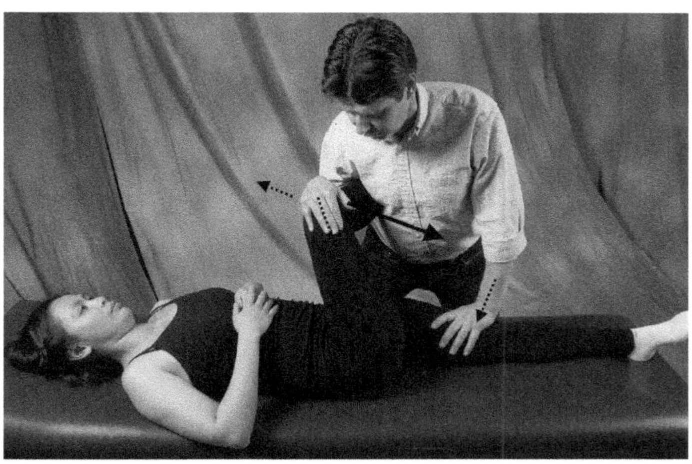

Figure 62.25 Muscle energy technique to lengthen the piriformis muscle. The practitioner position illustrated takes advantage of the abduction action of the piriformis when the hip is flexed and permits a very effective stretch that requires little effort to maintain. The hip is flexed to approximately 90° and is then slightly adducted. The practitioner should move close to the leg. A mild compressive force is placed down the axis of the femur (long dotted arrow) to stabilize the pelvis. Minor shifts in weight by the practitioner produce further adduction and external rotation (short dotted arrow) for a localized and effective stretch. The patient provides isometric effort by attempting to push the leg back to the midline (arrow) against the unyielding counterforce of the practitioner.

becomes an abductor of the hip when the hip is flexed. Effective stretching of this muscle using internal rotation is difficult because the hip joint limits the available rotation, so the use of adduction when the hip is flexed at approximately 90° is more effective (Fig. 62.25).

Acknowledgements

The author gratefully acknowledges the assistance of Rolena Stephenson as subject of the photos, of Kelly Rogers, ATSU photographer, and of Deborah Goggin MA, Scientific Writer, A.T. Still Research Institute, A.T. Still University, for reviewing this chapter.

References

Aparicio ÉQ, Quirante LB, Blanco CR, et al. 2009. Immediate effects of the suboccipital muscle inhibition technique in subjects with short hamstring syndrome. J Manipulative Physiol Ther 32: 262–269.

Bendova P, Ruzicka P, Peterova V, et al. 2007. MRI-based registration of pelvic alignment affected by altered pelvic floor muscle characteristics. Clin Biomech 22: 980–987.

Boyles RE, Ritland BM, Miracle BM, et al. 2009. The short-term effects of thoracic spine thrust manipulation on patients with shoulder impingement syndrome. Man Ther 14: 375–380.

Burns DK, Wells MR. 2006. Gross range of motion in the cervical spine: the effects of osteopathic muscle energy technique in asymptomatic subjects. J Am Osteopath Assoc 106: 137–142.

Chaitow L. 2013. Muscle energy techniques, 4th edn. Edinburgh: Churchill Livingstone.

Cleland JA, Childs JD, McRae M, et al. 2005. Immediate effects of thoracic manipulation in patients with neck pain: a randomized clinical trial. Man Ther 10: 127–135.

Coates G, O'Brodovich H, Goeree G. 1993. Hindlimb and lung lymph flows during prolonged exercise. J Appl Physiol 75: 633–638.

Cook C, Hegedus E, Showalter C, et al. 2006. Coupling behavior of the cervical spine: a systematic review of the literature. J Manipulative Physiol Ther 29: 570–575.

Di Fabio RP. 1999. Manipulation of the cervical spine: risks and benefits. Phys Ther 79: 50–65.

Dhinkaran M, Sareen A, Arora T. 2011. Comparative analysis of muscle energy technique and conventional physiotherapy in treatment of sacroiliac joint dysfunction. Indian J Physiother Occup Ther 5: 127–130.

Edmondston SJ, Henne SE, Loh W, et al. 2005. Influence of cranio-cervical posture on three-dimensional motion of the cervical spine. Man Ther 10: 44–51.

Fernández-de-las-Peñas C, Alonso-Blanco C, Miangolarra JC. 2007. Myofascial trigger points in subjects presenting with mechanical neck pain: a blinded, controlled study. Man Ther 12: 29–33.

Ferreira ML, Ferreira PH, Hodges PW. 2007. Changes in postural activity of the trunk muscles following spinal manipulative therapy. Man Ther 12: 240–248.

Fryer G. 2000. Muscle energy concepts: a need for change. J Osteopathic Med 3: 54–59.

Fryer G. 2003. Intervertebral dysfunction: a discussion of the manipulable spinal lesion. J Osteopathic Med 6: 64–73.

Fryer G. 2009. Research-informed muscle energy concepts and practice. In: Franke H (ed) Muscle energy technique: history – model – research (monograph). Ammersestr: Jolandos, pp 57–62.

Fryer G. 2011. Muscle energy technique: an evidence-informed approach. Int J Osteopathic Med 14: 3–9.

Fryer G. 2013. Muscle energy technique: research and efficacy. In: Chaitow L (ed). Muscle energy techniques, 4th edn. Edinburgh: Churchill Livingstone, pp 42–64.

Fryer G, Adams JH. 2011. Magnetic resonance imaging of subjects with acute unilateral neck pain and restricted motion: a prospective case series. Spine J 11: 171–176.

Fryer G, Fossum C. 2010. Therapeutic mechanisms underlying muscle energy approaches. In: Fernández-de-las-Peñas C, Arendt-Nielsen L, Gerwin RD (eds) Tension-type and cervicogenic headache: pathophysiology, diagnosis, and management. Sudbury, MA: Jones and Bartlett, pp 221–229.

Fryer G, Ruszkowski W. 2004. The influence of contraction duration in muscle energy technique applied to the atlanto-axial joint. J Osteopathic Med 7: 79–84.

Fryer G, Morris T, Gibbons P. 2004. Paraspinal muscles and inter-vertebral dysfunction: part 2. J Manipulative Physiol Ther 27: 348–357.

Fryette HH. 1954. Principles of osteopathic technic. Newark: American Academy of Osteopathy.

Gerwin R. 2005. Headache. In: Ferguson LW, Gerwin R (eds) Clinical mastery in the treatment of myofascial pain. Baltimore: Lippincott Williams & Wilkins, pp 1–29.

Gibbons P, Tehan P. 1998. Muscle energy concepts and coupled motion of the spine. Man Ther 3: 95–101.

Gibbons P, Tehan P. 2006. Manipulation of the spine, thorax and pelvis: an osteopathic perspective, 2nd edn. London: Churchill Livingstone.

González-Iglesias J, Fernández-de-las-Peñas C, Cleland JA, et al. 2009. Inclusion of thoracic spine thrust manipulation into an electro-therapy / thermal program for the management of patients with acute mechanical neck pain: a randomized clinical trial. Man Ther 14: 306–313.

Goodridge JP, Kuchera ML. 1997. Muscle energy treatment techniques for specific areas. In: Ward RC (ed) Foundations for osteopathic medicine. Baltimore: William & Wilkins, pp 697–761.

Greenman PE. 2003. Principles of manual medicine, 3rd edn. Philadelphia: Lippincott William & Wilkins.

Grip H, Sundelin G, Gerdle B, et al. 2007. Variations in the axis of motion during head repositioning: a comparison of subjects with whiplash-associated disorders or non-specific neck pain and healthy controls. Clin Biomech 22: 865–873.

Gupta S, Jaiswal P, Chhabra D. 2008. A comparative study between postisometric relaxation and isometric exercises in non-specific neck pain. J Exerc Sci Physiother 4: 88–94.

Haldeman S, Kohlbeck FJ, McGregor M. 2001. Unpredictability of cerebrovascular ischemia associated with cervical spine manipulation therapy: a review of sixty-four cases after cervical spine manipulation. Spine 27: 49–55.

Havas E, Parviainen T, Vuorela J, et al. 1997. Lymph flow dynamics in exercising human skeletal muscle as detected by scintography. J Physiol 504: 233–239.

Hossain M, Nokes LDM. 2005. A model of dynamic sacro-iliac joint instability from malrecruitment of gluteus maximus and biceps femoris muscles resulting in low back pain. Med Hypotheses 65: 278–281.

Hungerford B, Gilleard W, Lee D. 2004. Altered patterns of pelvic bone motion determined in subjects with posterior pelvic pain using skin markers. Clin Biomech 19: 456–464.

Ishii T, Mukai Y, Hosono N, et al. 2006. Kinematics of the cervical spine in lateral bending: in vivo three-dimensional analysis. Spine 31: 155–160.

Kuchera WA, Kuchera ML. 1992. Osteopathic principles in practice. Kirksville, MO: Kirksville College of Osteopathic Medicine Press.

Langevin HM, Cornbrooks CJ, Taatjes DJ. 2004. Fibroblasts form a body-wide cellular network. Histochem Cell Biol 122: 7–15.

Langevin HM, Bouffard NA, Badger GJ, et al. 2005. Dynamic fibroblast cytoskeletal response to subcutaneous tissue stretch ex vivo and in vivo. Am J Physiol Cell Physiol 288: C747–756.

Lederman E. 2005. The science and practice of manual therapy, 2nd edn. Edinburgh: Elsevier Churchill Livingstone.

Lee HY, Wang JD, Yao G, et al. 2007. Association between cervicocephalic kinesthetic sensibility and frequency of subclinical neck pain. Man Ther 13: 419–425.

Legaspi O, Edmond SL. 2007. Does the evidence support the existence of lumbar spine coupled motion? A critical review of the literature. J Orthop Sports Phys Ther 37: 169–178.

Leinonen V, Maatta S, Taimela S, et al. 2002. Impaired lumbar movement perception in association with postural stability and motor- and somatosensory- evoked potentials in lumbar spinal stenosis. Spine 27: 975–983.

Lenehan KL, Fryer G, McLaughlin P. 2003. The effect of muscle energy technique on gross trunk range of motion. J Osteopath Med 6: 13–18.

Liebenson C. 2007. Rehabilitation of the spine: a practitioner's manual, 2nd edn. Baltimore: Lippincott William & Wilkins.

Magnusson M, Simonsen EB, Dyhre-Poulsen P, et al. 1996a. Viscoelastic stress relaxation during static stretch in human skeletal muscle in the absence of EMG activity. Scand J Med Sci Sport 6: 323–328.

Magnusson SP, Simonsen EB, Aagaard P, et al. 1996b. Mechanical and physiological responses to stretching with and without preisometric contraction in human skeletal muscle. Arch Phys Med Rehabil 77: 373–377.

Malmstrom E, Karlberg M, Fransson PA, et al. 2006. Primary and coupled cervical movements. The effect of age, gender, and body mass index: a 3-dimensional movement analysis of a population without symptoms of neck disorders. Spine 31: E44–E50.

Malmstrom EM, Karlberg M, Holmstrom E, et al. 2010. Influence of prolonged unilateral cervical muscle contraction on head repositioning-decreased overshoot after a 5-min static muscle contraction task. Man Ther 15: 229–234.

Mitchell FL Jr, Mitchell PKG. 1995. The muscle energy manual. East Lansing, MI: MET Press.

Mitchell FL Jr, Mitchell PKG. 1998. The muscle energy manual: evaluation and treatment of the thoracic spine lumbar spine and rib cage. East Lansing, MI: MET Press.

Mitchell FL Jr, Mitchell PKG. 1999. The muscle energy manual: evaluation and treatment of the pelvis and sacrum. Vol 3. East Lansing, MI: MET Press.

Murphy DR, Hurwitz EL, Gregory AA. 2006. Manipulation in the presence of cervical spinal cord compression: a case series. J Manipulative Physiol Ther 29: 236–244.

Ogince M, Hall T, Robinson K, et al. 2006. The diagnostic validity of the cervical flexion-rotation test in C1 / 2-related cervicogenic headache. Man Ther 15: 15.

Osternig LR, Robertson R, Troxel RK, et al. 1987. Muscle activation during proprioceptive neuromuscular facilitation (PNF) stretching techniques. Am J Phys Med 66: 298–307.

Osternig LR, Robertson RN, Troxel RK, et al. 1990. Differential responses to proprioceptive neuromuscular facilitation (PNF) stretch techniques. Med Sci Sports Exercise 22: 106–111.

Palmgren PJ, Sandstrom PJ, Lundqvist FJ, et al. 2006. Improvement after chiropractic care in cervicocephalic kinesthetic sensibility and subjective pain intensity in patients with nontraumatic chronic neck pain. J Manipulative Physiol Ther 29: 100–106.

Patil PN, Chandu B, Metgud S, et al. 2010. Effectiveness of muscle energy technique on quadratus lumborum in acute low back pain-randomized controlled trial. Indian J Physiother Occupational Ther 4: 54–58.

Rana K, Bansal N, Savita HK. 2009. Comparative analysis on the efficacy of G.D. Maitland's concept of mobilization and muscle energy technique in treating sacroiliac joint dysfunction. Indian J Physiother Occupational Ther 3: 18–22.

Rogers RG. 1997. The effects of spinal manipulation on cervical kinesthesia in patients with chronic neck pain: a pilot study. J Manipulative Physiol Ther 20: 80–85.

Salvador D, Neto PED, Ferrari FP. 2005. Application of muscle energy technique in garbage collectors with acute mechanical lumbar pain. Fisioterapia Pesquisa 12: 20–27.

Schenk RJ, Adelman K, Rousselle J. 1994. The effects of muscle energy technique on cervical range of motion. J Man Manipulative Ther 2: 149–155.

Schenk RJ, MacDiarmid A, Rousselle J. 1997. The effects of muscle energy technique on lumbar range of motion. J Man Manipulative Ther 5: 179–183.

Selkow NM, Grindstaff TL, Cross KM, et al. 2009. Short-term effect of muscle energy technique on pain in individuals with non-specific lumbopelvic pain: a pilot study. J Man Manipulative Ther 17: E14–E18.

Simons DG, Travell JG, Simons LS. 1999. Myofascial pain and dysfunction: the trigger point manual. Vol 1, 2nd edn. Baltimore: William & Wilkins.

Sizer PS Jr, Brismee JM, Cook C. 2007. Coupling behavior of the thoracic spine: a systematic review of the literature. J Manipulative Physiol Ther 30: 390–399.

Souvlis T, Vicenzino B, Wright A. 2004. Neurophysiological effects of spinal manual therapy. In: Boyling JD, Jull GA (eds) Grieve's modern manual therapy: the vertebral column. Edinburgh: Elsevier Churchill Livingstone, pp 367–380.

Swart J. 1919. Osteopathic strap technic. Kansas City: Joseph Swart.

Trampas A, Kitsios A, Sykaras E, et al. 2010. Clinical massage and modified proprioceptive neuromuscular facilitation stretching in males with latent myofascial trigger points. Phys Ther Sport 11: 91–98.

Travell JG, Simons DG. 1992. Myofascial pain and dysfunction: the trigger point manual. Vol 2. Baltimore: Williams & Wilkins.

Wilson E, Payton O, Donegan-Shoaf L, et al. 2003. Muscle energy technique in patients with acute low back pain: a pilot clinical trial. J Orthop Sports Phys Ther 33: 502–512.

Chapter 63

Myofascial Induction Approaches

Andrzej Pilat

CHAPTER CONTENTS

Introduction	729
Fascia and its dynamics	730
Functions of the fascial system	730
Information transmission process	730
Anatomical considerations related to the continuity of the fascial system of the neck and upper extremity	732
Fascial anatomy of the cervical region	732
Fascial anatomy of the upper extremity	733
Anatomical considerations related to the continuity of the fascial system of the pelvis and lower extremity	738
Superficial and deep fascial anatomical links between the trunk and lower limbs	738
Deep fascial intermuscular links	740
Theoretical aspects related to the treatment of myofascial dysfunction syndrome	743
Mechanics of myofascial dysfunction syndrome formation	743
Proposed neurophysiological mechanisms of myofascial induction techniques	745
Scientific evidence related to the results in the myofascial approach	747
Research related to pathology	747
Clinical research in healthy subjects	747
Therapeutic strategies applied in the myofascial induction process	748
General observations related to the therapeutic process	748
Definition of the myofascial induction process	748
Bases for clinical applications	748
Examples of practical applications for upper quadrant disorders	749
Techniques related to the cervical spine	749
Techniques related to the shoulder girdle	750
Techniques related to the brachial and antebrachial fascia	752
Techniques related to the fascia of the hand	752
Examples of practical applications for lower quadrant disorders	753
Techniques related to the lumbopelvic region	753
Techniques related to the thigh region	755
Techniques related to the knee and the leg region	756
Contraindications	758
Conclusion	758

Introduction

Body movement involves fascial activity. An extensive definition of the fascia is needed to analyse body biomechanics and pathomechanics. However, there is a lot discrepancy in opinions on and definitions of what fascia is (Langevin & Huijing 2009; Kumka & Bonar 2012; Schleip et al 2012b; Swanson 2013). Kumka and Bonar (2012) defined fascia as an innervated, continuous, functional organ of stability and motion that is formed by three-dimensional collagen matrices. Fascia can be described as the body's dynamic unifying structure; it manifests as a continuum of fibres immersed in the ground substance that accompanies the body structures without any interruption (Pilat 2003). The fascial system represents a complex communicational architecture, which provides mechanoreceptive information; this process occurs as a result of not only its topographic distribution per se, but also mainly the pattern of *how* it inter-relates with other body structures, especially muscles. Its fibrous construction allows it to align with and accommodate to both intrinsic and extrinsic tensional body requirements. The tensional paths, created outside the correct biomechanical movement patterns, can thus redirect the body dynamics. The density, the distribution and the organoleptic characteristics of the system differ across the body, but its continuity is essential, allowing the fascia to act as a synergistic whole, absorbing and distributing local stimuli to the entire system. This inherent synergy of the structural fascial system helps the human body to be relatively independent of the gravitational force, and also gives it a great capacity to adapt according to changing external and internal requirements, for instance in relation to the availability of energy and nutrients in the immediate environment. Besides its structural role, the fascial system also distributes stimuli that the body receives: its sensor network registers thermal, chemical, pressure, vibrational and movement impulses, and it analyses, categorizes and transmits them to the central nervous system. The central nervous system then redirects the impulses and sends instructions to the organs. We can conclude therefore that the fascial system is not a passive and merely supporting structure, but rather a dynamic and mutable system (Swanson 2013).

This chapter discusses basic concepts involved in myofascial induction therapy applications to the musculoskeletal pain syndromes of the upper and lower quadrants. Special attention will be placed on:

- principles of fascial dynamics
  - biomechanics
  - innervations
  - impulse (information) transmission
- anatomical continuity along the upper and lower quadrants
- formation of fascial entrapment
- assessment principles
- basic treatment principles
- samples of treatment application
- indications and counterindications.

Fascia and its Dynamics

Fascia comprises the dense (both regular and irregular) connective tissue that is involved in different structures (e.g. aponeurosis, tendons, ligaments, joint capsules and nerve sheets) and forms a continuous bonding network between the elements of the musculoskeletal system, as well as the loose connective tissue that, by filling all the intermediate spaces of the body, creates links between all the anatomical components (vascular, nervous and visceral) (Langevin & Huijing 2009; Schleip et al 2012a). These connections may even exist at the cellular and intracellular levels (Chiquet et al 2009).

Functions of the fascial system

The fascial system not only forms anatomical connections through its continuous communication network, but also has a large variety of other functions, including (Pilat 2003):

- suspension
- support
- formation of functional units
- absorption and distribution of local stimuli as a synergistic whole
  - mechanical (pressure, vibration, movement)
  - chemical
  - thermal
- protection and autonomy of the muscles and viscera
- formation of compartments
- maintenance of body posture (Langevin 2006)
- tissue nutrition
- facilitation of body homeostasis
- participation in wound healing
- implication in control of afferent stimuli transmission.

Information transmission process

Some authors (Gerlach & Lierse 1990) have suggested an integrated body model named the 'bone–fascia–tendon system' ascribing to the fascia the bonding function of the muscular biomechanics. Such a complex and multitask system requires the ability to receive, process and transmit information related to body movement. The information can flow through the system, employing three different connexion patterns related to a specific purpose (Pilat & Testa 2009).

Mechanical (anatomical) pattern

These links are present at different anatomical levels (from macro- to microscopic) and could act hierarchically (Wang et al 2009). At the macroscopic level, observations of dissected unembalmed cadavers (Vleeming & Stoeckart 1997; Myers 2003; Stecco et al 2008; Pilat 2009) have demonstrated mechanical continuity of the fascia whereby all the muscles attached to a specific fascia act synergistically, creating myokinetic links (Stecco et al 2007; Pilat 2009). Recently Yaman et al (2013) presented evidence showing epimuscular myofascial force transmission through undissected muscles in situ, hence confirming the hypothesis that, in vivo, muscles are in principle not mechanically independent. In another in vivo experiment, Carvalhais et al (2013) observed myofascial force transmission between the latissimus dorsi and gluteus maximus muscles across the thoracolumbar fascia. Further, based on the observations made during endoscopic surgery, Guimberteau et al (2010) proposed that fascia not only surrounds muscle structures (epimysium), but also infiltrates the muscular mass and fat (in a very individual manner in each person), thus creating a three-dimensional interconnection within the body's network of macro- and micro-structures (Swartz et al 2001; Guimberteau et al 2010). Guimberteau et al (2005) have described the fascial system as an uninterrupted network, termed the 'multimicrovacuolar collagen dynamic absorption system' (MCDAS), that although seemingly a 'chaotic matrix' nevertheless maintains its form as a result of the actions of criss-crossing physical forces that impart a hierarchical and interdependent complexity, including both spatial and temporal relationships. This mechanical transverse force transmission through the fascia has also been extensively studied at microscopic level (Huijing 2009; Purslow 2010; Chi-Zhang & Gao 2012), with particular focus on the intermuscular fascia where the muscle fibres are inserted. Through these fascial connections, muscle fibres can participate in mechanical action even without directly inserting into the bone (Van der Wal 2009).

A mechanical model to explain the interactions described above is the tensegrity (tensorial integrity) model, which was proposed by Ingber (1998). This theory suggests a system of shared tensions at multiple body levels, and it can also explain the global reaction of the fascial system when it receives a mechanical stimulus (Chicurel et al 1998; Khalsa et al 2000; Ingber 2006). The research by Ingber (1998, 2003, 2005, 2006) and others (Parker & Ingber 2007; Stamenovic et al 2007; Wang et al 2009), on cellular dynamics and the active response of the cytoskeleton when mechanical forces are transmitted to it from the extracellular matrix, demonstrates the importance of tissue remodelling at both cellular and subcellular levels. This communication takes place through the extracellular matrix via integrins (molecular bridges between the matrix and the cytoskeleton), by which the cell 'senses' its environment and responds as required. The mechanical input can subsequently transfer to the nucleus membrane at the subcellular level (Maniotis et al 1997; Hu et al 2003), and finally can also modify gene expression (Chiquet et al 2009). Considering the fact that the human body is built up as a hierarchical design, these findings would suggest a similar principle in the increasing body's construction order. The dynamics of the fascial system's movements at cellular level are associated with contractions of myofibroblasts (a type of fibroblast containing dynamic actin microfilaments that contract in the manner of smooth muscle cells) (Gabbiani 2007).

Functional pattern

The fascia is considered to be a mechanosensitive structure (Langevin 2006; Vaticón 2009; Langevin et al 2011); however, neuroanatomical studies tend to focus mainly on discs, facet joints, muscles fibres, tendons or ligaments so there is a little information regarding fascial innervation. Our interest here focuses on the functional connection, which mainly takes place through the loose connective tissue structures between its unique network of mechanoreceptors, particularly the so-called interstitial mechanoreceptors (type III and IV free nerve endings). Each receptor has two subgroups, with low and high levels of mechanosensitivity related to the cell architecture. The presence of this kind of receptor was confirmed in recent studies:

- Group III muscle afferents are found in perimuscular fascia and the adventitia of muscle blood vessels and respond to a variety of stimuli, including pressure and stretch (which results in matrix deformation after mechanical impulse application (Lin et al 2009)).
- The thoracolumbar fascia (TLF) is a highly innervated tissue (Taguchi et al 2009).
- There is substantial innervation of non-specialized connective tissue through the Aδ and / or C-fibres (Corey 2011).
- There is a strong link between fascia and the autonomic nervous system (Haouzi et al 1999).
- Many fibres – especially in the superficial fascia – express tyrosine hydroxylase, an enzyme characteristic of postganglionic sympathetic fibres (dopamine secretion control). This finding may explain why patients with low back pain report increased intensities of pain when they are under psychological stress (Chou & Shekelle 2010).
- Neural action potential firing through nerve terminals is linked to specific mechanical deformation and extracellular matrix interactions (Lin et al 2009).
- Stimulation of group III and IV muscle afferents has been shown to have important reflex effects on both the somatic and the autonomic nervous systems. These include an inhibitory effect on α-motor-neurons, an excitatory effect on γ-motor-neurons and an excitatory effect on the sympathetic nervous system (Kaufman et al 2002).
- Specialized connective tissue structures are related to muscle structure (endomysium, perimysium, epimysium) and other body systems: circulatory (arterial, venous, lymphatic) and nervous. Remodelling of interstitial connective tissue may have important biomechanical, vasomotor and neuromodulatory effects.

It is suggested that the three-dimensional fascial network is also involved in the pain transmission process. The pain experienced in the extremities is often a referred pain (i.e. it is perceived in areas remote from the site of noxious stimulation). This kind of pain does not always follow the segmental pain pattern (Travell & Bigelow 1946). The central hyperexcitability theory (Mense 1994) explains the mechanism of pain from deep structures, but does not clarify the presence of non-segmental pain patterns from the superficial muscles such as the neck, the latissimus dorsi, the trapezius and limb muscles (Han 2009). In the subcutaneous tissue close to the outer level of the TLF, fibres are often found in the proximity of blood vessels. The location of most fibres around blood vessels suggests that at least parts of them are vasomotor fibres and, when activated, these fibres may cause ischaemic pain (Tesarz et al 2011). Free nerve endings have been found in all layers of the TLF (superficial, middle and deep); however, no corpuscular receptors such as pacinian and paciniform corpuscles or Golgi tendon organs have been found. Micro-injuries resulting from irritation of nociceptive nerve endings in the TLF may lead directly to back pain (Willard et al 2012). Tissue deformations due to injury, immobility or excessive loading could also impair proprioceptive signalling, which may lead to an increase in pain sensitivity via an activity-dependent sensitization of wide-dynamic-range neurons (Willard et al 2012). The 'barrier-dam' theory suggests that referred pain from the neck muscle, the pectoral girdle and the arm is peripheral in origin and is manifested by irritation of the peripheral nerves (Farasyn 2007). Langevin et al (2009) reported an abnormal connective tissue structure in the lumbar region in a group of subjects with chronic or recurrent low back pain, and suggested possible causes including abnormal movement patterns and chronic inflammation. Han (2009) has proposed an alternative hypothesis – termed the 'connective tissue theory'; considering the anatomical expansions of the fascia and the formation of the myokinetic links and chains, he suggests that the signalling mechanisms present in the loose connective tissue may be able to transmit noxious stimuli from the surface to the muscles and other deep structures, through the cells of the vascular and neural systems. Hence peripheral pain may also have a direct origin in the connective tissue.

Chemical pattern

Cells are fundamental units of living beings and they are immersed in the extracellular matrix, which constitutes their ecosystem. The extracellular matrix of the connective tissue is the medium in which the complex mechanotransduction process takes place – that is, the cells within it react dynamically, detecting and interpreting mechanical signals and converting them into chemical changes and / or modifications in gene expression (Ingber 2006; Ghosh & Ingber 2007; Parker & Ingber 2007; Chiquet 2009). Ingber (2006) considered the mediating structures of the mechanotransduction process to include both mechanosensitive proteins and structural hierarchical networks, from the organ down to the cellular level, and Vanacore et al (2009) identified networks of collagen IV present in the basement membrane that provided structural integrity to tissues and served as ligands for integrin cell-surface receptors. These networks mediate cell adhesion, migration, growth and differentiation. Shoham and Gefen (2012) demonstrated that adipocytes (also osteoblasts, chondroblasts and endothelial cells) are indeed mechanosensitive and mechanoreceptive. These mechanisms could help explain injury and disease that are related to changes in cell mechanics.

Anatomical Considerations Related to the Continuity of the Fascial System of the Neck and Upper Extremity

In the introduction we referred to the continuity of the body's fascial system. This continuous fascial linking is present in the mechanical connection between the head, the trunk and the upper limb. In this region, there is no clear division between muscular, nervous and vascular structures related to a single segment. Generally, from an anatomical perspective, less importance is given to the fascia than to the tissues related to it; however, it is this fascial structure that appears to ensure functional continuity throughout the body (Pilat 2003; Vanacore et al 2009).

Fascial anatomy of the cervical region

The fascial cervical system forms several spaces with a longitudinal orientation (Bienfait 1987; Upledger 1987; Bochenek & Reicher 1997; Pilat 2003), which divide, envelop, support and connect the muscles, bones, viscera, vascular vessels and peripheral nerves. They can be compared to a system of tubes concentrically placed inside one another, all of which are interconnected at different levels and in several ways (Pilat 2003) (Fig. 63.1). These interconnections unfold between the muscles, establishing mechanical links that determine the direction and the range of motion (Bochenek & Reicher 1997). The lubrication of these compartments, which is a result of the greater amount of fatty tissue or loose connective tissue present, allows for greater freedom of movement (particularly sliding) of the fascial system (Pilat 2009).

The fascial system is responsible for the transmission of dynamic (active) forces between the cranium, mandible, hyoid, sternum, clavicles, scapula, the first two ribs and the cervical spine. It enables communication between the endocranium and the endothorax, influencing not only the mechanics of the cervical region, the shoulder complex, the arm and the temporomandibular joint, but also the mechanics of the respiratory system and transmission in the vascular system between the mechanical input and the cephalic region (Pilat 2009).

The precise route and connection between fascial layers is different for each individual, and this is why it is difficult to classify its exact anatomy in relation to the transmission pathway and the inter-relations between various elements. However, most anatomists agree with the following classification and distribution of the fascial system (Pilat 2009):

- superficial fascia
- deep fascia
  - superficial lamina
  - prevertebral lamina.

This system forms complex links with the shoulder girdle and has continuity with the arm.

Superficial cervical fascia

The first structure in this continuity is the superficial fascia, located under the skin and forming a firm link (Pilat 2009). It closely surrounds the entire structure of the cervical spine (see Fig. 63.1A, Figs 63.2–63.3), varying in thickness, form, elasticity, resistance and fat content. It contains the platysma muscle, cutaneous nerves, capillaries and lymphatic vessels, and is an elastic structure. The dynamic activity of the superficial fascia is related to the platysma muscle, which expands

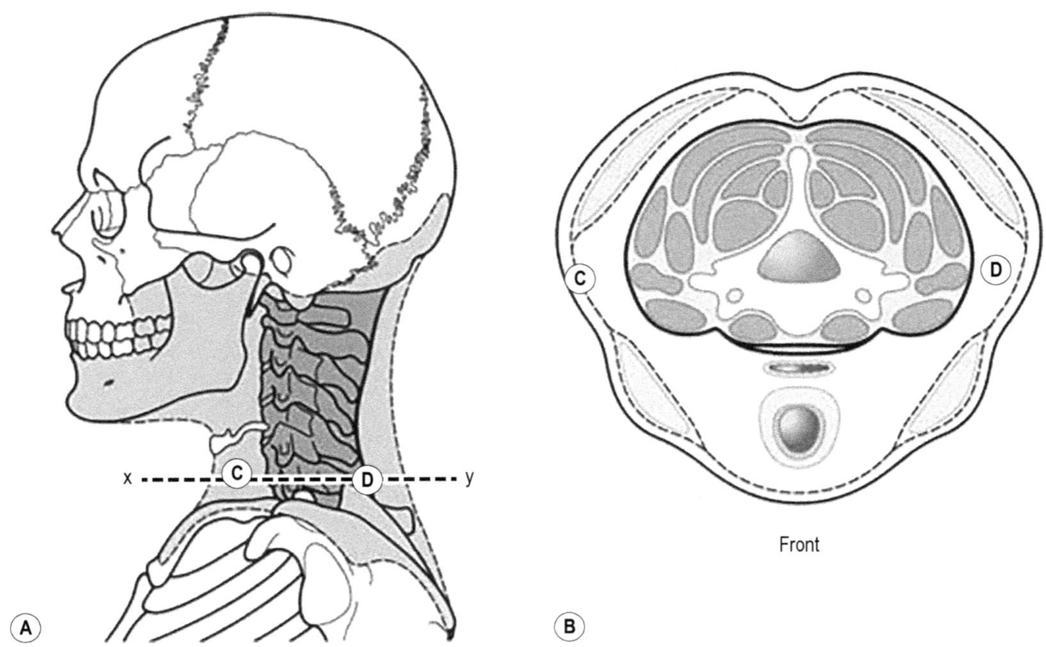

Figure 63.1 Scheme showing the continuity of the fascial system of the cervical region and its links with the scapular–thoracic region. (A) Sagittal projection. **(B)** Horizontal projection. **(C)** The superficial sheet of the deep cervical fasciae communicating the craneal structures and the chewing system with the scapular–thoracic region. **(D)** Prevertebral fascia creating the bond between the sub-occipital region and the shoulder girdle.

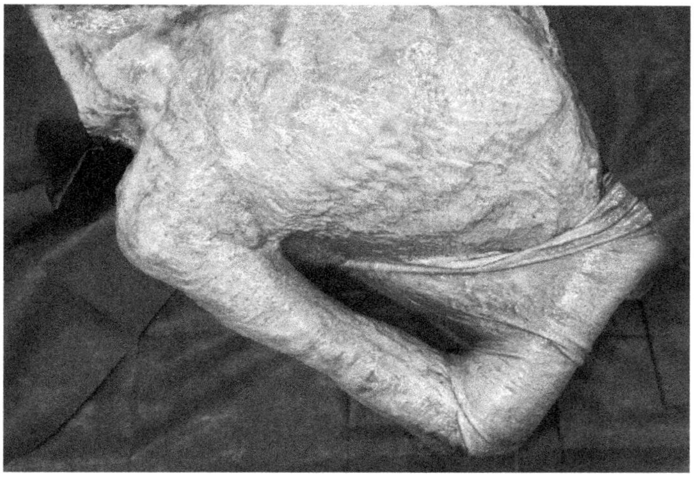

Figure 63.2 Continuity of the superficial fascia in the front part of the body, from the cervical region to the arm, from unembalmed cadaver dissection. Note the skin withdrawn at the level of the forearm as a glove. There is no independent movement between the superficial fascia and the skin.

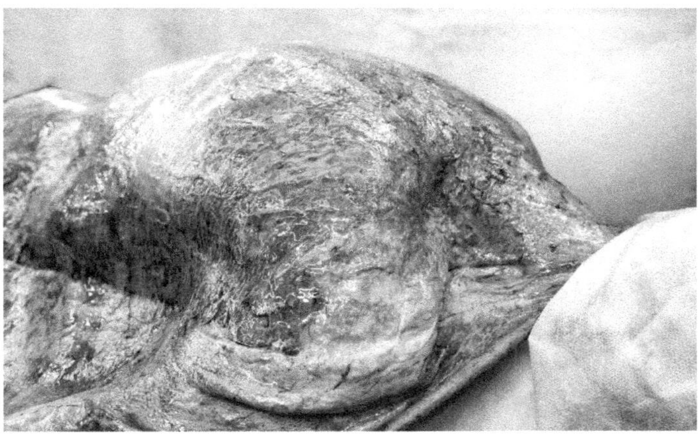

Figure 63.3 Continuity of the superficial fascia of the cervical, scapular and dorsal regions, from unembalmed cadaver dissection.

superficially over the anterolateral neck region. On the upper side, the superficial fascia along the platysma muscle envelops the mandible and continues to the superficial face muscles (i.e. the depressor anguli, depressor labii inferioris and orbicularis oris); on the lower side, it extends beyond the level of the clavicle and inserts into the second and third ribs; on the lateral side, it continues to the platysma insertions.

Deep cervical fascia

The deep cervical fascia is located under the skin, the superficial fascia and the platysma muscle. It is a thin lamina that envelops the neck structures like a collar. At the upper side the fascia inserts onto the periosteum of the occipital external protuberance, the mastoid process of the temporalis bone, the external acoustic meatus, the inferior border of the zygomatic arch and the masseter fascia. It inserts posteriorly onto the spinous processes of the cervical spine, and the nuchal and supraspinous ligaments.

From its posterior insertions, the superficial lamina of the deep cervical fascia divides bilaterally into two compartments enveloping first the upper trapezius and next the sternocleidomastoid muscle (see Fig. 63.1A). At the anterior border of the trapezius muscle, the fascia expands into a fibrotic lamina that attaches to the fascia of the scalene muscles. The sternocleidomastoid fascial envelope is asymmetric, with a deep layer that is thin and therefore low-load resistant. Its superficial layer is thicker and stronger, particularly at the superior part of the muscle belly. At the superior border, the cervical fascia of the sternocleidomastoid muscle forms several fibrotic trabeculae that cross the subcutaneous tissue and the dermis. The sternocleidomastoid and the upper trapezius muscles envelop the borders of the neck region, establishing several free spaces, which permit access to the deepest lamina of the cervical fascial system. Furthermore, on examination the cranial and clavicle insertions of both muscles appear as only one muscle, which may be due to the fact that both muscles arise from the same embryonic lamina, and / or that they are innervated by the same cranial nerve (XI). Finally, other structures that are mechanically associated with the superficial lamina of the deep cervical fascia include the submandibular glandule and the fibrotic capsule of the parotid glandule. This span forms a complex structure that integrates with the dynamics of the shoulder girdle.

The deepest level of the cervical fascia system is represented by the prevertebral fascia (see Fig. 63.1B), which envelops all the cervical muscles excluding the sternocleidomastoid, the upper trapezius and the infrahyoid. The inferior insertions, at the third thoracic vertebra, join the thoracolumbar fascia and continue up to the lumbar region. In its lateral trajectory, the prevertebral fascia runs bilaterally to the axillar fascia; at the anterior–inferior border, it continues towards the vertebral anterior longitudinal ligament and the posterior border of the mediastinum. It covers the three scalene muscles laterally, and the longus collis and longus cervicis muscles anteriorly. Finally, it rests over the transverse processes of the cervical vertebrae (Gallaudet 1931; Bochenek & Reicher 1997; Pilat 2009).

Fascial anatomy of the upper extremity

The upper limb fascia superficial layer

On the superficial level, the fascial continuity between the neck and the arm anatomically is clear (Figs 63.4– 63.5). Along the shoulder and arm region the fat content is high, particularly in women. In the forearm, this content depends on the physical build-up of the individual, though it gradually reduces towards the extremity (Fig. 63.6). In the hand, there is a marked difference between the dorsal and palmar regions, which probably results from the different functions assigned to each surface. In the dorsal area the fascia is loose and thin, which allows for greater mobility during manipulation such as finger-flexing (Fig. 63.7). The fascia of the palmar region is more firmly adhered to the skin (Fig. 63.8), although in the thenar and hypothenar eminence the superficial fascia is again more loose and thin, which facilitates manipulative and gripping actions in both these regions. The superficial fascia

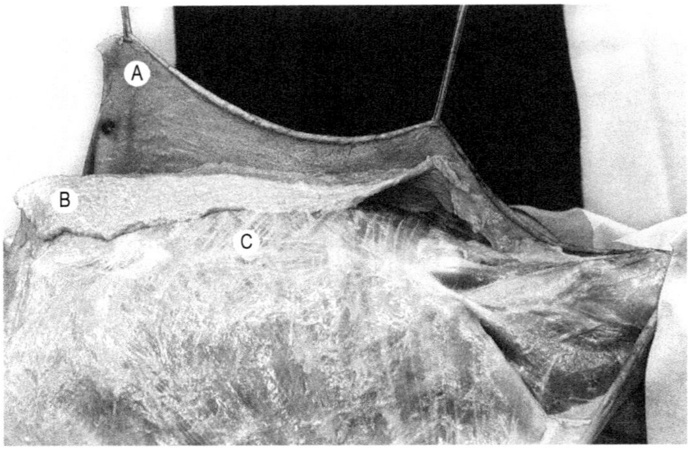

Figure 63.4 Superficial fascia of the cervical and pectoral region from unembalmed cadaver dissection. Note the continuity of the fascial structure and its considerable thickness with high fat content. A. Skin. B. Superficial fascia. C. Deep fascia at a pectoral region.

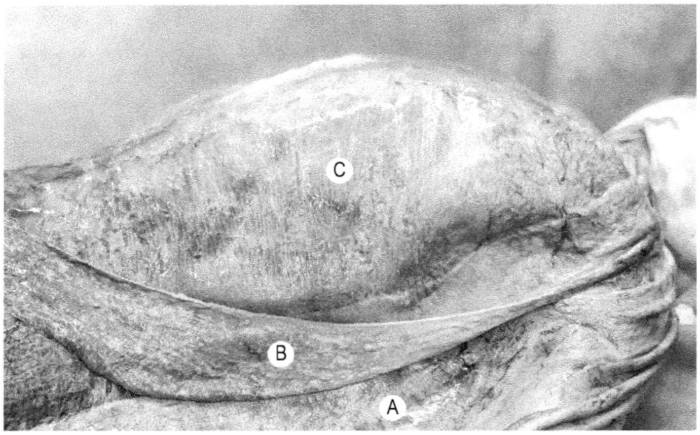

Figure 63.5 Superficial fascia of the scapular–thoracic region, from unembalmed cadaver dissection. Note the continuity of the fascial structure and its smaller thickness in relation to the pectoral region. A. Skin. B. Superficial fascia. C. Deep fascia at the dorsal region.

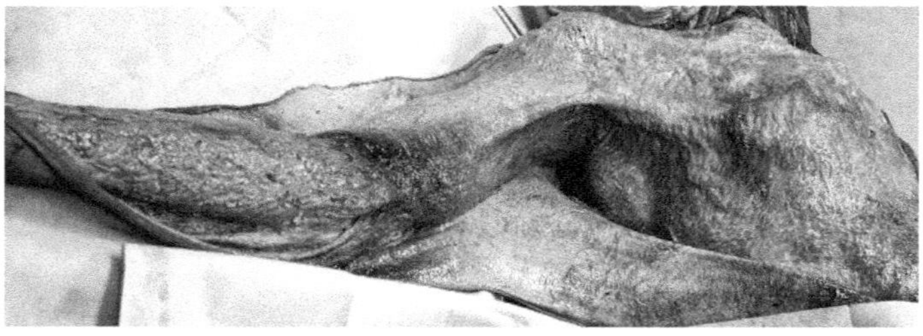

Figure 63.6 Superficial fascia in the forearm, from unembalmed cadaver dissection. Its thickness is smaller in comparison with the arm.

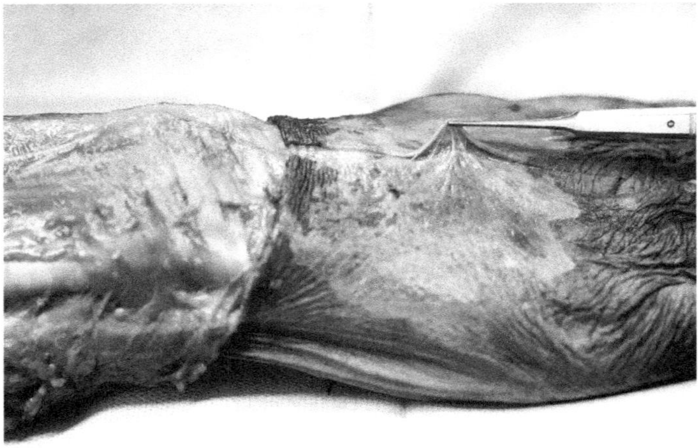

Figure 63.7 Areolar fascia in the dorsum of the hand, from unembalmed cadaver dissection. Note how easy it separates from the deep fascia.

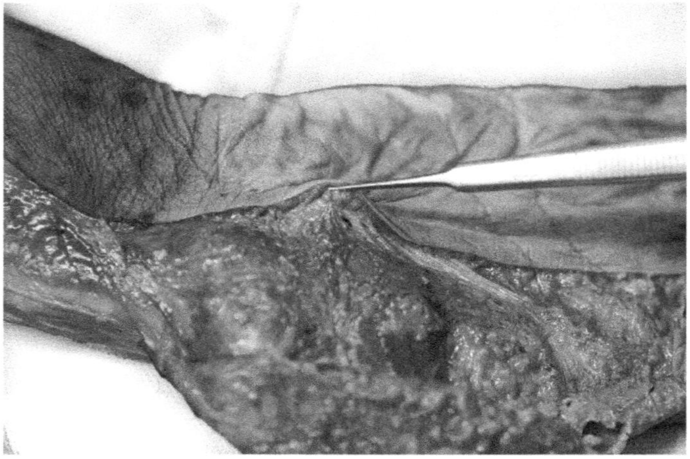

Figure 63.8 Superficial fascia in the palm of the hand from unembalmed cadaver dissection. Note how firmly it adheres to the skin.

has been given various names: subcutaneous fascia (Rouviere & Delmas 2005), cellular cutaneous tissue (Testut & Latarjet 2007) and subcutaneous adipofascial tissue (Avelar 1989). The characteristics of the hand fascia have been analysed mainly in relation to plastic surgery and the skin-healing process (Congdon et al 1946; Markmann & Barton 1987; Avelar 1989). Nevertheless, although the superficial fascia is a major anatomical structure, the dearth of exhaustive anatomical and biomechanical study makes it difficult to clarify its precise role in relation to body movements.

Arm fascia deep layer

The main dynamic fascial link between the cervical region and the upper limb is formed by the superficial sheet of the deep cervical fasciae (Fig. 63.9), which in its lower span extends along the length of the upper limb (Pilat 2003), forms numerous bonds and continues towards the spine of the scapula, the acromion process and the clavicle. These then form surface links to the pectoralis major, the deltoid, the trapezius, the infraspinatus, the teres minor, the teres major and the latissimus dorsi muscles (Fig. 63.10). The intermediate and deep levels (Figs 63.11–63.12) involve the pectoralis minor, the supraspinatus, the levator scapulae, and the rhomboid and

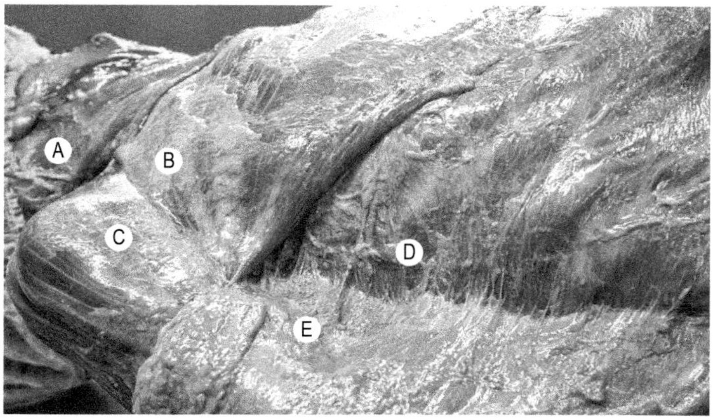

Figure 63.9 The anterior and lateral aspect of the deep fascia from unembalmed cadaver dissection. A. External lamina of the deep cervical fascia. B. Pectoral fascia. C. Deltoid fascia. D. Serratus anterior muscle fascia. E. Superficial fascia. The first four (A–D) form a continuous and thin lamina that infiltrates the muscle mass through fine expansions in the form of intramuscular septa.

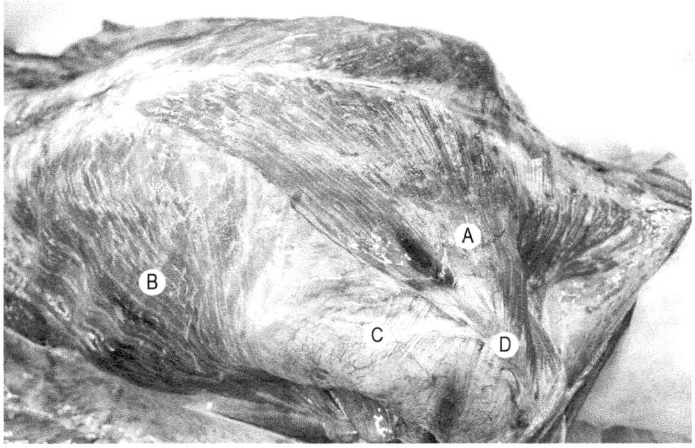

Figure 63.10 The posterior aspect of the deep fascia on the back, from unembalmed cadaver dissection. A. Trapezius muscle. B. Latissimus dorsi muscle. C. Infraspinatus fascia. Note a large density of the fibres of the insertions of the muscles on the spine of the scapula (D) and also the density, thickness and the multidirectional span of the infraspinatus fascia (C).

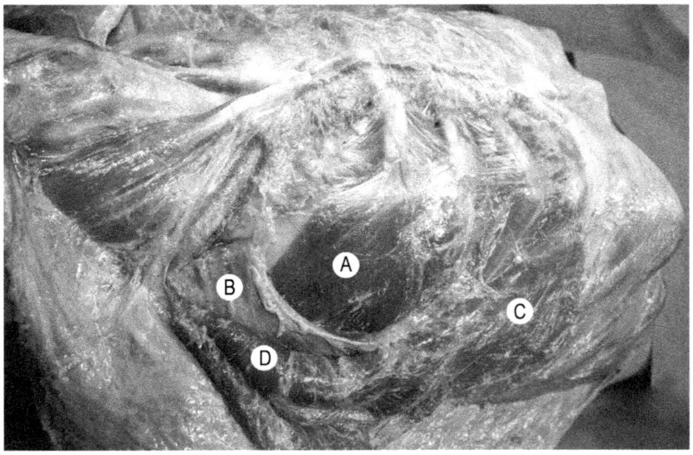

Figure 63.11 Clavipectoral fascia, from unembalmed cadaver dissection. A. Pectoralis minor muscle. B. Clavipectoral fascia. C. Serratus anterior muscle. D. The pectoralis major muscle is sectioned in its sternal and clavicular insertions, turned and resting on the arm.

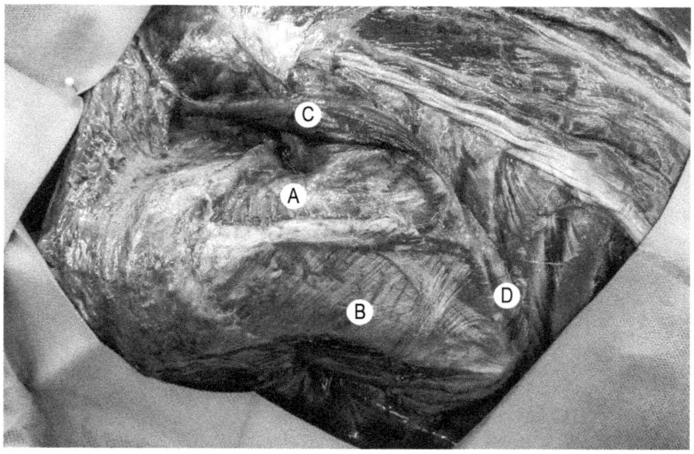

Figure 63.12 Deep aspect of the scapular region, from unembalmed cadaver dissection. A. Supraspinatus muscle. B. Infraspinatus muscle. C. Levator scapulae muscle. D. Rhomboid muscle is hidden under the scapula.

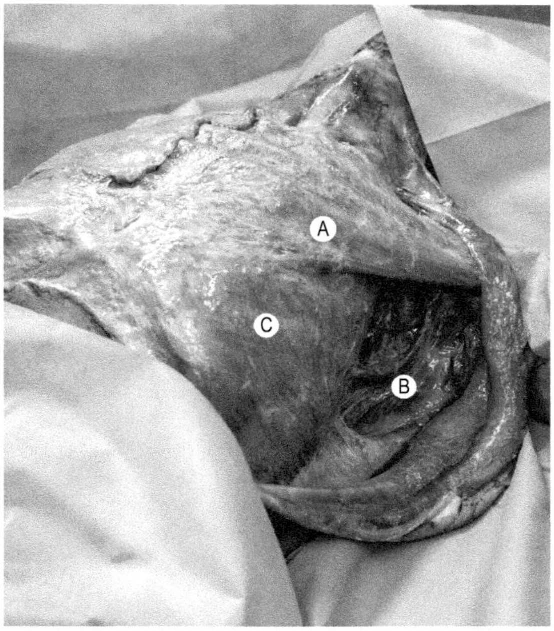

Figure 63.13 Panoramic view of the axillar fossa, from unembalmed cadaver dissection. A. Pectoralis major muscle. B. Latissimus dorsi muscle. C. Serratus anterior muscles.

subscapularis muscles. This span forms a complex structure that integrates with the dynamics of the shoulder girdle. It can be divided into two groups:

Front and anterior–lateral span

- The pectoralis fascia (Fig. 63.13) forms a thin sheet deployed over the front of the thorax, which in its medium span is firmly inserted into the sternum and continues, covering the front of the pectoralis major, to enfold over its lower edge, supporting the inner face. Under the pectoralis major it is continuous with the fascia of the anterior abdominal wall (Pilat 2003; Testut & Latarjet 2007).

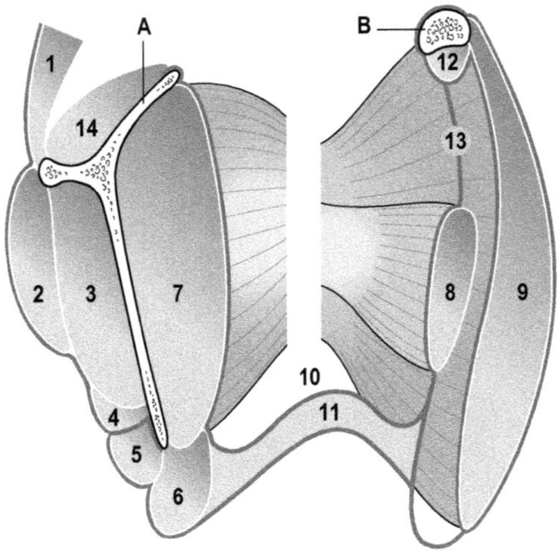

A Scapula
B Cavicle
1 Trapezius muscle
2 Deltoid muscle
3 Infraspinatus muscle
4 Teres minor muscle
5 Teres major muscle
6 Latissimus dorsi muscle
7 Subscapularis muscle
8 Pectoralis minor muscle
9 Pectoralis major muscle
10 Deep lamina of the axillar fascia
11 Superficial lamina of the axillar fascia
12 Subclavian muscle
13 Clavipectoral fascia
14 Supraspinatus muscle

Figure 63.14 Sagittal section of the axillar fossa, from fresh cadaver dissection.

- The deltoid fascia (see Fig. 63.9) extends as a direct lateral expansion of the pectoralis fascia. It enfolds the deltoid muscle and, in the posterior span, links to the infraspinatus muscle. The lower span continues with the brachial fascia.
- The clavipectoral fascia is suspended in the intermediate plane, starting at the front edge of the clavicle, the coracoid process and the coracoclavicular ligament. It enfolds the subclavian muscle, continues over the front part of the sternum and joins the deltoid fascia laterally. It also expands from its lower edge to enfold the pectoralis minor. In its deep span it is firmly integrated with the intercostal muscles and the ribs. Its lower end continues to the axillary fossa, where it joins the pectoralis fascia (see Fig. 63.11) (Gallaudet 1931; Bochenek & Reicher 1997).
- The serratus anterior fascia is very thin, and covers the muscle's entire surface (see Fig. 63.13).

Posterior and posterior–lateral span

- The trapezius fascia (see Fig. 63.10) is continuous with the superficial sheet of the deep cervical fasciae in its posterior length; from the spina of the scapula it becomes the trapezius fascia, covering its middle and lower fibres.
- The supraspinatus fascia (see Fig. 63.12) enfolds the supraspinatus muscle, enclosing it together with the osseous channel of the supraspinatus fossa within an osteofascial compartment (Rouviere & Delmas 2005).
- The infraspinatus fascia (see Fig. 63.12) is a very resistant structure that throughout its length, starting on the spine of the scapula, provides support to the infraspinatus, teres minor and teres major muscles, adjoining them at their insertions (Rouviere & Delmas 2005). It is firmly united to the medial and lateral borders of the scapula, with strong and multidirectional fibre connections.
- The latissimus dorsi fascia (see Figs 63.10–63.13) is continuous with the fascia of the teres major muscle and is strengthened inferiorly by the deep layer of the axillar fascia.
- The fascia of the levator of the scapulae muscle (see Fig. 63.12) comprises a thin sheet that accompanies the muscle throughout its length.
- The fascia of the subscapularis muscle covers the area of the subscapularis fossa, separating the subscapularis and the serratus major muscles.
- The rhomboid muscle fascia (see Fig. 63.12) is more robust in its span at the lower end, where it is continuous with the trapezius and the latissimus dorsi muscles.
- The axillary fascia (Figs 63.13–63.14) forms the axillar base. Throughout its surface it reaches from the lower border of the pectoralis fascia to the lower end of the teres major and latissimus dorsi muscles. It forms a sort of square that is suspended from the lower border of the pectoralis minor muscle, runs through the axillary edge of the scapula, enters the insertions of the subscapularis, teres major and teres minor muscles and finally approaches the glenoid cavity. In its medial span, it approaches the anterior serratus muscle (Bochenek & Reicher 1997; Rouviere & Delmas 2005; Testut & Latarjet 2007).

This very complex distribution of the myofascial system enables effective integration of the fascial structures of the cervical region with the brachial fascia, the antebrachial fascia and finally the hand structures.

- The brachial fascia forms a strong layer that envelops the structures of the arm like a glove. At the superior end, it is continuous with the pectoralis fascia (Fig. 63.15), the deltoid, the axillar and the dorsal fasciae, and then with the thoracolumbar fascia (Rouviere & Delmas 2005; Testut & Latarjet 2007) – thus linking the dynamics of the scapular girdle with those of the upper limb. Stecco et al (2008) identified these connections and fascial continuities in fresh cadaver specimens, and concluded that they cannot be assumed to be merely anatomical variations. They also noted the presence of a considerable number of muscular fibres that were somehow connected to the intramuscular septa; these septa were continuous with the fascia enveloping the overlying muscular fascia that

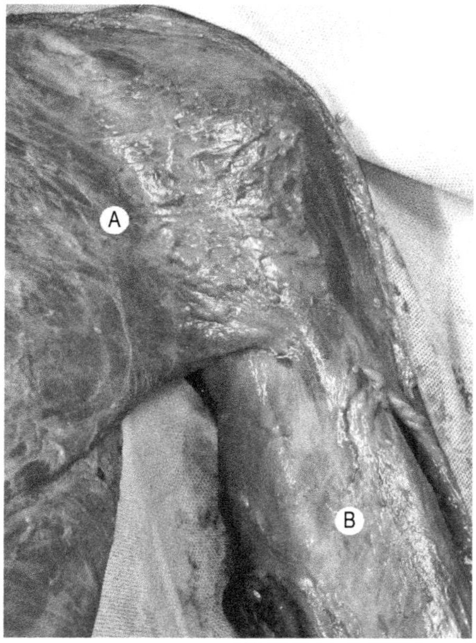

Figure 63.15 Detail of the interlinking of the fascia pectoralis with the brachial fascia, from unembalmed cadaver dissection. A. Pectoralis fascia. B. Brachial fascia.

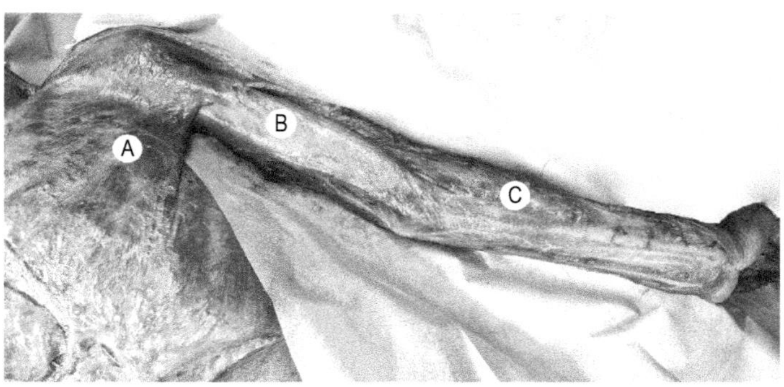

Figure 63.16 Fascial continuity of the anterior aspect of the upper limb, from unembalmed cadaver dissection. A. Pectoralis fascia. B. Brachial fascia. C. Antebrachial fascia.

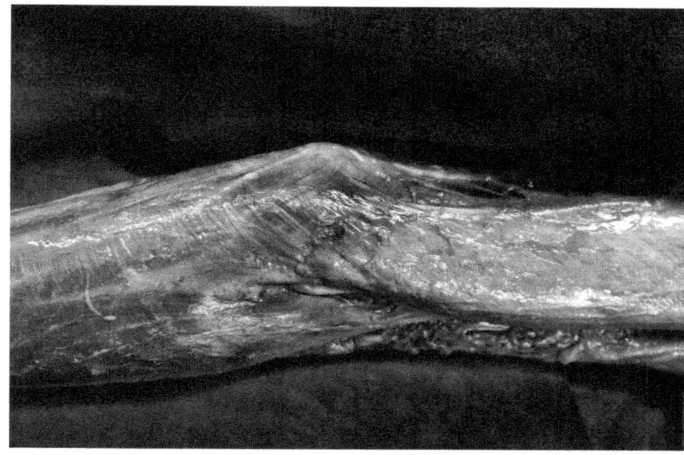

Figure 63.17 Lacertus fibrosus. Note the continuity between the brachial and antebrachial fascia, from unembalmed cadaver dissection.

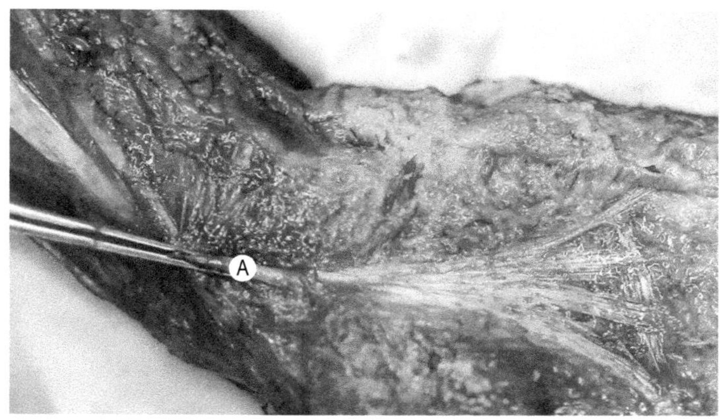

Figure 63.18 Palmar fascia, from unembalmed cadaver dissection. Note a dense and firm fibrotic union between the skin and the palmar fascia, evidenced by the presence of longitudinal and transverse fibres. A. The tendon of the palmaris longus muscle.

connected to the brachial fascia. This finding was confirmed in observations of transverse sections. When there is muscular contraction, some bundles will tense the intramuscular septa and indirectly strengthen the brachial fascia. Stecco et al (2008) further suggested that these expansions and insertions strengthen the anatomical design of the brachial fascia and place it under selective tension, which may increase the effectiveness of arm movement. The brachial fascia expands two fibrous sheets that are transversally oriented, forming the flexor and extensor compartments (Rouviere & Delmas 2005), which mainly involve the two main muscles of the arm: the triceps and biceps. In the upper third of the arm, there is a third compartment that contains the coracobrachial muscle.

- The antebrachial fascia arises as a direct continuation of the inferior section of the brachial fascia (Fig. 63.16). On the ventral surface, there is a very particular connection between the brachial and the antebrachial fasciae and the lower insertion of the brachial biceps muscle through the bicipital aponeurosis or lacertus fibrosus (Fig. 63.17). This fan-shaped structure (Testut & Latarjet 2007) extends from the lower tendon of the biceps to continue over the antebrachial fascia in the proximal end. It then inserts into the cubital region of the common mass of the epitrochlear muscles (Blemker et al 2005; Chew & Giuffrè 2005). The lacertus fibrosus connection is perhaps one of the best examples of the dynamic linkage whereby power is transmitted directly from fascia to fascia, reinforcing the bone–tendon connection. On the posterior of the limb is a direct link between the triceps muscle and the antebrachial fascia. One part of the triceps' tendon is firmly inserted into the olecranon and the other continues to attach to the antebrachial fascia.
- The palmar fascia extends in a fan pattern as a continuation of the antebrachial fascia. It is a thick structure reinforced by the long palmar muscle. It continues laterally to the thenar and hypothenar eminences (Fig. 63.18).

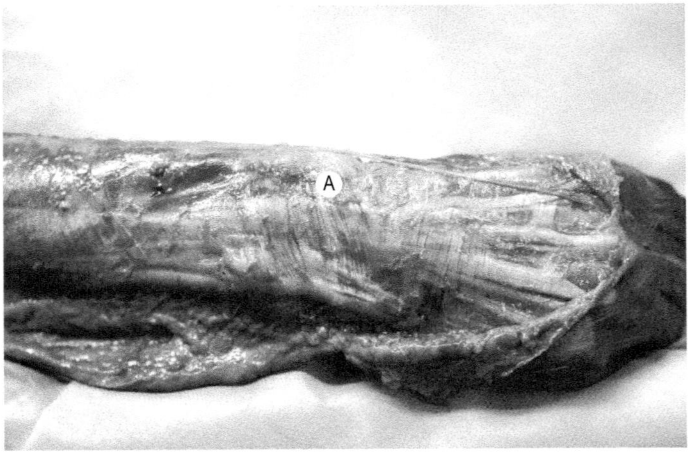

Figure 63.19 Dorsal fascia of the hand, from unembalmed cadaver dissection. A. Extensor retinaculum.

- The dorsal fascia of the hand is continuous with that of the forearm. It spreads to cover the tendons of the extensor muscles and then thickens to form the extensor retinaculum over a transverse span of the fibres (Fig. 63.19). The main function of the retinaculum is first to maintain the precise functional positioning of the extensors' tendons, and also to stop them becoming loose when in contraction.

Anatomical Considerations Related to the Continuity of the Fascial System of the Pelvis and Lower Extremity

Traditionally, the anatomical description of the fascia is related to the topography of the muscles attached to a specific part of the body. However, the adoption of a bipedal position and locomotion by humans has forced the development of a complementary support system for maintaining body weight and optimizing daily activities to rationalize the use of energy. For this reason, the anatomical analysis of the fascia of the lower quadrant focuses on the anatomical links comprising this system. The lumbar spine, for instance, is not alone capable of sustaining the normal loads that it carries daily (Crisco et al 1992; Willard et al 2012). Protecting the spine's fragile structures is a myofascial complex that surrounds the trunk (Bergmark 1989; Cholewicki et al 1997; Schuenke et al 2012; Willard et al 2012). The most important structure of this complex is the thoracolumbar fascia. Its principal functions are participation in the flexion and extension of the trunk (Gatton et al 2010), maintenance of upright body posture and also bipedal locomotion (Gracovetsky 2008; Willard et al 2012). Anatomically the thoracolumbar fascia appears as the largest body aponeurotic structure and dynamic connection bridging the trunk and limbs. Wood Jones (1944) considers that the topography and dynamics of fascia's lower extremity are linked to its ectoskeletal function, which has a role in maintaining the upright body position. Hence the architectural orientation of the fascial system is determined by its weight-bearing function; for example, the gluteus maximus and tensor fasciae latae muscles are mainly inserted into the deep fascia rather than onto the bone so as to maximize their mechanical efficiency. Within this framework, in the next section we analyse the continuity of the fascial system in consecutive layers of its construction and relate it to the force transmission during the basic tasks of the lower quadrant.

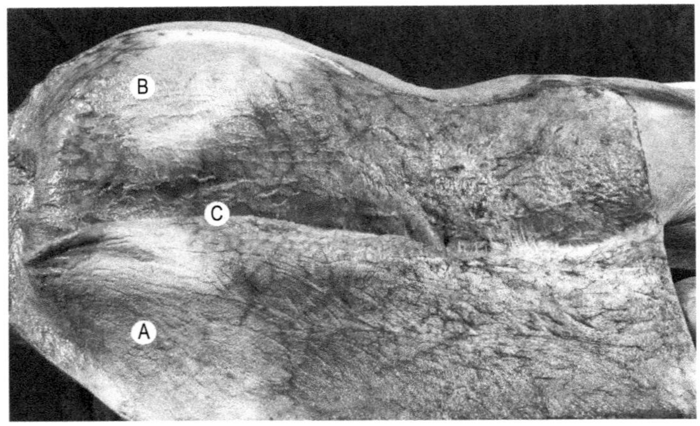

Figure 63.20 Back region from unembalmed cadaver dissection. A. Skin (inner view). B. Superficial fascia. C. Section line. Notes: Observe the differences of the vascularization intensity between the upper thoracic area (strongly vascularized), lower thoracic area (weakly vascularized) and lumbar area (again strongly vascularized). Note the mirror effect between the skin and superficial fascia areas.

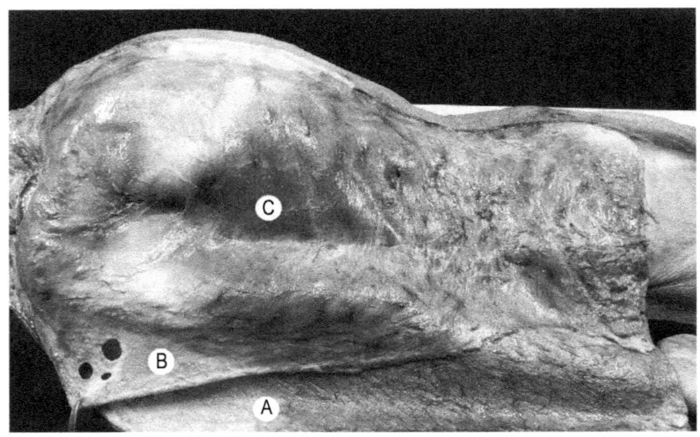

Figure 63.21 The superficial and deep fascia levels on the back from unembalmed cadaver dissection. A. Skin (inner view). B. Superficial fascia (inner view). C. Deep fascia.

Superficial and deep fascial anatomical links between the trunk and lower limbs

Superficial fascia (firmly attached to the skin)

On the posterior, the superficial fascia covers the thoracic and lumbar areas (see Fig. 63.3), then continues to the iliac crest (Figs 63.20–63.22) and runs without interruption down the length of the entire lower extremity up to the end of the foot structure (Fig. 63.23). On the anterior, it continues from the cervical segment through the pectoral and abdominal region to the inguinal area (see Fig. 63.2). There it becomes the fascia

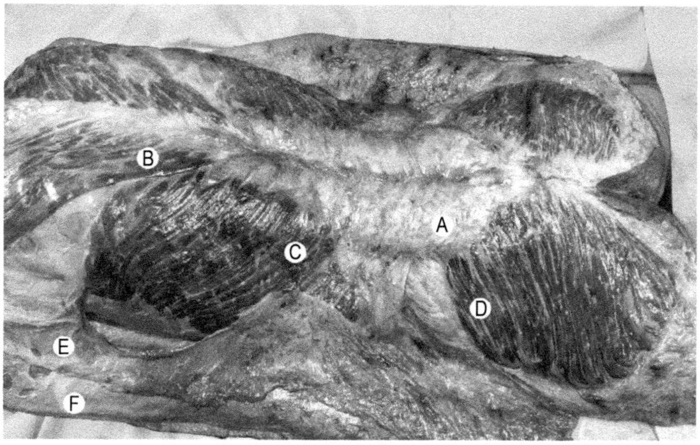

Figure 63.22 Thoracolumbar fascia as a bridge structure (image from unembalmed cadaver dissection). A. Thoracolumbar fascia (TLF). B. Trapezius muscle. C. Latissimus dorsi muscle (LD). D. Gluteus maximus muscle (GM). E. Deep fascia (inner view). F. Superficial fascia (inner view). Note the continuity between the LD and opposite GM across the TLF.

of the thigh and leg, continuing to the dorsum of the foot (see Figs 63.32, 63.38–63.39).

Deep fascia (located directly under the superficial fascia)

On the posterior, the deep fascia follows the same path as the superficial fascia from the cervical segment to the iliac crest (see Fig. 63.21), where it becomes the gluteal fascia and attaches to the iliac crest, sacrum and coccyx (Fig. 63.24). On the anterior, the abdominal fascia becomes the fascia lata at the iliac crest, groin and pubis levels (see Figs 63.32–63.33, 63.39).

Below the iliac crest and the inguinal area, the thoracolumbar fascia and abdominal fascia become the multilevel lower extremity fascial system (fascia lata, fascia of the leg, foot fascia).

Deep fascia of the thigh segment

The fascia lata surrounds the thigh. On the posterior, it is continuous with the gluteal fascia (Figs 63.24–63.25). On the anterior, its origin is in the inguinal ligament (see Figs 63.32–63.33, 63.39); it continues along the thigh and is inserted into the patella and tibia (see Figs 63.32, 63.39).

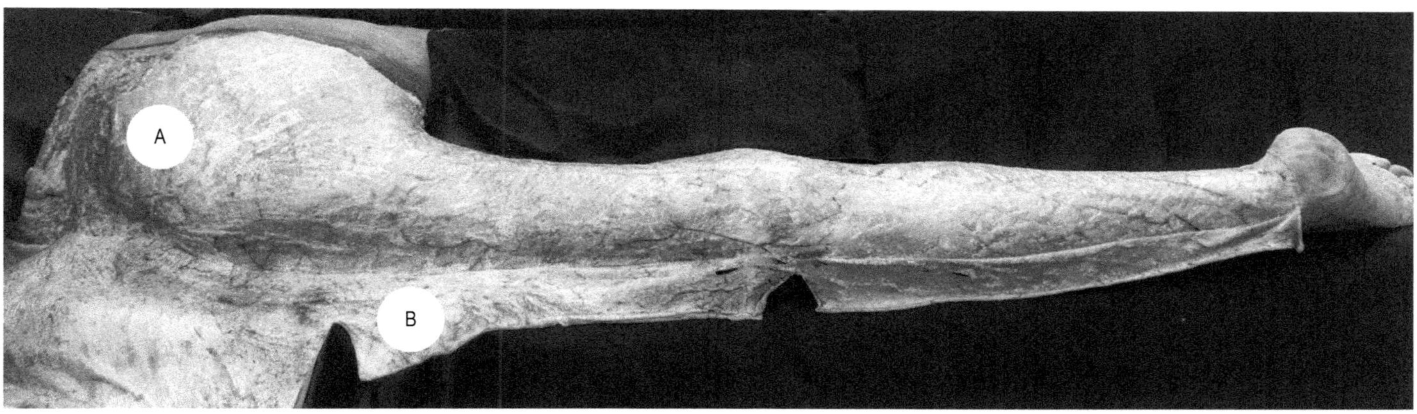

Figure 63.23 The continuity of the superficial fascia on lower extremity from unembalmed cadaver dissection (posterior view). A. The superficial fascia continuity. B. The skin (inner view).

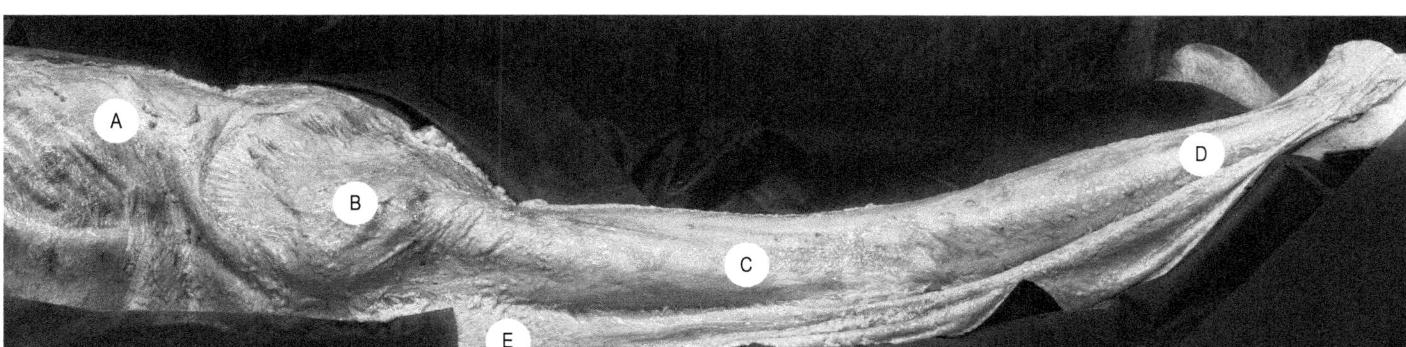

Figure 63.24 The continuity of the deep fascia on lower extremity from unembalmed cadaver dissection (posterior view). A. Back region. B. Gluteal region. C. Thigh region. D. Leg region. E. Skin in conjunction with the superficial fascia (inner view).

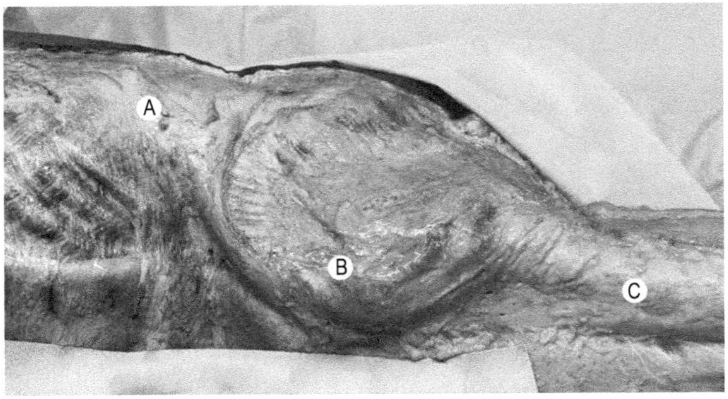

Figure 63.25 The continuity of the deep fascia on upper part of the lower extremity from unembalmed cadaver dissection (close-up view). Observe the fibrous appearance of the deep fascial tissue. A. Back region. B. Gluteal region (gluteal fascia). C. Thigh region (fascia lata).

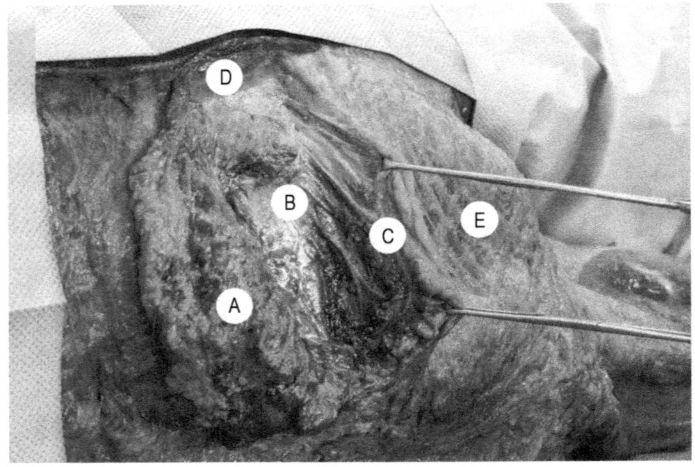

Figure 63.26 Cross-section of the gluteus maximus muscle from a unembalmed cadaver dissection. A. Cranial portion of the gluteus maximus muscle (inner view). B. Deep layer of the gluteal fascia. C. Caudal portion of the gluteus maximus muscle. D. Sacrum. E. Superficial layer of the gluteal fascia. Note the fibrous fascial connections.

On the inner side of the fascia lata there originate several fibrous expansions as the beginning of muscle fascias (fascial sheets) (see Fig. 63.33). In some places these sheets merge with ligaments (e.g. the iliopsoas fascia with the inguinal ligament) or tendons (e.g. the fascia of the tensor fasciae latae with its tendinous sheet).

Deep fascia of the leg segment

The fascia of the leg surrounds the leg structure with a strong insertion into the tibia merging with the periosteum (see Figs 63.39 and 63.75). On the posterior, it is continuous with the fascia lata (see Fig. 63.34). On the anterior, it attaches to fibula, the condyles and the tibial tuberosity (see Figs 63.39–63.40).

On the inner side of the fascia of the leg, an intermuscular septa (anterior and superior) originates, which together with the interosseous membrane form compartments that define and control the position of the leg muscles (see Fig. 63.70).

Deep fascia of the foot segment

At its lower end the leg fascia becomes fascia of the foot (see Fig. 63.34). The dorsal side covers the tendons of the long extensor muscles (see Fig. 63.39), whereas the plantar side covers the superficial muscles of the foot (see Fig. 63.34).

Deep fascial intermuscular links

Thoracolumbar segment

In the thoracolumbar segment the most relevant tissue is the thoracolumbar fascia and its connections. As mentioned earlier, the thoracolumbar fascia acts as a bridge structure between the muscles of the trunk and the extremities. At the most superficial level the most extensive connection is between the latissimus dorsi and gluteus maximus muscles (see Figs 63.22, 63.28), which is expressed in the activities of locomotion and trunk stabilization (see Fig. 63.29). Recently, Carvalhais et al (2013) demonstrated in vivo that manipulating the tension of the latissimus dorsi muscle also modified the passive hip variables, thus providing evidence of myofascial force transmission between the gluteus maximus and latissimus dorsi muscles on the opposite side. The deep lamina of

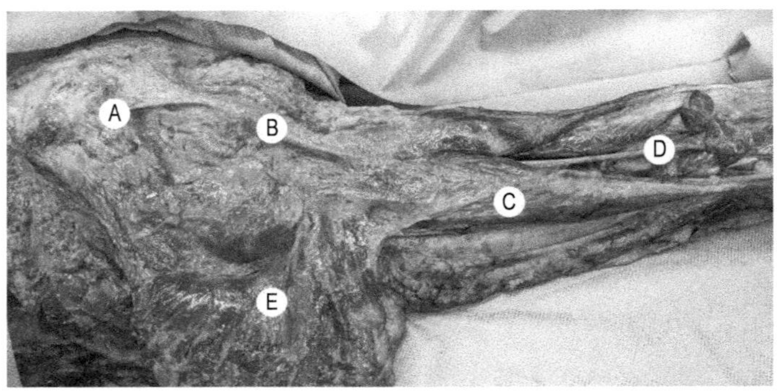

Figure 63.27 The posterior aspect of the gluteal region and the thigh from a unembalmed cadaver dissection. A. Sacrotuberous ligament. B. Tendon of the long head of the biceps femoris muscle. C. Biceps femoris muscle belly. D. Sciatic nerve. E. Gluteus maximus muscle (inner view). (Reproduced from Chaitow & Lovegrove Jones (2012). Chronic pelvic pain and dysfunction: practical physical medicine. Elsevier, with permission. Picture from the same author.)

the gluteal fascia (Fig. 63.26) communicates with the underlying muscles including the gluteus medius, piriformis, superior and inferior gemellus, obturatorius externus and quadratus femoris. There is a link between the sacrotuberous ligament and the tendon of the long head of biceps femoris muscle; it creates a deep connection between the biceps femoris and thoracolumbar fascia (Figs 63.27–63.28). The communication and transmission of mechanical impulses was found to be not only from and through the thoracolumbar fascia to the latissimus dorsi muscle, but also to the trapezius muscle and through both upper extremities (Fig. 63.29). In relation to the balance of force distribution through the fascial planes related to the thoracolumbar fascia, the interfascial lumbar triangle (LIFT) is important (Schuenke et al 2012; Willard et al 2012) (Fig. 63.30); this is the area of intersection of the fascia corresponding to the common extensor lumbar mass (i.e. the multifidus, longissimus and iliocostalis muscles), the abdominal muscles (i.e. the transversus abdominis, internal oblique and external oblique), the serratus posterior–inferior muscle, the latissimus dorsi and the quadratus lumborum. The authors suggested that this triangle may act to distribute laterally mediated tension in order to balance various viscoelastic modules, along either the middle or the posterior layers of the thoracolumbar fascia (Schuenke et al 2012).

Thigh segment

The deep fascia of the thigh initiates two intermuscular septa (medial and lateral), ordering the large muscles as well as the femoral vessels in its longitudinal path (see Fig. 63.31). It also initiates the muscle sheaths that define the positioning of individual muscles and their inter-relationship. On the posterior, it includes the continuity between the sacrotuberous ligament and the tendon of the long head of the biceps femoris muscle, as well as the path of the sciatic nerve (see Fig. 63.27). On the anterior, the fascia from the abdominal region crosses the inguinal ligament and covers the anterior thigh (Fig. 63.32). Note the fibrous appearance of the facial planes in Figure 63.33.

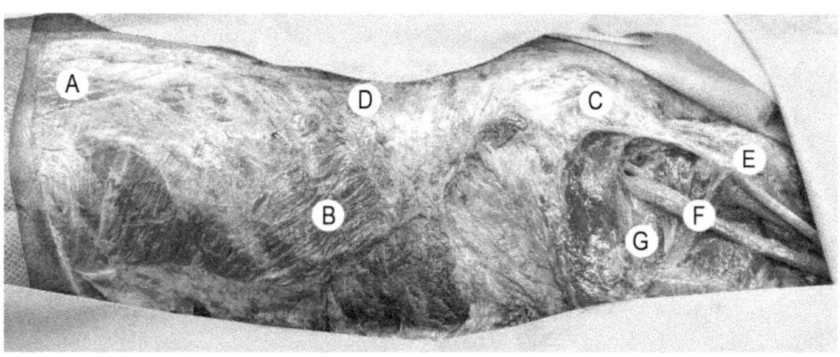

Figure 63.28 The posterior–lateral side of the back, pelvis and thigh from an unembalmed cadaver dissection. Deep aspect. A. Trapezius muscle. B. Latissimus dorsi muscle. C. Sacrotuberous ligament. D. Thoracolumbar fascia. E. Tendon of the long head of the biceps femoris muscle. F. Sciatic nerve. G. Piriformis muscle belly. (Reproduced from Chaitow & Lovegrove Jones (2012). Chronic pelvic pain and dysfunction: practical physical medicine. Elsevier, with permission. Picture from the same author.)

Leg and foot segment (Figs 63.34–63.39)

In the posterior aspect of the leg can be observed the fibrous aponeurotic expansions of gastrocnemius muscles and a long haul of Achilles tendon, with progressive densification of the fibres (see Fig. 63.35). Figure 63.36 shows the fascial plane between the gastrocnemius and soleus muscles. In a dissection of the plantar fascia (Fig. 63.37), the Achilles tendon and plantar fascia are seen to form a continuum interrupted by the

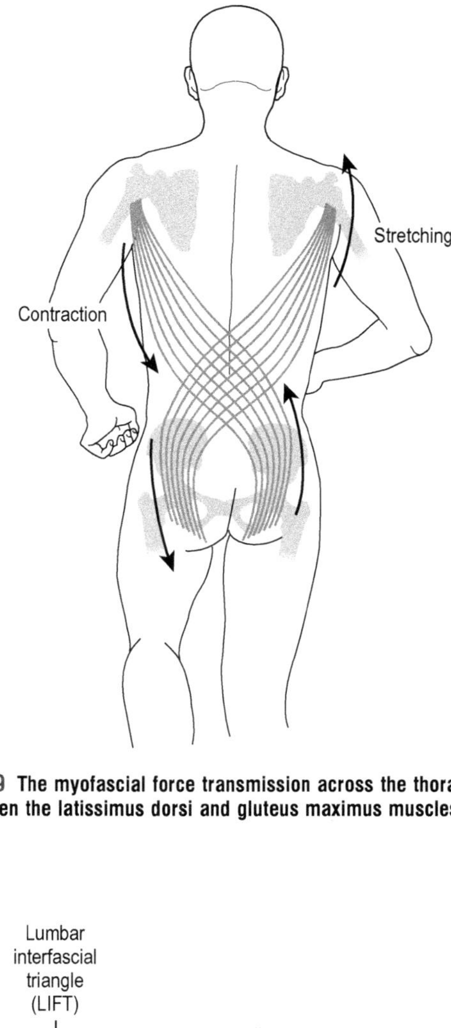

Figure 63.29 The myofascial force transmission across the thoracolumbar fascia between the latissimus dorsi and gluteus maximus muscles during running.

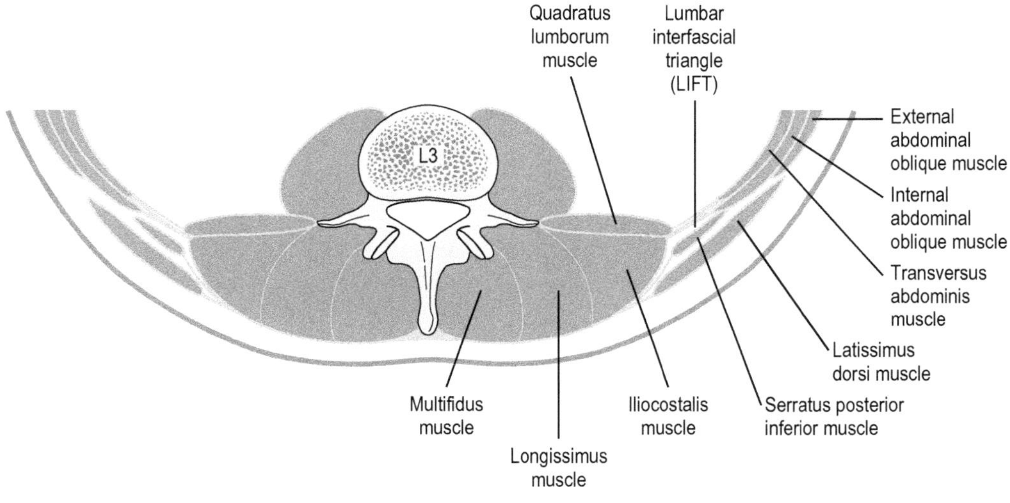

Figure 63.30 Cross-section at the L3 level.

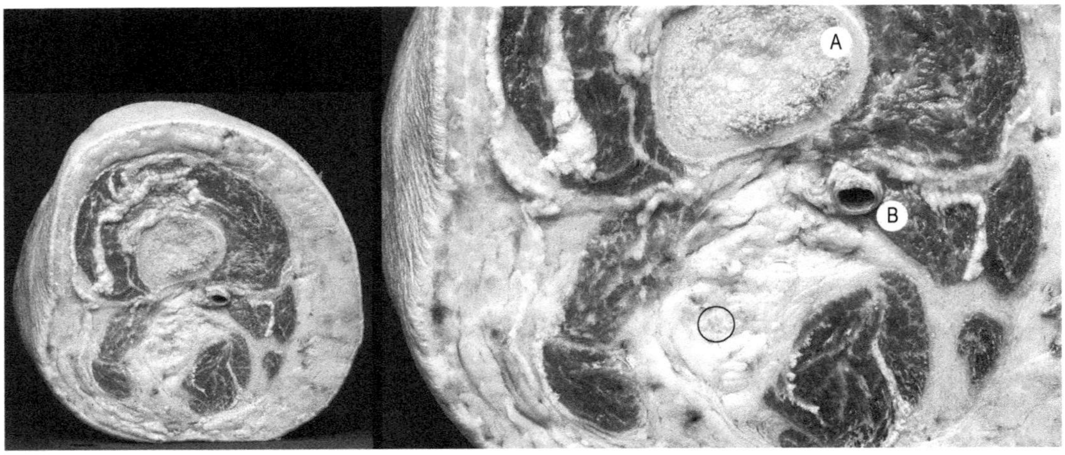

Figure 63.31 Cross-section of the third upper thigh from unembalmed cadaver dissection. A. Femur. B. Deep femoral artery. The circle shows the sciatic nerve.

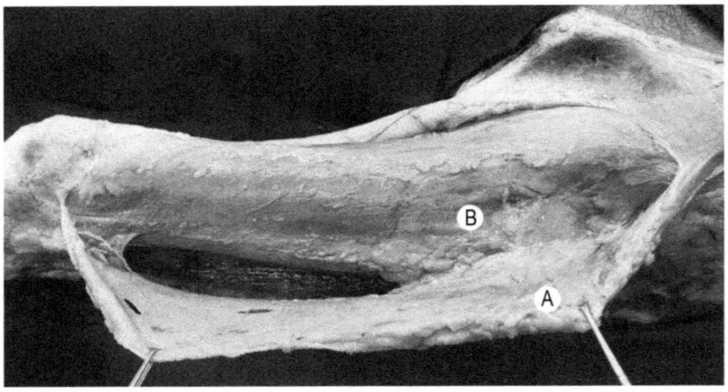

Figure 63.32 Close up of the fascial levels on the anterior aspect of the thigh from an unembalmed cadaver dissection. A. Superficial fascia (inner view). B. Deep fascia (fascia lata). (Reproduced from Chaitow & Lovegrove Jones (2012). Chronic pelvic pain and dysfunction: practical physical medicine. Elsevier, with permission. Picture from the same author.)

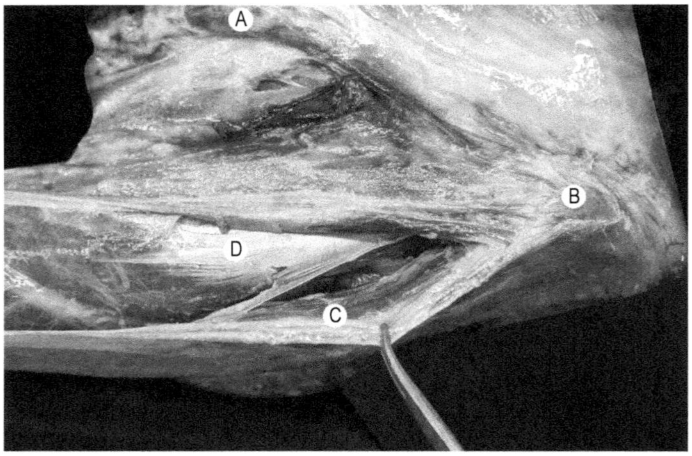

Figure 63.33 Incision of the deep fascia of the thigh from an unembalmed cadaver dissection. Note the aponeurotic expansion of the quadriceps muscle. A. Pubis. B. Anterior superior iliac crest. C. Deep fascia (fascia lata). D. Quadriceps muscle. (Reproduced from Chaitow & Lovegrove Jones (2012). Chronic pelvic pain and dysfunction: practical physical medicine. Elsevier, with permission. Picture from the same author.)

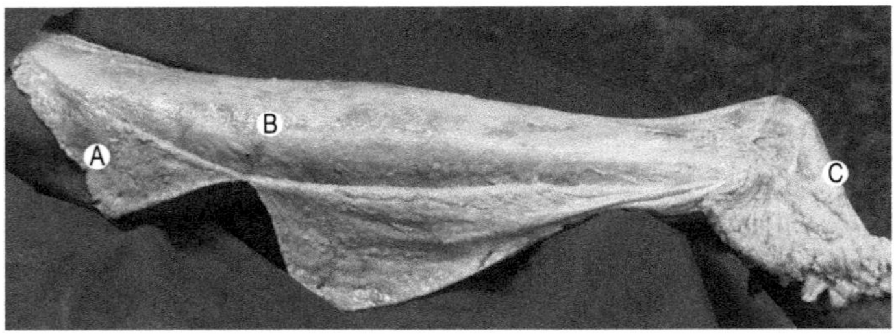

Figure 63.34 The deep fascia of the leg from an unembalmed cadaver dissection. A. Skin along with the superficial fascia and fat nodules. B. The deep fascia. C. The plantar fascia.

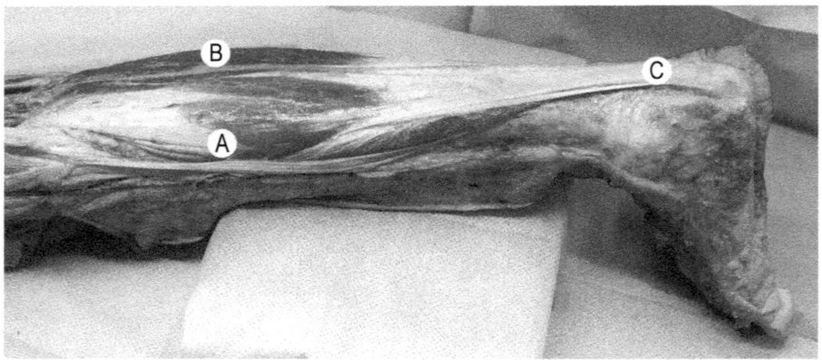

Figure 63.35 Muscles level of the posterior aspect of the leg from an unembalmed cadaver dissection. A. Medial gastrocnemius muscle. B. Lateral gastrocnemius muscle. C. Achilles tendon.

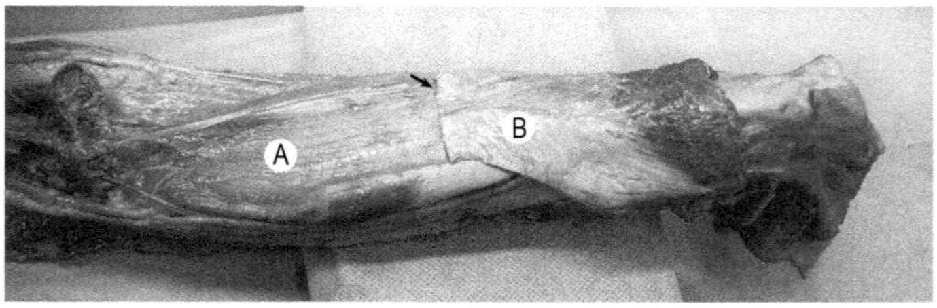

Figure 63.36 Deep aspect of posterior leg from a fresh cadaver dissection. A. Soleus muscle. B. Gastrocnemius muscles (inner view). Arrow: fascial connection.

periosteum of the calcaneus, with which both structures are merged. A similar phenomenon of fusion of the fascia with the periosteum can also be seen in the lateral aspect of the leg (see Fig. 63.75).

Knee joint and popliteal fossa segment

At the level of the knee joint, the fibrous stabilizing structure of the patella forms a multilevel and multidirectional complex web (Fig. 63.40). This network functions mainly in the positioning of the patella in between the quadriceps tendon, the infrapatellar ligament and the fascia lata; it also helps to control lateral patella movements (Figs 63.41–63.42).

In the popliteal fossa, the fascia system acts as a protection for the nerves and vessels passing through it (Fig. 63.42; see also Fig. 63.45). (Note the presence of abundant layer of loose connective tissue with a considerable amount of fat nodules in Fig. 63.45.)

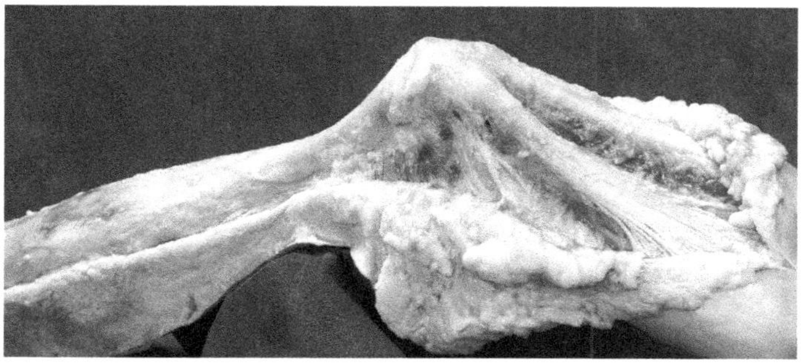

Figure 63.37 Plantar fascia from an unembalmed cadaver dissection. Observe the continuity between the plantar fascia and deep fascia of the leg.

Theoretical Aspects Related to the Treatment of Myofascial Dysfunction Syndrome

Mechanics of myofascial dysfunction syndrome formation

Fascial system dysfunction is defined as an alteration of the highly organized wave of specialized movements and as the incorrect transfer of information through the matrix (Pilat 2003). If there is impairment of proper fascial dynamics (i.e. gliding between endofascial fibres and interfascial planes) then optimal body functioning may be affected. This is connected to a suboptimal exchange of fluids; reduction in mobility alters the quality of blood circulation, which becomes slow and heavy, and leading in extreme cases to ischaemia and

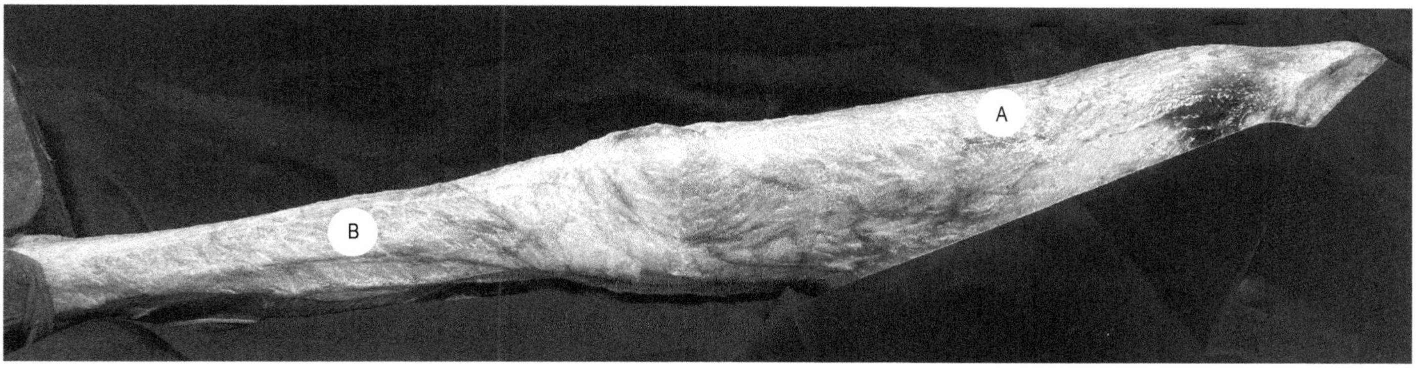

Figure 63.38 Superficial fascia path of the anterior aspect of lower extremity from an unembalmed cadaver dissection. A. Thigh region. B. Leg region.

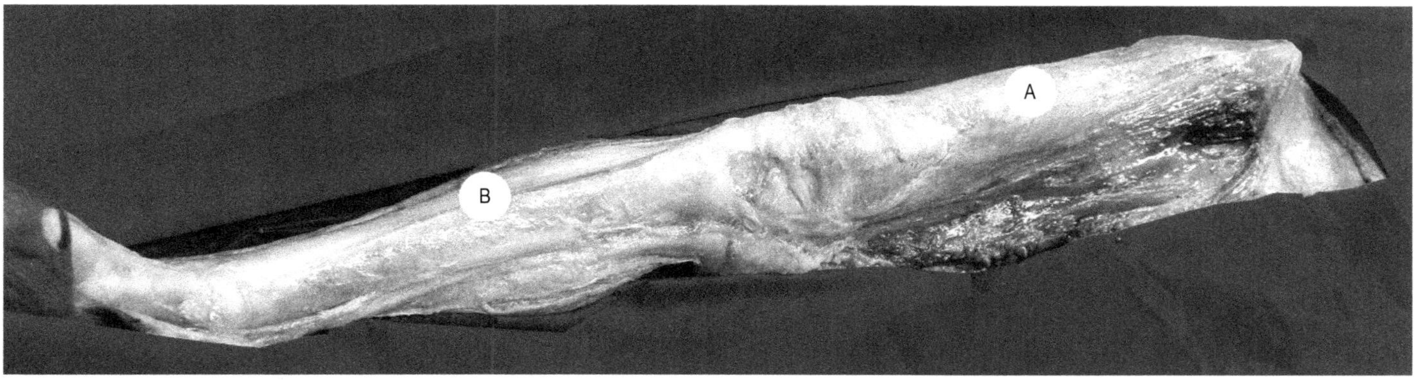

Figure 63.39 Deep fascia path of the anterior aspect of lower extremity from an unembalmed cadaver dissection. A. Thigh region (fascia lata). B. Leg region.

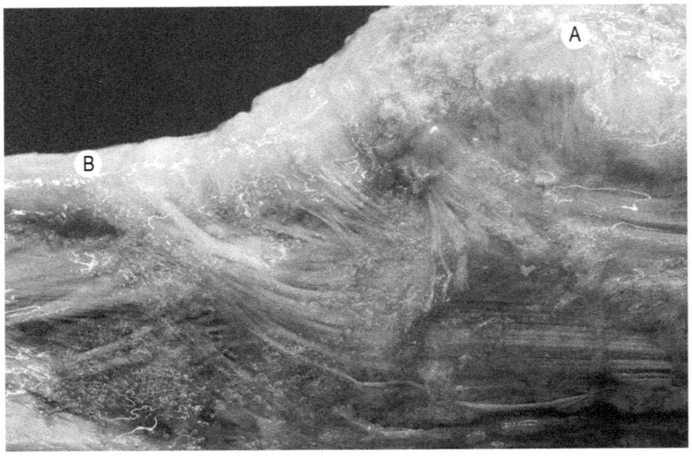

Figure 63.40 Close up of the anterior–lateral aspect of the knee joint from unembalmed cadaver dissection. A. Patella. B. Patellar tendon. Note the quite varied distribution of fascial fibres spread over the several levels.

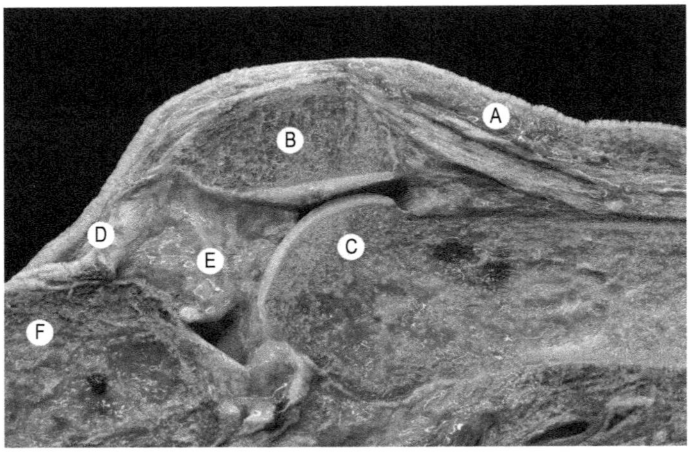

Figure 63.41 Cross-section of the knee joint in the sagittal plane. A. Suprapatellar fat body over the quadriceps femoris tendon. B. Patella. C. Femur. D. Patellar ligament. E. Infrapatellar fat pad. F. Tibia.

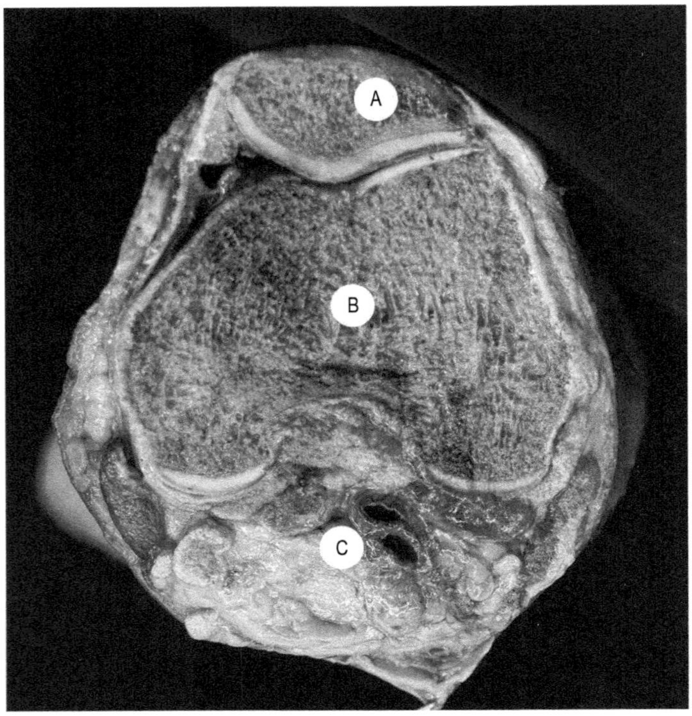

Figure 63.42 Cross-section over the patellofemoral joint from unembalmed cadaver dissection. A. Femur. B. Patella. C. Femoral artery.

deterioration of the quality of muscular fibres. Further, excessive stimulation of collagen fibre production facilitates the development of fibrosis in the myofascial system. The result is loss of matrix quality and consequently formation of entrapment areas (i.e. areas with reduced physiological movement with respect to amplitude, speed, resistance and coordination) (Pilat 2009).

Those fascial entrapments (Figs 63.43–63.44) promote the formation of compensatory (substitute) movement patterns. Regardless of the cause of the entrapment, if it persists for long periods of time, this eventually leads to excess load and ultimately dysfunction (Pilat 2003). These changes influence mostly the loose connective tissue structures and affect the specialized structures (dense regular and irregular connective tissue), producing overly dense tissue and reorientated fibres. These specialized structures include the tendons, ligaments and the articular capsules. Short-term changes will affect their function locally, and long-term changes may potentially result in global dysfunction patterns.

Fascial entrapment areas

In the locomotor system, the areas that are most vulnerable to fascial entrapment formation generally are:

- Bonding areas between fascial structures in places of extensive loads – for example, the bicipital aponeurosis (lacertus fibrosus) (see Fig. 63.17), in which the contracted muscle force is transmitted not only to the tendon and to the bone at its insertion point but also through the intrinsic and extrinsic connective tissue linked to the muscle (Huijing et al 1998; Huijing & Baan 2001a, 2001b). The bicipital aponeurosis appears not only as a structure that protects the neurovascular bundle, but also as one that dynamically stabilizes the biceps' tendon in its lower insertion (Eames et al 2007). It appears that it is because the traction force in the lower insertion of the biceps is so large – compared with that received by its two superior insertion tendons – that it requires this reinforcement.
  A similar anatomical design can be found in numerous structures, such as in the tendon of the quadriceps muscle with its insertion in patella (see Figs 63.40–63.41).
- Areas with excessive friction (e.g. tendons with tendinous sheaths reinforced by the retinaculum) (see Fig. 63.19) – an increase in the compression level between tendon and retinaculum leads to fibrocartilaginous changes (Benjamin 1995).
- Areas with numerous insertions of fascial structures with greater density of fibres (e.g. the scapular spine) (see Fig. 63.10) – these regions operate mechanically as movement linkage and distribution areas. When the entrapment occurs, this may result in altered local movement and / or a referred compensation process (Pilat 2009).

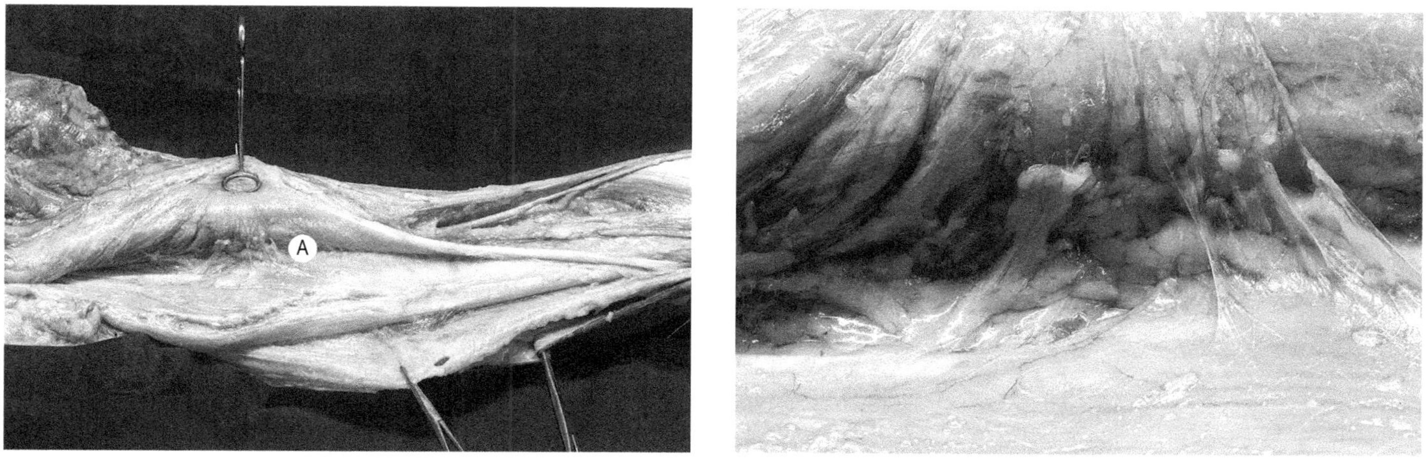

Figure 63.43 Fascial entrapments between two sliding planes. A. Location of the fascial entrapment.

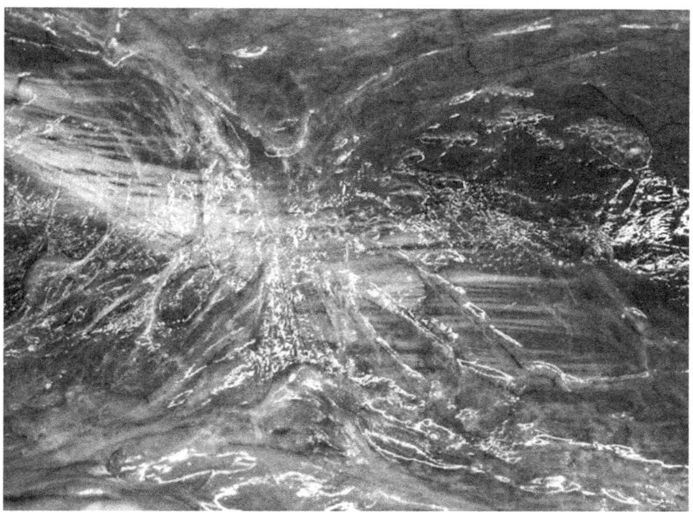

Figure 63.44 Fascial entrapment inside the movement plane. (Reproduced from Chaitow & Lovegrove Jones (2012). Chronic pelvic pain and dysfunction: practical physical medicine. Elsevier, with permission. Picture from the same author.)

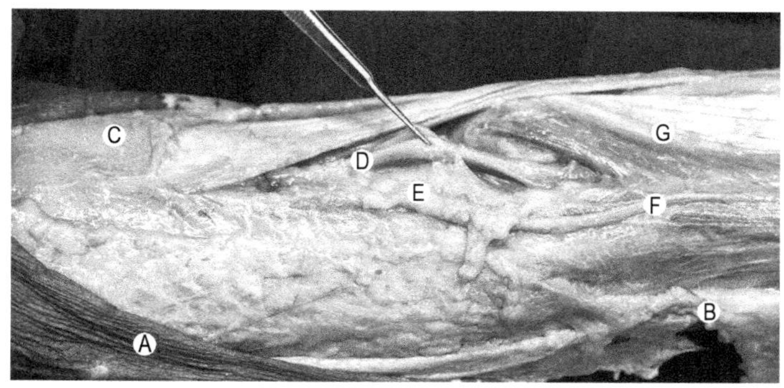

Figure 63.45 The deep aspect of the popliteal fossa, from unembalmed cadaver dissection. A. Skin. B. Superficial fascia. C. Deep fascia. D. Sciatic nerve. E. Loose connective tissue. F. Tibial nerve. G. Muscle fascia.

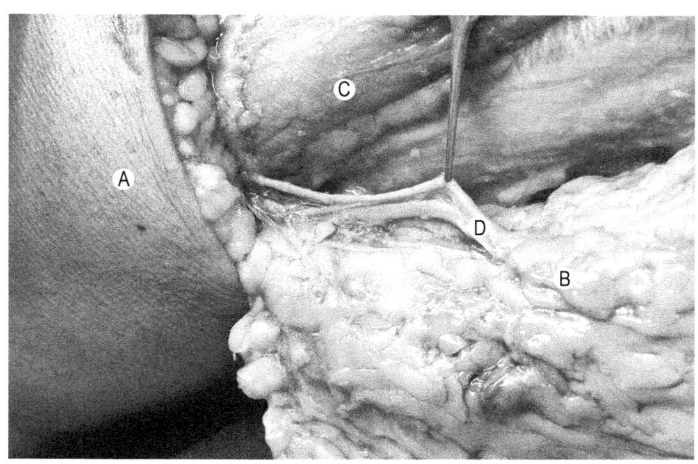

Figure 63.46 Forearm of the fat from fatty cadaver from unembalmed cadaver dissection. A. The skin. B. The superficial fascia with fat nodules. C. The deep fascia. D. Vein and cutaneous nerve. The left part was previously dissected. Normally both are embedded within the superficial fascia and fat tissue.

- Areas with prolonged and / or repeated hypomobility – for example, as a result of adjusting to inadequate postures.
- Body segments affected by traumatic or surgical processes.
- Structures involved in the protection of the neurovascular continuum – for example, the popliteal fossa (Fig. 63.45).
- Transit areas of perforating veins and nerves (Fig. 63.46).
- Places tending to bear excessive loads as a result of sustained and / or repeated emotional stress.

Proposed neurophysiological mechanisms of myofascial induction techniques

The fascia is proposed to act as a mechanosensitive system. During a treatment, the clinician stretches or / and compresses a specific body area in order to transmit a low-intensity mechanical stimulus. This input creates changes that spread through the body systems up to the molecular level. The outcome is a reciprocal reaction from the body, including biochemical, metabolic and finally physiological responses (Pilat 2014). This outcome may take place at any level of the system's structure (i.e. micro- or macroscopic) and responses may occur in any segment, and consequently the body's reactions can involve any musculoskeletal functional unit, organ, viscera or group of cells (Langevin 2006; Vaticón 2009).

Three mechanisms for the release and restructuring of the fascial system are proposed: (1) piezoelectricity, (2) the attitude of the interstitial mechanoreceptors with the consequential dynamics of the myofibroblasts and (3) viscoelasticity.

Piezoelectricity

Piezoelectricity is a phenomenon exhibited by certain crystals that, when a mechanical force is applied, become polarized within their structure, resulting in electrical potentials and loads on their surface (Pilat 2003). The crystals in the human body are liquid crystals (Szent-Gyorgyi 1941; Bouligand 1978) and, similarly, their response to a mechanical input is the generation of a minute electrical pulse; this occurs particularly in the matrix of the connective tissue, which becomes harmonic and oscillating. The information (impulse) is transmitted electrically through the matrix (Oschman 2003). As collagen is a semiconductor (Cope 1975), it is capable of forming an integrated electronic network that enables the interconnection of all the fascial system components (Bouligand 1978; O'Connell 2003; Ahn & Grodzinsky 2009; Rivard et al 2010). Thus, the basic properties of the system (i.e. elasticity, flexibility, elongation, resistance) will depend to a great extent upon the ability to maintain a continuous and correct information flow.

Myofibroblast dynamics

As the muscle is a contractile tissue that enables the body to move, the fascia should also be considered an intramuscular connective tissue that forms a functional unit along with the muscular fibres. The fascial system is richly innervated by an extensive network of mechanoreceptors included in the body's somatosensory system, as discussed above. It is proposed (Vaticón 2009) that there are two categories of reception / transmission / interpretation of each mechanical impulse:

- **Epicritical sensitivity:** This is knowledge, exploration, or quantitative information, transmitted through the lemniscal path from the pacinian and paciniform corpuscles, Golgi organs and Ruffini corpuscles.
- **Protopathic sensitivity:** This is qualitative and plastic information, transmitted through an extralemniscal path. The interstitial receptors (free nerves endings) are in charge of this sensitivity and act as a protection and alarm system. They are polymodal receptors that may also act as nociceptors.

Consequently, the mechanical impulse (e.g. manual pressure or traction) received by the mechanoreceptors creates a broad range of responses in the fascial system that may result in movement at both macro- and microscopic levels.

The possibility of inherent movement within the fascial system is still controversial. Some authors (Staubesand & Li 1997; Schleip et al 2005, 2007) believe that this phenomenon exists and is related to the dynamics of the myofibroblasts. They suggest that activation of actin microfilaments is the origin of movement, as demonstrated in the lumbar fascia of rats (Schleip et al 2007). More research on the dynamics of myofibroblasts in pathologies such as Dupuytren's contracture, plantar fasciitis, frozen shoulder or fibromyalgia, may confirm this observation. Several studies focusing mainly on the skin-healing process strongly support this line of reasoning (Fidzianska & Jablonska 2000; Gabbiani 2003, 2007; Satish et al 2008). Chaudhry et al (2008) formulated a three-dimensional mathematical model for deformation in human fasciae, and reported that the mechanical forces applied during manual techniques cannot modify the length of the structures of the dense connective tissue (e.g. plantar fascia), but can create mechanical changes in the loose connective tissue (e.g. superficial nasal fascia). The therapist's manual technique applied to the patient's body may stimulate fascial mechanoreceptors and triggers changes in skeletal muscle tone. This movement may be visible, or perceived only by carefully palpation.

Viscoelasticity

Viscoelasticity (viscosity and elasticity) defines the long-term behaviour of a material. A force applied to a material with viscoelastic properties causes it to deform. Over time, deformation can occur without any need to apply more force.

The viscoelastic properties of the fascia have been observed in numerous studies analysing certain fascial structures of the body – the TLF (Yahia et al 1993), fascia lata (Wright & Rennels 1964), subcutaneous fascia of rats (Iatridis et al 2003) – or global concepts of practical applications (Barnes 1990; Threlkeld 1992; Rolf 1997; Cantu & Grodin 2001; Pilat 2003; Schleip et al 2005, 2012b). Vaticón (2009) suggested that local mediators such as fibroblast growth factor (TGF-β1) participate in this process, and Langevin and Yandow (2002) proposed that metalloprotease has a role in regulating the collagen deposit/degradation balance in the remodelling of the fascial structure.

Viscoelasticity is linked to the remodelling process of the extracellular matrix, to changes in density and also to the correction orientation of the collagen fibres. Studies (ex vivo) conducted by Chaudhry et al (2007) in fascia lata, plantar fascia and nasal fascia confirm the viscoelastic properties of the tissue. Some of these observations are worth noting:

- The viscoelastic response begins 60 seconds after applying a constant traction or compression force.
- To avoid the blocking of the release response, it is suggested that the therapist does *not* gradually increase the applied force; rather, the force should be constant.
- Different fascial structures require different magnitudes of applied force; however, the time for response throughout the movement remains the same.

The three types of response in the fascial system are the result of applying a proper mechanical impulse, with the adequate force, time and speed. These response types occur at different levels of the body system (micro and / or macro) and also have different time scales (Langevin 2006; Huijing 2009; Pilat 2009; Vaticón 2009). Any of these mechanisms have the potential of influencing the behaviour of the other two (Langevin

2006). According to the response of the fascial system during the treatment, all the mechanisms may interact (Pilat 2003). Therefore, as a result of the myofascial induction techniques application, the clinician can:

- improve the circulation of the antibodies in the matrix
- increase blood flow to the restriction areas by releasing histamine
- improve fibroblast mechanics
- improve blood supply to the nervous tissue and increase the flow of metabolites to and from the tissue, thus accelerating the healing process (Evans 1980; Barnes 1990; Barlow & Willoughby 1992; Hamwee 1999; Pilat 2003).

Scientific Evidence Related to the Results in the Myofascial Approach (Pilat 2014)

A growing number of publications related to the clinical results of myofascial induction techniques have been reported in patients with pain syndromes compared with healthy subjects. A number of studies have shown significant changes linked to responses of the autonomic nervous system, as detailed below.

Research related to pathology

- An objective method for evaluating the effect of myofascial induction techniques applied to muscular lesions with dynamic sonoelastography was reported by Martínez and Galán-del-Río (2013).
- Leonard et al (2009) reported that connective tissue manipulation improved peripheral circulation and enhanced wound-healing processes in 20 patients with diabetic foot ulcers.
- Significant differences between pre- and post-treatment measurements of pressure pain thresholds with decreasing sensitivity to myofascial trigger points was reported in different strained muscles, including the adductor longus (Robb & Pajaczkowski, 2009), the upper trapezius muscle (Fryer & Hodgson 2005) and cervical muscle (Hou et al 2002).
- Marshall et al (2009) concluded that myofascial release helped to reduce the severity and intensity of muscle pain in people with chronic fatigue syndrome.
- Hicks et al (2009) reported that human fibroblasts secrete the soluble mediators of myoblast differentiation and that myofascial release can regulate muscle development.
- Tozzi et al (2012) investigated non-specific low back pain in relation to kidney mobility. Using real-time ultrasound, this study demonstrated that osteopathic fascial manipulation decreased pain perception and improved renal mobility.
- Useros and Hernando (2008) concluded that myofascial induction has beneficial effects in patients with brain damage, with special emphasis on automatic posture control.
- In patients with unilateral spatial neglect (an alteration of the head's position with respect to the median line), Vaquero Rodríguez (2013) observed significant results for the sensitivity variable in the experimental group treated with myofascial induction techniques, compared with those treated with Bobath therapy.
- Fernández-Lao et al (2011) applied myofascial release techniques in breast cancer survivors. The authors observed that myofascial release led to an immediate increase in salivary flow rates, suggesting the intervention had a parasympathetic effect.
- Vasquez (2011) reported the effectiveness of myofascial induction techniques in treating swimmers' shoulders with respect to articular balance and pain.
- Arguisuelas-Martínez (2010) demonstrated the effects of lumbar spine manipulation and thoracolumbar myofascial induction techniques on the spinae erector activation pattern.
- In a double-blind study, Urresti-López (2011) applied the suboccipital induction technique to 26 subjects with chronic neck pain. Electroencephalographic (EEG) changes were observed in latency reduction in the experimental group compared with the control group. This result suggests that improvements in cognitive processes including attention, memory activation and associative states are associated with the P300 wave. Lack of changes in other EEG parameters did not support the influence of vascular modifications.

Clinical research in healthy subjects

- Arroyo-Morales et al (2008a) reported that the heart rate variability and blood pressure recovery after a physically stressful situation were improved by myofascial release, compared with sham electrotherapy treatment.
- Arroyo-Morales et al (2008b) reported that application of an active recovery protocol using whole-body myofascial treatment reduced EMG amplitude and vigour when applied as a passive recovery technique after high-intensity exercise.
- Toro Velasco et al (2009) reported that the application of a single session of manual therapy (including myofascial induction techniques) produced an immediate increase of heart rate variability and a decrease in tension, anger status and perceived pain in patients with chronic tension-type headache.
- In a randomized single-blind placebo-controlled study, Arroyo-Morales et al (2009) reported that myofascial induction techniques might encourage recovery from a transient immune-suppressed state induced by exercise in healthy active women.
- Henley et al (2008) demonstrated quantitatively that cervical myofascial release shifted the sympathovagal balance from the sympathetic to the parasympathetic nervous system.
- In a study involving 41 healthy males randomly assigned to experimental or control groups, Fernandez-Pérez et al (2008) reported significantly decreased anxiety levels in healthy young adults after the application of myofascial induction treatment. Additionally, significantly lower systolic blood pressure values were observed, compared with baseline levels.

- Heredia-Rizo et al (2013) demonstrated that application of suboccipital muscle inhibition technique immediately improved the head position. Additionally, it immediately decreased the mechanosensitivity of the greater occipital nerve.
- Fernández-Pérez et al (2013) observed major immunological modulations, with an increased B-lymphocyte count 20 minutes after the craniocervical application of myofascial induction techniques.

Therapeutic Strategies Applied in the Myofascial Induction Process

General observations related to the therapeutic process

There are various concepts related to the treatment of the fascial system (Barnes 1990; Rolf 1997; Paoletti & Sommerfeld 1998; Cantu & Grodin 2001; Myers 2003; Chaitow & Delany 2002; Pilat 2003; Stecco 2004; Manheim 2008). Findings arising from the basic sciences on the mechanical and pathomechanical phenomena related to the therapeutic induction of the fascial system, as discussed above, provide a solid theoretical framework. However, there is a need to unify and validate clinical procedures (Remving 2007). The applications of myofascial induction techniques suggested below are based on the clinical experience of the author (Pilat 2003, 2007, 2009, 2011, 2012), and supported by the theoretical framework and research discussed above. The myofascial induction process may be combined with other manual therapy strategies.

Definition of the myofascial induction therapy process

Myofascial induction therapy is an assemblage of procedures focused on optimizing function and balance within the fascial system. The approach aims at local correction, recovery of global dynamics and pain-free body use. The treatment protocol is divided into two phases: (i) superficial (stroke) techniques and (ii) deep procedures.

Superficial (local) procedures are addressed to the surface and / or local restrictions detectable through direct palpation. These techniques consist of different strokes, applied from the most superficial to the deepest level. The main goal is the correction of subcutaneous restrictions (related to the superficial fascia) as well as those affecting muscles, tendons, ligaments that can be felt directly underneath the skin.

Deep myofascial induction therapy is a simultaneous evaluation and treatment process, which uses movements and three-dimensionally sustained pressures applied to the entire myofascial system and aimed at releasing of restrictions.

Bases for clinical applications

Assessment process

The assessment of fascial dysfunction is included in the clinical reasoning related to different manual therapy approaches to pathomechanics of the locomotor system. We suggest following the same techniques for investigating movement dysfunctions in each area treated. The suggested assessment sequence comprises:

- **Anamnesis including the patient's retrospective pathology (Pilat 2007):** Misuse – reduced coordination and / or stability; abuse – trauma; overuse – repetitive movements and / or excess load, all three becoming, in time, the fourth factor, that of disuse – atrophy or reduced load capacity (the disuse may become a pathology in itself).
- **Static evaluation of posture (observation):** Attention should be focused on the gravitational body behaviour.
- **Dynamic evaluation of posture:** Any test performed in manual therapy practice can be useful. It is also recommended that the examiner use global functional tests focusing on a movement quality analysis for basic daily activities, with special attention paid to the presence of any compensation movements. In addition, specific functional tests focused on the specific structure involved – for example, muscle (strength, elasticity) including tissue palpation and complementary tests – should be also included. (Ch 5 discusses clinical examination.)

Currently there is no specific and objective test available to isolate myofascial dysfunction from other musculoskeletal pathologies. This issue is confused by the close anatomical relationship between the muscular fibres and the fascia. However, recent research with high-resolution sonoelastography techniques (Martínez Rodríguez & Galán del Río 2013) anticipates the use of this procedure. For instance, alterations in motion pattern and modification of pain pattern will be useful indicators. Restrictions may occur in various directions and planes; they may even occur in different directions on the same plane, in the same direction in various planes, or in different planes in various directions. There is no need for the patient to perform active muscular contractions. The patient may be said to be in a state of active passiveness.

Clinical procedure principles (Pilat 2003, 2009, 2014)

- All procedures (protocols) must be individualized according to the treated dysfunction (pathology) and the patient's individual needs with regards their age, physical and emotional conditions, cultural aspects and gender. The specific technique chosen will also depend on the therapist's skills.
- Biomechanically, the myofascial system responds to compression and traction forces. These are the two mechanical strategies used when applying myofascial induction therapy.
- The direction of the releasing movement is towards facilitation. The clinician should refrain from performing movements in an arbitrary direction.
- The clinician selects the body region affected by myofascial dysfunction that may be associated with pain and / or dysfunction (hypo- / hypermobility, incoordination, lack of force, etc.). This region should be identified during the initial assessment process discussed above.

- Each body region affected by dysfunction requires a specific procedure application (Pilat 2003).
- The clinician tenses the tissue, referred to as the first restriction barrier, by applying a three-dimensional slow and gradual compression or traction. The pressure is constant during the first 60–90 seconds, which is the time required for releasing the first restriction barrier (i.e. beginning of the viscoelastic response).
- During the first phase of the application, the therapist barely moves the tissue.
- Overcoming the first restriction barrier, the therapist goes along with movement in the direction of the facilitation, pausing at each additional restriction barrier.
- In each technique, the therapist must overcome at least three to six consecutive barriers and the minimum time of application is 3–5 minutes.
- The tension applied to the tissue must be constant, but the pressure applied by the therapist may be modified until the first barrier is overcome. The pressure should be reduced when abundant activity and / or pain is perceived.

Examples of Practical Applications for Upper Quadrant Disorders

The following techniques are examples of the therapeutic strategies used in myofascial restrictions associated with the most common pathologies of the upper quadrant. They may be combined with other therapeutic strategies discussed in this textbook. Although we indicate those techniques most commonly used by clinicians, the choice is up to the clinical decision making of the therapist.

Techniques related to the cervical spine

Clinical considerations (Pilat 2003)

- A forward-head posture, with resulting overextension of the occipital muscles required to maintain a horizontal line of sight, causes continued tension on the hyoid muscles. The prolonged and repetitive tension leads to the jaw being depressed and moved backward, so forcing the person to open the mouth, which is countered by contraction of the temporal and masseter muscles, tensing the fascial system. This may result in temporomandibular joint movement limitation and / or distortion.
- The hyoid bone is involved in activities such as swallowing, talking, chewing, playing wind instruments, etc. The bone is fixed to the prevertebral and superficial fascia and, for this reason, fascial dysfunction may directly affect its proper functioning, resulting in dysfunctional dynamics of its 14 pairs of muscles.
- The three scalene muscles flex the lower cervical spine while the suboccipital muscles extend the head and contribute to protrusion. The scalenes, which must perform their duty of stabilizing the first rib, actually apply traction from the cervical vertebrae downwards and forwards.
- The muscles along the head and the length of the neck have a major role in maintaining the correct head position in the sagittal plane. Both groups are powerful flexors and have the role of counteracting the strong and prolonged tension of the paravertebral muscles and those of the common extensor mass.

Suboccipital induction (Fig. 63.47)

The patient is in supine position, and the clinician is seated on a chair at the patient's head. The clinician places both hands under the head, and then touches the suboccipital space with the second to the fifth fingertips, trying to place the fingers vertically. Applying the pressure towards the ceiling, the therapist follows the induction principles. The minimum application time should be 4 minutes.

Suprahyoid region induction (Fig. 63.48)

The patient is in supine position and the clinician stands at one side. The clinician places the caudal hand above and around the hyoid bone. The endings of the index and middle fingers of the cranial hand should be placed on the soft part

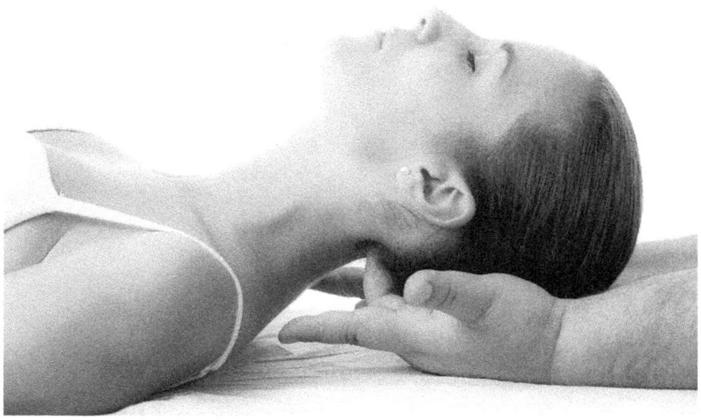

Figure 63.47 Suboccipital myofascial induction.

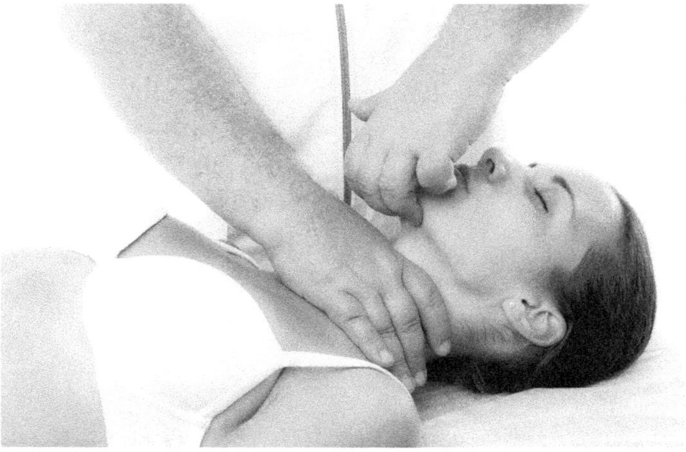

Figure 63.48 Suprahyoid region induction.

of the mandible directly under the chin. With the caudal hand the clinician applies slight traction in the caudal direction, while with the cranial hand applying traction towards the head. Applying a three-dimensional pressure, the clinician follows the induction principles.

Induction of the scalene muscles (Fig. 63.49)

The patient is in supine position and the clinician is seated on a chair at the patient's head. The clinician places both thumbs along the supraclavicular space, and maintains that position for approximately 60–90 seconds until there is a rotation of the head to one side. The therapist then makes contact from the side the head turned towards, while with the thumb of the other hand continuing the releasing manoeuvre. Pressure over the brachial plexus should be avoided. If any sensation of pins and needles is felt towards the upper limb, the fingers must release the hold on the brachial plexus.

Induction of the prevertebral fascia (Fig. 63.50)

With the patient in supine position, the clinician slightly turns the patient's head to one side and then places the fingers underneath the muscular mass of the sternocleidomastoid muscle (over the scalene and above the transverse process of the vertebral bodies of the middle and low cervical vertebrae) following the principles of induction. At no time should pressure be applied over the trachea and / or carotid artery.

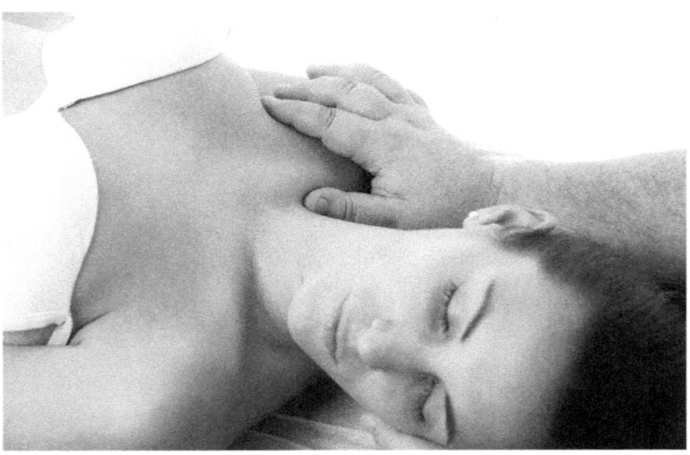

Figure 63.49 Myofascial induction of the scalene muscles.

Techniques related to the shoulder girdle

Clinical considerations (Pilat 2003)

The shoulder girdle connects the trunk with the hand via the small sternoclavicular joint. Without this joint connection, the dynamic continuity would be maintained by the myofascial structures alone. The trapezius, infraspinatus, supraspinatus and deltoid muscles connect to the spine of the scapula and represent the most important muscular connection for the dynamics of shoulder motion. The fascial insertions form a fibrous link (see Fig. 63.12). A fascial entrapment can change the distribution of tensional lines in the scapular region. The dysfunctional scapular movements alter the dynamics of the thoracoscapular and scapulohumeral movements, contributing to the dysfunction and shoulder pain.

Induction of the pectoralis and deltoid fascia (Fig. 63.51)

The patient is in supine position, and the clinician crosses the hands, placing the cranial hand over the front of the shoulder and the caudal hand over the ipsilateral edge of the sternum. Applying three-dimensional force, the clinician follows the principles of induction.

Induction of the clavipectoral and the pectoralis minor muscle fascia (Fig. 63.52)

The patient is in supine position, and the clinician holds the patient's arm with the cranial hand, abducting it approximately at 90° while applying a very gentle traction. The caudal hand, in prone position, is introduced into the space between the pectoralis major and the ribs and slowly directs the fingers medially and cranially. Applying a three-dimensional force, the clinician follows the principles of induction.

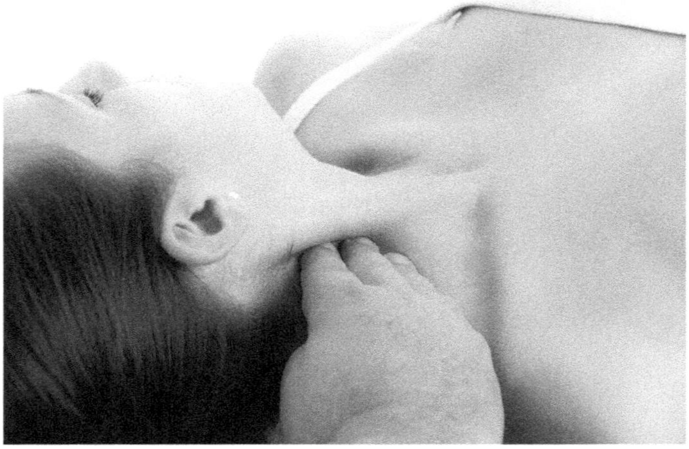

Figure 63.50 Induction of the prevertebral fascia.

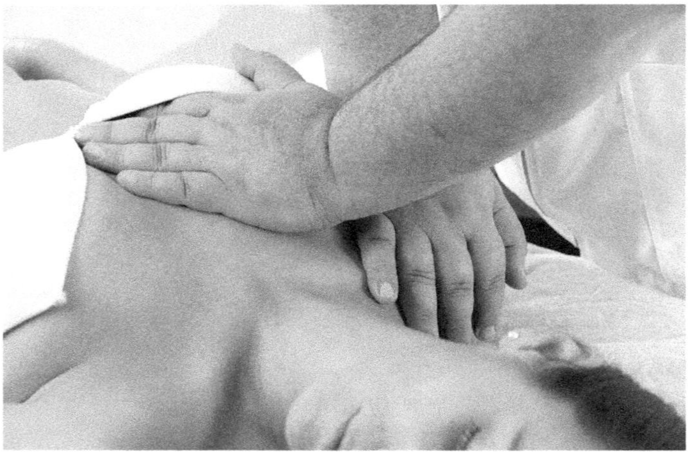

Figure 63.51 Induction of the pectoralis and deltoid fascia.

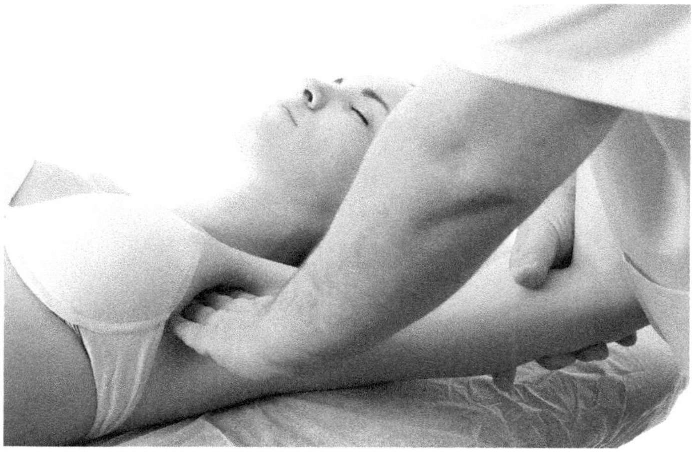

Figure 63.52 Induction of the clavipectoral and pectoralis minor muscle fascia.

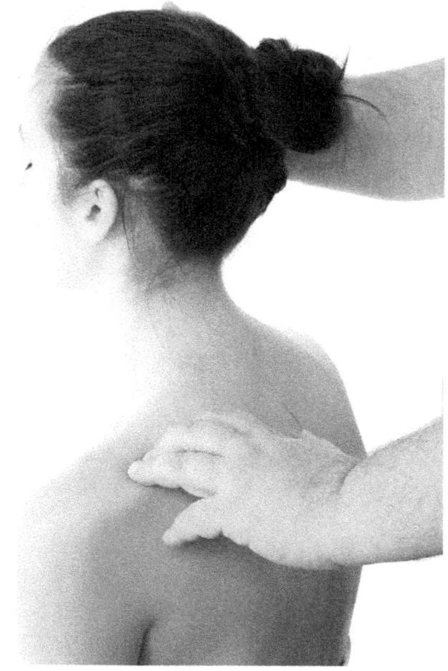

Figure 63.54 Myofascial induction of the spine of the scapula.

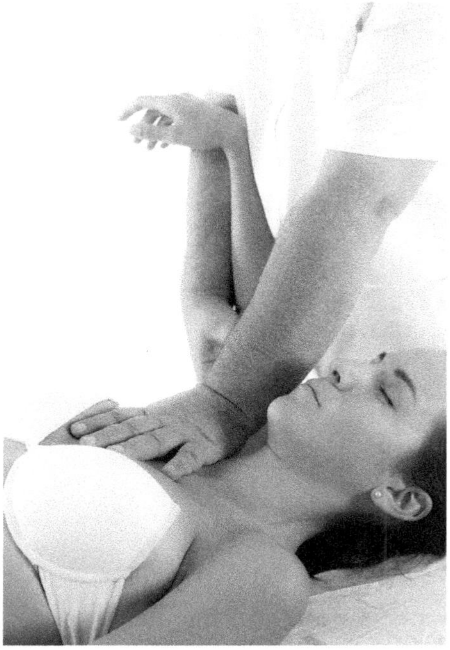

Figure 63.53 Integrated myofascial induction of the arm.

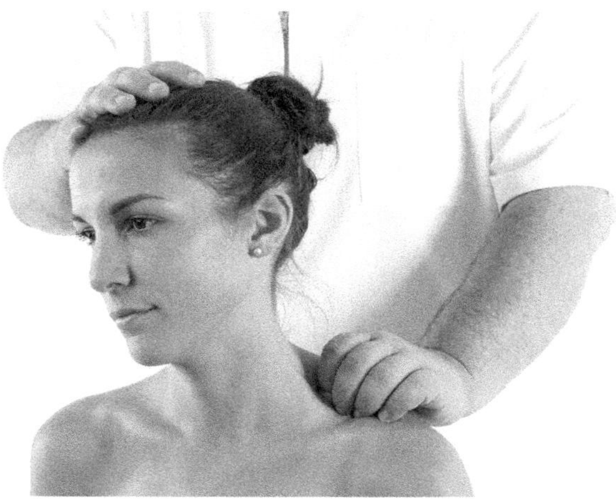

Figure 63.55 Myofascial induction of the trapezius muscle.

Integrated induction of the arm (Fig. 63.53)

The patient is in supine position, and the clinician places the caudal hand at the level of the sternum and with the cranial hand holds the patient's arm at an elevation of approximately 120°, applying a very gentle traction. Applying the three-dimensional force, the clinician follows the principles of induction. Facilitated movement of the upper limb should be allowed.

Induction of the spine of the scapula (Fig. 63.54)

The patient is seated and the therapist stands behind him / her. The clinician's external hand contacts the supraspinous fossa, pressing with the fingers in the direction of the spine at the scapula without causing pain. The other hand of the therapist is placed on the patient's head, simply to hold it. Applying a three-dimensional force, the clinician follows the principles of induction. It is normal to note head movement and the therapist should follow this.

Induction of the trapezius muscle (Fig. 63.55)

This technique follows the same principles as previously described. The leading hand of the therapist changes position as the fingers are placed on the upper edge of the trapezius muscle and contact the upper fibres. Painful reactions should be avoided and treated with special care.

Techniques related to the brachial and antebrachial fascia

Clinical considerations

Lateral epicondylalgia, or tennis elbow, is the most common pathology in the elbow region; it is generally associated with an excessive traction generated by the extensor musculature, and numerous tendons are fixed in the epicondyle. The muscle most often involved in this pathology is the extensor carpi radialis brevis. It is believed that the pathology is caused by the exaggerated traction of its tendon. (See Ch 39 for further discussion on lateral epicondylalgia.) However, Briggs and Elliott (1985) have demonstrated, by dissecting 139 upper limbs, that in only 29 cases was there a direct insertion of its tendon into the epicondyle. In the other cases, the tendon was fixed on the fascia of the extensor carpi radialis longus, extensor digitorum communis, supinator and the radial collateral ligament, forming a kind of fan. This example reveals the need to analyse and focus the therapy to the broad fascial bonds. Finally, the connection of the brachial biceps fascia with the antebrachial fascia through the lacertus fibrosus is also important (see Fig. 63.17).

Induction of the brachial and antebrachial fascia link (Fig. 63.56)

The patient is in supine position, with the arm abducted at approximately 90°, and the forearm flexed and in relaxed supination. The therapist places the outer hand (with palm down) over the ventral face of the medium third of the forearm. The inner hand (with palm up) is placed underneath, embracing the elbow and the near end of the forearm. Both hands softly press the forearm and perform a traction intention – the upper in caudal direction and the lower in cranial direction. The principles of induction are followed.

Induction of the bicipital fascia (Fig. 63.57)

With the patient in supine position and the forearm supine, the therapist places the hands (without crossing them) so that the fingers contact both ends of the bicipital fascia. The therapist presses with both hands towards each other. The principles of induction are followed.

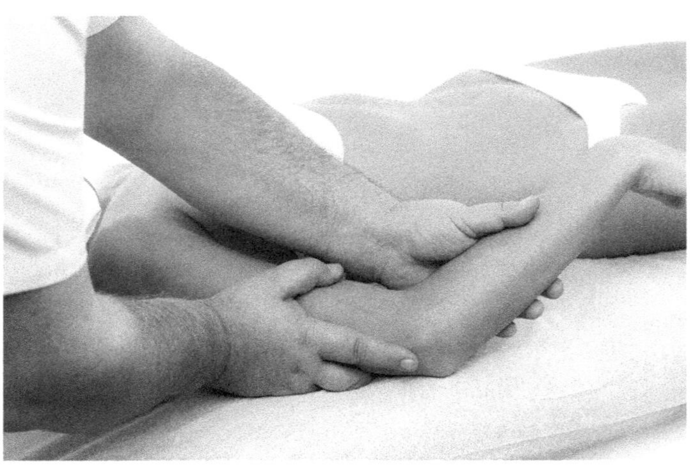

Figure 63.56 Induction of the connection of the brachial and antebrachial fascia.

Induction of the extensor retinaculum (Fig. 63.58)

With the patient in supine position and the forearm pronated, the therapist crosses the hands and places the caudal hand at the retinaculum region and the cranial hand on the back of the distal part of the forearm. The therapist then uses both hands to apply pressure towards the limb in both cranial and caudal directions. The principles of induction are followed.

Techniques related to the fascia of the hand

Clinical considerations

The studies of Kalin and Hirsch (1987) show that only 8 of 69 analysed interosseous muscles had bone insertions. In the other cases they attach to fascial structures. Further, the palmar fascia and its link to the palmar major muscle represent another fascial link that is directly related to functional integrity.

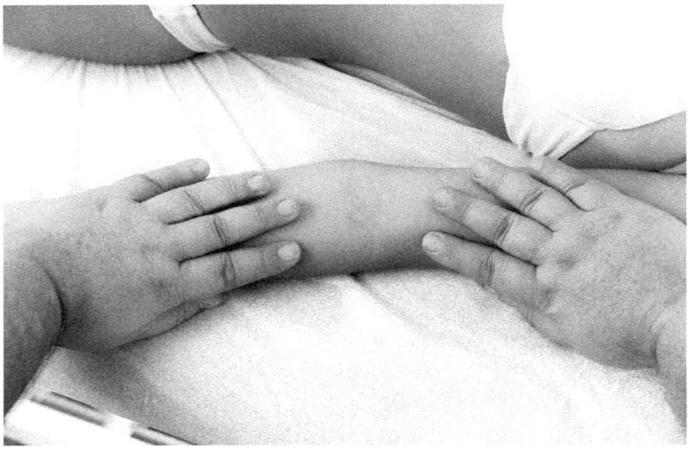

Figure 63.57 Induction of the bicipital fascia.

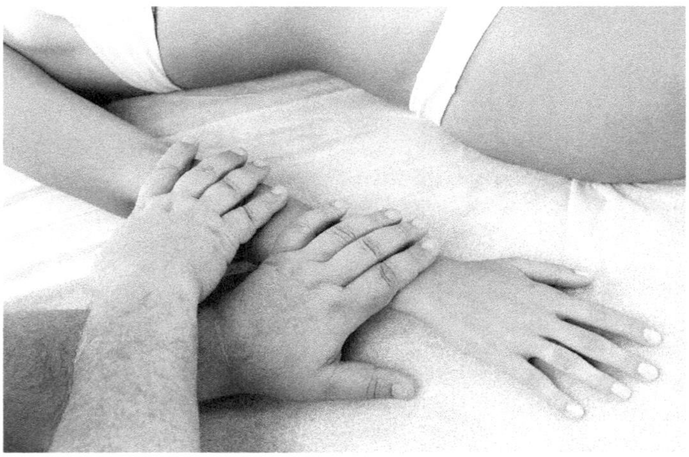

Figure 63.58 Myofascial induction of the extensor retinaculum.

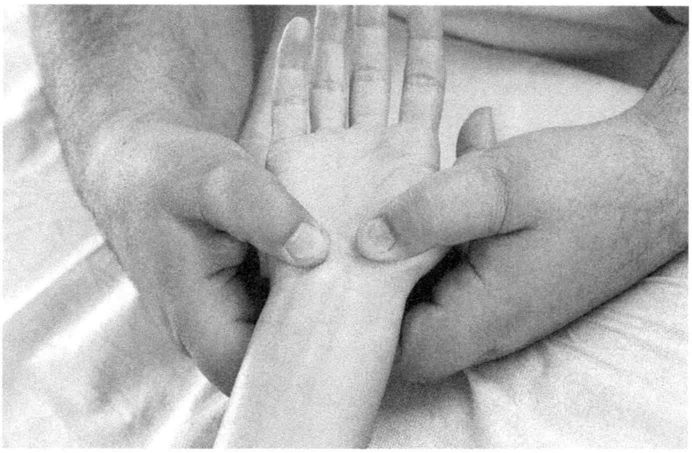

Figure 63.59 **Induction of the carpal tunnel and palmar fascia.**

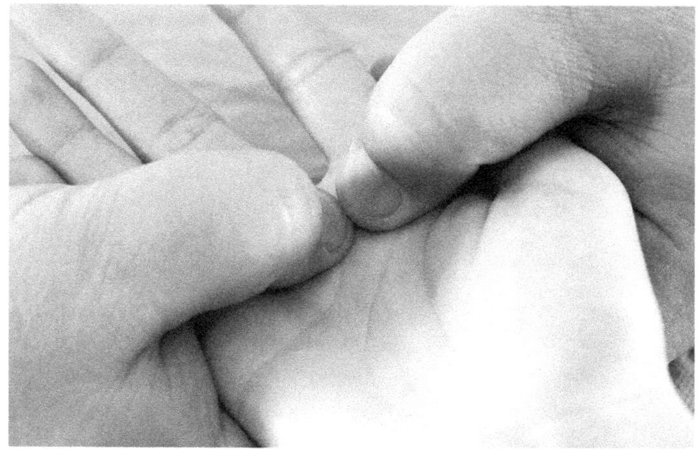

Figure 63.61 **Interosseous myofascial induction.**

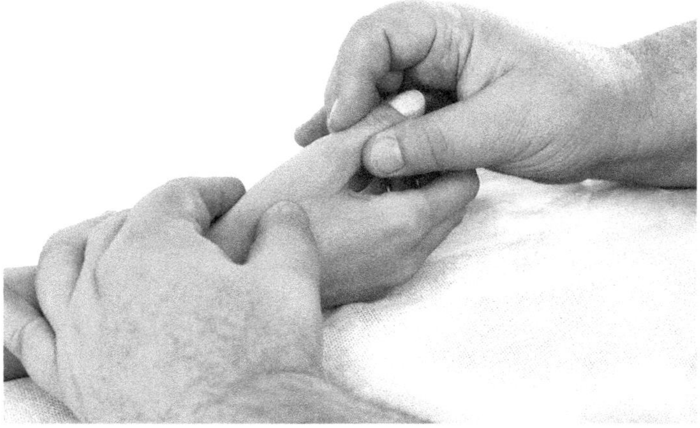

Figure 63.60 **Telescopic myofascial induction.**

Induction of the carpal tunnel and palmar fascia (Fig. 63.59)

The clinician places the thumbs on the region of the carpal tunnel and the flexed index fingers over the back of the wrist, forming a clamp. Holding the patient's wrist, the clinician then performs a telescopic three-dimensional traction while slightly extending the wrist. The principles of induction are followed. Considerable pressure should be maintained and the therapist's fingers not allowed to slip over the patient's skin. The same strategy is used to treat the palmar fascia, modifying the position of the fingers.

Telescopic three-dimensional induction (Fig. 63.60)

The clinician uses the non-dominant hand to stabilize the metacarpal bone or phalanx of the finger to be treated. The level of the stabilization will depend on the place of the pathology. With the other hand, the clinician holds the distal phalanx of the patient's finger between the thumb, the index and the middle fingers. A global treatment may be performed (simultaneously at all articular levels) or one only over a given level. The facilitated movement is followed.

Interosseous induction (Fig. 63.61)

The clinician places the thumbs over the palmar face of the metacarpophalangeal joints, so that he may separate the proximal phalanxes of the patient's fingers. The other fingers stabilize the patient's hand. With the thumbs, the therapist exercises a three-dimensional pressure. The same strategy may be applied over the dorsal interosseous after changing the position of the hands.

Examples of Practical Applications for Lower Quadrant Disorders

Techniques related to the lumbopelvic region

To protect the fragile structures of the lumbar spine, the support of the myofascial complex that surrounds the trunk is needed (Bergmark 1989; Cholewicki et al 1997; Willard 2007; Schuenke et al 2012; Willard et al 2012). One of the most important structures is the thoracolumbar fascia, which assists with lumbopelvic stability, static posture and movement. This fascial complex is continuous with the paraspinal muscles in the thoracic and cervical regions and even reaches to the cranial base (Willard et al 2012). In the lower end, the thoracolumbar fascia is anchored to the iliac crest. From there it continues with the gluteal fascia and fascia lata complex, linking to the lower extremity fascial system. The critical point on the lumbar region is the lumbar interfascial triangle (LIFT) region (see Fig. 63.30), which includes aponeurotic structures from almost all the muscles in this area (Schuenke et al 2012). Research (Stecco 2004; Schleip et al 2012a) has shown interesting observations related to the dynamics of fascial mechanoreceptors and their importance in pain perception. The innervation of the thoracolumbar fascia has important implications for current concepts of back pain and opens a new avenue for therapeutic strategies. Particularly interesting is the presence of substance-P-containing free nerve endings considered as nociceptive. The data suggest that the thoracolumbar fascia is a potential source of back pain.

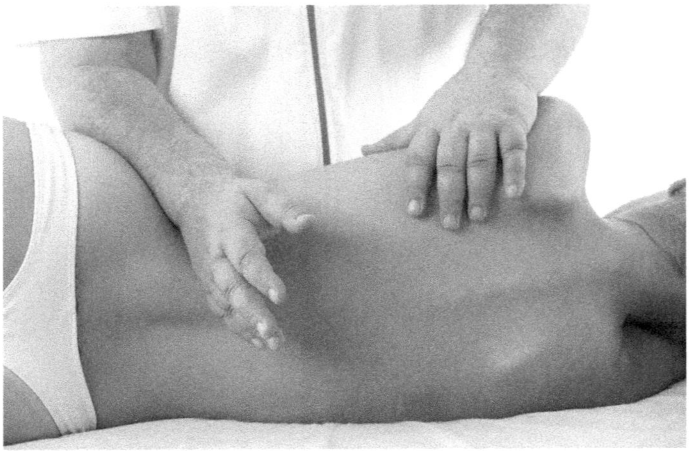

Figure 63.62 Induction of the lumbar interfascial triangle region (stroke application).

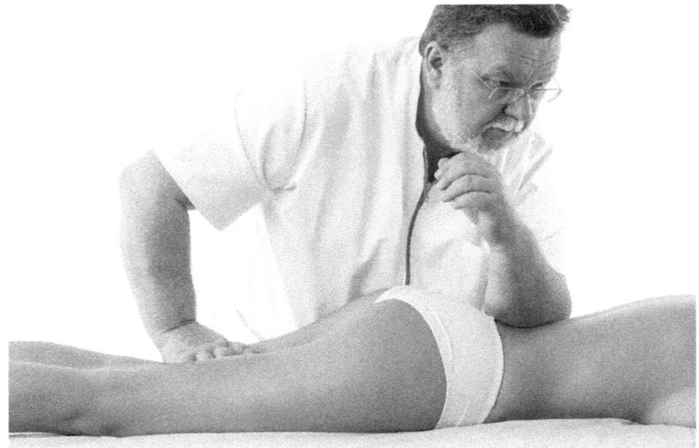

Figure 63.63 Induction of the lumbar interfascial triangle region (deep induction application).

In the anterior aspect, the fascial system bifurcates in the direction of the oblique abdominal muscles and at the front it is inserted into the linea alba. The fascia continues caudally to the pubis through the insertion of the external oblique muscles of the abdomen. The fascia at a deep transverse level communicates with the transversus abdominis and subsequently joins the iliac fascia. In the inferior part, it inserts into the inguinal canal by connecting to the fascial system in the lower extremity and continuing to the anterior thigh (Gallaudet 1931; Bochenek & Reicher 1997).

Induction of the lumbar interfascial triangle area (see Fig. 63.30) (Pilat 2003, 2011)

Stroke application (Fig. 63.62)

The patient is side-lying. The clinician stands in front of the patient and, with the cranial hand, stabilizes the trunk. The caudal forearm (with the thumb up) is placed in the space between the last rib and the iliac crest. The clinician (while avoiding sliding the forearm over the skin) applies a stroke backwards and forwards (i.e. with flexion and extension of the clinician's arm) over the underlying structures. The length of displacement is about 10 cm. The entire manoeuvre is repeated in three sets of 15 strokes each set. The clinician performs a very gentle pressure toward the table but avoids causing pain. Between the applications, the clinician can separate the patient's forearm from the body but should do so slowly.

Deep induction application (Fig. 63.63)

The patient is in prone position and the clinician stands at the level of the pelvis, facing the patient's head. The clinician places his / her elbow over the ipsilateral lumbar region between the last rib, the iliac crest and laterally to the paravertebral muscles. Next, the therapist presses the elbow towards the table. The other hand is placed over the patient's tight tissues in a cranial direction. This manoeuvre shortens the quadratus lumborum and facilitates access. The clinician should take advantage of his / her body weight. This position is held for approximately 3–5 minutes, and the principles of induction are followed.

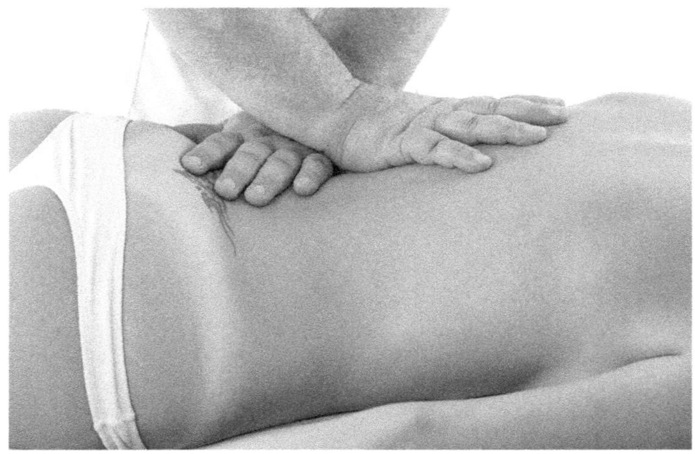

Figure 63.64 Cross-hands myofascial induction of the lumbar spine.

Cross-hands induction of the lumbar spine (Fig. 63.64) (Pilat 2003, 2011)

The patient is in prone position and the clinician is standing at the level of the patient's back. The clinician crosses both hands and places them on the patient's back and then presses with a slight force towards the table and in craniocaudal direction. The principles of induction are followed. This procedure can be performed in various ways: placing the hands directly on the line of the spinous processes (as in the figure), longitudinally on one side, or transversely above the iliac crests. The choice depends on the patient's symptoms.

Hip flexor region induction (Fig. 63.65) (Pilat 2003)

The patient is in supine position, and the clinician places his / her cranial hand on the anterior superior iliac spine and the other hand on the anterior upper third of the thigh. The clinician then presses with a slight force towards the table and in a craniocaudal direction. This position is held for approximately 3–5 minutes, and the principles of induction are followed. The hand placed on the anterior–superior iliac spine

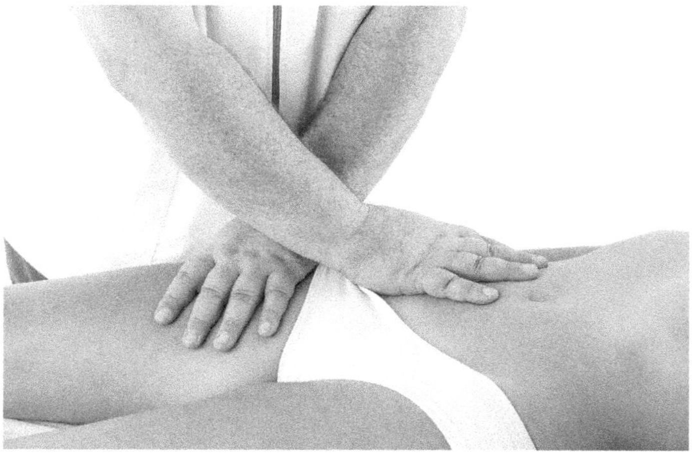

Figure 63.65 **Hip flexor region myofascial induction.**

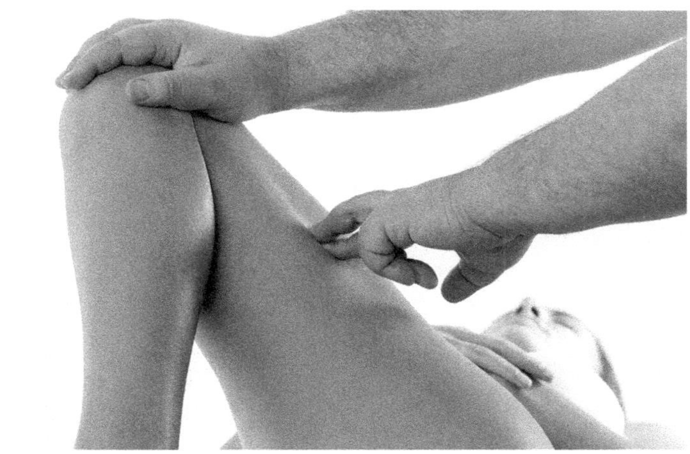

Figure 63.66 **Stroke on the iliotibial band.**

is for reference only. The therapist should avoid applying pressure directly on the bone.

Techniques related to the thigh region

Clinical considerations

Maintenance of a standing position requires equilibrium between the compartments of the thigh. Any imbalance is reflected not only in the muscles corresponding to each compartment, but also in the dynamics of the knee and particularly the patellofemoral joint. Rebalancing of the thigh compartments with respect to gravitational load transfer is recommended.

Stroke on the iliotibial band (Fig. 63.66) (Pilat 2003)

The patient is in supine position, with the thigh flexed and the foot supported over the table. The clinician with his / her cranial hand stabilizes the patient's knee, then, with the cranial hand, performs a stroke on the posterior edge of the iliotibial band from the knee level to the trochanteric region. Contact can be made with one finger reinforced by the other, with the knuckle, or with the elbow (the choice depends on the tissue resistance perceived). The therapist should avoid causing excessive pain. The stroke movement should cease for 6–7 seconds at each entrapment site (which is manifested by a sudden increase in resistance) and a constant force maintained. The therapist should not separate the hands before reaching the end of the stroke. This procedure is repeated three times. If pain results from friction on the skin, a small amount of water-based lubricant can be used. The procedure is repeated three times on the same area.

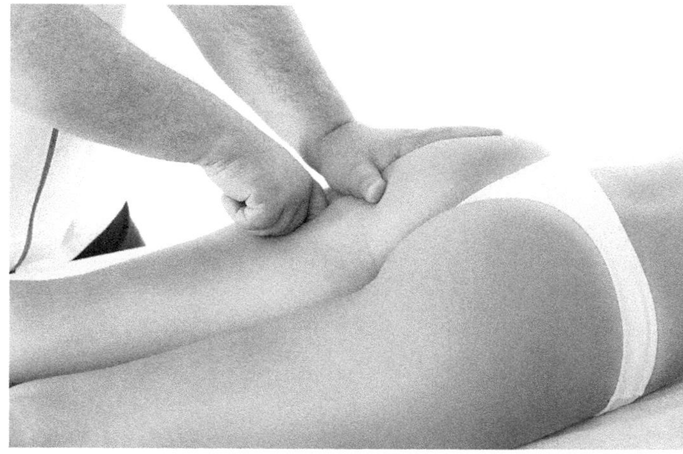

Figure 63.67 **Stroke on the isquiotibial path.**

Stroke on the isquiotibial path (Fig. 63.67) (Pilat 2003)

The patient is in prone position, and the clinician fixes the gluteal fascial area with his / her cranial hand, while with the other hand performs a longitudinal stroke. Contact can be made with one finger reinforced by the other with the knuckle or elbow (the choice depends on the tissue resistance perceived). The stroke pathway is from the ischial tuberosity to the entrance to the popliteal fossa. The therapist should avoid pressing in the region of the fossa itself, and avoid precipitating excessive pain. The stroke movement should cease for 6–7 seconds in each entrapment site (which is manifested by a sudden increase in resistance) while a constant force is maintained. The therapist should not separate the hands before reaching the end of the stroke. This procedure is repeated three times. If pain results from friction on the skin, a small amount of water-based lubricant can be used. The procedure is repeated three times along the same route.

Adductor path stroke (Fig. 63.68)

The patient is in prone position, and the clinician is standing at the level of the patient with the thigh of the ipsilateral leg flexed to 90°; with the caudal hand the clinician holds this position and places the cranial hand over the posterior part of the patient's thigh. The clinician then introduces the fingertips within the mass of the adductor muscles in the most hypomobile area and performs the stroke perpendicular to

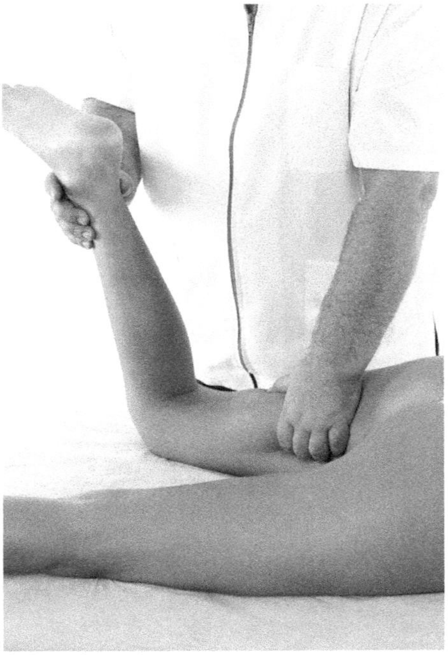

Figure 63.68 Adductor path stroke.

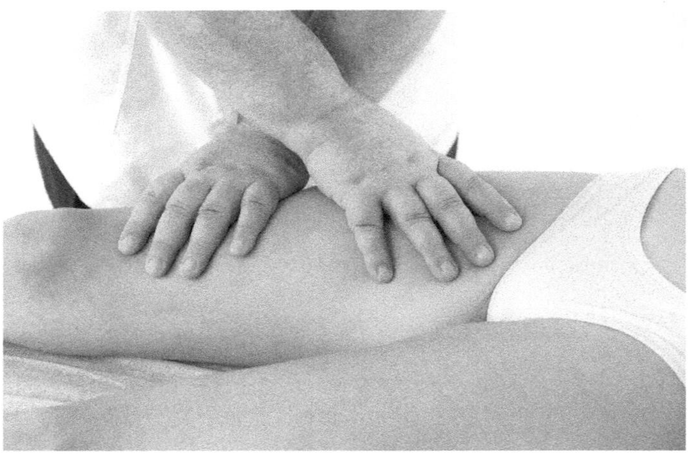

Figure 63.69 The knee extensor fascia induction.

the thigh line. The therapist should be cautious of pain. Three sets of 15 strokes are made, with the amplitude of the slip ranging between 3 and 4 cm.

The knee extensor fascia induction (Fig. 63.69) (Pilat 2003)

The patient is in supine position, and the clinician places his / her hands on the mass of the quadriceps so that the cranial hand is just above the patella and the other hand is on the upper third of the thigh. The clinician then presses with a slight force towards the table and in a craniocaudal direction. This position is held for approximately 3–5 minutes. The principles of induction are followed.

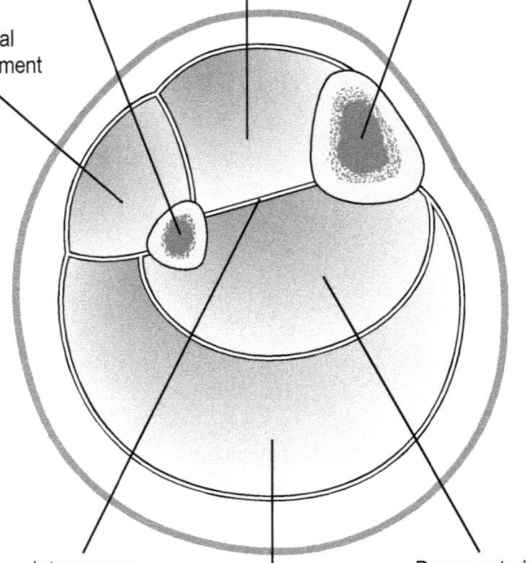

Figure 63.70 Schematic cross-section of the leg.

Techniques related to the knee and the leg region

Clinical considerations

The knee joint allows the lower limb to perform with both maximal stability and efficient mobility. On dissections of the popliteal region (see Fig. 63.45), it can be observed that the interconnection between the tendons of the hamstrings and gastrocnemius creates a cross-link. This relationship varies depending on whether the knee is being flexed or extended. The fascial structure is very dense and tough in the centre, but thin and elastic on the sides, whereas the tendons of the muscles are as mentioned above. The deep layer protects the great vessels and vital lower leg nerves, forming a femoral canal (Bochenek & Reicher 1997). Decompression of this region is the main focus of the treatment.

The fascial system of the leg is linked to the dynamics of its compartments (Fig. 63.70). Myofascial restrictions on the internal compartment are related to jogging and rapid-walking activities, especially if this is done on rigid surfaces. Pain often develops on the inner edge of the tibia and involves the origin of the posterior tibialis muscle. In extreme cases, sustained and repetitive traction on this area can lead to mechanical stress, causing difficulty in walking, cramps, night-time pain and even tibial fracture (Tucker 1990). Restrictions in the lateral compartment are rarer, and usually occur several hours after intense exercise. The posterior compartment can be affected by overuse and prolonged periods of inactivity; the resulting pain may be referred to the plantar fascia, affecting the proper functioning of the Achilles complex, and may even lead to total rupture. The Achilles tendon inserts into the calcaneus, forming a small loop. Therefore the plantar fascia may create some functional problems in

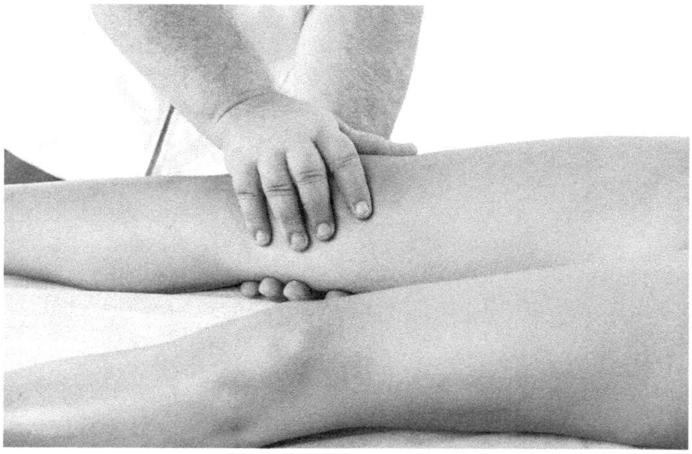

Figure 63.71 Transverse myofascial induction on the knee complex.

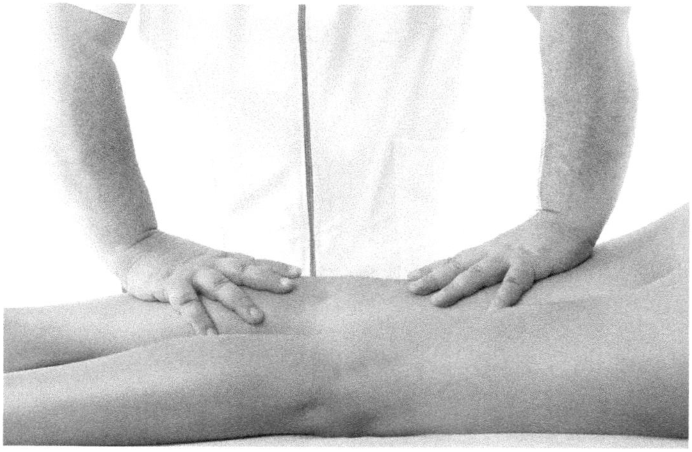

Figure 63.72 The popliteal fossa myofascial induction.

plantarflexion; it has therefore been suggested that treatment of myofascial restrictions be directed into the posterior compartment and the plantar fascia as a unit (Tucker 1990).

The plantar fascia includes the extrinsic and the intrinsic muscles of the foot. It is responsible for monitoring the integrity of the plantar arches, as well for stabilizing the foot in the last phase of walking. The fascia takes excessive loads during ambulation and climbing stairs, or taking the first steps in the morning. The performance of myofascial induction therapy may enable increased mobility and improved function of the entire complex of the plantar arches.

Transverse induction on the knee complex (Fig. 63.71) (Pilat 2003)

The patient is in supine position, and the clinician puts one hand below the patient's knee. The other hand is placed over the patella. The therapist then applies gentle pressure towards the table. This position is held for approximately 3–5 minutes and the principles of induction are followed. The expectation is for a positional adjustment movement of the patella. Sometimes slight knee flexion may occur, with subsequent tibiofemoral joint adjustments. The clinician should follow these movements.

The popliteal fossa induction (Fig. 63.72)

The patient is in prone position, and the clinician places the hands (without crossing them) on the thigh and leg, without directly contacting the popliteal fossa. The therapist then applies pressure with both hands towards the extremity and the fossa. The principles of induction are followed.

The posterior compartment of the leg release (Fig. 63.73) (Pilat 2003)

The patient is in prone position, with the knee flexed at 90° and the clinician sitting on the table behind the patient on the treated side. The clinician flexes all his / her fingers (excluding the thumbs) of both hands and contacts the space between the two gastrocnemius muscles at the level of the middle third of the leg. The clinician then attempts to move apart the fingers of both hands (without sliding on the skin) and hold the pressure for 3 to 5 minutes. The principles of induction should be followed.

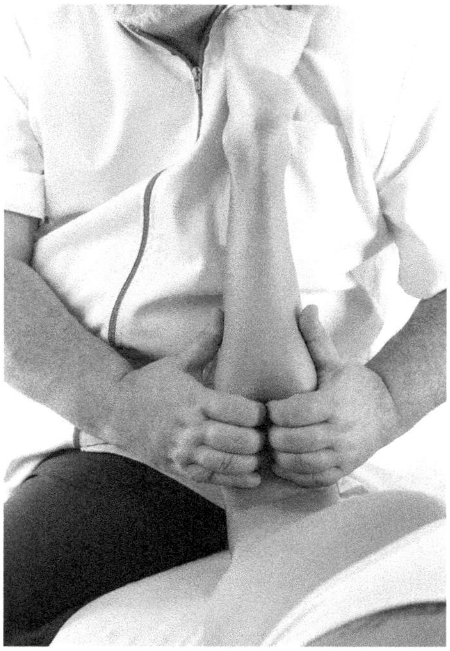

Figure 63.73 The posterior compartment myofascial induction.

The lateral compartment of the leg release (Pilat 2003)

Stroke application (Fig. 63.74)

The patient is in supine position, and the clinician grasps the calcaneus and, with the index finger of the other hand (reinforced by the middle finger), contacts the outer edge of the tibia. The finger should slide directly on the conversion line of the fascia to the periosteum (Fig. 63.75). A slow and smooth technique is performed in a cranial direction over the deep fascia close to the periosteum while monitoring for pain. Three repeat strokes are performed.

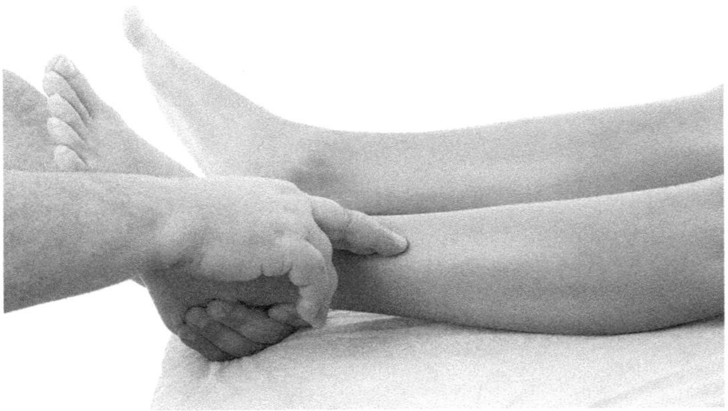

Figure 63.74 **External compartment release (stroke application).**

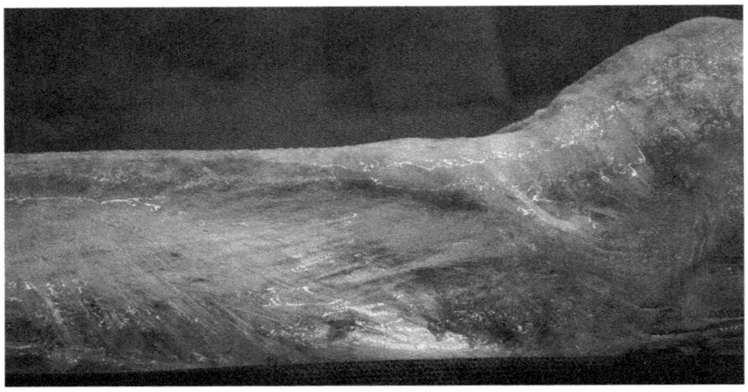

Figure 63.75 **The lateral aspect of the leg from unembalmed cadaver dissection.** Note the fibrosus insertion of the fascia.

Deep induction application (Fig. 63.76)

The clinician crosses the hands to perform this procedure. The cranial hand contacts below the knee and the caudal hand is over the external malleolus.

Plantar fascia induction (Fig. 63.77) (Pilat 2003)

The clinician holds the patient's foot on the medial side and places one hand on the heel and the other on the metatarsal region at the level of the hallux. The thumbs should be orientated longitudinally. The clinician then applies pressure towards the foot and in a longitudinal direction. The clinician follows the facilitated movement three-dimensionally for at least 3–5 minutes. During the course of treatment, the hand placed on the metatarsus must control the position of the hallux and change the degree of flexion and extension to allow a more complete treatment. During the application of the technique, the clinician's thumbs should move to the direction of the release without sliding over the skin.

Contraindications

The general contraindications to myofascial induction therapy are similar to those in any manual therapy procedure. However, a few should be emphasized:

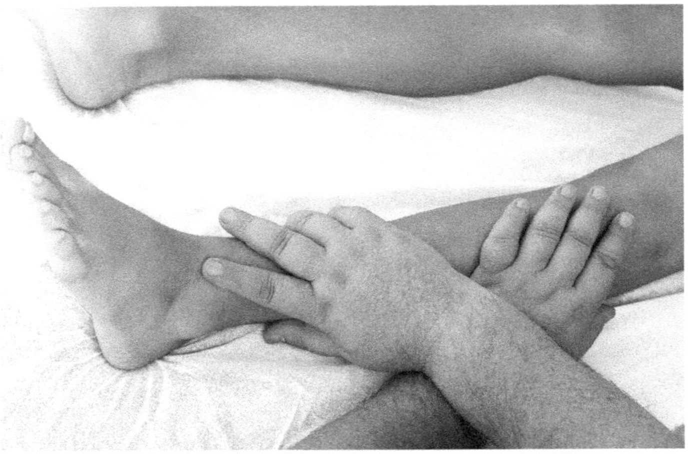

Figure 63.76 **External compartment release (deep induction application).**

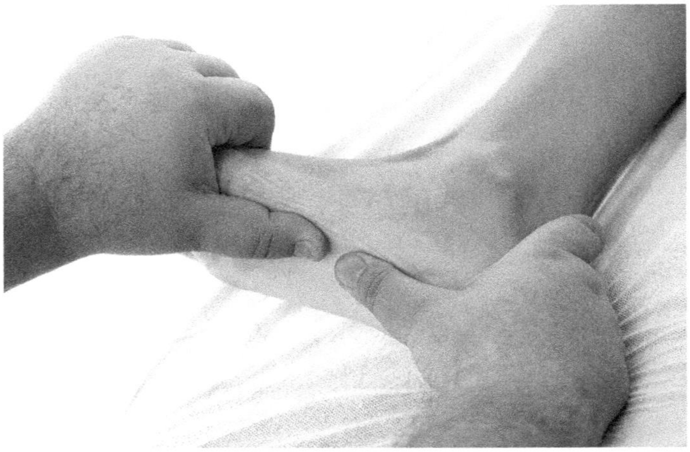

Figure 63.77 **Plantar fascia induction.**

- aneurysm
- systemic disease
- inflammatory soft tissue process in the acute phase
- acute circulatory deficiency
- advanced diabetes
- anticoagulant therapy.

Conclusion

From the anatomical and functional viewpoint, the dynamics of the fascia constitute a unifying structure that may contribute to numerous body systems. The applications of myofascial induction techniques may be of benefit in the treatment of some musculoskeletal diseases. We suggest the inclusion of myofascial induction techniques into the therapeutic process. Research related to the scientific basis of myofascial induction treatment is vast. However, there is still only limited clinical evidence for the technique, although this has been accumulating over the past few years. One factor is the difficulty of quantifying treatment outcomes, in isolation from other collateral phenomena. The development of new assessment methods (e.g. sonoelastography) will help in this challenge.

Preliminary evidence suggests that there may be some value, in terms of reducing pain and improving function, in the use of myofascial induction techniques for patients with chronic pain. However, future research is clearly needed to determine the benefits of myofascial induction techniques (Remvig 2007).

References

Ahn AC, Grodzinsky AJ. 2009. Relevance of collagen piezoelectricity to 'Wolff's Law'. Med Eng Phys 31: 733–741.

Arguisuelas-Martínez MD. 2010. Effects of lumbar spine manipulation and thoracolumbar myofascial induction technique on the spinae erector activation pattern. Fisioterapia 32: 250–255. [Article in Spanish.]

Arroyo-Morales M, Olea N, Martinez M, et al. 2008a. Effects of myofascial release after high-intensity exercise. J Manipulative Physiol Ther 31: 217–223.

Arroyo-Morales M, Olea N, Martínez M, et al. 2008b. Psychophysiological effects of massage-myofascial release after exercise. J Altern Complement Med 14: 1223–1229.

Arroyo-Morales M, Olea N, Ruíz C, et al. 2009. Massage after exercise – responses of immunologic and endocrine markers: a randomized single-blind placebo-controlled study. J Strength Cond Res 23: 638–644.

Avelar J. 1989. Regional distribution and behavior of the subcutaneous tissue concerning selection and indication for liposuction. Aesthetic Plastic Surgery 13: 155–162.

Barlow Y, Willoughby S. 1992. Pathophysiology of soft tissue repair. Br Med Bulletin 48: 698–711.

Barnes J. 1990. Myofascial release. Paoli: MFR Seminars.

Benjamin M. 1995. Fibrocartilage associated with human tendons and their pulleys. J Anat 187: 625–633.

Bergmark A. 1989. Stability of the lumbar spine: a study in mechanical engineering. Acta Orthop Scand Suppl 230: 1–54.

Bienfait M. 1987. Estudio e tratamento do esqueleto fibroso: fascias e pompages. Sao Paulo: Summus Editorial.

Blemker SS, Pinsky PM, Delp SL. 2005. A 3D model of muscle reveals the causes of nonuniform strains in the biceps brachii. J Biomech 38: 657–665.

Bochenek A, Reicher M. 1997. Anatomia czlowieka. Warszawa: PZWL.

Bouligand Y. 1978. Liquid crystals and their analogs in biological systems. Solid State Phys 14: 259–294.

Briggs CA, Elliott BG. 1985. Lateral epicondylitis. A review of structures associated with tennis elbow. Clin Anatomy 7: 149–153.

Cantu TL, Grodin AJ. 2001. Myofascial manipulation: theory and clinical application. Maryland: Aspen.

Carvalhais VO, Ocarino Jde, Araújo VL, et al. 2013. Myofascial force transmission between the latissimus dorsi and gluteus maximus muscles: an in vivo experiment. J Biomech 46: 1003–1007.

Chaitow L, Delany J. 2002. Clinical application of neuromuscular techniques. The lower body. Vol 2. London: Churchill Livingstone.

Chaitow L, Lovegrove Jones R (eds). 2012. Chronic pelvic pain and dysfunction: practical physical medicine. London: Elsevier Churchill Livingstone.

Chaudhry H, Huang C, Schleip R, et al. 2007. Viscoelastic behavior of human fasciae under extension in manual therapy. Bodywork Mov Ther 11: 159–167.

Chaudhry H, Schleip R, Ji Z, et al. 2008. Three-dimensional mathematical model for deformation of human fasciae in manual therapy. J Am Osteopath Assoc 108: 379–390.

Chew ML, Giuffrè B. 2005. Disorders of the distal biceps brachii tendon. Radiographics 25: 1227–1237.

Chi-Zhang C, Gao Y. 2012. Finite element analysis of mechanics of lateral transmission of force in single muscle fiber. J Biomech 45: 2001–2006.

Chicurel ME, Chen CS, Ingber DE. 1998. Cellular control lies in the balance of forces. Curr Opin Cell Biol 10: 232–239.

Chiquet M. 2009. How do fibroblasts translate mechanical signals into changes in extracellular matrix production? Matrix Biol 22: 73–80.

Chiquet M, Gelman L, Lutz R, et al. 2009. From mechanotransduction to extracellular matrix gene expression in fibroblasts. Biochim Biophys Acta 1793: 911–920.

Cholewicki J, Panjabi MM, Khachatryan A. 1997. Stabilizing function of trunk flexor–extensor muscles around a neutral spine posture. Spine 22: 2207–2212.

Chou R, Shekelle P. 2010. Will this patient develop persistent disabling low back pain? JAMA 303: 1295–1302.

Congdon ED, John Edson J, Yanitelli S. 1946. Gross structure of subcutaneous layer of anterior and lateral trunk in the male. Am J Anat 79: 399–429.

Cope FW. 1975. A review of the applications of solid state physics concepts to biological systems. J Biol Physics 3: 1–41.

Corey SM. 2011. Sensory innervation of the nonspecialized connective tissues in the low back of the rat. Cells Tissues Organs 194: 521–530.

Crisco JJ, Panjabi MM, Yamamoto I, et al. 1992. Euler stability of the human ligamentous lumbar spine. Part II: Experiment. Clin Biomech 7: 27–32.

Eames MH, Bain GI, Fogg QA, et al. 2007. Distal biceps tendon anatomy: a cadaveric study. Am J Bone Joint Surg 89: 1044–1049.

Evans P. 1980. The healing process at cellular level: a review. Physiotherapy 66: 256–259.

Farasyn A. 2007. Referred muscle pain is primarily peripheral in origin: the 'barrier-dam' theory. Med Hypotheses 68: 144–150.

Fernández-Lao C, Cantarero-Villanueva I, Fernández-de-las Peñas C, et al. 2011. Widespread mechanical pain hypersensitivity as a sign of central sensitization after breast cancer surgery. Pain Med 12: 72–78.

Fernández-Pérez AM, Peralta-Ramírez MI, Pilat A, et al. 2008. Effects of myofascial induction techniques on physiologic and psychologic parameters: a randomized controlled trial. J Altern Complem Med 14: 807–811.

Fernández-Pérez AM, Peralta-Ramírez MI, Pilat A, et al. 2013. Can myofascial techniques modify immunological parameters? J Altern Complem Med 19: 24–28.

Fidzianska A, Jablonska S. 2000. Congenital fascial dystrophy: abnormal composition of the fascia. J Am Acad Dermatol 43: 797–802.

Fryer G, Hodgson L. 2005. The effect of manual pressure release on myofascial trigger points in the upper trapezius muscle. J Bodywork Mov Ther 9;4: 248–255.

Gabbiani G. 2003. The myofibroblast in wound healing and fibrocontractive diseases. J Pathol 200: 500–503.

Gabbiani G. 2007. Evolution and clinical implications of the myofibroblast concept. In: Findley TW, Schleip R (eds) Fascia research: basic science and implications for conventional and complementary health care. Munich: Urban and Fischer, pp 56–60.

Gallaudet BB. 1931. A description of the planes of fascia of the human body. New York: Columbia University Press.

Gatton ML, Pearcy MJ, Pettet GJ, et al. 2010. A three-dimensional mathematical model of the thoracolumbar fascia and an estimate of its biomechanical effect. J Biomech 43: 2792–2797.

Gerlach UJ, Lierse W. 1990. Functional construction of the superficial and deep fascia system of the lower limb in man. Acta Anatomica 139: 11–25.

Ghosh K, Ingber DE. 2007. Micromechanical control of cell and tissue development: Implications for tissue engineering. Adv Drug Deliv Rev 59: 1306–1308.

Gracovetsky S. 2008. Is the lumbodorsal fascia necessary? J Bodywork Mov Ther 12: 194–197.

Guimberteau JC, Sentucq-Rigall J, Panconi B, et al. 2005. Introduction to the knowledge of subcutaneous sliding system in humans. Ann Chir Plast Esthet 50: 19–34.

Guimberteau JC, Delage JP, McGrouther DA, et al. 2010. The microvacuolar system: how connective tissue sliding works. J Hand Surg Eur Vol 35: 614–622.

Hamwee J. 1999. Zero balancing: touching the energy of bone. North Atlantic Books: Berkeley

Han DG, 2009. The other mechanism of muscular referred pain: the 'connective tissue' theory. Med Hypotheses 73: 292–295.

Haouzi P, Hill JM, Lewis BK, et al. 1999. Responses of group III and IV muscle afferents to distension of the peripheral vascular bed. J Appl Physiol 87: 545–553.

Henley CE, Ivins D, Mills M, et al. 2008. Osteopathic manipulative treatment and its relationship to autonomic nervous system activity as demonstrated by heart rate variability. Osteopath Med Prim Care 2: 7.

Heredia-Rizo AM, Oliva-Pascual-Vaca A, Rodríguez-Blanco C, et al. 2013. Immediate changes in masticatory mechanosensitivity, mouth opening, and head posture after myofascial techniques in pain-free healthy participants. J Manipulative Physiol Ther 36: 310–318.

Hicks M, Meltzer K, Cao T, et al. 2009. Human fibroblast (HF) model of repetitive motion strain (RMS) and myofascial release. In: Huijing PA, Hollander P, Findley TW, et al. (eds) Fascia research II: basic science and implications for conventional and complementary health care. Munich: Elsevier, p 259.

Hou CR, Tsai LC, Cheng KF, et al. 2002. Immediate effects of various physical therapeutic modalities on cervical myofascial pain and trigger point sensitivity. Arch Phys Med Rehabil: 83: 1406–1414.

Hu S, Chen J, Fabry B, et al. 2003. Intracellular stress tomography reveals stress focusing and structural anisotropy in cytoskeleton of living cells. Am J Physiol Cell Physiol 285: C1082–1090.

Huijing PA. 2009. Epimuscular miofascial force transmission: a historical review and implications for new research. J Biomech 42: 9–21.

Huijing PA, Baan GC. 2001a. Extramuscular myofascial force transmission within the rat anterior tibial compartment: proximo-distal differences in muscle force. Acta Physiol Scand 173: 297–311.

Huijing PA, Baan GC. 2001b. Myofascial force transmission causes interaction between adjacent muscles and connective tissue: effects of blunt dissection and compartmental fasciotomy on length force characteristics of rat extensor digitorum longus muscle. Arch Physiol Biochem 109: 97–109.

Huijing PA, Baan GC, Rebel GT, et al. 1998. Non-myotendinous force transmission in rat extensor digitorum longus muscle. J Exp Biol 201: 683–691.

Iatridis JC, Wu J, Yandow JA, et al. 2003. Subcutaneous tissue mechanical behavior is linear and viscoelastic under uniaxial tension. Connect Tissue Res 44: 208–217.

Ingber DE. 1998. The architecture of life. Sci Am 278: 48–57.

Ingber DE. 2003. Mechanobiology and diseases of mechanotransduction. Ann Med 35: 564–577.

Ingber DE. 2005. Tissue adaptation to mechanical forces in healthy, injured and aging tissues. Scand J Med Sci Sports 15: 199–204.

Ingber DE. 2006. Cellular mechanotransduction: putting all the pieces together again. FASEB J 20: 811–827.

Kalin PJ, Hirsch BE. 1987. The origins and function of the interosseous muscles of the foot. J Anat 152: 83–91.

Kaufman MP, Hayes SG, Adreani CM, et al. 2002. Discharge properties of group III and IV muscle afferents. Adv Exp Med Biol 508: 25–32.

Khalsa PS, Zhang C, Sommerfeldt D, et al. 2000. Expression of integri alpha-2beta1 in axons and receptive endings of neurons in rat, hairy skin. Neurosci Lett 293: 13–16.

Kumka M, Bonar B. 2012. Fascia: a morphological description and classification system based on a literature review. J Can Chiropr Assoc 56: 179–191.

Langevin, HM. 2006. Connective tissue: a body-wide signaling network? Med Hypotheses 66: 1074–1077.

Langevin HM, Huijing PA. 2009. Communicating about fascia: history, pitfalls, and recommendations. Int J Ther Massage Bodywork 2: 3–8.

Langevin HM, Yandow JA. 2002. Relationship of acupuncture points and meridians to connective tissue planes. Anat Rec 269: 257–265.

Langevin HM, Stevens-Tuttle D, Fox JR, et al. 2009. Ultrasound evidence of altered lumbar connective tissue structure in human subjects with chronic low back pain. BMC Musculoskeletal Disorders 10: 151.

Langevin HM, Bouffard NA, Fox JR, et al. 2011. Fibroblast cytoskeletal remodeling contributes to connective tissue tension. J Cell Physiol 226: 1166–1175.

Leonard JH, Teng SC, Gan JH, et al. 2009. Physiological effects of connective tissue manipulation on diabetic foot ulcer. In: Huijing PA, Hollander P, Findley TW, et al. (eds) Fascia research II: basic science and implications for conventional and complementary health care. Munich: Elsevier, p 95.

Lin YW, Cheng CM, LeDuc FR, et al. 2009. Understanding sensory nerve mechanotransduction through localized elastomeric matrix control. PLoS One 4: e4293.

Manheim C. 2008. The myofascial release manual. Thorofare, NJ: Slack Inc.

Maniotis A, Chen C, Ingber DE. 1997. Demonstration of mechanical connections between integrins, cytoskeletal filaments, and nucleoplasm that stabilize nuclear structure. Proc Natl Acad Sci USA 94: 849–854.

Markmann B, Barton FE. 1987. Anatomy of the subcutaneous tissue of the trunk and lower extremity. Plastic Reconst Surg 80: 248–254.

Marshall R, Paul L, Mc Fadyen AK. 2009. Evaluating the effectiveness of myofascial release to reduce pain in people with chronic fatigue syndrome (CFS). In: Huijing PA, Hollander P, Findley TW, Schleip R (eds) Fascia research II: basic science and implications for conventional and complementary health care. Munich: Elsevier, p 305.

Martínez Rodríguez R, Galán del Río F. 2013. Mechanistic basis of manual therapy in myofascial injuries. Sonoelastographic evolution control. J Bodywork Mov Ther 17: 221–234.

Mense S. 1994. Referral of muscle pain. J Pain 3: 1–9.

Myers T. 2003. Anatomy trains. Amsterdam: Elsevier.

O'Connell JA. 2003. Bioelectric responsiveness of fascia. Techniques Orthopaed 18: 67–73.

Oschman J. 2003. Energy medicine in therapeutics and human performance. Dover, NH: Nature's Own Research Association.

Paoletti S, Sommerfeld P. 1998. Les fascias: role des tissus dans la mécanique humaine. Paris: Sully.

Parker KK, Ingber DE. 2007. Extracellular matrix, mechanotransduction and structural hierarchies in heart tissue engineering. Philos Trans R Soc Lond B Biol Sci 362: 1267–1279.

Pilat A. 2003. Inducción miofascial. Madrid: McGraw-Hill.

Pilat A. 2007. El lenguaje del dolor (el proceso de interpretación del dolor en fisioterapia). Libro de Ponencias XV Jornadas de Fisioterapia.

Pilat A. 2009. Myofascial induction approaches for headache. In: Fernández-de-las-Peñas C, Arendt-Nielsen L, Gerwin RD (eds) Tension type and cervicogenic headache: pathophysiology, diagnosis and treatment. Boston: Jones & Bartlett.

Pilat A. 2011. Myofascial induction. In: Chaitow L (ed) Practical physical medicine approaches to chronic pelvic pain (CPP) and dysfunction. Edinburgh: Elsevier.

Pilat A. 2012. Myofascial induction approaches. In: Schleip R, Findley T, Chaitow L, et al. (eds) Fascia: the tensional network of the human body. Edinburgh: Elsevier Churchill Livingstone, pp 311–318.

Pilat A. 2014. Myofascial induction therapy (MIT®). In: Chaitow L (ed) Fascial dysfunction: manual therapy approaches. Pencaitland, Scotland: Handspring, Ch 14, pp 179–193.

Pilat A, Testa M. 2009. Tensegridad: el sistema craneosacro como la unidad biodinámica. Libro de Ponencias XIX Jornadas de Fisioterapia 95–111.

Purslow P. 2010. Muscle fascia and force transmission. J Bodywork Mov Ther 14: 411–417.

Remvig L. 2007. Fascia research. Myofascial release: an evidence based treatment concept? In: First International Fascia Research Congress Proceedings. New York: Elsevier Urban & Fischer. Online. Available: http://www.fasciacongress.org/2007/abstract_pdf/Remvig%20(39)%20-%20Myofascial%20Release%20An%20Evidence%20Based%20Treatment%20Concept.pdf. [Poster.]

Rivard M, Laliberté M, Bertrand-Grenier A, et al. 2010. The structural origin of second harmonic generation in fascia. Biomed Opt Express 2: 26–36.

Robb A, Pajaczkowski J. 2009. Prospective investigation on hip adductor strains using myofascial release. In: Huijing PA, Hollander P, Findley TW, Schleip R (eds) Fascia research II: basic science and implications for conventional and complementary health care. Munich: Elsevier, p 96.

Rolf I. 1997. La integración de las estructuras del cuerpo humano. Barcelona: Ediciones Urano.

Rouviere H, Delmas A. 2005. Anatomía humana. Barcelona: Masson.

Satish L, LaFramboise WA, O'Gorman DB, et al. 2008. Identification of differentially expressed genes in fibroblasts derived from patients with Dupuytren's contracture. BMC Med Genomics 1: 1–10.

Schleip R, Duerselen L, Vleeming A, et al. 2012a. Strain hardening of fascia: static stretching of dense fibrous connective tissues can induce a temporary stiffness increase accompanied by enhanced matrix hydration. J Bodywork Mov Ther 16: 94–100.

Schleip R, Jäger H, Klinler W. 2012b. What is 'fascia'? A review of different nomenclatures. J Bodywork Mov Ther 16: 496–502.

Schleip R, Klingler W, Lehmann-Horn F. 2005. Active fascial contractility: fascia may be able to contract in a smooth muscle-like manner and thereby influence musculoskeletal dynamics. Med Hypotheses 65: 273–277.

Schleip R, Klingler W, Lehmann-Horn F. 2007. Fascia is able to contract in a smooth muscle-like manner and thereby influence musculoskeletal mechanics. In: Findley TW, Schleip R (eds) Fascia research: basic science and implications for conventional and complementary health care. Munich: Urban and Fischer, pp 76–77.

Schuenke M, Vleeming A, Van Hoof T, et al. 2012. A description of the lumbar interfascial triangle and its relation with the lateral raphe: anatomical constituents of load transfer through the lateral margin of the thoracolumbar fascia. J Anatomy 221: 568–576.

Shoham N, Gefen A. 2012. Mechanotransduction in adipocytes. J Biomech 45: 1–8.

Stamenovic D, Rosenblatt N, Montoya-Zavala M, et al. 2007. Rheological behavior of living cells is timescale dependent. J Biophys 93: 39–41.

Staubesand J, Li Y. 1997. Begriff und Substrat der Fazienssklerose bei chronisch-venöser Insuffizienz. Phlebologie 26: 72–77.

Stecco L. 2004. Fascial manipulation for musculoskeletal pain. Padova: Piccin.

Stecco C, Gagey O, Belloni A, et al. 2007. Anatomy of the deep fascia of the upper limb. Second part: study of innervation. Morphologie 91: 38–43.

Stecco C, Porzionato A, Macchi V, et al. 2008. The expansions of the pectoral girdle muscles onto the brachial fascia: morphological aspects and spatial disposition. Cells Tiss Organs 188: 320–329.

Swanson RL. 2013. Biotensegrity: a unifying theory of biological architecture with applications to osteopathic practice, education, and research. J Am Osteop Assoc 113: 34–52.

Swartz MA, Tschumperlin DJ, Kamm RD, et al. 2001. Mechanical stress is communicated between different cell types to elicit matrix remodeling. Proc Natl Acad Sci USA 98: 6180–6185.

Szent-Gyorgyi A. 1941. The study of energy levels in biochemistry. Nature 148: 157–159.

Taguchi T, Hoheisel U, Mense S. 2009. Dorsal horn neurons having input from low back structures in rats. Pain 138: 119–129.

Tesarz J, Hoheisel U, Wiedenhofer B, et al. 2011. Sensory innervation of the thoracolumbar fascia in rats and humans. Neuroscience 194: 302–308.

Testut L, Latarjet A. 2007. Compendio de anatomía descriptiva. Madrid: Masson.

Threlkeld AJ. 1992. The effects of manual therapy on connective tissues. J Phys Ther 72: 893–902.

Toro Velasco C, Arroyo-Morales M, Fernández-de-las-Peñas C, et al. 2009. Short-term effects of manual therapy on heart rate variability, mood state, and pressure pain sensitivity in patients with chronic tension-type headache: a pilot study. J Manipulative Physiol Ther 32: 527–535.

Tozzi P, Bongiorno D, Vitturini C. 2012. Low back pain and kidney mobility: local osteopathic fascial manipulation decreases pain perception and improves renal mobility. J Bodywork Mov Ther 16: 381–391.

Travell J, Bigelow NH. 1946. Referred somatic pain does not follow a simple 'segmental' pattern. Fed Proc 5: 106.

Tucker C. 1990. The mechanics of sport injuries. Oxford: Blackwell, pp 321–326.

Upledger J. 1987. Craniosacral therapy II. Seattle, WA: Eastland Press.

Urresti-López FJ. 2011. Miodural bridge stimulation via suboccipital inhibition technique modifies the electroencephalogram significantly in reaction times producing cognitive changes do not occur in the control group. [DO Thesis for diploma in Osteopathy, SEFO-EOM.]

Useros AI, Hernando A. 2008. Liberación miofascial aplicada en un paciente adulto con daño cerebral. Biociencias 6: 1–7.

Van der Wal JC. 2009. The architecture of connective tissue as parameter for proprioception – an often overlooked functional parameter as to proprioception in the locomotor apparatus. Int J Ther Massage Bodywork 2: 9–23.

Vanacore R, Ham AJ, Voehler M, et al. 2009. Sulfilimine bond identified in collagen IV. Science 325: 1230–1234.

Vaquero Rodríguez A. 2013. Influence of myofascial therapy applied to the cervical region of patients suffering from unilateral spatial neglect and head deviation with respect to the median line. CSIC (ICNR 2012) Converging Clinical and Engineering Research on Neurorehabilitation. Biosystems and Biorobotics. Vol 1. Berlin: Springer, pp 371–374. Online. Available: http://link.springer.com/chapter/10.1007/978-3-642-34546-3_59. doi: 10.1007/978-3-642-34546-3_59.

Vasquez C. 2011. Effectiveness of the myofascial induction technique in the swimmer shoulder with respect to the articular balance and pain (Spanish). Cuestiones Fisioterapia 40: 177–184.

Vaticón D. 2009. Sensibilidad myofascial: el sistema craneosacro como la unidad biodinámica. Libro de Ponencias XIX Jornadas de Fisioterapia 24–30.

Vleeming A, Stoeckart R. 1997. The role of the pelvic girdle in coupling the spine and legs: a clinical–anatomical perspective on pelvic stability. In: Vleeming A (ed) Movement, stability and lumbopelvic pain. London: Elsevier, pp 113–138.

Wang N, Tytell J, Ingber DE. 2009. Mechanotransduction at a distance: mechanically coupling the extracellular matrix with the nucleus. Science 10: 75–81.

Willard FH. 2007. The muscular, ligamentous, and neural structure of the lumbosacrum and its relationship to low back pain. In: Vleeming A, Mooney V, Stoeckart R (eds) Movement, stability and lumbopelvic pain, 2nd edn. Edinburgh: Churchill Livingstone Elsevier, p 5.

Willard FH, Vleeming A, Schuenke MD, et al. 2012. The thoracolumbar fascia: anatomy, function and clinical considerations. J Anat 221: 507–536.

Wood Jones F. 1944. Structure and function as seen in the foot. London: Baillière, Tindall and Cox.

Wright DG, Rennels DC. 1964. A study of the elastic properties of plantar fascia. J Bone Joint Surg Am 46: 482–492.

Yahia LH, Pigeon P, DesRosiers EA. 1993. Viscoelastic properties of the human lumbodorsal fascia. J Biomed Eng 15: 425–429.

Yaman A, Ozturk C, Huijing PA, et al.. 2013. Magnetic resonance imaging assessment of mechanical interactions between human lower leg muscles in vivo. J Biomech Eng 135: 91003.

PART 11

Neurodynamics in the Upper and Lower Quadrants

64 Peripheral Nerve Mechanisms of Chronic Upper Limb Pain: Dynamics, Inflammation and Neurophysiology 765
Jane Greening and Andrew Dilley

65 Clinical Neurodynamics of the Upper and Lower Quadrants 781
Emilio J. Puentedura, Paul E. Mintken and Adriaan Louw

Chapter 64

Peripheral Nerve Mechanisms of Chronic Upper Limb Pain: Dynamics, Inflammation and Neurophysiology

Jane Greening, Andrew Dilley

CHAPTER CONTENTS

Introduction	765
Anatomy of a peripheral nerve	765
Mechanical properties of a peripheral nerve	766
Physical tests of nerve movement	767
In vivo measurements of nerve movement	768
Median nerve	768
Ulnar nerve	770
Nerve movement studies in patients	770
Inflammation of a peripheral nerve	771
Causes of inflammation	772
Inflammation and the microenvironment of the nerve	772
Animal models of nerve inflammation	772
Physiological role of inflammatory mediators	775
Disruption of axoplasmic transport	775
Nervi nervorum	776
Imaging nerve inflammation	776
Conclusion	776

Introduction

Chronic upper limb pain represents a significant social economic healthcare problem. The Health and Safety Executive in the UK places upper limb pain second only to low back pain in terms of incidence and lost work days. To the frustration of clinicians and patients, too little is known about the causes of chronic upper limb pain. Treatments tend not to be evidence based and are often focused on diagnostic labels rather than on individual patient presentations. Diffuse repetitive strain injury (RSI), which is also referred to as non-specific arm pain, chronic arm pain following whiplash injury and complex regional pain syndrome type 1 (CRPS1) that affects the upper limb are common conditions seen in the clinic. Despite differences in the initial cause of symptoms, many of these patients experience ongoing pain in their upper limbs with little sign of tissue injury. Patients describe spontaneous pain, pain with limb movements, deep muscle aches, paraesthesia, hyperalgesia (i.e. increased sensitivity to noxious stimuli), allodynia (i.e. increased sensitivity to non-noxious stimuli) and difficulties with the coordination of fine movement – all of which suggest a neuropathic contribution to the symptoms. Studies have also shown subtle changes in upper limb peripheral nerve function in both whiplash patients and those with RSI (Chien et al 2008; Greening & Lynn 1998; Greening et al 2003). However, nerve conduction studies have shown that there is often no objective sign of a frank nerve injury (Alpar et al 2002; Harrington et al 1998; Rodriquez et al 2004; Wallis et al 1998). Central nervous system changes account for some of these symptoms, although there is no evidence that such changes are the primary cause.

In these patient groups, previous investigations of cytokine levels suggest that inflammation affecting nerve tissue may contribute to symptoms (Carp et al 2007; Uceyler et al 2007a; Gerdle et al 2008). Animal studies have shown that nerve inflammation can result in significant peripheral and central changes that may account for painful symptoms described by these patients (Bove et al 2003; Dilley et al 2005; Carp et al 2007; Elliott et al 2008). It has also been suggested that increased nerve strain and changes to neural dynamics may contribute to symptoms (Quintner 1989; Byng 1997; Lynn et al 2002; Sterling et al 2002; Dilley et al 2005; Greening 2005; Greening et al 2005). Following an overview of peripheral nerve trunk anatomy, this chapter will review studies in the upper limb that have used ultrasound imaging and magnetic resonance imaging (MRI) to measure nerve movement and identify possible nerve inflammation in these patient populations. We will also review the now compelling evidence for altered nerve function, morphology and neuropathic symptoms following nerve inflammation.

Anatomy of a Peripheral Nerve

The peripheral nerve trunk has been described as consisting of an inner 'neural core' and an outer connective tissue tube or sheath (Ushiki & Ide 1990; Walbeehm et al 2004). The inner core consists of the endoneurium and perineurium, whereas the outer connective tissue sheath is formed of the epineurium (Fig. 64.1). The axons are located within the endoneurium of a peripheral nerve and are arranged into bundles called

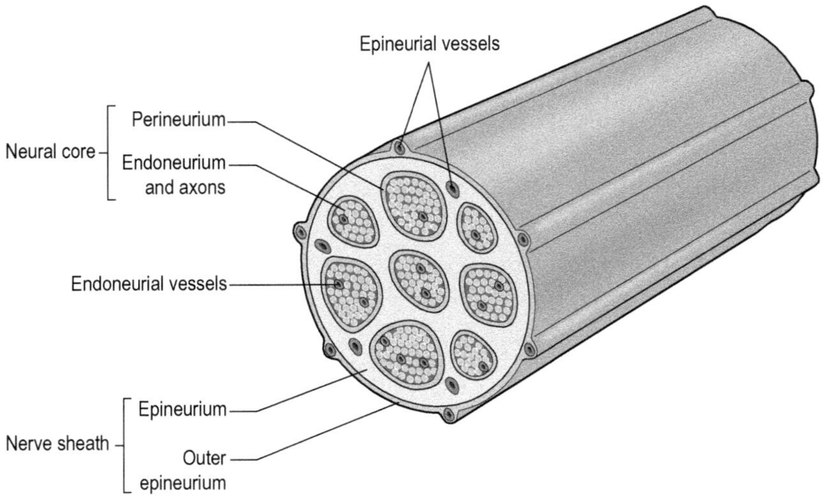

Figure 64.1 Cross-sectional diagram of a peripheral nerve trunk.

fascicles, which are surrounded by the perineurium. Axons are closely associated with Schwann cells, either individually (myelinated axons) or in small groups (unmyelinated axons in Remak bundles). The axons and cells of the endoneurium (i.e. Schwann cells, fibroblasts, macrophages and mast cells) plus the extensive endoneurial capillary network are supported by longitudinally aligned collagen fibrils that form the endoneurial connective tissue. The axons follow an undulating course that is supported by these endoneurial fibrils (Haninec 1986). The undulations appear as a light / dark optical effect under light microscopy and are referred to as bands of Fontana. This wave-like alignment of the axons may represent a reserve length during nerve elongation that protects the axons from high strain levels.

The perineurium is a highly specialized connective tissue structure formed of a tightly woven network of myofibroblasts. In humans it is up to 15 cells deep (Thomas et al 1993) and contains collagen fibrils that run longitudinally, obliquely and circumferentially to provide strength (Gamble & Eames 1964; Sunderland 1978). Although not as effective as the blood–brain barrier, the perineurium act as a diffusion barrier that helps maintain the endoneurial microenvironment surrounding the axons. A positive fluid pressure within the endoneurium is maintained by the impermeability of the perineurium and its circular arrangement of collagen fibrils (Sunderland 1978; Walbeehm et al 2004). When the nerve is under strain, the increased pressure within the endoneurium will act to resist the reduction in nerve cross-sectional area and will contribute to nerve stiffness. A movement plane exists between the perineurium and the epineurium. Bridging these layers is a series of viscoelastic connections that increase in stiffness as nerve strain is increased (Tillett et al 2004). Also passing obliquely between the perineurium and endoneurium are transperineurial blood vessels, which may contribute to this mechanical connection.

The epineurium forms the outer sheath of the nerve and consists of axially arranged undulating, thick collagen bundles (Ushiki & Ide 1990). It provides some degree of nerve extensibility and will cushion against external trauma. The epineurium is surrounded by a loose thin connective tissue, the adventitia, which, although connecting the peripheral nerve trunk to adjacent tissue, allows considerable nerve movement.

Both axonal conduction and axoplasmic transport are metabolic processes that require an uninterrupted blood supply. This is provided by the extensive interconnected vascular systems within the endoneurium, perineurium and epineurium. Extrinsic longitudinal vessels run along the loose adventitia in a sinuous course that allows the nerve considerable mobility. These connect to the intrinsic vessels within the epineurium, which follow a similar sinuous course. These epineurial vessels communicate in turn with the endoneurial vessels (Lundborg 1988).

The connective tissue of the nerve trunk is itself innervated by the nervi nervorum. There is also a contribution from axons forming the perivascular plexus (Hromada 1963). These unmyelinated axons (Thomas 1963) contain both substance P and calcitonin gene-related peptide, which classifies them as C-fibre axons (Sauer et al 1999; Zochodne & Ho 1992, 1993). Activation of these axons in response to nerve damage or capsaicin application to the nerve sheath causes nerve hyperaemia (i.e. increased blood flow) (Zochodne & Ho 1992). Electrophysiological studies have also demonstrated the nociceptive function of the nervi nervorum (Bove & Light 1995).

Whereas peripheral nerves have a thick layer of epineurium, the nerve roots are bathed in cerebrospinal fluid and have a thin pial covering. Compared with the peripheral nerve trunks, nerve roots are relatively vulnerable to mechanical stress and the effects of inflammatory mediators. The distal part of the nerve root is surrounded by a dural sleeve that is continuous with the thin epineurium of the spinal nerve. Although dural connections to the intervertebral foramina ensure that strain is not transmitted to the nerve roots during limb movements, movements of the cervical spine will impose a degree of strain on these structures.

Mechanical Properties of a Peripheral Nerve

Since most peripheral nerves pass across joints at some distance from the centre of joint rotation, their path length will change as the joint is rotated. Consequently, peripheral nerves have to move to accommodate changes in their path length.

Nerve movements can be longitudinal or transverse and can also occur in response to changes in surrounding soft tissues. When the nerve path is shortened, peripheral nerves will become slack and are said to be unloaded. In this shortened position, nerves tend to run a tortuous course (Sunderland 1978). When the nerve path is lengthened, the nerve will initially straighten. This is referred to as 'loading' the nerve (i.e. tensioning the nerve). Further lengthening of the nerve path (beyond the length of the nerve) will result in elongation (i.e. stretch) of the nerve. These increases in the nerve length usually occur without any detrimental effect on nerve function. The measure of elongation is strain, which is often expressed as a percentage increase in the nerve length. The greatest increase in nerve strain occurs in the segments closest to the joint that is moving (Dilley et al 2003).

Stress–strain curves have been described for excised nerves undergoing stress (Fig. 64.2). Stress is defined as the force / load applied divided by the area over which it acts (e.g. a larger diameter nerve is under less stress compared with a smaller diameter nerve when the same load is applied). Stress can be applied to the nerve trunk as longitudinal, compressive or shear stress, or any combination of these forces (Topp & Boyd 2006). In excised nerves, when load is initially applied to a nerve it is seen to elongate considerably (i.e. increase in strain) with minimal increase in longitudinal stress (the toe region on the stress–strain curve) (Kwan et al 1992) (see Fig. 64.2). With increasing load, the nerve continues to elongate at a steady rate, with a linear increase in longitudinal stress in what is termed the linear region of the stress–strain curve, until the nerve mechanically fails. The slope of the curve relates to the inherent stiffness of the nerve (a steeper slope indicating increased stiffness). The 'toe' region has been proposed as a region that protects axons against loading damage and may reflect the initial straightening of the neural connective tissue and axons (Rydevik et al 1990; Kwan et al 1992). However, the stress–strain curve of excised nerves may not completely apply to nerves in situ (Walbeehm et al 2004).

The positive fluid pressure within the endoneurium provides a mechanism to protect excessive loading of the mechanically weaker inner neural core during nerve elongation (Walbeehm et al 2004). This endoneurial fluid pressure (Lundborg 1988), which is maintained by the arrangement of collagen fibrils and impermeability of the perineurium, causes the inner neural core to act as a relatively incompressible inner chamber. Such a mechanism would resist a decrease in epineurial diameter during elongation and act to increase nerve stiffness.

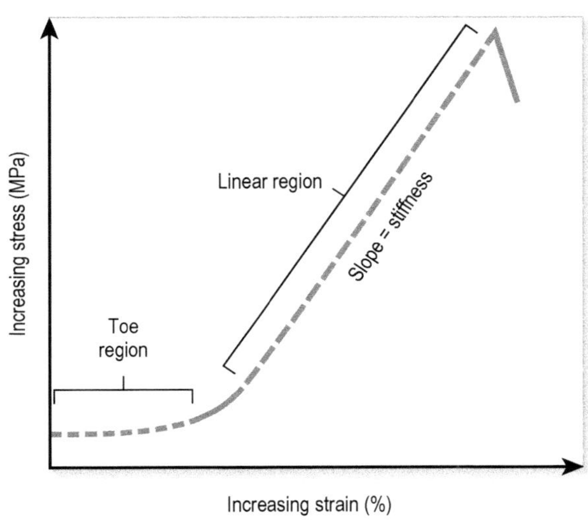

Figure 64.2 Stress–strain curve for an excised peripheral nerve.

Should the ability of nerves to elongate and slide freely become compromised by adhesion to surrounding tissues, then limb movements would result in a localized increase in nerve strain that may lead to a loss of function, fibrosis and painful symptoms (Millesi et al 1990; Mackinnon 2002). Studies have investigated the limits to which nerves can be stretched before their function is compromised. Levels of strain exceeding 6% can lead to changes in blood supply and therefore nerve function (Grewel et al 1996). Since nerves have to slide and stretch during limb movements, the inherent mechanical properties of the nerve are of extreme importance.

Physical tests of nerve movement

As well as tests of nerve function and nerve conduction, clinicians use physical tests (both active and passive) to apply strain and pressure (palpation) to nerve plexuses and peripheral nerve trunks. Historically, tests that apply nerve strain have been used to look for mechanical change in the peripheral nervous system. However, more recently it has become clear that nerve mechanical sensitivity will result in positive responses to these physical tests. In the upper limb, tests of nerve movement and nerve trunk palpation are particularly useful in cases where a neuropathic contribution is suspected and there is no overt sign of nerve injury (e.g. in RSI and chronic arm pain following whiplash injury). Movement tests of the brachial plexus and median, ulnar and radial nerves are considered to give a positive response when upper limb movements that apply strain to these nerve trunks and the brachial plexus result in symptom reproduction and consequent loss of joint rotation due to a protective flexor withdrawal response. Moderate digital pressure applied over nerve trunks is also shown to produce painful symptoms in patients with RSI or arm pain following whiplash injury (Greening et al 2005).

Positive responses to upper limb nerve movement tests are expected in patients where there is an obvious impairment of nerve movement. An impairment of nerve movement could result from frank compression or nerve transection (Lundborg 1988). Such restrictions in nerve movement in the presence of ongoing movements of the upper extremity could lead to local increases in nerve strain sufficient to affect the local nerve blood supply and nerve function. An increase in nerve strain may lead to epineurial bleeding and oedema, perpetuating a vicious circle of scarring and further increases in strain. Severe injury would result in axon degeneration with complete conduction block. In the upper limb there are well-documented sites where the peripheral nerve trunk may be more susceptible to 'irritation' and 'entrapment'. Lundborg (1988) describes these sites as where the nerve passes through a fibrous or fibro-osseous tunnel (e.g. thoracic aperture, carpal tunnel, cubital tunnel), under a constricting fibrous band or fascial edge (e.g. ulnar nerve under the flexor carpi ulnaris; median nerve through the pronator teres) or through any repetitively contracting muscle (e.g. with repeated forearm, finger or wrist movements).

The sensitivity and specificity of applying additional strain to individual cords of the brachial plexus and peripheral nerves during these upper limb nerve movement tests has been measured in cadaveric studies (Kleinrensink et al 2000). Interestingly, only the median nerve upper limb tension test (ULTT) was shown to be specific with regards applying strain to the medial cord of the brachial plexus and the median nerve trunk alone. Other nerve movement tests apply substantial strain to all the cords of the brachial plexus and to all peripheral nerve trunks.

In Vivo Measurements of Nerve Movement

It is important to understand how peripheral nerves cope with limb movements and normal levels of strain before examining neural dynamics in patients. Until fairly recently, the pattern of longitudinal nerve movement in vivo was not well understood, most information having been obtained from cadavers.

Cadaveric studies examined longitudinal movement of the median, ulnar and radial nerves in response to shoulder, elbow and wrist movements (Wilgis & Murphy 1986; Kleinrensink et al 1995; Wright et al 1996, 2001, 2005). Early observations of longitudinal movement of the median nerve were also reported in vivo using a microneurography recording electrode inserted into the nerve (McLellan & Swash 1976). These studies indicated that movements of 5–10 mm are readily produced. It was also claimed that strain values for the median nerve of over 10% are obtained for joint movement within the physiological range (Wright et al 1996) – values that are likely to cause reduced blood flow and impaired nerve conduction (Grewel et al 1996).

We have examined nerve movements in the upper limb in detail using high-frequency ultrasound imaging. In these studies, sequences of ultrasound images were analysed using a frame-by-frame cross-correlation algorithm that measured pixel shifts between images (Dilley et al 2001, 2003). With this technique, we have measured median and ulnar nerve movement and strain during neck and upper limb movements (Dilley et al 2003, 2007; Julius et al 2004).

Median nerve

Longitudinal nerve movement

Median nerve movement values that we obtained for wrist, shoulder and elbow movements were consistent with values obtained from cadavers (Wilgis & Murphy 1986; Wright et al 1996). When the upper limb was fully extended (i.e. 90° shoulder abduction, elbow extended and wrist in 40° extension) with contralateral neck side flexion – a position that was similar to the median nerve upper limb tension test positive (ULTT+) (Kleinrensink et al 2000) – the nerve strain in the forearm was estimated to be only 2.5–3%. This is very different from the 10% strain measured in cadavers (Wright et al 1996) and, although this may reflect the difference in method, our results indicate that, even with the limb extended, median nerve strain is at a level that is unlikely to produce pathological change.

Nerve compliance

Peripheral nerves are well adapted to cope with large changes in their path length. This means that high strain levels that would be detrimental to nerve function are never reached. Importantly, ultrasound studies show that the median nerve is easily unloaded (Dilley et al 2003, 2007). This unloading is due to localized regions of high compliance that exist at the shoulder and elbow joints (Fig. 64.3) – that is, where nerves follow a non-linear course when unloaded and / or exhibit less stiffness.

Evidence for a region of compliance through the shoulder was obtained from nerve movement data during neck and shoulder movements. First, during the first 50° of shoulder abduction with the elbow extended, there is virtually no median nerve movement in the arm and forearm. Nerve movement occurs only towards the end of abduction, once the nerve is loaded and begins to elongate along its whole length

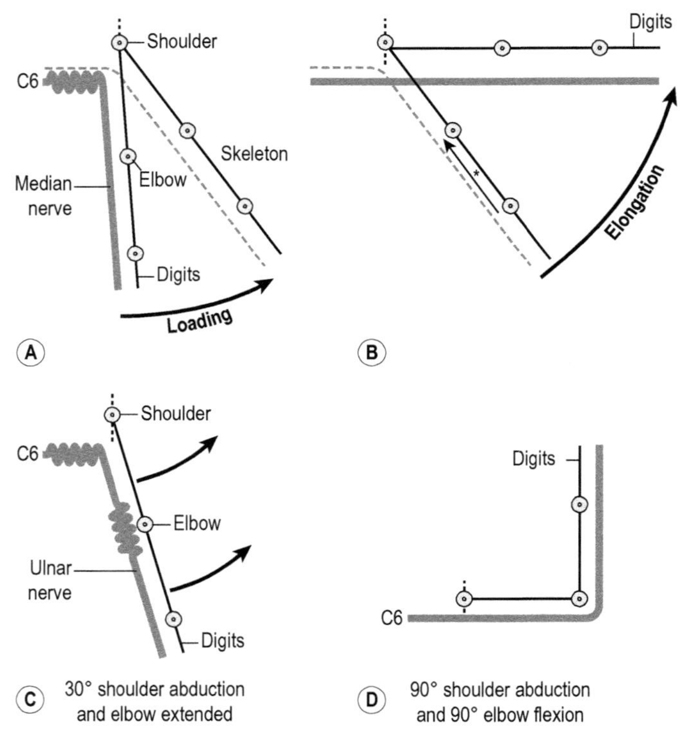

Figure 64.3 Nerve compliance at shoulder and elbow. (**A**) and (**B**) The pattern of median nerve movement during shoulder abduction: (**A**) 10–50° shoulder abduction. The median nerve at 10° shoulder abduction showing a region of high compliance (i.e. slack) in its proximal segment. As the shoulder is abducted to 50°, the nerve will initially straighten from its proximal segment as it becomes loaded. (**B**) 50–90° shoulder abduction. At approximately 50°, the nerve will start to elongate (stretch) as the shoulder is abducted to 90°. During stretching, the nerve will elongate towards the moving joint (indicated by the starred arrow). (**C**) and (**D**) The pattern of ulnar nerve movement during elbow flexion: (**C**) 30° shoulder abduction and elbow extended. The ulnar nerve at 30° shoulder abduction and the elbow straight showing regions of high compliance at the shoulder and across the elbow. (**D**) 90° shoulder abduction and 90° elbow flexion. As the shoulder is abducted to 90° and the elbow flexed to 90°, the nerve straightens at the proximal segment and across the elbow with negligible movement in the arm and forearm. (A and B from Dilley et al 2003, with permission.)

(see Fig. 64.3A,B). Secondly, during contralateral cervical lateral flexion with the shoulder adducted (i.e. shortened nerve path length), there is no nerve movement in the arm at the start of cervical movement. In contrast, with the shoulder at 90° abduction (i.e. extended nerve path length), nerve movement occurs throughout contralateral cervical lateral flexion. Thirdly, as the elbow joint is extended from 90° flexion to 45° with the shoulder in 90° abduction, the nerve moves in the arm but not in the forearm. At 45° with the shoulder in 90° abduction of elbow extension, slack is taken up through the shoulder region and the nerve becomes loaded. At this point, the nerve also moves in the forearm. This pattern of nerve movement is also accounted for by extensive folding of the median nerve in the arm with the elbow flexed (Fig. 64.4A–E). Examination of median nerve movement during elbow flexion reveals a region of compliance proximal to the elbow that exists even with the shoulder in 90° abduction (see Fig. 64.4A–C).

As well as folding and bowing of the nerve trunk as a mechanism for preventing excessive loading, the fascicles themselves are also able to bow independently of the outer connective tissue sheath (i.e. the epineurium and adventitia). The fascicles are likely to undergo loading at a later stage during stretch of the connective tissue sheath. This forms a protective mechanism that prevents excessive stretching of the axons. Fascicular folding is readily observed from ultrasound images of the median nerve when the nerve is unloaded (see Fig. 64.4F–I).

Nerve loading

It is only when the limb is extended that the median nerve will become loaded and behave like a continuous spring (i.e. the linear region of a stress–strain curve) (see Fig. 64.2). During normal physiological joint movements, the maximum strain in the median nerve is unlikely to exceed 4%. Therefore, the median nerve is well designed to cope with changes in its path length caused by limb movements. Any stretching that does occur is unlikely to threaten the intraneural blood supply or nerve conduction.

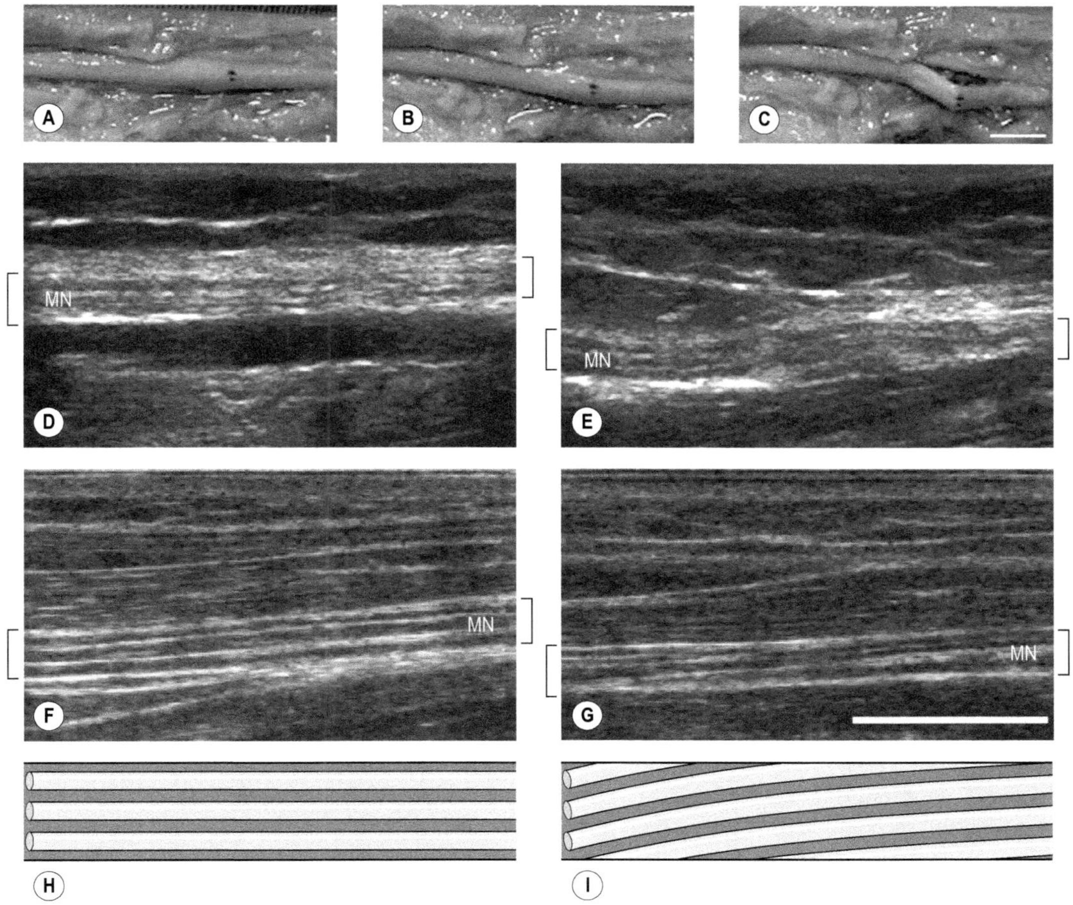

Figure 64.4 Median nerve folding in elbow flexion and shoulder abduction: (**A**) to (**C**) Images showing median nerve folding (just proximal to the bicipital aponeurosis) during elbow flexion with the shoulder in 90° abduction: (**A**) elbow extended with the median nerve stretched; (**B**) elbow at 45° flexion with slight nerve bowing as it unloads; (**C**) elbow at 90° flexion with clear folding of the nerve. A similar pattern can be seen with the shoulder adducted. Note that during dissection of the median nerve, the surrounding adventitia has been cut. (**D**) and (**E**) Ultrasound images of the median nerve just proximal to the bicipital aponeurosis: in (**D**) the elbow is extended and the median nerve appears straight; in (**E**) the elbow is flexed to 90° and the nerve follows a non-linear course. (**F**) and (**G**) Ultrasound images of the median nerve in the forearm showing the clearly defined fascicular structure: in (**F**), the limb is in an extended position (with the wrist and elbow extended) and the fascicles appear straight; in a flexed position (**G**), the fascicles appear curved. (**H**) and (**I**) represent the fascicular structure in the extended (**H**) and flexed (**I**) positions. (F and G from Dilley et al 2003, with permission.)

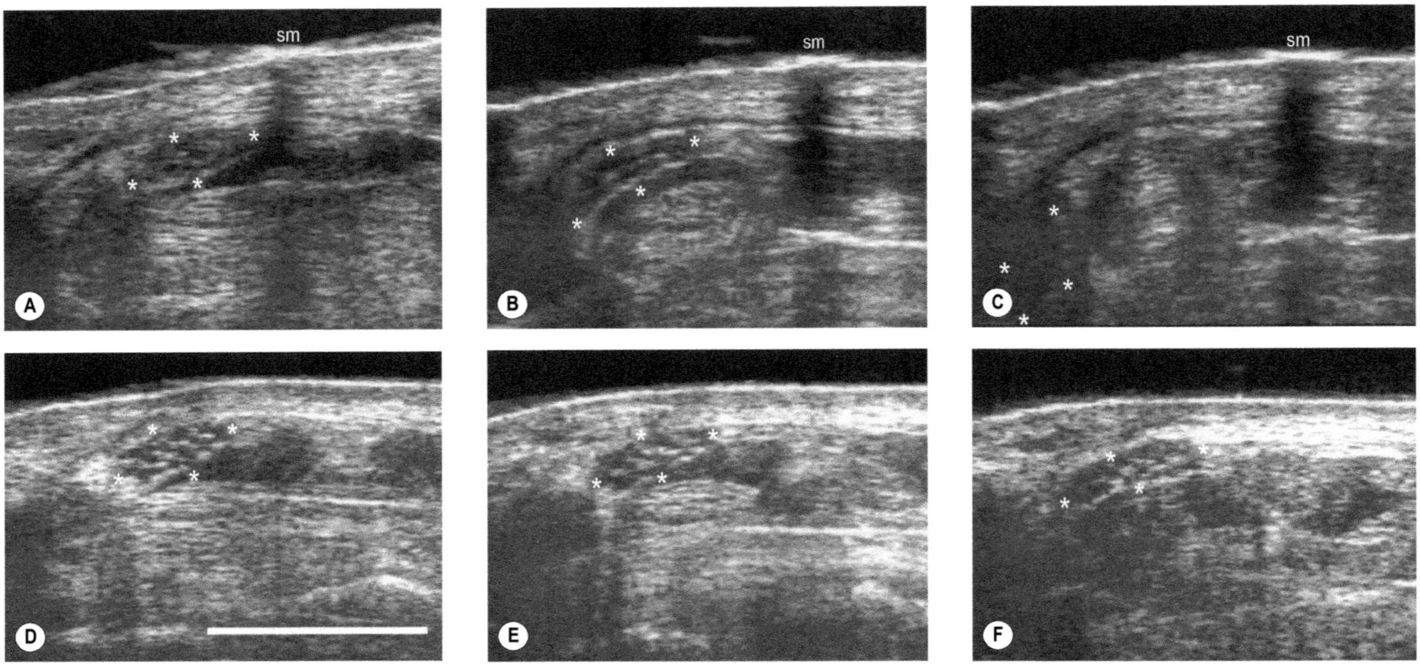

Figure 64.5 Cross-sectional (transverse) ultrasound images of the median nerve (outlined *) at the proximal carpal tunnel. (**A**) to (**C**) Images of the *non-symptomatic* side in a patient with RSI during wrist flexion: (**A**) wrist 30° extension, (**B**) mid position and (**C**) wrist 30° flexion, showing median nerve excursion in a lateral and posterior direction during wrist flexion. (**D**) to (**E**) Images of the *symptomatic* side in a patient with RSI during wrist flexion: (**D**) wrist 30° extension, (**E**) mid position and (**F**) wrist 30° flexion, showing very little transverse movement of the median nerve. (**F**) In the flexed wrist position, the nerve remains compressed between the flexor retinaculum and the flexor tendons. sm=skin marker.

Transverse median nerve movement

Transverse nerve movements occur during limb movements in response to deformation of adjacent soft tissues. This is not an active movement; rather, the nerve is pushed by movement of the adjacent soft tissue into a new position. For example, at the wrist the median nerve is observed to slide transversely in a lateral direction during wrist or digit flexion (Greening et al 2001). During this movement, the flexor tendons move anteriorly towards the roof of the carpal tunnel, which causes the median nerve to slide transversely (laterally) and in some cases posteriorly (Fig. 64.5A–C). In this instance, transverse sliding ensures that the nerve is not compressed between the tendons and the flexor retinaculum in positions of wrist and finger flexion.

Ulnar nerve

Ultrasound studies of longitudinal ulnar nerve movement (Dilley et al 2007) suggest that, similar to the median nerve, the ulnar nerve is unloaded in most functional upper limb positions. Nerve movement observations indicate a similar region of high compliance at the shoulder and elbow joint (see Fig. 64.3C,D). For example, shoulder abduction, with the elbow flexed, produces only negligible movement of the ulnar nerve in the arm or forearm. Elbow movements also cause negligible movement of the ulnar nerve in the arm or forearm (Dilley et al 2007). The latter result is surprising as elbow flexion produces an increase of approximately 18 mm in nerve path length, since the nerve lies approximately 12 mm from the centre of rotation of this joint. However, with the elbow flexed and the shoulder adducted, the ulnar nerve appears to be folded proximal to elbow joint, which indicates a region of high compliance at this joint. Unfortunately the above study did not measure transverse movement of the nerve at the cubital tunnel during elbow flexion, which would probably bring the nerve closer to the centre of rotation. Additionally, transverse movement could also explain the small degree of longitudinal nerve movement observed.

Nerve Movement Studies in Patients

Using ultrasound imaging, we have investigated median nerve movement in the most common nerve entrapment syndrome – carpal tunnel syndrome (CTS) – in patients after repair surgery for median nerve transection, as well as those with RSI and chronic arm pain after whiplash injury. All patients examined had painful symptoms with the application of the median nerve ULLT, apart from those with nerve repair following complete transection, where this test was not applied.

In RSI, painful symptoms are spread throughout the upper limb and therefore it has been postulated that longitudinal median nerve movement might be restricted at multiple sites. These sites include the shoulder region, the pronator teres muscle and the carpal tunnel. However, ultrasound studies of longitudinal nerve movement revealed no significant difference through the shoulder, the forearm or carpal tunnel in the RSI patients studied, compared with control subjects (Dilley et al 2008). We have also failed to find a reduction in longitudinal median nerve movement through the carpal tunnel in patients with CTS (Erel et al 2003), despite its being labelled clinically as an entrapment neuropathy. Similarly at surgery, longitudinal median nerve movement remained unchanged following carpal tunnel release (Tuzuner et al 2004). Using laser Doppler imaging, a small reduction in median nerve movement in CTS patients was noted when the nerve was loaded (i.e. wrist and elbow extension), but no change when the nerve was unloaded (i.e. elbow flexion) (Hough et al 2007). This small reduction in the loaded position by no means indicates a longitudinal entrapment of the median nerve.

Interestingly, studies of median nerve movement in patients with RSI and those with arm symptoms following whiplash injury do indicate a reduction in proximal longitudinal movement of the median nerve in the forearm during deep inspiration (Greening et al 2005). This decrease is, however, insufficient to cause detrimental increases in nerve strain; instead, it may be caused by a restriction in motion of the first rib. In RSI patients, poor and prolonged cervical spine posture might result in shortening of the scalene muscles (Pascarelli & Hsu 2001), causing an elevated first rib. During whiplash injury the first rib may also be elevated (based on clinical observations), possibly owing to the excessive stretch applied to the scalene muscles and their subsequent reflex shortening. Elevation of the first rib will compromise the space available to the trunks of the brachial plexus within the scalene triangle, possibly leading to neurogenic thoracic outlet syndrome.

Further, patients with RSI and CTS have a reduction in lateral transverse median nerve movement at the proximal carpal tunnel, and there is a significantly altered pattern of movement in patients with arm pain following whiplash (Nakamichi & Tachibana 1995; Allmann et al 1997; Greening et al 1999, 2001, 2005; Lynn et al 2002; Erel et al 2003) (see Fig. 64.5D–F). The lack of lateral transverse nerve movement of the median nerve at this osseous fibrous tunnel would, as previously described, subject the nerve to increasing pressure and irritation during wrist and finger movements. This would account for painful symptoms experienced by these patients during functional hand activities.

Although it is important to understand that small reductions in longitudinal and transverse nerve movement are unlikely to cause significant increases in longitudinal nerve strain, symptoms may occur as a result of nerve pathology at the first rib and within the carpal tunnel. The only example to date that we have of a reduction in longitudinal nerve sliding of the median nerve was found in patients who had undergone median nerve repair following traumatic nerve transection (Erel et al 2009). In these patients there was an 8% reduction of median nerve movement in the forearm during metacarpal extension on the repaired side compared with that on the uninjured side. The observed reduction on the repaired side was mainly due to three of the ten patients who showed a substantial change (up to 54% reduction compared with the uninjured side). Of particular interest was a correlation between a reduction in nerve sliding and time until surgery. Since nine of the ten patients had surgery within 1 week of injury, a delay (of days) may result in excessive scar formation and subsequent impairment in nerve movement.

In vivo measurement of ulnar nerve movement in conditions such as cubital tunnel syndrome and that of the radial nerve in radial tunnel syndrome, for example, remains to be evaluated. In the patients we have examined, namely RSI and arm pain following whiplash injury, despite 'positive' results for the median nerve ULTT and / or digital pressure over the nerve trunk, these patients do not show significant changes in longitudinal nerve movement. Clearly, these patients have a painful response to neural mechanical stimulation and have therefore developed nerve mechanical sensitivity. This poses some important questions. First, why should elongating a nerve within its normal physiological range or applying digital pressure over the nerve trunk cause painful symptoms – that is, how has the nerve become mechanically sensitive? Secondly, how does this inform our understanding of the aetiology of these conditions and modify treatment and rehabilitation?

Inflammation of a Peripheral Nerve

Trauma, either repetitive or a defined insult, underlies the onset of symptoms in patients with RSI, arm pain following whiplash and CRPS1. It is interesting to speculate that, although there is no indication of frank nerve injury, a more minor neural injury such as inflammation may be a cause of ongoing symptoms.

Despite differences in the mechanism of trauma, symptoms appear similar in these patients. Patients complain of spontaneous pain, pain with limb movements, deep muscle aches, paraesthesia, hyperalgesia, allodynia and difficulties with the coordination of fine movement. Importantly, all of the patients that we have examined have clear signs of nerve mechanical sensitivity (i.e. painful responses to nerve movement tests and to digital pressure over affected nerve trunks). The lack of sufficient evidence for restricted, or altered, longitudinal nerve movement in patients, coupled with the inherent biomechanical compliance of the upper limb peripheral nerves, suggests that strain increases into the pathological range are not an obvious cause of these symptoms. The lack of frank nerve injury on clinical testing also suggests that significant axonal degeneration and demyelination are an unlikely cause of symptoms for many patients. Therefore, what are the mechanisms that lead to pain in these patients?

The physiological mechanisms underlying symptoms in patients with chronic upper limb pain, including those with RSI, arm pain following whiplash and also CRPS1, are undoubtedly complex and will involve central neuropathic changes. Neuropathic symptoms that include clinical signs of nerve mechanical sensitivity suggest a mechanism of symptom production that extends beyond the central nervous system to the periphery. A peripheral mechanism is further supported by evidence of changes to Aβ-, Aδ- and C-fibre sensory and autonomic function in the peripheral nerves of patients with RSI and whiplash injury (Greening & Lynn 1998; Greening et al 2003; Chien et al 2008). Examination of sera from these patient groups reveals raised levels of inflammatory mediators, which is indicative of an inflammatory component (Kivioja et al 2001; Huygen et al 2002; Carp et al 2007; Uceyler et al 2007a; Gerdle et al 2008). Mediators that are up-regulated in RSI, CRPS1 and arm pain following whiplash include cytokines such as tumour necrosis factor (TNF)-α, interleukin (IL)-1β and IL-6. Cytokines are a group of signalling molecules secreted by immune cells that help regulate the inflammatory response. Cytokine levels frequently correlate with patient symptoms (Maihofner et al 2005; Carp et al 2007), indicating a role for inflammation in the pathophysiology of these chronic pain conditions. Physiological studies performed in animals have shown that inflammation can affect peripheral nerve function (see below). Together with reports of raised levels of immune mediators, these findings indicate a major role for inflammation in chronic pain.

Causes of inflammation

Inflammation of a peripheral nerve is triggered by a direct insult to the nerve itself, by infection or by local inflammation of adjacent tissues. In the last situation, the nerve is an innocent bystander, where the diffusion of inflammatory mediators released at a neighbouring injury site will cause disruption to, or cross, the blood–nerve barrier to reach the endoneurium. Examples of pathologies where peripheral nerves are vulnerable to indirect insult include muscle injury, disc herniation and tumours growing close to nerve trunks. It is important to remember that many patients with chronic upper limb pain do not clinically show signs of frank nerve injury. Therefore, the trauma associated with such conditions will be subtle, sufficient to cause inflammation but without significant axonal degeneration and demyelination. In whiplash injury, for example, nerve roots and spinal nerves may be subjected to a direct traction injury as well as to the effects of inflammatory mediators from adjacent injured structures. In CRPS1, which usually occurs as a complication following injury or surgery (Janig & Baron 2003), peripheral nerves may also be subjected to the effects of inflammatory mediators from adjacent injured tissues.

In RSI, the prolonged repetitive motion of the forearm muscles is considered sufficient to induce inflammation of the median nerve. Evidence for this mechanism has been provided by an animal model of the condition (Clark et al 2003). In this model, animals were trained to perform a high- or low-repetition, negligible force task over a period of up to 12 weeks. This task involved repeated reaching and grasping of food pellets. Both high- (8 reaches / min) and also low-repetition (3 reaches / min) tasks were sufficient to cause inflammation of the median nerve and the forearm tendons and muscles (Barbe et al 2003; Clark et al 2003; Elliott et al 2008). Inflammation occurred from 4 weeks on as macrophages that are activated by the immune response invaded the peripheral tissues. Cytokines (IL-1α, IL-1β, IL-6, IL-10 and TNF-α) were also expressed within the endoneurium by resident cells (Al-Shatti et al 2005).

Inflammation and the microenvironment of the nerve

Subtle changes in the endoneurial microenvironment underlie the development of neuropathic symptoms (Sommer et al 1993). The endothelial wall of the endoneurial capillaries and the perineurium comprise the blood–nerve barrier. The role of this barrier is to maintain the microenvironment of the endoneurium. It helps regulate the entry of molecules into the endoneurium and maintains the ionic milieu that is essential for normal axonal conduction. Although not as effective as the blood–brain barrier, circulating cells and proteins cannot easily cross the blood–nerve barrier (Olsson 1990). Activated T-lymphocytes are, however, an exception and these cells circulate freely between the capillaries and the endoneurium (Watkins & Maier 2002). Many of the resident cells within the endoneurium function as immune cells and, when activated, can secrete inflammatory mediators. These cells include fibroblasts, Schwann cells, macrophages, dendritic cells and mast cells (Watkins & Maier 2002; Moalem & Tracey 2006). Immediately following nerve trauma, the calcium-activated protease calpain causes the release of early proinflammatory cytokines such as TNF-α and IL-1β (Uceyler et al 2007b). These cytokines are secreted within the endoneurium by resident immune cells. The release of cytokines (e.g. TNF-α) and growth factors (e.g. vascular endothelial growth factor) triggers the breakdown of the blood–nerve barrier (Creange et al 1997) to allow immune cells and proteins that could not previously cross this barrier to enter the endoneurium. Chemokines such as chemokine (C-C motif) ligand 2 (CCL2) attract neutrophils and macrophages to the inflammatory site (Toews et al 1998), further enhancing the inflammatory response.

Animal models of nerve inflammation

A number of animal models have been developed that result in sensory behavioural changes similar to those observed in patients. These models include the chronic constriction injury model (CCI) (Bennett & Xie 1988), the spinal nerve ligation model (SNL) (Kim & Chung 1992) and the neuritis model (Bennett 1999). Laboratory studies using these models have shown that inflammation can alter the physiological properties of sensory axons. Many of these studies have focused on the development of ongoing activity (i.e. spontaneous firing of axons) and axonal mechanical sensitivity (i.e. responses of axons to direct mechanical stimulation), both of which are likely to contribute to a peripheral mechanism leading to production of painful symptoms. In particular, the development of axonal mechanical sensitivity provides a mechanism for pain in response to nerve movement tests and direct palpation of peripheral nerve trunks.

Both the CCI and the SNL model produce marked mechanical allodynia and thermal hyperalgesia (Bennett & Xie 1988; Kim & Chung 1992) as well as ongoing activity (Kajander & Bennett 1992; Tal & Eliav 1996; Chen & Devor 1998; Wu et al 2001, 2002; Djouhri et al 2006) and axonal mechanical sensitivity (Chen & Devor 1998; Dilley & Bove 2008b). In the SNL model, intact axons within the sciatic nerve co-mingle with injured axons that are undergoing the processes of Wallerian degeneration. Wallerian degeneration is the degeneration of injured axons and involves the recruitment of macrophages for the removal of axonal debris. The presence of activated macrophages implies the release of inflammatory mediators, which would induce a form of intraneural neuritis. A major finding in the SNL model is that uninjured C-fibre axons develop ongoing activity and respond to direct mechanical stimulation (Wu et al 2001; Dilley & Bove 2008b). However, both the CCI model and the SNL model cause significant neuropathy owing to extensive Wallerian degeneration and therefore do not reflect the subtle injury that is possibly associated with RSI, arm pain following whiplash injury or CRPS1.

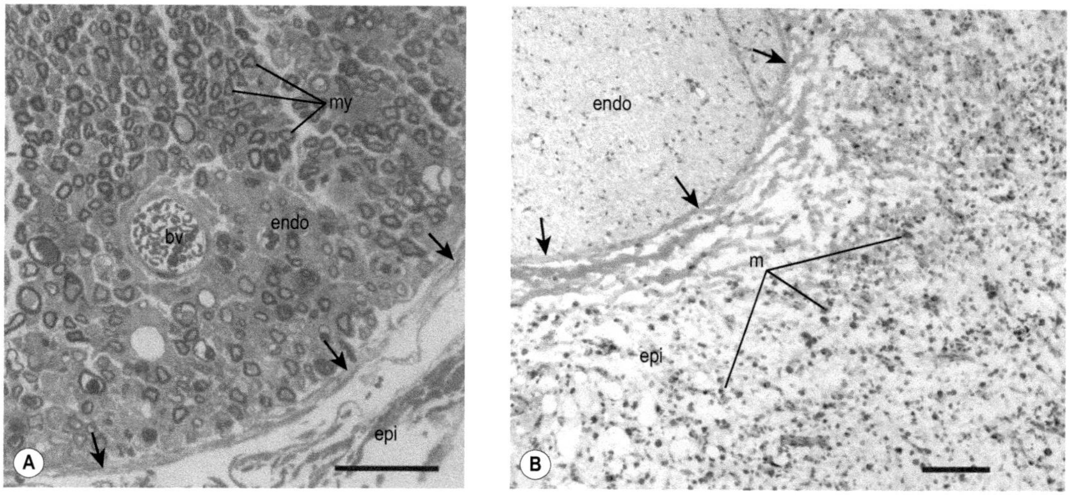

Figure 64.6 Microscopic appearance of the neuritis site: (**A**) Toluidine-blue-stained transverse section through the neuritis showing the relatively normal appearance of the myelinated axons (examples labelled 'my') with very few abnormal axons. Note the oedematous, less-consolidated appearance of the perineurium (arrows). (**B**) Haematoxylin-and-eosin-stained transverse section immunoreacted against activated macrophages (ED1+) at the neuritis. There are considerable numbers of macrophages in the epineurium (dark stain; examples labelled with 'm') with only minimal numbers in the endoneurium. Note the oedematous, less-consolidated appearance of the perineurium (arrows). endo=endoneurium; arrows=perineurium; epi=epineurium; bv=blood vessel. Scale bar in (**A**)=50 μm and in (**B**)=100 μm.

Neuritis model

The neuritis model is an animal model of localized peripheral nerve inflammation that more closely resembles the clinical presentation in many patients with chronic upper limb pain. It produces a minor nerve injury with inflammation in the absence of gross neuropathology – that is, degeneration or demyelination (Eliav et al 1999; Chacur et al 2001; Bove et al 2003; Dilley et al 2005) (Fig. 64.6A). In this model, an immunostimulant (either complete Freund's adjuvant (killed bacterial cell wall) or zymosan (killed yeast cell wall)) is applied locally around the sciatic nerve or nerve of interest. Over a period of days, a robust local inflammatory response occurs that is confined mainly to the epineurium (Bove et al 2009) (Fig. 64.6B). Within hours, activated macrophages, neutrophils and T-lymphocytes begin to congregate outside of the perineurium, their numbers eventually peaking at 4 weeks (Eliav et al 1999; Gazda et al 2001; Bove et al 2003, 2009). Surprisingly, the immune cells do not penetrate the perineurium to enter the endoneurium (Bove et al 2009), which is likely to reflect the diffusion properties of the perineurium. In contrast, very small numbers of T-lymphocytes have been reported within the endoneurium that have probably entered from the endoneurial vessels (Eliav et al 1999). Within the first week, the perineurium becomes oedematous, but by 4 weeks it has thickened to become consolidated (Bove et al 2009). The early oedematous, less-consolidated appearance of the perineurium provides a short window that allows inflammatory factors to diffuse across the barrier into the endoneurium. Following induction of the neuritis, animals develop cutaneous hypersensitivity with signs of mechanical allodynia (Eliav et al 1999; Chacur et al 2001; Bove et al 2003), as well as heat and mechanical hyperalgesia and cold allodynia (Eliav et al 1999). Interestingly, in the zymosan-induced model, mechanical allodynia was reported to be bilateral, which infers that a central mechanism is initiated by the localized peripheral nerve inflammation (Gazda et al 2001). Therefore, it is possible that a single inflammatory site may cause contralateral symptoms in patients.

These studies of locally induced inflammation in the absence of axonal degeneration result in significant neuropathic signs that are consistent with neuropathic pain in patients. However, the mechanisms underlying these sensory changes are unclear. Much of the current work on the neuritis model has focused on the physiological effects of inflammation on peripheral axons. These studies have shown that inflammation causes the development of ongoing activity in both unmyelinated (C-) and myelinated (A-) axons (Eliav et al 2001; Bove et al 2003, Dilley et al 2005). Most of the myelinated axons that develop ongoing activity are the Aδ-fibres (Eliav et al 2009), which, like C-fibre axons, are largely nociceptive. The observation of ongoing activity in nociceptors corresponds to the painful sensations described by patients, especially the symptoms of apparent unevoked spontaneous pain. Such increases in ongoing activity may also contribute to centrally driven neuropathic symptoms. Although central sensitization is considered to play a significant role in the development of neuropathic symptoms (Campbell et al 1988; Campbell & Meyer 2006), central sensitization is dependent upon the continued firing of peripheral axons into the central nervous system (LaMotte et al 1991; Gracely et al 1992). It has been shown that central neuropathic changes can be reversed by blocking the firing of axons from an irritated peripheral nerve (Gracely et al 1992).

The neuritis model was the first to show that inflammation causes otherwise normally conducting C- and A-fibre axons to develop mechanical sensitivity that is localized to the site of inflammation (Eliav et al 2001; Bove et al 2003; Dilley et al 2005; Dilley & Bove 2008b). Axonal mechanical sensitivity was tested both with direct pressure and by applying short stretches to the inflamed nerve (Fig. 64.7). Less than 5% stretch is sufficient to cause firing of axons in inflamed nerves (Dilley et al 2005), with the most sensitive axons responding to less than 3% stretch. Importantly, these stretch values are

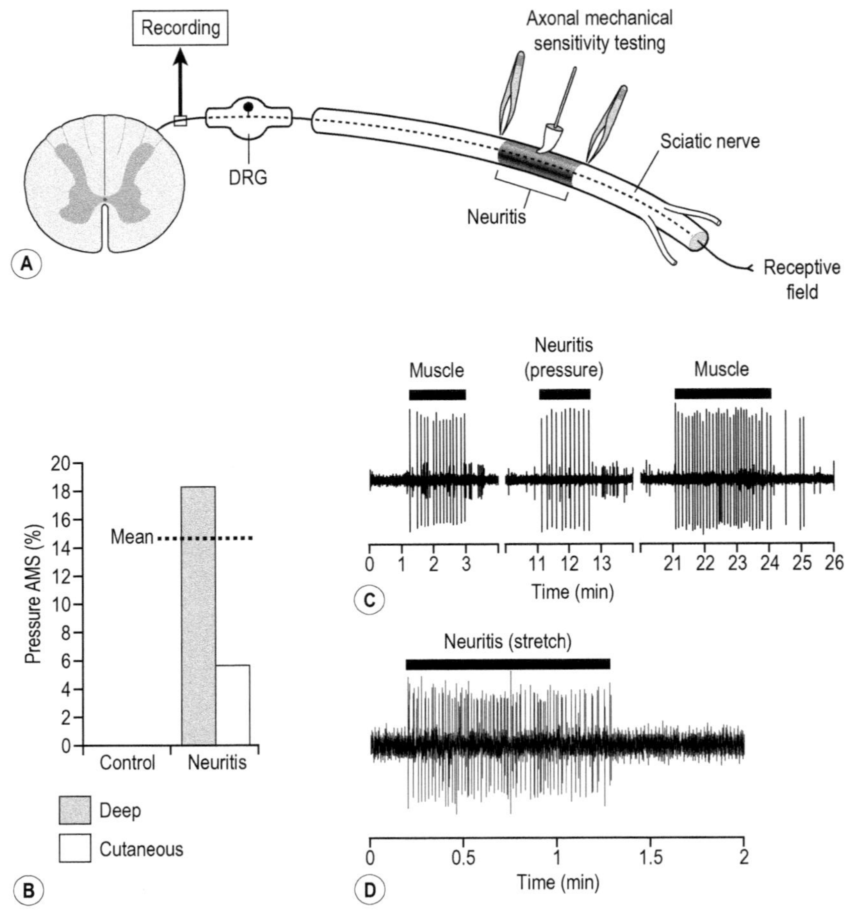

Figure 64.7 Electrophysiological recordings of axonal mechanical sensitivity in C-fibre axons: (**A**) Diagram of the experimental set-up. The sciatic nerve trunk is locally inflamed (neuritis) mid-thigh. Recordings are made from isolated C-fibre axons within the L5 dorsal root (recording) that pass through the neuritis. The nerve is mechanically stimulated at the neuritis either by direct pressure using a silicone-tipped probe or by stretching with fine forceps. Note the relationship of the L5 dorsal root to the dorsal root ganglion (DRG) and also the spinal cord. (**B**) The percentage of deep and cutaneous C-fibre axons that responded to pressure at the neuritis at 1 week. The average number of C-fibre axons that responded to pressure was 14.5% (9 of 62 axons) following neuritis (denoted by heavy horizontal line) compared with 0% (0 of 36 axons) in untreated animals. The majority of axons that developed axonal mechanical sensitivity innervated deep (8 of 44 axons) rather than cutaneous (1 of 18 axons) structures. (**C**) Typical response to pressure at the neuritis from an axon innervating the gastrocnemius muscle. Short horizontal lines above the responses represent the duration of the mechanical stimuli. The gastrocnemius muscle was mechanically stimulated initially to show that the axon had a functioning peripheral field (denoted by 'Muscle'). This was followed by mechanical stimulation of the nerve at the test site (denoted by 'Neuritis'). Mechanical responses from the periphery after stimulating the nerve demonstrated that the mechanical stimulus did not adversely affect the conduction of the axon. (**D**) Typical response to stretch across the neuritis site. The short horizontal line above the response represents the duration of the stretch. (B and C from Dilley & Bove 2008b; D from Dilley et al 2005, with permission.)

consistent with those obtained from human studies of median nerve stretch when the arm is fully extended in a position similar to the median nerve movement ULTT (Dilley et al 2003). This finding also suggests that, in patients, pathological increases in nerve strain are not a prerequisite for symptoms and that, in the presence of nerve mechanical sensitivity, arm pain may be experienced during normal physiological limb movements.

Normally, it is only the terminals of peripheral nerves that respond to mechanical stimulation by transduction through mechanically sensitive ion channels. It is important to state that mechanical sensitivity and ongoing activity originating part way along an axon do not occur in the absence of inflammation. It should be noted that these observations of axonal mechanical sensitivity contrast with the original findings reported in the CCI model, in which it was the tips of degenerated axons that became mechanically sensitive (Tal & Eliav 1996; Chen & Devor 1998). The neuritis model instead provides an inflammatory environment in the absence of axonal degeneration that is likely to be comparable to that in patients.

It is reported that C- and Aδ-fibre axons are more susceptible to the development of axonal mechanical sensitivity (Bove et al 2003). The increased susceptibility of these axons to the effects of inflammation is consistent with the nociceptive properties of these nerve fibres and also the symptoms of pain described by patients. Interestingly, mechanically sensitive axons mainly innervate deep structures such as muscles and joints (Bove et al 2003; Dilley & Bove 2008b) (see Fig. 64.7B). These findings fit well with the 'deep ache' described by patients and which is frequently complained of when nerve movement tests are applied. Localized peripheral nerve inflammation may also contribute to sympathetic changes in patients with CRPS1. In the neuritis model, the rate of ongoing activity in postganglionic sympathetic axons passing through the inflammatory site is reduced (Bove 2009).

In the neuritis model, axonal mechanical sensitivity is a relatively short-lived phenomenon and peaks within 1 week of developing neuritis (Dilley & Bove 2008b). By 2 months the axonal mechanical sensitivity has resolved. Despite the resolution of abnormal sensory responses, macrophages and T-lymphocytes still persist in the epineurium at 2 months (Bove et al 2009). It is likely that consolidation of the perineurium soon after the peak of the axonal mechanical sensitivity prevents inflammatory components released by these cells from entering the endoneurium.

It is evident from these laboratory studies that localized inflammation can be detrimental to axonal physiology. It has already been suggested that inflammation-induced increases in axonal excitability appear to drive central mechanisms, leading to central sensitization. Localized neuritis also triggers physiological changes to peripheral neurons that extend beyond the site of inflammation. Following neuritis, phenotypic changes (i.e. the expression of new proteins) occur in the cell bodies of sensory neurons (Dilley et al 2005). It is not yet clear what these changes represent. It is possible that they correspond to the up-regulation of ion channels that contribute to the ongoing activity and axonal mechanical sensitivity. Accordingly, in other models of nerve injury, there are reports of the up-regulation of sodium channels and mechanically sensitive channels that contribute towards painful symptoms (Black et al 2004; Pertin et al 2005; Duan et al 2007). Following neuritis, physiological changes also occur along the length of the axon. A reduction in the conduction velocity of C-fibre axons proximal to the neuritis has been reported that actually recovers at a similar time to the axonal mechanical sensitivity (Dilley & Bove 2008b). Local neuritis has also been shown to reduce the number of functioning peripheral nerve terminals (Dilley et al 2005). This is consistent with findings in patients with RSI, where peripheral nerve function is altered (Greening & Lynn 1998; Greening et al 2003).

Physiological Role of Inflammatory Mediators

It is apparent that local nerve inflammation can alter the properties of peripheral sensory axons, inducing ongoing activity and axonal mechanical sensitivity, both of which may contribute to painful symptoms in patients. However, it is important to understand which inflammatory components are responsible for these physiological changes and the neuronal mechanisms that lead to such changes.

The lack of large numbers of activated macrophages, T-cells and neutrophils within the endoneurium following neuritis suggests that the physiological effects are probably due to diffusible inflammatory mediators produced during the inflammatory response. In the neuritis model, raised levels of cytokines IL-1, IL-6 and TNF-α are reported at the inflammatory site within hours of induction (Gazda et al 2001; Eliav et al 2009). These cytokines are secreted by inflammatory cells that congregate outside of the perineurium and by resident cells (e.g. Schwann cells and fibroblasts). As well as orchestrating the immune response, cytokines also play an important physiological role. Nerve growth factor (NGF), which is better known for its role supporting the development of peripheral neurons, is also up-regulated during inflammation (McMahon et al 2005) and has a similar physiological role to that of cytokines. The administration of small doses of cytokines IL-1β, IL-6 and TNF-α causes hyperalgesia and allodynia in animals (Cunha et al 1992; Sorkin & Doom 2000; Schafers et al 2003a, 2003b; Zelenka et al 2005; Eliav et al 2009).

The acute perineural exposure of TNF-α to the sciatic nerve also increases ongoing activity in C-fibre axons (Sorkin et al 1997; Leem & Bove 2002). IL-1β is similarly reported to induce ongoing activity in myelinated axons following direct exposure (Ozaktay et al 2006), and both IL-1β and IL-6 sensitize heat-activated (Obreja et al 2002, 2005) and sodium channels (Liu et al 2006). The cytokines IL-1β and IL-6 have both been implicated in the development of axonal mechanical sensitivity and ongoing activity (Eliav et al 2009). The administration of NGF causes hyperalgesia in animals (Lewin et al 1993). It also induces ongoing activity (Kitamura et al 2005) and sensitizes peripheral terminals (Rueff & Mendell 1996) following its direct exposure to sensory neurons. From this data it can be seen that elevated levels of cytokines and NGF close to a peripheral nerve can lead to changes in the physiological function of sensory axons that may contribute towards painful symptoms in patients.

Chemokines are a group of inflammatory mediators with similar properties to cytokines. Along with cytokines, chemokines are also able to interact with both the immune and nervous systems. Of particular interest is the chemokine CCL2, which is up-regulated following nerve injury (White et al 2005). Administration of CCL2 rapidly induces mechanical allodynia in animals (Tanaka et al 2004). Its acute exposure also directly excites neurons (Oh et al 2001; Sun et al 2006) and sensitizes the transient receptor potential vanilloid 1 channel (TRPV1) (Jung et al 2008). TRPV1 is a channel that is widely expressed on nociceptive axons and is sensitive to capsaicin and mechanical stimulation. It is thought to play a significant role in the development of neuropathic pain.

The mechanisms by which these inflammatory mediators interact with peripheral neurons are unclear. Following nerve injury, cytokine and chemokine receptors located on sensory neurons are up-regulated (Schafers et al 2003a; Bhangoo et al 2007). Therefore, cytokines and chemokines may interact with their receptors on neurons to alter axonal function. Cytokines, chemokines and NGF also act to change the sensitivity and expression of ion channels that are associated with an increase in axonal excitability (e.g. TRPV1 and sodium channels) (Tanaka et al 1998; Gould et al 2000; Zhang et al 2005; Zhu & Oxford 2007; Jung et al 2008).

Disruption of axoplasmic transport

Mechanically sensitive ion channels at the peripheral terminals of axons are constantly being replaced by newly synthesized ion channels. New ion channel components are synthesized within cell bodies in the dorsal root ganglia and transported to the terminals by fast axoplasmic transport (Koschorke et al 1994). Inflammatory mediators can disrupt axoplasmic transport (Amano et al 2001; Armstrong et al 2004). This is consistent with the disruption of axoplasmic transport without Wallerian degeneration of axons following acute nerve trunk compression (Kitao et al 1997). It has been shown that the disruption of axoplasmic transport in the sciatic nerve can cause axonal mechanical sensitivity to develop at the site of disruption (Dilley & Bove 2008a). It is therefore hypothesized that, in patients, local nerve inflammation may disrupt axoplasmic transport in sensory axons to cause the accumulation and insertion of mechanosensitive ion channel components at the inflamed site (Dilley & Bove 2008a) (Fig. 64.8). The lack of functioning peripheral terminals in some conducting axons might have also resulted from a disruption of axonal transport at the neuritis (Dilley et al 2005). Therefore, axoplasmic transport disruption may have widespread effects on the health of the neuron. Changes to axoplasmic transport develop over days and therefore represent a chronic pathway that can lead to altered axonal physiology. This chronic mechanism contrasts with the acute effects of

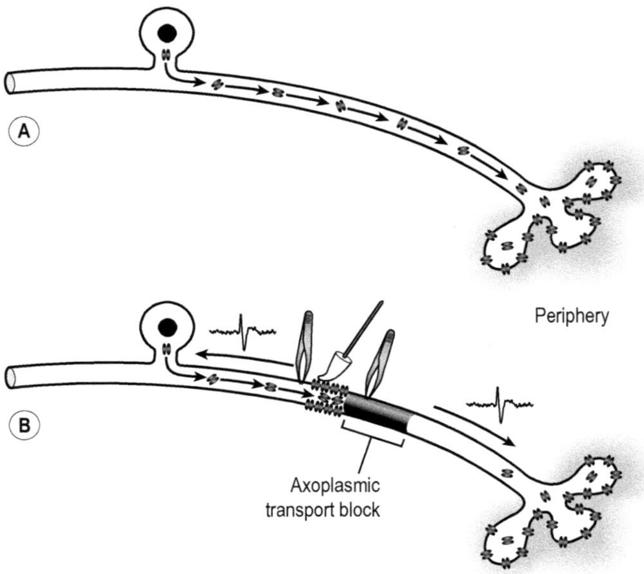

Figure 64.8 Inflammation-induced disruption of axoplasmic transport as a mechanism for the development of axonal mechanical sensitivity: (**A**) The components required for mechanical sensitivity are transported from the cell body of a sensory axon to the periphery for insertion at the terminal. (**B**) Inflammation-induced disruption of axoplasmic transport leads to the accumulation and insertion of mechanosensitive components proximal to the site of axoplasmic blockade. Mechanical stimulation of the axon membrane at the inflamed site (by pressure or stretch) will result in the generation of action potentials (denoted by arrows).

inflammatory mediators on peripheral sensory axons. Therefore, in patients, the peripheral mechanisms are likely to involve multiple pathways that ultimately contribute to painful symptoms.

Nervi Nervorum

The nervi nervorum also provides a potential mechanism that may account for nerve mechanical sensitivity, as axons of the nervi nervorum respond to mechanical stimulation of the nerve trunk (Bove & Light 1995). However, innervation of the nerve sheath by the nervi nervorum is sparse and mechanical stimulation of the sciatic nerve in untreated (control) animals has failed to find these axons (Eliav et al 2001; Bove et al 2003; Dilley et al 2005; Dilley & Bove 2008a). Sensitization of the nervi nervorum is therefore unlikely to be a major contributor to symptom production.

Imaging Nerve Inflammation

Magnetic resonance imaging (MRI) has been used as an indicator of inflammation in peripheral nerves (Filler et al 1993, 1996, 2004; Koltzenburg & Bendszus 2004). As part of the inflammatory process, the water content in neural tissues increases, which causes the nerve to appear hyperintense on T2-weighted MRI (Filler et al 1996; Koltzenburg & Bendszus 2004). For example, in CTS, the median nerve appears abnormally bright at the carpal tunnel on T2-weighted MRI – a change that suggests local nerve inflammation in this region (Cudlip et al 2002). We have demonstrated an increase in median and ulnar nerve signal intensity at the carpal tunnel and distal forearm in two patients with RSI, and also ulnar nerve signal intensity at the cubital tunnel in a patient with CRPS1 (Fig. 64.9). Prior to imaging, all three patients had painful responses to nerve movement tests, as well as palpation over the nerve trunks, at the hyperintense sites. These findings fit well with the theory of inflammation-induced nerve mechanical sensitivity and an underlying peripheral mechanism for the painful symptoms experienced by these patients.

Conclusion

Peripheral nerves are extremely well adapted to cope with limb movements within the physiological range. The only evidence that we have of altered longitudinal nerve sliding is in a small proportion of patients after median nerve repair. Patients with RSI, whiplash injury and CRPS1 have raised levels of inflammatory mediators, which indicates a role for inflammation. There is also some clinical evidence from MRI of peripheral nerve inflammation in RSI and CRPS1. In these patient groups and perhaps others, such as non-specific back pain and fibromyalgia, axons may become mechanically sensitive following exposure to inflammatory mediators. Animal studies using a model of localized nerve inflammation clearly demonstrate nerve mechanical sensitivity. This would suggest a peripheral neuropathic mechanism contributing to painful symptoms and a painful response to nerve movement tests.

Tests that demonstrate nerve mechanical sensitivity clinically (i.e. nerve movement tests and digital palpation) provide the clinician with the rationale to focus treatment, at an early date, towards alleviating a neuropathic condition. Treatment strategies should include drugs that can reduce the excitability of neurons (e.g. pregabalin, amitriptyline, carbamazepine and lidocaine). Symptom production is likely to involve complex mechanisms, which means that simple analgesics and non-steroidal anti-inflammatory drugs may not be effective. Future treatments may include inflammatory mediator receptor antagonists and neutralizing antibodies to reduce the effects of the inflammatory response. It is important that normal pain-free movement patterns are re-established in these chronic pain patients. There are many physical and cognitive treatment strategies available that may be helpful in achieving this. However, techniques that are applied to 'mobilize' the peripheral nervous system are not effective in CTS (O'Connor et al 2009) and are therefore unlikely to be of any benefit in these chronic pain patients. Nerve mobilization exercises may, in fact, be detrimental if they result in further noxious input. Sliding techniques that claim not to increase nerve strain have been suggested to reduce intraneural oedema and even affect nerve physiology (Coppieters & Butler 2008). However, to date, there is no scientific evidence that sliding techniques improve the axonal microenvironment or alter axonal physiology, or that these techniques improve outcomes for patients over and above other treatment strategies.

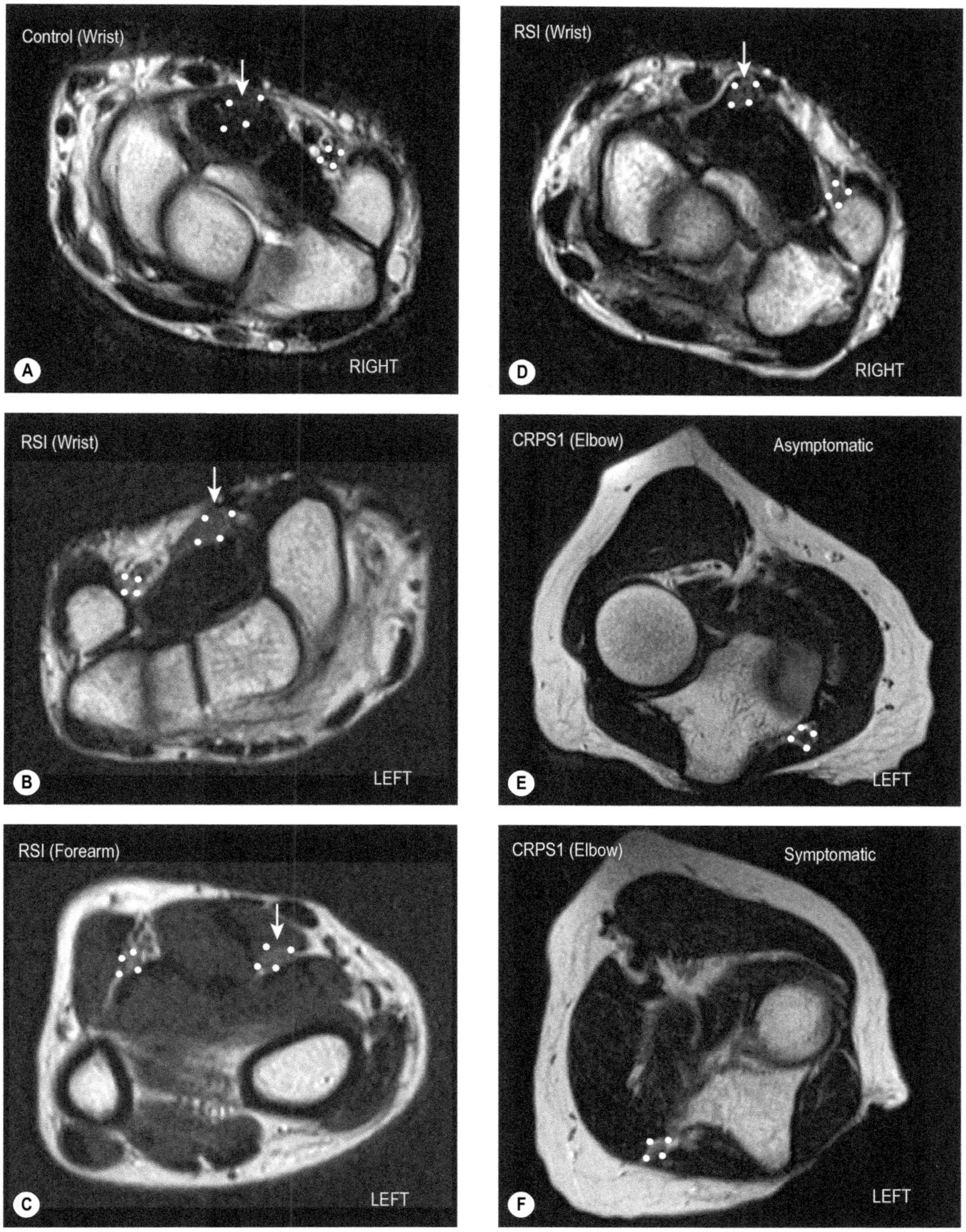

Figure 64.9 MRI scans of the wrist and elbow in patients with diffuse RSI and CRPS1. (**A**) to (**D**) T2-weighted images of the median and ulnar nerve: (**A**) at the carpal tunnel in a control subject, (**B**) at the carpal tunnel and (**C**) distal forearm on the symptomatic side in a patient with diffuse RSI, and (**D**) at the carpal tunnel on the symptomatic side of a second patient with diffuse RSI. Note the bright appearance of both the median and ulnar nerves in the patient images, which indicates inflammation. (**E**) to (**F**) T2-weighted images of the ulnar nerve on the (**E**) asymptomatic and (**F**) symptomatic side in a patient with CRPS1. Note the bright appearance of the ulnar nerve on the symptomatic side compared with the asymptomatic side. White dots represent the median and ulnar nerve boundaries. Arrows indicate the median nerve.

References

Al-Shatti T, Barr AE, Safadi FF, et al. 2005. Increase in inflammatory cytokines in median nerves in a rat model of repetitive motion injury. J Neuroimmunol 167(1–2): 13–22.

Allmann KH, Horch R, Uhl M, et al. 1997. MR imaging of the carpal tunnel. Eur J Radiol 25(2): 141–145.

Alpar EK, Onuoha G, Killampalli VV, et al. 2002. Management of chronic pain in whiplash injury. J Bone Joint Surg 84(6): 807–811.

Amano R, Hiruma H, Nishida S, et al. 2001. Inhibitory effect of histamine on axonal transport in cultured mouse dorsal root ganglion neurons. Neurosci Res 41(2): 201–206.

Armstrong BD, Hu Z, Abad C, et al. 2004. Induction of neuropeptide gene expression and blockade of retrograde transport in facial motor neurons following local peripheral nerve inflammation in severe combined immunodeficiency and BALB/C mice. Neuroscience 129(1): 93–99.

Barbe MF, Barr AE, Gorzelany I, et al. 2003. Chronic repetitive reaching and grasping results in decreased motor performance and widespread tissue responses in a rat model of MSD. J Orthop Res 21(1): 167–176.

Bennett GJ. 1999. Does a neuroimmune interaction contribute to the genesis of painful peripheral neuropathies? Proc Natl Acad Sci USA 96(14): 7737–7738.

Bennett GJ, Xie YK. 1988. A peripheral mononeuropathy in rat that produces disorders of pain sensation like those seen in man. Pain 33(1): 87–107.

Bhangoo S, Ren D, Miller RJ, et al. 2007. Delayed functional expression of neuronal chemokine receptors following focal nerve demyelination in the rat: a mechanism for the development of chronic sensitization of peripheral nociceptors. Mol Pain 3: 38.

Black JA, Liu S, Tanaka M, et al. 2004. Changes in the expression of tetrodotoxin-sensitive sodium channels within dorsal root ganglia neurons in inflammatory pain. Pain 108(3): 237–247.

Bove GM. 2009. Focal nerve inflammation induces neuronal signs consistent with symptoms of early complex regional pain syndromes. Exp Neurol 219(1): 223–227.

Bove GM, Light AR. 1995. Unmyelinated nociceptors of rat paraspinal tissues. J Neurophysiol 73(5): 1752–1762.

Bove GM, Ransil BJ, Lin HC, et al. 2003. Inflammation induces ectopic mechanical sensitivity in axons of nociceptors innervating deep tissues. J Neurophysiol 90(3): 1949–1955.

Bove GM, Weissner W, Barbe MF. 2009. Long lasting recruitment of immune cells and altered epi-perineurial thickness in focal nerve inflammation induced by complete Freund's adjuvant. J Neuroimmunol 213(1–2): 26–30.

Byng J. 1997. Overuse syndromes of the upper limb and the upper limb tension test: a comparison between patients, asymptomatic keyboard workers and asymptomatic non-keyboard workers. Man Ther 2(3): 157–164.

Campbell JN, Meyer RA. 2006. Mechanisms of neuropathic pain. Neuron 52(1): 77–92.

Campbell JN, Raja SN, Meyer RA, et al. 1988. Myelinated afferents signal the hyperalgesia associated with nerve injury. Pain 32: 89–94.

Carp SJ, Barbe MF, Winter KA, et al. 2007. Inflammatory biomarkers increase with severity of upper-extremity overuse disorders. Clin Sci 112(5): 305–314.

Chacur M, Milligan ED, Gazda LS, et al. 2001. A new model of sciatic inflammatory neuritis (SIN): induction of unilateral and bilateral mechanical allodynia following acute unilateral peri-sciatic immune activation in rats. Pain 94(3): 231–244.

Chen Y, Devor M. 1998. Ectopic mechanosensitivity in injured sensory axons arises from the site of spontaneous electrogenesis. Eur J Pain 2(2): 165–178.

Chien A, Eliav E, Sterling M. 2008. Whiplash (grade II) and cervical radiculopathy share a similar sensory presentation: an investigation using quantitative sensory testing. Clin J Pain 24(7): 595–603.

Clark BD, Barr AE, Safadi FF, et al. 2003. Median nerve trauma in a rat model of work-related musculoskeletal disorder. J Neurotrauma 20(7): 681–695.

Coppieters MW, Butler DS. 2008. Do 'sliders' slide and 'tensioners' tension? An analysis of neurodynamic techniques and considerations regarding their application. Man Ther 13(3): 213–221.

Creange A, Barlovatz-Meimon G, Gherardi RK. 1997. Cytokines and peripheral nerve disorders. Eur Cytokine Netw 8(2), 145–151.

Cudlip SA, Howe FA, Griffiths JR, et al. 2002. Magnetic resonance neurography of peripheral nerve following experimental crush injury, and correlation with functional deficit. J Neurosurg 96(4): 755–759.

Cunha FQ, Poole S, Lorenzetti BB, et al. 1992. The pivotal role of tumour necrosis factor alpha in the development of inflammatory hyperalgesia. Br J Pharmacol 107(3): 660–664.

Dilley A, Bove GM. 2008a. Disruption of axoplasmic transport induces mechanical sensitivity in intact rat C-fibre nociceptor axons. J Physiol 586(2): 593–604.

Dilley A, Bove GM. 2008b. Resolution of inflammation-induced axonal mechanical sensitivity and conduction slowing in C-fiber nociceptors. J Pain 9(2): 185–192.

Dilley A, Greening J, Lynn B, et al. 2001. The use of cross-correlation analysis between high-frequency ultrasound images to measure longitudinal median nerve movement. Ultrasound Med Biol 27(9): 1211–1218.

Dilley A, Lynn B, Greening J, et al. 2003. Quantitative in vivo studies of median nerve sliding in response to wrist, elbow, shoulder and neck movements. Clin Biomech 18(10): 899–907.

Dilley A, Lynn B, Pang SJ. 2005. Pressure and stretch mechanosensitivity of peripheral nerve fibres following local inflammation of the nerve trunk. Pain 117(3): 462–472.

Dilley A, Summerhayes C, Lynn B. 2007. An in vivo investigation of ulnar nerve sliding during upper limb movements. Clin Biomech 22(7): 774–779.

Dilley A, Odeyinde S, Greening J, et al. 2008. Longitudinal sliding of the median nerve in patients with non-specific arm pain. Man Ther 13(6): 536–543.

Djouhri L, Koutsikou S, Fang X, et al. 2006. Spontaneous pain, both neuropathic and inflammatory, is related to frequency of spontaneous firing in intact C-fiber nociceptors. J Neurosci 26(4): 1281–1292.

Duan B, Wu LJ, Yu YQ, et al. 2007. Upregulation of acid-sensing ion channel ASIC1a in spinal dorsal horn neurons contributes to inflammatory pain hypersensitivity. J Neurosci 27(41): 11139–11148.

Eliav E, Herzberg U, Ruda MA, et al. 1999. Neuropathic pain from an experimental neuritis of the rat sciatic nerve. Pain 83(2): 169–182.

Eliav E, Benoliel R, Tal M. 2001. Inflammation with no axonal damage of the rat saphenous nerve trunk induces ectopic discharge and mechanosensitivity in myelinated axons. Neurosci Lett 311(1): 49–52.

Eliav E, Benoliel R, Herzberg U, et al. 2009. The role of IL-6 and IL-1beta in painful perineural inflammatory neuritis. Brain Behav Immun 23(4): 474–484.

Elliott MB, Barr AE, Kietrys DM, et al. 2008. Peripheral neuritis and increased spinal cord neurochemicals are induced in a model of repetitive motion injury with low force and repetition exposure. Brain Res 1218(2): 103–113.

Erel E, Dilley A, Greening J, et al. 2003. Longitudinal sliding of the median nerve in patients with carpal tunnel syndrome. J Hand Surg 28(5): 439–443.

Erel E, Dilley A, Turner S, et al. 2009. Sonographic measurements of longitudinal median nerve sliding in patients following nerve repair. Muscle Nerve 41(3): 350–354.

Filler AG, Howe FA, Hayes CE, et al. 1993. Magnetic resonance neurography. Lancet 341(8846): 659–661.

Filler AG, Kliot M, Howe FA, et al. 1996. Application of magnetic resonance neurography in the evaluation of patients with peripheral nerve pathology. J Neurosurg 85(2): 299–309.

Filler AG, Maravilla KR, Tsuruda JS. 2004. MR neurography and muscle MR imaging for image diagnosis of disorders affecting the peripheral nerves and musculature. Neurol Clin 22(3): 643–647.

Gamble HJ, Eames RA. 1964. An electron microscope study of the connective tissues of human peripheral nerve. J Anat 98 655–663.

Gazda LS, Milligan ED, Hansen MK, et al. 2001. Sciatic inflammatory neuritis (SIN): behavioral allodynia is paralleled by peri-sciatic proinflammatory cytokine and superoxide production. J Peripher Nerv Syst 6(3): 111–129.

Gerdle B, Lemming D, Kristiansen J, et al. 2008. Biochemical alterations in the trapezius muscle of patients with chronic whiplash associated disorders (WAD): a microdialysis study. Eur J Pain 12(1): 82–93.

Gould HJ III, Gould TN, England JD, et al. 2000. A possible role for nerve growth factor in the augmentation of sodium channels in models of chronic pain. Brain Res 854(1–2): 19–29.

Gracely RH, Lynch SA, Bennett GJ. 1992. Painful neuropathy: altered central processing maintained dynamically by peripheral input. Pain 51(2): 175–194.

Greening J, 2005. How inflammation and minor nerve injury contribute to pain in nerve root and peripheral neuropathies. In: Boyling J, Jull G (eds) Grieve's modern manual therapy. The vertebral column. London: Churchill Livingstone, pp 205–215.

Greening J, Lynn B. 1998. Vibration sense in the upper limb in patients with repetitive strain injury and a group of at-risk office workers. Int Arch Occup Environ Health 71(1): 29–34.

Greening J, Smart S, Leary R, et al. 1999. Reduced movement of median nerve in carpal tunnel during wrist flexion in patients with non-specific arm pain. Lancet 354(9174): 217–218.

Greening J, Lynn B, Leary R, et al. 2001. The use of ultrasound imaging to demonstrate reduced movement of the median nerve during wrist flexion in patients with non-specific arm pain. J Hand Surg 26(5): 401–406.

Greening J, Lynn B, Leary R. 2003. Sensory and autonomic function in the hands of patients with non-specific arm pain (NSAP) and asymptomatic office workers. Pain 104(1–2): 275–281.

Greening J, Dilley A, Lynn B. 2005. In vivo study of nerve movement and mechano-sensitivity of the median nerve in whiplash and non-specific arm pain patients. Pain 115(3): 248–253.

Grewel R, Jiangming X, Sotereanos DG, et al. 1996. Biomechanical properties of peripheral nerve. Hand Clin 12(2): 195–204.

Haninec P. 1986. Undulating course of nerve fibres and bands of Fontana in peripheral nerves of the rat. Anat Embryol (Berl) 174(3): 407–411.

Harrington JM, Carter JT, Birrell L, et al. 1998. Surveillance case definitions for work related upper limb pain syndromes. J Occup Environ Med 55(4): 264–271.

Hough AD, Moore AP, Jones MP. 2007. Reduced longitudinal excursion of the median nerve in carpal tunnel syndrome. Arch Phys Med Rehabil 88(5): 569–576.

Hromada J. 1963. On the nerve supply of the connective tissue of some peripheral nervous tissue system components. Acta Anat (Basel) 55: 343–351.

Huygen FJ, De Bruijn AG, De Bruin MT, et al. 2002. Evidence for local inflammation in complex regional pain syndrome type 1. Mediators Inflamm 11(1): 47–51.

Janig W, Baron R. 2003. Complex regional pain syndrome: mystery explained? Lancet Neurol 2(11): 687–697.

Julius A, Lees R, Dilley A, et al. 2004. Shoulder posture and median nerve sliding. BMC Musculoskelet Disord 5: 23.

Jung H, Toth PT, White FA, et al. 2008. Monocyte chemoattractant protein-1 functions as a neuromodulator in dorsal root ganglia neurons. J Neurochem 104(1): 254–263.

Kajander KC, Bennett GJ. 1992. Onset of a painful peripheral neuropathy in rat: a partial and differential deafferentation and spontaneous discharge in A beta and A delta primary afferent neurons. J Neurophysiol 68(3): 734–744.

Kim SH, Chung JM. 1992. An experimental model for peripheral neuropathy produced by segmental spinal nerve ligation in the rat. Pain 50(3): 355–363.

Kitamura N, Konno A, Kuwahara T, et al. 2005. Nerve growth factor-induced hyperexcitability of rat sensory neuron in culture. Biomed Res 26(3): 123–130.

Kitao A, Hirata H, Morita A, et al. 1997. Transient damage to the axonal transport system without Wallerian degeneration by acute nerve compression. Exp Neurol 147(2): 248–255.

Kivioja J, Rinaldi L, Ozenci V, et al. 2001. Chemokines and their receptors in whiplash injury: elevated RANTES and CCR-5. J Clin Immunol 21(4): 272–277.

Kleinrensink GJ, Stoeckart R, Vleeming A, et al. 1995. Peripheral nerve tension due to joint motion. A comparison between embalmed and unembalmed human bodies. Clin Biomech 10(5): 235–239.

Kleinrensink GJ, Stoeckart R, Mulder PG, et al. 2000. Upper limb tension tests as tools in the diagnosis of nerve and plexus lesions. Anatomical and biomechanical aspects. Clin Biomech 15(1): 9–14.

Koltzenburg M, Bendszus M. 2004. Imaging of peripheral nerve lesions. Curr Opin Neurol 17(5): 621–626.

Koschorke GM, Meyer RA, Campbell JN. 1994. Cellular components necessary for mechanoelectrical transduction are conveyed to primary afferent terminals by fast axonal transport. Brain Res 641(1): 99–104.

Kwan MK, Wall EJ, Massie J, et al. 1992. Strain, stress and stretch of peripheral nerve. Rabbit experiments in vitro and in vivo. Acta Orthop Scand 63(3): 267–272.

LaMotte RH, Shain CN, Simone DA, et al. 1991. Neurogenic hyperalgesia: psychophysical studies of underlying mechanisms. J Neurophysiol 66(1): 190–211.

Leem JG, Bove GM. 2002. Mid-axonal tumor necrosis factor-alpha induces ectopic activity in a subset of slowly conducting cutaneous and deep afferent neurons. J Pain 3(1): 45–49.

Lewin GR, Ritter AM, Mendell LM. 1993. Nerve growth factor-induced hyperalgesia in the neonatal and adult rat. J Neurosci 13(5): 2136–2148.

Liu L, Yang TM, Liedtke W, et al. 2006. Chronic IL-1β signaling potentiates voltage-dependent sodium currents in trigeminal nociceptive neurons. J Neurophysiol 95(3): 1478–1490.

Lundborg G. 1988. Nerve injuries and repair. Edinburgh: Churchill Livingstone.

Lynn B, Greening J, Leary R. 2002. Sensory and autonomic function and ultrasound nerve imaging in RSI patients and keyboard workers (No. CRR 417/2002). London: Health and Safety Executive.

Mackinnon SE. 2002. Pathophysiology of nerve compression. Hand Clin 18(2): 231–241.

Maihofner C, Handwerker HO, Neundorfer B, et al. 2005. Mechanical hyperalgesia in complex regional pain syndrome: a role for TNF-alpha? Neurology 65(2): 311–313.

McLellan DL, Swash M. 1976. Longitudinal sliding of the median nerve during movements of the upper limb. J Neurol Neurosurg Psychiatry 39 566–570.

McMahon SB, Cafferty WB, Marchand F. 2005. Immune and glial cell factors as pain mediators and modulators. Exp Neurol 192(2): 444–462.

Millesi H, Zoch G, Rath T. 1990. The gliding apparatus of peripheral nerve and its clinical significance. Ann Hand Upper Limb Surg 9(2): 87–97.

Moalem G, Tracey DJ. 2006. Immune and inflammatory mechanisms in neuropathic pain. Brain Res Rev 51(2): 240–264.

Nakamichi K, Tachibana S. 1995. Restricted motion of the median nerve in carpal tunnel syndrome. J Hand Surg 20(4): 460–464.

O'Connor D, Marshall SC, Massy-Westropp N. 2009. Non-surgical treatment (other than steroid injection) for carpal tunnel syndrome. Cochrane Database Syst Rev (1): CD003219.

Obreja O, Rathee PK, Lips KS, et al. 2002. IL-1 beta potentiates heat-activated currents in rat sensory neurons: involvement of IL-1RI, tyrosine kinase, and protein kinase C. FASEB J 16(12): 1497–1503.

Obreja O, Biasio W, Andratsch M, et al. 2005. Fast modulation of heat-activated ionic current by proinflammatory interleukin 6 in rat sensory neurons. Brain 128(7): 1634–1641.

Oh SB, Tran PB, Gillard SE, et al. 2001. Chemokines and glycoprotein 120 produce pain hypersensitivity by directly exciting primary nociceptive neurons. J Neurosci 21(14): 5027–5035.

Olsson Y. 1990. Microenvironment of the peripheral nervous system under normal and pathological conditions. Crit Rev Neurobiol 5(3): 265–309.

Ozaktay AC, Kallakuri S, Takebayashi T, et al. 2006. Effects of interleukin-1 beta, interleukin-6, and tumor necrosis factor on sensitivity of dorsal root ganglion and peripheral receptive fields in rats. Eur Spine J 15(10): 1529–1537.

Pascarelli EF, Hsu YP. 2001. Understanding work-related upper extremity disorders: clinical findings in 485 computer users, musicians, and others. J Occup Rehabil 11(1): 1–21.

Pertin M, Ji RR, Berta T, et al. 2005. Upregulation of the voltage-gated sodium channel beta2 subunit in neuropathic pain models: characterization of expression in injured and non-injured primary sensory neurons. J Neurosci 25(47): 10970–10980.

Quintner JL. 1989. A study of upper limb pain and paraesthesiae following neck injury in motor vehicle accidents: assessment of the brachial plexus tension test of Elvey. Br J Rheumatol 28(6): 528–533.

Rodriquez AA, Barr KP, Burns SP. 2004. Whiplash: pathophysiology, diagnosis, treatment, and prognosis. Muscle Nerve 29(6): 768–781.

Rueff A, Mendell LM. 1996. Nerve growth factor NT-5 induce increased thermal sensitivity of cutaneous nociceptors in vitro. J Neurophysiol 76(5): 3593–3596.

Rydevik BL, Kwan MK, Myers RR, et al. 1990. An in vitro mechanical and histological study of acute stretching on rabbit tibial nerve. J Orthop Res 8(5): 694–701.

Sauer SK, Bove GM, Averbeck B, et al. 1999. Rat peripheral nerve components release calcitonin gene-related peptide and prostaglandin E-2 in response to noxious stimuli: Evidence that nervi nervorum are nociceptors. Neuroscience 92(1): 319–325.

Schafers M, Sorkin LS, Geis C, et al. 2003a. Spinal nerve ligation induces transient upregulation of tumor necrosis factor receptors 1 and 2 in injured and adjacent uninjured dorsal root ganglia in the rat. Neurosci Lett 347(3): 179–182.

Schafers M, Sorkin LS, Sommer, C. 2003b. Intramuscular injection of tumor necrosis factor-alpha induces muscle hyperalgesia in rats. Pain 104(3): 579–588.

Sommer C, Galbraith JA, Heckman HM, et al. 1993. Pathology of experimental compression neuropathy producing hyperesthesia. J Neuropathol Exp Neurol 52(3): 223–233.

Sorkin LS, Doom CM. 2000. Epineurial application of TNF elicits an acute mechanical hyperalgesia in the awake rat. J Peripher Nerv Syst 5(2): 96–100.

Sorkin LS, Xiao WH, Wagner R, et al. 1997. Tumour necrosis factor-alpha induces ectopic activity in nociceptive primary afferent fibres. Neuroscience 81(1): 255–262.

Sterling M, Treleaven J, Jull G. 2002. Responses to a clinical test of mechanical provocation of nerve tissue in whiplash associated disorder. Man Ther 7(2): 89–94.

Sun JH, Yang B, Donnelly DF, et al. 2006. MCP-1 enhances excitability of nociceptive neurons in chronically compressed dorsal root ganglia. J Neurophysiol 96(5): 2189–2199.

Sunderland S. 1978. Nerve and nerve injuries. Edinburgh: Churchill Livingstone.

Tal M, Eliav E. 1996. Abnormal discharge originates at the site of nerve injury in experimental constriction neuropathy (CCI) in the rat. Pain 64(3): 511–518.

Tanaka M, Cummins TR, Ishikawa K, et al. 1998. SNS Na^+ channel expression increases in dorsal root ganglion neurons in the carrageenan inflammatory pain model. Neuroreport 9(6): 967–972.
Tanaka T, Minami M, Nakagawa T, et al. 2004. Enhanced production of monocyte chemoattractant protein-1 in the dorsal root ganglia in a rat model of neuropathic pain: possible involvement in the development of neuropathic pain. Neurosci Res 48(4): 463–469.
Thomas PK. 1963. The connective tissue of peripheral nerve: a electron microscope study. J Anat 97(1): 35–44.
Thomas PK, Berthold CH, Ochoa J, et al. 1993. Microscopic anatomy of the peripheral nervous system. In: Dyck PJ, Thomas PK (eds) Peripheral neuropathy. Philadelphia: Saunders, pp 28–73.
Tillett RL, Afoke A, Hall SM, et al. 2004. Investigating mechanical behaviour at a core-sheath interface in peripheral nerve. J Peripher Nerv Syst 9(4): 255–262.
Toews AD, Barrett C, Morell P. 1998. Monocyte chemoattractant protein 1 is responsible for macrophage recruitment following injury to sciatic nerve. J Neurosci Res 53(2): 260–267.
Topp KS, Boyd BS. 2006. Structure and biomechanics of peripheral nerves: nerve responses to physical stresses and implications for physical therapist practice. Phys Ther 86(1): 92–109.
Tuzuner S, Ozkaynak S, Acikbas C, et al. 2004. Median nerve excursion during endoscopic carpal tunnel release. Neurosurgery 54(5): 1155–1160.
Uceyler N, Eberle T, Rolke R, et al. 2007a. Differential expression patterns of cytokines in complex regional pain syndrome. Pain 132(1–2): 195–205.
Uceyler N, Tscharke A, Sommer C. 2007b. Early cytokine expression in mouse sciatic nerve after chronic constriction nerve injury depends on calpain. Brain Behav Immun 21(5): 553–560.
Ushiki T, Ide C. 1990. Three-dimensional organization of the collagen fibrils in the rat sciatic nerve as revealed by transmission- and scanning electron microscopy. Cell Tissue Res 260(1): 175–184.
Walbeehm ET, Afoke A, de Wit T, et al. 2004. Mechanical functioning of peripheral nerves: linkage with the 'mushrooming' effect. Cell Tissue Res 316(1): 115–121.
Wallis BJ, Lord SM, Barnsley L, et al. 1998. The psychological profiles of patients with whiplash-associated headache. Cephalalgia 18(2): 101–105.
Watkins LR, Maier SF. 2002. Beyond neurons: evidence that immune and glial cells contribute to pathological pain states. Physiol Rev 82(4): 981–1011.
White FA, Sun J, Waters SM et al. 2005. Excitatory monocyte chemoattractant protein-1 signaling is up-regulated in sensory neurons after chronic compression of the dorsal root ganglion. Proc Natl Acad Sci USA 102(39): 14092–14097.
Wilgis EF, Murphy R. 1986. The significance of longitudinal excursion in peripheral nerves. Hand Clin 2 761–766.
Wright TW, Glowczewskie F, Wheeler D, et al. 1996. Excursion and strain of the median nerve. J Bone Joint Surg 78 1897–1903.
Wright TW, Glowczewskie F Jr , Cowin D, et al. 2001. Ulnar nerve excursion and strain at the elbow and wrist associated with upper extremity motion. J Hand Surg 26(4): 655–662.
Wright TW, Glowczewskie F Jr, Cowin D, et al. 2005. Radial nerve excursion and strain at the elbow and wrist associated with upper-extremity motion. J Hand Surg 30(5): 990–996.
Wu G, Ringkamp M, Hartke TV, et al. 2001. Early onset of spontaneous activity in uninjured C-fiber nociceptors after injury to neighboring nerve fibers. J Neurosci 21(8): RC140.
Wu G, Ringkamp M, Murinson BB, et al. 2002. Degeneration of myelinated efferent fibers induces spontaneous activity in uninjured C-fiber afferents. J Neurosci 22(17): 7746–7753.
Zelenka M, Schafers M, Sommer C. 2005. Intraneural injection of interleukin-1beta and tumor necrosis factor-alpha into rat sciatic nerve at physiological doses induces signs of neuropathic pain. Pain 116(3): 257–263.
Zhang N, Inan S, Cowan A, et al. 2005. A proinflammatory chemokine, CCL3, sensitizes the heat- and capsaicin-gated ion channel TRPV1. Proc Natl Acad Sci USA 102(12): 4536–4541.
Zhu W, Oxford GS. 2007. Phosphoinositide-3-kinase and mitogen activated protein kinase signaling pathways mediate acute NGF sensitization of TRPV1. Mol Cell Neurosci 34(4): 689–700.
Zochodne DW, Ho LT. 1992. Hyperemia of injured peripheral nerve: sensitivity to CGRP antagonism. Brain Res 598(1–2): 59–66.
Zochodne DW, Ho LT. 1993. Evidence that capsaicin hyperaemia of rat sciatic vasa nervorum is local, opiate-sensitive and involves mast cells. J Physiol 468: 325–333.

Chapter 65

Clinical Neurodynamics of the Upper and Lower Quadrants

Emilio J. Puentedura, Paul E. Mintken, Adriaan Louw

CHAPTER CONTENTS

Introduction to clinical neurodynamics 781
Appropriate terminology 781
Operational definitions 782
Neurophysiology in upper and lower quadrant pain 783
Nerve sensitivity 783
Central nervous system processing in neurodynamic tests 784
Clinical neuro-biomechanics in the upper and lower quadrants 784
Neurodynamic testing 785
Neurodynamic testing for the upper quadrant 786
Neurodynamic testing for the lower quadrant 791
Clinical application of neurodynamics in upper and lower quadrants 793
Treatment 795
Conclusion 796

Introduction to Clinical Neurodynamics

Manual therapy involves the selective examination and evaluation of the effects of movement, position and activities on the signs and symptoms of a neuromusculoskeletal disorder (Maitland 1986). This allows the clinician to formulate a working hypothesis regarding the movement problem, which can be confirmed or denied following careful reassessment during and after specific treatment applications. Manual therapy is therefore a useful approach to examining, evaluating and treating movement problems affecting the neuromusculoskeletal system. However, a key assumption made here is that there is a proportional input–output pain response, or, in other words, the musculoskeletal pain may be classified as either nociceptive or peripheral neuropathic and not centrally sensitized pain according to the pain mechanisms-based classifications (Smart et al 2012a, 2012b, 2012c). It is critically important in current manual therapy to determine which particular pain mechanism might be contributing to the clinical picture in order to appropriately direct management. (For more detail on pain mechanisms see Ch 6.)

It can be helpful to think of the mechanics of the body's moving parts in terms of components comprising a chassis (skeletal framework), articulations (joints and supporting ligaments), motors (muscles and tendons) and electrical wiring (nervous system). Each of the components that make up the neuro-musculoskeletal system plays an important and interdependent role in its overall health and function.

One could argue that many of the early manual therapy systems of the 1960s and 1970s placed a greater emphasis on the health and function of the articulations (joints) and, hence, 'manual therapy' became synonymous with 'passive joint mobilization' and 'joint manipulation' (Butler 1991). Despite an underlying awareness of the interdependency of the components of the neuro-musculoskeletal system, relatively little attention was paid to the physical health and movement of the nervous system. This changed dramatically following the published works of Gregory Grieve, Alf Breig, Geoffrey Maitland, Robert Elvey and David Butler. Their collective works opened a new frontier in manual therapy – the hypothesis that the entire nervous system is a mechanical organ that could develop 'adverse tension', or impaired mobility, which could then be treated with various movement therapies.

When the concept of mobilizing the nervous system took root within the physical therapy community in the late 1970s and early 1980s, it was met with some significant scepticism (Di Fabio 2001). The concept originally focused on the mechanical 'stiffness' within the nervous system, and it was thought at the time that this stiffness required aggressive stretching. Although a subset of patients benefited from treating this 'adverse neural tension' with 'stretching' and mobilization, many manual therapists soon found that some patients got significantly worse following these interventions, and therefore very quickly abandoned the use of these neural mobilization techniques.

Appropriate Terminology

'Adverse neural tension' has been defined as the abnormal physiological and mechanical responses produced by nervous system structures when testing their normal range of movement and stretch capabilities (Butler 1991). A 'neural tension test' is therefore designed to examine the physical (mechanical) abilities of the nervous system (Butler 2000). The use of the term 'tension' has significant limitations because it fails to take into account other aspects of nervous system function, such as movement, pressure, viscoelasticity and physiology

(Shacklock 1995a, 1995b, 2005a, 2005b). A more appropriate term is 'neurodynamic test' (Shacklock 2005b) and it is one that medical and healthcare professions should embrace.

The term 'neurodynamics' refers to the mechanics and physiology of the nervous system within the musculoskeletal system and how these systems relate to each other (Shacklock 1995b). It allows for the consideration of movement-related neurophysiological changes as well as the neuronal dynamics postulated to occur in the central nervous system (CNS) during physical and mental activity. A key tenet of this definition is that the nervous system is capable of movement and stretch, and that there is a 'normal' response (as well as 'abnormal') of the nervous system to movement and tension. Both Butler and Shacklock have advocated the transition to the term 'neurodynamic' as opposed to 'neural tension', because 'neurodynamics' places less emphasis on 'stretching' and 'tension' and more emphasis on the nervous system, the 'container' in which it lives and the mechanisms that can alter its function. These other mechanisms include changes to intraneural blood flow (Ogata & Naito 1986), neural inflammation (Zochodne & Ho 1991), mechanosensitivity (Calvin et al 1982; Nordin et al 1984) and muscle responses (Hall et al 1996; Van der Heide et al 2001).

Neurodynamic impairments should really be conceptualized as any specific physical dysfunction (be it neural, muscular or skeletal) that presumes to challenge physically the normal functioning of the nervous system. These impairments can arise from mechanical, chemical and / or sensitivity changes anywhere in the neuro-musculoskeletal system. Therefore, in neurodynamics, neural tissues may have a tension problem (mechanical), or be hypersensitive (a problem of pathophysiology), or it may be a combination of both (Shacklock 1995a). Instead of a length or 'tension' problem, the primary mechanical fault within the nervous system may be one of reduced sliding (neural sliding dysfunction) and / or could be a compression problem related to the tissues that form a mechanical interface to the nervous system. Therefore, the time has come for us to embrace the current nomenclature: 'neurodynamics'.

Operational definitions

In order to facilitate understanding of the rest of this chapter further, some operational definitions are now provided.

Clinical neurodynamics

This can be defined as the examination, evaluation and treatment of the mechanics and physiology of the nervous system as they relate to each other and are integrated with musculoskeletal function (Shacklock 1995b).

Neurodynamic test

The testing procedures used in clinical neurodynamics can be defined as a series of body movements that produce mechanical and physiological events in the nervous system according to the movements of the test (Shacklock 1995b). A neurodynamic test aims to challenge or test physically the mechanics and / or physiology of a part of the nervous system. For example, a mechanical component of a median neurodynamic test would be the ability of the median nerve tract to slide and glide in relation to surrounding tissues such as the lower cervical discs, scalenes, biceps and carpal tunnel. The physiological components may relate to blood flow within the median nerve tract, ion channel activity within axons of the median nerve, inflammation within various sections of the median nerve, and representational changes within the CNS of the median nerve, arm, forearm and their movements.

Neurogenic pain

This is pain that is initiated and / or caused by a primary lesion, dysfunction or transitory perturbation in the peripheral or central nervous system (Merskey & Bogduk 1994).

Sensitizing movements

These are movements that increase forces in the neural structures, in addition to movements employed in the standard neurodynamic test (Butler 2000; Shacklock 2005a). Sensitizing movements should not be confused with differentiating movements. Sensitizing movements can be useful in loading or moving the nervous system beyond the effects of the standard neurodynamic test (i.e. strengthening the test). However, they also load and move musculoskeletal structures and are therefore not as helpful in determining the existence of a neurodynamic problem as is a differentiating movement.

Differentiating movements

These are movements that emphasize or isolate the nervous system by producing movement in the neural structures in the area in question rather than by moving the musculoskeletal structures in the same area (Butler 2000; Shacklock 2005a). Differentiating movements place emphasis on the nervous system without affecting the other structures and so are used to help establish the existence of a neurodynamic problem. An example of a differentiating movement for a patient with carpal tunnel pain would be the addition of cervical ipsilateral side-bending (see later in this chapter for further examples).

Sliders

These are neurodynamic manoeuvres performed in order to produce a sliding movement of neural structures relative to their adjacent tissues (Butler 2000; Shacklock 2005a). Sliders involve application of movement / stress to the nervous system proximally while releasing movement / stress distally, and then reversing the sequence. Sliders allow larger ranges of motion, provide a means of distraction from the painful area and should provide multitissue, non-painful and, it would be hoped, fear-reducing novel inputs into the CNS (Butler 2000). Research has shown that sliders actually result in greater excursion than simply stretching the nerve (Coppieters & Butler 2008).

Tensioners

These are neurodynamic manoeuvres performed in order to produce an increase in tension (not stretch) in neural structures, which may improve neural viscoelastic and physiological functions (e.g. help neural tissue cope better with increased tension) (Butler 2000; Shacklock 2005a). Tensioners are the opposite of sliders in that movement / stress is applied proximally and distally to the nervous system at the same time, and then released. Tensioners may better challenge stiffness and more long-lasting physical dysfunction (Butler 2000).

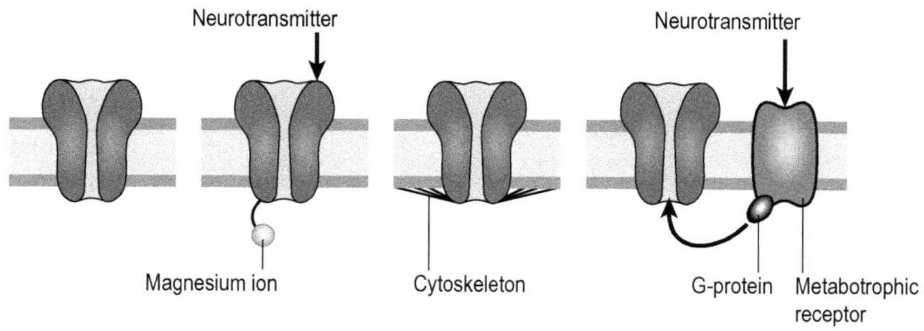

Figure 65.1 **Ion channels.**

Neurophysiology in Upper and Lower Quadrant Pain

Initially, manual therapists were more interested in the mechanical aspects of neurodynamics (Elvey 1986; Breig 1978; Butler 1991). Unfortunately this has led to a very 'mechanistic' view of the nervous system (Butler 2000). Most textbooks describe normal nerve mechanics related to various positions, postures or movements, subsequent abnormal mechanics (pathomechanics) and, finally, movement-based treatment aimed at restoring normal nerve movement (Butler 2000; Shacklock 2005a). None of this is disputed. However, increased knowledge in our understanding of nerve pain related to neurophysiological changes and the processing within the brain of nerve movement (and pain) warrants investigation and discussion.

Pathologies that affect peripheral nerves usually result in dysaesthetic pain and / or nerve trunk pain (Asbury & Fields 1984). Dysaesthetic pain (where light touch causes pain) often manifests as burning or tingling pain due to abnormal impulses from hyperexcitable afferent nerve fibres, which, due to injury, may become abnormal impulse-generating sites (AIGSs) (Asbury & Fields 1984; Woolf & Mannion 1999). AIGSs may fire spontaneously as the result of mechanical or chemical stimuli, such that dysaesthetic pain may present as very bizarre patterns – from bursts of pain in response to a stimulus to pain that presents spontaneously with no apparent stimulus.

In contrast, nerve trunk pain commonly presents as deep, achy pain arising from nociceptors within the nervous tissue that are sensitized to mechanical or chemical stimuli (Asbury & Fields 1984; Kallakuri et al 1998; Ozaktay et al 1998). Nerve trunk pain usually has a fairly straightforward stimulus–response relationship (Asbury & Fields 1984).

These two types of pain can be evoked by a variety of chemical or mechanical stimuli, and may lead to allodynia or hyperalgesia. Allodynia is a pain sensation that is evoked from stimuli that are not normally painful, whereas hyperalgesia is an exaggerated pain response to stimuli that would normally be painful (Asbury & Fields 1984; Woolf & Mannion 1999; Nee & Butler 2006).

Nerve sensitivity

In order to understand nerve sensitivity, knowledge of ion channels is required. Although the complexity of ion channel regulation is not yet properly understood and the research is based on animal studies, scientists and clinicians are using the information known about ion channels to improve patient care (Barry 1991; Butler 2000; Louw & Puentedura 2013). Ion channels are essentially proteins clumped together with an opening – to allow ions to flow in / out of the membrane (Devor 2006). They are synthesized in the dorsal root ganglion (DRG) based on a genetic coding, and are distributed along an axon to allow ions to flow in / out of the nerve to polarize and / or depolarize the membrane. Ion channels are not uniformly distributed along the axolemma, with certain areas known to have higher concentrations of ion channels – such as the DRG, axon hillock, nodes of Ranvier and areas where the axon has lost myelin (Devor et al 1993; Devor 1999, 2006). Adding to the complexity is the fact that there are countless types of ion channels, including channels that seem to respond to movement, pressure, blood flow, circulating adrenaline (epinephrine) levels, etc. (Fig. 65.1). From a survival perspective, this seems logical as a means for the nervous system to become 'sensitive' to various stimuli. However, the amount and type of ion channels found in the axolemma are in a constant state of change (Devor et al 1993; Devor 2006). Research has shown that the half-life of some ion channels may be as short as 2 days (Barry 1991), and ion channels that drop out of the membrane are not necessarily replaced by channels of the same type. Further, ion channel deposition is directly impacted by the environment in which the organism finds itself (Barry 1991). For example, changes in temperature around an animal with experimentally removed myelin produce higher concentrations of 'cold-sensing' channels in that area, animals in stressful environments produce higher concentrations of adrenosensitive channels, and animals that have joints with restricted movement cause up-regulation of movement-sensitive ion channels (Devor et al 1993; Devor & Seltzer 1999; Devor 2006). With higher concentrations of similar ion channels in an area, the chances for the nerve to depolarize and cause an action potential increase. In essence, the nerve may develop an AIGS. The nervous system can then become sensitive to various types of stimuli, such as temperature, movement, pressure, anxiety, stress, the immune system and more (Devor & Seltzer 1999; Butler 2000; Louw & Puentedura 2013) (Fig. 65.2). The nervous system can therefore be viewed as an alarm system beautifully designed to protect the organism, and the amount and type of ion channels at any given time may be a fair representation of what the brain computes is needed for survival (Butler & Moseley 2003; Louw & Puentedura 2013).

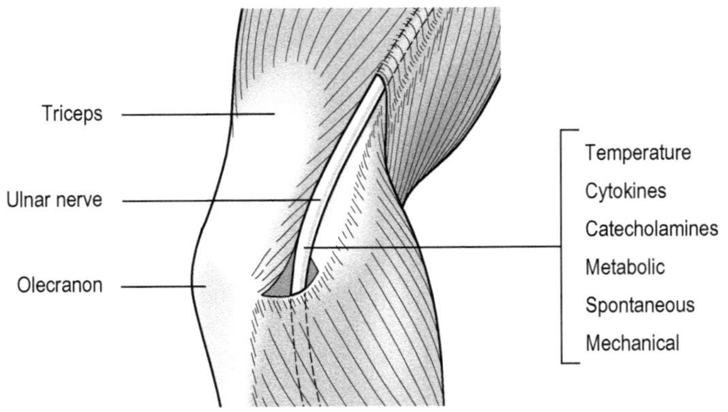

Figure 65.2 Ulnar nerve at the elbow – depicting types of ion channels.

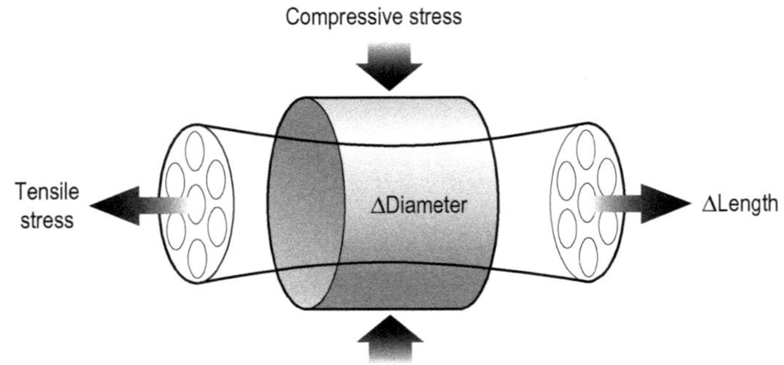

Figure 65.3 Stretching a nerve leads to increased intraneural pressure.

Central nervous system processing in neurodynamic tests

Many clinicians are familiar with the term 'central sensitivity'. Central sensitivity is defined as a condition in which peripheral noxious input into the CNS leads to an increased excitability where the response to normal inputs is greatly enhanced (Woolf 2007). Repeated painful stimuli, such as easily excitable AIGSs, may cause low-threshold neurons with large receptive fields to depolarize in response to stimuli that would normally be benign (Woolf 2007). It has been shown that injured neural tissue may alter its chemical makeup and reorganize synaptic contacts in the CNS such that innocuous stimuli are directed to cells that normally receive only noxious inputs (Woolf 2007). Hence, the CNS becomes 'hyperexcitable' owing to a combination of decreased inhibition and increased responsiveness (Mannion & Woolf 2000; Woolf 2000; Woolf & Salter 2000). This is analogous to turning up the volume on the system such that innocuous stimuli begin to generate painful sensations while noxious stimuli result in an exaggerated pain response. Woolf (2000) described this process as a change in both the software and the hardware of the CNS, and we would argue that clinicians have the tools to impact both of these.

Clinical Neuro-biomechanics in the Upper and Lower Quadrants

Neuro-biomechanics is the study of the normal and pathological range of motion of the nervous system. Unfortunately, what we know is based upon somewhat limited research, largely animal and cadaver studies. There is no doubt that this is an area in need of further research efforts, and the interest shown by researchers in this area is certainly helping to expand our knowledge. Readers are referred to other texts for further information on this topic (Kleinrensink et al 2000; Wright et al 2001; Dilley et al 2001, 2003, 2007, 2008; Erel et al 2003; Julius et al 2004; Ellis et al 2008; Coppieters et al 2009; Boyd et al 2012; Boyd & Dilley 2014).

A key issue in the understanding of neuro-biomechanics is the concept of the nervous system being a continuous tissue tract. The system is continuous mechanically via its continuous connective tissue formats, electrically via conducted impulses and chemically via its common neurotransmitters. The nervous system being a mechanical continuum is probably most relevant to the study of neurodynamics because it implies transmission of movement (sliding / gliding) and the development of tension (stretching) within and along the system. That is, wrist extension and elbow extension lengthen and move the median nerve distally within its neural pathway, and contralateral cervical lateral flexion adds a pull in the proximal direction. This has been demonstrated in cadaveric studies in which the nerve roots are marked with paper markers or pins. When the shoulder is depressed and abducted in external rotation, the cervical nerve roots are pulled out of the vertebral foramen.

Another key concept in neurodynamics is that of the mechanical interface. This interface is defined as that tissue or material adjacent to the nervous system that can move independently of the system (Butler 1991). Mechanical interfaces are central to an understanding of neurodynamics, because they represent the most likely sites for the development of movement / force transmission problems. Mechanical interfaces can be hard or bony (e.g. the ulnar nerve at the cubital tunnel), ligamentous (e.g. the ligament of Struthers in the forearm), joints (e.g. the zygapophyseal joints), or muscular (e.g. the supinator muscle in the forearm). Mechanical interfaces can be normal, where movement and function are optimal and symptom free, or they can be pathological, where something happens to restrict movement of the nervous system at the interface, or compress the nervous tissue. Examples would include osteophytes, extensive bruising, or swelling, which could occupy space at the mechanical interface resulting in restricted range of motion and independence of the nervous system and the interface. Numerous studies have shown that if the interface is injured or damage this may have repercussions for adjacent neural tissues. Examples include the cubital tunnel (Coppieters et al 2004), carpal tunnel (Erel et al 2003), intervertebral foramen and spinal canal (Chang et al 2006) and piriformis muscle (Kuncewicz et al 2006). If this happens, the range of motion of the nervous system can be impaired, and this would presumably lead to the abnormal mechanical response in our definition of neurodynamics.

As the nervous system winds its way through its anatomical course, it will be forced to stretch, slide (longitudinal or transverse), bend and become compressed. Stretch will be defined here as the elongation of the nerve relative to its starting length. However, nerves are not solid structures and stretch causes internal compression due to displacement of nerve tissue / fluid (Fig. 65.3). The physiological effects of stretch and compression of the nerve include changes to intraneural blood flow, conduction and axoplasmic transport. Studies have shown that if a peripheral nerve is held on an 8% stretch for 30 minutes it will cause a 50% decrease in blood flow, an 8.8% stretch for 1 hour will cause a 70% decrease in blood flow, and a 15% stretch for 30 minutes will cause an 80–100% blockage in blood flow (Ogata & Naito 1986; Driscoll et al 2002). Wall et al (1992) were able to demonstrate that a 6% stretch / strain of a peripheral nerve for 1 hour resulted in a 70% decrease in action potentials, and a 12% stretch / strain for 1 hour caused complete conduction block. Interestingly, in other studies, Millesi (1986) and Zoech et al (1991) reported that, from full wrist and elbow flexion to full wrist and elbow extension, the median nerve has to adapt to a nerve bed that becomes 20% longer. Similar data have been provided by Beith et al (1995) with respect to the sciatic / tibial nerve. Research by Breig and colleagues (Breig 1960, 1978; Breig & Marions 1963; Breig & El-Nadi 1966; Breig et al 1966; Breig & Troup 1979) has demonstrated that flexion of the cervical spine leads to tension in the dura and spinal cord, resulting in a cephalad movement of the cauda equina. This ultimately limits the available mobility of the sciatic nerve. Obviously, there must be some mechanical and physiological adaptations within peripheral nerves to accommodate such significant changes in length and to cope with prolonged stretching or strain. The effects of compression have also been studied, with as little as 20–30 mmHg causing decreased venous blood flow and 80 mmHg causing complete blockage of intraneural blood flow (Ogata & Naito 1986). Compression also is shown to alter axonal transport (Dahlin & Thambert 1993; Dahlin et al 1993) and conduction of action potentials (Fern & Harrison 1994a, 1994b).

Nerves can be seen to move relative to their adjacent tissues, and this motion has been described as 'sliding' or 'excursion' (McLellan & Swash 1976; Wilgis & Murphy 1986). Excursion is seen to occur both longitudinally and transversely. This sliding or excursion is considered an essential aspect of neural function because it serves to dissipate tension and distribute forces within the nervous system. Instead of stretching (and thereby developing tension), the nervous system can move longitudinally and / or transversely and distribute itself along the shortest course between fixed points; hence it can equalize tension throughout the neural tract.

As joints move, there is nerve bed elongation (increase in length of the neural container) on the convex side of the joint, and nerve bed shortening (decrease in length of the neural container) on the concave side of the joint. When there is nerve bed elongation, the nerve glides towards the joint that is moving and this is referred to as convergence. When there is nerve bed shortening, the nerve glides away from the joint that is moving and this is referred to as divergence. Dilley et al (2003) used real-time ultrasound to examine the effects of elbow extension on the median nerve and found the magnitude of excursion for the median nerve in the mid-upper arm to be 10.4 mm distally towards the elbow and in the mid-forearm to be 3.0 mm proximally towards the elbow. With the elbow held in extension while applying wrist extension, they recorded excursion of the median nerve at the mid-upper arm 1.8 mm distally towards the elbow, and in the mid-forearm 4.2 mm distally towards the wrist. It could be argued that some degree of excursion must also occur in the hand proximally towards the wrist.

Studies have shown that the starting position and the sequencing of limb movement during neurodynamic tests affect the degree of excursion along the nerve. In the same study referenced above, Dilley et al (2003) also examined the median nerve at the distal arm and mid-forearm using two different start positions – elbow in full extension, and shoulder at 45° or at 90° abduction – and then performed wrist extension from neutral to 45°. They found that greater excursion of the median nerve occurred when the shoulder was in a more-slackened position (45° abduction). For the shoulder at 45° abduction, excursion was 2.4 mm distally at the distal arm and 4.7 mm distally at the mid-forearm. For the shoulder at 90° abduction, excursion was 1.8 mm distally at the distal arm and 4.2 mm distally at the mid-forearm. The sequence of movements has also been shown to affect the distribution of symptoms in response to neurodynamic testing (Shacklock 1989; Zorn et al 1996); these authors reported a greater likelihood of producing a response that is localized to the region that is moved first or moved more strongly. Tsai (1995) conducted a cadaveric study in which strain in the ulnar nerve at the elbow was measured during ulnar neurodynamic testing in three different sequences: proximal to distal, distal to proximal and elbow first. The elbow-first sequence consistently produced 20% greater strain in the ulnar nerve at the elbow than the other two sequences. Therefore, it can be argued that greater strain in the nerves occurs at the site that is moved first – that is, the first component of a neurodynamic test or treatment technique.

Neurodynamic Testing

Butler (1991) proposed a base test system for neurodynamic evaluation. It is a clinically intuitive system that evolved for ease of handling and to fulfil a perceived clinical demand. It is based on existing tests and the basic principles of neurodynamics already discussed, and, in most clinical situations, the tests are refined or adapted based upon reasoned diagnoses and the clinical presentation of the patient with neck and arm symptoms. Nee and Butler (2006) described a positive neurodynamic test as one that reproduces a familiar symptom, is changed by the movement of a body segment away from the site of symptoms, or there are differences in the test response from side to side or from what is known to be normal in asymptomatic individuals. A positive test does not allow the identification of a specific area of injury, however; it is merely suggestive of increased mechanosensitivity somewhere along the neural tissue tract (Nee & Butler 2006).

It is recommended that all neurodynamic tests be performed actively before passively. This allows the therapist to gauge the patient's ability and willingness to move and provides an approximate measure of the range of motion likely to be encountered during the passive test. It also may decrease the patient's fears and anxieties about the test and symptoms likely to be elicited during the test. Finally, if the active movement is found to be extremely sensitive, a reasoned decision may be made not to perform the tests passively in order to avoid symptom exacerbation.

Some important handling issues with respect to performance of the neurodynamic tests include:

- Perform only if you have a clinical rationale for doing so.

- Establish clinical-reasoning hypotheses prior to the test regarding pathobiology, likely specific dysfunctions to be found on examination, precautions and sources of symptoms.
- Explain to patients exactly what you are going to do and what you want them to do. It is vital to have patients feel comfortable about reporting any responses to testing, anywhere in their body.
- Perform the test on the less-painful side or non-painful side first. If there is little difference between sides, perform the test on the left side first for consistency.
- Starting positions should be consistent each time, and any variations from normal practice should be noted / recorded (use of pillows, etc.).
- Note symptom responses including area and nature (type of response) with the addition of each component of the test.
- Watch for antalgic postures and other compensatory movements during the test (e.g. cervical movements or trapezius muscle activity).
- Test for symmetry between sides.
- Explain your findings to your patient.
- Repeat the test gently a number of times before recording an actual measurement.

Neurodynamic testing for the upper quadrant

The tests for the upper quadrant involve four varieties of the upper limb neurodynamic test (ULNT) and were evolved from Elvey's initial test (Elvey 1986). They include attention to the major neural pathways and the major sensitizing movements. The four tests will now be described in detail: they are ULNT1 (median nerve bias), ULNT2 (median nerve bias), ULNT2 (radial nerve bias) and ULNT3 (ulnar nerve bias) (Table 65.1). The numbers refer to the sensitizing movements where 1 is shoulder abduction, 2 is shoulder girdle depression and 3 is elbow flexion (Butler 2000). Two tests for the median nerve have been developed as this nerve is more commonly injured than the other nerves in the upper extremity, and it was felt that a test was required to evaluate shoulder girdle depression and glenohumeral elevation independently (Butler 2000). Additionally, ULNT2 is useful in patients that have limited glenohumeral abduction.

ULNT1 (median) active test

If the patient has described a symptom-provoking position or movement, have him / her demonstrate it for you and observe the mechanics involved. If possible, perform a quick structural differentiation. For example, if patients demonstrate a symptomatic position for their elbow pain, you could have them maintain that elbow position and then ask them to move their neck to see if that alters their elbow symptoms.

A simple protocol for the active evaluation of the median neurodynamic test (ULNT1) has been described (Butler 2000). Have the patient abduct and externally rotate the shoulder with the elbow flexed to 90° and the wrist flexed (Fig. 65.4A). Then ask the patient to extend the elbow and wrist, and finally tilt the head away from the affected side (Fig. 65.4B). Compare to the opposite side, and note symptom responses as well as what happens to the shoulder girdle. Where the nervous system is sensitive, the shoulder girdle will often elevate (Butler 2000).

ULNT1 (median) passive test

A detailed description of the ULNT1 test is available in previous texts (Butler 1991, 2000, Shacklock 2005a). The key points involved are that the patient lies in supine position, arms by the side, shoulder close to the edge of the examination table,

Table 65.1 Illustrating the major components, movements, sensitizing motions and differentiating motions for the four distinct upper limb neurodynamic tests

	ULNT1 median	ULNT2 median	ULNT2 radial	ULNT3 ulnar
Nerves tested	Median, anterior interosseous (C5, C6, C7)	Median, anterior interosseous (C5, C6, C7)	Radial	Ulnar, C8 and T1 nerve roots
Shoulder	Stabilized from elevating and abducted (90–110°)	Depressed and abducted (10°)	Depressed and abducted (10°)	Depressed and abducted (10–90°), hand to ear
Elbow	Extended	Extended	Extended	Flexed
Forearm	Supinated	Supinated	Pronated	Pronated
Wrist	Extended	Extended	Flexed and ulnarly deviated	Extended and radially deviated
Fingers and thumb	Extended	Extended	Flexed	Extended
Rotation of shoulder	Lateral	Lateral	Medial	Lateral
Cervical spine (sensitizing)	Contralateral side flexed	Contralateral side flexed	Contralateral side flexed	Contralateral side flexed
Cervical spine (differentiating)	Ipsilateral side flexed	Ipsilateral side flexed	Ipsilateral side flexed	Ipsilateral side flexed

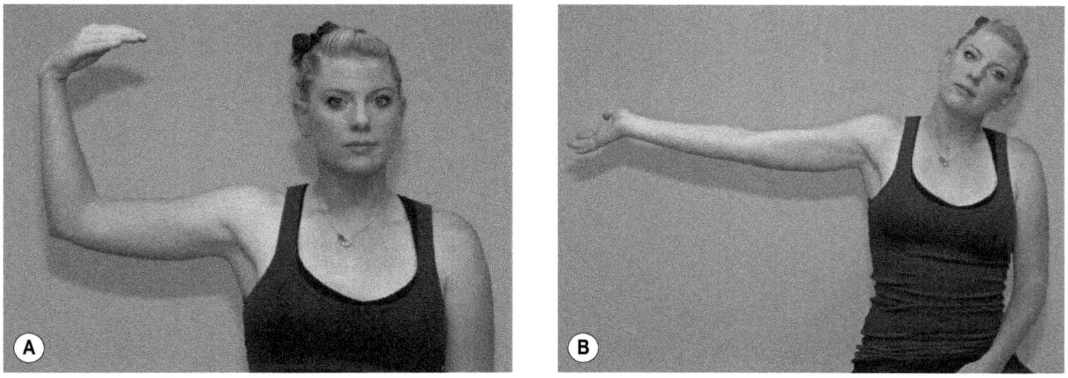

Figure 65.4 Active ULNT1 – median nerve. Have the patient abduct and externally rotate the shoulder with the elbow flexed to 90° and the wrist flexed (**A**). Then, have the patient extend the elbow, followed by wrist extension and cervical side-bending away from the affected side (**B**).

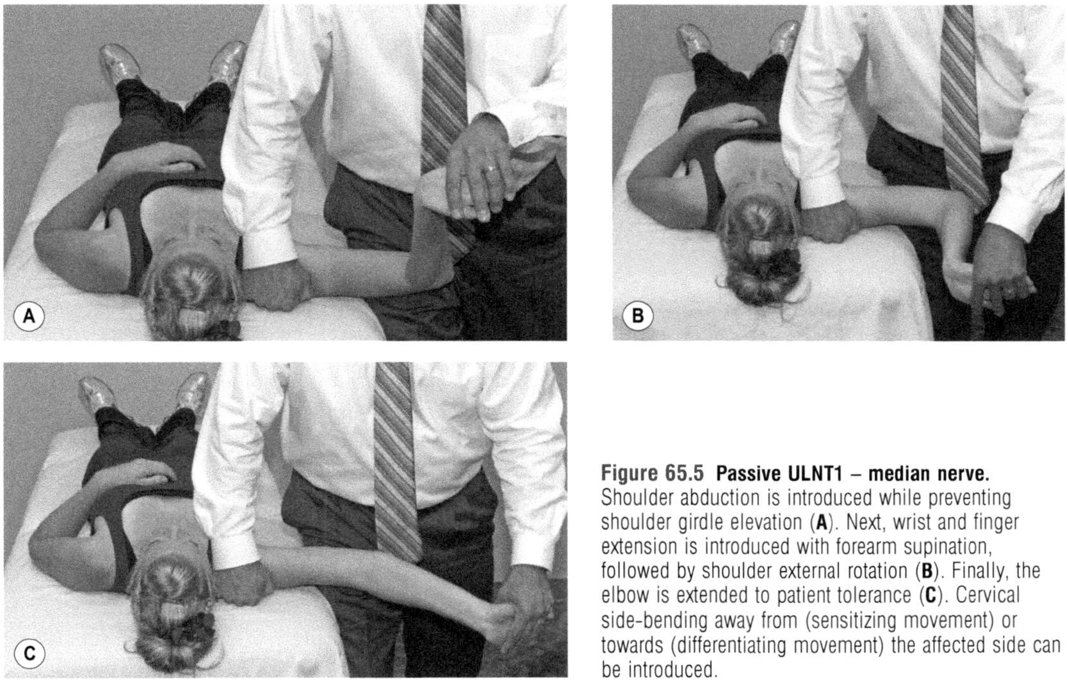

Figure 65.5 Passive ULNT1 – median nerve. Shoulder abduction is introduced while preventing shoulder girdle elevation (**A**). Next, wrist and finger extension is introduced with forearm supination, followed by shoulder external rotation (**B**). Finally, the elbow is extended to patient tolerance (**C**). Cervical side-bending away from (sensitizing movement) or towards (differentiating movement) the affected side can be introduced.

without a pillow if possible, and with body straight. The therapist stands with the near foot placed forward, near hip approximating the table and is facing the patient's head. The therapist's near hand presses on the table above the patient's shoulder in either a knuckle or fist position (Fig. 65.5A) but there should be no downward or caudad pressure on the superior aspect of the patient's shoulder. The focus is to maintain the shoulder position during the performance of the test and prevent any shoulder elevation rather than to depress the shoulder girdle passively. With the other hand, the therapist holds the patient's hand with the thumb extended to apply tension to the motor branch of the median nerve. The therapist's fingers wrap around the patient's fingers distal to the metacarpophalangeal joints. The patient's elbow is flexed at 90° and supported on the therapist's near (front) thigh (Fig. 65.5B).

The movements performed in sequence are glenohumeral abduction up to 90–110°, if available, in the frontal plane. This is followed by wrist and finger extension and forearm supination. Then, glenohumeral external rotation is added to the available range, although this is generally stopped at 90° if the patient is very mobile. The next component of the test is elbow extension and this should be done gently and with care not to cause any shoulder motion, especially adduction, which would thereby ease off the developing neurodynamic test (Fig. 65.5C). After the addition of each component the patient is asked to relate any and all symptoms that may be evoked. Attention is paid to differences in the test response between the involved and uninvolved sides, and may include asymmetries in the resistance perceived by the examiner in the range of motion available or the sensory response. The final component of the test involves structural differentiation with cervical spine movements. The selection of the proper structural differentiation motion will be based on where the symptoms (if any) are located. If distal symptoms have developed (e.g. forearm and wrist pain) and are to be differentiated, the neck is moved into contralateral lateral flexion and any change in the distal symptoms would constitute a positive structural differentiation. If cervical contralateral flexion increases the symptoms and cervical ipsilateral flexion decreases the symptoms, this would constitute a positive structural differentiation and perhaps lead to a positive neurodynamic test. If proximal symptoms have developed (e.g. neck and / or shoulder pain) and are to be differentiated, the wrist is released from its extended position and, again, any change in the proximal symptoms would constitute a positive structural differentiation.

A pattern of frequently reported and observed responses has been noted in young asymptomatic subjects (Kenneally 1985). 'Stretching', 'pulling', 'pain', 'tingling' and 'numbing' are commonly reported sensations even in subjects who are asymptomatic prior to the test. Kenneally and Rubenach (1988) summarized the responses of 400 asymptomatic individuals to the ULNT1 as follows:

- A deep stretch or ache was felt in the cubital fossa (99% of volunteers) extending down the anterior and radial aspect of the forearm and into the radial side of the hand.
- A definite tingling sensation was felt in the thumb and first three fingers.
- A stretch was felt (by a small percentage) in the anterior shoulder.
- Cervical lateral flexion away from the side tested increased evoked responses in 90% of subjects.
- Cervical lateral flexion towards the side tested decreased the test response in 70% of subjects.

Indications for the ULNT1

A therapist would consider using the ULNT1 in their clinic where, after detailed subjective evaluation, objective examination and evaluation, there is an hypothesis of neurogenic pain in the upper limb, or that the source of the disorder lies in the median nerve pathways and receptive fields. Alternatively, the patient may have indicated a pain-provoking movement or position that is similar to the test (e.g. hanging washing on the line) or a part of the test (e.g. forearm pronation and supination).

ULNT2 (median) active test

In some cases, it may not be possible or appropriate to abduct the shoulder and this is where the ULNT2 can be quite useful, as it uses shoulder girdle depression as the sensitizing movement. For the active test, the patient can hang their arm naturally by their side and look at the thumb (Fig. 65.6A). The therapist should have the patient point the thumb away, extend the wrist and then reach the hand down towards the floor (Fig. 65.6B). The patient can use the other hand to depress the shoulder girdle and, if necessary, can then side-bend the cervical spine away from the test side and compare responses with the other side.

ULNT2 (median) passive test

A detailed description of the ULNT2 test can be found in other texts (Butler 1991, 2000; Shacklock 2005a). Once again, the key points involved are that the patient lies supine on a slight diagonal with the shoulder just over the edge of the treatment table to allow for contact with the therapist's thigh. The therapist stands near the patient's shoulder and uses the thigh to depress the shoulder girdle carefully. The therapist's right hand cradles the patient's left elbow and the left hand controls the patient's wrist and hand. The patient's arm is in approximately 10° of abduction (Fig. 65.7A). The second component of the test is elbow extension and then whole-arm external rotation (Fig. 65.7B). Next, wrist and finger extension are added, and some specific handholds as suggested by various authors (Butler 2000; Shacklock 2005a) (Fig. 65.7C). Throughout this test, as each component is added, the patient is asked to relate any and all symptoms that may be evoked. Glenohumeral abduction is then added if necessary. In most cases, there will be sufficient symptoms evoked without adding abduction, and structural differentiation can be achieved through cervical contralateral lateral flexion. Once again, for positive structural differentiation, the therapist is looking for alteration of evoked symptoms by the addition or subtraction of test components distant to the symptoms. If symptoms were reported distally (e.g. in the forearm and / or wrist) then a change in the symptoms with cervical movements (increase with contralateral lateral flexion and decrease with ipsilateral lateral flexion) would represent positive structural differentiation.

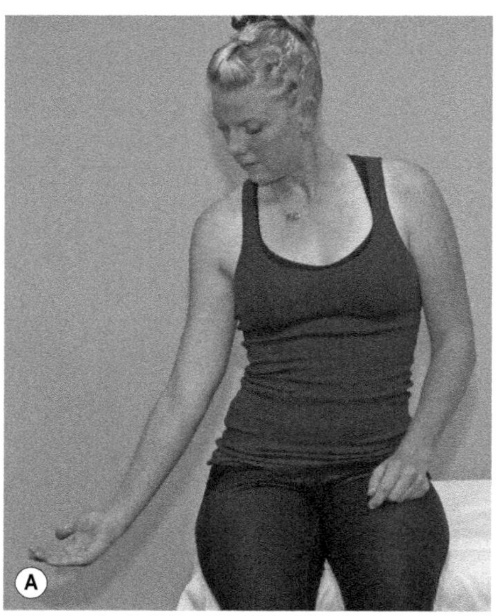

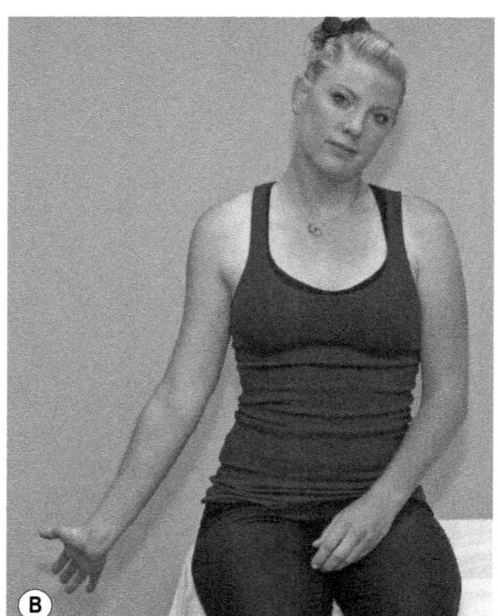

Figure 65.6 Active ULNT2 – median nerve. With the arm by the side, have the patient point the thumb away (**A**), then extend the wrist and reach the hand down towards the floor (**B**). Side-bending away from the affected side can be added, as well as shoulder depression and abduction.

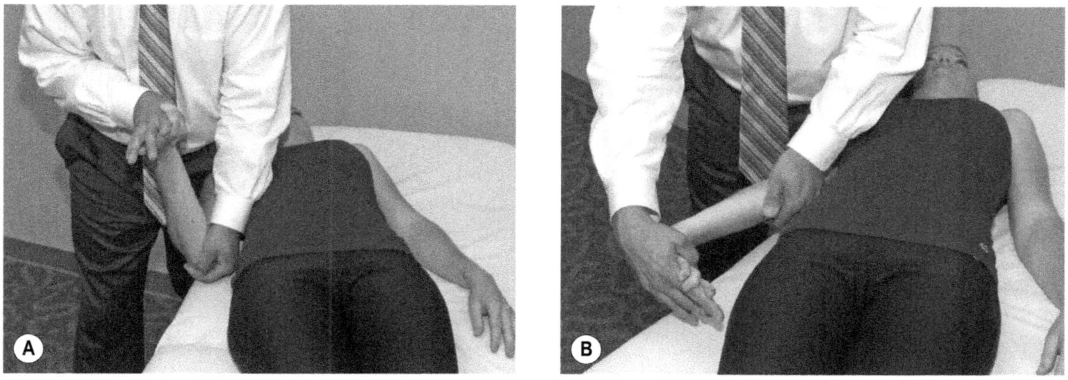

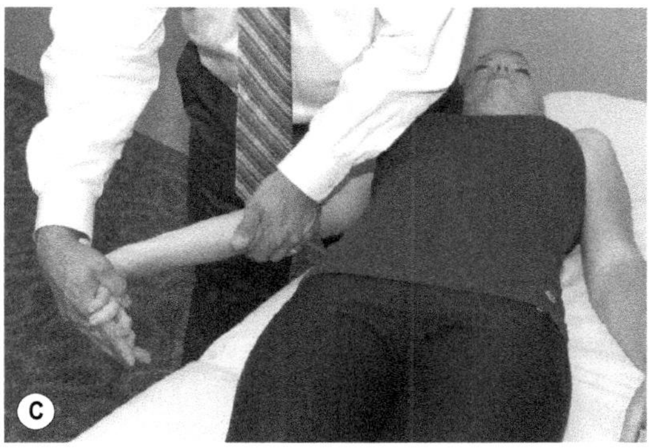

Figure 65.7 Passive ULNT2 – median nerve. Introduce shoulder girdle depression with the hip while supporting the patient's elbow with your inside hand and the patient's wrist and hand with your outside hand (**A**). The elbow is then extended, and the whole arm is externally rotated. Finally, the forearm is fully supinated, the wrist and fingers are extended (**B**) and the arm is slowly abducted (**C**) to symptom tolerance. Cervical side-bending away from (sensitizing movement) or towards (differentiating movement) the affected side can be introduced.

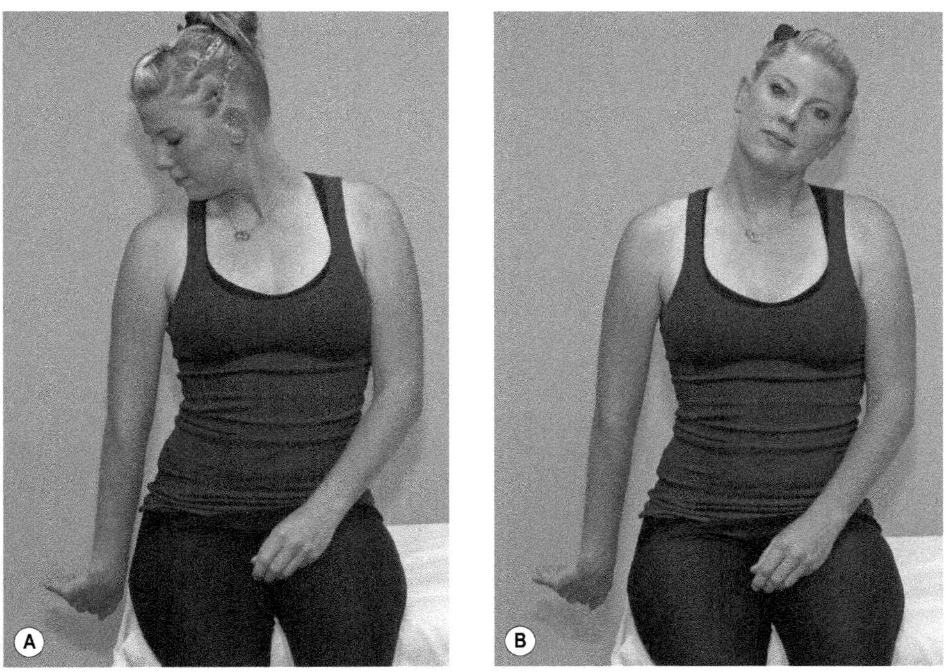

Figure 65.8 Active ULNT2 – radial nerve. With the arm by the side, have the patient flex the wrist, look at the palm and then internally rotate the arm so that he/she can look at the palm over the shoulder (**A**). Shoulder depression and abduction can be added, as well as contralateral cervical side-bending (**B**).

ULNT2 (radial) active test

There are many ways to have the patient perform an active ULNT2 (radial) test. The most common method is to have the patient hold the arm to their side, flex the wrist, look at the palm and then internally rotate the arm so that he / she can look at the palm over the shoulder (Fig. 65.8A). The patient can then depress and abduct the shoulder and look away to introduce contralateral cervical side-bending, if needed (Fig. 65.8B). Symptoms evoked during the performance of the active test may obviate the need for performing the test passively.

ULNT2 (radial) passive test

Further detailed descriptions of this test can be found in other texts (Butler 1991, 2000; Shacklock 2005a). The key points involved in this test, much like ULNT2 (median), are that the

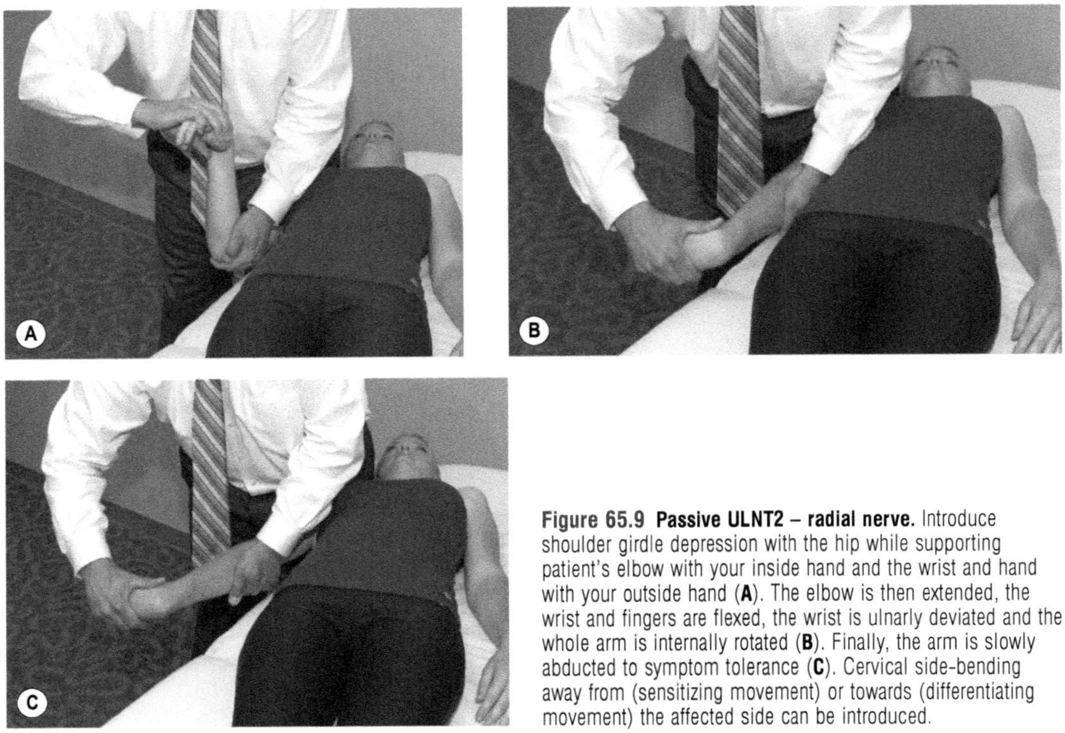

Figure 65.9 Passive ULNT2 – radial nerve. Introduce shoulder girdle depression with the hip while supporting patient's elbow with your inside hand and the wrist and hand with your outside hand (**A**). The elbow is then extended, the wrist and fingers are flexed, the wrist is ulnarly deviated and the whole arm is internally rotated (**B**). Finally, the arm is slowly abducted to symptom tolerance (**C**). Cervical side-bending away from (sensitizing movement) or towards (differentiating movement) the affected side can be introduced.

patient lies supine on a slight diagonal with the shoulder just over the edge of the treatment table to allow for contact with the therapist's thigh. The therapist stands near the patient's shoulder and uses the thigh to depress the shoulder girdle carefully. The therapist's right hand cradles the patient's left elbow and the left hand controls the patient's wrist and hand. The patient's arm is in approximately 10° of abduction (Fig. 65.9A). The second component of the test is elbow extension and then whole-arm internal rotation (Fig. 65.9B). Next, wrist and finger flexion is added, and it may be appropriate also to add in wrist ulnar deviation and thumb flexion (Fig. 65.9C). As with all the neurodynamic tests, as each component is added, the patient is asked to relate any and all symptoms that may be evoked. Glenohumeral abduction can be added if necessary, but, as with ULNT2 (median), in most cases there will be sufficient symptoms evoked without adding abduction, and structural differentiation can be achieved through cervical contralateral lateral flexion.

Yaxley and Jull (1991) investigated the most common responses to the ULNT2 (radial) test in 50 asymptomatic 18–30-year-old individuals. Their findings were a strong painful stretch over the radial aspect of the proximal forearm (84% of all responses), often accompanied by a stretch pain in the lateral aspect of the upper arm (32%), biceps brachii (14%) or the dorsal aspect of the hand (12%). Such a symptom response area would make the radial nerve at the elbow a candidate for a source of pain (Butler 2000).

ULNT3 (ulnar) active test

The active ULNT3 (ulnar) can be performed by asking the patient to look at the hand and hold it up as though holding a tray of drinks (in wrist extension) (Fig. 65.10A). Further loading can then be added by having the patient look away, add more elbow flexion, depress the shoulder girdle and add in forearm pronation (Fig. 65.10B). Cervical spine retraction is also thought to be another worthwhile sensitizing movement (Butler 2000). In patients with a good range of movement, and especially in younger flexible patients, the therapist can have them attempt the 'mask' position.

ULNT3 (ulnar) passive test

As with ULNT1 (median), this test has the patient lying supine, arms by the side, shoulder close to the edge of the examination table, without a pillow if possible, and with body straight. The therapist stands with the near foot placed forward, near hip approximating the table and facing the patient's head. The therapist's near hand presses on the table above the patient's shoulder in either a knuckled or fist position and this time applies a downward or caudad pressure on the superior aspect of the patient's shoulder to achieve shoulder girdle depression. With the other hand, the therapist holds the patient's hand, palm against palm, and the elbow starts in flexion (Fig. 65.11A). The wrist and fingers are extended (with perhaps some radial deviation) as the elbow is flexed. The forearm is then pronated and the shoulder taken into lateral rotation and abduction (Fig. 65.11B). This is achieved by the therapist 'walking' around the point of the patient's elbow within the groin. The final components added can be cervical contralateral lateral flexion or shoulder girdle depression, depending upon the symptoms evoked and structural differentiation. Flanagan (1993) reported normal values for this distal-to-proximal sequencing of the test and found that 82% of individuals reported responses in the hypothenar eminence and medial two fingers, and 64% reported pins and needles in the same area.

The ULNT3 (ulnar) test is often performed from proximal to distal, with shoulder girdle depression and shoulder abduction followed by shoulder external rotation, then elbow

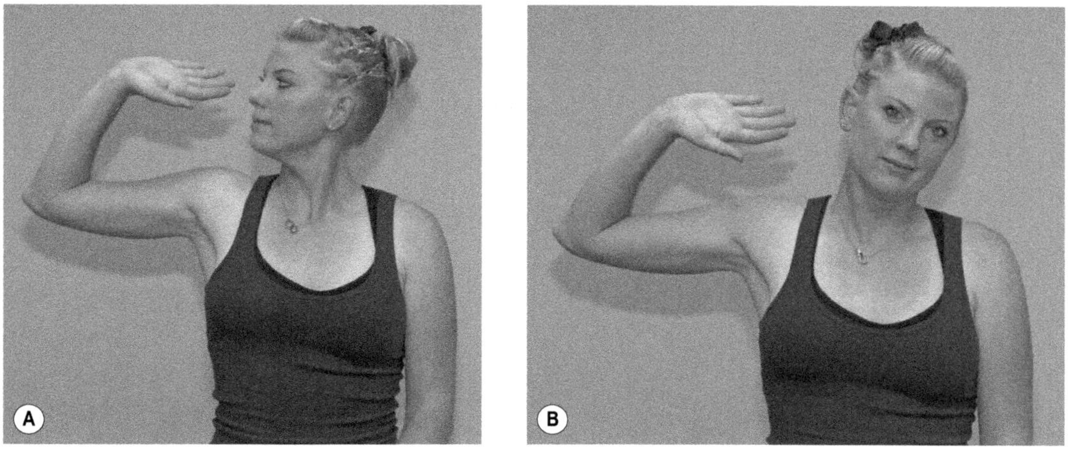

Figure 65.10 Active ULNT3 – ulnar nerve. The patient is asked to look at the hand and hold it up as though holding a tray of drinks (in wrist extension, as depicted in **A**). The nerve can be further challenged by increasing elbow flexion and contralateral cervical side-bending (**B**).

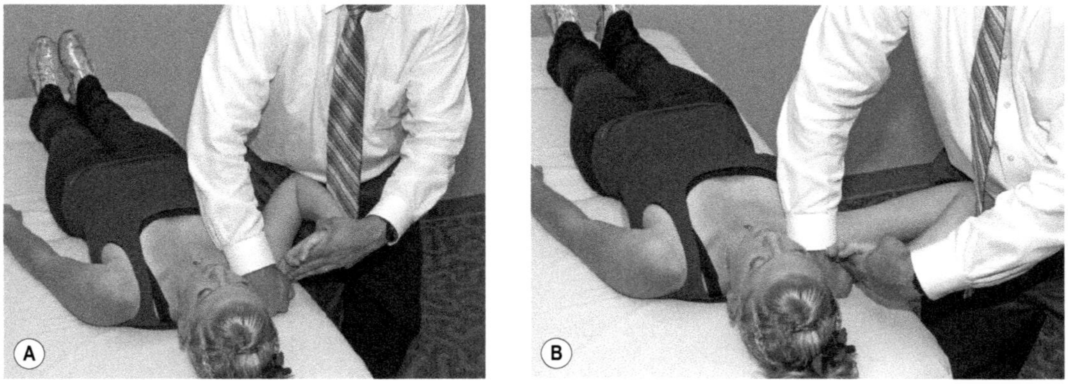

Figure 65.11 Passive ULNT3 – ulnar nerve. Face the patient and block the shoulder to prevent shoulder girdle elevation. The elbow is then flexed and stabilized by the therapist's hip. Wrist and finger extension is then introduced along with full pronation, radial deviation and shoulder external rotation (**A**). The shoulder is then abducted through the frontal plane to tolerance (**B**). Cervical side-bending away from (sensitizing movement) or towards (differentiating movement) the affected side can be introduced.

flexion and finally wrist and finger extension with forearm pronation. Butler (2000) has suggested that, in order to standardize the base test system, clinicians should make all the tests start from the shoulder girdle.

Neurodynamic testing for the lower quadrant

The tests for the lower quadrant include the slump test and the straight leg raise (SLR) test with multiple variations. They have been derived through attention to the major neural pathways and the major sensitizing movements, just as in the upper quadrant. Three specific tests will now be described in detail: the SLR, the slump test and the side-lying slump test.

Straight leg raise active test

If the patient has described a symptom-provoking position or movement, the therapist should have him / her demonstrate it and observe the mechanics involved. In this case, a patient may report posterior thigh symptoms associated with kicking the leg forward. If possible, a quick structural differentiation is performed. For example, the patient may demonstrate a symptomatic position for the posterior thigh pain, and the patient could be asked to maintain that thigh position and then to move the neck to see whether that alters the thigh symptoms.

A simple protocol for the active evaluation of the SLR test would be to have the patient walking or swinging the leg; alternatively, one could have the patient lay supine and actively elevate the leg while keeping the knee extended.

Straight leg raise passive test

A detailed description of the SLR test is available in other texts (Butler 2000; Shacklock 2005a). The key points involved are that the patient lies in supine position, with arms by the side, and tested side close to the edge of the examination table, without a pillow if possible, and with body straight. The therapist should face the patient and then place one hand under the ankle and the other hand above the patella (Fig. 65.12A). Care should be taken to avoid pressure on the superficial peripheral nerves about the ankle. Keeping the knee extended, the therapist should flex the hip in the perpendicular plane (avoiding hip abduction or adduction) (Fig. 65.12B). The patient's leg should be taken short of, to, or into sensory or motor responses depending on clinical reasoning (Butler 2000). The final component of the test (structural differentiation) may often be overlooked by clinicians. If distal symptoms have developed (e.g. calf or heel) and are to be differentiated, the patient can be asked to flex or an assistant could passively flex the cervical spine (Fig. 65.12C) and any change in the distal symptoms would constitute a positive structural differentiation. If cervical flexion increases these symptoms and cervical extension decreases these symptoms, this would constitute a positive structural differentiation and perhaps lead to a positive neurodynamic test. If proximal symptoms have developed (e.g. buttock or posterior thigh)

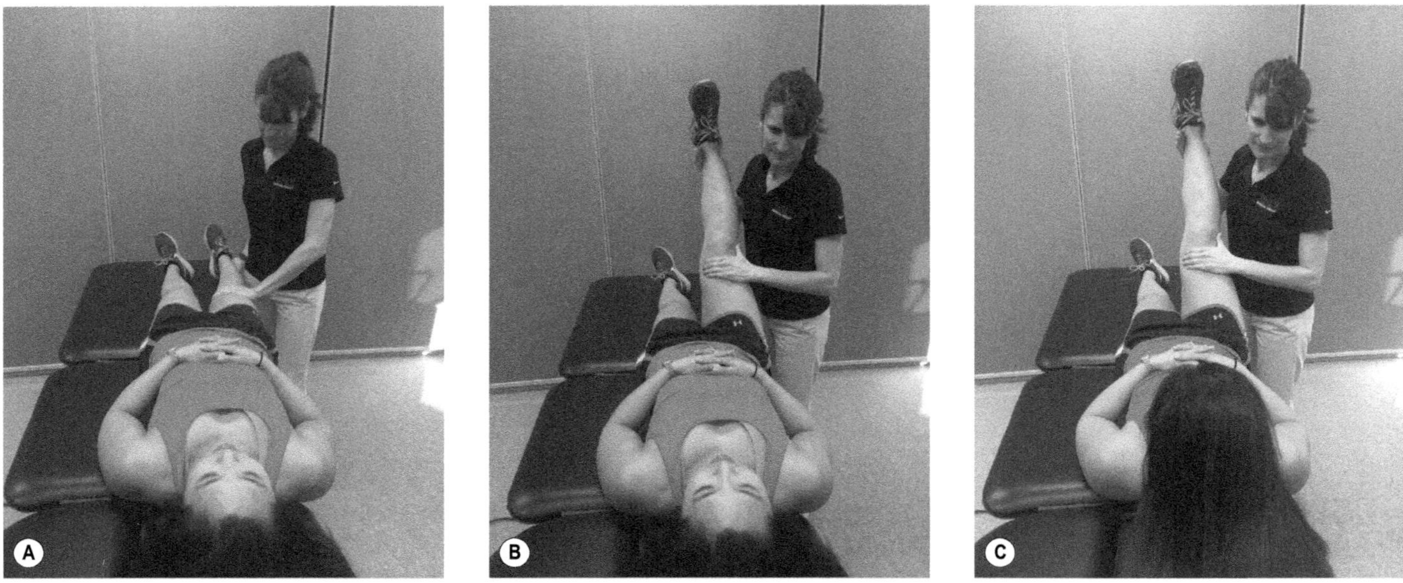

Figure 65.12 Passive straight leg raise. Face the patient and place the inside hand under the ankle and the outside hand above the patella (**A**). Slowly raise the leg into hip flexion without moving in the frontal plane (avoid hip abduction or adduction) to symptom tolerance (**B**). Cervical flexion (sensitizing movement) may be added (**C**); alternatively, cervical extension (differentiating movement) may be added.

and are to be differentiated, the ankle may be dorsiflexed and, again, any change in the proximal symptoms would constitute a positive structural differentiation.

Other frequently used sensitizing movements include hip adduction and / or hip medial rotation (which are thought to lengthen the sciatic nerve as it exits the sciatic foramen), ankle dorsiflexion (which is thought to lengthen the tibial and plantar nerves) and ankle plantarflexion with inversion (which is thought to lengthen the superficial fibular nerve). However, there is little evidence that these sensitizing movements create any greater tension or stress on the peripheral nerves that they target.

A pattern of frequently reported and observed responses includes posterior thigh, posterior knee and posterior calf symptoms extending to the foot (Slater et al 1994). These responses may indicate neural mechanosensitivity and result in protective muscle contraction of the hamstrings. In a recent review article, Weppler and Magnusson (2010) suggested that observed changes in tissue flexibility following hamstring stretching may result, not from affecting the mechanical properties of the muscle being stretched, but from changes in the individual's perception of stretch or pain.

Indications for the straight leg raise test

A therapist would consider using the SLR test in the clinic where, after detailed subjective evaluation, objective examination and evaluation, there is an hypothesis of neurogenic pain in the lower limb, or that the source of the disorder lies in the sciatic nerve pathways and receptive fields. Alternatively, the patient may have indicated a pain-provoking movement or position that is similar to the test (e.g. kicking a football).

Slump test

A detailed description of the slump test is available in other texts (Butler 1991, 2000; Shacklock 2005a). It is sometimes thought of as the SLR test in a seated position, so that head, neck and trunk movements can be added to load tissues further and input into the CNS. The test components should be performed actively with instruction from the therapist, and, if required, some components may be performed passively.

The key points involved are that the patient should start by sitting up straight with thighs well supported and ankles uncrossed (Fig. 65.13A). Hands behind the back are not absolutely necessary, but this may help with consistency of test performance. The patient is then asked to slump or 'sag in the middle back' while still looking forward (Fig. 65.13B). This is the first component of the test and should be performed without cervical motion to assess symptom response, if any. The second component is cervical flexion and the patient should be asked to move as far into his / her range as possible (Fig. 65.13C). No therapist overpressure need be applied at all. The response, if any, is assessed. Now the patient is asked to extend the knee (on the less- or non-painful side first) and again the symptom response is assessed (Fig. 65.13D). In most cases, patients may report central T8–T9 area symptoms when cervical flexion is added; they will be unable to extend their leg fully into knee extension owing to symptoms in the posterior thigh, and knee symptoms will ease when the cervical spine is extended (Fig. 65.13E) (Butler 1991).

The slump test may be sensitized by the addition of foot and ankle dorsiflexion, hip flexion and performing the test with the other leg already extended. The order of movements can also be varied to suit clinical reasoning.

Side-lying slump test

The side-lying slump test can be considered an extension of the prone knee bend (PKB) test. In the PKB test, the patient is prone close to the side of the treatment table and is asked to flex the knee actively without flexing the hip. Some studies have reported a positive PKB in the presence of upper lumbar disc herniation (Asquier et al 1996; Kreitz et al 1996); however,

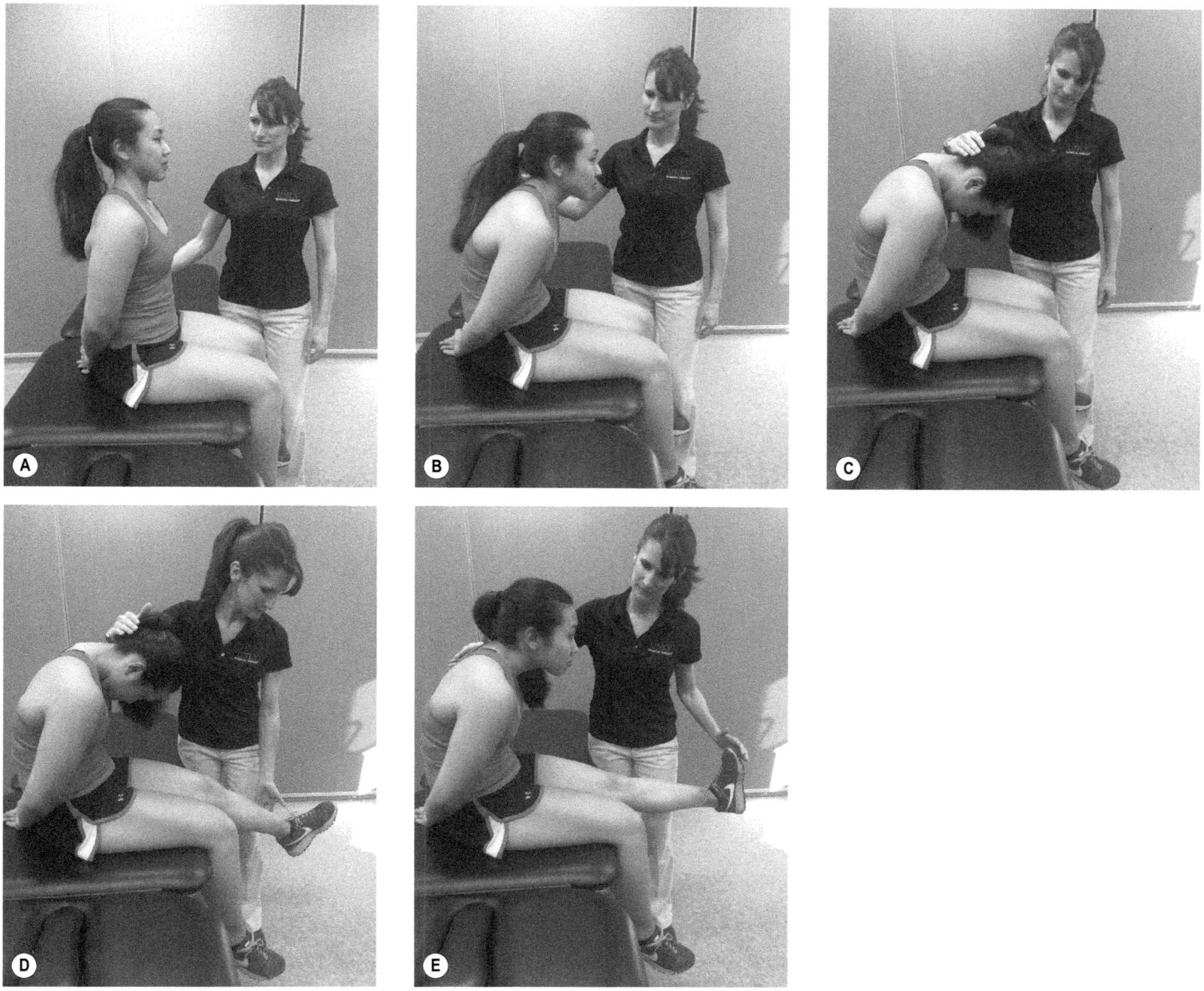

Figure 65.13 Slump test. The patient should be sitting upright with thighs well supported, ankles uncrossed and hands comfortably behind the back (**A**). Have the patient slump or 'sag the middle back' while still looking forward (**B**) and note the symptom response. Next, have the patient flex the cervical spine (**C**) and note the symptom response. Then, ask the patient to extend the knee (less- or non-painful side first) and again assess the symptom response (**D**). The final component is the release of cervical flexion (**E**) and noting any change in symptoms. The therapist should apply only light contact throughout the movement components.

the test is limited by the inability to differentiate symptom responses structurally. By placing the patient in side-lying, additional loading can be placed on the PKB by spinal flexion.

The patient is asked to hold the knee on the side on which he / she is lying, and is encouraged to touch it with the forehead to prompt cervical flexion (Fig. 65.14A). The therapist stands behind the patient and flexes the superior-side knee so that the ankle is resting on the hip and places a hand under the knee to support the leg. The therapist then stabilizes the pelvis with the other hand, and introduces hip extension to the point of evoked symptoms (Fig. 65.14B). If that position is held, the therapist can then assess symptom response to changes in head and neck movements (cervical extension) (Fig. 65.14C).

Clinical Application of Neurodynamics in Upper and Lower Quadrants

An important consideration always to keep in mind is that healthy mechanics of the nervous system enables pain-free posture and movement. In the presence of mechanical impairment (pathomechanics) of neural tissues (e.g. nerve entrapment), symptoms may be provoked during activities of daily living such as combing one's hair or bending down to reach the floor. The aim of using neurodynamic tests in assessment is to stimulate the nervous system mechanically by moving

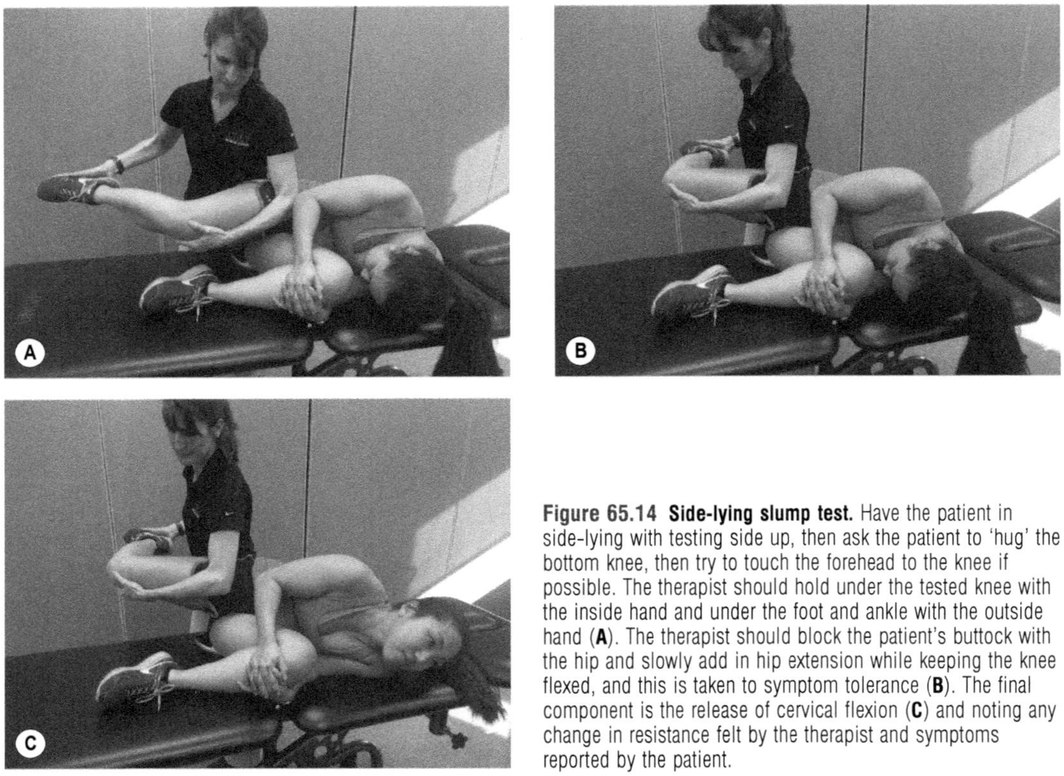

Figure 65.14 Side-lying slump test. Have the patient in side-lying with testing side up, then ask the patient to 'hug' the bottom knee, then try to touch the forehead to the knee if possible. The therapist should hold under the tested knee with the inside hand and under the foot and ankle with the outside hand (**A**). The therapist should block the patient's buttock with the hip and slowly add in hip extension while keeping the knee flexed, and this is taken to symptom tolerance (**B**). The final component is the release of cervical flexion (**C**) and noting any change in resistance felt by the therapist and symptoms reported by the patient.

neural tissues in order to gain an impression of their mobility and sensitivity to mechanical stresses. The purpose of treatment via these tests is to improve their mechanical and physiological function (Shacklock 2005a).

Mechanosensitivity is the chief mechanism that enables nerves to cause pain with movement. If a nerve is not mechanically sensitive, then it won't respond (cause pain) to mechanical forces applied to it. Mechanosensitivity can be defined as the ease with which impulses can be activated from a site in the nervous system when a mechanical force is applied. Normal nerves can be mechanosensitive (given sufficient force) and therefore respond to applied forces (Lindquist et al 1973). This is a key fact to keep in mind when making judgements about whether or not the neural tissues within the cervical spine and upper limb are a problem. Responses to neurodynamic tests in the upper limb are either normal or abnormal, and then either relevant or irrelevant (Shacklock 2005a). Normal neurodynamic test responses would be considered to be those that are in a normal location (relative to normative data), with normal quality of symptoms, and with normal range of movement for the upper / lower extremity. Abnormal neurodynamic test responses would be considered as those that are in a different location to normal, with different quality of symptoms and / or with a lesser range of movement of the limb than in the uninvolved side. In most cases, there may be reproduction of the patient's symptoms. The second clinical question to consider would be whether the test responses are relevant or irrelevant. Relevance, in this case, would mean that the test responses are causally related to the patient's current problem, and an irrelevant finding would be where the test responses are not causally related to the patient's current problem. Many times this can be elucidated by asking the patient 'Is that a familiar symptom to you?'

The symptoms evoked on a neurodynamic test can be inferred to be neurogenic (positive test in a clinical sense):

- if structural differentiation supports a neurogenic source
- if there are differences left to right and to known normal responses
- if the test reproduces the patient's symptoms or associated symptoms
- if there is support from other data such as history, area of symptoms, imaging tests, etc.

The greater the number of 'ifs' present, the stronger is the case for a clinically relevant test. Clinically, the information required from neurodynamic tests is symptom response, resistance encountered and changes to symptom response and resistance encountered as each component of the test is added or subtracted. This information, along with the patient history, subjective and objective examination, etc., should give the clinician the ability to diagnose provisionally the site of neuropathodynamics and then reassess this diagnosis after whatever treatment might be administered. It is important to realize that the treatment need not be a mobilizing technique for the nervous system, as the clinician may decide to mobilize or treat the mechanical interface, or may perhaps decide that the problem is not peripheral neurogenic in nature, but rather a 'central-processing enhancement' in which patient education / reassurance / discussion may be the treatment of choice. It is also important to remember that sensitivity to a neurodynamic test could be from a combination of primary (tissue-based) and secondary (CNS-based) processes (reference).

Treatment

In a randomized controlled trial, Tal-Akabi and Rushton (2000) compared neural mobilizations, joint mobilizations and no treatment in patients with carpal tunnel syndrome (CTS), and found that both interventions were more effective than no treatment at reducing pain and ultimate need for surgery. In contrast to the above study, Heebner and Roddey (2008) reported that the addition of neural mobilization to standard care did not result in improved outcomes in patients with CTS. Neural mobilizations in the upper quarter as part of a multimodal treatment approach have also been utilized with success in patients with cervical radiculopathy (Coppieters et al 2003a, 2003b; Cleland et al 2005; Costello 2008; Young et al 2009), lateral epicondylalgia (Vicenzino et al 1996, 1998, 1999a) and cubital tunnel syndrome (Coppieters et al 2004).

Management of a neuropathic arm should focus on reducing mechanosensitivity and restoring normal movement to both the nervous tissue and its mechanical interface (De-la-Llave-Rincón et al 2011). Reassessment should be continual, and include clinical evaluation along with patient feedback. We believe that patient education is paramount, and should include a brief discussion of neurodynamics, the neurobiology of pain and the continuity of the nervous system. Additionally, if there is a central sensitization component to the symptoms, this should also be addressed, along with any perceived or real fear of movement the patient may have. This info can reduce the threat value associated with their pain experience. (See Ch 6 for further information on patient education.)

Next, we have found it useful to treat any impairment in non-neural tissues so as to reduce any mechanical forces the 'container' may be placing on the nervous tissue. Interventions utilized may include joint mobilization / manipulation, stretching, soft tissue work and therapeutic exercise. Detailed discussion of these interventions is beyond the scope of this chapter and is covered in other chapters of the current textbook. Any of the above interventions, if utilized, should be followed by a reassessment of the provocative neurodynamic test to determine whether change has occurred. If it has, then treatment may be discontinued for that day, or specific neurodynamic interventions (either active or passive) may be added to the treatment.

We like to break neurodynamic interventions down further into one of two approaches –'sliders' and 'tensioners' – each of which has its own indications and clinical usefulness (Nee & Butler 2006; Coppieters & Butler 2008). With a sliding or gliding technique, combined movements of at least two joints are alternated in such a way that one movement elongates the nerve bed while the other movement shortens the nerve bed. This results in a situation where the nerve is mobilized through a large degree of longitudinal excursion with a minimum amount of tension. These techniques should be non-provocative, and may be more tolerable to patients than tensioning techniques. For example, abundant literature supports the use of cervical lateral glide mobilizations (Fig. 65.15) to effect changes in neck and / or arm symptoms (Vicenzino et al 1998, 1999a, 1999b; Cowell & Phillips 2002; Coppieters et al 2003b; Cleland et al 2005; Costello 2008; Young et al 2009) as this intervention has been shown to produce immediate

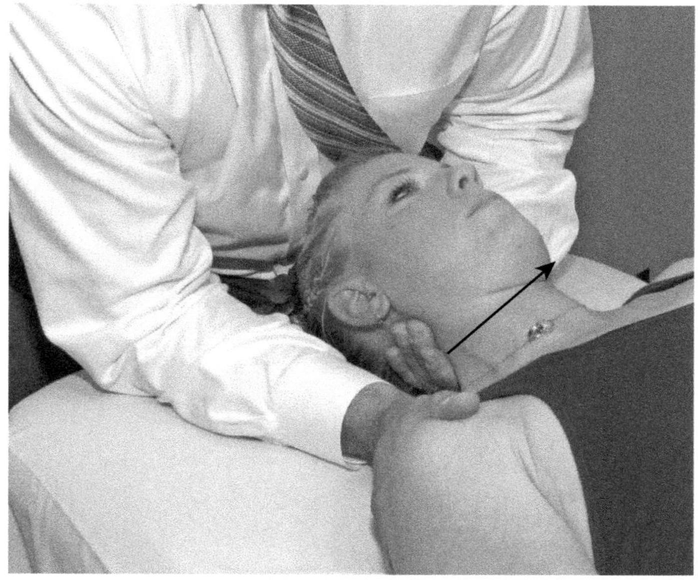

Figure 65.15 The cervical lateral glide technique (Elvey 1986). The hand used to perform the lateral glides is the hand opposite to the patient's affected side. The motion (arrow) should be purely transverse, away from the affected side, and the clinician's other hand is used to stabilize (rather than depress) the scapula on the affected side. The arm can also be placed in a ULNT position (Vicenzino et al 1999).

reductions in mechanosensitivity and pain in patients with lateral epicondylalgia (Vicenzino et al 1996) and cervicobrachial pain (Elvey 1986; Cowell & Phillips 2002; Coppieters et al 2003b). This can be done with or without the arm in the ULNT position.

Elvey (1986) reported that gliding techniques were more effective than no intervention at reducing pain and disability in patients with cervicobrachial pain, and was more effective than manual therapy directed at the shoulder and thoracic spine in reducing pain in these patients. Furthermore, Rozmaryn et al (1998) reported in a non-randomized controlled trial that the addition of neural gliding techniques to conservative management of patients with CTS reduced the need for surgery by 29.8%. An example of a passive slide mobilization for the median nerve would include positioning the patient's arm in 90–110° of abduction with 90° of shoulder external rotation, with the elbow flexed to 90°, and with wrist and finger extension and forearm supination (Fig. 65.16A). Next, to 'slide' the median nerve passively, wrist extension could be relaxed as the elbow is extended (distal slider), or the cervical spine could be actively side-bent to the ipsilateral side as the elbow is extended (proximal slider) (Fig. 65.16B). This could also be given as an active technique to be performed by the patient at home (Fig. 65.17A–B). Similarly, there is growing preliminary evidence that lower extremity neurodynamic sliding interventions lead to short-term increases in posterior thigh flexibility (Castellote-Caballero et al 2013).

With a tensioning technique, elongation of the nerve bed is obtained by moving one or several joints such that the 'tension' within the nerve is elevated (Coppieters & Butler 2008). These techniques are, by nature, more stressful to the neural tissue and should be used with caution as they may irritate the mechanosensitive patient. They are not static

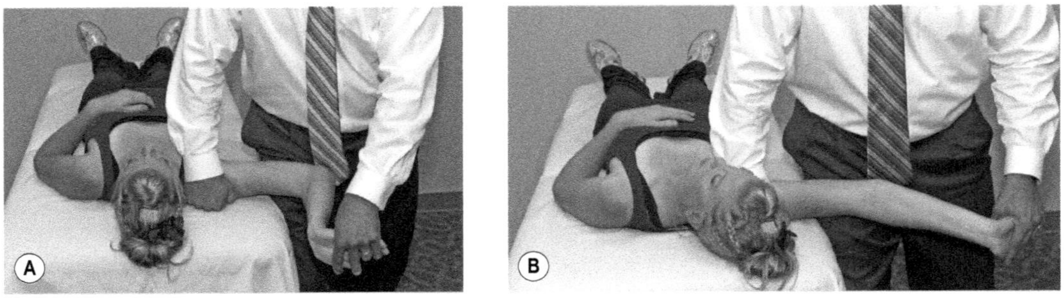

Figure 65.16 Passive 'slider' technique for the median nerve utilizing ULNT1 (median nerve). The patient is set up just prior to the onset of symptoms as per the passive ULNT1 (median nerve) passive test (**A**). Next, to 'slide' the median nerve, the cervical spine is actively side-bent to the ipsilateral side as the clinician extends the elbow (**B**). These movements are then reversed in sequence.

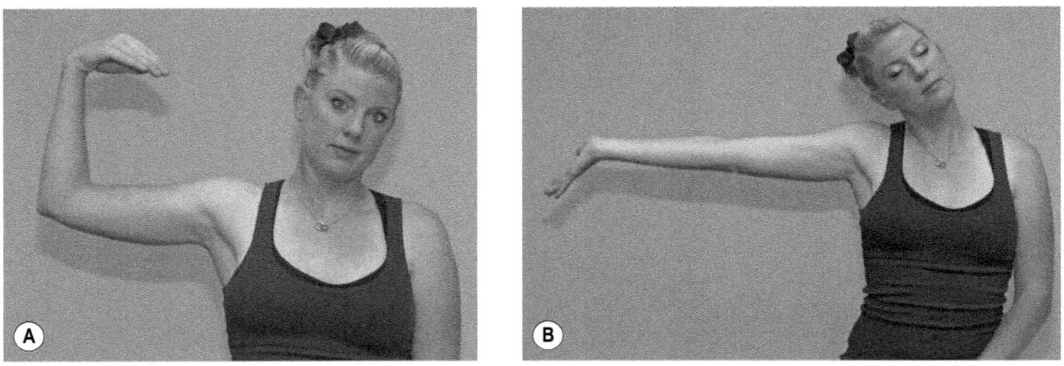

Figure 65.17 Active 'slider' technique for the median nerve utilizing ULNT1 (median nerve). The patient's arm is positioned in 90–110° of abduction with 90° of shoulder external rotation, with the elbow flexed to 90°, and with the wrist and fingers flexed with forearm supination (**A**). Next, to 'slide' the median nerve, the cervical spine is actively side-bent to the ipsilateral side as the patient actively extends the elbow and the wrist (**B**).

stretches and always involve gentle oscillations into and out of resistance. These techniques are generally indicated for patients who experience symptoms as a result of impairments in the neural tissue's ability to elongate; hence the goal is to restore the physical capabilities of the neural tissue to tolerate movement. The tension is increased to the point of a mild stretching sensation, or, in the case of non-irritable patients, may be taken to the onset of mild symptoms at the end of the oscillation. Any of the active or passive neurodynamic tests can be used as 'tensioners'. Kornberg and Lew (1989) conducted a comparative study involving 28 Australian Rules football players with grade I hamstring injuries. Sixteen were treated according to traditional methods, while 12 were given slump stretching (tensioners) as an addition to the traditional treatments. Results indicated that players receiving slump stretching returned to full function sooner.

Sets and repetitions are determined by the irritability of the patients as well as the response (positive or negative) to the interventions. We have found that starting with one to three sets of ten oscillations is useful, followed by a reassessment of the ULNT to determine whether the interventions have had any effect. Finally, techniques aimed at non-neural structures can be combined with neurodynamic interventions, such as the cervical lateral glide technique while holding the arm in a ULNT position (Vicenzino et al 1998, 1999b; Cowell & Phillips 2002; Coppieters et al 2003b; Cleland et al 2005; Young et al 2009).

Conclusion

Clinicians should keep in mind the underlying principles of neurobiomechanics – that is, the nervous system is a continuous tract that is subject to slide, glide, bend and stretch as it travels through its mechanical interface. Symptoms can arise as a result of intrinsic or extrinsic impairments anywhere along this tortuous course. Clinicians can render meaningful interventions that have a direct impact on the space, movement and blood supply for the nervous system, in addition to producing beneficial neurophysiological effects. Neurodynamic interventions (either passive or active) should involve smooth, controlled, gentle, large-amplitude movements. Sustained stretching is rarely indicated. Finally, we caution readers that neurodynamic interventions are but a small part of an overall patient-centred treatment approach that encompasses multiple interventions.

References

Asbury AK, Fields HL. 1984. Pain due to peripheral nerve damage: an hypothesis. Neurology 34: 1587–1590.

Asquier C, Troussier B, Chirossel JP, et al. 1996. Femoral neuralgia due to degenerative spinal disease: a retrospective clinical and radio-anatomical study of one hundred cases. Rev Rhum Engl Ed 63: 278–284.

Barry SR. 1991. Clinical implications of basic neuroscience research. I: Protein kinases, ionic channels, and genes. Arch Phys Med Rehabil 72: 998–1008.

Beith ID, Robins EJ, Richards P. 1995. An assessment of the adaptive mechanisms within and surrounding the peripheral nervous system, during changes in nerve bed length resulting from underlying joint movement. In: Shacklock MO (ed) Moving in on pain. Melbourne, Australia: Butterworth-Heinemann, pp 194–203.
Boyd BS, Dilley A. 2014. Altered tibial nerve biomechanics in patients with diabetes mellitus. Muscle Nerve 50(2): 216–223. doi:10.1002/mus.24155.
Boyd BS, Gray AT, Dilley A, et al. 2012. The pattern of tibial nerve excursion with active ankle dorsiflexion is different in older people with diabetes mellitus. Clin Biomech 27: 967–971.
Breig A. 1960. Biomechanics of the central nervous system. Stockholm: Almqvist and Wiksell.
Breig A. 1978. Adverse mechanical tension in the central nervous system. Stockholm: Almqvist and Wiksell.
Breig A, El-Nadi AF. 1966. Biomechanics of the cervical spinal cord. Relief of contact pressure on and overstretching of the spinal cord. Acta Radiol Diagn (Stockh) 4: 602–624.
Breig A, Marions O. 1963. Biomechanics of the lumbosacral nerve roots. Acta Radiol Diagn (Stockh) 1: 1141–1160.
Breig A, Troup J. 1979. Biomechanical considerations in the straight leg raising test. Spine 4: 242–250.
Breig A, Turnbull I, Hassler O. 1966. Effects of mechanical stresses on the spinal cord in cervical spondylosis: a study on fresh cadaver material. J Neurosurg 25: 45–56.
Butler DS. 1991. Mobilisation of the nervous system. Melbourne: Churchill Livingstone.
Butler DS. 2000. The sensitive nervous system. Adelaide: NOI Publications.
Butler DS, Moseley GL. 2003. Explain pain. Adelaide: NOI Publications.
Calvin WH, Devor M, Howe JF. 1982. Can neuralgias arise from minor demyelination? Spontaneous firing, mechanosensitivity, and after discharge from conducting axons. Exp Neurol 75: 755–763.
Castellote-Caballero Y, Valenza MC, Martin-Martin L, et al. 2013. Effects of a neurodynamic sliding technique on hamstring flexibility in healthy male soccer players: a pilot study. Phys Ther Sport 14: 156–162.
Chang SB, Lee SH, Ahn Y, et al. 2006. Risk factor for unsatisfactory outcome after lumbar foraminal and far lateral microdecompression. Spine 31: 1163–1167.
Cleland JA, Whitman JM, Fritz JM, et al. 2005. Manual physical therapy, cervical traction, and strengthening exercises in patients with cervical radiculopathy: a case series. J Orthop Sports Phys Ther 35: 802–811.
Coppieters MW, Butler DS. 2008. Do 'sliders' slide and 'tensioners' tension? An analysis of neurodynamic techniques and considerations regarding their application. Man Ther 13: 213–221.
Coppieters MW, Stappaerts KH, Wouters LL, et al. 2003a. Aberrant protective force generation during neural provocation testing and the effect of treatment in patients with neurogenic cervicobrachial pain. J Manipul Physiol Ther 26: 99–106.
Coppieters MW, Stappaerts KH, Wouters LL, et al. 2003b. The immediate effects of a cervical lateral glide treatment technique in patients with neurogenic cervicobrachial pain. J Orthop Sports Phys Ther 33: 369–378.
Coppieters MW, Bartholomeeusen KE, Stappaerts KH. 2004. Incorporating nerve-gliding techniques in the conservative treatment of cubital tunnel syndrome. J Manipul Physiol Ther 27: 560–568.
Coppieters MW, Hough AD, Dilley A. 2009. Different nerve-gliding exercises induce different magnitudes of median nerve longitudinal excursion: an in vivo study using dynamic ultrasound imaging. J Orthop Sports Phys Ther 39: 164–171.
Costello M. 2008. Treatment of a patient with cervical radiculopathy using thoracic spine thrust manipulation, soft tissue mobilization, and exercise. J Manual Manipul Ther 16: 129–135.
Cowell IM, Phillips DR. 2002. Effectiveness of manipulative physiotherapy for the treatment of a neurogenic cervicobrachial pain syndrome: a single case study experimental design. Man Ther 7: 31–38.
Dahlin LB, Thambert C. 1993. Acute nerve compression at low pressures has a conditioning lesion effect on rat sciatic nerves. Acta Orthop Scand 64: 479–481.
Dahlin LB, Archer DR, McLean WG. 1993. Axonal transport and morphological changes following nerve compression. An experimental study in the rabbit vagus nerve. J Hand Surg 18: 106–110.
De-la-Llave-Rincón AI, Puentedura EJ, Fernández-de-las-Penas C. 2011. Clinical presentation and manual therapy for upper quadrant musculoskeletal conditions. J Man Manipul Ther 19: 201–211.
Devor M. 1999. Unexplained peculiarities of the dorsal root ganglion. Pain Su 6: S27–S35.
Devor M. 2006. Sodium channels and mechanisms of neuropathic pain. J Pain 7: S3–S12.
Devor M, Govrin-Lippmann R, Angelides K. 1993. Na^+ channel immunolocalization in peripheral mammalian axons and changes following nerve injury and neuroma formation. J Neurosci 13: 1976–1992.
Devor M, Seltzer Z. 1999. Pathophysiology of damaged nerves in relation to chronic pain. In: Wall PD, Melzack R (eds) Textbook of pain. Edinburgh: Churchill Livingstone, pp 129–164.
Di Fabio R. 2001. Neural mobilization: the impossible. J Orthop Sports Phys Ther 31: 224–225.
Dilley A, Greening J, Lynn B, et al. 2001. The use of cross-correlation analysis between high-frequency ultrasound images to measure longitudinal median nerve movement. Ultrasound Med Biol 27: 1211–1218.
Dilley A, Lynn B, Greening J, et al. 2003. Quantitative in vivo studies of median nerve sliding in response to wrist, elbow, shoulder and neck movements. Clin Biomech 18: 899–907.
Dilley A, Summerhayes C, Lynn B. 2007. An in vivo investigation of ulnar nerve sliding during upper limb movements. Clin Biomech 22: 774–779.
Dilley A, Odeyinde S, Greening J, et al. 2008. Longitudinal sliding of the median nerve in patients with non-specific arm pain. Man Ther 13: 536–543.
Driscoll PJ, Glasby MA, Lawson GM. 2002. An in vivo study of peripheral nerves in continuity: biomechanical and physiological responses to elongation. J Orthop Res 20: 370–375.
Ellis R, Hing W, Dilley A, et al. 2008. Reliability of measuring sciatic and tibial nerve movement with diagnostic ultrasound during a neural mobilisation technique. Ultrasound Med Biol 34: 1209–1216.
Elvey RL. 1986. Treatment of arm pain associated with abnormal brachial plexus tension. Aust J Physiother 32: 225–230.
Erel E, Dilley A, Greening J, et al. 2003. Longitudinal sliding of the median nerve in patients with carpal tunnel syndrome. J Hand Surg Br 28: 439–443.
Fern R, Harrison PJ. 1994a. The contribution of ischaemia and deformation to the conduction block generated by compression of the cat sciatic nerve. Exp Physiol 79: 583–592.
Fern R, Harrison PJ. 1994b. The relationship between ischaemic conduction failure and conduction velocity in cat myelinated axons. Exp Physiol 79: 571–581.
Flanagan M. 1993. Normative responses to the ulnar nerve bias tension test. Adelaide: University of South Australia.
Hall T, Zusman M, Elvey R. 1996. Manually detected impediments in the straight leg raise test. Clinical solutions. In: Proceedings of the Ninth Biennial Conference of the Manipulative Physiotherapists' Association of Australia, 22–25 November 1995, Gold Coast, Queensland. St Kilda: MPAA.
Heebner ML, Roddey TS. 2008. The effects of neural mobilization in addition to standard care in persons with carpal tunnel syndrome from a community hospital. J Hand Ther 21: 229–240.
Julius A, Lees R, Dilley A, et al. 2004. Shoulder posture and median nerve sliding. BMC Musculoskelet Disord 5: 23.
Kallakuri S, Cavanaugh JM, Blagoev DC. 1998. An immunohistochemical study of innervation of lumbar spinal dura and longitudinal ligaments. Spine 23: 403–411.
Kenneally M. 1985. The upper limb tension test. In: Proceedings, Fourth Biennial Conference, Manipulative Therapists Association of Australia. Brisbane: Manipulative Therapists Association of Australia.
Kenneally M, Rubenach H. 1988. The upper limb tension test: the SLR of the arm. In: Grant R (ed) Physical therapy of the cervical and thoracic spine. New York: Churchill Livingstone, p 10.
Kleinrensink GJ, Stoeckart R, Mulder PG, et al. 2000. Upper limb tension tests as tools in the diagnosis of nerve and plexus lesions: anatomical and biomechanical aspects. Clin Biomech 15: 9–14.
Kornberg C, Lew P. 1989. The effect of stretching neural structures on grade one hamstring injuries. J Orthop Sports Phys Ther 10: 481–487.
Kreitz BG, Cote P, Yong-Hing K. 1996. Crossed femoral stretching test: a case report. Spine 21: 1584–1586.
Kuncewicz E, Gajewska E, Sobieska M, et al. 2006. Piriformis muscle syndrome. Ann Acad Med Stetin 52: 99–101.
Lindquist C, Nilsson BY, Skoglund CR. 1973. Observations on the mechanical sensitivity of sympathetic and other types of small-diameter nerve fibers. Brain Res 49: 432–435.
Louw A, Puentedura EJ. 2013. Therapeutic neuroscience education: teaching patients about pain: a guide for clinicians. Minneapolis: OPTP.
Maitland GD. 1986. Vertebral manipulation, 5th edn. Ontario: Butterworth.
Mannion RJ, Woolf CJ. 2000. Pain mechanisms and management: a central perspective. Clin J Pain 16: S144–S156.
McLellan DL, Swash M. 1976. Longitudinal sliding of the median nerve during movements of the upper limb. J Neurol Neurosurg Psychiatry 39: 566–570.

Merskey H, Bogduk N. 1994. Classification of chronic pain. Seattle, WA: IASP Press.
Millesi H. 1986. The nerve gap: theory and clinical practice. Hand Clin 2: 651–663.
Nee RJ, Butler DS. 2006. Management of peripheral neuropathic pain: integrating neurobiology, neurodynamics, and clinical evidence. Phys Ther Sport 7: 36–49.
Nordin M, Nystrom B, Wallin U, et al. 1984. Ectopic sensory discharges and paresthesiae in patients with disorders of peripheral nerves, dorsal roots and dorsal columns. Pain 20: 231–245.
Ogata K, Naito M. 1986. Blood flow of peripheral nerve: effects of dissection, stretching and compression. J Hand Surg Br 11B: 10–14.
Ozaktay AC, Kallakuri S, Cavanaugh JM. 1998. Phospholipase A2 sensitivity of the dorsal root and dorsal root ganglion. Spine 23: 1297–1306.
Rozmaryn LM, Dovelle S, Rothman ER, et al. 1998. Nerve and tendon gliding exercises and the conservative management of carpal tunnel syndrome. J Hand Ther 11: 171–179.
Shacklock MO. 1989. The plantarflexion / inversion straight leg raise test. An investigation into the effect of cervical flexion and order of component movements on the symptom response. Adelaide: University of South Australia.
Shacklock MO. 1995a. Clinical application of neurodynamics. In: Shacklock MO (ed) Moving in on pain. Melbourne, Australia: Butterworth-Heinemann, pp 123–131.
Shacklock MO. 1995b. Neurodynamics. Physiotherapy 81: 9–16.
Shacklock MO. 2005a. Clinical neurodynamics: a new system of musculoskeletal treatment. Sydney: Elsevier Butterworth-Heinemann.
Shacklock M. 2005b. Improving application of neurodynamic (neural tension) testing and treatments: a message to researchers and clinicians. Man Ther 10: 175–179.
Slater H, Butler DS, Shacklock MO. 1994. The dynamic nervous system: examination and assessment using tension tests. In: Boyling JD, Palastanga N (eds) Grieve's modern manual therapy, 2nd edn. Edinburgh: Churchill Livingstone.
Smart KM, Blake C, Staines A, et al. 2012a. Mechanisms-based classifications of musculoskeletal pain: symptoms and signs of central sensitisation in patients with low back (+ / – leg) pain. Man Ther 17: 336–344.
Smart KM, Blake C, Staines A, et al. 2012b. Mechanisms-based classifications of musculoskeletal pain: symptoms and signs of peripheral neuropathic pain in patients with low back (+ / – leg) pain. Man Ther 17: 345–351.
Smart KM, Blake C, Staines A, et al. 2012c. Mechanisms-based classifications of musculoskeletal pain: symptoms and signs of nociceptive pain in patients with low back (+ / – leg) pain. Man Ther 17: 352–357.
Tal-Akabi A, Rushton A. 2000. An investigation to compare the effectiveness of carpal bone mobilisation and neurodynamic mobilisation as methods of treatment for carpal tunnel syndrome. Man Ther 5: 214–222.
Tsai YY. 1995. Tension change in the ulnar nerve by different order of upper limb tension test. Chicago: Northwestern University. [MSc thesis.]
Van der Heide B, Allison GT, Zusman M. 2001. Pain and muscular responses to a neural tissue provocation test in the upper limb. Man Ther 6: 154–162.
Vicenzino B, Collins D, Wright A. 1996. The initial effects of a cervical spine manipulative physiotherapy treatment on the pain and dysfunction of lateral epicondylalgia. Pain 68: 69–74.
Vicenzino B, Collins D, Benson H, et al. 1998. An investigation of the interrelationship between manipulative therapy-induced hypoalgesia and sympathoexcitation. J Manipul Physiol Ther 21: 448–453.
Vicenzino B, Cartwright T, Collins D. 1999a. An investigation of stress and pain perception during manual therapy in asymptomatic subjects. Eur J Pain 3: 13–18.
Vicenzino B, Neal R, Collins D, et al. 1999b. The displacement, velocity and frequency profile of the frontal plane motion produced by the cervical lateral glide treatment technique. Clin Biomech 14: 515–521.
Wall EJ, Massie JB, Kwan MK, et al. 1992. Experimental stretch neuropathy. J Bone Joint Surg 74B: 126–129.
Weppler CH, Magnusson SP. 2010. Increasing muscle extensibility: a matter of increasing length or modifying sensation? Phys Ther 90: 438–449.
Wilgis EF, Murphy R. 1986. The significance of longitudinal excursion in peripheral nerves. Hand Clin 2: 761–766.
Woolf CJ. 2000. Pain. Neurobiol Dis 7: 504–510.
Woolf CJ. 2007. Central sensitization: uncovering the relation between pain and plasticity. Anesthesiology 106: 864–867.
Woolf CJ, Mannion RJ. 1999. Neuropathic pain: aetiology, symptoms, mechanisms, and management. Lancet 353: 1959–1964.
Woolf CJ, Salter MW. 2000. Neuronal plasticity: increasing the gain in pain. Science 288: 1765–1769.
Wright TW, Glowczewskie F Jr, Cowin D, et al. 2001. Ulnar nerve excursion and strain at the elbow and wrist associated with upper extremity motion. J Hand Sur Am 26: 655–662.
Yaxley G, Jull G. 1991. A modified upper limb tension test: an investigation of responses in normal subjects. Aust J Physiother 37: 143–152.
Young IA, Michener LA, Cleland JA, et al. 2009. Manual therapy, exercise, and traction for patients with cervical radiculopathy: a randomized clinical trial. Phys Ther 89: 632–642.
Zochodne DW, Ho LT. 1991. Stimulation-induced peripheral nerve hyperemia: mediation by fibers innervating vasa nervorum? Brain Res 546: 113–118.
Zoech G, Reihsner R, Beer R, et al. 1991. Stress and strain in peripheral nerves. Neuro-orthopedics 10: 73–82.
Zorn P, Shacklock MO, Trott P, et al. 1996. The effect of sequencing the movements of the upper limb tension test on the area of symptom reproduction. Clinical solutions. In: Proceedings of the Ninth Biennial Conference of the Manipulative Physiotherapists' Association of Australia, 22–25 November 1995, Gold Coast, Queensland. St Kilda: MPAA, pp 166–167.

Index

Page numbers followed by "*f*" indicate figures, "*t*" indicate tables, and "*b*" indicate boxes.

A

AB-IGHL. *see* Anterior bands of inferior glenohumeral ligaments (AB-IGHL).
Abdominal curl-up, for mechanical low back pain, 261, 261*f*
Abdominal draw-in manoeuvre, for mechanical low back pain, 259–260, 259*f*
Abdominal-bracing manoeuvre, for low back pain, 196
Abduction mobilization, 460–461, 461*f*
Abductor pollicis longus, 552, 552*f*, 577
  differential diagnosis, 552
  testing of, 552
Abnormal impulse-generating sites (AIGS), 783
Acceleration, of overhead throw, 324, 324*f*
Acetabular labral tears, 17
Achilles muscle, stretch reflex, testing of, 57*f*
Achilles tendinopathy, 19, 44, 646–649
  anatomy of, 647
  background, 646
  diagnosis of, 647–648, 647*f*–648*f*
  pathology and patho-biomechanics of, 647
  prevalence of, 19*t*
  treatment and prognosis of, 648–649
Achilles tendon, 647
Achilles tendon ruptures, 628–635
  consideration of forces applied on, 633–634, 634*t*
  diagnosis of, 629–630
  early range of motion *versus* immobilization, 631–632
  early weight-bearing *versus* late weight-bearing, 632
  epidemiology of, 629
  manual therapy techniques for, 634
  muscle endurance after, 634–635
  plantarflexion after, 634
    with an elastic band, 632, 632*f*
  post-surgical rehabilitation treatment of, 632–635
    protocols for, 634, 635*t*
  proprioception and, limitations of, 633
  range of motion exercises after, 633
  rerupture of
    after surgery, 631
    early mobilization and, 631
  risk factors of, 629
  scar tissue in, 633, 633*f*
  subtalar lateral glide joint motion in, 633, 633*f*
  surgical *versus* nonsurgical treatment for, 630–631, 630*f*
  swelling in, 633
  tendon elongation after, 631, 634
ACJ. *see* Acromioclavicular joint (ACJ).
ACL. *see* Anterior cruciate ligament (ACL).
ACR. *see* American College of Rheumatology (ACR).
Acromegaly, carpal tunnel syndrome and, 567
Acromioclavicular joint (ACJ), 293–301
  anatomy of, 293, 294*f*
  biomechanics of, 293–294
  diagnosis of, 295–298
  dysfunction and, 8*t*–9*t*
    injury of, 299
  management of, 298–299
  pathology of, 294–295, 294*b*, 295*f*
  physical examination tests for, 298*t*
Acromioclavicular resisted extension test, 295–296, 297*f*, 298*t*
Active compression test, 295–296, 296*f*, 298*t*, 337–338
Active movements, 63
Active straight leg raise test, for pelvic girdle pain, 281, 281*f*
Activity/exercise, in whiplash-associated disorders, 115
Acupuncture, for osteoarthritis, 488
Acute injuries, to acromioclavicular joint, 294
Acute loading, patellofemoral pain, 499
Acute low back pain, *versus* chronic low back pain, 236–237
Acute myocardial infarction, diagnosis of, 25, 25*t*, 27, 27*t*
Acute rib dysfunction, MET for, 719–720, 720*f*
Adaptive carpal instability (CIA), 561
Adduction mobilization, combined extension, 460*f*–461*f*
Adductor brevis muscle, TrPs in, 672, 672*f*
  dry needling of, 701, 701*f*
Adductor longus muscle, TrPs in, 672, 672*f*
  dry needling of, 701, 701*f*
Adductor magnus muscle, TrPs in, 672, 672*f*
  dry needling of, 701–702, 702*f*
Adductor path stroke, 755–756, 756*f*
Adductor tendinopathy, 405–407
  diagnosis of, 406
  epidemiology of, 405
  pathomechanics of, 405
  patient history of, 405–406
  treatment of, 406–407, 406*b*
Adhesive capsulitis, 8*t*–9*t*, 344
  see also Frozen shoulder
Adjunct exercises, for sternoclavicular joint, 307
Adson test, 137
'Adverse neural tension,' definition of, 781–782
Aα-fibre axons, mechanical sensitivity of, 774
Age, upper extremity disorders and, 10
Ageing, Achilles tendon and, 628–629
AIGS. *see* Abnormal impulse-generating sites (AIGS).
AIN. *see* Anterior interosseous nerve (AIN).
Alcohol use, excessive, 28
Allodynia, 765, 783
  TrPs and, 661
American College of Occupational and Environmental Medicine, 82*t*
American College of Rheumatology (ACR), 485
American Physical Therapy Association (APTA) Guideline, 82*t*
Analgesic effects, after thoracic spine manipulation, 150
Anamnesis, 748
Angiofibroblastic hyperplasia changes, 446
Ankle
  anterior cruciate ligament, 470
  biomechanics of, 606–607
    arthrokinematics in, 607
    axes of rotation in, 607
    open-packed and closed-packed positions, 607
    osteokinematics of, 607
    range of motion in, 607
  fractures, manipulation/mobilizations for, 638
  instability of
    chronic, 608
    functional, 608
    mechanical, 608
  stability of, role of ligaments in, 606*t*
  tendinopathies, manipulation/mobilization for, 639
Ankle arthritis, gait deviations in, 624
Ankle arthrodesis, *versus* arthroplasty, 624
Ankle disorders, lumbar spine treatment for, 223, 224*t*
Ankle dorsiflexion (L4), 56*f*
  mobility, limitation in, 637–638
Ankle eversion (S1-S2), 57*f*
Ankle sprains, 18, 605–615
  anatomy and physiology of, 605–607
    distal tibiofibular joint in, 605–606
    subtalar joint, 606
    talocrural joint in, 606
  biomechanics of ankle in, 606–607
    arthrokinematics in, 607
    axes of rotation in, 607
    open-packed and closed-packed positions, 607
    osteokinematics of, 607
    range of motion in, 607
  and chronic ankle instability, 608
  conservative treatment for, 610–613
  examination of, 608–610
    anterior drawer test in, 609, 609*f*
    figure-of-eight test in, 609–610, 610*f*
    functional testing in, 610
    medial talar tilt test in, 609, 609*f*
    Ottawa ankle rules in, 608
    range of motion in, 609
    subjective history in, 608–609
  incidence of, 605
  lateral, 607
  manipulation/mobilizations for, 637–639
  medial, 607–608
  non-thrust mobilization in, 610–612
    anterior-posterior, 611
    distal tibiofibular joint, 612
    lateral-medial, 611
  prevalence of, 19*t*
  stability and, role of collateral ligaments in, 606*t*
  syndesmotic injuries, 607–608
  therapeutic exercise for, 613
    mobility exercises in, 613
    proprioceptive, 613
    strengthening, 613
  thrust mobilization in, 610–612
    cuboid whip, 612, 613*f*
    proximal tibiofibular joint, 612, 612*f*
    rearfoot distraction, 611, 611*f*
  weight-bearing dorsiflexion mobilization with movement in, 612, 612*f*
Ankylosing spondylitis, 33*t*
Antebrachial fascia, 737, 737*f*
  myofascial induction of, 752, 752*f*
Anterior apprehension manoeuvre, 338, 339*f*
Anterior bands of inferior glenohumeral ligaments (AB-IGHL), 321–322
Anterior cruciate ligament (ACL), 467–470
  anatomy of, 467
  biomechanical/neuromuscular risk factors of, 468–470
    ankle/foot, 470
    hip, 469–470
    knee, 470
    trunk, 468–469
  biomechanics, 467–468
  incidence/prevalence of injury, 468
  risk factors for, 468*b*, 469*f*
  special tests for, 473*t*
  surgical management of, 477
Anterior cruciate ligament (ACL) reconstruction, 514–516
  bracing/weight-bearing, 514–515
  modalities in, 514
  neuromuscular re-education, 516
  range of motion exercises, 515
  rehabilitation goals of, 515*t*
  therapeutic exercise, 516
Anterior disc/manubrial rotation mobilization, left shoulder, 306, 306*f*

Anterior drawer test, 609, 609*f*
Anterior fontanel bone, 421–425
differential diagnosis of, 422–423
features of, 421–425
genesis of, 421
management for, 422
ossification of, 421, 422*f*
prognosis for, 422
Anterior interosseous nerve (AIN), 581
Anterior interosseous nerve (AIN) syndrome
common differential diagnosis of, 579*t*
special tests for, 579*t*
symptoms and signs of, 578*t*
Anterior knee pain, from patellofemoral pain syndrome, 18
Anterior scapular slide test, 337
Anterior slide test, 338, 339*f*
Anterior sling, in force closure, 277
Anterior superior iliac spine (ASIS), 438
Anterior tibialis muscle, 483
Anterior-posterior non-thrust mobilization, 611
Anteroposterior/lateral-medial glide, of glenohumeral joint, at end-of-range elevation, 352, 352*f*
Anterosuperior glenoid labrum, 334–335, 335*f*
Aortic aneurysms, 38–39
Apprehension test, for glenohumeral instability, 326
Arcade of Frohse, 576–577
Arm
fascia, deep layer of, 734–738, 735*f*
integrated myofascial induction of, 751, 751*f*
motions, for cervical neutral during limb load, 181
Arthritic conditions, of elbow, 455–456
anatomy review for, 455
diagnosis of, 456
incidence/prevalence of, 455–456
pathology/pathoanatomy of, 456
patient presentation with, 456*t*
prognosis and treatment planning for patients with, 456
Arthrofibrosis, of knee, 522
treatment of, after total knee arthroplasty, 522*t*
Arthrokinematics, in ankle sprains, 607
Arthroplasty, 488–489
Arthroscopic procedures, for hip disorders
for cam-type impingement, 414
for capsular and ligamentous structures, 414
for chondral defects, 414
for femoroacetabular impingement, 413–414
for pincer-type impingement, 413–414
postoperative considerations for, 415
precautions for, 415–416
capsular modification, 416
femoroplasty, 415
labral debridement with/without rim trimming, acetabular, 415
micro-fracture, 416
Articular cartilage, human, 483–484
Articular dysfunctions, 78*t*, 86*t*, 87–88
Articular system, postural correction exercises for, 186
ASIS. *see* Anterior superior iliac spine (ASIS).
Associative phase, of motor pattern retraining, 266–267
Asterisk sign, 639
Asymmetric weakness, side-flexion/rotation exercises for, 179–180, 180*f*–181*f*
'Athletic hernia', 407
Atlanto-axial (C1-C2) segment
MET for, 715–716, 715*f*
primary movement at, 715
Atraumatic swelling, 49
Attenuated muscle stretch reflexes (MSRs), 53
Audible pop, in spinal manipulative therapy, 248
Augmented pain, in whiplash, 112–113
Autonomous phase, of motor pattern retraining, 267
Axes of rotation, in ankle sprains, 607
Axillary fascia, 735*f*–736*f*, 736
Axonal mechanical sensitivity, in neuritis model, 774
Axonotmesis, 577
Axons, 765–766, 766*f*

B
Babinski sign, 59, 59*f*, 122
Back pain, 13
Balance
after total ankle arthroplasty, 628
dynamic, 508*f*
exercises, 508*f*
for mechanical low back pain, 268–269, 268*f*
neuromotor control, 431–432
Balance error scoring system (BESS), 506–507
'Barrel hug' exercise, 155
'Barrier-dam' theory, 731
Baseline data, 22–23
Bassett's ligament, 605–606
BCTQ. *see* Boston Carpal Tunnel Questionnaire (BCTQ).
Bennett fracture, 596
Bent knee sit-up, for mechanical low back pain, 261, 261*f*
BESS. *see* Balance error scoring system (BESS).
Biceps brachii muscle, TrPs in, 666, 667*f*
dry needling of, 696, 696*f*
Biceps femoris muscle
reflex activity of, 112
TrPs in, dry needling of, 704–705, 705*f*
Biceps load test, 337
Biceps muscle stretch reflex, testing of, 57*f*
Biceps-labrum complex, 335–336
Bicipital fascia, myofascial induction of, 752, 752*f*
Bicipital injury, 314
Blood flow, pulsatile, 498
Blood pressure examination, 49*t*
Blood supply
of labrum, 334
to patellar tendon, 535
Blood vessels, fibres in, 731
Blood-nerve barrier, 772
Blood-oxygenation-level-dependent (BOLD) signal, in chronic low back pain, 238
BOLD signal. *see* Blood-oxygenation-level-dependent (BOLD) signal.
Bonar scale, for tendinopathy, 548
Bone and Joint Initiative, 13
'Bone-fascia-tendon system', 730
Bony ingrowth, of the prosthesis, in total ankle arthroplasty, 624–625
Boston Carpal Tunnel Questionnaire (BCTQ), 569
BOSU squat with ball toss exercise, 439*f*
Botulinum toxin injection, trigger point dry needling and, 508–509
Botulinum toxin type A (Botox), 509
Bowler's squat exercises, 440*f*
Bowstring sign, in lumbar radiculopathy, 203
Boxers fracture, 595
Brachial fascia, 736–737, 737*f*
myofascial induction of, 752, 752*f*
Brachialis muscle
TrPs in, dry needling of, 696, 696*f*
Brachioradialis muscle
stretch reflex, testing of, 57*f*
TrPs in, 667, 668*f*
dry needling of, 696, 696*f*
Brain, in chronic pain
changes in, 66–70
descending pathways of, 69–70
functional changes in, 69, 69*f*
structural changes in, 68
treatment of, 66–75
Breathing patterns, in thoracic outlet syndrome, 138
Bridge exercises, in supine, for mechanical low back pain, 262, 263*f*–264*f*
Buford complex, 334–335
Bursa, of hip, disorders of, 397–412

C
C0-C1 (occipito-atlanto) segment
MET for, 716, 716*f*
primary movement at, 716
C1-C2 (atlanto-axial) segment
MET for, 715–716, 715*f*
primary movement at, 715
C2-C7 cervical segments, typical, MET for, 714–715, 715*f*
C2-C7 disc traction
seated, 162, 162*f*
in supine, 162, 162*f*
CAD. *see* Cervical arterial dysfunction (CAD).
Calcific tendonitis, 538
Calcifying tendinopathy, 314
Calcitonin-related gene peptide, 548
Calgary-Cambridge guides, 37
Calvarium, 421
Cam-type impingement, definition of, 414
Canadian C-spine rule, 31, 33*f*
CANS classification. *see* 'Complaints of the arm, neck and/or shoulder' (CANS) classification.
Capsular (superior) ligament, 303
Capsular/ligamentous structures, arthroscopic procedures for, 414
Capsular modification, 415–416
Carpal glide manipulation
with distal fixation, 591, 591*f*
with proximal fixation, 590–591, 590*f*
Carpal instability, 558–565
aetiopathogenesis of, 560–561
anatomy of, 559–560
biomechanics of, 559–560
classification of, 561
clinical tests for, 561–563
diagnostic dynamic ultrasound and arthroscopy as, 563
distal radioulnar joint and triangular fibrocartilage complex tests as, 563
general mid-carpal tests as, 561–562
lunotriquetral tests as, 562–563, 563*f*
radiological tests as, 563
scaphoid stress test as, 562*f*
scapholunate, second and third carpometacarpal joints and capitolunate tests as, 562
diagnostic considerations for, 561
examination and diagnosis of, 561–563
incidence and aetiology of, 558–559
ligamentous anatomy and stabilization of, 559–560
muscular anatomy of, 560
osseous anatomy of, 559
pathogenesis of, 561
patterns of, 560–561
recognized, 560–561
treatment and prognosis for, 563–564
conservative, 563–564
surgical, 564
wrist instability and, 558–559
defining, 558
functional stability, 558
Carpal instability combined (CIC), 561
Carpal instability dissociative (CID), 561
Carpal instability non-dissociative (CIND), 561
Carpal tunnel, scheme of, 567*f*
Carpal tunnel fascia, myofascial induction of, 753, 753*f*
Carpal tunnel syndrome (CTS), 8*t*–9*t*, 566–574, 770
anatomy in, 566, 567*f*
clinical examination of, 568–569
diagnosis of, 568–569
electrodiagnostic evaluation of, 569
incidence of, 566
manual therapy for, 585
patho-biomechanism of, 567–568
patient history in, 569
pregnancy and, 571–572
prevalence of, 566
prognosis of, 570–571
questionnaires for, 569
sensory and motor aspects in, 568
therapy for, 571
treatment of, 795
ultrasound assessment of, 569–570, 570*f*
untreated, prognosis of, 570–571
Carpometacarpal (CMC) I joint, 586, 596, 600
glides of, 592, 592*f*
osteoarthritis of, diagnosis of, 601
traction of, 591, 591*f*
Carpometacarpal (CMC) II-V joints, 586
traction of, 591*f*
Carpometacarpal (CMC) V joint, 586
Cartesian model of pain, 66, 70
Cauda equina syndrome, 51
Caudal glide self-mobilization, 417, 417*f*
Cavitation, 159
Cavovarus foot, 650
CCSI. *see* Clinical cervical spine instability (CCSI).
Cells, 731

Central carpal dorsal glides, 590
Central carpal palmar glides, 590, 590*f*
Central hyperexcitability
presence of, 112
theory, 731
Central nervous system
neurobiomechanics and, 784
in neurodynamic test, 784
Central sensitivity, definition of, 784
Central sensitization (CS), 42
Centralization, 76, 80, 256
in lumbar radiculopathy, 206
Cerebrovascular accidents, MET and, 712
Cervical arterial dysfunction (CAD), 102–103
screening for, 49–50
Cervical arterial system, vascular disorders of, 49
Cervical distraction, 56–58, 58*f*
Cervical distraction test, 123, 123*f*
Cervical extension, with overpressure, 61*f*
Cervical flexion (C1-C2), 54*f*
with overpressure, 61*f*
Cervical lateral glide technique, 795, 795*f*
Cervical mobilization, posterior-anterior, 168–169
transverse unilateral mid-cervical, 169, 169*f*
unilateral mid-cervical, 168–169, 169*f*
unilateral upper, 168, 168*f*
Cervical myelopathy, 102
active and passive movements of, 121
clinical signs and symptoms of, 119–120
confirmation tests of, 121–122
conservative approaches of, 127
current best evidence with regard to prognosis in, 126
differential diagnosis and treatment of, 118–131
essential aspects of, 126
electromyogram/electroneurogram of, 125
imaging of, 124–125
initial symptoms of, 51
nerve condition responses in, 125–126
observation of, 121
outcome measures of, 121
patient history in, 120–121
physical examination of, 121
review of proposed pathology and patho-biomechanics of, 119
surgical approaches of, 128–129
anterior, 128
posterior, 128–129
Cervical myeloradiculopathy
clinical signs and symptoms of, 120
confirmation tests of, 124
conservative approaches of, 127
current best evidence with regard to prognosis in, 126
differential diagnosis and treatment of, 118–131
essential aspects of, 126
imaging of, 124–125
nerve condition responses in, 125–126
outcome measures of, 124
patient history in, 124
physical examination of, 124
review of proposed pathology and patho-biomechanics of, 119
surgical approaches of, 128–129
anterior, 128
posterior, 128–129
Cervical nerve roots, manual muscle testing for, 53*t*
Cervical neutral, during limb load, 180–181, 181*f*
Cervical radicular pain, 100
Cervical radiculopathy, 100
active and passive movements of, 122–123
clinical signs and symptoms of, 120
confirmation tests of, 123–124
conservative approaches of, 127
current best evidence with regard to prognosis in, 126
definition of, 118
differential diagnosis and treatment of, 118–131
essential aspects of, 126
imaging of, 124–125
nerve condition responses in, 125–126
neurological testing of, 123
observation of, 122
outcome measures of, 122
patient history in, 122
physical examination of, 122–123
provocation tests of, 123–124
review of proposed pathology and patho-biomechanics of, 119
surgical approaches of, 128–129
anterior, 128
posterior, 128–129
Cervical rotation, with overpressure, 62*f*
Cervical rotation lateral flexion test (CRLF), 149
Cervical side-bending (C3), 54*f*
with overpressure, 61*f*
Cervical spine
assessment of, 714
innervated structure in, 99
manipulation and mobilization of, 158–173
adverse reactions to, 160–161
atlanto-axial separation of zygapophyseal articular joint, manipulative procedures for, 170, 170*f*
C2-C6 separation of zygapophyseal articular joint, manipulative procedures for, 169, 170*f*
contraindications to, 160
evidence for, 158–159
factors associated with poor outcomes in, 170*b*
hypothesized mechanisms of effect of, 159
manipulative procedures for, 169–170
patients for, selecting, 160
posterior-anterior mobilization, 168–169
specificity of, 159–160
versus thoracic spine manipulation, 158–159
translatoric. *see* Translatoric cervical manipulation and mobilization
MET for, 714–716
nociceptive stimulation of, 100, 101*f*
pain, 118
posterior-anterior mobility of, 62*f*
self-report measures of pain and function, 105–107, 106*t*
Cervical spine muscles, morphological changes to, 112
Cervical system, fascial, 732, 732*f*
Cervicogenic headache, thoracic spine manipulation for, 147
C-fibre axons
mechanical sensitivity of, 774, 774*f*
SNL model and, 772
Chemokines, 775
blood-nerve barrier and, 772
Child's pose, with side-flexion, for mechanical low back pain, 257*f*, 258
Chondral defects, arthroscopic procedures for, 414
Chondromalacia patellae, 498
Chop exercises, for mechanical low back pain, 269, 269*f*
Chronic constriction injury (CCI) model, 772
Chronic low back pain, 236–244
versus acute low back pain, 236–237
altered nociceptive transmission in, 237
interventions for, 239–241
efficacy of, factors associated with, 241–242
expectation in, 241
patient-clinician relationship in, 242
patient preference in, 241–242
joint-biased manual therapies for, 239–240
nerve-biased manual therapies for, 240–241
neuroimaging in, 237–239
soft-tissue-biased manual therapies for, 240
Chronic pain, 78*t*
changes in nervous system and brain in people with, 66–70
descending pathways, 69–70
functional changes, 69, 69*f*
neuromatrix, 66–68, 67*f*–68*f*
structural changes, 68
treating brain in, 66–75
treatment of, 70–73, 70*f*
graded motor imagery-restructuring brain/body maps, 73
therapeutic neuroscience education, 71–73, 72*f*
Chronic pelvic pain (CPP), 227–228
case reports on, 232, 232*b*–233*b*
conservative management of, 228–229, 228*f*–229*f*
clinical-reasoned approach for, 230–231
movement system dysfunction in, 230
pelvic floor muscle function in, 230–231, 231*f*–232*f*
understanding pain science in, 230, 230*f*
Clam shell exercise, 417, 417*f*, 428*f*, 505*f*
Claudication pain, 38–39
Clavipectoral fascia, 735*f*, 736
myofascial induction of, 750, 751*f*
Client-specific impairment measure (CSIM), 352–353
Clinical cervical spine instability (CCSI), 103
Clinical lumbar instability, 43
Clinical neurobiomechanics, of upper and lower quadrant, 784–785, 784*f*
Clinical neurodynamics, of upper and lower quadrants, 781–798
clinical application of, 793–794
definition of, 782
neurobiomechanics and, 784–785, 784*f*
neurophysiology, 783–784
central nervous system in neurodynamic tests, 784
nerve sensitivity, 783, 783*f*–784*f*
operating definitions in, 782
terminology in, 781–782
treatment in, 795–796
Clinical prediction rules (CPRs), 246–248, 526
in cervical spine manipulation, 160
for PFP, 503
patellar taping, 503
in treatment-based classification system, 218
Clinical special tests, 64
Clinical-reasoning process, 22
Clonus, 59, 60*f*
Closed kinetic chain
exercises, 475, 516
proprioceptive training in, 486*f*
Closed-packed positions, in ankle sprains, 607
Cocaine, 28
Cognitive behavioural therapy (CBT), studies of, 71–73
Cognitive phase, of motor pattern retraining, 266
Cold hyperalgesia, 113
Collateral ligaments, special tests for, 473*t*
Colles' fracture, management of, 585–586
Combination therapies, 485
'Complaints of the arm, neck and/or shoulder' (CANS) classification, 5
Compression
of anterior-lateral leg muscles, 687, 687*f*
of supraspinatus muscle, 681–682, 682*f*
of TrPs, 679–680
Compression test, for sacroiliac joint pathology, 280, 280*f*
Compressor, 136
Computed tomography (CT)
of acromioclavicular joint, 297–298
of cervical spine, 124–125
of Hill-Sachs lesion, 328–329
of lumbar radiculopathy, 204
of superior labrum anterior-to-posterior (SLAP) lesions, 340
Concave-convex rule, 350
Concavity compression, 311
Concomitant low back pain, 28
Concomitant neck pain, 28
Concordant sign, 22
Confirmatory tests, for lumbar spine instability, 217–218
Congruence angle (C-angle), 495
Connective tissue, of nerve trunk, 766
'Connective tissue theory', 731
Conservative management/treatment, 474–477
in lateral epicondylalgia, 447–448
versus surgical, 473–474
'Contract-relax' technique, 710
Contractile dysfunction, 78*t*, 86*t*, 88
of shoulder, 89
Contraction
of anterior-lateral leg muscles, 687, 687*f*
of supraspinatus muscle, 681–682, 682*f*
Controlled sit to stand exercise, 438*f*
Coracoacromial arch, 310
Coracoacromial ligament (CAL), anatomy of, 322, 322*f*
Coracohumeral ligament (CHL), 345, 345*f*
anatomy of, 322

Coracoid impingement, 313
Corticosteroids
for frozen shoulder, 347
injections, 447
Costoclavicular ligament, 303
Costoclavicular space, 134
Costoclavicular test, 137
CPP. *see* Chronic pelvic pain (CPP).
CPRs. *see* Clinical prediction rules (CPRs).
Cranial nerves, 60*t*–61*t*
examination of, 49*t*, 60, 60*t*–61*t*
Craniovertebral region, self-mobilization exercises for, 183–184, 183*f*
Crank test, 337–338
Crepitus, painful pretendinous, 647
CRLF. *see* Cervical rotation lateral flexion test (CRLF).
Cross-body adduction test, 295–296, 297*f*, 298*t*
Cross-sectional area (CSA), in evaluation of carpal tunnel syndrome, 570
Crossed straight leg raise test, for lumbar radiculopathy, 203
Crossed-hands technique, for segmental mobility testing, 149
Crossover tendinitis, 551
Cryotherapy, use of, 514
CSIM. *see* Client-specific impairment measure (CSIM).
CTS. *see* Carpal tunnel syndrome (CTS).
Cubital tunnel syndrome
common differential diagnosis of, 579*t*
special tests for, 579*t*
symptoms and signs of, 578*t*
Cuboid syndrome, manipulation/mobilization for, 638–639
Cuboid thrust manipulation, 642, 643*f*
Cuboid whip thrust manipulation, 612, 613*f*
Cyriax release test, 137
Cytokine(s)
blood-nerve barrier and, 772
neuritis model and, 775
repetitive strain injury and, 771–772

D

DALYs. *see* Disability-adjusted life years (DALYs).
Danish Health Technology Assessment, 82*t*
Data collection, in history taking, 22–23
De Quervain syndrome, multimodal management approach to, 586
De Quervain's tenosynovitis, 8*t*–9*t*, 552, 554–555
Deceleration, of overhead throw, 324, 324*f*
Deep fascia, 739, 739*f*–740*f*
cervical, 732*f*, 733
of foot segment, 740
intermuscular links of, 740–743
of leg segment, 740
of thigh segment, 739–740, 740*f*
Deep massage therapy, for plantar heel pain, 620
Deep neck extensors, recruitment of, 176, 176*f*–177*f*
Deep neck flexors (DNF), recruitment of, 175–176, 176*f*
Deep somatic pain, 24
Deep tendon reflexes, loss of, lumbar radiculopathy and, 200
Deep tissue friction massage, for wrist and hand tendinopathy, 553
Cyriax techniques of, 553
Deep-vein thrombosis (DVT), Wells' clinical decision rule for, 38–39, 39*t*
Default mode network (DMN), in chronic low back pain, 238–239
Degenerative joint disease, 389
Deltoid fascia, 735*f*, 736
myofascial induction of, 750, 750*f*
Deltoid ligament, injury to, 607–608
Deltoid muscle, TrPs in, 666, 666*f*
dry needling of, 695, 695*f*
dynamic transverse strokes of, 683, 683*f*–684*f*
Depression, symptoms associated with, 30–32, 31*b*
Derangement syndrome, 76, 78*t*, 86*t*
conceptual model of, 79
direction of loading strategies in, 87*f*
Dermatomes, 52, 52*f*
lumbar radiculopathy and, 200, 203*t*
Diagnostic accuracy, of test, 47–48
Differentiating movements, definition of, 782
Diffusion tensor imaging (DTI), in chronic low back pain, 238
Digital fractures, 594–598
anatomy of, 594
conservative treatment of, 596–598, 599*f*
diagnosis of, 596
epidemiology of, 594
metacarpal, 595
pathology of, 595–596
phalangeal, 595–596
prognosis for, 596
thumb, 596
treatment problems and treatment techniques associated with, 597*t*–598*t*
Digital osteoarthritis, 600–601
anatomy of, 600
conservative treatment of, 601
diagnosis for, 601
epidemiology of, 600
pathology of, 600
prognosis of, 601
Directional preference, 76, 256
Disability, associated with upper extremity pain, 9*t*
Disability-adjusted life years (DALYs), low back pain in, 210–211, 211*t*
Disc traction, in cervical spine manipulation, 160
C2-C7, 162, 162*f*
Discordant signs, 22
Distal carpal row, 559
Distal phalanx, fractures of, 595–596
Distal radioulnar joint, 559
dorsal glide radius, 587, 587*f*
mobilizations with movement, 587
ventral glide radius, 587
Distal sensory radial nerve syndrome
common differential diagnosis of, 579*t*
special tests for, 579*t*
symptoms and signs of, 578*t*
Distal tibiofibular joint, 605–606
non-thrust mobilization of, 612
Distal tibiofibular mobilization with movement, 'sprained ankle', 643, 643*f*
Distal tibiofibular non-thrust manipulation, 642, 642*f*
Distraction test, for sacroiliac joint pathology, 280, 280*f*
Divergence, of nerve, 785
DMN. *see* Default mode network (DMN).
Dorsal capitate-displacement test, 562
Dorsal intercalary segment instability (DISI), 561
splint, 564*f*
Double-crush syndrome, carpal tunnel syndrome and, 567
DRST. *see* Dynamic rotary stability test (DRST).
DRT. *see* Dynamic relocation test (DRT).
Dry needling
for plantar heel pain, 620–621, 620*f*
of TrPs, 690–709
in arm muscles, 693–697
description of, 691
general guidelines for, 692–693
in hip muscles, 700–707
in leg muscles, 700–707
in neck muscles, 693–697
risks of, 691
scientific evidence of, 691–692
in shoulder muscles, 693–697
in trunk muscles, 697–700
DTI. *see* Diffusion tensor imaging (DTI).
Dynamic balance, 508*f*
Dynamic instability, 560–561
Dynamic postural control, 431–432
Dynamic relocation test (DRT), 363, 367, 367*f*
Dynamic rotary stability test (DRST), 362–363, 366–367, 367*f*
Dynamic valgus torques, knee, 470
Dysaesthetic pain, 783
Dysfunction syndrome, 76–77
conceptual model of, 87–88

E

Early cocking, of overhead throw, 323–324, 324*f*
Early range of motion, Achilles tendon ruptures and, 631–632
Eccentric decline squat, 537*f*
Eccentric exercise, for tendinopathies, 554
Eccentric heel raises, bilateral and unilateral, for ankle tendinopathies, 648–649, 648*f*–649*f*
Eccentric lowers (Nordic hamstring-HS) exercise, 430*f*
Education, in whiplash-associated disorders, 115
Edwin Smith papyrus, 210–211
Eichhoff test, 552, 552*f*
Elbow, joint mobilization and manipulation of, 458–463
Elbow disorders, 451–457
Elbow extension (C7), 55*f*
Elbow flexion (C6), 55*f*
Elbow instability, 451–455
anatomy review for, 451
general treatment planning guidelines for, 451–452
lateral, 452–453
medial, 454–455
Elbow orthotics, 448
Elbow pain
lateral, 144
prevalence of, 7*t*
Elbow tendinopathy, lateral epicondylalgia, 445–450
considerations in conservative treatment, 447–448
diagnostic considerations of, 445–446
pathological considerations of, 446–447
prognostic considerations of, 447
Electromyography (EMG), of lumbar radiculopathy, 204–205
Electrophysical modalities, selected, 509–510
Electrophysiological reflexive tests, in chronic low back pain, 237
Elevated first-rib test, 137
Elevation, belt assisted, mobilization with movement, 354, 354*f*
EMG. *see* Electromyography (EMG).
EMS. *see* European Myelopathy Score (EMS).
Endoneurium, 766, 766*f*
microenvironment of, changes in, 772
β-endorphin, TrPs dry needling and, 692
Endotendon, 546
Endurance, motor function exercises for, 176–179
'Energy crisis hypothesis', 662
Enteropathic arthritis, 33*t*
Entrapment neuropathies, 575–583
anatomy in, 575–577
median nerve, 577
radial nerve, 576–577
ulnar nerve, 575–576
common differential diagnosis of, 579*t*
conservative treatment for, 581–582
general principles in, 581
radial nerve, 582
ulnar nerve, 581–582
diagnosis of, 577–581
median nerve, 580–581
radial nerve, 580
ulnar nerve, 578–580
epidemiology of, 575
pathology of, 577
prognosis of, 581
risk factors, 575
special tests for, 579*t*
symptoms and signs of, 578*t*
Epicondylalgia, lateral, 445
defined, 446
diagnostic considerations, 445–446
prognostic considerations of, 447
'Epicondylitis', 445
'Epicondylosis', 445
Epicritical sensitivity, of mechanical impulse, 746
Epidural steroid injections, for lumbar radiculopathy, 207
Epineurium, 766, 766*f*
Erector spinae muscles
stabilization exercises for, 219*t*
strengthening of, for lower back pain, 196
ESWT. *see* Extracorporeal shock-wave therapy (ESWT).
Ethnicity, in patient profile, 23
EULAR. *see* European League against Rheumatism (EULAR).
European League against Rheumatism (EULAR), 10–11, 485
European Myelopathy Score (EMS), 121
Examination, in glenohumeral instability, 325–326

Excessive alcohol use, 28
Excursion, of nerves, 785
Exercise progression model, 435f
Exercise therapy
for hip osteoarthritis, 393
for mechanical low back pain, 255
rotator cuff lesions shoulder impingement and, 316–317
Exercises
balance, 508f
designing an evidence-informed programme, 434–440
mobility, 435–437
muscle performance and neuromuscular control, 437–440
parameters, 440–441, 441t
rehabilitation, examples of, 506b
step-down, 507f
straight leg hip abduction, 518f
strengthening, 504–506
therapeutic, for lower quadrant, 426–442
Extension, restriction of, MET for
in lumbar spine, 721, 721f
in thoracic spine, 717–718, 717f–718f
Extension exercises
for mechanical low back pain, 256, 257f
mobilization, 155
in quadruped position, 196
Extension-oriented exercises, for low back pain, 195
Extensor carpi radialis brevis muscle, 550f, 551
differential diagnosis of, 551
testing of, 551
TrPs in, 668, 668f
Extensor carpi radialis longus muscle, 550f, 551
differential diagnosis of, 551
testing of, 551
TrPs in, 668, 668f
Extensor carpi ulnaris muscle, 550–551, 550f, 577
differential diagnosis of, 551
subluxation of, 555
testing of, 551
TrPs in, 668, 668f
Extensor digiti minimi muscle, 550f, 551–552, 577
differential diagnosis for, 552
testing of, 552
Extensor digitorum communis muscle, TrPs in, 668, 668f
Extensor digitorum longus muscle, TrPs in, 673, 673f
Extensor hallucis longus muscle, TrPs in, 673, 673f
Extensor indices muscle, 577
Extensor indicis proprius muscle, 550f, 551
differential diagnosis for, 551
testing of, 551
Extensor pollicis brevis muscle, 552, 552f
differential diagnosis, 552
testing of, 552
Extensor pollicis longus muscle, 552–553, 552f, 577
differential diagnosis for, 553
testing of, 553
Extensor progressions, higher load, 178–179, 179f–180f
Extensor retinacle, myofascial induction of, 752, 752f
External oblique muscle, TrPs in, dry needling of, 699–700, 699f
External rotation, end-range elevation, mobilization with movement, 354, 354f
Extracellular matrix
of connective tissue, 731
viscoelasticity and, 746–747
Extracorporeal shock-wave therapy (ESWT), 447–448
Extremity musculoskeletal pain conditions, brief epidemiology of, 85–86
Extremity problems
Mechanical Diagnosis and Therapy for, 85–91
medical diagnosis for, 86
Eye examination, 49t

F

FABERE's position stretch, 436
Facet gliding, in cervical spine manipulation, 160
Facet separation, in cervical spine manipulation, 160
Fascia, 730
anatomy of
cervical region, 732–733, 732f
upper extremity, 733–738
chemical pattern of, 731
dynamics of, 730–731
functional pattern of, 731
functions of, 730
information transmission process in, 730–731
inherent movement in, 746
mechanical (anatomical) pattern of, 730–731
as mechanosensitive system, 745–746
Fascial system
anatomical considerations in
of neck and upper extremity, 732–738
of pelvis and lower extremity, 738–743
classification and distribution of, 732
dysfunction of, definition of, 743–744
functions of, 730
release and restructuring of, 746
Fascicles, 546
Fatty infiltrate, magnetic resonance imaging of, 112
Fear-avoidance Beliefs Questionnaire, 38t, 106t, 107
Fear-of-movement beliefs, chronic whiplash and, 113
Femoral cutaneous nerve, posterior, in pelvic floor muscles, 226–227
Femoral nerve tension test, for lumbar radiculopathy, 203–204
Femoroacetabular impingement, arthroscopic procedures for, 413–414
Femoroplasty, 415
Fibrils, 546
Fibroblasts, 535
Fibrocartilage degeneration, 390
Fibular groove, 650
Fibularis (peroneus) brevis muscle, TrPs in, dry needling of, 707, 707f
Fibularis (peroneus) longus muscle, TrPs in, dry needling of, 707, 707f
'Figure 4' position, posterior to anterior mobilization, 394, 394f
Figure-4 stretch exercise, 436, 436f
Figure-of-eight test, 609–610, 610f
Finger abduction (T1), 55f
Finger extensor muscles, TrPs in, dry needling of, 697, 697f
Finger joint
glides, 592
mobilizations with movement, 592
traction, 592, 592f
Finger/thumb, pathology of, 594–602
digital fractures, 594–598
osteoarthritis of the digits, 600–601
rheumatoid arthritis affecting the digits, 601
ulnar collateral ligament (UCL) injury of thumb, 598–600
Finkelstein's test, 552, 552f
First metatarsal phalangeal non-thrust/thrust manipulation, 643, 643f
First-metatarsal rise sign, 653
First rib
elevated, MET for, 719, 719f
hypomobility, 155
Flexibility exercises, for low back pain, parameters for, 270
Flexion, restriction of, MET for
in lumbar spine, 720, 721f
in thoracic spine, 717, 717f
Flexion abduction external rotation (FABER) test, 403
Flexion-extension movement, 560
'Flexion mobilization' exercise, 155
Flexion-oriented exercises, for low back pain, 195
Flexion resistance test, for type II SLAP lesions, 337
Flexor carpi radialis muscle, 550f, 553, 577
differential diagnosis for, 553
testing of, 553
TrPs in, 669, 669f
Flexor carpi ulnaris muscle, 550, 550f, 575–576
differential diagnosis for, 550
testing of, 550
TrPs in, 669, 669f
Flexor digitorum longus muscle, TrPs in, dry needling of, 706–707
Flexor digitorum profundus muscle, 575–577
Flexor digitorum superficialis muscle, 577
TrPs in, 669, 669f
Flexor hallucis longus (FHL) tendon, 654
Flexor pollicis brevis muscle, 576
Flexor progressions, higher load, 176–178, 177f–178f
Flexor tendons, lacerations of, 600
Fluoroquinolone, Achilles tendon rupture and, 629
Follow-through phase, of overhead throw, 324, 324f
Fontanel bone, anterior, 421–425
differential diagnosis of, 422–423
features of, 421–425
genesis of, 421
management for, 422
ossification of, 421, 422f
prognosis for, 422
Foot/ankle
anterior cruciate ligament of, 470
conditions, 18–19
prevalence of, 19t
deep fascial intermuscular links in, 741–743
manipulation of, 637–645
clinical decision making for, 639
passive joint manipulation/mobilization, 641–642
self-mobilization interventions in, 643–644
talocrural joint of, passive manipulation of, 639–640
Foot/ankle disorders
lumbar spine treatment for, 223, 224t
postoperative management of, 623–636
Achilles tendon ruptures, 628–635
total ankle arthroplasty, 623–628
Foot/ankle tendinopathy, 646–656
Achilles tendinopathy, 646–649
anatomy of, 647
background, 646
diagnosis of, 647–648, 647f–648f
pathology and patho-biomechanics of, 647
treatment and prognosis of, 648–649
other, 654–655
anatomy of, 654
background, 654
diagnosis of, 654–655
pathology and patho-biomechanics of, 654
treatment and prognosis of, 655
peroneal tendinopathy, 649–651
anatomy of, 649–650
background of, 649
diagnosis of, 650–651
pathology and patho-biomechanics of, 650
presentation of pain and dysfunction in, 651t
treatment and prognosis of, 651
tibialis anterior tendinopathy, 651–653
anatomy in, 652
background of, 651–652
diagnosis of, 652
pathology and patho-biomechanics of, 652
treatment and prognosis of, 652–653
tibialis posterior tendinopathy, 653–654
anatomy of, 653
background of, 653
diagnosis of, 653–654
pathology and patho-biomechanics of, 653
stages of, 653
treatment and prognosis of, 654
Force alternatives, 76
Force closure, of pelvic ring, 277
Force progression, 76
Forefoot, disorders of, manipulation/mobilization for, 639
Form closure, of pelvic ring, 277
Forward head posture (FHP), 185
Forward step-down exercises, 437f, 438–439
Forward step-down test, 398
Four-point kneeling, 362, 365–366, 366f
Fractures
Bennett, 596
Boxers, 595
digital, 594–598
anatomy of, 594
conservative treatment of, 596–598, 599f
diagnosis of, 596
epidemiology of, 594
pathology of, 595–596
phalangeal, 595–596
prognosis for, 596
thumb, 596
treatment problems and treatment techniques associated with, 597t–598t
of distal phalanx, 595–596
low back pain and, 40

metacarpal, 595
of metacarpal head, 595
micro, 416
phalangeal, 595–596
shaft, 595
spinal, 102
vertebral compression, 40
Frank herniation, 79
Freezing phase, of frozen shoulder, 346
physical examination of, 347
treatment of, 347–348
Froment's sign, 580
Front plank, for mechanical low back pain, 264, 265*f*
Frontal plane force couple, 310–311, 310*f*
Frontal plane movement, in McKenzie assessment, 79
Frozen phase, of frozen shoulder, 346
physical examination of, 347
treatment of, 348
Frozen shoulder (FS), 344–349
diagnosis of, 346–347
history in, 346
physical examination for, 347, 347*f*
incidence of, 344
natural history of, 345–346, 346*f*
pathology of, 344–345
prevention of, 348
prognosis of, 345–346
recalcitrant, 348
stages of, 346*b*
treatment of, 347–348, 347*f*
Functional exercises, for shoulder region, 381–383, 382*f*–383*f*
Functional integration
dissociation task exercise, 440*f*
in mechanical low back pain, 266–267
neuromotor control, 431–432
Functional magnetic resonance imaging (fMRI), of low back pain, 67*f*, 72*f*
Functional movement testing, for gluteus medius tendinopathy, 402–403
Functional positional test
cervical extension, 49*t*
cervical rotation, 49*t*
Functional Rating Index (FRI), 38*t*
Functional testing, 398
F-wave, in lumbar radiculopathy, 205

G
Gaenslen's test, for sacroiliac joint pathology, 280, 281*f*
Gait
after total ankle arthroplasty, 627–628
disturbances, 119
Gas bubbles, release of, during manipulation, 159
Gastrocnemius muscle, 647
TrPs in, 672–673, 673*f*
dry needling of, 705–706, 706*f*
GBD. *see* Global Burden of Disease (GBD).
Gender
neck pain and, 98
upper extremity disorders and, 9–10
General health status, checklist for review of, 30*b*
General population, neck pain in
prevalence of, 98–99
prognostic factors of, 99, 99*b*
risk factors of, 99*b*
Glenohumeral capsuloligamentous structures, 310–311
Glenohumeral instability, 321–332
anatomy of, 321–322
biomechanics of, 322–323
diagnosis of, 325–329
examination in, 325–326
history in, 325
imaging for, 328–329
laxity tests for, 326–328
stability tests for, 326
management of, 330–331
pathology of, 323–325
prognosis of, 329–330
anatomical risk factors, 330
clinical risk factors, 329–330
Glenohumeral joint
altered motor control, 360
anatomy of, 334–335, 335*f*
passive mobilization interventions of, 350–352
Glenohumeral ligaments, 335*f*
Glenohumeral rotation test, 361, 365*f*
in supine and prone position, 364–365
Glenoid labrum, anatomy of, 334
Global Burden of Disease (GBD) study, 13–14, 95–96
in low back pain, 210–211
Global Rating of Change scale (GRC), 106*t*, 107
Gluteal muscles, 427
Gluteus maximus (GMax) muscle, 427
TrPs in, dry needling of, 700, 700*f*
during various therapeutic exercises, 429*t*
Gluteus medius (GMed) muscle, 427, 505*f*
MET for, 726, 727*f*
side-lying hip abduction in, 506*f*
TrPs in, 671, 671*f*, 726
dry needling of, 700, 700*f*
during various therapeutic exercises, 429*t*
Gluteus medius tendinopathy, 401–405
clinical examination of, 402–403
diagnosis of, 402–403
epidemiology of, 401
pathomechanics of, 401–402
patient history of, 402
prognosis for, 404–405
treatment of, 403–404, 404*f*
Gluteus minimus muscle
MET for, 726, 727*f*
TrPs in, 671–672, 672*f*, 726
dry needling of, 700, 701*f*
GMI. *see* Graded motor imagery (GMI).
Gracilis muscles, TrPs in, 672, 672*f*
Graded motor imagery (GMI), 73
GRC. *see* Global Rating of Change scale (GRC).
Greater trochanteric pain syndrome (GTPS), 17
prevalence of, 16*t*
GTPS. *see* Greater trochanteric pain syndrome (GTPS).
Guyon's tunnel syndrome
common differential diagnosis of, 579*t*
special tests for, 579*t*
symptoms and signs of, 578*t*
Gymnastics, medical, 373

H
Hallux extension (L5), 56*f*
Hamstring
dominance, 437
strengthening exercises, 430–431
tendinopathies of, 531
wall stretch exercise, 433*f*
Hand, dorsal fascia of, 738, 738*f*
Hand behind back, mobilization with movement, 355–356
belt assisted, 355–356, 356*f*
Hand dominance, upper extremity disorders and, 10
Handheld Doppler ultrasound, 49*t*
Headache, cervicogenic, thoracic spine manipulation for, 147
Healthcare, utilization and impact of
in lower extremity pain disorders, 19–20
in upper extremity pain syndromes, 9
Healthcare system, cervical spine disorders challenges to, 97
Heart, pain originating in, 25
Hebbian theory, 67–68
Heel pain, 44
Higher load extensor progressions, 178–179, 179*f*–180*f*
Higher load flexor progressions, 176–178, 177*f*–178*f*
Hill-Sachs lesion, 330, 330*f*
computed tomography of, 328–329
magnetic resonance arthrography of, 328–329
magnetic resonance imaging of, 328–329, 329*f*
plain radiographs of, 328
Hip
anterior cruciate ligament, 469–470
exercises recommended for activation of, 505*t*
external rotation of, 506*f*
pathology of, 43
posterior to anterior mobilization of, 394, 394*f*
Hip abduction
provocation test, for pelvic girdle pain, 281, 282*f*
strength testing, 403, 403*f*
Hip adduction angle, 469*f*
Hip conditions, 16–17
incidence of, 17
prevalence of, 16*t*
symptoms and osteoarthritis, 16
Hip disorders, 397–412
arthroscopic procedures for, in postoperative management, 413–416
capsular and ligamentous structures, 414
chondral defects, 414
femoroacetabular impingement, 413–414
postoperative considerations for, 415
precautions of, 415–416
lumbar spine treatment for, 221–222, 224*t*
phases of rehabilitation for, , in postoperative management, 416–418
maximum protection phase, 416
minimal protection phase, 417–418
moderate protection phase, 416–417
return to sport or daily life activities phase, 418
postoperative management of, 413–420
Hip flexion (L2-L3), 55*f*
Hip flexor muscle
MET for, 726, 726*f*
TrPs in, 726
Hip flexor region, myofascial induction of, 754–755, 755*f*
Hip flexor tendinopathy, 400–401
clinical examination of, 400
diagnosis of, 400
epidemiology of, 400
pathomechanics of, 400, 400*f*
prognosis for, 401
treatment for, 400–401
Hip joint, 426
Hip myofascial stretch exercise, 435*f*
Hip osteoarthritis, 43, 389–396
anatomy of, 390
characteristics of, 389
clinical presentation of, 392
definition of, 390
description of, 389
diagnosis of, 390–392
economic impact of, 390
epidemiological research in, 389
non-pharmacological treatment of, 392–394
exercise therapy for, 393
manual therapy for, 393–394
patient education for, 393
pathomechanics of, 390
prevalence of, 16*t*, 389
prognosis of, 392
risk factors of, 391–392
treatment of, 392–394
Hip pain, prevalence of, 16*t*
'Hip-spine syndrome', 221
Hip syndromes, 78*t*
History taking, 22–35
content of, 23*b*
in glenohumeral instability, 325
location and description of symptoms, 24–26, 25*f*–26*f*, 25*t*
medical history in, 28–29, 29*b*
patient profile in, 23, 24*t*
for patients with lower extremity syndromes, 36–46
symptom behaviour in, 26–27, 27*t*
symptom history in, 27–28
systems review in, 29–34, 30*b*–31*b*, 31*t*–33*t*, 33*f*
Hoffmann's reflex (H-reflex), 59, 59*f*
in cervical myelopathy, 126
in lumbar radiculopathy, 205
Hoffmann's test, 121, 122*f*
Horizontal adduction motion, 356–357
Horizontal side support exercise, 196
for mechanical low back pain, 263–264
Hornblower sign, 314
H-reflex. *see* Hoffmann's reflex (H-reflex).
Human articular cartilage, 483–484
Human knee, neurosensory mapping of, 497*t*
Hyperabduction syndrome, 134
Hyperactive muscle stretch reflexes, 53
Hyperalgesia, 765, 783
TrPs and, 661
Hypoalgesia, MET and, 711

Hypothyroidism, carpal tunnel syndrome and, 567
Hypoxia, 662

I

IAP. *see* Intra-abdominal pressure (IAP).
IGHL. *see* Inferior glenohumeral ligaments (IGHL).
Iliacus muscle, TrPs in, dry needling of, 703, 703*f*
Iliococcygeus, in male pelvic pain, 228–229
Iliotibial band, stroke on, 755, 755*f*
Iliotibial band syndrome (ITBS), 397–399, 532–535
  anatomy of, 533
  clinical examination of, 398
  conservative treatment and prognosis, 534–535
  diagnosis of, 398, 534
  epidemiology of, 397
  general anatomy of, 533*f*
  manual therapy treatment for, 398–399
  pathology and patho-biomechanics, 534
  pathomechanics of, 397–398
  prognosis for, 399
  two regions of, 533*f*
'Iliotibial friction syndrome', 534
Imaging, for glenohumeral instability, 328–329
Immobilization
  Achilles tendon ruptures and, 631–632
  for ulnar collateral ligament (UCL) injury, 600
Impact of Events Scale (IES), 113
Impingement
  cam-type, 414
  pincer-type, 413–414
  shoulder, rotator cuff lesions, 309–320
In-shoe orthoses, 510
Inclinometer, 149
Indirect distraction manipulation, 394, 394*f*
Indirect osteopathic manipulative technique (IOMT), 554
Infective spondylitis, 38
Inferior clavicular/disc glide, right shoulder, 306, 307*f*
Inferior glenohumeral ligaments (IGHL), 321–322
Inferior glide
  and anterior glide, of glenohumeral joint, 352, 352*f*
  end-range elevation, mobilization with movement, 354–355, 355*f*
  of glenohumeral joint, 351, 351*f*
Inferior labrum, anatomy of, 334
Inflammatory mediators, physiological role of, 775–776
Infraspinatus fascia, 735*f*, 736
Infraspinatus muscle
  anatomy of, 309
  therapeutic exercises for, 379–380, 380*f*
  TrPs in, 664–665, 664*f*
    dry needling of, 694, 694*f*
Injection, for lumbar radiculopathy, 207
Injury
  incidence/prevalence of
    anterior cruciate ligament, 468
    lateral collateral ligament, 471
    medial collateral ligament, 471
    meniscus, 472
    posterior cruciate ligament, 470
  progression, elbow instability, 451
Innominate anterior rotation, pelvic, restriction of, MET for, 722, 722*f*
Innominate posterior rotation, pelvic, restriction of, MET for, 722, 723*f*
Instability
  glenohumeral, 321–332
    anatomy of, 321–322
    biomechanics of, 322–323
    diagnosis of, 325–329
    management of, 330–331
    pathology of, 323–325
    prognosis of, 329–330
  lateral elbow, 452–453
    anatomy review for, 452
    diagnosis of, 452–453
    incidence/prevalence of, 452
    orthopaedic examination techniques for, 453*t*
    pathology/pathoanatomy of, 452
    prognosis and treatment planning for patients with, 453
  lumbar spine, 210–220
    clinical management of, 214–216
    proposed clinical examination for, 216–218
Instability catch sign, in lumbar spine instability, 217
Integrins, 547, 730–731
Interclavicular ligament, 303
Interlaminar epidural injection, for lumbar radiculopathy, 207
Interleukin-1 (IL-1), in neuritis model, 775
Interleukin-6 (IL-6), in neuritis model, 775
Internal carotid artery dissection, pain from, 25
'Internal derangement', 295
Internal oblique muscle, TrPs in, dry needling of, 699–700, 699*f*
Internal pelvic trigger point wand, 231, 232*f*
Internal snapping hip syndrome, 400–401
  clinical examination of, 400
  diagnosis of, 400
  epidemiology of, 400
  pathomechanics of, 400, 400*f*
  prognosis for, 401
  treatment for, 400–401
International Association for the Study of Pain (IASP), 99–100
Interossei, 595
Interosseous membrane, 606
Interosseous myofascial induction, 753, 753*f*
Interosseous sacroiliac ligament (ISL), 276
Interscalene space triangle, 133–134, 134*f*
Intersection syndrome, 551
  surgery for, 555
Interspinous muscles, 101*f*
Interstitial mechanoreceptors, in fascia, 731
Intervertebral discs, referral patterns from, 100*f*
Intervertebral foramen, 200
Interview, patient, in management of lumbar spine instability, 214
Intra-abdominal pressure (IAP), pelvic floor muscles and, 226
Intra-articular inclusions, 87
Intra-articular injection, fluoroscopic-guided, for sacroiliac joint pain, 277–278
Intra-articular ligament, 303
Intra-articular steroid injections, 485
Intra-rater reliability, 47
Intracapsular ligaments, 559
Intra-class correlation coefficients (ICCs), 47
Intravenous drug, causing bloodborne infections, 28
'Inverse C7-T1 relationship', 143
Inverted supinator sign, 121–122, 122*f*
Ion channels, 783, 783*f*–784*f*
Irradiation technique, abdominal draw-in manoeuvre and, 260
Irritability, 27, 42
Ischaemia, 498
Ischaemic compression technique, for TrPs, 679
Isolated adductor tenotomy, 407
Isolation exercises, 437–438
Isometric exercise, of shoulder, 378, 379*f*
Isometric strength, 52–53
Isotonic exercise, of shoulder, 378–381
Isotope bone scanning, of acromioclavicular joint, 297–298
Isquiotibial path, stroke on, 755, 755*f*
Isthmic spondylolisthesis, 78*t*
ITBS. *see* Iliotibial band syndrome (ITBS).

J

Jackknife stretch, for mechanical low back pain, 257*f*, 258
Japanese Orthopaedic Association (JOA) score, 121
Jobe relocation test, 338, 339*f*
Johnston County Osteoarthritis (JoCo OA) Project, 16
Joint(s)
  acromioclavicular, 293–301
  carpometacarpal (CMC) I, 586, 596, 600
  carpometacarpal (CMC) II-V, 586
  distal radioulnar, 559
  distal tibiofibular, 605–606
  glenohumeral, 334–335, 335*f*
  hip, 426
  knee, 756
  mid-carpal, 559
  patellofemoral, 493–495
  radiocarpal, 559
  sacroiliac, 78*t*, 426
  sternoclavicular, 302–308
  subtalar, 606–607
  talocrural, 606
  zygapophyseal, 100*f*
Joint mobilization, 158–173
  definitions and clinical applications of, 459–460
  evidence-based decision making, 458–459
  interventions of knee, 527–529
  for low back pain, 195
  and manipulation, 584–593
    of elbow, 458–463
    grades of movement, 584, 585*f*
    of knee, 525–530
    of wrist and hand, 586–592
  of shoulder, 350–357
Joint stability, motor control and, 358–359
Joint stiffness, in thoracic outlet syndrome, 139
Joint-biased manual therapies, for chronic low back pain, 239–240
Journal of Family Practice Guideline, 82*t*

K

Kaltenborn concept, 586
Kaltenborn technique, 585
Kappa (κ) coefficients, 47
Kettlebell lift exercise, for mechanical low back pain, 269, 269*f*
Kinaesthetic awareness, exercises for, 186–187, 187*f*
Kleinman's shear test, 562–563
Knee
  anterior cruciate ligament, 470
  arthrofibrosis of, 522
  articular structures of, 467
  complex, transverse myofascial induction in, 757, 757*f*
  conditions, 17–18
    prevalence of, 17*t*
    symptoms and osteoarthritis, 17–18
  disorders, lumbar spine treatment for, 222–223, 224*t*
  dynamic valgus torques on, 470
  evidence of manual therapy in, 525–527
  extensor fascia, myofascial induction of, 756, 756*f*
  flexion
    bilateral squat exercise, 475*f*
    split squat exercise, 476*f*
  human, neurosensory mapping of, 497*t*
  joint, 756
    deep fascial intermuscular links in, 743, 744*f*
  joint mobilization and manipulation of, 525–530
    interventions, 527–529
  lateral view of, 494*f*
  ligament rupture and meniscal tear, management, 473–477
  ligamentous and meniscal injuries of, 467–481
  menisci, 471–472
  pain, 493
    prevalence of, 17*t*
  postoperative management of, 514–524
    anterior/posterior cruciate ligament reconstruction, 514–516
    medial collateral ligament repair/reconstruction, 516–517
    meniscus, 517–520
    partial meniscectomy, 519–520
    total knee arthroplasty (TKA), 520–521
  problems, 86
  Q-angle of, 495*f*
  valgus angle, 469*f*
Knee extension (L3-L4), 55*f*
Knee ligamentous injury, 44
Knee meniscal injury, 44
Knee osteoarthritis, 43, 482–492, 498
  biomechanics of, 484
  incidence of, 18
  lumbar spine treatment for, 222–223
  prevalence of, 17*t*
  skin rolling, 487*f*
  specific pain mechanisms in, 483
Knee Outcome Survey, 38*t*
Knee tendinopathy, 531–541
  of hamstrings, 531
  iliotibial band syndrome, 532–535
  patellar, 535–537

popliteal, 537–538
quadriceps, 538–539
semimembranosus, 532
Kneeling, four-point, 362, 365–366, 366*f*

L

Labral debridement, with/without rim trimming, 415
Labral tears, 17
prevalence of, 16*t*
Labrum, of hip, disorders of, 397–412
Lactation, carpal tunnel syndrome during, 10
Laser therapy, rotator cuff lesions shoulder impingement and, 316
Late-cocking phase, of overhead throw, 323–324, 324*f*
Lateral box jumping, 476*f*
Lateral collateral ligament, 471
anatomy of, 471
biomechanics of, 471
incidence/prevalence of injury, 471
mechanism of injury/risk factors of, 471
surgical management of, 477
Lateral elbow instability, 452–453
anatomy review for, 452
diagnosis of, 452–453
incidence/prevalence of, 452
orthopaedic examination techniques for, 453*t*
pathology/pathoanatomy of, 452
prognosis and treatment planning for patients with, 453
Lateral elbow pain, 144
Lateral epicondylalgia, 445, 752
defined, 446
diagnostic considerations, 445–446
prognostic considerations of, 447
Lateral epicondylitis, 8*t*–9*t*
Lateral glide mobilization with movement, 462
Lateral glides, at 90° of flexion, 416, 417*f*
Lateral meniscus, 472
Lateral pivot shift test, 453*t*
Lateral shift exercises, for low back pain, 195
Lateral side-step exercise, 428*f*
Lateral trunk displacement, 469*f*
Lateral-medial non-thrust mobilization, 611
Latissimus dorsi fascia, 735*f*, 736
Latissimus dorsi muscle
MET for, 725, 725*f*
TrPs in, dry needling of, 695, 695*f*
Laxity tests, for glenohumeral instability, 326–328
LBP. *see* Low back pain (LBP).
LEFS. *see* Lower Extremity Functional Scale (LEFS).
Leg
deep fascial intermuscular links in, 741–743, 742*f*–743*f*
fascial system of, 756–757
lateral compartment of, release of, 757–758, 758*f*
pain, 42
posterior compartment of, release of, 756*f*–757*f*, 757
Levator scapulae muscle
fascia of, 735*f*, 736
MET for, 724, 724*f*
Lhermitte's sign, 60
Lichtman splint, 564, 564*f*
LIFT. *see* Lumbar interfascial triangle (LIFT).
Ligamentous, acute phase after, and meniscal injury, 474–475
Likelihood ratios (LRs), 48
Limb fascia, superficial layer of upper, 733–734, 734*f*
Limb pain, chronic upper, 765
physiological mechanisms of, 771–772
Linscheid test, 562
Loaded exercises, for contractile dysfunction, 89
Long dorsal ligament, 276
palpation of, for pelvic girdle pain, 282, 283*f*
Long-leg distraction manipulation, for sacroiliac joint, 286–287, 287*f*
Longissimus thoracis muscle, TrPs in, dry needling of, 698, 698*f*
Longitudinal massage, stretching, of adductor muscle taut band, 687, 687*f*
Longitudinal stroke
dynamic
of biceps brachii muscle taut band, 683, 684*f*
of gluteus medius muscle taut band, 686, 686*f*
of hand/wrist extensor muscle taut band, 684
of triceps brachii muscle taut band, 683, 684*f*
of scalene muscle taut band, 681, 681*f*
stretching
of gluteus medius muscle taut band, 686, 686*f*
of quadriceps muscle taut band, 687, 687*f*
Low back pain (LBP), 77
chronic, 236–244
versus acute low back pain, 236–237
altered nociceptive transmission in, 237
interventions for, 239–241
joint-biased manual therapies for, 239–240
nerve-biased manual therapies for, 240–241
neuroimaging in, 237–239
soft-tissue-biased manual therapies for, 240
in DALYs, 211*t*
definition of, 210–211, 236
diagnostic challenge of, 211–212
functional magnetic resonance imaging study of, 67*f*, 72*f*
guideline adherence for, 211
barriers to, 211*t*
historical appreciation of, 210–211
mechanical, 191–198
examination items for, 196
intervention for, 196
manipulation for, 194, 194*f*
screening for, 191–192, 192*t*
specific exercise group for, 194–195
spinal manipulation group for, 193–194
stabilization group for, 195–196
staging process in, 192–197, 192*t*
traction group for, 197
treatment-based classification system for, 191, 192*t*
medical expenditures in, 211*f*
MET for, 710–711
non-specific, 211–212
practice variability for, 211
during pregnancy, 227
prevalence of, 14*t*, 15, 199
red flags in patients with, 40*t*
spinal manipulative therapy for, 246
treatment-based classification system for, 212, 213*t*
Low-back-associated musculoskeletal pain syndromes, 42–43
Lower extremity, musculoskeletal conditions in, 13, 14*f*
Lower Extremity Functional Scale (LEFS), 38*t*
Lower extremity neurodynamics, lumbar spine treatment for, 223
Lower extremity pain disorders
epidemiology of, 13–21
healthcare utilization and impact in, 19–20
musculoskeletal conditions in, 13, 14*f*
prevalence and incidence of, 13–19
foot and ankle conditions, 18–19
greater trochanteric pain syndrome, 17
hip conditions, 16–17
knee conditions, 17–18
labral tears, 17
lumbar conditions, 13–16
Lower extremity syndromes
history taking for patients with, 36–46
associated with musculoskeletal pain syndromes and, 43–44
cardiovascular screen in, 38–39
communication style and approach in, 37
gastrointestinal screen in, 39
medical interview content in, 37
nature and behaviour of problem in, 41–42
neurological screen in, 38
non-mechanical pathologies differential diagnosis in, 39–40
psychosocial factors in, 40
purpose of interview in, 36
questions specific in, 42
red flags in, 40, 40*t*
specific low-back-associated musculoskeletal pain syndromes and, 42–43
symptom investigation in, 40–41
systems review and differential diagnosis inquiry in, 37–40, 39*t*
intake information for, 41*t*
self-reported outcome measures for, 38*t*
Lower limb challenges, for mechanical low back pain, 260–261, 260*f*
Lower quadrant, therapeutic exercises for, 426–442
activation levels of gluteus medius and gluteus maximus during, 429*t*
case study of, 426*b*–427*b*
designing an evidence-informed programme, 434–440
dynamic/functional assessment, 427
exercise parameters, 440–441, 441*t*
mobility, myofascial and articular impairments, 432–434
muscle performance, 427–431
neuromotor control, 431–432
physical examination of, 426
Lower quadrant pain, neurophysiology in, 783–784
Low-level LASER therapy, 447–448
LSS. *see* Lumbar spinal stenosis (LSS).
Lumbar conditions, 13–16
incidence of, 15–16
prevalence of, 13–15, 14*t*
Lumbar disc herniation, 43
radiculopathy and, 201
Lumbar extension, with overpressure, 62*f*
combined, 62*f*
Lumbar flexion, with overpressure, 62*f*
Lumbar interfascial triangle (LIFT), 740–741, 741*f*
myofascial induction of, 754, 754*f*
Lumbar manipulation, patellar mobilizations and, 503–504
Lumbar multifidus muscle, TrPs in, dry needling of, 697, 697*f*–698*f*
Lumbar nerve roots, manual muscle testing for, 54*t*
Lumbar radiculopathy, 199–209
active and passive movements in, 202
aetiology and background of, 199–200
anatomy of, 200–201
definitions of, 199–200
description of, by severity, 200*t*
differential diagnosis of, 201
evidence-based clinical examination of, 201–205
imaging in, 204
outcome measures in, 204
patient history in, 201–202
physical examination in, 202
provocation tests in, 202–204
natural history of, 200
neurological testing for, 202
observation of, 202
pain associated with, 51
pathogenesis of, 201
prevalence of, 199
signs and symptoms of, 200
treatment of, 205–208
conservative approaches in, 205–207
injection in, 207
surgical approaches in, 207–208
Lumbar side-bending, with overpressure, 62*f*
Lumbar spinal stenosis (LSS), 15, 42–43
prevalence of, 14*t*
Lumbar spine, 426
anatomy of, 200
assessment of, 720
cross-hands myofascial induction of, 754, 754*f*
in lower extremity pain syndromes, 221–225
lower extremity pain syndromes in, 221–225
MET for, 720–721
posterior-anterior mobility of, 63*f*
treatment
for ankle disorders, 223
for foot disorders, 223
for hip disorders, 221–222
for knee disorders, 222–223
for lower extremity neurodynamics, 223
Lumbar spine instability, 210–220
clinical management of, 214–216
first level of classification in, 214
patient interview in, 214
pattern recognition in, 214–215, 215*b*
physical examination in, 215, 216*f*
second level of classification in, 215
self-reported symptoms in, 214–215, 215*b*
proposed clinical examination for, 216–218
clinical prediction rules, 218
confirmatory tests, 217–218
screening tests, 216–217

Lumbar spine joint mobilization/manipulation, 245–254
audible pop in, 248
clinical prediction rules in, 246–248
contraindications for, 249–250, 249*b*
evidence for, 246
locking in, 248–249
nomenclature in, standardizing, 245
positioning in, 248–249
precautions for, 249–250, 250*b*
safety in, 249–250
techniques in, 249–250
central posterior-to-anterior mobilization, 250, 250*f*
lumbar rotation in flexion manipulation, 252–253, 253*f*
lumbar rotation in neutral or extension manipulation, 252, 253*f*
lumbar rotation mobilization, 251, 251*f*–252*f*
lumbopelvic regional manipulation, 251–252, 252*f*
unilateral posterior-to-anterior mobilization, 250–251, 250*f*
Lumbar spine thrust, high-velocity rotational, 205, 205*f*
Lumbar vertebrae, anatomy of, 200
Lumbopelvic cylinder, pelvic floor muscles in, 226
Lumbopelvic pain, pelvic floor muscles and, 227
Lumbricals, 595
Lunate, 559
Lunge backward exercise, 439*f*
Lunge test, for pelvic girdle pain, 281, 282*f*
Lunotriquetral ligament (LTL), 559–560, 559*f*
Lunotriquetral tests, 563*f*

M
Magnetic resonance arthrography (MRA)
of Hill-Sachs lesion, 328–329
of rotator cuff lesions shoulder impingement, 315
of superior labrum anterior-to-posterior (SLAP) lesions, 340, 340*f*
Magnetic resonance imaging (MRI)
for Achilles tendon rupture, 630
of acromioclavicular joint, 297–298
of cervical spine, 124–125, 125*f*
of fatty infiltrate, 112
functional, in chronic low back pain, 238
of Hill-Sachs lesion, 328–329, 329*f*
of lumbar radiculopathy, 204
of peripheral nerve inflammation, 776, 777*f*
for plantar heel pain, 617–618
of rotator cuff lesions shoulder impingement, 315
of superior labrum anterior-to-posterior (SLAP) lesions, 340
for tendinopathy, 549–550
for tibialis anterior tendinopathies, 652
Magnetoencephalography (MEG), in chronic low back pain, 238
Major adverse events, after cervical spine manipulation, 161
Manipulation
definition of, 161
joint mobilization and
of elbow, 458–463
of knee, 525–530
in lateral glide of elbow, 462, 462*f*
for low back pain, 194, 194*f*
lumbar, patellar mobilizations and, 503–504
varus thrust, 462, 462*f*
Manual activities, carpal tunnel syndrome and, 567–568
Manual muscle testing, 52–53
for cervical nerve roots, 52–53
for lumbar nerve roots, 54*t*
for lumbar radiculopathy, 202
Manual therapy
evidence, of knee, 525–527
for hip osteoarthritis, 393–394
for osteoarthritis, 486–488
for wrist and hand tendinopathy, 553, 555
Manubriosternal motion, 302
Marital status, in patient profile, 23
Massage therapies, for TrPs, 680
Matles test, for Achilles tendon rupture, 629–630, 630*f*
Maximum protection phase, of postoperative rehabilitation, 416
Maximum tensile strength, of ACL, 468
McKenzie, Robin, 76, 85
MCL. *see* Medial collateral ligament (MCL).
MDT. *see* Mechanical Diagnosis and Therapy (MDT).
Mechanical allodynia, 773
Mechanical Diagnosis and Therapy (MDT)
for extremity problems, 85–91
anatomy and biomechanics in, 86–87, 86*t*, 87*f*
brief epidemiology of, 85–86
diagnosis in, evidence regarding, 88
medical diagnosis for, 86
prognosis in, evidence regarding, 88
proposed pathological model in, 87–88
treatment of, evidence regarding, 88–89
for spine, 76–84
anatomy and biomechanics in, review of, 78–79
conservative treatment with, evidence regarding, 80–82, 81*t*–82*t*
diagnosis in, evidence regarding, 80
epidemiological perspective of, 77–78
literature base for, 77, 78*t*
prognosis in, evidence regarding, 80
proposed pathology and anatomy in, review of, 79–80
Mechanical interface, definition of, 784
Mechanical low back pain, 191–198
examination items for, 196
intervention for, 196
manipulation for, 194, 194*f*
screening for, 191–192, 192*t*
specific exercise group for, 194–195
spinal manipulation group for, 193–194
stabilization group for, 195–196
staging process in, 192–197, 192*t*
stage 1, 192–197, 193*t*
stage II and III, 197
therapeutic exercise for, 255–273
abdominal curl-up, 261, 261*f*
abdominal draw-in manoeuvre, 259–260, 259*f*
for balance, 268–269, 268*f*
bent knee sit-up for, 261, 261*f*
bridge exercises, in supine, 262, 263*f*–264*f*
evidence for, 255–256
front plank, 264, 265*f*
for functional integration, 266–267
high level strengthening, 269–270, 269*f*–270*f*
horizontal side support, 263–264
lower limb challenges, 260–261, 260*f*
for mobility, 256–259, 257*f*, 258*b*
for motor control, 259
for motor pattern retraining, 266–267
multifidus activation exercises, 262, 263*f*
parameters for, 270–271, 271*t*
pilates/yoga, 267–268
prone bridge, 264
for proprioception, 268–269
quadruped, 262, 264*f*
side plank, 263–264, 265*f*
on unstable surfaces, 264–266, 266*f*
traction group for, 197
treatment-based classification system for, 191, 192*t*
Mechanical neck pain, 95–109
causes of, 99–100
cervical spine self-report measures of, 105–107, 106*t*
Fear-avoidance Beliefs Questionnaire, 106*t*, 107
Global Rating of Change scale, 106*t*, 107
Neck Disability Index, 106, 106*t*
Numerical Pain Rating Scale, 106, 106*t*
Patient Specific Functional Scale, 106–107, 106*t*
classification of, 104–105
categories, 105
clinical presentation of, 100, 100*f*–101*f*
conceptual model of, 96*f*
definition of, 95–96, 96*f*
financial impact of, 97
in general population
prevalence of, 98–99
prognostic factors of, 99, 99*b*
risk factors of, 99*b*
and mobility, therapeutic exercise for, 182–185
articular/self-mobilization, 183–184, 183*f*
generalized active range of motion, 182–183
neurodynamics, 185
and motor function, therapeutic exercise for, 175–182
motor control, 180–182
recruitment, 175–176
side-flexion/rotation exercises for asymmetric weakness, 179–180, 180*f*–181*f*
strength and endurance, 176–179
postural correction and, therapeutic exercise for, 185–186, 186*f*
articular system, 186
muscle imbalance, 185
neuromeningeal system, 186
prevalence of, 96–99, 97*t*
prognosis in, 97–99
proposed management of, 100–105
first level of classification, 101
red flag screening, 101–103
second level of classification, 103–105, 104*f*
yellow flag screening, 103
review of anatomy specific to, 99
risk factors of, 97–99
therapeutic exercise for, 174–188
and somatosensory dysfunction, 186–187, 187*f*
treatment-based classification of, 105
in working individuals
prevalence of, 98
prognostic factors of, 98, 98*b*
risk factors of, 98*b*
Mechanically inconclusive syndromes, 78*t*
Mechanosensitivity, definition of, 794
Mechanotransduction, 547
Medial collateral ligament (MCL), 471
anatomy of, 471
biomechanics of, 471
incidence/prevalence of injury, 471
mechanism of injury/risk factors, 471
repair/reconstruction, 516–517
bracing/weight-bearing, 516
range of motion exercises of, 516
therapeutic exercise of, 516–517
surgical management of, 477
Medial elbow instability, 454–455
anatomy review for, 454
diagnosis of, 454–455
incidence/prevalence of, 454
orthopaedic examination techniques for, 455*t*
pathology/pathoanatomy of, 454
prognosis and treatment planning for patients with, 455
Medial epicondylitis, 8*t*–9*t*
Medial meniscus, 472
injury, 468*b*
Medial talar tilt test, 609, 609*f*
Medial talocalcaneal interosseus ligaments, 606
Median nerve, 768–770
anatomy of, 577
compliance of, 768–769, 768*f*–769*f*
diagnosis for, 580–581
loading of, 769
movement of
longitudinal, 768
studies of, 771
transverse, 770, 770*f*
Medical conditions, observation and screening for, 48–50, 49*t*, 50*f*
Medical gymnastics, 373
Medical history, 28–29, 29*b*
Medical interview, content of, 37
Medical screening. *see* Systems review.
MEG. *see* Magnetoencephalography (MEG).
Meniscal injury
acute phase after ligamentous and, 474–475
functional phase of ligamentous and, 477
ratio of male to female, 472
recovery phase of ligamentous and, 475–477
special tests for ligament and, 473*t*
surgical management of, 477
Meniscal repair/transplantation, 517–519
bracing/weight-bearing of, 518
modalities of, 517
neuromuscular re-education of, 519
postoperative intervention strategies for, 517*t*
range of motion exercises of, 518
therapeutic exercise of, 518–519, 519*f*

Meniscal tear, knee ligament rupture and, management of, 473–477
Meniscectomy, partial, 519–520
modalities of, 519
range of motion exercises of, 520
therapeutic exercises of, 520
Meniscus, 471–473, 517–520
anatomy of, 471–472
biomechanics of, 472
incidence/prevalence of injury, 472
injury in, 18
mechanism of injury/risk factors, 472–473
repair/transplantation, 517–519, 517*t*
special tests for, 473*t*
tear in, prevalence of, 17*t*
MET. *see* Muscle energy technique (MET).
Metacarpal fractures, 595
intra-articular, 595
Metacarpal head, fractures of, 595
Metacarpophalangeal (MCP) I mobilizations with movement, 592
MGHL. *see* Middle glenohumeral ligaments (MGHL).
Michigan Quality Improvement Consortium Guideline, 82*t*
Micro-fracture, 416
Midbrain periaqueductal grey (PAG), 69–70
activation of, 72*f*
Mid-carpal joint, 559
Mid-cervical spine, self-mobilization exercises for, 184
Middle glenohumeral ligaments (MGHL), 321–322
Mild adverse events, after cervical spine manipulation, 161
Milking test, 455*t*
Minimal protection phase, of postoperative rehabilitation, 417–418
Mobility exercises, 435–437
for mechanical low back pain, 256–259, 257*f*, 258*b*
for mechanical neck pain, 182–185
articular/self-mobilization, 183–184, 183*f*
generalized active range of motion, 182–183
neurodynamics, 185
Mobility testing, of first rib, 149
Mobilization
cervical, posterior-anterior, 168–169
definition of, 161
joint
definitions and clinical applications of, 459–460
evidence-based decision making, 458–459
and manipulation of elbow, 458–463
of knee
interventions, 527–529
manipulation, 525–530
non-thrust, 610–612
anterior-posterior, 611
distal tibiofibular joint, 612
lateral-medial, 611
in pronation/supination combined flexion, 461, 461*f*
of radiohumeral joint, 461, 462*f*
thrust, 610–612
cuboid whip, 612, 613*f*
proximal tibiofibular joint, 612, 612*f*
rearfoot distraction, 611, 611*f*
tibiofemoral, 515
Mobilization with movement (MWM), 584–585
distal radioulnar joint, 587
elevation, 353–354, 353*f*
belt assisted, 354, 354*f*
shoulder girdle, 355, 355*f*
end-range elevation
external rotation, 354, 354*f*
inferior glide, 354–355, 355*f*
finger joint, 592
hand behind back, 355, 356*f*
belt assisted, 355–356, 356*f*
horizontal adduction (AC/SC joints), 356, 357*f*
lateral glide, 462
metacarpophalangeal (MCP) I, 592
radiocarpal, 589
of shoulder complex, 352–357
for talocrural joint, 640–641
non-weight-bearing talocrural posterior glide, 641, 641*f*
weight-bearing talocrural posterior glide, 641, 641*f*
Moderate adverse events, after cervical spine manipulation, 161
Moderate protection phase, of postoperative rehabilitation, 416–417
Modified Jobe relocation test, 337
Motivational interviewing (MI), 37
Motor control
exercises for, 259
facilitation techniques, 262*b*
in mechanical neck pain, 180–182
cervical neutral, during limb load, 180–181, 181*f*
segmental control, during neck motion, 181–182, 182*f*
MET for, 714
of shoulder region, 358–372
and joint stability, 358–359
management of, through patient examples, 368–371
tests for, 361*b*–363*b*
Motor dysfunction, 111–112
Motor function, exercises for, in mechanical neck pain, 175–182
and motor control, 180–182
recruitment, 175–176
side-flexion/rotation exercises for asymmetric weakness, 179–180, 180*f*–181*f*
strength and endurance, 176–179
Motor pattern retraining, 266–267
motor control exercises for, 259
Motor vehicle crash (MVC), 110–111
Motor weakness, associated with radiculopathy, 120
Movar scale, for tendinopathy, 548
Movement awareness
of scapula, 362, 365*f*
of shoulder girdle, 361–364
Movement impairments, of shoulder girdle, 361–364
Movement repatterning, neuromotor control, 431–432
Moving valgus stress test, 455*t*
MRA. *see* Magnetic resonance arthrography (MRA).
MRI. *see* Magnetic resonance imaging (MRI).
Mulligan techniques, 585–586
mobilization with movement (MWM), 435–436
Multifidus
activation exercises, for mechanical low back pain, 262, 263*f*
stabilization exercises for, 219*t*
Multimodal treatment, for PFJ, 503–506
Multiplanar directional lunges exercise, 518*f*
Multiple sutural synostosis, 421, 422*f*
Muscle(s)
exercises recommended for activation of, 505*t*
of hip, disorders of, 397–412
of lower quadrant, MET for, 726–727
of upper quadrant, MET for, 724–725
weakness of, lumbar radiculopathy and, 202
Muscle energy technique (MET), 710
cautions for, 712
common errors in, 713*b*
contraindications to, 712
evidence of effectiveness of, 710–711
integrated approach to, 711–712
for myofascial tissues, 723–727
for pelvic girdle, 721–723
physiological mechanisms of, 711
principles of, 712
recruitment, 176*f*
for rib cage, 718–720
for spine, 713–714
Muscle flexibility, 426
Muscle imbalance
postural correction exercises for, 185
in thoracic outlet syndrome, 138–139
Muscle performance
activation, endurance and strength, 427–431
and neuromuscular control exercises, 437–440
phase 1 of, 437, 441*t*
phase 2 of, 437–439, 441*t*
phase 3 of, 439–440, 441*t*
Muscle recruitment, altered patterns of, 111–112
Muscle strength, 426
Muscle trigger points. *see* Myofascial trigger points.
Muscle-referred pain, 482
Musculoskeletal diseases, 13
Musculoskeletal pain, associated with age, 10
Musculoskeletal problems, 85
Musculoskeletal ultrasound (MSKUS), for plantar heel pain, 617–618
MWM. *see* Mobilization with movement (MWM).
Myelopathy, cervical
active and passive movements of, 121
clinical signs and symptoms of, 119–120
confirmation tests of, 121–122
conservative approaches of, 127
current best evidence with regard to prognosis in, 126
differential diagnosis and treatment of, 118–131
essential aspects of, 126
imaging of, 124–125
nerve condition responses in, 125–126
observation of, 121
outcome measures of, 121
patient history in, 120–121
physical examination of, 121
review of proposed pathology and pathobiomechanics of, 119
surgical approaches of, 128–129
anterior, 128
posterior, 128–129
Myeloradiculopathy, cervical
clinical signs and symptoms of, 120
confirmation tests of, 124
conservative approaches of, 127
current best evidence with regard to prognosis in, 126
differential diagnosis and treatment of, 118–131
essential aspects of, 126
imaging of, 124–125
nerve condition responses in, 125–126
outcome measures of, 124
patient history in, 124
physical examination of, 124
review of proposed pathology and pathobiomechanics of, 119
surgical approaches of, 128–129
anterior, 128
posterior, 128–129
Myofascial dysfunction syndrome, formation of, mechanics of, 743–745
fascial entrapment areas, 744–745, 745*f*
Myofascial extensibility, self-mobilization exercises for, 184–185, 184*f*–185*f*
Myofascial induction
approaches to, 729–761
assessment process in, 748
clinical applications of, 748–749
clinical research in healthy subjects, 747–748
contraindications to, 758
definition of, 748
general observations related to therapeutic process of, 748
for lower quadrant disorders, 753–758
knee and leg region, 756–758
lumbopelvic region, 753–755
thigh region, 755–756
neurophysiological mechanisms of, 745–747
procedure principles of, 748–749
research related to pathology, 747
results of, scientific evidence of, 747–748
therapeutic strategies applied in, 748–749
for upper quadrant disorders, 749–753
brachial and antebrachial fascia, 752
cervical spine, 749–750
fascia of hand, 752–753
shoulder girdle, 750–751
Myofascial tissues, MET for, principles of, 723–724
Myofascial trigger points, 347, 660–662
definition of, 660
exploration of, related to
lower quadrant pain syndromes, 670–673
upper quadrant pain syndromes, 662–670, 663*f*
manual identification of, 660
manual therapies for, 679–680
best evidence of, 679
clinical applications of, 681–687
compression, 679–680
dynamic interventions, 680
massage, 680
stretching, 680

neurophysiological basis of, 661–662
central sensitization mechanisms, 661
integrated hypothesis, 662
peripheral sensitization, 661
sympathetic nervous system, 661–662
referred pain elicited by, characteristics of, 660
treatment interventions for, 678
Myofibroblast dynamics, 746
Myotomes, 52–53
lumbar radiculopathy and, 200, 203*t*

N

NAIOMT. *see* North American Institute of Orthopaedic Manual Therapy (NAIOMT).
National Health and Nutrition Survey (NHANES), 16
NCS. *see* Nerve conduction studies (NCS).
NDI. *see* Neck Disability Index (NDI).
Neck Disability Index (NDI), 106, 106*t*
for cervical radiculopathy, 122
Neck pain
cervical spine manipulation for, 158–159
mechanical, 95–109 *see also* Mechanical neck pain
causes of, 99–100
cervical spine self-report measures of, 105–107, 106*t*
classification of, 104–105
clinical presentation of, 100, 100*f*–101*f*
conceptual model of, 96*f*
definition of, 95–96, 96*f*
financial impact of, 97
prevalence of, 96–99, 97*t*
prognosis in, 97–99
proposed management of, 100–105
review of anatomy specific to, 99
risk factors of, 97–99
treatment-based classification of, 105
MET for, 711
prevalence of, 7*t*
thoracic spine manipulation for, 144–147, 145*t*–146*t*
Neck Pain Task Force, 95
Neck-shoulder muscles, TrPs in, 662–663
Neck/upper limb disorders, 5
Neer impingement test, 314
Negative likelihood ratio (-LR), 48
Neighbouring neural circuits, primary pain map influencing, 67, 68*f*
Nerve
irritation, symptoms from, 135*t*
median, 768–770
mobilization, 582
peripheral. *see* Peripheral nerve
recovery, 581
sensitivity, 783, 783*f*–784*f*
trauma, conditions causing, 135*t*
trunk pain, 783
ulnar, 770
Nerve bed
elongation, 785
shortening, 785
Nerve conduction studies (NCS), of lumbar radiculopathy, 204–205
Nerve conduction velocity (NCV) test, for lumbar radiculopathy, 205
Nerve growth factor (NGF), 775
Nerve root compression / radiculopathy, 43
Nerve root examination, 51–59
of myotomes, 52–53
neurodynamic assessment and, 56–59
of reflexes, 53–56
of sensation, 52
'Nerve-sliding' techniques, 581
Nerve-biased manual therapies, for chronic low back pain, 240–241
Nervi nervorum, 568, 776
Nervous system, changes in, with chronic pain, 66–70
Neural mobilization exercises, for plantar heel pain, 620
'Neural tension test', 781–782
Neuritis model, 773–775, 773*f*–774*f*
Neurobiomechanics, definition of, 784
Neurodynamic assessment, 56–59
Neurodynamic test, 785–793
in assessment, 793–794
central nervous system processing in, 784
definition of, 782
handling issues in, 785–786
for lower quadrant, 791–793
neurogenic symptoms evoked in, 794
responses to, 794
for upper quadrant, 786–791
Neurodynamics
definition of, 782
lower extremity, lumbar spine treatment for, 223
mechanical interface and, 784
mobility exercises and, 185
Neurogenic pain
definition of, 782
in thoracic outlet syndrome, 139
Neuroimaging, in chronic low back pain, 237–239
Neurological deficits, screening for, 51–60
Neurological testing, for lumbar radiculopathy, 202
Neuromatrix, 66–68, 67*f*–68*f*
Neuromeningeal system, postural correction exercises for, 186
Neuromotor control, 431–432
proprioception, 431–432
retraining programme, 432*t*
Neuromuscular control
balance training and, 506–507
exercises, muscle performance and, 437–440
Neuromuscular electrical stimulation (NMES), 488
Neuropathic arm, management of, 795
Neuropathic pain, 24
Neuropraxia, 577
Neurotmesis, 577
Neutral zone, 181
NGF. *see* Nerve growth factor (NGF).
NHANES. *see* National Health and Nutrition Survey (NHANES).
NIH-Chronic Prostatitis Symptom Index (NIH-CPSI), 230–231, 231*f*–232*f*
NIH-CPSI. *see* NIH-Chronic Prostatitis Symptom Index (NIH-CPSI).
90/90 active hamstring muscle stretch exercise, 433*f*, 436
NMES. *see* Neuromuscular electrical stimulation (NMES).
Noble compression test, 534
for iliotibial band syndrome, 398
Nociceptive transmission, altered, in chronic low back pain, 237
Nociceptive withdrawal reflex (NWR), in chronic low back pain, 237
Non-articular soft tissue disorders, 3
Non-mechanical syndromes, 76–77
Non-neural tissues, impairment in, treatment of, 795
Non-neuro-musculoskeletal pathology, signs of, 48–49
Non-specific low back pain, 211–212
Non-steroidal anti-inflammatory drugs (NSAIDs)
for frozen shoulder, 347
for hip flexor tendinopathy, 400–401
for iliotibial band syndrome, 398–399
for internal snapping hip syndrome, 400–401
Non-thrust manipulation
prone mid-thoracic, 151–152, 151*f*
prone or side-lying ribs, 154, 154*f*
for sacroiliac joint pathology, 286
seated first-rib, 153–154, 153*f*
supine first-rib, 154, 154*f*
Non-thrust mobilization, 610–612
anterior-posterior, 611
distal tibiofibular joint, 612
lateral-medial, 611
thrust manipulation *versus*, 247
Non-weight-bearing talocrural posterior glide mobilization with movement, 641, 641*f*
North American Institute of Orthopaedic Manual Therapy (NAIOMT)
IGHL test, 327, 327*f*
MGHL test, 327, 327*f*
posterior capsule test, 327, 328*f*
SGHL/CHL test, 326, 327*f*
sulcus stability test, for IGHL-AB/PB and inferior labrum, 328, 328*f*
NPRS. *see* Numerical Pain Rating Scale (NPRS).
NSAIDs. *see* Non-steroidal anti-inflammatory drugs (NSAIDs).
Numeric analogue scale, for cervical radiculopathy, 122
Numerical Pain Rating Scale (NPRS), 106, 106*t*
Nutritional status, medical history and, 28–29
NWR. *see* Nociceptive withdrawal reflex (NWR).

O

OA. *see* Osteoarthritis (OA).
Ober test, 403, 534
Obesity, associated with upper extremity disorders, 10
Oblique abdominals, stabilization exercises for, 219*t*
O'Brien test, for type II SLAP lesions, 337
Occipito-atlanto (C0-C1) segment
MET for, 716, 716*f*
primary movement at, 716
Occlusive arterial disease, 38–39
Occupational workplace exposures, upper extremity pain disorders and, 10
ODI. *see* Oswestry Disability Index (ODI).
OLBDQ. *see* Oswestry Low Back Disability Questionnaire (OLBDQ).
Open-packed positions, in ankle sprains, 607
Opponens roll, 589
Optimal neuromuscular control, 427*f*
ORAI. *see* Osteoporosis Risk Assessment Instrument (ORAI).
Orthopaedic examination techniques
for lateral elbow instability, 453*t*
for medial elbow instability, 455*t*
Orthopaedic manual therapy (OMT), 350
Orthoses, in-shoe, 510
Orthotics, elbow, 448
Osteoarthritis (OA), 467
animal models of, 482
digital, 600–601
anatomy of, 600
conservative treatment of, 601
diagnosis for, 601
epidemiology of, 600
pathology of, 600
prognosis of, 601
end-stage, management of, 624
fractures and, latency time between, 624
hallmark of, 483–484
hip, 389–396
anatomy of, 390
characteristics of, 389
clinical presentation of, 392
definition of, 390
description of, 389
diagnosis of, 390–392
economic impact of, 390
epidemiological research in, 389
non-pharmacological treatment of, 392–394
pathomechanics of, 390
prevalence of, 389
prognosis of, 392
risk factors of, 391–392
treatment of, 392–394
hip symptoms and, 16
joint replacement and, 623–624
knee, 482–492, 498, 525
biomechanics of, 484
lumbar spine treatment for, 222–223
skin rolling, 487*f*
specific pain mechanisms in, 483
knee symptoms and, 17–18
pathophysiology and biochemistry of, 483–484
post-traumatic, mechanism of, 624
sensitization in, 483
sensory manifestations in, 482
Osteoarthritis-related pain, challenges in management of, 484–489
arthroplasty, 488–489
non-pharmacological, 485–488
pharmacological, 484–485
Osteokinematics, of ankle sprains, 607
Osteopathic treatment, in sacroiliac joint pathology, 287–288
Osteophytes, 390
Osteoporosis, secondary causes of, 29*b*
Osteoporosis Risk Assessment Instrument (ORAI), 32, 32*t*
Oswestry Disability Index (ODI), 204
Oswestry Low Back Disability Questionnaire (OLBDQ), 38*t*

Ottawa ankle rules, 608
Overhead elevation
mobilizations with movement, 353–354
progression of range of motion, 354–355
Overhead throw, 323–324, 324*f*

P

Pain
bidirectional top-down and bottom-up approach to, 70*f*
drawing, lumbar radiculopathy and, 202
groin, in sports hernia, 407
in impingement, 314
knee, 493
lower extremity syndromes, in lumbar spine, 221–225
map, in sacroiliac joint pathology, 278
muscle-referred, 482
patellofemoral, 496–497
clinical assessment of, 499–502
conservative treatment of, 502–510
history of complaint for patients with, 500*t*
objective assessment for patients with, 502*t*
pathophysiology of, 498
patient profile, demographics and clinical history for patients with, 501*t*
remote and local factors in, 499
risk and associated factors for, 498*t*
risk factors for, 498–499
subjective complaint for patients with, 500*t*
radicular, definition of, 199–200
referral patterns, of thoracic spine, 143
referred, 496–497
Pain neuromatrix, 66, 67*f*
Pain sensitivity tests, in chronic low back pain, 237
Painful arc sign, 314, 549
Painful neuropathies, 24
PAIVM. *see* Passive accessory intervertebral motion (PAIVM).
Palmar fascia, 737, 737*f*
myofascial induction of, 753, 753*f*
Palmaris longus muscle, TrPs in, 669, 669*f*
Palpation, 64
Palpation test, positional, for sacroiliac joint pathology, 279
Panic disorder, diagnosis of, 30–32, 30*b*
Parameters, exercises, 440–441, 441*t*
Parasympathetic innervation, of pelvic floor muscles, 227
Paratendon, 546
Paratenonitis, 548
and tendinosis, combined, 548–549
Passive accessory intervertebral motion (PAIVM), in lumbar spine instability, 217
Passive accessory techniques, for sacroiliac joint pathology, 279
Passive compression test, 338, 338*f*
Passive knee flexion stretch, 515*f*
Passive lumbar extension test, for lumbar spine instability, 217
Passive mobilization interventions, of glenohumeral joint, 350–352
Passive movements, 63–64
Passive physiological intervertebral movements (PPIVM), in lumbar spine instability, 217
Passive translatoric accessory mobilizations, 350
Patella, 493
angles, 496*f*
medial-lateral position of, 494–495
muscular forces around, 495*f*
palpation of inferior pole of, 536*f*
Patellar mobility tests, 502*f*
Patellar mobilizations, 515
and lumbar manipulation, 503–504
Patellar muscle stretch reflex, testing of, 57*f*
Patellar taping, position for, 503, 503*f*
Patellar tendinopathy, 535–537
anatomy of, 535
conservative treatment and prognosis of, 536–537
diagnosis of, 535–536
pathology and patho-biomechanics of, 535
Patellar tendon, 535
blood supply to, 535
Patellar tilt angle (PT-angle), 495
Patellofemoral joint, anatomy of, 493–495
Patellofemoral mobilization
caudal and cephalad, 529, 530*f*
medial and lateral, 529, 530*f*
Patellofemoral pain, 496–497
clinical assessment of, 499–502
conservative treatment of, 502–510
disorders, classification system of, 498*t*
history of complaint for patients with, 500*t*
objective assessment for patients with, 502*t*
pathophysiology of, 498
patient profile, demographics and clinical history for patients with, 501*t*
remote and local factors in, 499
risk and associated factors for, 498–499, 498*t*
subjective complaint for patients with, 500*t*
Patellofemoral pain syndrome (PFPS), 18, 43–44, 493–513, 525
lumbar spine treatment for, 222
open-packed position of, 494
prevalence of, 17*t*
symptoms of, 497
Patient education, of hip osteoarthritis, 393
Patient interview, in management of lumbar spine instability, 214
Patient profile, in history taking, 23, 24*t*
Patient Specific Functional Scale (PSFS), 38*t*, 106–107, 106*t*
Patients, for cervical spine manipulation and mobilization, 160
Patrick's test, for pelvic girdle pain, 281, 282*f*
Patte sign, 314
Paxinos sign, 295–296, 297*f*, 298*t*
PB-IGHL. *see* Posterior bands of inferior glenohumeral ligaments (PB-IGHL).
PBU. *see* Pressure biofeedback unit (PBU).
PCL. *see* Posterior cruciate ligament (PCL).
Peak hip adduction angles, 469
Pectineus muscle, TrPs in, dry needling of, 702, 702*f*
Pectoralis fascia, 735–736, 735*f*
myofascial induction of, 750, 750*f*
Pectoralis major muscle
MET for, 724, 725*f*
TrPs in, 665–666, 666*f*, 724
dry needling of, 693, 694*f*
Pectoralis minor muscle
fascia, myofascial induction of, 750, 751*f*
MET for, 724–725, 725*f*
TrPs in, 663–664, 664*f*
dry needling of, 693, 693*f*
Pelvic drop exercise, 429*f*
Pelvic floor muscles
anatomy of, 226–227
and lumbopelvic pain, 227
neural control of, 226–227
pelvic pain and, 226–235
Pelvic girdle, MET for, 721–723
Pelvic girdle pain, 274
classification of, 281
Pelvic pain, pelvic floor muscles and, 226–235
chronic, 227–228
case reports on, 232, 232*b*–233*b*
clinical-reasoned approach for management of, 230–231
management of, 228–229, 228*f*–229*f*
Pelvic ring, 275
Pelvic somatic dysfunctions, 721
Percussion test, for lumbar spine instability, 217
'Peri-arthrite scapulo-humerale', 344
see also Frozen shoulder
Perineurium, 766, 766*f*, 773
Peripheral nerve(s)
anatomy of, 765–766, 766*f*
disruption of axoplasmic transport, 775–776, 776*f*
inflammation of, 771–775
animal models of, 772–775
causes of, 772
imaging of, 776
in microenvironment, 772
neuritis model of, 773–775, 773*f*–774*f*
inflammatory mediators and, physiological role of, 775–776
mechanical properties of, 766–768, 767*f*
movement of
in patients, 770–771
physical tests of, 767–768
in vivo measurements of, 768–770
pathologies of, 783
stretch of, 784–785
Peripheral nerve sensitization, 42
Peripheral nervous system, central sensitization mechanism and, 568
Peripheral sensitization, TrPs as focus of, 661
Peritendinitis crepitans, 551
Peroneal tendinitis, 650
Peroneal tendinopathy, 649–651
anatomy of, 649–650
background of, 649
diagnosis of, 650–651
pathology and patho-biomechanics of, 650
presentation of pain and dysfunction in, 651*t*
treatment and prognosis of, 651
Peroneal tendon stability test, 650–651
Peroneal tubercle, 649
classification of, 649
computed tomography of, 651
dimensions of, 649
enlarged, 650
Peroneus quartus, 650
Peroneus tertius, 650
Pes planus deformity, and iliotibial band syndrome, 398
PFPS. *see* Patellofemoral pain syndrome (PFPS).
Phalangeal fractures, 595–596
Phalen test, 569, 569*f*
Photoplethysmography (PPM), 498
Physical disability, musculoskeletal diseases causing, 13
Physical examination, 47–65
clearing of spine in, 60–63
in differentiating vasculogenic head and neck pain, 49*t*
history taking and, 22
for neurological deficits, 51–60
cranial nerve examination, 60, 60*t*–61*t*
nerve root examination, 51–59
upper motor neuron examination, 59–60
observation and screening for medical conditions in, 48–50, 50*f*
region-specific examination, 63–64
for severe injuries to spine, 50–51, 50*f*
Physical therapy
after total ankle arthroplasty, 625
examination in, 22
for radiculopathy, 127
Physical workplace exposures, upper extremity pain disorders and, 10
Piano-key test, 563
Piezoelectricity, 746
Pilates, for mechanical low back pain, 267–268
Pincer-type impingement, definition of, 413–414
Piriformis muscle, 434
activation, high, 430
MET for, 726–727, 727*f*
TrPs in, 671, 671*f*, 726–727
dry needling of, 700–701, 701*f*
weakness of, 430
Piriformis syndrome, 671
Pisiform, 560
Pisotriquetral grind test, 550
PIT. *see* Prone instability test (PIT).
Plain film radiograph
of cervical spine, 124
of Hill-Sachs lesion, 328
of lumbar radiculopathy, 204
of rotator cuff lesions shoulder impingement, 315
Plantar fascia, 616, 617*f*, 757
myofascial induction of, 758, 758*f*
soft tissue mobilization of, 618*f*
Plantar fasciitis, 19, 44, 616
prevalence of, 19*t*
Plantar heel pain, 616–622, 673
anatomical considerations for, 616, 617*f*
diagnosis of, 617–618
imaging of, 617–618
invasive manual therapy for, 620–621, 620*f*
management of, 618–621
manipulation/mobilizations for, 638

non-invasive manual therapy for, 618–620, 618*f*, 619*t*
origin of, 616
pathology of, 616–617
prevalence of, 616
prognosis of, 618
risk factors of, 618
signs of, 617
symptoms of, 617
Plantarflexion (L5-S1), 56*f*
Plyometric exercise, 476*f*
PNF stretching. *see* Proprioceptive neuromuscular facilitation (PNF) stretching.
Popliteal fossa
deep fascial intermuscular links in, 742*f*, 743, 744*f*
myofascial induction of, 757, 757*f*
Popliteal tendinopathy, 537–538
anatomy of, 537–538
conservative treatment and prognosis of, 538
diagnosis of, 538
pathology and patho-biomechanics of, 538
Popliteus muscle, 537–538
Population, upper extremity pain syndromes and, 5
Positional palpation test, for sacroiliac joint pathology, 279
Positions, for cervical neutral during limb load, 181
Positive likelihood ratio (+LR), 48
Posterior bands of inferior glenohumeral ligaments (PB-IGHL), 321–322
Posterior clavicular/disc glide, right shoulder, 306–307, 307*f*
Posterior cruciate ligament (PCL), 470
anatomy of, 470
biomechanics of, 470
incidence/prevalence of injury, 470
mechanism of injury/risk factors of, 470
reconstruction, 514–516
bracing/weight-bearing, 514–515
modalities in, 514
neuromuscular re-education, 516
range of motion exercises, 515
rehabilitation goals of, 515*t*
therapeutic exercise, 516
special tests for, 473*t*
surgical management of, 477
Posterior disc/manubrial rotation mobilization, left shoulder, 306, 306*f*
Posterior glide, of glenohumeral joint, 351, 351*f*
in flexion, 352, 352*f*
Posterior inferior tibiofibular ligament (PITFL), 605–606
Posterior interosseous nerve (PIN), 576–577
Posterior interosseous nerve (PIN) syndrome, 577, 580
common differential diagnosis of, 579*t*
special tests for, 579*t*
symptoms and signs of, 578*t*
Posterior sacroiliac ligament (PSL), 276
Posterior sling, in force closure, 277
Posterior to anterior mobilization
'figure 4' position, 394, 394*f*
of hip, 394, 394*f*
'Posteriorly subluxed' rib dysfunction technique, modification of, 719–720, 720*f*
Posterolateral instability test, 453*t*
Posterolateral rotatory instability (PLRI), 451–452
Posterosuperior glenoid impingement, 312–313, 312*f*
Post-isometric relaxation technique, 710
of quadratus lumborum muscle taut band, 685–686, 686*f*
Post-traumatic arthritis, 456*t*
Post-traumatic stress
psychological factor of, 114
symptoms of, 113
whiplash and, 113
Post-traumatic Stress Diagnostic Scale (PDS), 113
Postural correction, exercises for, 185–186, 186*f*
Postural screen, of thoracic spine and rib cage, 148–149
Postural syndrome, 76–77, 78*t*, 86*t*, 88
Posture
dynamic evaluation of, 748
of shoulder region, 376
static evaluation of, 748
PPIVM. *see* Passive physiological intervertebral movements (PPIVM).
PPM. *see* Photoplethysmography (PPM).
Predynamic instability, 560–561
Pregnancy
carpal tunnel syndrome during, 10, 567, 571–572
low back pain during, 227
pelvic pain and, 283–284
Pressure biofeedback unit (PBU), abdominal draw-in manoeuvre and, 260
Pressure pain thresholds (PPT), carpal tunnel syndrome and, 568
Prevertebral fascia, 732*f*, 733
myofascial induction of, 750, 750*f*
Primary degenerative osteoarthritis, 456*t*
Primary frozen shoulder, 344
Primary impingement, 311
risk factors for, 313
Primary neoplastic conditions, 102
Primary pain map, influencing neighbouring neural circuits, 67, 68*f*
Primary skin lesions, during observation, 48–49
Primary somatosensory cortex (S1), 69
Profundus muscles, TrPs in, 669, 669*f*
Pronation, mobilization, 461, 461*f*
Pronator syndrome, 580–581
Pronator teres muscle, 577
TrPs in, 669, 669*f*
Prone bridge exercise, for mechanical low back pain, 264
Prone heel squeeze exercise, 416, 416*f*, 430*f*
Prone instability test (PIT)
for low back pain, 196
for lumbar spine instability, 218
Prone knee bend (PKB) test, 792–793
Prone mid-thoracic thrust and non-thrust manipulation, 151–152, 151*f*
Prone ribs non-thrust manipulation, 154
Prone upper thoracic thrust manipulation, 151, 151*f*
Proprioception
Achilles tendon rupture and, 633
after total ankle arthroplasty, 628
exercises for, in mechanical low back pain, 268–269
MET for, 714
neuromotor control, 431–432
Proprioceptive neuromuscular facilitation (PNF) stretching, 258, 331
parameters for, 270
Proteoglycans, 547
Protopathic sensitivity, of mechanical impulse, 746
Protrusion, of cervical spine, 79
Provocation tests, 337, 549
for cervical radiculopathy, 123–124
for lumbar radiculopathy, 202–204
for sacroiliac joint pathology, 279–280
for thoracic outlet syndrome, 136–137
Proximal carpal row, 559
Proximal phalanx
condyle of, fractures in, 595
intra-articular fractures of, 595
shaft fractures of, 595
Proximal tibiofibular joint thrust manipulation, 529, 529*f*, 612, 612*f*, 642, 642*f*
PSFS. *see* Patient Specific Functional Scale (PSFS).
Psoas major muscle, TrPs in, dry needling of, 702–703, 703*f*
Psoas muscles, TrPs in, 670–671, 670*f*
Psoriatic arthritis, 33*t*
Psychological distress, chronic whiplash associated with, 113
Psychometric data, for superior labrum anterior-to-posterior (SLAP) lesions, 338*t*
Psychosocial health, in neck pain, 99
Pubalgia, athletic, 407
Pubic symphysis, 275
Pubic symphysis compression test, for pelvic girdle pain, 281–282, 282*f*
Pubococcygeus, in male pelvic pain, 228–229
Pudendal nerve
entrapment, 230
in pelvic floor muscles, 226–227
Pulmonary system, local thoracic and chest pain in, 25
Pulsatile abdominal mass, presence of, 49
Pulsatile blood flow, 498
Push-up sign (from floor), 453*t*

Q

Q-angle. *see* Quadriceps angle (Q-angle).
Quadratus lumborum muscle
MET for, 726, 726*f*
stabilization exercises for, 219*t*
TrPs in, 670, 670*f*
dry needling of, 698, 698*f*
Quadratus plantae muscles, 616, 617*f*
Quadriceps angle (Q-angle), 495
dynamic, 496*f*
of knee, 495*f*
Quadriceps femoris muscle
strengthening, non-weight exercise for, 486*f*
TrPs in, 672, 672*f*
dry needling of, 703–704
Quadriceps muscle imbalance, 509
Quadriceps muscle strengthening, 475
leg press exercise, 475*f*
Quadriceps tendinopathy, 538–539
anatomy of, 538
conservative treatment and prognosis of, 539
diagnosis of, 539
pathology and patho-biomechanics of, 538–539
Quadruped arm/lower extremity lift, 507*f*
Quadruped exercises, for mechanical low back pain, 262, 264*f*
Quadruped gluteus medius strengthening exercise, 439*f*
Quadruped sit-back exercise, 435–436, 436*f*
Quantitative sensory testing
in chronic low back pain, 237
for whiplash-associated disorders, 114
Quebec CLIP guidelines, 82*t*
Quebec Task Force (QTF) system, 111

R

Radial carpal dorsal glides, 590
Radial nerve
anatomy of, 576–577
conservative treatment for, 582
diagnosis for, 580
Radial sensory nerve (RSN), entrapment of, 577
Radial tunnel syndrome, 580
common differential diagnosis of, 579*t*
special tests for, 579*t*
symptoms and signs of, 578*t*
Radial-ulnar deviation, 560
Radicular pain, definition of, 199–200
Radiculopathy
cervical
active and passive movements of, 122–123
anterior surgical approach for, 128
clinical signs and symptoms of, 120
confirmation tests of, 123–124
conservative approaches of, 127
current best evidence with regard to prognosis in, 126
definition of, 118
differential diagnosis and treatment of, 118–131
imaging of, 124–125
nerve condition responses in, 125–126
neurological testing of, 123
observation of, 122
outcome measures of, 122
patient history in, 122
physical examination of, 122–123
posterior surgical approach for, 128–129
provocation tests of, 123–124
review of proposed pathology and patho-biomechanics of, 119
surgical approaches of, 128–129
lumbar, 199–209
active and passive movements in, 202
aetiology and background of, 199–200
anatomy of, 200–201
definitions of, 199–200
description of, by severity, 200*t*
differential diagnosis of, 201
evidence-based clinical examination of, 201–205
natural history of, 200
neurological testing for, 202

observation of, 202
pathogenesis of, 201
prevalence of, 199
signs and symptoms of, 200
treatment of, 205–208
Radiocarpal dorsal glides, 588, 588*f*–589*f*
Radiocarpal joint, 559
Radiocarpal mobilizations with movement, 589
Radiocarpal palmar glide, 588, 588*f*
Radiocarpal radial glide, 588, 589*f*
Radiocarpal traction, 587, 587*f*–588*f*
Radiography
of acromioclavicular joint, 297–298
of hip osteoarthritis, 390–391
of lumbar radiculopathy, plain film, 204
of superior labrum anterior-to-posterior (SLAP) lesions, 340
Radiohumeral joint, mobilization of, 461, 462*f*
Radioscaphocapitate ligament (RSCL), 559*f*, 560
Radioscapholunate ligament (RSLL), 559*f*, 560
Range of motion
in ankle sprains, 607
generalized active, mobility exercises for, 182–183
of thoracic spine, 149
Reactive tendinopathy, 446
Rearfoot distraction thrust manipulation, 611
Receiver-operating characteristics (ROC), of pain sensitivity tests, 237
Recency effect, 216
Recruitment, exercises for, 175–176
Rectus abdominis muscle, TrPs in, dry needling of, 698–699, 699*f*
Rectus femoris muscle, TrPs in, 672, 672*f*
dry needling of, 703–704, 703*f*
Red flags, in low back pain, 191, 192*t*
Reference standard, 215
Referred pain, 496–497
description of, 659
differentiation of, 126*t*
from myofascial trigger points, 659–677
characteristics of, 660
patterns, 24
Reflex receptive fields (RRF), in chronic low back pain, 237
Reflexes, 53–56
Regional interdependence, lower extremity, 221, 224*t*
Rehabilitation exercises, examples of, 506*b*
Reiter syndrome, 33*t*
Release phenomenon, 136
Release test, for glenohumeral instability, 326
Releaser, 136
Reliability, 47
Relocation test
dynamic, 363, 367, 367*f*
for glenohumeral instability, 326
Repetitive strain injury (RSI), 765, 770–772
Research, for treatment-based classification system, 213
Resistance, for cervical neutral during limb load, 181
Resisted hip abduction provocation test, for pelvic girdle pain, 281, 282*f*
Resisted hip external rotation exercise, 437*f*
Retraction, of cervical spine, 79
Return to sport/daily life activities phase, of postoperative rehabilitation, 418
Rheumatoid arthritis, 456, 456*t*
affecting the digits, 601
carpal tunnel syndrome and, 567
Rhomboid ligament, 303
Rhomboid major muscle, TrPs in, dry needling of, 694, 695*f*
Rhomboid minor muscle, TrPs in, dry needling of, 694, 695*f*
Rhomboid muscle, fascia of, 735*f*, 736
Rib cage
assessment of, 718
manual therapy interventions for, 150–155
exercise to augment, 154–155
MET for, 718–720
regional interdependence of, 143–144
in upper quarter pain syndromes
evidence for manual therapy management of, 144–148
examination and screening of, 148–150
interpretation of examination and reassessment of, 149–150
mobility testing of first rib in, 149
postural screen of, 148–149
segmental mobility testing of, 149
Rib exhalation, restriction of, MET for, 718*f*, 719
Rib inhalation, restriction of, MET for, 718–719, 718*f*
RMQ. *see* Roland Morris Disability Questionnaire (RMQ).
Roland Morris Disability Questionnaire (RMQ), 38*t*, 204
Romberg test, 59, 60*f*
Roos test, 137
Rotation, cervical spine manipulation in, 169, 170*f*
Rotational lumbar spine thrust, high-velocity, 205, 205*f*
Rotational manipulation, of sacroiliac joint, 286, 286*f*–287*f*
Rotator cuff
anatomy of, 309
disorder, 8*t*–9*t*
pathology of, 311–313
tears, descriptions of, 309
Rotator cuff lesions shoulder impingement, 309–320
anatomy of, 309–310
biomechanics of, 310–311
diagnosis of, 313–315
management of, 315–318
pathology of, 311–313
prognosis of, 315, 316*b*
Rotator cuff tendinitis, 8*t*–9*t*
RRF. *see* Reflex receptive fields (RRF).
RSI. *see* Repetitive strain injury (RSI).

S

Sacral thrust test, for sacroiliac joint pathology, 280, 280*f*
Sacroiliac belts, for pelvic pain, 288
Sacroiliac 'gapping' technique, 723, 723*f*
Sacroiliac joint (SIJ), 78*t*, 426
as source of pain
anatomy of, 275–277
biomechanics of, 275–277
clinical examination in, 283
diagnosis of, 277–283
economic impact of, 275
exercise therapy for, 284–286, 284*f*–286*f*
management of, 274–290
manual therapy for, 286–288, 286*f*–287*f*
medical, 277–278
pathology of, 277
pathomechanics of, 277
physical examination in, 278–283
prevalence of, 274–275
prognosis of, 283–284
sacroiliac belts for, 288
subjective examination in, 278
treatment of, 284–288
Sacroiliac joint dysfunctions (SIJD), 274
Sacroiliac joint pain (SIJP) syndromes, 274
Sacroiliac thrust manipulation, 286–287, 287*f*
Sacrospinous ligament, 276
Sacrotuberous ligament, 276
palpation of, for pelvic girdle pain, 282, 283*f*
Sacrum, 275
Sarcomeres, compression of, 679
SAT. *see* Scapular assistance test (SAT).
Scalene muscles
MET for, 724, 724*f*
myofascial induction of, 750, 750*f*
TrPs in, 663, 663*f*, 724
dry needling of, 693, 693*f*
Scaphoid stress test, 562, 562*f*
Scapholunate ligament (SLL), 559, 559*f*
Scapula
altered motor control around, 359–360, 364–366
extension, control of, evaluation of, 366
movement awareness, 362, 365*f*
retraining of, 363, 370*f*
PNF patterns, 365, 365*f*
upward rotation, 362, 365, 365*f*
retraining of, 363, 369*f*
Scapular assistance test (SAT), 361, 361*f*
Scapular motions, 311, 312*f*
Scapular retraction test (SRT), 361, 364*f*
Scapulohumeral reflex, 59–60
Scapulothoracic motion, role of, 315–316
Sciatica, 15
definition of, 199–200
prevalence of, 14*t*
Screening tests, 48
for lumbar spine instability, 216–217
Seated first-rib thrust/non-thrust manipulation, 153–154, 153*f*
Seated mid-thoracic thrust manipulation, 151, 151*f*
Seated upper thoracic thrust manipulation, 150–151, 150*f*
SEBT. *see* Star excursion balance test (SEBT).
Secondary frozen shoulder, 344
Secondary impingement, 311–312
Segmental control, during neck motion, 181–182, 182*f*
Segmental extension, from slump, 177*f*
Segmental mobility testing, of thoracic spine and rib cage, 149
Selective diagnostic nerve root block (SNRB), 126
Selective tissue tension testing (STT), 549
Self-mobilization exercise, 183–184, 183*f*
for mechanical low back pain, 256–257
parameters for, 270
Self-stretch programme, for plantar heel pain, 620
Semimembranosus muscle, TrPs in, dry needling of, 705, 705*f*
Semimembranosus tendinopathy, 532
anatomy of, 532
diagnosis of, 532
pathology and patho-biomechanics of, 532
treatment and prognosis of, 532
Semitendinosus muscle, TrPs in, dry needling of, 705, 705*f*
Sensation, 52
Sensibility testing, for lumbar radiculopathy, 202
Sensitivity (true positive rate), 47–48
Sensitizing movements, definition of, 782
Sensorimotor control dysfunction, 111–112
Sensory axons, peripheral, local nerve inflammation and, 775
Sensory hypersensitivity, 112
Seronegative spondyloarthropathies, clinical findings in, 33*t*
Serratus anterior fascia, 735*f*, 736
Serratus anterior muscle, therapeutic exercises for, 381, 382*f*
SGHL. *see* Superior glenohumeral ligaments (SGHL).
Shaft fractures, 595
of proximal phalanx, 595
Sharp-Purser test, 50–51, 50*f*
Shockwave, 509–510
therapy to vastus lateralis muscle and tendon, 510*f*
Short Form 36 (MOS SF-36), 38*t*
Shoulder
frozen, 344–349
left
anterior disc/manubrial rotation mobilization of, 306, 306*f*
posterior disc/manubrial rotation mobilization of, 306, 306*f*
pathology, 86
right
inferior clavicular/disc glide of, 306, 307*f*
posterior clavicular/disc glide of, 306–307, 307*f*
Shoulder abduction (C5), 54*f*
Shoulder elevation (C4), 54*f*
Shoulder girdle
elevation, mobilization with movement, 355, 355*f*
motor control of
evaluation of, 360–367
management of, 367–371
postural assessment, 360–366
movement awareness of, 361–364
movement impairments of, 361–364
Shoulder impingement, rotator cuff lesions, 309–320
anatomy of, 309–310
biomechanics of, 310–311
diagnosis of, 313–315
management of, 315–318
pathology of, 311–313
prognosis of, 315, 316*b*
Shoulder pain
prevalence of, 7*t*
thoracic spine manipulation for, 148

Shoulder region
motor control of, 358–372
around glenohumeral joint, altered, 360
around scapula, altered, 359–360
isolated, 366–367
and joint stability, 358–359
management of, through patient examples, 368–371, 368*b*–370*b*
tests for, 361*b*–363*b*
therapeutic exercises for, 373–385
clinical background, 373
evidence of, 374
functional, 381–383, 382*f*–383*f*
indications for, 373, 374*b*
infraspinatus muscle, 379–380, 380*f*
isometric, 378, 379*f*
isotonic, 378–381
posture and, 376
principles of, 374–376, 375*f*
serratus anterior muscle, 381, 382*f*
stretching and, 376–378, 377*f*–378*f*
subscapularis muscle, 380, 380*f*
supraspinatus muscle, 379, 380*f*
teres minor muscle, 379–380, 380*f*
trapezius muscle, 380–381, 381*f*
Shoulder shrug, 361, 364, 364*f*
Side bridge, 507*f*
Side plank exercise, 196
for mechanical low back pain, 263–264, 265*f*
Side-flexion/rotation exercises, for asymmetric weakness, 179–180, 180*f*–181*f*
Side-glide in standing, 79
'Side-lying arm sweep' exercise, 155
Side-lying ribs non-thrust manipulation, 154, 154*f*
Side-lying slump test, 792–793, 794*f*
'Sign of the penis' (SOP), 230
SIJ. *see* Sacroiliac joint (SIJ).
SIJD. *see* Sacroiliac joint dysfunctions (SIJD).
Single- and double-legged bridge exercises, 430
Single-leg dead lift exercise, 439*f*
Single-leg squat test, 402, 402*f*
Single-leg squats exercise, 418, 418*f*, 438, 438*f*
Single-leg stance
perturbation training induced by, 476*f*
proprioceptive training, 476*f*
Single-leg stance test, 402
Single-leg vertical jump landing exercise, 440*f*
Single-leg wall squat exercise, 428*f*
Single-limb balance, 610
Sit-up, bent knee, for mechanical low back pain, 261, 261*f*
Sitting, low back pain and, 267
S-LANSS questionnaire, for whiplash-associated disorders, 114
SLAP lesions. *see* Superior labrum anterior-to-posterior (SLAP) lesions.
SLAP-prehension test, 337
Sliders, 782, 795, 796*f*
SLR. *see* Straight leg raise (SLR).
Slump test, 58–59, 59*f*, 792, 793*f*
for lumbar radiculopathy, 203
side-lying, 792–793, 794*f*
Smoking, cardiovascular health risks of, 28
SMT. *see* Spinal manipulative therapy (SMT).
Social situation, in patient profile, 23
Soft tissue massage, and trigger point therapy, 507
Soft tissue mobilization, for wrist and hand tendinopathies, 553
Soft-tissue-biased manual therapies, for chronic low back pain, 240
Soleus muscle
TrPs in, 672–673
dry needling of, 706, 706*f*–707*f*
Somatic innervation, of pelvic floor muscles, 227
Somatosensory dysfunction, exercises for, in mechanical neck pain, 186–187, 187*f*
Somatosensory homunculus, 69*f*
Southampton examination schedule, 5, 5*f*
Specific exercise group, for low back pain, 194–195
Specificity (true negative rate), 47–48
Speed test, for type II SLAP lesions, 337
Spinal cord, dynamic movements of, 119
Spinal cord compression, 119
Spinal coupled motion, 713
Spinal fractures, 102
Spinal manipulation group, for low back pain, 193–194
Spinal manipulative therapy (SMT), 245
audible pop in, 248
clinical prediction rules in, 246–248
contraindications for, 249–250, 249*b*
evidence for, 246
locking in, 248–249
nomenclature of, standardizing, 245
positioning in, 248–249
precautions for, 249–250, 250*b*
safety in, 249–250
techniques in, 249–250
central posterior-to-anterior mobilization, 250, 250*f*
lumbar rotation in flexion manipulation, 252–253, 253*f*
lumbar rotation in neutral or extension manipulation, 252, 253*f*
lumbar rotation mobilization, 251, 251*f*–252*f*
lumbopelvic regional manipulation, 251–252, 252*f*
unilateral posterior-to-anterior mobilization, 250–251, 250*f*
Spinal mobilization, with upper extremity movement-horizontal adduction, 356–357, 357*f*
Spinal nerve, 201
Spinal nerve ligation (SNL) model, 772
Spinal pain, 77
Spinal stenosis, 78*t*
Spine
clearing of, 60–63
Mechanical Diagnosis and Therapy for, 76–84
MET for, 713–714
in acute dysfunctions, 714
principles of, 713
for proprioception and control, 714
spinal coupled motion and, 713
variations of, 713–714
of scapula, myofascial induction of, 751, 751*f*
screening for severe injuries to, 50–51, 50*f*
Spine zygapophyseal joints, referral patterns from, 100*f*
Splinting, for carpal instability, 563–564
Sports hernia, 407–409
clinical examination of, 408–409
diagnosis of, 408–409
epidemiology of, 407
pathomechanics of, 408
prognosis for, 409
tissues related to, 407, 408*f*
treatment of, 409
Spurling's sign, 123, 123*f*
Spurling's test, 56–58
Squeaker's wrist, 551
SRT. *see* Scapular retraction test (SRT).
Stability tests
dynamic rotary, 362–363, 366–367, 367*f*
for glenohumeral instability, 326
Stabilization, motor control exercises for, 259
Stabilization exercises
with criteria for progression, 218, 219*t*
for sacroiliac joint pathology, 284
Stabilization group, for low back pain, 195–196
Standing iliotibial band stretch exercise, 434*f*
Standing quadriceps stretch, 504*f*
Star excursion balance exercise, 431*f*, 439
Star excursion balance test (SEBT), 402, 402*f*, 431–432, 499, 610
Static instability, 560–561
Stener lesion, 599
Step-down exercise, 507*f*
Step-down test, 398
Step up (L3-L4), 56*f*
Sternoclavicular joint, 302–308
adjunct exercises for, 307
anatomy of, 302–303
biomechanics of, 304
diagnosis of, 305–306
management of, 306–307
pathology of, 304–305
patients requiring medical/surgical consultation, 304–305
patients with indication for physical therapy intervention, 304–305
Steroid injection, for cervical radiculopathy, 127
Straight leg hip abduction exercise, 518*f*
Straight leg raise (SLR), 58–59, 58*f*
test
active, 791
indications for, 792
for lumbar radiculopathy, 202–203
passive, 791–792, 792*f*
Strain/counter-strain technique, for TrPs, 680
Strength
motor control exercises for, 259
motor function exercises for, 176–179
Strengthening exercises, 504–506
Stress shielding, 547
Stress-strain curve, of peripheral nerve, 767, 767*f*
Stretching
compression
of gastrocnemius muscle taut band, 687, 687*f*
of levator scapulae muscle taut band, 681, 681*f*
of psoas major muscle taut band, 686, 686*f*
of subscapularis muscle taut band, 683, 683*f*
of teres major muscle taut band, 682, 683*f*
of thumb muscles taut band, 684–685, 685*f*
exercises, for low back pain, 256
parameters for, 270
patella position, 504
of shoulder region, 376–378, 377*f*–378*f*
stroke
of infraspinatus muscle taut band, 682, 682*f*
longitudinal, of infraspinatus muscle taut band, 682, 682*f*
of TrPs, 680
Suboccipital myofascial induction, 749, 749*f*
Subpectoralis minor space, 134
Subscapularis muscle
anatomy of, 309
fascia of, 736
MET for, 725, 725*f*
therapeutic exercises for, 380, 380*f*
TrPs in, 665, 665*f*, 725
dry needling of, 694–695, 695*f*
Subscapularis tendon, anatomy of, 309–310
Substance P, 548
Subtalar joint, 606–607
articulation of, 607
lateral glide, 611
Subtalar joint lateral glide non-thrust manipulation, 641–642, 641*f*
Subtalar lateral glide self-mobilization, 639, 644, 644*f*
Sulcus angle (S-angle), 495
Superficial fascia
attached to skin, 738–739, 738*f*–739*f*
cervical, 732–733, 732*f*–733*f*
Superior glenohumeral ligaments (SGHL), 321–322
Superior labrum, anatomy of, 334
Superior labrum anterior-to-posterior (SLAP) lesions, 333–343
anatomy of, 334–335
biomechanics of, 335–336
classification of, 333
description of, 333
diagnosis of, 337–340
management of, 340–341
pathology of, 336–337
prognosis of, 341
psychometric data for, 338*t*
type II, subtypes of, 333, 334*f*
types of, 333, 334*f*
Supination combined flexion mobilization, 461, 461*f*
Supinator muscle, TrPs in, 667, 668*f*
dry needling of, 696–697, 697*f*
Supine first-rib thrust and non-thrust manipulation, 154, 154*f*
Supine passive straight leg raise test, for low back pain, 196
Supine ribs thrust manipulation, 154, 154*f*
Supine sign, in lumbar spine instability, 217
Suprahyoid region myofascial induction, 749–750, 749*f*
Suprascapular nerve block, for frozen shoulder, 347
Supraspinatus fascia, 735*f*, 736
Supraspinatus muscle
anatomy of, 309
compression of, 681–682, 682*f*

contraction of, 681–682, 682*f*
therapeutic exercises for, 379, 380*f*
TrPs in, 664, 664*f*
dry needling of, 693, 694*f*
Surgical decompression, for carpal tunnel syndrome, 572
Surgical techniques, for acute injuries, of acromioclavicular joint, 299
Surprise test, for glenohumeral instability, 326
Surrogate markers, upper extremity pain syndromes and, 5–6
Swiss ball exercise, for mechanical low back pain, 264–265, 266*f*
Sympathetic innervation, of pelvic floor muscles, 227
Sympathetic nervous system, TrPs and, 661–662
Sympathetic-mediated pain, in thoracic outlet syndrome, 136
Symptom behaviour, 26–27, 27*t*
Synovial irritation sign, 562
Systems review, in history taking, 29–34, 30*b*–31*b*, 32*t*–33*t*, 33*f*
for patients with lower extremity syndromes, 37–40
purposes of, 29–30
suggested questions for, 31*t*

T

'T4 syndrome', 143
Table-top relocation test, 453*t*
Talocrural distraction thrust manipulation, 639, 640*f*
Talocrural dorsiflexion self-mobilization, 644, 644*f*
Talocrural joint, 606
lateral glide, 611, 611*f*
mobilization with movement (MWM) techniques of, 640–641
non-weight-bearing talocrural posterior glide mobilization with movement, 641, 641*f*
weight-bearing talocrural posterior glide mobilization with movement, 641, 641*f*
passive joint manipulation/mobilization techniques of, 639–640
distraction thrust manipulation of, 639, 640*f*
lateral glide non-thrust manipulation of, 640, 640*f*
posterior glide non-thrust manipulation of, 640, 640*f*
Talocrural lateral glide non-thrust manipulation, 640, 640*f*
Talocrural posterior glide non-thrust manipulation, 640, 640*f*
Tampa Scale of Kinesiophobia (TSK), 22–23, 30–32
Taping
patellar, position, 503*f*
for rotator cuff lesions shoulder impingement, 316, 317*f*
Telescopic tridimensional induction, 753, 753*f*
Temporomandibular joint disorder (TMD), 483
Tenderness, of ACJ, test for, 295–296, 298*t*
Tendinitis, 548
Tendinopathy
adductor, 405–407
aetiology of, 546
calcifying, 314
classification of, 548–549
combined paratenonitis and tendinosis, 548–549
paratenonitis, 548
tendinitis, 548
tendinosis, 548
continuum model of presentation of, 448
definition of, 545–546
elbow, lateral epicondylalgia, 445–450
examination and diagnosis of, 549–550
gluteus medius, 401–405
hip flexor, 400–401
for the knee, 531–541
of hamstrings, 531
iliotibial band syndrome, 532–535
patellar, 535–537
popliteal, 537–538
quadriceps, 538–539
semimembranosus, 532
severity of, 548
Tendinosis, 445, 548
and paratenonitis, combined, 548–549
Tendon
anatomy of, 546–548
basic components of, 546
blood and nerve supply of, 546–547
pathoanatomy of, 547–548
healing of, 547–548
injury of, 547
matrix, 547
structure, basic, 546*f*
Tendonitis, calcific, 538
Tennis elbow. *see* Lateral epicondylalgia.
Tennis elbow bands, 448
Tenoblasts, 547
Tenocytes, 547
Tenosynovitis, 8*t*–9*t*
TENS. *see* Transcutaneous electrical nerve stimulation (TENS).
Tensegrity model, 730–731
Tensioners, 782, 795
Teres major muscle, TrPs in, 665, 665*f*
dry needling of, 694
Teres minor muscle
anatomy of, 309
therapeutic exercises for, 379–380, 380*f*
TrPs in, 665, 665*f*
dry needling of, 694
Terminal branches, 576
TFCC. *see* Triangular fibrocartilage complex (TFCC).
Thawing phase, of frozen shoulder, 346
physical examination of, 347
treatment of, 348
Therapeutic exercises, 373
activation levels of gluteus medius and gluteus maximus during, 429*t*
in early stages of rehabilitation, 516
for lower quadrant, 426–442
for mechanical low back pain, 255–273
abdominal curl-up, 261, 261*f*
abdominal draw-in manoeuvre, 259–260, 259*f*
for balance, 268–269, 268*f*
bent knee sit-up for, 261, 261*f*
bridge exercises, in supine, 262, 263*f*–264*f*
evidence for, 255–256
front plank, 264, 265*f*
for functional integration, 266–267
high level strengthening, 269–270, 269*f*–270*f*
horizontal side support, 263–264
lower limb challenges, 260–261, 260*f*
for mobility, 256–259, 257*f*, 258*b*
for motor control, 259
for motor pattern retraining, 266–267
multifidus activation exercises, 262, 263*f*
parameters for, 270–271, 271*t*
pilates/yoga, 267–268
prone bridge, 264
for proprioception, 268–269
quadruped, 262, 264*f*
side plank, 263–264, 265*f*
on unstable surfaces, 264–266, 266*f*
for osteoarthritis, 485–486
for shoulder region, 373–385
clinical background, 373
evidence of, 374
functional, 381–383, 382*f*–383*f*
indications for, 373, 374*b*
of infraspinatus muscle, 379–380, 380*f*
isometric, 378, 379*f*
isotonic, 378–381
posture and, 376
principles of, 374–376, 375*f*
of serratus anterior muscle, 381, 382*f*
stretching and, 376–378, 377*f*–378*f*
of subscapularis muscle, 380, 380*f*
of supraspinatus muscle, 379, 380*f*
of teres minor muscle, 379–380, 380*f*
of trapezius muscle, 380–381, 381*f*
Therapeutic modalities, for osteoarthritis, 488
Therapeutic neuroscience education (TNE), 71–73
Thigh segment, deep fascial intermuscular links in, 741, 742*f*
Thigh thrust test, for sacroiliac joint pathology, 280, 280*f*
Thomas test, 534
Thompson test, for Achilles tendon rupture, 629–630
Thoracic extension, evaluation of, 366
Thoracic flexion, role of, 315–316
Thoracic multifidus muscle, TrPs in, dry needling of, 697, 697*f*–698*f*
Thoracic outlet region, 132–133, 133*f*
Thoracic outlet syndrome (TOS), 132–141
aetiology of, 134, 135*t*
breathing patterns in, 138
clinical symptoms of, 134–136
arterial symptoms, 135
neurological symptoms, 135
venous symptoms, 135–136
clinical treatment and management of, 138–140
diagnosis of, 136–138
differential diagnosis of, 136, 137*b*
history of, 132, 133*f*
imaging assessment of, 138
intervention for, 139–140
joint stiffness in, 139
muscle imbalance in, 138–139
neurogenic pain in, 139
pathoanatomical causes of, 132–134
entrapment sites of, 133–134
functional causes of, 133
provocative test for, 136–137, 137*t*
sympathetic-mediated pain in, 136
therapy evaluation of, 138
Thoracic spine
assessment of, 716
biochemical relationship between upper quarter and, 143
impairments, association between upper quarter pain syndromes and, 143–144
manipulation of, 142–157
analgesic effects after, 150
versus cervical spine manipulation, 158–159
contraindications for, 150
for mechanical neck pain, 144, 145*t*–146*t*
manual therapy interventions for, 150–155
exercise to augment, 154–155
MET for, 716–718
pain referral patterns of, 143
regional interdependence of, 143–144
in upper quarter pain syndromes
active range of motion of, 149
evidence for manual therapy management of, 144–148
examination and screening of, 148–150
interpretation of examination and reassessment of, 149–150
postural screen of, 148–149
segmental mobility testing of, 149
Thoracic thrust manipulation
for mechanical neck pain, 144
prone mid-thoracic, 151–152, 151*f*
prone upper, 151, 151*f*
seated mid-thoracic, 151, 151*f*
seated upper, 150–151, 150*f*
supine upper and middle, 152–153, 152*f*–153*f*
Thoracolumbar fascia, 738, 740–741, 753
Thoracolumbar segment, deep fascial intermuscular links in, 740–741, 741*f*
Thorax
assessment of, 712
treatment of, 712
Thrust manipulation
versus non-thrust mobilizations, 247
for sacroiliac joint pathology, 286
seated first-rib, 153–154, 153*f*
supine ribs, 154, 154*f*
thoracic
for mechanical neck pain, 144
prone mid-thoracic, 151–152, 151*f*
prone upper, 151, 151*f*
seated mid-thoracic, 151, 151*f*
seated upper, 150–151, 150*f*
supine upper and middle, 152–153, 152*f*–153*f*
Thrust mobilization, 610–612
cuboid whip, 612, 613*f*
proximal tibiofibular joint, 612, 612*f*
rearfoot distraction, 611, 611*f*
Thumb, and finger, pathology of, 594–602
digital fractures, 594–598
osteoarthritis of the digits, 600–601

rheumatoid arthritis affecting the digits, 601
ulnar collateral ligament (UCL) injury of thumb, 598–600
Thumb abduction (C8), 55*f*
Tibial collateral ligament. *see* Medial collateral ligament.
Tibialis anterior muscle, 483
TrPs in, 673, 673*f*
dry needling of, 705, 705*f*
Tibialis anterior tendinopathy, 651–653
anatomy in, 652
background of, 651–652
diagnosis of, 652
pathology and patho-biomechanics of, 652
treatment and prognosis of, 652–653
Tibialis posterior tendinopathy, 653–654
anatomy of, 653
background of, 653
diagnosis of, 653–654
pathology and patho-biomechanics of, 653
stages of, 653
treatment and prognosis of, 654
Tibiofemoral anterior accessory glide, 527, 527*f*
Tibiofemoral joint, posterior-to-anterior accessory mobilization technique, 487*f*
Tibiofemoral knee extension physiological mobilization, 528, 528*f*
variation, 528, 528*f*
Tibiofemoral knee flexion physiological mobilization, 527–528, 527*f*
Tibiofemoral long-axis distraction manipulation, 528, 528*f*
Tibiofemoral mobilization, 515
with movement, 528–529, 529*f*
Tibiofemoral posterior accessory glide, 527, 527*f*
Tinel's test, 569
for entrapment neuropathies, 580
TKA. *see* Total knee arthroplasty (TKA).
T-lymphocytes, blood-nerve barrier and, 772
TMD. *see* Temporomandibular joint disorder (TMD).
TNE. *see* Therapeutic neuroscience education (TNE).
TNF-α. *see* Tumour necrosis factor-α (TNF-α).
Too-many-toes sign, 653
TOS. *see* Thoracic outlet syndrome (TOS).
Total ankle arthroplasty, 623–628
versus ankle arthrodesis, 623–624
balance and proprioception in, 628
changes in range of motion from, 627
efficacy of, 627–628
functional outcomes before and after, 628*t*
gait and, 627–628
history and physical examination in, 625
immediate postoperative phase of, 625–626, 626*f*
later postoperative phase of, 626–627
postoperative rehabilitation treatment for, 625–627
rehabilitation protocol for, 627*b*
self-reported outcomes of, 628
surgical procedures, 624–625
Total knee arthroplasty (TKA), 520–521
activities of daily living, 521
gait training and transfer training, 521
manual therapy and range of motion expectations, 521
modalities of, 521
procedures of, 520–521
therapeutic exercise of, 521
treatment of, 521
Trabecular pattern, patella, 493
Traction, for lumbar radiculopathy, 206, 206*f*
Traction group, for low back pain, 197
Transcutaneous electrical nerve stimulation (TENS), 509
Transforaminal epidural injections, for lumbar radiculopathy, 207
Translaminar epidural injection, for lumbar radiculopathy, 207
Translatoric articular/facet separation techniques, for cervical manipulation and mobilization, 162–165
atlanto-axial (AA) separation, in side-lying, 163, 163*f*
C2-C7 facet separation
seated, 163–164, 164*f*
in supine contralateral gap, 164–165, 165*f*
C7 facet separation, in supine, 165, 165*f*
occipito-atlanto (OA) separation, in supine, 163, 163*f*
Translatoric cervical manipulation and mobilization
translatoric articular/facet separation techniques in, 162–165
translatoric facet-gliding techniques in, 165–168
translatoric traction techniques in, 161–162
Translatoric facet-gliding techniques, for cervical manipulation and mobilization, 165–168
C2-C6 facet dorsal-caudal glide, seated, 167, 167*f*
C2-C6 facet ventral-cranial glide
seated, 166–167, 166*f*
in supine, 166, 166*f*
C7 facet dorsal-caudal glide, seated, 168, 168*f*
C7 facet ventral-cranial glide
seated, 167–168, 167*f*
in supine, 167, 167*f*
occipito-atlanto unilateral dorsal glide, in supine, 166, 166*f*
Translatoric traction techniques, for cervical manipulation and mobilization, 161–162
Transverse carpal ligament, 566, 567*f*, 576
Transverse ligament of the atlas (TLA), 50–51
Transverse massage
of hand/wrist flexor muscle TrPs, 684, 685*f*
of quadratus lumborum muscle taut band, 685, 685*f*
Transverse plane force couple, 310–311, 311*f*
Transverse strokes, dynamic, of deltoid muscle TrPs, 683, 683*f*–684*f*
Transversus abdominis
stabilization exercises for, 219*t*
training of, for low back pain, 196
Trapezius fascia, 735*f*, 736–738
Trapezius muscle
myofascial induction of, 751, 751*f*
therapeutic exercises for, 380–381, 381*f*
upper
MET for, 724, 724*f*
TrPs in, 724
Trauma
carpal instability and, 558–559
repetitive strain injury and, 771
Treadmill running exercise, 431*f*
Treatment-based classification system, for low back pain, 191, 192*t*, 212, 213*t*
clinical prediction rules in, 218
focusing on stabilization subgroup, 213–214
research investigating, 213
Trendelenburg test, 398
for gluteus medius tendinopathy, 402
for pelvic girdle pain, 281, 282*f*
Triangular fibrocartilage complex (TFCC)
central articular disc of, 560
tears of, 561
Triceps brachii muscle, TrPs in, 666–667, 667*f*
Triceps muscle stretch reflex, testing of, 57*f*
Trigger point dry needling, and botulinum toxin injection, 508–509
Trigger point therapy
massage and myofascial point, 508*f*
for plantar heel pain, 619–620
soft tissue massage and, 507
Trigger points (TrPs)
active, 660
definition of, 660
diagnosis, 660
dry needling of, 690–709
in arm muscles, 693–697
description of, 691
general guidelines for, 692–693
in hip muscles, 700–707
in leg muscles, 700–707
in neck muscles, 693–697
risks of, 691
scientific evidence of, 691–692
in shoulder muscles, 693–697
in trunk muscles, 697–700
latent, 660
palpation of, 662
Triquetrocapitatoscaphoid ligament, 559*f*, 560
Tropocollagen, 546
TrP pressure release technique, 679–680
TrPs. *see* Trigger points (TrPs).
True visceral pain, 24
Trunk, anterior cruciate ligament, 468–469
Trunk rotation control, for mechanical low back pain, 270*f*
Tumour necrosis factor-α (TNF-α)
in neuritis model, 775
TrPs dry needling and, 692
Tumours, carpal tunnel syndrome and, 567

U

Ulnar carpal dorsal glides, 590
Ulnar carpal palmar glides, 590
Ulnar collateral ligament (UCL) injury, of thumb, 598–600
anatomy of, 598–599
conservative treatment of, 600
diagnosis for, 599
epidemiology of, 598
pathology of, 599
prognosis for, 600
Ulnar link, 560
Ulnar nerve, 770
anatomy of, 575–576
conservative treatment for, 581–582
diagnosis for, 578–580
movement of, in vivo measurement of, 771
Ulnar snuffbox compression test, 563
Ulnomeniscotriquetral (UMT) dorsal glide test, 563
ULNT. *see* Upper limb neurodynamic test (ULNT).
Ultrasound
of acromioclavicular joint, 297–298
of rotator cuff lesions shoulder impingement, 315
of superior labrum anterior-to-posterior (SLAP) lesions, 340
for tendinopathy, 549–550
tibialis posterior tendinopathy and, 654
ULTT. *see* Upper limb tension test (ULTT).
Unicompartmental arthroplasty, 520
Uniplanar motions, in lumbar spine, restriction of, MET for, 720, 720*f*
Upper cervical spine instability, 50
Upper cut test, 314
Upper extremity, fascial anatomy of, 733–738
Upper extremity pain syndromes
causes of, 4*b*
epidemiological issues of, 3–6
classification criteria, 4–5, 5*f*
measurement of exposure, 5–6
non-specific pain, 4
population, 5
study design, 5
terminology, 3–4
healthcare utilization and impact in, 9, 9*t*
occurrence of, 6–7
prevalence, 6–7, 7*t*–9*t*
risk factors for, 9–11
age, 10
anthropometry, 10
gender, 9–10
hand dominance, 10
hormonal factors, 10
physical/mechanical factors, 10
psychosocial factors, 10–11
Upper limb neurodynamic test (ULNT), 137, 786, 786*t*
median active test
ULNT1, 786, 786*t*, 787*f*
ULNT2, 786*t*, 788, 788*f*
median passive test
ULNT1, 786–788, 786*t*, 787*f*
ULNT2, 786*t*, 788, 789*f*
radial
active test (ULNT2), 786*t*, 789, 789*f*
passive test (ULNT2), 786*t*, 789–790, 790*f*
ulnar
active test (ULNT3), 786*t*, 790, 791*f*
passive test (ULNT3), 786*t*, 790–791, 791*f*
Upper limb tension test (ULTT), 56–58, 58*f*, 123, 124*f*, 768
Upper motor neuron examination, 59–60
Upper quarter
biochemical relationship between thoracic spine and, 143
regional interdependence of, 143–144

Upper quarter pain syndromes, thoracic spine and rib cage in
active range of motion of, 149
evidence for manual therapy management of, 144–148
examination and screening of, 148–150
interpretation of examination and reassessment of, 149–150
postural screen of, 148–149
segmental mobility testing of, 149
Upward rotation, of scapula, 362, 365, 365*f*

V
Val158Met (rs4680) polymorphism, carpal tunnel syndrome and, 567
Valgus mobilization, 460–461
Valgus stress test, 455*t*
Varus mobilization, 460*f*–461*f*
Varus stress test, 453*t*
Vascular referral patterns, 26*f*
Vascular system, compression of, 132
Vasculogenic head/neck pain, physical examination procedures for differentiating, 49, 49*t*
Vastus lateralis muscle, TrPs in, 672, 672*f*
dry needling of, 704, 704*f*
Vastus lateralis tendon complex, 509–510
Vastus medialis muscle, TrPs in, 672, 672*f*
dry needling of, 704, 704*f*
Vastus medialis oblique (VMO), 494
VBM. *see* Voxel-based morphometry (VBM).
Vertebral canal, 200
Vertebral compression fractures, 40
Victorian Institute of Sports Assessment-Achilles (VISA-A) questionnaire, 647–648
Video surveillance, upper extremity pain syndromes and, 5–6
Visceral referral patterns, 24, 25*f*
Viscoelasticity, of fascia, 746–747
Visual analogue scale (VAS), for cervical radiculopathy, 122
V-ligament system, 560
VMO. *see* Vastus medialis oblique (VMO).
Volar intercalary segment (VISI), 561
Voxel-based morphometry (VBM), in chronic low back pain, 238

W
WAD. *see* Whiplash-associated disorders (WAD).
Waiter's bow exercise, for mechanical low back pain, 267, 267*f*
Wall press exercises, 429*f*
Wallerian degeneration, 772
Wartenberg's syndrome, 577, 580
common differential diagnosis of, 579*t*
special tests for, 579*t*
symptoms and signs of, 578*t*
Weight-bearing
Achilles tendon rupture and, 632
dorsiflexion mobility assessment, 643–644, 644*f*
resisted hip rotation exercise, 438*f*
talocrural posterior glide mobilization with movement, 641, 641*f*
Well leg raise test, for lumbar radiculopathy, 203
Western Ontario and McMaster Universities Arthritis Index (WOMAC), 38*t*, 526
Whiplash-associated disorders (WAD), 110–117
assessment of, 114
classification of, 111
condition of, 111
management of, 114–115
physical/psychological characteristics of, 111–113
augmented pain-processing mechanisms, 112–113
motor and sensorimotor control dysfunction, 111–112
prediction of outcome following, 113–114
psychological factors in, 113
Whiplash injury, neck pain after, thoracic spine manipulation for, 144–147, 145*t*–146*t*
Widespread hypoaesthesia, 112
Wind-up phase, of overhead throw, 323–324, 324*f*
WOMAC. *see* Western Ontario and McMaster Universities Arthritis Index (WOMAC).
Work Loss Data Institute, 82*t*
Working individuals, neck pain in
prevalence of, 98
prognostic factors of, 98, 98*b*
risk factors of, 98*b*
Wormian bones, 421
Wright's test, 137
Wrist extensor muscles, TrPs in, dry needling of, 697, 697*f*
Wrist-flexion finger extension manoeuvre, 562
Wrist flexion test, 580
Wrist/hand, tendinopathies of, 545–557
examination and diagnosis of, 549–550
clinical tests for, 549
diagnostic imaging and invasive testing in, 549–550
prognosis for, 553–555
tendinopathic entities of, 550–553
abductor pollicis longus and extensor pollicis brevis, 552, 552*f*
extensor carpi radialis longus and brevis (distal tendons), 550*f*, 551
extensor carpi ulnaris, 550–551, 550*f*
extensor digiti minimi, 550*f*, 551–552
extensor indicis proprius, 550*f*, 551
extensor pollicis longus, 552–553, 552*f*
flexor carpi radialis, 550*f*, 553
flexor carpi ulnaris, 550, 550*f*
treatment of, 553–555
conservative, 553–554, 554*f*
non-conservative, 554–555
Wrist/hand joint mobilization and manipulation, 586–592
carpal glide manipulation
with distal fixation, 591, 591*f*
with proximal fixation, 590–591, 590*f*
carpometacarpal (CMC) I
glides, 592, 592*f*
traction, 591, 591*f*
central carpal
dorsal glides, 590
palmar glides, 590, 590*f*
distal radioulnar joint
dorsal glide radius, 587, 587*f*
mobilizations with movement, 587
ventral glide radius, 587
finger joint
glides, 592
mobilizations with movement, 592
traction, 592, 592*f*
metacarpophalangeal (MCP) I mobilizations with movement, 592
opponens roll, 589
radial carpal
dorsal glides, 590
palmar glides, 589–590
radiocarpal
dorsal glide, 588, 588*f*–589*f*
mobilizations with movement, 589
palmar glide, 588, 588*f*
radial glide, 588, 589*f*
traction, 587, 587*f*–588*f*
ulnar glide, 588–589, 589*f*
scientific evidence for, 585–586
transverse carpal extension, 589
ulnar carpal
dorsal glides, 590
palmar glides, 590
Wrist/hand pain, prevalence of, 7*t*
Wrist-to-forearm ratio (WFR), in evaluation of carpal tunnel syndrome, 570

Y
Y-balance test, 610
Yoga, for mechanical low back pain, 267–268

Z
Zygapophyseal joints, spine, referral patterns from, 100*f*